eleventh edition

Maingot's

ABDOMINAL OPERATIONS

NOTICE

eleventh edition

Maingot's

ABDOMINAL OPERATIONS

Editors

Michael J. Zinner, MD, FACS
Surgeon-in-Chief and Chairman
Department of Surgery
Brigham and Women's Hospital
Clinical Director
Dana-Farber/Brigham and Women's Cancer Center
Moseley Professor of Surgery
Harvard Medical School
Boston, Massachusetts

Stanley W. Ashley, MD, FACS
Senior Surgeon and Vice Chairman
Department of Surgery
Brigham and Women's Hospital
Staff Surgeon
Dana-Farber/Brigham and Women's Cancer Center
Sawyer Professor of Surgery
Harvard Medical School
Boston, Massachusetts

Mc Graw Hill **Medical**

New York Chicago San Francisco Lisbon London Madrid Mexico City
Milan New Delhi San Juan Seoul Singapore Sydney Toronto

The McGraw-Hill Companies

Maingot's Abdominal Operations, Eleventh Edition

2 3 4 5 6 7 8 9 0 CCW/CCW 0 9 8 7

ISBN-13: 978-0-07-144176-6
ISBN-10: 0-07-144176-X

This book was set in New Baskerville by Silverchair Science + Communications, Inc.
The editors were Joe Rusko, Robert Pancotti, and Regina Brown.
The production supervisor was Catherine Saggese.
The cover designer was Cathleen Elliott.
The indexer was Jerry Ralya.
Courier Westford was printer and binder.

This book is printed on acid-free paper.

Library of Congress Cataloging-in-Publication Data

Maingot, Rodney, 1893–1982.
Maingot's abdominal operations. — 11th ed / editors, Michael J. Zinner, Stanley W. Ashley.
p.; cm.
Includes bibliographic references and index.
ISBN 0-07-144176-X (alk. paper)
1. Abdomen—Surgery. I. Zinner, Michael. II. Ashley, Stanley W. III. Title. IV. Title: Abdominal operations.
[DNLM: 1. Abdomen—surgery. 2. Digestive System Surgical Procedures—methods. 3. Surgical Procedures, Minimally Invasive—methods. WI 900 M225a 2007]
RD540.M24 2007
617.55059–dc22

200644955

CONTENTS

■ SECTION VII. LIVER

■ SECTION VIII. GALLBLADDER AND BILE DUCTS

■ SECTION IX. PANCREAS

■ SECTION X. SPLEEN

■ SECTION XI. MINIMALLY INVASIVE SURGERY

CONTRIBUTORS

Gina Adrales, MD
Assistant Professor of Surgery
Department of Surgery
Medical College of Georgia
Augusta, Georgia

Peter J. Allen, MD
Associate Professor of Surgery
Department of Surgery
Memorial Sloan-Kettering Cancer Center
New York, New York

Bardia Amirlak, MD
Department of Surgery
Creighton University School of Medicine
Omaha, Nebraska

Stanley W. Ashley, MD, FACS
Senior Surgeon and Vice Chairman
Department of Surgery
Brigham and Women's Hospital
Staff Surgeon
Dana-Farber/Brigham and Women's Cancer Center
Sawyer Professor of Surgery
Harvard Medical School
Boston, Massachusetts

Barbara Lee Bass, MD, FACS
John F. and Carolyn Bookout Distinguished Endowed Chair
Department of Surgery
The Methodist Hospital
Houston, Texas

Robert W. Beart, Jr., MD, FACS
Department of Colorectal Surgery
Keck School of Medicine
University of Southern California
Los Angeles, California

James M. Becker, MD, FACS
James Utley Professor of Surgery
Chairman and Surgeon-in-Chief
Department of Surgery
Boston University Medical Center
Boston, Massachusetts

Monica M. Bertagnolli, MD
Associate Surgeon
Brigham and Women's Hospital
Center for Sarcoma and Bone Oncology
Dana-Farber Cancer Institute
Associate Professor of Surgery
Harvard Medical School
Boston, Massachusetts

Ronald Bleday, MD
Chief, Division of Colon and Rectal Surgery
Brigham and Women's Hospital
Associate Professor of Surgery
Harvard Medical School
Boston, Massachusetts

Ricardo M. Bonnor, MD
Clinical Associate
Duke University Medical Center
Durham, North Carolina

Murray F. Brennan, MD
Chairman, Department of Surgery
Memorial Sloan-Kettering Cancer Center
Professor of Surgery
Weill Medical College of Cornell University
New York, New York

Stacy A. Brethauer, MD
Advanced Laparoscopic and Bariatric Surgery
Department of General Surgery
The Cleveland Clinic Foundation
Cleveland, Ohio

Timothy J. Broderick, MD, FACS
Associate Professor of Surgery and BME
Chief, Division of Gastrointestinal and Endocrine Surgery
University of Cincinnati College of Medicine
Cincinnati, Ohio

David C. Brooks, MD
Senior Surgeon
Director, Minimally Invasive Surgery
Brigham and Women's Hospital
Associate Professor of Surgery
Harvard Medical School
Boston, Massachusetts

Bryan M. Burt, MD
Department of Surgery
Brigham and Women's Hospital
Clinical Fellow in Surgery
Harvard Medical School
Boston, Massachusetts

John L. Cameron, MD, FACS
Alfred Blalock Distinguished Service Professor
Department of Surgery
The Johns Hopkins Medical Institutions
Baltimore, Maryland

Bipan Chand, MD
Director, Surgical Endoscopy
Department of General Surgery
The Cleveland Clinic Foundation
Cleveland, Ohio

Kathleen K. Christians, MD
Associate Professor of Surgery
Department of Surgery
Medical College of Wisconsin
Milwaukee, Wisconsin

Thomas E. Clancy, MD
Associate Surgeon
Brigham and Women's Hospital
Instructor in Surgery
Harvard Medical School
Boston, Massachusetts

Kevin C. P. Conlon, MB, MA, MCh, MBA, FACS, FRCSI
Professorial Surgical Unit
The Adelaide and Meath Hospital
The National Children's Hospital Dublin
University of Dublin–Trinity College Dublin
Dublin, Ireland

Zara Cooper, MD
Department of Surgery
Brigham and Women's Hospital
Harvard Medical School
Boston Massachusetts

Kimberly Moore Dalal, MD
Surgical Oncology Fellow
Memorial Sloan-Kettering Cancer Center
New York, New York

Michael M. Davies, MS, FRCS
Division of Colon and Rectal Surgery
Mayo Clinic and Medical Center
Rochester, Minnesota

Amy R. Evenson, MD
Department of Surgery
Beth Israel Deaconess Medical Center
Boston, Massachusetts

B. Mark Evers, MD
Professor and Robertson-Poth Distinguished Chair in General Surgery
Department of Surgery
The University of Texas Medical Branch
Galveston, Texas

Buckminster J. Farrow, MD
Department of Surgery
The University of Texas Medical Branch
Galveston, Texas

Stephen J. Ferzoco, MD
Assistant Chief of Surgery
Faulkner Hospital
Associate Surgeon
Brigham and Women's Hospital and Faulkner Hospital
Assistant Professor of Surgery
Harvard Medical School
Boston, Massachusetts

Alessandro Fichera, MD
Assistant Professor of Surgery
University of Chicago
Pritzker School of Medicine
Chicago, Illinois

Aaron S. Fink, MD
Professor of Surgery
Emory University School of Medicine
Manager, Surgical and Perioperative Care
Atlanta Veterans Affairs Medical Center
Decatur, Georgia

Josef E. Fischer, MD, FACS
Mallinckrodt Professor of Surgery
Harvard Medical School
Boston, Massachusetts;
Chair, Department of Surgery
Surgeon-in-Chief
Beth Israel Deaconess Medical Center
Boston, Massachusetts

Robert J. Fitzgibbons, Jr., MD, FACS
Harry E. Stuckenhoff Professor of Surgery
Associate Chairman, Department of Surgery
Chief, Division of General Surgery
Creighton University School of Medicine
Omaha, Nebraska

James W. Fleshman, Jr., MD
Chief, Section of Colon and Rectal Surgery
Professor of Surgery
Department of Surgery
Washington University School of Medicine
St. Louis, Missouri

Yuman Fong, MD
Murray F. Brennan Chair in Surgery
Department of Surgery
Memorial Sloan-Kettering Cancer Center
New York, New York

Frank A. Frizelle, MB ChB, MMedSc, FRACS, FACS
Professor of Colorectal Surgery
Colorectal Unit
Department of Surgery
Christchurch Hospital
Christchurch, New Zealand

Robert D. Fry, MD
Emilie and Roland T. deHellenbranth Professor of Surgery
Chief, Division of Colon and Rectal Surgery
University of Pennsylvania
Philadelphia, Pennsylvania

Thomas R. Gadacz, MD
Charbonnier Professor
Department of Surgery
Medical College of Georgia
Evans, Georgia

Atul A. Gawande, MD, MPH
Surgeon
Brigham and Women's Hospital
Assistant Professor of Surgery
Harvard Medical School
Boston, Massachusetts

Caprice C. Greenberg, MD, MPH
Associate Surgeon
Brigham and Women's Hospital
Instructor in Surgery
Harvard Medical School
Boston, Massachusetts

J. Michael Henderson, MB ChB, FRCS
Professor of Surgery
Cleveland Clinic Lerner College of Medicine of Case Western Reserve University
Chairman, Department of General Surgery
The Cleveland Clinic Foundation
Cleveland, Ohio

Oscar Joe Hines, MD
Section of Gastrointestinal Surgery
David Geffen School of Medicine
University of California at Los Angeles
Los Angeles, California

Scott G. Houghton, MD
Research Fellow
Department of Surgery
Gastroenterology Research Unit
Mayo Clinic College of Medicine
Rochester, Minnesota

Ralph H. Hruban, MD
Department of Pathology
The Johns Hopkins Medical Institutions
Baltimore, Maryland

John G. Hunter, MD
Mackenzie Professor and Chair
Department of Surgery
Oregon Health and Science University
Portland, Oregon

Roger D. Hurst, MD
Associate Professor of Surgery
University of Chicago
Pritzker School of Medicine
Chicago, Illinois

Danny O. Jacobs, MD, MPH
Professor and Chairman
Department of Surgery
Duke University Medical Center
Durham, North Carolina

Patrick J. Javid, MD
Department of Surgery
Brigham and Women's Hospital
Clinical Fellow in Surgery
Harvard Medical School
Boston, Massachusetts

Andreas M. Kaiser, MD, FACS
Assistant Professor of Clinical Surgery
Department of Colorectal Surgery
Keck School of Medicine
University of Southern California
Los Angeles, California

Edward Kelly, MD, FACS
Associate Surgeon
Brigham and Women's Hospital
Assistant Professor of Surgery
Harvard Medical School
Boston, Massachusetts

Michael S. Kent, MD
Clinical Instructor
Division of Thoracic and Foregut Surgery
University of Pittsburgh Medical Center
UMPC Presbyterian
Pittsburgh, Pennsylvania

Ira J. Kodner, MD, FACS, FASCRS
Solon & Bettie Gershman Professor of Surgery
Section of Colon and Rectal Surgery
Washington University School of Medicine
St. Louis, Missouri;
Department of Surgery
Barnes-Jewish Hospital
St. Louis, Missouri

Simon Law, MS, MA(Cantab), MBBChir, FRCS(Edin), FACS
Professor of Surgery
Department of Surgery
University of Hong Kong Medical Centre
Queen Mary Hospital
Hong Kong, People's Republic of China

Keith D. Lillemoe, MD
Jay L. Grosfeld Professor of Surgery and Chairman
Department of Surgery
Indiana University School of Medicine
Indianapolis, Indiana

Edward Lin, DO
Assistant Professor of Surgery
Emory Endosurgery Unit
Division of Gastrointestinal and General Surgery
Emory University School of Medicine
Atlanta, Georgia

Philip A. Linden, MD
Surgical Associate, Thoracic Surgery
Division of Thoracic Surgery
Brigham and Women's Hospital
Assistant Professor of Surgery
Harvard Medical School
Boston, Massachusetts

Jennifer K. Lowney, MD
Assistant Professor of Surgery
Section of Colon and Rectal Surgery
Washington University School of Medicine
St. Louis, Missouri

James D. Luketich, MD
Professor of Surgery
Chief, Division of Thoracic and Foregut Surgery
University of Pittsburgh Medical Center
UMPC Presbyterian
Pittsburgh, Pennsylvania

Najjia N. Mahmoud, MD
Assistant Professor of Surgery
Division of Colon and Rectal Surgery
University of Pennsylvania
Philadelphia, Pennsylvania

Michael R. Marohn, DO
Department of Surgery
The Johns Hopkins Medical Institutions
Baltimore, Maryland

Jeffrey B. Matthews, MD, FACS
Christian R. Holmes Professor of Surgery
Chairman, Department of Surgery
University of Cincinnati College of Medicine
Cincinnati, Ohio

David W. McFadden, MD, FACS
Professor and Chairman
Department of Surgery
West Virginia University
Surgeon-in-Chief
West Virginia University Hospital
Morgantown, West Virginia

Genevieve B. Melton, MD
Department of Surgery
The Johns Hopkins Medical Institutions
Columbia, Maryland

Fabrizio Michelassi, MD
Lewis Atterbury Stimson Professor of Surgery
Chairman, Department of Surgery
Weill Medical College of Cornell University
Surgeon-in-Chief
New York Presbyterian Hospital
Weill Cornell Medical Center
New York, New York

Sumeet K. Mittal, MD
Assistant Professor of Surgery
Department of Surgery
Creighton University School of Medicine
Omaha, Nebraska

Francis D. Moore, Jr., MD
Chief, General and Gastrointestinal Surgery
Brigham and Women's Hospital
Professor of Surgery
Harvard Medical School
Boston, Massachusetts

Michael W. Mulholland, MD, PhD
Department of Surgery
University of Michigan
Ann Arbor, Michigan

Alexander P. Nagle, MD
Assistant Professor of Surgery
Division of Gastrointestinal/Endocrine Surgery
Department of Surgery
Northwestern University
Feinberg School of Medicine
Chicago, Illinois

Heidi Nelson, MD
Department of Surgery
Mayo Clinic and Medical Center
Rochester, Minnesota

Ankesh Nigam, MD, FACS
Associate Professor
Section of Surgical Oncology
Department of Surgery
Albany Medical College
Albany, New York

Joseph W. Nunoo-Mensah, BM BS, FRCS(Eng)
Department of Surgery
Manchester Royal Infirmary
Manchester, United Kingdom

Brant K. Oelschlager, MD
The Swallowing Center and
Department of Surgery
The University of Washington Medical Center
Seattle, Washington

Theodore N. Pappas, MD, FACS
Professor, Department of Surgery
Duke University Medical Center
Durham, North Carolina

Subroto Paul, MD
Department of Surgery
Brigham and Women's Hospital
Clinical Fellow in Surgery
Boston, Massachusetts

Jeffrey H. Peters, MD, FACS
Professor and Chairman
University of Rochester School of Medicine and Dentistry
Surgeon-in-Chief
Strong Memorial Hospital
Department of Surgery
Rochester, New York

Henry A. Pitt, MD
Professor of Surgery
Indiana University
Indianapolis, Indiana

Antonio Ramos De la Medina, MD
Department of Surgery
Mayo Clinic College of Medicine
Rochester, Minnesota

Thomas E. Read, MD, FACS, FASCRS
Chief, Division of Colon and Rectal Surgery
Program Director, Colon and Rectal Surgery Residency
Western Pennsylvania Hospital
Clinical Campus of Temple University School of Medicine
Pittsburgh, Pennsylvania;
Associate Professor of Surgery
Temple University School of Medicine
Philadelphia, Pennsylvania

Howard A. Reber, MD
Section of Gastrointestinal Surgery
David Geffen School of Medicine
University of California at Los Angeles
Los Angeles, California

Angela T. Riga, MD, MSc, AFRCS
Professorial Surgical Unit
Royal Surrey Hospital
Guildford, Surrey
United Kingdom

Malcolm K. Robinson, MD
Surgeon
Director, Metabolic Support Service
Director, Program for Weight Management
Brigham Women's Hospital
Assistant Professor of Surgery
Harvard Medical School
Boston, Massachusetts

Michael Rosen, MD
General Surgery
Massachusetts General Hospital
Boston, Massachusetts

Michael G. Sarr, MD
James C. Masson Professor of Surgery
Department of Surgery
Gastroenterology Research Unit
Mayo Clinic College of Medicine
Rochester, Minnesota

Philip R. Schauer, MD
Director, Advanced Laparoscopic and Bariatric Surgery
Department of General Surgery
The Cleveland Clinic Foundation
Cleveland, Ohio

Richard D. Schulick, MD, FACS
Associate Professor of Surgery, Oncology, Gynecology, and Obstetrics
The Johns Hopkins Medical Institutions
Baltimore, Maryland

Seymour I. Schwartz, MD
Distinguished Alumni Professor of Surgery
University of Rochester School of Medicine and Dentistry
Rochester, New York

Patrick Schweder, BA, MA, MB ChB
Auckland City Hospital
Grafton, Auckland
New Zealand

Andrew A. Shelton, MD
Assistant Professor
Department of Surgery
Stanford University School of Medicine
Stanford, California

Ketan R. Sheth, MD
Clinical Associate
Duke University Medical Center
Durham, North Carolina

Gautam Shrikhande, MD
Department of Surgery
Beth Israel Deaconess Medical Center
Boston, Massachusetts

Diane M. Simeone, MD
Department of Surgery
University of Michigan
Ann Arbor, Michigan

Douglas S. Smink, MD, MPH
Department of Surgery
Brigham and Women's Hospital
Instructor in Surgery
Harvard Medical School
Boston, Massachusetts

Christopher J. Sonnenday, MD, MHS
Department of Surgery
The Johns Hopkins University School of Medicine
Baltimore, Maryland

Nathaniel J. Soper, MD
James R. Hines Professor of Surgery
Department of Surgery
Northwestern University
Feinberg School of Medicine
Chicago, Illinois

David I. Soybel, MD
Senior Staff Surgeon
Brigham and Women's Hospital
Associate Professor of Surgery
Harvard Medical School
Boston, Massachusetts

Arthur F. Stucchi, PhD
Associate Research Professor
Departments of Surgery, Pathology, and Laboratory Medicine
Boston University School of Medicine
Boston, Massachusetts

David J. Sugarbaker, MD
Chief, Division of Thoracic Surgery
Brigham and Women's Hospital
Phillip E. Lowe Senior Surgeon
Chief, Department of Surgical Services
Dana-Farber Cancer Institute
Richard E. Wilson Professor of Surgical Oncology
Harvard Medical School
Boston, Massachusetts

Richard S. Swanson, MD
Senior Surgeon
Brigham and Women's Hospital
Associate Professor of Surgery
Harvard Medical School
Boston, Massachusetts

Ali Tavakkolizadeh, MB, BS
Associate Surgeon
Brigham and Women's Hospital
Instructor in Surgery
Harvard Medical School
Boston, Massachusetts

James C. Thompson, MD
Ashbel Smith Professor of Surgery
Department of Surgery
The University of Texas Medical Branch
Galveston, Texas

Courtney M. Townsend, Jr., MD
John Woods Harris Distinguished Chairman
Department of Surgery
The University of Texas Medical Branch
Galveston, Texas

Thadeus L. Trus, MD, FRCS(C)
Associate Professor of Surgery
Department of Surgery
University of Rochester School of Medicine and Dentistry
Rochester, New York

Douglas J. Turner, MD
Assistant Professor of Surgery
Division of General Surgery
University of Maryland Medical Center
Baltimore, Maryland

Ashley Haralson Vernon, MD
Associate Surgeon
Brigham and Women's Hospital
Instructor in Surgery
Harvard Medical School
Boston, Massachusetts

Andrew L. Warshaw, MD, FACS
Chairman, Department of General Surgery
Massachusetts General Hospital
Boston, Massachusetts

Angus J. M. Watson, BSc, MB ChB, FRCS(Edin)
Colorectal Unit
Department of Surgery
Christchurch Hospital
Christchurch, New Zealand

Mark Lane Welton, MD
Associate Professor
Chief, Colon and Rectal Surgery
Department of Surgery
Stanford University School of Medicine
Stanford, California

Edward E. Whang, MD
Associate Surgeon
Brigham and Women's Hospital
Assistant Professor of Surgery
Harvard Medical School
Boston, Massachusetts

John A. Windsor, BSc, MB ChB, MD, FRACS, FACS
Professor of Surgery
Head, Department of Surgery
Faculty of Medical and Health Sciences
University of Auckland
Auckland, New Zealand

Todd Woltman, MD
The Swallowing Center and
Department of Surgery
The University of Washington Medical Center
Seattle, Washington

John Wong, MD, PhD, FRACS, FACS
Professor of Surgery
Department of Surgery
University of Hong Kong Medical Centre
Queen Mary Hospital
Hong Kong, People's Republic of China

Charles J. Yeo, MD, FACS
Professor and Chairman
Samuel D. Gross
Department of Surgery
Thomas Jefferson University
Philadelphia, Pennsylvania

Michael J. Zinner, MD, FACS
Surgeon-in-Chief and Chairman
Department of Surgery
Brigham and Women's Hospital
Clinical Director
Dana-Farber/Brigham and Women's Cancer Center
Moseley Professor of Surgery
Harvard Medical School
Boston, Massachusetts

PREFACE

Maingot's Abdominal Operations has always filled a unique niche. For many surgeons, including the editors, the text has consistently offered a comprehensive discussion of surgical diseases of the abdomen with a focus on operative strategy and technique. The book has served as a needed reference to refresh our knowledge before a common operation or in preparation for a novel one. Our intended audience for this edition is the same as the original publication—the surgical trainee as well as the practicing surgeon. It is both an honor and a privilege to have the opportunity to edit the eleventh edition of this classic textbook.

Abdominal surgery has clearly changed since Rodney Maingot's first edition, published in 1940. Not only has our knowledge base increased substantially, but the procedures themselves have become more complex. The current subspecialization in abdominal surgery, a consequence of these changes, might even challenge the need for such a comprehensive text. Abdominal disease is now being increasingly parceled up between foregut, hepatobiliary, pancreatic, colorectal, endocrine, vascular, and minimally invasive surgeons. For this edition, we have recognized this specialization and have chosen to eliminate sections on abdominal trauma and vascular disease, focusing instead on disorders of the gastrointestinal tract. We continue to believe, however, that for the digestive diseases, the basic principles of surgical care in each of the anatomical regions have more similarities than differences. Experience in any one of these organs can inform and strengthen the approach to each of the others. Few would question the need for the abdominal surgeon to be well versed in dealing with any unexpected disease encountered in the course of a planned procedure. For many of us, *Maingot's Abdominal Operations* has consistently filled that need. We also intend for this textbook to remain disease-focused in addition to its organ/procedure format.

The new edition of this textbook is a *total* revision—a completely new book. We have attempted to focus the book on operative procedures as well as on new concepts in diagnosis and management of abdominal disease. Consistent with the trend for many other clinical texts, we have reduced the length of this edition considerably. Although the text is condensed, we continue to present the opinions and knowledge of a number of experts. We continue to maintain the international flavor and have included a cross-section of both seasoned senior contributors and new leaders in gastrointestinal surgery.

An extensive artwork program was undertaken for this edition. Many line drawings have been recreated to reflect the contributors' preferred method for performing certain surgical procedures. Some of these drawings are new and give the book a more modern look and a greater overall consistency.

Although this edition is more focused than previous editions, many topics have been added or expanded, such as a new chapter examining gastrointestinal stromal tumors and an entire section on contemporary laparoscopic techniques—an increasingly dominant operative tool for the practicing abdominal surgeon. In many sections, there are deliberate duplications to bring more than one perspective to an important disease entity. We continue to believe that these varying viewpoints strengthen a textbook as important as *Maingot's*.

In the preface to the sixth edition, Rodney Maingot noted, "As all literature is personal, the contributors have been given a free hand with their individual sections. A certain latitude in style and expression is stimulating to the thoughtful reader." We have similarly tried to maintain consistency for the reader, but the authors have also been given a free hand in their chapter submissions.

We truly appreciate the contributions of the previous editor, Dr. Seymour Schwartz, for his assistance in the preparation of this edition. Without his support and guidance, we would not have been able to publish this book.

We would also like to thank the publisher, McGraw-Hill, and in particular Marc Strauss, Joe Rusko, and Robert Pancotti, for their unwavering support during the lengthy time of development of this project. Their guidance was invaluable for completing this project into a single comprehensive volume. Their suggestions and attention to detail made it possible to overcome the innumerable problems that occur in publishing such a large textbook.

We have been fortunate to deal with an outstanding illustrator during the creation of this book. As in the last edition, Mr. Philip Ashley was able to maintain the high standard of illustration needed to create and maintain the theme and consistency throughout the entire book.

This book could not have been completed without the wisdom and assistance of our faculty colleague, Dr. Ali Tavakkolizadeh, who helped oversee the completion of the book.

Finally, to our editorial assistant who has survived the trials of this book, Karen "Kit" Giffen has been invaluable, and we never would have been able to do it without her. Patrina Tucker, Linda Smith, Suzee Vicente, and Doreen Kontos have also stepped up and made this project possible. We owe them a great debt of gratitude for helping with every step of the work—typing manuscripts, editing and reading galleys and page proofs, and providing encouragement during the prolonged dry periods and preparation of this textbook.

To all of those who have participated in the creation and publication of this text, we thank you very much.

Michael J. Zinner, MD, FACS
Stanley W. Ashley, MD, FACS

Section I

INTRODUCTION

1

A Focused History of Surgery

Seymour I. Schwartz

The word *surgery* derives from the French term "chirurgien," which came from the Latin and in turn from the Greek words "cheir," meaning "hand" and "ergon," meaning work. Surgery has a long history beginning with what is said to be the earliest scientific document known, *The Edwin Smith Surgical Papyrus,* dating from the 17th century before Christ, actually a copy of an Egyptian manuscript originally written circa 3000–2500 BC. The document deals with a variety of wounds and cauterization for breast cancer. No abdominal surgery is mentioned.

Although *Maingot's Abdominal Operations* had its genesis in England, elective abdominal operations had their beginning in Danville, Kentucky, a town of 1000 at the time, with the removal of a 22½-pound ovarian tumor by Ephraim McDowell on December 25, 1809. By the end of the 19th century, the German school dominated abdominal surgery, but throughout the 19th century surgeons from Great Britain and the United States, the two countries that would eventually play major roles in the development of the multiple editions of *Maingot's Abdominal Operations,* contributed significantly to the evolution of abdominal operations. In 1804, Sir Astley Cooper published a *Treatise on Hernia.* On October 16, 1846, at the Massachusetts General Hospital, the birth of ether anesthesia took place and ushered in a new generation of possibilities for all of surgery. In 1867, John Stough Bobbs of Indianapolis reported the first successful elective operation on the gallbladder, a cholecystostomy with removal of stones and closure of the organ. The patient remained relatively asymptomatic for over 40 years. But as the 19th century came to a close the German schools of surgery became increasingly dominant, in large part related to Theodor Billroth and the surgeons he trained. Billroth is often referred to as "the father of abdominal surgery" based on his first resection of cancer of the pylorus in 1881 and also the numerous intestinal resections and enterorrhaphies that he performed.

As the 21st century is evolving, in regard to the current edition of *Maingot's Abdominal Operations,* it is appropriate to focus on the developments that took place during the preceding 20th century, by dividing this period into two time spans: one before 1940, the year that the first edition of *Maingot's Abdominal Operations* was published, and the other considering the progress that has taken place in the ensuing 60 years.

In discussing the history of surgical advances pertaining to the gastrointestinal tract per se, it is reasonable to proceed aborally from esophagus to rectum. Although in 1935 Winkelstein first defined the clinical picture of esophageal reflux and indicted the erosive action of gastric juice as the culprit, the issue of a functioning gastroesophageal sphincter was not appreciated. Consequently, no corrective operation was devised prior to publication of *Maingot's* first edition.

The surgical treatment of reflux esophagitis was first popularized by Allison, who defined a repair in 1951, mainly consisting of correction of the hiatal herniation. The high recurrence rate associated with that operation led to a consideration of fundoplication procedures, which were introduced in 1966 by Nissen and subsequently modified by Belsey, Hill, and Toupet. Since the advent of minimally invasive surgery in 1989, the majority of these fundoplications have been performed laparoscopically.

During the first four decades of the 20th century, there was considerable interest in the surgical treatment of peptic ulcer disease. Gastric resection was often the most commonly performed indexed operative procedure in a residency program. The operations were outgrowths of the procedures that were initially applied by Billroth and his associates for gastric cancer. In the early decades of the 20th century, excision of a gastric ulcer was widely practiced. When the excision, as was frequently the case, was extensive, there were problems with gastric emptying, prompting William Mayo in 1911 to add a complemental gastrojejunostomy. Then as now, the indications for surgical intervention in patients with peptic ulcer were obstruction, bleeding, perforation, and intractability. Pyloroplasty and gastrojejunostomy were the most frequently performed procedures for obstruction, and as early as 1925 Lewisohn reported a 34% incidence of neostomal ulcer after gastrojejunostomy. Before 1940, the surgeons at the Mayo Clinic continued to champion the procedure for duodenal ulcer. In 1937, R.R. Graham introduced his patch procedure for perforation. Gradually partial gastrectomy became the preferred surgical treatment for the complications of peptic ulcer disease.

The modern era of vagotomy in the management of peptic ulcer was ushered in on January 1943, when Dragstedt performed a subdiaphragmatic resection of the vagal trunks in a patient with an active duodenal ulcer. Dragstedt's earlier approach was transthoracic. Later, when he appreciated that a significant percentage of his patients developed gastric stasis, Dragstedt added a drainage procedure, either gastroenterostomy or pyloroplasty, as an accompaniment to the truncal vagotomy. Farmer and Smithwick recommended a two-pronged attack against the ulcer diathesis, combining truncal vagotomy with hemigastrectomy. In 1960, Griffith introduced the concept of selective gastric vagotomy, preserving the nerve of Laterjet and thereby obviating the need for a gastric drainage procedure.[1]

The applicability of vagotomy and partial gastric resection has been greatly reduced over the past two decades by the introduction of acid suppressive pharmaceuticals, including the histamine receptor antagonists and proton pump inhibitors. The use of these preparations has also generally obviated total gastrectomy for the previously intractable ulcers associated with the Zollinger-Ellison syndrome. Perhaps the most dramatic discovery to result in a marked reduction in the need for surgical management of peptic ulcer disease and a modification in treatment is the discovery by Warren and Marshall in 1983 of an association between *Helicobacter pylori* and peptic ulcer that is readily treatable with the hopes of totally eradicating peptic ulcer disease. This transition of gastric surgery from the 19th-century understanding of anatomy, to the 20th-century understanding of physiology and pathophysiology, to the 21st-century understanding of pharmacology mirrors the growth, development, and progress of the understanding of surgical diseases.[2]

The greatest increase in gastric surgery since 1940 is the application of gastric reduction for obesity. The initial surgical approach to the management of extreme obesity, jejunoileal bypass, was introduced by Kremen, Linner, and Nelson in 1954. The procedure was popularized by Payne and DeWind in 1969, but had many hazardous consequences and has been essentially discarded. Gastric bypass, introduced by Mason in 1966, has been the preferred method of surgical management for the past four decades and has become increasingly popular with the advent of minimally invasive surgery.

The principles of intestinal anastomosis are in large part based on Halsted's late-19th century studies on the importance of the submucosa as the layer providing strength for the suture line. Most of the early-20th century procedures on the small intestine were related to the treatment of obstruction. In 1932, Crohn, Ginzburg, and Oppenheimer introduced a newly recognized pathologic entity they called regional ileitis, which has come to be known as Crohn's disease or regional enteritis.

The major operative changes in small intestinal surgery that have taken place over the past two decades have been brought about by the introduction of stapling techniques. Mechanical suture instruments using staples began with Humer Hültl of Budapest, who in 1908 described an instrument for use in distal gastrectomy. It was modified by von Petz in 1924 and enjoyed a period of popularity in many centers. The next major step in stapling was the result of the dedicated efforts of the Scientific Research Institute for Experimental Surgical Apparatus and Instruments in Moscow. The investigators developed magazine-loaded instruments for vascular anastomosis, side-to-side intestinal anastomosis, and end-to-end intestinal anastomosis. These were imported to the United States and modified, beginning in 1958, largely due to the leadership of Ravitch and Steichen.[3] The introduction and widespread application of stapling devices helped revolutionize the technical aspects of surgery that have allowed minimally invasive procedures to be developed.

In the realm of colorectal surgery, although in 1883 Czerny introduced a technique for combined abdominal-peritoneal excision of rectal tumors, Miles' method, reported in 1907, popularized the procedure. The advent of stapling techniques during the past two decades has allowed for more anal preservation operations. The ileal pouch procedure represents a significant advance in the management of ulcerative colitis and familial polyposis. In 1947, Ravitch and Sabiston performed total colectomy, proximal proctectomy, mucosal distal proctectomy, and ileal anal anastomosis, but the results were generally not satisfactory with regard to frequency of defecation. The introduction in 1978 of a valveless ileal reservoir anastomosed to the anus addressed the problem and has become the standard.[4]

The first successful elective hepatic resection for tumor was performed by Langenbuch in 1888. The first collective review of hepatic resections for tumor was reported by Keen in 1899 and included only 20 cases. In 1911, Wendell reported the first case of near total right lobectomy for a primary hepatic tumor, but the modern age of hepatic resection is generally dated to the 1952 report of Lortat-Jacob and Robert that detailed a right lobectomy using a technique designed to control hemorrhage with ligation of the blood vessels and bile ducts to the right lobe in the hepatoduodenal ligament followed by extrahepatic ligation of the right hepatic vein prior to transection of the hepatic parenchyma. In 1967, using corrosion casts, Couinaud demonstrated that the liver is made up of eight distinct segments, thereby opening the door for segmental hepatic resections. The recent application of new instruments such as the harmonic scalpel and LigaSure vessel sealing system have expedited the performance of major hepatic resections without a need for transfusion.[5]

The year 1945 marked the beginning of the modern era of surgical intervention for portal hypertension with the report by Whipple and associates of the performance of end-to-side portacaval anastomoses and end-to-end splenorenal anastomoses. In 1953 Marion and in 1955 Clatworthy and colleagues independently described a shunt between the proximal transected end of the inferior vena cava and the side of the superior mesenteric vein. In 1967, Gleidman performed the first Dacron interposition mesocaval shunt, and the same year Warren and colleagues introduced the selective (distal) splenorenal shunt as a method of preserving flow to the liver. The shunt procedures are now performed infrequently, and are generally reserved for patients with massively bleeding esophagogastric varices and normal hepatocellular function. By contrast, in patients with uncontrollable bleeding varices and significant hepatocellular dysfunction, a TIPS (transjugular intrahepatic portosystemic shunt) procedure is generally used as a bridge to orthotopic liver transplantation. In 1959, Kasai and Suzuki introduced hepatic portoenterostomy for the management of biliary atresia. More recently orthotopic liver transplantation has been employed for these patients because of uncorrectable hepatocellular dysfunction.

Fifteen years elapsed between Bobbs' cholecystotomy and the first successful cholecystectomy, which was performed by Carl Langenbuch in 1882. By 1919, William J. Mayo was able to report on 2147 cholecystectomies. In 1923, Graham and Cole introduced cholecystography leading to a marked increase in biliary surgery. Operations for injuries and strictures of the common duct have undergone many refinements over the past century. An obstructed common bile duct was first successfully drained by a lateral anastomosis to the duodenum by Sprengel in 1891. A variety of plastic procedures and intestinal flap advancements were applied to bridge a gap between the common duct and the duodenum with minimal success. Beginning in 1941, Vitallium tubes were inserted into bile ducts as conduits, but all the tubes eventually became obstructed with sludge. The groups at the Mayo Clinic and Lahey Clinic, who both had extensive experience with these procedures, expressed a preference for choledochoduodenostomy, while most surgeons now employ a mucosal-to-mucosal anastomosis between the proximal duct and a Roux limb of jejunum.

Operations on the pancreas directed at the management of pancreatitis and neoplasms generally evolved subsequent to the publication of the first edition of Maingot's textbook. In 1958, Puestow introduced the popular lateral pancreaticojejunostomy. In 1965, Fry and Child reported their results with a 95% distal pancreatectomy. In 1985, Beger proposed resection of the head of the pancreas with duodenal preservation for pathology that was most marked in the head of the pancreas. In regard to the neuroendocrine tumors of the pancreas, Roscoe Graham performed the first successful resection of an insulinoma in 1929. In 1955, Zollinger and Ellison reported that non-beta islet cell tumors produced an "ulcerogenic humoral factor." The pathophysiology often mandated total gastrectomy to control the massive gastric hypersecretion, but the therapy has been markedly altered with the advent of proton pump inhibitors.[6]

Although in 1912 Kausch successfully performed a partial pancreatectomy in two stages, the name of Allen O. Whipple has achieved eponymic status as far as resection of pancreatic neoplasms is concerned. In 1935, Whipple initially carried out a two-stage operation for carcinoma of the ampulla consisting of an initial cholecystojejunostomy followed by total duodenectomy. By 1945, he advocated a one-stage pancreatoduodenectomy as the treatment of choice.

Splenectomy is performed for trauma or hematologic disorders. The first recorded successful splenectomy for trauma is credited to a British naval surgeon,

E. O'Brien, in 1816, who tied off the pedicle and removed a protruding spleen while stationed in San Francisco. In 1892, Reigner performed the first successful intraperitoneal splenectomy for trauma. In 1867, Péan successfully removed a spleen containing a large cyst. In 1911, Micheli reported the first splenectomy for a hematologic disorder in a patient with hemolytic anemia. Five years later, at the suggestion of Kaznelson, a Czech medical student, Schloffer performed the first splenectomy for idiopathic thrombocytopenic purpura, the most common hematologic indication. The most recent changes in splenic surgery relate to an increased willingness to observe patients, particularly children, with blunt trauma to the spleen, and the fact that elective splenectomies are generally being performed laparoscopically, as championed by Phillips and Carroll, Cuschieri and associates, and Thibault and coworkers.[7]

Intra-abdominal vascular surgery traces its modern origin to Dubost and colleagues' 1951 resection of an abdominal aortic aneurysm with reestablishment of continuity. The introduction of a prosthetic material to create a conduit is credited to Voorhees, Jaretzki, and Blakemore, who used Vinyon "N" cloth in 1969. The same year, Wylie and associates described autogenous tissue revascularization techniques for correction of renovascular hypertension.

The major advances in abdominal surgery that took place in the second half of the 20th century relate to the fields of organ transplantation and minimally invasive procedures. On December 23, 1954, Murray, Merrill, and Harrison performed the first renal transplant in identical twins. Eight years later the first successful cadaveric kidney transplant was performed by Murray in an immunosuppressed patient. The liver was the second visceral organ to be transplanted. In 1963, Starzl performed the first human liver transplant in a patient with biliary atresia. The patient died as did four other patients operated on by Starzl and one by Moore that year. In 1968, Starzl achieved the first success. The field recently has been extended by the use of live donors who provide a lobe for the recipient.

The first successful clinical pancreas transplant was performed by Kelly and Lillehei in 1966. In 1973, Gliedman and associates suggested using the ureter for exocrine pancreatic drainage. In 1982, the group at the University of Wisconsin developed the technique of direct drainage of the pancreas into the urinary bladder. Now, most whole organ pancreas transplants use the intestine for drainage. Recently improved results have been reported with islet cell transplants.

The small intestine was the last of the abdominal organs to be transplanted successfully. In 1987, Strazl and associates performed a multivisceral organ transplant, including the small intestine. The following year, the same group performed a successful combined liver and small intestine transplant, and Grant reported a successful isolated intestinal transplant from a live donor. In 1989, the Pittsburgh group performed the first successful cadaveric small intestinal transplant.

Doubtless, the most dramatic development in abdominal surgery is the introduction and expansion of laparoscopic procedures. Kelling was the first to examine the peritoneal cavity with an endoscope. In 1901, using a Nitze cystoscope, he entered and visualized the peritoneal cavity of a dog and referred to the procedure as "Koelioskopie." The first major series of laparoscopies in humans is attributed to Jacobaeus, who in 1911 reported examining both the abdominal and thoracic cavities with a "Lapaothorakoscopie." In 1937, Ruddock published a paper on "Peritoneoscopy" in which he detailed his experience with 500 cases including 39 in which biopsies were performed.

Laparoscopy essentially remained a procedure performed by gynecologists for many years. In fact it was a gynecologist, Mouret, who in 1987 performed the first laparoscopic cholecystectomy, using four trocars. But credit is generally assigned to Dubois, who described the procedure in 1988, for initiating interest in the procedure. In the brief 16 years that have ensued, there has been an explosive increase in the use of laparoscopic techniques for abdominal operations. Basic laparoscopic procedures include cholecystectomy, appendectomy, and hernia repair. Advanced procedures include fundoplication, Heller myotomy, gastrectomy, bariatric surgery, esophagectomy, enteral access, bile duct exploration, partial pancreatectomy, colectomy, splenectomy, adrenalectomy, and nephrectomy in addition to the standard gynecologic applications.[8]

The most recent refinement has been the addition of robotics, or more currently, computer-assisted remote mechanical devices. The appropriateness of the application of robotics to cholecystectomy has not been demonstrated. An advantage, however, has been ascribed to robotics for adrenalectomy.[9] Paralleling the expansion of laparoscopic surgery, there has been an increased application of endovascular techniques for the repair of aneurysm of the abdominal aorta. Endovascular abdominal aortic repair was introduced independently by Parodi and associates and Volodos and coworkers in 1991. Over a dozen endovascular grafts have been developed, and in 2002 there were more abdominal aortic aneurysms repaired in the state of New York by endovascular procedures than open operations.[10]

Over six decades have elapsed since the first edition of *Maingot's Abdominal Operations* was published. As is true for all of the sciences, growth recently has been geometric. During the time from the initial publication to the present, there have been more new and refined operations introduced than throughout the preceding years. The accelerated rate of change can only ensure the viability of future editions.

REFERENCES

1. Nyhus LM, Wastell C (eds). *Surgery of the Stomach and Duodenum.* Boston, MA: Little Brown and Co; 1986
2. Modlin IM. *The Evolution of Therapy in Gastroenterology.* Montreal, Canada: Axcan Pharma; 2002
3. Steichen FM, Ravitch MM. *Stapling in Surgery.* Chicago, IL: Year Book Medical; 1971
4. Goligher J. *Surgery of the Anus Rectum and Colon,* 5th ed. London, England: Baillière Tindall; 1984
5. McDermott WV. *Surgery of the Liver.* Cambridge, England: Blackwell Scientific; 1988
6. Schwartz SI, et al. *Principles of Surgery,* 7th ed. New York, NY: McGraw-Hill; 1989
7. Hiatt JR, Phillips EH, Morgenstern L. *Surgical Diseases of the Spleen.* New York, NY: Springer; 1997
8. Laparoscopy for the general surgeon. *Surg Clin North Am* 1992;72:997–1186
9. Jacob BP, Gagner M. Robotics and general surgery. *Surg Clin North Am* 2003;83:1405–1419
10. Krupinski WC, Rutherford RB. Update on open repair of abdominal aortic aneurysms: The challenges for endovascular repair. *J Am Coll Surg* 2004;199:946–960

2

Preoperative and Postoperative Management

Zara Cooper ■ Edward Kelly

Modern advances in patient care have enabled surgeons to treat more challenging and complicated surgical problems. In addition, surgical treatment can be offered to more fragile patients, with successful outcomes. In order to achieve these good results, it is vital to master the scientific fundamentals of perioperative management. The organ system–based approach allows the surgeon to address the patient's pre- and postoperative needs, and ensures that these needs are part of the surgical plan.

■ MANAGEMENT OF PAIN AND DELIRIUM

The most common neuropsychiatric complications following abdominal surgery are pain and delirium. Moreover, uncontrolled pain and delirium prevent the patient from contributing to vital aspects of his or her care such as walking and coughing, and promote an unsafe environment that may lead to the unwanted dislodgment of drains and other supportive devices, with potentially life-threatening consequences. Pain and delirium frequently coexist, and each can contribute to the development of the other. Despite high reported rates of overall patient satisfaction, pain control is frequently inadequate in the perioperative setting[1] with high rates of complications such as drowsiness and unacceptable levels of pain. Therefore it is mandatory that the surgical plan for every patient include control of postoperative pain and delirium and regular monitoring of the efficacy of pain control.

Pain management, like all surgical planning, begins in the preoperative assessment. In the modern era, a large proportion of surgical patients will require special attention with respect to pain control. Patients with preexisting pain syndromes, such as sciatica or interspinal disc disease, or patients with a history of opioid use may have a high tolerance for opioid analgesics. Every patient's history should include a thorough investigation for chronic pain syndromes, addiction (active or in recovery), and adverse reactions to opioid, nonsteroidal, or epidural analgesia. The pain control strategy may include consultation with a pain control anesthesiology specialist, but it is the responsibility of the operating surgeon to identify complicated patients and construct an effective pain control plan.

OPIOID ANALGESIA

Postoperative pain control using opioid medication has been in use for thousands of years. Hippocrates advocated the use of opium for pain control. The benefits of postoperative pain control are salutary, and include improved mobility and respiratory function, and earlier return to normal activities. The most effective strategy for pain control using opioid analgesia is patient-controlled analgesia (PCA), wherein the patient is instructed in the use of a preprogrammed intravenous pump that delivers measured doses of opioid (usually morphine or meperidine). In randomized trials, PCA has been shown to provide superior pain control and patient satisfaction compared to interval dosing,[2] but

PCA has not been shown to improve rates of pulmonary and cardiac complications[3] or length of hospital stay,[4] and there is evidence that PCA may contribute to postoperative ileus.[5] In addition, PCA may be unsuitable for patients with a history of substance abuse, high opioid tolerance, or those with atypical reactions to opioids.

EPIDURAL ANALGESIA

Due to the limitations of PCA, pain control clinicians have turned to epidural analgesia as an effective strategy for the management of postoperative pain. Postoperative epidural analgesia involves the insertion of a catheter into the epidural space of the lumbar or thoracic spine, enabling the delivery of local anesthetics or opioids directly to the nerve roots. The insertion procedure is generally safe, with complication rates of motor block and numbness between 0.5 and 7%,[6] and an epidural abscess rate of 0.5 per thousand.[7] Potential advantages of epidural analgesia include elimination of systemic opioids, and thus less respiratory depression, and improvement in pulmonary complications and perioperative ileus. There have been several large trials,[8–10] a meta-analysis,[6] and a systematic review[11] comparing PCA with epidural analgesia in the setting of abdominal surgery. These studies indicate that epidural analgesia provides more complete analgesia than PCA throughout the postoperative course. Furthermore, in randomized prospective series of abdominal procedures, epidural analgesia has been associated with decreased rates of pulmonary complications[12,13] and postoperative ileus.[14,15] Epidural analgesia requires a skilled anesthesia clinician to insert and monitor the catheter and adjust the dosage of neuraxial medication. Some clinicians may prefer correction of coagulopathy before inserting or removing the catheter, although the American Society of Anesthesiologists (ASA) has not issued official guidelines on this issue.

ANALGESIA WITH NONSTEROIDAL ANTI-INFLAMMATORY DRUGS

Oral nonsteroidal anti-inflammatory drugs (NSAIDs) have long been used for postoperative analgesia in the outpatient setting, and with the development of parenteral preparations, have come into use in the inpatient population. This class of medication has no respiratory side effects and is not associated with addiction potential, altered mental status, or ileus. In addition, these medications provide effective pain relief in the surgical population. However, use of NSAIDs has not been universally adopted in abdominal surgery due to concerns regarding the platelet dysfunction and erosive gastritis associated with heavy NSAID use. In prospective trials, NSAIDs were found to provide effective pain control without bleeding or gastritis symptoms following laparoscopic cholecystectomy,[16] abdominal hysterectomy,[17] and inguinal hernia repair.[18,19] NSAIDs have also been shown to improve pain control and decrease morphine dosage when used in combination following appendectomy.[20]

The sensation of pain is very subjective and personal. Accordingly, the surgeon must individualize the pain control plan to fit the needs of each patient. The pain control modalities discussed above can be used in any combination, and the surgeon should not hesitate to use all resources at his or her command to provide adequate relief of postoperative pain.

POSTOPERATIVE DELIRIUM

Delirium, defined as acute cognitive dysfunction marked by fluctuating disorientation, sensory disturbance, and decreased attention, is an all too common complication of surgical procedures, with reported rates of 11–25%, with the highest rates reported in the elderly population.[21,22] The postoperative phase of abdominal surgery exposes patients, some of whom may be quite vulnerable to delirium, to a large number of factors that may precipitate or exacerbate delirium (Table 2–1). These factors can augment each other: postoperative pain can lead to decreased mobility, causing respiratory compromise, atelectasis, and hypoxemia. Escalating doses of narcotics to treat pain can cause respiratory depression and respiratory acidosis. Hypoxemia and delirium can cause agitation, prompting

TABLE 2–1. CAUSES OF PERIOPERATIVE DELIRIUM

Pain
Narcotic analgesics
Sleep deprivation
Hypoxemia
Hyperglycemia
Acidosis
Withdrawal (alcohol, narcotics, benzodiazepines)
Anemia
Dehydration
Electrolyte imbalance (sodium, potassium, magnesium, calcium, phosphate)
Fever
Hypotension
Infection (pneumonia, incision site infection, urinary tract infection)
Medication (antiemetics, antihistamines, sedatives, anesthetics)
Postoperative myocardial infarction

treatment with benzodiazepines, further worsening respiratory function and delirium. This vicious cycle can play out right before the house officer's eyes, and if not interrupted, can result in serious complications or death. Preoperative recognition of high-risk patients and meticulous monitoring of every patient's mental status are the most effective ways to prevent postoperative delirium; treatment can be remarkably difficult once the vicious cycle has begun.

Patient factors that are associated with high risk of perioperative delirium include age greater than 70 years, preexisting cognitive impairment or prior episode of delirium, history of alcohol or narcotic abuse, and malnutrition.[21,23] Procedural factors associated with high delirium risk include operative time greater than 2 hours, prolonged use of restraints, presence of a urinary catheter, addition of more than three new medications, and reoperation.[22]

Once the patient's risk for postoperative delirium is identified, perioperative care should be planned carefully to decrease other controllable factors. Epidural analgesia has been associated with less delirium than PCA after abdominal surgery.[24] Sedation or "sleepers" should be used judiciously, if at all, with high-risk patients. If the patient requires sedation, neuroleptics such as haloperidol and the atypical neuroleptics such as olanzapine are tolerated much better than benzodiazepines.[25] The patient's mental status, including orientation and attention, should be assessed with every visit, and care should be taken to avoid anemia, electrolyte imbalances, dehydration, and other contributing factors.

Once the diagnosis of postoperative delirium is established, it is important to recognize that some of the causes of delirium are potentially life-threatening, and immediate action is necessary. Evaluation begins with a thorough history and physical examination at the bedside by the surgeon. The history should focus on precipitating events such as falls (possible traumatic brain injury), recent procedures, use of opioids and sedatives, changes in existing medications (e.g., withholding of thyroid replacement or antidepressants), and consideration of alcohol withdrawal. The vital signs and fluid balance may suggest sepsis, hypovolemia, anemia, or dehydration. The exam should include brief but complete sensory and motor neurological examinations to differentiate delirium from stroke. Pay attention to common sites of infection such as the surgical wound, the lungs, and intravenous catheters. Urinary retention may be present as a result of medication or infection. Deep venous thrombosis may be clinically evident as limb swelling. Postoperative myocardial infarction may often present as acute cardiogenic shock.

The history and physical examination should then direct the use of lab tests. Most useful are the electrolytes, blood glucose, and complete blood cell count. Pulse oximetry and arterial blood gases may disclose hypercapnia or hypoxemia. Chest x-ray may disclose atelectasis, pneumonia, acute pulmonary edema, or pneumothorax. Cultures may be indicated in the setting of fever or leukocytosis, but will not help immediately. Electrocardiogram (ECG) and cardiac troponin may be used to diagnose postoperative myocardial infarction.

Resuscitative measures may be required if life-threatening causes of delirium are suspected. Airway control, supplemental oxygen, and fluid volume expansion should be considered in patients with unstable vital signs. The patient should not be sent out of the monitored environment for further tests, such as head computed tomography (CT), until the vital signs are stable and the agitation is controlled. Treatment of postoperative delirium depends on treatment of the underlying causes. Once the underlying cause has been treated delirium may persist, especially in the elderly or critically ill patients, who regain orientation and sleep cycles slowly. In these patients it is important to provide orienting communication and mental stimulation during the day, and to promote sleep during the night. The simplest ways are the most effective: contact with family members and friends, use of hearing aids, engagement in activities of daily living, and regular mealtimes. Sleep can be promoted by keeping the room dark and quiet throughout the evening, and preventing unnecessary interruptions. If nighttime sedation is required, atypical neuroleptics or low-dose serotonin reuptake inhibitors such as trazodone are better tolerated than benzodiazepines. If agitation persists, escalating doses of neuroleptics (or benzodiazepines in the setting of alcohol withdrawal) can be used to control behavior, but hidden causes of delirium must be considered.

▪ CARDIAC EVALUATION

RISK ASSESSMENT

It has been estimated that 1 million patients have a perioperative myocardial infarction (MI) each year, and the contribution to medical costs is $20 billion annually.[26] Thoracic, upper abdominal, neurological, and major orthopedic procedures are associated with increased cardiac risk. Diabetes, prior MI, unstable angina, and decompensated congestive heart failure (CHF) are most predictive of perioperative cardiac morbidity and mortality, and patients with these conditions undergoing major surgery warrant further

TABLE 2–2. CLINICAL PREDICTORS OF INCREASED RISK FOR PERIOPERATIVE CARDIAC COMPLICATIONS

MAJOR
- Recent myocardial infarction (within 30 days)
- Unstable or severe angina
- Decompensated congestive heart failure
- Significant arrhythmias (high-grade atrioventricular block, symptomatic ventricular arrhythmias with underlying heart disease, supraventricular arrhythmias with uncontrolled rate)
- Severe valvular disease

INTERMEDIATE
- Mild angina
- Prior myocardial infarction by history or electrocardiogram
- Compensated or prior congestive heart failure
- Diabetes mellitus
- Renal insufficiency

MINOR
- Advanced age
- Abnormal electrocardiogram
- Rhythm other than sinus (e.g., atrial fibrillation)
- Poor functional capacity
- History of stroke
- Uncontrolled hypertension (e.g., diastolic blood pressure >10 mm Hg)

evaluation[27] (Table 2–2). Patient factors conferring intermediate risk include mild angina and chronic renal insufficiency with baseline creatinine ≥ 2 mg/dL.[28] It is worth noting that women were underrepresented in the studies on which the American College of Cardiology and the American Heart Association (ACC/AHA) guidelines are based.[29] A retrospective study in gynecological patients found that hypertension and previous MI were major predictors of postoperative cardiac events, as opposed to the ACC/AHA guidelines, which indicate that they are minor and intermediate criteria, respectively.[30] Vascular surgical patients are at highest risk because of the prevalence of underlying coronary disease in this population.[27,31] Other high-risk procedural factors include emergency surgery, long operative time, and high fluid replacement volume; these are associated with a more than 5% risk of perioperative cardiac morbidity and mortality. Intraperitoneal procedures, carotid endarterectomy, thoracic surgery, head and neck procedures, and orthopedic procedures carry an intermediate risk, and are associated with a 1–5% risk of a perioperative cardiac event.[28]

Perioperative evaluation to identify patients at risk for cardiac complications is essential in minimizing morbidity and mortality. Work-up should start with history, physical exam, and ECG to determine the existence of cardiac pathology. Screening with chest radiographs and ECG is required for men over 40 and women over 55. According to the ACC/AHA guidelines, indications for preoperative cardiac testing should mirror those in the nonoperative setting.[32] The preoperative evaluation should include the surgeon, anesthesiologist, primary care physician, and possibly a cardiologist. Cardiology consultations are recommended for patients with major clinical predictors, those with intermediate clinical predictors and poor functional status undergoing intermediate-risk procedures, or those undergoing high-risk procedures with poor functional status or intermediate clinical predictors (Table 2–3). Overall functional ability is the best measure of cardiac health. Patients who can exercise without limitations can generally tolerate the stress of major surgery.[33] Limited exercise capacity may indicate poor cardiopulmonary reserve and the inability to withstand the stress of surgery. Poor functional status is the inability to perform activities such as driving, cooking, or walking less than 5 km/h.

Intraoperative risk factors include operative site, inappropriate use of vasopressors, and unintended hypotension. Intra-abdominal pressure exceeding 20 mm Hg during laparoscopy can decrease venous return from the lower extremities and thus contribute to decreased cardiac output,[34] and Trendelenburg positioning can results in increased pressure on the diaphragm from the abdominal viscera, subsequently reducing vital capacity. Intraoperative hypertension has not been isolated as a risk factor for cardiac morbidity, but it is often associated with wide fluctuations in pressure, and has been more closely associated with cardiac morbidity than intraoperative hypotension. Preoperative anxiety can contribute to hypertension even in normotensive patients. Those patients with a history of hypertension, even medically controlled hypertension, are more likely to be hypertensive preoperatively. Those with poorly controlled hypertension are at greater risk of developing intraoperative ischemia, arrhythmias, and blood pressure derangements, particularly at induction and intubation. Twenty-five percent of patients will exhibit hypertension during laryngoscopy. Patients with chronic hypertension may not necessarily benefit from lower blood pressure during the preoper-

TABLE 2–3. FACTORS THAT INCREASE THE RISK OF PERIOPERATIVE CARDIAC COMPLICATIONS

Risk Variable	Odds Ratio (95% Confidence Interval)
Poor functional status	1.8 (0.9–3.5)
Ischemic heart disease	2.4 (1.3–4.2)
Heart failure	1.9 (1.1–3.5)
Diabetes	3.0 (1.3–7.1)
Renal insufficiency	3.0 (1.4–6.8)
High-risk surgery	2.8 (1.6–4.9)

ative period because they may depend on higher pressures for cerebral perfusion. Those receiving antihypertensive medications should continue them up until the time of surgery. Patients taking beta-blockers are at risk of withdrawal and rebound ischemia. Key findings on physical examination include retinal vascular changes and an S_4 gallop consistent with left ventricular hypertrophy. Chest radiography may show an enlarged heart, also suggesting left ventricular hypertrophy.

Noninvasive cardiac testing is used to define risk in patients known to be at high or intermediate risk, and detect those with congestive heart failure or dyspnea. It is most useful in intermediate-risk patients. No special laboratory tests are necessary unless there is evidence of active ischemia. A baseline ECG is necessary to identify any new ECG findings, to rule out active ischemia, and as a baseline for comparison during the postoperative period. The baseline ECG will be normal in 25–50% of patients with coronary disease, but no history of MI. A 12-lead ECG should be obtained in patients with chest pain, diabetes, prior revascularization, prior hospitalization for cardiac causes, all men age 45 or older, and all women aged 55 with two or more risk factors. High- or intermediate-risk patients should also have a screening ECG. A lower-than-normal ejection fraction demonstrated on echocardiography is associated with the greatest perioperative cardiac risk, and should be obtained in all patients with symptoms suggesting heart failure or valvular disease. Tricuspid regurgitation indicates pulmonary hypertension and is often associated with sleep apnea. The chest x-ray is used to screen for cardiomegaly and pulmonary congestion, which may signify ventricular impairment.

Exercise testing demonstrates a propensity for ischemia and arrhythmias under conditions that increase myocardial oxygen consumption. Numerous studies have shown that performance during exercise testing is predictive of perioperative mortality in noncardiac surgery. ST-segment changes during exercise including horizontal depression greater than 2 mm, changes with low workload, and persistent changes after 5 minutes of exercise are seen in severe multivessel disease. Other findings include dysrhythmias at a low heart rate, an inability to raise the heart rate to 70% of predicted, and sustained decrease in systolic pressure during exercise.

Unfortunately, many patients are unable to achieve adequate workload in standard exercise testing because of osteoarthritis, low back pain, and pulmonary disease. In this case pharmacological testing is indicated with a dobutamine echocardiogram. Dobutamine is a beta-agonist that increases myocardial oxygen demand and reveals impaired oxygen delivery in those with coronary disease. Echocardiography concurrently visualizes wall motion abnormalities due to ischemia. Transesophageal echocardiography may be preferable to transthoracic echocardiography in obese patients because of their body habitus, and has been shown to have high negative predictive value in this group.[35] Nuclear perfusion imaging with vasodilators such as adenosine or dipyridamole can identify coronary artery disease and demand ischemia. Heterogeneous perfusion after vasodilator administration demonstrates an inadequate response to stress. Wall motion abnormalities indicate ischemia and an ejection fraction lower than 50% increases the risk of perioperative mortality. Angiography should only be performed if the patient may be a candidate for revascularization.

CORONARY DISEASE

Most perioperative myocardial infarctions are caused by plaque rupture in lesions that do not produce ischemia during preoperative testing.[36] This presents an obvious challenge for detecting patients at risk. Stress testing has a low positive predictive value in patients with no cardiac risk factors, and has been associated with an unacceptably high rate of false-positives.[37]

Preoperative optimization may include medical management, percutaneous coronary interventions (PCI), or coronary artery bypass grafting (CABG).[38] The ACC/AHA guidelines (Fig 2–1) recommend coronary revascularization prior to noncardiac surgery in the following situations:

1. The combined risk of the two procedures does not exceed the risk of the surgical procedure alone.
2. Revascularization should reduce the risk of the noncardiac surgery more than the risk of the revascularization procedure itself.
3. Revascularization should not unduly delay the noncardiac surgery, especially if it is urgent.

Patients warranting emergent CABG will be at greatest risk for that procedure. A recent study from the Veterans Administration Hospitals recommends against revascularization in patients with stable cardiac symptoms.[39] Preoperative PCI does not decrease the risk of future MI or mortality in patients with stable coronary disease, and only targets stenotic lesions, rather than those most likely to rupture. One retrospective study found no reduction in morbidity or perioperative MI after percutaneous transluminal coronary angioplasty, and the authors proposed that surgery within 90 days of balloon angioplasty increased the risk of thrombosis.[40] However, PCI done more than 90 days before surgery did provide benefit when compared to those who had

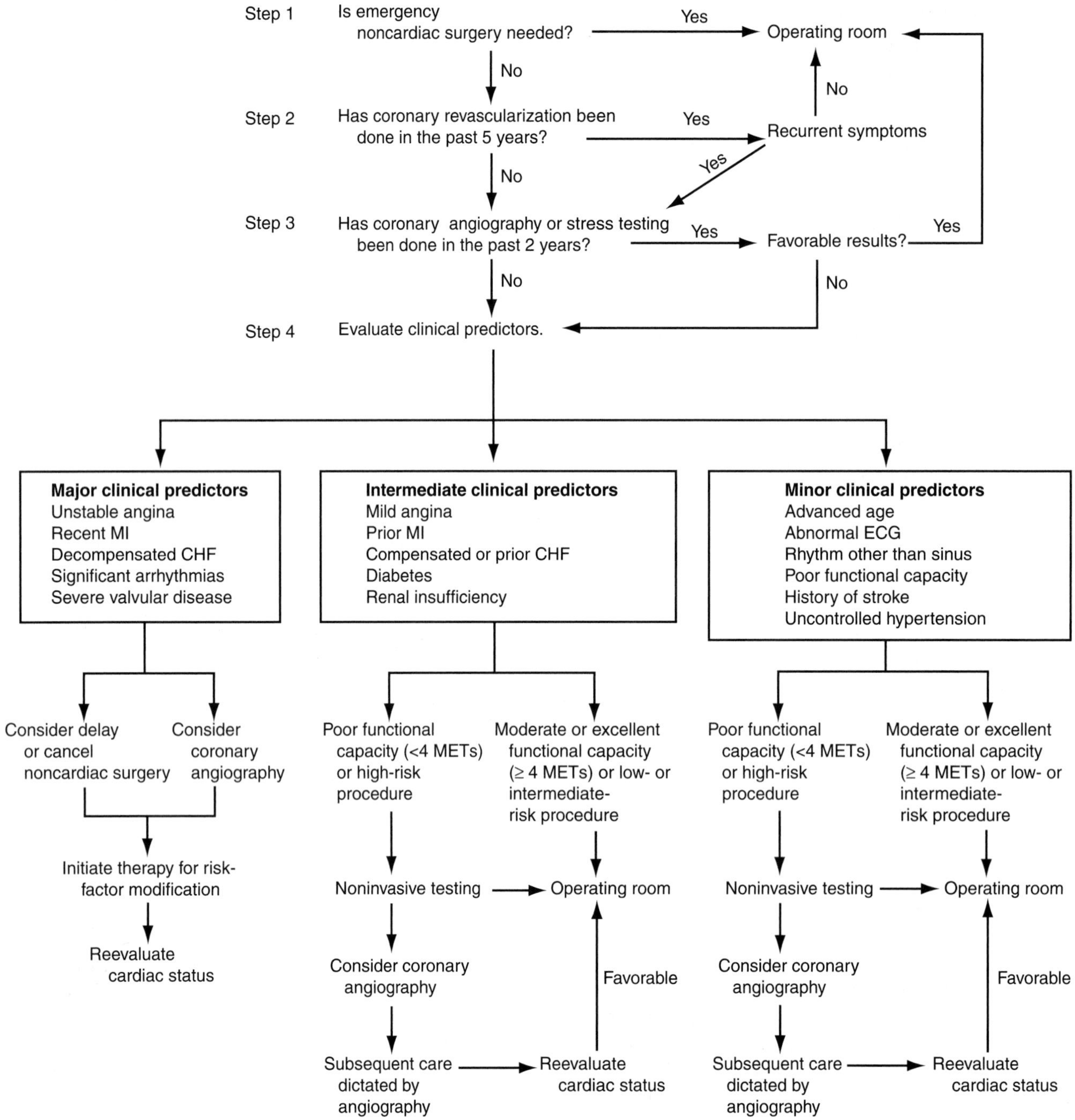

Figure 2–1. Preoperative cardiac risk assessment algorithm suggested by the ACC/AHA. (Adapted with permission from Eagle KA, Brundage BH, Chaitman BR, et al. Guidelines for perioperative cardiovascular evaluation for noncardiac surgery. Report of the American College of Cardiology/American Heart Association Task Force on Practice Guidelines [Committee on Perioperative Cardiovascular Evaluation for Noncardiac Surgery]. *J Am Coll Cardiol* 1996;27:921.) MI, myocardial infarction; CHF, congestive heart failure; ECG, electrocardiography; METs, metabolic equivalents.

no intervention at all. Another retrospective study found that patients who have surgery within 2 weeks of stenting had a high incidence of perioperative MI, major bleeding, or death.[41] Although a retrospective review from the Coronary Artery Surgery Study registry showed a lower mortality rate in patients with coronary artery disease who were post-CABG than those without CABG (0.09% versus 2.4%), this benefit did not include the morbidity associated with CABG itself. Unfortunately, the benefit was overwhelmed by the 2.3% morbidity rate seen with CABG in this cohort.[42] Survival benefit of CABG over medical management is realized for 2 years after surgery[43] so that preoperative mortality may decrease overall short-term survival. Revascularization and bypass grafting should be restricted to patients who would benefit from the procedure independent of their need for noncardiac surgery. One of the disadvantages of PCI in the preoperative setting is the need for anticoagulation to prevent early stent occlusion.

Catecholamine surges can cause tachycardia, which may alter the tensile strength of coronary plaques and incite plaque rupture.[44,45] Catecholamine surges can also increase blood pressure and contractility, contributing to platelet aggregation and thrombosis after plaque rupture and increasing the possibility of complete occlusion of the arterial lumen.[46] Perioperative beta-blockade mitigates these effects and has been shown to reduce MI and mortality from MI by over 30% in vascular surgical patients with reversible ischemia.[44] Furthermore, the benefits of perioperative beta-blockade continue for 2 years after surgery.[47] Beta-blockade is safe in patients with heart failure and moderate asthma, and it should be considered in all patients with cardiac risk factors regardless of preoperative testing results. Stress testing is only sensitive enough to predict three-fourths of patients who will suffer perioperative MI or death.[48] Thus, selective administration of beta-blockade can miss 25% of surgical patients who would benefit. Patients at highest risk still have a cardiac event rate of 10%, even with adequate perioperative beta-blockade.[37] Beta-blockade should be started days or weeks before surgery and adequate postoperative follow-up with an internist or cardiologist should be arranged in order to receive maximum benefit.

CONGESTIVE HEART FAILURE AND ARRHYTHMIA

Congestive heart failure is associated with coronary disease, valvular disease, ventricular dysfunction, and all types of cardiomyopathy. These are all independent risk factors that should be identified prior to surgery. Even compensated heart failure may be aggravated by fluid shifts associated with anesthesia and abdominal surgery and deserves serious consideration. Perioperative mortality increases with higher New York Heart Association class and preoperative pulmonary congestion. CHF should be treated to lower filling pressures and improve cardiac output before elective surgery. Beta-blockers, angiotensin-converting enzyme inhibitors, and diuretics can be employed to this end. The patient should be stable for 1 week before surgery.[49]

Arrhythmias and conduction abnormalities elicited in the history, on exam, or on ECG, should prompt investigation into metabolic derangements, drug toxicities, or coronary disease. In the presence of symptoms or hemodynamic changes, the underlying condition should be reversed and then medication given to treat the arrhythmia. Indications for antiarrhythmic medication and cardiac pacemakers are the same as in the nonoperative setting. Nonsustained ventricular tachycardia and premature ventricular beats contractions have not been associated with increased perioperative risk and do not require further intervention.[50,51]

VALVULAR DISEASE

Valvular disease should be considered in patients with symptoms of CHF, syncope, and a history of rheumatic heart disease. Aortic stenosis (AS) is a fixed obstruction to the left ventricular outflow tract, limiting cardiac reserve and an appropriate response to stress. History should elicit symptoms of dyspnea, angina, and syncope; examination may reveal a soft S_2, a late peaking murmur, or a right-sided crescendo-decrescendo murmur radiating to the carotids. AS is usually caused by progressive calcification or congenital bicuspid valve. Critical stenosis exists when the valve area is less than 0.7 cm^2 or transvalvular gradients are greater than 50 mm Hg, and is associated with an inability to increase cardiac output with demand. If uncorrected, AS is associated with a 13% risk of perioperative death. Valve replacement is indicated prior to elective surgery in patients with symptomatic stenosis.[52] Myocardial ischemia may occur in the absence of significant coronary artery occlusion in the presence of aortic valve disease. Perioperative management should include optimizing the heart rate to between 60 and 90 beats per minute and avoiding atrial fibrillation if possible. Because of the outflow obstruction, stroke volume may be fixed and bradycardia will lower cardiac output. Similarly, hypotension is also poorly tolerated.

Aortic regurgitation (AR) is associated with backward flow into the left ventricle during diastole and reduced forward stroke volume. Bradycardia facilitates regurgitation by increased diastolic time. Chronic AR causes massive LV dilatation (cor bovinum) and hypertrophy, which is associated with decreased LV function at later stages. AR is most often caused by rheumatic disease or congenital bicuspid valve. Medical treatment includes rate control and afterload reduction. Without valve replacement, survival is approximately 5 years once patients become symptomatic. This is an obvious consideration when planning any other surgical procedures.

Tricuspid regurgitation is usually caused by pulmonary hypertension secondary to severe left-sided failure. Other causes include endocarditis, carcinoid syndrome, and primary pulmonary hypertension. Hypovolemia, hypoxia, and acidosis can increase right ventricular afterload and should be avoided in the perioperative period.

Mitral stenosis is an inflow obstruction that prevents adequate left ventricular filling. The transvalvular pressure gradient depends on atrial kick, heart rate, and diastolic filling time. Tachycardia decreases filling time and contributes to pulmonary congestion. Mitral regurgitation is also associated with pulmonary hypertension with congestion, as the pathologic valve prevents forward flow, causing left atrial dilatation, and subsequent atrial arrhythmias. History and physical exam should focus on signs of congestive heart failure such as orthopnea, pedal edema, dyspnea, reduced exercise tolerance, and auscultatory findings such as murmurs and an S_3 gallop. Neurological deficits may signify embolic sequelae of valve disease. Perioperative rate control is essential for maintaining adequate cardiac output. ECG findings will reflect related arrhythmias and medications, but will not be specific for valve disease. Laboratory studies should identify secondary hepatic dysfunction or pulmonary compromise. Left ventricular hypertrophy is an adaptive response, which may cause subsequent pulmonary hypertension and diastolic dysfunction.

Patients with atrial fibrillation and prosthetic valves will be on anticoagulation preoperatively, and will need close monitoring in the perioperative period. Anticoagulation should be discontinued for a number of days preoperatively until the coagulation profile is suitable for surgery, and then resumed once it is safe from a hemostatic standpoint. Operative bleeding risk must be balanced against thromboembolic risk for the patient off of anticoagulation, and requires careful judgment. Heparin can be used as a bridge prior to surgery, and may require preoperative hospitalization. Thromboembolic risk increases with the amount of time that the patient's anticoagulation is subtherapeutic. Prosthetics in the mitral position pose the greatest risk for thromboembolism, and the risk increases with valve area and low flow. Mechanical valves pose a higher risk than tissue valves in patients with a history of valve replacement. Diuretics and afterload-reducing agents will enhance forward flow and minimize cardiopulmonary congestion. Patients with mitral valve prolapse should receive antibiotics.

Mitral regurgitation may also impair left ventricular function and lead to pulmonary hypertension. Stroke volume is reduced by backward flow into the atrium during systole. The left ventricle dilates to handle increasing end-systolic volume, eventually causing concentric hypertrophy and decreased contractility. The end result may be decreased ejection fraction and CHF. A decrease in systemic vascular resistance and increase in atrial contribution to the ejection fraction can both improve forward flow and reduce the amount of regurgitation. Echocardiography can clarify the degree of valvular impairment. Medical treatment centers on afterload reduction with vasodilators and diuretics. Mitral valve prolapse (MVP) is present in up to 15% of women, and is usually associated with a midsystolic click and late systolic murmur on physical exam. Murmur is indicative of prolapse. Although MVP is associated with connective tissue disorders, it usually occurs in otherwise healthy, asymptomatic patients. Echocardiography is used to confirm the diagnosis and evaluate the degree of prolapse. Chronically, MVP may be associated with mitral regurgitation, emboli, and increased risk of endocarditis. Prolapse may be aggravated by decreased preload, which should be minimized in the perioperative period. Patients with MVP are at risk of ventricular arrhythmias with sympathetic stimulation and endocarditis, which can be addressed with pain control and antibiotic prophylaxis, respectively.

Individuals with underlying structural cardiac defects are at increased risk for developing endocarditis after invasive procedures. Surgical procedures involving mucosal surfaces or infected tissues may cause transient bacteremia that is usually short-lived. Certain procedures are associated with a greater risk of endocarditis and warrant prophylaxis (Table 2–4). Abnormal valves, endocardium, or endothelium can harbor the bloodborne bacteria for a longer period of time, and infection and inflammation can ensue. While there are no randomized trials regarding endocarditis prophylaxis, the American Heart Association recommends prophylaxis for those[53] at high and moderate risk for developing the condition. Highest-risk patients have prosthetic heart valves, cyanotic congenital heart disease, or a history of endocarditis (even without structural abnormality).[54] Conditions associated with moderate risk include congenital septal defects, patent ductus arteriosus, coarctation of the aorta, and bicuspid aortic valve. Hypertrophic cardiomyopathy and acquired valvular disease

TABLE 2–4. AHA ENDOCARDITIS PROPHYLAXIS RECOMMENDATIONS

ANTIBIOTIC COVERAGE RECOMMENDED:

Respiratory: Tonsillectomy/adenoidectomy; rigid bronchoscopy; procedures involving respiratory mucosa

Gastrointestinal tract: Sclerotherapy for esophageal varices; esophageal dilation; ERCP; biliary tract surgery; procedures involving intestinal mucosa

Genitourinary tract: Prostatic surgery; cytoscopy; urethral dilation

ANTIBIOTIC COVERAGE NOT RECOMMENDED:

Respiratory: Endotracheal intubation; flexible bronchoscopy; tympanostomy tube insertion

Gastrointestinal tract: Transesophageal echocardiography; endoscopy without biopsy

In uninfected tissue: Urethral catheterization; uterine dilation and curettage; therapeutic abortion; manipulation of intrauterine devices

Other: Cardiac catheterization; pacemaker placement; circumcision; incision or biopsy on prepped skin also fall into this category. Mitral valve prolapse is a prevalent and often situational condition. Normal valves may prolapse in the event of tachycardia or hypovolemia, and may reflect normal growth patterns in young people. Prolapse without leak or regurgitation seen on Doppler studies is not associated with risk greater than that of the general population and no antibiotic prophylaxis is necessary.[55,56] However, the jet caused by the prolapsed valve increases the risk of bacteria sticking to the valve and subsequent endocarditis. Leaky valves detected by physical exam or Doppler warrant prophylactic antibiotics.[56] Those with significant regurgitation are more likely to be older and men, and other studies have shown that older men are more likely to develop endocarditis.[57–59] Some advocate prophylaxis for men older than 45 years with mitral valve prolapse even in the absence of audible regurgitation.[59] Prolapse secondary to myxomatous valve degeneration also warrants prophylactic antibiotics.[60,61] Prophylaxis is indicated in cases in whom mitral regurgitation cannot be determined.[62]

For patients at risk the goal should be administration of antibiotics in time to attain adequate serum levels during and after the procedure. For most operations, a single intravenous dose given 1 hour prior to incision will achieve this goal. Antibiotics should generally not be continued for more than 6–8 hours after the procedure to minimize the chance of bacterial resistance. In the case of oral, upper respiratory, and esophageal procedures, alpha-hemolytic streptococcus is the most common cause of endocarditis, and antibiotics should be targeted accordingly. Oral amoxicillin, parenteral ampicillin, and clindamycin for penicillin-allergic patients are suitable medications. Erythromycin is no longer recommended for penicillin-allergic patients because of gastrointestinal side effects and variable absorption.[63] Antibiotics given to those having genitourinary and nonesophageal gastrointestinal procedures should target enterococci.[63] While gram-negative bacteremia can occur, it rarely causes endocarditis. Parenteral ampicillin and gentamicin are recommended for highest-risk patients. Moderate-risk patients may receive amoxicillin or ampicillin. Vancomycin may be substituted in patients allergic to penicillin.

▪ PULMONARY EVALUATION

Pulmonary complications are common after surgery, and can prolong hospital stay for 1–2 weeks.[64] Complications include atelectasis, pneumonia, exacerbations of chronic pulmonary disorders, and respiratory failure requiring mechanical ventilation. Smoking, underlying chronic obstructive pulmonary disease (COPD), and poor exercise tolerance are the greatest risk factors for postoperative pulmonary complications. Physicians should ask about a history of smoking, decreased exercise capacity, dyspnea, and chronic cough. Examination should note pursed lip breathing, clubbing, and chest wall anatomy that could impair pulmonary function. Pulmonary testing is unnecessary in patients without a clear history of smoking or pulmonary disease. The predictive value of screening spirometry is unclear, and no threshold value has been identified to guide surgical decision making. Forced expiratory volume in 1 second less than 50% of predicted is indicative of exertional dyspnea and may herald the need for further testing. Preoperative chest x-ray abnormalities are associated with postoperative pulmonary complications,[64] but to this point there are no recommendations for screening radiographs in patients without pulmonary disease. Any preoperative chest x-ray must be examined for signs of hyperinflation consistent with COPD. While compensated hypercapnia has not been shown to be an independent predictor for postoperative ventilatory insufficiency in patients undergoing lung resection, preoperative arterial blood gas analysis provides useful baseline information for perioperative management of patients with chronic CO_2 retention. Transverse and upper abdominal incisions are associated with a higher rate of postoperative pulmonary complications than longitudinal midline incisions and lower abdominal incisions.[65] Surgery longer than 3 hours is also associated with higher risk.[66] General anesthesia is also associated with a higher risk of pulmonary complications than spinal, epidural, or regional anesthesia.[67]

Physiologic changes can be seen in the postoperative period, especially after thoracic and upper abdominal procedures. Vital capacity may decrease by 50–60%, and is accompanied by an increased respiratory rate to maintain tidal volumes. Normally, functional residual capacity usually exceeds the closing capacity of the alveoli so they remain open throughout the respiratory cycle. Prolonged effects of anesthetics and narcotics reduce functional reserve capacity postoperatively, causing alveolar collapse. These changes can last for weeks to months. A distended abdomen can impair diaphragmatic excursion; painful incisions around the diaphragm and other respiratory muscles contribute to splinting and inadequate pulmonary toilet. Narcotics can inhibit sighing and coughing reflexes, which normally prevent alveolar collapse during periods of sleep and recumbency. Analgesics must be titrated carefully to permit deep breathing and avoid impairing respiratory effort.

Inspired nonhumidified oxygen and halogenated anesthetics are cytotoxic and interfere with surfactant production and mucociliary clearance. Depressed respiratory reflexes, diaphragm dysfunction, and decreased functional reserve capacity all contribute to alveolar collapse and pooling of secretions. Aspiration risk is also increased. Excess secretions cause further alveolar collapse and create a milieu ripe for bacterial infection and pneumonia. Intubated patients should receive antacid prophylaxis and gastric drainage to minimize the risk of aspiration.

Multiple analyses have found that poor exercise tolerance is the greatest predictor of postoperative pulmonary impairment. The ASA risk classification is a gauge of general status, and is highly predictive of both cardiac and pulmonary complications.[68,69] Although advanced age is associated with increased incidence of chronic pulmonary disease and underlying impairment, it is not an independent risk factor for pulmonary complications.

Clearly, all smokers should be urged to stop before surgery. Even in the absence of coexisting pulmonary disease, smoking increases the risk of perioperative complications. Smoking confers a relative risk of 1.4–4.3, but a reduced risk of pulmonary complications has been shown in patients who stop smoking at least 8 weeks before cardiac surgery.[70] Even 48 hours of abstinence can improve mucociliary clearance, decrease carboxyhemoglobin levels to those of nonsmokers, and reduce the cardiovascular effects of nicotine. A nicotine patch may help some patients with postoperative nicotine withdrawal, but may not be advisable in patients at risk for poor wound healing.

COPD confers a relative risk of 2.7–4.7 in various studies. Symptoms of bronchospasm and obstruction should be addressed before surgery and elective procedures should be deferred in patients having an acute exacerbation. Preoperative treatment may include bronchodilators, antibiotics, steroids, and physical therapy to increase exercise capacity. Patients with active pulmonary infections should have surgery delayed if possible. Asthmatics should have peak flow equivalent to their personal best or 80% of predicted, and should be medically optimized to achieve this goal. Pulse corticosteroids may be used without an increased risk of postoperative infection or other complication.[71,72]

Malnourished patients may not be able to meet the demands of increased work of breathing, increasing their risk for respiratory failure. Obese patients have higher rates of oxygen consumption and carbon dioxide production, which increases their work of breathing. They may also exhibit restrictive physiology due to a large, stiff chest wall. A complete history should inquire about sleeping difficulty and snoring. Obesity increases the amount of soft tissue in the oropharynx, which can cause upper airway obstruction during sleep. Fifty-five percent of morbidly obese patients may have sleep-related breathing disorders such as obstructive sleep apnea and obesity-hypoventilation syndrome.[73] Symptoms include snoring and daytime sleepiness, and formal sleep studies are employed for definitive diagnosis. Sleep-disordered breathing is associated with hypoxia, hypercapnia, changes in blood pressure, nocturnal angina, and increased cardiac morbidity and mortality including stroke and sudden death.[74] Arterial blood gas with partial arterial oxygen pressure less than 55 mm Hg or partial arterial carbon dioxide pressure greater than 47 mm Hg confirms the diagnosis. An increased incidence of pulmonary hypertension and right-sided heart failure is seen in patients with obesity-hypoventilation syndrome and these patients should have an echocardiogram before surgery. In severe cases, intraoperative monitoring with a pulmonary artery catheter may be prudent.

In the patient who is awake, postoperative care should include coughing and deep breathing exercises, and in nonambulatory patients, early mobilization should include turning every 2 hours. Early ambulation prevents atelectasis and pooling of secretions, and increases the ventilatory drive. Upright position distributes blood flow and minimizes shunting. Preoperative medications should be resumed expeditiously. Incentive spirometry and pulmonary toilet are pulmonary expansion maneuvers, which reduce the relative risk of pulmonary complications by 50%.[75] Patients should receive preoperative education about these techniques. Inhaled ipratropium and beta-agonists, used together, may prevent postoperative wheezing and bronchospasm, and should be prescribed in patients at risk. Intermittent positive pressure ventilation and nasal bilevel positive airway pressure may be enlisted for secondary prevention. Epidural analgesia is superior to parenteral narcotics in abdominal and thoracic procedures for preventing pulmonary complications.

▪ GASTROINTESTINAL EVALUATION

Stress ulceration has been a well-recognized complication of surgery and trauma since 1832, when Cushing reported gastric bleeding accompanying head injury. With later research in gastric physiology and shock, it has been recognized that the appearance of gastric erosion results from failure of the protective function of gastric mucosa and back diffusion of hydrogen ion, enabling gastric acid to injure the mucosa. Once the mucosa is injured, the defenses are further weakened, leading to further injury in a vicious cycle. The protective functions of the mucosa rely on the stomach's rich blood flow to maintain high oxygen saturation. The most critical factor in the development of erosive ulceration now appears to be mucosal ischemia. Once the rich blood supply of the mucosa is compromised, the protective mechanisms are impaired, and gastric acid causes erosion, bleeding, and perforation.

In the late 1970s the incidence of gastric bleeding in critically ill patients was 15%. Recognition of the importance of organ perfusion has resulted in decreased rates of erosive stress gastritis. Factors often cited for this observation are: improvement in resuscitation and monitoring technology, nutritional support, and effective agents for medical prophylaxis. The prophylactic medicines are targeted to reduce gastric acidity. Antacids have been shown to provide effective protection against erosive ulceration; however, there is some risk of aspiration pneumonia. Antagonists of the histamine-2 (H_2) receptors of the parietal cells impair gastric acid secretion and also are effective prophylaxis for erosive ulceration. Due to ease of use, H_2-blockers have become the mainstay of stress ulcer prophylaxis in abdominal surgery.[76]

In the setting of elective operations when the patients are not critically ill, the incidence of stress ulceration is now very low and routine use of ulcer prophylaxis medication has been questioned. In addition, the routine use of H_2-antagonists in this setting may lead to increased risk of pneumonia because of failure of the gastric juices to kill bacteria.

POSTOPERATIVE ILEUS

Ileus is a condition of generalized bowel dysmotility that frequently impairs feeding in the postoperative setting. Ileus typically occurs after abdominal surgery, even if the bowel itself is not altered. It has been shown that laparotomy alone, without intestinal manipulation, leads to impaired gastrointestinal motility. The small bowel is typically affected the least, and can maintain organized peristaltic contractions throughout the perioperative period. The stomach usually regains a normal pattern of emptying in 24 hours, and the colon is last to regain motility, usually in 48–72 hours.

The exact mechanism that causes postoperative ileus is not known; however, physiologic studies have demonstrated the significant contribution of both inhibitory neural reflexes and local mediators within the intestinal wall. Inhibitory neural reflexes have been shown to be present within the neural plexuses of the intestinal wall itself, and in the reflex arcs traveling back and forth from the intestine to the spinal cord. These neural pathways may account for the development of ileus during laparotomy without bowel manipulation. In addition, inflammatory mediators such as nitric oxide are present in manipulated bowel and in peritonitis and may play a role in development of ileus.

Ileus can be recognized from clinical signs, such as abdominal distension, nausea, and the absence of bowel sounds and flatus, which should prompt the diagnosis. Abdominal x-ray imaging typically shows dilated loops of small bowel and colon. Bowel obstruction must also be considered with these clinical findings, however, and CT or other contrast imaging may be required to rule out obstruction.

Ileus can also appear following nonabdominal surgery, and can result from effects of medications (most often narcotics), electrolyte abnormalities (especially hypokalemia), and a wide variety of other factors.

Occasionally, the patient sustains a prolonged period of postoperative ileus. This can be due to a large number of contributing factors, such as intra-abdominal infection, hematoma, effects of narcotics and other medications, electrolyte abnormalities, and pain. In addition, there can be prolonged dysmotility from certain bowel operations, such as intestinal bypass.

The role of laparoscopic surgery in prevention of ileus is controversial. In theory, with less handling of the bowel laparoscopically and with smaller incisions, there should be less stimulation of the local mediators and neural reflexes. Animal studies comparing open and laparoscopic colon surgery indicate earlier resumption of normal motility studies and bowel movements with the laparoscopic approach. Human trials have not been conclusive. Several series demonstrate earlier tolerance of postoperative feeding with the laparoscopic approach to colon resection; however, these have been criticized for selection bias, and such studies are impossible to conduct in a blind fashion.

Early mobilization has long been held to be useful in prevention of postoperative ileus. While standing and walking in the early postoperative period have been proven to have major benefits in pulmonary function and prevention of pneumonia, mobilization has no demonstrable effect on postoperative ileus.

In the expected course of uncomplicated abdominal surgery, the stomach is frequently drained by a nasogastric tube for the first 24 hours after surgery, and the patient is not allowed oral intake until there is evidence that colonic motility has returned, usually best evidenced by the passage of flatus. Earlier feeding and no gastric drainage after bowel surgery can be attempted for healthy patients undergoing elective abdominal surgery, and has a high rate of success provided clinical symptoms of ileus are not present. In such patients, the use of effective preventive strategies is highly effective. These include maintenance of normal serum electrolytes, use of epidural analgesia, and avoidance of complications such as infection and bleeding. The routine use of nasogastric tubes for drainage in the postoperative period after abdominal surgery has come into question since the mid 1990s.

The most effective strategy for management of postoperative ileus following abdominal surgery has been the development of epidural analgesia. Randomized trials have shown that the use of non-narcotic (local anesthetic–based) epidural analgesia at the thoracic level in the postoperative period results in a decreased period of postoperative ileus in elective abdominal surgery. Ileus reduction is not seen in lumbar level epidural analgesia, suggesting that inhibitory reflex arcs involving the thoracic spinal cord may play a major role in postoperative ileus.

Narcotic analgesia, while effective for postoperative pain, has been shown to lengthen the duration of postoperative ileus, especially when used as a continuous infusion or as patient-controlled analgesia (PCA). Patients report better control of postoperative pain with continuous infusion or PCA as compared to intermittent parenteral dosing. Many studies have been done comparing various types of opioid analgesics, in attempts to find a type that does not prolong ileus. There has been no clearly superior drug identified; all currently available opioids cause ileus. Opioid antagonists such as naloxone have been used in trials to decrease ileus in chronic narcotic use, and there is evidence that antagonists are effective in that setting; however, in postoperative ileus the antagonists have not been shown to be clinically useful, again suggesting that other mechanisms are contributing to postoperative ileus.

EARLY POSTOPERATIVE BOWEL OBSTRUCTION

Early postoperative bowel obstruction refers to mechanical bowel obstruction, primarily involving the small bowel, which occurs in the first 30 days following abdominal surgery. The clinical picture may frequently be mistaken for ileus, and these conditions can overlap. The clinical presentation of early postoperative bowel obstruction is similar to that of bowel obstruction arising de novo: crampy abdominal pain, vomiting, abdominal distention, and obstipation. The incidence of early postoperative bowel obstruction has been variable in published series, due to difficulty in differentiating ileus from early postoperative bowel obstruction, but the reported range is from 0.7–9.5% of abdominal operations.

Retrospective large series show that about 90% of early postoperative bowel obstruction is caused by inflammatory adhesions. These occur as a result of injury to the surfaces of the bowel and peritoneum during surgical manipulation. The injury prompts the release of inflammatory mediators that lead to formation of fibrinous adhesions between the serosal and peritoneal surfaces. As the inflammatory mediators are cleared and the injury subsides, these adhesions eventually mature into fibrous, firm, bandlike structures. In the early postoperative period, the adhesions are in their inflammatory, fibrinous form, and as such do not usually cause complete mechanical obstruction.

Internal hernia is the next most common cause of early postoperative bowel obstruction, and can be difficult to diagnose short of repeat laparotomy. Internal hernia occurs when gaps or defects are left in the mesentery or omentum, or blind gutters or sacs are left in place during abdominal surgery. The typical scenario is colon resection involving extensive resection of the mesentery for lymph node clearance. If the resulting gap in the mesentery is not securely closed, small bowel loops may go through the opening and not be able to slide back out. A blind gutter may be constructed inadvertently during the creation of a colostomy. When the colostomy is brought up to the anterior abdominal wall, there is a space between the colon and the lateral abdominal wall, which may also trap the mobile loops of small bowel. Defects in the closure of the fascia during open or laparoscopic surgery can cause obstruction from incarcerated early postoperative abdominal wall hernia. Fortunately, internal hernia is a rare occurrence in the early postoperative period; however, it must be suspected in cases in whom bowel anastomoses or colostomies have been constructed. Unlike adhesive obstruction, internal hernia requires operative intervention due to the high potential for complete obstruction and strangulation of the bowel.

Intussusception is a rare cause of early postoperative bowel obstruction in adults, bur occurs more frequently in children. Intussusception occurs when peristalsis carries a segment of the bowel (called the lead point) up inside the distal bowel like a rolled up stocking. The lead point is usually abnormal in some way, and typically has some intraluminal mass, such as a tumor or the stump of an appendix after appendectomy. Other rare causes for early postoperative bowel obstruction include missed causes of primary obstruction at the index laparotomy, peritoneal carcinomatosis, obstructing hematoma, and ischemic stricture.

Management of early postoperative bowel obstruction depends on differentiation of adhesive bowel obstruction (the majority) from internal hernia and the other causes, and from ileus. Clinicians generally rely on radiographic imaging to discern ileus from obstruction. For many years plain x-ray of the abdomen was used: if the abdominal plain film showed air-distended loops of bowel and air-fluid levels on upright views, the diagnosis of obstruction was favored. However, plain radiographs can be misleading in the postoperative setting, and the overlap of ileus and obstruction can be confusing. Upper GI contrast studies using a water-soluble agent has better accuracy, and abdominal CT using oral contrast has been shown to have 100% sensitivity and specificity in differentiating early postoperative bowel obstruction from postoperative ileus.

Once the diagnosis is made, management is tailored to the specific needs of the patient. Decompression via nasogastric tube is usually indicated, and ileus can be treated as discussed. Adhesive bowel obstruction warrants a period of expectant management and supportive care, as the majority of these problems will resolve spontaneously. Most surgical texts recommend that the waiting period can be extended to 14 days. If the early bowel obstruction lasts longer than 14 days, less than 10% resolve spontaneously, and exploratory laparotomy is indicated. The uncommon causes of early postoperative bowel obstruction, such as internal hernia, require more early surgical correction, and should be suspected in the setting of complete obstipation, or when abdominal CT suggests internal hernia or complete bowel obstruction.

RENAL EVALUATION

Patients without a clinical history suggesting renal disease have a low incidence of significant electrolyte disturbances on routine preoperative screening.[77] However, those patients with renal or cardiac disease who are taking digitalis or diuretics, or those with ongoing fluid losses (i.e., diarrhea, vomiting, fistula, and bleeding) do have an increased risk of significant abnormalities and should have electrolytes measured and replaced preoperatively.

Preoperative urinalysis can be a useful screen for renal disease. Proteinuria marks intrinsic renal disease or congestive heart failure. Urinary glucose and ketones are suggestive of diabetes and starvation in the ketotic state, respectively. In the absence of recent genitourinary instrumentation, microscopic hematuria suggests calculi, vascular disease, or infection. A few leukocytes may be normal in female patients, but an increased number signifies infection. Epithelial cells are present in poorly collected specimens.

Patients with renal insufficiency or end-stage renal disease often have comorbidities that increase their overall risk in the perioperative period. Hypertension and diabetes correlate with increased risk of coronary artery disease and postoperative myocardial infarction, impaired wound healing, wound infection, platelet dysfunction, and bleeding. Preoperative history should note the etiology of renal impairment, preoperative weight as a marker of volume status, and timing of last dialysis and the amount of fluid removed routinely. Evaluation should include a cardiac risk assessment. Physical exam should focus on signs of volume overload such as jugular venous distention and pulmonary crackles. A full electrolyte panel (calcium, phosphorus, magnesium, sodium, and potassium) should be checked preoperatively, along with blood urea nitrogen and creatinine levels. Progressive renal failure is associated with catabolism and anorexia. Such patients need aggressive nutritional support during the perioperative periods to minimize the risk of infection and poor healing.

Dialysis-dependent patients should have dialysis within 24 hours before surgery, and may benefit from monitoring of intravascular volume status during surgery. Blood samples obtained immediately after dialysis, before equilibration occurs, should only be used in comparison to pre-dialysis values to determine the efficacy of dialysis.[78]

Postoperatively, patients with chronic renal insufficiency or end-stage renal disease will need to have surgical volume losses replaced, but care should be taken to avoid excess. Replacement fluids should not contain potassium, and early dialysis should be employed to address volume overload and electrolyte derangements. Patients with impaired creatinine clearance should have their medications adjusted accordingly. For example, meperidine should be avoided because its metabolites accumulate in renal impairment and can lead to seizures.

The choice of postoperative fluid therapy depends on the patient's comorbidities, the type of surgery, and conditions that affect the patient's fluid balance. There is no evidence that colloid is better than crystalloid in the postoperative period, and it is considerably more expensive.[79] Sepsis and bowel obstruction will require ongoing volume replacement rather than maintenance. Ringer's solution provides six times the intravascular volume as an equivalent amount of hypotonic solution. In patients with normal renal function, clinical signs such as urine output, heart rate, and blood pressure should guide fluid management. Once the stress response subsides, fluid retention subsides and fluid is mobilized from the periphery, and fluid supplementation is unnecessary. This fluid mobilization is evident by decreased peripheral edema and increased urine output. Diuretics given in the period of fluid sequestration may cause intravascular volume depletion and symptomatic hypovolemia.

Postoperative management includes close monitoring of urine output and electrolytes, daily weight, elimination of nephrotoxic medications, and adjustment of all medications that are cleared by the kidney. Hyperkalemia, hyperphosphatemia and metabolic acidosis may be seen and should be addressed accordingly. Indications for renal replacement therapy include severe intravascular overload, symptomatic hyperkalemia, metabolic acidosis, and complicated uremia (pericarditis and encephalopathy) (Table 2–5).

Postoperative renal failure increases perioperative mortality. Risk factors for postoperative renal failure include intraoperative hypotension, advanced age, congestive heart failure, aortic cross-clamping, administration of nephrotoxic drugs or radiocontrast, and preoperative elevation in renal insufficiency. Up to 10% of patients may experience acute renal failure after aortic cross-clamping. Postoperative renal failure rates are higher in hypovolemic patients, so preoperative dehydration should be avoided. Contrast nephropathy is a common cause of hospital-acquired renal failure, and manifests as a 25% increase in serum creatinine within 48 hours of contrast administration.

Nephropathy is caused by ischemia and direct toxicity to the renal tubules. Diabetes and chronic renal insufficiency are the greatest risk factors for dye nephropathy. Recent trials[80] have shown that patients receiving contrast have a lower incidence of contrast-induced nephropathy when treated with a sodium bicarbonate infusion. N-acetylcysteine given orally on the day prior to contrast exposure also decreases the incidence of radiocontrast nephropathy.[81]

Rising blood urea nitrogen and creatinine and postoperative oliguria (<500 mL/d) herald the onset of postoperative renal failure. Management is determined by the cause of renal insufficiency. Acute renal failure is classified into three categories: prerenal, intrarenal, and postrenal. Prerenal azotemia is common in the postoperative period. It is caused by decreased renal perfusion seen with hypotension and intravascular volume contraction. Intrarenal causes of oliguric renal failure include acute tubular necrosis (from aortic cross-clamping, shock, or renal ischemia), and less commonly, acute interstitial nephritis from nephrotoxic medication. Postrenal causes include obstruction in the collecting system (from bilateral ureteral injury, Foley catheter occlusion, or urethral obstruction). Work-up should include urinalysis, serum chemistries,

TABLE 2–5. INDICATIONS FOR HEMODIALYSIS

Serum potassium >5.5 mEq/L
BUN >80 mg/dL
Persistent acidosis
Acute volume overload
Uremic symptoms

and measurement of the fractional excretion of sodium. Invasive monitoring and cardiac echocardiogram may be employed to evaluate volume status. Ultrasound is indicated if obstruction is suspected.

Initial management of oliguria in adults includes placement of a bladder catheter, and a challenge with isotonic fluids (500 mL of normal saline or Ringer's lactate). If a bladder catheter is already present, it should be checked to ensure that it is draining properly. A urinalysis should be obtained with special attention to specific gravity, casts, and evidence of infection. Hematocrit should be evaluated to exclude bleeding and blood pressure measured to rule out hypotension as causes. The fractional excretion of sodium can help determine the etiology of the renal failure (Table 2–6). Serum creatinine is used to follow the course of acute renal failure. Patients who have been adequately resuscitated or who are in congestive heart failure require evaluation to rule out cardiogenic shock. Urinary retention can be treated with a Foley catheter, and ureteral obstruction can be addressed with percutaneous nephrostomy.

Intravascular volume depletion adversely affects cardiac output, tissue perfusion, and oxygen delivery. Monitoring includes total body weight, urine output, vital signs, and mental status. However, body weight should not be used alone because total volume overload can be seen in the setting of intravascular volume depletion. Invasive monitoring to measure cardiac filling pressures may be utilized when clinical assessment is unreliable.

Fluid overload may be seen in patients with renal, hepatic, and cardiac disease, and is associated with increased morbidity.[82] Critically ill patients may develop anasarca. It is difficult to determine volume status by observation alone, and invasive monitoring may be required.

Electrolyte abnormalities are common in the perioperative period. Serum sodium reflects intravascular volume status. Hyponatremia signifies excess free water in the intravascular space, and is caused by excess antidiuretic hormone in the postoperative period. It occurs in the setting of normo-, hypo-, or hypervolemia. It may be avoided by judicious use of isotonic fluids. Conversely, hypernatremia suggests a relative deficit of intravascular free water. Patients who are unable to drink, or those with large insensible losses, are most at risk. Treatment includes free water replacement.

Diuretics, malnutrition, and gastrointestinal losses may cause postoperative hypokalemia. Metabolic alkalosis shifts potassium into the intracellular compartment. Serum potassium levels less than 3 mEq/L warrant ECG monitoring and replacement in patients who are not anuric. Replacement in patients with renal insufficiency may be complex. Hyperkalemia is more commonly seen

TABLE 2–6. OLIGURIA IN THE PERIOPERATIVE PATIENT

	Prerenal	Intrarenal	Postrenal
Causes	Bleeding Hypovolemia Cardiac failure Dehydration	Drugs Contrast medium Sepsis Myoglobinuria	Obstruction
UOsm	>500 mOsm/L	Equal to plasma	Variable
U_{Na}	<20 mOsm/L	>50 mOsm/L	>50 mOsm/L
Fe_{Na}	<1%	>3%	Indeterminate

Fe_{Na}, fractional excretion of sodium; U_{Na}, urinary sodium concentration; UOsm, urinary osmolality.

in renal patients. It may also be seen in myonecrosis, hemolysis, and acidosis. Cardiac arrhythmias are seen at levels above 6.5 mEq/L and death is associated with levels greater than 8 mEq/L. These patients should have cardiac monitoring until their levels normalize. ECG will show widened QRS interval, peaked T waves, and absent P waves. Hyperkalemia should be treated with sodium bicarbonate to stimulate acidosis, as well as intravenous calcium and insulin with glucose to drive potassium into the intracellular compartment. Cation exchange resins can be administered orally or per rectum to bind ions in the gastrointestinal tract, but care should be taken for the patient who is post–GI surgery or has underlying gastrointestinal problems. Dialysis can by employed if other measures fail.

■ HEMATOLOGICAL EVALUATION

A complete preoperative evaluation should include assessment of hematological disorders, which can increase the risk for postoperative bleeding or thromboembolism. Patients should be asked about a family history of bleeding disorders and personal history of bleeding problems, especially after procedures. Excessive bleeding after dental procedures and menorrhagia in women can alert the physician to undiagnosed hematologic disease. Risk factors for postoperative hemorrhage include known coagulopathy, trauma, hemorrhage, or potential factor deficiency.[83] Factor deficiencies can be seen with a history of liver disease, malabsorption, malnutrition, or chronic antibiotic use. Even high-risk patients have only a 1.7% risk of postoperative hemorrhage and a 0.21% risk of death related to postoperative hemorrhage.[83,84]

Routine tests may include a complete blood count, prothrombin time (PT), activated partial thromboplastin time (PTT), and International Normalized Ratio (INR), but are not required in the asymptomatic patient with no associated history. The complete blood count will reveal leukocytosis, anemia, and thrombocytopenia or thrombocytosis. A baseline hematocrit is useful for postoperative management when anemia is suspected. Platelet count also provides a useful baseline, but does not provide information about platelet function. A bleeding time may be required to provide more information in select patients. However, bleeding time results are operator-dependent and highly variable, making it a poor screening tool for identifying high-risk patients.[85,86] An abnormal bleeding time is not associated with increased postoperative bleeding,[87] nor has it proven useful in identifying patients taking nonsteroidal anti-inflammatory medication or aspirin.[85] None of the aforementioned tests can be used to diagnose hereditary bleeding disorders. However, an elevated PTT may be seen in factor XI deficiency, and should be obtained in patients at risk for this deficiency. Low-risk patients are very unlikely to have bleeding complications even if the PTT is abnormal,[86] and have an increased risk of false-positives that can lead to unnecessary testing. PTT is not a reliable predictor of postoperative bleeding,[88] and should not be used to screen for bleeding abnormalities in patients without symptoms or risk factors.[89,90]

A platelet count of 20,000 or greater is usually adequate for normal clotting. Aspirin causes irreversible impairment of platelet aggregation, and is commonly prescribed in patients at risk of cardiovascular and cerebrovascular disease. The clinical effect of aspirin lasts 10 days, and it is for this reason that patients are asked to stop taking aspirin 1 week before elective surgery. Desmopressin can be used to partially reverse platelet dysfunction caused by aspirin and uremia. Other NSAIDs cause reversible platelet dysfunction and should also be held before surgery. Glycoprotein IIb-IIIa inhibitors prevent platelet-fibrin binding and platelet aggregation, and are used for 2–4 weeks after coronary angioplasty. Elective surgery should be avoided during these 2–4 weeks, as stopping treatment increases the risk of thrombosis. Patients who do not receive 4 weeks of antiplatelet therapy are at risk of stent thrombosis.[91]

Von Willebrand's disease (VWD) is an autosomal dominant disorder characterized by variable deficiency in Von Willebrand's factor (VWF). VWF is a cofactor for factor VIII, and plays a significant role in platelet adhesion. It is the most common congenital bleeding disorder, although its true prevalence is unknown because of its variable penetrance. Laboratory findings include a low VWF antigen, factor VIII activity <10% of normal, and abnormal ristocetin cofactor. It is associated with epistaxis, easy bruising, and postprocedure bleeding. Prolonged bleeding time in the setting of normal platelet count, PT, and PTT suggests an inherited platelet disorder. Platelet aggregation studies, including a test using the agonist ristocetin, can confirm the diagnosis. Myeloproliferative disorders, recent cardiopulmonary bypass, uremia, and drug therapy (e.g., glycoprotein IIb-IIIa inhibitors or aspirin) may cause acquired platelet disorders and must be considered as well.

Hemophilia A (factor VIII deficiency) and hemophilia B (factor IX deficiency) can cause spontaneous bleeding and are associated with severe and prolonged postoperative and traumatic bleeding. Intravenous or intranasal desmopressin releases VWF and factor VIII from endothelial storage sites and can be useful in achieving hemostasis in patients with hemophilia A and VWD. However, not all patients are responsive, and some patients with VWD may develop thrombocytopenia when VWF from storage sites binds to circulating platelets. Therefore, patients who may require desmopressin should be tested before surgery. Cryoprecipitate may be used in patients with VWD unresponsive to desmopressin or bleeding patients with fibrinogen levels less than 100 mg/dL. Aminocaproic acid may also be used in conjunction with desmopressin for VWD, hemophilia, and a variety of factor deficiencies. Aminocaproic acid is an antifibrinolytic agent that promotes clot formation and is useful for stopping acute bleeding when given as a continuous infusion. Most other factor deficiencies can also be treated with fresh frozen plasma.

Indications for red blood cell transfusion remain somewhat controversial and are often empirical in practice. Transfusing one unit of red blood cells or whole blood can increase the hematocrit by approximately 3% or hemoglobin by 1 g/dL. Multiple studies have demonstrated that overutilizing transfusion may adversely affect patient outcome and increase risk of infection. ASA guidelines[92] suggest that transfusion should be based on risks of inadequate oxygenation, rather than a threshold hemoglobin level. Generally transfusion is rarely indicated when the hemoglobin level exceeds 10 g/dL, but is almost always indicated when it is less than 6 g/dL, especially in the setting of acute anemia. Healthy individuals can usually tolerate up to 40% of blood loss without requiring blood cell transfusion, and blood products should not be used solely to expand volume or to improve wound healing. The decision to transfuse red cells or whole blood should be based on the patient's risk of complications associated with impaired oxygen delivery, including hemodynamic indices, history of cardiopulmonary disease, rate of blood loss, and preexisting anemia.

Conditions associated with abnormal platelets and low platelet counts can be treated with platelet transfusions. The usual dose, one unit of platelet concentrate/10 kg body weight, can be expected to increase the platelet count by approximately 5000–10,000 in an average adult. In patients without increased risk of bleeding, prophylactic platelet administration is not indicated until counts fall below 20,000, when spontaneous bleeding can be seen. Higher thresholds may be indicated for patients at increased risk of bleeding, known platelet dysfunction, and microvascular bleeding. Platelet transfusion is not helpful when bleeding is secondary to platelet destruction as in heparin-induced thrombocytopenia and autoimmune thrombocytopenia. Desmopressin can augment platelet function in uremia and incite release of VWF from the endothelium, which can improve platelet function. In surgical patients, platelet transfusion is rarely indicated with counts greater than 100,000, and usually is indicated when counts are less than 50,000. The decision to transfuse platelets should be based on the amount of bleeding expected, the ability to control bleeding, and the presence of platelet dysfunction or destruction.

Transfusion of fresh frozen plasma (FFP) is indicated to reverse warfarin before procedures or in the presence of active bleeding, for inherited or acquired coagulopathy that can be treated with FFP, and for massive transfusion of more than one whole blood volume. Microvascular bleeding can be seen if the PT/PTT is greater than 1.5 times normal, and FFP can be used to reverse bleeding in this setting. Warfarin reversal can be achieved with doses of 5–8 mL/kg, and 30% factor concentration can be achieved with 10–15 mL/kg. FFP should not be used to address volume depletion alone. Cryoprecipitate contains factors VIII, VWF, XIII, fibrinogen, and fibronectin, and can be used preventively in patients with these factor deficiencies and uremia.

Endothelial injury and venous stasis are the greatest risk factors for venous thromboembolism (VTE). The patient with hereditary thrombophilia, or a personal history of venous thromboembolism, cancer, or recent surgery (within 4 weeks) has an increased risk of VTE.[93] Preventive measures include external pneumatic leg compression, early mobilization after surgery, and anticoagulation. Compression devices are contraindicated in patients with severe peripheral vascular disease, venous stasis, or risk of tissue necrosis. Inferior vena cava (IVC) filters are indicated in patients who cannot take anticoagulation or who have failed anticoagulation therapy. Patients with a history of VTE benefit from IVC filter placement in the short term, but IVC filter placement is accompanied by an increased incidence of deep venous thrombosis over the long term.[94] Systemic anticoagulation is the preferred long-term option. Low-molecular-weight heparin (LMWH) and unfractionated heparin are equally effective for prevention of pulmonary embolism in patients with deep venous thrombosis.[94] Recent venous thromboembolism, atrial fibrillation, and mechanical heart valves are common indications for warfarin treatment.

Clinically, unfractionated heparin activity is measured by PTT and the therapeutic goal is usually 2.0–2.5 times normal. LMWH is a relatively stronger inhibitor of factor Xa and does not have the same effect on the PTT. The anticoagulant effect of LMWH is measured by factor Xa activity. Protamine can reverse the effects of heparin, but may cause allergic reactions and induce hypercoagulability, and should be used cautiously. FFP will not reverse heparin, and can actually increase heparin activity because it contains antithrombin III. Direct thrombin inhibitors can also prolong the PTT. Direct thrombin inhibitors are not reversible with protamine and may require large amounts of FFP for reversal.

At higher doses, heparin can also affect platelet function. Heparin must be administered subcutaneously or intravenously, as it is not absorbed enterally. Only one-third of administered heparin has anticoagulant activity, and heparin is highly bound to plasma proteins, accounting for its unpredictable response. The therapeutic goal is usually PTT 1.5–2.0 times normal.

Heparin can be used for the prevention and treatment of VTE. Surgical patients over age 40 or those at increased risk for VTE should receive 5000 U SC every 8–12 hours, depending on their weight. High-risk patients with a history or VTE, cancer, morbid obesity, or those having orthopedic procedures should either receive SC heparin with a goal of high range of normal or LMWH. In the event of acute venous thromboembolism intravenous heparin should be started promptly with a therapeutic goal of PTT 1.5–2.0 times normal. Oral anticoagulation should be started within 24 hours and continued for 3–6 months.[93]

Warfarin inhibits synthesis of vitamin K–dependent clotting factors (II, VII, IX, X, and proteins C and S). Poor diet, prolonged antibiotic use, and fat malabsorption can also cause vitamin K deficiency and cause abnormal coagulation. Except for Von Willebrand's factor and factor VIII, which are synthesized in the endothelium, all other coagulation factors are made in the liver, which also clears activated coagulation factors and coagulation degradation products. Liver disease can lead to multiple coagulation abnormalities including factor deficiencies, vitamin K deficiency, fibrinolysis, and elevated levels of fibrin degradation products. All patients with known or suspected liver disease should be tested for coagulopathy. Vitamin K can be administered subcutaneously or intravenously in deficient patients. The initiation of warfarin therapy is associated with a transient thrombotic state because plasma concentrations of protein C fall approximately 24 hours before concentrations of other clotting factors.

Heparin is the drug of choice for VTE during pregnancy because it does not cross the placenta. Adverse effects of heparin therapy may include hemorrhage, thrombocytopenia, and osteoporosis. Heparin-induced thrombocytopenia is an immune disorder seen in patients with prior exposure to heparin, which may cause thrombosis. Treatment includes cessation of heparin and utilization of alternative anticoagulants such as lepirudin, danaparoid, or argatroban. These should be given until platelet counts recover.

A thorough personal and family history is the best screening test for hypercoagulability. Clinical suspicion should be raised in the event of recurrent thrombosis, spontaneous abortions, thrombosis in a young patient, family history of thrombosis, and repeated exposure to heparin. Resistance to activated protein C, conferred by a mutation in factor V Leiden, is the most common heritable clotting disorder.

Anticoagulation is commonly employed to minimize the risk of embolic disease in patients with atrial fibrillation, recent or recurrent venous thromboembolism, and mechanical heart valves. Interrupting chronic therapy can transiently increase the risk of thromboembolism and the surgeon must weigh the risks of embolism versus the risk of postoperative bleeding when determining when to stop and resume anticoagulation.

If possible the INR should be 1.5 or lower before elective surgery. After warfarin is discontinued, it takes about 4 days for an INR in the range of 2.0–3.0 to spontaneously reach 1.5, and about 3 days for the INR to reach 2.0 after it is restarted. If therapy is withheld preoperatively, most patients will have a window of 2–4 days when they are not anticoagulated and at risk for venous thrombosis. This risk is compounded by the increased risk of thromboembolism associated with surgery.[95,96] It has been estimated that surgery increases the risk of venous thromboembolism by 100-fold in patients with recurrent disease.[97] Without anticoagulation, there is a 50% chance of recurrence within the 3 months after the first episode of venous thrombosis. Warfarin therapy reduces the risk to 10% after 1 month and 5% after 3 months. It is not advisable to interrupt anticoagulation within 1 month after an event of VTE, and if possible, surgery should be deferred until the patient has completed 3 months of therapy.[97] Chronic anticoagulation lowers the risk of thromboembolism in patients with atrial fibrillation and mechanical heart valves by 66% and 75%, respectively.[97]

Patients with prior embolic episodes are at increased risk for recurrence. Six percent of episodes of VTE and 20% of arterial thromboembolism may be fatal,[97] and a significant percentage cause disability. Alternatively, the risk of death after postoperative hemorrhage is less than 1%,[98] so the judicious use of postoperative anticoagulation can be relatively protective. Preoperative heparinization is not required during the second and third months of warfarin treatment for DVT because the risk is sufficiently low. Such patients have increased VTE risk after surgery and should receive postoperative anticoagulation. Patients who are at risk for recurrent DVT, and are within 2 weeks of the first episode, or who cannot tolerate anticoagulation are candidates for an IVC filter.[94]

Elective surgery should be deferred for the first month after arterial embolism because of the high risk of recurrence during this period. If necessary, patients should receive perioperative heparin while oral anticoagulation is held. Patients on long-term anticoagulation to prevent arterial thromboembolism do not need perioperative heparin because the risk of bleeding outweighs the risk of arterial embolism during this period.

Heparin should be titrated to a goal PTT of 1.5–2.0 times normal and given as a continuous intravenous infusion. It should be stopped 6 hours prior to a procedure, and can be restarted 12 hours after surgery if there was no evidence of bleeding at the end of the case. Heparin can be restarted without a bolus at the anticipated maintenance infusion rate.[97,98]

▪ INFECTIOUS COMPLICATIONS

Infectious complications can be most unwelcome and difficult to control after major abdominal surgery, yet they are surprisingly frequent despite all modern prophylactic measures. Reported surgical wound infection rates in elective operations vary from 2% for inguinal hernia repair,[99] to 26% for colectomy,[100] and is even higher for emergency surgery.[101] Surgical site infections (SSIs) increase overall mortality and morbidity, and increase hospital length of stay and overall costs. Therefore prevention and treatment of infectious complications should be included in surgical decision making for all abdominal procedures.

Prevention of SSIs begins with preoperative evaluation and identification of patients at high risk for SSI. Patient factors implicated in risk of SSI include age, diabetes mellitus, smoking, steroid use, malnutrition, obesity, active distant infection, prolonged hospital stay, and nasal colonization with *Staphylococcus aureus*.[102–105]

Standard basic surgical rules should be followed with every patient. These were codified as formal guidelines by the Centers for Disease Control and Prevention in 1999[106] and include recommendations for skin preparation with alcohol or iodophor, surgical barriers such as drapes and gowns, careful hand scrubbing, and appropriate selection of prophylactic antibiotics. Preoperative hair removal and antiseptic shower have not been shown to decrease SSI rates, and shaving and clipping of hair can increase SSIs. The CDC recommendations are summarized in Table 2–7. (See Table 4–3 for extended recommendations.)

Antibiotic prophylaxis may be indicated for patients at high risk, or in contaminated surgical procedures, but antibiotics should not be used indiscriminately. Overuse of antibiotics is associated with emergence of multidrug-resistant bacteria and increased rates of hospital-acquired infections. Selection of patients for antimicrobial prophylaxis requires stratification of patient risk factors as discussed above and procedure-specific risk factors. The degree of contamination in the surgical site has long been recognized as an independent risk factor for SSI,[107] leading to the wound classification system (Table 2–8) in use since 1983.

Patients undergoing class I (clean) procedures have a very low infection rate and generally do not benefit from prophylactic antibiotics, unless there is some suspicion at the start of the procedure that some contamination may occur, such as unplanned enterotomy in a patient with many previous abdominal procedures. In addition, many surgeons prefer to use antibiotic prophylaxis in class I procedures when a prosthesis is implanted; examples include hernia repair and vascular bypass. In this setting, the risk of SSI is low, but the morbidity and mortality of an infected prosthesis are great, and prophylaxis may decrease the risk. To date,

TABLE 2–7. CDC CATEGORY 1 RECOMMENDATIONS FOR REDUCTION OF SURGICAL SITE INFECTIONS

These are strongly recommended based on best clinical evidence:
Identify and treat distant infections prior to surgery
Do not remove hair routinely; if hair must be removed, use electric clippers immediately prior to surgery
Control hyperglycemia in the perioperative period
Cease tobacco smoking 30 days prior to surgery
Antiseptic shower the night prior to surgery
Antiseptic skin preparation
Surgery team should practice hand scrubs
Administer appropriate antimicrobial prophylaxis
Surgical barriers (gown, gloves, hat, mask)
Do not close contaminated skin incisions

TABLE 2–8. SURGICAL WOUND CLASSIFICATION

Class I. Clean
Uninfected wounds without contamination
Class II. Clean/contaminated
Uninfected wounds in procedures where the respiratory, gastrointestinal, or genitourinary tracts are entered in a controlled fashion without gross spillage
Class III. Contaminated
An operation with major breaks in sterile technique, gross spillage, or incisions into inflamed but not suppurating infections; fresh accidental wounds
Class IV. Dirty/infected
Wounds with necrotic or devitalized infected tissue

large prospective trials have not shown benefit of antibiotic prophylaxis in preventing prosthetic infections,[108,109] but smaller trials have suggested a decrease in site infection without change in implant infection rate.[110,111] Therefore, there is no strict guideline for the use of systemic antibiotics for implant surgery, and the surgeon must tailor the use of antibiotics to the individual patient's risk.

Patients with class II (clean/contaminated) surgical wounds do benefit from systemic antibiotic prophylaxis. The most studied example of this class of wound is elective colon resection. Most current guidelines recommend systemic broad-spectrum antibiotic coverage using a second-generation cephalosporin plus metronidazole if the parenteral route is used, and neomycin plus metronidazole or erythromycin base (both as nonabsorbable antibiotics), if the oral route is used.[112] Published evidence supports administration of antibiotics preoperatively in order to achieve maximum therapeutic levels at the time of incision, and repeat dosing to maintain therapeutic levels during a long procedure. There is no documented study showing benefit to additional doses of antibiotics after the procedure is over and the skin is closed, and prolonged use of prophylactic antibiotics contributes to emergence of resistant bacteria.[113,114]

Patients with class III (contaminated) wounds are a mixed population. Some of these wounds are the result of inadvertent entry into a contaminated field, some result from traumatic injury, and some are planned operations for débridement of infected tissue. In the latter case, antibiotic therapy is indicated for specific therapy rather than prophylaxis. In the case of penetrating traumatic injury to the colon, there is strong evidence to support single-dose antibiotic prophylaxis at the time of laparotomy, similar to elective colon resection.[115,116] Surgical judgment must be individualized in these cases as to whether the risk of skin closure can be justified due to the high rate of wound infection despite antibiotic prophylaxis.

Patients with class IV (dirty) wounds are generally undergoing débridement of already infected and necrotic tissue, and should be receiving antibiotic therapy targeted to the relevant organisms. Skin wound closure is generally not advised in these patients.

The wound classification system does not take into account patient risk factors or site-specific risk factors. Various physiologic scoring systems including the acute physiology score and the Acute Physiology, Age, and Chronic Health Evaluation index have been used to predict perioperative infection risk with some success. In an effort to provide more accurate risk stratification, the CDC's National Nosocomial Infection Surveillance project has developed a risk index that accounts for patient risk factors such as malnutrition and chronic medical conditions, and operative factors including duration and site of procedure.[117] Enlightened risk assessment of perioperative infections should be included in the discussion for informed surgical consent.

▪ NUTRITIONAL EVALUATION

The importance of proper nutritional assessment and management cannot be overstressed. In surgical patients, malnutrition increases risk for major morbidity,[118,119] including wound infection, sepsis, pneumonia, delayed wound healing, and anastomotic complications. Careful preoperative clinical assessment can identify those patients at increased nutritional risk. The assessment should include a thorough history and physical exam with attention paid to usual weight, recent weight loss, changes in eating and bowel habits, changes in abdominal girth, loss of muscle bulk, and the presence of diseases that carry a risk of malnutrition such as COPD, diabetes mellitus, inflammatory bowel disease, and psychiatric conditions such as bulimia and anorexia nervosa. The history and physical exam should identify those patients with nutritional risk; that risk can be stratified by calculation of the Nutritional Risk Index (NRI). The NRI is a simple calculation ($15.19 \times$ serum albumin (g/dL) + $41.7 \times$ present weight/usual weight) which has been shown in prospective studies to correlate with increased rates of mortality and complications from major abdominal surgery.[120,121] NRI less than 83 indicates a significantly increased rate of mortality and complications, especially wound dehiscence and infection. Severely malnourished patients have been shown to benefit from preoperative nutritional support.[122,123]

Malnutrition can be classified into protein deficiency (kwashiorkor), calorie deficiency (marasmus), or mixed protein calorie deficiency. In order to complete the nutritional assessment and to guide nutritional support, it is useful to classify the patient's specific nutritional state (Table 2–9). Malnutrition states are much more common than is generally acknowledged, with 30–55% of hospital inpatients meeting criteria for one of these diagnoses.[124]

Some interval of deficient nutritional intake is expected after an abdominal operation. In uncomplicated cases, this is usually the result of postoperative adynamic ileus and resolves promptly, in less than 7 days. Traditional surgical management includes provision of dextrose-containing intravenous fluids. The goal of this therapy is not to provide sufficient calories for complete nutritional support, but simply to provide enough carbohydrate to prevent breakdown of lean body mass. Certain organs, including the heart and brain, have an obligate requirement for carbohydrate as a primary energy source, and do not store energy in the form of fat or glycogen. If intake is insufficient to meet this requirement, the body breaks down hepatic glycogen to provide glucose to the circulation, and ultimately the brain and heart. Once hepatic glycogen stores have been depleted (after about 1 day of no intake) lean muscle mass is converted to glucose via gluconeogenesis to produce carbohydrate. Provision of only 100 g of exogenous glucose per day is sufficient to prevent breakdown of lean muscle mass in otherwise healthy subjects.

In already malnourished patients, or in patients who do not return to normal bowel function promptly, nutritional support is indicated. As in the preoperative setting, a thorough evaluation of the patient's nutritional status is necessary, as is the identification of the cause of bowel dysfunction. In the postoperative setting, there are many potential causes of bowel dysfunction (Table 2–10), and nutritional support should be individualized for each patient's needs. Some patients may respond to enteral support and some may require parenteral support. Whenever available, the enteral route is the preferred route of support, as it has been shown to cause less morbidity and mortality.[125]

Enteral nutritional support is effective in patients that have functional small bowel; examples include esophageal or gastric resection, patients with postoperative delirium or dysphagia, and patients who have gastroparesis. In the short term, if the dysfunction is expected to respond to treatment, nasogastric tubes can be used effectively to deliver full support. Patients that need long-term enteral support are best served with gastrostomy or jejunostomy tubes, which may be placed operatively or percutaneously. With good preoperative nutritional assessment and sound surgical judgment, these patients' needs for long-term postoperative sup-

TABLE 2–9. ASSESSMENT OF NUTRITIONAL STATUS

PROTEIN DEFICIENCY CRITERIA
Albumin <2.2 g/dL
Total lymphocyte count 800/mm^3 or less
Weight maintained
Peripheral edema
Inadequate protein intake (<50% of goal for 3 days or <75% for 7 days)
Four criteria out of these five establish the diagnosis of protein deficiency

CALORIE DEFICIENCY CRITERIA
Weight loss: 5% over 1 month or 7.5% over 3 months or 10% over 6 months
Underweight: less then 94% ideal body weight
Clinically measurable muscle wasting
Serum protein maintained
Inadequate calorie intake (50% for 3 days or <75% for 7 days)
Three criteria out of these five establish diagnosis of calorie deficiency

MIXED PROTEIN CALORIE MALNUTRITION CRITERIA

	Mild	Moderate	Severe
Weight loss	5–9%	10–15%	10–15% over 6 months
Underweight	94–85%	84–70%	<70% ideal weight
Albumin	2.8–3.4 g/dL	2.1–2.7 g/dL	<2.1 g/dL
Total lymphocytes	1499–1200/mm^3	1199–800/mm^3	<800/mm^3
Transferrin	199–150 mg/dL	149–100 mg/dL	<100 mg/dL
			Muscle wasting
			Deficient intake (at least 3 days)

To establish the diagnoses of mild or moderate protein calorie malnutrition, two of the five criteria shown must be met; to establish the diagnosis of severe protein calorie malnutrition, three of the seven criteria must be met.

port can often be anticipated, and long-term feeding access can be included in the operative plan. Enteral support may not suitable for some patients; examples include early postoperative bowel obstruction, fistula, or intestinal insufficiency (short-gut syndrome). In such patients parenteral support is indicated, and should be initiated without delay, and futile attempts to use the enteral route should be avoided.

Irrespective of the route of support, every patient on nutritional support should have his or her nutritional needs assessed and provided. The assessment begins with the calorie requirement. There are several formulas and nomograms that estimate basal energy expenditure, taking into account height, weight, age, gender, stress factors, and activity factors.[126] All of these methods are estimations, and may underfeed or overfeed certain subgroups, especially the obese. The method in most common clinical use bases basal energy expenditure on adjusted body weight (ABW). Using this method, ABW is defined as the patient's ideal body weight plus the difference between actual body weight (BW) and the ideal body weight divided by two:

$$ABW = IBW + .5\ (BW - IBW)$$

The baseline caloric requirement for weight maintenance based on ABW is 25 kcal/kg/d. This target may be adjusted upwards in patients with extreme metabolic demands, as is the case in burns or head injury.[125] Furthermore, the ABW can be used to establish the protein requirement. In unstressed normal subjects, the minimum daily protein requirement is 0.8 g protein/kg/d. In postoperative patients with healing wounds, this target is adjusted to 1.0–1.5 g/kg/d, and in severely ill patients to 2.0 g/kg/d. The highest requirements are seen in severe burn and bone marrow transplant patients.

Essential nutritional components must be provided, again irrespective of the route of support. These include water- and lipid-soluble vitamins, trace elements such as zinc and selenium, essential fatty acids such as linoleic and linolenic acids, and the eight essential amino acids. These trace elements are provided in abundance in all enteral feeds, and are part of the standard additives in parenteral formula.

Once nutritional support has been initiated, the patient's response to support must be followed closely, especially in parenteral support and in patients with preexisting metabolic conditions such as diabetes. Blood glucose should be monitored regularly during the first few days of support. Recent evidence has linked hyperglycemia in the postoperative setting, especially in critically ill patients, with increased risk of death and infection.[127,128] In addition, electrolyte abnormalities (especially those of potassium, magnesium, and phosphate) are often seen in the early period of nutritional support, and should be corrected.

TABLE 2–10. POSTOPERATIVE CAUSES OF DEFICIENT NUTRITIONAL INTAKE

Ileus
Bowel obstruction
Colitis (ischemic, infectious)
Fistula
Dysphagia
Gastric dysmotility
Intestinal insufficiency (short-gut syndrome)

It is also important to follow the markers of nutrition repletion to ensure that the calories and protein provided (based on the initial estimate) are sufficient, and the patient is not mobilizing lean body mass due to inadequate support. Serum markers such as prealbumin, retinol binding protein, and transferrin can be useful in this regard. They are serum proteins with short (2–7 days) turnover times that reflect the body's ability to synthesize new protein.[126] Unfortunately, the serum concentrations of these proteins are also affected by acute disease states and renal and hepatic failure, and can be difficult to interpret in postoperative patients. Nitrogen balance can also be used to monitor nutritional support and reflects the ability to synthesize new protein. Nitrogen balance is calculated by subtracting nitrogen excretion from nitrogen intake. Nitrogen intake is calculated from the protein intake, where each gram of protein/6.25 = the number of grams of nitrogen. Nitrogen excretion has two components: urinary urea nitrogen and insensible loss. Urinary urea nitrogen (UUN) can be measured in a 24-hour urine collection; insensible loss is generally accepted to be 4 g per day, unless there is another source of loss, such as abdominal drainage of proteinaceous ascites, enterocutaneous fistula, or nephrotic syndrome. Thus in most cases, nitrogen balance can be simplified to:

$$\text{Nitrogen balance} = \text{protein intake}/6.25 - 24\text{ hour UUN} - 4\text{ g (insensible loss)}$$

A patient that takes in more nitrogen than he or she excretes in the urine and feces is in positive nitrogen balance and is synthesizing new protein. On the other hand, a patient that is excreting more nitrogen than he or she is receiving in nutritional support is in negative nitrogen balance, and is therefore losing lean body mass, becoming more malnourished. These patients should be re-evaluated for nutritional needs and for sources of nutritional depletion, such as uncontrolled diabetes mellitus, sepsis, and organ failure.

By itself, uncontrolled diabetes mellitus can be viewed as a perioperative nutritional complication, as it results in nutritional depletion, interferes with delivery of parenteral and enteral nutrition, and is associated with increased infectious morbidity.[127,128] Randomized prospective trials in cardiac surgery patients and in the surgical intensive care unit population have shown that strict control of blood glucose in the normal range improves mortality and infectious morbidity.[129]

REFERENCES

1. Bauer M, Bohrer H, Aichele G, et al. Measuring patient satisfaction with anaesthesia: perioperative questionnaire versus standardised face-to-face interview. *Acta Anaesthesiol Scand* 2001;45:65–72
2. Ballantyne JC, Carr DB, Chalmers TC, et al. Postoperative patient-controlled analgesia: meta-analyses of initial randomized control trials. *J Clin Anesth* 1993;5:182–193
3. Nitschke LF, Schlosser CT, Berg RL, et al. Does patient-controlled analgesia achieve better control of pain and fewer adverse effects than intramuscular analgesia? A prospective randomized trial. *Arch Surg* 1996;131:417–423
4. Kenady DE, Wilson JF, Schwartz RW, et al. A randomized comparison of patient-controlled versus standard analgesic requirements in patients undergoing cholecystectomy. *Surg Gynecol Obstet* 1992;174:216–220
5. de Leon-Casasola OA, Karabella D, Lema MJ. Bowel function recovery after radical hysterectomies: thoracic epidural bupivacaine-morphine versus intravenous patient-controlled analgesia with morphine: a pilot study. *J Clin Anesth* 1996;8:87–92
6. Block BM, Liu SS, Rowlingson AJ, et al. Efficacy of postoperative epidural analgesia: a meta-analysis. *JAMA* 2003;290:2455–2463
7. Wang LP, Hauerberg J, Schmidt JF. Incidence of spinal epidural abscess after epidural analgesia: a national 1-year survey. *Anesthesiology* 1999;91:1928–1936
8. Boylan, JF, Katz J, Kavanagh BP, et al. Epidural bupivacaine-morphine analgesia versus patient-controlled analgesia following abdominal aortic surgery: Analgesic, respiratory, and myocardial effects. *Anesthesiology* 1998; 89:585–593
9. Bois S, Couture P, Boudreault D, et al. Epidural analgesia and intravenous patient-controlled analgesia result in similar rates of postoperative myocardial ischemia after aortic surgery. *Anesth Analg* 1997;85:1233–1239
10. Wu CL, Naqibuddin M, Fleisher LA. Measurement of patient satisfaction as an outcome of regional anesthesia and analgesia: a systematic review. *Reg Anesth Pain Med* 2001;26:196–208
11. Werawatganon T, Charuluxanun S. Patient controlled intravenous opioid analgesia versus continuous epidural analgesia for pain after intra-abdominal surgery. *Cochrane Database Syst Rev* 2005;(1):CD004088.
12. Hendolin H, Lahtinen J, Lansimies E, et al. The effect of thoracic epidural analgesia on respiratory function after cholecystectomy. *Acta Anaesthesiol Scand* 1987;31: 645–651
13. Cuschieri RJ, Morran CG, Howie JC, McArdle CS. Postoperative pain and pulmonary complications: comparison of three analgesic regimens. *Br J Surg* 1985;72:495–498
14. Scheinin B, Asantila R, Orko R. The effect of bupivacaine and morphine on pain and bowel function after colonic surgery. *Acta Anaesthesiol Scand* 1987;31:161–164
15. Bredtmann RD, Herden HN, Teichmann W, et al. Epidural analgesia in colonic surgery: results of a randomized prospective study. *Br J Surg* 1990;77:638–642
16. Horattas MC, Evans S, Sloan-Stakleff KD, et al. Does preoperative rofecoxib (Vioxx) decrease postoperative pain with laparoscopic cholecystectomy? *Am J Surg* 2004; 188:271–276
17. Bikhazi GB, Snabes MC, Bajwa ZH, et al. A clinical trial demonstrates the analgesic activity of intravenous parecoxib sodium compared with ketorolac or morphine after gynecologic surgery with laparotomy. *Am J Obstet Gynecol* 2004;191:1183–1191
18. Lau H, Wong C, Goh LC, et al. Prospective randomized trial of pre-emptive analgesics following ambulatory inguinal hernia repair: intravenous ketorolac versus diclofenac suppository. *ANZ J Surg* 2002;72:704–707
19. Mixter CG 3rd, Meeker LD, Gavin TJ. Preemptive pain control in patients having laparoscopic hernia repair: a comparison of ketorolac and ibuprofen. *Arch Surg* 1998; 133:432–437
20. Morton NS, O'Brien K. Analgesic efficacy of paracetamol and diclofenac in children receiving PCA morphine. *Br J Anaesth* 1999;82:715–717
21. Litaker D, Locala J, Franco K, et al. Preoperative risk factors for postoperative delirium. *Gen Hosp Psychiatry* 2001;23:84–89
22. Moller JT, Cluitmans P, Rasmussen LS, et al. Long-term postoperative cognitive dysfunction in the elderly ISPOCD1 study. ISPOCD investigators. International Study of Post-Operative Cognitive Dysfunction. *Lancet* 1998;351:857–861
23. Inouye SK, Charpentier PA. Precipitating factors for delirium in hospitalized elderly persons. Predictive model and interrelationship with baseline vulnerability. *JAMA* 1996;275:852–857
24. Mann C, Pouzeratte Y, Boccara G, et al. Comparison of intravenous or epidural patient-controlled analgesia in the elderly after major abdominal surgery. *Anesthesiology* 2000;92:433–441
25. Skrobik YK, Bergeron N, Dumont M, Gottfried SB. Olanzapine vs haloperidol: treating delirium in a critical care setting. *Intensive Care Med* 2004;30:444–449
26. Mangano DT, Goldman L. Preoperative assessment of patients with known or suspected coronary disease. *N Engl J Med* 1995;333:1750–1756
27. Eagle KA, Brundage BH, Chaitman BR, et al. Guidelines for perioperative cardiovascular evaluation for noncardiac surgery: report of the ACC/AHA Task Force on practice guidelines. *J Am Coll Cardiol* 1996;27:910–948
28. Park KW. Perioperative cardiology consultation. *Anesthesiology* 2003;98:754–762

29. Liu LI, Wiener-Kronish JP. Preoperative cardiac evaluation of women for noncardiac surgery. *Cardiol Clin* 1998; 16:59–66
30. Shackleford DP, Hoffman MK, Kramer PR Jr, et al. Evaluation of preoperative cardiac risk index values in patients undergoing vaginal surgery. *Am J Obstet Gynecol* 1995;173:80–84
31. Mangano DT, Hollenberg M, Fegert G, et al. Perioperative myocardial ischemia in patients undergoing noncardiac surgery—I: Incidence and severity during the 4 day perioperative period. The study of perioperative ischemia (SPI) research group. *J Am Coll Cardiol* 1991;4: 843–850
32. ACC/AHA task force report: Special report: guidelines for perioperative cardiovascular evaluation for non-cardiac surgery. *Circulation* 1996;93:1278–1317
33. Mukherjee D, Eagle KA. Perioperative cardiac assessment for non cardiac surgery, eight steps to the best possible outcome. *Circulation* 2003;107:2771–2774
34. Chui PT, Gin T, Oh TE. Anesthesia for laparoscopic surgery. *Anaesth Intensive Care* 1993;21:163–171
35. Madu EC. Transesophageal dobutamine stress echocardiography in the evaluation of myocardial ischemia in morbidly obese subjects. *Chest* 2000;117:657–661
36. Dawood MM, Gupta DK, Southern J, et al. Pathology of fatal perioperative myocardial infarction: implications regarding pathophysiology and prevention. *Int J Cardiol* 1996;57:37–44
37. Boersma E, Poldermans D, Bax JJ, et al. Predictors of cardiac events after major vascular surgery: role of clinical characteristics, dobutamine echocardiography, and beta-blocker therapy. *JAMA* 2001;285:1865–1873
38. Gersh BJ, Braunwald E, Bonow RO. Chronic coronary artery disease. In: Braunwald E, Zipes DP, Libby P (eds). *Heart Disease.* Philadelphia, PA: WB Saunders; 2001: 1272–1363
39. McFalls EO, Ward HB, Moritz TE, et al. Coronary artery revascularization before elective major vascular surgery. *N Engl J Med* 2004;352:2795–2804
40. Posner KL, Van Norman GA, Chan V. Adverse cardiac outcomes after noncardiac surgery in patients with prior percutaneous transluminal coronary angioplasty. *Anesth Analg* 1999;89:553–560
41. Kaluza GL, Joseph J, Lee JR, et al. Catastrophic outcomes of noncardiac surgery soon after coronary stenting. *J Am Coll Cardiol* 2000;35:1288–1294
42. Foster ED, Davis KB, Carpenter JA, et al. Risk of noncardiac operation in patients with defined coronary disease: The Coronary Artery Surgery Study (CASS) registry experience. *Ann Thorac Surg* 1986;14:42–50
43. Yusuf S, Zucker D, Peduzzi P, et al. Effect of coronary artery bypass graft surgery on survival: Overview of 10-year results from randomized trials by the Coronary Artery Bypass Graft Surgery Trialists Collaboration. *Lancet* 1994;344:563–570
44. Selzman CH, Miller SA, Zimmerman MA, Harkin AH. The case for beta-adrenergic blockade as prophylaxis against perioperative cardiovascular morbidity and mortality. *Arch Surg* 2001;136:286–290
45. Lee RT, Grodinsky AJ, Frank EH, et al. Structure dependent dynamic mechanical behavior of fibrous caps from human atherosclerotic plaques. *Circulation* 1991;83: 1764–1770
46. Rabbani R, Topol EJ. Strategies to achieve coronary arterial plaque stabilization. *Cardiovasc Res* 1999;4:402–417
47. Poldermans D, Boersma E, Bax JJ, et al. Dutch echocardiographic cardiac risk evaluation applying stress echocardiography study group. Bisoprolol reduces cardiac death and myocardial infarction in high-risk patients as long as 2 years after successful major vascular surgery. *Eur Heart J* 2001;22:1353–1358
48. Heller GV, Shehata AR. Pharmacological stress testing with technetium-99m single photon emission computerized tomography imaging in the perioperative assessment of patients undergoing non-cardiac surgery. *Am J Card Imaging* 1996;10:120–127
49. Detsky AS, Abrams HB, McLaughlin JR, et al. Predicting cardiac complications in patients undergoing non-cardiac surgery. *J Gen Intern Med* 1986;1:211–219
50. O'Kelly B, Browner WS, Massie B, et al. Ventricular arrhythmias in patients undergoing noncardiac surgery: The study of perioperative ischemia research group. *JAMA* 1992;268:217–221
51. Mahla E, Rotman B, Rehak P, et al. Perioperative ventricular dysrhythmias in patients with structural heart disease undergoing non cardiac surgery. *Anesth Analg* 1998;86:16–21
52. Eagle KA, Berger PB, Calkins H, et al. ACC/AHA guideline update for perioperative cardiac evaluation for noncardiac surgery—executive summary. A report of the American College of Cardiology/American Heart Association Task Force on Practice guidelines (Committee to update the 1996 guidelines on perioperative cardiac evaluation for noncardiac surgery). *J Am Coll Cardiol* 2002;39:542–553
53. Dajani AS, Taubert KA, Wilson W, et al. Prevention of bacterial endocarditis: Recommendations by the American Heart Association. *JAMA* 1997;227:1794–1801
54. Steckelberg JM, Wilson WR. Risk factors for infective endocarditis. *Infect Dis Clin North Am* 1993;7:9–19
55. Boudoulais H, Wooley CF. Mitral valve prolapse. In: Emmanouilides GC, Riemenschneider TA, Allen HD, Gutgesell HP (eds). *Moss and Adams Heart Disease in Infants, Children and Adolescents including the Fetus and Young Adult*, 5th ed. Baltimore, MD: Williams & Wilkins; 1995: 1063–1086
56. Carabello BA. Mitral valve disease. *Curr Probl Cardiol* 1993;7:423–478
57. Devereux RB, Hawkins I, Kramer-Fox R, et al. Complications of mitral valve prolapse. Disproportionate occurrence in men and older patients. *Am J Med* 1986;81:751–758
58. MacMahon SW, Roberts JK, Kramer-Fox R, et al. Mitral valve prolapse and infective endocarditis. *Am Heart J* 1987;113:1291–1298.
59. Devereux RB, Kramer-Fox R, Kligfield P. Mitral valve prolapse: Causes, manifestations, and management. *Ann Intern Med* 1989;111:305–317

60. Marks AR, Choong CY, Sanfillipo AJ, et al. Identification of high-risk and low-risk subgroups of patients with mitral valve prolapse. *N Engl J Med* 1989;320:1031–1036
61. Nishimura RA, McGoon MD, Shub C, et al. Echocardiographically documented mitral-valve prolapse. Long-term follow up of 237 patients. *N Engl J Med* 1985;313:1305–1309
62. Cheitlin MD, Alpert JS, Armstong WF, et al. ACC/AHA guidelines for the clinical application of echocardiography: A report of the American College of Cardiology/American Heart Association Task Force Guidelines (Committee on Clinical Application of Echocardiography). *Circulation* 1997;95:1686–1744
63. Durak DT. Prevention of infective endocarditis. *N Engl J Med* 1995;332:38–44
64. Lawrence VA, Dhanda R, Hilsenbeck SG, Page CP. Risk of pulmonary complications after elective abdominal surgery. *Chest* 1996;110:744–750
65. Becquemin JP, Piquet J, Becquemin MH, et al. Pulmonary function after transverse or midline incision in patients with obstructive pulmonary disease. *Intensive Care Med* 1985;11:247–251
66. Celli BR, Rodriguez KS, Snider GL. A controlled trial of intermittent positive pressure breathing, incentive spirometry, and deep breathing exercises in preventing pulmonary complications after abdominal surgery. *Am Rev Respir Dis* 1984;130:12–15
67. Tarhan S, Moffitt EA, Sessler AD, et al. Risk of anesthesia and surgery in patients with chronic bronchitis and chronic obstructive pulmonary disease. *Surgery* 1973;74:720–726
68. Gerson MC, Hurst JM, Hertzberg VS, et al. Prediction of cardiac and pulmonary complications related to elective abdominal and noncardiac thoracic surgery in geriatric patients. *Am J Med* 1990;88:101–107
69. Williams-Russo P, Charlson ME, Mackenzie CR, et al. Predicting postoperative pulmonary complications: Is it a real problem? *Arch Intern Med* 1992;152:1209–1213
70. Warner MA, Offord KP, Warner MA, et al. Role of preoperative cessation of smoking and other factors in postoperative pulmonary complications: A blinded prospective study of coronary artery bypass patients. *Mayo Clin Proc* 1989;64:609–616
71. Pien LC, Grammer LC, Patterson R. Minimal complications in a surgical population with severe asthma receiving prophylactic corticosteroids. *J Allergy Clin Immunol* 1988;82:696–700
72. Kabalin CS, Yarnld PR, Grammer LC. Low complication rate of corticosteroid-treated asthmatics undergoing surgical procedures. *Arch Intern Med* 1995;155:1379–1384
73. Flancbaum L, Choban PS. Surgical implications of obesity. *Annu Rev Med* 1998;49:215–234
74. Shepherd JW. Hypertension, cardiac arrhythmias, myocardial infarction and stroke in relation to obstructive sleep apnea. *Clin Chest Med* 1992;13:459–479
75. Brooks-Brunn JA. Postoperative atelectasis and pneumonia. *Heart Lung* 1995;24:94–115
76. Zinner MJ, Zuidema GD, Smith PA, et al. The prevention of upper gastrointestinal tract bleeding in patients in an intensive care unit. *Surg Gynecol Obstet* 1981;153:215–220
77. Kaplan EB, Sheiner LB, Boeckmann AJ, et al. The usefulness of preoperative laboratory screening. *JAMA* 1985;253:3576–3581
78. Ifudu O. Care of patients undergoing hemodialysis. *N Engl J Med* 1998;339:1054–1062
79. Cochrane Injuries Group Albumin Reviewers. Human albumin administration in critically ill patients: systematic review of randomized controlled trials. *BMJ* 1998;317:235
80. Merten GJ, Burgess WP, Gray LV, et al. Prevention of contrast-induced nephropathy with sodium bicarbonate. A randomized controlled trial. *JAMA* 2004;291;2328–2334
81. Tepel M, van der Giet M, Schwarzfeld C, et al. Prevention of radiographic-contrast-agent-induced reductions in renal function by acetylcysteine. *N Engl J Med* 2000;343:180–184
82. Lobo DN, Bostock KA, Neal KR, et al. Effect of salt and water balance on recovery of gastrointestinal function after elective colonic resection: a randomized controlled trial. *Lancet* 2002;359:1812–1818.
83. Suchman AL, Mushlin AI. How well does the activated partial thromboplastin time predict postoperative hemorrhage? *JAMA* 1986;256:750–753
84. Houry S, Georgeac C, Hay JM, et al. A prospective multicenter evaluation of preoperative hemostatic screening tests. The French Associations for Surgical Research. *Am J Surg* 1995;170:19–23
85. Burns ER, Lawrence C. Bleeding time. A guide to its diagnostic and clinical utility. *Arch Pathol Lab Med* 1989;113:1219–1224
86. Peterson P, Hayes TE, Arkin CF, et al. The preoperative bleeding time lacks clinical benefit: College of American Pathologists and American Society of Clinical Pathologists' position article. *Arch Surg* 1998;133:134–139
87. Gewirtz AS, Miller ML, Keys TF. The clinical usefulness of the preoperative bleeding time. *Arch Pathol Lab Med* 1996;120:353–356
88. Robbins JA, Rose SD. Partial thromboplastin time as screening test. *Ann Intern Med* 1979;90:796–797
89. Eisenberg JM, Goldfarb S. Clinical usefulness of measuring prothrombin time as a routine admission test. *Clin Chem* 1976;22:1644–1647
90. Robbins JA, Mushlin AI. Preoperative evaluation of the healthy patient. *Med Clin North Am* 1979;63:1145–1156
91. Kaluza GL, Joseph J, Lee JR, et al. Catastrophic outcomes of noncardiac surgery soon after coronary stenting. *J Am Coll Cardiol* 2000;35:1288–1294
92. American Society of Anesthesiologists Task Force on Blood Component Therapy. Practice guidelines for blood component therapy: A report by the American Society of Anesthesiologists Task Force on Blood Component Therapy. *Anesthesiology* 1996;84:732–747
93. Ginsburg SJ. Management of venous thromboembolism. *N Engl J Med* 1996;335:1816–1828
94. Decousus H, Leizorovicz A, Parent F, et al. A clinical trial of vena caval filters in the prevention of pulmonary embo-

lism in patients with proximal deep-vein thrombosis. Prevention du Risque d'Embolie Pulmonaire par Interruption Cave Study Group. *N Engl J Med* 1998;338:409–415
95. Flanc C, Kakkar VV, Clarke MB. The detection of venous thrombosis of the legs using 125 I-labelled fibrinogen. *Br J Surg* 1968;55:742–747
96. Carter CJ. The pathophysiology of venous thrombosis. *Prog Cardiovasc Dis* 1994;36:439–446
97. Kearon C, Hirsch J. Management of anticoagulation before and after elective surgery. *N Engl J Med* 1997;336:1506–1512
98. Hirsch J, Rasche R, Warkentin TE, et al. Heparin: Mechanism of action, pharmacokinetics, dosing considerations, monitoring, efficacy, and safety. *Chest* 1995;108(Suppl):258S–275S
99. Sanchez-Manuel FJ, Seco-Gil JL. Antibiotic prophylaxis for hernia repair. *Cochrane Database Syst Rev* 2004;(4):CD003769
100. Smith RL, Bohl JK, McElearney ST, et al. Wound infection after elective colorectal resection. *Ann Surg* 2004;239:599–605
101. O'Neill PA, Kirton OC, Dresner LS, et al. Analysis of 162 colon injuries in patients with penetrating abdominal trauma: concomitant stomach injury results in a higher rate of infection. *J Trauma* 2004;56:304–312
102. Christou NV, Nohr CW, Meakins JL. Assessing operative site infection in surgical patients. *Arch Surg* 1987;122:165–169
103. Perl TM, Cullen JJ, Wenzel RP, et al. Mupirocin and the Risk of *Staphylococcus aureus* Study Team. Intranasal mupirocin to prevent postoperative *Staphylococcus aureus* infections. *N Engl J Med* 2002;346:1871–1877
104. Gil-Egea MJ, Pi-Sunyer MT, Verdaguer A, et al. Surgical wound infections: a prospective study of 4,486 clean wounds. *Infect Control* 1987;8:277–280
105. Forse RA, Karam B, MacLean LD, Christou NV. Antibiotic prophylaxis for surgery in morbidly obese patients. *Surgery* 1989;106:750–756
106. Mangram AJ, Horan TC, Pearson ML, Silver LC, Jarvis WR. Guidelines for prevention of surgical site infection. *Infect Control Hosp Epidemiol* 1999;20:247–278
107. Polk HC Jr, Simpson CJ, Simmons BP, Alexander JW. Guidelines for prevention of surgical wound infection. *Arch Surg* 1983;118:1213–1217
108. Perez AR, Roxas MF, Hilvano SS. A randomized, double-blind, placebo-controlled trial to determine effectiveness of antibiotic prophylaxis for tension-free mesh herniorrhaphy. *J Am Coll Surg* 2005;200:393–397
109. Darouiche RO. Antimicrobial approaches for preventing infections associated with surgical implants. *Clin Infect Dis* 2003;36:1284–1289
110. Yerdel MA, Akin EB, Dolalan S, et al. Effect of single-dose prophylactic ampicillin and sulbactam on wound infection after tension-free inguinal hernia repair with polypropylene mesh: the randomized, double-blind, prospective trial. *Ann Surg* 2001;233:26–33
111. Bratzler DW, Houck PM. Antimicrobial prophylaxis for surgery: An advisory statement from the National Surgical Infection Prevention Project. *Clin Infect Dis* 2004;38:1706–1715
112. Hecker MT, Aron DC, Patel NP, et al. Unnecessary use of antimicrobials in hospitalized patients: current patterns of misuse with an emphasis on antianaerobic spectrum of activity. *Arch Intern Med* 2003;163:972–978
113. Eggiman P, Pittet D. Infection control in the ICU. *Chest* 2001;120:2059–2093
114. Fullen WD, Hunt J, Altemeier WA. Prophylactic antibiotics in penetrating wounds of the abdomen. *J Trauma* 1972;12:282–289
115. Thadepelli H, Gorbach SL, Broido PW, et al. Abdominal trauma, anaerobes, and antibiotics. *Surg Gynecol Obstet* 1973;137:270–276
116. Dellinger EP. Antibiotic prophylaxis in trauma: Penetrating abdominal injuries and open fractures. *Rev Infect Dis* 1991;13:S847–S857
117. Gaynes RP, Culver DH, Horan TC, et al. Surgical site infection (SSI) rates in the United States, 1992–1998: the National Nosocomial Infections Surveillance System basic SSI risk index. *Clin Infect Dis* 2001;33(Suppl 2):S69–S77
118. Sungurtekin H, Sungurtekin U, Balci C, et al. The influence of nutritional status on complications after major intraabdominal surgery. *J Am Coll Nutr* 2004;23:227–232
119. Rey-Ferro M, Castano R, Orozco O, et al. Nutritional and immunologic evaluation of patients with gastric cancer before and after surgery. *Nutrition* 1997;13:878–881
120. Bozzetti F, Gavazzi C, Miceli R, et al. Perioperative total parenteral nutrition in malnourished, gastrointestinal cancer patients: a randomized, clinical trial. *JPEN J Parenter Enteral Nutr* 2000;24:7–14
121. The Veterans Affairs Total Parenteral Nutrition Cooperative Study Group. Perioperative total parenteral nutrition in surgical patients. *N Engl J Med* 1991;325:525–532
122. Reilly JJ Jr, Hull SF, Albert N, et al. Economic impact of malnutrition: A model system for hospitalized patients. *JPEN J Parenter Enteral Nutr* 1988;12:371–376
123. Moore FA, Moore EE, Jones TN, et al. TEN versus TPN following major abdominal trauma-reduced septic morbidity. *J Trauma* 1989;29:916–922
124. Kudsk KA, Croce MA, Fabian TC, et al. Enteral versus parenteral feeding. Effects on septic morbidity after blunt and penetrating abdominal trauma. *Ann Surg* 1992;215:503–511
125. Demling RH, Seigne P. Metabolic management of patients with severe burns. *World J Surg* 2000;24:673–680
126. Haider M, Haider SQ. Assessment of protein-calorie malnutrition. *Clin Chem* 1984;30:1286–1299
127. Pomposelli JJ, Baxter JK 3rd, Babineau TJ, et al. Early postoperative glucose control predicts nosocomial infection rate in diabetic patients. *JPEN J Parenter Enteral Nutr* 1998;22:77–81
128. Furnary AP, Zerr KJ, Grunkemeier GL, Starr A. Continuous intravenous insulin infusion reduces the incidence of deep sternal wound infection in diabetic patients after cardiac surgical procedures *Ann Thorac Surg* 1999;67:352–360
129. van den Berghe G, Wouters P, Weekers F, et al. Intensive insulin therapy in the critically ill patients. *N Engl J Med* 2001;345:1359–1367

3

Endoscopy and Endoscopic Intervention

Edward Lin ■ *Aaron S. Fink*

There has been tremendous progress in the discipline of flexible endoscopy in the last decade. Fully flexible endoscopic systems can now reach virtually every portion of the gastrointestinal tract. With the addition of therapeutic channels to the flexible endoscope, endoscopy now offers both diagnostic and therapeutic capabilities. Ultrasound systems can be attached to the end of a flexible endoscope, affording views of the layers of the gastrointestinal wall as well as of adjacent organs and structures. The ever-expanding development of new endoscopic interventions continues to offer new therapeutic options for diseases conventionally treated with transabdominal surgery. This chapter will address the indications and techniques for gastrointestinal endoscopy and intervention specifically related to the use of a flexible endoscope. Fundamental techniques for upper, small bowel, and lower endoscopy will be discussed, along with some of the most frequently performed diagnostic and therapeutic procedures.

■ THE FLEXIBLE ENDOSCOPE

In all flexible endoscopic systems, light is transmitted down the endoscope shaft to illuminate the surface to be examined. The reflected image is conveyed back to the endoscopist via one of two different modalities: fiberoptics or electronics. In the former, a fixed lens at the end of the instrument shaft focuses the image on internal fiberoptic bundles. The image is then carried to an adjustable lens on the instrument head through which it is directly viewed. The fiberoptic bundle is 2–3 mm wide and is composed of 20,000–40,000 individual fine glass fibers, each approximately 10 micrometers in diameter. The image undergoes a series of internal reflections within each fiber as it is transmitted up the bundle (Fig 3–1). By ensuring identical orientation ("coherent") of the fibers at each end of the bundle, the image is faithfully transmitted back to the viewer. This process requires that each fiber be coated with low optical density glass to prevent escape of light from within. This "packing material" creates the characteristic meshed image seen in fiberoptic endoscopes, which inherently results in a lower resolution than that seen with rigid lens systems. The image can be directly viewed through the eyepiece at the instrument head, or transmitted to a video monitor by connecting the eyepiece to a video camera. When portions of the fiberoptic bundle are damaged from wear and tear or mishandling (i.e., fractures), light is not transmitted through that bundle and the view can be significantly compromised. However, these instruments are extremely flexible and are reasonably portable. Indeed, in many parts of the world, fiberoptic systems are still the standard.

Most endoscopes currently produced are electronic. In these systems, the image is reflected onto a charge-coupled device (CCD) chip mounted on the end of the instrument shaft. These chips contain thousands of light-sensitive points ("pixels"); the greater the number of pixels, the better the resolution. Current chips contain 100,000 to 300,000 pixels (fiberoptic endoscopes have resolution equivalent to 30,000 pixels). The image is then transmitted through wires instead of light bundles to additional electronics in the instrument head.

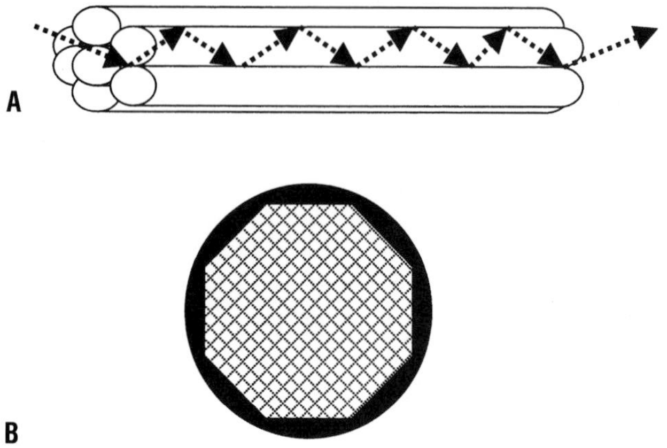

Figure 3–1. A. Identical orientation of fiberoptic bundles at both ends and internal reflections within each coated fiber result in optical coherence. **B.** Cross-section of the spatial arrangement of the bundles of a fiberoptic endoscope (usually 20,000–40,000 fibers) creates the meshed images.

The controls for maneuvering the tip of the endoscope are located on the headpiece, with a larger rotating knob controlling up or down deflection, and a smaller knob controlling left or right deflection. Locks accompany each knob to hold the deflection in position when needed. Two depressible buttons are located on the headpiece; the upper button produces suction, and the lower button produces air insufflation as well as water for cleaning the lens during the procedure (Fig 3–2). Most endoscopists hold the headpiece in the left hand, with the thumb on the up/down knob and the index and middle fingers on the suction and air/water button. The right hand operates the right/left knob and is used to hold the endoscope shaft. While it is intuitive to attempt rotating the shaft of the scope with the right hand, rotation is often limited by the torque resistance of the shaft and hand fatigue. Significant scope rotation can be achieved by altering the endoscopist's stance or by rotating the headpiece while inserting or withdrawing the shaft of the endoscope. The flexible shaft of an upper endoscope is usually 110–120 cm long with a working channel that can vary from 2.8–3.7 mm in diameter. Therapeutic endoscopes for endoscopic retrograde cholangiopancreatography (ERCP) can have diameters up to 4.2 mm.

Efforts to improve endoscopic training have led to the development of computer simulators for teaching endoscopic skills. Currently, simulators are available for training in flexible sigmoidoscopy, gastroscopy, ERCP, endoscopic ultrasound (EUS), and colonoscopy.

▪ PATIENT SEDATION AND MONITORING

Cardiopulmonary issues are the most commonly reported complications with endoscopic procedures. These complications include aspiration, oversedation, hypotension, hypoventilation, arrhythmia, bradycardia (vasovagal), and airway obstruction. Many of the latter are associated with use of intravenous moderate (formerly "conscious") sedation, defined as decreased consciousness associated with preservation of protective reflexes. Elderly patients or those with preexisting cardiopulmonary conditions are at increased risk for these complications, as are those undergoing more extensive endoscopic interventions. Patients with diseases associated with the oropharynx or trachea, and those with morbid obesity, sleep apnea, or neuromuscular degenerative diseases require extra vigilance during endoscopic procedures.

Most endoscopic procedures are performed in a darkened room, which limits the endoscopist's ability to monitor the patient by visual inspection. Familiarity with equipment location such as the suction apparatus, oxygen supply, and resuscitation carts is critical. The room should be free of clutter that may create obstacles to reaching the patient or providing assistance during the procedure. This is particularly true in performing bedside endoscopy in intensive care units, where the endoscopy consoles compete for space with ventilators and infusion pumps. Endoscopy should be performed with a dedicated assistant standing at the patient's head; this individual should assist in monitoring the patient and recording vital signs. As with any procedure requiring anesthesia, patients require a functioning intravenous access for medications and resuscitation if needed. A suction catheter tip should always be immediately available at the bedside to assist in clearing of oropharyngeal secretions.

Monitoring should be performed before, during, and after the procedure. Signs that are usually moni-

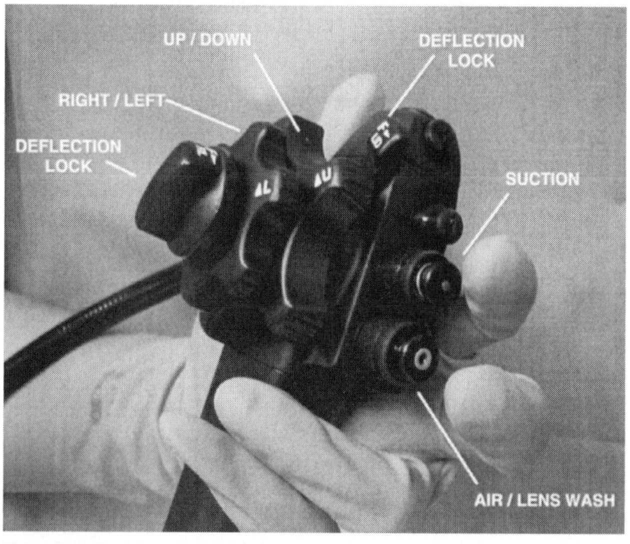

Figure 3–2. Headpiece of a digital endoscope, conventionally supported by the left hand.

tored include the patient's level of consciousness and comfort, vital signs, and ventilatory status. The patient's oxygenation status and cardiac electrical activity are also monitored; the latter requires electronic monitoring devices such as pulse oximeters that emit an audible beat corresponding to each heartbeat. These monitors are equipped with alarms that trigger if vital signs go above or fall below the normal range. These alarms should never be turned off.

Supplemental nasal oxygen is required to decrease the frequency of desaturation during endoscopic procedures. While the American Society for Gastrointestinal Endoscopy and the American College of Gastroenterology currently endorse the use of propofol due to its rapid onset of action and short half-life, not all endoscopy centers have adopted to its use given the expense and the need for a trained assistant (e.g., anesthetist or intensivist) to administer the drug. Therefore, benzodiazepines (for sedation and amnesia) combined with a narcotic analgesic are commonly used by the endoscopists to provide conscious sedation during endoscopic procedures (Table 3–1). Propofol sedation is often reserved for patients requiring deeper sedation; it is frequently used in an operating room setting with an anesthetist. Benzodiazepine antagonists can be used to reverse the effects of midazolam or diazepam; such agents are rarely needed if sedation is administered judiciously. It should be remembered that older patients often require less intravenous sedation than younger patients.

TABLE 3–1. ADVANTAGES AND DISADVANTAGES OF AGENTS COMMONLY USED FOR CONSCIOUS SEDATION DURING ENDOSCOPY

Drug	Advantages	Disadvantages
Diazepam	Antianxiety Amnestic Minimal cardiovascular effects Flat dose-response curve	Pain at injection site Chemical phlebitis
Midazolam	Rapid onset Stronger amnestic than diazepam Less phlebitis and injection pain	High potency Dose adjustment required for the elderly
Meperidine	Analgesic	Minimal amnesia Cardiopulmonary
Fentanyl	Analgesic	High potency Dose adjustments required for the elderly Hypoventilation risk
Propofol	Rapid onset Rapid clearance Amnestic	Pain with injection Bradycardia Hypotension Expensive

▪ DOCUMENTATION OF FINDINGS

Video endoscopes produce digital signals that can be recorded on a variety of media, including film, hardcopy printout, or disk. During the procedure, it is important to visually document important findings and their location for comparison with previous or follow-up studies. This practice allows other members of the health care team to understand and interpret the findings and plan appropriate treatment. Additional documentation on anatomic diagrams will also facilitate interpretation. Pertinent negative findings should also be documented.

▪ UPPER GASTROINTESTINAL ENDOSCOPY

INDICATIONS

Diagnostic esophagogastroduodenoscopy (EGD) is used for evaluating upper gastrointestinal disorders (Table 3–2). Patients being evaluated for mucosal lesions, upper GI bleeding, dysphagia, or odynophagia usually undergo EGD. Abnormal or inconclusive radiographic studies are also indications for endoscopy. Follow-up evaluations for ulcers or surveillance for patients with Barrett's esophagus are also indications. Potential contraindications to performing EGD include the lack of functioning equipment, a lack of trained endoscopists, and patient refusal. In cases in whom perforation is suspected or caustic chemicals are ingested, EGD should be postponed until the risk of perforation is reduced. Finally, coagulopathy, thrombocytopenia, or recent use of medications that inhibit proper clotting may be reasons for postponing EGD. In an era of direct referral of patients to the endoscopist without an initial office-based consultation (open-access endoscopy), a clearer understanding of indications and contraindications is necessary.

PATIENT PREPARATION

Upper gastrointestinal endoscopy usually does not require extensive preparation. Patients should be fasted for at least 4–6 hours before the examination. More time may be required in the presence of esophageal or gastric outlet obstruction. Occasionally, the latter will mandate pre-endoscopic passage of a large-bore tube for esophageal aspiration or gastric lavage. Before the study dentures and eyeglasses should be removed. If intervention is anticipated, a recent coagulation profile and platelet count should be within safe ranges.

Prophylactic antibiotics are rarely indicated; the most compelling indications include performance of esophageal sclerotherapy or dilatation in patients with prosthetic heart valves, previous endocarditis, systemic pul-

TABLE 3–2. INDICATIONS FOR APPROPRIATE USE OF ESOPHAGOGASTRODUODENOSCOPY

1. Abdominal symptoms not responsive to appropriate medical treatment
2. Abdominal symptoms with constitutional changes (e.g., weight loss, early satiety)
3. Abdominal symptoms age ≥ 45
4. Odynophagia or dysphagia
5. Gastroesophageal reflux disease not responsive to medical therapy
6. Nausea and vomiting
7. Familial adenomatous polyposis syndromes
8. Confirmation and tissue sampling of radiologic findings (e.g., strictures, ulcers)
9. Acute GI bleeding and treatment
10. Chronic GI anemia with normal colonoscopy
11. Tissue or fluid sampling
12. Document or treat esophageal and gastric varices
13. Assess esophageal or gastric injury
14. Removal of foreign bodies
15. Enteral access procedures
16. Management of achalasia and benign and malignant stenosis

Adapted with permission, from the ASGE Guidelines Statement 2004.

monary shunts, or recent vascular prostheses. For percutaneous endoscopic gastrostomy (PEG) tube placement, intravenous cephalosporins administered prior to the procedure decrease the rate of skin infections.

Many endoscopists spray topical pharyngeal anesthesia onto the posterior pharyngeal wall in order to suppress the gag reflex. This practice, as well as use of a small-diameter endoscope, is particular helpful if minimal or no intravenous sedation is to be used. The patient is usually in the left lateral decubitus position, with the head slightly elevated on a pillow. For PEG tube placements, the patient should be in the supine or semi-Fowler position. Once the patient is properly positioned and monitoring devices are in place, sedation is administered as needed.

DIAGNOSTIC AND THERAPEUTIC TECHNIQUES

Diagnostic Technique

The 120-cm forward-viewing endoscope is preferred for routine diagnostic endoscopy. Smaller-diameter pediatric endoscopes are available for use in small children or patients with strictures; their use may facilitate routine adult diagnostic examinations as well.

After adequately preparing the patient and confirming that the equipment is in proper working order, the endoscope tip is lubricated and then inserted directly into the esophagus. Intubation is best accomplished under direct vision by advancing the endoscope over the tongue, past the uvula and epiglottis, and then posterior to the cricoarytenoid cartilage on either side. This maneuver will impact the endoscope tip at the cricopharyngeal sphincter, which will relax and allow entry into the cervical esophagus if the patient swallows. Alternatively, the endoscope can be introduced blindly, guiding the tip into the midline of the patient's pharynx with the previously inserted second and third fingers of the left hand. Obviously this latter technique is more dangerous for both patient and endoscopist.

Once in the esophagus, the instrument is advanced under direct vision to the desired endpoint (usually the proximal duodenum), taking care to survey the mucosa both during insertion and withdrawal. Inspection is often easier during withdrawal, when the viscera are well distended with air; this is often the best time to pursue detailed examination and/or sampling of lesions noted during insertion.

The endoscope is advanced to the esophagogastric (EG) junction, noting the "Z-line," where the white squamous esophageal mucosa meets the red columnar gastric epithelium. This line should be within 2 cm of the diaphragmatic "pinch zone," which marks the diaphragmatic esophageal hiatus. This point can be accentuated by asking the patient to sniff while the area is visualized. Accurately identifying the location of the Z-line and hiatus is important because many subsequent diagnostic or treatment modalities are based on the location of this anatomic landmark (e.g., pH probe placement or endoscopic anti-reflux procedures). Furthermore, the Z-line can often be used to determine if an EG junction lesion is gastric or esophageal in origin.

After aspirating any gastric contents, the four gastric walls are surveyed using combinations of tip deflection and shaft rotation, insertion, or withdrawal. The endoscope is next advanced parallel to the longitudinal gastric folds along the greater curvature; entry into the antrum usually requires "corkscrewing" around the vertebral column. This affords an end-on view of the pylorus, which is approached directly. Passage through the pylorus can usually be seen and felt; this maneuver is facilitated by use of the single-handed technique. Entry into the duodenal bulb is recognized by the typical granular, pale mucosa. Finally, the second portion of the duodenum is entered by advancing to the superior duodenal angle, and then simultaneously deflecting the tip and rotating the shaft to the right. Paradoxically, withdrawal of the endoscope at this point usually advances the endoscope down the duodenum as the tip is "corkscrewed" around the superior duodenal angle. All areas should be carefully surveyed again as the endoscope is withdrawn.

It should be noted that with a forward-viewing endoscope in the stomach, it is particularly difficult to visualize the cardia, proximal fundus, and the lesser curvature. Thus, when in the antrum, either prior to entering or after withdrawing from the duodenal bulb, the endoscope should be retroflexed by simultaneously flexing the tip up 180° while advancing the shaft (Fig 3–3). In this position, the tip can then be rotated through 180° in either

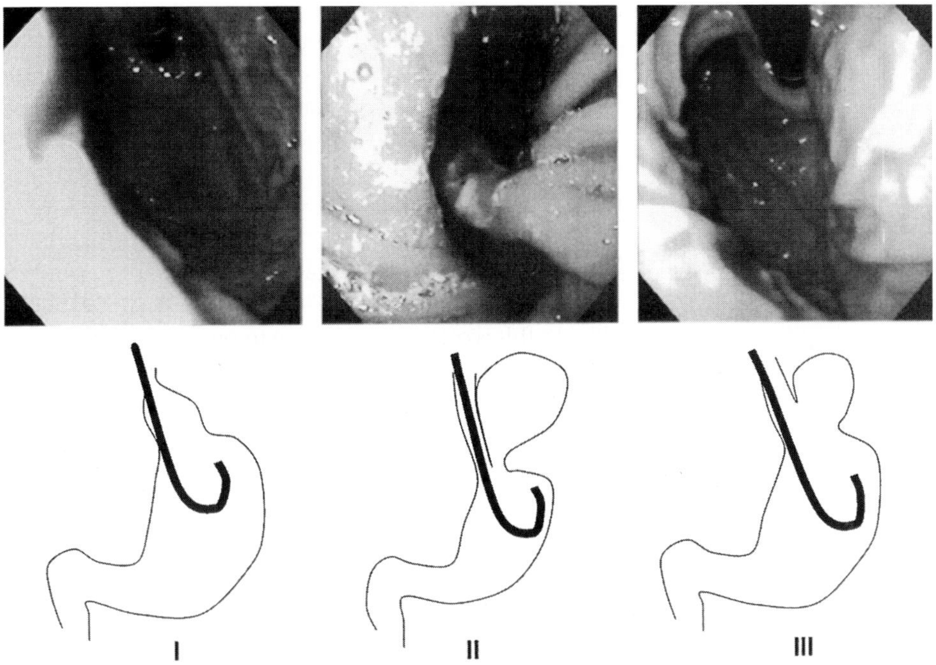

Figure 3–3. Retroflexed view of the gastric cardia and gastroesophageal junction. In this view, hiatal and paraesophageal hernias can be identified.

direction in order to adequately visualize the cardia and fundus. In the retroflexed position, the endoscope can be withdrawn to more closely inspect the cardia.

Techniques of Tissue Sampling

When desired, tissue sampling is most frequently obtained by directed biopsy. These are taken with cupped forceps (Fig 3–4) passed through the endoscope's therapeutic channel. Ideally, lesions should be biopsied from an "en-face" position. However, spiked biopsy forceps may facilitate biopsy of lesions which must be approached tangentially (e.g., esophagus). In either case, the forceps are applied with open jaws; once properly located, they are gently closed and withdrawn. Multiple biopsies should usually be obtained. For ulcers, one should biopsy the rim in all four quadrants, as well as the base or ulcer crater. Standard biopsy rarely penetrates the muscularis mucosa. Deeper biopsy can be obtained by using the jumbo forceps or with a diathermy snare loop.

Lesions can also be sampled by brush cytology. In this technique, a sleeved brush (Fig 3–5) is passed

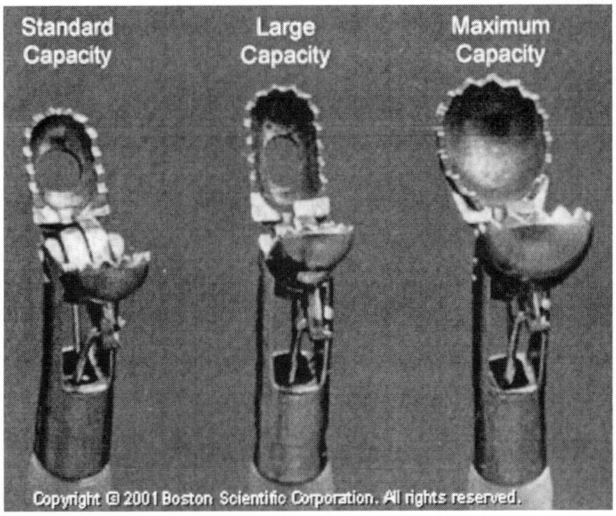

Figure 3–4. Examples of endoscopic biopsy forceps. (Courtesy of Boston Scientific Corporation, Natick, MA.)

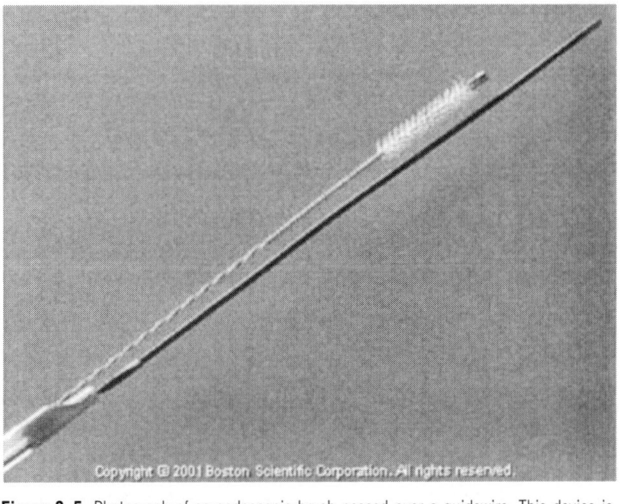

Figure 3–5. Photograph of an endoscopic brush passed over a guidewire. This device is commonly used for biliary tract tissue sampling. (Courtesy of Boston Scientific Corporation, Natick, MA.)

through the therapeutic channel towards the lesion. Once over the lesion, the brush head is advanced out of the sleeve and rubbed repeatedly over the lesion; the brush is then pulled back into the sleeve and both are withdrawn together. When convenient, the brush head is extended and wiped across several glass slides. These are rapidly fixed and sent for cytologic processing. When using disposable cytology brushes, the brush head should be transected and dropped into fixative; analysis of this fluid often provides a good cytology specimen.

Various staining techniques are in development to enhance the sensitivity of detecting mucosal abnormalities (chromoendoscopy) (Fig 3–6). Most involve spraying with dyes (e.g., methylene blue, indigo carmine, or Congo red) which stain or react with the mucosa. Chromoendoscopy requires high-resolution endoscopes with CCD chips containing up to 850,000 pixels which allow detection of minute lesions. These procedures are often facilitated by use of high-magnification endoscopes, which have thumb-operated levers or foot-operated pedals that zoom into or out of the magnified view without loss of focus. Using such systems, views can be magnified 50- to 115-fold when viewed on a standard 20-inch monitor.

Nonvariceal Bleeding Sources

Endoscopy plays a critical role in evaluation and treatment of this disorder and should be performed soon after the patient has stabilized. Upper GI endoscopy will accurately identify the bleeding source in 80–95% of patients. If possible, the upper gastrointestinal tract should first be lavaged free of all blood and clots. The endoscopic exami-

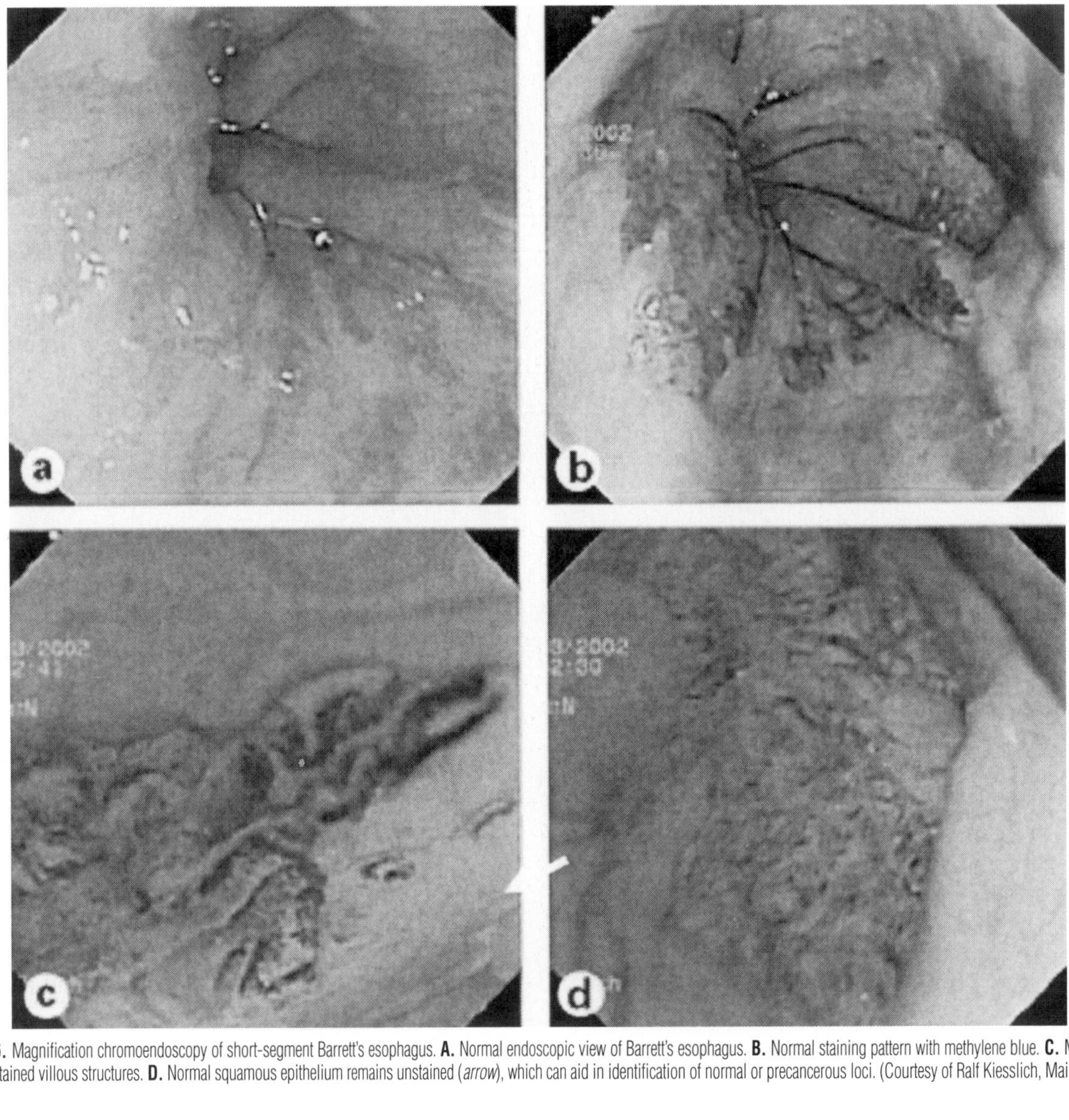

Figure 3–6. Magnification chromoendoscopy of short-segment Barrett's esophagus. **A.** Normal endoscopic view of Barrett's esophagus. **B.** Normal staining pattern with methylene blue. **C.** Magnified view (~150×) of stained villous structures. **D.** Normal squamous epithelium remains unstained (*arrow*), which can aid in identification of normal or precancerous loci. (Courtesy of Ralf Kiesslich, Mainz, Germany.)

nation is then performed, seeking active bleeding or stigmata of recent hemorrhage such as clot, black spots, or a visible vessel. Attempts should be made to obtain complete visualization of the esophagus, EG junction, fundus, antrum, pylorus, and proximal duodenum.

Before pursuing hemostatic therapy, one should be cognizant of the fact that 70–85% of patients stop bleeding spontaneously without further intervention, provided that coagulopathy is corrected. However, therapy is appropriate in actively bleeding lesions or those with a nonbleeding visible vessel or a sentinel clot. The latter factor is associated with a smaller risk of rebleeding when compared to actively bleeding lesions or those with visible vessels. Mallory-Weiss tears and Dieulafoy's lesions are less common nonvariceal lesions that may be treated with endoscopic intervention. Options for endoscopic hemostatic treatment include injection therapy, thermal energy, and endoscopic clipping.

Injection therapy is performed with a 4-mm 23-gauge needle passed through the operating channel of the endoscope. The sclerosant is injected submucosally at three or four sites surrounding a bleeding vessel and at an additional three or four sites 1–2 cm from the vessel. The amount injected varies with different agents, but should be small enough to avoid extension or damage to surrounding tissues, yet large enough to induce tamponade (and possibly sclerosis) by compressing adjacent tissue. This may take 5–10 mL at each site. Agents available include epinephrine (alone or with normal or hypertonic saline), absolute alcohol, thrombin in normal saline, sodium tetradecyl sulfate, and polidocanol. These agents all appear to be effective in most cases (90%) with very low complication rates.

Thermal therapies use heat to control hemorrhage by inducing tissue coagulation, collagen contraction, and vessel shrinkage. The two main types of thermal energy used are laser light and electric current.

Monopolar electrocoagulation transfers electric current from a generator to the tissues and then to the patient's ground plate. Because of the high energy density, the electric current is converted to heat at the small area of contact between the electrode and the tissue. The current is applied circumferentially around the artery until the bleeding stops. The heat generated, which can reach several thousand degrees, is sufficient to cause full-thickness tissue damage, so care is required when using this modality.

Bipolar probes use two active electrodes to concentrate current density close to the probe tip. This allows effective coagulation at lower temperatures, approximately 100°C. The probe is placed against the bleeding site, tamponading the bleeding. A 50-watt current is then passed in several 2-second pulses. This will bond the intimal surfaces of the bleeding vessels (coaptation).

The heater probe applies heat to the vessel by conduction. Coaptation is achieved by tamponading the vessel with the probe and applying three or four sequential pulses of 20–30 J each.

The laser generates heat that is absorbed by the tissues. Two types of lasers are currently used for hemostasis: the argon laser and the Nd:YAG (neodymium-yttrium-aluminum-garnet) laser. The argon laser is of limited use in the severely bleeding patient since the light is absorbed by red blood cells, thus decreasing the amount of energy applied to the vessel. Disadvantages of laser therapy include extreme heat (the Nd:YAG laser carries a greater risk of full-thickness injury), expense, and lack of portability.

Thermal therapies are successful in 80–95% of cases, with a rebleed rate of 10–20%. These techniques are easy to use and safe, with a perforation rate of 0.5%.

Endoscopic clipping is an effective method to control bleeding. Frequently, more than one clip is necessary at one site. These clips can effectively control bleeding, and usually fall off in 7–10 days, when the bleeding site heals (Fig 3–7). However, there are anecdotal reports of clips remaining at the site 2 months after placement.

It is also possible to treat bleeding with combined modalities such as coagulation and injection or clipping and injection. However, there are no studies to demonstrate the superiority of combined over single hemostatic therapy. Given the relatively high success rates of controlling upper GI bleeding by endoscopic modalities, it is appropriate to pursue endoscopic means whenever available before seeking surgical or interventional radiology options.

Variceal Bleeding Sources

Bleeding esophageal varices remain a significant clinical problem with hospital mortality rates approaching 30%. Without some form of intervention, it is well known that two-thirds of patients who survive an initial episode of bleeding will rebleed.

The patient's condition should be optimized before sclerotherapy. This should include repletion of volume and coagulation factors. The stomach should also be lavaged to clear blood clots. In the presence of massive bleeding, it may be necessary to begin vasopressin infusion or pass a Sengstaken-Blakemore tube for 12–24 hours before attempting sclerotherapy. If possible, however, sclerotherapy without prior tamponade is favored, since this approach is equally effective and lessens blood requirements and major complications.

The most commonly used sclerosants in the United States are 0.7–3.0% sodium tetradecyl sulfate and 5% sodium morrhuate. In Europe, ethanolamine is more commonly used. All of these agents can cause tissue damage and inflammation.

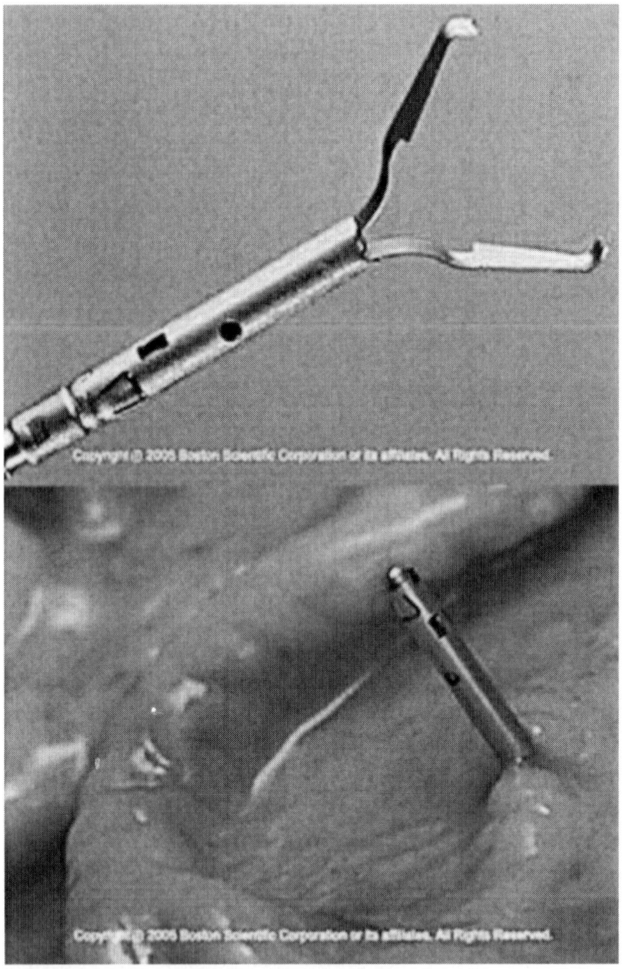

Figure 3–7. Endoscopic clips (Resolution Clip Device) can be passed through the endoscope's working channel and applied to bleeding sites and visible vessels, as well as mucosal tears. (Courtesy of Boston Scientific Corporation, Natick, MA.)

Sclerosants can be injected either intravariceally or paravariceally. Intravariceal injection is preferred since it controls acute variceal bleeding more effectively (90% versus 19% success). For gastric varices, injections are begun just above the gastroduodenal junction. Once the needle is placed into a varix, a 0.5-mL test dose is given to ensure intravariceal placement. After placement is confirmed, an additional 1.5 mL is injected at that site. This technique is repeated in a circular fashion until all varices at this level have been treated. Injections are continued by moving proximally, injecting at 2- to 3-cm intervals until small-caliber vessels are encountered. The total amount of sclerosant used varies with the agent used, but in general should not exceed 20 mL per session. If active variceal bleeding is encountered, injections are begun just proximal to the bleeding site and continued until bleeding subsides. A second session of sclerotherapy should be performed 5 days later. Sclerotherapy is usually repeated at 1- to 3-week intervals until varices are ablated.

Sclerotherapy controls acute variceal hemorrhage in at least 85% of episodes and probably lowers the rate of recurrent bleeding. Propranolol may decrease the rate of recurrent bleeding while awaiting variceal obliteration. While endoscopic control of variceal bleeding is pursued, other options such as transjugular intrahepatic portosystemic shunt (TIPS) or other portosystemic shunting should be considered because of the significant risks of rebleeding.

Endoscopic ligation is an alternative method for variceal eradication (Fig 3–8). In this technique, varices are ligated with elastic bands similar to those used during hemorrhoidal ligation. When compared to sclerotherapy, this method appears to be as effective and may improve morbidity and mortality. However, there is a learning curve associated with accurate placement of the bands.

When there is no evidence of bleeding, prophylactic endoscopic variceal eradication should not be performed because of the high risks of complications associated with the procedures.

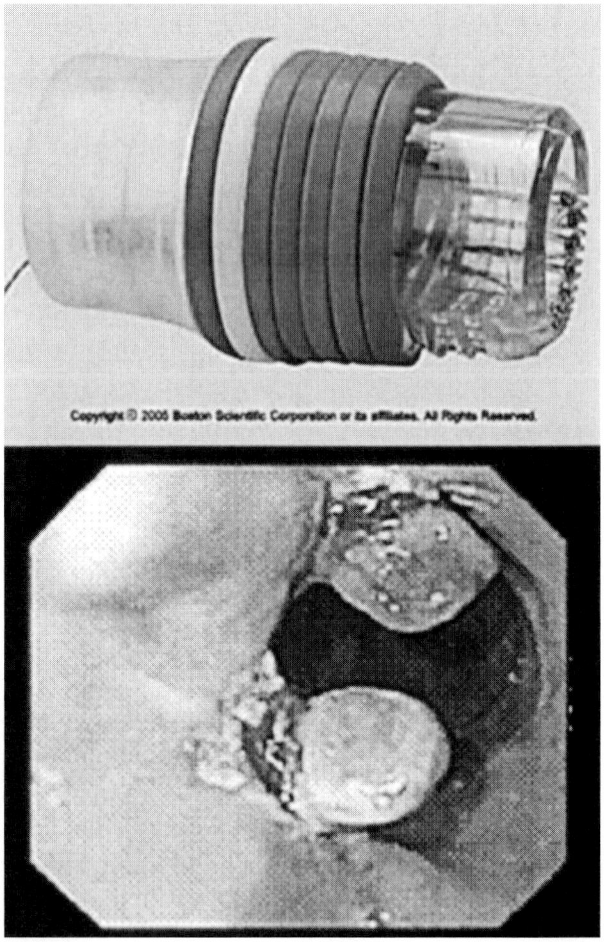

Figure 3–8. Photograph of a multiple-load variceal banding device; the cup is fitted over the end of a gastroscope. The device is placed over the intended site for banding, suction is applied for several seconds, and the bands are deployed. (Courtesy of Boston Scientific Corporation, Natick, MA.)

Percutaneous Endoscopic Gastrostomy and Jejunostomy

Percutaneous endoscopic gastrostomy (PEG) is now the preferred method for long-term feeding in patients who are unable to swallow or who require supplemental nutrition or chronic gastric decompression. PEG may be preferable to surgical gastrostomy since it is safe, less expensive, and less invasive. PEG and percutaneous endoscopic jejunostomy are contraindicated only in patients with total esophageal obstruction, massive ascites, or intra-abdominal sepsis.

Prior to the procedure, a single dose of prophylactic cephalosporin (or equivalent) should be given intravenously. The patient is placed in the supine or semi-Fowler position, after which the abdomen is prepared and draped using sterile technique. The endoscope is then passed into the stomach, which is distended with air insufflation. The assistant then presses on the abdomen with a finger and the impact against the anterior gastric wall should be noted. Ideally, this point should be 2–3 cm below the left costal margin. It is critical that the assistant's finger be clearly observed to indent the stomach. In patients with thin abdominal walls, light transillumination from within the stomach to the skin surface may aid in identifying a safe landmark.

A polypectomy snare is passed through the endoscope channel. The selected site on the abdominal wall is then infiltrated with local anesthesia. If desired, the fine needle used to anesthetize the skin can be inserted into the abdomen at the intended gastrostomy site; observation of the needle's clean entry into the stomach suggests the position is adequate. After making a small incision (approximately 5 mm) in the skin, the assistant then inserts a 14-gauge intravenous cannula through the incision; the intravenous cannula must be seen to enter the stomach. The snare is then tightened around the cannula and the inner stylet is removed. In the "pull technique," a long looped suture is placed through the cannula, after which the snare is released. The suture is then firmly grasped with the polypectomy snare. The endoscope and the tightened snare are removed together, bringing the suture out of the patient's mouth. The suture is secured to a well-lubricated 20F or 24F gastrostomy tube at its tapered external end. The assistant then pulls on the suture until the attached tube exits the abdominal wall (Fig 3–9). The endoscope is then reinserted and used to view the tube's inner bolster as the stomach is loosely seated against the abdominal wall and the tube is properly positioned. The endoscope is then removed and the tube is secured in place on the abdominal wall, usually with an external Silastic cross-bar or disc.

Two other techniques can be used for PEG placement. In the "push technique," in lieu of a suture a guidewire is inserted through the cannula and pulled out the patient's mouth. The gastrostomy tube is then pushed over the wire until it exits the abdominal wall. Finally, in the "introducer technique," the stomach is inflated, the site of insertion selected, and the intravenous cannula introduced into the stomach as described above. A J-tipped guidewire is then passed through the cannula into the stomach after which the cannula is removed. An introducer with a peel-away sheath is then passed over this wire, allowing removal of the wire and introducer. A Foley catheter or other similar gastrostomy tube is then placed through the sheath, its balloon inflated, and the sheath is removed. The catheter is then secured to the abdominal wall.

The PEG procedure can be extended to include jejunostomy (PEG-J) in patients who fail to tolerate gastric

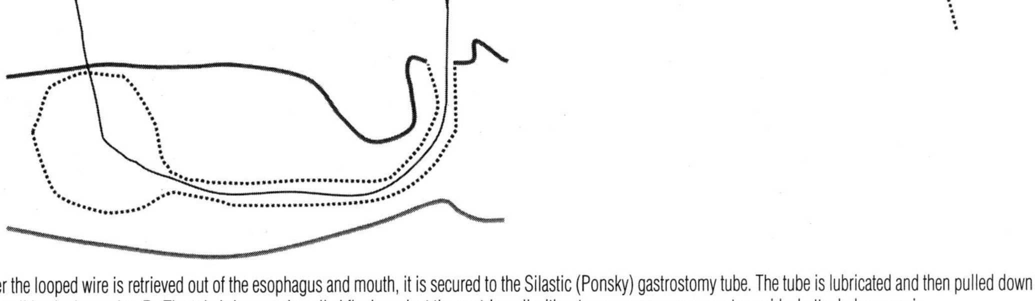

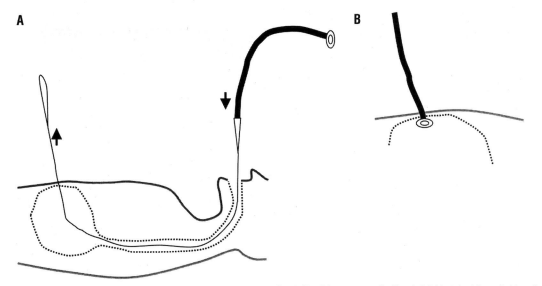

Figure 3–9. A. After the looped wire is retrieved out of the esophagus and mouth, it is secured to the Silastic (Ponsky) gastrostomy tube. The tube is lubricated and then pulled down the esophagus and out of the abdominal wall by the loop wire. **B.** The tube's bumper is pulled flush against the gastric wall without excess pressure so as to avoid a buttonhole necrosis.

feedings due to severe gastroesophageal reflux or gastroparesis. While enteral feeding by PEG-J is intuitively believed to decrease the incidence of aspiration when compared with PEG feedings, most series report aspiration pneumonia to occur in only 0–5% of patients with PEG feedings—even for the neurologically impaired patient.

PEG-J placement is achieved by passing a jejunal feeding tube through the PEG lumen (a 24F PEG tube accommodates up to a 12.5 F J-tube; a standard 20F PEG tube accommodates an 8.5F J-tube). Patients generally require deeper sedation of longer duration when a PEG-J is to be placed. The jejunal feeding tube can then be placed into the duodenum or jejunum under endoscopic or fluoroscopic guidance. Endoscopically, the jejunal tube is grasped with the foreign-body forceps and guided into the duodenum under direct vision. However, the limited length of the gastroscope makes the endoscopic guidance into the jejunum nearly impossible, and jejunal tubes placed in the duodenum are prone to recoil back into the stomach. Some have recommended anchoring the tip of the jejunal extension tube with endoscopic clips, but the clips will slough off with mucosal regeneration and the jejunal tube will recoil back into the stomach. The pediatric colonoscope with a 160-cm flexible shaft is most ideal for the PEG-J procedure. When the jejunal extension tube is delivered into the distal duodenum or proximal jejunum with forceps, the scope is withdrawn while leaving the forceps in position. Once the scope is back in the stomach, the forceps is then opened and withdrawn, leaving the jejunal extension tube in place.

Foreign Body Extraction

Foreign bodies are ingested predominantly by two groups of patients: children (ages 1–5 years) who accidentally swallow an object, and adults who are obtunded or inebriated, have a psychiatric disorder, or are prisoners. Most objects (80–90%) will pass spontaneously, but 10–20% must be removed endoscopically; approximately 1% require surgical intervention. Removal is usually necessary if the object has failed to move in 48–72 hours. Objects wider than 2 cm or longer than 5 cm will rarely pass and usually require endoscopic intervention. Signs of respiratory compromise or inability to handle secretions constitutes a true emergency and requires immediate extraction of the object.

When performing endoscopic extraction, protection of the airway is of vital importance. Thus the procedure should be performed with the patient in the Trendelenburg position to prevent the object from falling into the trachea during removal. Rarely, endotracheal intubation is required. An endoscopic overtube should be considered when removing sharp objects or multiple fragments.

Coins are the most common objects swallowed by children. Coins lodged in the esophagus should be removed promptly since the risk of pressure necrosis and fistula formation increases the longer the coin remains lodged. Endoscopic extraction is accomplished after adequate sedation with the patient in the Trendelenburg position. The coin is localized and grasped with a polypectomy snare or rat-tooth or tenaculum forceps. A Foley catheter is not recommended since it does not control the object well during removal. The coin will usually pass if it reaches the stomach.

In the adult population, meat impaction represents the most common foreign body. These should be removed if they remain longer than 12 hours. If the bolus should pass, esophagoscopy is still required since an obstructing esophageal lesion will be found in 70–95% of patients.

Sharp objects such as toothpicks, fish or chicken bones, needles, and razor blades should be removed if accessible because of the small but real risk of perforation. Use of an overtube may greatly facilitate removal of sharp objects. If the object has a single sharp end (e.g., an open safety pin), it can be pushed into the stomach, rotated to point the sharp end distally, and then removed. Items for which endoscopic extraction appears to carry an excessive risk are probably best removed surgically. If the object has passed beyond endoscopic access, a trial of spontaneous passage is reasonable with daily radiographic monitoring. If the object fails to progress after 2–3 days, or if the patient becomes symptomatic, surgical removal is warranted.

Ingested button batteries can injure the esophagus by direct corrosive action. In the stomach, they can erode and release toxic components. These batteries usually pass readily in other parts of the gastrointestinal tract without causing harm. After endoscopically removing a battery from the esophagus, it is important to inspect the esophagus to assess possible damage.

When encountered, cocaine-filled packets should never be removed endoscopically because of the risk of breakage; expectant management is more appropriate. Patients so managed should be closely monitored since they may require surgery for bowel obstruction.

Stricture Dilatation

Most commonly, a patient with an esophageal stricture complains of dysphagia or odynophagia. A barium swallow is usually obtained before endoscopy to demonstrate the structure and length of the obstructing lesion. Endoscopy should then be performed to identify the nature and character of the stricture, being prepared to perform dilation or stenting. Multiple biopsies and cytologic brushings of the area should always be obtained.

The most common cause of esophageal strictures is benign peptic stenosis secondary to gastroesophageal reflux (Fig 3–10). Most peptic and many radia-

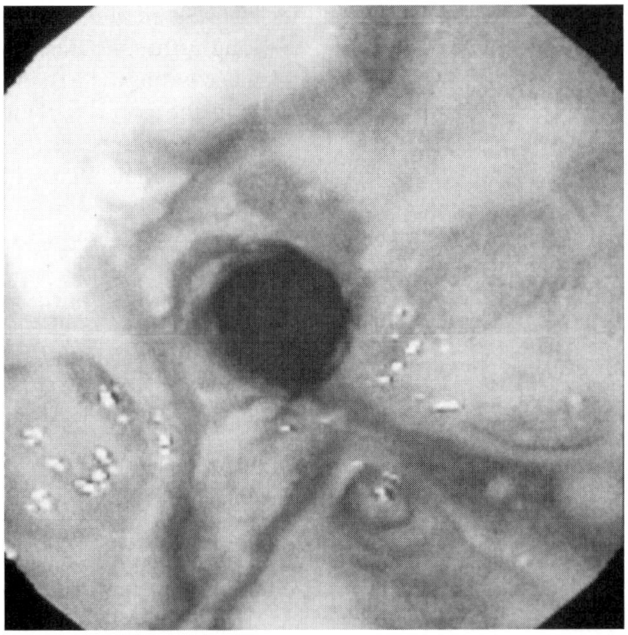

Figure 3–10. Endoscopic view of distal esophageal stricture. Multiple biopsies are taken of the stricture site prior to dilation maneuvers.

tion strictures are amenable to dilation therapy (close to 90% success rate), which is usually performed on an outpatient basis. The goal of esophageal dilation is to achieve a 14–15 mm diameter (45F), but it is prudent not to dilate a very narrow stricture to the desired diameter in one session. Treatment is safer when performed by incremental dilations over successive sessions. A general approach is to limit the number of dilations to three successive balloon or dilator sizes in one session. Injection of steroid solutions into the stricture may reduce the severity of postdilation inflammation, scarring, and restricture. The frequency of dilation will depend on the severity of the stricture and the patient's symptoms.

Although several types of dilators have been used (Fig 3–11), the two most common dilators used are the guidewire-driven type, which applies both axial and radial forces, and the balloon type, which applies only radial forces. Guidewire-driven dilators are easy to pass and offer the added safety of the guidewire; balloon dilators can be monitored endoscopically.

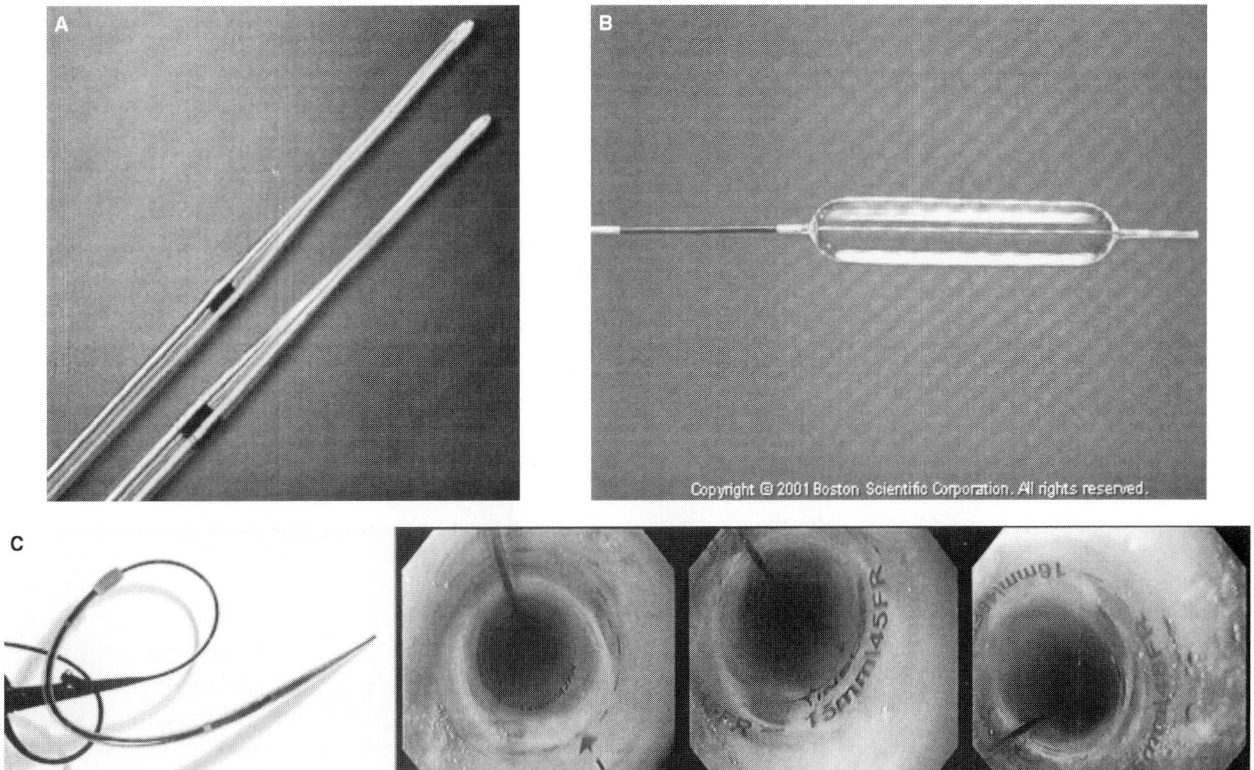

Figure 3–11. Examples of various dilators for strictures or luminal narrowings. **A.** Modified Savary dilator sets range from 21F to 60F in diameter and are usually 70 cm or 100 cm long. Savary dilators have a tapered end and a hollow core which allows passage over a rigid guidewire. Direct visualization of the dilation process is not possible with the Savary. (Courtesy of Wilson-Cook Medical, Winston-Salem, NC.) **B.** Balloon dilators, which provide radial force only, can be passed through the working channel of a standard endoscope, allowing dilatation to be visually monitored. (Courtesy of Boston Scientific Corporation, Natick, MA.) **C.** The Optical Dilator (Courtesy of Ethicon Endo-Surgery, Cincinnati, OH) is similar to a Savary in design, but has gradual size progressions on each dilator. A standard gastroscope is passed through the hollow tubing to offer rigidity and direct visualization. In this example, the stricture was sequentially dilated from 14 to 16 mm in 1-minute intervals.

Guidewire-driven dilators are suitable for use with tight strictures or when other dilators cannot be used. These are fairly rigid devices made of polyvinyl chloride (Savary). Each dilator has a hollow core and can be passed over an endoscopically or fluoroscopically placed guidewire. Although there are no controlled trials, some endoscopists maintain that fluoroscopic control increases the safety and effectiveness of guidewire-driven dilatation. Guidewire-driven metal olive dilators (Eder-Puestow) and mercury-filled dilators are rarely if ever used anymore.

Balloon dilators are used for short strictures, stenotic stomas, and achalasia. These dilators can be passed over a guidewire or through the endoscope's therapeutic channel. Balloon dilation of achalasia provides short-term (<6 months) success in approximately 75% of cases, and therefore repeat sessions are frequently required. Alternative treatments for achalasia include botulinum injections, which result in less tissue inflammation and fibrosis than repeated dilatations, and laparoscopic esophageal myotomy, which can be performed very successfully in skilled hands. While balloon dilatation has also been utilized for treatment of corrosive strictures, the rupture rate may be increased in this setting.

Endoscopic intervention is frequently required for malignant esophageal strictures. Patients with unresectable tumors or tracheoesophageal fistula may require palliative dilation and, occasionally, placement of an esophageal stent (Fig 3–12). Placement of these devices requires initial esophageal dilation followed by endoscopic assessment of tumor location and length. Under fluoroscopic guidance, the prosthesis is placed so that the distal end is 3–5 cm beyond the tumor or fistula. Most stents are delivered to the site of obstruction using the wider working channel of a colonoscope. Laser ablation and electrocoagulation therapy have also provided reasonable palliation.

Endoluminal Treatment of GERD

Since 2000, several endoluminal treatments for gastroesophageal reflux disease (GERD) have been introduced in the United States. Some have attained FDA approval, while others remain in various stages of testing. At present, these technologies are either based on suturing or energy delivery (Fig 3–13). All of these procedures are performed in the outpatient setting, and usually with conscious sedation. Examples of each of these modalities are described below.

EndoCinch (Bard, Billerica, MA). This device requires placement of an overtube in the oropharynx, a suction-suturing device at the end of a gastroscope, and a second gastroscope for suture knot tying and cutting. The mucosa is suctioned into a chamber within the suturing device at the end of the gastroscope and sutures are driven into the mucosa. Adjacent sutures are approximated creating a pleat. This procedure can be performed circumferentially to close the aperture of the gastroesophageal junction. It is generally labor intensive and requires multiple passages of the gastroscopes

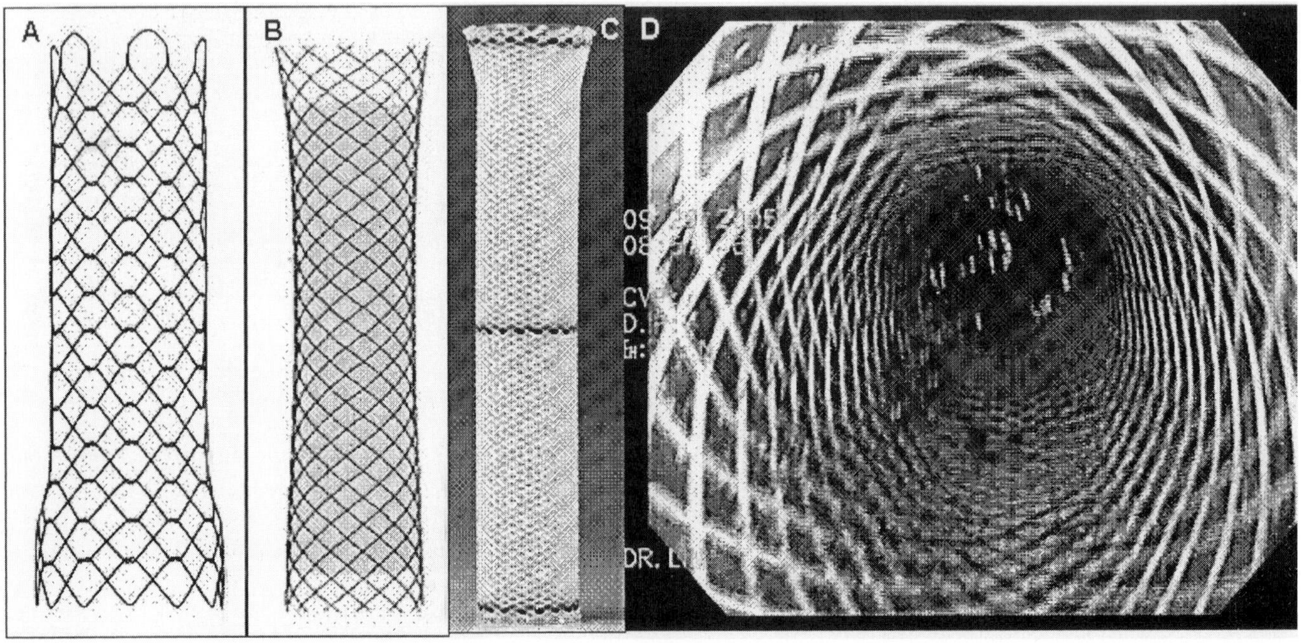

Figure 3–12. A. Self-expanding metallic stents compressed over delivery catheters are passed endoscopically through the working channels of colonoscopes or fluoroscopically over guidewires. These stents are permanent once placed. **B.** Another metallic stent with a synthetic covering to thwart tumor ingrowth. **C.** Silicone esophageal stents are removable and are used frequently in benign strictures. (Courtesy of Boston Scientific Corporation, Natick, MA.) **D.** A removable silicone stent placed in a patient undergoing radiation treatment for potentially resectable esophageal cancer.

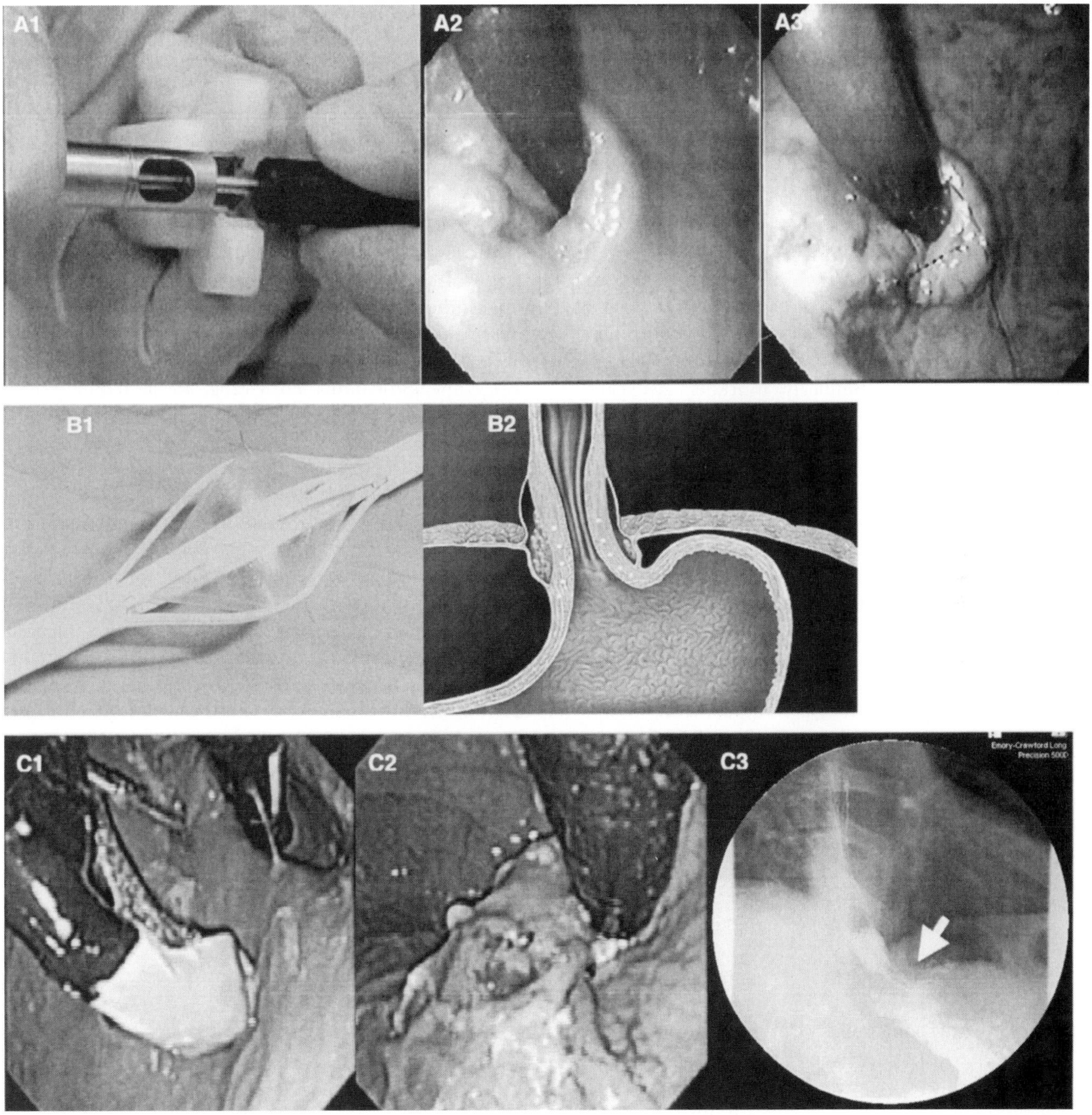

Figure 3–13. A1. EndoCinch gastroplasty sewing device placed at the tip of a gastroscope. (Courtesy of C.R. Bard, Inc, Murray Hill, NJ.) EndoCinch gastroplasty before (**A2**) and after (**A3**) the procedure. **B1.** The Stretta radio frequency energy delivery device (Courtesy of Curon Medical) treats the gastroesophageal junction at multiple levels to induce thickening of this region (**B2**). **C1.** The Plicator suture implant device (NDO Surgical) creates a full-thickness anterior gastric cardia fold that serves as a barrier against gastric reflux (**C2**). Upper GI contrast study demonstrates the tissue fold (*arrow*; **C3**).

for each suture application. The sutures capture the mucosa only and are not full thickness.

Plicator (NDO Surgical, Mansfield MA). The Plicator is also a suture-based technology that utilizes tissue graspers at the end of a suture implant device to draw the anterior gastric cardia into suture implant cartridges. The sutures create a full-thickness flap at the gastroesophageal junction, and are intended to serve as a barrier against reflux. The procedure is performed under direct visualization by placing a 5-mm gastroscope into the working channel of the suture implant device.

Stretta (Curon Medical, Sunnyvale CA). This is the only device that involves delivery of radio frequency energy to the lower esophageal sphincter muscles. Multiple applications at several levels are required to complete the treatment. The procedure is performed blindly after endoscopically confirming the location of the LES. The intention is to induce collagen deposition to the lower esophageal sphincter (LES), thereby adding more bulk and reducing the compliance of the LES. The effects are generally not immediate, but are realized over time.

COMPLICATIONS

Diagnostic upper gastrointestinal endoscopy is a safe procedure with complications reported in approximately 0.1% of cases. Similarly, mortality is exceedingly rare. As alluded to above, cardiopulmonary problems are the most common complications of endoscopy and are usually attributable to oversedation.

Procedure-related complications are also unusual following upper gastrointestinal endoscopy. Perforation is of greatest concern and occurs more frequently following emergency interventions and therapeutic procedures including dilation, sclerotherapy, and thermal hemostasis. When dilating or ablating esophageal lesions with laser, perforation may occur in as many as 10% of cases. For clinically stable patients, nonsurgical treatment of well-contained perforations can be considered. Other unique complications include ulceration and stricture following esophageal sclerotherapy. Finally, local wound infection (including necrotizing fasciitis) can occur with PEG tubes, especially if the incision is too small or the tube is pulled too tightly against the gastric wall, leading to gastric necrosis and leaks around the tube. Occasionally, a PEG can separate from the abdominal wall with resultant peritonitis or colonic erosion. In cases of coloenteric or gastrocolonic fistula without peritonitis, the PEG tube should be left in place for several days to allow the fistula tract to mature; the tubes can then be removed. Most low-output colonic fistulae will spontaneously close.

Pneumoperitoneum is sometimes present 1–2 days following PEG tube placement, and is most commonly discovered on chest x-rays made for unrelated reasons. In these situations, patients are usually asymptomatic. The pneumoperitoneum generally resolves with little intervention beyond bowel rest.

▪ ENDOSCOPY OF THE PANCREATICOBILIARY TREE

INDICATIONS

William McKune—a surgeon—introduced endoscopic retrograde cholangiopancreatography (ERCP) in 1968 when he described endoscopic guidance of a catheter into the ampulla of Vater. This technical achievement allowed precise imaging of the pancreatic ductal system. In 1974, German and Japanese physicians described endoscopic sphincterotomy. This therapeutic extension of ERCP greatly expanded the ability to treat diseases of the pancreaticobiliary system.

Indications for ERCP are summarized in Table 3–3. Unlike conventional endoscopy, access to ERCP may not always be readily available; when necessary, surgeons should efficiently utilize alternative methods (e.g., radiological or surgical) of accessing and treating diseases of the pancreaticobiliary tract. Conversely, the availability of ERCP should not be an indication for its liberal use. The surgeon managing the patient should weigh the indications and diagnostic and therapeutic yield, as well as the risks when determining the most efficacious approach.

PATIENT PREPARATION

Patient preparation, sedation, and monitoring for ERCP are similar to those for upper endoscopy. Intravenous access is required for administration of analgesia, intestinal paralytics, and other medications. Since the procedure is most commonly performed with the patient in the prone position with the head turned right, the intravenous access is preferred in the right arm so that the intravenous tubing does not lie under the patient and can be freely accessed. Normal coagulation profiles are more relevant in ERCP, especially if sphincterotomy or endoprosthesis insertion is contemplated.

TABLE 3–3. INDICATIONS FOR ENDOSCOPIC RETROGRADE CHOLANGIOPANCREATOGRAPHY

BILIARY
1. Choledocholithiasis without spontaneous resolution
2. Management of strictures
3. Obtaining tissue samples
4. Stenting
5. Evaluate sphincter of Oddi dysfunction
6. Ductal injury or leaks
PANCREATIC
1. Ampullary adenoma
2. Recurrent acute pancreatitis
3. Chronic pancreatitis
4. Duct leak
5. Duct strictures/obstructions
6. Pancreatic fluid/cyst
7. Cytology
8. Intraductal ultrasound

Adapted, with permission, from Adler DG, Baron TH, Davila RE et al, and the Standards of Practice Committee of the American Society for Gastrointestinal Endoscopy. ASGE guideline: The role of ERCP in diseases of the biliary tract and the pancreas. *Gastrointest Endsoc* 2005;62:1–8.

Prophylactic antibiotics are usually administered before the procedure.

The patient's oropharynx is anesthetized with local anesthesia. In addition to standard intravenous sedation and analgesia, other medications commonly used are glucagon (0.5–1.0 mg) or hyoscyamine sulfate (0.2–0.5 mg), administered intravenously to decrease duodenal motility. While some endoscopists initiate the procedure with the patient in the prone position, most position the patient on the fluoroscopy table in the left lateral decubitus position with the left arm behind the back, anticipating conversion to the prone position once the endoscope is appropriately located in the descending duodenum. For patients who are critically ill, assistance from the anesthesiology team in the endoscopy suite or in the operating room should be arranged.

DIAGNOSTIC AND THERAPEUTIC TECHNIQUES

ERCP is performed using a 90-degree side-viewing scope. The scope is passed blindly into the esophagus and rapidly advanced into the proximal stomach where any residual secretions should be aspirated. The scope rides along the greater curvature towards the pylorus. In order to enter the pylorus with a side-viewing scope, it is vital to keep the scope within the central axis of the antrum with the pylorus viewed in the 6-o'clock position. Visualization of the pylorus is often limited, and passage into the duodenal bulb is frequently felt rather than seen.

To manipulate around the superior duodenal angle, the endoscope is turned to the right, and the tip is deflected down to reach the second portion of the duodenum. The endoscope is usually withdrawn during this maneuver, leaving the scope in the ideal "short-scope" position, 60–70 cm from the incisors, facing the medial duodenal wall (Fig 3–14). If the endoscope is passed into the duodenum by continually advancing, steering, and rotating, a big loop or the "long-scope" position usually results in the stomach. The long-scope position is not preferred because it is uncomfortable to the patient and also reduces control of the endoscope tip.

With the "short-scope" position, the endoscopist views the papilla directly along the medial duodenal wall. If not, very minute movements of the tip will bring the papilla into view. Intermittent doses of glucagon should be given to induce and maintain duodenal paralysis. A scout radiograph is obtained to verify adequate radiologic technique, as well as to identify calcifications or other findings present before contrast injection. The papilla is then cannulated using one of the various types of catheters available, usually beginning with a 7F diagnostic catheter. Catheters with radiopaque tips are often preferred, since the radiologic marker facilitates radiologic identification of the catheter tip. Once the papilla has been successfully cannulated, contrast is injected under radiologic control so as to avoid overfilling the biliary and/or pancreatic ductal systems. If dilated ducts are encountered, use of diluted (half-strength) contrast may prevent obscuring small stones.

Selective cannulation of the biliary and pancreatic ducts depends on the angle of the catheter. The pan-

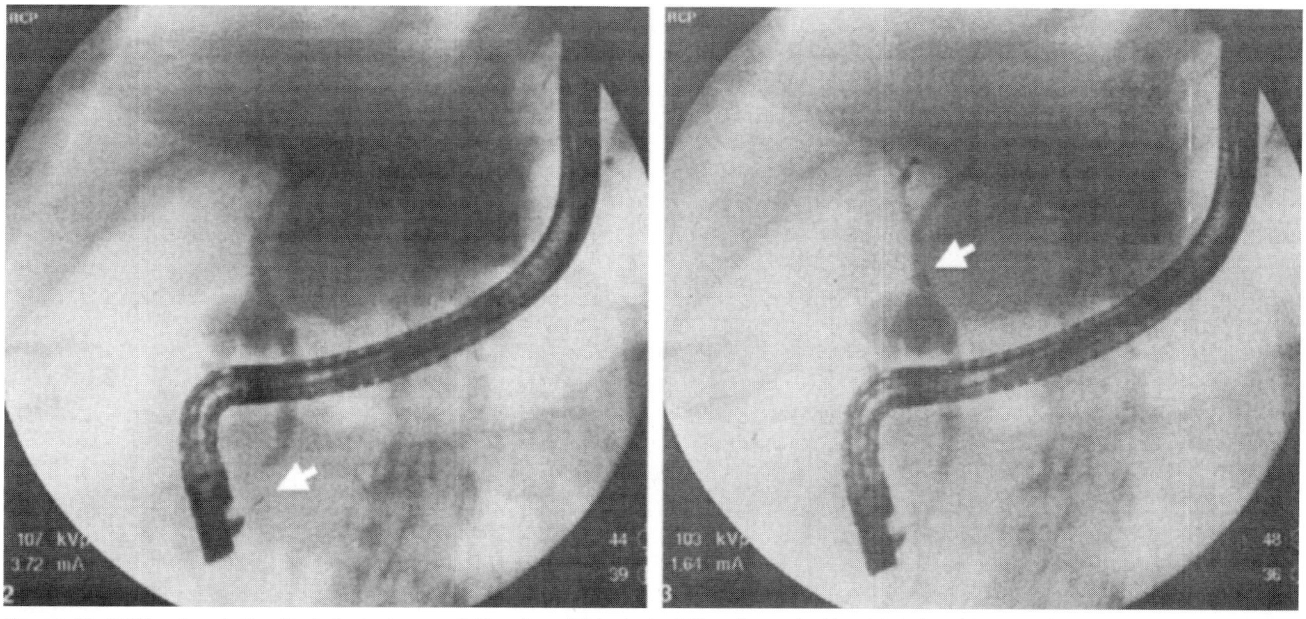

Figure 3–14. ERCP is performed with a side-viewing duodenoscope that faces the medial duodenal wall. The radiopaque tip of the guidewire (*arrow*) is seen passing the ampulla and riding up the common bile duct. The duodenoscope is in the "short-scope" position, without looping in the stomach.

creatic duct tends to enter the papilla in a relatively perpendicular fashion at the 3- or 4-o'clock position. In contrast, the bile duct runs towards 11 o'clock from the lower right aspect of the papilla. When the ampulla is difficult to cannulate, a rendezvous technique can be used in which biliary access is achieved by percutaneous transhepatic passage of a guidewire into the common bile duct and the ampulla with fluoroscopy or ultrasound guidance.

Proper radiologic technique is critical to obtaining interpretable radiographs. Artifacts such as air bubbles, streaming and layering of contrast, and contrast spillage into the duodenum should be recognized. With the currently available expertise, the greatest risk posed by ERCP may well be misinterpretation. Indeed, while surgeons are relatively familiar with cholangiograms, pancreatograms remain more difficult to interpret. This task has been facilitated by consensus agreement on the endoscopic classification of chronic pancreatitis (Fig 3–15 and Table 3–4).

If endoscopic sphincterotomy is indicated, the diagnostic cannula is removed over a 0.035-inch guidewire that is deeply inserted into the bile duct. The sphincterotome is then inserted over the indwelling guidewire (Fig 3–16). The sphincterotome consists of a standard cannula containing a continuous wire loop, 2–3 cm of which is exposed near the tip. Sphincterotomy must not be attempted until the sphincterotome has been clearly demonstrated to be within the bile duct and not the pancreatic duct.

Once proper ductal cannulation is verified, the sphincterotome is withdrawn until approximately half of the wire is visible outside of the papilla, pointing toward 11 or 12 o'clock. The wire is then tightened, bowing it against the papillary roof. Current is then applied

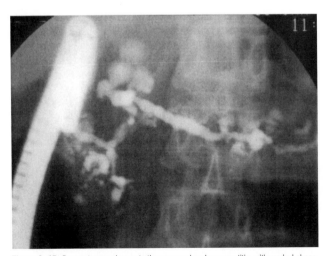

Figure 3–15. Pancreatogram demonstrating severe chronic pancreatitis, with marked abnormality of the main pancreatic duct as well as filling of several large cystic cavities.

TABLE 3–4. CAMBRIDGE CLASSIFICATION OF ENDOSCOPIC PANCREATOGRAPHIC CHANGES IN CHRONIC PANCREATITIS

Terminology	Main Pancreatic Duct	Abnormal Main Pancreatic Duct Branches	Additional Features
Normal	Normal	None	None
Equivocal	Normal	<3	None
Mild	Normal	≥ 3	None
Moderate	Abnormal	≥ 3	None
Severe	Abnormal	≥ 3	One or more of: Large cavity Obstruction Filling defects Severe dilation Irregularity

Adapted from permission, from Fink AS. Endoscopic intervention for pancreatic disorders. In: Hunter JG, Sackier J (eds). *High Tech Surgery: New Approaches to Old Diseases.* New York, NY: McGraw-Hill; 1993:245–254.

in short bursts while maintaining gentle upward force on the wire and gently lifting the sphincterotome, making the incision in small increments. Only a small (e.g., 5-mm) incision is needed to facilitate subsequent therapeutic interventions (e.g., endoprosthesis insertion), while larger incisions are usually made when dealing with choledocholithiasis (based on the size of the largest stone). The maximum incision length should not pass the first transverse duodenal fold.

The most common indications for endoscopic sphincterotomy are choledocholithiasis, sphincter of Oddi dysfunction, acute cholangitis, stent placement, and acute gallstone pancreatitis.

Choledocholithiasis. Retained or recurrent common bile duct stones represent the most common indication for endoscopic sphincterotomy, and ERCP with sphincterotomy successfully treats 95% of these cases. In expert hands, over 90% of bile ducts can be subsequently cleared of calculi with balloon catheters or Dormia baskets, resulting in an overall ductal clearance rate approximating 85%. Stone size is often a limiting factor, as stones greater than 2 cm in diameter often require fragmentation prior to removal.

It is recommended that ductal clearance be attempted at the time of endoscopic sphincterotomy, since relying on spontaneous stone passage increases the risk of cholangitis, pancreatitis, and stone impaction, as well as the need for repeated endoscopic interventions. Adequate ductal drainage must be ensured if all stones cannot be removed. The latter can be accomplished with nasobiliary drainage or endoscopic stent insertion.

Routine preoperative ERCP and sphincterotomy are not warranted in patients undergoing biliary opera-

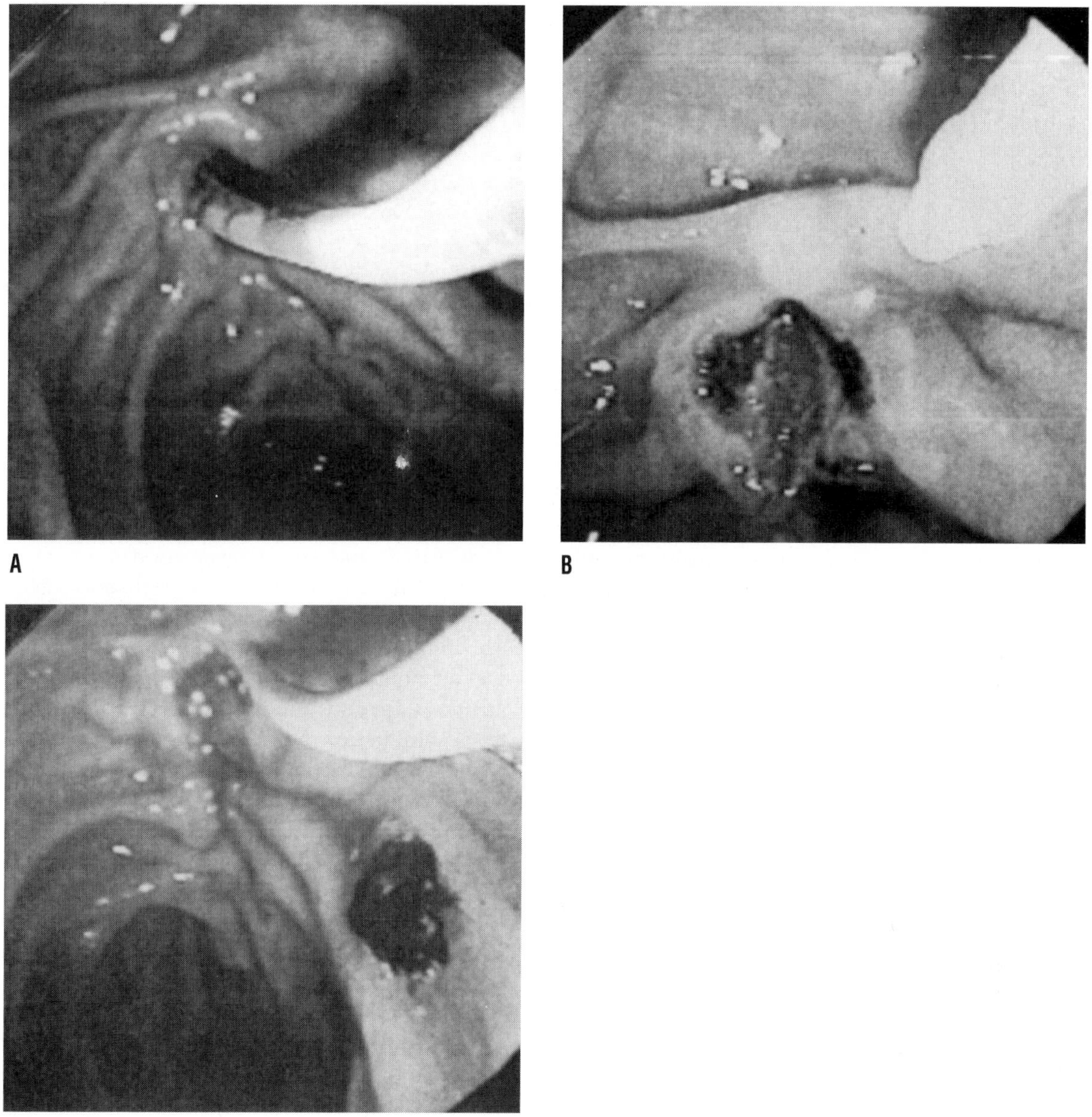

A

B

C

Figure 3–16. A. A sphincterotome has been inserted into the bile duct and is positioned for sphincterotomy. **B.** View of the completed sphincterotomy. Note that the choledochal epithelium is clearly seen. **C.** The bile duct is being swept with a balloon catheter. Note the previously removed common bile duct stone lying in the duodenum.

tions for symptomatic cholelithiasis. Transient rise in liver function tests is not an indication for ERCP. It is often more prudent to follow the liver function tests and clinical signs and symptoms for these patients. ERCP can always be performed after a cholecystectomy if stones are discovered intraoperatively. Over the last two decades, data have evolved to aid surgeons in predicting the probability of common bile duct stones; this information should be utilized in determining the need for performing ERCP for biliary stones (Table 3–5). Other options include use of a choledochoscope or ureteroscope during laparoscopic common bile duct exploration. These scopes can accommodate lithotripsy probes, as well as balloons and baskets for stone extraction.

Sphincter of Oddi Dysfunction. Sphincter of Oddi dysfunction must be entertained in patients with unexplained biliary colic or acute pancreatitis. While multiple noninvasive tests have been evaluated in this disorder (e.g., ultrasonography and scintigraphy), they all appear to lack adequate sensitivity or specificity. The development of endoscopic manometric techniques now allows direct measurement of motility and intraluminal pres-

TABLE 3–5. RISKS OF CHOLEDOCHOLITHIASIS IN DETERMINING THE NEED FOR ENDOSCOPIC RETROGRADE CHOLANGIOPANCREATOGRAPHY

Clinical Diagnosis	Choledocholithiasis	Cholecystitis, Pancreatitis, or Resolving CBD Stones	Cholecystitis, Pancreatitis, or Resolving CBD Stones	Biliary Colic
CBD diameter	≥ 5 mm	≥ 5 mm	< 5 mm	< 5mm
Liver function tests (≥2 categories.)	TB ≥ 1.5 Alk phos ≥ 150 AST≥ 100 ALT ≥ 100	TB ≥ 1.5 Alk phos ≥ 150 AST ≥ 100 ALT ≥ 100	TB ≥ 1.5 Alk phos ≥ 150 AST ≥ 100 ALT ≥ 100	TB <1.5 Alk phos <150 AST <100 ALT <100
Risk of CBD stones	93%	32%	4%	1%

Alk phos, alkaline phosphatase; AST< aspartate aminotransferase; ALT, alanine aminotransferase; CBD, common bile duct; TB, total bilirubin.

Adapted, with permission, from Liu et al. Patient evaluation and management with selective use of magnetic resonance cholangiography and endoscopic retrograde cholangiopancreatography before laparoscopic cholecystectomy. *Ann Surg* 2001;234:33–40.

sures within both the biliary and pancreatic segments of the sphincter of Oddi.

Symptoms of biliary colic, elevated liver function tests, dilated common bile duct (>12 mm), and delayed biliary drainage (>45 min) are most consistent with sphincter of Oddi dysfunction, and manometry is generally not warranted. The common thread in patients with this disorder is elevated basal sphincter pressure. Criteria for abnormal manometry include basal pressure >40 mm Hg, peak sphincter pressure >240 mm Hg, >50% retrograde contractions, no relaxation with cholecystokinin administration, and contraction waves >8 per minute. Sphincter of Oddi manometry is technically challenging to perform and relatively few centers perform it routinely. Pancreatitis is the most common complication following sphincter manometry studies.

Acute Cholangitis. Urgent endoscopic intervention has now been clearly shown to be the procedure of choice for patients with acute suppurative cholangitis. In these patients it is especially prudent to aspirate bile before performing cholangiography. The latter, in turn, should be performed with minimal contrast injection. After abnormalities have been identified, sphincterotomy and stone extraction can be attempted in stable patients. In critically ill patients, simple nasobiliary drainage or stenting without sphincterotomy should be performed, reserving sphincterotomy and duct clearance to a later session when the patient is more stable. Alternatively, percutaneous transhepatic biliary drainage by the interventional radiologist can be an excellent method of decompressing the biliary tree, which is the primary goal in treating acute cholangitis. One significant advantage to the radiologic approach is being able to perform the procedure with the critically ill patient in the supine position. Morbidity and mortality can be significantly reduced when the obstructing stone is removed once the patient is stable.

Acute Gallstone Pancreatitis. Most patients with biliary pancreatitis can be managed conservatively. Following improvement, laparoscopic cholecystectomy should be performed prior to discharge. In carefully selected patients, urgent endoscopic sphincterotomy for acute gallstone pancreatitis may be performed safely. Indeed, early ERCP and sphincterotomy for severe gallstone pancreatitis can significantly reduce morbidity and mortality. Therefore, if experienced endoscopic support is available, urgent ERCP and sphincterotomy should be considered for patients with severe disease and definite gallstones, especially if clinical deterioration continues or rapid resolution fails to occur. Urgent ERCP should also be considered in patients with severe disease but equivocal radiological studies, in whom the presence of gallstones is still suspected based on biochemical criteria.

Endoprosthesis Insertion. Currently available endoprostheses vary in their composition, shape, size, length, and method of anchorage. The small-caliber (6–7F) pig-tailed endoprostheses initially used were associated with a high incidence of early occlusion from sludge, resulting in recurrent jaundice and/or cholangitis. Subsequent improvements led to development of straight 10 and 11.5F endoprostheses with side flaps for retention, as well as self-expandable metal stents. The larger-caliber stents (10F or greater) provide best functional results.

The large-caliber plastic stents are inserted using a three-layer technique (Fig 3–17). Initially, a diagnostic cholangiogram or pancreatogram is obtained to identify the lesion's extent and to determine the length of endoprosthesis required. If desired, a small sphincterotomy can then be performed to facilitate subsequent manipulations; this maneuver is often unnecessary. An atraumatic guidewire and an overlying Teflon catheter are then passed well up the desired duct, passing any stricture. Various independent manipulations of the guidewire and catheter may be required to obtain the desired position. Once these accessories are in the proper location, the endoprosthesis is pushed into place

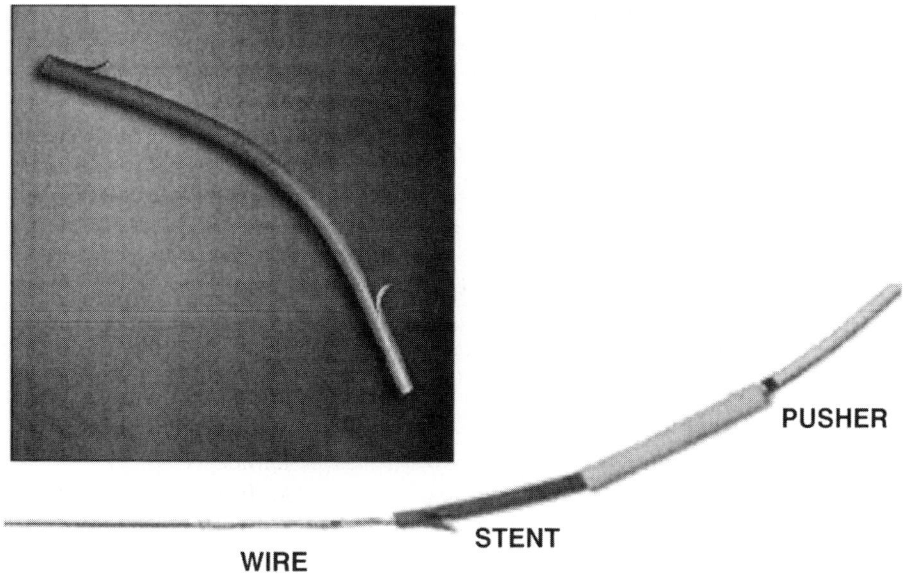

Figure 3–17. Biliary stent with flaps at each end for anchoring (Wilson-Cook, Inc, Winston-Salem, NC). The stent is loaded over a guidewire and pushed into position in the standard three-layer technique.

using a pusher tube. Ideally, the endoprosthesis will be located with its upper flap above the stricture and its lower flap just outside the papilla.

A special delivery system is used to insert self-expanding metal stents in a collapsed state (9F diameter). After release, the stent shortens in length and expands to 8–10 mm diameter (30F). Self-expanding stents appear to be significantly less prone to sludge occlusion, and are therefore longer-lived than straight plastic stents. Despite their longer patency, these stents become unremovable after a few days due to resultant tissue reaction and fibrosis. Indeed, some stents become completely incorporated into the bile duct wall. Furthermore, these stents can be plagued by tumor ingrowth, which is usually treated by subsequent insertion of a plastic stent through the metal stent.

Biliary endoprostheses have been utilized for multiple indications and the technical feasibility depends on the location of the disease. Malignant strictures below the bifurcation (Fig 3–18) can be successfully stented in as many as 90% of cases, with acceptable morbidity and mortality rates, approximating 2–5% each. Success rates decline steeply as the stricture's location climbs above the bifurcation. Lesions at the hilum or above may require insertion of more than one endoprosthesis.

In addition to malignant obstruction, endoscopically-inserted endoprostheses have been utilized increasingly in treating benign biliary disorders, including strictures. Most benign strictures or bile duct leaks are the result of penetrating or operative trauma, and endoprostheses have been successful in managing the majority of these patients. However, if these stents are placed long-term, frequent obstruction and cholangitis are commonly encountered, requiring additional intervention. Most of the stents have patency duration of 3–6 months. In patients whose injuries do not respond to short-term stent placement, definitive surgical reconstruction should be considered.

Similar endoscopic maneuvers have proven useful in other benign biliary conditions including sclerosing cholangitis, choledochoceles, and complications following orthotopic liver transplantation. Several preliminary reports even describe endoscopic access to the gallbladder via the cystic duct, allowing diagnosis and treatment of gallbladder disorders.

In addition to biliary disorders, ERCP has been employed in the management of benign pancreatic disorders. Pancreatic duct stenting can be used successfully to decompress the ductal system, bypass ductal leaks and strictures, and to treat pancreatic fistulas. Patients with pancreatic divisum may be treated with minor papilla stenting or sphincterotomy. Pancreatic stents are smaller than biliary stents and they contain side holes for drainage.

ERCP for pancreatic ductal stone extraction is technically difficult. Some clinicians have reported success with the use of contact lithotripsy and/or extracorporeal shock wave lithotripsy to manage pancreaticolithiasis. Such patients may be better served with surgical pancreaticojejunal drainage or partial pancreatectomy.

Pancreatic pseudocysts have also been approached endoscopically. When cysts are in communication with the main pancreatic duct, stent placement can sometimes facilitate cyst drainage. In patients with pseudocysts that lie immediately posterior to the stomach, stents can be passed from the stomach into the pseudocyst endoscopically. However, these stents often

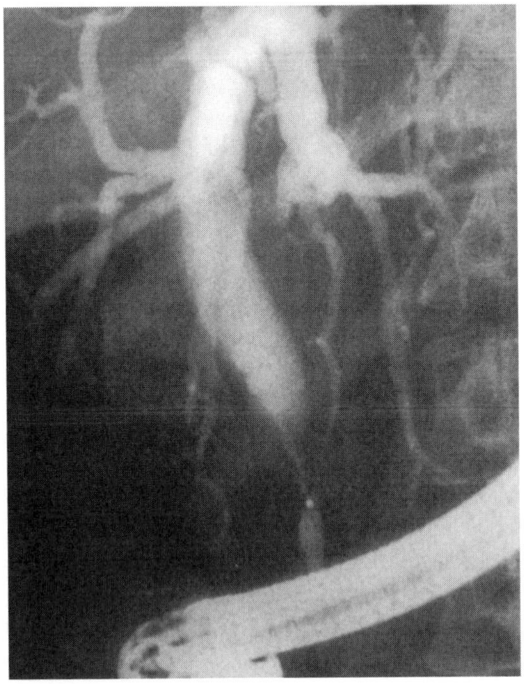

A

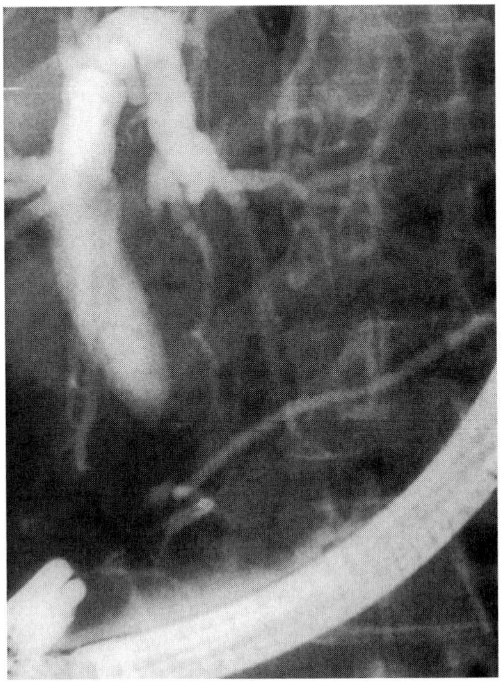

B

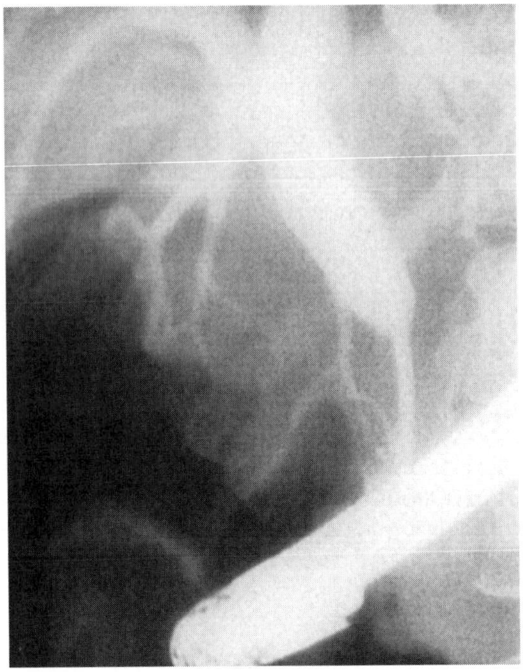

C

Figure 3–18. A. Endoscopic cholangiogram demonstrating high-grade distal common bile duct obstruction consistent with cholangiocarcinoma or pancreatic carcinoma. **B.** On a subsequent injection, the pancreatic duct is visualized and found to be normal, confirming the diagnosis of cholangiocarcinoma. **C.** An endoprosthesis is being inserted into the bile duct to relieve the obstructive jaundice.

become occluded by debris and pseudocysts that were once sterile are now contaminated by gut flora. With minimally invasive transluminal surgery on the horizon, the role of transluminal stent placement for pancreatic pseudocysts will require reappraisal.

Palliation of unresectable malignant biliary obstruction in elderly high-risk patients appears to be one of the most significant indications for biliary endoprostheses. In these circumstances, endoscopically inserted stents are superior to percutaneous stents and at least as good—and possibly better than—biliary enteric bypass. Furthermore, endoscopic intervention is less expensive, requires a shorter hospital stay, and incurs less patient discomfort. These results are discounted somewhat by the subsequent need to replace occluded stents or to bypass duodenal obstruction in those patients (approximately 10–15%) who survive long enough to develop these complications.

COMPLICATIONS

The complications uniquely associated with pancreaticobiliary cannulation are most notably pancreatitis and sepsis. Post-ERCP pancreatitis is associated with multiple forceful pancreatic duct injections, usually while struggling during a difficult bile duct cannulation. While the reported incidence of this complication is definition-dependent, it probably occurs in no more than 2–3% of cases. Although most cases are mild, severe life-threatening pancreatitis can occur. When intervention is performed with ERCP, the rate of pancreatitis obviously rises. Despite numerous trials, there remains no definitive evidence supporting prophylactic administration of somatostatin or enzyme inhibitors.

Bacteremia and sepsis can be documented in 15% of patients undergoing diagnostic ERCP, and is the most common cause of death following this procedure. The risk of cholangitis or sepsis is particularly increased following attempted endoscopic therapy in the presence of infected bile. Sepsis is also more common with malignant obstruction than with strictures. Protocols that may reduce post-ERCP sepsis include antibiotic administration until the biliary tree is completely decompressed, minimizing contrast injection volume and pressure, and ensuring adequate drainage at the procedure's completion, preferably at the same time as sphincterotomy, stone extraction, and/or endoprosthesis placement.

Following endoscopic sphincterotomy, serious complications can occur and may require surgical intervention. These complications include hemorrhage, perforation, cholangitis, and pancreatitis. Complications occur in 5–6% following endoscopic sphincterotomy and death occurs in 1%. Approximately 75–80% of complications can be managed without surgery.

Hemorrhage is the most common complication seen after endoscopic sphincterotomy and can be avoided by slow, controlled incisions. Epinephrine injection or balloon tamponade may be useful if endoscopic vision is not obscured by the bleeding. If surgical intervention is necessary, it is probably best to include ligation of the feeding vessel. Alternatively, interventional radiology may be employed to embolize the bleeding vessel.

Perforation is the least common complication, and usually requires surgical intervention. The diagnosis is usually made upon discovering air or contrast in the retroperitoneal space. CT scan may also be helpful if differentiation from post-sphincterotomy pancreatitis proves difficult. If diagnosed early and the bile duct has been cleared, many patients can be managed with nasobiliary decompression, nasogastric suction, and intravenous antibiotics.

Pancreatitis and cholangitis can also follow endoscopic sphincterotomy. The former may be decreased by minimizing trauma during cannulation and avoiding coagulation near the pancreatic duct. Cholangitis should be extremely uncommon if adequate biliary drainage has been achieved.

Stent occlusion is inevitable and is usually heralded by recurrent cholangitis unless stents are routinely changed before the onset of sepsis (e.g., every 3 months). Most cases of endoprosthesis occlusion can be successfully treated with antibiotics and stent replacement.

▪ SMALL BOWEL ENTEROSCOPY

The third portion of the duodenum can be reached during standard upper gastrointestinal endoscopy and the most distal ileum can be accessed via the ileocecal valve during colonoscopy. If necessary, the distal duodenum and very proximal jejunum can be reached by oral passage of a long (160-cm) colonoscope. However, this approach is technically demanding and may inflict moderate patient discomfort.

Obscure gastrointestinal bleeding, accounting for less than 5% of gastrointestinal bleeding, is the most frequent indication for small bowel endoscopy. The latter is best performed at laparotomy, since nonoperative "push" endoscopy utilizing long endoscopes will make a diagnosis in only 50% of patients.

For intraoperative enteroscopy, a long colonoscope is inserted per os or per anus. The endoscope is then advanced down from the duodenum or up from the colon into the small bowel. This is performed under endoscopic vision, taking care to minimize air insufflation. The surgeon guides the endoscope tip, telescoping the bowel over the endoscope and applying pressure to reduce loops in the stomach or colon. Intraoperative endoscopy has also been recommended for other indications including selection of the appropriate extent of intestinal resection. One of the most difficult challenges following a long procedure involving small bowel enteroscopy is the significant bowel distention that results, making abdominal fascia closure difficult if not impossible without a mesh.

Although intraoperative enteroscopy is considered the gold standard for endoscopic evaluation of the small bowel, nonsurgical endoscopic alternatives have been proposed. The Sonde flexible endoscope, a very long endoscope with no tip deflection capabilities, is passed down into the small bowel by passive peristalsis. Interest in this technology is more of historical interest than a practical one. Of more current interest, capsule or pill endoscopy has become a substitute for small bowel endoscopy. In this technique, after swallowing the capsule, 50,000 images are digitally recorded over an 8-hour period as the pill traverses distally into the small bowel. Capsule endoscopy does not require endoscopic skills but relies on interpretation and estimation of where pathology exists. Reported sensitivity and specificity of capsule endoscopy spans a wide range, but most studies report 50–60% yield for detecting recent bleeding sites and far lower yield rates for remote bleeding. Capsule endoscopy is perhaps more appropriate for diagnosing inflammatory bowel disease. When the capsule does not pass into the rectum, surgical retrieval is necessary.

In 2000, double-balloon endoscopy (DBE) was introduced as a means of examining the entire small bowel (Fig 3–19). The system consists of a thin endoscope with an 8.5-mm diameter and 200-cm working length, and a 145-cm soft overtube with an outer diameter of 12.2 mm. A soft latex balloon attached to the tip of the endoscope can be inflated or deflated with a mechanical pump. The soft overtube also has a balloon at the tip that can be inflated or deflated. The role of the mechanical pump is to tightly regulate the pressure of the balloon, so as to distribute consistent force against the bowel wall. There is also a newer therapeutic scope with a wider diameter and a 2.8-mm working channel.

The DBE endoscope is inserted into the duodenum and the balloon is inflated. The overtube, which has previously been loaded on the endoscope, is then advanced into the duodenum and the overtube balloon is inflated to anchor the small bowel. The endoscope's balloon is deflated and advanced further to a distal location, followed by balloon reinflation. The overtube balloon is deflated and advanced to the level of the endoscope tip. Gentle simultaneous withdrawal of the scope and the overtube will telescope the small bowel onto the overtube. This sequence is repeated several times until the small bowel examination is completed. This procedure can also be performed in retrograde fashion from the colon into the small bowel (Fig 3–20).

While DBE holds tremendous diagnostic and therapeutic promise, it is labor intensive and may take 1–3 hours to complete. As anticipated, it may be associated with significant discomfort for the patient. Some endoscopists have even performed the procedure under general anesthesia and with fluoroscopic guidance. DBE may prove to be particularly helpful in patients who have altered small bowel anatomy (e.g., patients who require ERCP following Roux-en-Y gastric bypass) or in patients with redundant or tortuous colon who have failed previous attempts at colonoscopy.

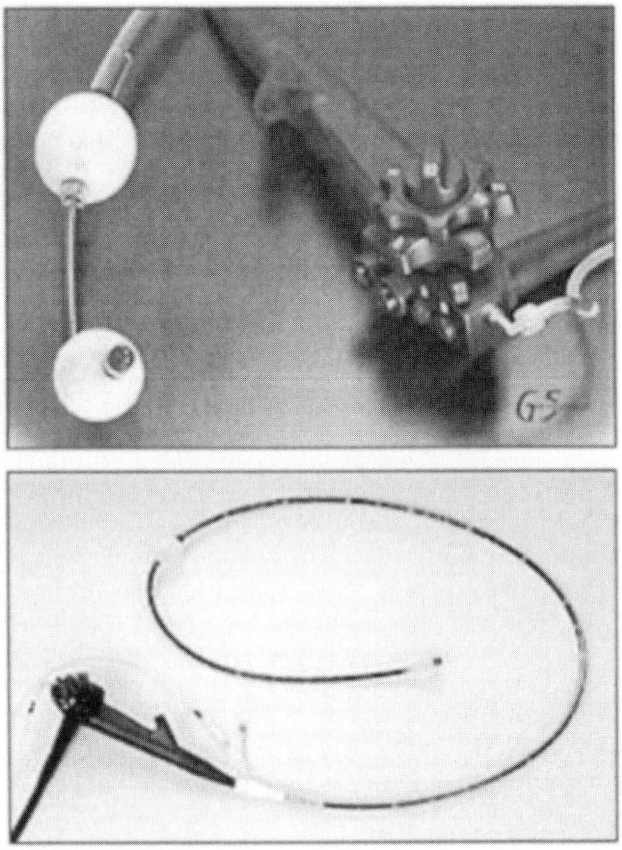

Figure 3–19. The double-balloon endoscopy (DBE) system places a 200-cm endoscope within a soft overtube. Both the soft overtube and the endoscope have a pressure-controlled inflatable balloon that is used to telescope the small bowel during examination. (Courtesy of Fujinon Inc., Wayne, NJ.)

▪ ENDOSCOPY OF THE LOWER GASTROINTESTINAL TRACT

INDICATIONS

This section will focus on flexible sigmoidoscopy and colonoscopy, which constitute the majority of lower gastrointestinal endoscopic procedures. While multiple indications are listed for flexible sigmoidoscopy (Table 3–6), the majority of examinations are performed to screen for rectosigmoid neoplasia in asymptomatic patients. Originally, the American Cancer Society, the National Cancer Institute, and the American College of Physicians all recommended that every person over 50

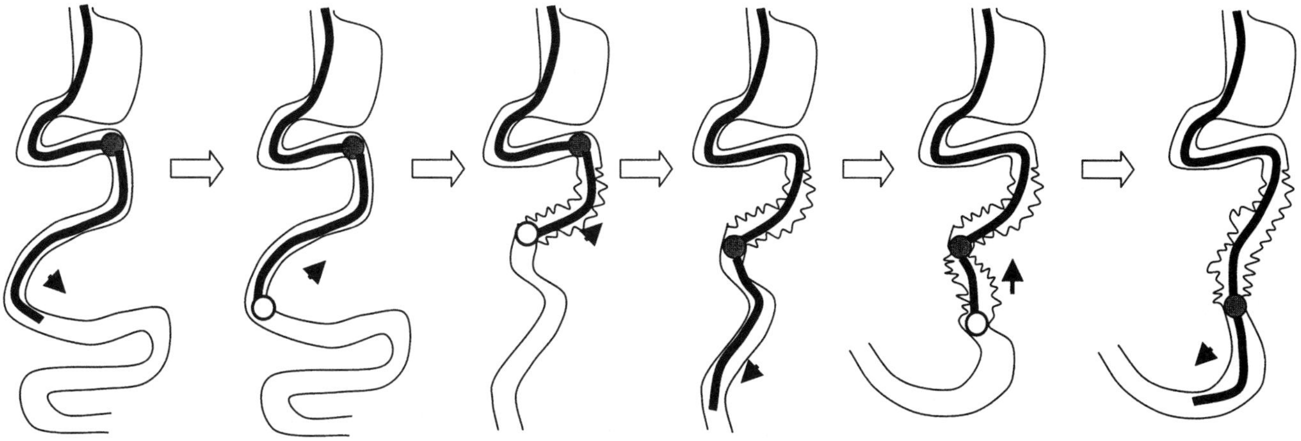

Figure 3–20. Schematic depicting antegrade insertion of the double-balloon endoscope. The overtube balloon (*dark balloon*) anchors the proximal small bowel. The endoscope is advanced to a point and its balloon inflated. This is followed by withdrawal of the endoscope with the inflated balloon to the previous site anchored by the overtube balloon. The bowel is anchored again by deflating and re-inflating the overtube's balloon. The same maneuver is repeated until the examination is completed. A similar technique can be used for redundant colon examination as well as for retrograde insertion into the distal small bowel.

years of age should undergo annual fecal occult blood tests and screening flexible sigmoidoscopy at 3- to 5-year intervals. However, sigmoidoscopy screening cannot define the status of the proximal colon. Proximal lesions found without associated rectosigmoid lesions occur in 20–50% of cases. Thus the role of flexible sigmoidoscopy in screening for colorectal neoplasia remains unclear. However, for the examination of known distal colorectal disease or for follow-up examination of the distal colon, flexible sigmoidoscopy—which can easily be performed in the office without sedation—is ideal.

Other indications for flexible sigmoidoscopy include hematochezia and bloody diarrhea. In the former circumstance, etiologies are most frequently discovered if the procedure is performed soon after passage of the bright red bloody stool. The proximal colon does not need to be examined if a fissure or hemorrhoid is discovered in association with fresh blood in the perianal area. When evaluating bloody diarrhea, flexible sigmoidoscopy may reveal characteristic findings of viral colitis in immunocompromised patients or pseudomembranous colitis in patients who have recently received antibiotics. In practice, flexible sigmoidoscopy is easily performed using a regular colonoscope, and if more proximal disease is suspected, the scope is simply advanced.

Table 3–7 describes the indications for colonoscopy. While surgical societies (SAGES and ASCRS) tend to be more aggressive in their recommendations for screening or surveillance colonoscopies than medical gastroenterology societies, particularly in patients who have had previous cancer or polyps, there are no scientific data to promote one society's recommendations over another (Table 3–8).

TABLE 3–6. INDICATIONS FOR FLEXIBLE SIGMOIDOSCOPY

DIAGNOSTIC
1. Polyp or cancer screening with fecal occult blood testing
2. When colonoscopy is not indicated
3. Polyp/cancer surveillance in between scheduled colonoscopies
4. Evaluate radiologic findings of the distal colon and rectum
5. Follow-up examination for inflammatory bowel disease
6. Inspect distal colonic anastomosis
7. Evaluate strictures for malignancy

THERAPEUTIC
1. Detorsion of sigmoid volvulus
2. Remove foreign body
3. Distal stricture management

Adapted, with permission, from the American Society of Colon and Rectal Surgeons and Society of American Gastrointestinal and Endoscopic Surgeons guidelines, 2004.

TABLE 3–7. INDICATIONS FOR COLONOSCOPY

DIAGNOSTIC
1. Evaluate and confirm radiographic findings
2. Polyps
3. Unexplained GI bleeding or iron deficiency anemia
4. Colon cancer screening
5. Follow-up after intervention for polyp or cancer
6. Inflammatory bowel disease
7. Significant diarrhea
8. Intraoperative localization of lesions

THERAPEUTIC
1. Control bleeding
2. Polypectomy
3. Remove foreign body
4. Reduce sigmoid volvulus
5. Decompress pseudo-obstruction (Ogilvie's)
6. Dilate or stent strictures (malignant and benign)

Adapted, with permission, from the Society of American Gastrointestinal and Endoscopic Surgeons guidelines, www.colonoscopy.info, 2002; and the American Society of Colon and Rectal Surgeons parameters, 2004.

TABLE 3–8. COMPARATIVE RECOMMENDATIONS FOR SURVEILLANCE COLONOSCOPY FOLLOWING POLYPECTOMY

Polyp Type	Gastroenterology Consortium (1997)	ASGE (1997)	American Cancer Society (1997)	ASCRS (1999)	SAGES (1997)
Hyperplastic polyp	NR	NRM	NRM	NR	NRM
Single adenoma (<1 cm)	NRM	q3–5 years	q3 years, then regular schedule	q3–5 years	q3–5 years
Single adenoma (≥ 1 cm)	q3 years, then q5 years	q3 years	q3 years, then q5 years	q1 year, then q5 years	q3–5 years
Multiple adenomas (≥ 2 cm)	q3 years	q3 years, then q5 years	q3 years, then q5 years	q1 years, then q5 years	q3–5 years

ASGE, American Society for Gastrointestinal Endoscopy; ASCRS, American Society of Colon and Rectal surgeons; SAGES, Society of American Gastrointestinal Endoscopic Surgeons; NR, not recommended; NRM, no recommendations made.
Adapted, with permission, from Mysliwiec PA et al. Are physicians doing too much colonoscopy? A national survey of colorectal surveillance after polypectomy. *Ann Intern Med* 2004;141:264–271.

The high accuracy and therapeutic potential of colonoscopy render it superior to flexible sigmoidoscopy and barium enema. Due to cost issues, however, the latter combination is frequently recommended in lieu of colonoscopy, even in high-risk patients.

Both ulcerative colitis and Crohn's disease of the colon are high-risk conditions for colorectal cancer. Colorectal cancer screening should begin 8–10 years after the onset of colitis with multiple biopsies taken every 10 cm, resulting in 30–40 biopsy specimens per examination.

Finally, surveillance is indicated following polypectomy or resection of colon cancer. Current recommendations suggest that patients with single or only a few adenomas should have colonoscopy within 3 years after polypectomy. After one negative 3-year follow-up examination, subsequent colonoscopy can be repeated at 5-year intervals. Follow-up endoscopies may be necessary at 1 and 4 years in those patients with multiple polyps or suboptimal initial clearing examination. Following resection of colorectal carcinoma, similar surveillance regimens have been proposed, with an initial clearing examination 1 year after resection.

PATIENT PREPARATION

Most endoscopic evaluations of the lower gastrointestinal tract can be done as outpatient procedures. For flexible sigmoidoscopy of the non-strictured colon, limited preparation is needed. This can usually be accomplished by administration of one or two phosphate enemas 20–30 minutes before the examination; no dietary restrictions are required. If the procedure is performed promptly, the colon is usually clean up to the level of the transverse colon or even the hepatic flexure in young patients. In the presence of severe diverticular or other narrowing, antispasmodics may be required during enema administration. Alternatively, the patient may be prepared with oral lavage.

For colonoscopy, all iron-containing medications should be stopped at least 3 days prior to the procedure since these compounds produce a dark, sticky stool which interferes with inspection and is difficult to clear. The patient should begin a light diet (preferably clear liquids) the day before the examination.

The most common bowel preparation for colonoscopy utilizes a sodium sulfate–based electrolyte solution containing polyethylene glycol as an osmotic agent (e.g., GoLYTELY). Patients often do not like the taste and the volume required (close to 4 L). Fleet Phospho-soda is an alternative that is better tolerated, particularly in the newly introduced tablet form (Visicol). However, the latter oral regimens must be accompanied by adequate fluid intake to facilitate colonic lavage.

While transient bacteremia occurs during colonoscopy, prophylactic antibiotics are usually not required. Exceptions to this include patients with mechanical heart valves, mitral valve prolapse, and vascular grafts.

DIAGNOSTIC AND THERAPEUTIC TECHNIQUES

Flexible Colonoscopy

There are several general principles that should be remembered whenever performing flexible sigmoidoscopy or colonoscopy. These include: (1) insufflate as little as possible and aspirate excess air; (2) push as little as possible so as to avoid unnecessary loops; (3) withdraw the endoscope frequently in order to shorten the colon; (4) correlate the shaft length inserted with the anticipated location (e.g., 50 cm should be at the splenic flexure); and (5) respond to patient discomfort, which usually indicates excessive looping or insufflation.

Endoscopic examination of the lower gastrointestinal tract should always be preceded by digital rectal examination. This procedure both lubricates the anus and relaxes the anal sphincters. Thereafter, having verified that all functions (especially air insufflation) are working properly, the endoscope is introduced either by pressing it sideways into the rectum until the sphincter relaxes or by pushing the tip alongside the forefinger as the latter is withdrawn.

Only limited maneuvers of the endoscope are possible during a colonoscopy, which include insertion, withdrawal, or twisting (with or without tip deflection). In addition, the patient's abdomen can be compressed or the position can be changed. Empirical trials of various manipulations are often necessary to maximize insertion.

The initial view obtained usually reveals a "red-out." This is remedied by withdrawing the scope and insufflating air until the lumen is visualized. The endoscope is then progressively advanced into the bowel until the maximum desired insertion is achieved. Various combined manipulations usually allow the endoscope to be advanced well into the descending colon, and occasionally beyond the splenic flexure. Clockwise torque may prove helpful in passing the sigmoid–descending colon junction. Occasionally it is helpful to have an assistant advance and withdraw the colonoscope (Fig 3–21).

Upon reaching the splenic flexure, the colonoscope should be straightened (usually by withdrawal combined with torque) prior to continued insertion. This not only increases the endoscope's mechanical efficiency, but also facilitates deeper insertion. Again, combined manipulations are utilized until the splenic flexure is passed and the transverse colon is entered. External pressure on the sigmoid loop by an assistant may be needed to enter the transverse colon. The scope deflection should be reduced to less than 90° as it is advanced past the splenic flexure. The transverse colon is then passed, usually with little difficulty; repeated in-and-out maneuvers as well as external pressure are occasionally required to telescope a redundant transverse colon.

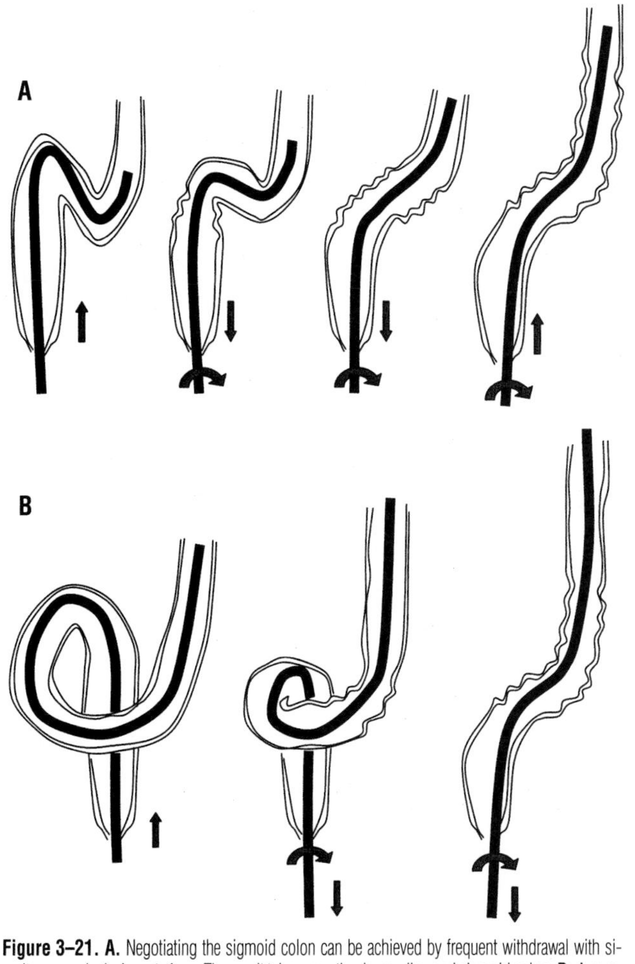

Figure 3–21. A. Negotiating the sigmoid colon can be achieved by frequent withdrawal with simultaneous clockwise rotations. The result telescopes the descending and sigmoid colon. **B.** A common approach for straightening a sigmoid "alpha" loop is to narrow the radius of the loop by withdrawing the scope and providing clockwise rotation. When the loop is straightened, the scope usually pushes forward.

Trials of various combined maneuvers are usually required to pass the hepatic flexure into the ascending colon. Deflation, withdrawal, external pressure, and change of the patient's position may all prove useful. Once the ascending colon is intubated, one should not conclude that insertion is complete until the ileocecal valve or the appendiceal orifice is identified. Transillumination or palpation in the right iliac fossa may be used, but this is not always accurate. The terminal ileum can be intubated by deflecting the tip towards the ileocecal valve, gently withdrawing the scope, and prying open the upper lip of the valve. Throughout this maneuver, air insufflation is used.

During colonoscopy, intubation of the cecum is the usual goal; photodocumentation of the landmarks (crow's feet appearance of the tenia confluence, appendiceal orifice, and/or the ileocecal valve) is important. Withdrawal of the colonoscope is as important, if not more important, than insertion because a careful mucosal examination is best performed at this time. Patients may be turned from the left lateral decubitus position into the prone position in order to gain a different perspective of the colon. When the colonoscope is 20 cm from the anal verge, a retroflexed view within the rectal vault is important to document anorectal disease not seen on insertion. Again, photodocumentation of this critical landmark is recommended.

Hemostasis

Patients with lower gastrointestinal bleeding present with chronic bleeding, recent severe bleeding, or active bleeding. Chronic bleeding is associated with a history of melena, hematochezia, or blood-streaked stools; alternatively, the patient is found to have occult fecal blood, with or without anemia. Flexible endoscopy will diagnose the source of bleeding in most of these patients. Although sigmoidoscopy will often identify the cause, the remaining colon usually needs to be examined, either radiologically or endoscopically. Therefore, it may be desirable to proceed directly to colonoscopy, especially if colonic neoplasm is a significant risk. If colonoscopy is negative in this setting, many would recommend upper gastrointestinal endoscopy.

Colonoscopy is indicated in the patient with recent severe, but currently inactive, bleeding. The patient should be adequately resuscitated, coagulation parameters should be corrected, and the colon should be prepared. During colonoscopy stigmata of recent hemorrhage are sought, including active bleeding, adherent clot in a single diverticulum or on an ulcerative lesion, or a nonbleeding visible vessel in an ulcer. If the site of bleeding is found, it may be directly treated using the same techniques as described for the upper gastrointestinal tract.

Examination of active severe lower gastrointestinal bleeding usually requires urgent lavage followed by colonoscopy. This approach will frequently identify angiodysplasia as the source of hemorrhage. Caution is appropriate when using thermal techniques (mono- or bipolar electrocautery, heated probe, or laser) to treat angiodysplasias, since they tend to occur in the thin-walled proximal colon.

Polypectomy

Most colonic polyps are asymptomatic and are usually discovered on screening or diagnostic barium radiographs or endoscopic examinations. While colonic polyps can ulcerate and bleed, or rarely cause partial bowel obstruction, neoplastic polyps (adenomas) are of clinical concern due to their malignant potential. Nonneoplastic polyps (hyperplastic, hamartomas, lymphoid aggregates, and inflammatory polyps) have no malignant potential and only need to be distinguished from their neoplastic counterparts.

Adenomas occur in a variety of shapes, sizes, and histologic patterns. Polyps are described as pedunculated or sessile, depending on whether they contain a discrete stalk. According to the World Health Organization, neoplastic polyps can be classified as tubular (<25% villous tissue), tubulovillous (25–75% villous tissue), or villous adenomas (>75% villous tissue). Tubular adenomas are the most common (80%), while tubulovillous (15%) and villous adenomas (5%) are much less frequently encountered. Some degree of dysplasia occurs in all polyps and is reported as low-grade or high-grade (severe). Increasing dysplasia correlates with increasing adenoma size, extent of villous component, and patient age. The risk of invasive cancer also increases with increasing polyp size.

Although most polyps larger than 1 cm can be detected by double, but not single, contrast barium enema, colonoscopy offers the advantage of biopsy and removal of most of these lesions with minimal morbidity (1–2%) and virtually no mortality. In many instances polypectomy, which ensures no residual disease, is the definitive treatment for early colon cancer and is therefore a life-saving procedure. Such patients should have repeat surveillance colonoscopy within 1 year.

Options for managing polyps include hot biopsy, electrocoagulation, and excision. Regular biopsy forceps should not be used since they will leave residual adenomatous fragments which can lead to polyp recurrence. In contrast, hot biopsy will conduct thermal energy to the polyp base, destroying any remaining polypoid tissue. Hot biopsy should not be used on lesions larger than 6 mm, since excessive thermal energy is required. Additional caution should also be used when delivering thermal energy to the proximal colon with its thinner wall. Ulcerated, indurated sessile lesions may be malignant and are best removed surgically.

Polypectomy technique has become reasonably standardized (Fig 3–22), such that most pedunculated polyps can be removed endoscopically in one piece. If safe, most polyps should be removed when visualized, since they may not be as easily located upon withdrawing the endoscope. However, the priority should be to complete the colonoscopic examination. Most polyps over 1 cm in diameter can usually be easily visualized, allowing polypectomy to be deferred until instrument withdrawal. Polypectomy can be performed at a different session when more time can be dedicated to eradicating the polyps from the colon.

Typically, a snare is placed around the head of the polyp and then maneuvered down the stalk, taking care to place the catheter tip at the desired transection site. When the snare is in proper position, the polyp is transected by progressively closing the snare while applying continuous coagulation current. Sessile polyps less than 2 cm in diameter can usually be removed in one piece. The snare is placed around the polyp with the wire directly on the mucosa. The snare is then closed as the polyp is lifted, entrapping the mucosa and minimal submucosa, creating a "pseudostalk." Electrocautery is then applied while the polyp is continuously lifted away from the colonic wall. Larger polyps may require piecemeal removal in 1- to 1.5-cm segments. Following successful endoscopic resection of a large sessile polyp, follow-up colonoscopy should be done in 3–6 months to verify completeness of the resection. Extremely large polyps may require more than one endoscopic session or an operation for complete removal. Injection of saline (up to 30–40 mL) below the mucosa of a polyp can also be used to elevate the polyp for endoscopic snaring.

It is important to constantly move the polyp during excision so as to avoid conducting current into, and thus injuring, the opposite colonic wall. It is also important to retrieve resected polyps for pathological examination. While some small polyps can be suctioned into a specimen trap,

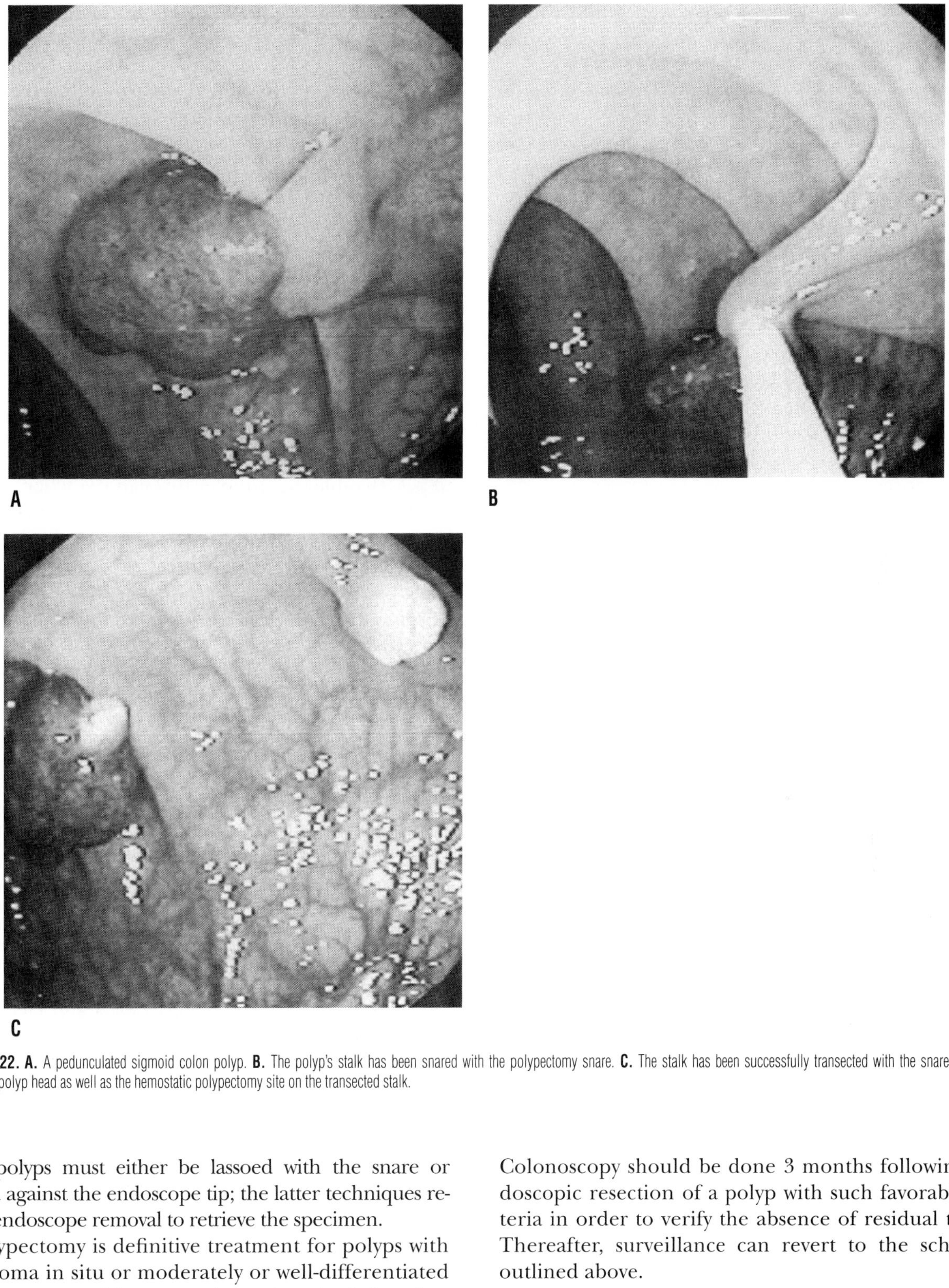

Figure 3–22. A. A pedunculated sigmoid colon polyp. **B.** The polyp's stalk has been snared with the polypectomy snare. **C.** The stalk has been successfully transected with the snare. Note the transected polyp head as well as the hemostatic polypectomy site on the transected stalk.

large polyps must either be lassoed with the snare or sucked against the endoscope tip; the latter techniques require endoscope removal to retrieve the specimen.

Polypectomy is definitive treatment for polyps with carcinoma in situ or moderately or well-differentiated invasive cancer without vascular or lymphatic invasion in which the cancer is removed from the excisional margin. Assuming acceptable surgical risk, colectomy is usually indicated following endoscopic resection of malignant polyps that do not meet these criteria. Colonoscopy should be done 3 months following endoscopic resection of a polyp with such favorable criteria in order to verify the absence of residual tissue. Thereafter, surveillance can revert to the schedule outlined above.

Colonic Decompression

Acute pseudo-obstruction of the colon was first described by Ogilvie in 1948. This syndrome is characterized by acute massive dilation of the cecum and right colon without organic obstruction. If untreated, the distension can lead to perforation, peritonitis, and death.

Conservative treatment is indicated in patients with cecal diameters less than 9–10 cm, since the risk of perforation is minimal. Nothing should be given by mouth, and nasogastric suction should be initiated; gentle enemas and insertion of a rectal tube may also prove beneficial, as may change of the patient's position if possible. Fluid and electrolyte abnormalities should be corrected, narcotics should be stopped, and any infections or associated conditions treated as soon as possible. Serial abdominal examinations and repeat abdominal radiographs should be performed every 12–24 hours. If the cecal diameter continues to increase and exceeds 12 or 13 cm, or if there is no improvement in 48–72 hours, the colon should be decompressed or neostigmine therapy considered.

Decompression can be a tedious procedure, requiring patience and experience. Air insufflation should be kept to a minimum or turned off completely. Frequent irrigation through the suction channel may be necessary to clear the channel and maintain visibility. Although the cecum is the optimal endpoint, successful decompression has been achieved with passage to the hepatic flexure. The colonic lumen should be collapsed by applying intermittent suction as the endoscope is withdrawn. If desired, a decompressive tube can be left in the ascending colon. Colonoscopy will prove successful in 80–85% of patients with Ogilvie's syndrome. However, if a second decompression is required, 40% of these patients will experience yet another recurrence of colonic dilation. Bloody colonic contents or dark-blue or black mucosa suggests ischemia or necrosis; these findings are indications for surgery.

Colonic volvulus is common in elderly institutionalized patients and is another potential indication for colonoscopic decompression. Colonoscopic decompression of a sigmoid volvulus can be a useful temporizing measure, allowing the colon to be prepared for elective surgery. Colonoscopy can also provide assessment of bowel viability, the most important prognostic indicator. Visualization of ischemic mucosa mandates operative intervention. Although colonoscopy will decompress the volvulus in most patients, recurrence is frequent (50–70%) without operative treatment. Cecal volvulus is generally not responsive to colonoscopic decompression and operative treatment is warranted.

Stricture Dilatation

In hopes of avoiding surgical resection, nonoperative treatment of colonic strictures is being pursued with increasing frequency. Both radiologic and endoscopic approaches have been utilized; the latter, however, is technically easier and allows visual inspection and histologic evaluation of the stricture. While strictures of diverse etiology have been addressed endoscopically, anastomotic strictures appear to offer the best results.

Once the stricture has been identified, one must determine its cause. This usually requires biopsy and/or mucosal brushing. The pediatric colonoscope may aid in visualizing the colon proximal to the stricture.

The dilators used for these procedures are the same or similar to those used in the upper gastrointestinal tract. Balloon dilators are most commonly used, since they can be placed anywhere in the colon. Ideally, they are positioned under direct vision via the colonoscope, once the latter is correctly positioned distal to the stricture. Silicone lubrication is usually necessary in order to pass the dilating catheter through the scope. Longer (8 cm) and wider (diameters greater than 51F) balloons may be used. If angulation precludes insertion through the scope, the balloon dilators can be positioned under fluoroscopic guidance via a colonoscopically-placed guidewire. In the left colon, hollow-core rigid dilators can also be inserted under fluoroscopic control over previously inserted guidewires. Some suggest that balloon dilatation may be a reasonable option in patients with recurrent Crohn's strictures within reach of the colonoscope.

Endoscopic Nd:YAG lasers have been used to relieve malignant obstruction, allowing luminal recanalization and bowel preparation prior to resection or providing palliation in over 85% of patients with advanced disease. Prior to attempting this procedure, the endoscopist should have experience with laser therapy elsewhere in the gastrointestinal tract.

Lastly, stenting of malignant colonic obstructions is an appealing method to decompress the bowel, allowing for subsequent bowel preparation and elective resection without a temporary colostomy. Stenting may also serve as definitive therapy in patients with unresectable or terminal disease. This technique is performed in conjunction with fluoroscopic guidance.

COMPLICATIONS

Fluid and electrolyte imbalance can occur during bowel preparation. Dehydration and hypovolemia are more common than fluid overload. The risk of these complications has been decreased by the introduction of oral purge solutions containing sodium sulfate and nonabsorbable solutes such as polyethylene glycol. Cardiopulmonary complications can also occur following analgesia administration. These reactions have been described above.

Complications specifically related to colonoscopy include hemorrhage and perforation. The former is most unusual following diagnostic colonoscopy, occurring in 0–0.07% of cases. Hemorrhage in this setting is usually intra-abdominal, resulting from the use of excessive force during manipulation. Serosal or mucosal tears are the most common sources.

Although still uncommon, hemorrhage is seen more often following polypectomy (1–3%). Postpolypectomy bleeding can be immediate or delayed. Most hemorrhage occurring immediately following polypectomy is due to inadequate coagulation of the feeding vessel; this complication can usually be handled during colonoscopy either by re-snaring and recoagulating the polypectomy stump or by standard hemostatic techniques. Approximately 2% of polypectomies are complicated by delayed bleeding which usually stops without need for transfusion. This complication can be managed expectantly with typical supportive therapy.

Perforation is the most common complication of diagnostic colonoscopy, occurring in <1% of cases. These injuries are caused by mechanical or pneumatic pressure and are most common at the rectosigmoid or sigmoid–descending colon junctions. While surgery is often required, patients with limited, confined perforations of the left colon can sometimes be managed conservatively with bowel rest, intravenous fluids and antibiotics, and close observation.

Therapeutic colonoscopy, including polypectomy or hemostasis, can also be complicated by perforation. Reported incidences are rare (<1%), with the greatest risks occurring with the removal of sessile polyps. Following polypectomy, patients occasionally develop localized peritoneal irritation, fever, tachycardia, and leukocytosis without overt perforation. This syndrome has been labeled transmural burn, postpolypectomy coagulation syndrome, or serositis, and is probably attributable to a transmural electrocoagulation injury. Patients with this complication can also be treated conservatively with uneventful recovery expected within 48–72 hours.

▪ ENDOSCOPIC ULTRASOUND

Given its diagnostic and therapeutic utility (Table 3–9), endoscopic ultrasound (EUS) is now a commonly performed procedure in everyday endoscopic practice. Individual layers of the gastrointestinal wall are visualized as five distinct layers of alternating hyper- and hypoechogenicity (Fig 3–23). The first two layers correspond to the interface and the mucosa, the third layer represents the submucosa, the fourth the muscularis mucosa, and the fifth the adventitia/serosa. EUS can distinguish structures as small as 2 mm in diameter and can also evaluate adjacent organs or structures that are outside of the gastrointestinal tract.

TABLE 3–9. INDICATIONS FOR ENDOSCOPIC ULTRASOUND

PANCREATIC
1. Fine-needle aspiration and cytology of malignancy
2. Drainage of fluid collections
3. Lymph node sampling (to determine resectability)
4. Assess portal venous system
5. Intraductal ultrasound
6. Ampullary mass
HEPATOBILIARY
1. Detect stones (in conjunction with or in lieu of ERCP)
2. Intraductal ultrasound
3. Periportal lymph node sampling
4. Biopsy of liver mass
MEDIASTINAL
1. Aortopulmonary window lymph node sampling (in lieu of mediastinoscopy)
2. Bronchial and carinal tissue sampling/cytology
3. Lung cancer staging
ESOPHAGEAL
1. Esophageal cancer staging
2. Follow-up of hiatal hernia repair and antireflux surgery (under investigation)
GASTRIC
1. Gastric cancer staging
2. Evaluation of submucosal masses
RETROPERITONEAL
1. Adrenal cytology
2. Celiac axis nerve blocks
3. Retroperitoneal biopsies
4. Renal biopsies
COLORECTAL
1. Anorectal cancer staging
2. Anorectal lymph node evaluation
3. Anal sphincter evaluation
4. Perirectal abscess detection and management

The procedure is performed much like routine diagnostic endoscopy. Preparation, medication, and endoscope passage are performed in the usual fashion. Once the endoscope is in the desired position, acoustic coupling is usually achieved by filling both the lumen and a balloon on the endoscope tip with deaerated water. When performing EUS, artifacts due to excess air insufflation are the greatest impediment to obtaining proper images.

INSTRUMENTATION

EUS employs a probe with higher frequency (7.5, 12, 15, and 20 MHz) than conventional extracorporeal probes. These higher frequencies afford greater resolution and shorter depth of penetration (7.5 MHz = 7-cm penetra-

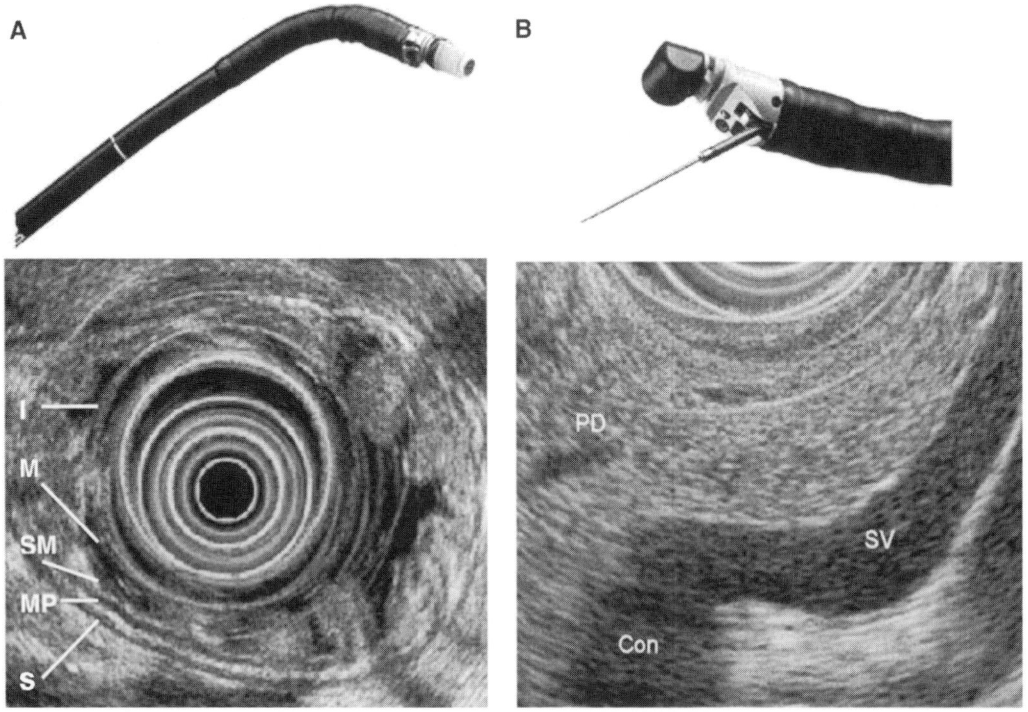

Figure 3–23. Endoscopic ultrasound can be performed with either a radial (**A**) or a linear (**B**) probe. The procedure can also be used to perform directed needle biopsy (**B**). I, interface between probe and mucosa (hyperechoic or white); M, mucosa (hypoechoic or black); SM, submucosa (white); MP, muscularis propria (black); S, serosa (white); PD, pancreatic duct; SV, splenic vein; Con, confluence of SV and SMV. (Courtesy of Olympus Medical Systems, Melville, NY.)

tion; 12 MHz = 3-cm penetration). The transducer is attached to a standard endoscope, which can either be a 360-degree radial probe or a 90- to 180-degree linear probe. Doppler capability has now been added to transducers, facilitating identification of vascular structures.

Miniature probes are also available. These thin catheters have transducers attached to their tips and can be inserted into the 2.8-mm working channels of regular endoscopes to allow ultrasonographic examination of areas of concern, including the biliary tree. A three-dimensional probe is under development; it will enable reconstruction of the entire bowel wall and adjacent structures.

INTERVENTION AND THERAPEUTICS

When a lesion is found, the working port of a linear probe allows for fine-needle aspiration biopsies. In general, cytology technicians should be available to confirm the samples' adequacy prior to terminating the procedure. Injection and sclerotherapy (e.g., celiac axis neurolysis) may be facilitated by the use of EUS guidance.

Esophageal Cancer

EUS for locoregional staging of esophageal cancer may affect treatment. EUS has a role in detecting tracheal invasion in proximal esophageal cancers. Lymph node involvement, particularly in the celiac plexus, can also assist in tumor staging.

Pancreatic Cancer

EUS has high accuracy rates for detection or exclusion of pancreatic masses, particularly for very small lesions. It is possible to perform transmural aspiration biopsies of these lesions through the posterior gastric wall or the duodenum. With different positions of the EUS scope, the entire pancreas and its ductal system can be examined.

Colorectal Cancer

EUS for colorectal cancer usually requires a larger-diameter probe. This modality has been instrumental in differentiating mucosal from deeper tumors, and may alter treatment based on its findings, especially for rectal cancer. For example, patients with only mucosal cancer of the rectum rarely have lymph node involvement and may be amenable to mucosal resections. Cancers invading less than halfway through the submucosal layer have a 10% chance of lymph node involvement and can usually be resected with a standard low anterior resection.

▪ ENDOSCOPIC TRANSLUMINAL SURGERY

Endoscopic transluminal surgery represents yet another extension of endoscopic techniques. While many aspects of this new approach are evolving, recent reports have described the use of the gastroscope, EUS, and even the side-viewing endoscope to perform transluminal surgery in animals. Some of the procedures described include oophorectomy, gastrojejunostomy, and crural closure in hiatal hernias. In humans, endoscopic transluminal appendectomies and cholecystectomies have been performed.

▪ SELECTED READINGS

THE FLEXIBLE ENDOSCOPE

Axon ATR. Working party report to the World Congresses of Gastroenterology, Sydney, 1990. Disinfection and endoscopy: summary and recommendations. *J Gastroenterol Hepatol* 1991;6:23–24

Bottrill PM, Axon ATR. Cleaning and disinfection of flexible endoscopes and ancillary equipment: use of automatic disinfectors. *J Gastroenterol Hepatol* 1991;6:45–47

Brown GJ, Saunders BP. Advances in colonic imaging: technical improvements in colonoscopy. *Eur J Gastroenterol Hepatol* 2005;17:785–792

Schembre D. Smart endoscopes. *Gastrointest Endosc Clin N Am* 2004;14:709–716

Dunkin BJ. Flexible endoscopy simulators. *Semin Laparosc Surg* 2003;10:29–35

PATIENT SEDATION AND MONITORING

Training committee. American Society for Gastrointestinal Endoscopy. Training guideline for use of propofol in gastrointestinal endoscopy. *Gastrointest Endosc* 2004;60: 167–172

Rex DK, Heuss LT, Waler JA, Qi R. Trained registered nurses/endoscopy teams can administer propofol safely for endoscopy. *Gastroenterology* 2005;129:1384–1391

Faulx AL, Vela S, Das A et al. The changing landscape of practice patterns regarding unsedated endoscopy and propofol use: a national Web survey. *Gastrointest Endosc* 2005;62:9–15

Arrowsmith JB, Gerstman BB, Fleischer DE, Benjamin SB. Results from the American Society for Gastrointestinal Endoscopy/US Food and Drug Administration collaborative study on complication rates and drug use during gastrointestinal endoscopy. *Gastrointest Endosc* 1991;37: 421–427

Waring JP, Baron TH, Hirota WK, et al, and the American Society for Gastrointestinal Endoscopy, Standards of Practice Committee. Guidelines for conscious sedation and monitoring during gastrointestinal endoscopy. *Gastrointest Endosc* 2003;58:317–322

Faigel DO, Baron TH, Goldstein JL et al and the Standards of Practice Committee, American Society for Gastrointestinal Endoscopy. Guidelines for the use of deep sedation and anesthesia for GI endoscopy. *Gastrointest Endosc* 2002;56:613–617

2003 American Society for Gastrointestinal Endoscopy Technology Status Evaluation Report. Monitoring equipment for endoscopy. *Gastrointest Endosc* 2004;59:761–765

Patel S, Vargo JJ, Khandwala F et al. Deep sedation occurs frequently during elective endoscopy with meperidine and midazolam. *Am J Gastroenterol* 2005;100:2689–2695

Rey JR, Axon A, Budzynska A, Kruse A, Nowak A. Guidelines of the European Society of Gastrointestinal Endoscopy (E.S.G.E.) for antibiotic prophylaxis for gastrointestinal endoscopy. *Endoscopy* 1998;30:318–324

UPPER GASTROINTESTINAL ENDOSCOPY

Repici A, Conio M, DeAngelis C et al. Temporary placement of an expandable polyester silicone-covered stent for treatment of refractory benign esophageal strictures. *Gastrointest Endosc* 2004;60:513–519

Cipolletta L, Bianco MA, Marmo R et al. Endoclips versus heater probe in preventing early recurrent bleeding from peptic ulcer: a prospective and randomized trial. *Gastrointest Endosc* 2001;53:147–151

American Society for Gastrointestinal Endoscopy Guideline. The role of endoscopy in the surveillance of premalignant conditions of the upper gastrointestinal tract. Guidelines for clinical application. *Gastrointest Endosc* 1998;48:663–668

Adler DG, Leighton JA, Davila RE et al and the American Society for Gastrointestinal Endoscopy. ASGE guideline: The role of endoscopy in acute non-variceal upper-GI hemorrhage. *Gastrointest Endosc* 2004;60:497–504

Lee SD, Kearney DJ: A randomized controlled trial of gastric lavage prior to endoscopy for acute upper gastrointestinal bleeding. *J Clin Gastroenterol* 2004;38:861–865

Lee JG, Turnipseed S, Romano PS et al. Endoscopy-based triage significantly reduces hospitalization rates and costs of treating upper GI bleeding: a randomized controlled trial. *Gastrointest Endosc* 1999;50:755–761

Lo GH, Lai KH, Cheng JS et al. Prophylactic banding ligation of high-risk esophageal varices in patients with cirrhosis: a prospective, randomized trial. *J Hepatol* 1999;31:451–456

2003 American Society for Gastrointestinal Endoscopy Technology Status Evaluation Report. Tools for endoscopic stricture dilation. *Gastrointest Endosc* 2004;59:753–760

Lutfi RE, Torquati A, Richards WO. Endoscopic treatment modalities for gastroesophageal reflux disease. *Surg Endosc* 2004;18:1299–1315

Triadafilopoulos G. Ten frequently asked questions about endoscopic therapy for gastroesophageal reflux disease. *American Society for Gastrointestinal Endoscopy Clinical Update* 2004;12

American Society for Gastrointestinal Endoscopy Guideline. The role of endoscopy in the management of variceal hemorrhage, updated July 2005. *Gastrointest Endosc* 2005;62:651–655

American Society for Gastrointestinal Endoscopy Guideline. Esophageal dilation. *Gastrointest Endosc* 1998;48:702–704

Nguyen V, Huang IP, Lin E. Esophageal dilation using a single-use direct optical viewing technique. (in press 2006)

Canto MI. Chromoendoscopy and magnifying endoscopy for Barrett's esophagus. *Clin Gastroenterol Hepatol* 2005;3: S12–S15

Reed WP, Kilkenny JW, Dias CE, Wexner SD and the society of American Gastrointestinal and Endoscopic Surgeons EGD Outcomes Study Group. A prospective analysis of 3525 esophagogastroduodenoscopies performed by surgeons. *Surg Endosc* 2004;18:11–21

Bosco JJ, Barkun AN, Isenberg GA et al and the American Society for Gastrointestinal Endoscopy Technology Assessment Committee. Endoscopic enteral nutritional access devices *Gastrointest Endosc* 2002;56:796–802

American Society for Gastrointestinal Endoscopy. Guideline for the management of ingested foreign bodies. *Gastrointest Endosc* 1995;42:622–625

ENDOSCOPY OF THE PANCREATICOBILIARY TREE

Adler DG, Baron TH, Davila RE et al and the Standards of Practice Committee of the American Society for Gastrointestinal Endoscopy. ASGE guideline: The role of ERCP in diseases of the biliary tract and the pancreas. *Gastrointest Endosc* 2005;62:1–8

Rosch T, Hofrichter K, Frimberger E et al. ERCP or EUS for tissue diagnosis of biliary strictures? A prospective comparative study. *Gastrointest Endosc* 2004;60:390–396

Fogel EL, Debellis M, McHenry L et al. Effectiveness of a new long cytology brush in the evaluation of malignant biliary obstruction: a prospective study. *Gastrointest Endosc* 2006;63:71–77

Acosta JM, Katkhouda N, Debian KA et al. Early ductal decompression versus conservative management for gallstone pancreatitis with ampullary obstruction: a prospective randomized clinical trial. *Ann Surg* 2006;243:33–40

Liu CL, Fan ST, Lo CM et al. Comparison of early endoscopic ultrasonography and endoscopic retrograde cholangiopancreatography in the management of acute biliary pancreatitis: a prospective randomized study. *Clin Gastroenterol Hepatol* 2005;3:1238–1244

Shiozawa S, Tsuchiya A, Kim DH et al. Useful predictive factors of common bile duct stones prior to laparoscopic cholecystectomy for gallstones. *Hepatogastroenterology* 2005;52:1662–1665

Morgenthal CB, Lin E. The evolution of flexible endoscopy: the impact on surgical practice. Surg Endosc (in press 2006)

Mallery JS, Baron TH, Dominitz JA et al. Complications of ERCP. *Gastrointest Endosc* 2003;57:633–638

Disario JA, Freeman ML, Bjorkman DJ et al. Endoscopic balloon dilation compared with sphincterotomy for extraction of bile duct stones. *Gastroenterology* 2004;127:1291–1299

Zhou MQ, Li NP, Lu RD. Duodenoscopy in treatment of acute gallstone pancreatitis. *Hepatobiliary Pancreat Dis Int* 2002;1:608–610

Fazel A, Quadri A, Catalano MF, Meyerson SM, Geenen JE. Does a pancreatic duct stent prevent post-ERCP pancreatitis? A prospective randomized study. *Gastrointest Endosc* 2003;57:291–294

Andriulli A, Clemente R, Solmi L et al. Gabexate or somatostatin administration before ERCP in patients at high risk for post-ERCP pancreatitis: a multicenter, placebo-controlled, randomized clinical trial. *Gastrointest Endosc* 2002;56:488–495

Folsch UR, Nitsche R, Ludtke R, Hilgers RA, Creutzfeldt W. Early ERCP and papillotomy compared with conservative treatment for acute biliary pancreatitis. The German Study Group on Acute Biliary Pancreatitis. *N Engl J Med* 1997;336:237–242

Fan ST, Lai EC, Mok FP et al. Early treatment of acute biliary pancreatitis by endoscopic papillotomy. *N Engl J Med* 1993;328:228–232

Neoptolemos JP, London N, Slater ND et al. A prospective study of ERCP and endoscopic sphincterotomy in the diagnosis and treatment of gallstone acute pancreatitis. A rational and safe approach to management. *Arch Surg* 1986;121:697–702

Fink AS, Perez de Ayala V, Chapman M, Cotton PB. Radiologic pitfalls in endoscopic retrograde pancreatography. *Pancreas* 1986;1:180–187

Axon AT, Classen M, Cotton PB et al. Pancreatography in chronic pancreatitis: international definitions. *Gut* 1984;25:1107–1112

Ahearne PM, Baillie JM, Cotton PB et al. An endoscopic retrograde cholangiopancreatography (ERCP)-based algorithm for the management of pancreatic pseudocysts. *Am J Surg* 1992;163:111–115

Misra SP, Dwivedi M. Long-term follow-up of a prospective randomized study of endoscopic versus surgical treatment of bile duct calculi in patients with gallbladder in situ. *Br J Surg* 1996;83:708–709

Targarona EM, Ayuso RM, Bordas JM et al. Randomised trial of endoscopic sphincterotomy with gallbladder left in situ versus open surgery for common bile duct calculi in high-risk patients. *Lancet* 1996;347:926–929

Hammarstrom LE, Holmin T, Stridbeck H, Ihse I. Long-term follow-up of a prospective randomized study of endoscopic versus surgical treatment of bile duct calculi in patients with gallbladder in situ. *Br J Surg* 1995;82:1516–1521

Howden JK, Baillie J. Preoperative versus postoperative endoscopic retrograde cholangiopancreatography in mild to moderate pancreatitis: a prospective randomized trial. *Gastrointest Endosc* 2001;53:834–836

Chang L, Lo S, Stabile BE et al. Preoperative versus postoperative endoscopic retrograde cholangiopancreatography in mild to moderate gallstone pancreatitis: a prospective randomized trial. *Ann Surg* 2000;231:82–87

Toouli J, Roberts-Thomson IC, Kellow J et al. Manometry based randomised trial of endoscopic sphincterotomy for sphincter of Oddi dysfunction. *Gut* 2000;46:98–102

Geenen JE, Hogan WJ, Dodds WJ, Toouli J, Venu RP. The efficacy of endoscopic sphincterotomy after cholecystectomy in patients with sphincter-of-Oddi dysfunction. *N Engl J Med* 1989;320:82–87

Lai EC, Mok FP, Tan ES et al. Endoscopic biliary drainage for severe acute cholangitis. *N Engl J Med* 1992;326:1582–1586

Smith AC, Dowsett JF, Russell RC, Hatfield AR, Cotton PB. Randomised trial of endoscopic stenting versus surgical bypass in malignant low bile duct obstruction. *Lancet* 1994;344:1655–1660

Andersen JR, Sorensen SM, Kruse A, Rokkjaer M, Matzen P. Randomised trial of endoscopic endoprosthesis versus operative bypass in malignant obstructive jaundice. *Gut* 1989;30:1132–1135

Speer AG, Cotton PB, Russell RC et al. Randomised trial of endoscopic versus percutaneous stent insertion in malignant obstructive jaundice. *Lancet* 1987;2:57–62

Dite P, Ruzicka M, Zboril V, Novotny I. A prospective, randomized trial comparing endoscopic and surgical therapy for chronic pancreatitis. *Endoscopy* 2003;35:553–558

SMALL BOWEL ENTEROSCOPY

Kaffes AJ, Koo JH, Meredith C. Double-balloon enteroscopy in the diagnosis and the management of small-bowel diseases: an initial experience in 40 patients. *Gastrointest Endosc* 2006;63:81–86

Berson LB. Double-balloon enteroscopy: the new gold standard for small-bowel imaging? *Gastrointest Endosc* 2005; 62:71–75

Yamamoto H. Double-balloon endoscopy. *Clin Gastroenterol Hepatol* 2005;3:S27–S29

Carey EJ, Fleischer DE. Investigation of the small bowel in gastrointestinal bleeding-enteroscopy and capsule endoscopy. *Gastroenterol Clin North Am* 2005;34:719–734

Matsumoto T, Moriyama T, Esaki M, Nakamura S, Iida M. Performance of antegrade double-balloon enteroscopy: comparison with push enteroscopy. *Gastrointest Endosc* 2005;62:392–398

Marmo R, Rotondano G, Piscopo R, Bianco MA, Cipolletta L. Meta-analysis: capsule enteroscopy vs. conventional modalities in diagnosis of small bowel diseases. *Aliment Pharmacol Ther* 2005;22:595–604

Essen GM, Dominitz JA, Faigel DO et al. Enteroscopy. *Gastrointest Endosc* 2001;53:871–873

ENDOSCOPY OF THE LOWER GASTROINTESTINAL TRACT

Rodriguez-Bigas MA, Boland CR, Hamilton SR et al. A National Cancer Institute workshop on hereditary nonpolyposis colorectal cancer syndrome: Meeting highlights and Bethesda guidelines. *J Natl Cancer Inst* 1997; 89:1758–1762

Winawer S, Fletcher R, Rex D et al. Colorectal cancer screening and surveillance: Clinical guidelines and rationale—Update based on new evidence. *Gastroenterology* 2003; 124:544–560

Davila RE, Rajan E, Adler D et al. American Society for Gastrointestinal Endoscopy guideline: the role of endoscopy in the diagnosis, staging, and management of colorectal cancer. *Gastrointest Endosc* 2005;61:1–7

Anthony T, Simmang C, Hyman N et al. Practice parameters for the surveillance and follow-up of patients with colon and rectal cancer. *Dis Colon Rectum* 2004;47:807–817

Dominitz JA, Eisen GM, Baron TH et al. Complications of colonoscopy. *Gastrointest Endosc* 2003;57:441–445

Dunlop MG. Guidance on gastrointestinal surveillance for hereditary non-polyposis colorectal cancer, familial adenomatous polyposis, juvenile polyposis, and Peutz-Jeghers syndrome. *Gut* 2002;51(Suppl 5):V21–V27

Eaden JA, Mayberry JF. Guidelines for screening and surveillance of asymptomatic colorectal cancer in patients with inflammatory bowel disease. *Gut* 2002;51(Suppl 5):V10–V12

Rex DK, Bond JH, Winawer S et al. Quality in the technical performance of colonoscopy and the continuous quality improvement process for colonoscopy: recommendations of the U.S. Multi-Society Task Force on Colorectal Cancer. *Am J Gastroenterol* 2002;97:1296–1308

Green BT, Rockey DC, Portwood G et al. Urgent colonoscopy for evaluation and management of acute lower gastrointestinal hemorrhage: a randomized controlled trial. *Am J Gastroenterol* 2005;100:2395–2402

Segnan N, Senore C, Andreoni B et al. Randomized trial of different screening strategies for colorectal cancer: patient response and detection rates. *J Natl Cancer Inst* 2005;97:347–357

Mandel JS, Church TR, Bond JH et al. The effect of fecal occult-blood screening on the incidence of colorectal cancer. *N Engl J Med* 2000;343:1603–1607

Winawer SJ, Stewart ET, Zauber AG et al. A comparison of colonoscopy and double-contrast barium enema for surveillance after polypectomy. National Polyp Study Work Group. *N Engl J Med* 2000;342:1766–1772

Schoen RE, Corle D, Cranston L et al. Is colonoscopy needed for the nonadvanced adenoma found on sigmoidoscopy? The Polyp Prevention Trial. *Gastroenterology* 1998; 115:533–541

American Society for Gastrointestinal Endoscopy Guideline: The role of endoscopy in the patient with lower-GI bleeding. *Gastrointest Endosc* 2005;62:656–660

Nelson DB, Barkun AN, Block KP et al. Technology status evaluation report. Colonoscopy preparations. *Gastrointest Endosc* 2001;54:829–832

Targarona EM, Balague C. Stenting of obstructing colonic cancer. *Surg Endosc* 2005;19:745–746

ENDOSCOPIC ULTRASOUND

Gopal DV, Chang EY, Kim CY et al. EUS characteristics of Nissen fundoplication: normal appearance and mechanisms of failure. *Gastrointest Endosc* 2006;63:35–44

Preston SR, Clark GW, Martin IG, Ling HM, Harris KM. Effect of endoscopic ultrasonography on the management of 100 consecutive patients with oesophageal and junction carcinoma. *Br J Surg* 2003;90: 1220–1224

Hunt GC, Faigel DO. Assessment of EUS for diagnosing, staging, and determining respectability of pancreatic cancer: a review. *Gastrointest Endosc* 2002;55:232–237

Gress F, Schmitt C, Sherman S, Ikenberry S, Lehman G. A prospective randomized comparison of endoscopic ultrasound- and computed tomography-guided celiac plexus block for managing chronic pancreatitis pain. *Am J Gastroenterol* 1999;94:900–905

Siemsen M, Svendsen LB, Knigge U et al. A prospective randomized comparison of curved array and radial echoendoscopy in patients with esophageal cancer. *Gastrointest Endosc* 2003;58:671–676

Savides T, Perricone A. Impact of EUS-guided FNA of enlarged mediastinal lymph nodes on subsequent thoracic surgery rates. *Gastrointest Endosc* 2004;60:340–346

ENDOSCOPIC TRANSLUMINAL SURGERY

Ikeda K, Fritscher-Ravens A, Mosse CA et al. Endoscopic full-thickness resection with sutured closure in a porcine model. *Gastrointest Endosc* 2005;62:122–129

Gostout CJ. The evolution of endoluminal intervention. *Gastrointest Endosc* 2005;62:130–131

Kantsevoy SV, Jagannath SB, Niiyama H et al. Endoscopic gastrojejunostomy with survival in a porcine model. *Gastrointest Endosc* 2005;62:287–292

Section II

ABDOMINAL WALL

4

Incisions, Closures, and Management of the Abdominal Wound

Bryan M. Burt ■ *Ali Tavakkolizadeh* ■ *Stephen J. Ferzoco*

■ INCISIONS

A well-calculated and well-performed incision is of paramount importance to abdominal surgery. Of equal importance is a proper method of wound closure. Any error, such as a poorly chosen incision, unsatisfactory means to close, or unsuitable selection of suture material, may result in serious complications including hematoma, hernia, wound infection, stitch abscess, unpleasant scar, and the dreaded wound dehiscence and evisceration.

In the most recent previous edition of this book, Ellis outlined three basic principles to guide selection of the incision and closure of the wound. These are accessibility, flexibility, and security.[1]

- Accessibility. The incision should provide direct and timely exposure to the diseased or injured anatomy and must provide sufficient space for the procedure to be well performed. Exposure is greatly facilitated not only by a well-made incision, but also by the apt use of retractors and packs, correct posture of the patient on the operating room table, and optimized lighting.
- Flexibility. The incision should be amenable to extension if the complexity of the procedure demands greater exposure than originally anticipated. It should, however, interfere as little as possible with the function of the abdominal wall, limiting sacrifice of nerve supply to the abdominal musculature, preferably the sacrifice of only a single segmental nerve trunk.
- Security. Closure of the wound must be strong and reliable. Ideally, it should leave the abdominal wall with integrity comparable to or superior to its preoperative state.

TYPES OF INCISIONS

Abdominal incisions can be divided into four main anatomic categories.

- Vertical. Vertical incisions may be midline or paramedian. They may be supraumbilical or infraumbilical and can be extended superiorly or inferiorly in either direction. For optimal exposure of the entire abdominal cavity, as in the case of abdominal trauma, a midline vertical incision can be taken superiorly to the xiphoid process and inferiorly to the symphysis pubis.
- Transverse and oblique. These incisions can be placed in any of the four quadrants of the abdomen. Common incisions include the Kocher subcostal incision for biliary surgery, the Pfannenstiel infraumbilical incision for gynecologic surgery, the McBurney incision for appendectomy, and the transverse or oblique lateral incision for exposure of the colon.
- Abdominothoracic. This incision provides superior exposure of the upper abdominal organs by joining the peritoneal cavity, pleural space, and mediastinum into a single operative field.

It is particularly useful for extensive exposure of the liver and esophagogastric junction.

- Retroperitoneal and extraperitoneal. These incisions are ideal for surgery of the kidney, adrenal gland, aorta, and for renal transplantation.

CHOICE OF INCISION

Many factors influence the choice of incision for abdominal surgery. These include the organ of interest and anticipated procedure, the body habitus of the patient and degree of obesity, the urgency of the operation and whether speed is a pressing consideration, the presence of previous abdominal incisions, and the preference and experience of the operating surgeon.

Most surgeons prefer a midline or paramedian approach to the abdominal viscera. In emergency operations, the midline incision undoubtedly provides the most rapid access to the abdominal cavity, and if necessary can be extended swiftly to the whole length of the abdominal wall. Re-entry into the abdomen should be achieved through the previous incision, if possible. If the previous incision is weak or a site of incisional hernia, the abdominal wall can be repaired at this time. A new incision should never be made closely parallel (within 5 cm) to the site of any previous incision without understanding the distinct risk of ischemic necrosis of intervening skin and fascial bridges. Future surgical prospects are considered and the incision should be placed so that it will not interfere with planned procedures, for example, to avoid or incorporate colostomies, fistulas, and the like. Similarly if the patient has the potential for recurrent disease requiring re-exploration, consideration of location is important.

Midline versus Transverse Incisions

In thin patients with narrow subcostal angles, a transverse or oblique incision has little advantage; however, in obese patients with wide subcostal angles, a subcostal incision provides excellent exposure of the upper abdominal viscera, biliary tract, spleen, and pancreas. There are many occasions, however, in which either a vertical or transverse incision would provide appropriate an equal exposure.

Some authors feel that transverse incisions in abdominal surgery are based on better anatomic and surgical principles than vertical incisions and should be preferred.[2,3] Anatomically, the fascial fibers of the anterior abdominal wall lie in a transverse direction and are therefore divided by a vertical incision. Suture closure of a vertically placed wound places suture material between these fibers, as opposed to the placement of suture material around these fibers as would be done in closing a transverse incision. Furthermore, tension lines lie mediolateral in vertically placed incisions and craniocaudal in transversely placed incisions. For these reasons, many surgeons believe that sutures placed perpendicularly to muscle fibers in transverse incisions are more secure and less liable to cut through fascia.

A number of retrospective clinical studies and a meta-analysis have concluded that the transverse incision is superior to the vertical incision with regard to long-term and short-term outcomes, including postoperative pain, pulmonary complications, and frequencies of incisional hernia and burst abdomen.[3] However, the vertical incision is still the most commonly performed incision in general surgery. This discrepancy is explained by a number of deficits in study design and analysis such as the underpowering of clinical trials, lack of standardization of abdominal wall closure, nonblinded methods, and study inhomogeneities in meta-analysis.[4] Clearly, only carefully designed randomized clinical trials can compare one incision to another.

The only randomized controlled trial that has been performed that focused on the frequency of burst abdomen (i.e., evisceration) could find no benefit of transverse incision (0%) over midline incision (0.69%).[5] Likewise, controlled clinical trials demonstrate no significant differences in incisional hernias when comparing transverse (0.85%) to midline incisions (3.85%),[5] and transverse (14%) to paramedian incisions (14%).[6] With regard to postoperative wound infections, there are no data to support a difference in infectious wound complications among these incisions.[3] Data on early-onset pulmonary complications are conflicting but in randomized trials they are equally distributed in each group.[7]

Midline versus Paramedian Incisions

The vertical incision can be divided into three main subtypes: midline, medial paramedian, and lateral paramedian. The theoretical advantage of the paramedian incision over a midline incision is a diminished risk of wound dehiscence and incisional hernia. The paramedian incision enters the abdomen through dissection of the rectus muscle from its anterior and posterior sheaths. Upon closure, the rectus muscle should resume its original place and splint the defects in the anterior and posterior rectus fascia. In actuality, however, when these incisions are reopened, the medial edge of the rectus muscle is invariably noted to be adherent by scar to the posterior sheath incision and does not effectively buttress the wound. The speculative advantages of the paramedian incision have been investigated in prospective randomized trials demonstrating that the conventional (medial) paramedian incision offers no advantage in wound failure rates when compared to midline or transverse incisions.[6]

In 1980, Guillou described a modified paramedian incision, "the lateral paramedian incision," that is created several centimeters lateral to the traditional paramedian incision.[8] Randomized prospective data show a statistically significantly decrease in incidence of incisional hernia in lateral paramedian incisions (0%) when compared to medial paramedian incisions (14.9%)[8] and midline incisions (6.9%).[9] The main disadvantage of the paramedian incision is the length of time needed to create the wound, which increases as the distance from the midline increases.

Cold Blade versus Electrocautery

Although it has become common practice for many surgeons to use electrocautery to create abdominal incisions, it is often taught that sharp dissection is superior to electrocautery for creation of the abdominal incision. These claims were supported by early animal data demonstrating higher wound infection rates and poorer wound strength in incisions made with elecrocautery.[10] More recent randomized data have put this issue to rest. Six prospective randomized clinical trials have compared cold blade scalpel to electrocautery for wound creation through skin and though the subcutaneous layer.[11–16] These trials differ with respect to incision (cholecystectomy, midline laparotomy, and thoracic incision), wound classification, and timing of surgery (elective or emergent). Their data have demonstrated that incisions made with electrocautery are created significantly quicker, produce less blood loss, allow for less postoperative pain, and produce no difference in short-term and long-term wound complications when compared to scalpel incisions.

DESCRIPTION OF INDIVIDUAL INCISIONS

Vertical Incisions

Midline Incisions. The midline incision is the fastest approach toward the peritoneal cavity and has a number of advantages. It offers adequate exposure to almost every region of the abdominal cavity and retroperitoneum. It is nearly bloodless and does not require division of muscle fibers or sectioning of nerves. It is unsurpassed when speed is of the essence. The upper midline incision, or the epigastric midline incision, provides exposure for most operations on the esophageal hiatus, abdominal esophagus and vagus nerves, stomach, duodenum, gallbladder, pancreas, and spleen (Fig 4–1). The lower midline incision, or infraumbilical incision, is similar to the upper midline incision and may extend superiorly to join it. It provides exposure for most operations on the lower abdominal and pelvic organs.

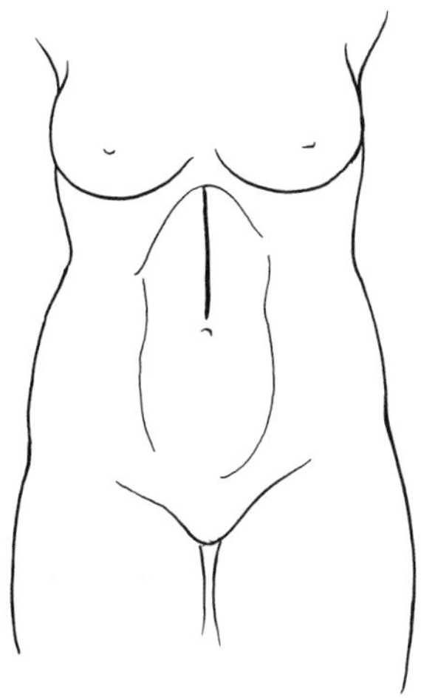

Figure 4–1. Epigastric midline incision: surface markings.

The upper midline incision is made exactly in the midline of the abdomen and extends from the tip of the xiphoid process to approximately 1 cm above the umbilicus. The operating surgeon and assistant apply lateral opposing traction on the skin and a scalpel firmly sweeps along the course of the incision with the initial stroke cutting deeply well into the subcutaneous fat. Gauze pads are applied to provide lateral opposing traction on the edges of the subcutaneous fat. Using either electocautery or a cold blade, the incision is carried down to the linea alba, identified by observing the decussation of fascial fibers in the upper abdomen. The linea alba, extraperitoneal fat, and peritoneum are then divided in series. In the upper half of the incision, the extraperitoneal fat is abundant and vascular, requiring coagulation of its vessels with diathermy. A subumbilical incision or a full-length midline laparotomy incision is made in a similar manner. When negotiating the umbilicus, the vertical incision is carried around it in a curvilinear manner. Alternatively, the skin may be held taught by an assistant towards him- or herself, allowing the surgeon to carry the midline incision in a continuous and straight direction while avoiding the retracted umbilicus and yet staying in the midline.

The peritoneum should be opened with the greatest care to avoid injury to underlying viscera, particularly when operating on patients with distended loops of bowel. The falciform ligament is best avoided by entering the peritoneum well to the left, or preferably to the right of the midline, beneath the belly of the rectus muscle. To avoid injuring the bladder, the peritoneum is entered in the upper portion of the incision. A safe method of entry involves picking up a fold of peritoneum with a pair of toothed forceps, palpating the fold to ensure that there are no underlying viscera, and carefully and sharply incising the side of the raised fold, avoiding any loop of intestine that may be gripped by the forceps. The small opening is enlarged to admit two fingers that are then used to protect the underlying viscera as the peritoneum is further divided along the length of the wound (Fig 4–2). Special attention must be given when operating on the patient with intestinal obstruction to avoid distended bowel immediately beneath the line of incision. Likewise, when reopening the abdomen following a previous surgery, it is critical to suspect and avoid loops of bowel adherant to the abdominal wall. If possible, the incision should start several centimeters beyond the previous scar so that the peritoneum can be opened where it is relatively free of adhesions. In difficult entries, it is wise to attempt division of the peritoneum at the opposite end of the incision. Once the peritoneum has been opened, the fascia and peritoneum can be held up with a hemostat and Kocher clamps so that the line of adhesions can be visualized and divided under direct vision. The falciform ligament can be clamped in two places, divided, and ligated if it interferes with exposure of the field or agility of the surgeon.

Paramedian Incisions. A paramedian incision is a vertical incision that is made 2.5–5 cm from the midline on either the right or left side of the abdomen. Like the midline incision, the paramedian incision avoids injury to nerves and limits trauma to the rectus muscle. It provides a secure, anatomic closure with good restoration of function. When necessary, it can also be extended from xiphisternum to pubis, allowing excellent exposure of the abdomen. It is, however, considerably more time-consuming than a midline incision.

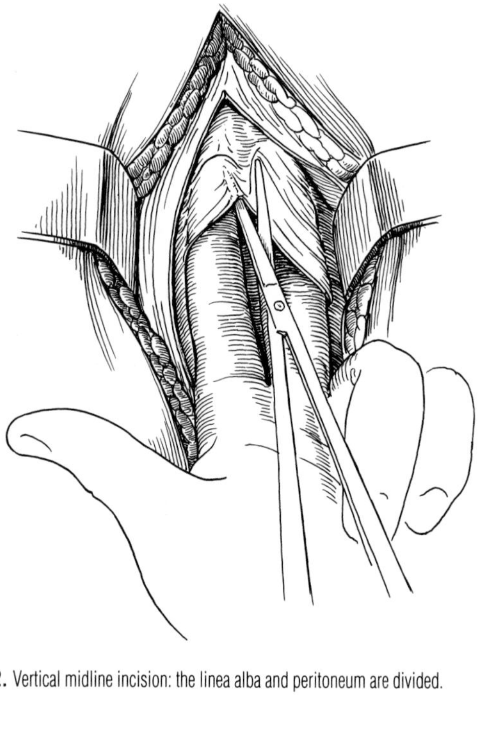

Figure 4–2. Vertical midline incision: the linea alba and peritoneum are divided.

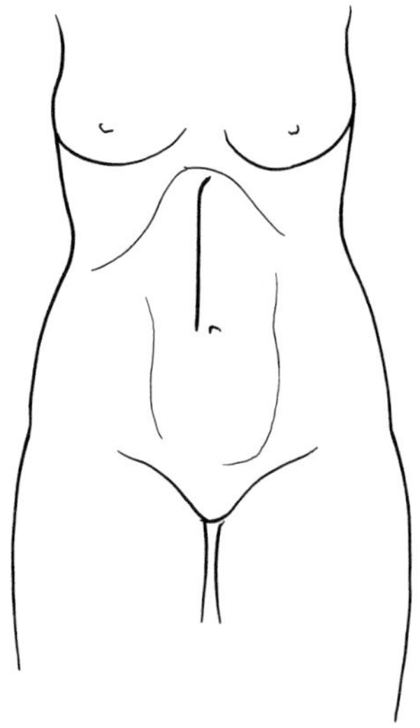

Figure 4–3. Upper paramedian incision: surface markings. Additional exposure can be obtained by sloping the upper portion of the incision upward toward the xiphoid process.

Medial Paramedian Incision. An upper paramedian incision is begun at the costal margin and carried to about 2–8 cm below the umbilicus. Additional access can be obtained by sloping the upper portion of the incision upward toward the xiphoid (Fig 4–3). The lower paramedian incision is similar and indeed can be continuous with an upper paramedian incision, enabling exposure of the abdomen from the costal margin to the pubis.

The anterior border of the rectus sheath is exposed and incised for the entire length of the wound. The medial aspect of the anterior rectus fascia is then dissected off the rectus muscle to its medial edge (Fig 4–4). Particular care must be taken in the upper abdomen because of the tendinous inscriptions that attach the rectus muscle to the anterior fascia. These are located just inferior to the xiphoid process, at the umbilicus, and occasionally halfway between these two points. Segmental vessels will be encountered at these three points and must be electrocoagulated or clamped and ligated. Once free anteriorly and medially, the rectus muscle is easily retracted laterally because it is not adhered to the posterior rectus fascia. The posterior sheath and peritoneum are then incised vertically for the length of the skin incision.

The lower paramedian incision differs in only two respects from the upper paramedian incision. The inferior epigastric vessels will be encountered in dissection and should be divided and tied where they run across the inferior portion of the incision. Addition-

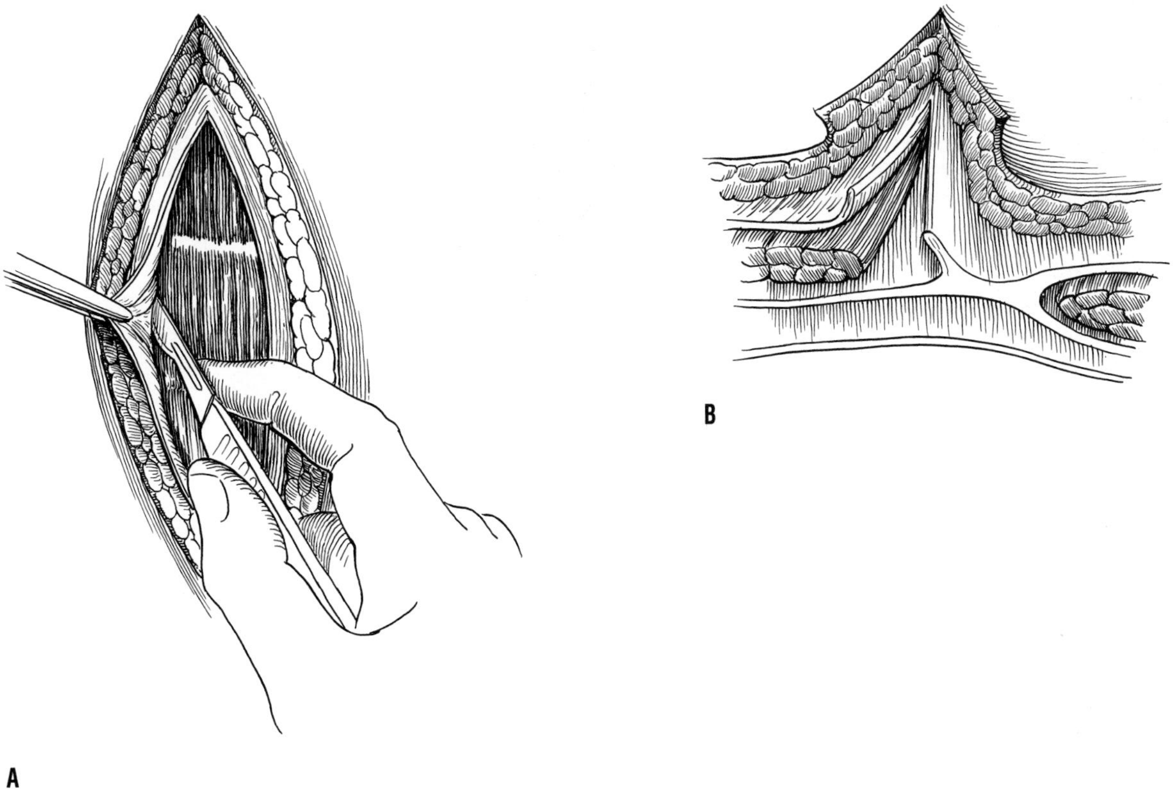

Figure 4–4. A. Paramedian incision: dissection of the rectus muscle from the anterior rectus sheath. **B.** Paramedian incision in transverse section.

ally, the posterior sheath of the rectus fascia is deficient inferior to the semilunar fold of Douglas in this region (Fig 4–5).

Lateral Paramedian Incision. The lateral paramedian incision is a modification of the standard paramedian incision. Originally described by Guillou,[8] it entails a vertical incision placed at the junction of the middle and outer thirds of the width of the rectus sheath. The anterior sheath, at this level containing two layers, is dissected from the rectus muscle. The rectus muscle is retracted laterally in the usual fashion and the posterior sheath and peritoneum are divided in the same plane as the anterior sheath. The wound is splinted by the rectus muscle and allows for a "wide-shutter" mechanism to reinforce the closure of the abdominal wall. As necessary to augment exposure, the upper margin or lower margin of the incision can be angled inward toward the xiphoid process or pubic symphysis (Fig 4–6).

Vertical Muscle-Splitting Incision. The vertical muscle-splitting incision is made in much the same way as the traditional paramedian incision except the rectus muscle is split longitudinally in its median one-third to one-sixth. The posterior rectus sheath and peritoneum are then incised in the same line. This wound can be opened and closed quickly and is of particular value in reopening the scar of a previous paramedian incision where dissecting the rectus muscle from scar tissue can be virtually impossible. An extensive incision is to be avoided, however, because it results in significantly more bleeding and sectioning of nerves that may cause weakening of the corresponding area of the abdominal wall.

Transverse and Oblique

There are several variations of transverse and oblique incisions. Transverse incisions can be strictly horizontal or they may curve to varying degrees. Likewise, oblique incisions may be curved or straight and will vary in angle. The wound may be limited to the lateral abdominal wall oblique muscles, or may divide a portion of one rectus muscle, the entire rectus muscle, or can even divide the complete width of both rectus muscles. Transverse and oblique incisions generally follow Langer's lines of tension and result in better cosmesis than vertical incisions. Sectioning of nerves is usually limited to one and rarely two nerves. A properly placed infraumbilical transverse incision can provide satisfactory exposure to the pelvic organs and the rectosigmoid and rectum. Exposure is limited, however, when pathology is located in both the upper and lower abdomen.

Kocher Subcostal Incision. A right subcostal incision is used commonly for open operations of the gallbladder and biliary tree. It is particularly valuable in obese or muscular patients with wide subcostal angles. The left-sided subcostal incision is used less often, mainly for elective splenectomy. The incision may be carried across the midline as a bilateral subcostal incision. This "arrowhead" or "bucket handle" incision provides excellent exposure of the upper abdomen and is frequently employed in extensive hepatic resections and liver transplantation, in performing total gastrectomy in obese patients, and for anterior access to both adrenal glands.

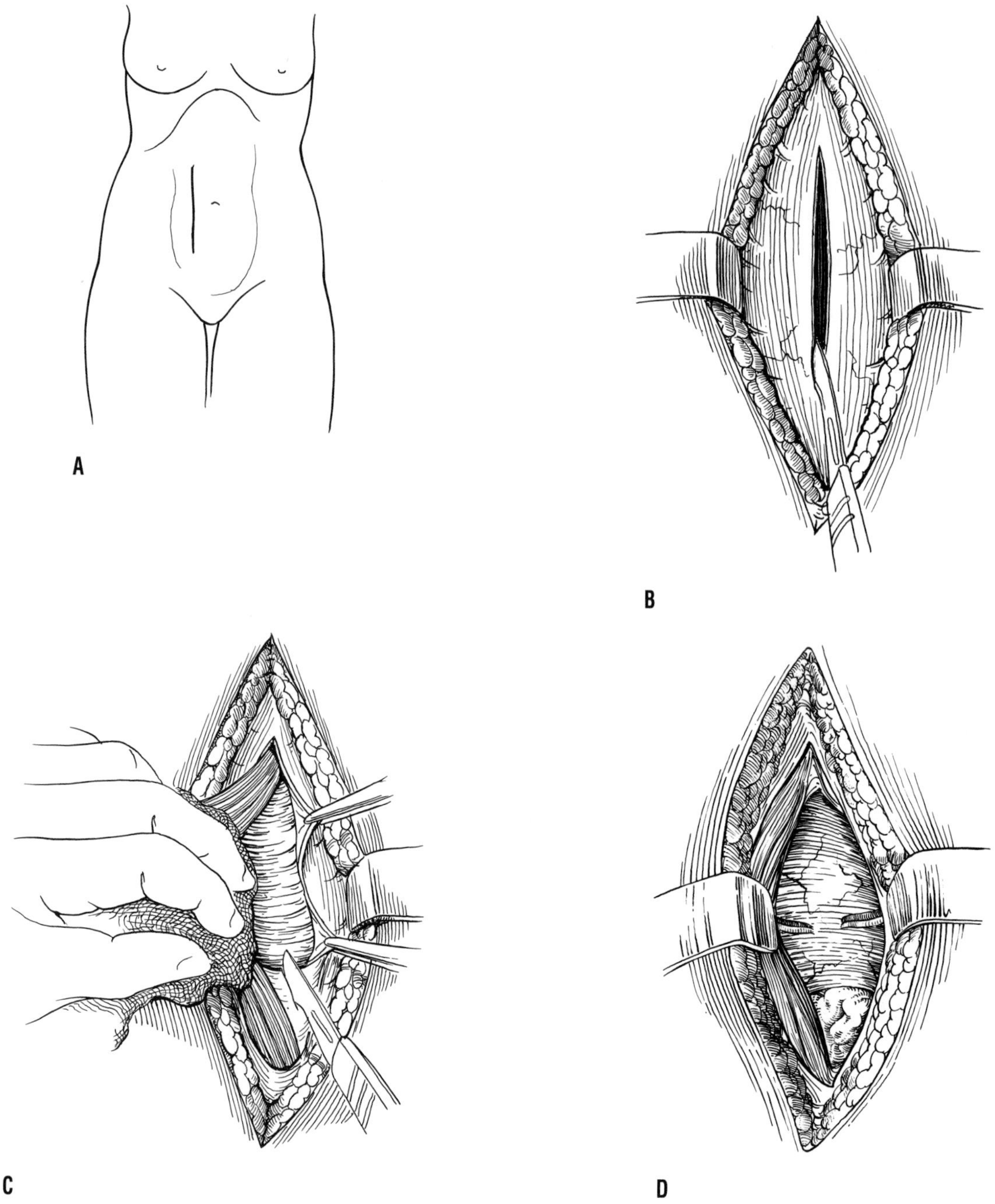

Figure 4–5. Lower paramedian incision. **A.** Surface markings. **B.** Incision of the rectus sheath. **C.** Retraction of the rectus abdominis muscle. **D.** Location of the branches of the inferior epigastric vessels that run across the lower portion of the incision. *Continued*

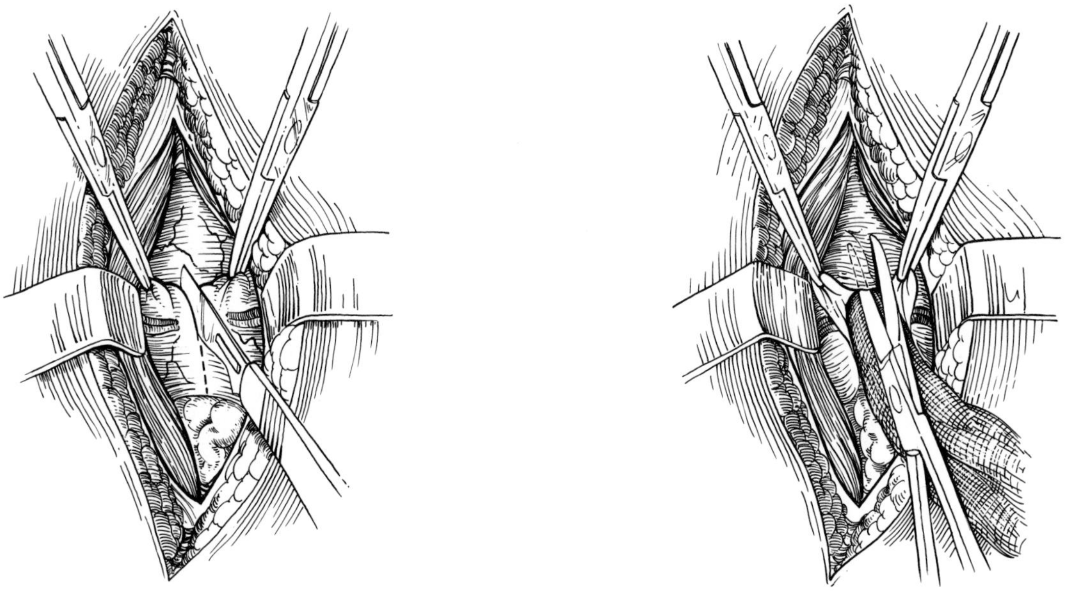

E F

Figure 4–5, cont'd. E. Peritoneum opened. **F.** The peritoneum is incised for the full length of the wound.

The standard subcostal incision commences in the midline about 2.5–5 cm below the xiphoid process (approximately one-third of the way between the xiphoid and the umbilicus). It is extended laterally and inferiorly about 2.5 cm below the costal margin for approximately 12 cm, although the length will vary with the build of the patient (Fig 4–7). The incision should leave sufficient room from the costal margin that if a hernia develops, adequate superior abdominal wall tissues are available for repair. The incision can be placed more inferior if the liver is enlarged. Following incision of the rectus sheath along the plane of the skin incision, the rectus muscle is divided using electrocautery or ligatures to control branches of the superior epigastric artery. The incision can be continued on to the lateral abdominal muscles for a short distance without ill effect. The eighth intercostal nerve may be encountered and divided, though care should be taken to preserve the ninth nerve. The incision is then taken through the peritoneum in the plane of the skin incision.

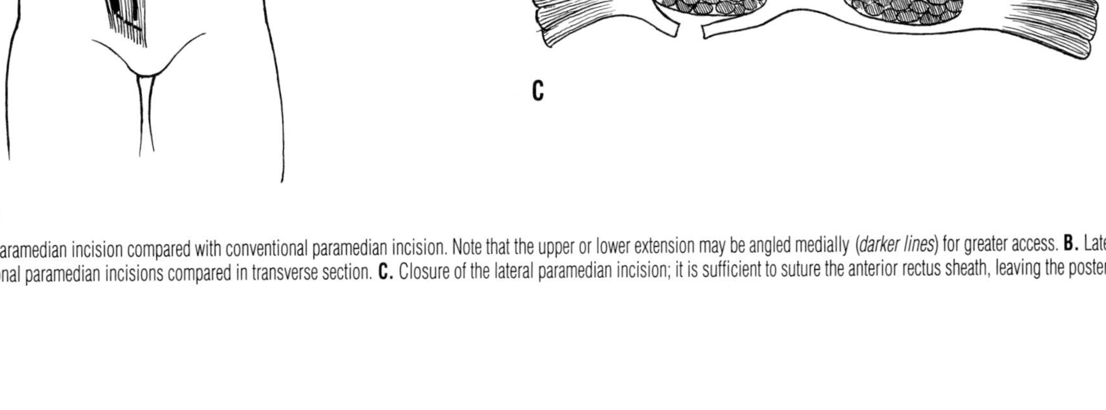

A B C

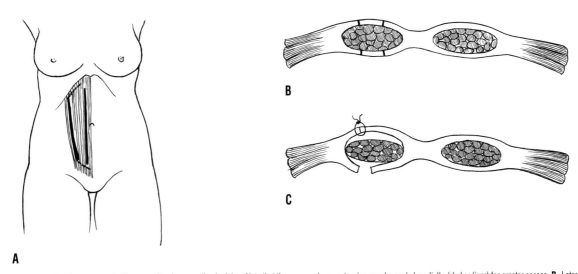

Figure 4–6. A. Lateral paramedian incision compared with conventional paramedian incision. Note that the upper or lower extension may be angled medially (*darker lines*) for greater access. **B.** Lateral paramedian and conventional paramedian incisions compared in transverse section. **C.** Closure of the lateral paramedian incision; it is sufficient to suture the anterior rectus sheath, leaving the posterior sheath open.

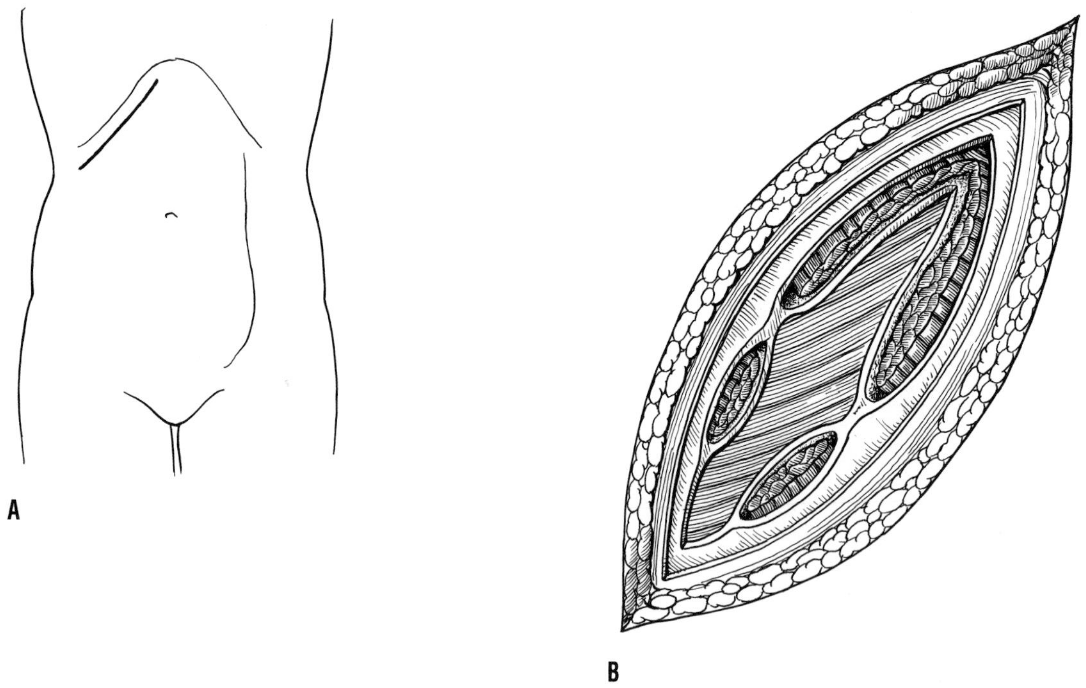

Figure 4–7. Kocher incision. **A.** Surface markings. **B.** Division of the rectus and medial portions of the lateral abdominal muscles.

The rectus muscle has a segmental nerve supply and a transverse or slightly oblique incision passes between adjacent nerves without injuring them. Provided its anterior and posterior sheaths are closed, the rectus muscle can be divided transversely without major weakness of the abdominal wall because it is not deprived of the distal part of its innervation. Healing of the incision results, effectively, in the formation of additional iatrogenic fibrous inscriptions of the muscle.

McBurney Gridiron and Rockey-Davis Muscle Splitting Incisions. Originally described by Charles McBurney in 1894,[17] the muscle-splitting right iliac fossa incision is well suited for appendectomy. The classic McBurney incision is made in an oblique direction. Most surgeons today use the Rockey-Davis incision. It is a modification of the time-honored McBurney incision that employs a cosmetically superior transverse incision in the line of the skin crease (Fig 4–8).

The suspected position of the appendix and the thickness of the abdominal wall will determine the level of the incision as well as its length. Careful palpation of a fully anesthetized patient will often reveal a mass, facilitating placement of the incision directly over the diseased appendix. If no mass is palpable, the incision is centered over McBurney's point at the junction of the middle and outer thirds of the line projecting from the umbilicus to the anterior superior iliac spine. If the patient is obese, or if extension of the incision is anticipated, the incision should be placed obliquely, better enabling lateral extension as a muscle-cutting incision.

Each muscular layer of the abdominal wall is sequentially split in the direction of its muscle fibers. This is accomplished with the use of closed Kelly hemostats inserted in the center of each muscle and opened perpendicular to the direction of fibers. The surgeon's index finger can also be used to gingerly open the muscles. After skin and subcutaneous tissues are incised, the external oblique aponeurosis is ex-

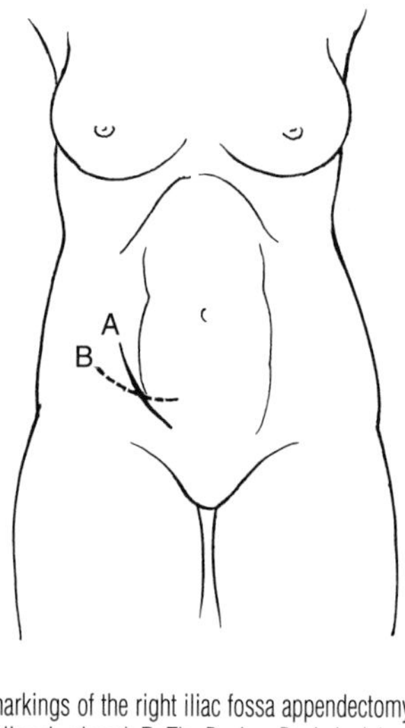

Figure 4–8. Surface markings of the right iliac fossa appendectomy incisions. **A.** The classic McBurney incision is obliquely placed. **B.** The Rockey-Davis incision is transversely placed in a skin crease.

posed and divided in the "hands-in-pockets" direction of its fibers to reveal the underlying internal oblique muscle. At a point adjacent to the lateral border of the rectus sheath, a small incision is made in the internal oblique muscle which is then opened in the direction of its fibers. Once the underlying transversalis muscle is exposed, it is split in a similar manner to reveal the transversalis fascia and peritoneum. The peritoneum is entered by picking up a fold of its tissue and nicking it with a blade. It is stretched with inserted index fingers and the appendix and cecum are exposed (Fig 4–9).

If further exposure is necessary, the wound can be enlarged by dividing the anterior sheath in line with

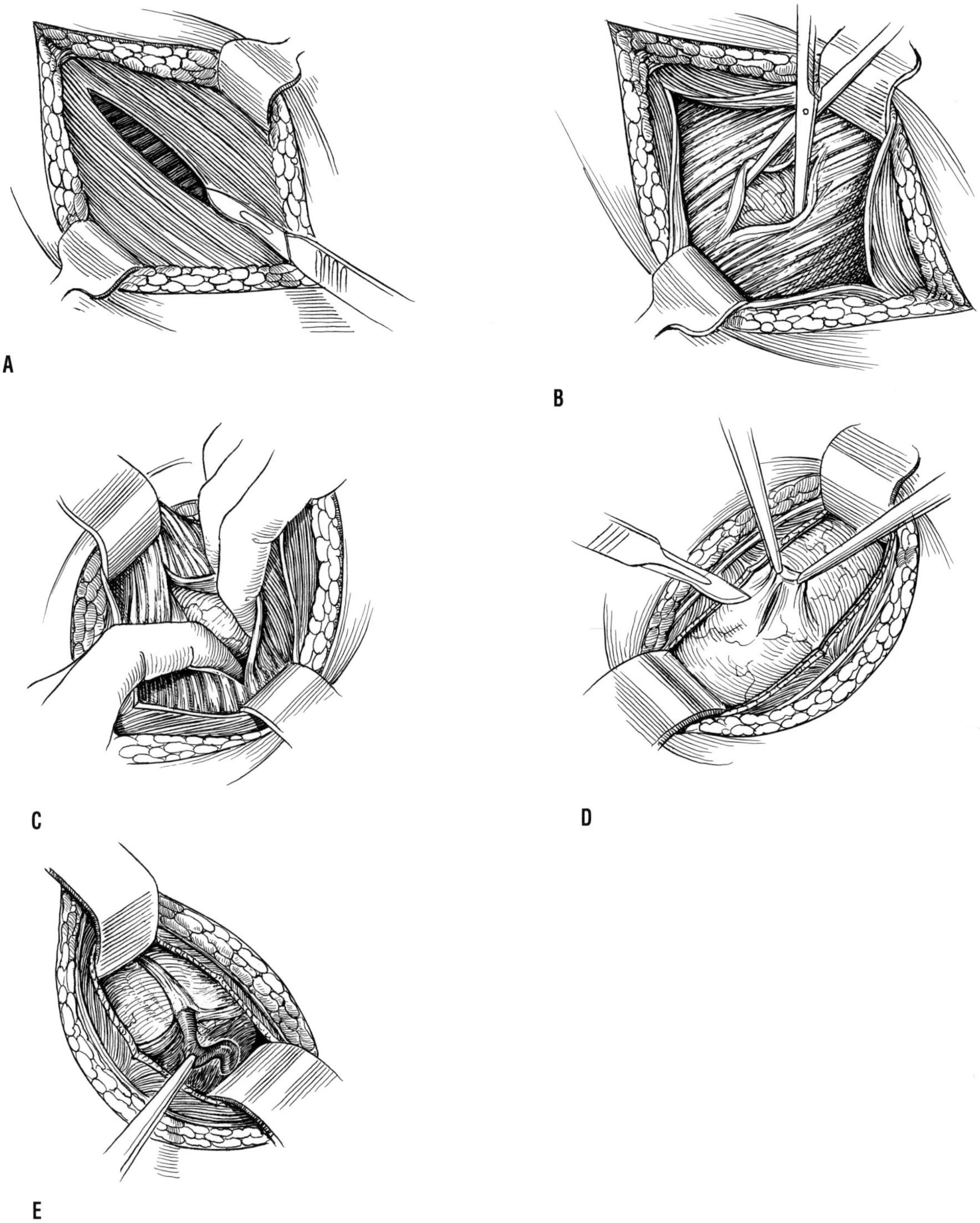

Figure 4–9. McBurney muscle-splitting incision. **A.** Division of the external oblique aponeurosis. **B.** The internal oblique and transversus muscles are split. **C.** The index fingers of each hand enlarge the opening. **D.** Incision of the peritoneum. **E.** Exposure of the appendix.

the incision, retracting the rectus muscle medially, and extending the peritoneal defect medially into the posterior rectus sheath. If the operation demands enlargement of the wound laterally (Weir extension), this can be accomplished by division of the oblique muscles superolaterally. This incision provides good access to the iliac fossa and can be exercised for a right- or left-sided hemicolectomy, cecostomy, or sigmoid colostomy. Medial and lateral extension of the McBurney incision bears the name the Rutherford-Morrison incision.

Pfannenstiel Incision. The Pfannenstiel incision is used frequently for gynecologic operations and for access to the retropubic space in the male for extraperitoneal retropubic prostatectomy. The skin incision is placed in the curving interspinous crease that lies approximately 5 cm superior to the symphysis pubis. It usually carried out for about 12 cm in length. Both anterior rectus sheaths are exposed and divided transversely for the entire length of the wound. Hemostat clamps are applied to the superior and inferior leaflets of the divided sheath that are widely separated from the underlying rectus muscles superiorly to the umbilicus and inferiorly to the pubic symphysis. The recti are retracted laterally and the peritoneum is opened vertically in the midline. Care must be taken to protect the bladder at the lower end of the wound (Fig 4–10). Exposure provided by the Pfannenstiel incision is somewhat limited and it should not be used when a procedure outside of the pelvis is anticipated. An advantage of this incision is

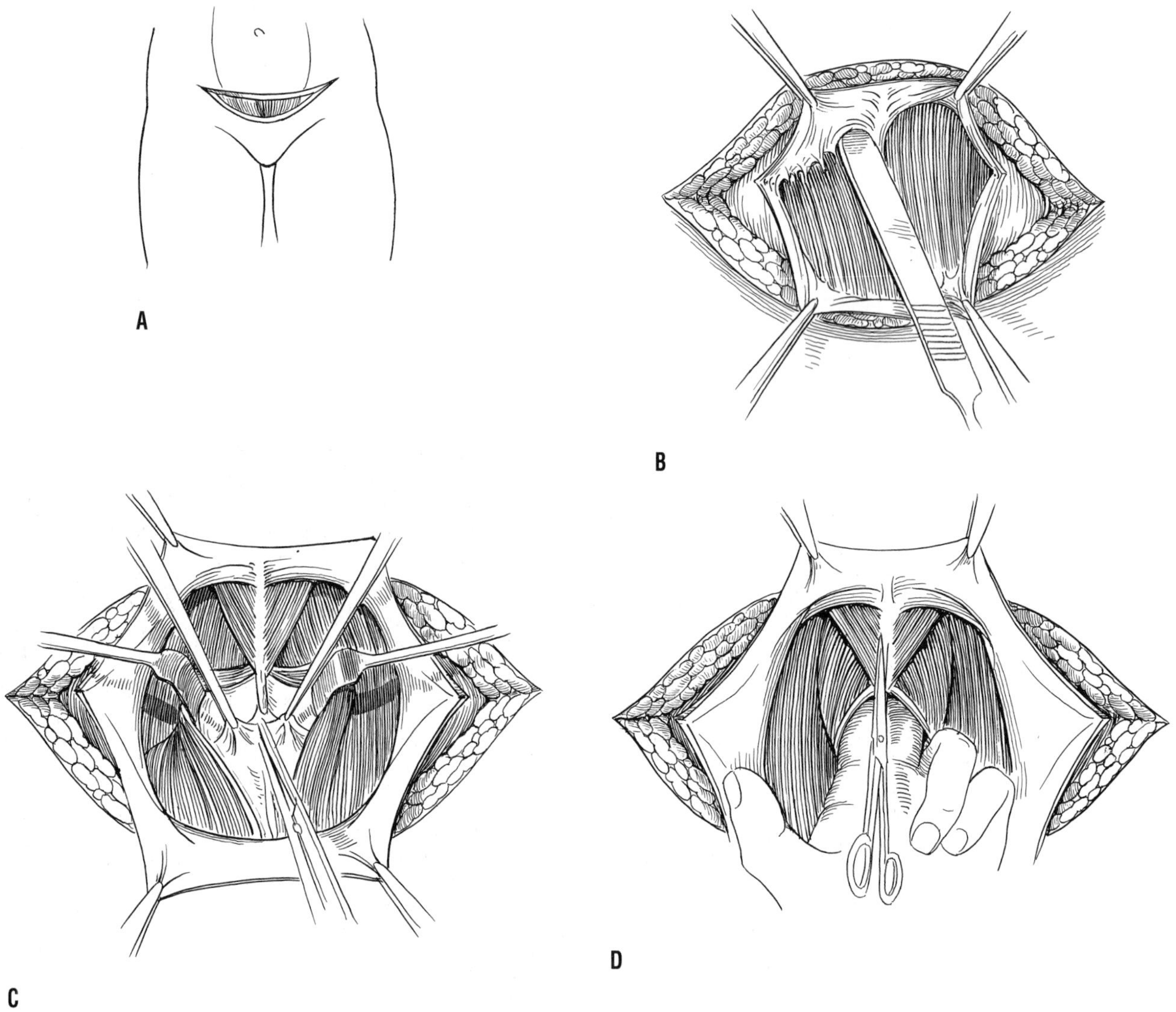

Figure 4–10. Pfannenstiel incision. **A.** Skin incision. **B.** Horizontal division of the anterior rectus sheath and developing fascial flap. **C.** Dividing in the midline and entering the peritoneal cavity. **D.** Opening midline. *Continued*

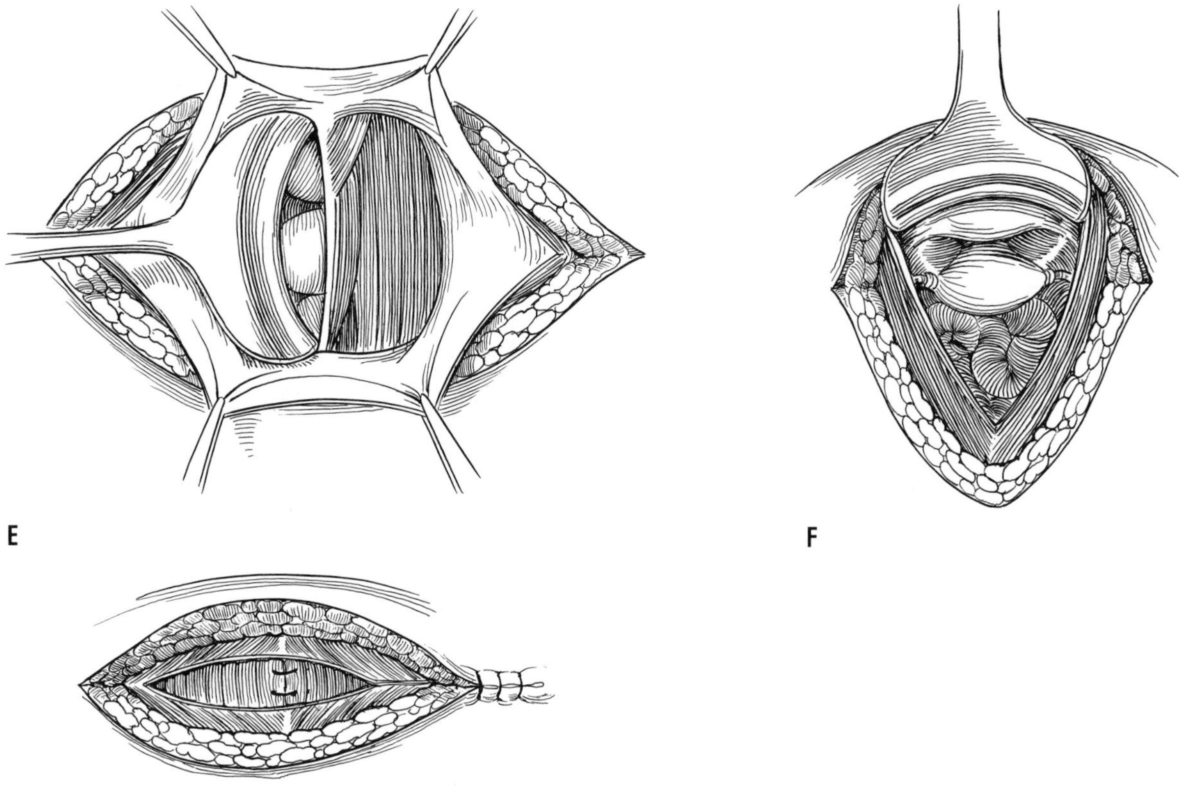

E

F

G

Figure 4–10, cont'd. E. Lateral retractors are placed for exposure. **F.** Inferior retractors placed for exposure. **G.** Closure midline and inferior rectus.

that it leaves an almost invisible scar because it is placed in a skin crease and is partially hidden by pubic hair.

Abdominothoracic Incisions

The thoracoabdominal incision provides excellent exposure by converting the peritoneal and pleural spaces into one common cavity. The left thoracoabdominal incision is particularly useful for access to the left hemidiaphragm, gastroesophageal junction, gastric cardia and stomach, distal pancreas and spleen, left kidney and adrenal gland, and aorta. The right thoracoabdominal incision is used effectively for operations on the right hemidiaphragm, upper esophagus, liver, hepatic triad, inferior vena cava, right kidney and adrenal gland, and the proximal pancreas. When the operation can safely be performed through an abdominal incision, this is preferable, as morbidity is increased with the opening of the two cavities. Some of the more commonly encountered anatomic complications to be avoided include splenic injury and phrenic nerve injury with subsequent diaphragmatic dysfunction.

The patient is placed in the "corkscrew" position on the operating room table for maximal access into both the abdominal and thoracic cavities. The abdomen is tilted approximately 45 degrees from the horizontal by using sandbags, and the thorax is twisted into the full lateral position (Fig 4–11A). The abdominal part of the incision may consist of a midline or upper paramedian incision, which allows preliminary exploration of the abdomen. In patients with cancer of the lower esophagus or stomach, completion of the abdominal portion of the incision is advised to determine resectability before extending the incision to enter the thorax. An obliquely placed limb of the abdominal incision is then added to continue along the line of the eighth interspace, identified easily where it is immediately caudal to the inferior pole of the scapula (Fig 4–11B). Alternatively, an oblique upper abdominal incision can be used and continued directly into the thoracic incision.

After the abdomen is explored, the chest incision is deepened through the latissimus dorsi and serratus anterior muscles, and then the external oblique muscle and aponeurosis. The intercostal muscles of the eighth interspace are divided to enter the pleural cavity and the incision is continued across the costal margin, which is divided with a scalpel. It is often useful at this point to resect a short segment of costal cartilage

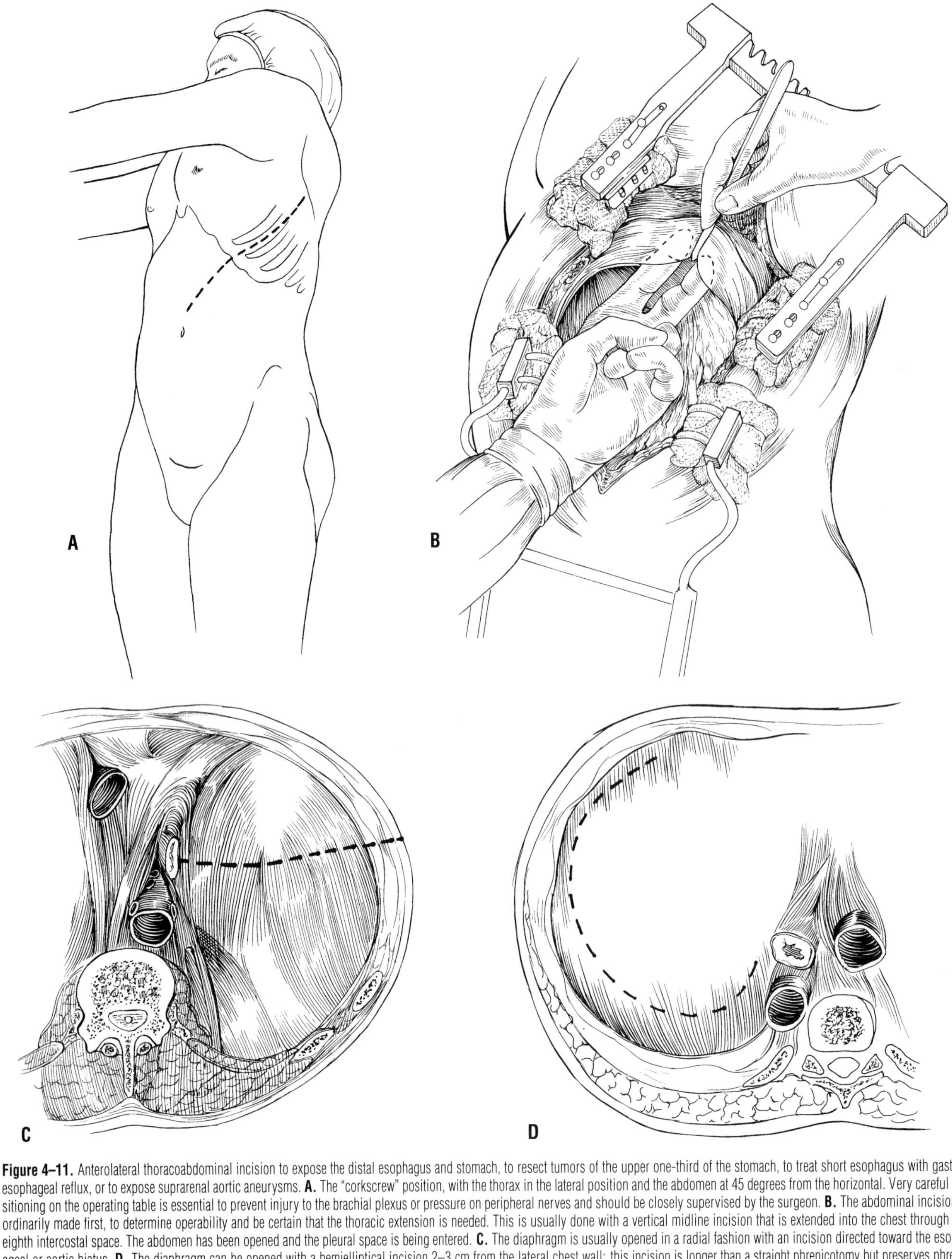

Figure 4–11. Anterolateral thoracoabdominal incision to expose the distal esophagus and stomach, to resect tumors of the upper one-third of the stomach, to treat short esophagus with gastroesophageal reflux, or to expose suprarenal aortic aneurysms. **A.** The "corkscrew" position, with the thorax in the lateral position and the abdomen at 45 degrees from the horizontal. Very careful positioning on the operating table is essential to prevent injury to the brachial plexus or pressure on peripheral nerves and should be closely supervised by the surgeon. **B.** The abdominal incision is ordinarily made first, to determine operability and be certain that the thoracic extension is needed. This is usually done with a vertical midline incision that is extended into the chest through the eighth intercostal space. The abdomen has been opened and the pleural space is being entered. **C.** The diaphragm is usually opened in a radial fashion with an incision directed toward the esophageal or aortic hiatus. **D.** The diaphragm can be opened with a hemielliptical incision 2–3 cm from the lateral chest wall; this incision is longer than a straight phrenicotomy but preserves phrenic nerve function, of importance in patients with chronic pulmonary disease or less than optimal pulmonary function. (Reproduced, with permission, from Penn I, Baker RJ. Abdominal wall incisions and repair. In: Baker RJ, Fischer JE (eds). *Mastery of Surgery*, 4th ed. Philadelphia, PA: Lippincott Williams & Wilkins; 2001:197.)

to facilitate closure of the chest wall. A Finochietto self-retaining rib retractor is inserted and the intercostal space and is gently spread. Rib resection to gain exposure is rarely necessary. The diaphragm is incised radially toward the esophageal or aortic hiatus, isolating and tying branches of the phrenic vessels before their division. If the operation does not require a radial incision of the diaphragm to the esophageal hiatus, the diaphragm should be divided in a curvilinear fashion 2–3 cm from its attachment to the chest wall. This hemielliptical incision will preserve phrenic nerve function and is useful for patients with less than optimal pulmonary function.[18]

At completion of the operation, chest tubes placed in the pleural cavity are brought out of the thorax through separate stab incisions. The diaphragm is repaired in two layers using nonabsorbable mattress sutures. Pericostal sutures are passed around the ribs and the chest muscles and abdominal wall are closed in layers.

Retroperitoneal and Extraperitoneal Incisions

Retroperitoneal and extraperitoneal approaches to the abdomen have several advantages over intraperitoneal exposures. Manipulation and retraction of intraabdominal viscera is limited and postoperative ileus is reduced. Hemorrhage is more likely to be tamponaded in the retroperitoneum than when it occurs in the peritoneal cavity. Infection and extravasation of urine are more frequently localized here than within the peritoneal cavity and are more readily drainable. Retroperitoneal and extraperitoneal approaches can be used for operations on the kidney, ureter, adrenal gland, bladder, splenic artery and vein, groin hernias, vena cava, lumbar sympathetic chain, abdominal aorta, and common, internal, and external iliac vessels.

Retroperitoneal Approach to the Lumbar Area. The retroperitoneal approach to the lumbar area is frequently used in aortic surgery, nephrectomy, lumbar symphathectomy, and ureterolithomy. The patient is positioned with the operative side elevated 30–45 degrees with knee and hip flexed. The incision is carried from the level of the umbilicus at the lateral margin of the rectus sheath toward the twelfth rib for approximately 12–14 cm (Fig 4–12). A portion of the twelfth rib is resected if further exposure is required, taking care not to injure

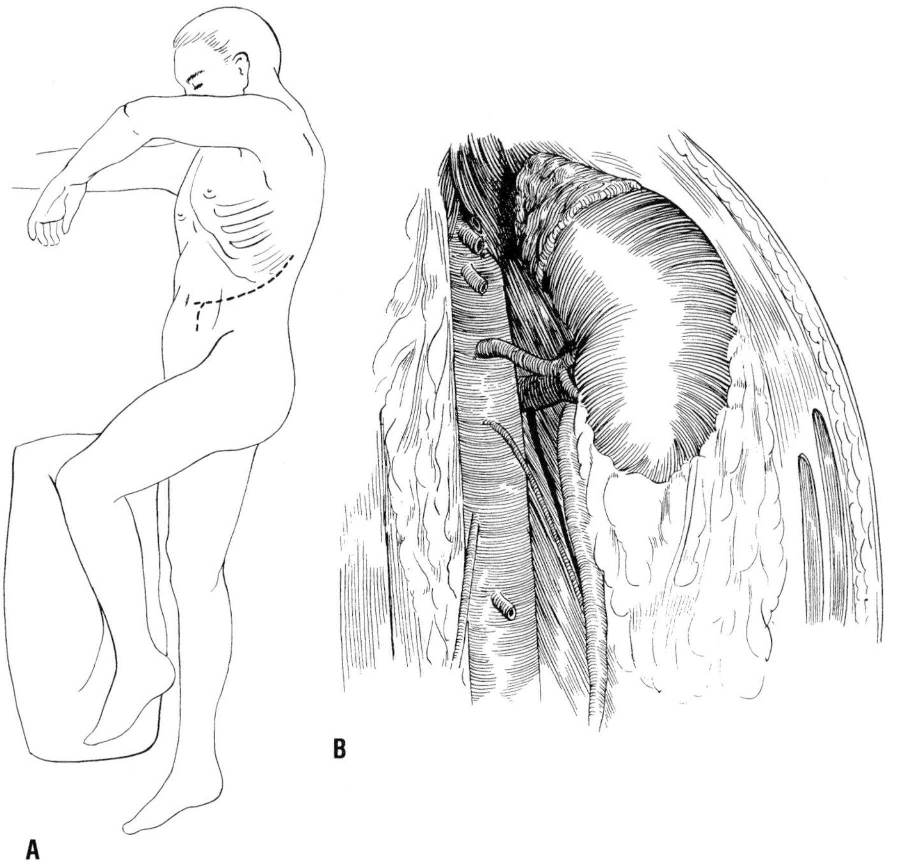

Figure 4–12. A. Left lumbar approach to the retroperitoneum, specifically for exposing the kidney, adrenal, and infrarenal abdominal aorta. **B.** The peritoneum has been bluntly dissected from the retroperitoneal structures with the preperitoneal fat and soft tissue. Origins of the celiac, superior mesenteric, left renal, and inferior mesenteric arteries are shown. (Reproduced, with permission, from Penn I, Baker RJ. Abdominal wall incisions and repair. In: Baker RJ, Fischer JE (eds). *Mastery of Surgery*, 4th ed. Philadelphia, PA: Lippincott Williams & Wilkins; 2001:194.)

the underlying pleura. The external oblique, internal oblique, and transversalis muscles are exposed, undermined, and opened in the direction of their fibers. The retroperitoneum is entered and the peritoneum and retroperitoneal fat are moved anteriorly by blunt dissection, being mindful to not dissect behind the psoas muscle. The lower pole of the kidney, ureter, and sympathetic chain are easily identified. The vena cava is exposed on the right and the aorta on the left. If the peritoneum is unintentionally entered, it is closed immediately with continuous absorbable suture. At the conclusion of the procedure, the retroperitoneal fat and viscera fall back into place and the muscles of the abdominal wall are repaired in layers.

Posterior Approach to the Adrenal Glands. With the posterior approach, dissection is performed entirely in the retroperitoneal space. Excellent exposure of the right adrenal vein and inferior vena cava is achieved. Inadvertent injury to the viscera or spleen is minimized and postoperative ileus is rare. Importantly, patients have decreased pain, fewer pulmonary complications, and shorter hospital stays than patients undergoing transabdominal adrenalectomy.

The patient is laid in the prone jackknife position. A curvilinear incision is made beginning on the tenth rib approximately three fingerbreadths lateral to the midline and carried inferiorly and laterally toward the iliac crest, ending approximately four fingerbreadths lateral to the midline (Fig 4–13). The subcutaneous tissues are divided to reveal the posterior layer of the lumbodorsal fascia. This fascia and the fibers of the latissimus dorsi muscle which originate from it are divided. The erector spinae muscle is exposed and retracted medially to uncover the twelfth rib and the glistening middle layer of the lumbodorsal fascia. The attachments of the erector spinae to the twelfth rib are divided with electrocautery, securing with clamps and ligating the vessels and nerves that penetrate the fascia to enter the erector spinae muscle. The twelfth rib is then resected periosteally, taking care not to injure the underlying pleura. Gerota's fascia is exposed by incising the lumbodorsal fascia along the lateral margin of the quadratus lumborum muscle. The intercostal neurovascular bundle should now become visible directly below the bed of the resected twelfth rib. The intercostal vessels are clamped, divided, and ligated and the intercostal nerve is gently retracted downward. The posterior fibers of the diaphragm where they insert on the periosteum of the twelfth rib are identified and divided. The lower margin of the lung will enter the field with hyperinflation. The pleura is pushed gently away. If it is inadvertently entered, the resulting pneumothorax is handled at closure by insertion of a large-bore rubber catheter into the pleural cavity and exiting through the wound. After closure of the fascial fibers around the catheter, the lung is hyperinflated evacuating all air from the pleural space, and the catheter is briskly removed.

Retroperitoneal Approach to the Iliac Fossa. The retroperitoneal approach to the iliac fossa provides access to the bladder, distal ureter, and common, internal, and external iliac vessels. It is often employed for surgery on the iliac arteries and for kidney transplantation into the iliac fossa. It is also used to drain psoas or retrocecal abscesses and to resect localized retroperitoneal tumors. The skin incision is an oblique incision extending from approximately 2 cm above the anterosuperior iliac spine to just lateral to the pubic symphysis (Fig 4–14) and can be extended superiorly as far as the costal margin if necessary. The external oblique, internal oblique, and transverse abdominis muscles are divided in line with the skin incision. The external and internal inguinal rings lie inferior to the lower edge of the incision and are not visualized. The retroperitoneal area is entered and the retroperitoneal fat and peritoneum are bluntly dissected and retracted superomedially. If the peritoneum is inadvertently entered, it is closed immediately. Closure of each muscular and fascial layer is achieved with absorbable or nonabsorbable suture in either continuous or interrupted fashion.

▪ CLOSURE OF THE ABDOMINAL INCISION

Closure of the abdominal wall is a common denominator of all abdominal surgery. It is one of the first things that a surgeon is taught during his or her training. The methods of closure are often based on local traditions and the preferences of the teacher, and the surgeon is often reluctant to change these methods later on in his or her career. Abdominal closure is performed in a multitude of fashions and there are an abundance of differently tailored studies on this matter.

The goal of wound closure is to restore function of the abdominal wall after a surgical procedure. The optimal method should be so technically simple that its results are as good for the hands of the trainee as they are for the experienced surgeon. It should leave the patient with a reasonably aesthetic scar, and most importantly, it should minimize the frequency of wound rupture, incisional hernia, wound infection, and sinus formation.

CLOSURE OF THE PERITONEUM

Traditional surgical dogma has taught that because all tissue layers of the abdominal wall are violated when an abdominal incision is made, all layers should be approximated when the incision is closed. Closure of the peritoneum is based on the premise that normal anatomy will be restored, the risks of infection and wound herniation

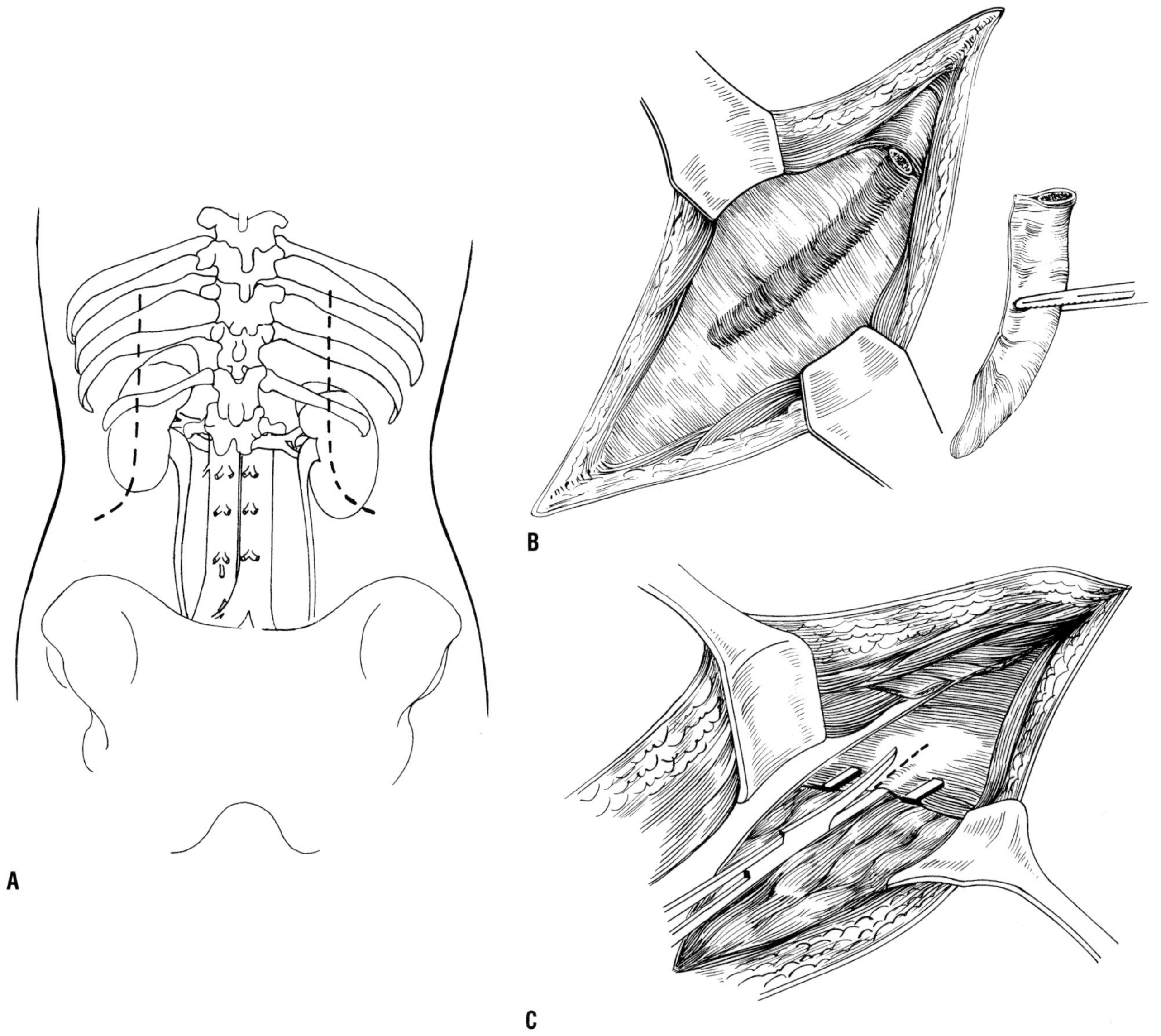

Figure 4–13. The posterior approach to the kidney and adrenal. **A.** J-shaped incision over the tenth to twelfth ribs, extending inferiorly 6–10 cm below the twelfth rib. **B.** Resection of the twelfth rib facilitates exposure. **C.** The diaphragmatic attachment to the twelfth rib is taken down, with care taken not to enter the pleura. If the pleura is opened, the wound closure is done over a pleural suction catheter, which is removed with simultaneous positive airway pressure by the anesthetist as the skin is being closed. (Reproduced, with permission, from Penn I, Baker RJ. Abdominal wall incisions and repair. In: Baker RJ, Fischer JE (eds). *Mastery of Surgery*, 4th ed. Philadelphia, PA: Lippincott Williams & Wilkins; 2001:195.)

will be reduced, and adhesions will be minimized. Experience has questioned these surgical principles in the face of randomized controlled clinical trials. In 1977, Ellis and Heddle first reported their results of a randomized study comparing closure and nonclosure of the parietal peritoneum in a vertical laparotomy incision. No difference was found in the incidence of wound dehiscence or hernia between the nonclosure arm (3.0% and 4.3%, respectively) and the closure arm (2.5% and 4.3%, respectively).[19] Similar results are found in randomized trials comparing closure versus nonclosure of the peritoneum in open cholecystectomy incisions,[20] lateral paramedian incisions,[21] and gynecologic and obstetric incisions.[22] It is concluded that closure of the peritoneum is unnecessary and not recommended. It is associated with a slightly longer operative time and more postoperative pain, and there are some suggestions that it may cause increased formation of adhesions.[22]

CLOSURE OF THE FASCIA

Closure of the abdomen can be done in layers or en mass. A layered closure technique reconstructs the anterior and posterior aponeurotic sheaths in two different layers with the posterior layer generally incorporating the peritoneum. Mass closure involves a single-layer closure of all musculofascial layers and may or may not

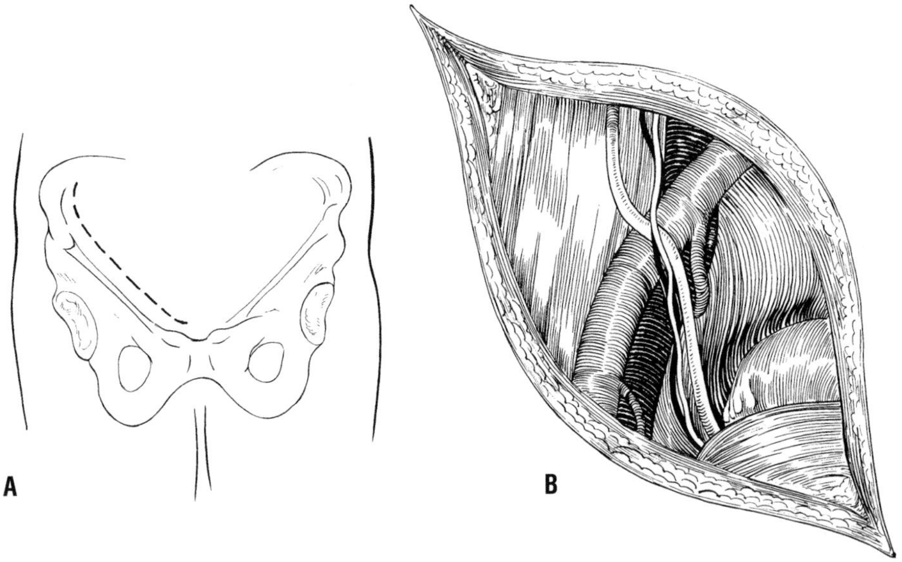

Figure 4–14. Right lower quadrant extraperitoneal approach to the iliac vessels, ureter, and bladder, used for renal transplant, but also very useful to expose the iliac artery and vein, drain psoas or retrocecal abscesses, or resect localized retroperitoneal tumors. **A.** The skin incision may be shorter than depicted in thinner patients or if an abscess is to be drained. **B.** Peritoneum is retracted medially by blunt dissection, which exposes the psoas muscle and gonadal artery and vein, shown anterior to the ureter. (Reproduced, with permission, from Penn I, Baker RJ. Abdominal wall incisions and repair. In: Baker RJ, Fischer JE (eds). *Mastery of Surgery*, 4th ed. Philadelphia, PA: Lippincott Williams & Wilkins; 2001:196.)

include the peritoneum. Numerous clinical trials have compared layered to mass abdominal closure. Some studies have shown an increased incidence of burst abdomen and incisional hernia with layered closure,[23–25] and some studies show no difference in these complications,[26] but no studies demonstrate an advantage of layered over mass closure. Rates of wound sepsis and sinus formation have also been studied in randomized trials and do not depend on closure technique.

It has been claimed that a continuous, running suture will result in more secure wound closure than a series of sutures placed in an interrupted fashion. The theoretical advantage of a continuous closure is the distribution of tension differences across the suture line and the ability of the wound to adjust to the stresses and strains of the postoperative period. This should minimize tissue strangulation and wound rupture from suture under strain cutting through fascia. The disadvantage of the continuous closure method is that a single thread holds the fascia together and its breakage jeopardizes the entire wound. Clinical evidence, however, demonstrates that continuous and interrupted closures of the abdomen are responsible for similar incidences of wound dehiscence, incisional hernia, wound infection, wound pain, and suture fistula.[27–31]

The use of resorbable versus nonresorbable suture in closing the fascia has long been debated. Rates of 17% for scar pain and 8% for suture fistula using permanent suture[27] have stirred interest in the use of resorbable sutures. Resorbable sutures, however, bear an intrinsic loss of tensile strength during the vulnerable postoperative period, and may result in an increase in wound disruption and ventral hernia. The early use of the absorbable catgut suture has been shown to lead to a high incidence of wound rupture and incisional hernia due to its early degradation.[26] To overcome this problem, synthetic absorbable sutures with delayed degradation were introduced to combine the advantages of absorbability with strength comparable to nonabsorbable materials. There are conflicting reports in the literature about wound failure when nonabsorbable and absorbable suture are compared in randomized clinical trials. The resorbable sutures polyglycolic acid (Dexon), polyglactic acid (Vicryl), polydioxanone (PDS), and polyglyconate (Maxon) have been shown to be equally as effective as nonabsorbable suture with respect to wound dehiscence and incisional hernia.[32–35] Other studies, however, demonstrate that polydioxanone and polyglactic acid polymer absorbable suture may be associated with an increased incidence of incisional hernia when weighed against nonabsorbable suture.[25,27]

Another choice is monofilament versus multifilament suture. Multifilament suture is known to provide a better growth environment for bacteria and is associated with a higher incidence of wound sepsis when compared to monofilament suture.[25,33] Bacteria are drawn into the fibers of multifilament suture by capillary action and thrive there by escaping phagocytosis. Wound sepsis is a major risk factor for incisional hernia, but despite these considerations, multifilament suture has not been shown to result in a greater incidence of wound failure over monofilament closure.[23,30] Monofilament catgut suture also deserves special consideration. It is a reactive material that causes a marked inflammatory reaction and is associated with a higher incidence of wound infection than other monofilament materials.[36]

Our experience and interpretation of the literature is that the optimal surgical method of closing the abdominal wound is a continuous mass closure. This technique appears to reduce the incidence of wound rupture, is considerably less time consuming,[28,37] is less expensive, and does not increase the incidence of incisional hernia, wound infection, or sinus formation. The choice of suture material is more complex. We prefer to use a resorbable suture with delayed degradation, such as polydioxanone. Other resorbable materials are appropriate as well, but catgut should not be used. Among nonresorbable sutures, monofilament suture is recommended.

Method of Mass Closure of the Abdomen

Whether the incision is vertical or transverse, the steps for closure are more or less the same. It is now fully realized that healing of the wound takes place by formation of a dense fibrous scar that unites the opposing faces of the wound en mass. The purpose of the suture is to approximate the wound edges while this dense fibrous scar deposits and matures.

For closure of the midline laparotomy incision, we employ two size 0 looped polydioxanone (PDS) sutures. One loop is used at the upper extremity and one at the lower extremity of the wound so that only one knot need be tied at the middle of the incision. The needle is passed securely through the vertex of the fascial incision and by passing the needle though the loop, the end of the suture line is anchored firmly to the abdominal wall. A medium-width metal ribbon is often placed into the peritoneal cavity to ensure a clear field for suturing and to avoid incorporating visceral structures into the suture line. The suture is run in a continuous manner, taking full-thickness bites of the linea alba fascia incorporating components of the anterior and posterior rectus aponeuroses (Fig 4–15). The peritoneum need not be incorporated into the closure. Wide bites are taken a minimum of 1 cm from the wound edge and placed at 1-cm intervals. To reserve an adequate length of suture in the wound, the suture length should measure at least four times the length of the wound.[38] This should prevent the cutting out of sutures that may occur during abdominal distention and dynamic tensile changes that occur on the postoperative wound.

A similar technique is used for closure of the paramedian incision. The anterior and posterior rectus sheaths are picked up and included in one bite (Fig 4–16). A transrectus incision will incorporate the medial sliver of rectus muscle into the suture loops. Mass closure of a lateral paramedian incision is not possible. For this incision, the anterior and posterior rectus sheaths are closed separately. We prefer to close the Kocher subcostal incision in two layers, closing the posterior rectus sheath with a continuous absorbable suture and the anterior sheath with a separate, running nonabsorbable suture. Rockey-Davis muscle-splitting incisions are also closed in layers. The peritoneum can be closed with continuous absorbable suture to exclude the viscera from the field. The internal oblique and transversalis muscles are closed as a single layer with interrupted absorbable suture and the aponeurosis of the external oblique is then closed with a continuous absorbable suture. The skin is left open if intraperitoneal purulence or a gangrenous appendix was present.

SUBCUTANEOUS TISSUE CLOSURE

With the high prevalence of obesity in developed countries, treatment of the subcutaneous tissues in abdominal wound closure becomes increasingly important. The vascular supply to the subcutaneous tissue of the abdominal wall is poor, rendering it susceptible to soft-tissue infection. Likewise, if this level of the abdominal wall contains a potential space promoting accumulation of seroma, the risk of infection increases.

Only one prospective randomized trial has been conducted to determine the value of suturing the subcutaneous fat. Using a subcostal incision for cholecystectomy, the authors demonstrated no significant differences in complications between closure and nonclosure of the subcutaneous tissues.[39] Wound seepage, however, was reduced in incisions in which the subcutaneous layer was closed. Two randomized controlled clinical trials of cesarean section incisions have produced different results. Suture closure of the subcutaneous layer resulted in a significant decrease in the rates of wound disruption (14.5%) when compared to wounds in which the subcutaneous layer is left open (26.6%).[40] A separate trial failed to demonstrate any benefit of suture closure in wounds with less than 2 cm of subcutaneous tissue, but confirm the reduction in wound disruption in wounds with greater than 2 cm of tissue.[41]

Some authors have speculated that reduction of serous fluid in the subcutaneous dead space by placement of closed-system subcutaneous tissue drains would reduce the risk of wound complications. Prospective ran-

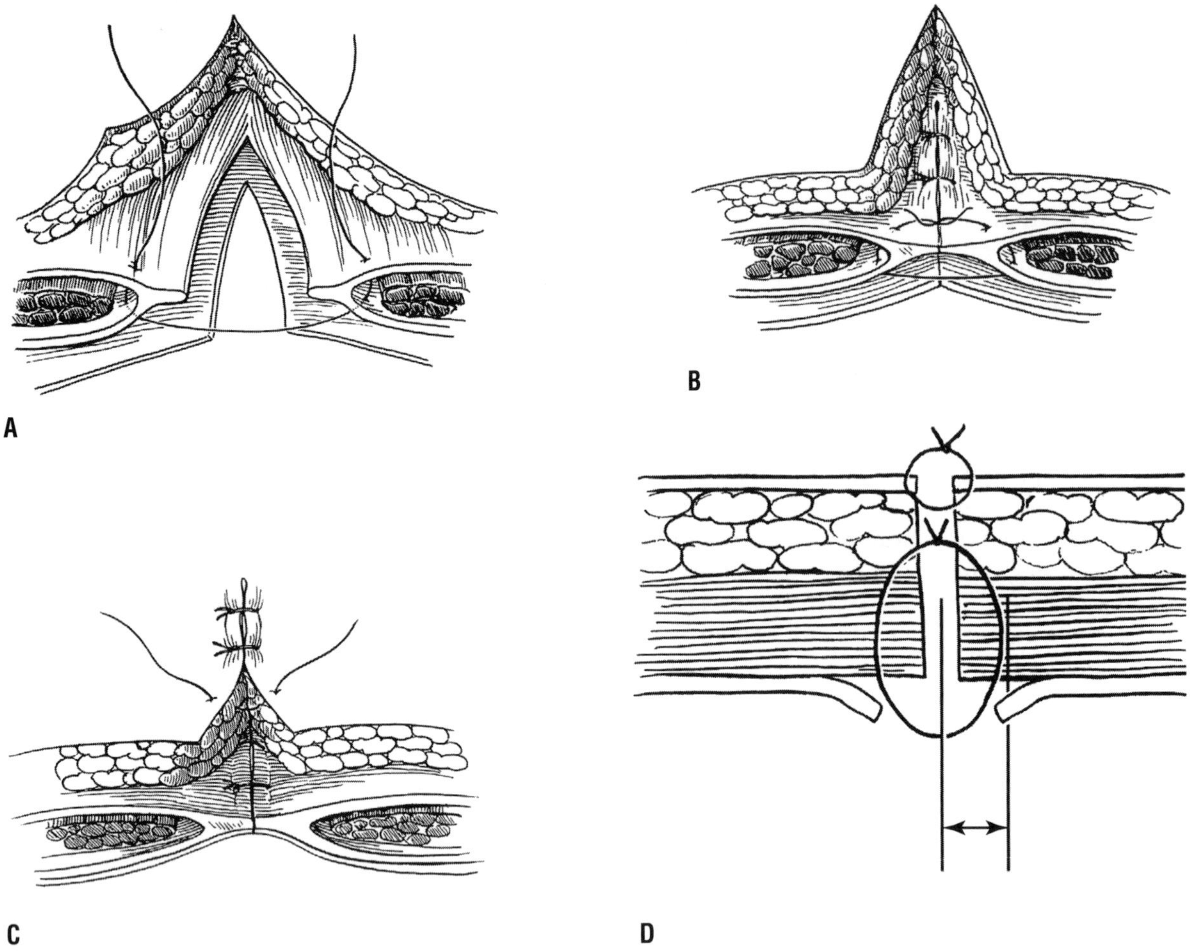

Figure 4–15. Stages in the mass closure of the midline abdominal incision.

domized clinical data from the general surgical literature do not support the use of these devices.[42,43]

We do not routinely close the subcutaneous layer of the wound. On some occasions, in obese patients, we will employ the use a series of simple, interrupted, absorbable polyglactic acid (vicryl) sutures to reapproximate the subcutaneous layer. These stitches are inverted to bury the knots within the wound.

SKIN CLOSURE

If the surgical site is heavily contaminated (class III or class IV wound), the skin should be left open to heal by secondary intention or by delayed primary skin closure.[44] A number of closure techniques for clean (class I) and clean-contaminated (class II) wounds are available for the skin. These include interrupted suture, subcuticular suture, surgical staples, surgical tape, and adhesive glues. Goals of skin closure are tissue approximation, minimizing wound infection, acceptable cosmesis, and minimizing postoperative pain. These goals should be achieved with a simple, rapid, and cost-effective method.

Three randomized controlled studies have compared skin staples to subcuticular sutures. In all studies, no difference in the rate of wound infection could be demon-

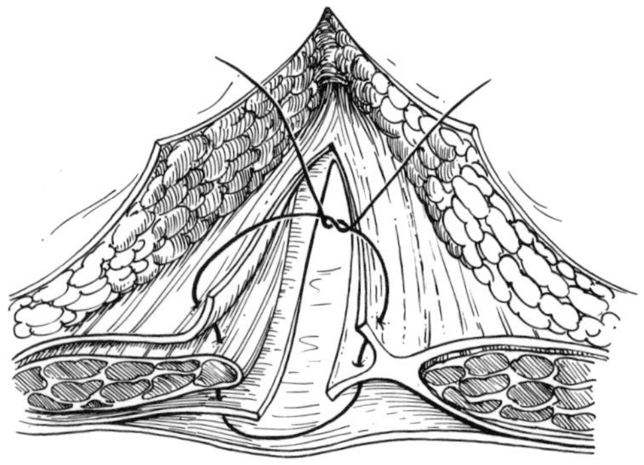

Figure 4–16. Mass closure of the paramedian incision.

strated.[45–47] Two of these studies revealed less postoperative pain and less postoperative analgesia requirement in wounds closed with subcuticular suture.[45,46] Two of these studies also demonstrated a superior cosmetic result in subcuticular closures over surgical staples; however, this cosmetic difference narrowed over time and became insignificant by 6 months.[46,47]

Adhesive tapes are often used to reapproximate skin edges in simple lacerations. Following abdominal surgery, adhesive tapes are useful to cover skin incisions closed by subcuticular suture, where they serve to further reapproximate skin edges and to dress the wound. The use of adhesive tape without suture closure was compared to interrupted silk skin suturing of abdominal wounds in one early trial. No difference in the rates of wound infection could be found. The tapes were significantly more comfortable and patients preferred them over sutures, but wide scarring occurred more frequently with surgical tapes.[48]

Synthetic glues are gaining popularity in skin closure of surgical wounds. When compared with traditional skin-closing devices including sutures, staples, or adhesive tapes, some cyanoacrylate glues have been found to be comparable in effectiveness and safety for repair of lacerations. They are applied more rapidly and decrease the amount of required wound care by serving as their own dressings. In elective abdominal procedures with small and large (>4 cm) incisions, these glues have been shown in clinical trials to have similar outcomes with respect to wound durability when compared to traditional techniques,[49,50] although there are conflicting data on wound healing, cosmesis, and postoperative pain.[50,51]

We prefer to close skin with a running, nonbraided, absorbable suture in a subcuticular technique. Adhesive tapes are placed over the closed incision without the use of skin glues.

PROPHYLACTIC DRAINAGE OF THE ABDOMEN

Prophylactic operative drains are employed to remove intraperitoneal collections such as blood, bile, ascites, chyle, and pancreatic or intestinal juice. Drains are also placed to signal early complications such as postoperative hemorrhage and leakage of intestinal suture lines. Prophylactic drainage of the abdomen is used routinely by gastrointestinal surgeons around the world. There are, however, good randomized controlled data to question their utility.

A recent systematic review and meta-analyses were performed to determine the evidence-based value of prophylactic drainage in gastrointestinal surgery.[52] There is evidence of level 1 quality that operatively-placed drains do not reduce complications after elective hepatic resection,[52–55] cholecystectomy,[56] pancreatic resection for cancer,[57] elective colonic or rectal resection with primary anastomosis,[52] and appendectomy for any stage of appendicitis.[52] One randomized controlled trial (evidence level 2b) has failed to show any benefit of prophylactic drainage after subtotal or total gastrectomy with extended lymph node dissection for gastric cancer.[58] However, in the absence of more complete prospective data on the use of abdominal drainage in upper gastrointestinal surgery, consensus opinion (evidence level 5) recommends that drains should be used in esophageal or gastric resections due to the potentially fatal outcome of anastomotic leak in these procedures.

When drains are used in abdominal surgery, they should be placed through stab wounds separate from the main incision. Drains placed through the operative wound increase the risk of incisional surgical site infection.[44] Additionally, closed suction drains should be used to avoid the increase in surgical site infection risk of open drainage systems. The duration of drainage will vary with the purpose for which they have been inserted, and there are no evidence-based rules to guide timing of removal. Generally, drains that have been introduced to vent oozing or bleeding should be withdrawn after 24–48 hours, while drains placed where a localized abscess has been drained may need to remain in situ for more than 3 days. Drains should be removed as soon as they have served their purpose.

RETENTION CLOSURE OF THE ABDOMEN

The incidence of fascial disruption after major abdominal operations is 1–3% and is associated with a mortality rate of 15–20%.[59] Several patient-related factors are associated with an increased risk of fascial dehiscence. These include advanced age, male gender, hypoproteinemia, malnutrition, anemia, malignant disease, jaundice, azotemia, and treatment with steroids. More important than systemic factors in fascial disruption are local mechanical factors and a sound initial surgical closure.[59] Bringing drains or ostomies through the main incision clearly compromises fascial integrity. Wound sepsis is a major predisposing factor for both fascial disruption as well as incisional hernia. Increased intra-abdominal pressure is almost uniformly incriminated as a cause of fascial dehiscence. It may be secondary to abdominal complications such as vomiting, ileus, or bowel obstruction, pulmonary complications such as atelectasis, pneumonia, or bronchitis, or the nature of the operation, as in repair of diaphragmatic hernia.

Most authors would agree on the use of retention sutures for repair of fascial dehiscence. However, the indications for prophylactic placement of retention sutures at initial operation have not been well examined prospectively and are not well agreed upon. The purpose of using retention sutures in this setting is to relieve tension along the primary suture line to prevent wound disruption and allow normal relaxed wound healing. They are sometimes employed for initial laparotomy closure when poor wound healing is anticipated, as in obese, cirrhotic, and cachectic patients, those receiving corticosteroids, or when increased intra-abdominal pressure is anticipated, as in postoperative ileus.

There has been only one randomized trial of full-thickness retention suture placement in midline laparotomy closure. In this trial, Hubbard and associates could not identify a benefit of retention suture closure over standard mass closure of the abdominal wall.[60] The disadvantages of retention sutures, however, are well known and include the potential hazard of caught viscera, significant postoperative pain, a residual cross-hatched scar, and leakage of intraperitoneal fluid through the wound.[61] For these reasons, retention suture closure has largely fallen out of favor by many surgeons during primary laparotomy closure. Others recommend primary closure with retention sutures in certain circumstances. In a retrospective comparison of midline abdominal wound dehiscence, Makela and colleagues identified several preoperative variables that are significantly associated with fascial disruption: hypoalbuminemia, anemia, malnutrition, chronic pulmonary disease, and emergency procedure. For patients with three or more of these preoperative risk factors, this group recommends internal retention suture closure.[62]

The technique of placing retention sutures varies from surgeon to surgeon and many methods have been described. We employ 2-0 nylon simple, interrupted sutures to transfix all layers of the abdominal wall including skin and peritoneum. They are inserted via a long cutting needle approximately 2.5 cm from the margin of the wound and approximately 2.5 cm apart. Various methods have been devised in an attempt to protect the skin and subcutaneous tissue from damage. At the skin level, the sutures are threaded through 5-cm rubber tubing bolsters to prevent skin breakdown (Fig 4–17). They are removed in approximately 14 days. If the skin is closed, it is done with staples.

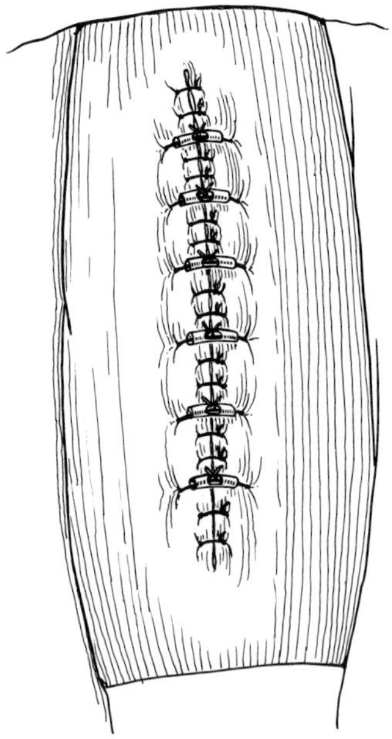

Figure 4–17. Retention sutures tied and held in position supported by rubber tubing.

TEMPORARY CLOSURE OF THE ABDOMEN

Severe abdominal trauma with hemorrhagic shock and ongoing resuscitation can cause massive edema of the bowel, abdominal wall, and retroperitoneum that may preclude a safe primary closure of the abdominal wound. Primary closure of the abdomen under tension leads to fascial necrosis and dehiscence, aggravates tissue injury, and promotes wound infection.[63] In these instances and in the setting of major abdominal wall tissue loss, alternative temporary abdominal closure devices are utilized to achieve a tension-free closure, facilitate "damage control," allow planned re-exploration, and prevent abdominal compartment syndrome.

The principles of management of temporary closure of the abdomen require a closure technique that protects and maintains the viscera within the abdomen while minimizing tension of the abdominal wall. Since the original description of temporary abdominal closure in Bogota, Columbia in 1984,[64] various closure devices have been used including silos, towel-clip skin closures, various prosthetic meshes, retention sutures, and the vacuum-assisted closure (VAC) pack.[65] There are no well designed trials comparing the superiority of one technique over the others. Two techniques that have proven efficacious include absorbable mesh closure and the vacuum-assisted Bogota bag. Both of these methods provide effective temporary coverage of the abdominal wall with a low fistula rate and allow for delayed definitive fascial closure.[66,67]

We commonly employ the vacuum-assisted Bogota bag dressing for difficult abdominal wall closures. This technique involves placement of a sterile saline bag beneath the fascia of the open abdomen. A sponge and suction tubing are placed over the subfascial bag and a second sterile saline bag is placed over this dressing and sutured to the skin. Subsequently, an occlusive dressing is placed over the superficial bag (Fig 4–18). This dressing is changed every 24–72 hours, either in the ICU or the operating room, until the fascia can be closed. The VAC dressing allows for containment and protection of the viscera, containment of fluid loss, prevention of wound contamination, prevention of abdominal compartment syndrome, and maintenance of constant medial tension on the fascial edges, making late medial mobilization of the fascia possible.

▪ MANAGEMENT OF THE POSTOPERATIVE WOUND

ROUTINE CARE

The most common practice is to keep wounds covered postoperatively. Studies dating back to the 1960s have documented that clean, surgically closed wounds, managed by a technique of early exposure on postoperative day two do not have an increased incidence of infection.[68] By the second postoperative day, carefully approximated wound edges are sufficiently sealed by coagulum and epithelial regrowth to resist contamination. There are several advantages to early exposure of the wound: the healing wound remains clean and dry, daily inspection or palpation of the wound is possible, and the patient does not have the annoyance of tape and bandages with the associated risk of allergic skin reactions. This approach also eliminates the expense of replacing dressings.

The ideal dressing should be inexpensive, absorptive, nonadherent, and allow moist healing. Traditionally, wounds have been covered with a piece of dry sterile gauze applied with tape, and despite the claims of manufacturers of commercially available dressings, none has proved superior. The application of an occlusive nonporous strip of adhesive tape is sometimes indicated, in particular if a nearby stoma or drain site may soak the gauze dressing. In the previous edition of this book, Ellis refers to an unpublished study that was carried out in which abdominal wounds were one-half dressed with conventional gauze and the other half covered with a completely waterproof occlusive dressing. The experiment was abandoned rapidly when a large number of stitch abscesses in the occluded portion of the wounds were seen. Others, however, have not found an increased incidence of wound infection with such dressings and they may be used when indicated.[69] Clean and dry wounds may even be left exposed immediately postoperatively. In a randomized study of patients undergoing either inguinal hernia repair or high saphenous ligation, there were no significant differences in terms of wound infection, pain, or quality score when immediately-exposed wounds were compared to those that were covered with a dry gauze dressing or an occlusive film dressing.[70]

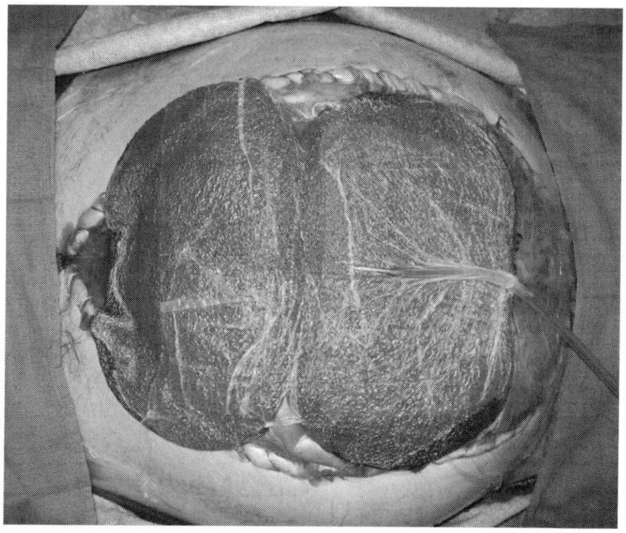

Figure 4–18. Vacuum-assisted Bogota bag dressing.

We routinely take down dressings on the morning of postoperative day two, after re-epithelialization has taken place. Because the wound is water resistant at this time, patients are allowed to shower, and the washing helps to reduce the bacterial count at the surgical site.

WOUND COMPLICATIONS

Surgical Site Infections

Some degree of erythema at the surgical site is normal and reflects the inflammatory process that leads to wound healing. In suspicious cases, wound erythema can be observed with the edges demarcated with ink. If the erythema is expanding, there is increased peri-incisional pain or tenderness, or purulent discharge from the wound is noted, the likelihood of an infective process is increased and further intervention and treatment should be considered.

Surgical site infections (SSIs) are the most common nosocomial infections in surgical patients. It has been estimated that each SSI results in 7.3 additional inpatient days and adds over $3000 to the hospital charges.[44] One of the important risk factors in developing a wound infection is the bacterial colony count at the surgical site. The threshold above which the risk is thought to increase substantially is greater than 10^5 colony counts per gram of tissue. In the presence of foreign bodies, however, a much lower count may result in development of an infection. Key goals are the use of good surgical technique to avoid tissue trauma and avoidance of excessive use of sutures whenever possible. Other risk factors for development of wound infections include advanced age, obesity, diabetes mellitus, smoking, malnutrition, altered immune response, preoperative hospitalization, presence

TABLE 4–1. CRITERIA FOR DEFINING SURGICAL SITE INFECTIONS (SSIs)

Incisional SSI		Organ/Space SSI
SUPERFICIAL INCISIONAL Infection occurring within 30 days of surgery; **and** Infection involves only skin and subcutaneous tissue; **and** At least one of the following: 1. Purulent discharge 2. Organisms isolated from aseptically cultured fluid or tissue 3. At least one sign of infection: pain or tenderness, localized swelling, redness, or heat **and** the incision is deliberately opened by surgeon unless the incision is culture-negative 4. Diagnosis of SSI by the surgeon or attending physician	DEEP INCISIONAL Infection occurring within 30 days of surgery, or within 1 year of operation if implants are in place; **and** Infection involves deep soft tissue; **and** At least one of the following: 1. Purulent discharge 2. Deep incision spontaneously dehisces or is deliberately opened by a surgeon when the patient has at least one of the following symptoms: fever (>38°C), localized pain or tenderness unless the site is culture-negative 3. Evidence of deep infection on direct examination, during reoperation, or on radiological examinations 4. Diagnosis of SSI by the surgeon or attending physician	Infection occurs within 30 days of surgery, or within 1 year of operation if implants are in place; **and** Infection involves any part of anatomy that was manipulated during an operation, other than the incision; **and** At least one of the following 1. Purulent drainage that is placed through a stab wound into the organ space 2. Organism isolated from and aseptically cultured fluid or tissue 3. Evidence of deep infection on the direct examination, during reoperation, or on radiological examinations 4. Diagnosis of SSI by surgeon or attending physician

of infection at a remote body site, length of operation, and use of surgical drains.[44]

SSIs are subdivided into two categories: incisional and organ/space, each with a specific definition and diagnostic criteria (Table 4–1).[44] Incisional SSIs are those in which the infectious process is limited to the surgical site. They are further divided into superficial SSIs involving the skin and subcutaneous tissue, and deep SSIs involving fascial and muscle layers. Organ/space SSIs are those in which the infectious process involves any part of the anatomy that was manipulated during the surgery.

The risk of a postoperative SSI is in part related to the surgical wound classification. However, several studies have indicated that assessing the risk of an SSI based on wound classification alone is inaccurate, with a wide variation in infection rates (Table 4–2).[71,72] Thus, other risk-scoring systems have been developed to better calculate the risk of wound infections. Examples of such scoring systems are the SENIC (Study of the Efficacy of Nosocomial Infection Control) and NNIS (National Nosocomial Infection Surveillance) risk indexes. These scoring systems take into account the factors that have been shown to influence wound infection rates. The SENIC system scores four markers to assess infection risks: (1) abdominal surgery, (2) an operation lasting longer than 2 hours, (3) wound classification of contaminated or dirty, and (4) an operation on a patient with three or more discharge diagnoses.[71] The NNIS system calculates risk of SSI by scoring three risk factors: (1) an American Society of Anesthesiologists preoperative assessment score of greater than 2, (2) a wound classification of contaminated or dirty, and (3) increased duration of the operation.[72] Using these scoring systems, a more accurate preoperative forecast of the likelihood of an SSI can be made. High-risk wounds should be left open. These systems also allow a more precise comparison of outcomes among surgeons and operative centers.

The organisms most commonly responsible for SSIs are *Staphylococcus aureus* and coagulase-negative staphylococci. After abdominal surgery, enteric organisms (*Escherichia coli* and *Enterobacter* spp.) are the most common pathogens. For most SSIs, the source of the responsible pathogen is the patient's endogenous flora.

It is important that surgeons take measures to prevent SSIs. The Centers for Disease Control and Prevention recommendations for the prevention of SSIs are summarized in Table 4–3.[44] The use of preoperative prophylactic antibiotics in all clean-contaminated, and clean cases with associated risk factors is recommended. The antibiotic of choice for most upper gastrointestinal procedures is cefazolin or a comparable first-generation cephalosporin that is cheap and effective. For colorectal surgery, metronidazole is added to this regimen and mechanical bowel preparation should be undertaken. The administration of nonabsorbable oral antibiotics is also recommended prior to colorectal surgery, although this practice has been questioned and abandoned by some. Preoperative intravenous antibiotics should be administered 30–60 minutes before the incision is made to allow the agent to reach maximal tissue concentration. In obese patients, the antibiotic dose will need to be increased accordingly. For long procedures, it is important to repeat the dose of antibiotics after every two half-lives to maintain an effective serum concentration.

The treatment for incisional SSIs involves removal of several contiguous skin stitches or staples to relieve tension and drainage of any underlying collection. Antibiotics are indicated in the presence of any surrounding cellulitis. The effective use of antibiotics depends on

TABLE 4–2. CLASSIFICATION OF SURGICAL WOUNDS

Type of Wound	Definition	Risk of SSI
Class I: Clean	An uninfected operative wound in which no inflammation is encountered and respiratory, alimentary, genital, or uninfected urinary is not entered. They are primarily closed, and if necessary drained with close drainage	1–5%
Class II: Clean-contaminated	An operative wound in which the respiratory, alimentary, genital, or urinary tracts are entered under controlled conditions and without unusual contamination. In particular, surgery involving the biliary tract, appendix, vagina, and oropharynx are included in this category provided no evidence of infection or a major break in technique is encountered.	2–9%
Class III: Contaminated	Open fresh accidental wounds. In addition, surgery with major breaks in sterile technique (e.g., open cardiac massage) or gross spillage from the gastrointestinal tract, and incisions in which acute, nonpurulent inflammation is encountered are included in this category	3–13%
Class IV: Dirty-infected	Old traumatic wounds with retained devitalized tissue and those that involve existing clinical infection or perforated viscera	3–13%

(1) knowledge of the organisms involved, (2) their sensitivities to the available antimicrobial agents, and (3) maintenance of an adequate tissue concentration of the drug. Cefazolin or an equivalent first- or second-generation cephalosporin is an appropriate agent if antimicrobial coverage is needed for an uncomplicated incisional SSI. It must be stressed that purulence requires drainage and no antibiotic can substitute for this fundamental surgical principle. Wound cultures are obtained only in the presence of purulence and are used to guide selection of appropriate antibiotics. Following abscess drainage, the wound is left open to provide further drainage.

Deep space SSIs also require drainage. This can be performed using carefully placed drains if the infection is localized. Increasingly, such drains are placed percutaneously under CT or ultrasound guidance. Deep space infections that are not safely amenable to interventional drainage will require operative drainage. Broad-spectrum antibiotics are indicated for intra-abdominal infections.

Necrotizing Wound Infections

Necrotizing soft tissue infections are often lethal complications. Their incidence in postoperative wounds is low but they represent a serious infection that requires early identification and treatment. Although necrotizing soft tissue infections are a heterogenous group consisting of several specific syndromes (Table 4–4),[73] the treatment principles are essentially the same for all. Patients often present early within 48 hours postoperatively with incisional pain and often become toxic as the infection progresses. With these infections, the incision may initially appear benign but will usually demonstrate serous drainage. Disproportionate incisional pain and edema may be present. These infections progress rapidly and result in deep tissue necrosis. In suspected cases, immediate surgical exploration and extensive débridement is recommended. Débridement of affected tissues and surrounding cellulitis is the most important single therapeutic factor. Necrotic tissue is resected until healthy bleeding tissue is encountered. Gram's stain and culture should be acquired from the drainage and from affected tissue. The wound is irrigated and antibiotics are administered. The infections are often caused by *Clostridium perfringens* or group A beta-hemolytic streptococci but can be the result of a mixed group of organisms. Initial therapy should include a broad spectrum of coverage. A recommended regimen is penicillin, clindamycin, and an aminoglycoside. Following débridement, the wound is loosely dressed with gauze and is inspected at least daily. Any evidence of extension of the gangrenous tissue is an indication for further débridement.

Although the initial management of these necrotizing infections is essentially the same, there are several specific disorders that deserve mentioning, as they may require specific therapy.

Gas Gangrene. When one considers how often abdominal wounds become contaminated with septic peritoneal fluid, it is surprising that gas gangrene infection of abdominal wounds is so rare. Gas gangrene infection following abdominal surgery results from liberation of clostridia contained within the alimentary tract or biliary system. Clostridia can almost invariably be recovered from normal stools, and they may occasionally be found when bile, gallbladder wall, or even gallstones are cultured anaerobically. The patients usually present with pain at the surgical wound site that is often severe and associated with a high temperature and rapid pulse rate, and it eventually progresses to profound shock. When such wounds are examined in the early stages, the edges are found to be edematous, red, and acutely inflamed. They later become dusky and necrotic. The patient looks ill. The wound is crepitant with purulent discharge containing gas bubbles and an irritating brownish, watery fluid that has a peculiar foul odor. Early surgical intervention is recommended in suspected cases with débridement of all infected and nonviable tissue.

Although there have been no controlled clinical trials, there is strong evidence that hyperbaric oxy-

TABLE 4–3. CDC RECOMMENDATIONS TO PREVENT SURGICAL SITE INFECTIONS

PREOPERATIVE FACTORS

Preparation of the patient:

1. Identify and treat all infections remote from the surgical site and postpone elective surgery until infection has resolved
2. Do not remove hair unless it interferes with surgery
3. If hair is to be removed, remove immediately preoperatively using clippers
4. Ensure good blood glucose control in diabetic patients and avoid hyperglycemia
5. Encourage cessation of tobacco use (at least for 30 days before surgery, if possible)
6. Do not withhold blood products, as transfusion does not affect rates of SSI
7. Require the patient to shower or bathe with an antiseptic solution the night before surgery
8. Remove gross contamination from the surgical site before performing antiseptic skin preparation
9. Use an appropriate antiseptic solution for skin preparation
10. Apply preoperative antiseptic solution for skin preparation in concentric circles moving outward toward the periphery
11. Keep the preoperative hospital stay as short as possible

Hand/forearm antisepsis for surgical team:

1. Keep nails short and do not wear artificial nails
2. Perform a preoperative scrub for at least 2–5 minutes up to the elbows
3. After performing the surgical scrub, keep the hands up and away from the body (elbows flexed) so that the water runs from the tips of fingers towards the elbows. Dry hands with a sterile towel and don a sterile gown and gloves
4. Clean underneath each fingernail
5. Do not wear hand or arm jewelry

Management of infected or colonized surgical personnel:

1. Educate and encourage surgical personnel who have signs and symptoms of a transmissible infectious illness to report promptly to their supervisor and occupational health personnel
2. Develop well-defined policies concerning patient care responsibilities when personnel have potentially transmissible infectious conditions. These policies should govern (1) responsibility of personnel in using health services and reporting illness, (2) work restrictions, and (3) clearance to resume work after an illness that required work restriction. The policies should also identify staff members that have the authority to remove personnel from duty
3. Obtain appropriate cultures and exclude from duty surgical personnel who have draining skin lesions until infections has been ruled out, or until these personnel have received adequate therapy and infection has been resolved
4. Do not routinely exclude surgical personnel who are colonized with organisms such as *Staphylococcus aureus* or group A streptococci, unless they have been linked epidemiologically to dissemination of the organism

Antibiotic prophylaxis:

1. Administer a prophylactic antimicrobial agent only when indicated, and select it based on its efficacy against the most common pathogens causing SSIs for a specific operation, and in accordance with published recommendations
2. Administer by the IV route the initial dose of prophylactic antimicrobial agent, timed such that bactericidal concentration of the drug is established in serum and tissue when the incision is made. Maintain therapeutic levels of the agent in serum and tissues throughout the operation, and for a few hours after the incision has been closed
3. Before elective colorectal operations, in addition to the above measures, mechanically prepare the bowel by using enemas and cathartic agents. Give nonabsorbable oral antimicrobial agents in divided doses on the day before the operation
4. For high-risk cesarean sections, administer the prophylactic antimicrobial agent immediately after the umbilical cord is clamped
5. Do not routinely use vancomycin for prophylaxis

INTRAOPERATIVE

Ventilation:

1. Maintain positive pressure ventilation in the operating room with respect to the corridors and adjacent area
2. Maintain a minimum of 15 air changes per hour, of which at least 3 should be fresh air
3. Filter all air, recirculated and fresh, through the appropriate filters per the American Institute of Architects' recommendations
4. Introduce all air at the ceiling, and exhaust air near the floor
5. Do not use ultraviolet radiation in the operating room
6. Keep operating suite doors closed except as need for passage of equipment, personnel, or patients
7. Consider performing orthopedic implant operations in an operating suite supplied with ultraclean air
8. Limit the number of personnel entering the operating room

Cleaning and disinfection of environmental surfaces:

1. When visible soiling or contamination of surfaces or equipment with blood or other body fluids occurs during an operation, use and EPA-approved hospital disinfectant to clean the affected areas before the next operation
2. Do not perform special cleaning (in addition to cleaning with routine Environmental Protection Agency-approved hospital disinfectant) or closing of operating rooms after contaminated or dirty operations
3. Do not use tacky mats at the entrance to the operating room suite or individual operating rooms for infection control
4. Wet vacuum the operating floor with an EPA-approved disinfectant after the last operation of the day or night

Microbiological sampling:

1. Do not perform routine environmental sampling of the operating room

Continued

TABLE 4–3. (CONTINUED) CDC RECOMMENDATIONS TO PREVENT SURGICAL SITE INFECTIONS

Sterilization of surgical instruments:
1. Sterilize all surgical instruments according to published guidelines
2. Perform flash sterilization only for patient care items that will be used immediately. Do not flash sterilize for reasons of convenience or to save time

Surgical attire and drapes:
1. Wear a surgical mask that fully covers the mouth and nose when entering the operating room if an operation is about to begin or is underway, or if sterilized instruments are exposed. Wear the mask throughout the operation
2. Wear a cap or hood to fully cover hair on the head and face
3. Do not wear shoe covers for prevention of SSIs
4. Wear sterile gloves if scrubbed as a surgical team member. Put on gloves after donning the sterile gown
5. Use surgical gowns and drapes that are effective barriers when wet
6. Change scrub suits that are visibly soiled, contaminated, and/or are penetrated by blood or other potentially infectious material

Asepsis and surgical technique:
1. Adhere to principles of asepsis when placing intravascular devices, spinal or epidural anesthesia catheters, or when dispensing or administering IV drugs
2. Assemble sterile equipment and solutions immediately prior to use
3. Handle tissue gently, maintain effective hemostasis, minimize devitalized tissue and foreign bodies and eradicate dead space at the surgical site
4. Use delayed primary skin closure or leave an incision open if the surgeon considers the surgical site to be heavily contaminated
5. If drain is necessary, use closed suction drain, and place it through a separate incision distant from the operating incision. Remove the drain as soon as possible

POSTOPERATIVE INCISION CARE

1. Protect an incision that has been closed primarily with a sterile dressing for 24–48 hours postoperatively
2. Wash hands before and after dressing changes and before and after any contact with surgical site
3. When an incision dressing must be changed, use sterile technique
4. Educate the patient and family regarding proper incision care, symptoms of SSI, and the need to report such symptoms

SURVEILLANCE

1. Use CDC definitions of SSI without modification for identifying SSIs among surgical inpatients and outpatients
2. For inpatient cases, use direct prospective observation, indirect prospective detection, or a combination of both for the duration of the patient's hospitalization
3. When postdischarge surveillance is performed for detecting SSIs following certain operations, use a method that accommodates available resources and data needs
4. For outpatient cases, use a method that accommodates available resources and data needs
5. Assign a surgical wound classification upon completion of an operation. A surgical team member should make the assignment
6. For a patient undergoing an operation chosen for surveillance, record those variables shown to be associated with increased risk of SSI
7. Periodically calculate operation-specific SSI rates stratified by variables shown to be associated with increased risk of SSI
8. Report appropriately stratified operation-specific SSI rates to surgical team members. The optimum frequency and format of such rate computations will be determined by stratified case-load sizes and the objectives of local, continuous quality improvement initiatives

gen is of considerable value in treating clostridial infection, and reduces the mortality rate by some reports from 66–23%.[74] The high oxygen pressure within the chamber improves tissue oxygenation, promotes healing, and increases free radical formation by neutrophils.[75]

Necrotizing Fasciitis. This syndrome has been divided into two groups depending on the responsible organisms. Type I necrotizing fasciitis is a polymicrobial infective process with slower progress. Type II necrotizing fasciitis is caused by group A streptococci and has a more rapid progression.[73,76]

Type I (Polymicrobial). This type of necrotizing infection is a slowly progressive lesion that affects the total thickness of the skin, but does not involve the deep fascia. Pus formation is variable and it usually presents as nonspecific cellulitis around the wound and slowly extends over the next few days. Its central area becomes purple and then develops all of the features of gangrene. When affecting the perineum, the disease is referred to as Fournier's gangrene.

The organisms involved are usually a mixture of anaerobes, gram-negative rods, and enterococcus. Treatment is begun with a broad-spectrum regimen of antibiotics and then tailored pending the result of microbiological cultures. Hyperbaric oxygen has also been shown to be effective in treatment of Fournier's gangrene.

Type II (Group A Streptococci). This infection presents as a progressive and rapidly necrotizing process affecting the subcutaneous fat, the superficial fascia, and the superior surface of the deep fascia. Initially, the skin is intact, but later becomes gangrenous secondary to interruption of its deep blood supply. The condition is readily distinguished from gas gangrene because of the absence of crepitus, the absence of muscle involvement, and the failure to isolate clostridia from tissues or exudate. Necrotizing fasciitis occurs postoperatively, particularly after abdominal or perineal operations. Although CT or MRI imaging has been proposed by some, early opera-

TABLE 4–4. TYPES OF NECROTIZING SOFT TISSUE INFECTIONS

	Predisposing Factors	Microbiology	Dominant Features
Necrotizing fasciitis type I (polymicrobial)	Surgery, trauma, diabetes mellitus	Anaerobes, gram-negative aerobic bacilli	Necrosis of fat and fascia; may have gas
Necrotizing fasciitis type II (group A streptococcal)	Surgery, minor trauma, *Varicella*	*Streptococcus pyogenes*	Rapidly progressive necrosis of multiple tissue layers; no gas; shock
Clostridial myonecrosis (gas gangrene)	Trauma, surgery, spontaneous (cancer patient)	Clostridial species	Myonecrosis; prominent gas formation

tive exploration is recommended in suspected cases. Frozen section can be sent intraoperatively and Gram's stain performed to confirm the diagnosis.

The organism involved is group A *Streptococcus*, which is usually very sensitive to penicillin. However, it has been suggested that the combination of penicillin and clindamycin is superior to the use of penicillin alone.[76] Treatment principles are as highlighted above, namely high clinical suspicion, early surgical exploration with extensive débridement, and administration of antibiotics.

HEMATOMA

It is difficult to accurately estimate the incidence of postoperative wound hematomas, but in clean operative wounds it is thought to be about 2%. The risk is increased in patients with a bleeding diathesis, the most common cause of which is iatrogenic following the use of anticoagulants. With the ever-increasing use of heparin as prophylaxis against thromboembolic complications, the prevalence of wound hematomas has increased. Studies that have compared unfractionated heparin (UFH) to low-molecular-weight heparin (LMWH) have shown a wound hematoma rate of around 4–8% following abdominal surgery. These studies have suggested that the use of LMWH is at least as safe as UFH with regard to wound hematomas and major bleeding complications.[77,78] It has also been assumed that the use of aspirin and nonsteroidal anti-inflammatory therapy prior to surgery increases the risk of postoperative hematoma formation, and many surgeons recommend discontinuing these agents 1 week prior to surgery. However, there are few published data to defend this practice.

Hematomas are caused by faulty hemostasis of the layers of the abdominal wall, but they are not serious complications unless they become infected. They usually give rise to an aching pain in the wound that is accompanied by a slight rise in temperature. Small hematomas may be difficult to detect unless wounds are palpated carefully. Since these small hematomas usually resolve, they may be left alone. If large, and particularly if soft, they should be aspirated with a wide-bore needle, or the edges of the wound that overlies them should be separated with a probe and the contents evacuated. If there is considerable extravasation of blood giving rise to a fluctuating mass, it is best to return the patient to the operating room. There the wound is opened, clot is evacuated, and any visible bleeding vessels are ligated or coagulated with diathermy. The wound is then closed and consideration is given to placing a suction drain.

STITCH ABSCESS

Stitch abscesses are usually seen about postoperative day 10, but may occur earlier or weeks after the wound has apparently healed. Stitch abscesses may be superficial or deep. When superficial, they may appear as brown or mauve-colored fluctuating circumscribed blisters more or less in the line of the incision. They produce a certain amount of uneasiness and pain in the wound and are best evacuated by incising the blistered area and expressing the contents. Antibiotic treatment rarely will be necessary. Such sinuses heal rapidly as soon as the offending stitch is removed, leaving only a slight scar.

When deep, stitch abscesses may be felt as rounded, indurated masses in the depths of the wound and are painful to touch. The use of nonabsorbable sutures such as polypropylene to close the abdominal wound has been associated with increasing incidence of deep stitch abscesses when compared to closure with a slowly absorbing suture such as polydioxanone.[79,80] When polypropylene has been used, treatment for persistent stitch sinuses requires removal of the offending suture.

ABDOMINAL WOUND DEHISCENCE AND EVISCERATION

Disruption of an abdominal wound may be limited to the deep fascia with the skin remaining intact. When it is complete, all the layers of the abdominal wall have burst apart with or without associated protrusion of a viscus (evisceration). Historically, dehiscence rates of up to 10% have been reported. With recent advances in suture material and the use of mass closure technique the rate of dehiscence has generally been less than 1%,[81] although a recent report from the Veterans Affairs national quality program has documented a rate of 3.2%.[82]

The mean time to wound dehiscence is 8–10 postoperative days.[80,83] There are several clinical presentations of wound disruption. The patient may have an abrupt rush of pink serosanguineous discharge from the wound. This pink discharge is almost pathognomonic of dehiscence and when noted the wound should be examined. A small portion of the skin incision is opened, and using a probe the deeper layers are inspected to determine if fascial union is satisfactory. Sometimes this pink discharge is associated with a large subcutaneous hematoma or a soft and tympanitic boggy swelling that distends the wound. Both these findings should be investigated in the operating room. If a large hematoma has formed, it should be evacuated and the depths of the wound examined to see if any separation has occurred. The soft boggy swelling generally indicates that a knuckle of bowel has herniated through the abdominal wall and lies beneath the skin incision.

Another presentation of wound dehiscence is one in which the wound appears clean and dry, but following some excessive strain the patient feels a sudden "give" in the wound, which when examined will be found to have dehisced with the gut eviscerated. It is surprising how painless this condition is, and how little if any shock results. Dehiscence can occur in infected wounds, in which case the onset is usually gradual. An abscess forms which is usually drained but results in gradual weakening and separation of the deeper layers. Matted omentum and intestine are often adherent to the edges of the muscle, and evisceration in such circumstances is uncommon.

Abdominal dehiscence is a morbid complication. The mortality rate following wound dehiscence has ranged from 9–43%, with a recent review reporting a mortality rate of 16%.[84] Prevention is therefore an important issue, and a cornerstone of this is meticulous surgical technique. Several technical considerations are worth mentioning:

1. *Incisions.* Although it had been suggested that midline incisions, particularly in the upper abdomen, are more prone to disruption than paramedian incisions, several randomized studies have shown this to be an incorrect assumption.
2. *Technique of laparotomy closure.* Several randomized studies and meta-analyses have now shown that a technique of mass closure with a running suture is the best method for closure of midline wounds.

   Several technical failures following laparotomy closure can lead to wound dehiscence. The suture material may rupture because it is too weak for the tension placed upon it and thus sutures of appropriate strength should be used. This usually means a suture of 0 or 1 caliber. The sutures may also cut through the tissues, either because the sutures are placed too close to the wound edge or because of excessive weakening of tissues. A general guideline is to place sutures 1 cm apart with 1-cm bites of fascia. Another frequent technical error is improper knot tying which may lead unraveling.

Several papers have specifically looked at the nontechnical risk factors for dehiscence in the postoperative period. They form a heterogeneous group of studies using different techniques of laparotomy closure. From these studies, several important risk factors have been revealed: age (>65 years), hypoalbuminemia, wound infection (increases the risk by more than five times), ascites, obesity, steroid use, chronic obstructive pulmonary disease, current pneumonia, cerebrovascular accident with residual deficit, anemia (hematocrit <30), prolonged ileus, coughing, emergency operation, operative time greater than 2.5 hours, and postgraduate year 4 resident as surgeon.[62,82,84]

The largest study among the group analyzed over 570 cases of dehiscence in the Veterans Affairs population. Data were subject to multivariate analysis and resulted in identification of several independent risk factors for this complication (Table 4–5). Together, these data were used to develop an abdominal wound dehiscence risk index for prediction of development of postoperative wound dehiscence (Table 4–6).[82] Whether placement of retention sutures in those at high risk is

TABLE 4–5. RISK FACTOR SCORES FOR ABDOMINAL WOUND DEHISCENCE

Risk Factor	Score
Cerebrovascular accident/stroke without deficit	4
History of chronic obstructive pulmonary disease	4
Current pneumonia	4
Emergency procedure	6
Operative time >2.5 hours	2
Postgraduate year 4 as surgeon	3
Clean wound classification	–3
Superficial wound infection	5
Deep wound infection	17
Failure to wean	6
One or more complications	7
Return to the operating room	–11

TABLE 4–6. RISK CATEGORIES FOR WOUND DEHISCENCE

Risk Category	Total Score	Predicted Rate of Dehiscence
Low	≤3	1.47%
Medium	4–10	2.70%
High	11–14	4.53%
Very High	>14	10.90%

helpful in preventing dehiscence has not been determined. Many surgeons place retention sutures at laparotomy closure in those with several risk factors that put a patient at high risk for fascial dehiscence.

The basic treatment principle for repair of the disrupted wound is re-suturing of wound edges. It is recommended for the majority of cases, especially for those in whom the accident has occurred early in the postoperative period in whom the edges of the wound, although they may be frayed and torn, are relatively clean. The objective of surgery is to replace the eviscerated organs into the abdominal cavity, and to prevent recurrent dehiscence and later development of ventral hernias. As soon as the condition is recognized, the wound and protruding viscera should be freely bathed with warm normal saline solution and covered with large sterile dressing. When the patient has been moved to the operating room, general anesthesia should be administered and a nasogastric tube placed to decompress the stomach. The edges of the abdominal wall are then lifted upward, and the prolapsed bowel is replaced below the level of the peritoneal edges. At this stage, fragments of suture material are extracted, and the wound edges are freshened by snipping away necrotic tissue and edematous skin tags. It will be noted in many cases that the fascial edges are swollen and retracted outward, highlighting the need for immediate repair of the dehisced wound to prevent further retraction of the wound edges. If only a very small area of the wound has been disrupted, this portion alone should be sutured. However, if more than half of the wound has been disrupted, the correct procedure is to open the remaining portion of the wound and suture the whole wound afresh.

Resuturing should be performed using a strong monofilament nonabsorbable suture such as polypropylene. There are several technical considerations when closing such a wound, such as whether to use continuous or interrupted sutures, and whether or not to use retention sutures. Continuous closure has the theoretical advantages of evenly distributing the tension along the length of the wound and being quicker to perform. However, the tissue at the site of dehiscence is often weakened, and if one of the sutures cuts through the fascia the wound will open. There may therefore be a benefit in closing the fascia with interrupted sutures. Two retrospective analyses, however, have shown no significant reduction in the incidence of late ventral hernia following interrupted closure of a dehisced wound.[83,85] Whether retention sutures need to be placed is another unresolved issue. Retrospective analysis of data does not show any benefits in placement of retention sutures in terms of later development of an incisional hernia. Some surgeons suggest that the incidence of evisceration would be reduced and recommend the use of retention sutures. It has been shown, however, that placement of retention sutures results in increased pain and discomfort for the patient, and some have proposed abandoning their use altogether.[61]

Retention sutures, if placed, can be internal (wide bites of the fascia deep to the skin), or external (full-thickness bites of fascia and skin are taken together). One technique to place external retention sutures consists of placing strong monofilament nylon stitches 2.5 cm from the margin of the wound and about 2.5 cm apart that transfix all the layers of the abdominal wall on both margins of the wound. As they are introduced, the free ends are clipped with hemostats. The fascia is then closed with a running nonabsorbable suture before the retention sutures are threaded though 5-cm pieces of protective rubber tubing and firmly tied. These retention sutures are generally kept in place for 2–4 weeks.

Despite these measures, repaired dehisced laparotomy wounds have a 69% hernia development risk over a 10-year period, the majority of which develops over the first 2 years. Dehisced wounds associated with evisceration, or those in patients that had undergone abdominal aneurysm repair had an even higher rate of hernia development.[85] Because of such high hernia rates, there has been recent interest in closure of dehisced wounds using nonabsorbable mesh. In a retrospective review, fascial dehiscence closed in this fashion had a trend towards lower incidence of ventral hernia development, although this did not reach statistical significance.[83]

If the size of defect is small, the patient is critically ill, and there is no evisceration of viscera, then the dehiscence can be dealt with conservatively. This will result in the development of an incisional hernia that can be repaired later, when the patient has recovered. This technique involves packing the open wound with a moist sterile dressing and generous strips of elastic adhesive tape placed transversely across the abdomen. An abdominal binder can be used for further support, and the patient should avoid excessive physical activity. The dressing should be changed at regular intervals until healing takes place. In some cases, a secondary suture of the skin can be carried out at this stage, but in other instances one may elect to allow the wound to heal entirely by granulation. Recent introduction of vacuum-assisted wound closure devices (VAC devices) has been helpful in such cases. By applying such dressings the wounds are kept clean, and the controlled negative pressure helps to evacuate fluid and stimulate healing.[86]

INCISIONAL HERNIA

An incisional hernia is one that develops in the scar of a surgical incision. It may be small and insignificant, or it may bulge through the wound to become a large, unsightly, and uncomfortable hernia. Only hernias with narrow necks and large sacs are at risk of strangulation; those with a wide neck are a nuisance but not usually a danger. The topic of incisional hernias has been covered extensively in Chapter 5.

REFERENCES

1. Ellis H. *Maingot's Abdominal Operations.* New York, NY: McGraw-Hill; 1997:395
2. Penn I, Baker R. *Mastery of Surgery.* New York, NY: Lippincott Williams & Wilkins; 2001
3. Grantcharov TP, Rosenberg J. Vertical compared with transverse incisions in abdominal surgery. *Eur J Surg* 2001;167:260
4. Reidel MA, Knaebel HP, Seiler CM, et al. Postsurgical pain outcome of vertical and transverse abdominal incision: design of a randomized controlled equivalence trial. *BMC Surg* 2003;3:9
5. Greenall MJ, Evans M, Pollock AV. Midline or transverse laparotomy? A random controlled clinical trial. Part I: Influence on healing. *Br J Surg* 1980;67:188
6. Ellis H, Coleridge-Smith PD, Joyce AD. Abdominal incisions—vertical or transverse? *Postgrad Med J* 1984;60:407
7. Greenall MJ, Evans M, Pollock AV. Midline or transverse laparotomy? A random controlled clinical trial. Part II: Influence on postoperative pulmonary complications. *Br J Surg* 1980;67:191
8. Guillou PJ, Hall TJ, Donaldson DR, et al. Vertical abdominal incisions—a choice? *Br J Surg* 1980;67:395
9. Cox PJ, Ausobsky JR, Ellis H, et al. Towards no incisional hernias: lateral paramedian versus midline incisions. *J R Soc Med* 1986;79:711
10. Rappaport WD, Hunter GC, Allen R, et al. Effect of electrocautery on wound healing in midline laparotomy incisions. *Am J Surg* 1990;160:618
11. Kearns SR, Connolly EM, McNally S, et al. Randomized clinical trial of diathermy versus scalpel incision in elective midline laparotomy. *Br J Surg* 2001;88:41
12. Hussain SA, Hussain S. Incisions with knife or diathermy and postoperative pain. *Br J Surg* 1988;75:1179
13. Johnson CD, Serpell JW. Wound infection after abdominal incision with scalpel or diathermy. *Br J Surg* 1990;77:626
14. Pearlman NW, Stiegmann GV, Vance V, et al. A prospective study of incisional time, blood loss, pain, and healing with carbon dioxide laser, scalpel, and electrosurgery. *Arch Surg* 1991;126:1018
15. Telfer JR, Canning G, Galloway DJ. Comparative study of abdominal incision techniques. *Br J Surg* 1993;80:233
16. Groot G, Chappell EW. Electrocautery used to create incisions does not increase wound infection rates. *Am J Surg* 1994;167:601
17. McBurney C. The incision made in the abdominal wall in cases of appendicitis, with a description of a new method of operating. *Ann Surg* 1894;20:38
18. Lumsden AB, Colbourn GL, Sreeram S, et al. The surgical anatomy and technique of the thoracoabdominal incision. *Surg Clin North Am* 1993;73:633
19. Ellis H, Heddle R. Does the peritoneum need to be closed at laparotomy? *Br J Surg* 1977;64:733
20. Dorfman S, Rincon A, Shortt H. Cholecystectomy via Kocher incision without peritoneal closure. *Invest Clin* 1997;38:3
21. Gilbert JM, Ellis H, Foweraker S. Peritoneal closure after lateral paramedian incision. *Br J Surg* 1987;74:113
22. Tulandi T, Al-Jaroudi D. Nonclosure of peritoneum: a reappraisal. *Am J Obstet Gynecol* 2003;189:609
23. Wadstrom J, Gerdin B. Closure of the abdominal wall; how and why? Clinical review. *Acta Chir Scand* 1990;156:75
24. Goligher JC, Irvin TT, Johnston D, et al. A controlled clinical trial of three methods of closure of laparotomy wounds. *Br J Surg* 1975;62:823
25. Bucknall TE, Ellis H. Abdominal wound closure—a comparison of monofilament nylon and polyglycolic acid. *Surgery* 1981;89:672
26. Leaper DJ, Pollock AV, Evans M. Abdominal wound closure: a trial of nylon, polyglycolic acid and steel sutures. *Br J Surg* 1977;64:603
27. Wissing J, van Vroonhoven TJ, Schattenkerk ME, et al. Fascia closure after midline laparotomy: results of a randomized trial. *Br J Surg* 1987;74:738
28. Trimbos JB, Smit IB, Holm JP, et al. A randomized clinical trial comparing two methods of fascia closure following midline laparotomy. *Arch Surg* 1992;127:1232
29. Richards PC, Balch CM, Aldrete JS. Abdominal wound closure. A randomized prospective study of 571 patients comparing continuous vs. interrupted suture techniques. *Ann Surg* 1983;197:238
30. Larsen PN, Nielsen K, Schultz A, et al. Closure of the abdominal fascia after clean and clean-contaminated laparotomy. *Acta Chir Scand* 1989;155:461
31. Fagniez PL, Hay JM, Lacaine F, et al. Abdominal midline incision closure. A multicentric randomized prospective trial of 3,135 patients, comparing continuous vs interrupted polyglycolic acid sutures. *Arch Surg* 1985;120:1351
32. Carlson MA, Condon RE. Polyglyconate (Maxon) versus nylon suture in midline abdominal incision closure: a prospective randomized trial. *Am Surg* 1995;61:980
33. Irvin TT, Koffman CG, Duthie HL. Layer closure of laparotomy wounds with absorbable and non-absorbable suture materials. *Br J Surg* 1976;63:793

34. Corman ML, Veidenheimer MC, Coller JA. Controlled clinical trial of three suture materials for abdominal wall closure after bowel operations. *Am J Surg* 1981;141:510
35. Cameron AE, Parker CJ, Field ES, et al. A randomised comparison of polydioxanone (PDS) and polypropylene (Prolene) for abdominal wound closure. *Ann R Coll Surg Engl* 1987;69:113
36. Murray DH, Blaisdell FW. Use of synthetic absorbable sutures for abdominal and chest wound closure. Experience with 650 consecutive cases. *Arch Surg* 1978;113:477
37. Martyak SN, Curtis LE. Abdominal incision and closure. A systems approach. *Am J Surg* 1976;131:476
38. Jenkins TP. The burst abdominal wound: a mechanical approach. *Br J Surg* 1976;63:873
39. Hussain SA. Closure of subcutaneous fat: a prospective randomized trial. *Br J Surg* 1990;77:107
40. Naumann RW, Hauth JC, Owen J, et al. Subcutaneous tissue approximation in relation to wound disruption after cesarean delivery in obese women. *Obstet Gynecol* 1995;85:412
41. Cetin A, Cetin M. Superficial wound disruption after cesarean delivery: effect of the depth and closure of subcutaneous tissue. *Int J Gynaecol Obstet* 1997;57:17
42. Farnell MB, Worthington-Self S, Mucha P Jr, et al. Closure of abdominal incisions with subcutaneous catheters. A prospective randomized trial. *Arch Surg* 1986;121:641
43. Shaffer D, Benotti PN, Bothe A Jr, et al. A prospective, randomized trial of abdominal wound drainage in gastric bypass surgery. *Ann Surg* 1987;206:134
44. Mangram AJ, Horan TC, Pearson ML, et al. Guideline for Prevention of Surgical Site Infection, 1999. Centers for Disease Control and Prevention (CDC) Hospital Infection Control Practices Advisory Committee. *Am J Infect Control* 1999;27:97
45. Ranaboldo CJ, Rowe-Jones DC. Closure of laparotomy wounds: skin staples versus sutures. *Br J Surg* 1992;79:1172
46. Frishman GN, Schwartz T, Hogan JW. Closure of Pfannenstiel skin incisions. Staples vs. subcuticular suture. *J Reprod Med* 1997;42:627
47. Zwart HJ, de Ruiter P. Subcuticular, continuous and mechanical skin closure: cosmetic results of a prospective randomized trial. *Neth J Surg* 1989;41:57
48. Webster DJ, Davis PW. Closure of abdominal wounds by adhesive strips: a clinical trial. *Br Med J* 1975;20:696
49. Singer AJ, Quinn JV, Clark RE, Hollander JE. Closure of lacerations and incisions with octylcyanoacrylate: a multicenter randomized trial. *Surgery* 2002;131:270
50. Blondeel PN, Murphy JW, Debrosse D, et al. Closure of long surgical incisions with a new formulation of 2-octylcyanoacrylate tissue adhesive versus commercially available methods. *Am J Surg* 2004;188:307
51. Harold KL, Goldstein SL, Nelms CD, et al. Optimal closure method of five-millimeter trocar sites. *Am J Surg* 2004;187:24
52. Petrowsky H, Demartines N, Rousson V, et al. Evidence-based value of prophylactic drainage in gastrointestinal surgery: a systematic review and meta-analyses. *Ann Surg* 2004;240:1074
53. Fong Y, Brennan MF, Brown K, et al. Drainage is unnecessary after elective liver resection. *Am J Surg* 1996;171:158
54. Belghiti J, Kabbej M, Sauvanet A, et al. Drainage after elective hepatic resection. A randomized trial. *Ann Surg* 1993;218:748
55. Liu CL, Fan ST, Lo CM, et al. Abdominal drainage after hepatic resection is contraindicated in patients with chronic liver diseases. *Ann Surg* 2004;239:194
56. Lewis RT, Goodall RG, Marien B, et al. Simple elective cholecystectomy: to drain or not. *Am J Surg* 1990;159:241
57. Conlon KC, Labow D, Leung D, et al. Prospective randomized clinical trial of the value of intraperitoneal drainage after pancreatic resection. *Ann Surg* 2001;234:487
58. Kim J, Lee J, Hyung WJ, et al. Gastric cancer surgery without drains: a prospective randomized trial. *J Gastrointest Surg* 2004;8:727
59. Poole GV Jr. Mechanical factors in abdominal wound closure: the prevention of fascial dehiscence. *Surgery* 1985;97:631
60. Hubbard TB Jr, Rever WB Jr. Retention sutures in the closure of abdominal incisions. *Am J Surg* 1972;124:378
61. Rink AD, Goldschmidt D, Dietrich J, et al. Negative side-effects of retention sutures for abdominal wound closure. A prospective randomised study. *Eur J Surg* 2000;166:932
62. Makela JT, Kiviniemi H, Juvonen T, et al. Factors influencing wound dehiscence after midline laparotomy. *Am J Surg* 1995;170:387
63. Saxe JM, Ledgerwood AM, Lucas CE. Management of the difficult abdominal closure. *Surg Clin North Am* 1993;73:243
64. Burch JM, Ortiz VB, Richardson RJ, et al. Abbreviated laparotomy and planned reoperation for critically injured patients. *Ann Surg* 1992;215:476
65. Brock WB, Barker DE, Burns RP. Temporary closure of open abdominal wounds: the vacuum pack. *Am Surg* 1995;61:30
66. Stone PA, Hass SM, Flaherty SK, et al. Vacuum-assisted fascial closure for patients with abdominal trauma. *J Trauma* 2004;57:1082
67. Jernigan TW, Fabian TC, Croce MA, et al. Staged management of giant abdominal wall defects: acute and long-term results. *Ann Surg* 2003;238:349
68. Hermann RE, Flowers RE, Wasylenki EW. Early exposure in the management of the postoperative wound. *Surg Gynecol Obstet* 1965;120:503
69. Hulten L. Dressings for surgical wounds. *Am J Surg* 1994;167:42S
70. Law N, Ellis HE. Exposure of the wound—a safe economy in the NHS. *Postgrad Med J* 1987;63:27
71. Haley RW, Morgan WM, Culver DH, et al. Update from the SENIC project. Hospital infection control: recent progress and opportunities under prospective payment. *Am J Infect Control* 1985;13:97
72. Culver DH, Horan TC, Gaynes RP, et al. Surgical wound infection rates by wound class, operative procedure, and patient risk index. National Nosocomial Infections Surveillance System. *Am J Med* 1991;91:152S
73. Urschel J. Necrotizing soft tissue infections. *Postgrad Med J* 1999;75:645

74. Riseman JA, Zamboni WA, Curtis A, et al. Hyperbaric oxygen therapy for necrotizing fasciitis reduces mortality and the need for debridements. *Surgery* 1990;108:847
75. Clark L, Moon R. Hyperbaric oxygen in the treatment of life-threatening soft-tissue infections. *Respir Care Clin N Am* 1999;5:203
76. Bisno A, Stevens D. Streptococcal infections of skin and soft tissues. *N Engl J Med* 1996;334:240
77. Nurmohamed MT, Verhaeghe R, Haas S, et al. A comparative trial of a low molecular weight heparin (enoxaparin) versus standard heparin for the prophylaxis of postoperative deep vein thrombosis in general surgery. *Am J Surg* 1995;169:567
78. Kakkar VV, Boeckl O, Boneu B, et al. Efficacy and safety of a low-molecular-weight heparin and standard unfractionated heparin for prophylaxis of postoperative venous thromboembolism: European multicenter trial. *World J Surg* 1997;21:2
79. Hodgson NC, Malthaner RA, Ostbye T. The search for an ideal method of abdominal fascial closure: a meta-analysis. *Ann Surg* 2000;231:436
80. van't Riet M, Steyerberg EW, Nellensteyn J, et al. Meta-analysis of techniques for closure of midline abdominal incisions. *Br J Surg* 2002;89:1350
81. Bucknell TE, Cox PJ, Ellis H. Burst abdomen and incisional hernia: a prospective study of 1129 major laparotomies. *BMJ* 1982;284:931
82. Webster C, Neumayer L, Smout R, et al. Prognostic models of abdominal wound dehiscence after laparotomy. *J Surg Res* 2003;109:130
83. Gislason H, Viste A. Closure of burst abdomen after major gastrointestinal operations—comparison of different surgical techniques and later development of incisional hernia. *Eur J Surg* 1999;165:958
84. Pavlidis TE, Galatianos IN, Papaziogas BT, et al. Complete dehiscence of the abdominal wound and incriminating factors. *Eur J Surg* 2001;167:351
85. van't RM, De Vos Van Steenwijk PJ, Bonjer HJ, et al. Incisional hernia after repair of wound dehiscence: incidence and risk factors. *Am Surg* 2004;70:281
86. Schimp VL, Worley C, Brunello S, et al. Vacuum-assisted closure in the treatment of gynecologic oncology wound failures. *Gynecol Oncol* 2004;92:586

5

Hernias

Patrick J. Javid ■ David C. Brooks

A hernia is defined as an area of weakness or complete disruption of the fibromuscular tissues of the body wall. Structures arising from the cavity contained by the body wall can pass through, or herniate, through such a defect. While the definition is straightforward, the terminology is often misrepresented. It should be clear that *hernia* refers to the actual anatomic weakness or defect, and *hernia contents* describe those structures that pass through the defect.

Hernias are among the oldest known afflictions of humankind, and surgical repair of the inguinal hernia is the most common general surgery procedure performed today.[1] Despite the high incidence, the technical aspects of hernia repair continue to evolve.

■ INGUINAL HERNIA

HISTORY

The word "hernia" is derived from a Latin term meaning "a rupture." The earliest reports of abdominal wall hernias date back to 1500 BC. During this early era, abdominal wall hernias were treated with trusses or bandage dressings. The first evidence of operative repair of a groin hernia dates to the first century AD. The original hernia repairs involved wide operative exposures through scrotal incisions requiring orchiectomy on the involved side. Centuries later, around 700 AD, principles of operative hernia repair evolved to emphasize mass ligation and en bloc excision of the hernia sac, cord, and testis distal to the external ring. The first report of groin hernia classification based on the anatomy of the defect (ie, inguinal versus femoral) dates to the 14th century, and the anatomical descriptions of direct and indirect types of inguinal hernia were first reported in 1559.

Bassini revolutionized the surgical repair of the groin hernia with his novel anatomical dissection and low recurrence rates. He first performed his operation in 1884, and published his initial outcomes in 1889.[2] Bassini reported 100% follow-up of patients over a 5-year period, with just 5 recurrences in over 250 patients. This rate of recurrence was unheard of at the time and marked a distinct turning point in the evolution of herniorraphy. Bassini's repair emphasizes both the high ligation of the hernia sac in the internal ring, as well as suture reinforcement of the posterior inguinal canal. The operation utilizes a deep and superficial closure of the inguinal canal. In the deep portion of the repair, the canal is repaired by interrupted sutures affixing the transversalis fascia medially to the inguinal ligament laterally. This requires an incision through the transversalis fascia. The superficial closure is provided by the external oblique fascia.

In addition to Bassini's contributions, the first true Cooper's ligament repair, which affixes the pectineal ligament to Poupart's ligament and thereby repairs both inguinal and femoral hernia defects, was introduced by Lotheissen in 1898. McVay further popularized the Cooper's ligament repair with the addition of a relaxing incision to reduce the increased wound tension.

The advances in groin hernia repair in the century following Bassini have shared the primary goal of reducing long-term hernia recurrence rates. To this end, efforts have been directed at developing a repair that imparts the least tension on the tissues that are brought together to repair the hernia defect. Darn repairs were first introduced in the early 20th century to reduce wound tension by using either autologous tissue or synthetic suture to bridge the gap between fascial tissues. Muscle and fascial flaps were attempted without consistent success. In 1918, Handley introduced the first use of silk as a prosthetic darn and nylon followed several years later. However, it was found that heavy prosthetic material increased the risk of wound infection, and the silk suture ultimately lost its strength over time. The use of autologous or synthetic patches was also attempted in order to reduce wound tension and improve rates of recurrence. The first patches, beginning in the early 20th century, consisted of silver wire filigree sheets that were placed along the inguinal canal. Over time, the sheets suffered from metal fatigue leading to hernia recurrence. Reports of the wire patches eroding into adjacent inguinal structures and even the peritoneal cavity itself caused even more concern with this technique. The modern synthetic patch, made of a plastic monofilament polymer (polyethylene), was introduced by Usher in 1958. Lichtenstein, who developed a sutureless hernia repair using a plastic mesh patch placed across the inguinal floor, further popularized this technique.

In the search for a technical means to reduce recurrence, emphasis was also placed on a meticulous dissection that would avoid placement of a prosthetic mesh. The most popular version was the Shouldice technique, initially introduced in 1958, and in essence a modification of the Bassini operation. This technique involves meticulous dissection of the entire inguinal floor and closure of the inguinal canal in four layers. The transversalis fascial layer itself is closed in two layers, as opposed to the single layer of interrupted suture advocated by Bassini. While the operation can be technically challenging to the beginner, it has been associated with excellent long-term outcomes and low recurrence rates.

Today, laparoscopic techniques have been validated as safe and effective in the treatment of groin hernias and have become commonplace. The laparoscopic approaches were initially developed in the early 1990s as laparoscopic techniques diffused throughout other specialties of general surgery.

EPIDEMIOLOGY

Seventy-five percent of all abdominal wall hernias are found in the groin, making it the most common location for an abdominal wall hernia. Of all groin hernias, 95% are hernias of the inguinal canal with the remainder being femoral hernia defects. Inguinal hernias are nine times more common in men than in women. Although femoral hernias are found more often in women, the inguinal hernia is still the most common hernia in women.[3] The overall lifetime risk of developing a groin hernia is approximately 15% in males and less than 5% in females. There is clearly an association between age and hernia diagnosis. After an initial peak in the infant, groin hernias become more prevalent with advancing age. In the same way, the complications of hernias (incarceration, strangulation, and bowel obstruction) are found more commonly at the extremes of age.

Currently in this country, approximately 700,000 operations for inguinal hernia repair are performed annually.[4]

ANATOMIC CLASSIFICATION

A thorough classification system has been developed to assist in the proper diagnosis and management of the inguinal hernia. All hernias can be broadly classified as congenital or acquired, and it is thought that the vast majority of inguinal hernias are congenital in nature. Acquired groin hernias develop after surgical incision and manipulation of the involved abdominal wall tissues. Given the paucity of primary groin incisions utilized in modern general surgery, acquired hernias of the inguinal or femoral region are rare.

Inguinal hernias are further divided by anatomical location into direct and indirect types. This differentiation is based on the location of the actual hernia defect in relation to the inferior epigastric vessels. The inferior epigastric vessels are continuous with the superior epigastric vessels that originate from the internal mammary artery cephalad and ultimately course caudally into the common femoral artery and vein. These vascular structures make up the lateral axis of Hesselbach's triangle, which includes the lateral border of the rectus sheath as its medial border and the inguinal (Poupart's) ligament itself as the inferior border. Hernias that develop lateral to the inferior epigastric vessels are termed *indirect* inguinal hernias, and those that develop medial to the vessels are *direct* inguinal hernias. In this way, direct hernia defects are found *within* Hesselbach's triangle. Hernias of the femoral type are located caudal or inferior to the inguinal ligament in a medial position.

The indirect inguinal hernia develops at the site of the internal ring, or the location where the spermatic cord in men and the round ligament in women enters the abdomen. While they may present at any age, indirect inguinal hernias are thought to be congenital in etiology. The accepted hypothesis is that these hernias arise from the incomplete or defective obliteration of the processus vaginalis during the fetal period. The processus is the peritoneal layer that covers the testicle or ovary as it passes through the inguinal canal and into the scrotum in men or the broad ligament in women. The internal ring closes, and the processus vaginalis becomes obliterated following the migration of the testicle into the inguinal canal. The failure of this closure provides an environment for the indirect inguinal hernia to develop. In this way, the remnant layer of peritoneum forms a sac at the internal ring through which intra-abdominal contents may herniate, thereby resulting in a clinically detectable inguinal hernia. Anatomically, the internal ring is lateral to the external ring and the remainder of the inguinal canal, and this explains the lateral relationship of the indirect inguinal hernia to the inferior epigastric vessels. It is noteworthy that indirect inguinal hernia develops more frequently on the right, where descent of the gonads occurs later during fetal development.

Direct inguinal hernias, in contrast, are found medial to the inferior epigastric artery and vein, and within Hesselbach's triangle. These hernias are acquired and only rarely found in the youngest age groups. They are thought to develop from an acquired weakness in the fibromuscular structures of the inguinal floor, so that the abdominal wall in this region can no longer adequately contain the intra-abdominal contents. The exact relationship between direct inguinal hernias and heavy lifting or straining remains unclear, and some studies suggest that the incidence of direct hernia is no greater in people in professions that routinely involve heavy manual labor.[5]

While femoral hernias account for less than 10% of all groin hernias, their presentation can be more acute in nature. In fact, it is estimated that up to 40% of femoral hernias present as emergencies with hernia incarceration or strangulation.[3] In this way, femoral hernias may also present with bowel obstruction. The empty space through which a femoral hernia forms is medial to the femoral vessels and nerve in the femoral canal and adjacent to the major femoral lymphatics. The inguinal ligament forms the cephalad border of the empty space. However, while the empty space is inferior to the ligament, the herniated contents may present superior to the ligament, thereby making an accurate diagnosis difficult.

Femoral hernias are much more common in females than males, although inguinal hernias are still the most common hernia in women. The predilection for femoral hernias in women may be secondary to less bulky groin musculature or weakness in the pelvic floor tissues from previous childbirth. It has been shown that previous inguinal hernia repair may be a risk factor for the subsequent development of a femoral hernia.[3]

ANATOMY OF THE GROIN

The boundaries of the inguinal canal must be understood to comprehend the principles of hernia repair. In the inguinal canal, the anterior boundary is the external oblique aponeurosis; the posterior boundary is composed of the transversalis fascia with some contribution from the aponeurosis of the transversus abdominis muscle; the inferior border is imparted by the inguinal and lacunar ligaments; and the superior boundary is formed by the arching fibers of the internal oblique musculature.

The internal (or deep) inguinal ring is formed by a normal defect in the transversalis fascia through which the spermatic cord in men and the round ligament in women passes into the abdomen from the extraperitoneal plane. The external (or superficial) ring is inferior and medial to the internal ring and represents an opening of the aponeurosis of the external oblique. The spermatic cord passes from the peritoneum through the internal ring and then caudally into the external ring before entering the scrotum in males.

From superficial to deep, the surgeon first encounters Scarpa's fascia after incising the skin and subcutaneous tissue. Deep to Scarpa's layer is the external oblique aponeurosis, which must be incised and spread to identify the cord structures. The inguinal ligament represents the inferior extension of the external oblique aponeurosis, and extends from the anterior superior iliac spine to the pubic tubercle. The medial extension of the external oblique aponeurosis forms the anterior rectus sheath. The iliohypogastric and ilioinguinal nerves, which provide sensation to the skin, penis, and the upper medial thigh, lie deep to the external oblique aponeurosis in the groin region. The internal oblique aponeurosis is more prominent cephalad in the inguinal canal, and its fibers form the superior border of the canal itself. The cremaster muscle, which envelops the cord structures, originates from the internal oblique musculature. The transversalis abdominis muscle and its fascia represent the true floor of the inguinal canal. Deep to the floor is the preperitoneal space, which houses the inferior epigastric artery and vein, the genitofemoral and lateral femoral cutaneous nerves, and the vas deferens, which traverses this space to join the remaining cord structures at the internal inguinal ring.

ETIOLOGY

The indirect inguinal hernia, the most common form of groin hernia across all ages and both genders, is thought to be congenital in etiology. The processus vaginalis is the pocket of peritoneum that forms around the testicle as it descends through the internal ring and along the inguinal canal into the scrotum during the 28th week of gestation. The primary etiology behind the indirect inguinal hernia is believed to be a patent processus vaginalis, which in essence represents a hernia sac. In this way, the hernia defect is the internal ring itself, and the sac is preformed but never closes at the end of gestation. Once intra-abdominal contents find their way into the sac, an indirect inguinal hernia is formed.

It is likely, however, that every person with a patent processus vaginalis does not develop an inguinal hernia during his or her lifetime. Thus, other predisposing factors must aid in indirect inguinal hernia formation. It is commonly thought that repeated increases in intra-abdominal pressure contribute to hernia formation; hence, inguinal hernias are commonly associated with pregnancy, chronic obstructive pulmonary disease, abdominal ascites, patients who undergo peritoneal dialysis, laborers who repeatedly flex the abdominal wall musculature, and individuals who strain from constipation. It is also thought that collagen formation and structure deteriorates with age, and thus hernia formation is more common in the older individual.

Several inborn errors of metabolism can lead to hernia formation. Specifically, conditions such as Ehlers-Danlos syndrome, Marfan's syndrome, Hunter's syndrome, and Hurler's syndrome can predispose to defects in collagen formation. There is evidence that cigarette smoking is associated with connective tissue disruption, and hernia formation is more common in the chronic smoker.

CLINICAL MANIFESTATIONS

The groin hernia can present in a variety of ways, from the asymptomatic hernia to frank peritonitis in a strangulated hernia. Many hernias are found on routine physical examination or on a focused examination for an unrelated complaint. These groin hernias are usually fully reducible and chronic in nature. Such hernias are still referred for repair since they invariably develop symptoms, and asymptomatic hernias still have an inherent risk of incarceration and strangulation.

The most common presenting symptomatology for a groin hernia is a dull feeling of discomfort or heaviness in the groin region that is exacerbated by straining the abdominal musculature, lifting heavy objects, or defecating. These maneuvers worsen the feeling of discomfort by increasing the intra-abdominal pressure and forcing the hernia contents through the hernia defect. Pain develops as a tight ring of fascia outlining the hernia defect compresses intra-abdominal structures with a visceral neuronal supply. With a reducible hernia, the feeling of discomfort resolves as the pressure is released when the patient stops straining the abdominal muscles. The pain is often worse at the end of the day, and patients in physically active professions may experience the pain more often that those who lead a sedentary lifestyle.

Overwhelming or focal pain from a groin hernia is unusual and should raise the suspicion of hernia incarceration or strangulation. An incarcerated hernia occurs when the hernia contents are trapped in the hernia defect so that the contents cannot be reduced back into the abdominal cavity. The tight circumferential pressure applied by the hernia defect serves to impede the venous outflow from the hernia contents, resulting in congestion, edema, and tissue ischemia. Ultimately, the arterial inflow to the hernia contents is compromised as well, resulting in tissue loss and necrosis, termed strangulation of the hernia.

All types of groin hernias are at risk for incarceration and strangulation, although the femoral hernia seems to be predisposed to this complication. Incarceration and strangulation of a groin hernia may present as a bowel obstruction when the tight hernia defect constricts the lumen of the viscus. Hence, all patients presenting with bowel obstruction require a thorough physical examination of the groin region for inguinal and femoral hernias. If there is no bowel in the hernia sac, an incarcerated groin hernia may alternatively present as a hard, painful mass that is tender to palpation.

The physical exam differs between an incarcerated and a strangulated hernia. The incarcerated hernia may be mildly tender due to venous congestion from the tight defect. The strangulated hernia will be tender and warm and may have surrounding skin erythema secondary to the inflammatory reaction from the ischemic bowel. The patient with the strangulated hernia may have a fever, hypotension from early bacteremia, and a leukocytosis. The incarcerated hernia requires operation on an urgent basis within 6–12 hours of presentation. If the operation is delayed for any reason, serial physical exams are mandated to follow any change in the hernia site indicating the onset of tissue loss. The strangulated hernia clearly requires emergent operation immediately following diagnosis.

It may also be difficult to differentiate fat from bowel contents in the hernia sac. It is important to recognize that incarcerated omental fat alone can produce significant pain and tenderness on physical exam.

PREGNANCY AND GROIN HERNIA

Not surprisingly, groin hernias during pregnancy may become symptomatic. This is related to the increased intra-abdominal pressure from the growing fetus and enlarging uterus. The symptomatic groin discomfort may become positional later in pregnancy as the uterus shifts location with movement. While the risk of complications of groin hernias still exists during pregnancy, the enlarging uterus may in theory protect against incarceration by physically blocking the intra-abdominal contents from the inlet of the defect.

In general, elective repair of groin hernias during pregnancy is not recommended, even if they become increasingly symptomatic. Emergent repair of the incarcerated or strangulated hernia is undertaken as needed.

PHYSICAL EXAMINATION

As with any hernia, the groin hernia should be properly examined with the patient in the standing position. This allows the hernia contents to fill the hernia sac and make the hernia obvious on physical examination. Some hernias, however, may be easily identifiable in the supine position. It should be noted that the exact anatomical classification of the inguinal hernia (ie, indirect versus direct) is impossible to accurately predict based on physical exam alone.

In the male patient, using the second or third finger, the examiner should invaginate the scrotum near the external ring and direct the finger medial towards the pubic tubercle. The examiner's finger will thus lie on the spermatic cord with the tip of the finger within the external ring. The patient is then asked to cough or perform a Valsalva maneuver. A true inguinal hernia will be felt as a silk-like sensation against the gloved finger of the examiner. This is the infamous "silk glove" sign.

The female patient does not have the long and stretched spermatic cord to follow with the examiner's finger during the physical examination. Instead, two fingers can be placed along the inguinal canal, and the patient is asked to cough or strain. If present, the examiner should feel the sensation of the hernia sac against the gloved finger. Particular attention in the female patient should be paid to the location of the sensation; femoral hernia sacs will present medial and just inferior to the lower border of the inguinal ligament.

While the physical examination does not differ in the infant, it can be more challenging to elicit the hernia impulse given the compressed groin anatomy of the young child. It is well known that a groin hernia can be more readily diagnosed in the infant who is actively crying and hence increasing the intra-abdominal pressure through flexion of the abdominal wall musculature.

The examination for the femoral hernia in both genders involves palpation of the femoral canal just below the inguinal ligament in the upper thigh. In this way, the most easily palpable landmark is the femoral artery, which is located lateral in the canal. Medial to the femoral artery is the femoral vein, and the femoral empty space is just medial to the vein. This area can be located easily, palpated with two fingers, and then examined closely while the patient coughs or strains. In general, a focused groin hernia examination should involve the investigation for both inguinal and femoral hernias in both genders.

TREATMENT

The treatment of all hernias, regardless of their location or type, is surgical repair. Elective repair is performed to alleviate symptoms and to prevent the significant complications of hernias, such as incarceration or strangulation. While the limited data available on the natural history of groin hernias show that these complications are rare, the complications are associated with a high rate of morbidity and mortality when they occur. At the same time, the risks of elective groin hernia repair, even in the patient with a complicated medical history, are exceedingly low. Outcomes of surgical repair are generally excellent with minimal morbidity and relatively rapid return to baseline health.

The major risk with delayed surgical repair is the risk of incarceration and/or strangulation. It is not possible to reliably identify those hernias that are at an increased risk for these complications. It is known that the risk of incarceration of a hernia is greatest soon after the hernia manifests itself. This is likely due to the fact that at the early stage of the hernia, the defect is small and fits tightly around the hernia sac; therefore any contents that fill the sac may quickly become trapped within the hernia. Over time, the hernia defect stretches due to the tissue that enters and leaves the sac with changes in intra-abdominal pressure. After 6 months, the risk of hernia incarceration decreases from 5% per year to 1–2% per year. In general, the larger the palpable defect on physical examination, the lower the risk of incarceration. Clearly, all risks of tissue loss aside, elective hernia repair is still preferred over emergent repair.

ANESTHESIA

Groin hernia repair can be performed using a variety of anesthesia options, including general, regional (such as spinal or epidural), and local anesthesia.[6] Laparoscopic repairs usually require general anesthesia in order to provide the complete muscle relaxation needed to achieve insufflation of the preperitoneal or peritoneal space.

Open groin hernia repairs are most often performed using either regional or local anesthesia. Local anesthesia with controlled intravenous sedation, referred to as monitored anesthesia care, is often preferred in the repair of the reducible inguinal hernia. Its advantages include the ease of induction and awakening, the short postanesthesia recovery period, and the fact that its intensity can easily be titrated up or down based on patient comfort levels intraoperatively. The only major disadvantage to this approach is in patients who experience considerable pain during repairs of large groin hernias.

In groin hernia repair, local anesthesia can be administered as a direct infiltration of the tissues to be incised or as a local nerve block of the ilioinguinal and iliohypogastric nerves. The latter is associated with improved local pain control, but may be difficult to achieve. The local nerve block also spares the soft tissue of edema from diffuse infiltration of local anesthesia.

Spinal or continuous epidural anesthesia allows the surgeon greater freedom to maneuver within the operative field since the anesthetized region is larger than in local anesthesia. However, these modes of anesthesia carry their own infrequent risks such as urinary retention, prolonged anesthetic effect, hypotension, and spinal headache. They may also be associated with longer in-hospital recovery times on the day of surgery.

A randomized trial of local, regional, and general anesthesia in 616 adult patients undergoing open inguinal hernia repair in 10 hospitals found that local anesthesia was superior in the early postoperative period.[7] Compared to those who received regional or general anesthesia, patients who received local anesthesia had less postoperative pain and nausea, shorter time spent in the hospital, and fewer unplanned overnight admissions (3% versus 14% and 22%, respectively).

OPERATIVE TECHNIQUES

Successful surgical repair of a hernia depends on a tension-free closure of the hernia defect to attain the lowest possible recurrence rate. Previous efforts to simply identify the defect and suture it closed resulted in unacceptably high recurrence rates of up to 15%. Modern techniques have improved upon this recurrence rate by placement of mesh over the hernia defect, or in the case of laparoscopic repair, behind the hernia defect. One exception to this rule is the classic Shouldice repair, which uses meticulous dissection and closure without mesh placement to obtain a consistently low recurrence rate. Another benefit of the tension-free closure is that it has been shown to cause the patient significantly less pain and discomfort in the short-term postoperative period.

Figure 5–1 illustrates the essential steps to the modern open inguinal hernia repair. All of the open anterior herniorraphy techniques begin with a transversely-oriented slightly curvilinear skin incision of approximately 6–8 cm positioned one to two fingerbreadths above the inguinal ligament. Dissection is carried down through the subcutaneous and Scarpa's layers. The external oblique aponeurosis is identified and cleaned so that the external ring is identified inferomedially. Being careful to avoid injury to the iliohypogastric and ilioinguinal nerves, the aponeurosis is incised sharply and opened along its length through the external ring with fine scissors. The nerves underlying the external oblique fascia are then identified and isolated for protection. The soft tissue is cleared off the posterior surface of the external oblique aponeurosis on both sides and the spermatic cord is mobilized. Using a combination of blunt and sharp dissection, the cremaster muscle fibers enveloping the cord are separated from the cord structures and the cord itself is isolated. At this point, it is possible to accurately define the anatomy of the hernia. An indirect hernia will present with a sac attached to the cord in an anteromedial position extending superiorly through the internal ring. A direct inguinal hernia will present as a weakness in the floor of the canal posterior to the cord. A pantaloon defect will present as both a direct and indirect defect in the same inguinal canal.

The specifics of the common modern techniques for hernia repair will be discussed further.

The Shouldice Technique

The Shouldice technique is commonly used for open repair of inguinal hernias and is the most popular pure tissue hernia repair. It is in essence the modern evolution of the Bassini repair performed in a multilayered fashion. Both operations use a tightening of the internal ring and closure of the transversalis fascia to the inguinal ligament as their primary tenets of hernia repair.[8]

Figure 5–2 illustrates the basic steps in the Shouldice repair. After suitable exposure and isolation of the cord, a pair of scissors is passed posterior to the transversalis fascia beginning at the medial pillar of the internal ring

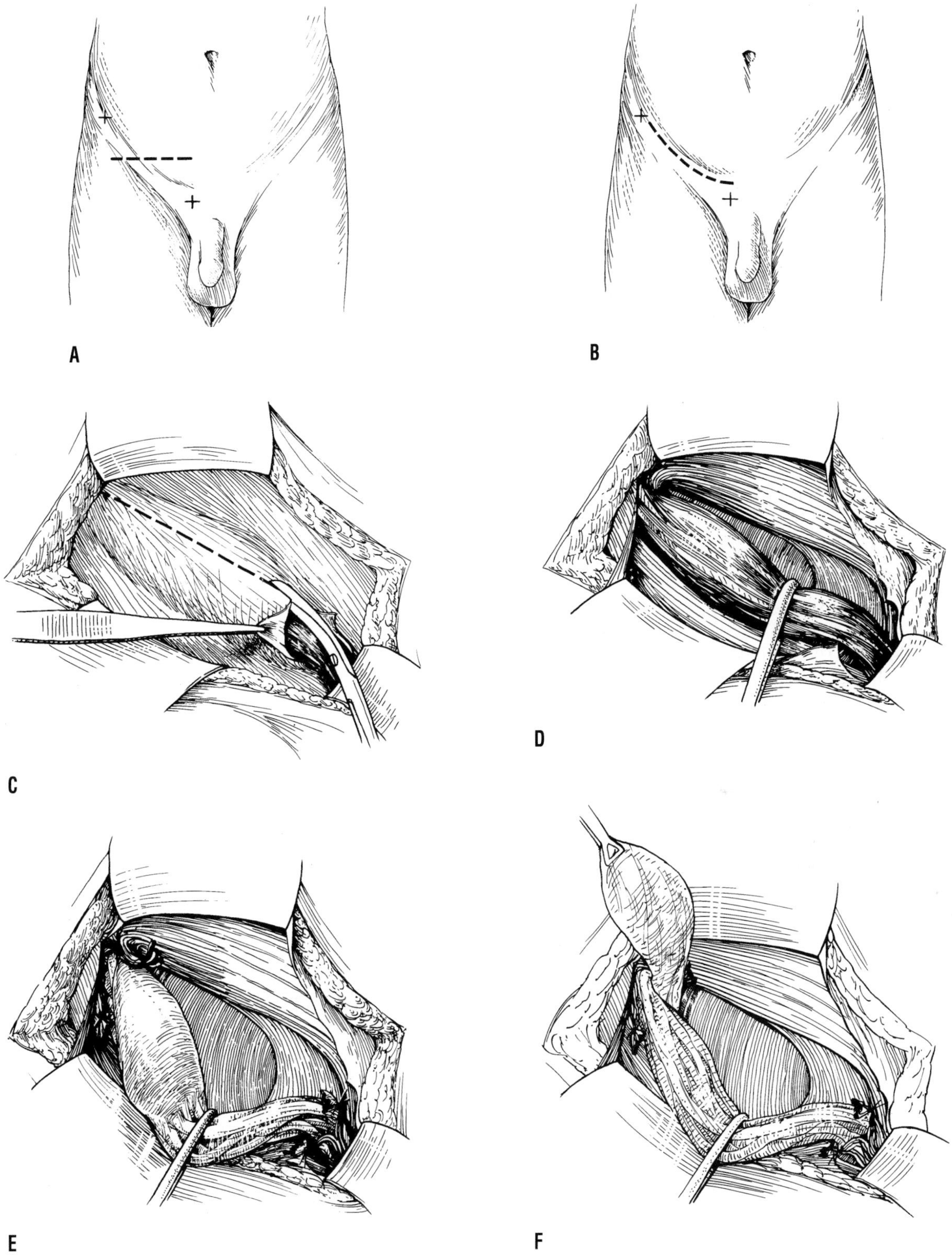

Figure 5–1. Adult hernia incision and dissection. **A.** Transverse incision. **B.** Curved skin crease incision. **C.** The aponeurosis of the external oblique is incised along the direction of its fibers. **D.** The inguinal canal is exposed and the spermatic cord mobilized. **E.** The spermatic cord has been skeletonized, and the internal ring and posterior wall of the canal (the transversalis fascia) have been defined. **F.** A medium-sized sac has been dissected free of the cord elements. *Continued*

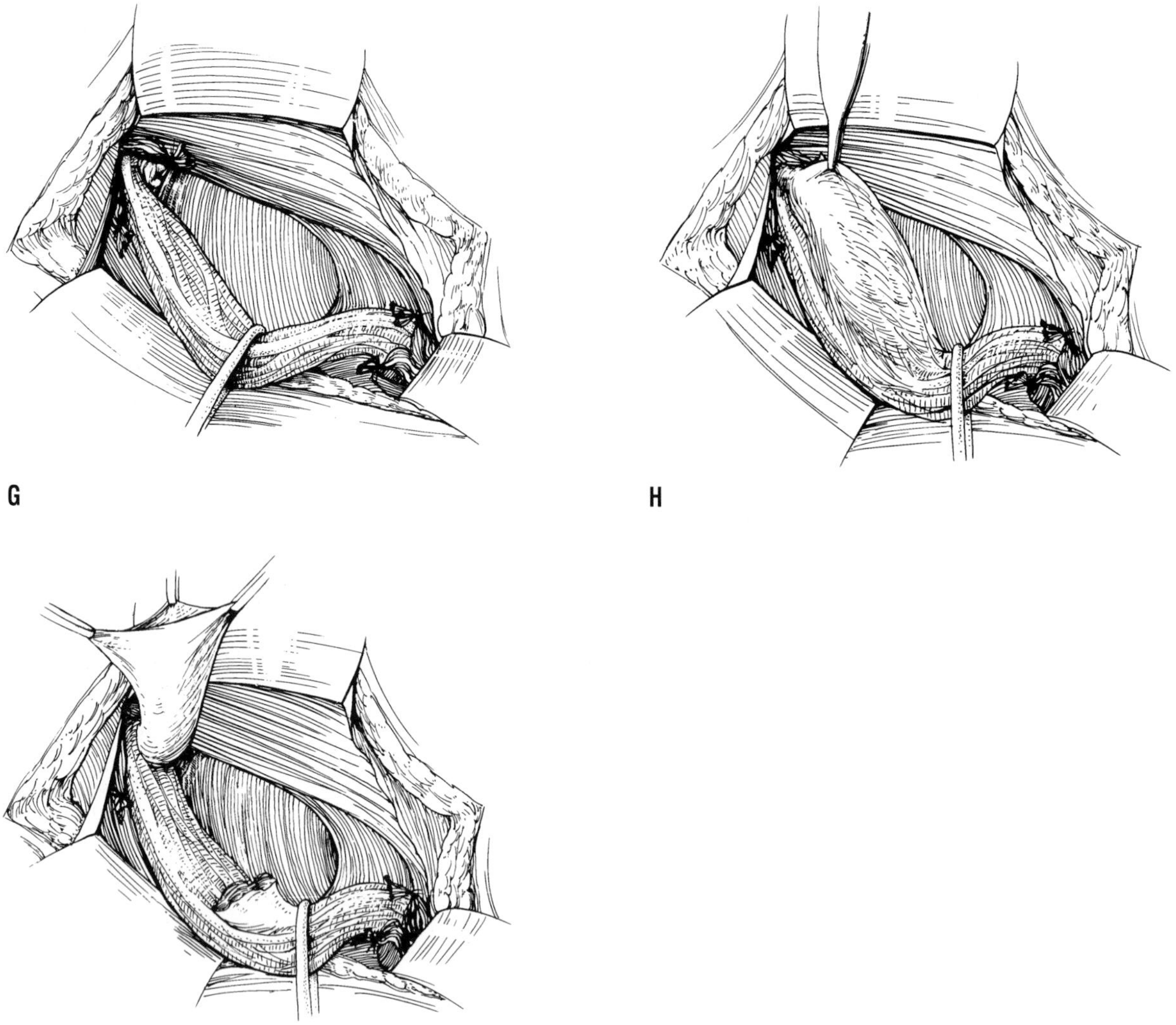

G

H

I

Figure 5–1, cont'd. G. The sac has been invaginated. **H.** A long or complete sac is being dissected free close to the internal ring. **I.** The sac has been transected. After Rejovitzky, MD.

and extending inferomedially to the pubic tubercle. In this way, the transversalis fascia is separated from the preperitoneal fat plane. Care must be taken at this stage to preserve the inferior epigastric vessels that reside in the preperitoneal space. The transversalis fascia is then opened with scissors along the entire inguinal floor from internal ring to pubic tubercle, and the posterior surface of the transversalis is cleaned of its preperitoneal attachments. As the first layer of the repair, the free edge of the lower transversalis flap is sutured in a continuous, imbricated fashion behind the upper flap to the posterior surface of the upper transversalis fascia and the lateral component of the posterior rectus sheath. This running suture layer is started medially at the pubic tubercle and carried up to and through the internal ring, thereby tightening the transversalis fascia around the cord at its entrance to the inguinal canal. The first layer is not tied but continued in a running fashion from lateral to medial as a second layer closing the upper transversalis flap to the base of the lower edge as well as the inguinal ligament. This second layer progresses medially to the pubic tubercle where it is tied to the original tail that started the first layer. The third layer of continuous suture starts at the tightened internal ring and brings together the conjoined tendon (the internal oblique and transversus abdominis aponeuroses) medially with the inguinal ligament laterally. This layer is run down to the pubic tubercle, and returns back to the internal ring as the fourth layer including the anterior rectus sheath medially with the posterior aspect of the external oblique aponeurosis laterally. The cord can now be relaxed gently on the new inguinal floor, and the external oblique aponeurosis is closed in one to two additional continuous layers extending down to the external ring to reapproximate this structure. The original descriptions of the operation by Shouldice used continuous stainless steel wire suture for

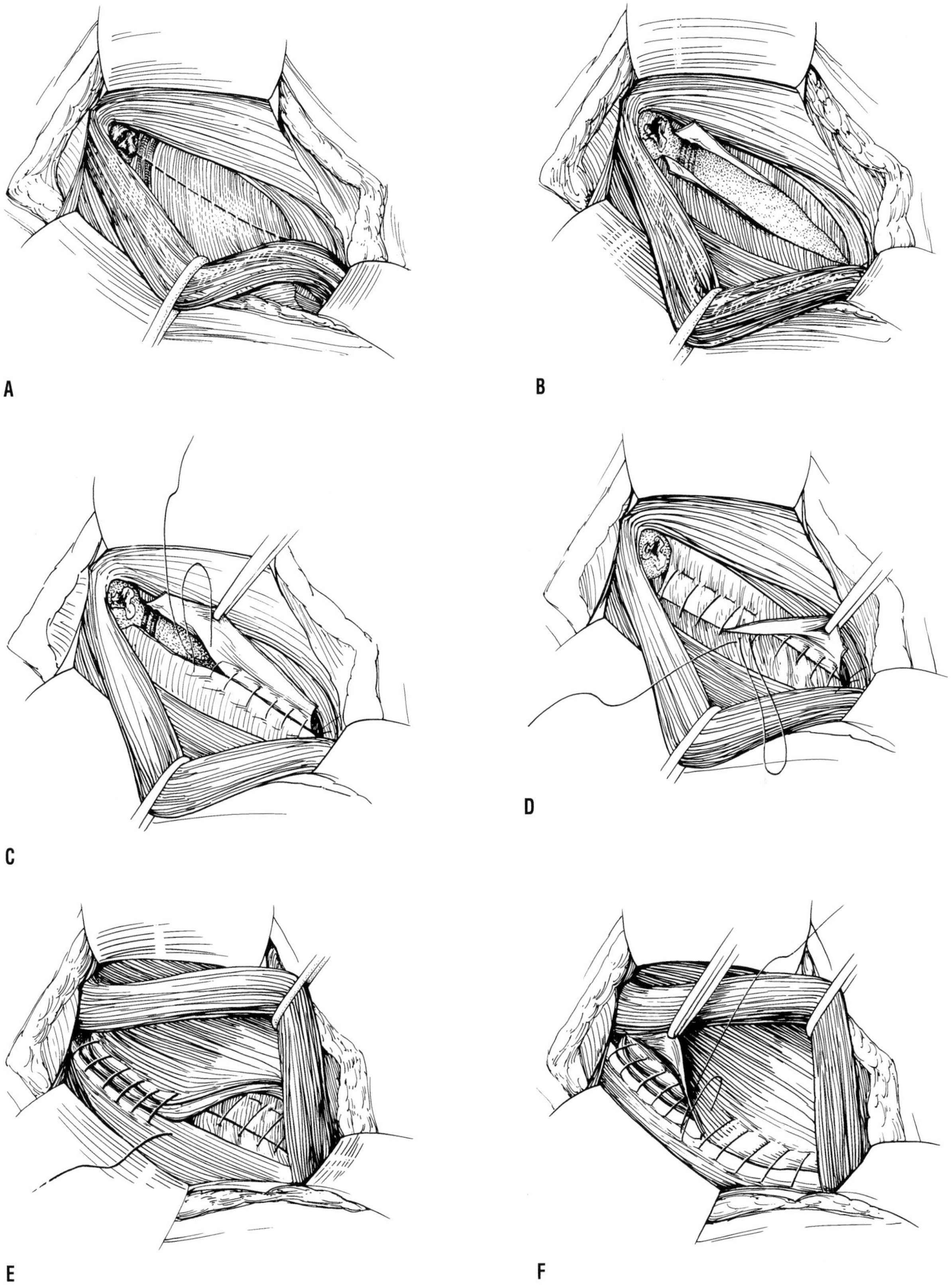

Figure 5–2. The Shouldice operation. **A.** The transversalis fascia is being incised. **B.** The upper and lower flaps of the transversalis fascia have been dissected free and elevated to expose the extraperitoneal fat and the inferior epigastric vessels. **C.** The first layer of the Shouldice operation. **D.** The second layer. **E.** The third layer. **F.** The fourth layer. *Continued*

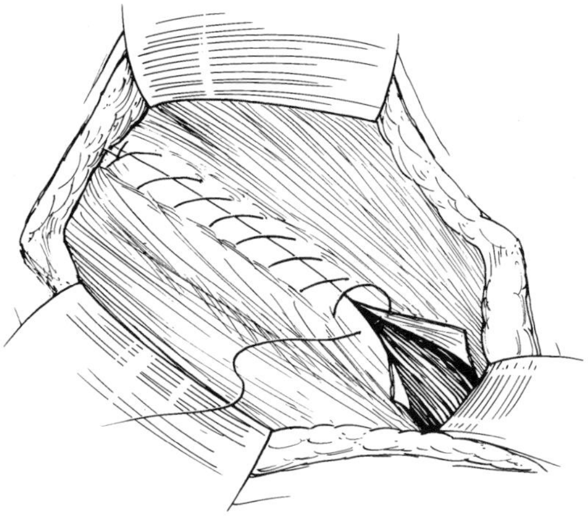

G

Figure 5–2, cont'd. G. The external oblique aponeurosis has been repaired anterior to the spermatic cord. After Rejovitzky, MD.

all four layers of repair, although surgeons commonly use permanent synthetic suture today.

The Shouldice Hospital reports excellent long-term outcomes from their operation with recurrence rates less than 1% in selected patients.[9,10] These results have not been achieved with any other pure tissue technique. The operation is well tolerated by most patients using local anesthesia only. From the multiple, overlapping, continuous suture lines, Shouldice proponents argue that any tension brought about in this type of closure is dispersed throughout the entire inguinal canal. The dissection is complicated, however, and requires excellent surgical technique and anatomic awareness. Moreover, other surgeons utilizing the Shouldice method have not achieved recurrence rates this low. Thus, the low rate of recurrence associated with the Shouldice technique likely depends on the level of surgical expertise and the patient selection. In one report of 183 inguinal hernia repairs using the Shouldice technique under local anesthesia, the recurrence rates for beginners versus more experienced surgeons were 9.4% versus 2.5%, respectively.[11]

The Cooper Ligament Repair

The Cooper ligament repair is the only technique that definitively repairs both the inguinal and femoral hernia defects in the groin. The operation is often named after Chester McVay, who popularized the operation in the 1940s and introduced the concept of the relaxing incision to decrease the tension from the repair. The repair is also a primary tissue repair in that no mesh is utilized.

The Cooper ligament repair begins similar to the Shouldice procedure, and exposure and isolation of the cord is performed. The transversalis fascia is then opened and cleaned posteriorly. At this time, Cooper's ligament is identified and dissected free of its fibrous and fatty attachments. The defects are repaired by using interrupted suture to affix the upper border of the transversalis fascia to Cooper's ligament beginning medially at the pubic tubercle and continuing until the femoral sheath is reached. At this point, the femoral canal is closed by carefully suturing Cooper's ligament to the femoral sheath. The repair is continued with interrupted sutures between the transversalis fascia and the iliopubic tract laterally until the entrance point of the cord is reached. In this way, the closure creates a new, and tighter, internal inguinal ring around the cord.

The Cooper ligament repair requires a relaxing incision because this pure tissue repair is associated with significant tension in closing all three groin hernia defects. After the transversalis fascia has been mobilized, and prior to the closure of the fascia to Cooper's ligament, a 2–4 cm vertical incision is made at the lateral border of the anterior rectus sheath beginning at the pubic tubercle and extending superiorly. The relaxing incision can be left open since the rectus muscle should protect against any herniation; alternatively, some surgeons argue for placement of a mesh over the relaxing incision since hernia formation can occur at this site.

The Cooper's ligament repair is an outstanding technique for a femoral hernia and is associated with excellent long-term results in experienced hands. Disadvantages of the repair include a longer operating time, a more extensive dissection, the potential for vascular injury and thromboembolic complications from the femoral vessels, and a longer postoperative recovery phase.

PROSTHETIC REPAIRS

Polypropylene mesh is the most common prosthetic used today in mesh repairs of the inguinal hernia. The two most common prosthetic repairs are the Lichtenstein[12] and the "plug and patch" repair as described by Gilbert[13] and popularized by Rutkow and Robbins.[14]

The type of mesh to be used during prosthetic inguinal hernia repairs deserves a brief discussion. The most common and preferred mesh for groin hernia repair is a polypropylene woven mesh marketed under a variety of names. Polypropylene is preferred because it allows for a fibrotic reaction to occur between the inguinal floor and the posterior surface of the mesh, thereby forming scar and strengthening the closure of the hernia defect. This fibrotic reaction is not seen to the same extent with other varieties of prosthetic, namely expanded polytetrafluoroethylene (PTFE) mesh. PTFE is often used for repair of ventral or incision hernias in which the fibrotic reaction with the underlying serosal surface of the bowel is best avoided.

There are limited prospective, randomized data comparing the recurrence rate of open prosthetic repairs versus open nonprosthetic repairs. An attempted meta-analysis concluded that mesh repair was associated with fewer overall recurrences, although the authors report that formal analysis was limited by the lack of available study data.[16] A review of 26,000 inguinal hernia repairs from Denmark found that mesh repairs had a lower reoperation rate than conventional open repairs.[17] The majority of groin hernia repairs performed in the United States in the modern era utilize mesh placement.

The Lichtenstein Technique

The Lichtenstein inguinal hernia repair was the first pure prosthetic, tension-free repair to achieve consistently low recurrence rates in long-term outcomes analysis. This operation begins with the incision of the external oblique aponeurosis, and the isolation of the cord structures. Any indirect hernia sac is mobilized off the cord to the level of the internal ring. At this point, a large mesh tailored to fit along the inguinal canal floor is placed so that the curved end lies directly on top of the pubic tubercle. The mesh patch extends underneath the cord until the spermatic cord and the tails of the mesh patch meet laterally. Here, an incision is made in the mesh, and the cord is inserted between the tails of the mesh, thereby creating a new, tighter, and more medial internal ring. The tails are sutured together with one nonabsorbable stitch just proximal to the attachment of the cord. The mesh is then sutured in a continuous or interrupted fashion to the pubic tubercle inferiorly, the conjoined tendon medially, and the inguinal ligament laterally.

Rutkow and Robbins have reported interesting and effective advances in the Lichtenstein technique. The "plug and patch" repair, as illustrated in Figure 5–3, represents a tension-free herniorraphy and can even be performed without sutures. In this technique, the patch is placed in a similar fashion to the modern Lichtenstein repair as it lies along the inguinal canal from the pubic tubercle medially to beyond the cord laterally. In addition, a mesh plug in the form of an umbrella or cone is snugly fit up and into the internal ring. In this way, the repair goes beyond just a tightening of the internal ring, but serves to close the ring around the spermatic cord. Modifications of this operation exist and are practiced commonly by general surgeons. The patch and plug can be sutured to the surrounding inguinal canal tissue in an interrupted or continuous fashion. Alternatively, both prostheses can be placed in appropriate position with no suture affixment. In this way, the body's natural scarring mechanism will hold both pieces of mesh in place over time. Wide internal ring defects, often caused by large or chronic indirect sacs, may require one or two sutures to tack the plug in place to avoid slippage into the canal anteriorly or the retroperitoneal space posteriorly.

The Preperitoneal Approach

The preperitoneal space is found between the transversalis fascia and the peritoneum itself. The actual groin hernia defect is located anterior to this space, whether the defect exists in the internal ring (indirect inguinal hernia) or through the transversalis floor of the inguinal canal (direct inguinal hernia). Several authors, including Rives, Nyhus, Stoppa, and Kugel, advocate the use of a preperitoneal or posterior approach to repair of the inguinal hernia. They argue that this approach is more effective than the traditional anterior herniorraphy because a repair in the preperitoneal plane fixes the hernia defect in the space between the hernia contents and the hernia defect. In contrast, the anterior approach does not keep the hernia contents from contact with the defect, but rather fixes the hernia defect anterior to the defective anatomy. The operation is also advocated for difficult inguinal hernia recurrences, since the posterior approach will usually remain open and without scar following a previous anterior hernia repair. The original operation as described by Nyhus repairs the hernia primarily with suture, although more recent modifications incorporate a mesh patch posterior to the floor of the inguinal canal. As described later in this chapter, the standard laparoscopic technique for inguinal hernia repair is based entirely on the preperitoneal hernia repair.

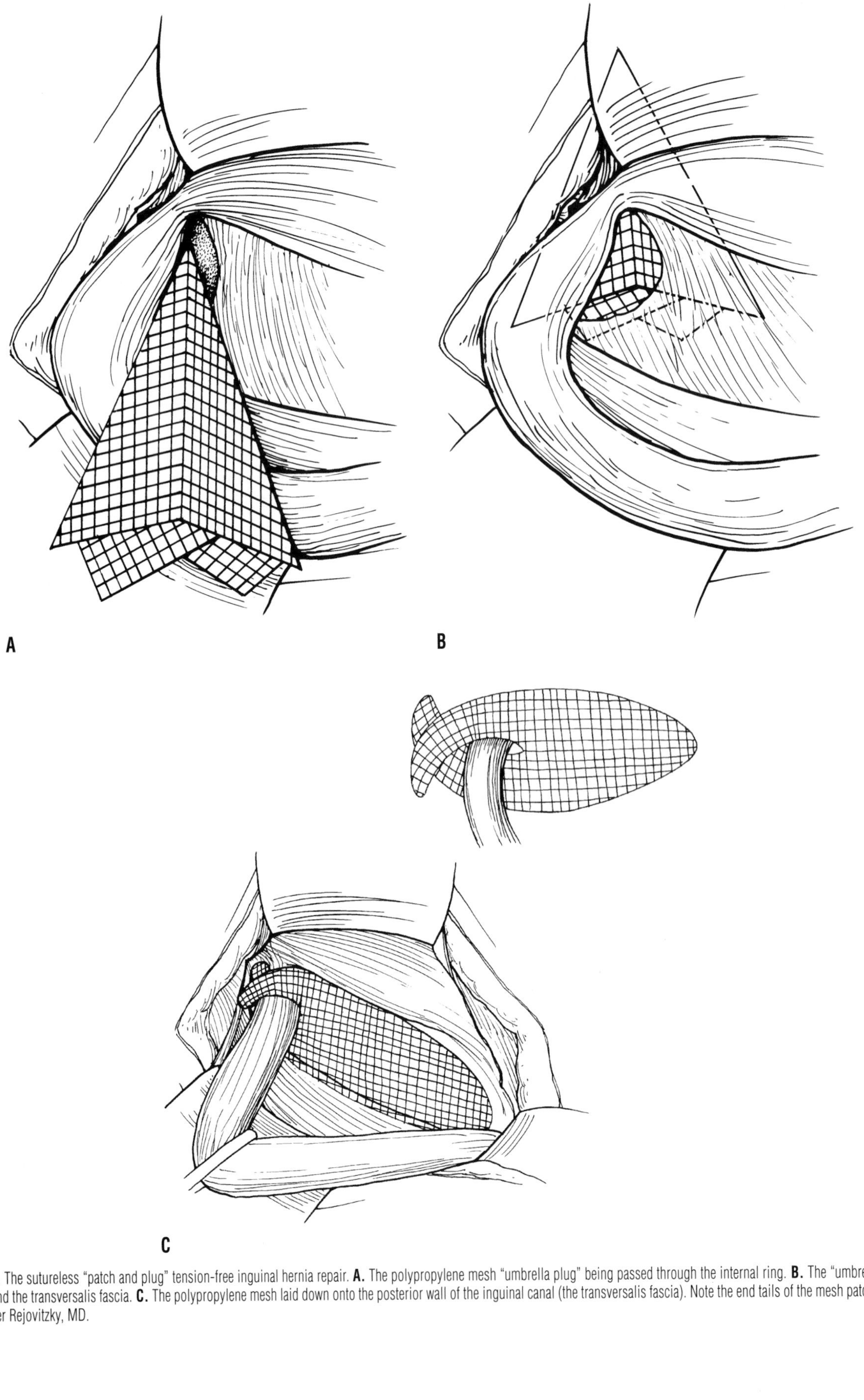

Figure 5–3. The sutureless "patch and plug" tension-free inguinal hernia repair. **A.** The polypropylene mesh "umbrella plug" being passed through the internal ring. **B.** The "umbrella plug" has opened behind the transversalis fascia. **C.** The polypropylene mesh laid down onto the posterior wall of the inguinal canal (the transversalis fascia). Note the end tails of the mesh patch embracing the cord. After Rejovitzky, MD.

Figures 5–4 and 5–5 illustrate the preperitoneal repair as described by Rives.[15] In the preperitoneal hernia repair, the incision is usually made transversely in the lower quadrant 2–3 cm cephalad to the inguinal ligament. The incision is made slightly more medial than the anterior approach so that the lateral border of the rectus muscle can be exposed after incising the anterior rectus sheath. Once the muscle is exposed, retraction of the rectus muscle medially allows for careful opening of the posterior rectus sheath and entry into the preperitoneal space. The inferior epigastric vessels and the cord can be visualized in this space. The cord usually does not require extensive manipulation or dissection since the usual cord attachments (lipoma and cremaster fibers) are found in the anterior layers of the inguinal canal. In this way, the approach also avoids exposure to the sensory nerves of the inguinal canal.

Once the preperitoneal space has been entered and exposed, the specific repair to be performed depends on hernia anatomy. For direct defects, the sac is inverted back into the peritoneal cavity but does not need to be excised. The transversalis fascia is then reapproximated over the inverted sac using interrupted sutures; in this way the upper border of the transversalis fascia is affixed to the lower border composed of the iliopubic tract. For indirect defects, the sac is reduced off of the cord and a high ligation of the sac is performed at the sac neck; ironically, with this ap-

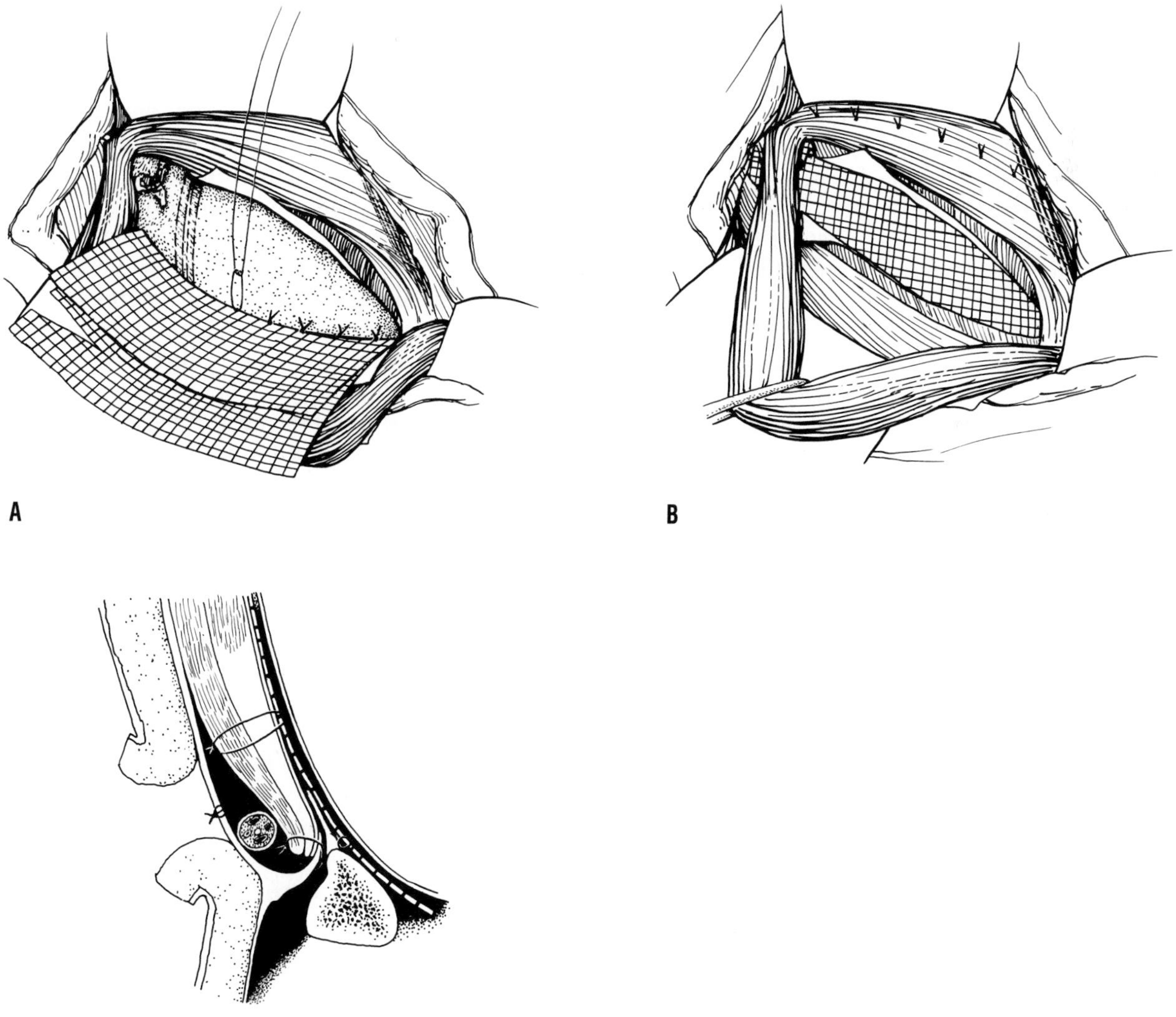

A

B

C

Figure 5–4. Rives prosthetic mesh repair. **A.** Lower line of fixation of the mesh. **B.** Lateral and upper points of fixation of the mesh. **C.** Preperitoneal placement of the mesh and the Bassini-type repair of the posterior wall of the inguinal canal anterior to the mesh. After Rejovitzky, MD.

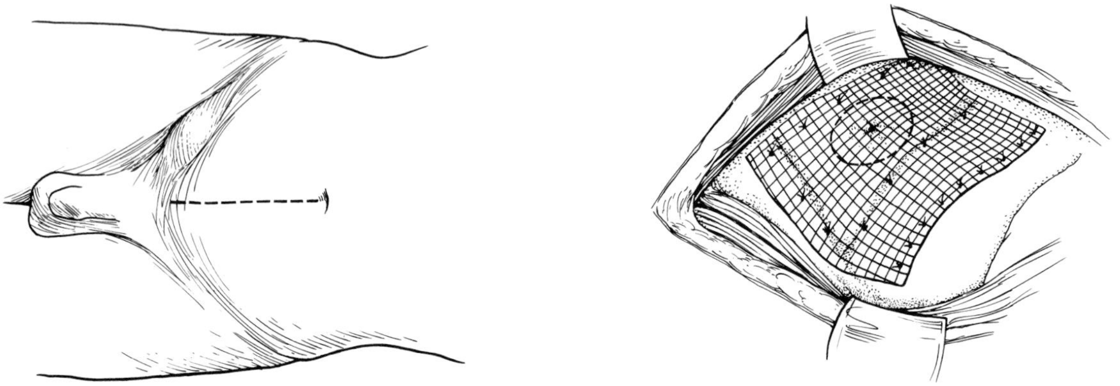

A B

Figure 5–5. A. The lower midline incision used for the preperitoneal approach to inguinal hernia repair. **B.** Another view of the points of attachment of the mesh in the preperitoneal plane. After Rejovitzky, MD.

proach, the "high ligation" is actually a "posterior" ligation, since the surgeon ideally should transect the sac just above the preperitoneal fat, which is situated along the inferior border of the exposed field. Once the sac has been ligated, the defect in the internal ring is repaired from the posterior plane using interrupted suture to affix the ring leaflets of the transversalis fascia to the iliopubic tract thereby tightening the ring itself.

Modifications of this approach using the prosthetic mesh patch are relatively straightforward. The mesh patch is placed underneath the transversalis fascia and directly on the preperitoneal fat. This patch, if placed completely over the inguinal region, covers any peritoneum that could potentially form a hernia sac through a direct or indirect fascial defect.

LAPAROSCOPIC REPAIR

Laparoscopic groin hernia repair was first performed by Ger in 1979, although it was only within the past decade and a half that laparoscopic hernia repair became more accepted. The laparoscopic approach to hernia repair has since evolved into a common and effective procedure. Today, the laparoscopic approach comprises approximately 20–25% of groin hernia operations and 80,000–100,000 laparoscopic hernia repairs are performed annually in the United States. The most important difference between the laparoscopic and open approaches for inguinal hernia repair is anatomical: the laparoscopic approach uses mesh to repair the hernia defect in a plane posterior to the defect (either in the preperitoneal space or from within the peritoneal cavity), whereas the open approaches repair the hernia anterior to the defect.

Three different techniques exist for laparoscopic repair of groin hernias. The transabdominal preperitoneal (TAP) repair involves standard laparoscopy with access into the peritoneal cavity and placement of a large mesh along the anterior abdominal wall, thereby repairing the hernia posterior to the defect. This technique was the first laparoscopic hernia repair to be performed. Ports are generally placed through the umbilicus and then laterally on either side of the rectus muscle. The hernia defect is usually well visualized from within the peritoneal cavity. After both inguinal regions have been inspected and laparoscopic adhesiolysis performed if necessary, the median umbilical ligament (the urachal remnant), the medial umbilical ligament (the remnant of the umbilical artery), and the lateral umbilical fold (the reflection of peritoneum over the inferior epigastric vessels) are identified. The parietal layer of peritoneum is then incised superior to the hernia defect and reflected inferiorly, thereby exposing the hernia defect, the epigastric vessels, Cooper's ligament, the pubic tubercle, and the iliopubic tract. The cord structures are then dissected free of their peritoneal attachments. In a direct hernia, the peritoneal sac is pulled back within the peritoneal cavity with gentle traction to separate the thin peritoneal layer from the equally thin layer of transversalis fascia anterior to it. In an indirect hernia, the peritoneal sac is retracted off of the cord structures and pulled back within the peritoneal cavity. Alternatively, in the setting of a large chronic indirect hernia, the sac can be divided distal to the internal ring so that only the proximal portion of the sac needs to be mobilized for the repair. A large polypropylene mesh patch is then placed between the peritoneum and the transversalis fascia that covers the inguinal floor, internal ring, and the femoral canal. The mesh is stapled or tacked to the pubic tubercle medially, Cooper's ligament inferiorly, and the anterior superior iliac spine laterally. The incised peritoneal flap is then closed over the mesh.

While the TAP repair has been shown to be effective, there is a risk that the prosthetic mesh will be in direct content with the bowel, and significant concern has been raised about the potential for intra-abdominal adhesions postoperatively.[18] Enthusiasm for this technique has waned in recent years with the advent of extraperitoneal laparoscopic approaches to inguinal hernia repair.

The total extraperitoneal (TEP) approach to laparoscopic inguinal hernia repair is currently the most popular laparoscopic technique. This repair is performed entirely within the preperitoneal space and does not involve the peritoneal cavity when performed correctly. In this technique, the surgeon carefully develops a plane between the peritoneum posteriorly and the abdominal wall tissues anteriorly and thus insufflates the preperitoneal space. An incision is made inferior to the umbilicus, and the anterior rectus sheath on the ipsilateral side is incised. The rectus muscle is retracted laterally, and the preperitoneal space is bluntly dissected to allow placement of a balloon port to facilitate insufflation. Once the space has been insufflated, two additional ports are placed in the midline between the umbilicus and the pubic symphysis. In experienced hands, this approach provides for excellent visualization of the groin anatomy, and the dissection proceeds in a similar fashion to the TAP. The TEP repair allows a large prosthetic mesh to be placed through a laparoscopic port into the preperitoneal space, and it is then positioned deep to the hernia defect to repair the hernia from a posterior approach.[19]

The intraperitoneal onlay mesh technique (IPOM) was developed as a simplified version of the TAP repair. In this technique, laparoscopic exposure is obtained directly into the peritoneal cavity as in the TAP. However, this technique does not require an extensive mobilization of the peritoneal flap and dissection of the preperitoneal space. Rather, a large mesh is simply stapled or sutured directly posterior to the peritoneum to repair the hernia. In theory, once the peritoneum scars to the mesh after allowing for connective tissue ingrowth, the peritoneum will not be mobile enough to herniate through the actual defect and intra-abdominal pressure will keep the abdominal contents posterior to the mesh patch. The disadvantage of this procedure is that there is direct exposure of mesh to the intra-abdominal contents and therefore a high risk of adhesion formation and possible erosion of the mesh into bowel contents. Another potential disadvantage of the IPOM is the fact that in large inguinal hernias, the mesh and peritoneum may herniate through the defect together, thereby negating any protective effect imparted by the mesh patch. Therefore at the present time, this procedure is thought to be experimental only.

There are few prospective, randomized data available to adequately judge short- and long-term results of the different laparoscopic inguinal hernia techniques. A recent systematic review found that among the several nonrandomized trials, TAP was associated with an increased rate of port site herniation and visceral organ injury. This review concluded that there are insufficient data from prospective, randomized trials to make firm conclusions about the relative effectiveness of the TEP and TAP procedures.[20]

There are emerging data comparing laparoscopic techniques to open inguinal hernia repair, although the evidence is far from definitive. While there are multiple meta-analyses in the literature, only two truly compare the laparoscopic hernia technique with a tension-free open repair. A meta-analysis of 29 randomized trials in 2003 found that laparoscopic hernia repair was associated with earlier discharge from the hospital, quicker return to normal activity and work, and fewer postoperative complications than open repair.[21] However, in these data there was a trend towards an increase in the risk of recurrence after laparoscopic repair. A separate meta-analysis reviewing 41 published randomized trials found no significant difference in risk of recurrence between the two approaches.[22] Laparoscopic repair was associated with a quicker return to function and less postoperative pain, but also was found to have a higher risk of visceral and vascular injuries. A more recent multicenter, randomized trial that analyzed long-term hernia results in over 2000 patients in 14 Veterans Affairs hospitals found that laparoscopic hernia repair was associated with a higher recurrence rate among primary hernias, but was equivalent to open repair in recurrent hernias.[23] In all of these studies, the laparoscopic repair was noted to take more time in the operating room. Finally, a recent study has reported a significant learning curve inherent in the laparoscopic approach.[24] Clearly, more definitive multicenter data from surgeons experienced in both procedures are needed to reach formal conclusions about the utility of both hernia approaches.

A separate issue that deserves further study in laparoscopic hernia repair is the anatomical disturbance of the space of Retzius. This area, first described by Retzius in the 19th century, is the prevesical space located anterior and lateral to the bladder. Suprapubic prostatectomy is performed with dissection through this space, and this operation may be made more difficult following laparoscopic hernia repair.

▪ SURGICAL COMPLICATIONS OF GROIN HERNIA

Although groin hernia repair is associated with excellent short- and long-term outcomes, complications of the procedure exist and must be recognized.

RECURRENCE

Recurrence of the hernia in the early postoperative setting is rare. When this does occur, it is often secondary to deep infection, undue tension on the repair, or tissue ischemia. Clearly, all of these etiologies raise the concern for a technical complication on the part of the surgeon, either in the handling of the groin tissues or the placement of mesh or suture. The patient who is overactive in the immediate postoperative setting may also be at risk for early hernia recurrence. In this way, it is thought that early exercise is performed before the suture or mesh in the repair has had an opportunity to hold tissue in place and promote scar tissue formation. In the initial postoperative setting, patients may also develop seromas along the planes of dissection as well as fluid in the obliterated hernia sac. These benign consequences of surgery must be differentiated from the more worrisome early recurrence.

Tension is an important, if not the primary, etiology of hernia recurrence. Tissues repaired under undue tension will tend to pull apart, even if sutures or mesh have been affixed to them. In addition, tension at the site of suture may lead to ischemia at the point where the suture pulls against the tissue, thereby further weakening the hernia repair. Sutures can also cut out or fall apart, especially if placed in a continuous fashion, when tensile force predominates. The role of excessive tissue tension in promotion of hernia recurrence is the basic rationale behind the modern, tension-free and increasingly suture-free hernia repairs advocated by hernia experts such as Lichtenstein and Rutkow.

The size of the hernia defect is proportional to the risk of hernia recurrence. Larger hernias have an increased rate of recurrence postoperatively. This is most likely due to the nature of the surrounding fascial tissues that are critical to the strength and reliability of the repair. As large hernias stretch and attenuate the surrounding fascial planes, these tissues are correspondingly weaker when repaired with suture or mesh. The weakened tissue may also be relatively ischemic at the time of hernia repair, although this has not been adequately studied.

An emergency operation for strangulated or incarcerated hernia may increase the risk of postoperative recurrence. It is likely that the strangulated hernia, with its inherent inflammation, tissue ischemia, and fascial edema, provides an environment in which the hernia repair is placed either at increased tension or through unhealthy tissue.

A hernia that is overlooked in the operating room represents a potential etiology of hernia recurrence, although this should not be a major concern for the modern hernia surgeon. Most of the repairs in the current era emphasize the repair of both an indirect and direct defect through strengthening of the internal ring and inguinal canal floor, respectively.

A final etiology of hernia recurrence pertains to tobacco use and smoking. The relationship between smoking and hernia formation as well as recurrence was first reported in 1981 and further research has identified proteolytic enzymes that may degrade the connective tissue components.[25]

INFECTION

Infection of the hernia wound or mesh is an uncommon postoperative complication but represents another etiology of hernia recurrence. In specialized hernia practices, the incidence of wound infection following inguinal hernia operation is 1% or less. When an infection does occur, skin flora are the most likely etiology, and appropriate gram-positive antibiotics should be initiated. Patients who undergo mesh placement during groin herniorraphy are at a slightly higher risk of postoperative wound infection. It is often difficult to determine whether the mesh itself is infected or if just the skin or soft tissue anterior to the layer of mesh is infected. However, even if mesh is present, most postoperative groin hernia infections can be treated with aggressive use of antibiotics after the incision is opened and drained expeditiously.[26] Mesh removal in this setting is rarely indicated; when this is mandated, primary closure or redo herniorraphy with a synthetic tissue substitute may be warranted and a preperitoneal approach may be necessary.

Seromas and hematomas are frequent complications in the postoperative setting. Seromas form in the dead space remaining from a wide dissection during the hernia repair or when fluid fills the distal remnant of the hernia sac. While the sac is often ligated or excised during open herniorraphy, it remains in place following laparoscopic repair, and the filling of the remnant sac with seroma-type fluid has been termed a pseudohernia. This must be differentiated from the more concerning complication of the early recurrent hernia. Defined fluid collections infrequently require drainage or aspiration, as most will reabsorb or drain through the incision on their own.

Hematoma formation must be assiduously avoided during groin hernia repair. This is especially true in the anticoagulated patient, and therefore it is recommended that patients temporarily stop taking aspirin and clopidogrel at least 1 week prior to their operation. Hematoma formation may be minor and lead only to ecchymoses and wound drainage. The ecchymosis often spreads inferiorly into the scrotal plane in a dependent fashion. The hematoma usually resolves in days to weeks following repair and supportive management for pain control including scrotal elevation and warm packs is all that is required. A large volume of hematoma is concerning, as it may serve as a nidus for infection deep in the hernia wound and may risk secondary infection of the prosthetic mesh. Therefore hemostasis at the end of a groin hernia repair is paramount to achieve effective wound healing.

NEURALGIA

Postoperative groin pain, or neuralgia, is common to varying degrees following groin herniorrhaphy.[27] Often, the neuralgia will follow the known distribution of the regional nerves, including the ilioinguinal, iliohypogastric, genital branch of the genitofemoral nerve, and the lateral femorocutaneous nerves. During open hernia repair, the ilioinguinal, iliohypogastric, and the genitofemoral nerves are most commonly injured, while the lateral femorocutaneous nerve is more commonly injured during laparoscopic herniorraphy. Nerve injury is usually due to entrapment of a portion of the nerve in the mesh or suture line placed in one of the soft tissue layers.

Neuralgias can be prevented by meticulously avoiding overt manipulation of the nerves during operative dissection. The ilioinguinal and iliohypogastric nerves are generally injured during elevation of the external oblique fascial flaps, while the genitofemoral nerve is most likely to be injured during the isolation of the cord and stripping of the cremaster muscle fibers. Often, once the nerve branches are identified, they are encircled with a vessel loop and retracted out of the operative field to avoid injury. The nerves can also be intentionally sacrificed at time of surgery. The result of this maneuver is a region of sensory deprivation in the distributions of these nerve structures, namely on the inner upper thigh and the hemiscrotum. However, the sensory deprivation is thought to be better tolerated by the patient than the chronic and persistent pain attributed to nerve entrapment in scar or mesh. In laparoscopic repair, nerve injury can be prevented by avoiding tack or staple placement below the iliopubic tract.

Neuralgia should first be managed conservatively, with attempts at local anesthetic injection in the affected groin. When local anesthesia is injected along the known course of a nerve, this modality may serve as both a diagnostic and therapeutic maneuver. In some cases, temporary control of the chronic pain with local anesthesia may reduce or altogether eliminate the sequelae of chronic groin pain. When this conservative approach does not succeed, groin re-exploration can be performed to ligate or excise affected nerve branches. This is clearly not the preferred first option, since the groin wound has abundant scar and previously undamaged nerve structures may be placed at additional risk. Occasionally, patients will present with postoperative neuralgia that does not match the distribution of any known inguinal nerve. Groin re-exploration should be avoided in this case since it is unlikely to ameliorate the pain and may damage additional structures.

Nerve injury during laparoscopic repair can occur during the tacking of the mesh to the anterior abdominal wall. Tacks should be avoided in the known areas of nerve structures. Some surgeons prefer to not place any tacking staples at all when performing laparoscopic herniorraphy to avoid this complication altogether.

BLADDER INJURY

The urinary bladder may be inadvertently injured during dissection of a direct inguinal hernia sac, but only rarely during repair of an indirect defect. The bladder can also participate in a sliding hernia, so that a portion of the bladder wall is adherent to the sac in a direct defect. Because of the potential for this complication, direct sacs should be inverted into the peritoneal cavity so that excessive dissection can be avoided. If bladder injury takes place, the sac should be opened, and the bladder injury repaired in two layers of an absorbable suture. In general, a urethral catheter is placed for a minimum of 7–14 days.

TESTICULAR INJURY

Testicular swelling and atrophy is seen after inguinal hernia repair. Edema of the scrotum or testis may be secondary to edema or hematoma of the inguinal canal that tracks inferomedially to the scrotum in a dependent fashion. Alternatively, a tender testicle or an atrophic testicle may be secondary to injury to the blood supply to the genitals during dissection and isolation of the cord. In most cases, this is not an emergency in the adult patient, and the testes will atrophy without significant infectious complications so that orchiectomy is rarely necessary. A testicle that is tender on examination may require ultrasonographic imaging to rule out testicular torsion or a corresponding abscess. Necrosis of the testes, a very rare complication of groin hernia repair, usually requires orchiectomy to avoid infectious complications.

In the pediatric patient, traction on the cord in the cephalad direction can cause the testes to migrate into the inguinal canal and out of the scrotum. For this reason, the scrotum is often prepped sterilely in the pediatric inguinal hernia operation, and the testes is confirmed to be in appropriate position by palpation at the end of the hernia repair. If the testes remains in the inguinal canal following herniorraphy, this may require manipulation of the testes further down the canal and into the scrotum using a long atraumatic forceps or a choker instrument.

VAS DEFERENS INJURY

Injury to the vas is a rare complication of groin hernia surgery in the male patient. Transection of the vas is the most serious form of this injury; this requires urologic consultation and likely immediate reanastomosis in the child or young adult, but may only require ligation of both ends in the older adult patient. Minor injuries to the vas can be avoided by using gentle, atraumatic traction only and by avoiding complete grasping or squeezing of the vas. The most worrisome sequela of vas deferens obstruction or transection is formation of antisperm antibodies in the serum, leading to infertility.

▪ THE STRANGULATED GROIN HERNIA

The strangulation of a groin hernia is a complication of the hernia itself rather than of a hernia repair. This pathophysiologic process is associated with a high rate of mortality and morbidity, especially in the elderly population with multiple comorbidities. The risk of strangulation is highest in the first months to years after the initial presentation of a reducible hernia. Gallegos and associates estimated the probability of inguinal hernia strangulation over time to be 2.8% over 3 months and 4.5% at 2 years.[28] It is likely that with time, the hernia contents weaken the hernia defect and widen the hernia neck so that the sac is no longer compressed as tightly, thereby decreasing the opportunity for incarceration and strangulation to take place.

The mortality from a strangulated hernia is related to the duration of the strangulation and the age of the patient. A longer duration of strangulation leads to a greater degree of tissue edema, ischemia, and risk of outright necrosis. Therefore, a strangulated hernia clearly represents a surgical emergency. The incarcerated hernia without overt signs of strangulation on examination and laboratory analysis should undergo attempts at reduction, often requiring conscious sedation to minimize discomfort. After the hernia is reduced, the repair can take place 1–2 days later, usually during the same inpatient hospitalization, to minimize risk of recurrent incarceration leading to strangulation.

Surgery for an incarcerated inguinal hernia is most often performed under general anesthesia given the high likelihood that bowel resection will need to be performed. Epidural or spinal anesthesia may suffice in select cases, but local anesthesia should not be employed. The location of the incision depends on the diagnosis and clinical assessment. In those patients who are unlikely to have ischemic bowel present within the hernia sac, an inguinal incision will likely be successful in both reducing the hernia contents and repairing the hernia defect. If nonviable bowel is found on exploration of the inguinal canal, the resection and anastomosis can take place deep to the transversalis fascia in the preperitoneal space or a midline incision can be made. If the initial physical examination yields signs of ischemic bowel that may necessitate resection, a midline laparotomy can be performed and the hernia repaired in the inguinal canal using a tissue repair after the laparotomy is closed. A helpful alternative is the preperitoneal hernia repair, which can be used to evaluate the bowel and repair the hernia defect, yet it can also be easily converted to an intraperitoneal exposure if extensive bowel resection and anastomosis is required. Placement of prosthetic mesh should be avoided when possible in strangulated hernia repair given the increased risk of bacterial translocation and wound infection.

▪ FEMORAL HERNIA

The femoral hernia is the second most common abdominal wall hernia, although it makes up only 5–10% of all hernias. The femoral hernia is more common in females than males, by a ratio of approximately 4:1.

ANATOMY AND ETIOLOGY

Figure 5–6 illustrates the anatomy of the femoral hernia. The defect through which a femoral hernia occurs is in the medial femoral canal. The anterior boundary of this defect is the inguinal ligament, the lateral boundary the femoral vein, the posterior boundary the pubic ramus and Cooper's ligament, and the medial boundary the lacunar portion of the inguinal ligament. This space is ob-

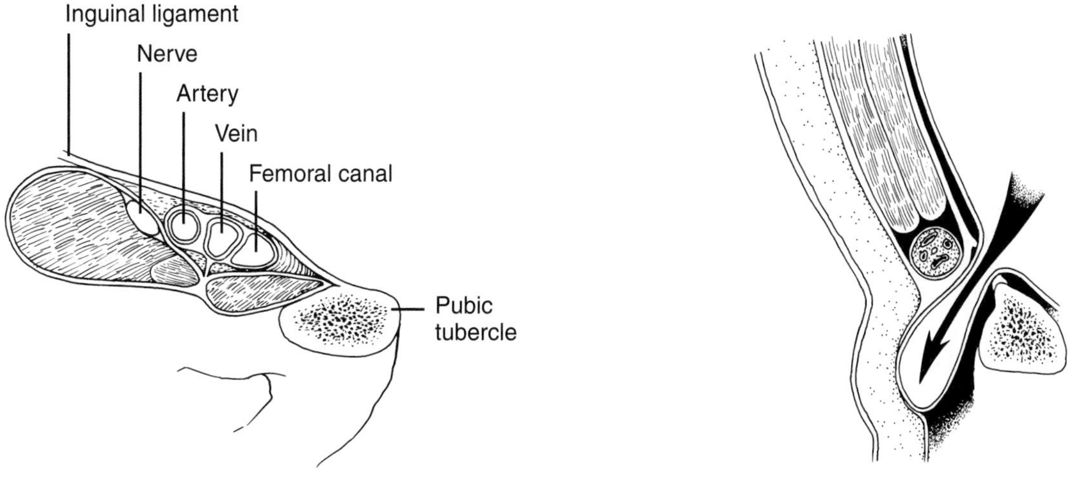

A B

Figure 5–6. The anatomy of the femoral hernia. **A.** The structures posterior to the inguinal ligament. **B.** The femoral hernia passing through the femoral canal and bulging in the groin below the inguinal ligament. After Rejovitzky, MD.

viously tight and does not have room to expand when hernia contents fill the sac since the boundaries are either ligamentous, bony, or the fibrous femoral sheath and its vessels. Therefore, femoral hernias have a high propensity for incarceration and strangulation. Gallegos and associates reported the cumulative probability of femoral hernia strangulation to be 22% in the first 3 months following diagnosis and 45% at nearly 2 years.[28] Therefore, repair of a known femoral hernia is mandatory to avoid this highly morbid complication.

In contrast to the inguinal hernia, the femoral hernia is unlikely to be of congenital etiology. The incidence of femoral hernia in infancy and childhood is exceedingly low, in the range of 0.5%. In addition, there is no embryologic mechanism for a preexisting sac of peritoneum in the femoral canal. The hernia defect most often presents in middle-aged to older women, suggesting that the natural loss of tissue strength and elasticity is a primary etiology.

CLINICAL PRESENTATION

The femoral hernia often presents as a small bulge just below the medial groin crease. It is often difficult to reduce on initial presentation.[29] The hernia usually extends caudad as the sac increases in size with abdominal contents but may extend up and over the inguinal ligament anteriorly. Not uncommonly, the femoral hernia presents acutely with strangulation given its anatomic limitations. The differential diagnosis for a femoral hernia includes femoral lymphadenopathy, groin lipoma, or a soft tissue mass of benign or rarely malignant nature.

TREATMENT

The operative approach to repairing the reducible femoral hernia differs from inguinal hernia repair in several ways. The incision is usually centered transversely just below the inguinal ligament, although a standard groin hernia incision may still afford exposure to the defect. The simplest approach is anterior to the inguinal ligament. Here, the sac can often be found, dissected, and reduced into the peritoneal cavity. Repair of the defect can be performed using a Cooper's ligament repair as described above, by affixing the transversalis fascia to the Cooper's ligament medially and the iliopubic tract laterally up to the internal ring. Alternatively, a simple suture repair can be performed by tacking the inguinal ligament anteriorly to Cooper's ligament posteromedially to close the defect. A third option is a purse-string suture placed first anteriorly into the inguinal ligament, then through the lacunar ligament medially, the pectineal ligament posteriorly, and finally through the fascia medial to the femoral vein and back to the inguinal ligament. All of these techniques can successfully close the femoral hernia defect.

However, a unique complication from suture repair of the femoral hernia defect is bleeding from an aberrant obturator artery. This vessel originates from the inferior epigastric rather than the internal iliac artery and traverses a space medial to the femoral hernia defect adjacent to the pubic ramus. The medial suture placed in femoral hernia repair can injure an aberrant obturator artery if present. A simple and possibly safer way to repair the femoral defect is a mesh plug placed from cephalad to caudad to obstruct the defect and promote scar tissue formation. This technique, shown in Figure 5–7, has been reported by Lichtenstein with excellent results and low rates of recurrence.[30]

If the femoral hernia sac is large and filled with voluminous intra-abdominal contents, a preperitoneal repair should be considered. In this way, the transversalis fascia is opened and the preperitoneal plane is entered. This approach is particularly useful during repair of a strangulated hernia since there is more space to allow for inspection of the bowel to ensure viability. Bowel resection, if needed, can also take place in the preperitoneal space prior to full reduction of the hernia contents.

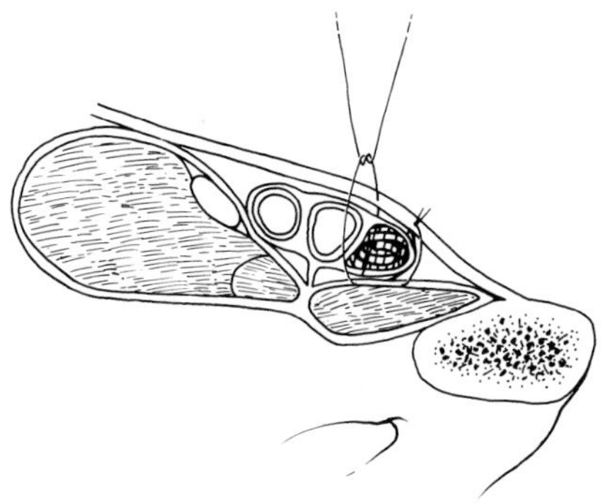

Figure 5–7. The Lichtenstein polypropylene plug for repair of a femoral hernia. After Rejovitzky, MD.

▪ UMBILICAL HERNIA

The umbilicus represents a midline opening in the linea alba. Umbilical hernia occurs when the umbilical scar closes incompletely in the child or fails and stretches in later years in the adult patient. The hernia becomes readily apparent once the abdominal contents move through the umbilical opening given the relative lack of soft tissue in the anterior body wall at the site of the umbilicus.

HISTORY

Umbilical hernias have been documented throughout history with the first references dating back to the ancient Egyptians with the first known record of a surgical repair by Celsus in the first century AD. Mayo in 1901 reported the first series of patients to undergo the classic overlapping fascia operation through a transverse umbilical incision using nonabsorbable suture.[31]

INCIDENCE

Estimates of umbilical hernia present at birth have a wide range. In Caucasian babies, the incidence has been reported at 10–30%, although for unknown reasons it may be several times greater in African-American children. Umbilical hernia is even more common in premature infants of all races and there is a tendency for familial inheritance.

The majority of congenital pediatric umbilical hernias are known to close over time, as the infant becomes a child. In this way, by school age, only 10% of umbilical hernias remain open on physical examination. Umbilical hernia repair in the child is therefore rarely performed electively before the age of 2 years, and incarceration in the child is rare. Current recommendations in the pediatric surgical literature advise the delay of umbilical hernia repair until at least 2–3 years of age given the likelihood that most umbilical hernias will spontaneously close in the young child.

The incidence of umbilical hernia in the adult is largely unknown but most cases are thought to be acquired rather than congenital. It is known to occur more commonly in adult females with a female:male ratio of 3:1. Umbilical hernia is also more commonly found in association with processes that increase intra-abdominal pressure, such as pregnancy, obesity, ascites, persistent or repetitive abdominal distention in bowel obstruction, or peritoneal dialysis. The etiology of umbilical hernia in the adult may be multifactorial, with increased intra-abdominal pressure working against a weak or incomplete umbilical scar.

EMBRYOLOGY AND ANATOMY

The fascial margins that make up the umbilical defect are formed by the third week of gestation, and the umbilical cord takes shape in the fifth week of gestation. In the sixth week, the intestinal tract migrates through the umbilicus and outside the coelom as intestinal growth outpaces the size of the abdominal cavity. The intestinal tract returns to the abdominal cavity through the umbilical defect as the midgut undergoes rotation at the tenth week of gestation, and subsequent to this, the four folds of the somatopleure begin to fuse inward. This, in turn, forms the tight umbilical defect which allows only the passage of the umbilical vessels. At birth, when the umbilical cord is manually ligated, the umbilical arteries and vein thrombose and the umbilical aperture closes. Any defect in the process of umbilical closure will result in an umbilical hernia through which omentum or bowel can herniate.

CLINICAL MANIFESTATIONS

The diagnosis of umbilical hernia is not difficult to make. The condition presents with a soft bulge located anterior or adjacent to the umbilicus. In most cases, the bulge will be readily reducible so that the actual fascial defect can be easily defined by palpation. The patient may provide a history of vague abdominal pain associated with herniation and reduction. The list of differential diagnoses is short and includes abdominal wall varices associated with advanced cirrhosis, umbilical granulomas, and metastatic tumor implants in the umbilical soft tissue (Sister Joseph's node). In clinical practice, there is usually little doubt as to the diagnosis of umbilical hernia on physical exam.

While the majority of umbilical hernias will close spontaneously in the infant, the clinical spectrum varies widely in the adult. The hernia in the adult is often symptomatic and does not show a tendency to close without intervention. As the hernia contents increase in size, the overlying umbilical skin may become thin and ultimately ulcerated by pressure necrosis. The umbilical hernia with incarcerated omentum may present with significant tenderness on exam, despite the fact that bowel integrity is not at risk. Alternatively, an umbilical hernia may be found incidentally in the adult on physical exam. This hernia is usually small and any hernia contents are usually readily reducible. The small, asymptomatic, reducible hernia in the adult can be observed without the need for immediate intervention.

Patients with umbilical hernia secondary to chronic, massive ascites require special consideration. The repair of such hernias is associated with significantly increased morbidity and mortality. Fluid shifts leading to hemodynamic instability, infection, electrolyte imbalance, and blood loss are all considerable risks for the patient in this clinical scenario. Umbilical hernia recurrence is also common in this setting given the persistently increased intra-abdominal pressure. Thus, hernia repair in this population should be reserved for those with progressively symptomatic or incarcerated umbilical hernias.

TREATMENT

In the pediatric patient with a small umbilical hernia, a short curvilinear (smile) incision is made just inferior to the umbilicus in the typical skin crease. A skin flap is then raised cephalad using blunt dissection and low-level electrocautery. Dissection is carried through the subcutaneous tissues and down to the fascial level. The neck of the sac is then encircled with a hemostat. After the sac is dissected free of its umbilical attachments, it can be reduced or inverted completely into the peritoneal cavity or incised to explore the contents of the hernia sac. In this way, the redundant portion of the sac can be excised using electrocautery. The fascial defect is then closed transversely with interrupted sutures in a horizontal mattress fashion, and the skin of the umbilicus is tacked to the fascia layer using a single suture. This operation is usually performed under general anesthesia as a day-surgery procedure.

In the adult patient, most small umbilical hernia repairs are performed using local anesthesia with the possible addition of intravenous sedation. The approach is also through a curvilinear incision, placed transversely on the inferior border of the umbilicus or vertically on one curved edge of the umbilicus (Fig 5–8). A skin flap is raised to elevate the umbilicus off the hernia sac. The sac is again dissected free of its fascial attachments to isolate the sac for complete reduction and to allow for an adequate width of fascia for suture closure. The sac contents are then reduced into the abdominal cavity and any excess sac can be excised. The defect is then closed with a strong, nonabsorbable suture (such as 0 polypropylene or nylon), usually in an interrupted fashion. The fascial edges are approximated through this technique. The traditional "vest-over-pants" technique originated by Mayo is less commonly utilized since overlapping fascial closures have been shown to weaken the overall wound strength in hernia repair.

In large defects that may close only with a significant degree of tension, a cone of polypropylene mesh can be fitted to fill the umbilical defect in place of a tissue repair. The mesh is then sutured circumferentially to the surrounding umbilical fascia to prevent migration.

▪ EPIGASTRIC HERNIA

An epigastric hernia is a defect in the abdominal wall in the midline junction of the aponeuroses of the abdominal wall musculature from the xiphoid process superiorly to the umbilicus inferiorly. The region of this midline raphe is termed the linea alba, and the rectus muscles are situated just lateral to the linea alba. In this area, there is no muscle layer to protect against herniation of intra-abdominal contents through defects in the midline fascia. A paraumbilical hernia is an epigastric hernia that borders on the umbilicus.

HISTORY

The epigastric hernia was first described by Villeneuve in 1285, but the term "epigastric hernia" was only first used to describe this condition in 1812 by Leville. The first successful repair of an epigastric hernia was reported in 1802 by Maunior.

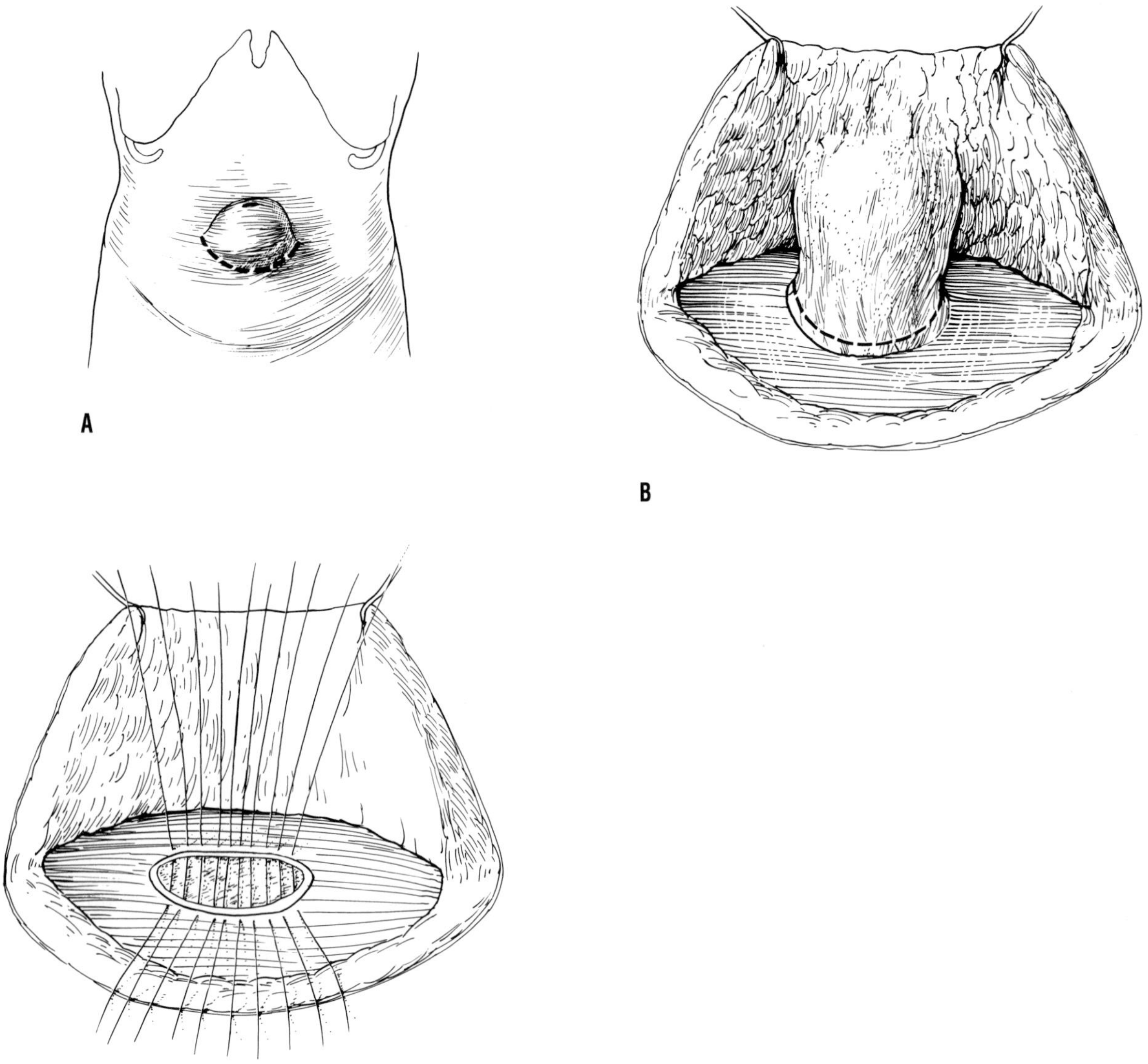

A B C

Figure 5–8. Repair of the small umbilical hernia. **A.** The "smile" curvilinear incision that allows for a skin flap to be raised. **B.** The incising of the hernia sac. **C.** The sutures in place. Mattress type sutures can also be used to alleviate undue tension in larger hernias. After Rejovitzky, MD.

INCIDENCE

Estimates of the frequency of epigastric hernia in the general population range from 3–5%. It is most commonly diagnosed in middle age, and congenital epigastric hernias are uncommon. The condition is more common in males by a ratio of 3:1. Twenty percent of epigastric hernias may be multiple, although most are associated with one dominant defect.

ANATOMY AND ETIOLOGY

The cause of epigastric hernia is largely unknown. Since the condition does not predominate in children, it is unlikely that the defect is entirely congenital in origin. Rather, the hernia is likely the result of multiple factors, such as a congenitally weakened linea alba from a lack of decussating midline fibers and subsequent increase in intra-abdominal pressure, surrounding muscle weakness, or chronic abdominal wall strain.

The midline defect is usually elliptical in nature, with the long axis oriented transversely. The width of the defect is generally a few millimeters to several centimeters, and larger defects are rare. In most cases, the hernia is filled by a small amount of preperitoneal fat only and no peritoneal sac is present. The hernia will often not be seen on laparoscopy owing to the lack of peritoneal involvement through the hernia defect. Epigastric hernias that involve a peritoneal sac usually contain only omentum and rarely small intestine.

CLINICAL MANIFESTATIONS

Epigastric hernia is often asymptomatic and represents a chance finding on physical exam. Patients with symptomatic hernias complain of vague abdominal pain above the umbilicus that is exacerbated with standing or coughing and relieved in the supine position. Severe pain may be secondary to incarceration or strangulation of preperitoneal fat or omentum. Bowel strangulation in epigastric hernias is a rare finding.

On examination, the hernia is diagnosed by palpating a small, soft, reducible mass in the midline superior to the umbilicus. The mass may protrude with a Valsalva maneuver or with standing. Palpation can be especially difficult in the obese patient. Rarely, imaging is needed to confirm the diagnosis, and computed tomography of the abdomen is the preferred technique.

TREATMENT

As illustrated in Figure 5–9, operative repair of the epigastric hernia can most often be performed as a day-surgery procedure under local anesthesia. General anesthesia should be reserved for the complicated patient, a very large hernia, or the pediatric population. The herniated contents are exposed through a small midline vertical or transverse incision. The defect in the linea alba and the surrounding fascia are cleared of subcutaneous fat. Effort is made to identify a peritoneal sac protruding through the defect. If identified, a small sac can be simply inverted back within the abdominal cavity. Alternatively, a larger sac can be opened, its contents reduced, and any excess peritoneum excised. It is usually not necessary to perform formal closure of the peritoneal sac. The defect is then closed transversely with a few interrupted sutures of polypropylene or nylon, taking generous bites of surrounding fascia.

This repair usually suffices with minimal recurrence. In general, it is not necessary to reconstruct the linea alba for a single epigastric hernia. Most patients will not develop a subsequent epigastric hernia at a separate site, and repair of an epigastric hernia is a minor ambulatory procedure that can be repeated easily if necessary.

■ OBTURATOR HERNIA

An obturator hernia is one of the rarest forms of hernia, and most surgeons will see few in an entire career. An obturator hernia occurs when there is protrusion of intra-abdominal contents through the obturator foramen in the pelvis.

INCIDENCE

The true incidence of obturator hernia is unknown. The largest reported series includes only 43 patients diagnosed with obturator hernia over a 30-year period.[32] It is thought that less than 1% of mechanical bowel obstructions arise from strangulated obturator hernias. The hernia is much more common in females, with a female:male ratio of 6:1. The gender discrepancy is often explained by differences in female pelvic anatomy, including a broader pelvis, a wide obturator canal, and the increase in pelvic diameter brought about by pregnancy. Most cases of obturator hernia present in the seventh and eighth decades, and this condition is clearly associated with advanced age. Bilateral obturator hernias have been reported in 6% of cases.

ANATOMY

The obturator foramen is formed by the ischial and pubic rami (Fig 5–10). The obturator membrane covers the majority of the foramen space, except for a small portion through which the obturator vessels and nerve pass. These vessels traverse the canal to leave the abdominal cavity and enter the medial aspect of the thigh. The boundaries of the obturator canal are the obturator groove on the superior pubic ramus superiorly and the upper edge of the obturator membrane inferiorly. The canal is approximately 3 cm in length, and the obturator vessels and nerve lie posterolateral to the hernia sac in the canal. The hernia sac usually takes the shape of the canal, so that it is long and narrow before ballooning in the upper thigh. The hernia lies deep to the pectineus muscle and therefore is difficult to palpate on exam. Small bowel is the most likely intra-abdominal organ to be found in an obturator hernia, although rare cases have been reported of the appendix, Meckel's diverticulum, omentum, bladder, and ovary incarcerated in the hernia.

CLINICAL MANIFESTATIONS

Obturator hernia is associated with four cardinal findings that assist in the difficult diagnosis. Rarely do all four physical findings occur together. The most common clinical manifestation is intestinal obstruction, which occurs in over 80% of patients. This is often in the form of acute obstruction secondary to hernia strangulation.[33] The second most common finding is

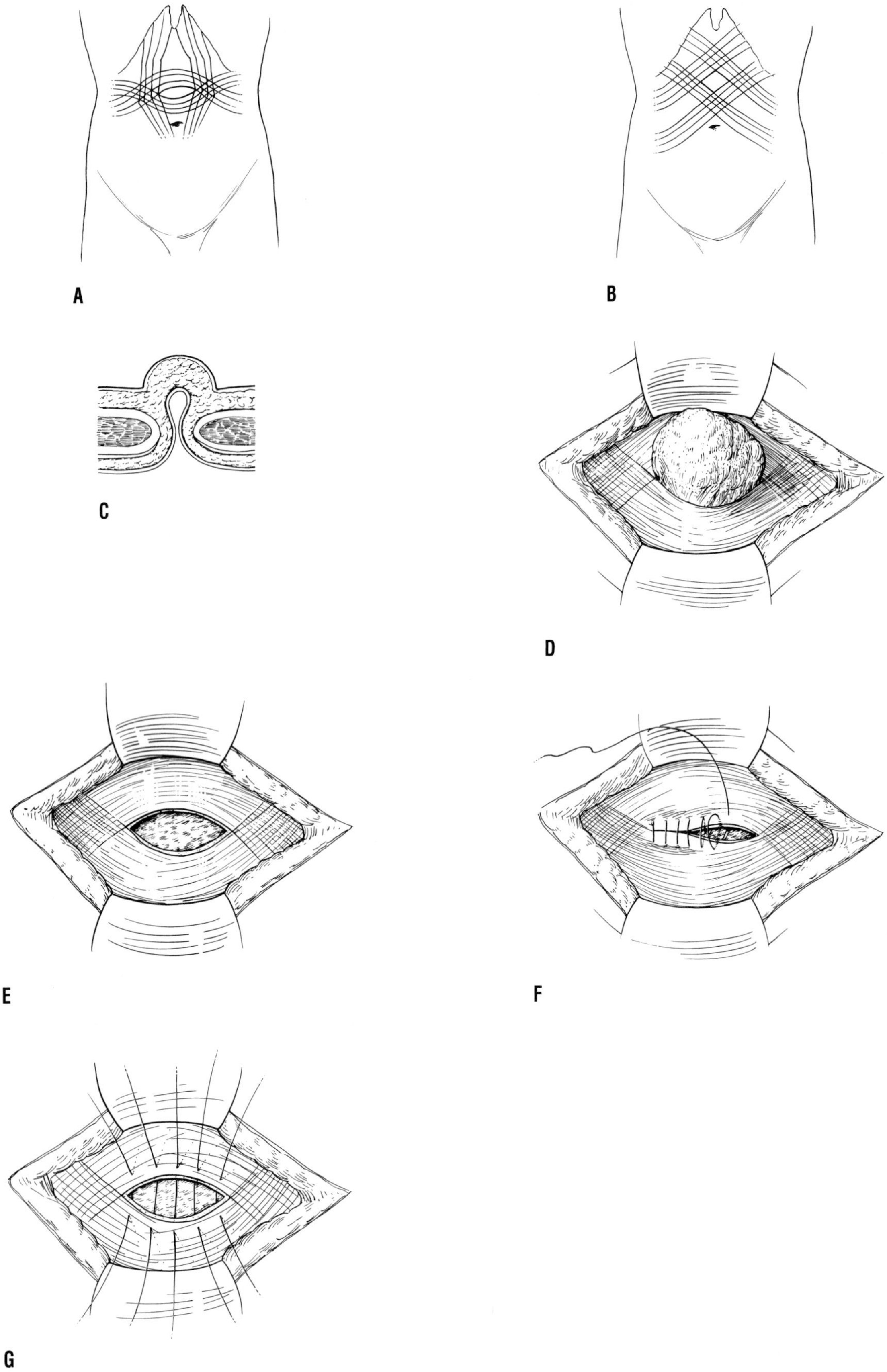

Figure 5–9. Repair of the epigastric hernia. **A.** The elliptical opening. **B.** The diamond-shaped opening. **C.** The small empty sac. **D.** Herniated fat exposed during dissection. **E.** Herniated fat and the sac have been excised. **F.** Repair of continuous suture technique. **G.** Repair using interrupted sutures. After Rejovitzky, MD.

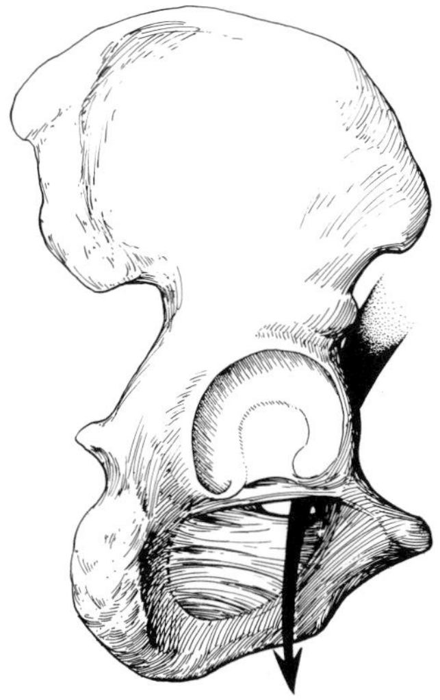

Figure 5–10. The direction of the obturator hernia through the obturator canal. After Rejovitzky, MD.

the Howship-Romberg sign, seen in about one-half of patients with obturator hernia. With this sign, patients characteristically complain of pain along the medial surface of the thigh that may radiate to the knee and hip joints. The finding is likely associated with compression of the obturator nerve between the canal and the hernia sac. The adductor reflex in the thigh may also be weakened or lost secondary to motor dysfunction from an entrapped obturator nerve. The third finding, observed in 30% of patients, is a history of repeated episodes of bowel obstruction that pass quickly and without intervention. This is likely due to periodic incarceration of the hernia sac in the obturator canal. Finally, a fourth finding is a palpable mass in the proximal medial aspect of the thigh at the origin of the adductor muscles. The palpable mass is only found in an estimated 20% of patients with obturator hernia. The mass is best palpated with the thigh flexed, abducted, and rotated outward.

In rare cases, ecchymoses may be noted in the upper medial thigh due to effusion from the strangulated hernia contents. The obturator hernia mass may also be palpated laterally on a vaginal exam.

TREATMENT

The only treatment for obturator hernia is surgical repair. All obturator hernias should be operated on soon after diagnosis given the high risk for bowel incarceration and strangulation. There is no role for conservative management given the location of the hernia and the fact that the strangulated obturator hernia is difficult to diagnose. A preoperative diagnosis of obturator hernia is rare indeed, and a diagnosis prior to presentation with bowel obstruction is even more uncommon. The typical case of obturator hernia presents as an acute small bowel obstruction with evidence of ischemic bowel on exam, laboratory analyses, or imaging. Therefore obturator hernia repair is often performed as a surgical emergency via a midline laparotomy.

There are three general operative approaches for obturator hernia repair: the lower midline transperitoneal approach, the lower midline extraperitoneal approach, and the anterior thigh exposure.

The lower midline transperitoneal approach is the most common method for repair of obturator hernias since most cases are encountered unexpectedly during exploratory laparotomy for small bowel obstruction of unknown etiology. Following laparotomy, the dilated small bowel is run deep into the pelvis where it is found to enter the obturator canal alongside the obturator vessels and nerve. A careful attempt should be made to reduce the incarcerated bowel with gentle traction. This maneuver may be augmented by palpation on the medial inner thigh to push the hernia sac into the abdominal cavity from the outside. This is difficult to perform without assistance since the thigh is rarely sterilely prepared for the exploratory laparotomy unless a preoperative diagnosis of obturator hernia has been made. The pelvic side of the obturator canal has a rigid opening that cannot be digitally dilated, making reduction of the hernia sac more difficult. If traction alone does not allow reduction of the bowel, the obturator membrane can be carefully incised from anterior to posterior to facilitate exposure. Care should be taken to avoid injury to both the incarcerated bowel and the obturator vessels. If these maneuvers are unsuccessful, a counter incision can be made in the medial groin to facilitate reduction from both sides of the canal. Once the hernia has been reduced, the intestine is assessed for viability and resected as needed. The hernia opening is then closed around the obturator vessels with a running layer of polypropylene or nylon suture applied in the thin layer of fascia that encircles the inner circumference of the canal. Alternatively, in a clean case without bowel contamination, a piece of mesh can be placed over the obturator foramen. Some hernia surgeons suture the mesh to Cooper's ligament to avoid migration.

The midline extraperitoneal approach is used when the diagnosis of obturator hernia has been made preoperatively. It allows complete exposure of the opening of the obturator canal. The incision is made in the midline from the umbilicus to the pubis. The preperitoneal plane is entered deep to the rectus muscle, and the bladder is peeled from the peritoneum. The space is opened so that the superior pubic ramus and the obturator internus muscle are exposed. The hernia sac is seen as a projection of peritoneum passing inferiorly into the obturator canal. The sac is incised at the base, the contents are reduced, and the neck of the sac is transected. Any remaining distal sac in the canal is extracted by traction or with long forceps. The internal opening to the obturator canal is closed with a continuous suture as described above. The bites of tissue should include the periosteum of the superior pubic ramus and the fascia on the internal obturator muscle. Care must be exercised at all times to avoid injury to the obturator vessels and nerve that run alongside the hernia defect. In addition to or in place of the suture closure of the obturator defect, preperitoneal mesh placement has been described to cover the defect.

The thigh approach begins with a vertical incision in the upper medial thigh placed along the adductor longus muscle (Fig 5–11). The muscle is retracted medially to expose the pectineus muscle, which is cut across its width to expose the sac. The sac is carefully incised, the contents inspected and reduced if viable, and the sac is excised. The hernial opening is closed with a continuous suture layer. If the bowel contents within the hernia sac do not appear viable, it is difficult to perform an adequate small bowel resection through the thigh incision and therefore midline laparotomy is usually performed.

Laparoscopic transperitoneal and extraperitoneal approaches have been recently described for obturator hernia repair with placement of prosthetic mesh to close the obturator opening.[34]

RESULTS

Mortality after obturator hernia repair has been much higher than with other hernias because it is associated with acute bowel obstruction in an elderly population with multiple comorbidities. Recent data show a mortality of less than 5% and a 25% incidence of small bowel resection during obturator hernia repair.[32] These reports emphasize the benefit in accuracy in the modern era afforded by computed tomographic imaging techniques. Recurrence rates are low in published series, although long-term follow-up has proved difficult in this patient population.

▪ PERINEAL HERNIAS

Hernias of the perineum are rare and composed of protrusions of the intra-abdominal contents through a weakened pelvic floor. They may also be termed pelvic hernias, ischiorectal hernias, pudendal hernias, subpubic hernias, or hernias of the pouch of Douglas. Perineal hernias should be differentiated from the more common rectocele or cystocele, which are related to pelvic floor relaxation, most often from childbirth, and do not represent true hernias.

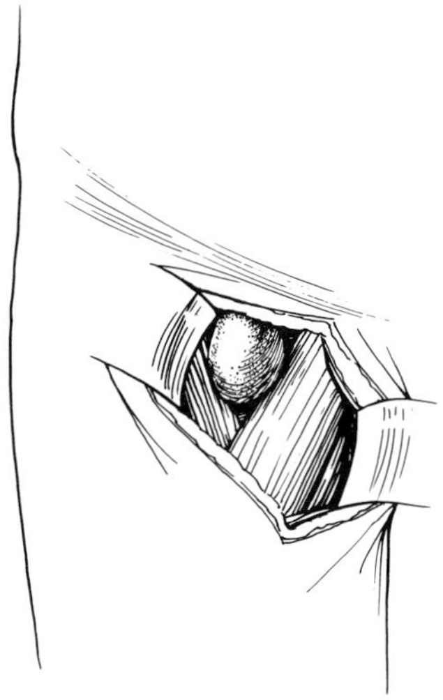

Figure 5–11. The thigh approach for repair of the obturator hernia. After Rejovitzky, MD.

Primary perineal hernias are extremely rare. The first reported case was by Scarpa in 1821. Secondary, or postoperative, perineal hernias are more commonly seen and occur in patients status post abdominoperineal resection in which the pelvic musculature is dissected to resect the distal rectum.

ETIOLOGY

Primary perineal hernias occur in the older population, usually between the fifth and seventh decades of life. They are at least five times more common in women than men, and this is thought to be associated with the broader pelvic floor in the female and long-term effects of pregnancy and childbirth. Factors that may predispose to a primary perineal hernia include a deep or elongated pouch of Douglas, obesity, chronic ascites, history of pelvic infection, and obstetric trauma.

Postoperative perineal hernia may occur in patients who have undergone abdominoperineal resection or pelvic exenteration. It is thought to form as a result of excision of the levator ani musculature and its surrounding fascia with incomplete repair of the pelvic floor. An excision of the coccyx is thought to be an additional aggravating factor in hernia formation. As in primary perineal hernias, women are affected more often than men. The condition, while more common than the primary perineal hernia, remains rare.

ANATOMY

The pelvic floor is formed by the levator ani and iliococcygeus muscles and their fascia. The pelvic outlet is bounded by the pubic symphysis and the subpubic ligament anteriorly, the pubic rami and ischial tuberosities laterally, and the coccyx and sacrotuberous ligaments posteriorly. The outlet is divided into anterior and posterior divisions by the superficial transversus perinei muscles. The anterior space is termed the urogenital triangle, and the posterior space is termed the ischiorectal fossa. Anterior and posterior perineal hernias are named according to the location of the hernia defect and subsequent sac protrusion, as shown in Figure 5–12.

The anterior perineal hernia occurs almost exclusively in women. The sac enters in front of the broad ligament and lateral to the bladder, emerging anterior to the transversus perinei musculature. The sac may pass between the ischiopubic bone and the vagina, thereby producing a swelling in the posterior portion of the labia majus. Posterior perineal hernias are found in both genders but remain more common in women. In men, the hernia sac emerges between the bladder and the rectum to present as a bulge in the perineum. In women, the hernia enters between the rectum and the uterus to pass posteriorly to the broad ligament. In this space, the hernia can push forward to present as a bulge in the posterior vagina or emerge posteriorly into the rectum. The hernia can pass through the levator ani muscle or between it and the iliococcygeus muscle. A lateral pelvic hernia may occur through the hiatus of Schwalbe when the levator ani muscle is not firmly attached to the internal obturator fascia. This type of perineal hernia can present anteriorly in the labium majus or posteriorly in the ischiorectal fossa.

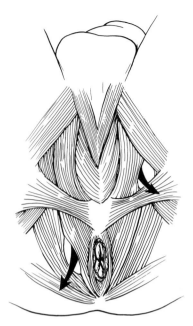

Figure 5–12. The anatomy of the perineal hernia showing the location of both anterior and posterior defects. After Rejovitzky, MD.

CLINICAL MANIFESTATIONS

The patient with a perineal hernia most often complains of a soft protuberance that is reduced in the recumbent position. In cases of anterior perineal hernia, minor urinary retention or discomfort may be reported. A soft bulge may be noted in the posterior vagina or the labia, thereby interfering with labor or intercourse. In posterior perineal hernias, the patient may describe a mass protruding between the gluteus muscles, thereby making sitting difficult after the hernia has emerged in a standing position. The patient may rarely complain of constipation or the feeling of incomplete defecation.

In general, symptoms from a perineal hernia are mild, and strangulation is rare since the hernia defect in the pelvic floor is large and surrounded by soft tissue and atrophied musculature. Rectal prolapse may be confused with a posterior perineal hernia, although the two can exist concomitantly. The perineal hernia, even when the defect involves the posterior pelvic floor, will present as a bulge anterior to the prolapsed rectum.

TREATMENT

Three options for repair of the perineal hernia exist including the transperitoneal, perineal, and the combined approaches. The transperitoneal approach is the preferred method for complete repair. In this technique, a lower midline abdominal incision is performed and the bowel retracted out of the pelvis with the patient in the Trendelenburg position. A defect in the muscular lining of the pelvic floor will be noted, and any remaining bowel in the defect can usually be easily reduced. The sac is everted and excess sac tissue can be excised. While small defects in the pelvic floor can be closed with interrupted sutures of nylon or polypropylene, this is usually not an adequate repair given the poor strength of the atrophied tissue that often surrounds the hernia defect. Therefore a repair with a large piece of nonabsorbable mesh is preferred and is usually tacked down to the pelvic floor tissues with interrupted nonabsorbable monofilament sutures.

The perineal approach to hernia repair is more direct and avoids a laparotomy but suffers from inadequate exposure of the actual hernia defect. In this technique, a transverse or longitudinal incision is made directly over the site of the hernia bulge. The sac is identified and dissected free of its attachments to the surrounding pelvic musculature and fascia. The sac is then excised and its contents are reduced within the abdominal cavity. The defect is repaired with interrupted nonabsorbable suture, as the exposure is usually not wide enough for proper placement of mesh. While this approach may be suitable for a small hernia defect in an unhealthy patient, the risk of recurrence is high.

In extraordinary cases in which the hernia contents cannot be reduced during a transperitoneal repair, a combined approach with dissection from the perineum can be considered. The actual repair of the hernia defect should take place from within the abdomen to obtain optimal exposure and facilitate placement of mesh to reinforce the closure.

Postoperative perineal hernia repairs may also be repaired by either a transperitoneal or perineal approach. However, the transperitoneal approach is preferred in this scenario, as the hernia contents may be difficult to completely reduce secondary to postoperative adhesion formation. In addition, given the previous operative dissection, the pelvic floor is already weakened and mesh placement is often necessary to achieve an adequate, tension-free closure of the defect.

▪ SPIGELIAN HERNIA

A spigelian hernia occurs along the semilunar line, which traverses a vertical space along the lateral rectus border from the costal margin to the pubic symphysis. Adriaan van der Spieghel (1578–1625), a pupil of Fabricius of Padua and a professor of anatomy and surgery, was the first to accurately describe the semilunar line. He described the spigelian fascia as the aponeurotic structure between the transversus abdominis muscle laterally and the posterior rectus sheath medially. This fascia is what makes up the semilunar line, and it is through this fascial layer that a spigelian hernia forms.

Spigelian hernia is well described, and almost 1000 cases have been reported in the medical literature. It is likely that more of these hernias will be diagnosed, as the spigelian hernia is readily seen on computed tomography scans as well as laparoscopic views of the anterior abdominal wall.

ANATOMY

In practice, the semilunar line is taken as the lateral border of the rectus sheath. Spieghel originally intended this structure to represent the line of transition from the muscular fibers of the transversus abdominis muscle to the posterior aponeurosis of the rectus. The semilunar line runs from the ninth rib cartilage superiorly to the pubic tubercle inferiorly. The spigelian fascia varies in width along the semilunar line, and it gets wider as it approaches the umbilicus. The widest portion of the spigelian fascia is the area where the semilunar line intersects the arcuate line of Douglas (the linea semicircularis; Fig 5–13). It is in this region, between the umbilicus and the arcuate line, where more than 90% of spigelian hernias are found.[35] It is thought that since the spigelian fascia is widest at this point, it is also weakest in this region. Below the arcuate line, all of the transversus abdominis aponeurotic fibers pass anterior to the rectus muscle to contribute to the anterior rectus sheath, and there is no posterior component of the rectus sheath. The rearrangement of muscle and fascial fibers at the intersection of the arcuate and semilunar lines is thought to cause an area of functional weakness that is predisposed to hernia formation. Hernias at the upper extremes of the semilunar line are rare and usually not true spigelian hernias since there is little spigelian fascia in these regions.

As the hernia develops, preperitoneal fat emerges through the defect in the spigelian fascia bringing an extension of the peritoneum with it (Fig 5–14). The hernia usually meets resistance from the external oblique aponeurosis, which is intact and does not undergo rearrangement of its aponeurotic fibers at the arcuate line. For this reason, almost all spigelian hernias are interparietal in nature, and only rarely will the hernia sac lie in the subcutaneous tissues anterior to the external oblique fascia. This fact makes the accurate diagnosis of spigelian hernias more challenging. The hernia also cannot develop medially due to resistance from the intact rectus muscle and sheath.

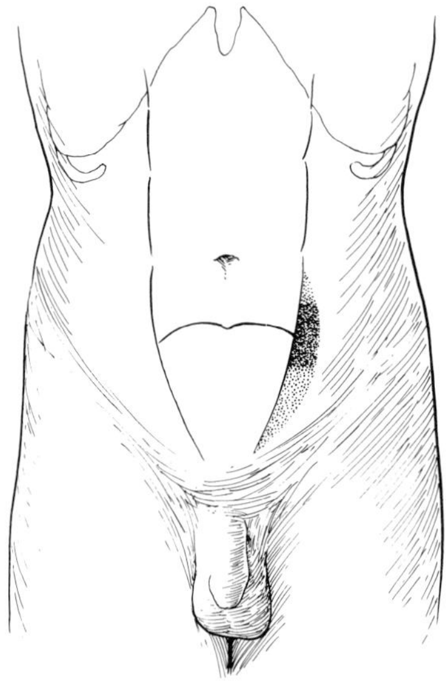

Figure 5–13. Anatomy of the spigelian hernia and the sites of most common occurrence. After Rejovitzky, MD.

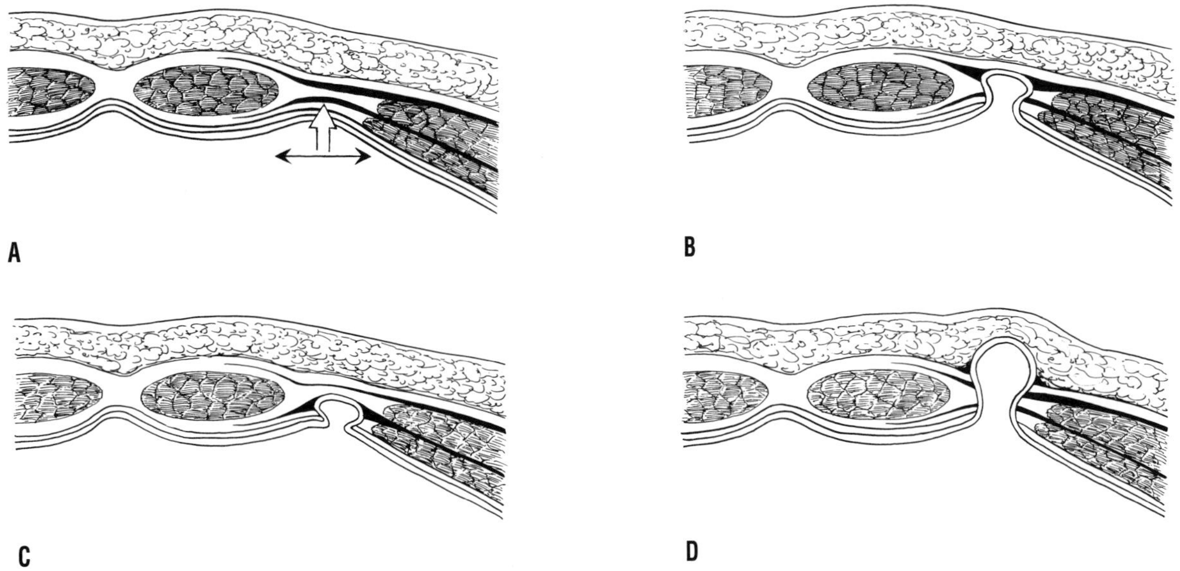

Figure 5–14. The spigelian hernia. **A.** Breaching the spigelian fascia. **B.** The most common type has passed through the transversus abdominis and the internal oblique aponeuroses and is spreading out in the interstitial layer posterior to the external oblique aponeurosis. **C.** The less common type in the interstitial layer between the transversus abdominis aponeurosis and the internal oblique muscle. **D.** The least common subcutaneous type. After Rejovitzky, MD.

Therefore, a large spigelian hernia is most often found lateral and inferior to its defect in the space directly posterior to the external oblique muscle.

CLINICAL MANIFESTATIONS

The patient most often presents with a swelling in the middle to lower abdomen just lateral to the rectus muscle. The patient may complain of a sharp pain or tenderness at this site. The hernia is usually reducible in the supine position. However, up to 20% of spigelian hernias will present incarcerated, and for this reason operative repair is mandatory once the hernia is confirmed on diagnosis. The reducible mass may be palpable, even if it sits below the external oblique musculature.

When the diagnosis is unclear, radiologic imaging may be necessary. Ultrasound examination has been shown to be the most reliable and easiest method to assist in the diagnostic work-up. Testa and colleagues found that abdominal wall ultrasonography was accurate in 86% of cases of spigelian hernia.[36] If the hernia is fully reduced during examination and no mass is palpable, ultrasound evaluation can show a break in the echogenic shadow of the semilunar line associated with the fascial defect. Ultrasound can also identify the nonreduced hernia sac passing through the defect in the spigelian fascia. Computed tomographic scanning of the abdomen will also confirm the presence of a spigelian hernia. As described above, the anatomy of the spigelian hernia should make it readily apparent on laparoscopic evaluation of the anterior abdominal wall.

TREATMENT

The treatment for spigelian hernia is operative repair once the diagnosis has been confirmed, given the risk for incarceration. This is usually performed under general anesthesia given the need for splitting of the external oblique muscle. A transverse incision is made directly over the palpable mass or fascial defect. A hernia in the subcutaneous space will reveal itself immediately, and an interparietal hernia will require further dissection. In this way, the external oblique fascia is incised and the external oblique muscle is split to identify the sac posterior to the muscle. The sac is freed from its surrounding attachments until the neck is isolated. The sac is opened, the intra-abdominal contents reduced, and the sac is either excised if sizable or simply inverted into the intra-abdominal cavity. Suturing the medial and lateral edges of the internal oblique and transversus abdominis aponeuroses closes the fascial defect. Essentially, this approximates the internal oblique and transversus fascia laterally to the rectus sheath medially. Prosthetic mesh is not required for this repair, although the use of mesh plugs to close the hernia defect has been described.[36] Recurrence is uncommon and the operation is usually well tolerated.

▪ LUMBAR HERNIA

The lumbar region is bordered by the twelfth rib superiorly, the iliac crest inferiorly, the erector spinae muscles of the back posteriorly, and a vertical line between the anterior tip of the twelfth rib and the iliac crest anteriorly. The region contains two anatomic triangles, through which the rare lumbar hernia can form. The inferior lumbar triangle of Petit is the more common of the two. Its anterior border is the posterior edge of the external oblique muscle, the posterior border is the anterior extent of the latissimus dorsi muscle, and the inferior border is the iliac crest (Fig 5–15). The anterior floor of the canal formed by this triangle is the lumbar fascia. Occasionally, the lower border of the latissimus dorsi muscle overlaps the external oblique muscle, and in this setting the triangle is absent. The superior lumbar triangle of Grynfeltt (see Fig 5–15) is deeper and is bounded by the twelfth rib and the serratus posterior inferior muscle, the posterior border of the internal oblique muscle, and by the quadratus lumborum and erector spinae muscles posteriorly. The floor of the superior triangle is composed of transversalis fascia and the entire triangular space is covered posteriorly by the latissimus dorsi muscle.

Congenital lumbar hernias are rare, but case reports can be found in the literature. Lumbar hernias most commonly present in adults older than 50 years of age. Two-thirds of the cases are reported in males, and left-sided hernias are thought to be more common. Bilateral lumbar hernias have been reported. Acquired lumbar hernias have been associated with back or flank trauma, poliomyelitis, back surgery, and the use of the iliac crest as a donor site for bone grafts.

Strangulation is rare in lumbar hernias since at least two of the three boundaries for the hernia defect are soft and muscular in origin. The hernia tends to increase in size over time and may assume large proportions and overhang the iliac crest. Symptoms range from a vague dullness in the flank or lower back to focal pain associated with movement over the site of the defect. On physical examination, a soft swelling in the lower posterior abdomen will be found that is usually reducible without difficulty. The hernia will increase in size with straining or a standard Valsalva maneuver. Ultrasonographic or computed tomographic imaging is usually obtained in the patient with a suspected lumbar hernia to confirm the diagnosis.

Operative repair of the lumbar hernia is performed with the patient under general anesthesia and in a modified lateral decubitus position. A kidney rest can be used to widen the lumbar space between the twelfth rib and iliac crest. An oblique skin incision is made in the region of the hernia and the sac is identified. The dissection may require takedown of the latissimus dorsi muscle to reach the deeper superior lumbar triangle. Once the sac is identified, it is opened and the contents carefully reduced. The empty sac can then be inverted or simply excised. While complicated procedures for lumbar hernia closure utilizing muscle flaps and grafts have been described, a small defect surrounded by healthy tissue can usually be closed primarily with an interrupted or continuous layer of nylon or polypropylene suture. If a large defect is found or the tissues appear weak, the hernia may be repaired with a large sheet of prosthetic nonabsorbable mesh placed between the peritoneal layer and the abdominal wall musculature. To prevent migration, the mesh is usually fixed to the peripheral tissues by a series of interrupted nonabsorbable sutures.

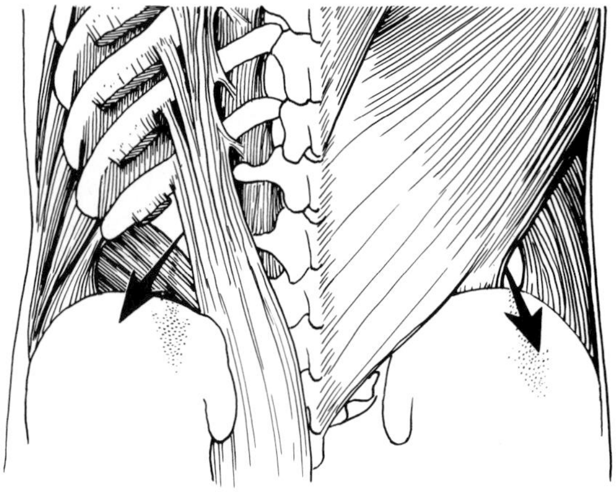

Figure 5–15. The anatomy of the lumbar hernia illustrating the superior and inferior lumbar triangles. After Rejovitzky, MD.

Recently, minimally invasive approaches to repair of lumbar hernias have been reported. These involve either intraperitoneal laparoscopy necessitating takedown of the lateral peritoneal reflection of the colon to facilitate exposure of the hernia defect,[37] or retroperitoneoscopy in which the lateral retroperitoneal space is entered and insufflated.[38] Initial results with the minimally invasive approaches are encouraging, although these case series contain small numbers of subjects.

▪ SCIATIC HERNIA

A sciatic hernia is defined as a protrusion of peritoneum and intra-abdominal contents through the greater or lesser sciatic notch (Fig 5–16). The greater sciatic notch is traversed by the piriformis muscle, and hernia sacs can protrude either superior or inferior to this muscle. There are classically three variants of the sciatic hernia that are defined by their anatomic site of exit from the pelvis. The suprapiriform defect is by far the most common and is thought to represent 60% of cases of sciatic hernia. Infrapiriform hernias are found in approxi-

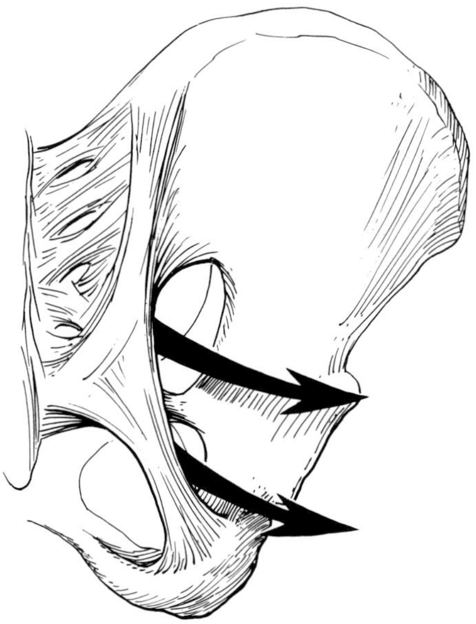

Figure 5–16. The superior and inferior sciatic foramina and the direction of sciatic hernias. After Rejovitzky, MD.

mately 30% of cases, and subspinous hernias (through the lesser sciatic foramen) occur in 10% of cases.

The hernia sac passes laterally, inferiorly, and ultimately posteriorly to lie deep to the gluteus maximus muscle. While case reports of this rare hernia exist in the pediatric age group, the majority of sciatic hernias are found in the adult population. The patient complains of pain deep in the buttock that may radiate down the leg in the sciatic nerve distribution. Alternatively, the patient may report a lump in the buttock or infragluteal area that is painful and tender. Rarely, ureteral obstruction occurs because the ipsilateral ureter is contained within the hernia contents. Physical examination often reveals a reducible mass deep to the gluteus maximus, although the actual hernia defect is rarely palpable given the anatomic depth and the thickness of the buttock musculature. Incarceration of the hernia can occur, and sciatic hernia has been known to present with bowel obstruction.

The treatment of a sciatic hernia is surgical. Both transperitoneal and transgluteal approaches have been described in depth, and the transperitoneal technique is preferred in the setting of bowel obstruction or incarceration. Rarely, a combined approach will be necessary to fully reduce the hernia contents. Even in the setting of incarceration, the bowel can usually be reduced from within the hernia with gentle traction. When necessary with the transperitoneal approach, the defect can be dilated with manual manipulation or the piriformis muscle may be partially incised. Full visualization of the structures is necessary and great care must be taken to avoid injury to the many nerves and vessels found in this region. After the sac has been excised, the defect is repaired using interrupted nonabsorbable suture or a prosthetic mesh plug or patch for larger hernia defects.

The posterior or transgluteal technique can be utilized for uncomplicated, reducible sciatic hernias diagnosed preoperatively. With this method the patient is placed in the prone position. The gluteus maximus muscle is approached through a gluteal incision starting at the posterior edge of the greater trochanter and is detached at its origin to expose the hernia defect. This exposure allows visualization of the piriformis muscle, the gluteal vessels and nerve, and the sciatic nerve. The sac is then isolated and opened. Following reduction of the hernia contents, the defect can be sutured closed using large nonabsorbable suture or repaired with a prosthetic mesh.

▪ POSTOPERATIVE VENTRAL WALL (INCISIONAL) HERNIA

A postoperative ventral abdominal wall hernia, more commonly termed incisional hernia, is the result of a failure of fascial tissues to heal and close following laparotomy. Such hernias can occur after any type of abdominal wall incision, although the highest incidence is seen with midline and transverse incisions.[39] Postoperative ventral hernias following paramedian, subcostal, McBurney, Pfannenstiel, and flank incisions have also been described in the literature. Laparoscopic port sites may also develop hernia defects in the abdominal wall fascia.

As the approximated fascial tissue separates, the bowel and omentum herniates through the opening, covered by a peritoneal sac. These hernias can increase in size to enormous proportions, and giant ventral hernias can contain a significant amount of small or large bowel. At the extreme end of the ventral hernia spectrum is the giant incisional hernia that leads to loss of the abdominal domain, which occurs when the intra-abdominal contents can no longer lie within the abdominal cavity.

INCIDENCE AND ETIOLOGY

Incisional hernias have been reported in up to 20% of patients undergoing laparotomy. Modern rates of incisional hernia range from 2–11%.[40–42] It is estimated that approximately 100,000 ventral incisional hernia repairs are performed each year in the United States alone. The incidence seems to be lower in smaller incisions, so that laparoscopic port site hernias are much less common than hernias following large midline abdominal incisions. While it was once believed that the majority of incisional hernias presented within the first 12 months following laparotomy, longer-term data indicate that at least one-third of these hernias will present 5–10 years postoperatively.

Multiple risk factors exist for the development of an incisional hernia. Some of these risks are under the control of the surgeon at the initial operation, while many others are patient-specific or related to postoperative complications. Patient-specific risks for postoperative ventral hernia include advanced age, malnutrition, presence of ascites, corticosteroid use, diabetes mellitus, cigarette smoking, and obesity.[39,43–45] Emergency surgery is known to increase the risk of incisional hernia formation. Wound infection is believed to be one of the most significant prognostic risk factors for development of an incisional hernia.[39,46] It is for this reason that many surgeons advocate aggressive and early opening of the skin closure to drain any potential infection at the fascial level. Postoperative sepsis has also been identified as a risk for subsequent incisional hernia.

Technical aspects of wound closure likely contribute to incisional hernia formation. Wounds closed under excessive tension are prone to fascial closure disturbance. Therefore, a continuous closure is advocated to disperse the tension throughout the length of the wound. In this way, 1-cm bites of fascia on either side of the incision are taken with each pass of the suture and the suture is advanced 1 cm at a time along the length of the incision. The type of incision may affect hernia formation. Studies have shown that transverse incisions are associated with a reduced incidence of incisional hernia compared to midline vertical laparotomies, although the data are far from conclusive.[44,47]

CLINICAL MANIFESTATIONS

The patient with an incisional hernia will complain of a bulge in the abdominal wall originating deep to the skin scar. The bulge may cause varying degrees of discomfort or may present as a cosmetic concern. Symptoms will usually be aggravated by coughing or straining as the hernia contents protrude through the abdominal wall defect. In large ventral hernias, the skin may present with ischemic or pressure necrosis leading to frank ulceration. Presentation of the incisional hernia with incarceration causing bowel obstruction is not uncommon. This may be associated with a history of repeated mild attacks of colicky dull abdominal pain and nausea consistent with incomplete bowel obstruction.

On examination the hernia is usually easy to identify and the edges of the fascial defect can often be defined by palpation. The entire abdominal wall along the length of the incision should be inspected and palpated carefully, as multiple hernias are often present in the setting of an incisional hernia. In the obese patient with a suspected incisional hernia that cannot be confirmed on examination, computed tomography of the abdomen is the best way to visualize intra-abdominal contents within the hernia sac. In extreme instances, laparoscopy may be required to diagnose a hernia defect that only intermittently contains intra-abdominal contents.

TREATMENT

The treatment of ventral incisional hernia is operative repair, and three general classes of operative repair have emerged in the modern era. These techniques include primary suture repair of the hernia, open repair of the hernia with prosthetic mesh, and laparoscopic incisional hernia repair. The major sequela from operative repair of the incisional hernia is hernia recurrence, and there are convincing data that placement of mesh to repair the hernia defect has decreased the high recurrence rate historically associated with primary suture repair to less than 25%.[48,49] Many advocates of the operation believe that laparoscopic incisional hernia repair will have the lowest rate of hernia recurrence and definitive studies are underway to assess this question.

In general, primary repair of incisional hernias can be performed for hernia defects less than 4 cm in diameter with strong, viable surrounding tissue. For larger hernias or hernias associated with multiple small defects, mesh repair is indicated. Even with mesh repair, hernia recurrence remains a significant complication. In one multicenter trial, for example, 200 patients were randomly assigned to suture or mesh repair of a primary hernia or a first recurrence of hernia at the site of a vertical midline incision.[50] The 3-year cumulative rates of recurrence among patients who had suture or mesh for repair of a primary hernia were 43% and 24%, respectively. The rates of second recurrence were 58% and 20%, respectively.

Primary Suture Repair

The operation is best performed with the patient under general anesthesia to achieve full relaxation of the abdominal wall musculature. The skin is opened through the previous incision and dissection is performed through the subcutaneous tissues. Care should be taken as the level of the anterior rectus sheath is approached since portions of the sac and its contents may lie at this level. The sac is identified and cleared of its attachments to the fascia using electrocautery. In this way, any peritoneal attachments to the anterior abdominal wall in the vicinity of the hernia are taken down and the sac is fully reduced into the abdominal cavity. The fascia is then cleared of soft tissue both anteriorly and posteriorly for at least a 3–4 cm margin. This allows for a margin of healthy fascia to bring together in the midline with suture closure.

The fascia is then closed using an interrupted layer of nonabsorbable suture by taking large bites of the clean fascia on both sides of the defect. The sutures are usually placed sequentially and then tied after the entire layer of suture has been placed. The fascia is then inspected to confirm that no additional defects are present and that the repair sutures are not pulling through the tissue due to excessive tension. The skin is closed over the fascia using either staples or a running subcuticular layer. If the hernia contents have created a large pocket in the soft tissue above the anterior fascia, placement of a closed suction drain for evacuation of early seroma fluid can be considered.

Mesh Repair

The use of sheets of nonabsorbable prosthetic mesh placed across the incisional hernia defect and sutured to the abdominal wall is routinely employed in the modern era. It is associated with a low incidence of perioperative complications and lower rates of recurrence than open, nonmesh repairs.

Many variations of mesh repair for the incisional hernia have been described (Fig 5–17). The mesh is cut to the shape of the hernia defect with a margin added circumferentially around the mesh to suture to healthy surrounding fascia. The mesh is sutured to the fascial layer either deep to the peritoneum or between the peritoneum and the abdominal wall. Alternative techniques have been described that suture pieces of mesh to fascia from both intra- and extraperitoneal planes.

The operation is performed under general anesthesia. The old scar is incised and the soft tissue dissected down to the level of the anterior rectus sheath. Here the defect is identified and the fascia is cleared of surrounding soft tissue attachments to allow a 3–4 cm rim of healthy fascia circumferentially. The sac is then freed from the fascia in order to reduce the hernia contents and prevent recurrence. This portion of the operation is often technically challenging, as significant adhesion formation may have occurred following the initial operation. It is often impossible to stay in an extraperitoneal plane in this situation, and dissection within the abdominal cavity may be necessary to fully excise the sac and reduce its contents. The mesh can now be placed either anterior to the fascia or posterior from within the intra-abdominal cavity. Effort should be made to protect the bowel from direct contact with the mesh patch, and a layer of omentum can often be placed be-

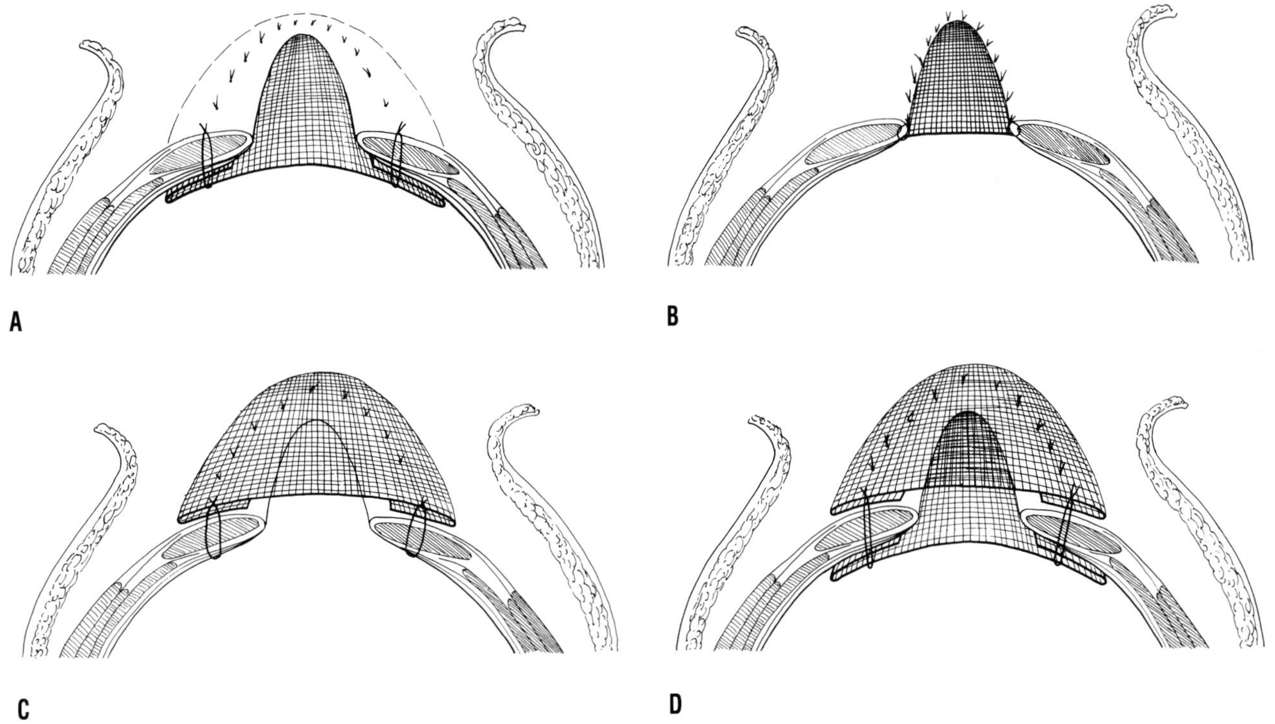

Figure 5–17. Variations of prosthetic mesh repair for incisional hernia. **A.** Underlay graft. **B.** Inlay graft. **C.** Overlay graft. **D.** Combined overlay and underlay grafts. *Continued*

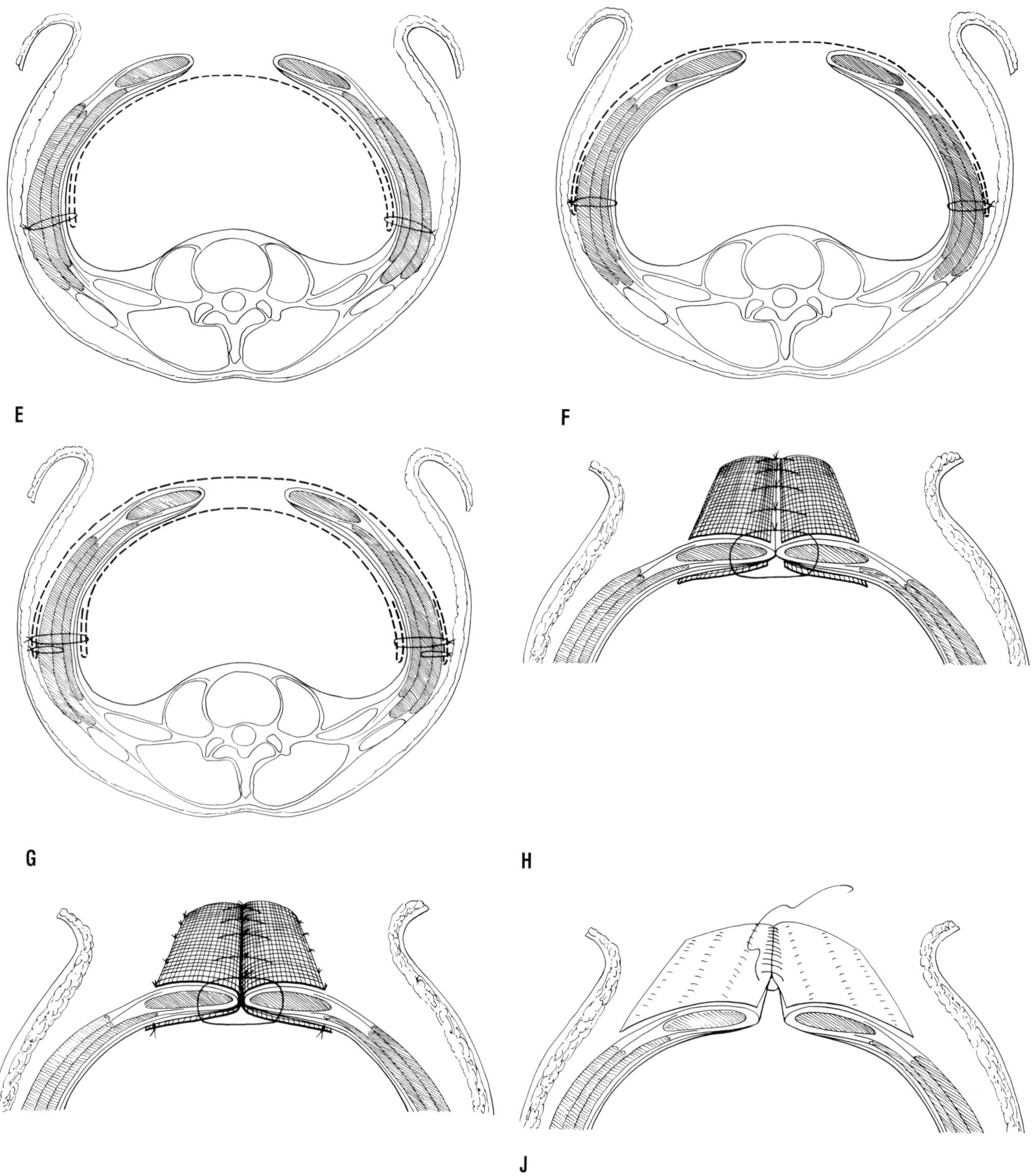

Figure 5–17, cont'd. E. Large underlay graft. **F.** Large overlay graft. **G.** Combined large overlay and underlay grafts. **H.** Reinforcing onlay and underlay strips of mesh. **I.** Wrap-around mesh reinforcement of wound edges. **J.** Two sheets of mesh sutured to abdominal wall, then sutured to each other to draw together the edges of the wound. After Rejovitzky, MD.

tween them. The mesh is sutured in an interrupted fashion in multiple sites throughout the entire circumference of the patch to ensure that any tension is distributed throughout the entire area of the repair. Large, nonabsorbable suture is used to affix the mesh to the fascia layer.

Laparoscopic Repair

The evolution of ventral hernia repair has advanced from open mesh repair to the application of mesh repair to the laparoscopic approach. In this technique, the defect is repaired posteriorly and no dissection within the scarred layer of anterior fascia is required. The laparoscopic approach may also allow for identification of additional hernia defects in the anterior abdominal wall during the repair.

One of the challenging aspects of laparoscopic repair is port access into a peritoneal cavity that has been previously operated upon. In general, access can be obtained for needle insufflation via the left upper quadrant, placing the port along the anterior axillary line to avoid injury to the more laterally positioned spleen. Once insufflation has been achieved and instruments inserted, the next challenge is the extensive laparoscopic lysis of adhesions that is often necessary to gain exposure to the entire hernia defect. The goal of the adhesiolysis is to provide a 3–4 cm circumferential area of overlap for the mesh patch beyond the edge of the ventral hernia defect.

After the appropriate adhesions have been taken down and the fascial edges of the defect confirmed, the sac is retracted and excised from within the hernia. The outline of the defect is then drawn on the anterior abdominal wall. Edges of the defect at the skin level can be confirmed from within the abdominal cavity using the laparoscope. The mesh is then cut to fit this defect with a margin of 3–4 cm on each side to provide adequate coverage and to minimize tension. Nonabsorbable sutures are placed around the circumference of the mesh and tied, but not cut. The mesh is rolled so that the anterior surface lies inside the roll, and the mesh is inserted into the abdomen through a large 10- or 12-mm port.

Once inside the abdominal cavity, the mesh is unrolled and positioned. A transfascial suture passer can be introduced through small stab incisions placed around the marked border of the defect. The suture passer retrieves the long ends of the suture that has been previously placed in the mesh, and the ends are tied at the skin level at 4–6 points around the repair and buried with the subcutaneous tissue in the stab incision. This affixes the mesh patch to the fascia layers around the circumference of the patch. After all sutures have been tied and cut, laparoscopically-placed tacks or staples can be used to further fasten the mesh to the anterior abdominal wall. Whether the strength of the repair is imparted by the transfascial sutures or the tacks or both remains controversial.

COMPLICATIONS

The major complication from open, nonmesh incisional hernia repair is recurrence. Rates of recurrence in this type of repair have approached 30–50% in some series. The risk of recurrence is likely related to the tension placed on the repair in large hernias, and for this reason incisional hernias with a diameter greater than 4 cm should be repaired with mesh.

Open incisional hernia repairs using mesh can also suffer from hernia recurrence, although the risk is far less than that of the nonmesh technique. Several studies have shown that the risk of recurrence in incisional hernia repair with mesh is approximately 10%. Recurrence in this setting is usually secondary to the appearance of an additional, unrecognized hernia site or an improperly placed prosthesis that pulls away from the fascia edge of the repair. Hematoma or seroma formation may occur in the cavity left behind following a hernia repair. For this reason, closed suction drains may be placed if a large amount of dead space remains following the repair. The drains should be managed judiciously, however, since they may be placed in proximity to the prosthetic mesh, thereby increasing the chance of secondary infection. Wound infection and infection of the mesh can be grave complications, often necessitating removal of the mesh and application of an allogenic tissue graft. Wound infection in open mesh repairs is thought to approximate 5%.

The laparoscopic approach to incisional hernia repair shares the general complications of laparoscopy, including the potential for port site herniation, vascular injury from trocar placement, and inadvertent bowel injury during laparoscopic adhesiolysis. The mesh placed during laparoscopic repair can also be prone to infection, although the incidence of mesh infection appears to be lower in laparoscopic than open mesh techniques. This may be related to the extensive tissue dissection required to place the mesh in the open procedure. Several nonrandomized studies have shown that the laparoscopic approach is associated with a low incidence of hernia recurrence, in the range of 0–11%.[51] Seroma formation in the retained sac above the mesh may occur but usually resolves spontaneously.

There are numerous prospective studies that provide data for the individual techniques, but data are scarce in the comparison between open and laparoscopic mesh repairs for incisional hernia. Nonrandomized, retrospective studies have provided ample evidence that the laparoscopic approach is associated with fewer postoperative complications, a lower incidence of wound and mesh infections, a lower rate of recurrence in long-term follow-up, and shorter in-hospital stays.[52] The only prospective, randomized study in the literature demonstrated reduced rates of perioperative complications and hernia recurrence in the laparoscopic group in a total cohort of 60 patients.[53] Larger scale, multicenter trials are currently underway to definitively evaluate the two approaches to incisional hernia repair.

REFERENCES

1. Rutkow IM, Robbins AW. Demographic, classificatory, and socioeconomic aspects of hernia repair in the United States. *Surg Clin North Am* 1993;73:413
2. Bassini E. Nouvo Metodo per la Cura Radicale dell' Ernia Inguinale. Padua, Italy: Prosperini; 1889
3. McIntosh A, Hutchinson A, Roberts A, et al. Evidence-based management of groin hernia in primary care—a systematic review. *Fam Pract* 2000;17:442
4. Schumpelick V, Treutner KH, Arlt G. Inguinal hernia repair in adults. *Lancet* 1994;344:375
5. Kang SK, Burnett CA, Freund E, et al. Hernia: is it a work-related condition? *Am J Ind Med* 1999;36:638
6. Young DV. Comparison of local, spinal, and general anesthesia for inguinal herniorrhaphy. *Am J Surg* 1987;153:560
7. Nordin P, Zetterstrom H, Gunnarsson U, et al. Local, regional, or general anaesthesia in groin hernia repair: multicentre randomised trial. *Lancet* 2003;362:853
8. Shouldice EE. The treatment of hernia. *Ontario Med Rev* 1953;20:670
9. Simons MP, Kleijnen J, van Geldere D, et al. Role of the Shouldice technique in inguinal hernia repair: A systematic review of controlled trials and a meta-analysis. *Br J Surg* 1996;83:734
10. Shouldice EB. The Shouldice repair for groin hernias. *Surg Clin North Am* 2003;83:1163
11. Klingsworth AN, Britton BJ, Morris PJ. Recurrent inguinal hernia after local anesthetic repair. *Br J Surg* 1982;68:273
12. Lichtenstein IL, Shulman AG, Amid PK. The cause, prevention, and treatment of recurrent groin hernia. *Surg Clin North Am* 1993;73:529
13. Gilbert AI. An anatomic and functional classification for the diagnosis and treatment of inguinal hernia. *Am J Surg* 1989;157:331
14. Rutkow IM, Robbins AW. "Tension-free" inguinal herniorrhaphy: a preliminary report on the mesh plug technique. *Surgery* 1993;114:3
15. Rives J. Major incisional hernias. In: Chevrel JP (ed). *Surgery of the Abdominal Wall.* New York, NY: Springer-Verlag; 1987:116
16. Scott NW, Webb K, Go PM, et al. Open mesh versus non-mesh repair of inguinal hernia. *Cochrane Database Syst Rev* 2001;(4):CD002197
17. Bay-Nielsen M, Kehlet H, Strand L, et al. Quality assessment of 26,304 herniorraphies in Denmark: a prospective nationwide study. *Lancet* 2001;358:1124
18. Vader VL, Vogt DM, Zucker KA, et al. Adhesion formation in laparoscopic inguinal hernia repair. *Surg Endosc* 1997;11:825
19. Ferzli G, Sayad P, Huie F, et al. Endoscopic extraperitoneal herniorrhaphy: A 5-year experience. *Surg Endosc* 1998;12:1311
20. Wake B, McCormack K, Fraser C, et al. Transabdominal pre-peritoneal (TAPP) versus totally extraperitoneal (TEP) laparoscopic techniques for inguinal hernia repair. *Cochrane Database Syst Rev* 2005;(1):CD004703
21. Memon MA, Cooper NJ, Memon B, et al. Meta-analysis of randomized clinical trials comparing open and laparoscopic inguinal hernia repair. *Br J Surg* 2003;90:1479
22. Collaboration EH. Laparoscopic compared with open methods of groin hernia repair: systematic review of randomized controlled trials. *Br J Surg* 2000;87:860
23. Neumayer L, Giobbie-Hurder A, Jonasson O, et al. Open mesh versus laparoscopic mesh repair of inguinal hernia. *N Engl J Med* 2004;350:1819
24. Neumayer LA, Gawande AA, Wang J, et al. Proficiency of surgeons in inguinal hernia repair: effect of experience and age. *Ann Surg* 2005;242:344
25. Read RC. A review: the role of protease-antiprotease imbalance in the pathogenesis of herniation and abdominal aortic aneurysm in certain smokers. *Postgrad Gen Surg* 1992;4:161
26. Gilbert AI, Felton LL. Infection in inguinal hernia repair considering biomaterials and antibiotics. *Surg Gynecol Obstet* 1993;177:126
27. Tverskoy M, Cozacov C, Ayache M, et al. Postoperative pain after inguinal herniorraphy with different types of anesthesia. *Anesth Analg* 1990;70:29
28. Gallegos NC, Dawson J, Jarvis M, Hobsley M. Risk of strangulation in groin hernias. *Br J Surg* 1991;78:1171
29. Corder AP. The diagnosis of femoral hernia. *Postgrad Med J* 1992;68:26
30. Lichtenstein IL, Shore JM. Simplified repair of femoral and recurrent inguinal hernia by a "plug" technique. *Am J Surg* 1974;128:439
31. Mayo WJ. An operation for the radical cure of umbilical hernia. *Ann Surg* 1901;31:276
32. Kammori M, Mafune K, Kirashima T, et al. Forty-three cases of obturator hernia. *Am J Surg* 2004;187:549
33. Skandalakis JE. Obturator hernia. In: Skandalakis JE, Gray SW, Mansberger AR, et al (eds). *Hernia Surgical Anatomy and Technique.* New York, NY: McGraw-Hill; 1989:174
34. Tucker JG, Wilson RA, Ramshaw BJ, et al. Laparoscopic herniorraphy: technical concerns in prevention of complications and early recurrence. *Am Surg* 1995;61:36
35. Montes IS, Deysine M. Spigelian and other uncommon hernia repairs. *Surg Clin North Am* 2003;83:1235
36. Testa T, Fallo E, Celoria G, et al. Spigelian hernia: its echotomographic diagnosis and surgical treatment. *G Chir* 1992;13:29
37. Sakarya A, Ayded H, Erhan MY, et al. Laparoscopic repair of acquired lumbar hernia. *Surg Endosc* 2003;17:1494
38. Habib E. Retroperitoneoscopic tension-free repair of lumbar hernia. *Hernia* 2003;7:150
39. Bucknall TE, Cox PJ, Ellis H. Burst abdomen and incisional hernia: a prospective study of 1129 major laparotomies. *Br Med J* 1982;284:931

40. Santora TA, Rosalyn JJ. Incisional hernia. *Surg Clin North Am* 1993;73:557
41. Mudge M, Hughes LE. Incisional hernia: a 10 year prospective study of incidence and attitudes. *Br J Surg* 1985; 72:70
42. Regnard JF, Hay JM, Rea S. Ventral incisional hernias: incidence, date of recurrence, localization, and risk factors. *Ital J Surg Sci* 1988;3:259
43. Read RC, Yoder G. Recent trends in the management of incisional herniation. *Arch Surg* 1989;124:485
44. Greenall MJ, Evans M, Pollack AV. Midline or transverse laparotomy? A random controlled clinical trial. Part I: influence on healing. *Br J Surg* 1980;67:188
45. Makela JT, Kiviniemi H, Juvonen T, et al. Factors influencing wound dehiscence after midline laparotomy. *Am J Surg* 1995;170:387
46. Gys T, Hubens A. A prospective comparative clinical study between monofilament absorbable and non-absorbable sutures for abdominal wall closure *Acta Chir Belg* 1989;89:265
47. Carlson MA, Ludwig KA, Condon RE. Ventral hernia and other complications of 1,000 midline incisions. *South Med J* 1995;88:450
48. Millikan KW, Baptisa M, Amin B, et al. Intraperitoneal underlay ventral hernia repair utilizing bilayer ePTFE and polypropylene mesh. *Am Surg* 2003;69:258
49. McLanahan D, King LT, Weems C, et al. Retrorectus prosthetic mesh repair of midline abdominal hernia. *Am J Surg* 1997;173:445
50. Luijendijk RW, Hop WC, van den Tol MP, et al. A comparison of suture repair with mesh repair for incisional hernia. *N Engl J Med* 2000;343:292
51. Thoman DS, Phillips ES. Current status of laparoscopic ventral hernia repair. *Surg Endosc* 2002;16:939
52. Cobb WS, Kercher KW, Heniford BT. Laparoscopic repair of incisional hernias. *Surg Clin North Am* 2005;85:91
53. Carbajo MA, Martin del Olmo JC, Blanco JI, et al. Laparoscopic treatment vs. open surgery in the solution of major incisional and abdominal wall hernias with mesh. *Surg Endosc* 1999;13:250

6

Intestinal Stomas

Ira J. Kodner ■ *Thomas E. Read*

An intestinal stoma is an opening of the intestinal or urinary tract onto the abdominal wall, constructed surgically or appearing inadvertently. A colostomy is a connection of the colon to the skin of the abdominal wall. An ileostomy involves exteriorization of the ileum on the abdominal skin. In rare instances, the proximal small bowel may be exteriorized as a jejunostomy. A urinary conduit involves a stoma on the abdominal wall that serves to convey urine to an appliance placed on the skin. The conduit may consist of an intestinal segment, or in some cases a direct implantation of the ureter, or even the bladder, on the abdominal wall.

Information about the types and numbers of stomas constructed, complications of stomas, and resultant impairment of an individual's life has been limited because the diseases for which stomas are constructed are not mandated as reportable in the United States. Therefore the United Ostomy Association (UOA), a voluntary group of 40,000 members with stomas of various types, undertook the mission of collecting data from patients in the United States and Canada who have an intestinal stoma. A review of 15,000 such entries shows the peak incidence for ileostomy construction owing to ulcerative colitis to occur in persons between 20 and 40 years of age, with a lower peak but in the same age range for patients with Crohn's disease. The second largest peak represents colostomies constructed because of colorectal cancer, and this peak is in patients 60–80 years of age. When complications were analyzed according to original indication for surgery, we found that many patients knew that they had complications but were not aware of the exact nature of the complication. Postoperative intestinal obstruction occurred in all categories of disease, as did retraction of the stoma and abscess formation. There was a preponderance of hernia formation in patients who had surgery for colorectal cancer, whereas abscess, fistula, and stricture formation were the major complications in the patients with Crohn's disease. As new surgical procedures are devised, a justification for their utilization is often the reduction of the level of handicap that exists among patients who have had construction of a conventional ostomy. The UOA survey revealed that patients resumed household activities 90% of the time, vocational activities 73% of the time, social activities 92% of the time, and sexual activities 70% of the time. It is taken into account that patients who have proctectomy for cancer frequently lose their sexual function because of autonomic denervation and not because of the presence of a stoma.

Changes that have improved the quality of life of the patient with a stoma include the development and availability of improved stoma equipment. Specialized surgical techniques, some of which are described in this chapter, have been developed that facilitate the subsequent maintenance of an ostomy. In addition, specialized nursing techniques applied both preoperatively and postoperatively have enhanced the care of the patient with a stoma.

The overall incidence of stoma construction appears to be decreasing and will probably continue to do so. There are now fewer abdominoperineal resections for cancer because of the advent of new surgical techniques, especially the use of stapling devices, as well as an increased use of local treatment for selected rectal tumors. The incidence of permanent ileostomies is decreasing because of the popularization of sphincter-saving procedures for patients with ulcerative colitis and familial polyposis. The surgical procedures that eliminate permanent stomas, however, have resulted in an increasing use of temporary loop ileostomies, which are usually more difficult stomas to manage.

■ COMMON COMPLICATIONS OF STOMAS

Each type of stoma is associated with a particular spectrum of complications, but some problems are common to all intestinal stomas. The specific ones are dealt with under each category of stoma. A common complication, regardless of the stoma type, is destruction of the peristomal skin, which is usually caused by poor location or construction of the stoma. In addition to the acute maceration and inflammation of the skin, pseudoepitheliomatous hyperplasia may arise at the mucocutaneous border of stomas subjected to chronic malfitting appliances. Appearance of a fistula adjacent to a stoma usually indicates recurrence of Crohn's disease. One of the difficult complications to handle, especially in an obese patient, is improper location of the stoma, which prohibits maintenance of the seal of an appliance. A special problem arises in the patient who has portal hypertension because the construction of a stoma results in the creation of a portosystemic shunt, and varices can form in the peristomal skin.

Other common problems include the need for precautions with medications, especially time-released enteric medications, which may pass through a shortened intestinal tract unabsorbed. Laxatives also can be devastating to patients with no colon or with a proximal colostomy. In some cases the ostomy patient has chronic difficulty maintaining proper fluid and electrolyte balance, and diuretics in these patients can be especially difficult to manage. The usual intestinal preparations prior to diagnostic testing should be altered for the patient with an intestinal stoma.

Data from the UOA registry indicate that patients have regained a good quality of life following construction of an intestinal stoma. Conventional ileostomy and sigmoid colostomy account for 73% of the patients in the UOA data registry. Colorectal cancer, chronic ulcerative colitis, and Crohn's disease account for 88% of the patient diagnoses. Ileostomy revisions are most commonly performed for Crohn's disease. The incidence of surgery to correct stoma complications was 10.5% for patients with a conventional ileostomy and 7.5% for patients with a sigmoid colostomy.

The data from the UOA registry suggest that emphasis should be placed on proper construction of standard stomas. The stoma location should be chosen and marked preoperatively, even if there is only a remote possibility of need for an intestinal stoma during the operative procedure.

■ COLOSTOMY

The most common indication for fashioning a colostomy is cancer of the rectum. Since a colostomy is an opening of the large intestine with no sphincteric control, its location would obviously be better on the abdominal wall than in the perineum, where an appliance cannot be maintained. A distal colorectal anastomosis in an elderly patient with a poorly functioning anal sphincter may result in what is essentially a "perineal colostomy." In these cases, it often behooves the surgeon to construct a good colostomy rather than to restore intestinal continuity to an incontinent anus. Colostomies are also constructed as treatment for obstructing lesions of the distal large intestine and for actual or potential perforations.

TYPE BY ANATOMIC LOCATION

Traditionally, the type of colostomy has been categorized by the part of the colon used in its construction. The most common type has been called an "end-sigmoid" colostomy. However, if the inferior mesenteric artery is transected during an operation for cancer of the rectum, the blood supply to the sigmoid colon is no longer dependable, and it should not be used for stoma construction. Therefore, an "end-descending" colostomy is usually preferable to an end-sigmoid colostomy. Other types of colonic stomas include the transverse colostomy and cecostomy. The physiology of the colon should be taken into account when considering stoma construction. The right side of the colon absorbs water and has irregular peristaltic contractions. Stomas made from the proximal half of the colon usually expel a liquid content. The left colon serves as a conduit and reservoir and has a few mass peristaltic motions per day. The content is more solid, and in many cases the stoma output can be regulated by irrigation. Proximal colostomies should be avoided, as they will combine the worst features of both a colostomy and an ileostomy: liquid, high-volume, foul-smelling effluent. The left colon should be used for a colostomy if possible; the distal transverse colon is also a reasonable choice.

DETERMINATION OF COLOSTOMY LOCATION

The location of the colostomy must be carefully selected preoperatively. It should avoid any deep folds of fat, scars, and bony prominences of the abdominal wall. The site is chosen by evaluating the patient in the standing, sitting, and supine positions. Often abdominal skin and fat folds are only noted with the patient in the sitting position. A stoma faceplate is applied to the abdominal wall with its medial margin at the midline; care is taken to not overlay any fold, scar, or prominence; and the stoma site is marked. If a sigmoid or descending colostomy is contemplated, the most desirable position is usually in the left lower quadrant of the abdomen. However, if the patient is obese, it may be preferable to site the colostomy in the left upper quadrant so that it is visible to the patient and not trapped on the undersurface of a panniculus. If a distal transverse colostomy is planned, the left upper quadrant is usually the preferable site. Please refer to the section on determination of the ileostomy location for more details regarding stoma site selection.

TYPE BY FUNCTION

More important than the anatomy of the colon is the function that the colostomy is intended to perform. There are two considerations: (1) to provide decompression of the large intestine, and (2) to provide diversion of the feces.

Decompressing Colostomy

A decompressing colostomy does not necessarily provide diversion of feces. These stomas are constructed most often for distal obstructing lesions causing massive dilation of the proximal colon without ischemic necrosis, severe sigmoid diverticulitis with phlegmon, and for select patients with toxic megacolon. Alternative treatments exist for these conditions: total abdominal colectomy with ileostomy or ileorectal anastomosis; segmental colectomy with construction of end colostomy; and segmental colectomy with intraoperative colonic lavage and primary anastomosis with or without temporary diverting loop ileostomy. However, temporary decompressing stomas are still useful and safe. The procedure acts as a bridge to definitive operation for toxic patients with benign disease and those with malignant distal obstruction. The major disadvantage of a decompressing stoma is that it does not necessarily provide complete fecal diversion and thus carries the risk of potentially fatal sepsis if there is distal perforation.

Types of Decompressing Stomas. There are three types of decompressing stomas: (1) the so-called "blow-hole" decompressing stoma constructed in the cecum or transverse colon, (2) a tube type of cecostomy, and (3) a loop-transverse colostomy.

Cecostomy and "Blow-Hole" Stoma. A cecostomy should be constructed only rarely because it is difficult to manage postoperatively. It should be reserved for the severely, acutely ill patient with massive distention and impending perforation of the colon. This is seen most often with distal obstructing cancer or in some of the pseudo-obstruction syndromes seen in elderly or immunocompromised patients. Because these operations are done on an urgent basis and the abdomen is usually distorted by intestinal dilation, the choice of site for an incision is over the dilated cecum. The location of this incision or of an intended decompressing transverse colostomy is selected by placing a marker on the umbilicus when an abdominal film is obtained.

A disadvantage of a cecostomy or loop colostomy done through a small incision is that one cannot evaluate other parts of the colon for potential ischemic necrosis due to massive dilation. The construction of a blow-hole cecostomy or transverse colostomy (Fig 6–1) is carried out by making a 4–6 cm transverse incision over the most dilated part of intestine and then placing a series of interrupted, seromuscular, absorbable sutures between the peritoneum and the seromuscular layer of the bowel to be decompressed. This should be done through an incision sufficient to allow subsequent incision of the intestine and suturing of the intestine to the skin. The bowel wall will be very thin, and it is not unusual to have leakage of gas as the sutures are being placed. It may be helpful to irrigate with a dilute solution of kanamycin throughout this procedure to prevent infection of the abdominal wall.

Once the first layer of sutures has been placed and the intestine is sealed from the remainder of the abdominal cavity, needle decompression of the gas-distended viscus is performed to reduce the tension on the intestinal wall. When this procedure is completed, a second layer of absorbable sutures is placed between the seromuscular layer of the intestine and the fascia of the abdominal wall. Subsequently, the colon is incised, usually with release of a large amount of liquid and gas. The full thickness of intestine then is sutured to the full thickness of skin, again with absorbable sutures, and an appliance is placed over the stoma. Postoperatively, it is not unusual for there to be significant inflammation in the abdominal wall around such a stoma, and after a period of weeks, significant prolapse may occur. Therefore these stomas should be used for short periods of time, with definitive resection performed as soon as possible.

A tube cecostomy (Fig 6–2) is constructed by making a similar incision or by approaching the cecum through a laparotomy incision. A purse-string suture is placed in the cecal wall, and a large mushroom-tipped or Malecot catheter is placed in the cecum. The purse-

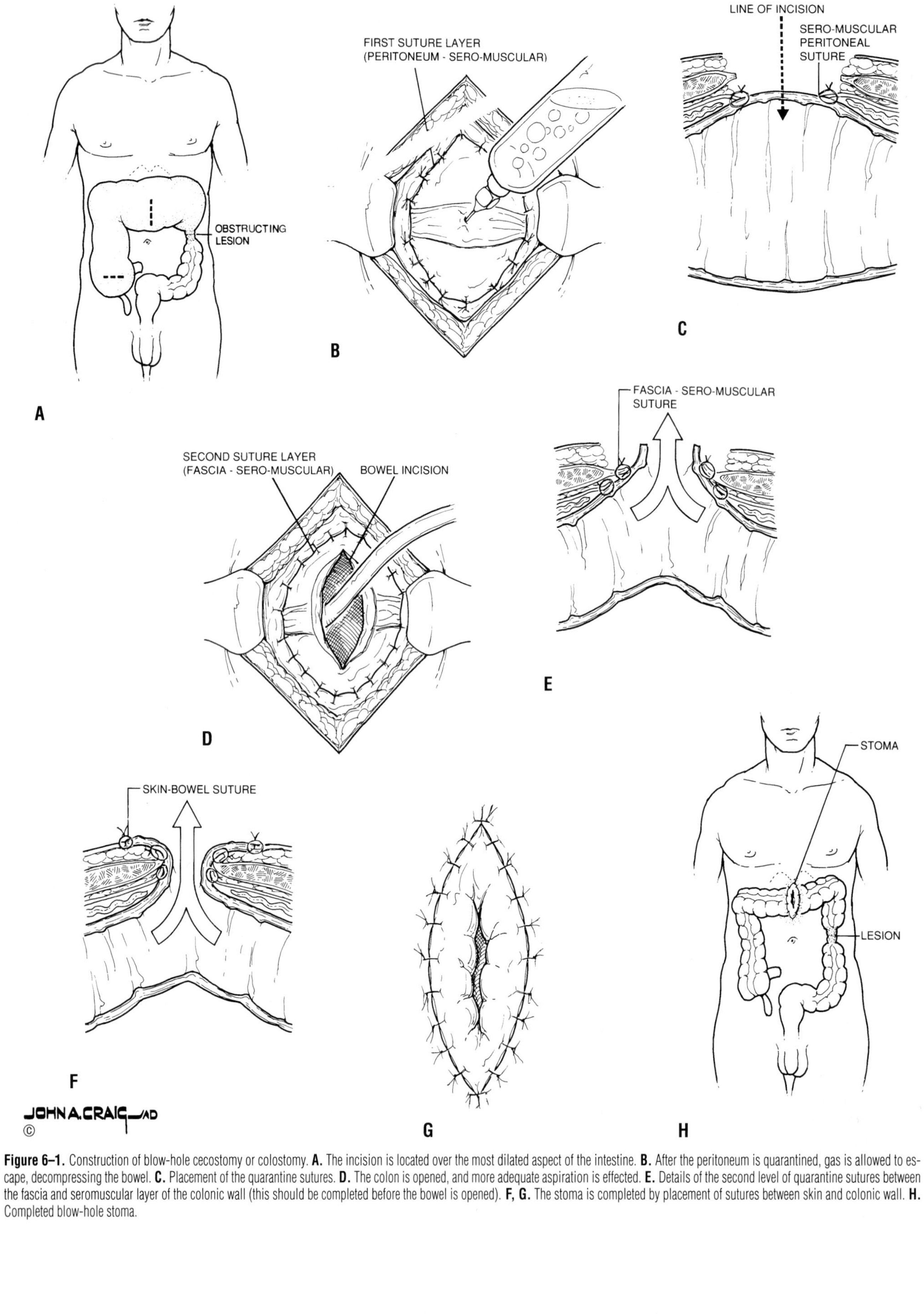

Figure 6–1. Construction of blow-hole cecostomy or colostomy. **A.** The incision is located over the most dilated aspect of the intestine. **B.** After the peritoneum is quarantined, gas is allowed to escape, decompressing the bowel. **C.** Placement of the quarantine sutures. **D.** The colon is opened, and more adequate aspiration is effected. **E.** Details of the second level of quarantine sutures between the fascia and seromuscular layer of the colonic wall (this should be completed before the bowel is opened). **F, G.** The stoma is completed by placement of sutures between skin and colonic wall. **H.** Completed blow-hole stoma.

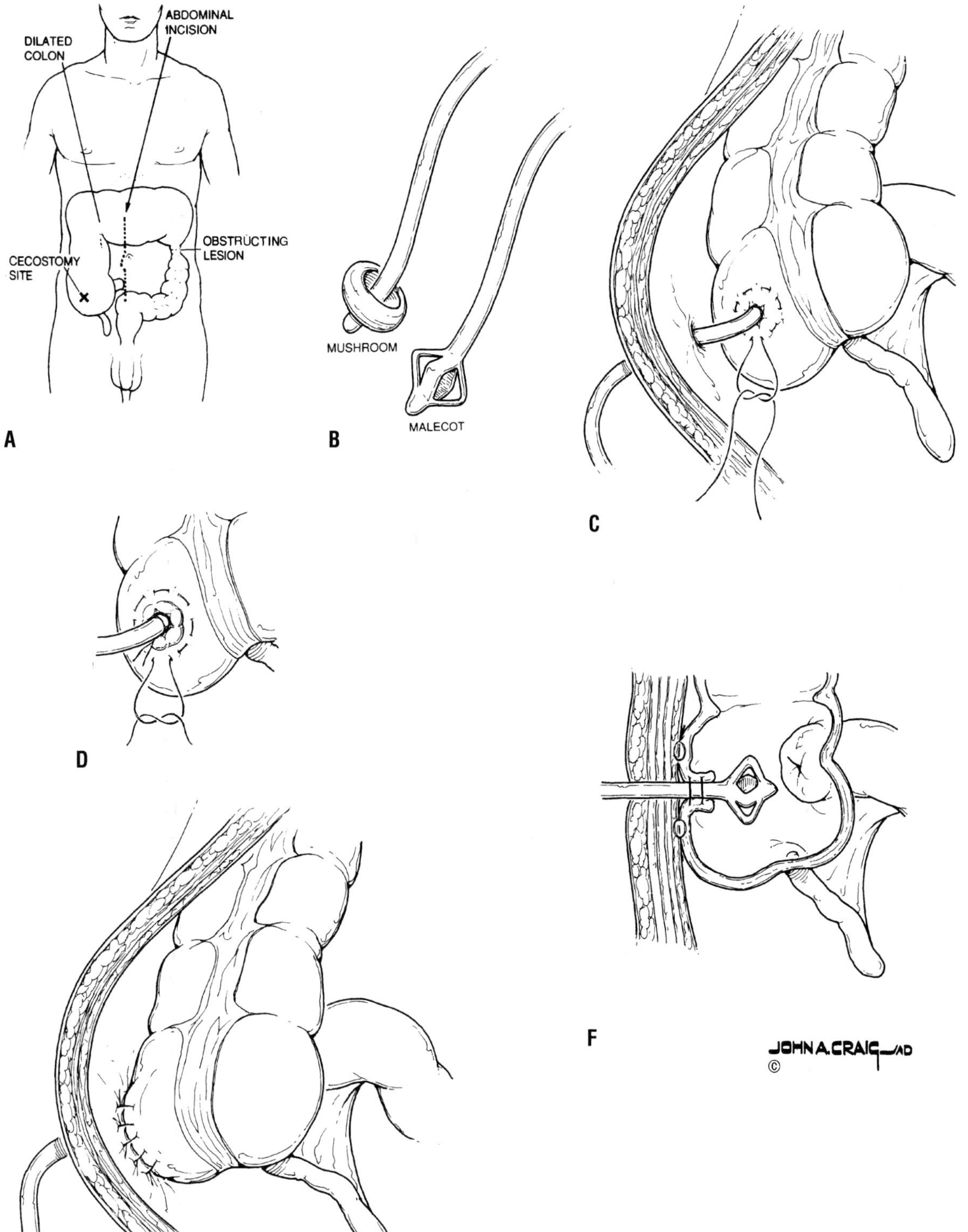

Figure 6–2. Construction of a tube cecostomy. **A.** The cecostomy is constructed over the most dilated aspect of the cecum. **B.** A very large Malecot or mushroom-tipped catheter is used. **C, D.** The catheter is secured within the cecum by two purse-string sutures. **E.** The cecum is sutured to the abdominal wall at the entry site of the catheter. **F.** Cross-section of the completed tube cecostomy.

string suture secures the catheter. Usually a second purse-string suture is placed, and the tube is brought through a right lower quadrant incision. The cecum then is sutured to the peritoneum of the abdominal wall. The advantage of this stoma is that there is less chance of prolapse. The major disadvantage is that the tubes usually become blocked with feces, drain poorly, and sometimes leak stool adjacent to the drain.

Loop-Transverse Colostomy. A loop-transverse colostomy (Fig 6–3) can be used as a decompressive stoma, although it will usually divert the flow of stool from the distal colon. Occasionally, the posterior wall of the stoma recesses far enough below the wall of the abdomen so that stool can enter the distal loop, although this is uncommon. These stomas are constructed for reasons similar to those described for the blow-hole type stoma and to provide temporary diversion for protection of complicated distal anastomoses. The other advantage is that when properly constructed, a loop-transverse colostomy can serve as a long-term stoma. The incidence of prolapse is not prohibitive. Parastomal hernias can occur if the fascia is not closed tightly enough, and these stomas usually cannot be regulated by irrigation techniques.

The site can be chosen for this stoma in an emergency situation as previously described, or it can be marked electively on the abdominal wall in preparation for potential construction in patients who are to have low colorectal anastomoses or in those in whom it is anticipated that inflammatory reaction will be encountered and will require temporary diversion of intestinal contents as a safeguard against contamination from a leaking anastomosis. This occurs occasionally in patients with severe diverticulitis. In an elective situation, the stoma can be placed through the rectus muscle either on the right or left side, depending on later intentions of closing or resecting the colostomy site in continuity with a cancer operation, or it can be brought through the midline (Fig 6–3A).

Construction of loop colostomy requires the colon to be mobile enough to be brought to the level of the abdominal wall (Fig 6–3B). If this cannot be done or if the colon is so massively dilated that loop colostomy is not safe, one should resort to the use of a blow-hole colostomy as previously described, in which only one wall of the intestine is utilized and tension on the mesentery is avoided. The loop-transverse colostomy is constructed by placing a tracheostomy tape around the colon at the site chosen for the colostomy. The transverse colon at this site is usually dissected free of the overlying omentum in the embryonic peritoneal fusion planes. The tracheostomy tape and colon are brought through an avascular window in the omentum to allow better sealing between the colon and the abdominal wall (Figs 6–3B and 6–3C). The fascia is then closed on either side of the loop of colon tightly enough to allow snug passage of one fingertip (Fig 6–3D). This usually seems frighteningly tight but is necessary to prevent postoperative hernia and prolapse.

The skin then is closed, also snugly, on either side of the loop of colon. The tracheostomy tape then is replaced by a T-shaped plastic rod that frequently has a suture through each end so that it can be easily repositioned should it be displaced (Fig 6–3E). The wound is protected, and attention is directed to the protruding loop of colon, which is incised either longitudinally or transversely to allow the best separation of the edges of the colon (Fig 6–3F). Full thickness of intestine is then sutured to full thickness of skin with absorbable suture material (Fig 6–3G). If this stoma is properly constructed, the posterior wall will bulge upward, providing the desired diversion as well as decompression. An appliance then is applied either over the rod or beneath the rod, depending on the tension of the stoma.

In the postoperative period, the appliance is emptied or changed as necessary, and the wound is kept clean. The rod is usually left in place for 1 week and then is easily removed. The colostomy appliance is fashioned as necessary as the contour of the stoma and skin opening change. Patients with this type of stoma usually are not taught to irrigate, because irrigation is infrequently successful. After the immediate postoperative period, the patient usually is instructed to empty the appliance as necessary and to change the entire appliance every 1 or 2 days, depending on the condition of the skin and the ability to maintain an adequate seal of the appliance to the skin.

Closure of a Temporary Colostomy. The most important consideration in dealing with closure of a temporary colostomy is deciding when it is safe to restore intestinal continuity. Distal integrity and adequacy of sphincter muscle function must be carefully evaluated before closure of the stoma is undertaken. The reason for constructing the stoma initially must be taken into account, and contrast studies and endoscopy should demonstrate clearly that the original reason for fecal diversion no longer exists.

Adequate function of the anal sphincter must be demonstrated before the temporary colostomy is closed. This can be done by formal manometric and electromyographic studies or by giving the patient a 500-mL enema and asking him or her to hold it until

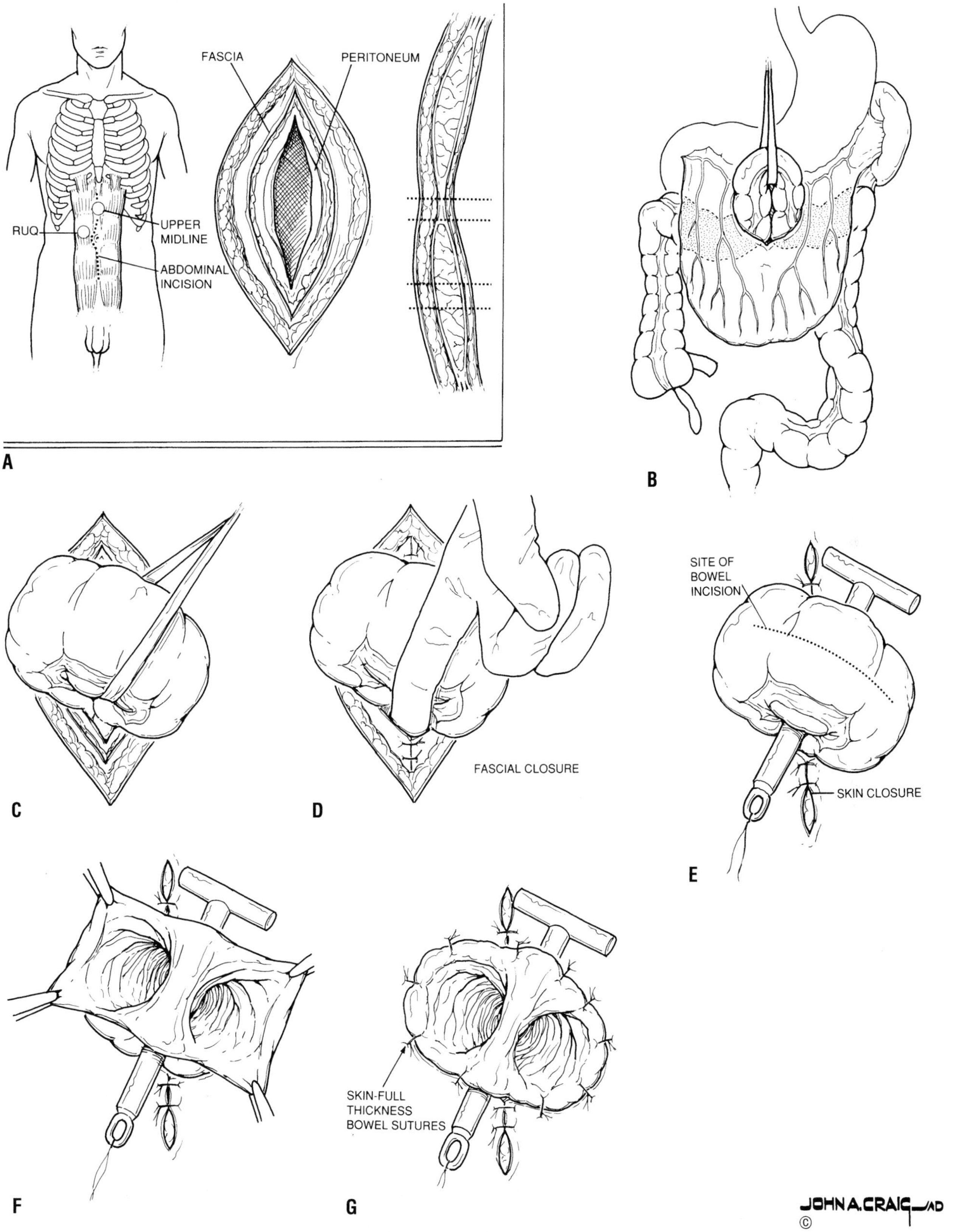

Figure 6–3. Construction of a loop-transverse colostomy. **A.** Choice of stomal location. **B, C.** Tracheostomy tape is used to pull the loop of colon through the incision. **D.** The fascia is closed tightly around the loop of intestine. **E, F, G.** The loop of colon is opened over a supporting rod and is sutured to the skin of the abdominal wall.

he or she can comfortably walk to a toilet and expel the enema. If the sphincter does not work and cannot be repaired, the patient will be better off with a properly constructed end colostomy than with attempts to preserve a nonfunctional sphincter. Once it is decided that it is safe to close the colostomy, the procedure should be undertaken with the same skill and precaution as that required for a colon anastomosis (Fig 6–4). The complication rate following colostomy closure is not insignificant, and is cited by some authors as a reason to avoid diverting colostomy construction at all costs. However, as with all issues in medicine, careful consideration of the potential risks and benefits of the procedure in the individual patient should be made prior to deciding on whether or not fecal diversion is indicated.

The closure is begun by making a circumferential incision around the stoma, including a small rim of skin (Fig 6–4A). If the stoma has been placed in the midline, the midline incision may be opened on either side of it to allow adequate mobilization. The circumferential incision is deepened until the peritoneal cavity is entered and the colon and surrounding omentum can be separated from the abdominal wall. The colon then is brought through the incision, and the serosal surface is clearly defined circumferentially (Figs 6–4B and 6–4C). This involves resecting omentum and fibrofatty tissue from the serosal surface. Once this step is completed, the stoma is ready for closure, which can be accomplished by a linear stapling device (Figs 6–4D and 6–4E), by a hand-sutured closure (Figs 6–4F and 6–4G), or if the bowel has been compromised in any way, by complete transection of the colon and construction of a formal end-to-end anastomosis. Caution must be taken to ensure that no small intestine has been injured and that no significant bleeding has been left unattended. Once this has been accomplished, the colon is returned to the abdominal cavity and the abdomen is closed. Usually the skin itself is left open for delayed primary closure.

Diverting Colostomy

A diverting colostomy is constructed to provide diversion of intestinal content. It is performed because the distal segment of bowel has been completely resected (as during abdominoperineal resection), because of known or suspected perforation or obstruction of the distal bowel (e.g., obstructing carcinoma, diverticulitis, leaking anastomosis, or trauma), or because of destruction or infection of the distal colon, rectum, or anus (e.g., Crohn's disease or failed anal sphincter reconstruction).

Choices for Construction. Although a completely diverting colostomy can be made only by complete transection of the colon, a well constructed loop-transverse or sigmoid colostomy may provide near complete fecal diversion. Stool and flatus will move preferentially toward the low-pressure side of any pressure gradient, and this usually means that it will flow into the stoma appliance which is at atmospheric pressure, rather than into the distal bowel. However, patients who have loop stomas must be counseled that if the stoma appliance becomes full and tense, stool and flatus can be forced distally. This discussion should take place prior to discharge from the hospital, as this phenomenon usually occurs late at night after the patient has slept and not emptied their appliance. The first passage of flatus or stool per anus in a patient who was under the impression that their fecal stream was completely diverted can prompt an emergent call to their surgeon.

If a colostomy is being performed proximal to an obstructing lesion, to decompress the colon and divert the flow of stool, it is critical that the distal limb of the colostomy be vented to the atmosphere and not closed. If the distal limb is closed and there is a complete obstruction distal to the colostomy, this will create a closed loop obstruction, and there is a substantial risk of distention and perforation.

If the rectum and anus have been completely resected, an end colostomy is created. If a partial colectomy/proctectomy has been performed, and an anastomosis is not constructed, an end colostomy is created and the distal bowel is closed (as in a Hartmann resection) or brought to the skin as a mucus fistula. The decision about whether to create a mucus fistula or to close the distal segment will hinge on whether there is concern regarding distal obstruction, the length of the distal segment, and the integrity of the distal segment. For example, in a patient undergoing sigmoid colectomy and colostomy for complicated diverticulitis, it is reasonable to close the rectal stump providing that proctoscopy reveals a normal rectum. Conversely, in a patient undergoing abdominal colectomy and ileostomy for toxic colitis, it may be preferable to bring the distal sigmoid to the skin level as a mucus fistula to avoid rectal stump blowout. A mucus fistula may be constructed as a separate stoma, opening just a corner of the closed end as a small vent. Alternatively, the mucus fistula can be constructed so that the small vent is matured (i.e., here, "mature" means that the colonic wall is sutured primarily to the skin) in a corner of the abdominal wall opening used to create the proximal stoma in the manner of Prasad and Abcarian (the "divided end-loop" stoma). This facilitates care in that the patient has only one stoma appliance, and facilitates stoma closure because both limbs of the bowel are located

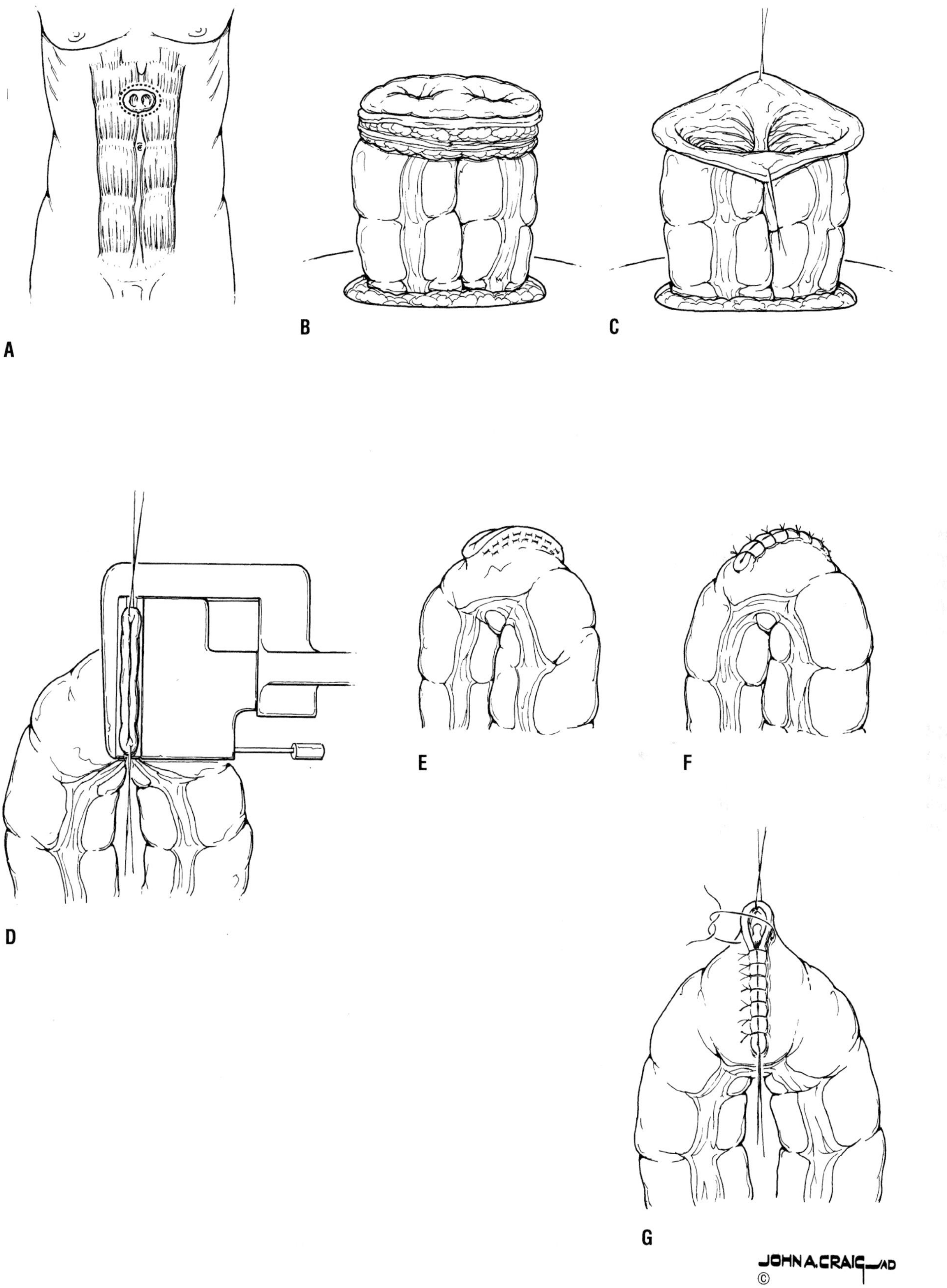

Figure 6–4. Closure of a loop-transverse colostomy. **A.** A circumferential incision is made around the stoma, with reopening of the midline incision if needed. **B, C.** The colon is mobilized adequately. **D, E.** Staple closure of the colostomy. **F, G.** Suture closure of the colostomy.

adjacent to one another. The old operation of the so-called Divine double-barreled colostomy should be abandoned because the adjacent full-diameter stomas make application of an appliance very difficult.

Construction of an End Colostomy (Fig 6–5). An end, completely diverting, colostomy usually is located in the left lower quadrant, where the site is chosen preoperatively by placing a vertical line through the umbilicus and another line transversely through the inferior margin of the umbilicus and by affixing a disk the size of a stoma faceplate to designate the stoma opening through the rectus muscle and on the summit of the infraumbilical fan fold (Fig 6–5A). An alternative location is through the midline fascia, not necessarily at the umbilicus. Although this site initially seems esthetically unappealing, it allows construction of a stoma with a lower incidence of symptomatic hernia formation because of the ability to tightly close the linea alba around the stoma.

Once a site is chosen, the patient should be evaluated in multiple body configurations to verify the adequacy of the stoma site. A common mistake is to choose the site with the patient supine and then find when the patient rises to a standing or sitting position that the chosen site is completely obscured by fat folds, scar tissue, or a protruding skeletal structure. The location should be adjusted up or down, even considering the use of upper quadrants of the abdomen if necessary, to allow proper fixation of an appliance and easy access by the patient. The site usually is marked with ink in the patient's room and then is scratched into the skin with a needle in the operating room after induction of anesthesia. This is totally painless for the patient and does not leave a permanent tattoo should colostomy not be needed.

An end colostomy most often is constructed after removal of the rectum for low-lying malignancy (see Chapter 25). The entire left colon is mobilized on its mesentery, and depending on mobility of the colon and thickness of the abdominal wall, may require mobilization of the splenic flexure (Fig 6–5B). If the patient has received neoadjuvant pelvic radiotherapy and/or the inferior mesenteric artery is transected at its origin at the aorta, the entire sigmoid colon should be removed because of concerns regarding ischemia and a descending colostomy created.

If the colostomy is to be brought through the left lower quadrant, an opening in the abdominal wall is made at the previously marked site by excising a 3-cm disk of skin. The undesirable oval configuration of a stoma is avoided by placing traction clamps in the dermis, the fascia, and the peritoneum. These clamps are held in alignment when the opening is made through the abdominal wall. This duplicates the configuration of the abdominal wall when the abdomen is closed and should allow construction of a desirable circular stoma.

The fat, fascia, muscle, and posterior peritoneum are then incised longitudinally (Fig 6–5A). No fat is excised. The opening is then dilated to allow passage of two fingers, and the closed end of the colon is pulled through the abdominal wall (Fig 6–5C). There, mesentery of the colon can be sutured to the lateral abdominal wall with a running suture, although the complication of small bowel obstruction due to torsion of the small bowel mesentery around the colon mesentery has not been proven to be reduced by this maneuver. After the wound is closed and protected, attention is directed to completing the colostomy (Figs 6–5C, 6–5D, and 6–5E). The stoma is completed by excising the staple or suture line and by placing chromic catgut sutures between the full thickness of colon and skin. If the stoma is constructed because of inflammatory bowel disease or radiated bowel, a spigot configuration is utilized by applying principles similar to those for ileostomy construction. This facilitates a good appliance seal for anticipated high-volume, liquid effluents.

If the colostomy will be brought through the midline, no fixation of the mesentery is necessary. The intended midline colostomy is brought through the abdominal incision, and the entire incision is closed, with the sutures adjacent to the colostomy being tied last. At least a few interrupted sutures are placed on either side of the colostomy even if a running closure of the abdominal wall is used. As the last sutures are tied, the colon is pulled through the abdominal wall, and the surgeon's finger is placed adjacent to the stoma as a spacer to avoid compromise of the blood supply to the stoma. The skin is closed and the wound is protected as attention is directed to the colostomy, where either the staple line is excised or the clamp is removed, and full thickness of colon is sutured to full thickness of skin with interrupted absorbable sutures.

Once the stoma construction is complete, an appliance is applied in the operating room. The simplest is a one-piece appliance with a skin barrier that can be cut to the appropriate size of the stoma. This same appliance can be used for colostomy and ileostomy. The pouch is allowed to fall to the patient's side, because in the postoperative period, the patient will be supine rather than upright the majority of the time. The appli ance, which need not be sterile, is held in place with the skin adhesive of the appliance and is secured with strips of nonallergenic tape placed in "picture-frame" fashion. The remaining wound dressing is applied. Tincture of benzoin should never be used to maintain adhesion of an appliance to the skin because it has a high risk of initiating contact dermatitis. If colostomy function does not begin within 4 or 5 days, the stoma

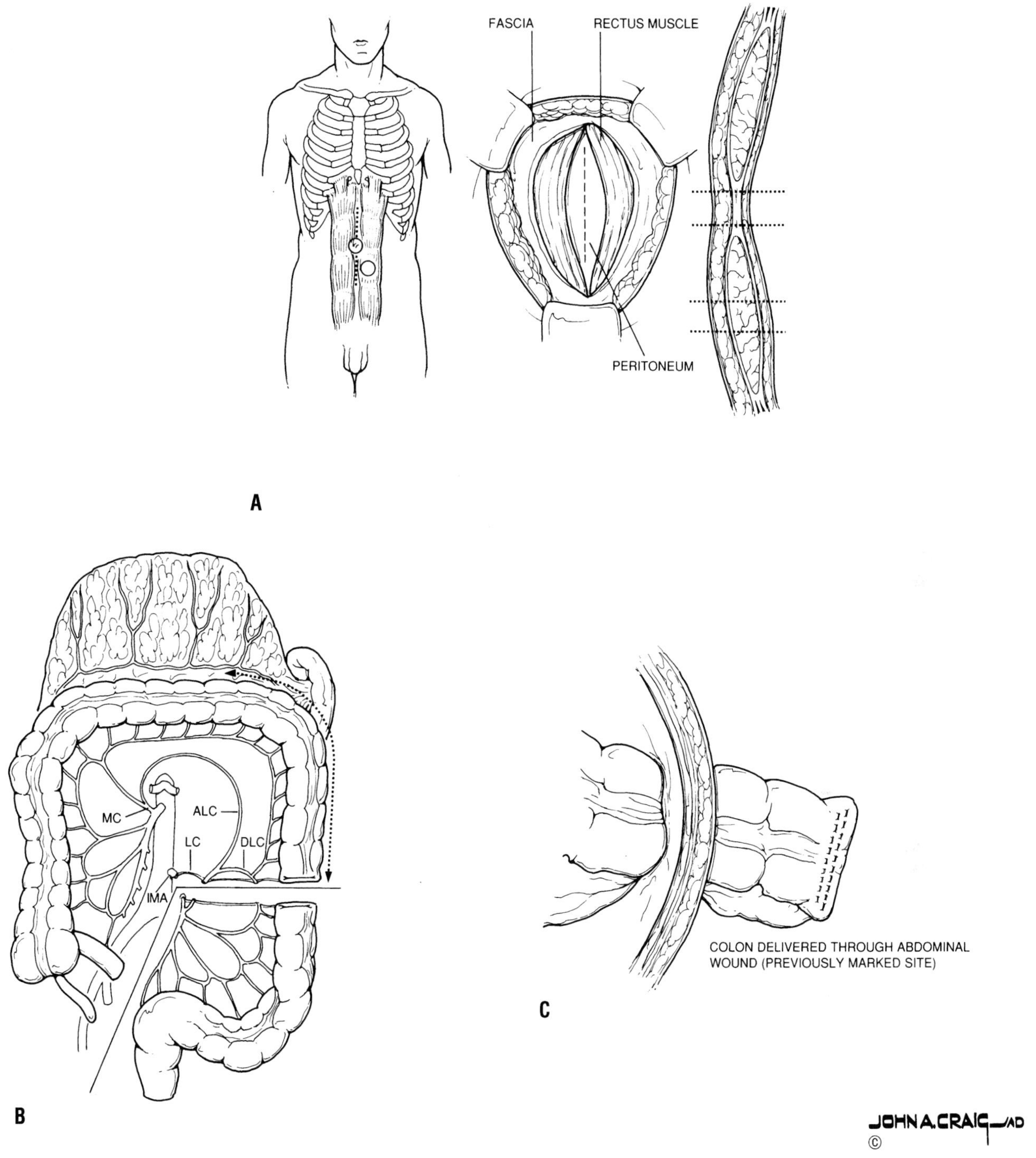

Figure 6–5. Construction of an end (diverting) colostomy. **A.** Selection of stoma location and technique of incision of the abdominal wall at the colostomy site. **B.** Technique of colonic mobilization and provision of adequate blood supply for the colostomy. **C, D, E.** Final stages of constructing a "mature" end colostomy. (LC, left colic artery; MC, middle colic artery; ALC, ascending left colic artery; DLC, descending left colic artery.) *Continued*

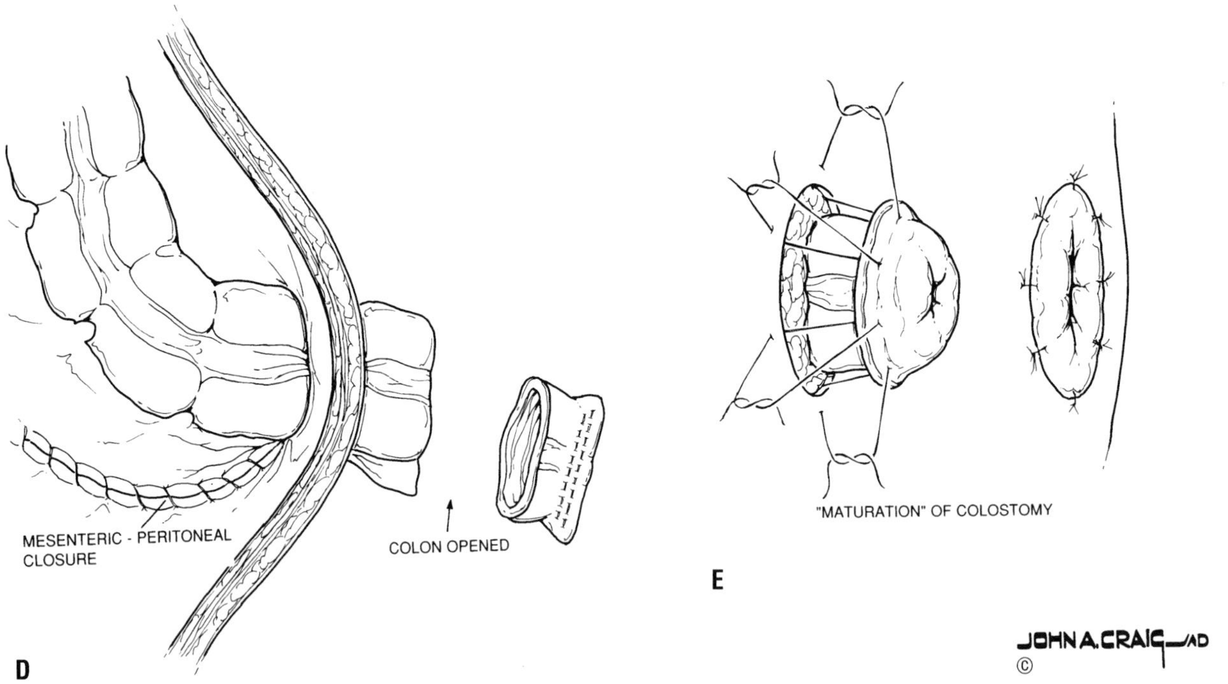

Figure 6–5, cont'd. C, D, E. Final stages of constructing a "mature" end colostomy. (LC, left colic artery; MC, middle colic artery; ALC, ascending left colic artery; DLC, descending left colic artery.)

can be irrigated with small volumes (250 mL) of normal saline to initiate stoma function. The enterostomal therapy nurses are involved early in the care of the stoma and in teaching the patient and family to provide long-term care of the colostomy. In most cases, the patient is taught the technique of stoma irrigation, and then each individual decides in the more distant postoperative course if she or he wishes to irrigate the stoma or not.

LONG-TERM COLOSTOMY MANAGEMENT

The patient with a properly-constructed, well-functioning colostomy may elect to irrigate once a day or every other day and to wear only minimal appliance in the intervening period, although the patient should be instructed to always carry an appliance should episodes of diarrhea occur. Simple appliances exist to allow absorption of mucus and deodorized passage of gas during the period between irrigations, if the patient elects to irrigate.

Irrigation

The advantages of irrigating the colostomy include the absence of need for wearing an appliance at all times, the provision of a more regulated lifestyle, the reduced passage of uncontrolled gas, less leakage of stool between irrigations, and the general feeling of comfort that some people experience after irrigating the colostomy. The disadvantages are that it is a time-consuming ritual and that some people feel discomfort when the bowel is distended during irrigation. Irrigation carries a minimal risk of perforation. Absorption of water during the irrigation process can be significant, and the patient with an irritable bowel syndrome will usually not achieve adequate control by irrigation and may be frustrated by attempting to do so. The principle of irrigation is based on the fact that the distal colon displays a few mass peristaltic motions each day and that these can be stimulated by distention of the intestine. It has been shown that 80% of people who irrigate daily can depend on the discharge from the colostomy being one or two movements per day. Poor results from irrigation can be anticipated if the patient has irritable bowel syndrome, a peristomal hernia, irradiated bowel, inflammatory bowel disease, poor eyesight, reduced manual dexterity, or simply fear of dealing with the intestine at the abdominal wall. A preoperative history of irritable bowel syndrome is most important because these patients must never be promised regular function of their colostomies.

The technique of irrigation, usually performed in the morning, uses a cone tip that fits into the stoma only enough to provide a seal and to allow the instillation of 500–1000 mL of water. It is not necessary to dilate the stoma, and a finger is inserted only periodically to determine the direction for placement of the cone tip. Once the water has been instilled, a drainage bag is applied, and the individual can proceed with morning chores while the colostomy empties in response to the stimulation. Between irrigations the patient usually wears a security pouch, which permits passage of gas through a charcoal filter and provides a small pad to absorb any mucus normally secreted by the colonic mucosa.

Ischemia or infection causing partial loss of the intestinal wall or separation of the stoma from the skin can result in stricture of the colostomy. A tight stricture makes irrigation impossible and frequently causes the patient significant discomfort because of the resulting partial obstruction. Because the stricture is always at skin level, its correction is simple and no patient should suffer because of a colostomy stricture.

COLOSTOMY COMPLICATIONS

General Considerations

A common problem experienced by the patient with a colostomy is irregularity of function, which most often is related to irritable bowel syndrome or irradiation of the intestine. Many problems are related to improper location of the stoma, which allows seepage of mucus and maceration of the skin because an appliance seal cannot be adequately maintained. Parastomal hernia formation is common, and prolapse less so. Patients experience episodes of diarrhea and constipation depending on their underlying disease, dietary habits, and episodic infections. Patients with colostomies are troubled with gas and odor problems because there is no sphincter around the stoma and gas can be passed uncontrollably. This problem is usually regulated by diet, and in some cases by administering mild antidiarrheal agents when social activity dictates. Minimal bleeding around a stoma is common because the mucosa is exposed to environmental trauma. Of course, prolonged bleeding should be evaluated to be sure that there is not a recurrence of the primary disease process. The same is true of cramps and diarrhea. These can be acceptable occasionally, but anything of a prolonged or severe nature must be evaluated.

Evaluation of the UOA data registry shows that hernia formation is the most common complication of end colostomy, with obstruction, abscess, and fistula presenting less frequently. Of all of the complications that occur, few require surgical correction. Fecal impaction does occur with a colostomy and can be managed by a combination of oil and detergent given as a retention irrigation in the hospital or by the simple combination of salad oil, warm water, and mild liquid detergent at home.

Stoma Stricture

The problem of stoma stricture can be minimized by suturing the full thickness of the colon to the skin of the abdominal wall at the time of initial construction. Stricture of stomas resulted from formation of serositis in previous times when it was believed unsafe to open the colon initially, and it was opened in a delayed fashion. Even for the transverse-loop colostomy, the colonic wall should be sutured primarily to the skin of the abdominal wall. The process has come to be called "maturation" of the colostomy. Another cause of colostomy stricture is ischemia, usually as a result of resection of too much mesentery during construction of the stoma. Repair may require a simple local procedure if the stricture is focal at the skin level, or revision of the stoma via a transabdominal approach if the stricture involves a longer segment.

Colostomy Necrosis

Ischemia or necrosis of the colostomy results from excessive resection of colonic mesentery, excessive tension on the mesentery leading to the stoma, creation of a fascial opening too small to accommodate the bowel and its mesentery, or poor perfusion due to low-flow states. The blood supply to an end colostomy is unidirectional, without collaterals; therefore it will be most sensitive to changes in visceral perfusion. If the necrosis is limited to the area of the stoma anterior to the fascia, it may be observed carefully, and stoma revision performed electively at a later date, if necessary. If the necrosis extends into the peritoneal cavity, the abdomen should be explored and the stoma re-created.

Paracolostomy Hernia

Paracolostomy hernia is a frequent complication of colostomy creation, even when all is done according to acceptable surgical principles. The creation of an abnormal opening in the abdominal wall that is then subjected on a daily basis to the pressures of Valsalva maneuvers may predispose the patient to suffer a gradual enlargement of the fascial opening. The relative weakness of the posterior rectus sheath in the inferior abdominal wall, with the potential space that exists alongside the rectus muscle, may also predispose the patient to develop a peritonealized sac in the rectus sheath without a large fascial defect. Although it is surgical dogma to create stomas in the rectus sheath to lessen the development of parastomal hernias, there are no definitive data to support this contention.

Asymptomatic parastomal hernias should be observed because the rate of recurrence after repair or relocation of the stoma is high. Patients should be counseled to seek immediate medical attention if they develop symptoms or signs of intestinal incarceration in the hernia. Symptomatic hernias may be relocated or repaired, although no technique has proven to be reliably successful. Local suture repair often fails, and although broad fascial mesh repair appears to be a more rigorous method of repair, there is still a substantial risk of recurrence and the added concern of mesh infection. Laparoscopic repair with intraperitoneal mesh is being used more frequently, although it would appear to offer no advantage over open mesh repair other than a potential reduction in wound complications and short-term postoperative recovery.

Colostomy Prolapse

Prolapse of the colostomy is seen most often with the transverse-loop colostomy. This is probably the result of several factors, most prominent being the lack of fixation of the transverse mesocolon to the retroperitoneum, and the size of the fascial opening necessary to bring both limbs of the colon and the mesocolon to the skin level. If the transverse loop colostomy is constructed to decompress a dilated colon, the fascial opening may need to be large initially, and then predispose the colostomy to prolapse later. The opening becomes excessive once the colon decompresses. The surgical treatment of this complication is difficult, and the best treatment is to rid the patient of the primary disease and restore intestinal continuity. If this is not possible, the loop colostomy should be converted to an end colostomy with mucous fistula. Prolapse of an end colostomy can be managed by a local procedure in which the mucocutaneous junction is disconnected, the redundant colon resected, and the mucocutaneous junction recreated.

Colostomy Perforation

Perforation of the colon just proximal to the stoma most often occurs during careless irrigation with a catheter or during contrast x-ray studies when a catheter is placed in the colostomy and a balloon is inflated. This occurrence represents a surgical emergency and must be dealt with by laparotomy and reconstruction of the colostomy with adequate drainage, if there is significant fecal or barium contamination. Cases of mild inflammation with extravasation of air only can be managed with antibiotics and localized drainage, and surgery can be avoided.

▪ ILEOSTOMY

An ileostomy is an opening constructed between the small intestine and the abdominal wall, usually by using distal ileum, but sometimes more proximal small intestine. The stoma is constructed on a permanent basis for patients who require removal of the entire colon, and usually the rectum, for inflammatory bowel disease, either Crohn's disease or ulcerative colitis. The use of a loop ileostomy is becoming more frequent because of the complex sphincter-preserving operations being performed for ulcerative colitis and familial polyposis. For these operations (restorative proctocolectomy), it is necessary to have complete diversion of intestinal flow while the pouches are allowed to heal and adapt. The loop ileostomy is also useful in cases where multiple and complex anastomoses must be performed distally, usually for Crohn's disease or rectal cancer. As sphincter-preserving operations are used more often, diminishing numbers of permanent ileostomies will be constructed, but similar principles and techniques will be utilized in constructing the temporary loop ileostomies. The same principles used in constructing an ileostomy can be applied to the construction of a urinary conduit.

The surgical construction of an ileostomy must be more precise than that for a colostomy because the content is liquid, high volume, and corrosive to the peristomal skin. Therefore, the stoma must be accurately located preoperatively, and it must have a spigot configuration to allow an appliance to seal effectively and precisely around the stoma.

Various types of ileostomies can be constructed. The most common has been the end ileostomy, using a technique popularized by Brooke and Turnbull. The loop ileostomy is used, as described, to protect diseased areas or surgical procedures distally. The loop-end ileostomy is a stoma that uses the principles of a loop ileostomy but is constructed as a permanent stoma when the mesentery and its blood supply need special protection. The continent ileostomy, a technique devised by the Swedish surgeon, Nils Kock, is an internal pouch that does not require the wearing of an external appliance. The urinary conduit is a stoma constructed of small intestine to provide a conduit to the outside for the urinary tract.

DETERMINATION OF ILEOSTOMY LOCATION

The location of the ileostomy must be carefully chosen before surgery (Fig 6–6). It should avoid any deep folds of fat, scars, and bony prominences of the abdominal wall. The site is chosen by drawing a vertical line through the umbilicus and a transverse line through the inferior margin of the umbilicus and applying a disk the size of a stoma faceplate (approximately 8 cm in diameter) to determine the location. The disk is allowed to abut on both of the lines in the right lower quadrant, and the site is marked with ink. The patient

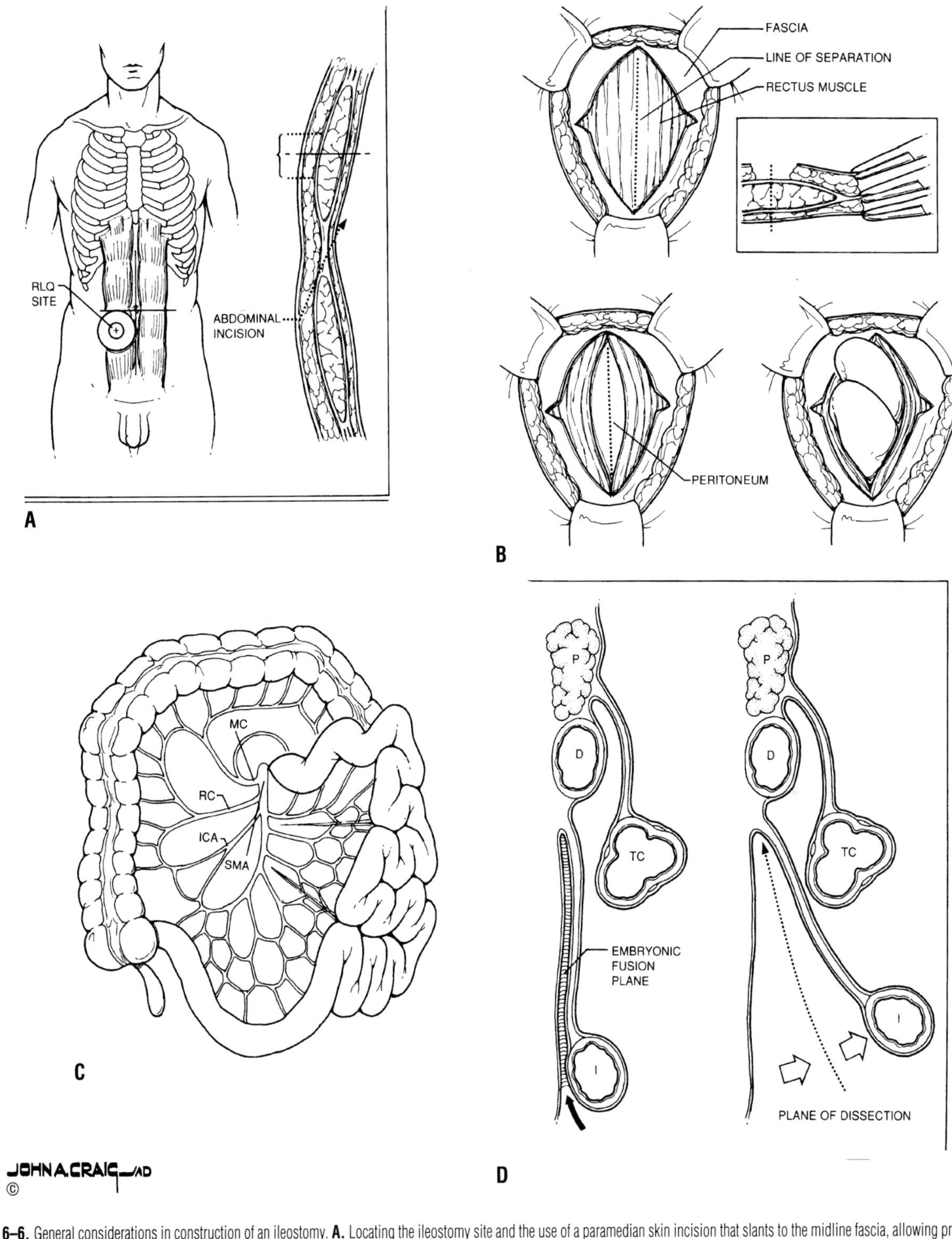

Figure 6–6. General considerations in construction of an ileostomy. **A.** Locating the ileostomy site and the use of a paramedian skin incision that slants to the midline fascia, allowing preservation of the peristomal skin. **B.** Technique for making the abdominal wall opening. **C.** Vascular supply of the distal ileum, which must be used to maintain viability of the ileostomy. (MC, middle colic artery; RC, right colic artery; ICA, ileocolic artery; SMA, superior mesenteric artery.) **D.** Plane of mobilization of the distal ileum to allow construction of an ileostomy without tension. (P, pancreas; D, duodenum; TC, transverse colon; I, ileum.)

then is brought to an exaggerated sitting position and allowed to turn in various directions to be sure the site is adequate in all positions. If not, the location should be adjusted to bring the stoma to the summit of the infraumbilical fat fold to be sure that there is clearance for fitting of an appliance. When the patient is in the operating room and anesthesia has been administered, the chosen site is scratched with a fine needle before preparation of the abdominal skin is carried out. The majority of complications arising from ileostomies can be avoided by taking these precautions in marking the site for the stoma preoperatively. Even in cases in which the use of a stoma seems remote, the precaution of marking the site preoperatively should be taken. In addition, whenever possible, patients should be seen by an enterostomal therapist and an ostomy visitor so that they can be given information about the stoma and its care. The visit from an ostomate (someone who has done well with a similar stoma) is helpful because it allows the patient to know that the surgery can be survived and that life can be continued productively and normally with the presence of a stoma. The discussion should avoid excessive details about types of equipment and types of stoma problems during the postoperative period.

When an ileostomy is anticipated, the choice of abdominal incision is a left paramedian skin incision, slanting the incision to the midline fascia (Fig 6–6A). This gives the advantage of opening the fascia through the midline to provide a simple, effective closure and at the same time preserve all the right lower quadrant peristomal skin for maintenance of the appliance seal.

End Ileostomy

The construction of the ileostomy begins early in the operative procedure. When the colon is mobilized for colectomy, as is the usual case when an ileostomy is to be constructed, full mobilization of the mesentery of the distal ileum should be carried out (Fig 6–6D). This is an important and often neglected part of the procedure. There is an embryonic fusion plane of the mesentery of the small intestine to the right posterior abdominal wall. The ileum can be elevated on this mesentery up to the duodenum, allowing extreme mobility of the terminal ileum. The ileocolic artery is then transected as part of the colectomy, and the remaining blood supply to the small intestine is preserved (Fig 6–6C). It is important to preserve the most distal arcade of vessels and mesenteric tissue on the ileum at the segment of the intended ileostomy. This blood supply is prepared early in the operative procedure so that if there is any question about the vascularity of the distal ileum, it will be known long before the abdomen is closed. The preservation of this distal bit of mesentery and fat on the ileum sometimes appears to cause excess bulk around the ileostomy, but this fat soon atrophies, allowing a well-vascularized stoma of appropriate size. The intestine is transected with a linear-cutting type of stapling instrument so that the end of the ileum can be easily pulled through the abdominal wall without increased risk of contamination. This can, of course, also be accomplished by suturing the end of the ileum.

When the colectomy has been completed, an opening is prepared in the right lower quadrant of the abdominal wall at the previously marked site (Fig 6–6B). This is accomplished by placing traction clamps on the dermis, fascia, and peritoneum so that the round configuration of the stoma will be maintained. A 3-cm disk of skin is excised, the fat is preserved, and a longitudinal incision approximately 3–4 cm long is made through all layers, with each layer being retracted with three small retractors as the incision is deepened. The fascia is incised longitudinally as well, and frequently a small lateral notch is placed on each side. The muscle is separated, and any vessels are coagulated. The posterior fascia and peritoneum then are incised, and the surgeon inserts two fingers through the opening to be sure that it will accommodate the intestine. The ileum is brought through the abdominal wall to the intended length, usually about 6 cm (Fig 6–7B). The mesentery of the distal ileum may be sutured to the right lateral abdominal wall, although there are no data to prove that this maneuver reduces the incidence of intestinal obstruction, stoma prolapse, or stoma retraction.

The abdomen is then closed. The incision is protected, and attention is directed to the ileostomy where the staple line or suture line is excised, verifying the adequacy of blood supply. If the blood supply of the stoma is questioned, more of the ileum should be resected.

The next objective is to make a protruding, everting stoma. This is accomplished by placing 3-0 chromic catgut sutures through the full thickness of intestine, the seromuscular area of the ileum at the base of the stoma, and the dermis (Fig 6–7E). Sutures through the skin should be avoided, because any stellate scarring will prevent the maintenance of the required seal of the appliance. Eight of these sutures should be placed, one in and one between each quadrant, and as traction is applied after they are all placed, the stoma should evert nicely.

After the stoma is completed, an ileostomy appliance is applied. A simple appliance in which the skin barrier can be cut to the size of the stoma is best. The pouch is allowed to hang to the side, and a stoma skin adhesive (not benzoin) is applied to the appliance if needed. The pouch is taped in position using a picture-frame configuration of nonallergenic tape. In the immediate postoperative period, if there is any question about leakage

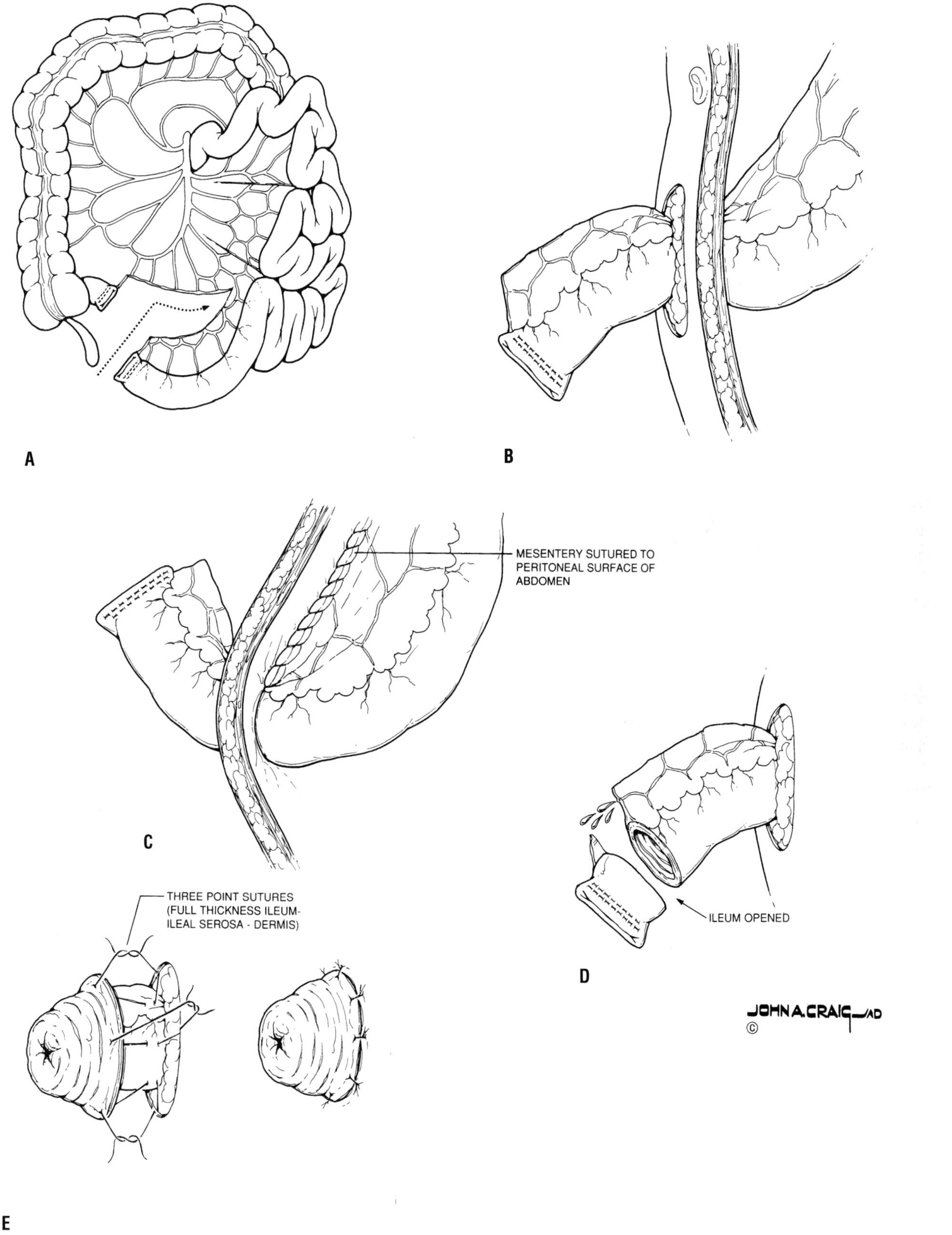

Figure 6–7. Construction of an end ileostomy. **A.** The distal arcade of vessels and some mesentery are preserved on the segment to be used for ileostomy construction. **B.** The closed ileum is pulled through the abdominal wall to a length of 6 cm. **C.** The mesentery of the ileum is fixed to the abdominal wall. **D.** The adequacy of the blood supply is verified. **E.** The spigot configuration is achieved by placing sutures to include full thickness of intestine, the seromuscular layer at the base of the stoma, and the dermis.

around the appliance or malfitting of the appliance, it should be changed and the skin cleaned immediately. It is important to preserve the integrity of the peristomal skin, and all the nursing staff should be aware of the importance of this. The leaking appliance should not be left for changing by the next shift or for the enterostomal therapist the next morning, because the skin can be damaged during this waiting period.

Loop Ileostomy

The loop ileostomy stoma is constructed when both diversion of the intestinal flow and decompression of the distal intestine are required. The location is chosen exactly as one would choose the site for an end ileostomy. The construction can then follow one of two techniques. The technique popularized by Turnbull at the Cleveland Clinic involves choosing the site in the intestine for the intended loop ileostomy and then placing orienting sutures proximally and distally (Fig 6–8A). A loose suture with one knot can be placed proximally and one with two groups of knots distally. It is important to maintain this orientation as the stoma is constructed.

The opening in the abdominal wall is made the same as for an end ileostomy (Fig 6–6B), but the loop of intestine is drawn through this abdominal opening by a tracheostomy tape placed through the mesentery and around the intestine (Fig 6–8A). Some surgeons recommend orienting the proximal functioning loop in the inferior position, placing a partial twist on the loop of intestine. Although this may help configure the spout of the ileostomy so that ileal effluent is less likely to undermine the appliance, this maneuver may be associated with a higher rate of intestinal obstruction. In massively obese patients with a shortened mesentery, it is necessary to make a conical configuration of the opening in the abdominal wall, with the internal opening being much larger than the external opening at the skin. If this maneuver is used, it is best to place a row of tacking sutures between the peritoneum and the loop of intestine to maintain position and orientation. Once the loop is drawn through the abdominal wall, the abdomen is closed, maintaining the orientation of the loop. It is usually not necessary to fix the mesentery of the ileum to the abdominal wall when constructing a loop ileostomy. The wound is then protected, and attention is directed to the stoma.

The tracheostomy tape is replaced by a small plastic rod, which is commercially available (Fig 6–8B). It is not sutured to the peristomal skin, but it often has a heavy suture tied around each side so that should the rod dislodge, it can be drawn back through the mesentery rather than being pushed through, with risk of injuring the mesentery. The loop of intestine is opened by making a four-fifths circumferential incision at the distal aspect of the loop, allowing 1 cm of ileum above the skin level in the superior aspect (Fig 6–8B). The recessive limb thus is formed distally, and sutures are placed between the full thickness of ileum and dermis at this level. As the proximal aspect of the stoma is constructed, sutures are placed as previously described between the full thickness of ileum, the seromuscular area at the base of the stoma, and the dermis. As these sutures are tied, the stoma should assume a spigot configuration supported by the rod. If their use is indicated, a few small pieces of Penrose drain can be placed in the subcutaneous tissue as the sutures are tied. These provide short-term drainage of the peristomal tissue and should be removed after 24 hours. The ileostomy appliance may be placed beneath the rod or over the rod, depending on the tension of the mesentery. The rod is left in place for 1 week, and the same ileostomy care is provided as previously described.

Another technique for constructing a completely diverting ileostomy is that popularized by Abcarian and Prasad that more recently has been used to protect the anastomosis for restorative proctocolectomy (Fig 6–9). This technique involves transecting the ileum with a linear-cutting stapling instrument. No compromise of the mesentery is involved. The opening in the abdominal wall is made in identical fashion to that previously described, but when the intestine is pulled through, the proximal component is excised, and the stoma is constructed as previously described for an end ileostomy. The recessive limb at the base of the stoma has one corner of the staple line excised, and the full thickness of ileum is sutured to the dermis at the superior aspect of the stoma. This allows a small recessive limb that serves to decompress the distal intestine.

Closure of Loop Ileostomy. When endoscopic procedures and contrast studies have shown that the pouch is intact or that the distal anastomoses have healed securely, consideration can be given to closing the loop ileostomy. If the primary procedure has involved the anal sphincter mechanism, careful physical examination and manometric studies should verify the adequacy of sphincter function before intestinal continuity is restored.

For closure of the loop ileostomy (Fig 6–10), a circumferential dissection is carried out, with a minimal rim of skin included, until the peritoneal cavity is entered and clean peritoneal surface of abdominal wall can be palpated circumferentially. Once this is accomplished, the loop of intestine can usually be brought easily through the circular incision in the abdominal wall. Closure then is completed by excising the rim of fibrous tissue, with care being taken to preserve as much of the viable intestinal wall as possible (Figs 6–10B and 6–10C). The choice of closure then varies between hand-sutured

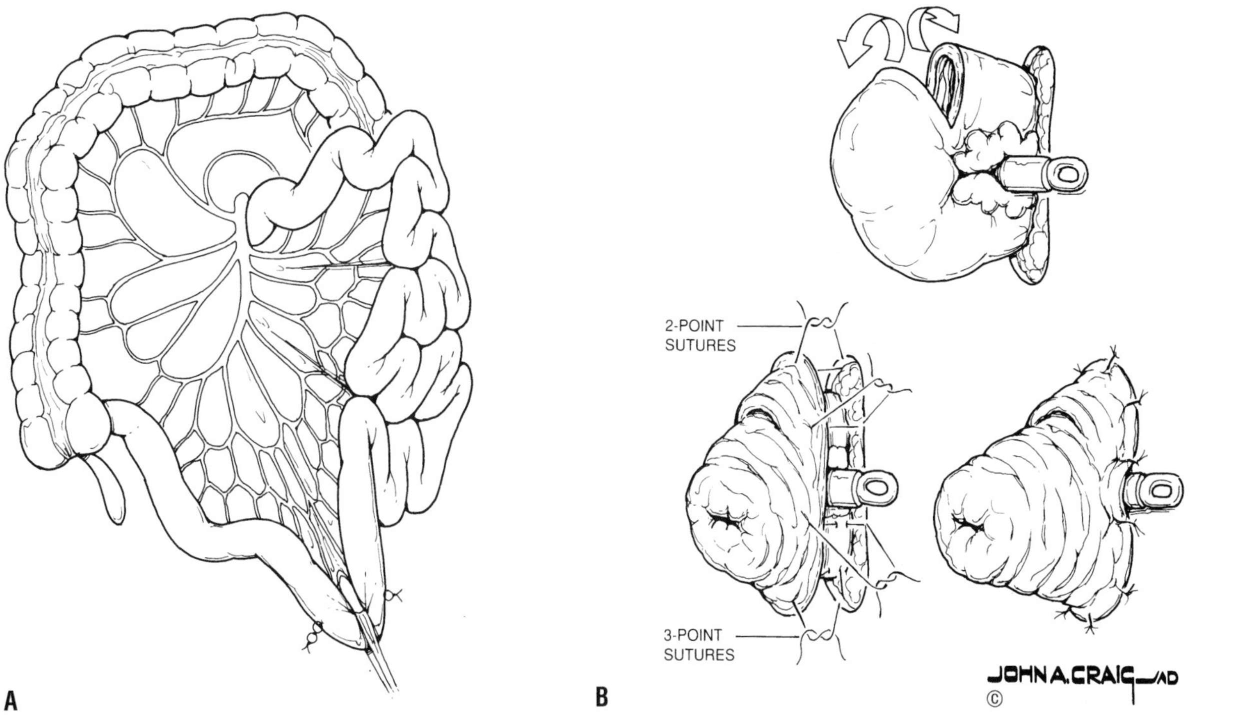

Figure 6–8. Construction of a loop ileostomy. **A.** A tracheostomy tape is placed at the segment for the intended ileostomy with sutures to identify proximal and distal limbs. **B.** The loop is pulled through the abdominal wall while its proper orientation is maintained. The tape is replaced by a plastic rod, and the spigot configuration is completed.

transverse closure (Figs 6–10D and 6–10E), stapled transverse closure (Figs 6–10F and 6–10G), or formal construction of an anastomosis.

For closure of the separated-loop ileostomy (Fig 6–11), the mobilization is carried out in similar fashion, and a functional end-to-end closure is performed. A linear-cutting stapler is applied and removed, and the enterotomy is closed transversely. The intestine should be rotated so that antimesenteric surfaces are used for the staple line. If this type of closure is utilized, it is important to offset the staple lines so that there is no possibility of their healing together and causing an obstruction. After intestinal continuity is restored, the abdominal wall is closed, and the skin is left open for delayed primary closure.

Loop-End Ileostomy

A loop-end ileostomy should be constructed in the rare circumstances in which it is unsafe to resect the mesentery of the distal ileum or when there is tension created on the mesentery as the ileum is brought to the abdominal wall for construction of the ileostomy. This occurs in the patient with a thickened mesentery or a very obese abdominal wall, or in a patient who has had multiple surgical procedures that altered the mesentery. These conditions preclude dealing with the usually pliable mobile tissue. This technique is especially useful in the obese patient who requires construction of a urinary conduit after cystectomy and radiation. The technique is especially helpful because a supporting rod can be placed beneath the stoma for 1 week to help avoid retraction through a thick abdominal wall (Fig 6–12).

Constructing a loop-end ileostomy involves transecting the ileum as previously described, but the closed end will remain closed (Fig 6–12A). The staple line is inverted with seromuscular sutures, or if it is to be used for a urinary conduit, only absorbable sutures are used to close the end of the ileum, because stone formation has been reported around staples (Fig 6–12B). The orienting sutures are then placed as described for construction of a loop ileostomy, and a tracheostomy tape is placed so that when the loop of ileum is pulled through the abdominal wall, the closed recessive end will be superior and just within the abdominal cavity (Fig 6–12C). The construction of the loop-end stoma then proceeds exactly as that described for the loop ileostomy (Figs 6–12D, 6–12E, and 6–12F). However, in this case in which the stoma will be permanent, the mesentery of the distal ileum is fixed to the abdominal wall (Fig 6–12D). If the stoma will be used as a urinary conduit, the loop of the conduit should be brought through the abdominal wall before the ureteral anastomoses have been carried out. It is a disconcerting problem to have the ureters fixed and then find there is an inadequate length of ileum to bring through the abdominal

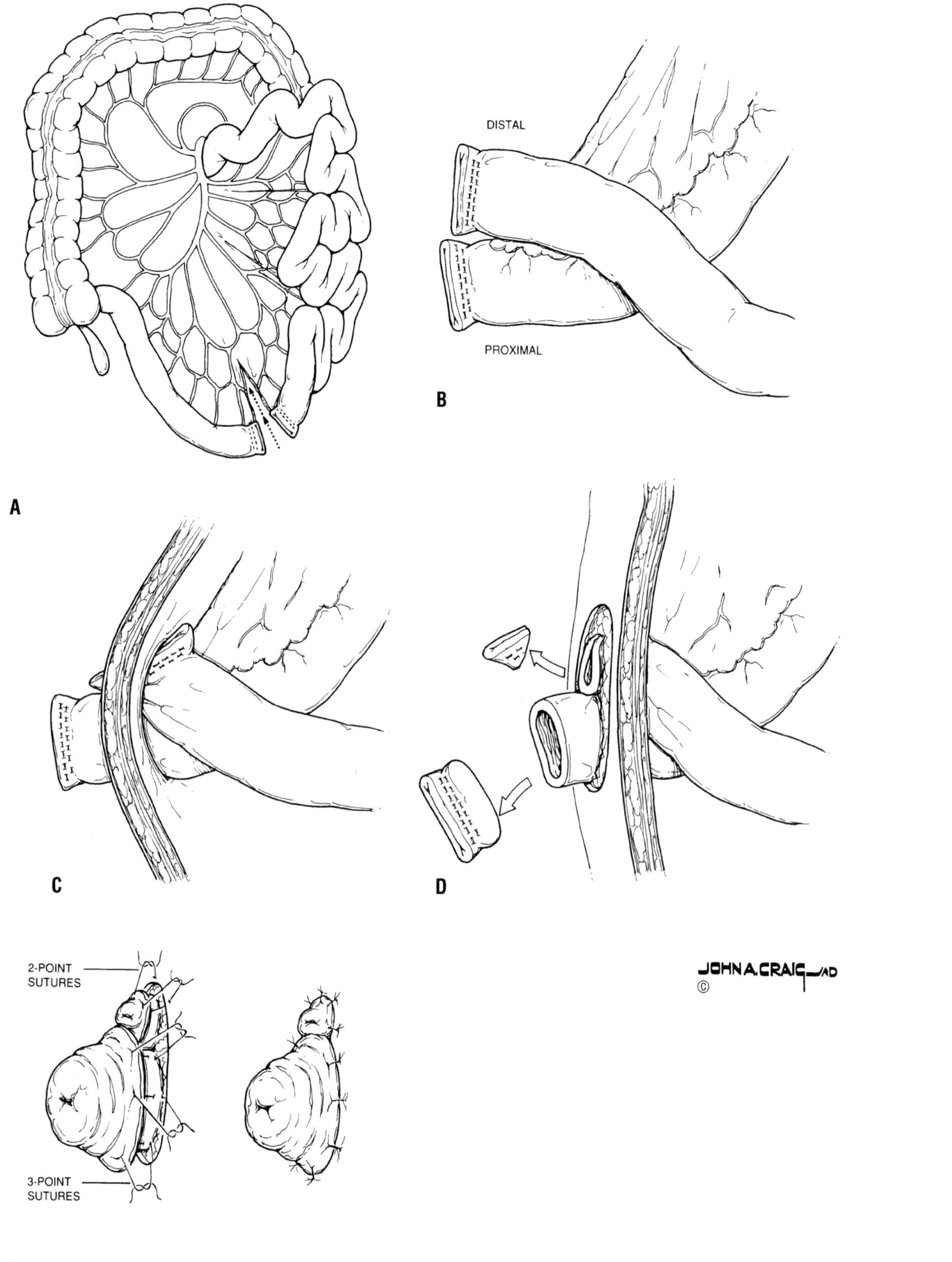

Figure 6–9. Construction of a separated loop ileostomy. **A.** The distal ileum, but very little of the mesentery, is transected, using a linear-cutting staple device, in preparation for constructing the ileostomy. **B, C.** The proximal, functioning component is brought through for spigot construction, whereas only the corner of the distal component is brought through. **D.** The entire staple line of the proximal component and a corner of the distal component are excised. **E.** The functioning spigot and nonfunctioning recessive opening are completed.

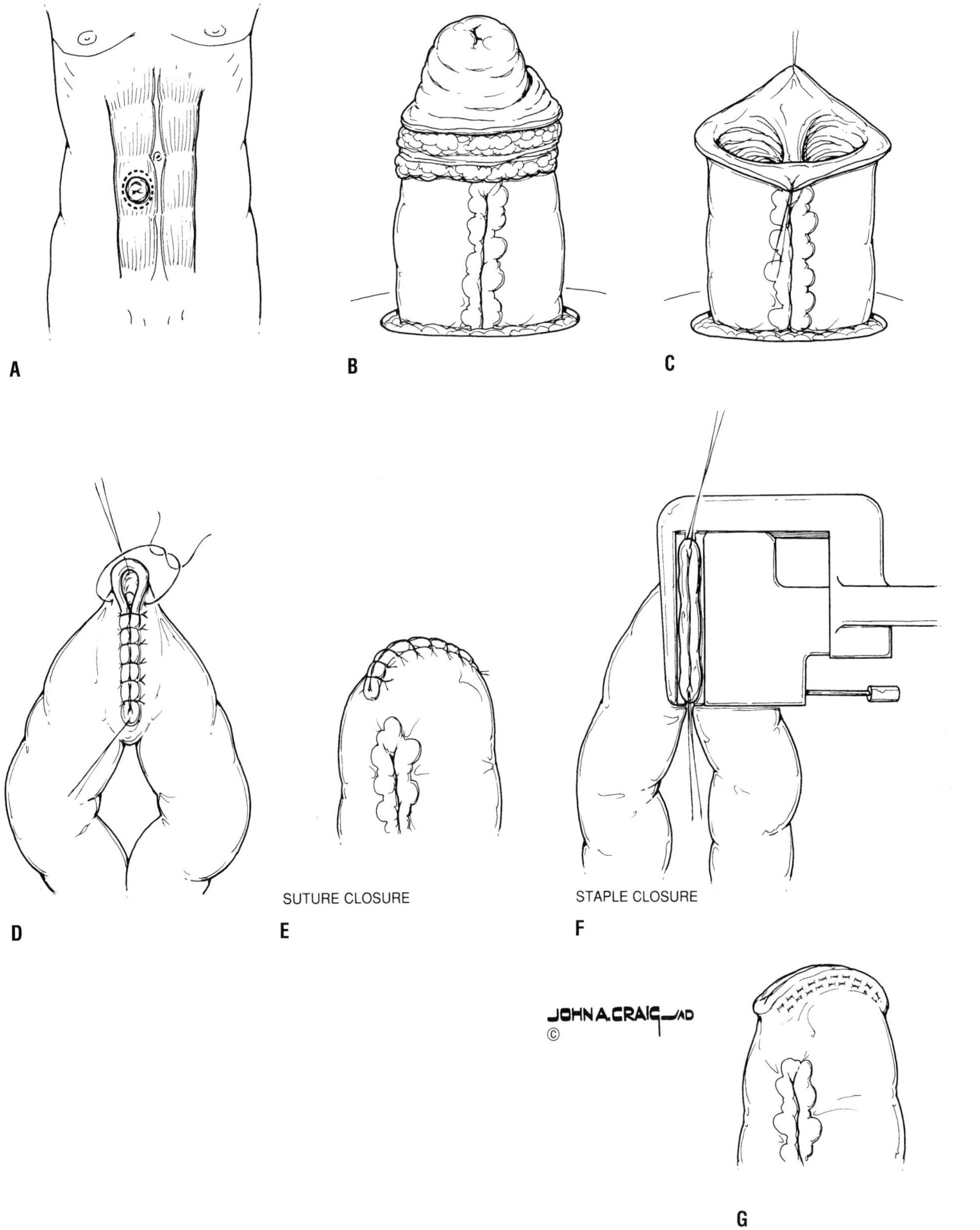

Figure 6–10. Closure of a loop ileostomy. **A.** A circumferential incision is made and carried into the peritoneal cavity. **B.** The loop of intestine is completely mobilized. **C.** The fibrofatty tissue is completely excised, preserving all the intestine. **D, E.** A suture closure can be performed, or a transverse stapled closure (**F, G**) can be performed.

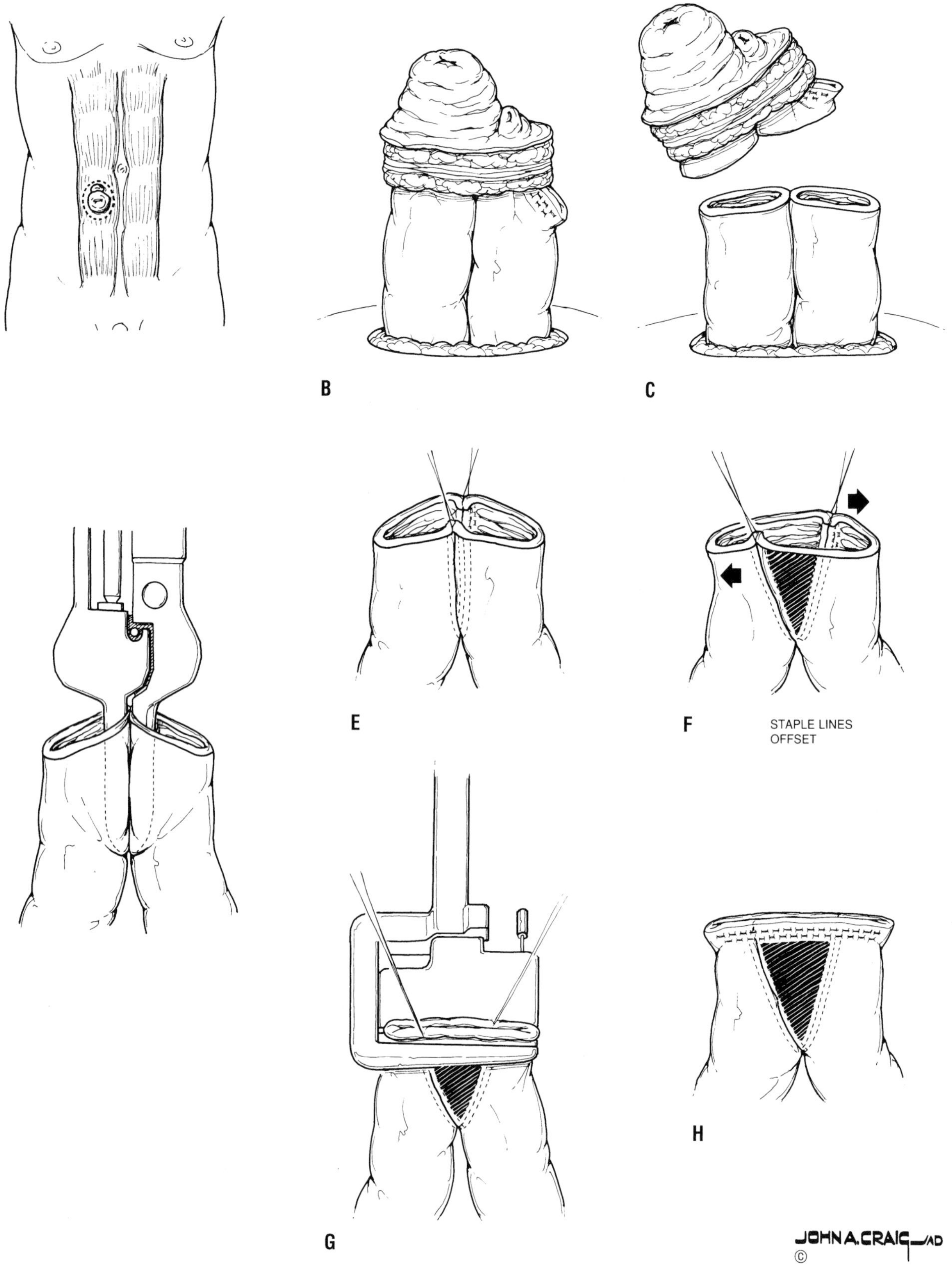

Figure 6–11. Closure of a separated loop ileostomy. **A.** A circumferential incision is made and carried into the peritoneal cavity. **B, C.** The stoma site and residual staples are excised. **D.** A linear-cutting stapler is applied to the antimesenteric side of the intestine. **E, F.** The components of the staple line are offset. **G, H.** The functional end-to-end closure is completed with a linear stapling instrument.

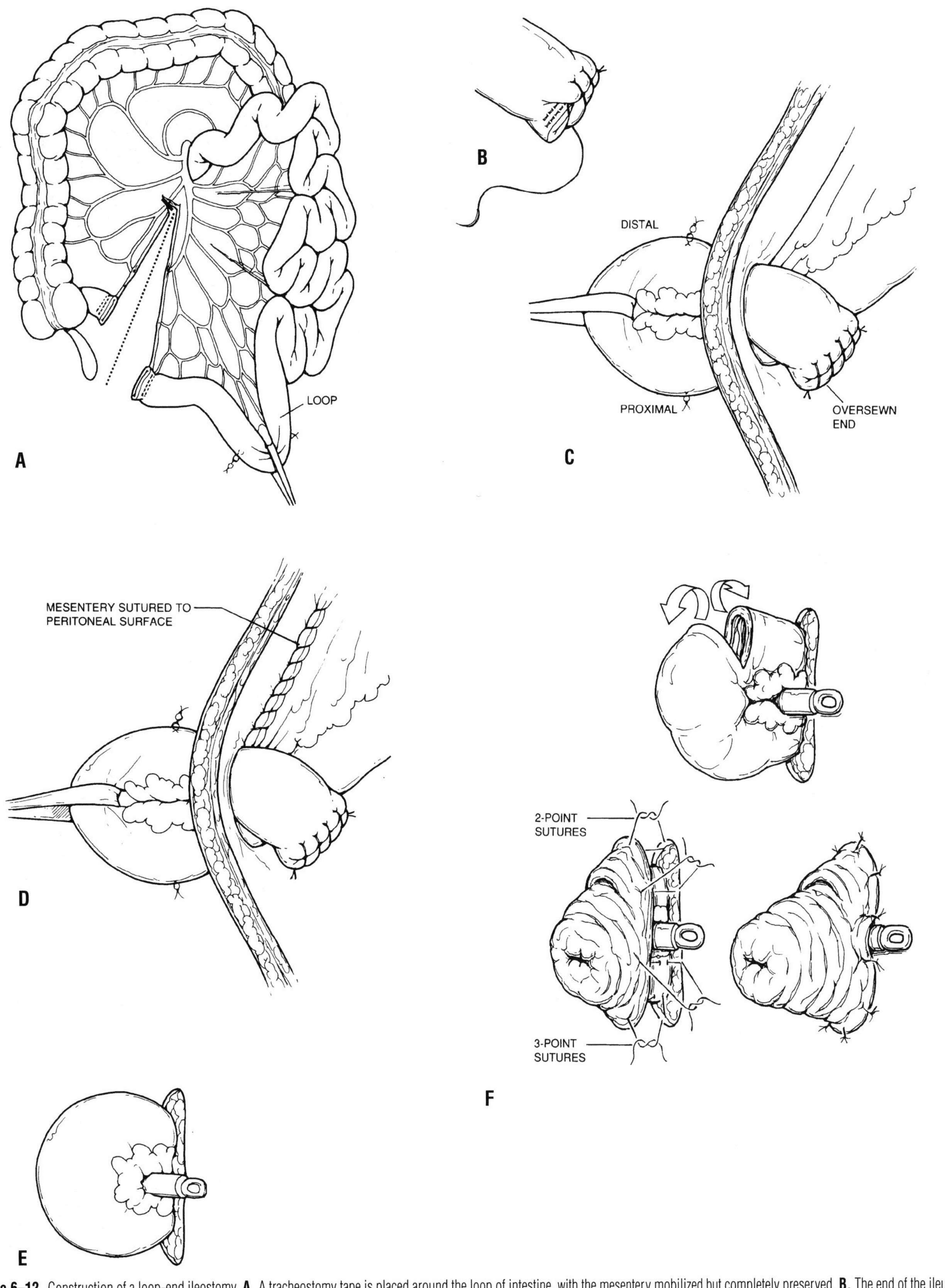

Figure 6–12. Construction of a loop-end ileostomy. **A.** A tracheostomy tape is placed around the loop of intestine, with the mesentery mobilized but completely preserved. **B.** The end of the ileum is inverted. **C.** The intestine is pulled through the abdominal wall so that the functional limb will be in the inferior position, and the closed end is allowed to reside just within the abdominal cavity. **D.** The mesentery of the ileum is fixed to the abdominal wall because this is meant to be a permanent stoma. **E.** The tracheostomy tape is replaced with a small plastic rod. **F.** The stoma construction is completed exactly the same as described for a loop ileostomy.

wall. It is also easier to place the ureteral stents when the construction is done in this fashion.

A special problem has been found in patients with a loop-end ileostomy in that there continues to be mucus secretion from the recessive limb, and after a period of several months, this secretion may interfere with the perfect seal of the ileostomy appliance. If interference does occur, it may become necessary to resect the distal limb and convert the stoma to a proper end ileostomy. This is a small price to pay, however, because it is an easy operation to remove the recessive limb, and it can be done without opening the abdominal cavity. Of more importance is the fact that the loop configuration during the initial procedure has allowed maintenance of blood supply and a protruding configuration under circumstances in which this otherwise may have been impossible, and that would have resulted in major complications.

Postoperative Care and Complications

The components of an ileostomy appliance are a skin barrier, some type of adhesive disk, a faceplate, and a drainable pouch. In fact, most ileostomy appliances are now commercially available as one-piece or semi-disposable two-piece units. The one in common use has a skin barrier with a fixed plastic ring so that the stoma opening can be cut precisely, the skin barrier applied, and the pouch snapped directly onto the plastic ring, thus allowing easy drainage and disposal of the pouch part of the appliance. The skin barrier component should need changing only every 4–5 days in a patient with a properly protruding and located stoma. A well-constructed ileostomy should allow the patient to display normal physical vigor, to eat a well-balanced palatable diet, and to engage in normal recreational and sexual activity. There should be no prolapse or retraction, the skin should remain normal, and the appliance should not leak. Between 500 and 800 mL of thick liquid content should be passed per day.

Before the concept of stoma eversion was conceived, in approximately 1960, the majority of patients who underwent construction of an ileostomy had serious postoperative complications, usually related to serositis, which caused a partial obstruction at the stoma itself. These patients suffered massive fluid and electrolyte imbalance and often death, which were related to the enormous sequestration of fluid secondary to the small bowel obstruction. This condition was called "ileostomy dysfunction" and was anticipated after the construction of each stoma. This devastating problem essentially has been eliminated, since stomas have been everted and serositis has been prevented as the result of using the Turnbull and Brooke technique. The output from an ileostomy should not be excessive, even in the immediate postoperative period.

Patients with ileostomies do have problems, most often related to maintenance of the seal of the appliance because of poor location or defective configuration of the stoma. In some cases, it is necessary either to revise the stoma locally to bring it into a spigot configuration, or to relocate it so an appliance can be securely applied. The more common problems experienced by ileostomy patients involve odor and gas control, because there is no sphincter in the ileostomy. The patients usually can manage these problems by paying attention to foods and medications ingested, by using various deodorant products, and by maintaining meticulous personal hygiene.

The only unusual long-term risk to the ileostomy patient is that of dehydration, which occurs especially in hot weather and during strenuous physical activity. The individuals should be instructed to maintain adequate intake of fluids and electrolytes. They should routinely have medications on hand for simple diarrhea so that control can be achieved before dehydration occurs. Many patients with ileostomies will at times present with acute blockage of the stoma, which is usually related to food indiscretion. It is hazardous to perform digital examination of an ileostomy, and this should rarely be done. Patients will have ingested some fibrous food with a high residual component and will present with cramping abdominal pain, dehydration, and vomiting. These patients should be admitted to the hospital and started on intravenous fluid replacement, and the stomal problem should be dealt with as follows. A 24F Foley catheter is placed in the stoma, and the balloon is inflated with 3–5 mL of saline just beneath the fascia. The stoma is then irrigated with 50 mL of saline. There will be either a clear return or return of food particles. If the return is clear, it suggests more proximal obstruction, and a water-soluble contrast study should be done for evaluation. If the problem is food blockage, the instillation of the contrast medium often will prove therapeutic. If it is due to a more proximal blockage, it must be dealt with as a small intestinal obstruction. If food particles are returned from the initial irrigation, the irrigation must be continued with warm saline until stoma function returns and the blockage is eliminated. This procedure often requires 12–24 hours and intravenous fluid supplementation. Figure 6–13 is an algorithm for the alleviation of ileostomy blockage.

Some patients develop a high ileostomy output because of dietary indiscretion, infectious disease, short bowel syndromes, or recurrence of inflammatory bowel disease. The cause must be determined and each problem dealt with individually. It is important to maintain fluid and electrolyte balance as these problems are being resolved. Special care must be provided for the patient with short bowel syndrome to maintain electrolyte balance and to compensate for the vitamin B_{12}, cal-

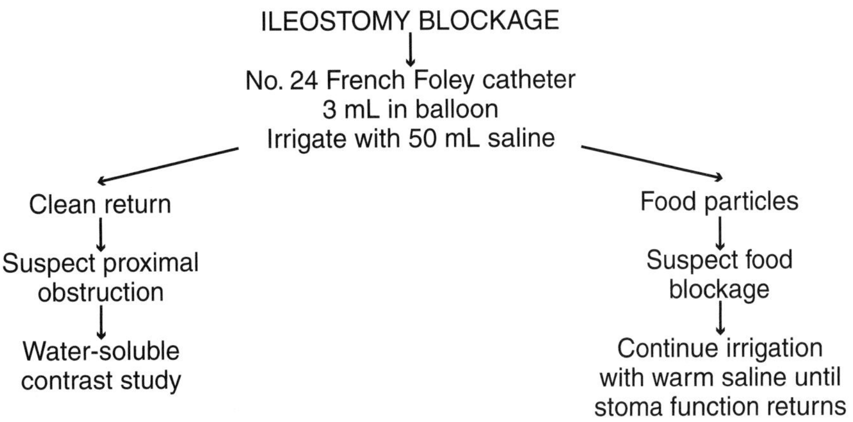

Figure 6–13. Ileostomy blockage algorithm. (Reproduced, with permission, from Kodner IJ. Stoma complications. In: Fazio VW (ed). *Current Therapy in Colon and Rectal Surgery.* Philadelphia, PA: BC Decker; 1990:420–425.)

cium, and fat malabsorption that occurs with absence of the distal ileum.

Another special problem that may occur with an ileostomy is the formation of a paraileostomy fistula. This usually represents recurrence of Crohn's disease and should be dealt with based on the extent of the Crohn's disease. While evaluation and treatment are being carried out, the appliance should be modified so that the fistula is allowed to drain into the appliance, and no attempt should be made to cover the fistula opening. This is usually achieved by modification of the configuration of the skin barrier component of the appliance.

Patients and those individuals aiding in the care of the ileostomy should be in the habit of observing the ileostomy for injury. There are no pain fibers in the ileum, and it is not unusual for a patient to lacerate the stoma with a malfitting appliance without noticing the injury, especially on the inferior aspect of the stoma.

Destruction of the peristomal skin can be so severe as to require split-thickness skin graft for definitive management. In these cases and in others in which the skin is injured around the stoma, a special ileostomy appliance may be utilized. It is based on maintenance of the seal to the mucosa of the ileum rather than to the peristomal skin. This appliance is used infrequently, when it is the only solution to complicated peristomal skin problems. Its use requires wearing supportive belts to maintain the appliance in place, but the skin can be treated with medicated pads during this period.

Review of the UOA data registry overall shows a low incidence of complications from ileostomy and an even lower incidence of need for corrective surgery. A study by McCleod showed that 72% of the patients with conventional ileostomies lead normal lives and that only 9% had a restricted lifestyle because of the stoma. Ninety percent of the patients spent <1 hour a day dealing with their stomas.

■ CONTINENT ILEOSTOMY

The continent ileostomy, or Kock pouch, has been used as an alternative to a conventional ileostomy for selected patients with ulcerative colitis or familial polyposis. It involves construction of an internal pouch with a continent nipple valve. The continent ileostomy allows placement of the stoma in an inconspicuous location and avoids the need for wearing an appliance permanently. It does require multiple intubations of the pouch daily to allow emptying. The complication rate for construction of this continent ileostomy has been high because of the difficulty in maintaining continence of the nipple valve and position of the pouch so that intubation can be easily accomplished. This operation should probably be done only in centers where it is performed frequently and where the complications are managed by an experienced team. The continent ileostomy can be constructed as a primary procedure for patients with ulcerative colitis. It may also be considered for patients who have an existing ileostomy that malfunctions, is poorly located, or causes severe injury to the peristomal skin because of allergic reaction to the ostomy equipment. However, the Kock pouch has been used infrequently as primary treatment for patients with familial polyposis and ulcerative colitis since the advent of the ileal-anal pull-through (ileal-anal anastomosis or "restorative proctocolectomy"). Most surgeons agree that the continent ileostomy is contraindicated for patients with Crohn's disease because of the significant risk of recurrent disease. It is also not to be recommended for patients who have a well-functioning end ileostomy.

The advantages of continent ileostomy are that a patient need not wear an appliance, the patient is continent between intubations, and she or he may experience a better quality of life. The disadvantages are that not all patients are continent, it does require multiple intubations during the day, there can be difficulty in intubation, and the surgery is prolonged and carries a substantial risk of complications. If the procedure fails, the individual will lose a significant amount of small intestine. Also, psychological factors may have been involved in the original motivation for choosing the internal ileostomy that are not alleviated by the more complicated surgical procedure.

CONSTRUCTION OF CONTINENT ILEOSTOMY

The construction of an intestinal reservoir for feces was first described in 1967 by Nils Kock. His original description of a U-shaped pouch was based on the theory that interruption of coordinated peristalsis would enhance capacity. Since then, J- and S-shaped pouches have been used with similar results. An S-shaped pouch is described here.

The construction of a continent ileostomy, or Kock pouch, can be broken into four components: (1) the creation of a pouch, (2) the creation of a nipple valve, which provides continence, (3) the suspension of the pouch from the abdominal wall in such a way as to prevent slippage of the nipple valve, and (4) the creation of a stoma.

The terminal ileum should be transected as close to the cecum as possible (Fig 6–14A). The S-shaped reservoir is fashioned from a 30- to 45-cm segment of distal ileum, starting 15 cm from the cut end (Fig 6–14B). The last 15 cm is used for the outlet (5 cm) and nipple valve (10 cm). The intestine is tacked in place in the shape of an S, using interrupted seromuscular sutures of 2-0 polyglycolic acid placed at the edge of the mesentery. Each limb of the S should be 10–15 cm long. The intestine is opened along the entire portion of the S, with the surgeon taking care to incise close to the mesenteric border on the outer limbs of the S and exactly at the antimesenteric surface of the central limb. A single-layer continuous suture line of 2-0 synthetic absorbable suture is first placed between the two walls of the central limb and the inner walls of the two outer limbs (Fig 6–14C). The sutures that begin on the posterior wall continue onto the anterior wall as the suture line reaches the outer wall of each of the two outer limbs of the S. The anterior wall is completed by continuing the suture from each direction, using an inverting full-thickness technique (either "baseball" or Connell) until the sutures meet in the middle. Before the pouch is closed, the nipple valve must be constructed.

The 15 cm of ileum distal to the pouch will become the nipple valve and stoma. Prior to the completion of the anterior wall suture, with the pouch mostly open, the nipple valve is made by intussuscepting the ileum into the pouch (Figs 6–14D and 6–14E). A Babcock clamp is passed into the distal ileum from within the pouch and is closed onto the full thickness of the bowel at a point 5 cm from the pouch. The clamp is drawn into the pouch, intussuscepting the bowel on itself to form the nipple valve. The valve is maintained in this position by placing a line of GIA staples on either side of the mesentery and a third row of staples on the antimesenteric aspect (Fig 6–14F). Occasionally it is possible to place four staple lines equidistant around the circumference of the nipple valve (Fig 6–14G). A linear-cutting stapling instrument with the cutting blade removed is used to place the staple lines. One arm of the instrument is inserted into the lumen of the nipple from within the pouch before closing and firing the instrument. These staple lines make a serosa-to-serosa fixation of the nipple valve and prevent its unfolding. The anterior wall of the pouch is then completed as previously described (Fig 6–15A). A 5-cm outlet of distal ileum remains that will pass through the abdominal wall and allow construction of a flush stoma.

The right lower quadrant stoma site is created as described earlier in this chapter, with the opening placed below the belt line and within the rectus muscle. Before the outlet is passed through the abdominal wall opening, a sling of soft synthetic mesh (1 × 10 cm) is passed through a window made in the mesentery of both the pouch and nipple valve under the major vessels as they fold into the nipple valve mesentery (Figs 6–15B and 6–15C). The strip of mesh maintains the nipple configuration and helps secure the pouch to the abdominal wall. Seromuscular absorbable sutures are used to fix the mesh to the base of the outlet (Fig 6–15D). The two ends of the sling are left long because they are sutured together at the antimesenteric surface of the outlet. This facilitates delivery of the outlet through the stoma site and allows a securing suture of nonabsorbable material to be placed through the sling into the anterior fascia. As the outlet is readied to be drawn through the abdominal wall, a row of three untied seromuscular sutures is placed on the shoulders of the pouch medial and lateral to the outlet (Fig 6–15E). These sutures, incorporating the posterior fascia and peritoneum, are used to fix the pouch to the anterior abdominal wall. The outlet is delivered through the stoma site and the pouch is drawn toward the abdominal wall. The sutures then are tied, first laterally and

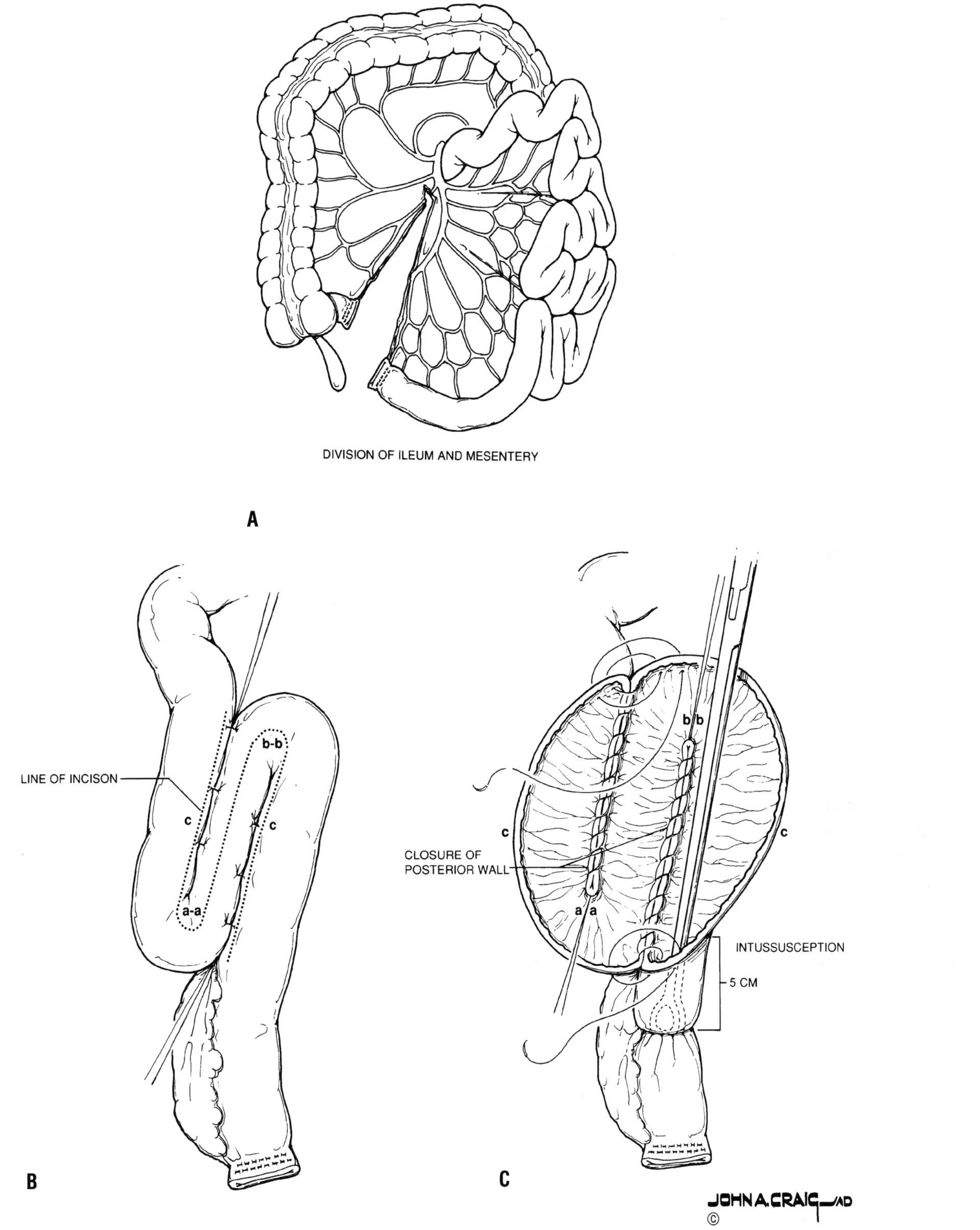

Figure 6–14. Construction of a continent ileostomy. **A.** The colectomy should be completed with as much distal ileum preserved as possible. **B.** Alignment of the components of the S-shaped pouch and nipple valve and the line of incision to open the pouch. **C.** The pouch construction is begun with continuous 2-0 synthetic absorbable suture material. *Continued*

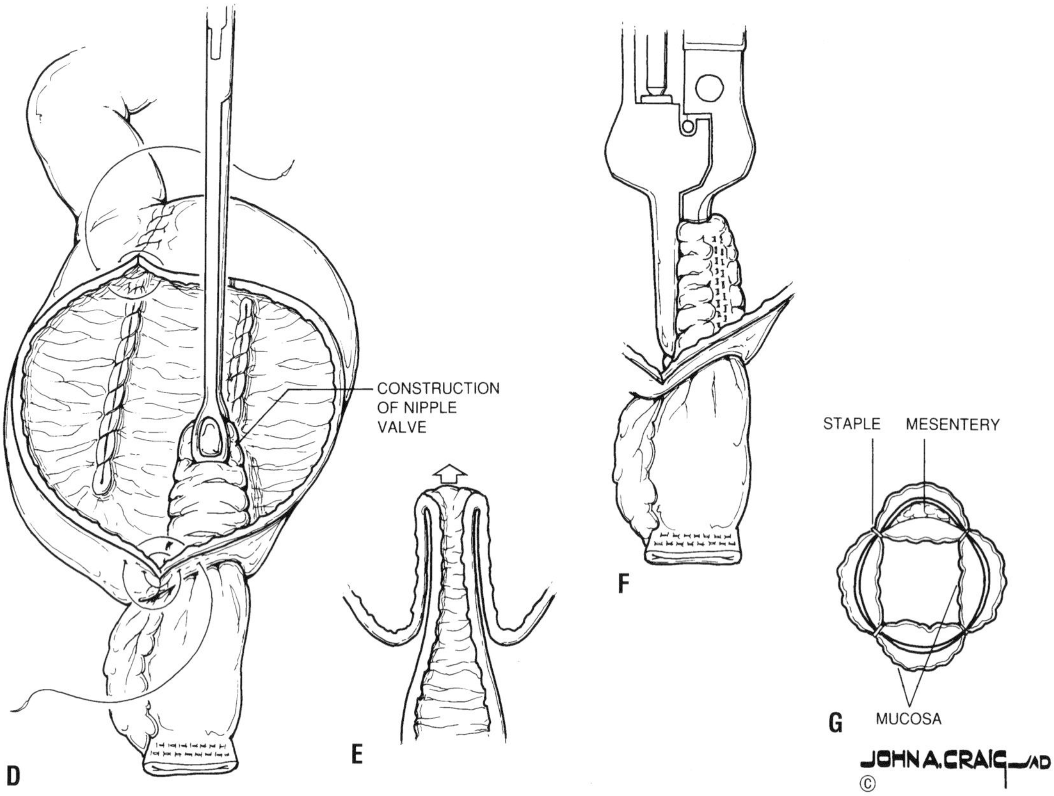

Figure 6–14, cont'd. D. The anterior wall of the pouch is formed by continuous suture from each corner, and the nipple valve is constructed before complete closure of the pouch. **E.** The ileum is intussuscepted to form the 5-cm long nipple valve. **F, G.** The intussusception is maintained by placement of multiple lines of staples adjacent to the mesentery and on the antimesenteric borders.

then medially (Fig 6–15F). A permanent securing suture is placed through the tails of the sling and the anterior fascia, and the ends of the mesh are trimmed.

If possible, the cut edge of the small intestine's mesentery is sutured to the anterior abdominal wall (Fig 6–15F). A continuous suture is placed from the outlet of the pouch to the falciform ligament. The pouch in its final position should rest at the right pelvic brim, with the antimesenteric surface (anterior wall) of the pouch directed inferiorly.

The terminal ileum at the outlet should be excised at skin level (Fig 6–15G). The stoma is finally completed by absorbable sutures between the subcuticular layer of the skin and the full thickness of the intestinal wall (Fig 6–15H). A Medina catheter is passed through the stoma into the pouch and is secured to the skin to prevent slippage of the tube into or out of the pouch (Fig 6–15I). There should be minimal resistance and no deviation from a straight passage. The pouch should be drained in this manner for 2 weeks before intermittent clamping is begun during the third week. Finally, the pouch should be extubated and reintubated every 4 hours until the intervals gradually increase to 6 or 8 hours.

The nipple valve provides increasing continence as pressure rises in the pouch. Should the nipple valve lose its configuration and prolapse or should it slip through the mesenteric aspect of the pouch (the weakest point), either incontinence or obstruction will result. These two problems, along with "pouchitis," are the most common complications following the continent ileostomy procedure. As a result, many variations of pouch construction have been used in attempts to prevent or correct these problems.

If a fistula should form from the nipple valve or if the nipple valve should slip, it may be possible to preserve the pouch and construct a new nipple valve (Fig 6–16). The technique involves resecting the pouch outlet, including the nipple valve, after fully mobilizing the pouch from the abdominal wall and pelvis (Fig 6–16B). The terminal ileum is transected 15 cm proximal to the pouch (Fig 6–16C). The pouch then is rotated 180 degrees on its mesentery (Fig 6–16D). A new nipple valve is created as previously described by intussuscepting the new outlet on itself and placing staple lines along the valve to secure the fold (Figs 6–16E, 6–16F, and 6–16G). The opening in the pouch wall created when the old outlet was resected serves as the entry to the pouch to perform this maneuver. The proximal ileum's cut edge is then anastomosed to the pouch through a second enterotomy in a position that allows the pouch to lie comfortably in the

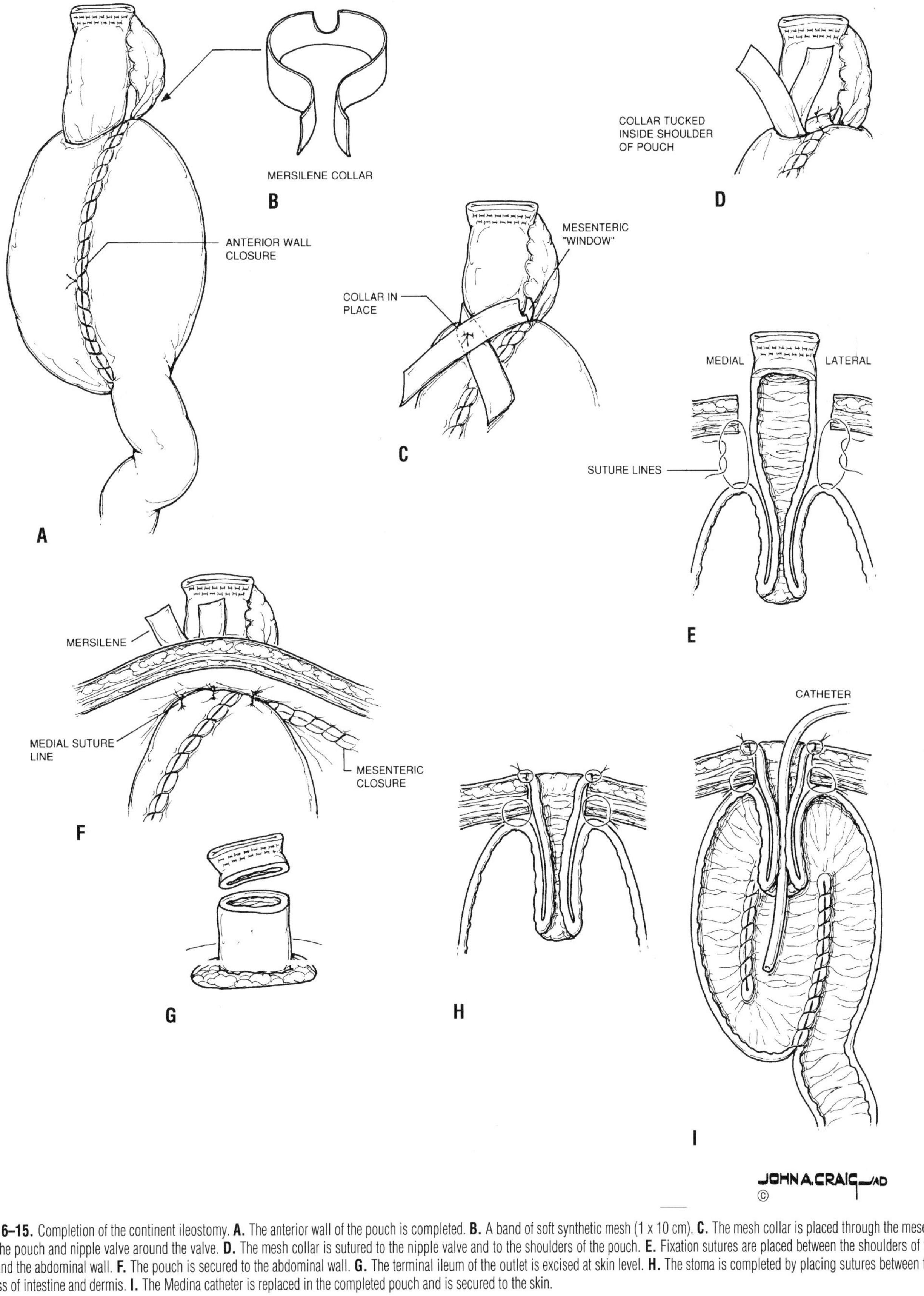

Figure 6–15. Completion of the continent ileostomy. **A.** The anterior wall of the pouch is completed. **B.** A band of soft synthetic mesh (1 x 10 cm). **C.** The mesh collar is placed through the mesentery of the pouch and nipple valve around the valve. **D.** The mesh collar is sutured to the nipple valve and to the shoulders of the pouch. **E.** Fixation sutures are placed between the shoulders of the pouch and the abdominal wall. **F.** The pouch is secured to the abdominal wall. **G.** The terminal ileum of the outlet is excised at skin level. **H.** The stoma is completed by placing sutures between full thickness of intestine and dermis. **I.** The Medina catheter is replaced in the completed pouch and is secured to the skin.

right lower quadrant as before (Fig 6–16D). If at all possible, the existing stoma site should be preserved and reused. The pouch then is resuspended by using a mesh sling as described above, and the stoma is constructed (Figs 6–16H and 6–16I). The pouch should be protected by constant drainage through an indwelling Medina catheter for at least 1 week. Because the pouch will not require expansion and the patient will not need education, the prolonged period of progressive clamping should not be necessary.

■ URINARY CONDUIT

The urinary conduit is constructed of a segment of intestine with well-maintained vascularity so that it can be connected to the urinary tract to allow egress of urine through the abdominal wall via a stoma constructed exactly like an ileostomy. It is not intended to have any type of reservoir capacity but merely to provide an open conduit. This urinary conduit is constructed most often after removal of the urinary bladder for invasive cancer. It is also used for management of severe obstructive uropathy, the congenital abnormalities of spina bifida, meningomyelocele, or bladder exstrophy, and for trauma to the spinal cord resulting in a severely neurogenic bladder. The incidence of this surgery for congenital and traumatic disorders is decreasing as other means of emptying the bladder are devised. The cystectomy, construction of the urinary conduit, and ureterointestinal anastomosis are most often carried out by urologists, but the construction of the stoma, as well as restoration of intestinal continuity, may be done by a surgeon more experienced in intestinal and stoma surgery.

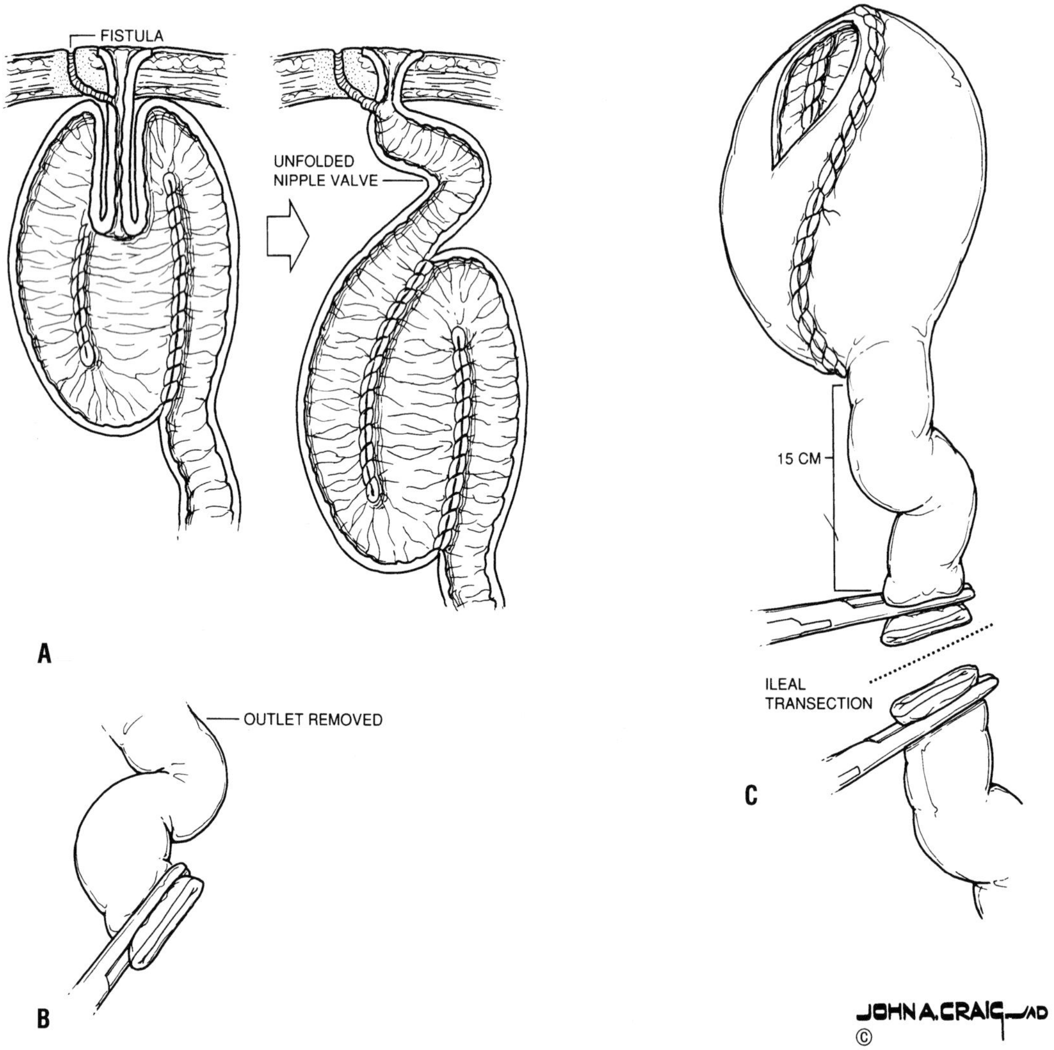

Figure 6–16. Preservation of the continent ileostomy after fistula formation or loss of the nipple configuration. **A.** Fistula between skin and nipple value *(left)* and slipped nipple value *(right)*. **B.** The faulty nipple valve and outlet are excised. **C.** The distal ileum is transected 15 cm proximal to pouch, leaving enough intestine to reconstruct the valve and stoma. *Continued*

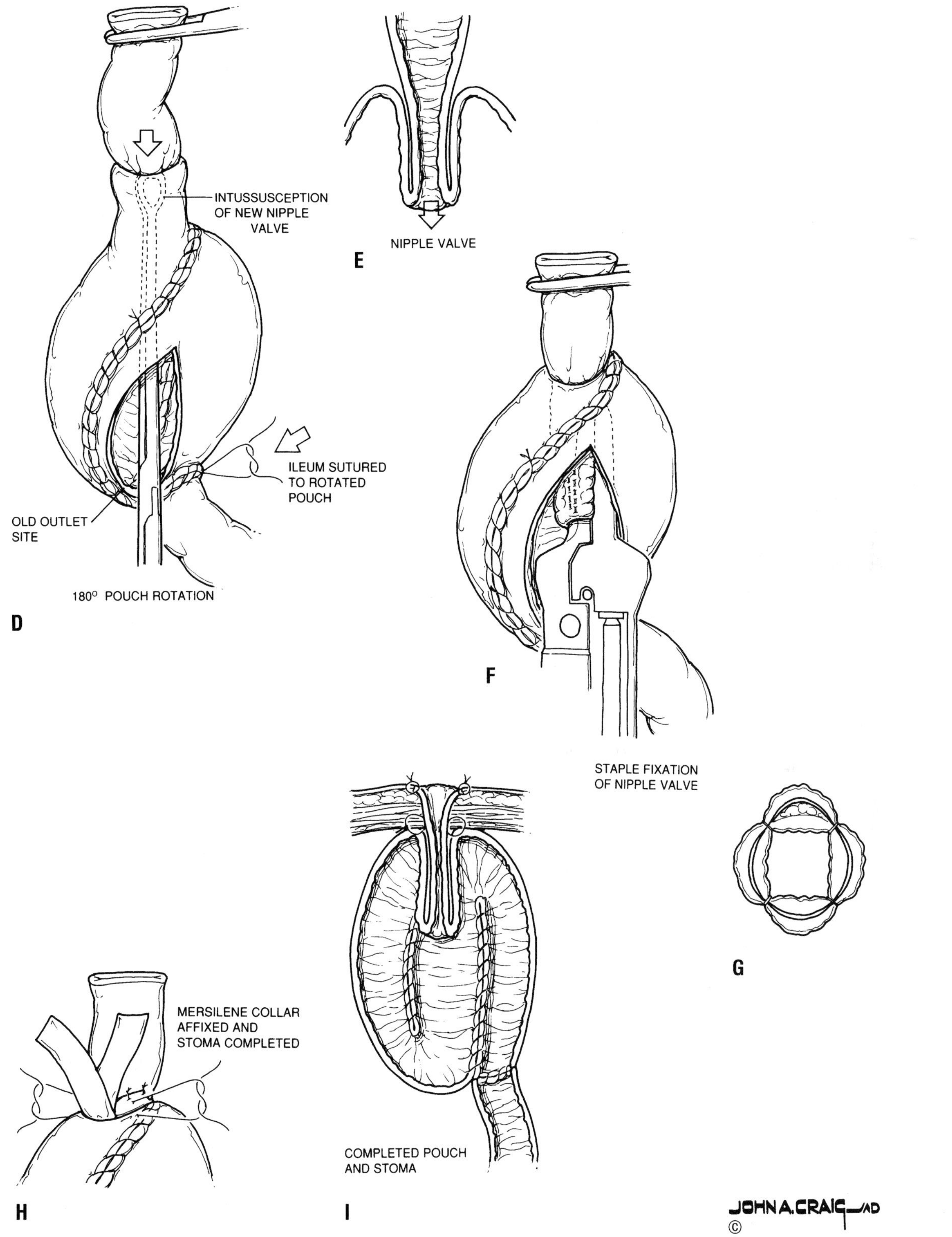

Figure 6–16, cont'd. D. The pouch is rotated 180 degrees, and the intestine is anastomosed to the pouch through a second enterostomy. **E, F, G.** The nipple valve is reconstructed as before, through the enterotomy made by resecting the old valve. **H, I.** The pouch is fixed to the abdominal wall, and the stoma is completed.

The basic principles of construction of the conduit and stoma involve isolation of a segment of intestine, with maintenance of the mesenteric blood supply and enough mobility to allow the distal end to be used as a stoma and the proximal end to serve as the site for ureteral implantation. It is most important to maintain the isoperistaltic direction of the intestine, especially if the conduit is constructed of sigmoid colon. The conduit must not be made of irradiated bowel, even if this requires using either colonic or proximal small intestinal conduits. If the stoma is improperly constructed, there may be a stasis of urine, resulting in reflux and damage to the proximal tract.

The surgical technique consists of choosing a long enough segment of small intestine to allow the stoma to be constructed at the level of the abdominal wall and still allow the proximal end to reach close enough to the retroperitoneum to preclude tension on the ureterointestinal anastomoses (Fig 6–17). Usually, 18–20 cm of intestine is enough, but this must be modified if there is a shortened mesentery or a massively obese abdominal wall. It is in these latter situations that the loop-end stoma, supported over a small rod, can be advantageous. After the segment of intestine is chosen, the mesentery at the distal point is incised to allow enough mobility for reaching the abdominal wall. The mesentery at the proximal site of transection is incised only in a limited fashion, and care must be taken to preserve a generous blood supply (Fig 6–17A). Intestinal continuity is restored, with the intended conduit positioned posterior to the restored intestine (Fig 6–17B). The ileoileal anastomosis may be completed in any fashion that uses sutures or staples. The conduit is then cleaned of intestinal content, and the proximal end is closed. Closure must be done with absorbable sutures, because staples can lead to stone formation. It is then preferable to make the opening in the abdominal wall to construct the stoma as previously described for an ileostomy (Fig 6–17C and 6–17D). This procedure ensures that the ureteral anastomosis will be completed with the conduit in its final position and without the need for applying tension to bring the intestine through the abdominal wall. The ureteral anastomoses are performed, and stents are placed (Fig 6–17E). All aspects of the stoma construction are the same as those for an ileostomy except that the appliance must contain a valve to allow constant drainage since the volume of urine is high and its weight would tend to pull the appliance off if constant drainage were not maintained. In the distant postoperative period, this problem is solved by the patient emptying the appliance frequently and by sleeping attached to a night drainage system.

COMPLICATIONS OF THE URINARY CONDUIT

The most common complication of a urinary conduit is a leaking appliance because of improper placement or construction of a flush rather than a protruding stoma. Although some urologists believe that a flush stoma is less susceptible to injury, most surgeons disagree with this concept and believe that a spigot configuration is best. Sometimes sutures are placed in the skin rather than in the dermis during stoma construction. This leads to a circumferential series of radial scars that preclude maintenance of the seal of the appliance. Because the stoma effluent is thin liquid, the appliance seal must be precise to avoid injury to the peristomal skin. If there is stasis in the conduit and poor seal of an appliance, an odor will develop and become the cause of great concern to the patient. It is not unusual to have to revise and sometimes relocate flush urinary conduit stomas. If this is done, care must be taken to ensure that the length of the conduit is adequate. If it is not, it is possible to add a segment of small intestine so that a proper stoma can be constructed without having to revise the ureterointestinal anastomoses.

The patient who does not maintain adequate personal hygiene and acidification of the urine may develop stone formation, with crystal formation around the stoma itself. This development can be alleviated by acidifying the urine or by placing a small amount of vinegar in the appliance. If the stoma has been constructed within the field of radiation, the radiation can break down the skin around the stoma. This requires relocation of the stoma to a nonirradiated location on the abdominal wall. Relocation should be done even if the upper quadrants need to be used. Recent advances have employed the principles of Kock pouch construction, previously described, to allow construction of a continent urinary diversion.

■ INTESTINAL FISTULA

The formation of an intestinal fistula is not planned by the surgeon. Therefore it must be dealt with as it occurs. Applying modern principles of stoma care to maintain the integrity of the peristomal skin until definitive treatment of the fistula can be carried out should prevent damage to the skin from primitive means of preventing severe destruction of the skin and abdominal wall. These stomal care techniques, coupled with intravenous nutritional supplementation, should alleviate forever uncontrolled intestinal drainage from abdominal wounds.

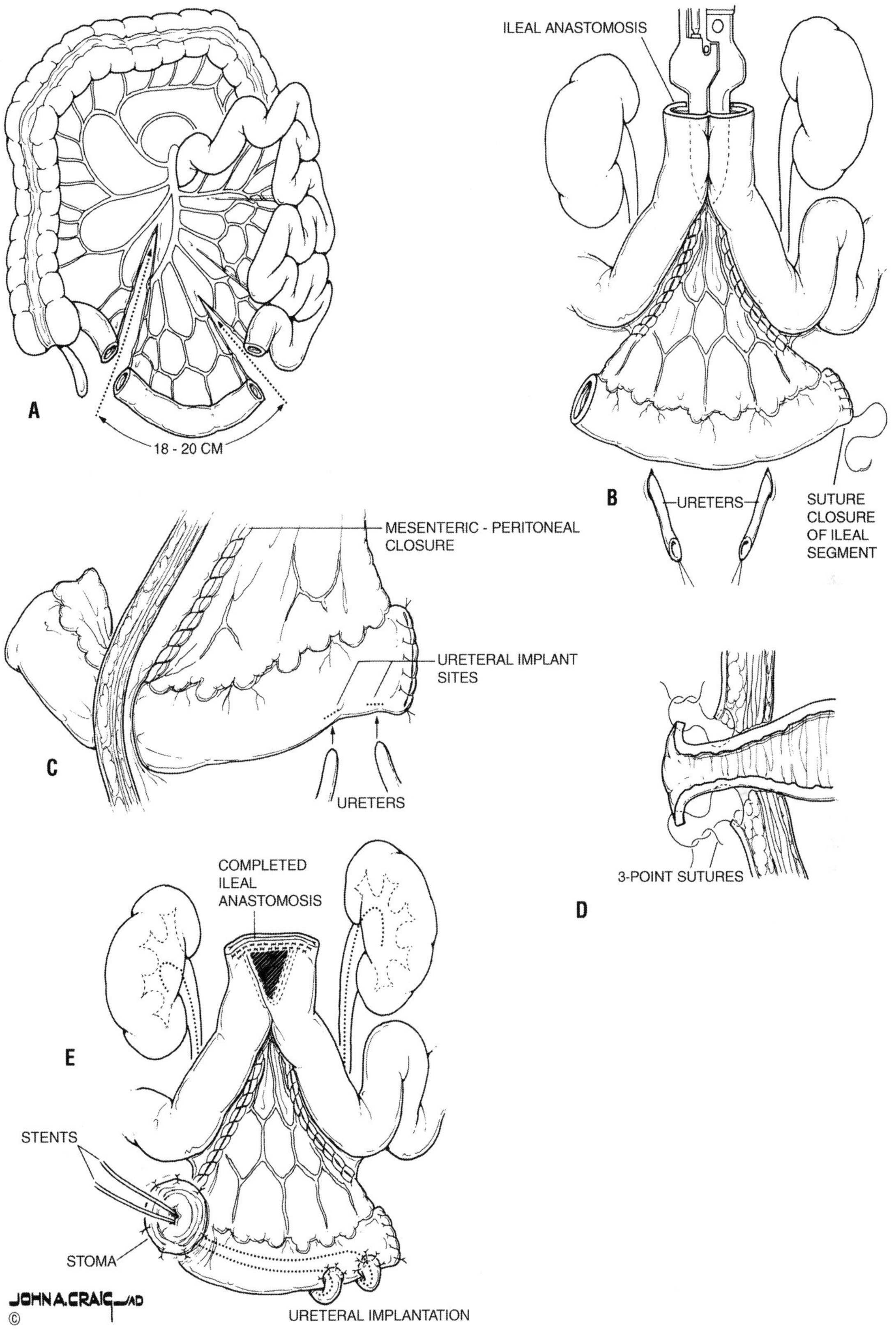

Figure 6–17. Construction of a urinary conduit. **A.** An 18- to 20-cm segment of distal ileum is taken out of continuity, and the blood supply is carefully preserved. **B.** Intestinal continuity is restored, and the intended conduit located posterior to the restored intestine. **C.** The ureteral conduit anastomoses are completed. **D.** The stoma is constructed with a spigot configuration. **E.** Stents are placed through the completed ureteral anastomoses.

■ LAPAROSCOPIC CREATION OF INTESTINAL STOMAS

The most appealing operation early on in the laparoscopic colorectal surgery experience was creation of a diverting intestinal stoma. Laparoscopic loop stoma creation does not require division of the bowel or anastomosis, and the only incision larger than 5 mm required is the stoma site incision itself. Thus the full benefits of the totally laparoscopic approach can be realized. Surgeons inexperienced in laparoscopic approaches to colorectal disease may find that creation of intestinal stomas is a relatively straightforward and rewarding method to begin their laparoscopic colorectal experience.

Laparoscopic creation of intestinal stomas was reported in the early 1990s and the technique was quickly adopted by many surgeons. Several case series demonstrating the safety and efficacy of the procedure have been reported in the literature. Although there has not been a prospective, randomized trial of laparoscopic versus open stoma creation, case-controlled series have demonstrated reduced duration of postoperative ileus and reduced length of hospital stay with the laparoscopic approach. The benefits of the laparoscopic approach to stoma creation become immediately obvious to surgeons, and thus it is unlikely that a prospective, randomized trial will ever be performed.

Laparoscopic ileostomy and colostomy creation have been performed for a plethora of indications, including obstructing rectal adenocarcinoma, rectal obstruction from extrarectal malignancies, fecal incontinence, penetrating rectal trauma, sacral pressure ulceration, obstructed defecation, perineal Crohn's disease, pelvic fracture, and lumbosacral burns. Virtually any disease process that is an indication for fecal diversion is an indication for consideration of the laparoscopic approach. Laparoscopic creation of diverting loop colostomy is particularly appropriate for patients suffering from symptomatic near-obstructing rectal carcinoma. The technique allows the surgeon to evaluate the liver and peritoneum for the presence of metastases that may be undetected on preoperative imaging studies, and institute fecal diversion without creating adhesions in the abdomen and pelvis that may increase toxicity of neoadjuvant radiotherapy and make future proctectomy more difficult. The absence of a laparotomy incision allows patients to recover rapidly, and allows them to begin neoadjuvant radiotherapy treatments almost immediately.

Some authors have argued that trephine stoma creation is an easier, quicker, and less expensive method of stoma creation than the laparoscopic technique. For the thin patient with a virgin abdomen who will not benefit from abdominal exploration, the trephine method does offer those advantages. However, for patients who are obese, those who have had multiple prior laparotomies, those who would benefit from abdominal exploration, or those who require mobilization of the intestine from its retroperitoneal attachments, the laparoscopic approach offers significant advantages.

In order to save time and expense in the operating room, we have developed an approach to the patient requiring fecal diversion that combines the advantages of both trephine and laparoscopic stoma creation. If the patient is thin and would not necessarily benefit from laparoscopic exploration of the peritoneal cavity, the patient is approached initially with the intention of creating a trephine stoma, with the laparoscopic approach held in reserve. The patient is positioned for a laparoscopic procedure, but the laparoscopic equipment is kept unopened in the operating room. The stoma incision is made, and if the bowel can be delivered in correct orientation to the skin level, the stoma is created and the laparoscopic equipment remains unopened. However, if trephine creation of the stoma is impossible, a Hasson trocar is placed through the stoma incision and the procedure proceeds laparoscopically.

TECHNIQUE OF LAPAROSCOPIC STOMA CREATION

Patients undergoing diverting colostomy should be placed in the dorsal lithotomy position in order to have access to the anorectum; patients undergoing ileostomy may be placed in the supine position. The preselected stoma site is opened, a purse-string suture is placed in the posterior rectus sheath, and a Hasson trocar is placed. A 5-mm trocar is placed in the contralateral abdomen and the peritoneal cavity explored. If the bowel to be used for the stoma is sufficiently mobile, no other trocars need to be placed. If mobilization is required, additional 5-mm trocars can be placed to facilitate the dissection. Mobility is usually adequate when the bowel will reach to the peritoneal surface at the stoma site, as the distance to the skin level will decrease when pneumoperitoneum is released. A 5-mm camera is then placed through one of the 5-mm port sites, and the bowel grasped in the correct orientation using an instrument placed through the Hasson trocar at the stoma site. It is occasionally useful to mark the bowel for orientation of the proximal and distal limbs with sutures or clips prior to delivery through the stoma site—this is especially true when creating an ileostomy. The pneumoperitoneum is then released and the posterior rectus sheath opened over the trocar, allowing the bowel to be delivered through the stoma opening.

If the bowel is to be divided and an end stoma fashioned, it is critical that orientation be confirmed. Left-sided colostomy orientation can be confirmed by insufflation of air through a proctoscope, instillation of povidone iodine or dye through a small opening in the distal limb of the stoma with confirmation of dye passage to the rectum via a proctoscope, or passage of a flexible sigmoidoscope to the stoma site. Alternatively, the colon can be divided with a linear cutting stapler, the distal end is allowed to retract into the peritoneal cavity, and direct visualization with a 5-mm laparoscope is performed to ensure that the distal bowel can be traced in continuity to the rectum.

The rapidity with which postoperative ileus resolves following laparoscopic creation of intestinal stomas may allow patients to return home within 1–2 days. This may create a problem for the patient and the enterostomal therapist, who has little time to perform in-hospital stoma care training. Therefore it is advantageous to have the patient meet with the enterostomal therapist preoperatively, not only for stoma site marking, but for stoma care teaching as well.

LAPAROSCOPIC STOMA CLOSURE

Laparoscopic techniques are most applicable to patients who have undergone colectomy with construction of a proximal colostomy. Although laparoscopic adhesiolysis is occasionally a beneficial adjunct to loop stoma closure, this is rarely required, as most loop stomas can be closed via a peristomal incision. The most common indication for a laparoscopic approach to the restoration of intestinal continuity is colostomy takedown and construction of coloproctostomy following sigmoid colectomy for complicated diverticular disease ("Hartmann reversal"). This procedure can either be straightforward or complicated, depending on the number and severity of intraperitoneal adhesions and the degree of pelvic fibrosis.

Several methods can be used to perform laparoscopic Hartmann reversal. Some surgeons establish laparoscopic access initially, perform adhesiolysis, mobilize the colon and rectum, take down the colostomy and insert the anvil of the end-to-end stapling device, re-establish pneumoperitoneum, and perform the anastomosis. A more common method is to take down the colostomy initially, and perform as much of the procedure as possible through the colostomy opening prior to establishing pneumoperitoneum. A substantial amount of adhesiolysis and mobilization can often be performed through the stoma incision, especially if there is a parastomal hernia present that has enlarged the fascial opening. The proximal colon can be prepared for anastomosis and the anvil of a circular stapling device inserted. Pneumoperitoneum is then established, either by closure of the fascia or insertion of a hand-assist device. The size of the fascial defect will determine which method is more advantageous for the patient and surgeon. The operation is then completed laparoscopically.

Prior to embarking on a laparoscopic reversal of a Hartmann procedure performed for diverticular disease, the surgeon should consider that it may be necessary to resect retained sigmoid colon and mobilize the splenic flexure to allow soft descending colon to reach easily into the pelvis for a colorectal anastomosis. Preoperative evaluation of the proximal colon and distal rectal stump with endoscopy and/or contrast enema will help the surgeon plan the operative procedure and exclude alternative diagnoses.

It is also possible to perform laparoscopic restoration of intestinal continuity following total abdominal or subtotal colectomy and ileostomy. The ileostomy can be taken down, and an end-to-end anastomosis performed laparoscopically using a surgical stapling device.

SELECTED READINGS

Arumugam PJ, Bevan L, et al. A prospective audit of stomas—analysis of risk factors and complications and their management. *Colorectal Dis* 2003;5:49–52

Birnbaum EH, Fleshman JW. Anal manometry. In: Juijpers HC (ed). *Colorectal Physiology: Fecal Incontinence.* Boca Raton, FL: CRC Press; 1993:111–118

Birnbaum EH, Myerson RJ, et al. Chronic effects of pelvic radiation therapy on anorectal function. *Dis Colon Rectum* 1994;37:909–915

Bricker EM. Bladder substitution after pelvic evisceration. *Surg Clin North Am* 1950;30:1511

Burch JM, Martin RR, et al. Evolution of the treatment of the injured colon in the 1980s. *Arch Surg* 1991;126:979–984

Butcher HR Jr, Sugg WL, et al. Ileal conduit method of ureteral urinary diversion. *Ann Surg* 1962;156:682

Byers JM, Steinberg JB, et al. Repair of parastomal hernias using polypropylene mesh. *Arch Surg* 1992;127:1246

Chappuis CW, Frey DJ, et al. Management of penetrating colon injuries: a prospective randomized trial. *Ann Surg* 1991;213:492

Chechile G, Klein EA, et al. Functional equivalence of end and loop ileal conduit stomas. *J Urol* 1992;147:582

Cheung MT. Complications of an abdominal stoma: an analysis of 322 stomas. *Aust N Z J Surg* 1995;65:808–811

Corman JM, Odenheimer DB. Securing the loop—historic review of the methods used for creating a loop colostomy. *Dis Colon Rectum* 1991;34:1014

Corman ML. *Colon and Rectal Surgery*, 3rd ed. Philadelphia, PA: JB Lippincott; 1993

Crile G Jr, Turnbull RB Jr. Mechanism and prevention of ileostomy dysfunction. *Ann Surg* 1954;140:459

Deol ZK, Shayani V. Laparoscopic parastomal hernia repair. *Arch Surg* 2003;138:203–205

Dinnick T. The origins and evolution of colostomy. *Br J Surg* 1934;22:142

Doughty D. Role of the enterostomal therapy nurse in ostomy patient rehabilitation. *Cancer* 1992;70(Suppl):1390

Edwards DP, Leppington-Clarke A, et al. Stoma-related complications are more frequent after transverse colostomy than loop ileostomy: a prospective randomized clinical trial. *Br J Surg* 2001;88:360–363

Fallon WF Jr. The present role of colostomy in the management of trauma. *Dis Colon Rectum* 1992;35:1094

Feinberg SM, McLeod RS, et al. Complications of loop ileostomy. *Am J Surg* 1987;153:102

Fleshman JW, Cohen Z, et al. The ileal reservoir and ileoanal anastomosis procedure: factors affecting technical and functional outcome. *Dis Colon Rectum* 1988;31:10

Fleshman JW, Kodner IJ, et al. Anal incontinence. In: Zuidema G (ed). *Shackelford's Surgery of the Alimentary Tract.* Philadelphia, PA: WB Saunders; 1993

Fleshman JW. Loop ileostomy. *Surg Rounds* 1992;Feb:129

Fleshman JW, Soper NJ. Medical management of benign anal disease. In: Quigley EMM, Sorrell MF (eds). *Medical Care of the Gastrointestinal Surgical Patient.* Baltimore, MD: Williams & Wilkins; 1994

Fry RD, Shemesh EI, et al. Perforation of the rectum and sigmoid colon during barium-enema examination: management and prevention. *Dis Colon Rectum* 1989;32:759

Fucini C, Wolff BG, et al. Bleeding from peristomal varices: perspectives on prevention and treatment. *Dis Colon Rectum* 1991;34:1073

Garcia D, Hita G, et al. Colonic motility: electric and manometric description of mass movement. *Dis Colon Rectum* 1991;34:577

Geraghty JM, Talbot IC. Diversion colitis: histological features in the colon and rectum after defunctioning colostomy. *Gut* 1991;32:1020

Gordon PH, Nivatvongs S. *Principles and Practice of Surgery for the Colon, Rectum, and Anus.* St. Louis, MO: Quality Medical; 1992

Gottlieb LM, Handelsman JC. Treatment of outflow tract problems associated with continent ileostomy (Kock pouch): report of six cases. *Dis Colon Rectum* 1991;34:936

Grundfest-Broniatowski S, Fazio V. Conservative treatment of bleeding stomal varices. *Arch Surg* 1983;118:981

Hasegawa H, Radley S, et al. Stapled versus sutured closure of loop ileostomy: a randomized controlled trial. *Ann Surg* 2000;231:202–204

Janes A, Cengiz Y, et al. Preventing parastomal hernia with a prosthetic mesh. *Arch Surg* 2004;139:1356–1358

Jayaprakash A, Creed T, et al. Should we monitor vitamin B_{12} levels in patients who have had end-ileostomy for inflammatory bowel disease? *Int J Colorectal Dis* 2004;19:316–318

Jeter KF. Perioperative teaching and counseling. *Cancer* 1992; 70(Suppl):1346

Jeter KF. *These Special Children. A Book for Parents of Children with Colostomies, Ileostomies, & Urostomies.* Palo Alto, CA: Bull; 1982

Kalady MF, Fields RC, et al. Loop ileostomy closure at an ambulatory surgery facility: a safe and cost-effective alternative to routine hospitalization. *Dis Colon Rectum* 2003;46:486–490

Kaveggia FF, Thompson JS, et al. Placement of an ileal loop urinary diversion back in continuity with the intestinal tract. *Surgery* 1991;110:557

Khoo RE, Cohen MM. Laparoscopic ileostomy and colostomy. *Ann Surg* 1995;221:207–208

Kodner IJ. Colostomy and ileostomy. *Clin Symp* 1978;30:1

Kodner IJ. Colostomy. Indications, techniques for construction, and management of complications. *Semin Colon Rectal Surg* 1991;2:73

Kodner IJ, Fleshman JW, et al. Intestinal stomas. In: Schwartz SI (ed). *Maingot's Abdominal Operations.* Stamford, CT: Appleton & Lange; 1989:1143

Kodner IJ, Fry RD, et al. Colon, rectum, and anus. In: Schwartz SI (ed). *Principles of Surgery.* New York, NY: McGraw-Hill; 1993:1191

Kodner IJ, Fry RD, et al. Current options in the management of rectal cancer. *Adv Surg* 1991;24:1

Kodner IJ, Fry RD, et al. Intestinal stomas: their management. In: Veidenheimer MC (ed). *Seminars in Colon & Rectal Surgery.* Philadelphia, PA: WB Saunders; 1991:65

Kodner IJ, Fry RD, et al. Intestinal stomas: their management. Philadelphia, PA: WB Saunders; 1991:65

Kodner IJ. Stoma complications. In: Fazio VW (ed). *Current Therapy in Colon and Rectal Surgery.* Hamilton, Ontario: BC Decker; 1989:420

Köhler LW, Pemberton JH, et al. Quality of life after proctocolectomy: a comparison of Brooke ileostomy, Kock pouch, and ileal pouch-anal anastomosis. *Gastroenterology* 1991;101:679

Leblanc KA, Bellanger DE, et al. Laparoscopic parastomal hernia repair. *Hernia* 2005;9:140–144

Ludwig KA, Milsom JW, et al. Laparoscopic techniques for fecal diversion. *Dis Colon Rectum* 1996;39:285–288

MacKeigan JM, Cataldo PA. *Intestinal Stomas: Principles, Techniques, and Management.* St. Louis, MO: Quality Medical; 1993

MacLeod JH. Colostomy irrigation—a transatlantic controversy. *Dis Colon Rectum* 1972;15:357

Marcello PW, Roberts PL, et al. Obstruction after ileal pouch-anal anastomosis: a preventable complication? *Dis Colon Rectum* 1993;36:1105–1111

Mazor A, Lacey D, et al. Angiogenesis, type IV collagen, and PCNA do not predict metastasis in localized colorectal cancer. *Soc Surg Oncol Symp* 1993;46:Abstract

McLeod RS, Fazio VW. Quality of life with the continent ileostomy. *World J Surg* 1984;8:90

McLeod RS, Lavery IC, et al. Patient evaluation of the conventional ileostomy. *Dis Colon Rectum* 1985;28:152

Moran BJ, Jackson AA. Function of the human colon. *Br J Surg* 1992;79:1132

Myerson RJ, Michalski JM, et al. Adjuvant radiation therapy for rectal carcinoma: predictors of outcome. *Radiology* 1993;189:214(Abstract)

Myerson RJ, Shapiro SJ, et al. Carcinoma of the anal canal. *Am J Clin Oncol* 1994;18:32–39

Nightingale JMD, Lennard-Jones JE, et al. Oral salt supplements to compensate for jejunostomy losses: comparison of sodium chloride capsules, glucose electrolyte solution, and glucose polymer electrolyte solution. *Gut* 1992;33:759

Oliveira L, Reissman P, et al. Laparoscopic creation of stomas. *Surg Endosc* 1997;11:19–23

Orsay CP, Kim DO, et al. Diversion colitis in patients scheduled for colostomy closure. *Dis Colon Rectum* 1993;36:366

Ortiz H, Sara MJ, et al. Does the frequency of paracolostomy hernias depend on the position of the colostomy in the abdominal wall? *Int J Colorectal Dis* 1994;9:65–67

Parks SE, Hastings PR: Complications of colostomy closure. *Am J Surg* 1985;149:672

Pearl RK, Prasad ML, et al. Early local complications from intestinal stomas. *Arch Surg* 1985;120:1145

Pearl RK, Prasad ML, et al. End-loop stomas: the new generation of intestinal stomas. *Contemp Surg* 1985;27:270

Pemberton JH, Philips SF, et al. Quality of life after Brooke ileostomy and ileal pouch-anal anastomosis: comparison of performance status. *Ann Surg* 1989;209:620(discussion)

Prasad ML, Pearl RK, et al. End-loop colostomy. *Surg Gynecol Obstet* 1984;158:380

Prasad ML, Pearl RK, et al. Rodless ileostomy. A modified loop ileostomy. *Dis Colon Rectum* 1984;27:270

Price AL, Rubio PA. Laparoscopic colorectal surgery: a challenge for ET nurses. *J Wound Ostomy Continence Nurs* 1994; 21:179–182

Remzi FH, Oncel M, et al. Current indications for blow-hole colostomy:ileostomy procedure. A single center experience. *Int J Colorectal Dis* 2003;18:361–364

Rieger N, Moore J, et al. Parastomal hernia repair. *Colorectal Dis* 2004;6:203–205

Rolstad BS, Wilson G, et al. Sexual concerns in the patient with an ileostomy. *Dis Colon Rectum* 1983;26:170

Rombeau JL, Wilk PJ, et al. Total fecal diversion by the temporary skin-level loop transverse colostomy. *Dis Colon Rectum* 1978;21:223

Rubin MS, Schoetz DJ Jr, et al. Parastomal hernia. Is stoma relocation superior to fascial repair? *Arch Surg* 1994;129:413–418; discussion 418–419

Sakai Y, Nelson H, et al. Temporary transverse colostomy vs loop ileostomy in diversion: a case-matched study. *Arch Surg* 2001;136:338–342

Shemesh EI, Kodner IJ, et al. Statistics from the ostomy registry. *Ostomy Quart* 1987;24:70

Shirley F, Kodner IJ, et al. Loop ileostomy: techniques and indications. *Dis Colon Rectum* 1984;27:382

Soliani P, Carbognani P, et al. Colostomy plug devices: a possible new approach to the problem of incontinence. *Dis Colon Rectum* 1992;35:969

Starke J, Rodriguez-Bigas M, et al. Primary adenocarcinoma arising in an ileostomy. *Surgery* 1993;114:125

Stephenson ER Jr, Ilahi O, et al. Stoma creation through the stoma site: a rapid, safe technique. *Dis Colon Rectum* 1997; 40:112–115

Svaninger G, Nordgren S, et al. Sodium and potassium excretion in patients with ileostomies. *Eur J Surg* 1991;157: 601

Swain BT, Ellis CN Jr. Laparoscopy-assisted loop ileostomy: an acceptable option for temporary fecal diversion after anorectal surgery. *Dis Colon Rectum* 2002;45:705–707

Thompson JS, Williams SM. Technique for revision of continent ileostomy. *Dis Colon Rectum* 1992;35:87

Trelford JD, Goodnight J, et al. Total exenteration, two or one ostomy. *Surg Gynecol Obstet* 1992;175:126

Turnbull RB Jr, Weakley F (eds). *Atlas of Intestinal Stomas.* St. Louis, MO: CV Mosby; 1967

Unti JA, Abcarian H, et al. Rodless end-loop stomas: seven-year experience. *Dis Colon Rectum* 1991;34:999

Wexner SD, Taranow DA, et al. Loop ileostomy is a safe option for fecal diversion. *Dis Colon Rectum* 1993;36:349

Wiesner RH, LaRusso NF, et al. Peristomal varices after proctocolectomy in patients with primary sclerosing cholangitis. *Gastroenterology* 1986;90:316

Winslet MC, Drolc Z, et al. Assessment of the defunctioning efficiency of the loop ileostomy. *Dis Colon Rectum* 1991;34: 699

Winslet MC, Poxon V, et al. A pathophysiologic study of diversion proctitis. *Surg Gynecol Obstet* 1993;177:57

Young CJ, Eyers AA, et al. Defunctioning of the anorectum: historical controlled study of laparoscopic vs. open procedures. *Dis Colon Rectum* 1998;41:190–194

7

Abdominal Abscess and Enteric Fistula

Amy R. Evenson ■ *Gautam Shrikhande* ■ *Josef E. Fischer*

■ ABDOMINAL ABSCESS

PERITONEAL CAVITY ANATOMY

A thorough understanding of peritoneal anatomy is required to understand the typical areas of abscess formation. Regions such as within the greater sac, the right subhepatic space, the right and left subphrenic spaces, the paracolic gutters, and the pelvis are particularly susceptible to fluid accumulation, and as a result, abscess formation. The anatomic boundaries of these regions can be seen in Figure 7–1. The right subphrenic space lies between the right hemidiaphragm and the right lobe of the liver. Posteriorly are the right triangular and coronary ligaments of the liver and medially is the falciform ligament. The left subphrenic space lies between the left hepatic lobe and the left hemidiaphragm. Laterally, the space extends between the spleen and liver and is bounded medially by the falciform ligament. The paracolic gutters lie between the body wall and either the descending colon on the left or the ascending colon on the right. Communication from the left paracolic gutter with the pelvis is limited due to the sigmoid colon and limited with the left subphrenic space due to the phrenicocolic ligament. On the other hand, there is unhindered communication with the right paracolic gutter and the right subphrenic space, the right subhepatic space, and the pelvis. These anatomic relationships are important in clinical situations in which abscess etiologies are unclear.

The right subhepatic space lies between the inferior surface of the liver and the hepatic flexure and transverse mesocolon. Medially lies the second portion of the duodenum and the hepatoduodenal ligament, and laterally lies the body wall. This space opens into Morison's pouch posteriorly, the most dependent portion of the abdominal cavity in the recumbent position. The pelvic cavity is the most dependent area of the peritoneal cavity in the upright position. The space is bounded by the urinary bladder anteriorly, and the rectum, bony pelvic wall, and the retroperitoneum posteriorly. This creates an anatomic area that can be difficult to access. Finally, the lesser sac is a space that lies posterior to the stomach and gastrohepatic ligament. Superiorly lies the caudate lobe of the liver, and inferiorly the transverse mesocolon. The lesser sac communicates with the greater sac through the foramen of Winslow.

PATHOPHYSIOLOGY

Abdominal abscesses are formed in areas of localized peritonitis in which the infection is walled off by a barrier such as omentum and parietal or visceral peritoneum. Infectious organisms that are capable of inciting a localized peritoneal response include various gram-negative enteric bacteria, *Enterococcus*, *Bacteroides*, and yeast. Once the peritoneum is activated secondary to both a local and systemic cytokine response, there are changes in blood flow, enhancement of bacterial phagocytosis, and fibrin deposition to trap bacteria. The bacterial sequestration by fibrin slows the systemic spread of bacteria thereby reducing the risk of over-

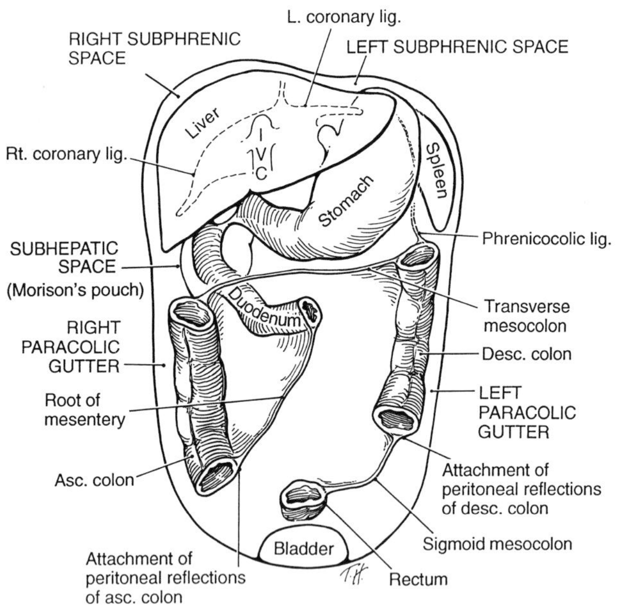

Figure 7–1. Diagram of intraperitoneal spaces.

whelming bacteremia. However, the deposition of fibrin may also protect the bacteria from usual host defenses, thus establishing a persistent infection that can result in abscess formation.[1]

Abdominal abscesses have been classically divided into three categories: intraperitoneal (anatomically described above), retroperitoneal, and visceral. Intraperitoneal abscesses generally develop one of two ways. The first is a result of diffuse peritonitis in which loculations of purulent material form in the most dependent areas. The second mode of formation is due to a contiguous disease process or injury in which the host defenses adequately prevented diffuse peritonitis and walled off the process.[2] Retroperitoneal abscesses form in the potential space between the peritoneum and the transversalis fascia lining the posterior aspect of the abdominal cavity. Visceral abscesses develop within the confines of one of the abdominal viscera such as the liver, pancreas, or gallbladder. These abscesses typically form as a result of hematogenous or lymphatic seeding from various sites, or in the case of the gallbladder, infectious cholecystitis.

Intra-abdominal abscesses are best treated quickly and effectively, as the mortality of patients with intra-abdominal abscesses ranges from 10–20%. Factors influencing outcome include organ failure, lesser sac abscesses, positive blood cultures, recurrent and/or persistent abscesses, multiple abscesses, age greater than 50 years, and subhepatic abscesses. Data show that the deaths from abdominal abscess are for the most part the consequence of ineffective or untimely drainage.[3]

CLINICAL PRESENTATION

In surgical practice, extravisceral abscesses form following failed anastomoses, infection of intraperitoneal fluid collections following abdominal surgery, contained leakage from a spontaneous visceral perforation, or residual loculations following diffuse peritonitis. High spiking fevers, chills, abdominal pain, anorexia, and delay of return of bowel function in the postoperative patient are typical presenting signs and symptoms of intraperitoneal abscess.

Subphrenic abscesses can present with vague upper quadrant abdominal pain, referred shoulder pain, and occasionally hiccoughs. Typically, paracolic and interloop abscesses present with localized tenderness and may manifest as a palpable mass on abdominal examination. Abscesses may also cause local irritation of the urinary bladder causing frequency, or of the rectum resulting in diarrhea and tenesmus.

DIAGNOSIS

Abdominal plain films can be helpful in identifying air-fluid levels in the upright or decubitus positions, extraluminal gas, or a soft tissue mass displacing the bowel. Chest radiographs may help to differentiate subphrenic from pleural fluid collections. Plain radiography may suggest the presence of an abscess, but other imaging modalities have essentially replaced plain films in the evaluation of intra-abdominal abscesses.

The initial use of ultrasound in the diagnosis of intra-abdominal fluid collections was found to have several advantages and disadvantages. The accuracy of ultrasound in the diagnosis of intra-abdominal abscesses was found to be 97% with a sensitivity of 93% and a specificity of 99%.[4] Ultrasonography allows for a rapid and complete examination of the abdomen, even in extremely ill patients. When one considers the cost of ultrasound, it remains an important tool. In addition, it usually does not require transportation of a critically ill patient, as it can be performed at the bedside, an important consideration.

The utility of ultrasound, however, is dependent on the skills and experience of the operator. These are several limitations to the utility of ultrasound. First, in regions other than the pelvis, the right upper quadrant, and the left upper quadrant when the spleen is present, optimal imaging is difficult to achieve[5] (Fig 7–2). Second, in patients with an ileus, a situation that is not uncommon with an intra-abdominal abscess, imaging is distorted by bowel gas. Other common issues in surgical patients that can impede ultrasound include staples, wound dressings, and stomas. Next, it was found that the

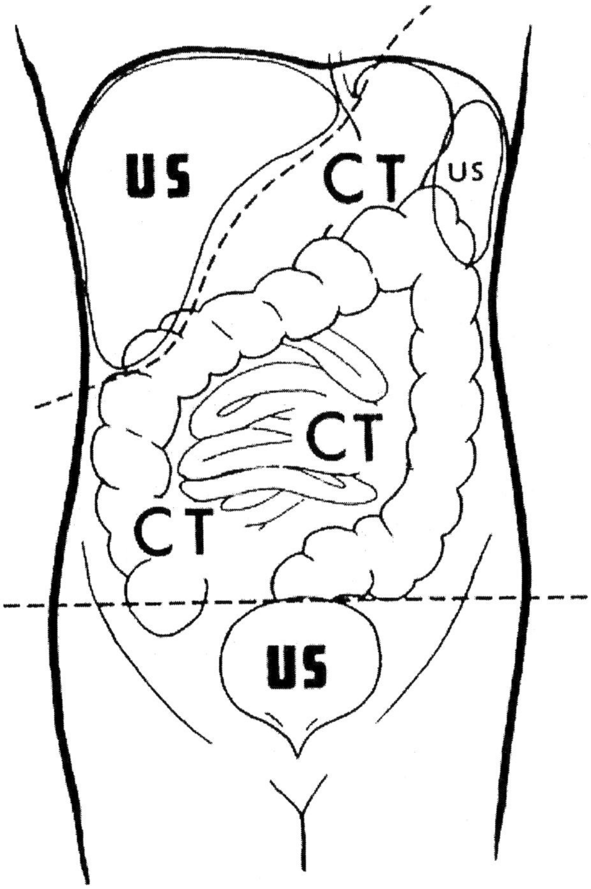

Figure 7–2. Schematic of areas in which ultrasound (*US*) and computed tomography (*CT*) scanning are most useful in the diagnosis of intra-abdominal abscesses. (Reprinted, with permission, from Mueller PR, Simeone JF. Intraabdominal abscesses. Diagnosis by sonography and computed tomography. *Radiol Clin North Am* 1983;21:425–443.)

ultrasonic characteristics of abscesses and hematomas overlapped. Furthermore, the nature of the fluid as determined by ultrasound could only occasionally help determine the composition of the fluid collection.[6]

Computed tomography (CT) scanning has rapidly emerged as an accurate and frequently used modality in this disease process. Detection of 97% of abdominal abscesses has been reported[7] (Table 7–1 and Figs 7–3 and 7–4). Criteria for identification of an abscess have been well described and include identification of an area of low CT attenuation in an extraluminal location or within the parenchyma of solid abdominal organs. The density of abscesses usually falls between that of water and solid tissue.[5] Other radiological signs of an abscess are mass effect that replaces or displaces normal anatomic structures, a lucent center that is not enhanced after the intravenous administration of a contrast medium, enhancing rim around the lucent center after contrast administration, and gas in the fluid collection.[7] One of the major advantages of CT over ultrasound is the ability to detect abscesses in the retroperitoneum and pancreatic area.

There are some disadvantages to CT scanning. Occasionally, there may be a solid-appearing collection that is really an abscess with a high leukocyte and protein content. Also, necrotic tumor and tissue can occasionally demonstrate intracavitary gas and not be infected. Next, septations and other signs of loculated abscesses can be seen much better with ultrasound than CT. Finally, CT scanning is sometimes unable to differentiate between subphrenic and pulmonic fluid, a relatively common situation in abdominal surgery.[5]

MANAGEMENT

The initial management of a patient with an intra-abdominal abscess includes preparation for potential operative or percutaneous management as well as initiating antibiotic therapy. Initially, antibiotic coverage should be broad with coverage for enteric aerobes and anaerobes. Following successful drainage of the abscess, however, one should quickly tailor the antibiotics to culture results. Depending on the clinical status of the patient, early discontinuation of antibiotic therapy should be considered if adequate drainage is achieved. Aggressive fluid resuscitation is appropriate for most patients, and correction of acid-base and electrolyte abnormalities should be undertaken. If the leukocyte count is elevated, standard evaluation should also include blood culture, urinalysis and urine culture, assessment of central venous catheter status, and routine chest imaging. The physician should also anticipate an ileus and the need for an alternative source of nutrition such as parenteral nutrition. Nasogastric tube placement is warranted if nausea and vomiting are present.

Percutaneous Drainage

Percutaneous drainage of abscesses has become an established technique and a safe alternative to surgery.

TABLE 7–1. COMPARISON OF ULTRASOUND AND COMPUTED TOMOGRAPHY IN DETECTION OF INTRA-ABDOMINAL ABSCESSES

	Advantages	Disadvantages
US	Rapid exam Lower cost No need for patient transport Good for evaluation of pelvis, RUQ, LUQ (if spleen present) Can demonstrate septations	Operator-dependent Poor for imaging bowel Limited by air in bowel (ileus), staples, dressings, stomas, excessive adipose tissue Cannot distinguish abscess from hematoma, lymphocele, biloma, seroma
CT	Good for entire abdomen, especially evaluation of retroperitoneum and pancreas	Can miss abscesses with high protein content May be difficult to differentiate subphrenic from pulmonic fluid

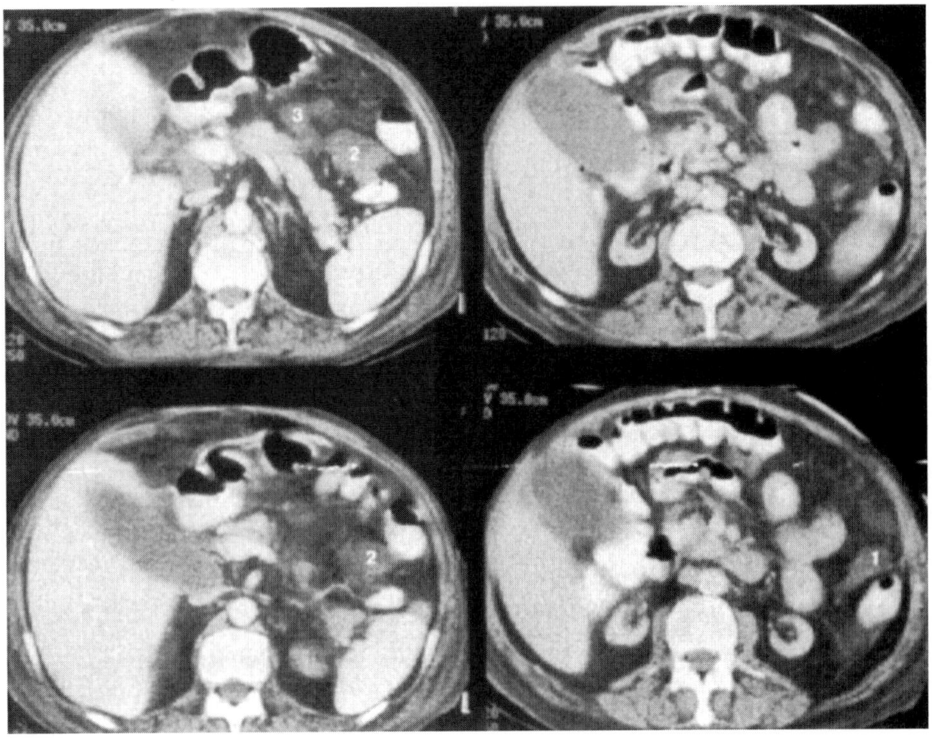

A

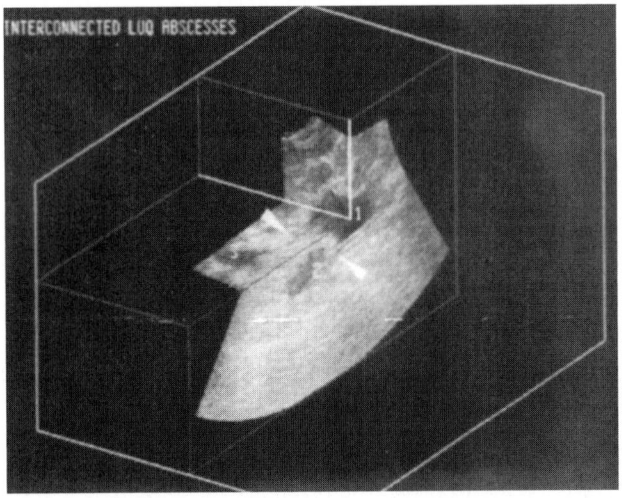

B

Figure 7–3. Imaging with CT and US may be complementary. **A.** CT demonstrates three apparently separate abscesses, *1* anterior to the descending colon and *2* and *3* in the lesser sac. **B.** Three-dimensional ultrasound demonstrating communication between all three abscesses. Two percutaneous drains were placed via a common access route to drain these abscesses. (Reprinted, with permission, from Rose SC, Roberts AC, Kinney TB et al. Three-dimensional ultrasonography for planning percutaneous drainage of complex abdominal fluid collections. *J Vasc Interv Radiol* 2003;14:451–459.)

Advantages of percutaneous techniques include avoidance of general anesthesia, lower costs, and the potential for fewer complications. Prerequisites for catheter drainage include an anatomically safe route to the abscess, a well-defined unilocular abscess cavity, concurring surgical and radiologic evaluation, and senior surgical back-up for technical failure. Contraindications to catheter drainage include absence of appropriate access routes, internal septations and loculations, and presence of a coagulopathy.[8] Multiple abscesses, abscesses with enteric connections as seen with enterocutaneous fistulas, and the need to traverse solid viscera are not contraindications.

It is unclear whether percutaneous drainage is best done with ultrasound or CT guidance. CT provides for more precise identification of organs and bowel loops and is more accurate for planning of drainage route.[8] Once the abscess is identified, initial diagnostic aspiration should be sent for Gram's stain and microbiological culture. The catheter used for drainage should be as small as possible for safety yet large enough that the tubing does not become obstructed. Most commonly

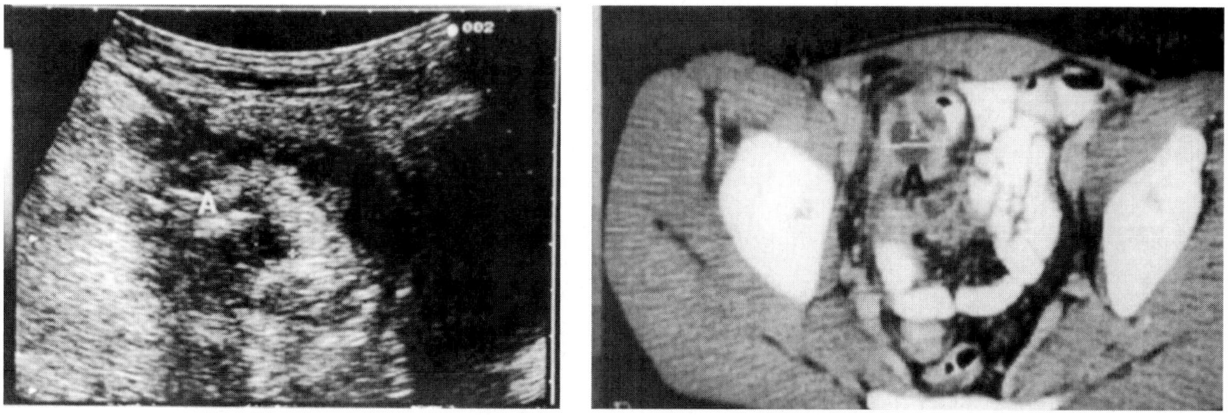

A B

Figure 7–4. Mesenteric abscess identified by US and CT. **A.** Deep mesenteric abscess (*A*) appears as a round hypoanechoic lesion with internal echoes and an irregular wall. **B.** CT demonstrates a collection of fluid (*A*) in the mesentery between small bowel loops. (Reprinted, with permission, from Maconi G, Sampietro GM, Parente F et al. Contrast radiology, computed tomography and ultrasonography in detecting internal fistulas and intra-abdominal abscesses in Crohn's disease: a prospective comparative study. *Am J Gastroenterol* 2003;98:1545–1555.)

used catheters range in size from 8.0–12.0F. With appropriate catheter placement, the abscess cavity typically decompresses and collapses. Irrigation of the catheter should be done once daily to ensure tube patency. As catheter drainage decreases, repeat CT scanning can be performed to evaluate for residual contents. If drainage increases over time or continues at a steady rate, the development of an enteric fistula must be suspected. The ultimate endpoint of catheter placement is clinical improvement of the patient. Potential complications of catheter placement include bacteremia, sepsis, vascular injury, enteric puncture, cutaneous fistula, or transpleural catheter placement.

Studies comparing outcomes of surgical and percutaneous drainage of intra-abdominal abscesses demonstrate that both methods have similar results. In one study, patients were matched for age, abscess location, and etiology, and had similar Acute Physiology, Age, and Chronic Health Evaluation II scores (APACHE II). There were no differences between percutaneous and surgical drainage in patient morbidity, mortality, or duration of hospital stay.[9] Another group retrospectively examined postoperative intra-abdominal abscesses after laparotomy. This study similarly demonstrated that use of either form of drainage resulted in similar cure rates for postoperative intra-abdominal abscesses.[10] Some authors contend that the method of drainage is not as important as the initial success in localization of the abscess.[11]

Subphrenic and Subhepatic Abscess. The majority of patients presenting with an abscess in these regions had a recent previous operation. Left colonic operations and gastric and splenic operations precede the development of left subphrenic abscesses. Right colonic, biliary, and hepatic surgery lead to the development of infrahepatic or suprahepatic abscesses. Anastomotic disruption secondary to technical error, excessive tension, hypothermia, or postoperative hypotension leads to subphrenic abscesses, as does accumulation of blood secondary to inadequate hemostasis.

Some have shown that subphrenic abscesses are more likely to have a successful outcome than abscesses in other locations, presumably due to their anatomic location.[12] In another study, successful catheter drainage was achieved in 85% of subphrenic abscesses with a complication rate of 4.8%.[13] Failure of catheter drainage occurred in patients with multiple loculations or those in whom the primary cause of the abscess required surgery as in the case of perforated ulcer or acute cholecystitis.[13]

Paracolic Abscess. Abscesses in this region typically occur as a result of colonic perforations. Commonly, abscesses extend inferiorly into the pelvis. Common clinical conditions encountered on the surgical service include perforated diverticulitis and appendicitis. When these abscesses have enteric communication, percutaneous drainage may be carried out without any significant risk of fistula formation. When the abscesses have cutaneous fistulous tracts, the preferred catheter drainage is through the tract. The fistulous tract can be identified with a fistulogram and a catheter can be placed through the tract for adequate drainage.

In the case of percutaneous drainage of periappendiceal abscesses, it has been reported that 90% of patients can be successfully treated by catheter drainage and antibiotic therapy alone.[14] In the case of diverticular abscesses, one study has reported that preoperative percutaneous drainage obviates the need for colostomy and multiple-stage surgery in 74% of patients. In this series, patients had large paracolic or pelvic abscesses with a mean size of 8.9 cm. Seventy-nine percent of the patients required catheter drainage for less than 3 weeks.[15]

Interloop Abscess. These abscesses are typically interspersed through loops of small bowel, mesentery, and omentum. Due to the ill-defined nature of these abscesses, surgical drainage is the usual method of treatment. The entire length of the bowel should be run and all adhesions should be freed. All abscesses should be aggressively débrided, especially for fibrin, which may contain entrapped bacteria, and the abdomen should be copiously irrigated.

Pelvic Abscess. Pelvic abscesses are the result of diffuse peritonitis, perforated diverticulitis and appendicitis, and various gynecologic processes. Some deep pelvic structures are unapproachable because of interposed structures such as the urinary bladder, loops of bowel, and skeletal and neurovascular structures. Abscesses near the anterior abdominal wall are usually easily drained by the percutaneous approach. Deeper abscesses have required more innovative approaches such as the transsciatic and translumbar approaches. In women, transvaginal sonographically-guided drainage can be an effective method. Transrectal sonographically-guided drainage of deep pelvic abscesses has been shown to be a safe and effective alternative to surgical transrectal and transgluteal approaches.[16]

Surgical Drainage

Surgical drainage is the preferred method of management of ill-defined abscesses, fungal abscesses, infected hematomas, necrotic tumor masses, and interloop abscesses. Open surgical drainage can be used for situations in which percutaneous techniques are unlikely to be successful or following failed attempts at minimally-invasive drainage.

The transperitoneal approach allows for examination of the entire abdominal cavity and allows for the drainage of multiple abscesses. Subphrenic abscesses and right subhepatic abscesses may be approached by lateral abdominal incisions. After the patient has been adequately hydrated and appropriate antibiotics have been given, an incision is made and meticulous attention is paid to protecting the wound with antibiotic-soaked sponges (or if large enough, antibiotic-soaked wound towels which are sewn in) to help prevent postoperative wound issues. Once abscess cavities are identified, they are entered and drained quickly to minimize spillage and contamination of the rest of the peritoneal cavity. The abscess cavity then should be widely opened. Specimens should be sent for Gram's stain and culture. In the case of resistant abscesses, a biopsy of the abscess cavity can be sent to pathology for further evaluation. Copious warm antibiotic irrigation must be used at the end of the operation to properly cleanse the abdominal cavity. Closed suction drains should be placed in dependent positions to reduce the risk of reaccumulation. In extremely contaminated cases, the incision may be left open and packed to prevent wound infection. However, there is little to be lost by a subcuticular closure after antibiotic irrigation of the abscess cavity and the wound, with a closed suction drain placed subcutaneously. Drains should be kept in for at least 10 days, as suppuration occurs late.

Postoperatively, antibiotics should be tailored to culture results and parenteral nutrition should be started if required. Since ileus is not uncommon in these patients, caloric requirements via the enteric route can be difficult to achieve. However, if possible, trophic tube feeds should be initiated to prevent atrophy of intestinal villi. It is extremely important to prevent the drains from becoming obstructed. Routine flushing with normal saline or antibiotic solution may be required.

▪ ENTERIC FISTULAS

Enterocutaneous fistulas represent a second group of complex intraperitoneal infectious processes. Even with recent advances in parasurgical management, critical care, and nutritional support, enterocutaneous fistulas remain great challenges to the general surgeon. Mortality remains high, between 10–30% in recent series, largely due to the frequent complications of sepsis and malnutrition. Electrolyte imbalances, initially identified by Edmunds and associates as a third key factor leading to mortality, are not as important in contributing to mortality in current practice.[17] Key to the management of these complex patients is an understanding of the pathophysiology and a sound, multidisciplinary team approach to diagnosis, physiologic support, and reconstruction of these fistulas.

CLASSIFICATION

Fistulas involving the alimentary tract can be classified by the anatomy of the structures involved, the amount and composition of drainage, and the etiology responsible for their formation. In addition to classification, these distinctions may provide important prognostic information about the physiologic impact of fistulas and the likelihood that they will close without surgical resection, the principal decision confronting the responsible surgeon.

Etiologic Classification

Enterocutaneous fistulas result from several processes: (1) diseased bowel extending to surrounding structures; (2) extraintestinal disease involving otherwise normal bowel; (3) trauma to normal bowel including inadvertent or missed enterotomies; or (4) anastomotic disruption following surgery for a variety of conditions. Fistulas between the alimentary tract and skin may be classified as postoperative or spontaneous. Approximately three-quarters of fistulas occur following an operation, most commonly subsequent to procedures performed for malignancy, inflammatory bowel disease, or adhesions.[18] Patient factors that increase the likelihood of developing a postoperative fistula include malnutrition, infection, and emergency operations with concomitant hypotension, anemia, hypothermia, and poor oxygen delivery. If possible, these conditions should be corrected prior to operation, but in emergency situations, optimization of resuscitation and performance of a technically meticulous procedure including adequate mobilization, good quality bowel with good blood supply, and no tension will provide the best chance of a good outcome. Postoperative enterocutaneous fistulas result from either disruption of the anastomosis or inadvertent (and often unrecognized) bowel injury during the dissection or abdominal closure. Attention to avoidance of tension or ischemia in the creation of anastomoses is paramount in minimizing postoperative enterocutaneous fistulas.

The remaining 25 percent of fistulas do not occur following a surgical procedure. These spontaneous fistulas often develop in patients with cancer or following radiation therapy. Fistulas occurring in the setting of malignancy or irradiation are unlikely to close without operative intervention. A second major group of patients with spontaneous fistulas are those with inflammatory conditions such as inflammatory bowel disease, diverticular disease, perforated ulcer disease, or ischemic bowel.[19] Of these, fistulas in patients with inflammatory bowel disease are most common; these fistulas often close following a prolonged period of parenteral nutrition, only to reopen when enteral nutrition resumes.[20] An understanding of the etiology of an enterocutaneous fistula may provide information about the ultimate need for surgical intervention.

Anatomic Classification

Fistulas may communicate with the skin (external fistulas) or other intraperitoneal or intrathoracic organs (internal fistulas). Internal fistulas that bypass only short segments of bowel may not be symptomatic; however, internal fistulas of bowel that bypass significant length of bowel or that communicate with either the bladder or vagina typically cause symptoms and become clinically evident. The identification and management of internal fistulas is beyond the scope of this review, but in general, internal fistulas should be resected if they are symptomatic or cause physiologic or metabolic complications.

Identification of the anatomic site of origin of external fistulas may provide further information on the etiology and likelihood of closure of the fistula.

Oral, Pharyngeal, and Esophageal Fistulas. Historically, the leading etiology of oropharyngeocutaneous fistulas had been advanced head and neck malignancies. In the current era, improved access to health care has resulted in identification and management of these tumors prior to such advanced states, but the radical resections and reconstructions performed are complicated by postoperative fistulas in 5–25% of cases.[21] Alcohol and tobacco use, poor nutrition, and preoperative chemoradiation therapy all contribute to poor wound healing and increase the risk of fistula formation. Failure of closure of the pharyngeal defect at the base of the tongue most commonly leads to fistula formation and free microvascular flaps are the preferred method for closure. Brown and colleagues reported a significantly decreased postoperative fistula rate in patients who underwent free flap closure versus those with pedicled pectoralis flap closure, 4.5% versus 21%, respectively.[22] Flaps should be positioned such that the vessels are flat and straight to avoid venous congestion and loss of the flap. In the setting of a radiated field, dissection should be minimized to prevent development of false planes and further devascularization.

Most esophagocutaneous fistulas result from either breakdown of the cervical anastomosis following resection of esophageal malignancy or following esophageal trauma. Treatment of cervical esophageal fistulas, similar to that of oropharyngeal fistulas, involves drainage of sepsis, débridement of devitalized tissue, and primary layered closure. In contrast, thoracic esophageal fistulas to the pleural space, bronchial tree, or trachea may rapidly lead to empyema, mediastinitis, and overwhelming sepsis, necessitating a more aggressive surgical approach including wide drainage, and if early enough, closure reinforced with a pleural or muscle flap. Due to the severity of leakage of esophageal contents within the thorax, these fistulas rarely result in spontaneous external drainage.

Less common causes of oropharyngeocutaneous or esphagocutaneous fistula include tuberculosis, laryngeal or thoracic surgery, trauma, congenital neck cysts, anterior cervical spine fusion, and foreign body perforations.[23–28] The principles of drainage, débridement, and layered closure often result in successful closure of these fistulas. Other reports suggest a role for tissue adhesive in the closure of these fistulas.[25,29]

Gastric Fistulas. The etiology of gastrocutaneous fistulas has changed in recent years. While most of these fistulas remain postoperative complications, the most commonly reported procedure associated with gastrocutaneous fistula formation is the removal of a gastrostomy feeding tube. The duration of gastrostomy tube placement appears to be related to the likelihood of development of a fistula after tube removal, with nearly 90% of children developing a fistula when the tube had been in situ for more than 9 months.[30] While the incidence of fistula formation after gastrostomy tube placement may be as high as 44% in recent studies,[30] there are numerous reports of resolution of these fistulas with fibrin-glue injection rather than operative closure.[29,31–34] While the rate of gastrocutaneous fistula following operations for nonmalignant processes such as ulcer disease, reflux disease, and obesity is between 0.5% and 3.9%,[33] the growing obesity epidemic in the United States and the recent rapid increase in bariatric procedures may also be expected to lead to an increase in the incidence of gastrocutaneous fistula following surgery for benign disease. Fistula formation following resection for gastric cancer remains a dreaded complication with significant mortality rates. Preservation of blood supply by maintaining the gastroepiploic arcade will reduce the risk of gastric necrosis and fistula formation. A tension-free anastomosis requires sufficient mobilization of the duodenum. Should tension occur, consideration of conversion to a Billroth II may be the preferred reconstruction. Careful closure of the edges of the anastamoses (the angle de mort) with a tripartite suture and postoperative nasogastric decompression will lessen the risk of suture-line dehiscence.

Spontaneous gastrocutaneous fistulas are uncommon, but can result from inflammation, ischemia, cancer, and radiation.

Duodenal Fistulas. The majority of duodenocutaneous fistulas develop after gastric resections or surgery involving the duodenum, pancreas, colon, aorta, kidney, or biliary tract. Spontaneous cases resulting from trauma, malignancy, Crohn's disease, and ulcer disease account for the remaining duodenal fistulas.[35,36] Prognostically, duodenal fistulas segregate into two groups: lateral duodenal fistulas and duodenal stump fistulas. Edmunds and associates and Malangoni and colleagues reported a decreased spontaneous closure rate with lateral duodenal fistulas when compared to duodenal stump fistulas.[17,37] Duodenal decompression via catheter duodenostomy may decrease the risk of fistula formation to less than 1%.[38]

Small Bowel Fistulas. The majority of gastrointestinal cutaneous fistulas arise from the small intestine. Seventy to ninety percent of enterocutaneous fistulas occur in the postoperative period.[20,39,40] Postoperative small bowel fistulas result from either disruption of anastomoses or injury to the bowel during dissection or closure of the abdomen. Operations for cancer, inflammatory bowel disease, and adhesiolysis are the most common procedures antecedent to small bowel fistula formation. During the course of a procedure, resection with end-to-end anastomosis is recommended for small bowel defects and injuries, especially when simple closure would be expected to reduce the luminal diameter. All sersosal injuries should be repaired with interrupted 3-0 silk sutures.

Spontaneous small bowel fistulas arise from inflammatory bowel disease, cancer, peptic ulcer disease, or pancreatitis. Crohn's disease is the most common cause of spontaneous small bowel fistula.[41] The transmural inflammation underlying Crohn's disease may lead to adhesion of the small bowel to the abdominal wall or other abdominal structures. Microperforation may then cause abscess formation and erosion into adjacent structures or the skin. Roughly half of Crohn's fistulas are internal and half are external.[42–44] Crohn's fistulas typically follow one of two courses. The first type represents fistulas that present in the early postoperative period following resection of a segment of diseased bowel. These fistulas arise in otherwise healthy bowel and follow a course similar to non-Crohn's fistulas with a significant likelihood of spontaneous closure. The other group of Crohn's fistulas arises in diseased bowel and has a low rate of spontaneous closure. Additionally, should spontaneous closure occur, these fistulas often reopen upon resumption of enteral intake. Early operative closure of these fistulas should be considered.

Colonic Fistulas. Spontaneous fistulas of the colon result from diverticulitis, malignancy, inflammatory bowel disease, appendicitis, and pancreatitis, while treatment of these conditions accounts for the majority of postoperative colocutaneous fistulas. Anastomotic breakdown or extension from inadequately resected disease bowel account for the majority of the postoperative fistulas. Additionally, as seen with gastrocutaneous fistulas, an increased incidence of colocutaneous fistulas has been reported following percutaneous gastrostomy placement.[45–48] Injuries at the time of gastrostomy placement as well as erosion of a properly placed gastrostomy tube have been proposed as mechanisms for this complication. Appendiceal fistulas may result from drainage of an appendiceal abscess or appendectomy in a patient with Crohn's disease.[49–51] In the case of the latter, the fistula often originates from the terminal ileum, not the cecum. The inflamed ileum adheres to the abdominal wall closure and subsequently results in fistula formation. Erosion of a percutaneous drain for spontaneous right lower quadrant abscess is also an increasing cause of gastrointestinal cutaneous fistula in Crohn's disease.

Radiation therapy contributes to both spontaneous and postoperative colocutaneous fistulas. Russell and Welch reported a 31% incidence of breakdown of primary anastomoses performed in irradiated tissues with resulting sepsis or fistula formation.[52] Techniques to provide additional protection and blood supply to anastomoses performed under these conditions include coverage of anastomoses with omentum, filling of dead space with muscle flaps, or sigmoid exclusion.[53,54] Proximal diverting colostomy or ileostomy may allow sufficient anastomotic healing prior to suture-line challenge with luminal contents. Clearly, operation or reoperation in an irradiated field is subject to recurrence of colocutaneous fistulas, and these fistulas are unlikely to undergo spontaneous closure.[55]

Fistula Tract Characteristics. In addition to describing the organs involved in fistulas, anatomic characteristics of fistula tracts may also be helpful in determining prognosis (Table 7–2). Due to anatomic considerations and the nature of effluent from different sites in the enteric tract, certain locations are more likely to undergo spontaneous closure. These favorable types include oropharyngeal, esophageal, duodenal stump, and jejunal fistulas. Unfavorable sites include the stomach, lateral duodenum, ligament of Treitz, and ileum. Anatomic factors suggesting low likelihood of spontaneous closure include fistulas associated with large abscesses, intestinal wall defects of greater than 1 cm, intestinal discontinuity, distal obstruction, diseased adjacent bowel, and fistulous tracts of less than 2 cm[19] (Fig 7–5). In contrast, fistulas with intestinal wall defects less than 1 cm and longer tracts are more likely to undergo spontaneous closure. However, in our experience, lateral duodenal fistulas are likely to close, and short fistula tracts are not a disadvantage if the intestinal epithelium has not grown to the surface. It is not just the length of the fistula but intestinal epithelium on the surface that results in non-closure. Once intestinal epithelium reaches to the surface, one has an enterostomy, which will not close spontaneously.

TABLE 7–2. PREDICTIVE FACTORS FOR SPONTANEOUS CLOSURE AND/OR MORTALITY

Factor	Favorable	Unfavorable
Organ of origin	Oropharyngeal Esophageal Duodenal stump Pancreaticobiliary Jejunal Colonic	Gastric Lateral duodenal Ligament of Treitz Ileal
Etiology	Postoperative Appendicitis Diverticulitis	Malignancy Inflammatory bowel disease
Output	Low (<200–500 mL/day)	High (>500 mL/day)
Nutritional status	Well-nourished Transferrin >200 mg/dL	Malnourished Transferrin <200 mg/dL
Sepsis	Absent	Present
State of bowel	Healthy adjacent tissue Intestinal continuity Absence of obstruction	Diseased adjacent bowel Distal obstruction Large abscess Bowel discontinuty Previous irradiation
Fistula characteristics	Tract >2 cm Bowel wall defect <1 cm^2	Tract <1 cm Defect >1 cm^2 Epithelialization Foreign body
Miscellaneous	Original operation performed at same institution	Referred from outside institution

Physiologic Classification

Enterocutaneous fistulas cause the loss of fluid, minerals, trace elements, and protein, as well as allow the release of irritating and caustic substances onto the skin and subcutaneous tissues. Accurate measurement of both the amount and nature of enterocutaneous effluent allows for accurate replacement and an understanding of the physiologic and metabolic challenges to the patient (Table 7–3). Fistulas may be divided into high-output (>500 mL per day), moderate-output (200–500 mL/day), and low-output (<200 mL/day) groups. Classification of enterocutaneous fistulas by the amount of daily output provides information regarding mortality, and in recent series may predict spontaneous closure.[17,56–58] In the classic series of Edmunds and associates, patients with high-output fistulas had a mortality rate of 54%, compared to a 16% mortality rate in the low-output group.[17] More recently, Levy and colleagues reported a 50% mortality rate in patients with high-output fistulas, while those with low-output fistulas had a 26% mortality.[56] In the largest series reported to date, Soeters and coworkers reported no association between fistula output and rate of spontaneous closure, while multivariate analysis by Campos and associates suggested that patients with low-output fistulas were three times more likely to achieve closure without operative intervention.[20,58] The reason for these different rates of closure is that high-output fistulas are likely to be of small-bowel origin, while low-output fistulas are likely to be of colonic origin. Moderate-volume fistulas tend to be of either colonic or mixed small- and large-bowel origin (see Table 7–2).

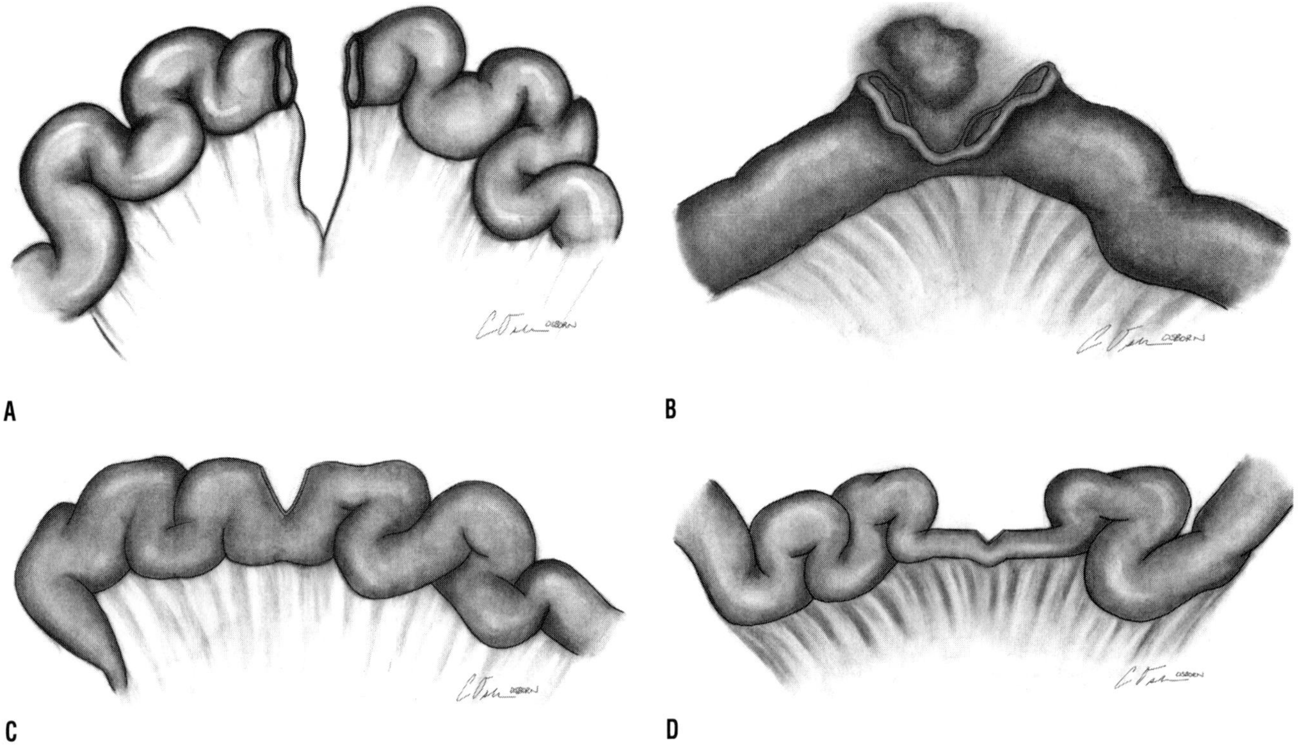

Figure 7–5. Types of bowel wall pathology in enterocutaneous fistulas. **A.** Total anastomotic disruption. **B.** Partial disruption with adjacent abscess. **C.** Lateral fistula with distal obstruction. **D.** Fistula in strictured intestine.

PREVENTION

Proper preoperative patient preparation and meticulous surgical technique will lessen the risk of postoperative fistula formation. In the elective setting, operation may be delayed to allow for normalization of nutritional parameters, thus optimizing wound healing and immune function. Several nutritional characteristics have been suggested to increase the risk of anastomotic breakdown:

1. Weight loss of 10–15% of total body weight over 3–4 months;
2. Serum albumin less than 3 mg/dL;
3. Serum transferrin less than 220 mg/dL;
4. Anergy to recall antigens; or
5. Inability to perform activities of daily living due to weakness or fatigue.[59]

Delay of elective procedures to allow for nutritional support to address these abnormalities may decrease the risk of anastomotic dehiscence and formation of postoperative fistulas.

Mechanical and antibiotic bowel preparation reduce the amount of particulate fecal material as well as colonic bacterial counts. In practice, mechanical bowel preparation for elective colon operations combined with systemic antibiotics with activity against enteric or-

TABLE 7–3. BODY FLUID ELECTROLYTE COMPOSITION

Source	Volume (mL/day)	pH	Na	K	HCO_3^-	Cl
Gastric	2000–2500	<4	60	10	—	90
		>4	100	10	—	100
Pancreatic	1000		140	5	90–110	30–45
Bile	1500		140	5	35	100
Small bowel	3500		100–130	15	25–35	100–140
Diarrhea	1000–4000		60	10–20	10	45–65
Urine	1500		20–40	20	—	20
Sweat			50	5	—	55

All values for sodium, potassium, bicarbonate, and chloride given in milliequivalents per liter.

ganisms provides adequate prophylaxis. A recent meta-analysis of studies examining mechanical and antibiotic bowel preparation suggests that bowel prep, especially with a polyethylene glycol preparation, may increase the risk of anastomotic leakage, but confirmatory studies are required before omission of preparation would be recommended in practice.[60]

In emergency operations, delays for optimization of nutritional status and bowel preparation are not possible. Instead, emphasis should be on adequate resuscitation and restoration of circulating volume, normalization of hemodynamics, provision of appropriate antibiotic therapy, and meticulous surgical technique. Performance of anastomoses in a healthy, well-perfused bowel without tension provides the best chance for healing, especially when one can easily see the performance of the anastomosis clearly. Careful hemostasis to avoid postoperative hematoma formation will decrease the risk of abscess, while inadvertent enterotomies and serosal injuries should be identified and repaired. If possible, an omental flap should be used to separate the anastomosis from the abdominal incision. Secure abdominal wall closure using healthy tissue and care to avoid injury to the underlying bowel are important to prevent postoperative fistula formation. In the postoperative period, further resuscitation may be required to ensure hemodynamic stability and avoid inadequate tissue oxygenation. It is essential to avoid periods of transient postoperative hypotension related to the anesthesia.

PATHOPHYSIOLOGY

Edmunds recognized the role of sepsis, malnutrition, and electrolyte abnormalities in contributing to the morbidity and mortality of enterocutaneous fistulas.[17] Leakage of intestinal contents results in the loss of electrolyte- and protein-rich fluid. Despite the ability to obtain rapid, accurate determinations of serum electrolytes, abnormalities persisting greater than 24 hours are not uncommon in these patients. While no longer a major contributor to the mortality of enterocutaneous fistulas, the persistence of aberrant values reflects the difficulty of successfully repleting ongoing losses in these complex patients. Knowledge of the source of the fistula, chemical analysis of fistula output, frequent serum electrolyte determinations, and aggressive replacement represent the best approach to maintenance of normal values.

The combination of malnutrition and sepsis remains the main challenge to fistula patients and those involved in their care. Patients with fistulas are often nutritionally depleted prior to the development of their fistulas. Patients with the spontaneous development of fistulas often have inflammatory bowel disease or cancer. Patients with postoperative fistulas likely have had limited enteral intake in the period preceding their operations due to the disease for which the operation is indicated (e.g., cancer or obstruction). Additionally, these patients have often had a period of bowel preparation prior to and limited enteral nutrition following surgery. Depending on the level of the fistula, more or less bowel is available for absorption of oral feeds. Finally, the hypercatabolic state induced by the presence of infection increases the nutritional challenge.

Bowel perforation may result in a localized abscess, generalized peritonitis, and/or fistula formation. Most recent series suggest that sepsis remains the leading cause of mortality in enterocutaneous fistula patients.[20,58,61] Early control of sepsis by drainage of abscesses and control of fistula drainage provides the fistula patient's best hope of recovery. The presence of infection adds to the stress on these patients and limits the ability to achieve positive nitrogen balance. In the series of Hill and colleagues, despite receiving parenteral nutrition, patients with uncontrolled sepsis lost 2% of body protein stores per day and up to 24% of total body protein within 2 weeks.[62] Until sepsis is controlled, it is almost impossible to put patients into positive nitrogen balance with nutritional support.

Nutritional status is also associated with mortality. Fazio reported no mortality in patients with serum albumin levels exceeding 3.5 g/dL, while a level of less than 2.5 g/dL resulted in a mortality rate of 42%.[61] Hypoalbuminemia has also been suggested to limit wound healing in burned rats[63] and to lead to bowel dysfunction manifesting as diarrhea in patients with chronically low levels.[64] Kuvshinoff assessed the utility of other serum markers of nutrition and demonstrated that serum transferrin predicts both mortality and rate of spontaneous closure, while retinol-binding protein and thyroxin-binding prealbumin are useful in predicting mortality alone.[39] Provision of nutritional support to normalize these serum markers leads to positive nitrogen balance and will aid in the ability to spontaneously heal an enterocutaneous fistula and support healing following operative resection and reconstruction.

Recent work on the mucosal immune hypothesis suggests that both the route and type of nutrition affect the maintenance of intestinal and respiratory integrity and the outcome of critically-ill patients.[65–67] According to the hypothesis, immune cells are sensitized to foreign antigens in the Peyer's patches of the distal small intestine. The sensitized cells are then distributed to submucosal locations in both the intestine and respiratory tract as well as mammary, salivary, and lacrimal glands, where IgA is secreted.[65] In animal studies, provision of a complex enteral formulation protected immune function better than total parenteral nutrition (TPN) or TPN fed intra-gastrically.[65,68] In critically ill patients, enteral feeding resulted in fewer infectious complications.[65,66,69] Enteral feeding, although clearly advantageous, may not always be possible. Further work has demonstrated that supplementing parenteral nutrition with glutamine provides an advantage over nonsupplemented TPN,[70–73] although our own laboratory has been unable to reproduce these findings. An immunosupportive role of nutrition, especially enteral nutrition, can aid in the prevention of sepsis in these patients. A vicious cycle of sepsis contributing to hypercatabolism and malnutrition leading to decreased immunity must be broken to successfully treat these patients.

The social and psychological impact of enterocutaneous fistula cannot be overlooked. Due to the complicated wound care required, malnutrition, and disability, patients with fistulas will be unlikely to be able to work and may lose their employment as well as their source of income and insurance. These patients may become dependent on others for financial support and medical assistance. Additionally, the psychological impact of a difficult, draining, foul-smelling wound and the major impact on the patient's daily activities of living cannot be underestimated.

DIAGNOSIS, EVALUATION, AND MANAGEMENT

Regardless of the etiology or specific nature of the fistula, the ultimate goals in treating patients with enterocutaneous fistula are the re-establishment of bowel continuity, the ability to achieve oral nutrition, and the closure of the fistula. These goals, however, are deceptively simple in these complex patients and can best be achieved through the use of a detailed, multidisciplinary management protocol. Given the metabolic and septic physiology often present with enterocutaneous fistulas, recognition of the development of an enterocutaneous fistula should prompt aggressive resuscitation and stabilization of the patient. Drainage of obvious septic sources must be undertaken and nutritional support commenced. Nutritional support should be delayed 24 hours for drainage, as hematogenous seeding of the catheter may result in catheter sepsis. If an abscess is pointing, one should do a fistulogram through the abscess before open drainage, using an angiocath to see where the water-soluble dye tracks to. Information obtained in this fashion is unlikely to be obtained in any other way. Upon stabilization of the patient, attention turns to diagnostic measures to determine the nature and course of the fistula. This information in combination with the patient's response to nonoperative measures determines the length of time before operative intervention is performed. If surgery is required, meticulous technique in combination with a well-prepared team approach will optimize the likelihood of a successful patient outcome. However, operative closure of the fistula does not end the surgical team's obligation to the patient, as continued nutritional support and physical and emotional rehabilitation are often required to return the patient to his or her pre-illness state. As in any complicated illness, care of the patient with an enterocutaneous fistula can be divided into several phases (Table 7–4).

Phase 1: Recognition and Stabilization

Identification and Resuscitation. The patient presenting with a postoperative enterocutaneous fistula may do well initially for the first few days after operation. Within the first week, however, the patient may suffer delayed return of bowel function and fever. Erythema of the wound develops and opening the wound reveals purulent drainage that is soon followed by enteric contents. The diagnosis is now clear and management shifts from routine postoperative care to the management of a potentially critically ill patient. The combined insults of the preoperative disease process, a bowel preparation, a week of minimal nutritional support, and a septic state often results in a profoundly volume-depleted patient. The first stage in management of the fistula patient, therefore, is the restoration of volume using crystalloid and colloid products as appropriate to restore oxygen-carrying capacity and plasma oncotic pressure. Several liters of crystalloid are usually required to replace fluid lost into the bowel and bowel wall. While maintenance of a specific target hematocrit is controversial, blood should be transfused to support oxygen-carrying capacity to a hematocrit of at least 30%. Similarly, albumin may aid in wound healing[63] and intestinal function[64] and is involved in the transport of certain nutrients and medications. Administration of albumin to a serum level of 3.0 mg/dL supports these functions and is used in our practice unless sepsis-induced capillary leak is present.

Control of Sepsis. The leakage of enteric contents outside of the bowel lumen may lead to generalized peritonitis or abscess in addition to fistula formation. As the leading cause of mortality in modern series of enterocutaneous fistula, aggressive management of sepsis is essential in these patients. Frankly septic patients should be explored to drain abscesses. During these procedures, consideration should be given to performing a fistulogram by injecting water-soluble contrast

TABLE 7–4. MANAGEMENT PHASES OF FISTULA

Phase	Goals	Time Course
Recognition/stabilization	Resuscitation with crystalloid, colloid, or blood Control of sepsis with percutaneous or open drainage and antibiotics Electrolyte repletion Provision of nutrition Control of fistula drainage Commencement of local skin care and protection	24–48 hours
Investigation	Fistulogram to define anatomy and characteristics of fistula	7–10 days
Decision	Evaluate the likelihood of spontaneous closure Decide duration of trial of nonoperative management	10 days to 6 weeks
Definitive management	Plan operative approach Refunctionalization of entire bowel Resection of fistula with end-to-end anastomosis Secure abdominal closure Gastrostomy and jejunostomy	When closure unlikely or after 4–6 weeks
Healing	Continue nutritional support until full oral nutrition achieved Zinc supplementation Psychological and emotional support	5–10 days after closure until full oral nutrition

into the abscess under fluoroscopic guidance. Percutaneous drainage of collections in nonseptic patients should also be performed. Placement of central venous catheters for parenteral nutrition should be delayed for 24 hours following drainage of septic foci, as bacteremia following these procedures may seed catheters, leading to line sepsis and further physiologic insult in these fragile patients.

The use of antibiotics in patients with enterocutaneous fistulas should be reserved for specific indications. Most large series of patients with fistulas demonstrate that patients received seven to nine antibiotics during their treatment.[17,20,74] In order to avoid selecting for resistant organisms, antibiotics should only be given for defined infections and for a set duration of therapy.

Control of Fistula Drainage and Skin Care. Concurrent with drainage of sepsis, a plan to control fistula drainage and provide local skin care will prevent continued irritation of the surrounding skin and abdominal wall structures. Should operation be required, an intact abdominal wall will allow for secure closure and improved chance for lasting resolution of the fistula. Very-low-output fistulas may appear to be adequately managed with dry dressings; however, should the skin close over the fistula tract, an abscess will result. In our experience, a sump constructed from a soft latex catheter (i.e., Robinson nephrostomy tube) may be placed in the wound (Fig 7–6). This tube is soft at body temperature and will not erode into the bowel or abdominal wall structures. The tube is connected to wall suction and vented with a 14-gauge catheter. Accurate recording of fistula output is facilitated by this drainage system.

Protection of the surrounding skin from enteric drainage and from frequent dressing changes can be achieved through a number of preparations including Karaya powder, ileostomy cement, Stomahesive, or ion exchange resins. A skilled enterostomal therapist can often provide useful insight into these issues. More recently, vacuum-assisted closure (VAC) devices have been reported to both

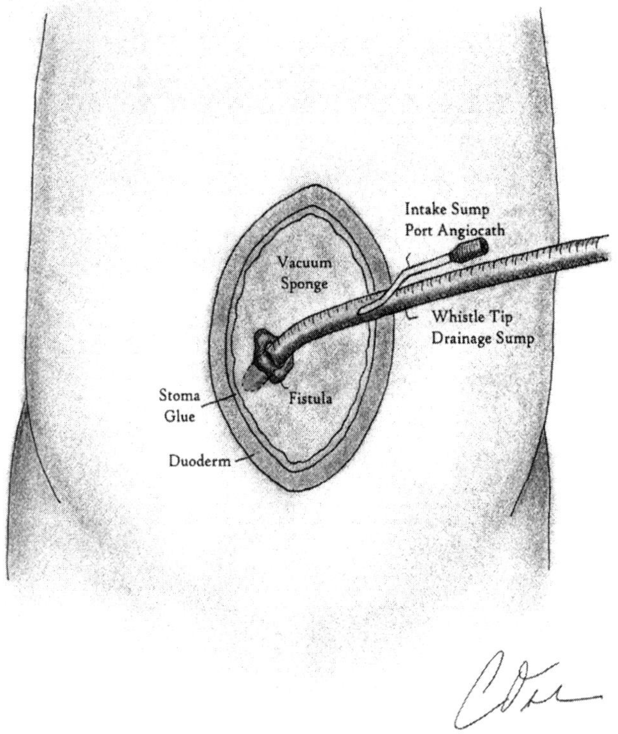

Figure 7–6. A sump drain system using a soft rubber catheter connected to suction and vented with an angiocath provides local control of fistula drainage.

aid in the care of these complicated wounds and promote nonoperative closure[75–77] (Fig 7–7). While there are no large series or randomized trials of the use of these devices in the management of enterocutaneous fistula, VAC dressings provide another option for wound care in these patients. The disadvantage of VAC dressings is the amount of time necessary to change these dressings, often 2–2.5 hours. However, these dressings need only be changed every 5 or so days.

Reduction of Fistula Output. While fistula output does not correlate with the rate of spontaneous closure, reduction of fistula drainage may facilitate wound management and decrease the time to closure. In the absence of obstruction, prolonged nasogastric drainage is not indicated and may even contribute to morbidity in the form of patient discomfort, impaired pulmonary toilet, alar necrosis, sinusitis or otitis media, and late esophageal stricture. Should obstruction be present, operative intervention to relieve the obstruction may be required. Measures to decrease the volume of enteric secretions include administration of histamine antagonists or proton pump inhibitors. Reduction in acid secretion will also aid in the prevention of gastric and duodenal ulceration as well as decrease the stimulation of pancreatic secretion. Sucralfate, a mucosal protective agent, may also reduce gastric acidity while also providing a constipating action that may decrease fistula output as well.

As inhibitors of the secretion of many gastrointestinal hormones including gastrin, cholecystokinin, secretin, insulin, glucagons, and vasoactive peptide, it has been hoped that somatostatin and octreotide may reduce time to closure and promote nonoperative closure of enterocutaneous fistulas. Somatostatin and its analogue octreotide may be used to reduce gastrointestinal secretions, fistula output, and time to closure; however, data that demonstrate an effect on the rate of nonoperative closure of enterocutaneous fistulas are lacking.[78–88] Potential side effects of the use of these agents include difficult glucose homeostasis and cholelithiasis. Large prospective, randomized trials are needed to further clarify the role of somatostatin and octreotide in the management of enterocutaneous fistulas. Octreotide may accelerate closure of pancreatic fistulas, however.

Infliximab, a monoclonal antibody to tumor necrosis factor-alpha, has been shown to be beneficial in inflammatory and fistulizing inflammatory bowel disease.[89–91] Use of infliximab in patients with fistulas following ileal pouch–anal anastomosis for ulcerative colitis resulted in clinical response in six of seven patients and fistula closure in five patients after three treatments.[89] In a study of 100 patients with fistulizing Crohn's disease, infliximab

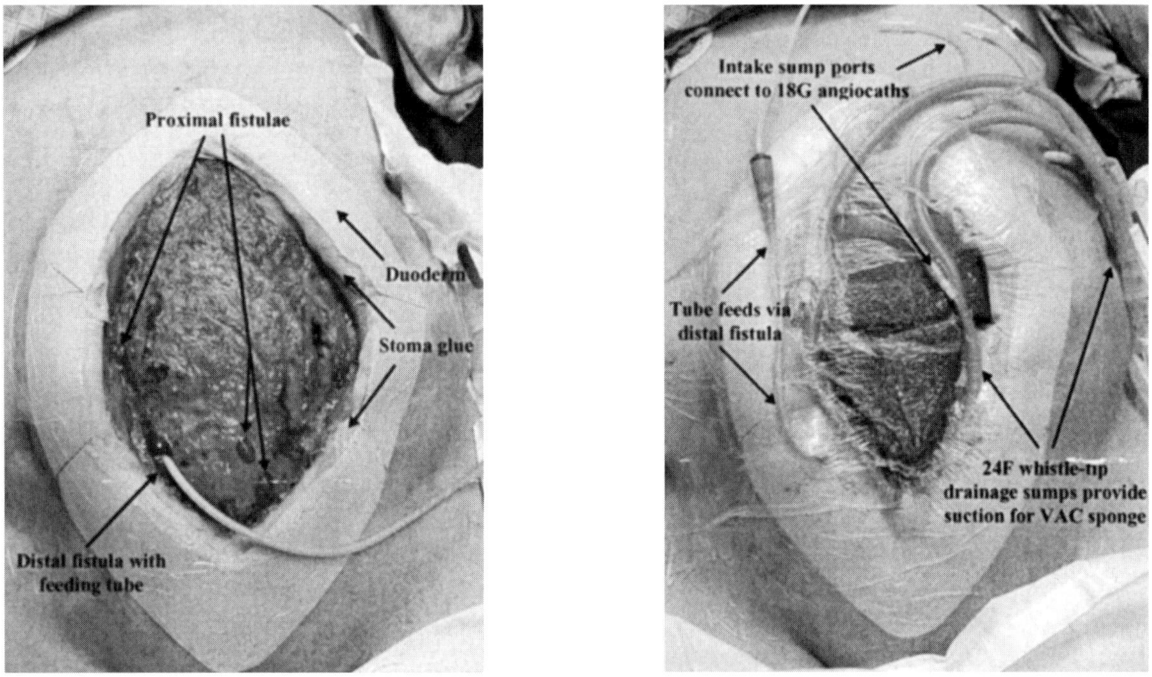

Figure 7–7. Use of a vacuum-assisted closure (VAC) dressing and sumps in the management of an enterocutaneous fistula. **A.** Duoderm was applied to the skin edges while a feeding tube was placed in the distal fistula. **B.** The VAC dressing was applied with sump drains in addition to the suction tubing. (Reprinted, with permission. Shrikhande GV, Fischer JE. Enterocutaneous Fistula. In: Cameron J (ed). *Current Surgical Therapy*, 8th ed. Philadelphia, PA: Elsevier; 2004:136–137.)

infusion resulted in complete response in 50 patients, partial response in 22 patients, and no response in 28 patients.[90] In a randomized trial of patients with chronic fistulas (duration greater than 3 months), administration of infliximab resulted in a significantly increased rate of closure of all fistulas when compared to placebo.[91] Adverse events in these trials were largely infectious complications, including abscess formation, pneumonia, varicella zoster, *Candida* esophagitis, and upper respiratory tract infection.[89–91] Evidence suggests a role of infliximab in treatment of fistulas complicating inflammatory bowel disease; whether this agent will be of use in patients without Crohn's disease or ulcerative colitis remains to be determined.

Nutritional Support. Provision of nutritional support may be all that is necessary for spontaneous healing of enterocutaneous fistulas. Alternatively, should operative intervention be required, normalization of nutritional parameters will provide the patient with the best chance for successful fistula resolution. Malnutrition, identified by Edmunds in 1960 as a major contributor to mortality in these patients, may be present in 55–90% of patients with enterocutaneous fistulas.[17,19] Patients with postoperative enterocutaneous fistulas are often malnourished due to a combination of poor enteral intake, the hypercatabolic septic state, and the loss of protein-rich enteral contents through the fistula. Proper nutrition may improve immune function, provide protein precursors for wound healing, and support the functions of the gastrointestinal tract.

Once sepsis has been controlled, attention to the metabolic and nutritional needs of the patient takes precedence. Assessment of the patient's nutritional status using elements of history via the Subjective Global Assessment,[92] laboratory values, anthropometric analysis, and newer techniques such as bioelectrical impedance anaylsis[93,94] provide a baseline and starting point for planning. Metabolic needs can be estimated using the Harris-Benedict equations and appropriate stress factors. Repeated use of metabolic cart analysis (indirect calorimetry) can provide ongoing assessment of the appropriateness of macronutrient balance. As a general guideline, we provide 25–32 kilocalories per kilogram per day with a calorie:nitrogen ratio of 150:1 to 100:1 and at least 1.5 grams per kilogram per day of protein. These are general principles of nutritional management and ongoing reassessment of each patient's clinical and laboratory values are required to optimize support for these complex patients.

Parenteral nutrition has long been the cornerstone of support for patients with enterocutaneous fistulas.[20,74,95] Parenteral nutrition can be commenced once sepsis has been controlled and appropriate intravenous access has been established. Transition to partial or total enteral nutrition has been advocated in recent reports to prevent atrophy of gastrointestinal mucosa as well as support the immunologic and hormonal functions of the gut and liver.[18] Additionally, parenteral nutrition is expensive and requires dedicated nursing care to prevent undue morbidity and mortality from line insertion, catheter sepsis, and metabolic complications. Thus, attempting enteral feeding is appropriate in most fistula patients. As achieving goal rates of enteral feeding may take several days, patients are often maintained on parenteral nutrition as tube feedings are advanced. Enteral feeding may occur per os, via feeding tubes placed nasogastrically or nasoenterically, or via the fistula itself (i.e., fistuloclysis). Enteral support typically requires 4 feet of small intestine and is contraindicated in the presence of distal obstruction. Drainage from the fistula may be expected to increase with the commencement of enteral feeding; however, spontaneous closure may still occur, often preceded by a decrease in fistula output. A recent report details the experience of an intestinal failure unit in using fistuloclysis in twelve patients prior to reconstructive surgery.[96] Gastrostomy tubes were placed into the bowel distal to the fistula and iso-osmotic polymeric tube feedings were commenced without reinfusion of chyme from the proximal fistula. Eleven of twelve patients were able to discontinue parenteral support and nutritional status was maintained until surgery in nine patients (19–422 days) and for at least 9 months in the two patients who did not undergo operative intervention.[96] Of note, surgeons in this study also reported improved bowel caliber, thickness, and ability to hold sutures in patients who had received enteral nutrition.[96]

Phase 2: Investigation

Once the patient has been stabilized with control of sepsis and commencement of nutritional support, investigation into the course and character of the fistula should be undertaken. This typically occurs 7–10 days after the identification of the fistula and allows time for the fistula tract to mature to the point where catheters can be placed in all orifices. Careful fistulography with water-soluble contrast provides information not obtainable through any other means. The senior surgeon responsible for the patient's care should be present with the most-senior available radiologist for the performance of the study. Particular attention should be paid to the length, course, and relationships of the fistula tract, the absence or presence of bowel continuity or distal obstruction, the nature of the bowel adjacent to the fistula, and the absence or presence of an abscess cavity in communication with the fistula[97] (see Fig 7–5). These details will help determine whether surgical intervention will be necessary, as well as aid in the planning of such a procedure. The early films, without a lot of dye, give the most information.

Computed tomography is most useful in the early management of patients with fistulas to identify abscesses and guide percutaneous interventions. Fistula tracts are not usually visible on axial CT imaging, although sagittal or reconstructed images may provide useful information. Barium contrast upper gastrointestinal studies and enemas rarely provide additional information. If multiple contrast studies are planned, the order of the tests should be carefully planned so that retained contrast will not interfere with subsequent examinations.

Phase 3: Decision

Ideally, provision of a period of sepsis-free nutrition will result in closure of enterocutaneous fistulas within 4–6 weeks. Spontaneous closure of fistulas restores intestinal continuity and allows resumption of oral nutrition. Unfortunately, complex fistulas undergo spontaneous closure in only one-third of cases. Therefore, once resuscitation, wound care, and nutritional support are assured, a decision must be made regarding the likelihood of spontaneous closure of a specific fistula.

Information obtained from imaging investigations provides anatomic details about the fistula, while the specifics of the clinical course of the patient, including weight gain, improvement in nutritional parameters, and decrease in fistula output provide prognostic details. Fistulograms demonstrating fistulas arising from diseased bowel, in proximity to large abscesses, in settings of disruption of intestinal continuity, in the presence of distal obstruction, and those with short tracts (less than 2 cm) are unlikely to close without operative intervention. Similarly, fistulas originating in the stomach, ileum, or near the ligament of Treitz have lower rates of spontaneous closure. In contrast, fistulas arising from biliary, pancreatic, or jejunal sources are more likely to resolve spontaneously (see Table 7–2). Fistulas associated with inflammatory bowel disease often close with nonoperative management only to reopen upon resumption of enteral nutrition. These fistulas should be formally resected once closed to prevent recurrence. Fistulas in the setting of malignancy or irradiated bowel are particularly resistant to closure and would suggest the need for earlier operative intervention.

The timing of operative intervention for fistulas that are unlikely to or fail to close is important. Early operation is indicated to control sepsis not amenable to percutaneous intervention. These early procedures are typically limited to drainage of abscesses and resection of phlegmona with definitive resection of fistulas deferred until the patient can be nutritionally and physiologically optimized. The common practice of waiting at least 4–6 weeks for definitive operative management of enterocutaneous fistulas is based on several factors. First, 90–95% of fistulas that will spontaneous close typically do so within 5 weeks of the original operation.[18,74] Furthermore, operation during the first 10 days to 6 weeks from diagnosis of postoperative fistulas is made more difficult by the "obliterative peritonitis" described by Fazio and associates.[61] In this series, reoperations within 10 days of or delayed at least 6 weeks from the original procedure resulted in mortality rates of 13% and 11%, respectively.[61] In contrast, patients undergoing reoperations between 10 days and 6 weeks of the original laparotomy suffered a mortality rate of 26%. Additionally, delaying operative intervention allows for nutritional support and normalization of serum albumin and transferrin, while delay also allows resolution of local abdominal wound sepsis and preparation of the abdominal wall for secure closure. Optimally, if operation is required, 4 months should elapse from the last operative procedure because the adhesions will have matured and will be easier to deal with after that interval.

Phase 4: Definitive Management

Just as the initial management and diagnosis of patients with gastrointestinal cutaneous fistulas is time- and labor-intensive, the definitive operative reconstruction of these complicated patients requires the commitment of significant time and resources. The surgical team should expect to be in the operating room for up to 7 or 8 hours. Should a complex abdominal wall closure be expected, a fresh team of plastic and reconstructive surgeons should be involved in the planning and performance of the procedure and should be consulted preoperatively with enough time to plan the reconstructive procedure.

The patient should have achieved optimal nutritional parameters and be free of all signs of sepsis. Through careful management of fistula drainage, a well-healed abdominal wall without inflammation should be present. Prophylactic antibiotics should be administered based on the patient's previous microbiological data, and tube feedings should be tapered in the days preceding operation to allow mechanical and antibiotic preparation of the bowel.

The operation should commence through a new incision distant from any potential sources of inflammation or infection. Often, a transverse incision offers the best opportunity to enter the abdomen in an area free of adhesions. If the prior midline incision must be used, entering the abdomen either above or below the limits of the previous incision reduces the risk of inadvertent entry into adherent bowel. Wound towels dipped in antibiotic solution or wound protectors should be used to prevent contamination of the abdominal wall tissues during the course of the operation.

Dissection to free the entire length of the bowel from the ligament of Treitz to the rectum is termed bowel refunctionalization. Refunctionalization identifies and allows resection of all areas of abscess and all sources of obstruction, thus ensuring the best possible chance of avoiding failure of the present operation. Dissection commences in the areas of least dense adhesions. Use of antibiotic-soaked laparotomy pads on areas of dense adhesions often creates edema that aids in further dissection. Use of the scalpel and scissors to sharply dissect adhesions prevents inadvertent damage to the bowel, as does approaching adhesions from the side, rather than head-on. Careful attention to dissection and closure of all enterotomies in the manner of Heineke-Mikulicz and serosal tears with Lembert sutures of 5-0 Prolene provides the patient with the best possible outcome.

Resection of the bowel involved in the fistula is preferred over bypass, Roux-en-Y drainage, or simple serosal patching, although these approaches may be necessary in extreme cases. Bowel anastomosis should be performed using a two-layer, interrupted, end-to-end anastomosis with nonabsorbable sutures in healthy bowel. Avoiding tension and ensuring adequate blood supply are principles of sound surgical practice that must be followed in these difficult reoperative cases. Both throughout and following the steps of dissection, resection, and anastomosis, frequent irrigation of the abdominal cavity with antibiotic solution should be performed, and constant vigilance for inadvertent bowel injury should be maintained. For duodenal fistulas, however, if operation is required, a direct attack on the fistula is less wise. Instead a gastrojejunostomy, with or without vagotomy, with gastrostomy, jejunostomy, and drainage is most likely to give a successful result.

Placement of a flap of omentum between the fresh anastomosis and the abdominal wall closure may prevent recurrence of fistulization. Use of Seprafilm may be an adjuvant therapy to aid in prevention of complications from future adhesions.[98,99] Consideration of placement of a decompressive gastrostomy using a no. 20 whistle-tip catheter obviates the need for prolonged postoperative nasogastric tube placement in the event of prolonged ileus, which may be expected. Nasogastric tubes are uncomfortable and may interfere with ambulation and pulmonary toilet. Similarly, placement of a feeding jejunostomy may also aid in the postoperative care of patients undergoing procedures of this scale.

Abdominal wall closure is the final operative step in the management of patients with enterocutaneous fistulas and is of utmost importance in preventing recurrence. If the abdominal wall has recovered from the previous inflammation and sepsis, a primary closure may be possible. If a difficult closure is anticipated, a complex myocutaneous flap procedure may be required. The involvement of the plastic and reconstructive surgical service is advised under these circumstances and the use of a fresh team will maximize the likelihood of a good outcome for the patient. Under no circumstances should mesh or Goretex be used for closure; intact native tissue should be at the bowel-peritoneal interface or refistulization will likely occur.

As the cumulative experience with complex laparoscopic procedures has increased, several groups have reported laparoscopic approaches to enteric and enterocutaneous fistulas.[100–105] The largest of these series reported 73 procedures in 72 patients, 20% of which were enterocutaneous fistulas.[104] The authors reported a mean operative time of 199 minutes with a 4.1% conversion rate.[104] Average postoperative length of stay was 5.2 days with a complication rate of 11%, consisting of postoperative bleeding, readmission for partial small bowel obstruction and cholecystitis, and infectious complications including pneumonia, urinary tract infection, central line sepsis, and wound infection.[104] In this series, there was one recurrence of a diverticular colovesical fistula 5 months postoperatively.[104] While the role of laparoscopy in managing enterocutaneous fistula patients will likely continue to evolve, the complex nature of many of these fistulas will demand an open approach in order to ensure the best outcome for the patient.

Phase 5: Healing

Whether closure of fistulas occurs spontaneously or through operative management, continuation of support is necessary to avoid recurrence. Nutritional support via tube feedings should be continued until the patient is consistently tolerating at least 1500 kilocalories per day orally. Healing of the surgical wound and anastomoses requires a positive nitrogen balance to avoid breakdown of newly formed proteins. Oral feeding typically commences 1 week postoperatively with a soft diet, rather than with the traditional progression from clear liquids to full liquids. The patient's family and nutritional support staff will play an important role in providing foods that are appealing to the patient, as it is often difficult to persuade these patients to eat. Zinc supplementation may improve patients' sense of taste and increase oral intake. Similarly, cycling tube feedings overnight may stimulate hunger and increase food intake during the day.

Delayed complications continue to be a risk for fistula patients even after healing of their fistulas. Postoperative complications such as anastomotic stricture and adhesive small bowel obstruction, as well as short-bowel syndrome due to multiple resections and recurrence of fistulization may all impede patient recovery. While reoperation in these patients remains a challenge, standard surgical principles should be followed in decision making and performance of any further procedures.

By the time their fistulas have closed, enterocutaneous fistula patients have often been hospitalized for several months with limited ambulation and have suffered from septic and metabolic challenges, thus leaving them physically deconditioned and emotionally fatigued. Physical and occupational therapists play a role throughout each patient's hospitalization, but their efforts become even more important during the healing phase as the focus shifts to reintroducing the patient to normal activities of daily living. Involvement of case management staff early in the patient's course will identify obstacles to the patient's successful reintroduction to an active lifestyle, while use of psychiatric consultation-liaison services will identify and address issues of depression and adaptive disorders. Finally, active involvement by the senior surgeon responsible for the patient's care to ensure a coherent treatment plan and adequate communication with the patient and family will help avoid confusion and fear while dealing with these challenging cases.

One complication not widely reported is the inability of these patients to think clearly and have appropriate decision making. This is particularly important for business owners and highly-placed executives. This is likely due to protein depletion in the brain. This complication normally takes 12–18 months to resolve. The patient should be reassured that this complication will resolve spontaneously with good nutrition.

CONCLUSIONS

Gastrointestinal cutaneous fistulas remain dreaded complications of cancer, inflammatory bowel disease, and general surgical operations. An understanding of the pathophysiology and risk factors for development of these fistulas may minimize their creation as well as provide a sound plan for their management. Early recognition and resuscitation of patients with fistulas combined with control of sepsis and provision of nutritional support may limit associated complications. Investigation into the anatomic and etiological characteristics of each fistula may provide information about the likelihood of spontaneous closure or suggest earlier operative management. Careful planning and technique during definitive surgical therapy and the involvement of a multidisciplinary team will provide the best possibility of resolution of the fistula. Finally, postoperative maintenance of adequate nutrition and physical and emotional support may allow restoration of the patient to a functional and productive role in society and ensures the durability of the repair.

REFERENCES

1. McRitchie DI, Girotti MJ, Glynn MFX et al. Effect of systemic fibrinogen depletion on intraabdominal abscess formation. *J Lab Clin Med* 1991;118:48
2. Altemeier WA, Culbertson WR, Fullen WD et al. Intraabdominal abscesses. *Am J Surg* 1973;125:70
3. Fry DE, Garrison RN, Heitsch RC et al. Determinants of death in patients with intraabdominal abscess. *Surgery* 1980;88:517
4. Taylor KJW, Wasson JF, Graaff C et al. Accuracy of greyscale ultrasound diagnosis of abdominal and pelvic abscesses in 220 patients. *Lancet* 1978;8055:83
5. Mueller PR, Simeone JF. Intraabdominal abscesses: diagnosis by sonography and computed tomography. *Radiol Clin North Am* 1983;21:425
6. Doust BD, Quiroz F, Stewart JM. Ultrasonic distinction of abscesses from other intra-abdominal fluid collections. *Radiology* 1977;125:213
7. Roche J. Effectiveness of computed tomography in the diagnosis of intra-abdominal abscess: a review of 111 patients. *Med J Aust* 1981;2:85
8. Clark RA, Towbin R. Abscess drainage with CT and ultrasound guidance. *Radiol Clin North Am* 1983;21:445
9. Hemming A, Davis NL, Robins RE. Surgical versus percutaneous drainage of intra-abdominal abscesses. *Am J Surg* 1991;161:593
10. Bufalari A, Giustozzi G, Moggi L. Postoperative intraabdominal abscesses: percutaneous versus surgical treatment. *Acta Chir Belg* 1996;96:197
11. Deveney CW, Lurie K, Deveney KE. Improved treatment of intra-abdominal abscess. *Arch Surg* 1988;123:1126
12. Jaques P, Mauro M, Safrit H et al. CT features of intraabdominal abscesses: prediction of successful percutaneous drainage. *AJR Am J Roentgenol* 1986;146:1041
13. Mueller PR, Simeone JF, Butch RJ et al. Percutaneous drainage of subphrenic abscess: a review of 62 patients. *AJR Am J Roentgenol* 1986;147:1237
14. Jeffrey RB, Tolentino CS, Federle MP et al. Percutaneous drainage of periappendiceal abscesses: review of 20 patients. *AJR Am J Roentgenol* 1987;149:59
15. Stabile BE, Puccio E, vanSonnenberg E et al. Preoperative percutaneous drainage of diverticular abscess. *Am J Surg* 1990;159:99
16. Alexander AA, Eschelman DJ, Nazarian LV et al. Transrectal sonographically guided drainage of deep pelvic abscesses. *AJR Am J Roentgenol* 1994;162:1227
17. Edmunds LH, Williams GM, Welch CE. External fistulas arising from the gastro-intestinal tract. *Ann Surg* 1960; 152:445
18. Berry SM, Fischer JE. Enterocutaneous fistulas. *Curr Probl Surg* 1994;31:474
19. Berry SM, Fischer JE. Classification and pathophysiology of enterocutaneous fistulas. *Surg Clin North Am* 1996;76:1009

20. Soeters PB, Ebeid AM, Fischer JE. Review of 404 patients with gastrointestinal fistulas: impact of parenteral nutrition. *Ann Surg* 1979;190:189
21. Myssiorek D, Becker GD. Extended single transverse neck incision for composite resections: does it work? *J Surg Oncol* 1991;48:101
22. Brown MR, McCulloch TM, Funk GF et al. Resource utilization and patient morbidity in head and neck reconstruction. *Laryngoscope* 1997;107:1028
23. Xavier S, Kochhar R, Nagi B et al. Tuberculous esophagocutaneous fistula. *J Clin Gastroenterol* 1996;23:118
24. Janssen DA, Thimsen DA. The extended submental island lip flap: an alternative for esophageal repair. *Plast Reconstr Surg* 1998;102:835
25. Eng J, Sabanathan S, Mearns AJ. Late esophageal fistula after pneumonectomy. *Ann Thorac Surg* 1994;57:1337
26. Fuji T, Kuratsu S, Shirasaki N et al. Esophagocutaneous fistula after anterior cervical spine surgery and successful treatment using a sternocleidomastoid muscle flap. A case report. *Clin Orthop* 1991;267:8
27. Lin JN, Wang KL. Persistent third branchial apparatus. *J Pediatr Surg* 1991;26:663
28. Laskin JL. Parotid fistula after the use of external pin fixation: report of a case. *J Oral Surg* 1978;36:621
29. Rabago LR, Ventosa N, Castro JL et al. Endoscopic treatment of postoperative fistulas resistant to conservative management using biological fibrin glue. *Endoscopy* 2002;34:632
30. Gordon JM, Langer JC. Gastrocutaneous fistula in children after removal of gastrostomy tube: incidence and predictive factors. *J Pediatr Surg* 1999;34:1345
31. Shand A, Pendlebury J, Reading S et al. Endoscopic fibrin sealant injection: a novel method of closing a refractory gastrocutaneous fistula. *Gastrointest Endosc* 1997;46:357
32. Lomis NN, Miller FJ, Loftus TJ et al. Refractory abdominal-cutaneous fistulas or leaks: percutaneous management with a collagen plug. *J Am Coll Surg* 2000;190:588
33. Papavramidis ST, Eleftheriadis EE, Papavramidis TS et al. Endoscopic management of gastrocutaneous fistula after bariatric surgery by using a fibrin sealant. *Gastrointest Endosc* 2004;59:296
34. Gonzalez-Ojeda A, Avalos-Gonzalez J, Mucino-Hernandez MI et al. Fibrin glue as adjuvant treatment for gastrocutaneous fistula after gastrostomy tube removal. *Endoscopy* 2004;36:337
35. Shorr RM, Greaney GC, Donovan AJ. Injuries of the duodenum. *Am J Surg* 1987;154:93
36. Pokorny WJ, Brandt ML, Harberg FJ. Major duodenal injuries in children: diagnosis, operative management, and outcome. *J Pediatr Surg* 1986;21:613
37. Malangoni MA, Madura JA, Jesseph JE. Management of lateral duodenal fistulas: a study of fourteen cases. *Surgery* 1981;90:645
38. Rodkey GV, Welch CE. Duodenal decompression in gastrectomy. *N Engl J Med* 1960262:498
39. Kuvshinoff BW, Brodish RJ, McFadden DW et al. Serum transferrin as a prognostic indicator of spontaneous closure and mortality in gastrointestinal cutaneous fistulas. *Ann Surg* 1993;217:615
40. Reber HA, Robert C, Way LW et al. Management of external gastrointestinal fistulas. *Ann Surg* 1978;188:460
41. Lindberg E, Jarnerot G, Huitfeldt B. Smoking in Crohn's disease: effect on localization and clinical course. *Gut* 1992;33:779
42. Hill GL, Bourchier RG, Witney GB. Surgical and metabolic management of patients with external fistulas of the small intestine associated with Crohn's disease. *World J Surg* 1988;12:191
43. Harper PH, Fazio VW, Lavery IC et al. The long term outcome in Crohn's disease. *Dis Colon Rectum* 1987;30:174
44. Pettit SH, Irving MH. The operative management of fistulous Crohn's disease. *Surg Gynecol Obstet* 1988;167:223
45. Smyth GP, McGreal GT, McDermott EW. Delayed presentation of a gastric colocutaneous fistula after percutaneous endoscopic gastrostomy. *Nutrition* 2003;19:905
46. Kim HS, Lee DK, Baik SK et al. Endoscopic management of colocutaneous fistula after percutaneous endoscopic gastrostomy. *Endoscopy* 2002;34:430
47. Yamazaki T, Sakai Y, Hatakeyama K et al. Colocutaneous fistula after percutaneous endoscopic gastrostomy in a remnant stomach. *Surg Endosc* 1999;13:280
48. Saltzberg DM, Anand K, Juvan P et al. Colocutaneous fistula: an unusual complication of percutaneous endoscopic gastrostomy. *JPEN J Parenter Enteral Nutr* 1987;11:86
49. Nanni G, Bergamini C, Bertoncini M et al. Spontaneous appendicocutaneous fistula: case report and literature review. *Dis Colon Rectum* 1981;24:187
50. Skaane P. Spontaneous appendicocutaneous fistula: report of a case and review of the literature. *Dis Colon Rectum* 1981;24:550
51. Hyett A. Appendicocutaneous fistula: a hazard of incomplete appendectomy. *Aust N Z J Surg* 1995;65:144
52. Russell JC, Welch JP. Operative management of radiation injuries of the intestinal tract. *Am J Surg* 1979;137:433
53. Lui RC, Friedman R, Fleischer A. Management of postirradation recurrent entero-cutaneous fistula by muscle flaps. *Am Surg* 1989;55:403
54. Aitken RJ, Elliot MS. Sigmoid exclusion: a new technique in the management of radiation-induced fistula. *Br J Surg* 1985;72:731
55. Donner CS. Pathophysiology and therapy of chronic radiation-induced injury to the colon. *Dig Dis* 1998;16:253
56. Levy E, Frileux P, Cugnenc PH et al. High-output external fistulae of the small bowel: management with continuous enteral nutrition. *Br J Surg* 1989;76:676
57. Campos ACL, Meguid MM, Coelho JCU. Surgical management of gastrointestinal fistulas. *Surg Clin North Am* 1996;76:1191
58. Campos ACL, Andrade DF, Campos GMR et al. A multivariate model to determine prognostic factors in gastrointestinal fistulas. *J Am Coll Surg* 1999;188:483
59. Shrikhande G, Fischer JE. Enterocutaneous fistula. In: Cameron J (ed). *Current Surgical Therapy*, 9th ed. Baltimore, MD: Mosby; 2003

60. Slin K, Vicaut E, Panis Y et al. Meta-analysis of randomized clinical trials of colorectal surgery with or without mechanical bowel preparation. *Br J Surg* 2004;91:1125
61. Fazio VW, Coutsoftides T, Steiger E. Factors influencing the outcome of treatment of small bowel cutaneous fistula. *World J Surg* 1983;7:481
62. Hill GL, Bourchier RG, Witney GB. Surgical and metabolic management of patients with external fistulas of the small intestine associated with Crohn's disease. *World J Surg* 1988;12:191
63. Kobayashi H, Nagai H, Yasuda Y et al. The early influence of albumin administration on protein metabolism and wound healing in burned rats. *Wound Repair Regen* 2004;12:109
64. Hwang TL, Lue MD, Nee YJ et al. The incidence of diarrhea in patients with hypoalbuminemia due to acute or chronic malnutrition during enteral feeding. *Am J Gastroenterol* 1994;89:376
65. Kudsk KA. Current aspects of mucosal immunology and its influence by nutrition. *Am J Surg* 2002;183:390
66. Kudsk KA, Croce MA, Fabian TC et al. Enteral versus parenteral feeding: effects on septic morbidity after blunt and penetrating abdominal trauma. *Ann Surg* 1992;215:503
67. Shou J, Lappin J, Daly JM. Impairment of pulmonary macrophage function with total parenteral nutrition. *Ann Surg* 1994;219:291
68. King BK, Kudsk HA, Li J et al. Route and type of nutrition influence mucosal immunity to bacterial pneumonia. *Ann Surg* 1999;229:272
69. Moore EE, Moore FA, Franciose RJ et al. Postischemic gut serves as a priming bed for circulating neutrophils that provoke multiple organ failure. *J Trauma* 1994;37:881
70. Burke DJ, Alverdy JC, Aoys E et al. Glutamine-supplemented total parenteral nutrition improves gut immune function. *Arch Surg* 1989;124:1396
71. Kudsk HA, Wu Y, Fukatsu K et al. Glutamine-enriched total parenteral nutrition maintains intestinal interleukin-4 and mucosal immunoglobulin A levels. *J Parenter Enteral Nutr* 2000;24:270
72. Li J, King KA, Janu PG et al. Glycyl-L-glutamine-enriched total parenteral nutrition maintains small intestine gut-associated lymphoid tissue and upper respiratory tract immunity. *J Parenter Enteral Nutr* 1998;22:31
73. DeWitt RC, Wu Y, Renegar KB et al. Glutamine-enriched total parenteral nutrition preserves respiratory immunity and improves survival to a *Pseudomonas* pneumonia. *J Surg Res* 1999;84:13
74. Rose D, Yarborough MF, Canizaro PC et al. One hundred and fourteen fistulas of the gastrointestinal tract treated with total parenteral nutrition. *Surg Gynecol Obstet* 1986;163:345
75. Erdmann D, Drye C, Heller L et al. Abdominal wall defect and enterocutaneous fistula treatment with the vacuum-assisted closure (VAC) system. *Plast Reconst Surg* 2001;108:2066
76. Alvarez AA, Maxwell GL, Rodriguez GC. Vacuum-assisted closure for cutaneous gastrointestinal fistula management. *Gynecol Oncol* 2001;80:413
77. Cro C, George KH, Donnelly J et al. Vacuum assisted closure system in the management of enterocutaneous fistulae. *Postgrad Med J* 2002;78:364
78. Torres AJ, Landa JI, Moren-Azcoita M et al. Somatostatin in the management of gastrointestinal fistulas: a multicenter trial. *Arch Surg* 1992;127:97
79. Nubiola-Calonge P, Badia JM, Sancho J et al. Blind evaluation of the effect of octreotide (SMS 201-995), a somatostatin analogue, on small-bowel fistula output. *Lancet* 1987;2:672
80. Scott NA, Finnegan S, Irving MH. Octreotide and postoperative enterocutaneous fistulae: a controlled prospective study. *Acta Gastroenterol Belg* 1993;56:266
81. Sancho JJ, di Costanzo J, Nubiola P et al. Randomized double-blind placebo-controlled trial of early octreotide in patients with postoperative enterocutaneous fistula. *Br J Surg* 1995;82:638
82. Hild P, Dobroschke J, Henneking K et al. Treatment of enterocutaneous fistulas with somatostatin. *Lancet* 1986;2:626
83. Ysebaert D, Van Hee R, Hubens G et al. Management of digestive fistulas. *Scand J Gastroenterol Suppl* 1994;207:42
84. di Costanzo J, Cano N, Martin J. Somatostatin in persistent gastrointestinal fistula treated by total parenteral nutrition. *Lancet* 1982;2:338
85. Nubiola P, Badia JM, Martinez-Rodenas F et al. Treatment of 27 postoperative enterocutaneous fistulas with the long half-life somatostatin analogue SMS 201-995. *Ann Surg* 1989;210:56
86. Isenmann R, Schielke DJ, Morl FK et al. Adjuvant therapy with somatostatin IV in post-operative fistulae of the pancreas, gall bladder, and small intestine: a multicenter, randomized study. *Akt Chir* 1994;29:96
87. Hernandez-Aranda JC, Gallo-Chico B, Flores-Ramirez LA et al. Treatment of enterocutaneous fistulae with or without octreotide and parenteral nutrition. *Nutr Hosp* 1996;11:226
88. Spiliotis J, Vagenas K, Panagopoulos K. Treatment of enterocutaneous fistulas with TPN and somatostatin, compared with patients who received TPN only. *Br J Clin Pract* 1990;44:616
89. Viscido A, Habib FI, Kohn A et al. Infliximab in refractory pouchitis complicated by fistulae following ileo-anal pouch for ulcerative colitis. *Aliment Pharmacol Ther* 2003;17:1263
90. Ricart E, Panaccione R, Loftus EV et al. Infliximab for Crohn's disease in clinical practice at the Mayo Clinic: the first 100 patients. *Am J Gastroenterol* 2001;96:722
91. Present DH, Rutgeerts P, Targan S et al. Infliximab for the treatment of fistulas in patients with Crohn's disease. *N Engl J Med* 1999;340:1398
92. Chintapatla S, Scott NA. Intestinal failure in complex gastrointestinal fistulae. *Nutrition* 2002;18:991
93. Wang XB, Ren JA, Li JS. Sequential changes of body composition in patients with enterocutaneous fistula during the 10 days after admission. *World J Gastroenterol* 2002;8:1149
94. Cox-Reijven PL, van Kreel B, Soeters PB. Bioelectrical impedance measurements in patients with gastrointestinal disease: validation of the spectrum approach and a comparison of different methods for screening nutritional depletion. *Am J Clin Nutr* 2003;78:1111

95. MacFadyen BV, Dudrick SJ, Ruberg RL. Management of gastrointestinal fistulas with parenteral hyperalimentation. *Surgery* 1973;74:100
96. Teubner A, Morrison K, Ravishankar HR et al. Fistuloclysis can successfully replace parenteral feeding in the nutritional support of patients with enterocutaneous fistula. *Br J Surg* 2004;91:625
97. Aguirre A, Fischer JE, Welch CE. The role of surgery and hyperalimentations in therapy of gastrointestinal-cutaneous fistulae. *Ann Surg* 1974;180:393
98. DeCherney AH, diZerega GS. Clinical problem of intraperitoneal postsurgical adhesion formation following general surgery and the use of adhesion prevention barriers. *Surg Clin North Am* 1997;77:671
99. Vrijland WW, Tseng LN, Eijkman HJ et al. Fewer intraperitoneal adhesions with use of hyaluronic acid-carboxymethylcellulose membrane: a randomized clinical trial. *Ann Surg* 2002;235:193
100. Hewett PJ, Stitz R. The treatment of internal fistulae that complicate diverticular disease of the sigmoid colon by laparoscopically assisted colectomy. *Surg Endosc* 1995;9:411
101. Joo JS, Agachan F, Wexner SD. Laparoscopic surgery for lower gastrointestinal fistulas. *Surg Endosc* 1997;11:116
102. Poulin EC, Schlachta CM, Mamazza J et al. Should enteric fistulas from Crohn's disease or diverticulitis be treated laparoscopically or by open surgery? A matched cohort study. *Dis Colon Rectum* 2000;43:621
103. Watanabe M, Hasegawa H, Yamamoto S et al. Successful application of laparoscopic surgery to the treatment of Crohn's disease with fistulas. *Dis Colon Rectum* 2002;45:1057
104. Regan JP, Salky BA. Laparoscopic treatment of enteric fistulas. *Surg Endosc* 2004;18:252
105. Garcia GD, Freeman IGH, Zagorski SM et al. A laparoscopic approach to the surgical management of enterocutaneous fistula in a wound healing by secondary intention. *Surg Endosc* 2004;18:554

Section III

ESOPHAGUS

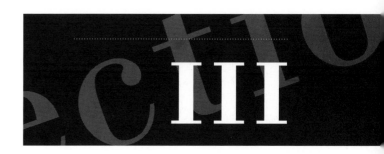

8

Benign Esophageal Disorders

Todd Woltman ▪ Brant K. Oelschlager

The esophagus is a muscular tube that transports ingested material from the pharynx to the stomach. Its function is complex and it is subject to a variety of disorders. This chapter deals with the most common benign disorders including paraesophageal hernia, esophageal diverticula, motility disorders and perforation. We hope to provide a simple and logical approach for the evaluation and treatment of these disorders. Reviews of esophageal malignancy and gastroesophageal reflux disease can be found elsewhere in this book.

▪ PARAESOPHAGEAL HERNIA

Paraesophageal hernias result from a defect of the diaphragmatic hiatus wherein gradual enlargement of the hiatal orifice allows abdominal contents to herniate into the mediastinum. This is usually a naturally acquired condition but similar clinical presentations may occur after trauma or after previous surgery on the gastroesophageal junction (i.e., fundoplication). The stomach by itself is most typically involved; however, other associated organs may be included within the hernia sac including the spleen, colon, pancreas, or liver. Surgical tradition has been that these defects are at high risk of causing serious morbidity and mortality. Consequently, in the past the mere existence of a paraesophageal hernia was thought significant enough to warrant operative intervention.[1–3] However, we now know that these hernias are not always symptomatic and that they are often discovered incidentally. Thus several controversies surrounding paraesophageal hernias exist, including which patients should undergo repair and how the repair should be carried out.

ETIOLOGY AND ANATOMIC CLASSIFICATION

Hiatal hernias are classified by the anatomic location of the gastroesophageal junction in relation to the diaphragmatic hiatus and by the composition of the hernia sac. Type I hiatal hernias represent the traditional "sliding" hiatal hernia. This is characterized by cephalad displacement of the gastroesophageal junction through the hiatus into the mediastinum (Fig 8–1). They represent the vast majority of hiatal hernias. Most of these hernias are small and asymptomatic, and are rarely the cause of severe problems. Herniation is the result of weakening and gradual attenuation of the phrenoesophageal membrane and diaphragmatic crura. They are usually reducible, but may become fixed above the hiatus if they become large. The presence of a type I hiatal hernia may predispose to gastroesophageal reflux, as there is loss of extrinsic contribution to the anti-reflux mechanism of the lower esophageal sphincter.

Type II hiatal hernias are characterized by superior migration of the fundus of the stomach along side the gastroesophageal junction and esophagus into the mediastinum (Fig 8–2). In these hernias the gastroesophageal junction remains in its normal intra-abdominal position. These hernias are also referred to as "rolling" hernias.

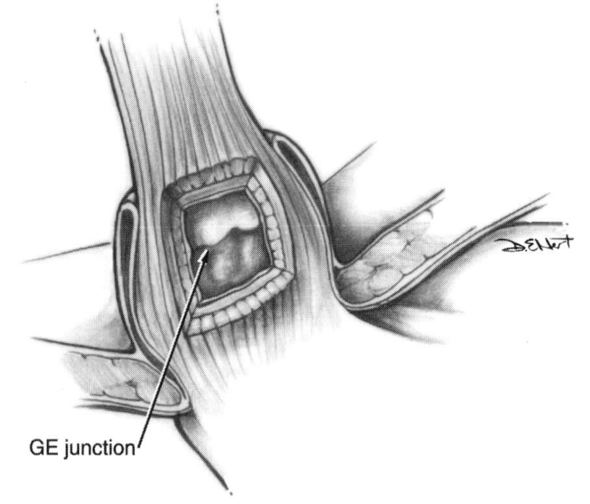

Figure 8–1. Type I hiatal hernia or sliding hiatal hernia.

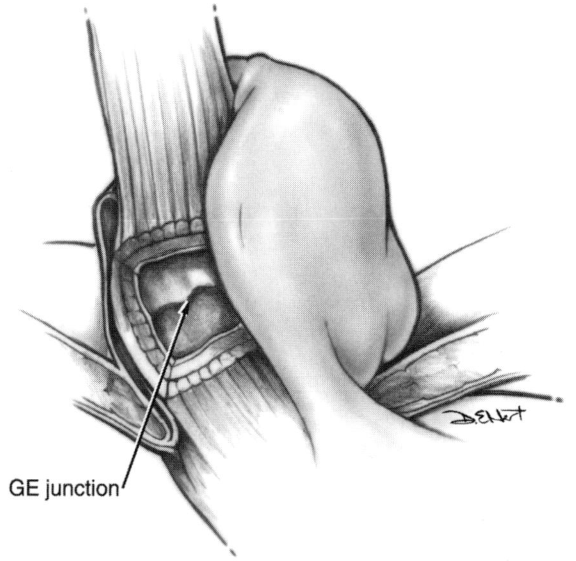

Figure 8–3. Type III hiatal hernia.

Type III hiatal hernias represent a combination of types I and II and are more common than a pure type II hernia. In this case both the gastroesophageal junction and the fundus migrate through the hiatus (Fig 8–3). There is a gradual and progressive lack of fixation of the gastroesophageal junction with attenuation of the intra-abdominal gastric attachment such as the gastrosplenic attachments. The defects may become quite large, with the entire stomach residing in the chest, being referred to as "giant" paraesophageal hernias. This mobility ultimately leaves the stomach susceptible to partial or complete outlet obstruction as well as to volvulus. Volvulus is typically organoaxial with twisting along the longitudinal axis of the stomach. However, mesoaxial volvulus may occur, in which the stomach folds anterior along its transverse axis.

Type IV hernias are distinguished by the presence of other abdominal viscera within the defect. This commonly includes omentum and transverse colon, but may also include others as previously stated.[4] These defects appear to have a higher incidence of serious results with 50% of the patients presenting emergently.[5]

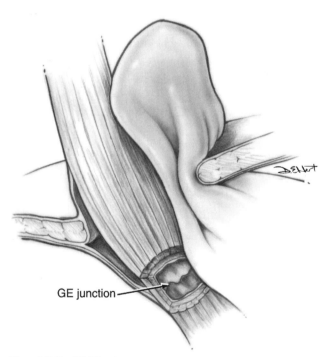

Figure 8–2. Type II hiatal hernia.

CLINICAL PRESENTATION

Paraesophageal hernias are not uniformly symptomatic, many are discovered incidentally on chest x-ray or during endoscopy performed for other reasons. This fact becomes important when deciding whether or not to operate on a patient with a paraesophageal hernia. The true incidence of paraesophageal hernia is unknown. The frequently asymptomatic nature of even sizable paraesophageal hernias makes estimation of the denominator difficult. In a review of 7310 patients with hiatal hernia, a paraesophageal hernia was identified in 14.3%.[6]

Commonly presenting symptoms include early satiety, postprandial bloating or pain, dysphagia, heartburn, and regurgitation. Additional symptoms include chest pain and dyspnea. Severe pain is usually as the result of volvulus or incarceration. Some patients may present with pneumonia secondary to recurring silent aspiration. Many patients' symptoms come to light only retrospectively through careful history taking.

There is a high incidence of iron deficiency anemia in this population. In fact, this problem affects more than one-third of patients with this condition.[7] This results from recurrent bleeding due to Cameron's ulcers and chronic ischemia of the gastric fundus secondary to extrinsic compression from the crura.

Historically it was reported that 20–45% of patients may present with acute onset of cataclysmic complications such as incarceration with strangulation or severe bleeding,[3,8] and with such acute presentation the operative mortality in some small series approached 50%.[3,8] A contributing factor to these unfortunate outcomes is that paraesophageal hernias tend to occur in older patients who frequently have multiple comorbidities. It was for this reason that many advocated repair of all these defects before acute volvulus occurred.

DIAGNOSIS AND EVALUATION

The physical exam is frequently unrevealing in these patients, especially when the presence of a paraesophageal hernia is unsuspected. Auscultation of the chest may reveal decreased breath sounds or the presence of bowel sounds. Chest percussion may reveal dullness secondary to space-occupying abdominal viscera within the thorax.

IMAGING STUDIES

Upright posteroanterior and lateral chest films can often confirm the diagnosis of paraesophageal hernia. In fact many paraesophageal hernias are discovered when chest films are obtained for wholly unrelated reasons. A retrocardiac air-fluid level due to the intrathoracic stomach is a classic finding. If a nasogastric tube is in place it may be observed coiling within the stomach above the diaphragm.

A barium upper GI series is an invaluable test in the evaluation of paraesophageal hernia. It gives accurate anatomic information about the extent of the hernia and the location of the gastroesophageal junction, delineating the type of hernia present. It also provides functional information, as it can assess gastric emptying and reveal evidence of gastroesophageal reflux.

Computed tomography is a secondary modality in the detection of paraesophageal hernia. However, it can provide valuable information about organ involvement in type IV hernias. Recent developments in 3-D reconstruction have enabled imaging with amazing detail. In the future, this technology may prove useful in evaluating the structure of the diaphragmatic crura and its anatomic relations to the stomach, aiding in preoperative planning.

ENDOSCOPY

Flexible endoscopy can be helpful in diagnosing and characterizing paraesophageal hernias. Technically, entrance into the stomach may be difficult due to the complex geometry of the hernia and the gastroesophageal junction. Using a retroflexed view the operator can evaluate the appearance of the gastroesophageal junction and the hernia. In a type II hernia there will be a separate orifice adjacent to the gastroesophageal junction extending cranially. With a type III hernia the scope will be seen entering the pouch itself, above a constriction caused by extrinsic compression from the hiatus. Additionally, endoscopy allows for inspection and biopsy of the esophageal and gastric mucosa. This is essential to evaluate for Barrett's esophagus, ulcers, and occult malignancy, especially in patients with chronic anemia.

MANOMETRY AND PH TESTING

While utilization of manometry in the evaluation of paraesophageal hernias is not mandatory, we routinely perform this study. It does provide useful information on esophageal peristalsis. Intubation of the lower esophageal sphincter (LES) may be difficult or impossible. If successfully intubated, information on LES pressures and relaxation are obtained. Identification of the LES also allows for accurate placement of pH probes if ambulatory pH testing is used to quantify acid exposure when reflux seems to be contributing to symptoms. Some groups who selectively perform fundoplications in concert with paraesophageal hernia repair use 24-hour pH studies to aid in patient selection. However, one could reasonably decide that pH testing is not absolutely necessary in the evaluation of the symptomatic patient.

THERAPY

Several controversies exist regarding the treatment for paraesophageal hernias, including operative indications, approaches, and technical details such as the use of prosthetic mesh and the importance of fundoplication. We believe that a correction of the hernia is indicated in patients with symptoms. There are widely divergent opinions with regard to the indications for surgery in patients with incidentally discovered paraesophageal hernias.

INDICATIONS FOR TREATMENT

Retrospective studies published in the late 1960s[3,9] reported a considerable incidence of severe complications in patients with mild symptoms due to paraesophageal hernias who were followed expectantly. Skinner and Belsey reported that nearly one-third of the 21 patients that they followed eventually died due to complications attributable to their hernia.[9] In their hands, elective paraesophageal hernia repair carried a 1% mortality, leading to the recommendation for elective repair of all paraesophageal hernias. More recently, this belief has been challenged. In a more recent report of 23 patients followed for up to 20 years (median 6.5 years) only 4 patients developed progressive symptoms.[10]

Early reports may have overestimated the rate of complications in patients followed expectantly, especially in patients with minimal or no symptoms. Since most paraesophageal hernias are asymptomatic and discovered incidentally, there are likely many more people who have hernias who never develop a problem than those who do. Many patients with paraesophageal hernias are elderly and have multiple comorbidities, thus they are more likely to have perioperative complications. In a study using a Markov Monte Carlo analysis, Stylopoulos and colleagues[11] estimated that patients undergoing a strategy of watchful waiting would develop acute symptoms requiring surgery at a rate of 1.1% per year. Using this estimate, they projected that less than 20% or patients would benefit from elective repair of asymptomatic or minimally symptomatic paraesophageal hernias.

CONTROVERSIES

Operative Approach

The approach and extent of the repair is also controversial. Regardless of the approach several goals should be accomplished: (1) reduction of the hernia contents into the abdomen, (2) excision of the hernia sac, and (3) repair of the diaphragmatic defect. Repairs can be carried out through the chest or through the abdomen, with each having its champions. Laparoscopic techniques allow repair without the morbidity of a thoracotomy or large abdominal incision.

The transthoracic approach has the major advantage of allowing for direct mobilization of the intrathoracic esophagus and well as for the potential to perform a gastroplasty. These techniques are required if a shortened esophagus is encountered (which is relatively common in paraesophageal hernias), allowing for tension-free closure of the crural defect. Several authors have suggested that tension due to esophageal shortening is a major contributor to hernia recurrence after repair.[12,13] Esophageal mobilization is more difficult with the open transabdominal approach. In contrast, the laparoscopic approach allows for extensive mobilization of the mediastinal esophagus and some believe that a true short esophagus is rarely encountered.[14,15] This has been our experience as well. Indeed we mobilize the esophagus to the aortic arch if required. Furthermore, if a gastroplasty is felt to be necessary, it can be accomplished laparoscopically. The transabdominal approach allows for more efficient reduction of the hernia contents and re-creation of the intra-abdominal anatomy. From the chest, reduction is accomplished by pushing the hernia within the abdomen followed by crural repair. The transabdominal approach avoids the need for single lung ventilation, a significant benefit in a frail patient with underlying pulmonary disease.

There has been much enthusiasm for laparoscopic repair of paraesophageal hernias. Potential advantages include small incisions, less pain, quicker recovery, and shorter hospital stays. When compared to the standard open abdominal approach, there is better visualization of the hiatus and the mediastinum with laparoscopy.

Prudence is necessary, as with paraesophageal hernias there is major distortion of the anatomy, making these operations technically challenging. One can become easily confused resulting in potentially disastrous complications. These operations should only be approached by surgeons with significant advanced laparoscopic foregut experience. Several experienced groups have sizable series demonstrating the feasibility and the safety of this approach for paraesophageal hernias.[12,16,17] However, recent reports suggesting a high recurrence rate has given some surgeons pause. Hashemi and associates[13] reported a 41% recurrence rate after a laparoscopic approach compared to a 15% recurrence rate after thoracotomy or laparotomy. In the laparoscopic group, the majority of the recurrences were radiographic recurrences, with two-thirds of the patients experiencing no or minimal symptoms.

Crural Repair

The durability of the crural repair depends on a tension-free closure. This may be difficult under certain circumstances. A large long-standing defect may make a tension-free cruroplasty impossible, such that even if the pillars are approximated, the persistent stress may lead to failure. With large defects the muscle of the crura becomes attenuated and weak, providing ineffective material to hold stitches. Even in normal circumstances, the hiatal repair is under constant assault. Every time the patient coughs, sneezes, or strains, stress is placed on the repair. Some surgeons routinely utilize pledgets to help prevent sutures from pulling through.

Many surgeons have advocated the use of prosthetic material to provide a tension-free closure or to buttress a primary repair. This approach has proven successful in preventing recurrence in other types of hernia repairs, such as inguinal or incisional hernias. Some surgeons perform a relaxing incision in the diaphragm followed by primary closure of the crura.[5] The prosthetic material is then used to repair the defect from the relaxing incision. This technique may aid in keeping the mesh from lying adjacent to the esophagus or stomach. Several potential disadvantages of routine use of these materials exist, including the potential for esophageal stricture, mesh migration, infection, and erosion into the esophagus or stomach. This has led to some reluctance about their use.[18,19] Polypropylene mesh in particular produces significant adhesions and should be avoided. Polytetrafluoroethylene has the benefit of producing fewer adhesions, but it still has the potential for erosion into the esophagus.

Recently, we proposed the use of a bioabsorbable collagen mesh derived from porcine small intestinal submucosa to buttress the crural repair.[20] It has the benefit of being biologically inert and completely resorbable within 6–12 months. It is designed to serve as a scaffold for fibroblast ingrowth and ultimately to promote a strong native tissue matrix. Short-term safety has been demonstrated but long-term success in preventing recurrence remains to be demonstrated.

Routine Fundoplication

Some surgeons propose the performance of an anti-reflux procedure only when there is preoperative evidence of gastroesophageal reflux disease.[21–23] They support this with the low incidence of postoperative reflux symptoms in their series. However, when 24-hour pH testing is performed, abnormal postoperative acid exposure is detected in up to 40% of patients.[19,24] Even in patients without abnormal reflux prior to operation, extensive dissection around the gastroesophageal junction disrupts external attachments that are important to the physiological anti-reflux barrier. Many surgeons, including our group, believe that the addition of a fundoplication and anchoring of the wrap to the hiatus may aid in preventing recurrence.

OPERATIVE TECHNIQUE: LAPAROSCOPIC PARAESOPHAGEAL HERNIA REPAIR

Positioning

The patient is positioned in the low lithotomy position with the anterior superior iliac spine 10 cm above the break. The patient is placed on a beanbag and a gel pad which are molded to form a seat to support the patient when placed in the reverse Trendelenburg position. Both arms are tucked. The surgeon stands between the legs with the assistant on the surgeon's right. The method of access is at the surgeon's discretion. Five ports are used and are placed as shown in Figure 8–4. After placement of the ports the patient is placed

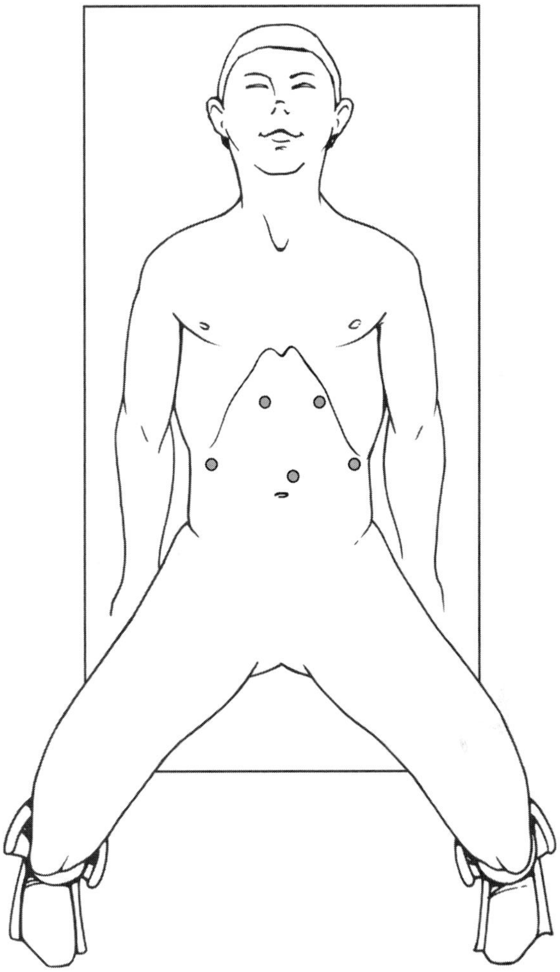

Figure 8–4. Laparoscopic port placement for a hiatal hernia repair.

in full reverse Trendelenburg position and a liver retractor is placed, held in place by self-retaining holder attached to the table.

Dissection

The operation is begun by gently reducing the hernia contents. We follow a left-crus approach as we have previously described.[16] The short gastric vessels are then divided using an ultrasonic shears, including any posterior attachments between the stomach and the retroperitoneum. Using an electrocautery hook the sac is the opened at its attachment to the left crus and gently dissected off the muscle (Fig 8–5). It is important to stay in the correct plane and preserve the fragile crural pillars. Dissection is continued anteriorly around the hiatus, while continually providing retraction of the sac, caudally mobilizing it out of the mediastinum. During this phase of the operation, care is taken to identify the esophagus and the anterior vagus nerve, which are easily obscured by the redundant sac. Identification of the esophagus and accurate dissection is aided by the

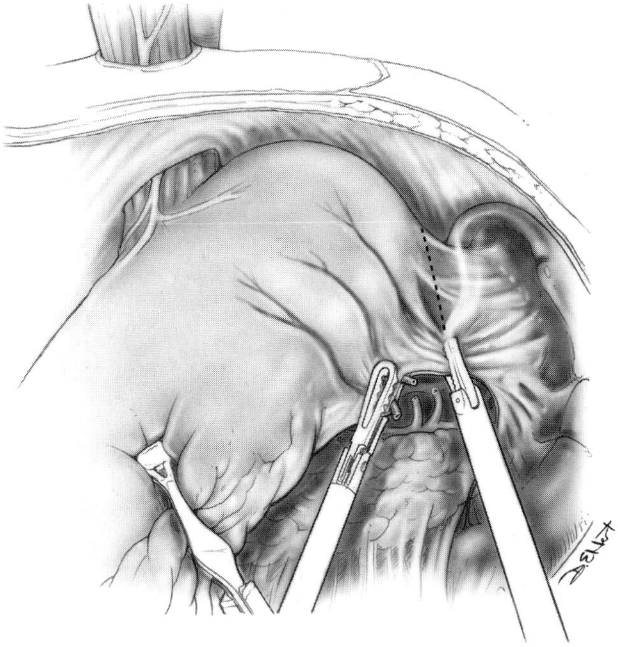

Figure 8–5. After the short gastric vessels are divided the phrenoesophageal membrane is easily exposed and divided.

use of a 52F lighted bougie. The bougie can constrain esophageal mobility, and thus is pulled back into the proximal esophagus and advanced when necessary.

The hepatogastric ligament is then opened. The right attachments of the sac to the crus are then divided and the posterior vagus nerve identified. The left gastric vessels may be drawn up through the hiatus. In this case the vessel is identified and preserved. A retroesophageal window is created to allow the passage of a 2.2-cm Penrose drain, which is used to encircle the esophagus at the gastroesophageal junction. The assistant grasps the Penrose and manipulates the esophagus and stomach to provide retraction and exposure.

Once the sac is fully reduced, mediastinal dissection is continued until the esophagus has at least 3-cm presenting in the abdomen without tension. There are frequently posterior aortoesophageal branches that will require division with the ultrasonic shears or clips. As stated previously, with the utilization of extensive esophageal mobilization we have found the occurrence of a true short esophagus to be infrequent. After full eversion of the sac, it is resected. The anterior vagus is identified and excision is begun just to the left of the nerve. We believe this will prevent recurrences. Furthermore, when the fundoplication is performed it prevents the inclusion of the often bulky sac within the wrap.

Crural Repair and Fundoplication

When mobilization is complete, attention is turned toward closure of the crural defect. This is accomplished with interrupted 2-0 nonabsorbable sutures. Closure is begun posterior to the esophagus at the decussation of the right and left crura (Fig 8–6). Lowering the pressure of pneumoperitoneum to 10 or 12 mm Hg or occasionally tying the knots externally as suggested by Way (Way, JACS) may aid in the cruroplasty. Infrequently we judge that complete posterior closure will produce excessive anterior angulation of the esophagus and we place one or two anterior sutures. The tightness of the repair is gauged using the 50F bougie, in order to avert postoperative dysphagia. After closing the hiatus, the bougie is withdrawn and a fundoplication is created. It is our preference to perform a Nissen fundoplication. This not only protects against gastroesophageal reflux disease (which occurs in up to 50% of patients if cruroplasty only is performed), but with our technique, it is also an effective gastropexy. A marking stitch is then placed 3 cm from the gastroesophageal junction and 2 cm medial to the greater curve. The surgeon pulls the fundus through the retroesophageal window and identifies the marking stitch. A mirror image portion of the anterior fundus is brought forward to the esophagus from left to right to join the posterior fundus at the 9 o'clock position. The geometry of the wrap is checked for symmetry by returning the posterior fundus back through the retroesophageal window. When constructed correctly, the divided vessels along the greater curve should lie in apposition to the left diaphragmatic crus, while the sutured fundoplication should be in the right side.

A total of four sutures are placed to create a 2.5- to 3-cm fundoplication over a 50F bougie. The anterior aspect should lie at 11 o'clock. We then place two coronal sutures that act to secure the wrap and gastroesophageal junction below the hiatus. The surgeon places a stitch through the top of the fundoplication on the

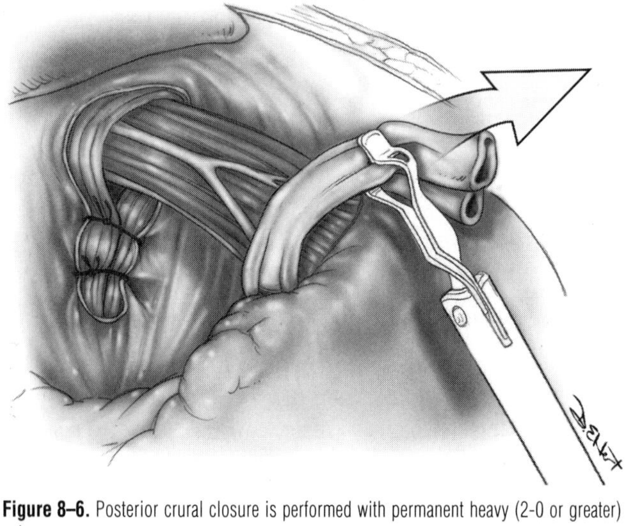

Figure 8–6. Posterior crural closure is performed with permanent heavy (2-0 or greater) suture.

right, through the lateral wall of the esophagus, and finally through the right crus. A similar suture is placed on the left. Two or three additional gastropexy sutures are placed to secure the wrap where it naturally lies, anteriorly and posteriorly, to the repaired hiatus.

For the open technique, essentially the same steps are taken but through a midline incision.

▪ MOTILITY DISORDERS

Swallowing is an elaborate coordination of events that results in propulsion of a food bolus from the oropharynx to the stomach, while simultaneously preventing aspiration of foodstuffs into the airway. Disruption of these complex mechanisms, usually referred to as motor disorders, can result in symptoms, most notably chest pain and/or dysphagia. Achalasia is the most frequently surgically treated of these entities. There are other "spastic" motility disorders of the esophagus such as diffuse esophageal spasm, hypertensive lower esophageal sphincter, and nutcracker esophagus, which share some of the characteristics of achalasia, and occasionally require surgical intervention. The main goal of surgical therapy in these motility disorders is the treatment of dysphagia by facilitating esophageal emptying. Medical therapy is usually ineffective in improving emptying; therefore a mechanical intervention of some sort is most often required. Chest pain, the other common symptom of motility disorders, is much more difficult to treat and does not always improve when dysphagia is corrected. The most common procedure to facilitate esophageal emptying is an esophageal myotomy, which is very effective in the treatment of achalasia. Esophagectomy is generally not a satisfactory option; it ultimately results in the replacement of the nonfunctioning esophagus with an inert tube (which lacks peristalsis) and it places the patient at a much higher risk.

SPASTIC MOTILITY DISORDERS

Patient Presentation and Evaluation

Dysphagia and chest pain are the hallmarks of esophageal spastic disorders, with chest pain often the predominant symptom. After appropriate investigation has eliminated coronary artery disease as the source, examination of the esophagus is often the most logical step. The evaluation of each of these disorders is similar, beginning with a careful history. This should include a psychological history, as psychiatric disorders may be discovered in many of these patients. A barium esophagogram and upper endoscopy are required to evaluate for structural etiologies or malignancy. Manometry is essential for characterizing the motility disorder in question. The treatment is typically based on the manometric findings of each disorder. While the patient may not have classic reflux symptoms, 24-hour pH monitoring should be considered if the above-mentioned work-up is unrevealing. Gastroesophageal reflux disease (GERD) is a common cause of noncardiac chest pain and should be considered in these patients. GERD and motility disorders can coexist; in fact, in some cases GERD may be a contributor to the underlying manometric abnormality. Abnormal reflux can be found in 20–50% of these patients with spastic motility disorders,[25–27] and pharmacological treatment of the patient's reflux may lead to improvement in symptoms.[27,28] Surgical anti-reflux therapy may also be performed in patients with GERD and motility disorders, and should not be considered a contraindication to a fundoplication. We recently reported successfully treating patients with GERD and various hypercontractile esophageal motility disorders (such as hypertensive lower esophageal sphincter and nutcracker esophagus) with a Nissen fundoplication with success similar to those without motility disorders.[29]

Diffuse Esophageal Spasm

Diffuse esophageal spasm (DES) was originally described by Osgood in 1889.[30] It is found in 3–5% of patients evaluated for esophageal motility disorders,[25] and is manometrically distinguished by relatively normal motility punctuated by simultaneous contractions. It is defined by the presence of these simultaneous contractions in greater than 20% of wet swallow. Manometry may also demonstrate long-duration contractions, high-amplitude waves, spontaneous contractions not associated with swallows, and elevated LES pressures. The etiology of DES is unknown. Patients are often hypersensitive to provocative agents such a cholinergic agonists and pentagastrin.[31] Barium esophagogram may be normal or may show disorganized peristalsis with the classic "corkscrew" esophagus. Upper endoscopy is typically unremarkable. Recent evidence suggests that there may be a defect in neural inhibition that is normally mediated by nitric oxide within the esophageal body.[32] Surgery plays a very limited role in the treatment of this problem.

Nutcracker Esophagus

Nutcracker esophagus (NE) was first described in 1977 by Pope and associates.[33] The term was coined by Benjamin and Castell[34] based on the characteristic high-amplitude (>180 mm Hg) waves that may be prolonged in nature (>6 s). As with DES, patients with NE may have a hypersensitive esophagus. Intraesophageal balloon distention reproduces the chest pain experienced by these patients.[35] LES pressures may be normal but are often elevated, with normal relaxation (Fig 8–7). As the pattern of peristalsis is not altered, barium esophagogram is usually unremark-

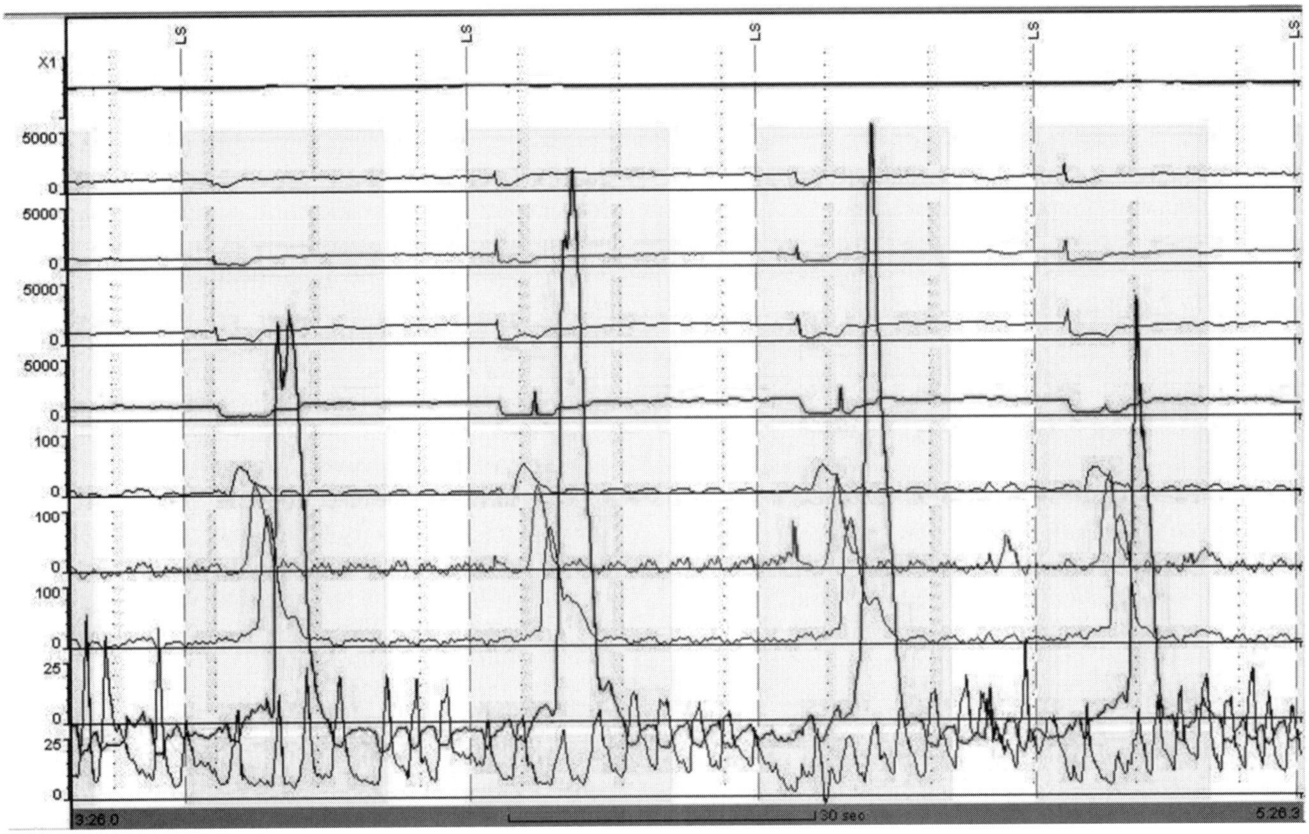

Figure 8–7. High-amplitude contractions (>180 mm Hg) consistent with nutcracker esophagus.

able. Upper endoscopy is normal but endoscopic ultrasonography may demonstrate thickening of the muscularis propria.[36] Interestingly, psychiatric disorders such as anxiety, depression, and somatoform disorders appear to be found in higher-than-predicted frequencies in this population, as first described by Clouse and associates.[37,38] As a note of caution, when performing manometry on patients with GERD, we often observe high-amplitude waves consistent with NE, particularly in the distal esophagus. Generally, these patients do not report symptoms consistent with NE. In these situations we do not feel it is advisable to direct therapy based on this manometric finding. Instead, therapy should be directed toward their underlying problem, reflux. Often we observe that the manometric findings will normalize with the prevention of ongoing insult to the esophagus from acid reflux. Rarely, these patients may present with dysphagia, in which case one may consider a myotomy of the distal esophagus and LES to improve esophageal emptying.

Hypertensive Lower Esophageal Sphincter

Hypertensive lower esophageal sphincter is an abnormality diagnosed when there is an elevated LES pressure (>45 mm Hg) in the absence of a concomitant disorder of esophageal body peristalsis. LES relaxation is usually normal.

THERAPY

The goal of therapy is to relieve symptoms, and not to reverse the motility disorder. This therapy depends on accurate diagnosis. Medical therapy is the first-line therapy for most spastic motility disorders, and is effective to some extent in up to 80% of patients.[39] As previously mentioned, if GERD is present, it should be treated and may provide good relief. Patients should also be reassured that they have no underlying cardiac disease or malignancy contributing to their symptoms. This has been shown to reduce patient anxiety, to reduce their utilization of health care,[40] and to produce some improvement in chest pain.[41]

Medical therapy consists of various pharmacological agents acting on smooth muscle, though none demonstrates superior efficacy.[42,43] These include nitroglycerin, isosorbide dinitrate, and calcium channel blockers. We usually begin with calcium channel blockers, as they are better tolerated.

As previously mentioned, a psychological component may be an important contributor in patients with esophageal angina. Therapy addressing this component has been shown to be helpful in several clinical trials.[44,45] Several psychoactive agents demonstrate some efficacy, possibly to a greater extent than smooth muscle agents. These include benzodiazepines, tricyclics, and trazodone.[38,46]

Botulinum toxin A (Botox) is a neurotoxin produced by *Clostridium botulinum.* Botox binds to cholinergic nerves and irreversibly inhibits acetylcholine release. This effect is eventually overcome by regeneration of new synapses. Botox injection has been used with some limited success.[48] However with DES and NE, where there is not a discrete abnormality, the question arises of where in the esophagus to focus the therapy.

The use of surgical myotomy in these aforementioned diseases is at present limited. There is a reluctance to use such an invasive procedure in a relatively benign group of disorders since they often can be managed with varying success medically. When GERD is present, anti-reflux procedures have been shown to be of help. In the absence of reflux and failure of medical therapy, esophageal myotomy may be considered. While myotomy may provide relief of chest pain in such patients, the subset of patients whose main problem is dysphagia and whose esophagus empties poorly seem to benefit the most. The recent advent of minimally invasive approaches has dramatically decreased the morbidity of esophageal myotomy, perhaps allowing a more liberal expansion of its indications to these entities. A thoracoscopic approach may be beneficial if a long esophageal myotomy is desired.[49] Under those circumstances, a distal myotomy as a first step is important to decrease the resistance to flow through the GE junction.

ACHALASIA

Achalasia is a primary esophageal motor disorder of unknown etiology and the most common of esophageal motility disorders. It is an uncommon ailment with a reported incidence of 0.5–1 per 100,000 in the United States. Achalasia affects both sexes equally, typically presenting between the ages of 20 and 50, though it can occur in all ages. It is characterized by ineffective relaxation of the LES combined with loss of esophageal peristalsis, leading to impaired emptying and gradual esophageal dilation. Dysphagia is the cardinal feature of achalasia, accompanied by varying degrees of aspiration, weight loss, and pain. The anatomic defect appears to be a decrease or loss of inhibitory nonadrenergic, noncholinergic ganglion cells in the esophageal myenteric plexus. Histological analysis of esophagi resected from patients with end-stage achalasia demonstrates myenteric inflammation and progressive depletion of ganglion cells and subsequent neural fibrosis.[50] There is also a significant reduction in the synthesis of nitric oxide and vasoactive intestinal peptide, the most important mediators of relaxation in the LES. Macroscopically there may often be thickening of the circular layer of the distal esophagus. Achalasia also carries a slight increased risk of cancer, in particular squamous cell carcinoma.

Patient Presentation

Most patients with achalasia present with progressive dysphagia to solids and liquids, although symptoms may be subtle and nonspecific early in its course. The mean duration of symptoms prior to presentation is 2 years, and the diagnosis often takes much longer, as the symptoms are often attributed to GERD or other disorders. Initially the patient may complain of the sensation of a retrosternal "sticking" of foodstuffs. Stress or cold liquids may exacerbate dysphagia. Patients may regurgitate undigested food, especially after meals or when lying supine. Patients may stand after eating or raise their arms over their head to enlist gravity and to increase the intrathoracic pressure in an attempt to aid esophageal emptying. If unable to force food into the stomach by the ingestion of liquids or other means, spontaneous or forced regurgitation are often employed to evacuate the esophagus. Occasionally, physicians even confuse the disease with an eating disorder. As a result of regurgitation, aspiration of esophageal contents may lead to pulmonary disease. In fact, up to 10% of patients with achalasia experience significant bronchopulmonary complications.[51]

Many patients express a sensation of heartburn, explaining why many patients are initially diagnosed with GERD. Though patients with achalasia may experience gastroesophageal reflux,[52] more often heartburn is secondary to fermentation of retained undigested food in the esophagus. Chest pain clearly distinguishable from heartburn occurs in 30–50% of patients. The etiology of this pain is unclear, and is unpredictably relieved by esophageal myotomy and other treatments. Weight loss is variable and tends to be insidious. The magnitude of weight loss tends to correlate with the severity of the underlying disease. Rapid onset of symptoms (≤6 months), advanced age (>50 years), or significant weight loss (>15 lb) should raise suspicion for pseudoachalasia, usually secondary to malignancy or extraluminal obstruction. In these cases a thorough work-up with a CT scan and/or endoscopic ultrasound must be performed before further therapy is considered.

Evaluation

A barium esophagogram is typically the first imaging study utilized in the evaluation of dysphagia. The scout film may demonstrate an air-fluid level in the esophagus with a paucity of gastric air. The classic appearance of achalasia on a barium study is the "bird's beak" tapering of the distal esophagus with a column of contrast medium in the esophageal lumen (Fig 8–8). Vari-

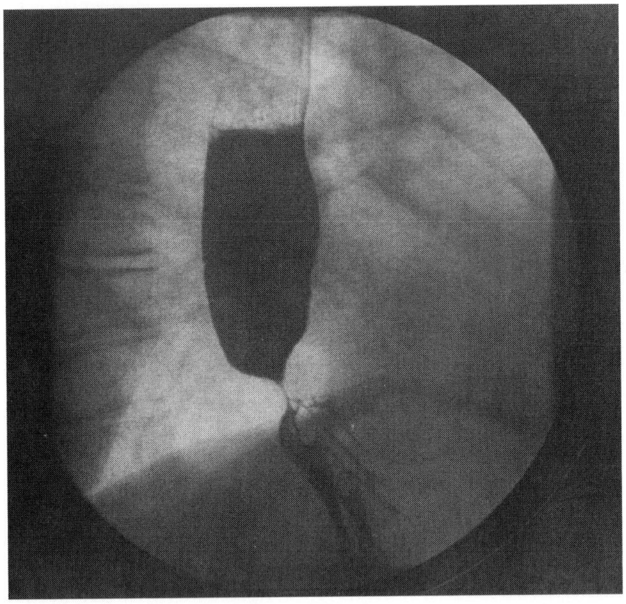

Figure 8–8. Barium study demonstrating a dilated esophagus and smooth, tapered gastroesophageal junction, typical of achalasia.

able esophageal dilation is seen, ranging from mild in the early stages to the massive sigmoid-shaped esophagus of end-stage achalasia. Fluoroscopic evaluation may also reveal nonpropulsive, tertiary contractions of the esophageal body with failure to clear the barium bolus from the esophagus.

Manometry is the gold standard for confirming the diagnosis of achalasia. The resting LES pressure may be elevated, but it may also be normal. The cardinal feature is failure of the LES to completely relax with swallowing. Complete absence of peristalsis is the sine qua non of achalasia. The waveforms are usually simultaneous and of low amplitude (Fig 8–9). When present, they are simultaneous and nonpropulsive in nature. A subset of patients with vigorous achalasia are found to have high-amplitude contractions. In patients with a dilated and tortuous esophagus, the LES may be difficult to intubate, requiring fluoroscopic guidance for manometry catheter placement. In the patient who will not tolerate esophageal manometry, nuclear scintigraphy can be used to evaluate esophageal transit.

Twenty-four-hour pH monitoring is neither required nor usually helpful. While patients with achalasia may experience some element of gastroesophageal reflux, it is not clinically relevant. Furthermore, acidification of esophageal contents secondary to fermentation of retained food may lead to a false-positive study.[53]

Endoscopic evaluation is used to rule out other processes that may mimic achalasia. The characteristic appearance is an atonic, dilated esophagus with a tightly closed LES that does not open with insufflation. With gentle pressure the scope is admitted through the LES with a "pop," in contrast to a peptic stricture or a malignancy, which does not yield. The gastroesophageal junction, including a retroflexed view of the gastric cardia, should be carefully inspected. Biopsies of any mucosal abnormality should be obtained. If pseudoachalasia cannot be ruled out, endoscopic ultrasound or a CT scan may prove informative.

Treatment

The treatment of achalasia is directed at the palliation of symptoms and does not change the underlying pathology. The neuromuscular defect is not corrected. The goal of all therapeutic options is to relieve the functional obstruction of the distal esophagus, thus improving esophageal emptying.

Drugs that relax smooth muscle and decrease LES pressure such as nitrates and calcium channel blockers have been used to treat achalasia. Unpredictable and incomplete absorption of oral formulations secondary to poor esophageal emptying is one limitation, thus sublingual administration is the most efficacious route. Relief from these agents is inconsistent and generally short-lived, with most patients showing continued progression of their disease.[54–56] Side effects such as headaches and peripheral edema are common, limiting their adoption. Their usefulness is limited to temporizing symptoms until more effective therapy can be implemented, or in those patients deemed too frail to undergo a more invasive treatment.

Botox is injected into the LES through the working port of a flexible endoscope, and can be accomplished with minimal incidence of immediate complications. Early enthusiasm has waned, as results have not proven to be durable. Botox injection is initially effective in 60–85% of patients, but 50% develop recurrent symptoms within 6 months.[57] Repeat administration is possible but efficacy is diminished with subsequent injections. As Botox is a relatively expensive therapy, the need for repeat treatment limits both its convenience and cost-effectiveness. Another problem with this therapy is that Botox injection can cause an intense inflammatory reaction of the gastroesophageal junction with subsequent fibrosis. This may impact future surgical therapy, as most patients have continued or progressive symptoms. Our experience during esophageal myotomy is that there is more difficulty in finding the submucosal plane in patients with prior Botox therapy versus untreated patients (53% versus 7%). Although there does not appear to be a difference in the ultimate relief of dysphagia, we did experience an increased rate of perforation (7% versus 2%) in patients with prior Botox therapy.[58] While not well understood, Botox appears to be more effective in older patients and in those with vigorous achalasia. Botox should be reserved for patients unwilling or deemed unfit to undergo an

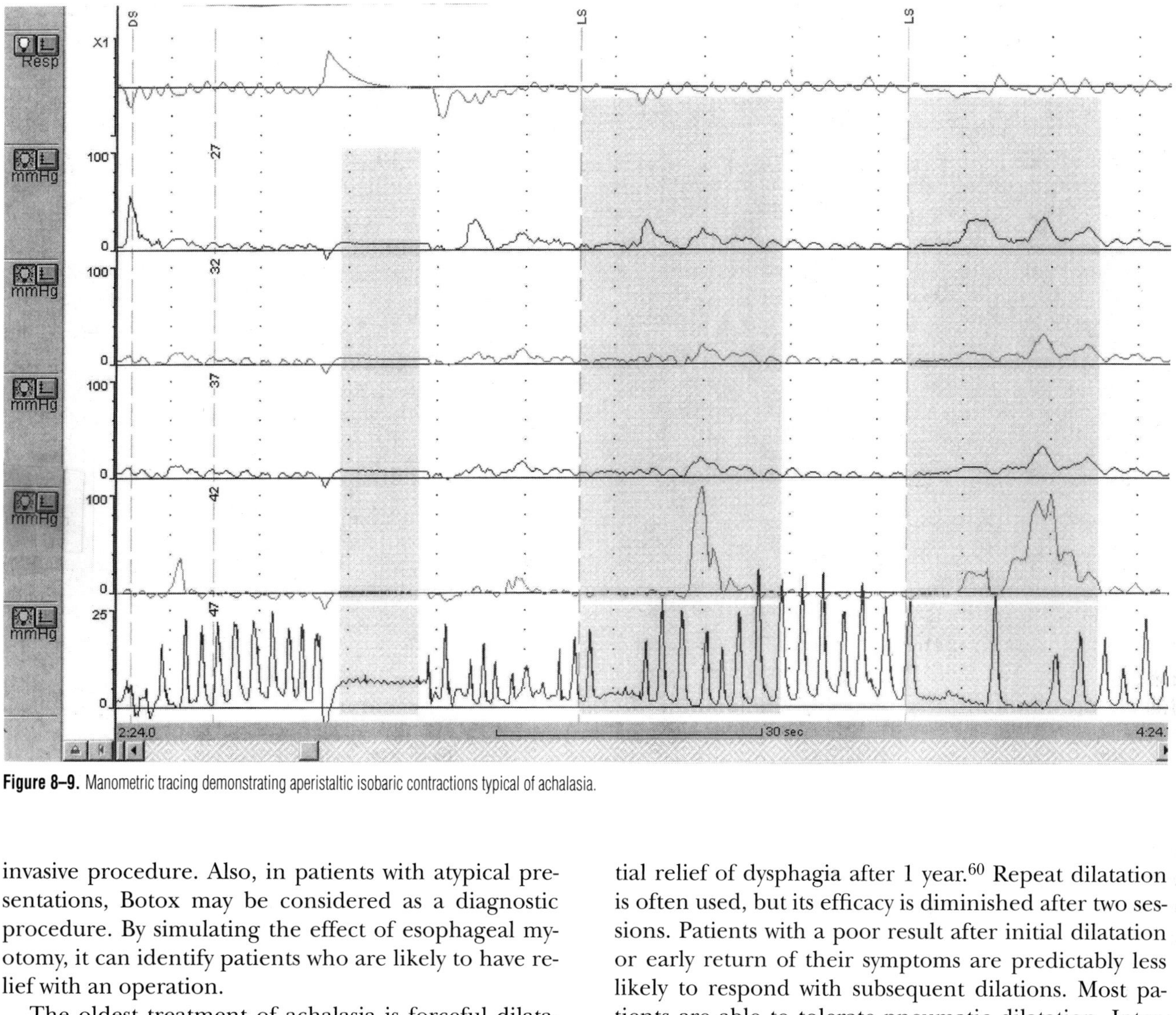

Figure 8–9. Manometric tracing demonstrating aperistaltic isobaric contractions typical of achalasia.

invasive procedure. Also, in patients with atypical presentations, Botox may be considered as a diagnostic procedure. By simulating the effect of esophageal myotomy, it can identify patients who are likely to have relief with an operation.

The oldest treatment of achalasia is forceful dilatation of the LES, originally accomplished by the passage of a piece of whalebone with a sponge affixed to the end.[59] This is essentially tearing of the esophageal muscle, resulting in an imprecise, uncontrolled myotomy. This therapy has become more effective with the development of graded pneumatic polyethylene balloons. Under fluoroscopic guidance, balloons (at least 30 mm in diameter) are passed through the LES and inflated, disrupting the fibers of the LES. The balloon is kept inflated from 1–3 minutes and then deflated. This is followed by an esophagram with water-soluble contrast to evaluate the LES diameter and to evaluate for perforation. If no extravasation is seen, the patient is observed for 6 hours and then discharged home. The "graded" approach refers to the use of serially larger balloons (up to 40 mm) with subsequent dilatations for initial nonresponders. Only a single dilatation is performed per session. Response rates of 60–90% can be achieved, with approximately 70% of patients obtaining substantial relief of dysphagia after 1 year.[60] Repeat dilatation is often used, but its efficacy is diminished after two sessions. Patients with a poor result after initial dilatation or early return of their symptoms are predictably less likely to respond with subsequent dilations. Most patients are able to tolerate pneumatic dilatation. Interestingly, younger patients do not respond as well as older patients.[61] This is thought to be due to their tissues being more compliant and simply stretching during dilatation rather that tearing. The presence of a hiatal hernia, significantly dilated esophagus (>7 cm), or an epiphrenic diverticulum increases the risk of perforation and are relative contraindications. While the likelihood of improving dysphagia increases with increasing balloon diameter, so does the likelihood of perforation. Overall, the incidence of perforation is about 2% per dilation attempt.[62] Whether to treat achalasia initially with pneumatic dilatation depends on physician and surgeon expertise, patient age and comorbidities, and patient preference. If dilation fails, a myotomy can usually be performed without additional difficulties.

Surgical therapy was originally described in 1914 by Ernest Heller, who performed the first cardiomyotomy for achalasia. His original description called for the performance of two myotomies along the gastroesophageal junction, one anterior and one posterior. This has subsequently been modified and now only an anterior myotomy is performed. Excellent results with cardiomyotomy can be achieved in 90–95% of patients. Extramucosal cardiomyotomy provides more reliable relief of dysphagia than pneumatic dilation, as it allows accurate division of LES muscle fibers rather than blind disruption. Traditionally, this was accomplished either by a transthoracic or a transabdominal approach. Each approach is associated with an obvious incision and postoperative stays of 7–10 days. For this reason, despite superior long-term results from surgical myotomy,[60] most patients were treated by less invasive therapies such a pneumatic dilatation. Recent developments in minimally invasive techniques now allow performance of cardiomyotomy by either a thoracoscopic[63] or a laparoscopic[64] approach. Reduction in postoperative pain and morbidity, as well as improved cosmesis, has made the surgical option more attractive. Some feel that a megaesophagus (>8 cm) is a contraindication to a myotomy because of poor relief of dysphagia. We feel that with laparoscopy there is little to lose by attempting a myotomy and reserving an esophagectomy for failures. Using this approach the majority of patients obtain relief and avoid subsequent esophagectomy.

The first approach using minimally invasive techniques was thoracoscopy.[63] Through a left thoracoscopic approach a long myotomy could be performed, extending approximately 0.5 cm across the gastroesophageal junction (similar to the open approach). The thought was that this would provide relief of dysphagia without rendering the cardia completely incompetent and resulting in significant reflux. Initial results were promising, with 89% of patients experiencing relief of dysphagia.[65] However, over time several patients (9/35) in our series required myotomy extension or postmyotomy dilation to relieve dysphagia.[66] Furthermore, over 60% had abnormal reflux when 24-hour pH monitoring was performed. Thus it became clear that successful relief of dysphagia often depends on extending the myotomy well onto the stomach, which can only be done from an abdominal approach. Also, even a limited gastric myotomy and hiatal dissection, such as is performed with a thoracoscopic myotomy, results in a high incidence of reflux.

For these reasons, most esophageal surgeons now perform a Heller myotomy via a laparoscopic approach. The advantages include excellent visualization of the distal esophagus and the stomach, so that an extended gastric myotomy and an antireflux procedure may be performed. Moreover, it avoids the anesthetic complexity of single-lung ventilation required for thoracoscopy. We have substantial experience with both approaches and have found that laparoscopy is more effective in relieving dysphagia (93% versus 85%) with a shorter hospital stay (48 versus 72 hours) and less postoperative reflux (17% versus 60%).[67]

There are two main controversies surrounding Heller myotomy. One is the extent of the esophageal myotomy, and the other is whether an anti-reflux procedure should be performed, and if so which one. While there is agreement that the proximal extent of the myotomy should reach 6–7 cm above the gastroesophageal junction, the distal extent of the myotomy is controversial. Some believe the goal in performing a myotomy is to adequately relieve dysphagia without unnecessarily disrupting the anti-reflux barrier. We have found that there is no length of esophageal myotomy that maximally relieves dysphagia and minimizes the occurrence of reflux. This is emphasized by the thoracoscopic approach that, despite a limited distal extension of the myotomy, produced GERD in most patients. We recently compared a more traditional approach (a 1.5–2 cm gastric myotomy) with an extended gastric myotomy (at least 3 cm). We found that the longer myotomy resulted in less dysphagia (1.2 versus 2.1 on a four-point frequency scale) and fewer interventions for recurrent dysphagia (3% versus 17%).[67] Since we advocate an extended gastric myotomy, we feel an anti-reflux procedure is prudent in most cases. Those who advocate not performing an anti-reflux procedure cite good clinical results and low incidence of heartburn.[68,69] However, few groups perform postmyotomy 24-hour pH monitoring to evaluate for the true incidence of gastroesophageal reflux without a fundoplication. Moreover, this practice results in intervention rates for dysphagia as high as 14%,[69] which we think is likely the result of a limited gastric myotomy.

Most surgeons find that performing an anti-reflux procedure in conjunction with laparoscopic myotomy does not add significant time or morbidity to the operation, and is not associated with increased postoperative dysphagia. Certainly, a partial fundoplication (Dor or Toupet) is the best option. A total fundoplication (e.g., Nissen fundoplication) may cause a functional obstruction for a nonpropulsive esophagus, resulting in a high incidence of dysphagia.[70] An anterior (Dor) fundoplication requires less posterior dissection, and thus is easier and theoretically preserves more of the anti-reflux barrier. Also, since the wrap is brought anterior to the myotomy, it potentially covers any undetected mucosal injuries. A posterior (Toupet) fundoplication is the preferred partial fundoplication when indicated for GERD. However, its superiority in preventing reflux after myotomy has not been demonstrated. Since it holds the edges of the myotomy open, a Toupet may provide protection against recurrent dysphagia. For these reasons it is our procedure of choice. While each of these anti-reflux techniques has its own theoretical benefits and champions, there is no strong evidence supporting one over the other.

Operative Technique

Two principles of operative therapy are important in treating motility disorders. The first is that the site and extent of the myotomy must be directed by the findings of the manometry study. If manometry shows the entire thoracic esophagus to be involved in the pathologic process (i.e., nutcracker esophagus), then a myotomy that spans the length of the thoracic esophagus may be required. The second issue is ablating the LES. Even if the LES pressure is normal, it should be disrupted. After an extensive myotomy of the esophageal body or with the aperistaltic esophagus of achalasia, the ability to transmit a bolus of food normally will be lost. Even a normal LES pressure could represent a functional obstruction to a myotomized esophagus. Our approach is to begin with a laparoscopic myotomy that extends as proximal as possible. For those with spastic motility disorders that are still symptomatic, we will then extend the myotomy, usually through the right chest.

Thoracoscopic Heller Myotomy. The patient should be instructed to take a liquid diet for 2 days prior to the operation if esophageal emptying is inhibited. With a dilated, sigmoid esophagus (i.e., S-shaped distended esophagus of advanced achalasia), we will extend this to 4 days. This will decrease the amount of solid debris in the lumen of the esophagus and lessen the chance of a severe aspiration event during intubation. A double-lumen endotracheal tube is necessary to allow single-lung ventilation. A bougie, preferably lighted, is needed for the operation. The bougie should be placed under direct vision during the operation, especially if a diverticulum is present, in order to reduce the chance of injury to the esophagus.

The patient is placed in the lateral decubitus position. Access to the lower esophagus and esophagogastric junction is achieved through a left-sided approach. Since most of the processes described above require disruption of the LES, the majority of myotomies will be performed from the left. The right-sided approach is necessary when a myotomy of the entire esophagus is required, except its most inferior aspect. This approach is also useful for an associated midesophageal diverticulum located on the right side. An anti-reflux procedure cannot be performed easily from this approach due to inaccessibility to the esophagogastric junction. The ports are placed to allow maximum visualization of the inferior thoracic esophagus and the superior esophagus if needed. The ports are placed in an equilateral triangle, notably much closer than what is normally done in the abdomen, with the videoendoscope located in the fifth intercostal space, just inferior to the scapular tip. The working ports should be located in the posterior axillary line. An additional fourth port in the anterior axillary line is used by the assistant to retract the lung. The surgeon and the assistant stand next to each other on the same side of the operating table. Thus both are standing at the patient's back, while the video cart monitor is in front of the patient. Carbon dioxide insufflation is not necessary for the procedure, as single-lung ventilation usually suffices.

The lung is retracted anteriorly after it is deflated. The inferior pulmonary ligament is divided with cautery and blunt dissection, avoiding the inferior pulmonary vein. Once this is accomplished, the pleural reflection over the esophagus is opened with cautery dissection so that the longitudinal muscle fibers of the esophagus may be identified. The lighted bougie is passed into the esophagus by the anesthesiologist. By splaying the muscle fibers of the esophagus over the bougie with one instrument, electrocautery is used to dissect down to the submucosa. Care is taken to identify and preserve the vagus nerve throughout the operation. A combination of blunt dissection, spreading, and cauterization is used to divide the muscular layers of the esophagus for the length of the myotomy. Flexible endoscopy should be used to verify the adequacy of the myotomy. If a left-sided approach is used, a partial wrap (Dor or Belsey) may be added. If the right-sided approach is used, then the anti-reflux procedure is not possible. If a diverticulum is present, it may be dissected to its neck and transected by an automatic stapling and cutting device.

After completion of the myotomy, two chest tubes are placed through trocar sites and the remaining sites are closed. The patient is allowed to consume a liquid diet on the day of the operation, unless a diverticulum was resected, in which case the diet is started on the third postoperative day. Hospital stay varies, but patients are usually discharged within 2 days of starting a diet.

The length of the myotomy varies with each of the disease processes and with the findings of the preoperative evaluation. If a hypertensive lower esophageal sphincter without concomitant esophageal body dysmotility is being treated, the myotomy is confined to the distal esophagus, LES, and cardia. If NE is being treated and preoperative manometry revealed high-amplitude contractions in the proximal esophagus, an extended myotomy should be performed, perhaps through a right thoracoscopic approach.

Laparoscopic Heller Myotomy. The set-up is the same as that for a Nissen fundoplication. The patient is placed in a modified lithotomy position with a standard five-port placement. We routinely mobilize the gastric fundus and short gastric vessels to minimize tension on the subsequent fundoplication. An extensive anterior and lateral hiatal and mediastinal esophageal dissection is performed to maximize the length of the myotomy. It is important to identify the left (anterior) vagus nerve and separate it from the esophagus to enable the performance of a continuous esophagogastric myotomy.

A lighted 50F bougie is passed into the body of the stomach. The bougie illuminates the esophagus, which helps with identification and stability when performing the myotomy. The fat pad overlying the cardioesophageal junction is excised, a step critical to accurately identifying the gastroesophageal junction. A Babcock clamp opened over the bougie just distal to the gastroesophageal junction provides exposure of the distal esophagus. We perform the myotomy with an L-shaped hook electrocautery device, although minimal energy is used so as to minimize mucosal injury. The appropriate plane may be more difficult to identify in patients who have previously undergone treatment with Botox or pneumatic dilatation. The longitudinal muscle fibers are divided first, exposing the inner circular muscle which is then separated from the mucosa. For this reason most submucosal bleeding should be controlled with pressure and time. The myotomy should be carried as proximal as safely possible (usually 6–8 cm) and 2–3 cm onto the stomach. As discussed previously, we routinely perform a 3-cm distal myotomy. The distal dissection is the most difficult because the muscular layers are poorly defined and the mucosa is thinner. Mucosal perforations should be repaired with fine (4-0 or 5-0) absorbable suture, and rarely require other intervention. Endoscopy may be used to check the completeness of the myotomy and for unrecognized mucosal injury. As we perform an extended distal myotomy, we routinely perform an anti-reflux procedure. We prefer a standard Toupet fundoplication, securing both edges of the fundus to each side of the myotomy as well as to the diaphragm (Fig 8–10). More recently robotic techniques have been used to perform Heller myotomy. The advantage of this approach is the excellent visualization of the muscular coat of the esophagus and its layers and the 3-D visualization which facilitates the performance of the fundoplication. The disadvantage of using robotic techniques is the cost associated with the robot and the difficulties associated with the use of such a large, complex apparatus in proximity with the assistant surgeon.

Postoperatively we do not recommend the use of a nasogastric tube. Nausea is aggressively treated with antiemetics, as retching and vomiting can have catastrophic results in the early postoperative period. Patients are generally started on liquids the night of the procedure and advanced to a soft diet prior to discharge. Average length of stay is 1–2 days, and resumption of normal diet and activities occurs within 2–3 weeks. We routinely request that patients undergo repeat manometry and pH studies 4–6 months after surgery. We mostly do this to evaluate for postoperative reflux, which may contribute to late failures (i.e., from peptic stricture). Patients with abnormal amounts of reflux are routinely prescribed a proton pump inhibitor.

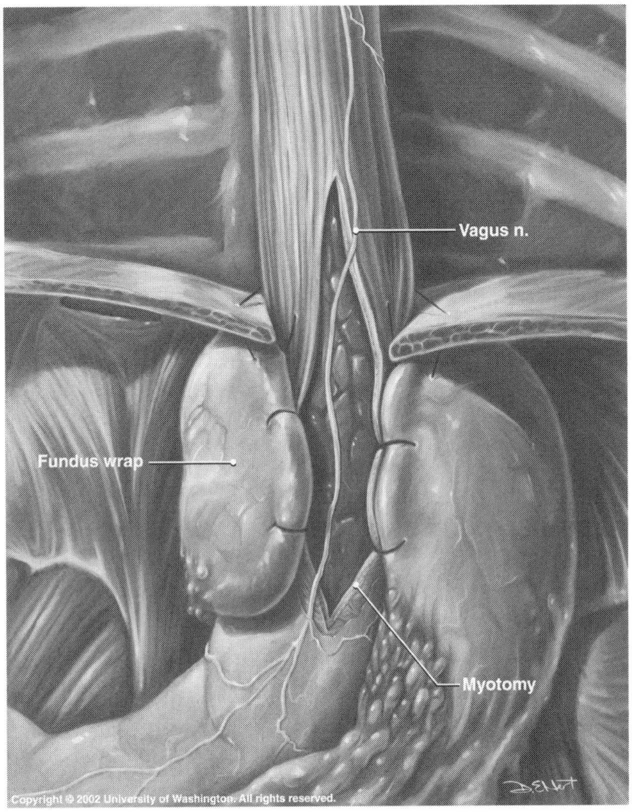

Figure 8–10. Completed Heller myotomy with Toupet fundoplication. (Reproduced, with permission, from the University of Washington, Seattle.)

SUMMARY

Esophageal motility disorders can produce troubling, and potentially life-threatening, symptoms for patients. With the exception of achalasia, medical therapy is the first-line treatment of these disorders. In contrast, surgical therapy (Heller myotomy) is the most effective treatment to relieve dysphagia associated with achalasia. The advent of minimally invasive techniques, specifically the laparoscopic approach, significantly reduced the morbidity of surgical therapy, making it the procedure of choice for most patients with achalasia who need surgical treatment. These techniques may allow for the expansion of indications for myotomy to include DES and NE in those patients who fail all medical therapy. For achalasia, pneumatic dilatation is a viable alternative, though it is associated with inferior results and a higher risk of esophageal perforation as compared with surgical therapy. Pharmacotherapy and Botox provide inferior results and should be reserved for temporizing therapy or in patients who are deemed too frail for surgical intervention. For best results, a laparoscopic myotomy should be carried at least 3 cm onto the stomach, and a partial fundoplication should be performed to reduce the incidence of postoperative gastroesophageal reflux.

Although we have described and prefer the laparoscopic/thoracoscopic techniques, the very same principles apply to the open techniques, whether through a midline laparotomy or fifth or sixth intercostal space thoracotomy.

■ ESOPHAGEAL DIVERTICULA

Esophageal diverticula are uncommon. They can be found at any level of the esophagus, but can generally be placed in one of three classifications: pharyngoesophageal, midesophageal, or epiphrenic. Those found proximally and distally in the esophagus are usually *pulsion* diverticula, caused by elevated intraluminal pressures. These are not true diverticula, as they are comprised only of mucosa. Midesophageal diverticula are typically *traction* diverticula, resulting from an extrinsic process, which occurs adjacent to the esophageal wall, pulling on it. These are true diverticula, commonly found near the carina. They used to be more common as a result of tubercular inflammation. This section will review Zenker's and epiphrenic diverticula, as traction diverticulum of the midesophagus rarely occurs anymore, and does not usually require surgical treatment.

PHARYNGOESOPHAGEAL DIVERTICULUM (ZENKER'S) AND CRICOPHARYNGEAL BAR

Zenker's diverticulum and cricopharyngeal bar (cricopharyngeal achalasia) are disorders of the upper esophageal sphincter (UES). Understanding the anatomy and function of the UES is essential to planning an operation to treat these disorders.

The pharynx meets the esophagus where the inferior pharyngeal constrictor joins the cricopharyngeus muscle. The inferior constrictor originates from the thyroid and cricoid cartilage, its fibers coursing obliquely and horizontally inserting on the median raphe of the posterior pharynx. The cricopharyngeus muscle arises from the cricoid cartilage, passes posteriorly to the pharyngoesophageal junction, and inserts on the contralateral side of the cricoid cartilage. The interlacing of muscle fibers at the posterior aspect of the pharynx leaves areas of potential weakness where herniation of the mucosa may occur. Killian's triangle is one of these areas and is found between the inferior constrictor and the cricopharyngeus muscle.[71] Two additional areas where the paucity of muscle fibers creates a relative weakness in the pharyngeal wall are the Killian-Jamieson area between the fibers of the cricopharyngeus, and Laimer's triangle between the junction of the cricopharyngeus and the first circular fibers of the esophagus (Fig 8–11).[72]

The inferior constrictor compresses the pharynx during swallowing, propelling the swallowed bolus downward. The cricopharyngeus muscle maintains tonic contraction, closing the inlet to the esophagus between swallows, and relaxes during swallowing to allow bolus entry into the esophagus. The cricopharyngeus muscle generates most, but not all of the pressure at the manometrically-identified UES, as the physiologic high-pressure zone is often found to be of greater length than the anatomically-identified muscle fibers. The function of the UES is to prevent the entrance of air into the esophagus and to prevent high gastroesophageal refluxate from entering the larynx.[73]

When a swallow is initiated, the UES relaxes while the oral and pharyngeal phases of deglutition proceed. As the tongue propels the bolus posteriorly, the larynx is elevated and compressed, preventing the bolus from entering the trachea. The bolus passes into the pharynx and the constrictors then contract to propel the bolus

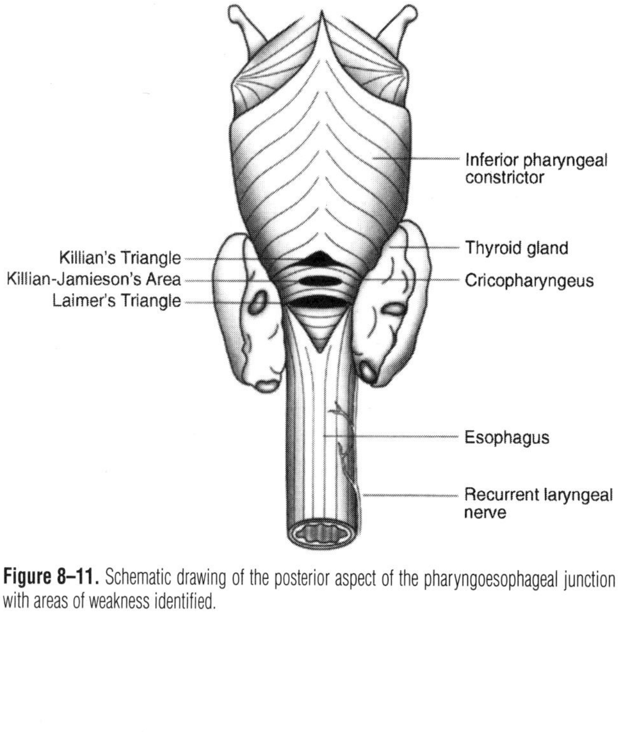

Figure 8–11. Schematic drawing of the posterior aspect of the pharyngoesophageal junction with areas of weakness identified.

into the esophagus. The tonic contraction of the UES is inhibited and the bolus proceeds into the esophagus. This is a conceptually simple interpretation of deglutition. However, extensive study of the physiology of the UES and the pathophysiology of the diseases that affect the UES have revealed the complexity of UES activity.

Zenker's Diverticulum

Since pharyngoesophageal diverticula occur in the late middle aged or elderly, it is felt to be an acquired condition. These are the most common types of esophageal diverticula. They are thought to arise from increased pressure within the pharynx, but the causes are unclear.[74] Manometry has demonstrated that the UES is capable of relaxing, but that the lack of coordination between bolus propagation and sphincter relaxation results in increased pressure in the pharynx. Manometric evaluation of the UES shows some degree of discoordination in more than two-thirds of patients.[75] The precise nature of the dysfunction can be difficult to assess with stationary manometry, as the UES is relatively narrow compared to the vertical distance it moves during normal swallowing. Use of fluoroscopy while performing manometry has helped elucidate this problem by ensuring proper placement of the manometry catheter at the UES, which shows that the sphincter does not relax completely.[76] There is also evidence suggesting that the muscles of the cricopharyngeus and the proximal esophagus are fibrosed and therefore do not function normally. Histological analysis of sphincter muscles showed that they were replaced by fibrotic tissue, possibly explaining the abnormal response of the sphincter to swallowing.[77–79] It is not known whether the fibrosis is a cause or effect of the disease.

Pharyngoesophageal diverticulum usually occurs in the seventh to eighth decades of life. Dysphagia and regurgitation are the most common complaints. Dysphagia may occur as a result of the dysfunctional UES. It may also be due to displacement or obstruction of the pharyngoesophageal junction caused by a large diverticulum. As the diverticulum enlarges, regurgitation of undigested food, particularly during recumbency, becomes more prevalent. Aspiration, halitosis, excessive salivation, and a "lump in the throat" may also occur. The physical exam is usually not helpful, but may reveal a palpable mass, most commonly on the left side of the neck.

A contrast esophagogram should be obtained. It will usually reveal the diverticulum and will help to exclude an esophageal tumor. Although a videoesophagogram will also demonstrate abnormal movement of the contrast during deglutition, it is probably not necessary to obtain one. Other studies that can confirm the diagnosis include esophagoscopy and manometry. Caution is essential during instrumentation of the esophagus in order to prevent iatrogenic perforation. A 24-hour pH study has been used to determine if there is associated gastroesophageal reflux, which is believed by some to contribute to the pathogenesis of the disease. None of the previous three tests is likely to alter the therapy, and they are probably not necessary in the typical patient with a pharyngoesophageal diverticulum.

Cricopharyngeal Bar

A cricopharyngeal bar is identified radiographically by a persistent posterior indentation of contrast. This is best seen on a lateral view during a videoesophagogram. Residual contrast may be seen above the cricopharyngeus well after the closure of the UES. Despite the presence of such a finding, no consistent clinical symptoms are usually identified in these patients; the etiology and the significance of a cricopharyngeal bar are unknown.

The persistent indentation has been speculated to result from either a failure to relax (thus the term UES achalasia) or an incoordination of the constrictors and the cricopharyngeus muscle. Dantas and associates investigated six patients with cricopharyngeal bars and eight controls without this finding on barium swallow.[80] The subjects were assessed using videofluoroscopy and UES manometry. The patients were found to have normal contraction of the pharynx, normal UES pressures, and normal bolus transit. When compared to the controls, the patients with cricopharyngeal bars had reduced UES relaxation and increased upstream bolus pressures. This suggests that cricopharyngeal bars arise as a result of failure of the muscle to completely relax. In contrast, others have found that resting, relaxation, and contraction pressures are normal in patients with cricopharyngeal bar.[81] These authors claim that the cricopharyngeal muscle is the only normal portion of the pharyngoesophageal segment, and that the inferior constrictor and the proximal esophagus are abnormally dilated.

Even when a cricopharyngeal bar can be demonstrated, the clinical significance of this finding is unknown. Asymptomatic patients may have similar degrees of narrowing as patients with cervical esophageal dysphagia.[80] Furthermore, cricopharyngeal bar is seen in greater than 50% of patients with gastroesophageal reflux.[82] Due to the ambiguity of these findings and the lack of symptoms attributable to this dysfunction, surgical intervention for cricopharyngeal bar is only appropriate for very selected patients. The patients should not have an underlying medical condition known to affect motility (myopathy, Parkinson's disease, or myasthenia gravis), neoplasia must be excluded, and gastroesophageal reflux should be eliminated as a cause of the cricopharyngeal bar. If these requirements are satisfied, and the patient has symptoms referable to the cervical esophagus, a cricopharyngeal myotomy may provide some relief.

Treatment and Controversies

Most patients with pharyngoesophageal diverticula who are able to tolerate an operation should probably be treated, as the natural history of the disease is one of progression leading to complications.[74] The exception is probably the patient whose diverticulum is relatively small and asymptomatic. However, since this disease occurs exclusively in the elderly, a considerate evaluation of perioperative risks should be done before a final decision is made to proceed with the operation. No medical therapy has been shown to be effective at treating these diverticula. Several elements of the surgical treatment have been topics of debate.

Operative Approach. The open cervical approach has been the treatment of choice in the United States for many years.[83–85] Many European surgeons have advocated some variant of the peroral approach for treating pharyngoesophageal diverticula for some time.[86–89] More recently, in the U.S. there has been a similar crossover in the approaches, though there have been no prospective, randomized trials comparing the transcervical and peroral approaches for treating pharyngoesophageal diverticula.

In fact, there are few studies comparing endoscopic and open treatment of Zenker's diverticulum. Smith and colleagues demonstrated in a retrospective analysis that the endoscopic stapling technique took less time (26 minutes versus 88 minutes). Due to higher equipment costs of the stapling technique the aggregate operative charges were equivalent ($5178 versus $5113).[90] The mean length of stay, however, was much shorter for the endoscopic procedure (1.3 days versus 5.2 days), thus the inpatient hospital charges were less for this procedure ($3589 versus $11,439). For patients with comorbidities and anatomy amenable to this approach, endoscopic stapling provides a reasonable alternative to the traditional transcervical approach. Long-term results and better comparative studies are needed.

Diverticulectomy versus Diverticulopexy. In an attempt to avoid infection due to leak from a resected diverticulum, some surgeons perform a diverticulopexy. The diverticulum is sutured to the precervical fascia so that the apex is cephalad to its neck. By not opening the mucosa, the incidence of infection would theoretically be less. In a nonrandomized study of 43 patients approached by a transcervical route, all patients had myotomies performed; 14 had diverticulectomy and 29 had diverticulopexy.[91] Two patients in both groups developed neck infections, and one patient in the diverticulectomy group developed mediastinitis. There was no statistical difference in the incidence of wound infection or mediastinitis between the two groups. It may be argued that the study did not have enough patients to detect a difference in septic complications, potentially obscuring any theoretical benefit of the diverticulopexy procedure. However, it should be noted that diverticulopexy was the procedure of choice in their most recent patients, as the authors discarded the use of diverticulectomy for treatment. Thus, no known difference exists between the two procedures with respect to outcome or complications. Although in the past some advocated diverticulectomy alone, the incidence of recurrence was so high that it is now inadvisable to treat the diverticulum without performing a myotomy.[83]

Treatment of Gastroesophageal Reflux. Other abnormalities of esophageal and gastric function may be found in up to 60% of patients with pharyngoesophageal diverticula.[92] The most common finding is gastroesophageal reflux disease. As with cricopharyngeal bar, the association between the two is thought to stem from an attempt by the UES to prevent gastric contents from reaching the pharynx. The concept of addressing both entities simultaneously has waxed and waned for the past 30 years, depending on the accepted explanation of the pathophysiology of pharyngoesophageal diverticulum.[93] Some surgeons believe that if abnormal gastroesophageal reflux is demonstrated preoperatively, it should be treated surgically during the same procedure as the pharyngoesophageal diverticulum. The rationale behind this approach is the assumption that once the cricopharyngeal myotomy is performed, the refluxate may more easily enter the larynx, causing laryngitis, hoarseness, and even aspiration. However, not all patients with Zenker's diverticulum have concomitant foregut pathology. The wisest approach is to address each entity based on its severity and the discomfort it creates for the patient. If heartburn, regurgitation of digested food, and esophagitis are the predominant findings in a patient who has a small Zenker's diverticulum on a contrast study, the reflux should be treated first.[94] Similarly, if the patient has cervical dysphagia, regurgitation of undigested food, and a mildly abnormal 24-hour pH study, the pharyngoesophageal diverticulum should be treated alone.

Operative Technique

Open Cervical Diverticulectomy. Prior to operative treatment of the diverticulum, the patient should be on a liquid diet for 1 or 2 days to minimize the amount of retained food particles in the diverticulum. Most diverticula originate in the posterior aspect of the pharynx. As they grow, about 25% project to the left side and 10% to the right side. Although the preoperative contrast study will help to determine which side of the neck will provide the best exposure for the procedure, the left side is usually preferred. The approach from the left is easier from an anatomic standpoint. The tracheoesophageal groove and the recurrent laryngeal nerve are more accessible due to the slight rightward shift of the trachea relative to the esophagus in the neck.

Access to the area is gained through a low transverse cervical incision along the anterior border of the sternocleidomastoid muscle. The dissection proceeds along the avascular plane anterior to the sternocleidomastoid muscle, which is retracted laterally. The carotid sheath is retracted laterally and the thyroid gland medially. The middle thyroid vein is ligated and transected, as is the omohyoid muscle to improve exposure. Care must be taken to avoid injuring the recurrent laryngeal nerve. With the posterolateral aspect of the esophagus exposed, a 50F bougie is carefully passed into the esophagus. The surgeon should guide the bougie to prevent it from entering the diverticulum and perforating it. With the bougie in place, a circumferential dissection of the esophagus is performed. The esophagus is then dissected cephalad along the posterior midline toward its junction with the pharynx. During this portion's dissection, the diverticulum will be encountered.

The diverticulum is grasped with a Babcock clamp and dissected free from adjacent structures, elevating it into the wound (Fig 8–12). The neck of the diverticulum is cleared of the surrounding tissues. This should reveal the triangle of Killian. At this point, a myotomy is performed. The cricopharyngeus muscle and the proximal few centimeters of the longitudinal and circular muscle of the esophagus are also transected, so that the mucosa pouches through the myotomy site (Fig 8–13).

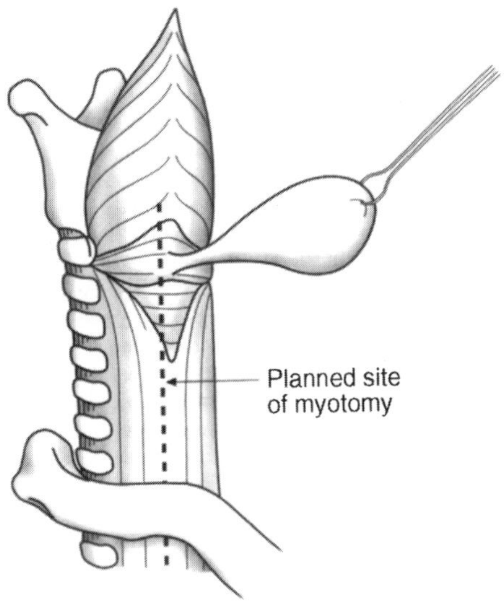

Figure 8–12. Diverticulum elevated from the dissection site. The site of the planned myotomy is marked by the dotted line.

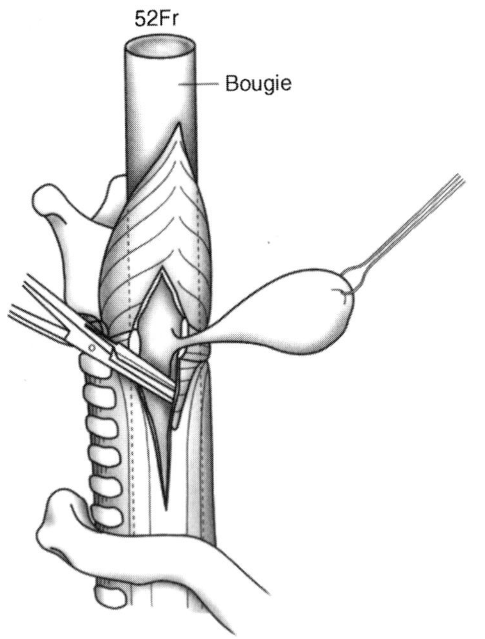

Figure 8–13. The myotomy is extended onto the esophagus for several centimeters.

The diverticulum should be excised whenever possible to reduce the amount of redundant mucosa at the pharyngoesophageal junction. To accomplish this, a linear stapler is placed across the neck of the diverticulum with a bougie inside the esophagus to prevent narrowing of the lumen (Fig 8–14). The platysma is closed loosely and the skin is approximated. Drainage of the wound is not necessary. The patient is allowed a liquid diet on the first postoperative day, and if no evidence of a leak is present, the diet may be advanced.

Resolution of dysphagia and regurgitation may be expected and has been reported in 82–100% of patients treated with this approach.[75,95,96] Despite the symptomatic improvement, the mechanism of deglutition is not entirely restored to normal. For example, postoperative video contrast studies show abnormalities in pharyngeal peristalsis, a visible cricopharyngeus, premature closure of the cricopharyngeus, and occasionally a residual diverticulum.[78]

Mortality from this procedure should be less than 1%. The most disturbing complication, esophagocutaneous fistula, occurs in 6–20% of cases but heals spontaneously.[96] Other potential complications include soft tissue infection, mediastinitis, recurrent laryngeal nerve injury, hematoma, and late stenosis. The frequency of these complications ranges between 1% and 6%.[77] Some authors feel that mucosal injury and recurrent laryngeal nerve injury may be reduced by operating with loupe magnification.[91] Recurrence rates are low, and if the diverticulum is excised while a bougie is in the esophagus, postoperative stenosis is rare.

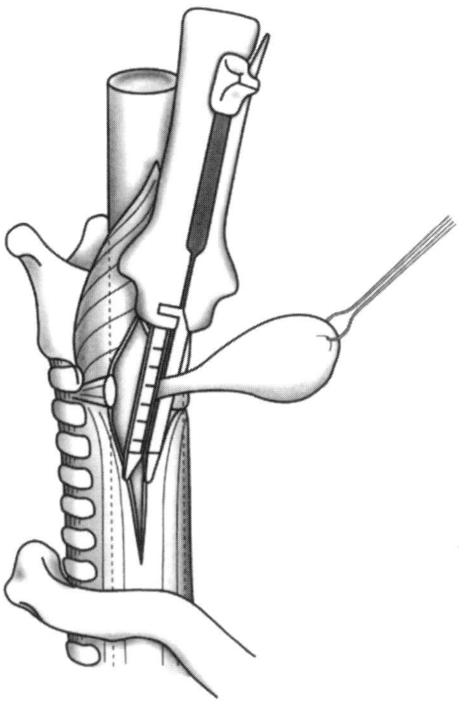

Figure 8–14. The linear stapler is placed across the neck of the diverticulum. Note that the bougie is in place before transecting the diverticulum.

Peroral or Endoscopic Approach. Most peroral methods of treating diverticula are variations of Dohlman's modification of Mosher's first description in 1917.[87] Rigid endoscopy is used to gain exposure to the pharynx while the patient is under general anesthesia. The esophageal lumen and the diverticular neck are identified. The intervening muscle between the lumen of the esophagus and the pouch of the diverticulum is divided. The diverticulum is no longer a blind-ended pouch, as the anterior wall of the diverticulum communicates with the esophageal lumen. Most surgeons who use this technique employ cautery or laser technology to divide the muscle between the diverticulum and the esophagus. One problem with this technique is that it allows communication between the lumen of the esophagus and the deep tissue planes of the neck. Although the potential complications of deep tissue infection and mediastinitis are concerns, they occurred in only 12 of 544 patients treated in one of the largest series.[97]

Another method of transecting the tissue between the two structures is to employ a commercially available automatic stapling and cutting device.[88] This has gained significant popularity in the last few years. One arm of the device is placed into the lumen of the esophagus and the other into the diverticulum. Four rows of staples are then fired into the tissue bridge, with a blade cutting between the inner two rows of staples (Figs 8–15A and 8–15B). Thus, the common wall is stapled and divided, theoretically preventing the escape of esophageal contents from the cut edges. Several series have shown this to be a safe and effective procedure with satisfaction rates in the 90% range.[73,98,99]

Limitations and contraindications to the procedure include restrictions in exposure (small oral cavity, prominent dentition, or cervical spine disease) and a very small diverticulum (<3 cm). Endoscopic stapling may also not be adequate for an extremely large diverticulum, as there is often persistent pooling in the diverticulum. The most serious complication is esophageal or pharyngeal perforation which occurs up to 10% of the time in some series.[73] Inadequate cricopharyngeal transection may also occur, leading to persistent or recurrent symptoms requiring surgical revision. The advantage is that it takes less time to complete, does not require an incision, and therefore may have less morbidity. This is an important consideration since this disease most commonly presents in the elderly.

Summary

Zenker's diverticula are the result of a dysfunctional UES and a weakness in the posterior muscular fibers of the pharyngoesophageal junction. Regurgitation and cervical dysphagia are the most common symptoms. Diagnostic work-up may be limited to a contrast study of the pharynx and the esophagus. Concurrent foregut pathology should be addressed on its own merit. No medical therapy is effective in the treatment of pharyngoesophageal diverticula. Surgical treatment, including resection of the diverticulum and cricopharyngeal myotomy, relieves symptoms and has excellent results.

EPIPHRENIC DIVERTICULA

Patients with esophageal diverticula may be asymptomatic or may present with dysphagia, regurgitation, chest pain, halitosis, chronic cough, aspiration pneumonia, or upper gastrointestinal bleeding.[100] Evaluation of these patients is aimed at defining the anatomy of the diverticulum itself and elucidating the underlying pathophysiology resulting in the diverticulum. The majority of, if not all, epiphrenic diverticula are the result of an underlying esophageal motility disorder.[101] Mondiere made the first attribution of esophageal dysmotility as the cause of esophageal diverticula in 1833.[102] These are not true diverticula, as they consist of only esophageal mucosa and submucosa herniating through the muscular wall of the esophagus. Epiphrenic diverticula are pulsion diverticula, resulting from high intraluminal pressure secondary to a relatively distal obstruction. As such, esophageal manometry is the most useful tool in assessing these patients.

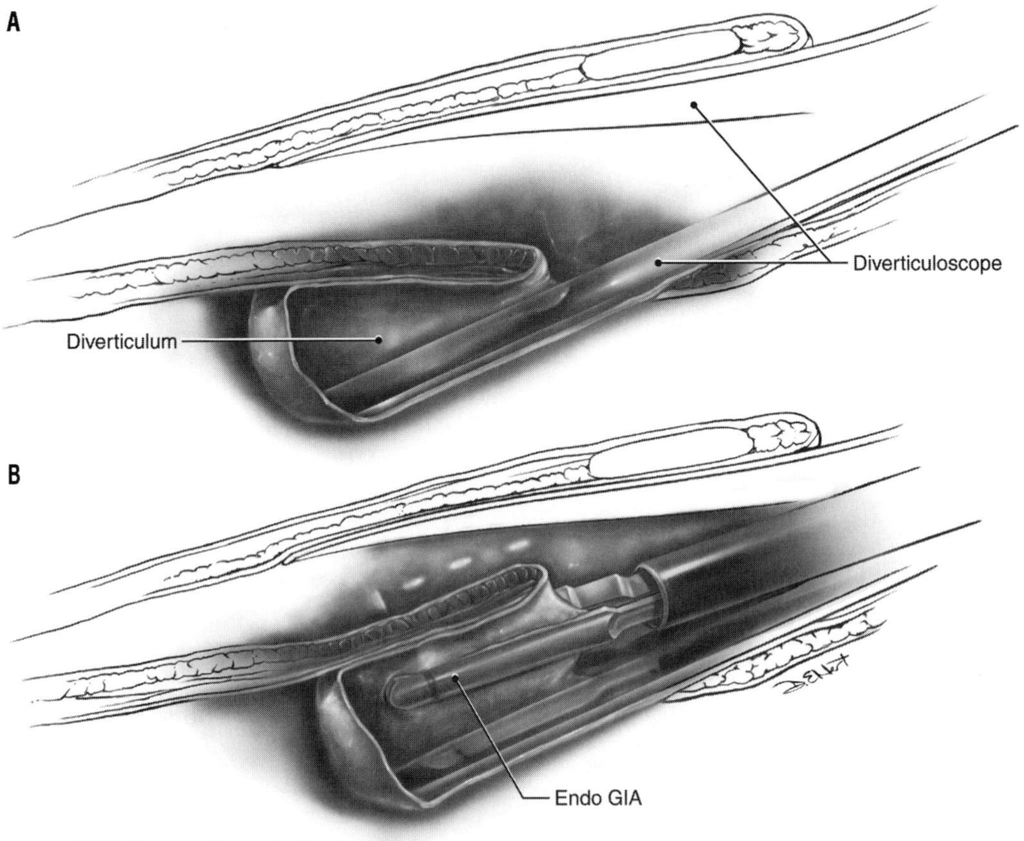

Figure 8–15. A. Exposure of the esophagus and diverticulum is gained with a diverticuloscope placed perorally. **B.** The linear stapler is placed across the cricopharyngeus muscle by placing a blade in the esophagus and the diverticulum. (Reproduced, with permission, from the University of Washington, Seattle.)

Passage of the manometry catheter may be difficult due to coiling in the diverticulum; however, this can be overcome with endoscopic assistance in placement of the catheter. While achalasia is the most common motility disorder identified, others may also be found including nutcracker esophagus, diffuse esophageal spasm, and hypertensive lower esophageal sphincter.[101] However, a specific motility disorder is not always identified on stationary manometry. Clinically, the severity of the patient's symptoms seems to best correlate with the magnitude of the underlying motility disorder, rather than the absolute size of the diverticula.[103] A chest CT would likely not provide further useful information. 24-Hour pH testing may demonstrate gastroesophageal reflux but this is not clinically relevant. Upper endoscopy provides information about the neck of the diverticulum, and other anatomic information that might be helpful in deciding the surgical approach. It also rules out any contributing functional obstruction or possible malignancy.

Management

The treatment in these cases is directed at the underlying pathophysiology and the functional obstruction of the distal esophagus, as well as dealing with the diverticulum. Several therapeutic approaches are available for treating esophageal motility disorders resulting in epiphrenic diverticula, such as pneumatic dilation, especially achalasia. (See motility disorder section.)

With any of the nonsurgical therapies, while treatment of the underlying motility disorder may be achieved, nothing has been done to address the diverticulum, which may still produce symptoms. In one series, aspiration pneumonia was identified in 45% of patients with untreated esophageal diverticula.[104] Thus surgical therapy is generally necessary for epiphrenic diverticulum. The surgical approach has in the past been a diverticulectomy via a left thoracotomy, with or without an associated esophageal myotomy. The diverticulum is dissected free and then resected with a stapler while a bougie of appropriate size is kept within the lumen of the esophagus to prevent narrowing (Fig 8–16). Postoperatively, a contrast study is obtained to rule out a leak.

Unless a myotomy is performed, however, the underlying motility disorder will not be treated. Indeed, the omission of a myotomy has been associated with

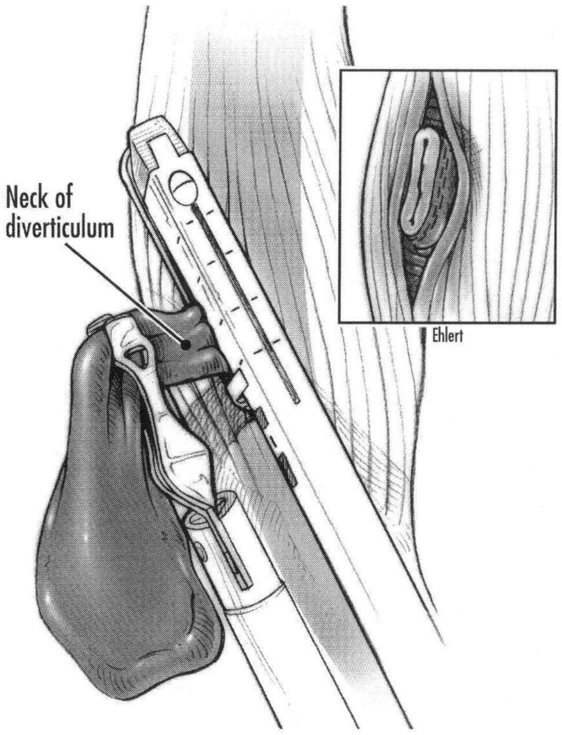

Figure 8–16. Epiphrenic diverticulum resected with a linear stapler. Inset: staple line. (Reproduced, with permission, from the University of Washington, Seattle.)

an increased incidence of recurrence and suture line leakage.[105] Excellent results with cardiomyotomy can be achieved in 90–95% of patients. Traditionally, this was accomplished either by a transthoracic or a transabdominal approach. Recent developments in minimally invasive techniques now allow performance of cardiomyotomy by either a thoracoscopic[63] or a laparoscopic[64] approach. The laparoscopic approach is now the preferred approach. Most diverticula of the lower third of the esophagus can easily be approached laparoscopically. In contrast to a thoracic approach, there is no need for single-lung ventilation or use of a chest tube postoperatively. Laparoscopy also avoids the morbidity of a painful thoracic incision. Using the laparoscopic approach, typical postoperative length of stays are 1–2 days, versus 7–10 days with thoracotomy. Thus, laparoscopic diverticulectomy and myotomy can be performed with less morbidity and likely provides some economic advantage versus traditional approaches. In addition, we are able to perform a longer gastric myotomy, which results in less dysphagia and fewer interventions for recurrent dysphagia.[67] We also add an anti-reflux procedure to prevent postmyotomy GERD. An added benefit in this case is that it buttresses the diverticulectomy staple line for additional protection. Esophagectomy is generally not necessary, and is reserved for those patients with end-stage achalasia and in those who have failed previous surgical management.

▪ ESOPHAGEAL PERFORATION

Esophageal perforation is an uncommon occurrence. This is fortunate, as it is a surgical emergency that is often difficult to manage, and has devastating sequelae if diagnosis and treatment are delayed. Historically, Hermann Boerhaave first described the entity of spontaneous esophageal rupture in 1723.[106] He documented the case of Baron Wassenaer, the Grand Admiral of Holland. In this case, the admiral self-administered emetics after a bout of overeating. This resulted in powerful vomiting which was soon followed by severe pain and subsequent death within 24 hours. Boerhaave performed the autopsy finding a ruptured esophagus and food contents within the chest. Esophageal perforation is a full-thickness injury to the esophagus that can occur during a number of situations, with the vast majority of injuries secondary to iatrogenic causes. However, other causes include spontaneous perforation, blunt or penetrating trauma, tumor rupture, injury from ingested foreign bodies, infection, and caustic injuries. Prior to the middle of the last century, esophageal perforation was a uniformly fatal entity. Advances in diagnosis, surgical therapy, antimicrobials, and intensive care now allow survival in the majority of cases diagnosed and treated in a timely manner.

ETIOLOGY

In a collective review of 559 patients, iatrogenic injury produced 59% of the esophageal injuries, followed by spontaneous perforations (15%), ingested foreign bodies (12%), trauma (9%), operative injury (2%), and tumor perforation (1%).[107]

With the increasing role for mechanical intubation of the esophagus for diagnostic and therapeutic purposes, perforation during these procedures is by far the leading cause. While the relative incidence of perforation is low, the absolute numbers of procedures being done results in a significant number of injuries. The incidence of injury during flexible endoscopy is estimated at 0.03%.[108] This risk is elevated slightly with the addition of bougienage and balloon dilatation. The incidence may approach or exceed 4% with the use of large pneumatic balloons to treat achalasia.[62] Other infrequent sources include thermal injury during therapy for gastrointestinal bleeding, injury during sclerotherapy or ligation of esophageal varices, and perforation during photodynamic therapy or stent placement during the palliation of malignancy.

Accidental perforation may also occur during the course of a surgical procedure, whether or not the esophagus is the organ of interest during the operation. This includes thyroidectomy, carotid procedures, tracheostomy, mediastinoscopy, cardiac valve repair, pneumonectomy or lung transplant, aortic aneurysm repair, cervical spine operations, and chest tube placement. Most frequently, injuries occur during operations directed at the esophagus or esophagogastric junction, such as anti-reflux operations, esophagogastric myotomies, and vagotomies. These injuries have become more frequent as increasing numbers of foregut operations are being performed since the advent of minimally invasive approaches.

Spontaneous perforations are the result of barotrauma secondary to a rapid increase in intraluminal pressure leading to transmural injury. Any action which produces a ballistic increase in pressure may produce this injury, such as during hyperemesis, heavy lifting, or Valsalva during childbirth.

Trauma-associated perforations are typically the result of penetrating injuries; however, perforation due to blunt force trauma, while rare (0.001%),[109] is not unknown. Blunt injuries are most commonly the result of increased intraesophageal pressure leading to rupture. Patients with blunt esophageal injury often have several associated injuries, making diagnosis difficult and delays in treatment common.

Foreign bodies result in perforations at points of physiological esophageal narrowing such as the cricopharyngeus or the aortic arch. These injuries may be the result of penetration from sharp objects (i.e., fish bones) or from gradual pressure necrosis and erosion of an impacted bolus.

Ingestion of caustic material, particularly lye, results in liquefaction necrosis of the esophageal wall and delayed necrosis. These injuries occur in children or in those who have ingested material during suicide attempts.

Medications may also cause injury resulting in perforations. Nonsteroidal anti-inflammatory drugs, etidronate, and potassium chloride are common culprits. Impaction secondary to motility disorders or prior stricture can be contributing factors.

CLINICAL PRESENTATION

The clinical presentation of esophageal perforation depends on the location of the injury, the size of the injury, and the time interval since the occurrence of the injury. The lack of a true serosa makes the esophagus more susceptible to perforation. Extravasation of luminal contents leads to mediastinal contamination. The esophageal contents spread through the potential space of the prevertebral fascia. Saliva, gastric acid, bile, and foodstuffs cause a severe inflammatory reaction in the mediastinum and chest, leading to massive fluid sequestration. Bacteria are also carried into this space, leading to polymicrobial infection. Ultimately, if untreated, this leads to sepsis and ultimately cardiovascular collapse. The presenting symptoms may mimic a variety of pathologies such as myocardial infarction, aortic dissection, and pancreatitis, among others. A recent history of esophageal intubation should quickly raise the possibility of perforation and necessitates further inspection.

Cervical injuries commonly present with subcutaneous emphysema, dysphagia or odynophagia, neck pain worsened with flexion, and bloody regurgitation. Symptoms may be initially relatively modest in comparison with more distal injuries. Thoracic injuries typically produce more immediate symptoms. There is usually free rupture of the visceral pleura, except in very localized perforations, resulting in extensive contamination of the pleural cavity as well as the mediastinum. Chest pain, fever, tachypnea, and tachycardia are common. Abdominal perforations produce signs or symptoms of an acute abdomen.

DIAGNOSIS

Early diagnosis of esophageal perforation, regardless of the location of injury, has been clearly shown to reduce morbidity and mortality.[107] As noted, the symptoms of perforation often mimic other pathologies, leading to unfortunate delays in diagnosis and treatment. Plain films of the neck, chest, or abdomen may show evidence of esophageal perforation. This may demonstrate free air within the neck, mediastinum, or abdomen. Pleural effusions or evidence of mediastinal widening may also be seen. If films are obtained soon after the onset of symptoms, radiographic findings may be absent or minimal.[110]

Plain films should be followed with a contrast esophagogram in the upright and lateral decubitus position (Fig 8–17). Gastrografin is advocated as the initial agent in suspected perforation because of the theoretical risk of inflammation due to extravasated barium. However, this risk has recently been called into question.[111,112] Use of water-soluble agents will detect 50% of cervical injuries and 75% of thoracic perforations.[113] Caution should be used with Gastrografin in patients at risk for aspiration, as it may lead to an intense pneumonitis. In these cases, or in cases of a negative study, dilute barium should be used. This results in detection of 60% of cervical and 90% of thoracic injuries confirmed with surgical exploration.[114,115]

Less frequently, CT may be useful. In patients with a negative esophagogram in whom there remains a high index of suspicion, this study may provide valuable information. Additionally, CTs can easily be obtained in the patient unable to undergo a standard esophagogram.

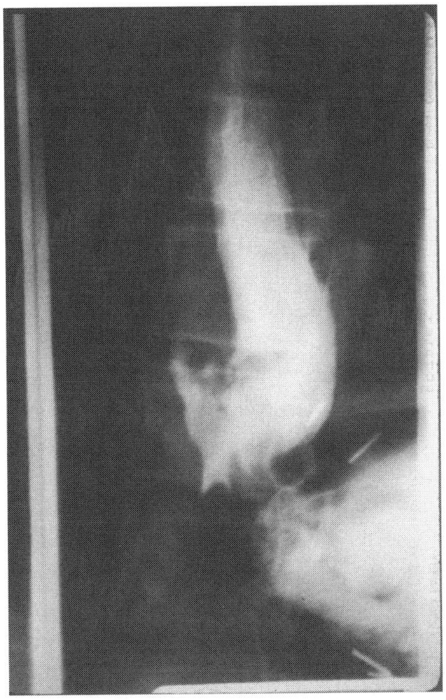

Figure 8–17. Contrast esophagogram with extravasation of contrast in the distal esophagus.

Endoscopy may occasionally be useful in evaluating difficult-to-diagnose injuries or to rule out injury after penetrating trauma. Endoscopy is also useful in determining the exact level of injury and its extension and can be helpful during surgery when one is uncertain of the extent of the mucosal injury. It is reported to have 100% sensitivity and 83% specificity.[116] However, caution is necessary, as air insufflation during examination may extend small tears, forcing operative intervention in a minor injury which otherwise could have been managed nonoperatively.

MANAGEMENT

Nonoperative Management

Nonoperative management may be attempted in select situations, such as in injuries that are small, contained, and without extensive contamination (i.e., no symptoms or signs of sepsis). Several series suggest that in carefully selected patients this approach can be used successfully.[117–121] Cameron and associates[121] and Altorjay and colleagues[117] have established the following criteria for conservative management of these injuries: (1) early diagnosis with mild symptoms and absence of sepsis; (2) containment of leakage within the neck or mediastinum that drains back into the esophagus; (3) absence of distal obstruction or malignancy; and (4) availability of a surgeon experienced with esophageal disease.

These patients receive broad-spectrum antibiotics, intravenous acid suppressors, and total parenteral nutrition. The patient should be frequently reassessed and the surgeon prepared to operate if it becomes necessary. Repeat imaging should be performed in any patient with clinical deterioration or signs of infection. Well-localized fluid collection can be managed with CT-guided percutaneous drainage if accessible. Serial esophagograms with water-soluble contrast are performed to evaluate healing. Oral restriction and intravenous antibiotics are continued for 7–14 days, depending on the serial imaging studies and the patient's clinical condition.

There have been recent reports of the successful use of endoscopically placed self-expanding coated stents to seal the perforation.[122,123] While appealing, especially in the case of disseminated malignancy or in the patient thought too frail to tolerate an operation, the role of this therapeutic option remains to be defined.

Operative Management

Cervical Perforations. Cervical perforations are approached through an incision along the anterior border of the left sternocleidomastoid. The incision is carried down through the strap muscles and the omohyoid. Care is taken to identify the recurrent laryngeal nerve and to protect it. After division of the middle thyroid vein, the trachea and larynx are retracted medially and the carotid sheath laterally, followed by careful inspection of the esophagus circumferentially. Once the injury is identified the injury is débrided and closed with a single layer of absorbable material. A closed suction drain is then placed and the incision closed. In the event no perforation can be clearly identified, wide drainage should be employed. In either scenario, the patient is given antibiotics preoperatively and they are continued for at least 5 days. A contrast esophagogram is then obtained. If there is no evidence of a leak, the patient is started on clear liquids and observed. Persistent leak is managed with continued drainage and intravenous nutrition.

Thoracic Perforations. These injuries are typically approached through a thoracotomy. The proximal and mid-esophagus are approached via a right thoracotomy and the distal esophagus via a left thoracotomy. The injured area needs to be identified (and if it is not clear, an intraoperative endoscopy may facilitate identification, location, and measurement of its extent). The esophagus is mobilized circumferentially with care not to injure the vagi and two Penrose drains are passed, one above and one below the injured area. This affords excellent exposure of the injury. Injuries identified within the first 24 hours are treated with mediastinal débridement, irrigation, and primary closure. The rent is carefully débrided; a small longitudinal myotomy is sometimes necessary to ensure identification of the extent of the mucosal injury. The mucosa is repaired with a single layer of absorbable suture. Most surgeons will reinforce the repair with a patch of pleura or intercostal muscle (Fig 8–18). A minimum of two large chest tubes are placed. One of the most common types of injuries is the perforation that occurs as a consequence of a pneumatic dilatation. In most instances the perforation manifests itself during the early stages and the great majority of these patients would benefit from an operative intervention. The primary goal of operation in these patients is to address the perforation (i.e., close it), following the principles outlined above, and secondarily to perform a myotomy on the contralateral side of the esophagus. If this is not done, the closure is at higher risk of rupture because of the persistent obstruction, but most importantly, the patient will remain symptomatic and it is unlikely that an endoscopic dilatation will again be considered. Returning to the site surgically after some time will be made much more difficult because of the resulting adhesions. Thus while not necessarily intuitive, the performance of a myotomy to address achalasia during the closure of an esophageal perforation is vital to the success of the operation.

For injuries encountered after the first 24 hours, primary repair may be difficult, as the tissue is friable and any repair is at high risk for breakdown. In this situation a T-tube may be inserted and the perforation closed around it, creating an esophagocutaneous fistula[124] (Fig 8–19).

The tube can be left in place for 4–6 weeks and then can usually be pulled without difficulty. An alternative for the unstable patient with severe contamination and delayed diagnosis is esophageal exclusion and diversion. This consists of creation of a cervical esophagostomy, drainage of the mediastinum, placement of a gastrostomy, and a feeding jejunostomy. The patient then typically undergoes esophagectomy and reestablishment of gastrointestinal continuity with a conduit once they are clinically stable and nutritionally replete.

For extensive injuries or in the case of perforation in the presence of malignancy, esophagectomy is an alterna-

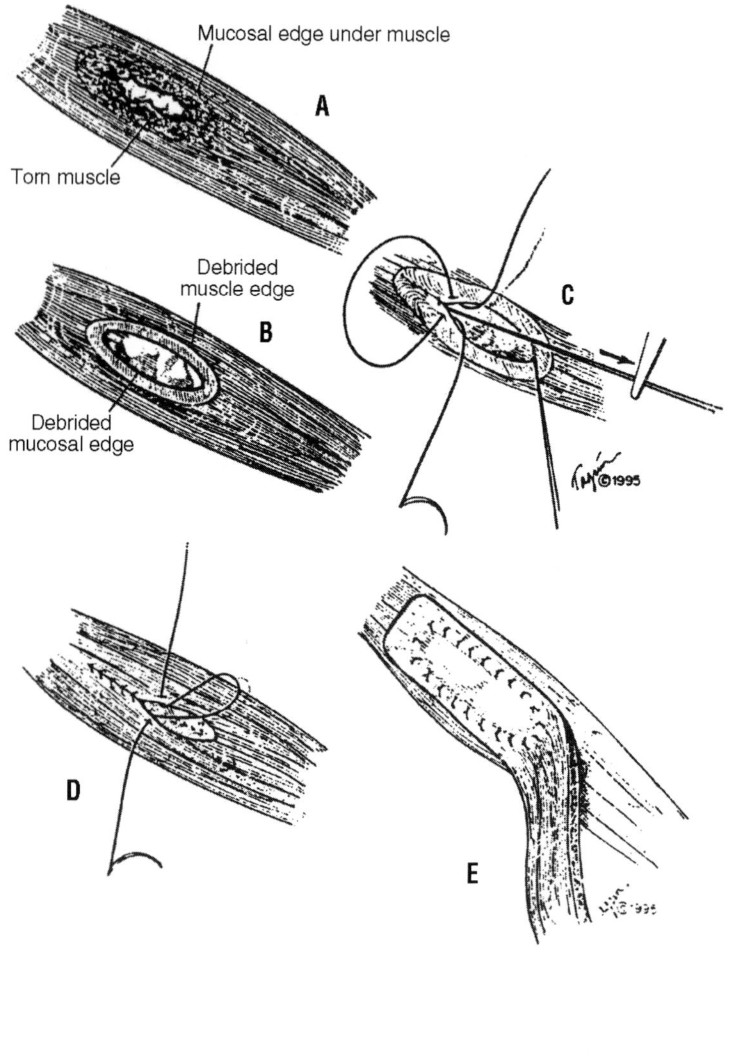

Figure 8–18. Technique of reinforced primary repair of esophageal perforation. **A.** Ragged partially necrotic muscle at the border of the tear hides the full extent of the mucosal injury. **B.** Necrotic muscle has been débrided back to fully expose the mucosal defect and the mucosal edge is trimmed to healthy tissue. **C.** Inverting interrupted fine 4-0 sutures are placed and tied so the knots remain inside. Inward traction on the previously placed suture facilitates proper mucosal inversion. Suturing is begun in each corner and finished in the middle. **D.** A second layer of interrupted fine 4-0 sutures is placed if possible in the muscle layer to cover the mucosal repair. **E.** A previously harvested intercostal muscle flap with an intact vascular bundle is swung on its posteriorly based pedicle to cover and buttress the repair. This is sutured over the closure with interrupted mattress sutures in a circumferential fashion to make a third watertight layer. All sutures are placed first before trying to facilitate an exact repair. (Reproduced, with permission, from Wright CD, et al. Reinforced primary repair of thoracic esophageal perforation. *Ann Thorac Surg* 1995;60:245.)

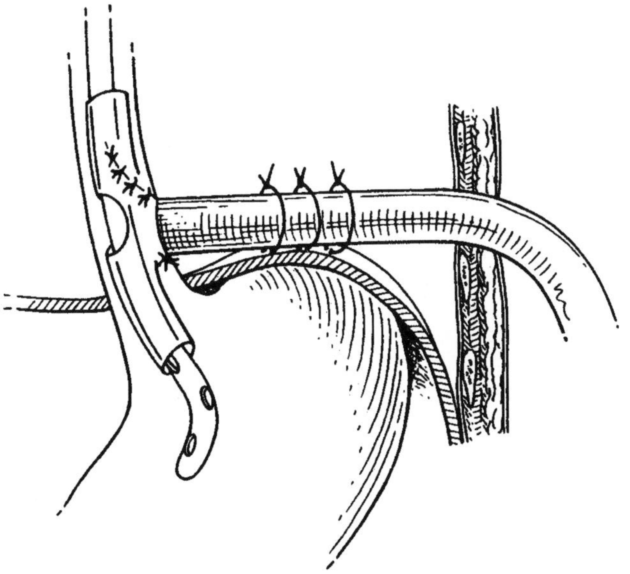

Figure 8–19. T-tube placed in the esophagus, secured on the diaphragm away from the aorta, and brought out through the chest wall. (Reproduced, with permission, from Bufkin BL, Miller JI Jr, Mansour KA. Esophageal perforation: emphasis on management. *Ann Thorac Surg* 1996;61:1447.)

tive if the patient is stable enough to undergo an operation. For cases with minimal contamination, transhiatal esophagectomy is a reasonable option. Patients with more extensive contamination are best approached via thoracotomy to ensure adequate débridement and drainage to control sepsis. Thoracic perforations, regardless of the final course of treatment, are treated with wide drainage, intravenous antibiotics, and nutrition. Nutrition is best provided through a feeding jejunostomy, reserving the stomach as a possible conduit in the future, as these patients tend to have protracted postoperative courses.

The extent of contamination and the condition of the patient will determine whether an immediate or staged reconstruction is carried out. Details of these operations can be found elsewhere in this text.

OUTCOMES

The mortality associated with esophageal perforations depends on the location of the injury and the interval between perforation and treatment. Cervical injuries tend to have a lower mortality. This is likely due to better control of contamination within the planes of the neck. In contrast, as described previously, thoracic and abdominal perforations may lead to widespread soilage of the chest or abdominal cavities. In a recent review by Brinster and associates[107] of 397 patients from several series, mortality from cervical perforations averaged 6% (0–16%), that from thoracic injuries 27% (0–44%), and that from abdominal injuries 21% (0–43%).

A time period of 24 hours between injury and treatment appears to be a line of distinction with respect to mortality after perforation. In the same review by Brinster and colleagues of 390 patients from 11 series, treatment within 24 hours resulted in a 14% (0–28%) mortality rate, whereas a delay in treatment of 24 hours resulted in a 27% (0–46%) mortality rate.

REFERENCES

1. Willwerth BM. Gastric complications associated with paraesophageal herniation. *Am Surg* 1974;40:366
2. Cloyd DW. Laparoscopic repair of incarcerated paraesophageal hernias. *Surg Endosc* 1994;8:893
3. Hill LD. Incarcerated paraesophageal hernia. *Am J Surg* 1973;126:286
4. Farrell B, Gerard PS, Bryk D. Paraesophageal hernia causing colonic obstruction. *J Clin Gastroenterol* 1991;13: 188
5. Huntington TR. Laparoscopic mesh repair of the esophageal hiatus. *J Am Coll Surg* 1997;184:399
6. Duranceau A, Jamieson GG. Hiatal hernia and gastroesophageal reflux. In: Sabiston DC Jr, Lyerly HK, (eds). *Textbook of Surgery, the Biologic Basis of Modern Surgical Practice,* 15th ed. Philadelphia, PA: WB Saunders; 1997:767
7. Cameron AJ, Higgins JA. Linear gastric erosion: a lesion associated with large diaphragmatic hernia and chronic blood loss anaemia. *Gastroenterology* 1986;91:338
8. Walther B, DeMeester TR, Lafontaine E, et al. Effect of paraesophageal hernia on sphincter function and its implication on surgical therapy. *Am J Surg* 1984;132:586
9. Skinner DB, Belsey RH. Surgical management of esophageal reflux and hiatus hernia. Long-term results with 1030 patients. *J Thorac Cardiovasc Surg* 1967;53:33
10. Allen MS, Trastek VF, Deschamps C, et al. Intrathoracic stomach. Presentation and results of operation. *J Thorac Cardiovasc Surg* 1993;105:253
11. Stylopoulos MD, Gazelle GS, Rattner DW. Paraesophageal hernias: operation or observation. *Ann Surg* 2002; 236:492
12. Luketich JD, Raja S, Fernando HC, et al. Laparoscopic repair of giant paraesophageal hernia: 100 consecutive cases. *Ann Surg* 2000;4:608
13. Hashemi M, Peters JH, DeMeester TR, et al. Laparoscopic repair of large type III hiatal hernia: objective follow-up reveals high recurrence rate. *J Am Coll Surg* 2000; 190:553
14. O'Rourke RW, Khajanchee YS, Urbach DR, et al. Extended transmediastinal dissection: an alternative to gastroplasty for short esophagus. *Arch Surg* 2003;138:735
15. Madan AK, Frantizides CT, Patsavas KL. The myth of the short esophagus. *Surg Endosc* 2004;18:31
16. Horgan S, Eubanks TR, Jacobsen G, et al. Repair of paraesophageal hernias. *Am J Surg* 1999;177:354
17. Kercher KW, Matthews BD, Ponsky JL, et al. Minimally invasive management of paraesophageal herniation in the high-risk surgical patient. *Am J Surg* 2001;182:510

18. Carlson MA, Condon RE, Ludwig KA, et al. Management of intrathoracic stomach with polypropylene mesh prosthesis reinforced transabdominal hiatus hernia repair. *J Am Coll Surg* 1998;187:227
19. Trus TL, Bax T, Richardson WS, et al. Complication of laparoscopic paraesophageal hernia repair. *J Gastrointest Surg* 1997;1:221
20. Oelschlager BK, Barreca M, Chang L, et al. The use of small intestine submucosa in the repair of paraesophageal hernias: initial observation of a new technique. *Am J Surg* 2003;186:4
21. Williamson WA, Ellis FH, Streitz JM, et al. Paraesophageal hiatal hernia: is an anti-reflux procedure necessary? *Ann Thorac Surg* 1993;56:447
22. Myers GA, Harms BA, Starling JR. Management of paraesophageal hernia with a selective approach to antireflux surgery. *Am J Surg* 1995;170:375
23. Geha AS, Massad MG, Snow NJ, et al. A 32-year experience in 100 patients with giant paraesophageal hernia: the case for abdominal approach and selective antireflux repair. *Surgery* 2000;128:623
24. Behrns KE, Schlinkert RT. Laparoscopic management of paraesophageal hernia: early results. *J Laparoendosc Surg* 1996;6:311
25. Richter JE, Bradley LA, Castell DO. Esophageal chest pain: current controversies in pathogenesis, diagnosis and treatment. *Ann Intern Med* 1989;119:66
26. Cherian P, Smith LF, Bardham KD, et al. Esophageal tests in the evaluation of non-cardiac chest pain. *Dis Esophagus* 1995;8:129
27. Achem SR, Kolts BE, Wears R, et al. Chest pain associated with nutcracker esophagus: A preliminary study of the role of gastroesophageal reflux. *Am J Gastroenterol* 1993;88:187
28. Fass R, Fennerty B, Johnson C, et al. Correlation of ambulatory 24-hour esophageal pH monitoring results with symptom improvement in patients with noncardiac chest pain due to gastroesophageal reflux diseases. *J Clin Gastroenterol* 1998;28:36
29. Barreca M, Oelschlager BK, Pellegrini CA. Outcomes of laparoscopic Nissen fundoplication in patients with "hypercontractile esophagus." *Arch Surg* 2002; 137:724
30. Osgood H. A peculiar form of esophagismus. *Boston Med Surg J* 1889;120:401
31. Richter JE. Oesophageal motility disorders. *Lancet* 2001; 358:823
32. Behar J, Biancani P. Pathogenesis of simultaneous esophageal contractions in patients with motility disorders. *Gastroenterology* 1993;105:11
33. Brand DL, Martin D, Pope CE. Esophageal manometrics in patients with anginal type chest pain. *Am J Dig Dis* 1977;23:300
34. Benjamin SB, Castell DO. The "nutcracker esophagus" and the spectrum of esophageal motor disorders. *Curr Concepts Gastroenterol* 1980;5:3
35. Mujica VR, Mudipall RS, Rao SS. Pathophysiology of chest pain in patients with nutcracker esophagus. *Am J Gastroenterol* 2001;96:1371
36. Melzer E, Tiomny A, Coret A, et al. Nutcracker esophagus: severe muscular hypertrophy on endosonography. *Gastrointest Endosc* 1995;42:366
37. Clouse RE, Lustman PJ. Psychiatric illness and contraction abnormalities of the esophagus. *N Engl J Med* 1983; 309:1337
38. Clouse RE, Lustman PJ, Eckert TC, et al. Low-dose trazodone for symptomatic patients with esophageal contraction abnormalities. A double-blind, placebo-controlled trial. *Gastroenterology* 1987;92:1027
39. Katada N, Hinder RA, Hinder PR, et al. The hypertensive lower esophageal sphincter. *Am J Surg* 1996;172: 439
40. Waterman DC, Dalton CB, Ott DJ, et al. Hypertensive lower esophageal sphincter: what does it mean? *J Clin Gastroenterol* 1989;11:139
41. Richter JE, Dalton CB, Bradley CA, et al. Oral nifedipine in the treatment of noncardiac chest pain in patients with the nutcracker esophagus. *Gastroenterology* 1987;93:21
42. Achem SR, Kolts BE, MacMath T, et al. Effects of omeprazole versus placebo in treatment of noncardiac chest pain and gastroesophageal reflux. *Dig Dis Sci* 1997;42: 2138
43. Clouse RE. Spastic disorders of the esophagus. *Gastroenterologist* 1997;5:112
44. Klimes I, Mayou RA, Pearce MJ, et al. Psychological treatment for atypical non-cardiac chest pain: a controlled evaluation. *Psychol Med* 1990;20:605
45. Mayou RA, Bryant BM, Sanders D, et al. A controlled trial of cognitive behavioral therapy for non-cardiac chest pain. *Psychol Med* 1997;27:1021
46. Beitman BD, Basha IM, Trombka LH, et al. Alprazolam in the treatment of cardiology patients with atypical chest pain and panic disorder. *J Clin Psychopharmacol* 1988;198:127
47. Peghini P, Katz P, Castell DO. Imipramine increases pain and sensation thresholds to esophageal balloon distention in humans. *Dig Dis Sci* 1995;40:1325
48. Miller LS, Parkman HP, Schiano TD, et al. Treatment of symptomatic nonachalasia esophageal motor disorders with botulinum toxin injection at the lower esophageal sphincter. *Dig Dis Sci* 1996;41:10
49. Shimi SM, Nathanson LK, Cuschieri A. Thoracoscopic long oesophageal myotomy for nutcracker oesophagus: initial experience of a new surgical approach. *Br J Surg* 1992;79:533
50. Goldblum JR, Rice TW, Richter JE. Histopathological features in esophagomyotomy specimens from patients with achalasia. *Gastroenterology* 1996;111:648
51. Howard PJ, Maher L, Pryde A, et al. Five year prospective study of the incidence, clinical features, and diagnosis of achalasia in Edinburgh. *Gut* 1992;33:1011
52. Shoenut JP, Trenholm BG, Micflickier AB, et al. Reflux pattern in patients with achalasia without operation. *Ann Thorac Surg* 1988;45:303
53. Smart HL, Foster PN, Evans DF, et al. Twenty four hour oesophageal acidity in achalasia before and after pneumatic dilatation. *Gut* 1987;28;883

54. Gelfond M, Rozen P, Keren S, et al. Effect of nitrates on LOS pressure in achalasia: a potential therapeutic aid. *Gut* 1981;22:312
55. Traube M, Dubovik S, Lange RC, et al. The role of nifedipine therapy in achalasia: results of a randomized, double-blind, placebo-controlled study. *Am J Gastroenterol* 1989;84:1259
56. Gelfond M, Rozen P, Gilat T. Isosorbide dinitrate and nifedipine treatment of achalasia: a clinical, manometric and radionuclide evaluation. *Gastroenterology* 1982;83:963
57. Vaezi MF, Richter JE. Current therapies for achalasia: comparison and efficacy. *J Clin Gastroenterol* 1998;27:21
58. Horgan S, Hudda K, Eubanks T, et al. Does botulinum toxin injection make esophagomyotomy a more difficult operation? *Surg Endosc* 1999;13:576
59. Willis T. In: *Hagae Comitis. Pharmaceutice Rationalis Sive Diatribe de Medicamentorum Operationibus in Human Corpore.* London, England; 1674
60. Csendes A, Braghett I, Hernriquez A, et al. Late results of a prospective randomized study comparing forceful dilatation and oesophagomyotomy in patients with achalasia. *Gut* 1989;30:299
61. Clouse RE, Abramson BK, Todorczuk JR. Achalasia in the elderly: Effects of aging on clinical presentation and outcome. *Dig Dis Sci* 1991;36:225
62. Reynolds JC, Parkman HP. Achalasia. *Gastroenterol Clin North Am* 1989;18:223
63. Pellegrini C, Wetter LA, Patti M, et al. Thoracoscopic esophagomyotomy: initial experience with a new approach for the treatment of achalasia. *Ann Surg* 1992;216:291
64. Cuschieri A, Shimi S, Nathanson LK. Laparoscopic cardiomyotomy for achalasia. *J R Coll Surg Edinb* 1991;36:152
65. Pelligrini CA, Leichter R, Patti M, et al. Thoracoscopic esophageal myotomy in the treatment of achalasia. *Ann Thorac Surg* 1993;56:680
66. Patti MG, Pellegrini CA, Horgan S, et al. Minimally invasive surgery for achalasia: an 8-year experience with 168 patients. *Ann Surg* 1999;230:587
67. Oelschlager BK, Chang L, Pellegrini CA. Improved outcome after extended gastric myotomy for achalasia. *Arch Surg* 2003;138:490
68. Sharp KW, Khaitan L, Scholz S, et al. 100 Consecutive minimally invasive Heller myotomies: lessons learned. *Ann Surg* 2002;235:631
69. Richards WO, Clements RH, Wang PC, et al. Prevalence of gastroesophageal reflux after laparoscopic Heller myotomy. *Surg Endosc* 1999;13:1010
70. Wills VL, Hunt DR. Functional outcome after Heller myotomy and fundoplication for achalasia. *J Gastrointest Surg* 2001;5:408
71. Agur A. *Grant's Atlas of Anatomy.* Baltimore, MD: Williams & Wilkins; 1991:650
72. Westrin KM, Ergun S, Carlsoo B. Zenker's diverticulum—a historical review and trends in therapy. *Acta Otolaryngol* 1996;116:351
73. Counter PR, Hilton ML, Baldwin DL. Long-term follow-up of endoscopic stapled diverticulotomy. *Ann R Coll Surg Engl* 2002;84:89
74. Ellis FH Jr. Pharyngoesophageal (Zenker's) diverticulum. *Adv Surg* 1995;28:171
75. D'Ugo D, Cardillo G, Granone P, et al. Esophageal diverticula. Physiopathological basis for surgical management. *Eur J Cardiothorac Surg* 1992;6:330
76. McConnel FM, Hood D, Jackson K, et al. Analysis of intrabolus forces in patients with Zenker's diverticulum. *Laryngoscope* 1994;104:571
77. Lerut T, van Raemdonck D, Guelinckx P, et al. Zenker's diverticulum: is a myotomy of the cricopharyngeus useful? How long should it be? *Hepatogastroenterology* 1992;39:127
78. Zaninotto G, Costantini M, Anselmino M, et al. Onset of oesophageal peristalsis after surgery for idiopathic achalasia. *Br J Surg* 1995;82:1532
79. Venturi M, et al. Biochemical markers of upper esophageal sphincter compliance in patients with Zenker's diverticulum. *J Surg Res* 1997;70:46
80. Dantas RO, Cook IJ, Dodds WJ, et al. Biomechanics of cricopharyngeal bars. *Gastroenterology* 1990;99:1269
81. Ekberg O. Cricopharyngeal bar: myth and reality. *Abdom Imaging* 1995;20:179
82. Brady AP, Stevenson GW, Somers S, et al. Premature contraction of the cricopharyngeus: a new sign of gastroesophageal reflux disease. *Abdom Imaging* 1995;20:225
83. Gregoire J, Duranceau A. Surgical management of Zenker's diverticulum. *Hepatogastroenterology* 1992;39:132
84. Louie HW, Zuckerbraun L. Staged Zenker's diverticulectomy with cervical esophagostomy and secondary esophagostomy closure for treatment of massive diverticulum in severely debilitated patients. *Am Surg* 1993;59:842
85. Nguyen HC, Urquhart AC. Zenker's diverticulum. *Laryngoscope* 1997;107:1436
86. Benjamin B, Innocenti M. Laser treatment of pharyngeal pouch. *Aust N Z J Surg* 1991;61:909
87. Bradwell RA, Bieger AK, Strachan DR, et al. Endoscopic laser myotomy in the treatment of pharyngeal diverticula. *J Laryngol Otol* 1997;111:627
88. Collard JM, Otte JB, Kestens PJ. Endoscopic stapling technique of esophagodiverticulostomy for Zenker's diverticulum. *Ann Thorac Surg* 1993;56:573
89. Ishioka S, Sakai P, Maluf FF, Melo JM. Endoscopic incision of Zenker's diverticula. *Endoscopy* 1995;27:433
90. Spiro SA, Berg HM. Applying the endoscopic stapler in excision of Zenker's diverticulum: a solution for two intraoperative problems. *Otolaryngol Head Neck Surg* 1994;110:603
91. Laccourreye O, Menard M, Cauchois R, et al. Esophageal diverticulum: diverticulopexy versus diverticulectomy. *Laryngoscope* 1994;104:889
92. Lerut T, VanRaemdonck D, Guelinckx P, et al. Pharyngo-oesophageal diverticulum (Zenker's). Clinical, therapeutic and morphological aspects. *Acta Gastroenterol Belg* 1990;53:330

93. Watemberg S, Landau O, Avrahami R. Zenker's diverticulum: reappraisal. *Am J Gastroenterol* 1996;91:1494
94. Collard JM, Romagnoli R, Lengele B, et al. Heller-Dor procedure for achalasia: from conventional to video-endoscopic surgery. *Acta Chir Belg* 1996;96:62
95. Barthlen W, Feussner H, Hannig C, et al. Surgical therapy of Zenker's diverticulum: low risk and high efficiency. *Dysphagia* 1990;5:13
96. Laing MR, Murthy P, Ah SKW, et al. Surgery for pharyngeal pouch: audit of management with short- and long-term follow-up. *J R Coll Surg Edinb* 1995;40:315
97. van Overbeek JJ. Meditation on the pathogenesis of hypopharyngeal (Zenker's) diverticulum and a report of endoscopic treatment in 545 patients. *Ann Otol Rhinol Laryngol* 1994;103:178
98. Narne S, Cutrone C, Bonavina L, et al. Endoscopic diverticulotomy for the treatment of Zenker's diverticulum: results in 102 patients with staple-assisted endoscopy. *Ann Otol Rhinol Laryngol* 1999;108:810
99. Stoeckli SJ, Schmid S. Endoscopic stapler-assisted diverticulo-esophagostomy for Zenker's diverticulum: patient satisfaction and subjective relief of symptoms. *Surgery* 2002;131:158
100. Matthews B, Nelms C, Lohr C, et al. Minimally invasive management of epiphrenic esophageal diverticula. *Am Surg* 2003;69:465
101. Nehra D, Lord RV, DeMeester TR, et al. Physiologic basis for the treatment of epiphrenic diverticulum. *Ann Surg* 2002;234:346
102. Mondiere J. Notes sur quelques maladies de l'oesophage. *Arch Gen Med Paris* 1833;3:28
103. Orringer M. Epiphrenic diverticula: fact and fable. *Ann Thorac Surg* 1993;55:1067
104. Altorki N, Sunagawa M, Skinner D. Thoracic esophageal diverticula: why is operation necessary? *J Thorac Cardiovasc Surg* 1993;105:260
105. Benacci J, Deschamps C, Trastek V, et al. Epiphrenic diverticulum: results of surgical treatment. *Ann Thorac Surg* 1993;55:1109
106. Boerhaave H. *Atrocis, nes descripti pruis, morbi historia: secundum meicae artis leges conscripta.* Lugundi Batavorum: Boutesteniana; 1724
107. Brinster CJ, Singhal S, Lee L, et al. Evolving options in the management of esophageal perforation. *Ann Thorac Surg* 2004;77:1475
108. Sivis SE, Nebel O, Roger G, et al. Endoscopic complications. Results of the 1974 American Society for Gastrointestinal Endoscopy Survey. *JAMA* 1976;235:928
109. Beal SL, Pottmeyer EW, Spisso JM. Esophageal perforation following external blunt trauma. *J Trauma* 1988;28:1425
110. Han SY, McElvein RB, Aldrete JS, et al. Perforation of the esophagus: correlation of site and cause with plain film findings. *Am J Roentgenol* 1985;145:537
111. Gollub MJ, Bains MS. Barium sulfate; a new (old) contrast agent for diagnosis of postoperative esophageal leaks. *Radiology* 1982;144:231
112. James AE Jr, Montali RJ, Chaffee V, et al. Barium or gastrograffin; which contrast media for diagnosis of esophageal tears? *Gastroenterology* 1975;68:1103
113. Foley MJ, Ghahremani GG, Rogers LF. Reappraisal of contrast media use to detect upper gastrointestinal perforations: comparison of ionic water-soluble media with barium sulfate. *Radiology* 1982;144:231
114. Sarr MG, Pemberton JH, Payne WS. Management of instrumental perforations of the esophagus. *J Thorac Cardiovasc Surg* 1982;84:211
115. Bladergroen MR, Lowe JE, Postlethwait RW. Diagnosis and recommended management of esophageal perforation and rupture. *Ann Thorac Surg* 1986;42:235
116. Horwitz B, Krevsky B, Buckman RF Jr, et al. Endoscopic evaluation of penetrating esophageal injuries. *Am J Gastroenterol* 1993;88:1249
117. Altorjay A, Kiss J, Voros A, et al. Nonoperative management of esophageal perforations. Is it justified? *Ann Surg* 1997;225:415
118. Shaffer HA Jr, Valenzuela G, Mittal RK. Esophageal perforation. A reassessment of the criteria for choosing medical or surgical therapy. *Arch Intern Med* 1992;152:757
119. Mengold L, Klassen KP. Conservative management of esophageal perforation. *Arch Surg* 1965;91:232
120. Larrieu AJ, Kieffer R. Boerhaave syndrome: report of a case treated non-operatively. *Ann Surg* 1975;181:452
121. Cameron JL, Kieffer RF, Hendrix TR, et al. Selective nonoperative management of contained intrathoracic esophageal disruptions. *Ann Thorac Surg* 1979;27:404
122. Morgan RA, Ellul JP, Denton ER, et al. Malignant esophageal fistulas and perforations: management with plastic-covered metallic endoprostheses. *Radiology* 1997;204:527
123. Mumtaz H, Barone GW, Ketel BL, et al. Successful management of a nonmalignant esophageal perforation with a coated stent. *Ann Thorac Surg* 2002;74:1233
124. Bufkin BL, Muller JI, Mansour KA. Esophageal perforation: emphasis on management. *Ann Thorac Surg* 1996;61:1447

8A

Gastroesophageal Reflux Disease

Thadeus L. Trus ■ *Jeffrey H. Peters*

■ THE EVOLUTION OF SURGICAL TREATMENT FOR GASTROESOPHAGEAL REFLUX DISEASE

Gastroesophageal reflux disease (GERD) was not recognized as a significant clinical problem until the mid 1930's and was not identified as a precipitating cause for esophagitis until after World War II.[1] Initially, the symptoms of gastroesophageal reflux were associated with a hiatal hernia. This led to the conclusion that the hernia itself was the cause of the symptoms. It seemed reasonable to attempt to correct these symptoms by surgically reducing the hernia with simple closure of the crura. The result of this first surgical effort was uniform failure.

Phillip Allison was the first to link the symptoms of hiatus hernia to the occurrence of gastroesophageal reflux. This contribution encouraged surgeons to improve the function of the cardia rather than simply reducing the hernia. The Allison repair, introduced in 1951, represented the first effort in this direction.[2] He emphasized the need to place the gastroesophageal junction in its normal intra-abdominal position to improve its function. Although the repair was associated with a high incidence of recurrence, Allison justly received the credit for initiating the modern era of antireflux surgery.[3]

The experience with the Allison repair demonstrated that relief from the symptoms of reflux occurred in those patients whose gastroesophageal junction remained in the intra-abdominal position. The problem was that in 50% of patients, the hernia recurred. Consequently, surgeons were stimulated to develop procedures designed to place and anchor the lower esophagus more effectively in the intra-abdominal position. Initially, these operations consisted of various forms of gastropexy in which an intra-abdominal esophagus was achieved by pulling the stomach down in the abdomen, whether it was herniated or not, and attaching it to the anterior abdominal wall or to any posterior peritoneal structure that seemed strong enough to maintain it there. The design of the gastropexy operation placed the stomach and esophagus under a great deal of continual tension which was further stressed by normal respiratory and swallowing movements. Consequently, dislodgement of the gastropexies occurred with the return of reflux symptoms.[4,5] The most popular of these operations was the **Hill procedure**, which anchors the gastroesophageal junction posteriorly to the median arcuate ligament.[6]

With the exception of the Hill procedure, these operations did not stand the test of time and were gradually abandoned as more durable methods were sought to achieve an intra-abdominal esophagus. One of these was the **Belsey Mark IV repair**[7] and the other the **Nissen fundoplication.**[8,9] Both procedures incorporate a portion of the distal esophagus into the stomach to ensure that it will be affected by changes in intra-abdominal pressure transmitted by the gastric conduit. The Belsey Mark IV procedure is, in essence, a partial fundoplication, or an enveloping of the distal esophagus with the gastric fundus over 280°, while the Nissen is a complete fundoplication, or a 360° enveloping of the distal esophagus by the gastric fundus.

With wider application of the Nissen procedure, it became evident that a successful Nissen fundoplication is not simply a matter of wrapping the stomach around the lower esophagus and sewing it in place. Rather, a good deal of judgement and experience is required to determine how tight and how long to make the fundoplication, what portion of the stomach should be used, and what conditions preclude the use of the operation. Consequently, Nissen fundoplications have contributed to a number of severe postoperative complications.[10] Most can be attributed to surgical technique and inaccurate selection of patients for operation. If the fundoplication is constructed too long or performed as a wrap rather than an enveloping of the esophagus by the fundus, permanent dysphagia, or odynophagia, may result. Such a fundoplication precludes physiologic belching and vomiting. Instead of performing the operation properly, surgeons began to introduce a variety of partial fundoplications to avoid these problems. They are usually constructed by covering either the anterior or the posterior wall of the distal esophagus with the stomach. This necessitates suturing the fundus of the stomach to the esophagus as the primary and most important portion of the procedure. This suture line is subject to a great deal of stress, and as a consequence, has a limited durability. Although the partial fundoplication operations are successful in preventing reflux and permitting physiologic belching when they remain intact, they disrupt with a distressing frequency.

The most durable of the partial fundoplication procedures is the Belsey Mark IV operation. In this procedure, the attachment of the esophagus to the stomach is more extensive than that advocated for the other partial fundoplications, and the procedure is performed transthoracically, so that the esophagus can be adequately mobilized to construct the repair without undue tension. In situations where the esophagus has shortened, aggressive mobilization does not give a tension-free repair and disruption or withdrawal of the repair into the chest is the rule, giving rise to the symptoms of recurrent heartburn or dysphagia. Recognition of this problem stimulated the development of an esophageal-lengthening technique, by making a tube about the diameter of the esophagus and 5 cm in length along the lesser curvature of the stomach and constructing a Belsey type partial fundoplication over the tube. This procedure is called a **Collis Belsey repair** in honor of Dr. J. Leigh Collis who designed the gastroplasty and Dr. Ronald Belsey who designed the antireflux repair.[11] Although effective as an esophageal lengthening technique, the Collis repair has many drawbacks, the most obvious of which is acid production within the tubularized portion of the stomach.

The main drawback of the Belsey Mark IV procedure is that, when universally applied by surgeons with varied skills, the antireflux protection achieved is not as predictable as with a complete Nissen fundoplication. This is because the Belsey procedure is difficult to teach and explain and has less margin for error. In experienced hands, the success of the Belsey operation appears similar to that of the Nissen.

These historical lessons have allowed improvements in antireflux surgery to the point that excellent results can be achieved in the majority of patients given proper patient selection and the meticulous performance of the appropriate procedure. It is hoped that in this era of minimally invasive surgery, mistakes of the past will not be repeated by those who are unfamiliar with the pathophysiology of the disease and history of antireflux surgery.

▪ DEFINITION AND SYMPTOMS OF GERD

Gastroesophageal reflux is a common disease that accounts for approximately 75% of esophageal pathology. It is now recognized as a chronic disease requiring lifelong medical therapy. Various endoscopic antireflux interventions, although innovative, have not been successful in consistently controlling gastroesophageal reflux. Antireflux surgery is the only effective and long-term therapy and is the only treatment that is able to modify the natural history of recurrent progressive reflux esophagitis. Despite the common prevalence of GERD, it can be one of the most challenging diagnostic and therapeutic problems in benign esophageal disease. A contributing factor to this is the lack of a universally accepted definition of the disease.

The most simplistic approach is to define the disease by its symptoms. However, symptoms thought to be indicative of gastroesophageal reflux disease, such as heartburn or acid regurgitation, are very common in the general population; many individuals consider these symptoms to be normal and do not seek medical attention. Even when excessive, these symptoms are not specific for gastroesophageal reflux. They can be caused by other diseases such as achalasia, diffuse spasm, esophageal carcinoma, pyloric stenosis, cholelithiasis, gastritis, gastric or duodenal ulcer, and coronary artery disease. A thorough, structured evaluation of the patient's symptoms is essential prior to any therapy, particularly any form of esophageal surgery.

The presence and severity of both typical symptoms of heartburn, regurgitation and dysphagia, and atypical symptoms of cough, hoarseness, chest pain, asthma and aspiration should be discussed with the patient in detail. Many of these atypical symptoms may not be esophageal–related and hence will not improve and may even worsen with antireflux surgery.

Heartburn is generally defined as a substernal burning type discomfort, beginning in the epigastrium and radiating upward. It is often aggravated by meals, spicy or fatty foods, chocolate, alcohol, or coffee and can be worse in the supine position. It is commonly, although not universally, relieved by antacids or antisecretory medications. Epidemiologic studies have shown that heartburn occurs monthly in as many as 40% to 50% of the Western population. The occurrence of heartburn at night, and its effect on quality of life have recently been highlighted by a Gallup poll conducted by the American Gastroenterologic Society (Table 8A–1).[12]

Regurgitation, the effortless return of acid or bitter gastric contents into the chest, pharynx, or mouth is highly suggestive of foregut pathology. It is often particularly severe at night when the patient is supine in bed or when he or she bends over and can be secondary to either an incompetent or obstructed gastroesophageal junction. With the later, as in achalasia, the regurgitant is often bland, as if food was put into a blender. When questioned, most patients can distinguish between the two. It is the regurgitation of gastric contents that may result in associated pulmonary symptoms, including cough, hoarseness, asthma, and recurrent pneumonia. Bronchospasm can be precipitated by esophageal acidification and cough by either acid stimulation or distention of the esophagus.

Dysphagia, or difficulty swallowing, is a relatively nonspecific term but arguably the most specific symptom of foregut disease. It is often a sign of underlying malignancy and should be aggressively investigated until a diagnosis is established. Dysphagia refers to the sensation of difficulty in the passage of food from the mouth to the stomach and can be divided into oropharyngeal and esophageal etiologies. **Oropharyngeal dysphagia** is characterized by difficulty transferring food out of the mouth into the esophagus, nasal regurgitation, and/or aspiration. **Esophageal dysphagia** refers to the sensation of food sticking in the lower chest or epigastrium. This may or may not be accompanied by pain (odynophagia), which will be relieved by the passage of the bolus.

Chest pain, although commonly and appropriately attributed to cardiac disease, is frequently secondary to esophageal pathology as well. As early as 1982, DeMeester et al. showed that nearly 50% of patients with severe chest pain, normal cardiac function, and normal coronary arteriograms had positive 24-hour pH studies, implicating gastroesophageal reflux as the underlying etiology.[13] Exercise-induced gastroesophageal reflux is well known to occur and may result in exertional chest pain similar to angina.[14] It can be quite difficult if not impossible to distinguish the two etiologies, particularly on clinical grounds alone.[15,16]

Nevens et al. evaluated the ability of experienced cardiologists to differentiate pain of cardiac versus esophageal origin.[17] Of 248 patients initially seen by cardiologists, 185 were thought to have typical angina and 63

TABLE 8A–1. AMERICAN GASTROENTEROLOGIC SOCIETY GERD SURVEY SUMMARY

- 50 million American have nighttime heartburn at least 1/wk
- 80% of heartburn sufferers had nocturnal symptoms—65% both day & night
- 63% report that it affects their ability to sleep and impacts their work the next day
- 72% are on prescription meds
- Nearly half (45%) report that current remedies do not relieve all symptoms

atypical pain. Forty eight (26%) of those thought to have classic angina had normal coronary angiogram s and 16 of the 63 with atypical pain had abnormal angiograms. *Thus the cardiologists' clinical impression was wrong 25% of the time.* Finally, Pope et al investigated the ultimate diagnosis in 10,689 patients presenting to an emergency room with acute chest pain.[18] Seventeen percent were found to have acute ischemia, 6% stable angina, 21% other cardiac causes, and 55% had noncardiac causes. They concluded that the majority of people presenting to the emergency room with chest pain do not have an underlying cardiac etiology for their symptoms. Chest pain precipitated by meals, occurring at night while supine, that is non-radiating and responsive to antacid medication or accompanied by other symptoms suggesting esophageal disease, such as dysphagia or regurgitation, should trigger the thought of possible esophageal origin. Further, the distinction between heartburn and chest pain is also difficult and largely dependent upon the individual patient. *One person's heartburn is another's chest pain.*

MECHANISMS OF ESOPHAGEAL SYMPTOMS

The precise mechanisms accounting for the generation of symptoms secondary to esophageal pathology remain unclear. Considerable insight has been acquired, however. Investigations into the effect of luminal content,[19,20] esophageal distention[20–22] and muscular function[23], neural pathways and brain localization,[24,25] have provided a basic understanding of the stimuli responsible for symptom generation. It is also clear that the viscero-neural pathways of the foregut are complexly intertwined with that of the tracheobronchial tree and heart. This fact accounts for the common overlap of clinical presentations with diverse disease processes in upper gastrointestinal, cardiac, and pulmonary systems.

Early investigations of the pathogenesis of esophageal symptomatology studied the effects of balloon distention and or esophageal acid infusion on symptom generation. Classic studies, reported as early as the 1930s, investigated the type and location of symptom

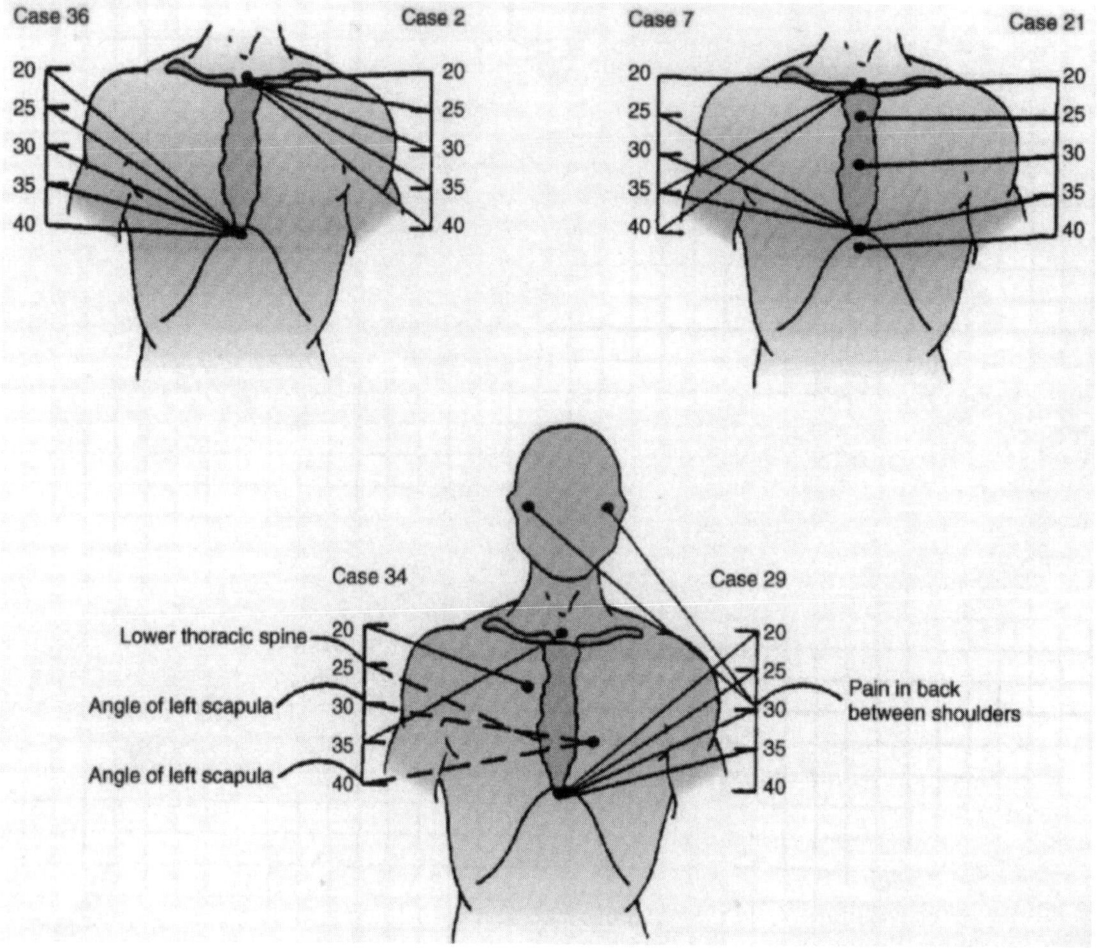

Figure 8A–1. Location of symptoms with esophageal balloon distention in six patients. The legend (20–40) indicates the level of balloon distention within the esophagus and the circles the location of the referred symptom. (From Polland WS et al. *J Clin Invest* 1931: 435–452.)

perception in patients following balloon distention at 5-cm increments in the esophagus.[26] These data revealed highly variable patient responses (Fig 8A–1). Patients rarely accurately localized the location of the stimulus, often perceiving the symptom in areas above, below, or quite distant from the location of the distending balloon. Some patients perceived chest pain, some heartburn, and others nausea. Symptoms occurring between the shoulder blades and base of the neck, and retrobulbar eye pain were also observed. These findings underscore the highly variable nature of symptom generation secondary to foregut epithelial stimuli. More recent studies have confirmed these findings. Taken together, they suggest considerable variability in individual sensory sensitivity and/or cerebral cortical processing.

Esophageal perfusion with either acid or bile salts can elicit various degrees of symptoms ranging from mild heartburn to severe angina-like chest pain. Symptom perception is dependent upon both the concentration and contact time of the offending agent and is highly variable from individual to individual. In general, discomfort becomes reproducible below pH 4, a fact demonstrated in the early years of esophageal pH testing. This was, in part, responsible for the selection of pH 4 as the threshold pH below which acid reflux was considered present on ambulatory esophageal pH testing. Acid perfusion was the basis for the Bernstein test used historically as a means to diagnose GERD. The test has largely fallen by the wayside, in part due to its poor sensitivity and specificity. Similarly, studies of the effects of bile salt perfusion of the esophagus have shown nociception with perfusion. Simultaneous measurement of pH, motility, and ultrasound has shown that sustained contraction of the esophageal longitudinal muscle correlated with the onset of chest pain.[23]

A number of studies have investigated the cortical response to esophageal balloon distention and acid perfusion. Responses have been detected via cortical evoked potential, positron emission tomography (PET), and magnetic resonance imaging (MRI). Kern & Shaker have recently reported the cerebral cortical MRI response to esophageal acid exposure and balloon distention in 10 healthy volunteers.[24] Intraesophageal perfusion of 0.1 N HCl for 10 minutes increased functional MRI signal intensity in all subjects with an average signal increase of 6.7% occurring approximately 5 minutes after perfusion, without inducing heartburn or chest pain. Saline perfusion elicited no detectable change. Similar changes were seen with balloon distention, although the response times were significantly longer for acid perfusion. Responses were seen in the posterior cingulate, parietal, and anterior frontal lobes. The authors concluded that esophageal mucosal acid contact produces a cerebral cortical response detectable by functional MRI and that the temporal characteristics of the acid response are different than balloon distention.

Studies on the natural history of GERD are difficult to perform because of the mobility of modern society. Those that have been done indicate that most patients have limited disease responsive to simple lifestyle, dietary and medical therapy and do not go on to develop complications. Investigations of the natural history of GERD in the absence of esophagitis have demonstrated return of symptoms in the majority of patients following cessation of medical therapy.[27] Furthermore, progression to a more severe form of the disease occurs in 10% to 20% of patients.[28] Increasingly, GERD is recognized as a chronic disease requiring lifelong medical treatment to prevent symptomatic recurrence, with the potential for progressive esophageal injury and end organ dysfunction. Surgery provides the only known means of altering the natural history of the disease.

The Swiss population tends to be less mobile and characterized by highly organized lifestyles. This has allowed the opportunity for physicians at the University of Laussanne, Switzerland to longitudinally follow a large number of patients with reflux esophagitis. In the Laussanne region, the prevalence of esophagitis at endoscopy rose from 190 per 100,000 population in 1970 to 1058 per 100,000 in 1980. Although the major reason for this increase is likely the wider availability and use of upper endoscopy, increased consumption of alcohol, tobacco, large fatty meals, and perhaps even antisecretory agents may have played a role. Savary and colleagues have investigated the natural history of grades 1 to 3 esophagitis in 701 patients receiving medical therapy including omeprazole. Forty-six percent of patients had an isolated episode of esophagitis, 31% had recurrent episodes of esophagitis but no increase in their severity, and 23% developed recurrent and progressive mucosal damage.

At present there is no reliable method to identify which patients will develop progressive disease. Although the concept of endoscopic surveillance has largely centered upon those patients with Barrett's esophagus, it seems prudent to suggest intermittent upper endoscopy as a means to detect patients with progressive or recurrent disease. Patients who fall into these categories should be offered early antireflux surgery as a means to prevent the development of the irreversible complication of Barrett's esophagus or the progressive deterioration of esophageal function. There is growing evidence to suggest antireflux surgery offers better protection against the dysplastic progression of Barrett's esophagus.[29]

▪ THE PATHOGENESIS OF GERD

In humans, a zone of high pressure can be identified at the junction of the esophagus and stomach. This lower esophageal "sphincter" provides the barrier between the esophagus and stomach that normally prevents gastric contents from entering the esophagus. It has no anatomical landmarks, but its presence can be identified by a rise in pressure over gastric baseline pressure as a pressure transducer is pulled from the stomach into the esophagus. This high pressure zone is normally present except in two situations: (a) after a swallow, when it momentarily relaxes to allow passage of food into the stomach, and (b) when the fundus is distended with gas, it is eliminated to allow venting of the gas (a belch). The common denominator for virtually all episodes of gastroesophageal reflux, whether physiologic or pathologic, is the loss of the normal high pressure zone and the resistance it imposes to the flow of gastric juice from an environment of higher pressure, the stomach, to an environment of lower pressure, the esophagus. In severe disease this is usually due to the permanent nonexistent or a reduced high pressure zone. In early disease or normal subjects, loss of the high pressure zone is transient.

THE LOWER ESOPHAGEAL SPHINCTER

Three characteristics of the lower esophageal sphincter maintain its resistance or "barrier" function to intragastric and intra-abdominal pressure challenges. These are its pressure, its overall length, and the length exposed to the positive pressure environment of the abdomen (Table 8A–2). The tonic resistance of the lower esophageal sphincter is a function of both its pressure and the length over which this pressure is exerted.[30] The shorter the overall length of the high pressure zone, the higher the pressure must be to maintain sufficient resistance to remain competent (Fig 8A–2). Consequently, a normal sphincter pressure can be nullified by a short overall sphincter length. Further, as the stomach fills, the

TABLE 8A–2. NORMAL MANOMETRIC VALUES OF THE DISTAL ESOPHAGEAL SPHINCTER, N = 50

Parameter	Median Value	2.5th Percentile	97.5th Percentile
Pressure (mmHg)	13.0	5.8	27.7
Overall length (cm)	3.6	2.1	5.6
Abdominal length (cm)	2.0	0.9	4.7

length of the sphincter decreases, rather like the neck of a balloon shortening as the balloon is inflated. If the overall length of the sphincter is abnormally short when the stomach is empty, then with minimal gastric distention there will be insufficient sphincter length for the existing pressure to maintain sphincter competency, and reflux will occur.

The third characteristic of the lower esophageal sphincter is its position, in that a portion of the overall length of the high pressure zone should be exposed to positive intra-abdominal pressure. During periods of increased intra-abdominal pressure, the resistance of the lower esophageal sphincter would be overcome if the abdominal pressure were not applied equally to the high pressure zone and stomach.[31] Think of sucking on a soft soda straw immersed in a bottle of coke; the hydrostatic pressure of the fluid and the negative pressure inside the straw due to sucking cause the straw to collapse instead of allowing the liquid to flow up the straw in the direction of the negative pressure. If the abdominal length is inadequate, the sphincter cannot respond to an increase in applied intra-abdominal pressure by collapsing and reflux is more liable to result.

If the pressure in the high pressure zone is abnormally low, the overall length is short, or the zone is minimally exposed to the abdominal pressure environment in the fasting state, then the lower esophageal sphincter resistance is permanently lost, and the reflux of gastric contents into the esophagus is unhampered throughout the circadian cycle. A *permanently defective sphincter* is thus identified by one or more of the following characteristics: resting pressure <6 mmHg, abdominal length <1 cm, or total length < 2 cm.

In comparison with values in normal subjects, these values are below the 2.5 percentile for each parameter. The most common cause of a permanently defective sphincter is an inadequate abdominal length, likely secondary to the near ubiquitous presence of a hiatal hernia in patients with GERD.[32]

For the clinician, the finding of a permanently defective sphincter has several implications. Foremost, it is almost always associated with esophageal mucosal injury[33] and predicts that the patient symptoms will be

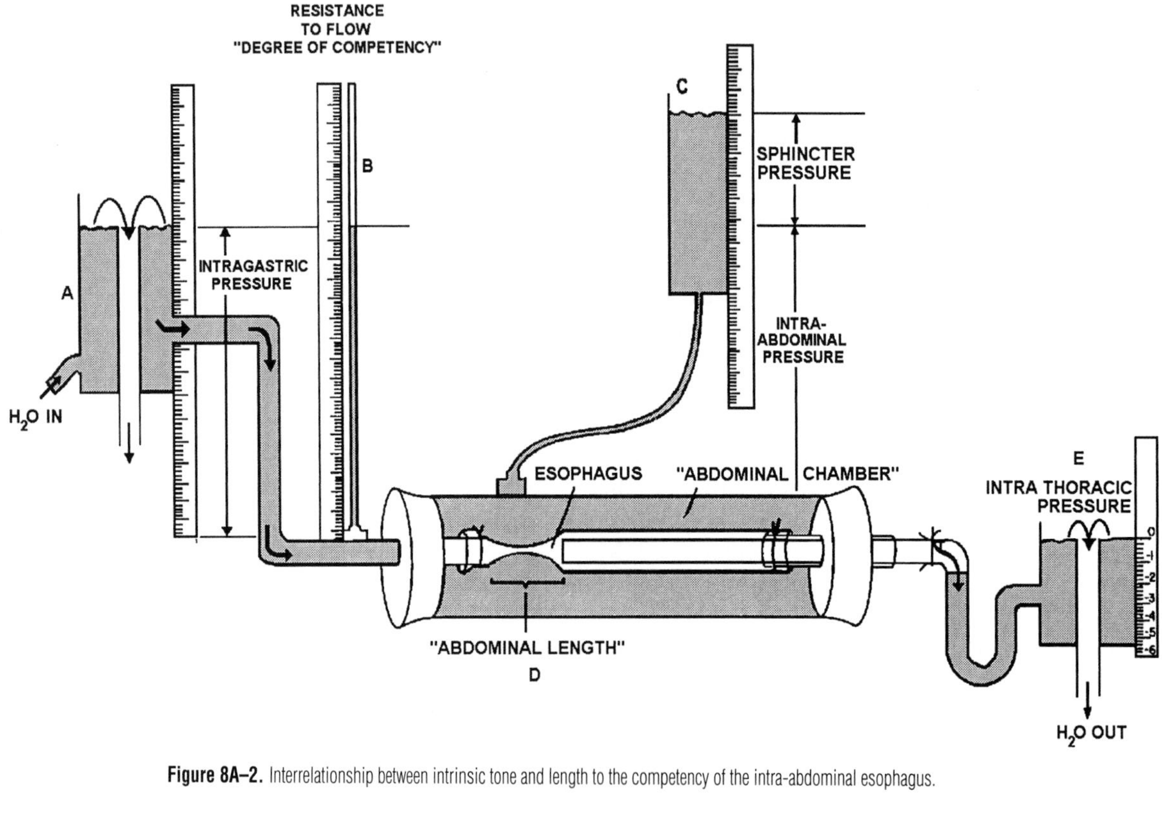

Figure 8A–2. Interrelationship between intrinsic tone and length to the competency of the intra-abdominal esophagus.

difficult to control with medical therapy.[34] It is a signal that surgical therapy is likely to be needed for consistent and long term control of the patient's symptoms. It is now accepted that when the sphincter is permanently defective, it is irreversible, even when the associated esophagitis is healed. The presence of a permanently defective sphincter is commonly associated with reduced esophageal body function and, if the disease is not brought under control, the progressive loss of effective esophageal clearance can lead to severe mucosal injury, repetitive regurgitation, aspiration, and pulmonary failure.[35,36]

A transient loss of the high pressure zone can also occur, and is usually due to a functional problem of the gastric reservoir.[37] Excessive air swallowing or food can result in gastric dilatation and, if the active relaxation reflex has been lost, an increased intragastric pressure. When the stomach is distended, the vectors produced by gastric wall tension pull on the gastroesophageal junction with a force that varies according to the geometry of the cardia; that is, the forces are applied more directly when a hiatal hernia exists than when a proper angle of His is present. The forces pull on the terminal esophagus causing it to be "taken up" into the stretched fundus, thereby reducing the length of the high pressure zone or "sphincter." This process continues until a critical length is reached, usually about 1 to 2 cm, when the pressure drops precipitously and reflux occurs. The mechanism by which gastric distention contributes to shortening of the length of the high pressure zone, so that its pressure drops and reflux occurs, provides a mechanical explanation for "transient relaxations" of the lower esophageal sphincter without invoking a neuromuscular reflex. Rather than a "spontaneous" muscular relaxation, there is a mechanical shortening of the high pressure zone, secondary to progressive gastric distention, to the point where it becomes incompetent. These "transient sphincter" shortenings occur in the initial stages of gastroesophageal reflux disease and are the mechanisms for the early complaint of excessive postprandial reflux. After gastric venting, the length of the high pressure zone is restored and competence returns until distention again shortens it and encourages further venting and reflux. This sequence results in the common complaints of repetitive belching and bloating in patients with GERD. The increased swallowing frequency seen in patients with GERD contributes to gastric distention and is due to their repetitive ingestion of saliva in an effort to neutralize the acid refluxed into their esophagus.[38] Thus, GERD may begin in the stomach, secondary to gastric distention due to overeating and the increased ingestion of fried foods which delay gastric emptying. Both characteristics are common in Western society and may explain the high prevalence of the disease in the Western world.

THE IMPORTANCE OF A HIATAL HERNIA

If mechanical forces set in play by gastric distention are important in pulling on the terminal esophagus and shortening the length of the high pressure zone or "sphincter," then the geometry of the cardia, that is the presence of a normal acute angle of His or the abnormal dome architecture of a sliding hiatus hernia, should influence the ease with which the sphincter is pulled open. A close relationship exists between the degree of gastric distention necessary to overcome the high pressure zone and the morphology of the cardia (Fig 8A–3).[39] Greater gastric dilatation, as reflected by a higher intragastric pressure, is necessary to "open" the sphincter in patients with an intact angle of His compared to those with a hiatus hernia.[40] This is what would be expected if the high pressure zone were shortened by mechanical forces and accounts for why a hiatal hernia is often associated with the presence of GERD.

A recent series of studies from Glasgow assesses the nature of the acid environment at the gastroesophageal junction,[41] including possible inciting factors in the development of cardia and distal esophageal adenocarcinoma. The studies were initiated to investigate a long-recognized observation that esophageal pH monitoring reveals postprandial esophageal acidification at the same time as the gastric contents are alkalinized. This paradox is hard to explain given the fact that reflux of gastric content into the esophagus is the primary mechanism underlying GERD.

Hypothesizing that acidic material must be present somewhere in the upper stomach, the investigators studied luminal pH at 1 cm increments across the upper stomach and lower esophagus in healthy volunteers before and after meals. Surprisingly, they identified a "pocket" of acid at the gastroesophageal junction unaffected by the buffering action of the meal, which extended across the squamocolumnar junction an average of 1.8 cm into the lumen of the esophagus (Fig 8A–4). The authors concluded that this was the source of postprandial esophageal acid exposure. They expanded these initial studies confirming that the same process occurs in patients with endoscopy negative dyspepsia and normal conventional esophageal pH monitoring 5 cm above the upper border of the lower esophageal sphincter.[42] Perhaps more importantly, they also identified that dietary nitrate consumed in the form of green vegetables results in the generation of concentrations of nitric oxide at the

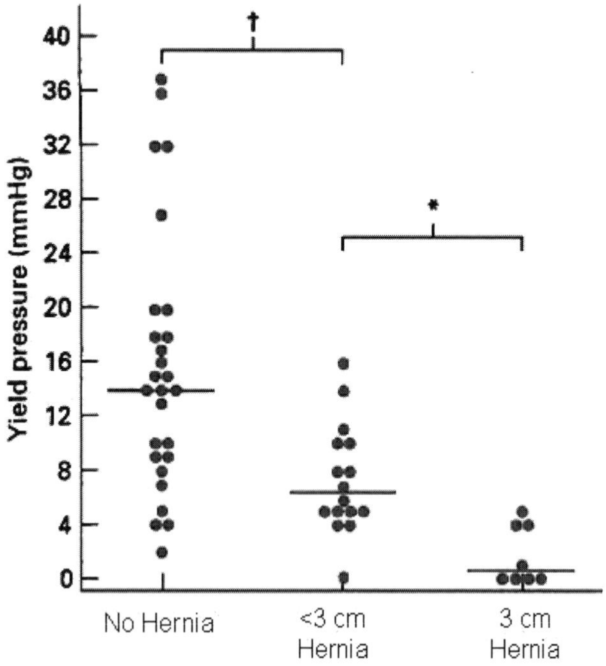

Figure 8A–3. The intragastric pressure at which the lower esophagus endoscopically opened in response to gastric distention by air during endoscopy. Note that the dome architecture of a hiatus hernia (HH) influenced the ease with which the sphincter can be pulled open by gastric distention. (From Ismail T, Bancewicz J, Barlow J. Yield pressure, anatomy of the cardia and gastro-oesophageal reflux. *Br J Surg* 1995;82:943–947.)

gastroesophageal junction high enough to be potentially mutagenic (Fig 8A–5).[43] These observations provide the fundamental basis for the observations of inflammation and other alterations in the epithelium long known to occur at the squamocolumnar junction in both overt and unrecognized GERD.

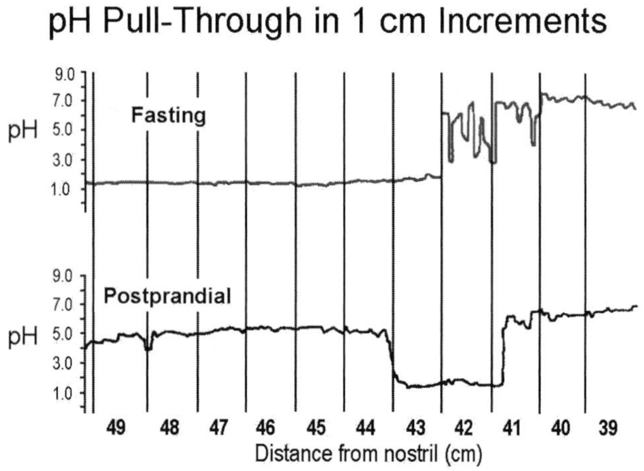

Figure 8A–4. Acid pocket at gastroesophageal junction. (From Fletcher J, Wirz A, Young J, Vallance R, McColl KEL. Unbuffered highly acidic gastric juice exists at the gastroesophageal junction after a meal. *Gastroenterology* 2001; 121:775–783.)

ESOPHAGEAL CLEARANCE

An important component limiting esophageal exposure to gastric juice once it has gained access is an effective esophageal pump.[44] Ineffective esophageal motility can result in an abnormal esophageal exposure to gastric juice in individuals who have a mechanically effective lower esophageal sphincter and normal gastric function but are unable to clear physiologic reflux episodes. This situation is relatively rare, and ineffectual clearance is more apt to be seen in association with a mechanically defective sphincter, where esophageal body function deteriorates from repetitive inflammation and augments the esophageal exposure to gastric juice by prolonging the duration of each reflux episode.

Four factors important in esophageal clearance are gravity, esophageal motor activity, salivation, and anchoring of the distal esophagus in the abdomen.[45,46] The loss of any one can augment esophageal exposure to gastric juice by contributing to ineffective clearance. The loss of gravity accounts for one reason why reflux episodes are more prolonged in the supine position. In this position, esophageal clearance depends almost completely on the peristalsis of the esophageal body. The bulk of refluxed gastric juice is cleared from the esophagus by a primary peristaltic wave initiated by a pharyngeal swallow. Secondary peristaltic waves, although able to be initiated by either distention of the esophagus or a drop in the intraesophageal pH, have been shown on ambulatory motility studies to be uncommon and have a smaller role in clearance than previously thought.[38] The esophageal contractions initiated by a drop in esophageal pH rarely have a normal peristaltic pattern and usually have are broad-based, powerful and synchronous. They reduce the efficiency of esophageal clearance by encouraging the regurgitation of refluxed material into the pharynx, predisposing the patient to aspiration. They may also cause chest pain that is commonly confused with angina pectoris.

Manometry of the esophageal body can detect failure of esophageal clearance by analysis of the contraction amplitude and speed of wave progression through the esophagus. The work of Kahrilas and Dodds has shown that the amplitude of an esophageal contraction required to clear the esophagus of barium varies according to the level.[47] Lower segments require a greater amplitude than upper segments and inadequate amplitude results in ineffective clearance.

Salivation contributes to esophageal clearance by neutralizing the minute amount of acid that is left following a peristaltic wave.[48] Return of esophageal pH to normal is significantly longer if salivary flow is reduced, such as after radiotherapy, and shorter if saliva is stimulated by sucking lozenges. Saliva production may also be

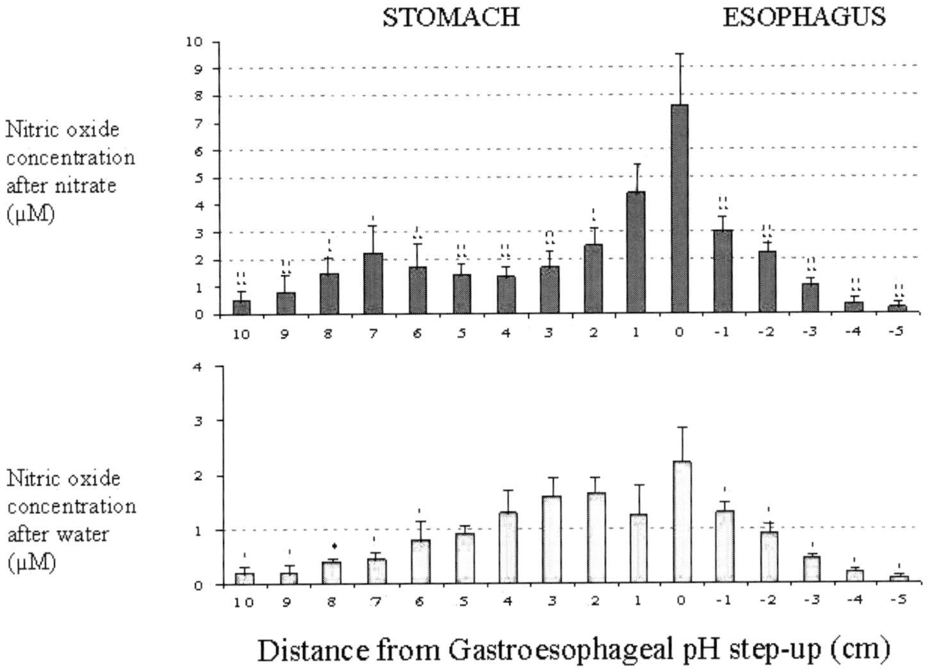

Figure 8A–5. Nitric oxide at GEJ. (From Iljima K. Henry E, Moriya A. Wirz A, Kelman AW, McColl KEL. Dietary nitrate generates potentially mutagenic concentrations of nitric oxide at the gastroesophageal junction. *Gastroenterology* 2002; 122:1248–1257.)

increased by the presence of acid in the lower esophagus and, when this occurs, the patient experiences excessive mucus in the throat. Clinically, this is referred to as "water brash."[49] The reduction in saliva flow during the night also contributes to the prolongation of reflux episodes while asleep in the supine position.

The presence of a hiatal hernia can also contribute to an esophageal propulsion defect due to loss of anchorage of the esophagus in the abdomen and results in a reduced efficiency of acid clearance (Fig 8A–6).[50] Sloan and Kahrilas have shown that complete esophageal emptying without retrograde flow was achieved in 86% of test swallows in control subjects without a hiatal hernia, 66% in patients with a reducing hiatal hernia, and only 32% of patients with a non-reducing hiatal hernia.[51] Impaired clearance in patients with non-reducing hiatal hernias is one of the ways a hiatal hernia contributes to the pathogenesis of GERD.

The data support the likelihood that GERD begins in the stomach. Fundic distention occurs because of overeating and delayed gastric emptying secondary to the high-fat Western diet. The distention causes the sphincter to be "taken up" by the expanding fundus, exposing the squamous epithelium with the high pressure zone, which is the distal 3 cm of the esophagus, to gastric juice. Repeated exposure causes inflammation of the squamous epithelium, the development of columnar epithelium and what can be termed carditis. This is the initial step and explains why in early disease the esophagitis is mild and commonly limited to the very distal esophagus. The patient compensates by increased swallowing, allowing saliva to bath the injured mucosa and alleviate the discomfort induced by exposure to gastric acid. Increased swallowing results in aerophagia, bloating, and repetitive belching. The distention induced by aerophagia leads to further exposure and repetitive injury to the terminal squamous ep-

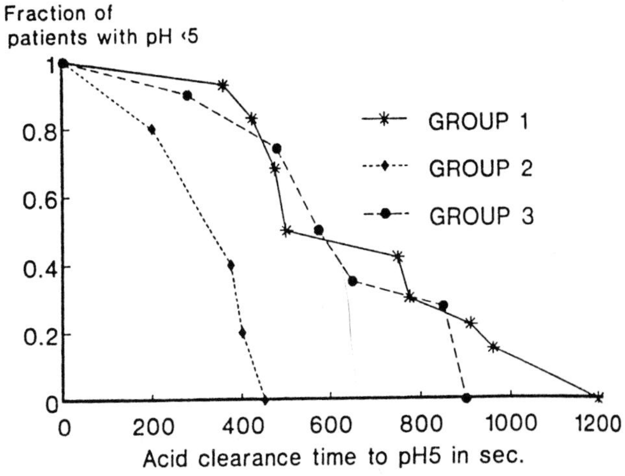

Figure 8A–6. Acid clearance in subjects with hiatal hernia and symptoms of gastroesophageal reflux disease (group 1). Subjects with no hiatal hernia but symptoms of gastroesophageal reflux disease (group 2), and subjects with hiatal hernia but no symptoms of gastroesophageal reflux disease (group 3). The y axis shows the number of patients who persist with esophageal pH less than 5. The acid clearance time to pH 5 or greater is significantly faster in group 2 (symptomatic, no hiatal hernia) compared with group 1 (symptomatic, hiatal hernia) and group 3 (asymptomatic, hiatal hernia). Groups 1 and 3 have similar acid clearance times. (From Mittal RK, Lange RC, McCallum RW. *Gastroenterology* 92:132, 1987, with permission.)

ithelium and the development of cardiac-type mucosa. This is an inflammatory process, commonly referred to as "carditis" and explains the complaint of epigastric pain so often registered by patients with early disease. The process can lead to a fibrotic mucosal ring at the squamocolumnar junction and explains the origin of a Schatzki ring. Extension of the inflammatory process into the muscularis propria causes a progressive loss in the length and pressure of the distal esophageal high pressure zone associated with an increased esophageal exposure to gastric juice and the symptoms of heartburn and regurgitation. The loss of the barrier occurs in a distal to proximal direction and eventually results in the permanent loss of lower esophageal sphincter resistance and the explosion of the disease into the esophagus with all the clinical manifestations of severe esophagitis. This accounts for the observation that severe esophageal mucosal injury is almost always associated with a permanently defective sphincter. At anytime during this process and under specific luminal conditions or stimuli, such as exposure time to a specific pH range, intestinalization of the cardiac type mucosa can occur and set the stage for malignant degeneration.

▪ COMPLICATIONS OF GERD

The complications of gastroesophageal reflux result from the damage inflicted by gastric juice on the esophageal mucosa, laryngeal or respiratory epithelium (Fig 8A–7). These can be conceptually divided into 1) mucosal complications such as esophagitis and stricture, 2) extra–esophageal or respiratory complications such as laryngitis, recurrent pneumonia and progressive pulmonary fibrosis and 3) metaplastic and neoplastic complications such as Barrett's esophagus, and esophageal adenocarcinoma. The prevalence and severity of complications is related to the degree of loss of the gastroesophageal barrier, defects in esophageal clearance and the content of refluxed gastric juice (Fig 8A–8).[33]

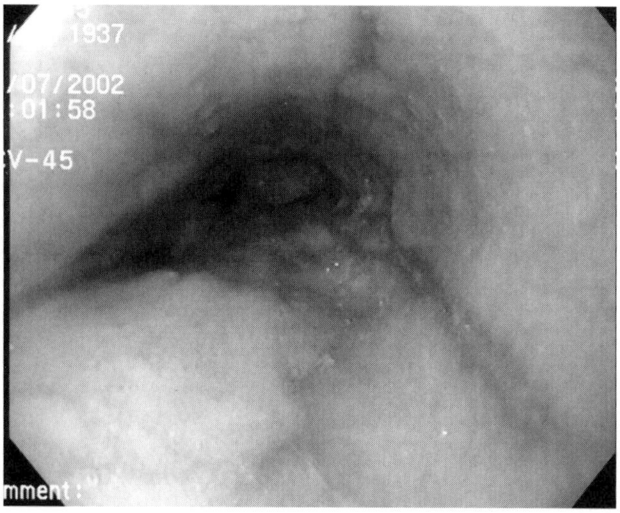

Figure 8A–7. Endoscopic appearance of esophagitis.

MUCOSAL COMPLICATIONS

The potential injurious components that reflux into the esophagus include gastric secretions, such as acid and pepsin, biliary and pancreatic secretions that regurgitate from the duodenum into the stomach, and toxic compounds generated in the mouth, esophagus and stomach by the action of bacteria on dietary substances.

Our current understanding of the role of the various ingredients of gastric juice in the development of esophagitis is based upon classic animal studies performed by Lillimoe, Harmon and others.[52,53] These studies have shown that acid alone does minimal damage to the esophageal mucosa, but the combination of acid and pepsin is highly deleterious. Hydrogen ion injury to the esophageal squamous mucosa occurs only at a pH below 2. In acid refluxate, the enzyme pepsin appears to be the major injurious agent. Similarly, the reflux of duodenal juice alone does little damage to the mucosa, while the combination of duodenal juice and gastric acid is particularly noxious. Reflux of bile and pancreatic enzymes into the stomach can either protect or augment esophageal mucosal injury. For instance, the reflux of duodenal contents into the stomach may prevent the development of peptic esophagitis in a pa-

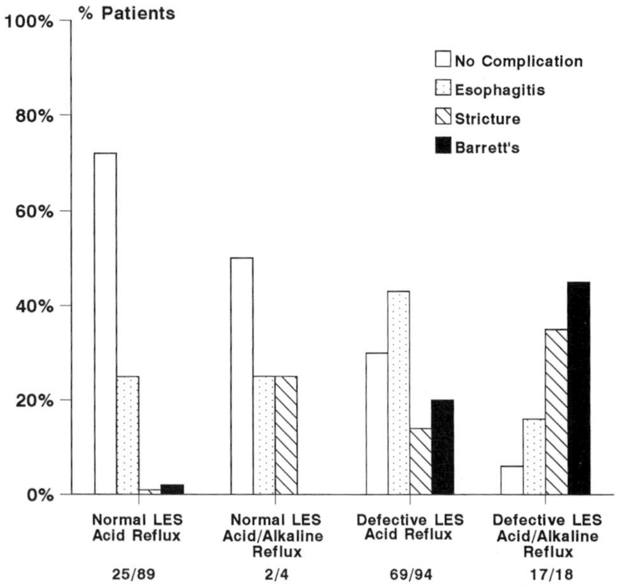

Figure 8A–8. Prevalence of esophageal mucosal injury related to the presence of a defective lower esophageal sphincter, esophageal body motility or both.

tient whose gastric acid secretion maintains an acid environment, because the bile salts would attenuate the injurious effect of pepsin and the acid would inactivate the trypsin. Such a patient would have bile-containing acid gastric juice that, when refluxed, would irritate the esophageal mucosa, but cause less esophagitis than if it were acid gastric juice containing pepsin. In contrast, the reflux of duodenal contents into the stomach of a patient with limited gastric acid secretion can result in esophagitis, because the alkaline intragastric environment would support optimal trypsin activity and the soluble bile salts with a high pK_a would potentiate the enzymes effect. Hence, duodenal-gastric reflux and the acid secretory capacity of the stomach interrelate by altering the pH and enzymatic activity of the refluxed gastric juice to modulate the injurious effects of enzymes on the esophageal mucosa.

This disparity in injury caused by acid and bile alone as opposed to the gross esophagitis caused by pepsin and trypsin provides an explanation for the poor correlation between the symptom of heartburn and endoscopic esophagitis. The reflux of acid gastric juice contaminated with duodenal contents could break the esophageal mucosal barrier, irritate nerve endings in the papillae close to the luminal surface, and cause severe heartburn. Despite the presence of intense heartburn, the bile salts present would inhibit pepsin, the acid pH would inactivate trypsin, and the patient would have little or no gross evidence of esophagitis. In contrast, the patient who refluxed alkaline gastric juice may have minimal heartburn because of the absence of hydrogen ions in the refluxate, but have endoscopic esophagitis because of the bile salt potentiation of trypsin activity on the esophageal mucosa. This is supported by recent clinical studies which indicate that the presence of alkaline reflux is associated with the development of mucosal injury.[54,55]

Although numerous studies have suggested the reflux of duodenal contents into the esophagus in patients with GERD, few have measured this directly. The components of duodenal juice thought to be most damaging are the bile acids and, as such, they have been the most commonly studied. Most studies have implied the presence of bile acids using pH measurements. Studies using either prolonged ambulatory aspiration techniques (Fig 8A–9) or spectrophotometric bilirubin measurement (Fig 8A–10) have shown that, as a group, patients with GERD have greater and more concentrated bile acid exposure to the esophageal mucosa than normal subjects.[56,57] This increased exposure occurs most commonly during the supine period while asleep, and during the upright period following meals. Most studies have identified the glycine conjugates of cholic acid, deoxycholic, and chenodeoxycholic acids

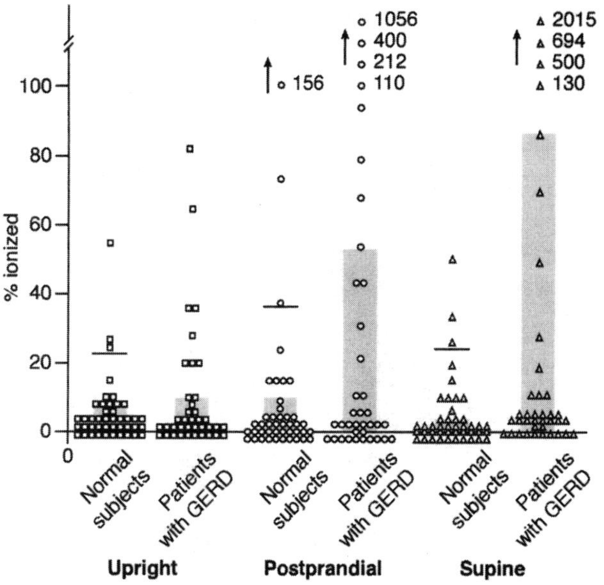

Figure 8A–9. Peak bile acid concentration (μmol/L) for patients and normal subjects during upright, postprandial and supine aspiration periods. The shaded area represents the mean and the bar the 95th percentile values.

as the predominant bile acids aspirated from the esophagus of patients with GERD, although appreciable amounts of taurine conjugates of these bile acids were also found. Other bile slats were identified but in small concentrations. This is as one would expect as glycine conjugates are three times more prevalent than taurine conjugates in normal human bile.

The potentially injurious action of toxic compounds either ingested or newly formed on the mucosa of the gastroesophageal junction and distal esophagus has long been postulated. Until recently however, few stud-

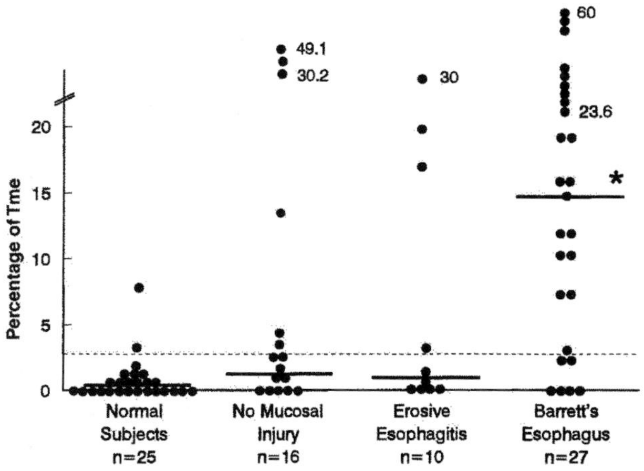

Figure 8A–10. Prevalence of abnormal esophageal bilirubin exposure in healthy subjects and in patients with gastroesophageal reflux disease with varied degrees of mucosal injury. (From Kauer WKH, Peters JH, DeMeester TR et al. Mixed reflux of gastric juice is more harmful to the esophagus than gastric juice alone. The need for surgical therapy reemphasized. *Ann Surg* 1995; 222:525–533.)

ies have substantiated this possibility. Expanding upon studies of acid exposure at the gastroesophageal junction, investigators from Glasgow, Scotland have recently shown that dietary nitrate consumed in the form of green vegetables and food contaminated by nitrate-containing fertilizers, results in the generation of nitric oxide at the gastroesophageal junction in concentrations high enough to be potentially mutagenic.[43] Previous studies have shown that nitrate ingested in food is reabsorbed in the small bowel with approximately 25% re-secreted into the mouth via the salivary glands. Oral bacterial chemically transforms the relatively innocuous nitrate to the more toxic nitrite which is swallowed and subsequently converted to nitric oxide and other toxic nitroso-compounds by acid and ascorbic acid in the stomach. Whether this mechanism in fact contributes to injury and or neoplastic transformation in the upper stomach, gastroesophageal junction and distal esophagus is currently unknown.

RESPIRATORY COMPLICATIONS

It is increasingly recognized that a significant proportion of patients with gastroesophageal reflux will have either primary respiratory symptoms or respiratory symptoms in association with more prominent heartburn and regurgitation.[58] For example, numerous studies have shown that up to 50% of asthmatics have either endoscopic evidence of esophagitis or increased esophageal acid exposure on 24 hour ambulatory pH monitoring.[59,60] This suggests that the frequency of dual pathology is higher than would be expected by chance alone.

Pathophysiology of Reflux-Induced Respiratory Symptoms

Two mechanisms have been proposed as the pathogenesis of reflux-induced respiratory symptoms. The first, the so-called "reflux" theory maintains that respiratory symptoms are the result of the aspiration of gastric contents. The second or "reflex" theory maintains that vagally-mediated bronchoconstriction follows acidification of the lower esophagus. The evidence supporting a reflux mechanism is fivefold. Firstly, clinical studies have documented a strong correlation between idiopathic pulmonary fibrosis and hiatal hernia. The presence of GERD was shown to be highly associated with several pulmonary diseases including asthma in a recent Department of Veterans Affairs study.[58] Secondly, pathological acid exposure in the proximal esophagus is often identified in patients with respiratory symptoms and reflux disease. Thirdly, scintigraphic studies have shown aspiration of ingested radio-isotope in some patients with reflux and respiratory symptoms. Fourthly, simultaneous tracheal and esophageal pH monitoring in patients with reflux disease have documented tracheal acidification in concert with esophageal acidification. Finally, animal studies have shown that tracheal instillation of hydrochloric acid profoundly increases airways resistance.[61]

A reflex mechanism is primarily supported by the fact that bronchoconstriction occurs following the infusion of acid into the lower esophagus.[62] This can be explained by the common embryologic origin of the tracheoesophageal tract and their shared vagal innervation. Secondly, patients with respiratory symptoms and pathological distal esophageal acid exposure but normal proximal esophageal acid exposure may experience an improvement in their respiratory symptoms after antireflux therapy.

The primary challenge in implementing treatment for reflux associated respiratory symptoms lies in establishing the diagnosis. In those patients with predominantly typical reflux symptoms and secondary respiratory complaints, the diagnosis may be straightforward. However, in a substantial number of patients with reflux-induced respiratory symptoms, the respiratory symptoms dominate the clinical scenario. Gastroesophageal reflux in these patients is often silent and is only uncovered when investigation is initiated. A high index of suspicion is required, notably in patients with poorly controlled asthma in spite of appropriate bronchodilator therapy. Supportive evidence for the diagnosis can be gleaned from endoscopy and stationary esophageal manometry. Endoscopy may show erosive esophagitis or Barrett's esophagus. Manometry may indicate a hypotensive lower esophageal sphincter or ineffective body motility, defined by 30% or more contractions in the distal esophagus of <30 mmHg in amplitude.

The gold standard for the diagnosis of reflux-induced respiratory complaints is ambulatory dual probe pH monitoring. One probe is positioned in the distal esophagus and the other at a more proximal location. Sites for proximal probe placement have included the trachea, pharynx, and proximal esophagus. Most authorities would agree that the proximal esophagus is the preferred site for proximal probe placement. While ambulatory esophageal pH monitoring allows a direct correlation between esophageal acidification and respiratory symptoms, the chronological relationship between reflux events and bronchoconstriction is complex.

Treatment

Once gastroesophageal reflux is suspected or thought to be responsible for respiratory symptoms, treatment may be with either prolonged proton pump inhibitor (PPI) therapy or antireflux surgery. A 3 to 6-month trial of high dose PPI therapy (BID or TID dosing) may help confirm (by virtue of symptom resolution) the fact that reflux is partly or completely responsible for the respira-

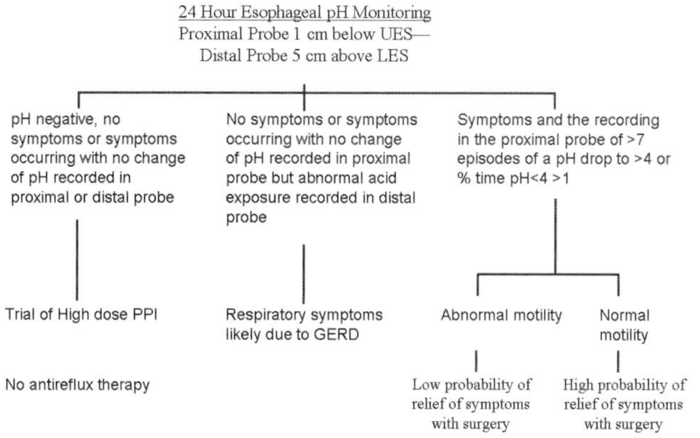
24 Hour Esophageal pH Monitoring
Proximal Probe 1 cm below UES—
Distal Probe 5 cm above LES
pH negative, no symptoms or symptoms occurring with no change of pH recorded in proximal or distal probe
No symptoms or symptoms occurring with no change of pH recorded in proximal probe but abnormal acid exposure recorded in distal probe
Symptoms and the recording in the proximal probe of >7 episodes of a pH drop to >4 or % time pH<4 >1
Trial of High dose PPI
Respiratory symptoms likely due to GERD
Abnormal motility
Normal motility
No antireflux therapy
Low probability of relief of symptoms with surgery
High probability of relief of symptoms with surgery

Figure 8A–11. Algorithm of clinical decision making based upon outcome of dual probe 24-hour pH testing and esophageal manometry in patients with respiratory symptoms thought secondary to gastroesophageal reflux disease.

tory symptoms. The persistence of symptoms despite PPI treatment, however, does not necessarily rule out reflux as being a potential contributor. The algorithm depicted in Fig 8A–11 bases clinical decisions on the results of dual probe 24 hour pH monitoring is and is a useful starting point.

Based upon reported observations, relief of respiratory symptoms can be anticipated for 25–50% of patients with reflux-induced asthma treated with anti-secretory medications.[63–65] Fewer than 15%, however, can be expected to have objective improvements in their pulmonary function. The reason for this apparent paradox may be that most studies employed relatively short courses of anti-secretory therapy (<3 months). This time period may have been sufficient for symptomatic improvement but insufficient for recovery of pulmonary function. The chances of success with medical treatment are likely directly related to the extent of reflux elimination. The conflicting findings of reports of anti-secretory therapy may well be due to inadequate control of gastroesophageal reflux in some studies. The literature indicates that anti-reflux surgery improves respiratory symptoms in nearly 90% of children and 70% of adults with asthma and reflux disease.[66,67] Improvements in pulmonary function were demonstrated in around one-third of patients. Comparison of the results of uncontrolled studies of each form of therapy and the evidence from the two randomized controlled trials of medical versus surgical therapy indicate that fundoplication is the most effective therapy for reflux-induced asthma.[66] The superiority of the surgical anti-reflux barrier over medical therapy is probably most noticeable in the supine posture, which corresponds with the period of acid breakthrough with PPI therapy and is the time in the circadian cycle when asthma symptoms and peak expiratory flow rates are at their worst.

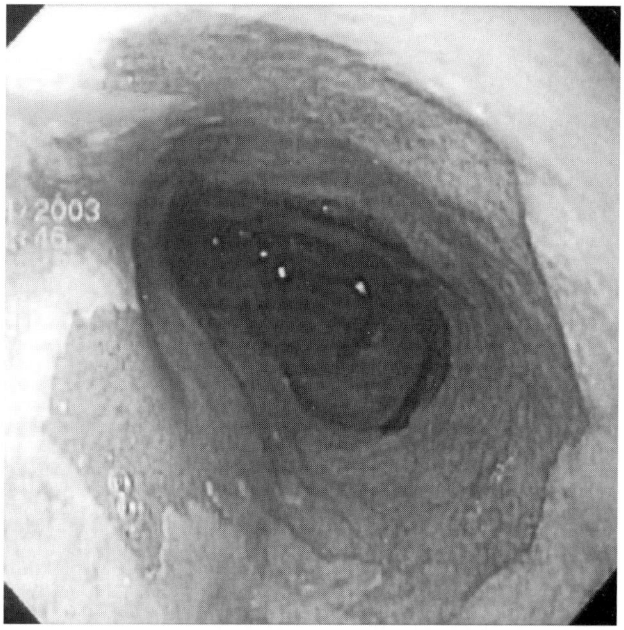

Figure 8A–12. Endoscopic appearance of Barrett's esophagus. Note the pink metaplastic mucosa as opposed to the normal whitish squamous lining of the esophagus.

It is also important to realize that, in asthmatic patients with a non reflux-induced motility abnormality of the esophageal body, performing an anti-reflux operation may not prevent the aspiration of orally regurgitated, swallowed liquid or food. This can result in respiratory symptoms and airway irritation that may elicit an asthmatic reaction. This factor may be the explanation why surgical results appear to be better in children than adults since disturbance of esophageal body motility is more likely in adult patients.

METAPLASTIC (BARRETT'S) AND NEOPLASTIC (ADENOCARCINOMA) COMPLICATIONS

The condition whereby the tubular esophagus is lined with columnar epithelium rather than squamous epithelium was first described by Norman Barrett in 1950 (Fig 8A–12).[68] He incorrectly believed it to be congenital in origin. It is now realized that it is an acquired abnormality, occurring in 7 to 10 percent of patients with GERD, and represents the end stage of the natural history of this disease.[69] It is also understood to be distinctly different from the congenital condition in which islands of mature gastric columnar epithelium are found in the upper half of the esophagus.

The definition of Barrett's esophagus has evolved considerably over the past decade.[70] Traditionally, Barrett's esophagus was identified by the presence of any columnar mucosa extending at least 3 cm into the esopha-

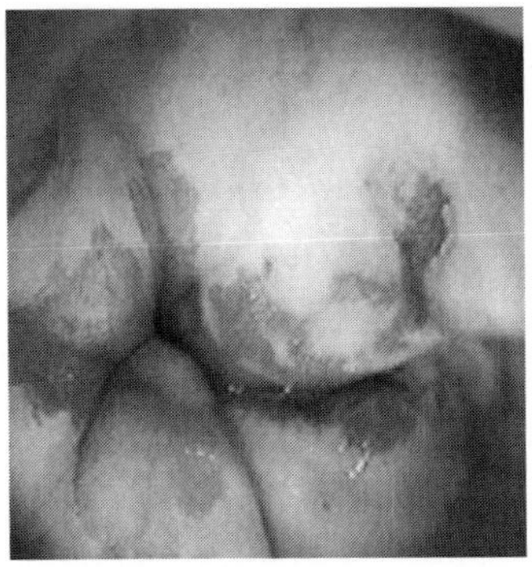

Figure 8A–13. Endoscopic appearance of short segment (< 3 cm) Barrett's esophagus.

gus. Recent data indicating that specialized intestinal type epithelium is the only tissue predisposed to malignant degeneration, coupled with the finding of a similar risk of malignancy in segments of intestinal metaplasia less than 3cm long, have resulted in the diagnosis of Barrett's esophagus given any length of endoscopically visible tissue that is intestinal metaplasia on histology (Fig 8A–13). Whether to call long segments of columnar mucosa without intestinal metaplasia Barrett's esophagus is unclear. The hallmark of intestinal metaplasia is the presence of goblet cells. Recent studies have identified a high prevalence of biopsy proven intestinal metaplasia at the cardia, in the absence of endoscopic evidence of a columnar-lined esophagus. The significance and natural history of this finding remains unknown. The term Barrett's esophagus should currently be used in the setting of an endoscopically visible segment of intestinal metaplasia of any length, or columnar replacement of the esophagus of 3 cm or more.

Factors predisposing to the development of Barrett's esophagus include early onset GERD, abnormal lower esophageal sphincter and esophageal body physiology and mixed reflux of gastric and duodenal contents into the esophagus.[71] Direct measurement of esophageal bilirubin exposure as a marker for duodenal juice, has shown that 58% of the patients with GERD have increased esophageal exposure to duodenal juice and that this exposure is most dramatically related to Barrett's esophagus.

Pathophysiology of Barrett's Metaplasia

Recent studies suggest that the metaplastic process at the gastroesophageal junction may begin by conversion of distal esophageal squamous mucosa to cardiac type epithelium, heretofore presumed to be a normal finding.[72] This is likely due to exposure of the distal esophagus to excess acid and gastric contents via prolapse of esophageal squamous mucosa into the gastric environment. This results in inflammatory changes at the gastroesophageal junction and/or a metaplastic process, both of which may results in the loss of muscle function and a mechanically defective sphincter, allowing free reflux with progressively higher degrees of mucosal injury. Intestinal metaplasia within the sphincter may result, as in Barrett's metaplasia of the esophageal body. This mechanism is supported by the finding that as the severity of GERD progresses, the length of columnar lining above the anatomic gastroesophageal junction is increased.

Treatment

The relief of symptoms remains the primary force driving antireflux surgery in patients with Barrett's esophagus. Healing of esophageal mucosal injury and the prevention of disease progression are important secondary goals. In this regard, patients with Barrett's esophagus are no different than the broader population of patients with gastroesophageal reflux. Antireflux surgery should be considered when patient factors suggest severe disease or predict the need for long term medical management, both of which are almost always true in patients with Barrett's esophagus.

Proton pump inhibitor (PPI) therapy, both to relieve symptoms and to control any co-existent esophagitis or stricture is an acceptable treatment option in patients with Barrett's esophagus. Once initiated, however, most patients with Barrett's will require life-long treatment. Complete control of reflux with PPI therapy can be difficult, however, as has been highlighted by studies of acid breakthrough while on therapy. Katzka, Castell, Triadafilopoulos and others have shown that 40-80% of patients with Barrett's esophagus continue to experience abnormal esophageal acid exposure despite up to 20 mg twice daily of PPI.[73,74] Ablation trials have shown that mean doses of 56 milligrams of omeprazole are necessary to normalize 24 hour esophageal pH studies.[75] Antireflux surgery likely results in more reproducible and reliable elimination of reflux of both acid and duodenal content, although long term outcome studies suggest that as many as 25% of patients post-fundoplication will have persistent pathologic esophageal acid exposure confirmed by 24 hour pH studies.[76]

An important consideration is that patients with Barrett's esophagus generally have severe GERD, with its attendant sequelae such as large hiatal hernia, stricture, shortened esophagus and poor motility. These anatomic and physiologic features make successful antireflux surgery a particular challenge in this population. Indeed, recent data suggest that antireflux surgery in patients with Barrett's esophagus may not be as successful in the long term as in those without Barrett's.

Studies focusing on the symptomatic outcome following antireflux surgery in patients with Barrett's esophagus document excellent to good results in 72–95% of patients at 5 years following surgery.[77,78] The outcome of

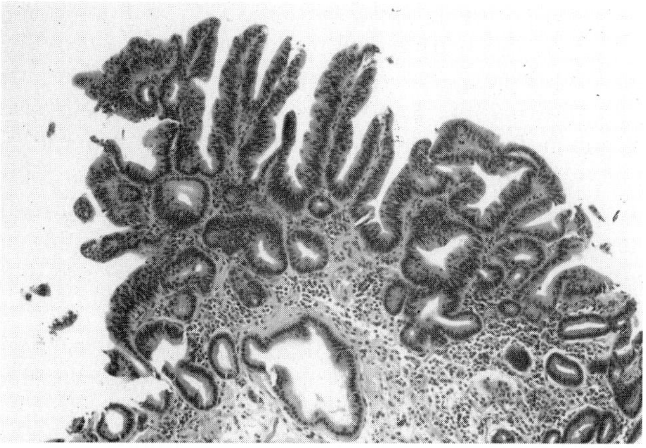

Figure 8A–14. Histologic appearance of high-grade dysplasia. The cellular architecture and structure of the glands is becoming disorganized.

laparoscopic Nissen fundoplication in patients with Barrett's esophagus has been assessed at 1–3 years after surgery. Hofstetter et al. reported the experience at the University of Southern California (USC) in 85 patients with Barrett's esophagus at a median of 5 years after surgery. Fifty-nine had long and 26 short segment Barrett's and fifty underwent a laparoscopic antireflux procedure.[76] Reflux symptoms were absent postoperatively in 79% of the patients. Postoperative 24-hour pH was normal in 17/21 (81%). Ninety-nine percent of the patients considered themselves cured or improved and 97% were satisfied with the surgery. Similar studies have been published from Emory University, the University of Washington and from Europe.[77,78]

The Development of Dysplasia in Barrett's Esophagus

The prevalence of dysplasia in patients presenting with Barrett's esophagus ranges from 15–25% if low grade dysplasia is included and 5–10% if only high grade dysplasia is considered. The identification of dysplasia in Barrett's epithelium rests upon histologic examination of biopsy specimens. The cytologic and tissue architectural changes are similar to those described in ulcerative colitis (Fig 8A–14). By convention, Barrett's metaplasia is currently classified into four broad categories:

1. No dysplasia
2. Indefinite for dysplasia
3. Low grade dysplasia
4. High grade dysplasia

There are few prospective studies documenting the progression of non-dysplastic Barrett's epithelium to low or high grade dysplasia. Those that are available suggest that 5–10%/yr will progress to dysplasia and 0.5–1%/yr to adenocarcinoma (Table 8A–3). Once identified, Barrett's esophagus complicated by dysplasia should undergo aggressive therapy (Table 8A–4). Patients whose biopsies are interpreted as indefinite for dysplasia should be treated with a medical regimen consisting of 60–80 mg of PPI therapy for 3 months and re-biopsied. Importantly, esophagitis should be healed prior to interpretation of the presence or absence of dysplasia. The presence of severe inflammation makes the microscopic interpretation of dysplasia difficult. The purpose of acid suppression therapy is to resolve inflammation that may complicate the interpretation of the biopsy specimen. If the diagnosis remains indefinite, the patient should be treated as if low grade dysplasia were present with continued medical therapy or antireflux surgery and repeat biopsy every 6 months. Patients with low grade dysplasia are perhaps the most difficult group. This is due to the potential difficulty in surveillance following antireflux surgery. Biopsies within the fundic wrap may be difficult for the inexperienced endoscopist. Either aggressive medical treatment or, given an experienced endoscopist, antireflux surgery is appropriate.

High grade dysplasia should be confirmed by two pathologists knowledgeable in GI pathology. Corroboration of dysplasia is important prior to consideration of esophagectomy. Most authorities would agree that the current standard of care is to proceed with esophagectomy in patients with high grade dysplasia who are physiologically fit enough to tolerate a major surgical undertaking. Recent less invasive options, including photodynamic therapy and endoscopic mucosal resection, have been reported with some success[79,80] though remain largely investigational or reserved for high-risk surgical candidates. On average, 45 to 50% of patients with the preoperative diagnosis of Barrett's esophagus with high-grade dysplasia will harbor invasive cancer when the specimen is removed and examined in its en-

TABLE 8A–3. DEVELOPMENT OF DYSPLASIA: PROSPECTIVE EVALUATION OF 62 PATIENTS

Initial Diagnosis	N	Metaplasia	Indeterminate/LGD	HGD	CA
Metaplasia	39	27	10	1	1
I/LGD	20	4	8	3	2
HGD	3			1	2

I = indeterminate, LGD = low grade dysplasia, HGD = high grade dysplasia.
Reid et al. *Gastroenterology* 102:1212, 1992.

TABLE 8A–4. MANAGEMENT OF BARRETT'S ESOPHAGUS WITH DYSPLASIA

Indefinite for Dysplasia
Aggressive antireflux therapy (60 mg/day PPI)
Re-biopsy in 3 months
Low-Grade Dysplasia
Aggressive antireflux therapy
Medical vs surgical
High-Grade Dysplasia
Confirmation by 2 experienced pathologists
Esophagectomy (? extent)

tirety. Thus, high grade dysplasia is a marker for the presence of invasive carcinoma in nearly half of patients. This fact has been confirmed in studies from the University of Southern California as well as those from the Mayo Clinic, Johns Hopkins and many other centers around the world.[81–84] It is not possible with present technology, including endoscopic ultrasound, to differentiate the patients who harbor a cancer from those who do not. Furthermore, esophageal adenocarcinoma associated with high grade dysplasia, identified by surveillance endoscopy, is generally highly curable. We and others have documented 5 year survival rates of 90% in this setting.

▪ PREOPERATIVE ASSESSMENT OF PATIENTS WITH GASTROESOPHAGEAL REFLUX DISEASE

ENDOSCOPIC EVALUATION

Endoscopy is a critical part of the pre-operative evaluation of patients with GERD. It's key function is to detect complications of gastroesophageal reflux, the presence of which may influence therapeutic decisions. The locations of the diaphragmatic crura, the gastroesophageal junction and the squamocolumnar junction should always be recorded.

Nonerosive esophagitis is difficult to reliably recognize endoscopically and is subject to wide observer variability. Its presence may be confirmed by biopsy that shows mucosal infiltration with polymorphs, lymphocytes, eosinophils, and the recently described balloon cells.[85] The extension of the relative height of the mucosal papillae and hyperplasia of the basal zone are further evidence of mucosal injury.[86] These microscopic signs, while providing corroborative evidence, do not prove the presence of increased exposure to gastric juice as they can occur from other forms of injury.[87,88]

The presence of mucosal breaks defines esophagitis. The severity of esophagitis is most often characterized by the Los Angeles classification[89]: The presence of 1 or more mucosal breaks which are less than or equal to 5 mm in length is classified as Grade A. Grade B esophagitis is identified by the presence of one or more mucosal breaks which are longer than 5 mm. Grade C esophagitis represents a more advanced stage where one or more mucosal breaks bridge the tops of folds but involve less than 75% of the esophageal lumen circumference. One or more mucosal breaks bridging the tops of folds and involving more than 75% of the esophageal lumen circumference are classified as Grade D. In the setting of a stricture, the severity of the esophagitis above it should be recorded. The absence of esophagitis above a stricture suggests a drug-induced injury or a neoplasm as a cause for the stricture. The latter should always be considered and is ruled out only by tissue biopsies.

Barrett's esophagus is suspected at endoscopy when there is difficulty in visualizing the squamocolumnar junction at its normal location and by the appearance of a redder, more luxuriant mucosa than is normally seen in the lower esophagus. Its presence is diagnostic of the reflux of gastric juice and must be confirmed by the finding of columnar epithelium with intestinalization on microscopic inspection of the biopsy. Multiple biopsies should be taken in a cephalad direction to determine the level at which the junction of Barrett's epithelium and normal squamous mucosa occurs. Barrett's esophagus is susceptible to ulceration, bleeding, stricture formation and malignant degeneration. Dysplasia is the earliest sign of malignant change. Because dysplastic changes typically occur in a random distribution within the distal esophagus a minimum of four biopsies (each quadrant) every 2-cm should be obtained from the metaplastic epithelium. Particular attention must be paid to the squamocolumnar junction in these patients, where a mass, ulcer, nodularity, or inflammatory tissue is always considered suspicious for malignancy and requires thorough biopsy.

A hiatal hernia is endoscopically confirmed by finding a pouch lined with gastric rugal folds lying 2 cm or more above the margins of the diaphragmatic crura. A prominent sliding hernia is frequently associated with increased esophageal exposure to gastric juice. When a paraesophageal hernia exists, particular attention is taken to exclude a gastric ulcer or gastritis within the pouch. The intragastric retroflex or "J" maneuver is important in evaluating the full circumference of the mucosal lining of the herniated stomach.

ROENTGENOGRAPHIC EXAMINATION

The roentgenographic definition of gastroesophageal reflux varies depending on whether the reflux of barium is spontaneous or induced by various maneuvers. In only about 40% of patients with classic symptoms of GERD is spontaneous reflux of barium observed by the radiologist, i.e., reflux of barium from the stomach into the esophagus with a patient in the upright position. In most patients who show spontaneous reflux of barium on roentgenography, the diagnosis of increased esophageal acid exposure is confirmed by 24-hour esophageal pH monitoring. Therefore, the roentgenographic demonstration of spontaneous regurgitation of barium into the esophagus in the upright position is a reliable indicator that reflux is present. Failure to see this does not, however, indicate the absence of disease.

A hiatal hernia is present in over 80% of patients with gastroesophageal reflux. The presence of a hiatal hernia is an important component of the underlying pathophysiology of gastroesophageal reflux. The assessment of peristalsis on video esophagram may add to, but by no means replaces, the information obtained by esophageal manometry studies. In dysphagic patients, barium impregnated marshmallow, bread, or hamburger is a useful adjunct, which can discern a functional esophageal transport disturbance not evident on the liquid barium study.

DETECTION OF GASTROESOPHAGEAL REFLUX

Ambulatory pH Monitoring

Preoperative pH monitoring off medications should be performed in the majority of patients being considered for antireflux surgery. The most direct method of measuring increased esophageal exposure to gastric juice is by an indwelling pH electrode.[90,91] Prolonged monitoring of esophageal pH is performed by placing a pH probe 5 cm above the manometrically measured upper border of the distal sphincter with the patient off all acid suppression. It quantitates the actual time the esophageal mucosa is exposed to gastric juice, measures the ability of the esophagus to clear refluxed acid and correlates esophageal acid exposure to the patient's symptoms. A 24-hour period is necessary so that measurements are made over one complete circadian cycle. This allows for measuring the effect of a physiological activity such as working, eating or sleeping on the reflux of gastric juice into the esophagus.

The measurement is expressed by the time the esophageal pH was below a given threshold during the 24-hour period. This single assessment, although concise, does not reflect how the exposure has occurred; that is, did it occur in a few long episodes or several short episodes? Consequently, two other assessments are necessary: the frequency of the reflux episodes and their duration.

The units used to express esophageal exposure to gastric juice are: 1) cumulative time the esophageal pH is below a chosen threshold expressed as the percent of the total, upright, and supine monitored time; 2) frequency of reflux episodes below a chosen threshold expressed as number of episodes per 24 hours; and 3) duration of the episodes expressed as the number of episodes greater than five minutes per 24 hours and the time in minutes of the longest episode recorded. Normal values for these six components of the 24-hour record at each whole number pH threshold were derived from 50 asymptomatic control subjects. The upper limits of normal were established at the 95th percentile. Most centers use pH 4 as the threshold. Using this threshold, there was a uniformity of normal values for the six components from centers throughout the world when compared at a Zurich conference. The normal values for the six components are shown in Table 8A–5. This indicated that esophageal acid exposure can be quantitated, and that normal individuals have similar values despite nationality or dietary habits.

TABLE 8A–5. NORMAL VALUES FOR ESOPHAGEAL EXPOSURE TO PH <4 (N = 50)

Component	Mean	Standard Deviation	95th Percentile
Total time pH <4	1.51	1.36	4.45
Upright time pH <4	2.34	2.34	8.42
Supine time pH <4	0.63	1.0	3.45
No. of episodes	19.00	12.76	46.9
No. >5 minutes	0.84	1.18	3.45
Longest episode	6.74	7.85	19.8

To combine the result of the six components into one expression of the overall esophageal acid exposure below a pH threshold, a pH score was calculated by using the standard deviation of the mean of each of the six components measured in the 50 normal subjects as a weighing factor.[92] By accepting an abstract zero level two standard deviations below the mean, the data measured in normal subjects could be treated as though it had a normal distribution. Thus, any measured patient value could be referenced to this zero point and in turn be awarded points based on whether it was below or above the normal mean value for that component. The formula used for performing the calculation illustrated in Fig 8A–15 was:

$$\text{Component score} = \frac{\text{Pt Value} - \text{Mean}}{\text{SD}} + 1$$

This formula was used to score each of the six components of the 24-hour pH record obtained from the 50 normal subjects. The score for each component was added to obtain a composite score for each of the 50 normal subjects and the upper level of a normal score was established at the 95th percentile. The upper limits of normal for the composite score for each whole number pH threshold is shown in Table 8A–6.

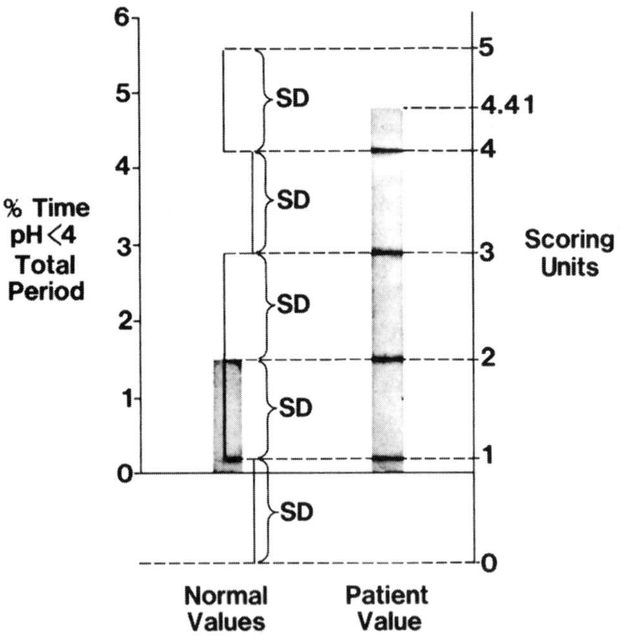

Figure 8A–15. Concept of using the standard deviation as the scoring unit to score the component percent time pH <4 for the total period. Note the establishment of an abstract zero point 2 SD below the mean value for total-period acid exposure measured in normals. Theoretically, this allows scoring the measurement in patients as though the normal values were parametric. By this method, a patient who had a total acid exposure below pH 4 of 4.8 percent would have a score for this component of 4.41.

When evaluated in a test population with an equal distribution of normal healthy subjects and patients with the classical reflux symptoms and a defective sphincter, 24-hour esophageal pH monitoring had a sensitivity and specificity of 96%. This gave a predictive value of a positive and a negative test of 96% and an overall accuracy of 96%. Based on these studies and extensive clinical experience, until recently, 24-hour esophageal pH monitoring has emerged as a gold standard for the diagnosis of gastroesophageal reflux disease.[93]

Catheter based 24-hour ambulatory esophageal pH monitoring does have a significant drawback of the physical presence of a transnasal catheter which must be worn for 24 hours. Although most ask patients to go about their normal activities of daily living, many do not comply due to embarrassment by the catheter or from discomfort. The recent development of a wireless capsule which can be implanted it the esophagus and record pH data for 48 hours has significantly changed patient satisfaction with the procedure.[94–95]

The Bravo™ pH Capsule measures pH levels in the esophagus and transmits continuous esophageal pH readings to a receiver worn on the patient's belt or waistband (Fig 8A–16).[96] Symptoms the patient experiences are recorded in a diary and/or by pressing buttons on the receiver unit. The capsule eventually detaches and pass through the digestive tract in 5–7 days.

TABLE 8A–6. NORMAL COMPOSITE SCORE FOR VARIOUS PH THRESHOLDS

pH Threshold	Upper Level of Normal Value (95th Percentile)
<1	14.2
<2	17.37
<3	14.10
<4	14.72
<5	15.76
<6	12.76
>7	14.90
>8	8.50

Source: DeMeester TR, Stein HJ: Gastroesophageal Reflux Disease, in Moody FG, Carey LC, Jones RS, Kelly KA, Nahrwold DL, Skinner DB (eds): *Surgical Treatment of Digestive Disease*, 2nd edition. Chicago: Year Book Medical Publishers, Inc., 1989, pp 65–108.

Combined Multichannel Intraluminal Impedance-pH

It is increasingly recognized that 24-hour pH monitoring as a historical gold standard for diagnosing and quantifying gastroesophageal reflux has significant limitations. During this study, reflux is defined as a drop in the pH below 4, which effectively "blinds" the test to reflux occurring at higher pH values. Furthermore, in patients with persistent symptoms on PPI therapy, pH monitoring has limited utility as it can only detect abnormal acid reflux (pH <4), the occurrence of which has been altered by the antisecretory medication. Given that PPI antisecretory therapy is highly effective in neutralizing gastric acid, the question of whether the patients' persistent symptoms are due to acid breakthrough (a well documented phenomenon) and persistent acid reflux, nonacid reflux or not due to reflux become key issues in the decision for potential surgical treatment. Until recently this differentiation could not be made. A reliable method for detecting both acid and nonacid reflux has at least theoretical potential to define these populations of patients and thus improve patient selection for antireflux surgery. The recent introduction of multichannel intraluminal impedance technology allows the measurement of both acid and non-acid reflux, with potential to significantly enhance diagnostic accuracy. It usefulness remains unproven however.[97]

Impedance is the measurement of electrical resistance between two electrodes. The environment between the two electrodes affects impedance (Fig 8A–17). For example, in a liquid, highly ionic environment the impedance goes down, in the presence of gas impedance goes up. By placing multiple electrodes along the length of an otherwise standard pH catheter, we are capable of simultaneously measuring pH and impedance at multiple levels in real time. Thus, a liquid reflux episode can be detected as a retrograde drop in impedance (Fig 8A–18). Multichannel impedance thus can

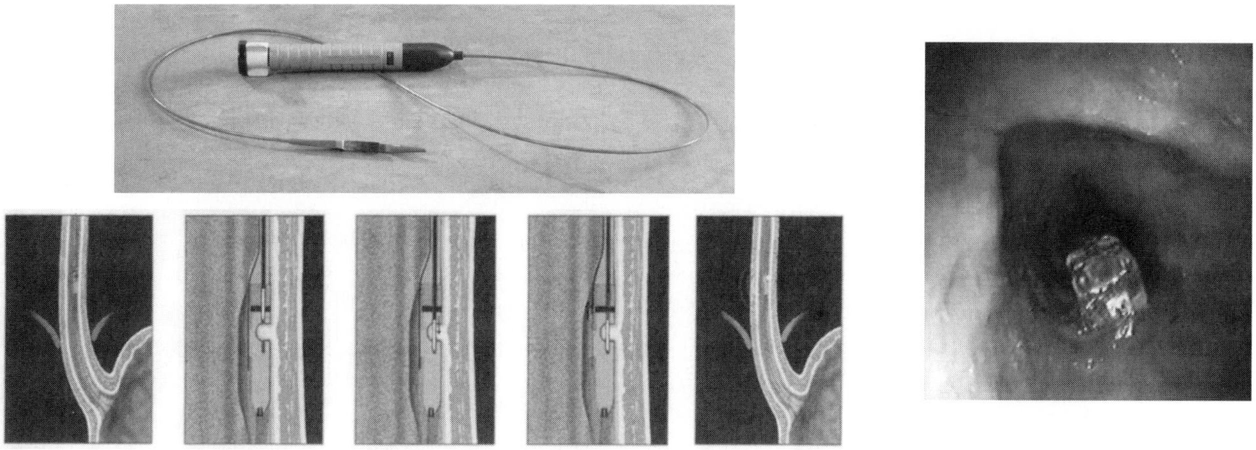

Figure 8A–16. Illustration of the Bravo indwelling 48 hour pH capsule and its receiver.

detect any material within the lumen of the esophagus (liquid, air or both) as well as the height or proximal extent of the reflux episode. Furthermore, the combination of impedance sensors and pH sensors in the same catheter allows for the measurement acid and nonacid reflux. Published data demonstrates the effectiveness of this technology in detecting refluxed material and their characteristics.[98,99]

Using this technology, Balaji et al. recently showed that most gastroesophageal reflux remains despite acid suppression. Impedance-pH may be particularly useful in evaluating patients with persistent symptoms despite PPI treatment, patients with respiratory symptoms, and postoperative patients who are having symptoms that are elusive to diagnosis.[100]

ASSESSMENT OF ESOPHAGEAL BODY AND LOWER ESOPHAGEAL SPHINCTER FUNCTION

Esophageal manometry is a widely used technique to examine the motor function of the esophagus and its sphincters. At present it is the most accurate method for assessing the function of the lower sphincter and body of the esophagus.[101] In patients with symptomatic GERD, manometry of the esophageal body can identify a mechanically defective lower esophageal sphincter and failure of esophageal clearance.

Manometry is an important component in the preoperative work up of patients who are candidates for antireflux surgery. First and foremost, it excludes named motility disorders such as achalasia which may be occasionally misdiagnosed as reflux. It also identifies the degree of lower esophageal sphincter incompetence, and/ or ineffective esophageal motility. Finally, it allows one to measure the precise location of the gastroesophageal junction for accurate pH probe placement.

Esophageal manometry is performed using electronic pressure-sensitive transducers or, less frequently now, water-perfused catheters with lateral side holes attached to transducers outside the body. Usually a train of five pressure transducers are bound together with the transducers placed at 5 cm intervals from the tip and oriented radially at 72 degrees from each other

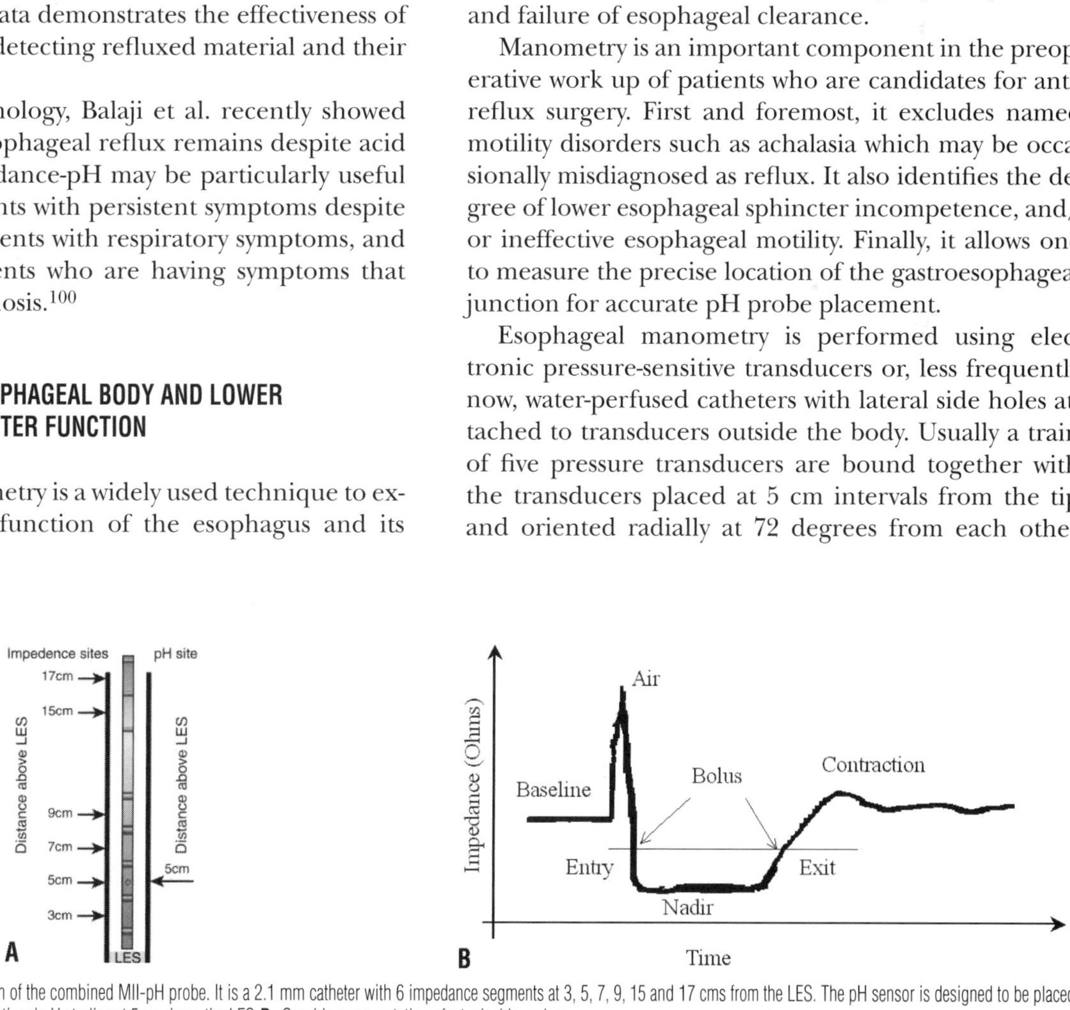

Figure 8A–17. A. Configuration of the combined MII-pH probe. It is a 2.1 mm catheter with 6 impedance segments at 3, 5, 7, 9, 15 and 17 cms from the LES. The pH sensor is designed to be placed in a similar position to the conventional pH studies at 5cm above the LES **B.** Graphic representation of a typical impedance curve.

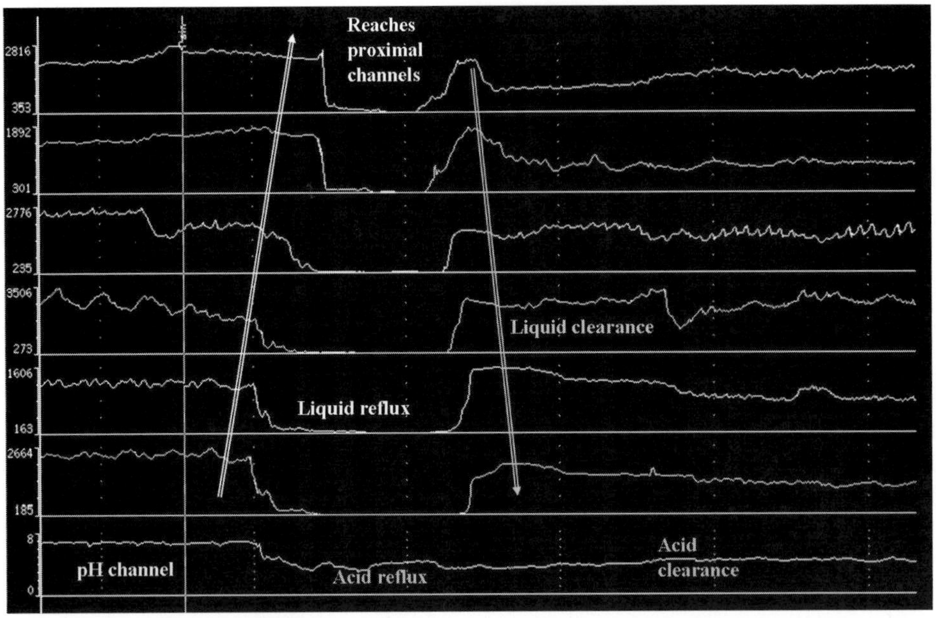

Figure 8A–18. Demonstration of an impedance detected acid reflux episode.

around the circumference of the catheter. A special catheter assembly consisting of four pressure transducers at the same level, oriented at 90 degrees to each other, is of special use in assessing three dimensional vector volume of the lower esophageal sphincter. Occasionally other specially designed catheters may be used to asses the upper sphincter.

As the pressure sensitive station is brought across the gastroesophageal junction, a rise in pressure from the gastric baseline identifies the beginning of the lower esophageal sphincter. The respiratory inversion point is identified when the positive excursions that occur with breathing in the abdominal cavity change to negative deflections in the thorax. The respiratory inversion point serves as a reference point at which the amplitude of lower esophageal sphincter pressure and the length of the sphincter exposed to abdominal pressure are measured. As the pressure sensitive station is withdrawn into the body of the esophagus, the upper border of the lower esophageal sphincter is identified by the drop in pressure to the esophageal baseline. From these measurements the pressure, abdominal length, and overall length of the sphincter are determined (Fig 8A–19). To account for the asymmetry of the sphincter (Fig 8A–20), the measurement is repeated with each of the five transducers and the average values for sphincter pressure above gastric baseline, overall sphincter length, and abdominal length of the sphincter are calculated.

The level at which incompetence of the lower esophageal sphincter occurs was defined by comparing the frequency distribution of these values in the 50 healthy volunteers to a population of similarly studied patients with symptoms of GERD. A lower esophageal sphincter is considered defective by having one or more of the following characteristics: an average lower esophageal sphincter pressure of less than 6 mm Hg, an average length exposed to the positive pressure environment in the abdomen of 1 cm or less, and an average overall sphincter length of 2 cm or less.

To assess the relaxation and post-relaxation contraction of the lower esophageal sphincter, a pressure transducer is repositioned within the high pressure zone, with a distal transducer located in the stomach and the proximal transducer within the esophageal body. Ten wet swallows (5 cc water) are performed. The normal

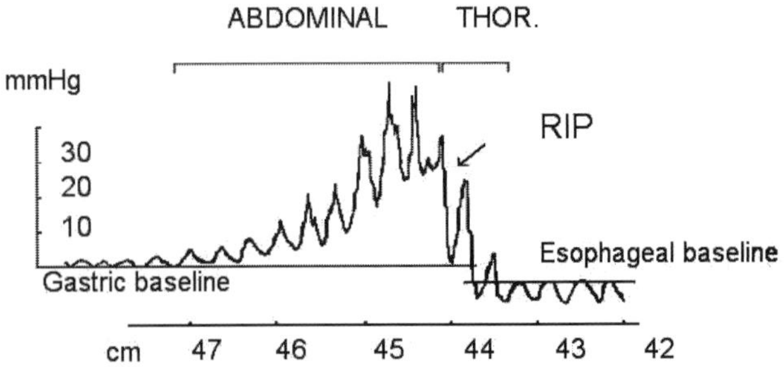

Figure 8A–19. Esophageal manometric pull trough tracing of the lower esophageal sphincter. The sphincter begins as the pressure rises off the gastric baseline. Positive and negative deflections reflect the pressure created by respiratory excursion. The RIP (respiratory inversion point) represents the transition from the intra-abdominal to intrathoracic portion of the sphincter and can be detected by the transition from positive to negative respiratory pressure excursions. The esophageal baseline pressure is normally 5 mmHG below gastric baseline reflecting the negative intrathoracic pressure.

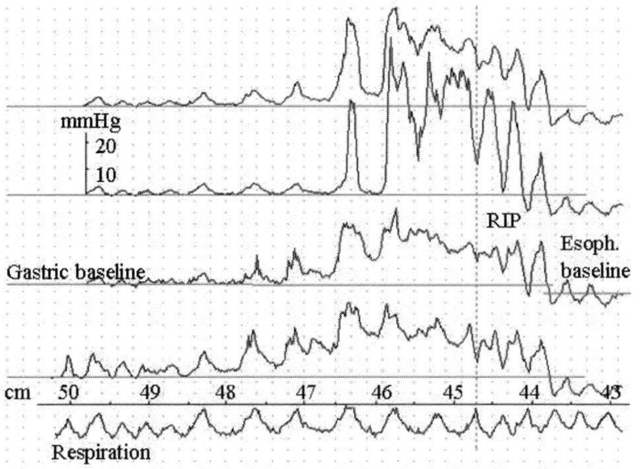

Figure 8A–20. Pull trough water perfused manometry of the lower esophageal sphincter using 4 radially oriented side holes all at the same level. The measuring ports are oriented every 90 degrees around the clock face. As the catheter is pulled through the sphincter the radial asymmetry of the LES is nicely seen. Both the beginning of the sphincter and the relative pressures differ from channel to channel.

pressure of the lower esophageal sphincter should drop to the level of gastric pressure during each wet swallow.

The function of the esophageal body is assessed with the 5 pressure transducers located in the esophagus. To standardize the procedure the most proximal pressure transducer is located 1 cm below the well-defined cricopharyngeal sphincter. By this method a pressure response throughout the whole esophagus can be obtained on one swallow. The study consists of recording ten wet swallows. Amplitude, duration, and morphology of contractions following each swallow are calculated at all recorded levels of the esophageal body. The delay between the onset or peak of esophageal contractions at the various levels of the esophagus is used to calculate the speed of wave propagation. The relationship of the esophageal contractions following a swallow are classified as peristaltic or simultaneous.

High Resolution Manometry

Evaluation using catheters with 5 pressure sensors described above has recently been challenged by high resolution manometry as a new standard in manometric evaluation.[102–103] High resolution catheters contain miniaturized pressure sensors positioned every centimeter along its length. The vast amount of data generated by these sensors is then processed and presented in traditional linear plots or as a visually enhanced spatiotemporal video tracing which is readily interpreted (Fig 8A–21). This enhanced spatial resolution allows simultaneous monitoring of contractile activity over the entire esophageal length.

High resolution manometry may allow the identification of focal motor abnormalities previously overlooked. It has enhanced the ability to predict bolus propagation and increased sensitivity in the measurement of pressure gradients. It is also faster and better tolerated since it eliminates the need for pull through positioning.

TESTS OF DUODENOGASTRIC FUNCTION

Esophageal disorders are frequently associated with abnormalities of the stomach and duodenum. Abnormalities of the gastric reservoir or increased gastric acid secretion can be responsible for increased esophageal exposure to gastric juice. Reflux of alkaline duodenal juice, including bile salts, pancreatic enzymes, and bicarbonate, is thought to have a role in the pathogenesis of esophagitis and complicated Barrett's esophagus. Furthermore, functional disorders of the esophagus often are not confined to the esophagus alone, but are associated with functional disorders of the rest of the foregut, i.e., stomach and duodenum. Tests of duodenogastric function that are helpful to investigate esophageal symptoms include gastric emptying studies, gastric acid analysis, and the use of cholescintigraphy for the diagnosis of pathologic duodenogastric reflux. The single test of 24-hour gastric pH monitoring can be used to identify gastric hypersecretion and imply the presence of duodenogastric reflux and delayed gastric emptying.

GASTRIC EMPTYING

Gastric emptying studies are performed with radionuclide-labelled meals. Emptying of solids and liquids can be assessed simultaneously when both phases are marked with different tracers. After ingestion of a labelled standard meal, gamma camera images of the stomach are obtained in 5–15 minute intervals for 1.5 to 2 hours. After correction for decay, the counts in the gastric area are plotted as percentage of total counts at the start of the imaging. The resulting emptying curve can be compared to data obtained in normal volunteers. In general normal subjects will empty 59% of a meal within 90 minutes.

▪ SURGICAL TREATMENT

INDICATIONS FOR ANTIREFLUX SURGERY

Antireflux surgery is indicated for the treatment of objectively documented, relatively severe GERD. Candidates for surgery include not only patients with erosive esophagitis, stricture and Barrett's esophagus, but also

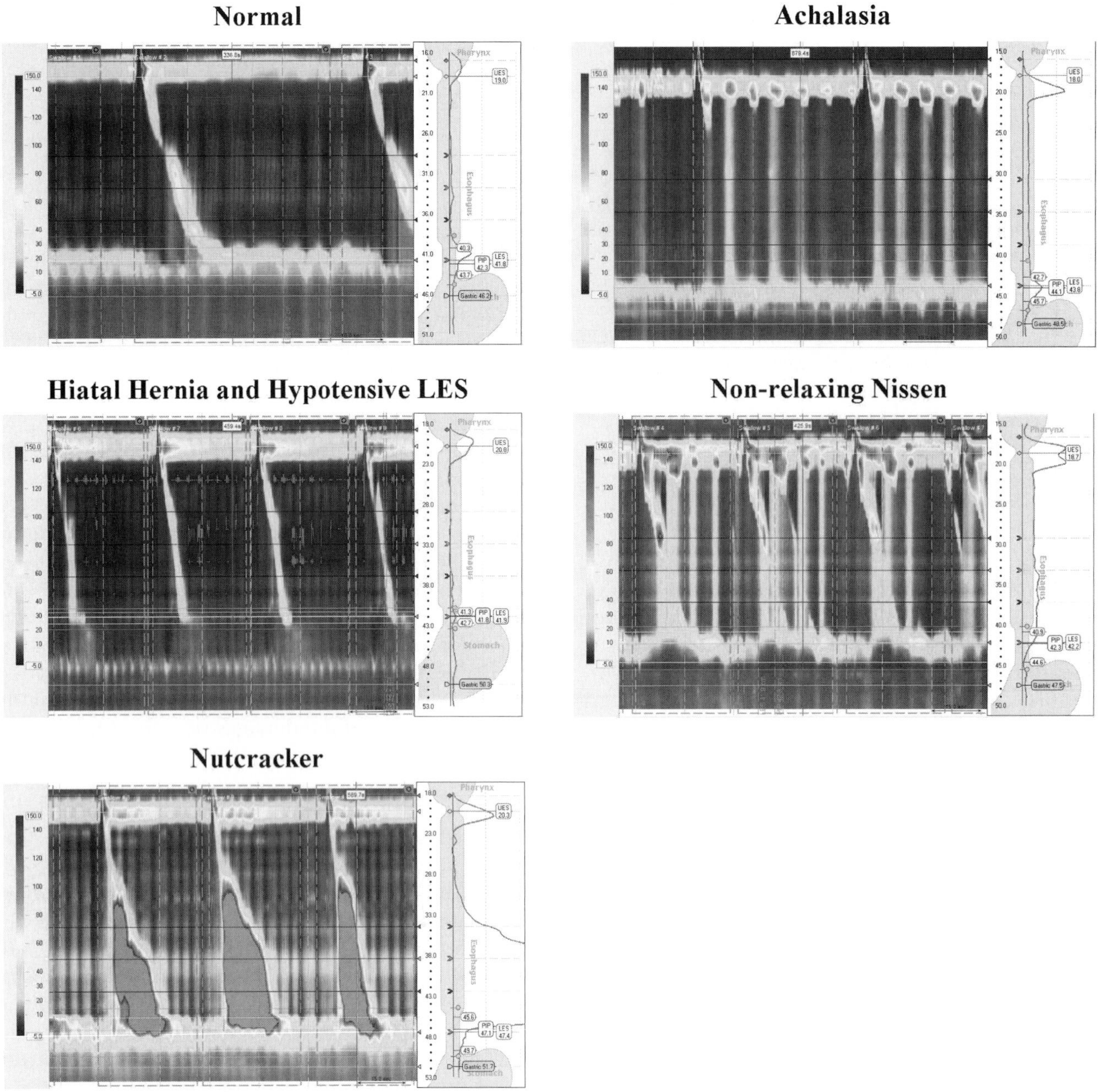

Figure 8A–21. Representative tracing of high resolution manometry from patients with various esophageal disease.

those without severe mucosal injury who show long term dependency on proton-pump inhibitors for symptom relief. Patients with atypical or respiratory symptoms who have a good response to intensive medical treatment are also candidates. Antireflux surgery is a reasonable treatment option in all patients who have demonstrated the need for long-term medical therapy, particularly if escalating doses of proton-pump inhibitors are needed to control symptoms and may be the preferred option in patients younger than 50 years of age, those who are noncompliant with their drug regimen, those for whom medications are a financial burden, and those who favor a single intervention over long-term drug treatment. It may be the treatment of choice in patients who are at high risk of progression despite medical therapy. Although this population is not well defined, risk factors that predict progressive disease and a poor response to medical therapy include: (1) nocturnal reflux on 24-hour esophageal pH study, (2) a structurally deficient lower esophageal sphincter, (3) mixed reflux of gastric and duodenal juice, and (4) mucosal injury at presentation.[103]

FACTORS TO CONSIDER PRIOR TO ANTIREFLUX SURGERY

Successful antireflux surgery is largely defined by two objectives—achieving the long-term relief of reflux symptoms and the absence of complications or complaints induced by the operation. In practice, achieving these two deceptively simple goals is difficult. Both are critically dependent upon establishing that the symptoms for which the operation is performed are due to excess esophageal exposure to gastric juice, as well as the proper performance of the appropriate antireflux procedure. Success can be expected in the vast majority of patients if these two criteria are met. The status of the lower esophageal sphincter is not as important a factor as in the days of open surgery. Patients with normal resting sphincters are often selected for antireflux surgery in the era of laparoscopic fundoplication. The outcome is not dependent upon sphincter function.[104]

The diagnostic approach to patients suspected of having gastroesophageal reflux disease and being considered for antireflux surgery has four important goals:

1. Establishing that GERD is the underlying cause of the patient's symptoms.
2. Estimating the risk of progressive disease.
3. Determining the presence or absence of esophageal shortening.
4. Evaluating esophageal body function, and occasionally, gastric emptying function.

OBJECTIVE DOCUMENTATION OF GASTROESOPHAGEAL REFLUX

The introduction of laparoscopic access, coupled with the growing recognition that surgery is a safe and durable treatment for GERD, has increased the number of patients being referred for laparoscopic fundoplication. The threshold for surgical referral is such that increasing numbers of patients without endoscopic esophagitis or other objective evidence of the presence of reflux are now considered candidates for laparoscopic antireflux surgery. These facts combine to underscore the importance of selecting patients for surgery who are likely to have a successful outcome. Although a Nissen fundoplication will reliably and reproducibly halt the return of gastroduodenal juice into the esophagus, little benefit is likely if the patient's symptoms are not caused by this specific pathophysiologic derangement. Thus, in large part, the anticipated success rate of laparoscopic fundoplication is directly proportional to the degree of certainty that GERD is the underlying cause of the patient's complaints.

Three factors predictive of a successful outcome following antireflux surgery have emerged (Table 8A–7).[105]

TABLE 8A–7. PREDICTORS OF OUTCOME AFTER LAPAROSCOPIC FUNDOPLICATION: STEPWISE LOGISTIC REGRESSION RESULTS OF 199 PATIENTS

Predictor		Adjusted Odds Ratio (95% Confidence Intervals)	Wald's p Value
Composite acid score	Increased	5.4 (1.9–15.3)	<0.001
	Normal	—	—
Symptom	Typical	5.1 (1.9–13.7)	<0.001
	Atypical	—	—
Response to medical therapy	Complete/Partial	3.3 (1.3–8.7)	=0.02
	Minor/None	—	—

Odds ratios and corresponding p values are adjusted for age and for all other factors in the model.
From: Campos GMR, Peters JH, DeMeester TR, et al. Multivariate analysis of the factors predicting outcome after Laparoscopic Nissen fundoplication. *J Gastrointest Surg* 1999; 3: 292–300.

These are (1) an abnormal score on 24-hour esophageal pH monitoring, (2) the presence of typical symptoms of GERD, namely heartburn or regurgitation, and (3) symptomatic improvement in response to acid suppression therapy prior to surgery. It is immediately evident that each of these factors helps to establish that GERD is indeed the cause of the patient's symptoms and that they have little to due with the severity of the disease.

Assessment of Esophageal Body Function

The propulsive force of the body of the esophagus should be evaluated by esophageal manometry to determine if it has sufficient power to propel a bolus of food through a newly reconstructed valve. Patients with normal peristaltic contractions do well with a 360° Nissen fundoplication. When peristalsis is absent, severely disordered, or the amplitude of the contraction is below 20 mm Hg in multiple levels of the esophageal body, a partial fundoplication may be offered to the patient. While a partial fundoplication may reduce the risk of postoperative dysphagia in the setting of a failed esophagus it is not as effective an antireflux barrier.[106] The majority of patients with ineffective esophageal motility and weak contraction amplitudes limited to a single segment tolerate a short, loose Nissen fundoplication.[107]

Detection of Esophageal Shortening

Anatomic shortening of the esophagus can compromise the ability to do an adequate repair without tension and lead to an increased incidence of breakdown or thoracic displacement of the repair (Fig 8A–22).[108] Esophageal shortening is identified radiographically by a sliding hiatal hernia that will not reduce in the upright

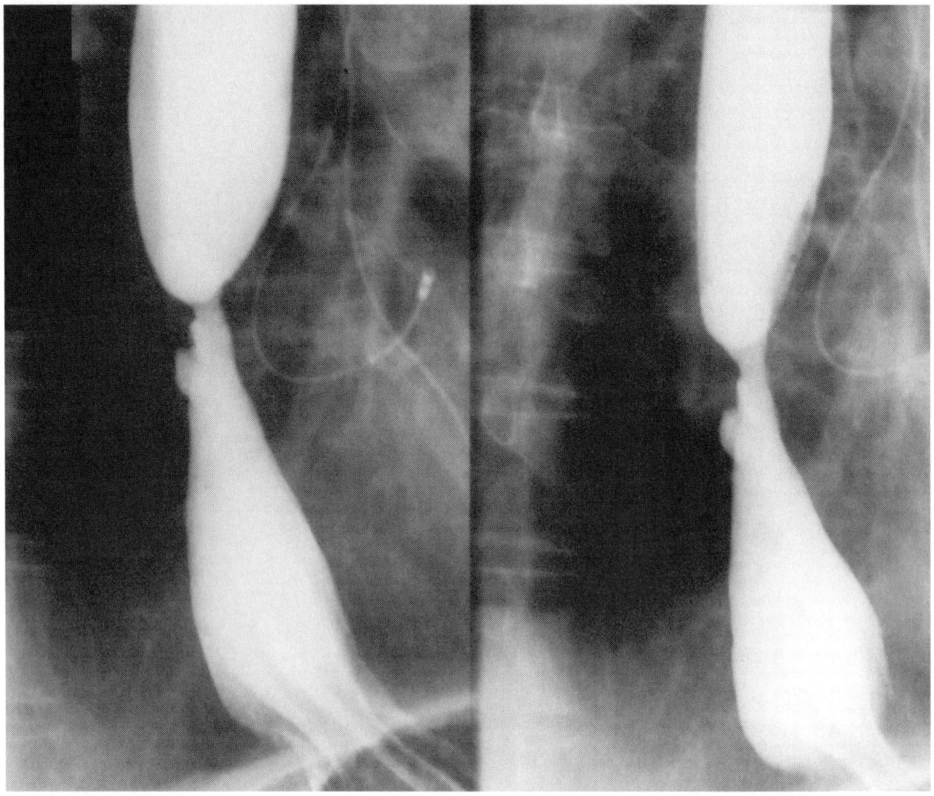

Figure 8A–22. Barium filled esophagogastric segment in a patient with a short esophagus. Note the gastroesophageal junction is well above the hiatus.

position or that measures larger than 5 cm between the diaphragmatic crura and gastroesophageal junction on endoscopy. When present, a transthoracic approach should be entertained. Laparoscopic access and a transabdominal gastroplasty or wedge fundectomy is an alternative although the long term outcome of these procedures is poorly documented and almost certainly not as good as a standard Nissen fundoplication.[109] In patients who have a motility study that shows the compete absence of contractility or more than 50% interrupted or dropped contractions or a history of several failed previous antireflux procedures, esophageal resection should be considered as an alternative.

Subclinical Gastric Pathology

Complaints of epigastric pain, nausea, vomiting, and loss of appetite may be an indication of overt or covert gastric motility abnormalities. When present, an assessment of gastric emptying should be considered. Delayed gastric emptying is found in approximately 10–20% of patients with GERD and can contribute to symptoms after an antireflux repair.[110] Usually, however, mild degrees of delayed gastric emptying are corrected by the antireflux procedure and only in patients with severe emptying disorders is there a need for an additional gastric procedure.

PRINCIPLES OF SURGICAL THERAPY

The primary goal of antireflux surgery is to safely reestablish the competency of the cardia by mechanically improving its function while preserving the patient's ability to swallow normally, to belch to relieve gaseous distention, and to vomit when necessary. Regardless of the choice of the procedure this goal can be achieved if attention is paid to five principles in reconstructing the cardia. First, the operation should restore the pressure of the distal esophageal sphincter to a level twice resting gastric pressure, i.e., 12 mm Hg for a gastric pressure of 6 mm Hg, and its length to at least 3 cm. This can be achieved by buttressing the distal esophagus with the fundus of the stomach. Preoperative and postoperative esophageal manometry measurements have shown that the resting sphincter pressure and the overall sphincter length can be surgically augmented over preoperative values, and that the change in the former is a function of the degree of gastric wrap around the esophagus.

Second, the operation should place an adequate length of the distal esophageal sphincter in the positive pressure environment of the abdomen by a method that ensures its response to changes in intra-abdominal pressure. The permanent restoration of 1.5–2 cm of abdominal esophagus in a patient whose sphincter pressure has been augmented to twice resting gastric pressure will maintain the competency of the cardia over various challenges of intra-abdominal pressure. Increasing the length of sphincter exposed to abdominal pressure will improve competency only if it is acted on by challenges of intra-abdominal pressure. Thus, the creation of a conduit that will ensure the transmission of intra-abdominal pressure changes around the abdominal portion of the sphincter is a necessary aspect of surgical repair. This is achieved by a properly constructed fundoplication.

Third, the reconstructed cardia should relax with swallowing. A vagally mediated relaxation of the distal esophageal sphincter and the gastric fundus occurs with swallowing normally. The relaxation lasts for approximately ten seconds and is followed by a rapid recovery to its former tonicity. To ensure relaxation of the sphincter occurs post fundoplication, three factors are important; firstly, only the fundus of the stomach should be used to buttress the sphincter since it is known to relax in concert with the sphincter,[111] second the fundoplication should be properly placed around the sphincter and not incorporate a portion of the stomach or be placed around the stomach itself since the body of the stomach does not relax with swallowing, and third, damage to the vagal nerves during dissection of the thoracic esophagus should be avoided because it may result in failure of the sphincter to relax.

Fourth, the fundoplication should not increase the resistance of the relaxed sphincter to a level that exceeds the peristaltic power of the body of the esophagus. The resistance of the relaxed sphincter depends on the degree, length, and diameter of the fundoplication and on the variation in intra-abdominal pressure. A 360° fundoplication should be no longer than 2 cm and constructed over a 60 French bougie. This will ensure that the relaxed sphincter will have an adequate diameter with minimal resistance that can easily be overcome by esophageal body contractions of normal amplitude. This is not necessary when constructing a partial fundoplication.

Fifth, the operation should ensure that the fundoplication can be placed in the abdomen without undue tension and maintained there by approximating the crura of the diaphragm above the repair. Leaving the fundoplication in the thorax converts a sliding hernia into a paraesophageal hernia with all the complications associated with that condition.[112] Maintaining the repair in the abdomen under tension predisposes to an increased incidence of recurrence. This occurs in patients who have a stricture or Barrett's esophagus and is probably due to shortening of the esophagus from the inflammatory process. This problem can be resolved by using a thoracic approach in certain instances of significant shortening. Liberal use of gastroplasty should be avoided to prevent persistent, albeit reduced, esophageal acid exposure.

PRIMARY ANTIREFLUX REPAIRS

The Nissen Fundoplication

The most common antireflux procedure is the Nissen Fundoplication. The procedure can be performed through the abdomen or the chest, but is most often approached laparoscopically. Rudolph Nissen described the procedure as a 360° fundoplication around the lower esophagus for a distance of 4–5 cm. Although this provided good control of reflux, it was associated with a number of side effects which have encouraged modifications of the procedure as originally described. These include taking care to use only the gastric fundus to envelope the esophagus in performing the fundoplication, sizing the fundoplication with a 60 French bougie, and limiting the length of the fundoplication to 1–2 centimeters.[113] The essential elements necessary for the performance of a transabdominal fundoplication are common to both the laparoscopic and open procedures and include the following:

1. Crural dissection, identification, and preservation of both vagi.
2. Circumferential dissection of the esophagus.
3. Crural closure.
4. Fundic mobilization by division of short gastric vessels.
5. Creation of a short, loose fundoplication by enveloping the anterior and posterior wall of the fundus around the lower esophagus.

LAPAROSCOPIC NISSEN FUNDOPLICATION

Laparoscopic fundoplication has become commonplace and has rapidly replaced traditional open Nissen fundoplication as the procedure of choice.[114,115]

Patient Positioning and Port Placement

The patient should be placed supine, in a modified lithotomy position, or with the legs abducted if a split leg table is available. The table is elevated 30 to 45 degrees. If lithotomy is used, the knees should be only slightly flexed so as not to interfere with the mobility of the instruments during the course of the procedure. The surgeon, should stand between the patients legs, allowing the right and left handed instruments to approach the hiatus form the respective upper abdominal quadrants. The assistant should stand on the patient's left side. Five ports (variously from 5–12 mm) are utilized (Fig 8A–23). The camera is placed slightly above the umbilicus and to the left of midline via a trans-rectus incision. In most patients, placement of the camera in the umbilicus will not allow adequate visualization of the hiatal structures once dis-

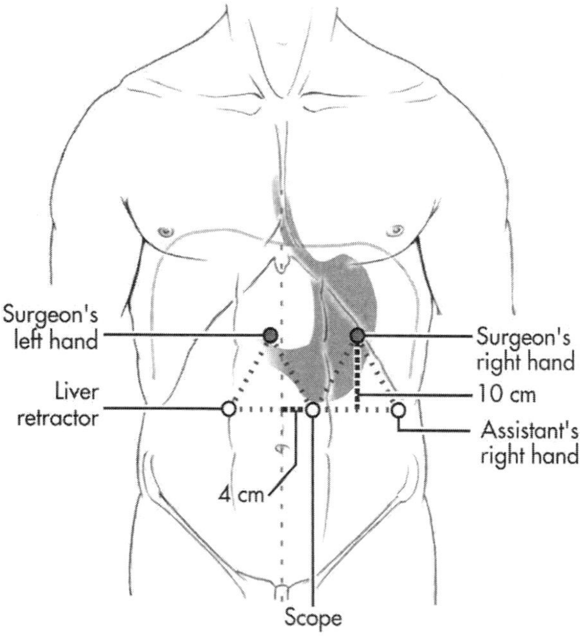

Figure 8A–23. Patient positioning and trocar placement for laparoscopic antireflux surgery. The patient is placed with the head elevated 45 degrees in the modified lithotomy position. The surgeon stands between the patient's legs and the procedure is completed via 5 abdominal access ports.

sected. Two lateral retracting ports are placed in the right and left anterior axillary lines respectively. The right sided liver retractor can be placed immediately subcostal in the right anterior axillary line or in the right mid-abdomen approximately even with the camera. Both allow an acute angle toward the left lateral segment of the liver and thus the ability to push the instrument toward the operating table, lifting the liver. A second retraction port is placed at the level of the umbilicus, in the left mid-clavicular line. The surgeon's right handed trocar is placed in the left midclavicular line, 2 to 3 inches below the costal margin and the left slightly to the left of the xiphiod. Placing the operating trocars on either side of the midline allows triangulation between the camera and the two instruments, avoiding the difficulty associated with the instruments being in direct line with the camera. The surgeon's left hand operating port should be long to allow passage through the falciform ligament. This technique eliminates the constant interference from the falciform ligament during instrument exchanges and keeps the port directed toward the hiatus.

One of the most important, and occasionally the most difficult elements of laparoscopic surgery, is adequate retraction and safe exposure of the necessary structures. A 5mm flexible end retractor is placed into the right anterior axillary port, the flexible end is stiffened into a triangular shape, and positioned to hold the left lateral segment of the liver towards the anterior abdominal wall. The retractor should be fixed into position using a table-mounted mechanical arm so as to minimize trauma to the elevated liver since bleeding from this area interferes with visualization of the operative field. Mobilization of the left lateral segment by division of the triangular ligament is not necessary.

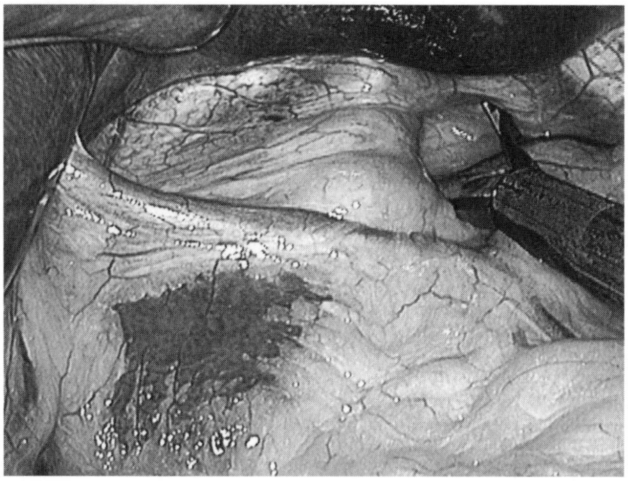

Figure 8A–24. Intraoperative photograph of the initial laparoscopic view of the esophageal hiatus after suitable retraction of the liver. Note the widened crura and hiatal hernia.

An atruamatic clamp is placed into the left anterior axillary port and the stomach is retracted toward the patients feet. This maneuver exposes the esophageal hiatus (Fig 8A–24). Commonly a hiatal hernia will need to be reduced. An atraumatic clamp should be used, and care taken not to grasp the stomach too vigorously, as gastric perforations can occur.

Hiatal Dissection. The key to the hiatal dissection is identification of the right crus (Fig 8A–25). In all except the most obese patients there is a very thin portion of the gas-

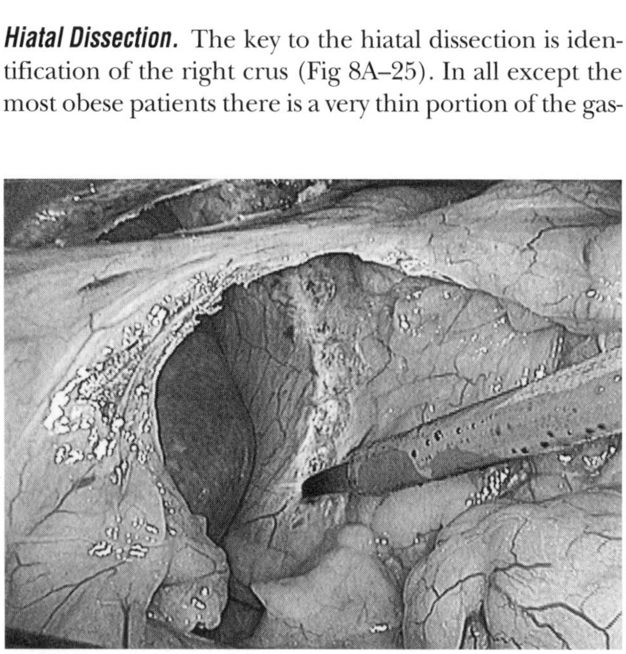

Figure 8A–25. Intraoperative photograph of the initial dissection of the esophageal hiatus. The right crus is identified, and the dissection begun by incising the peritoneum along its anterior border as shown in the photograph. This will allow dissection into the retroperitoneum and mediastinum.

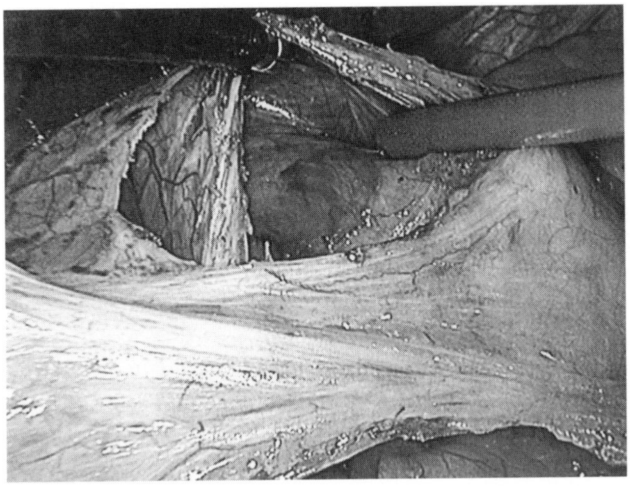

Figure 8A–26. Intraoperative photograph of division of the anterior crural fibers and mobilization of the esophagus off the left crus.

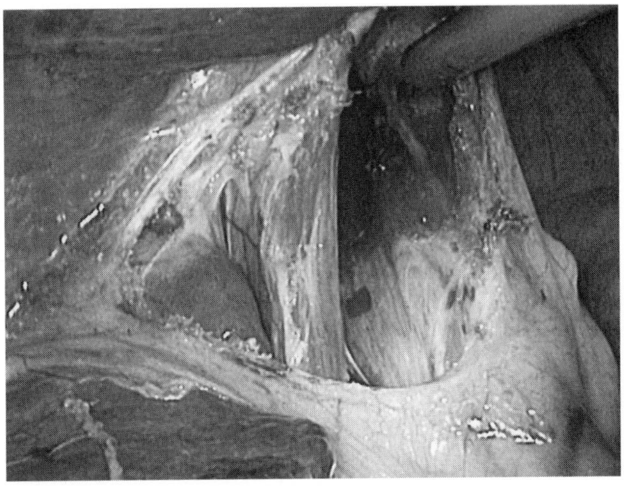

Figure 8A–27. Anterior dissection of the esophageal hiatus. The anterior (left) vagus nerve often "hugs" the inside of the left crus and can be injured if not dissected off prior to crural dissection.

trohepatic omentum overlying the caudate lobe of the liver. Dissection is begun by incision of this portion of the gastrohepatic omentum below the hepatic branch of the anterior vagal nerve. Using either ultrasonic shears or scissors with cautery, the gastrohepatic omentum is divided in a cephalad direction. Preservation of the hepatic branch of the anterior vagus nerve is not necessary but we tend to do so. A large left hepatic artery arising from the left gastric artery will be present in up to 25% of patients and should be identified and avoided. Once opened, the outside of the right crus will become evident. The inferior vena cava is usually protected behind the caudate lobe of the liver but may be in close proximity to the right crus, particularly if a large hiatal hernia is present. The peritoneum overlying the anterior aspect of the right crus is incised with scissors and electrocautery or ultrasonic shears. The medial portion of the right crus leads into the mediastinum, and is entered by blunt dissection with both instruments. At this juncture the esophagus usually becomes evident. The right crus is retracted laterally and the posterior or right vagus is identified and either dissected away from the esophagus for a distance of 3–4 centimeters or mobilized with the esophagus. The anterior or left vagus is left undisturbed.

Meticulous hemostasis is critical. Blood and fluid tends to pool in the hiatus and is difficult to remove. Irrigation should be kept to a minimum. Care must be taken not to injure the phrenic artery and vein as they course above the hiatus. Lifting the esophagus with a blunt-tipped grasper placed within the esophageal hiatus underneath the organ, the dissection is carried inferiorly and laterally exposing the medial and lateral aspects of the right crus. A large hiatal hernia often makes this portion of the procedure easier as it accentuates the diaphragmatic crura. On the other hand, dissection of a large mediastinal hernia sac can be difficult.

Following dissection of the right crus, attention is turned toward the anterior crural confluence. The left-handed grasper is used to hold up the tissues anterior to the esophagus, and sweep the esophagus downward and to the right, separating it from the left crus (Fig 8A–26). The anterior crural tissues are then divided and the left crus identified. The anterior vagus nerve often "hugs" the left crus and can be injured in this portion of the dissection if not carefully searched for and protected (Fig 8A–27). The left crus is dissected as completely as possible, including taking down the angle of His and the attachments of the fundus to the left diaphragm (Fig 8A–28). A complete dissection of the lateral and inferior aspect of the left crus and fundus of the stomach is the key maneuver allowing circumferential mobilization of the esophagus. Failure to do so will result in difficulty encircling the esophagus, particu-

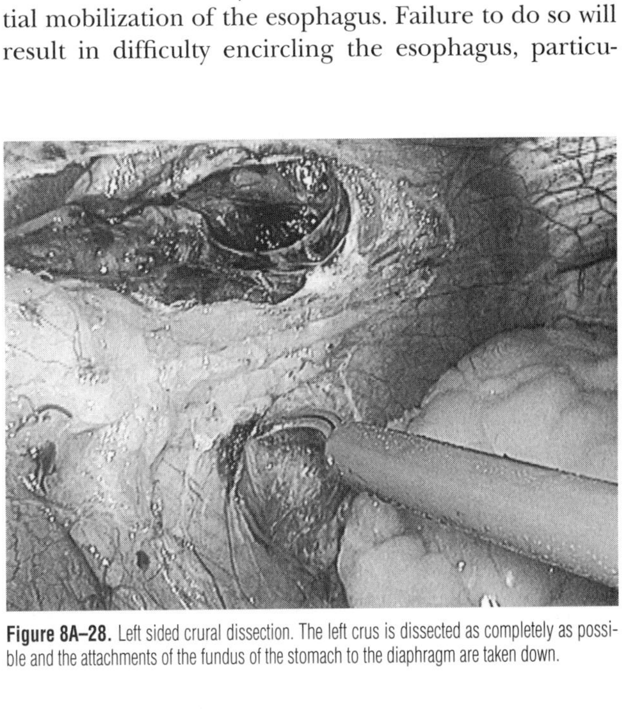

Figure 8A–28. Left sided crural dissection. The left crus is dissected as completely as possible and the attachments of the fundus of the stomach to the diaphragm are taken down.

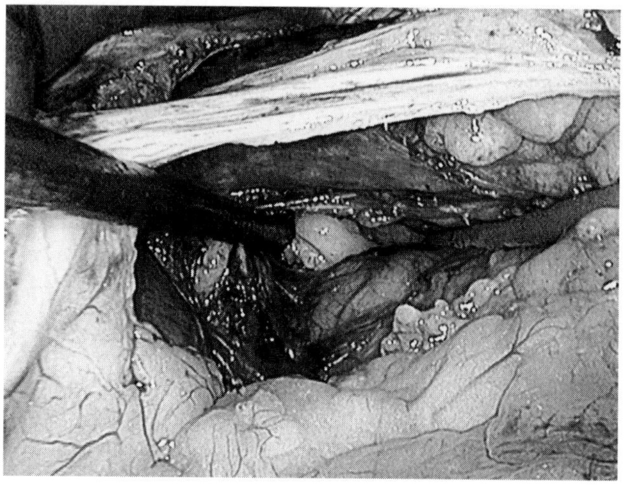

Figure 8A–29. A window behind the gastroesophageal junction is created to allow passage of a Penrose drain and later the fundoplication. The posterior vagus nerve should be identified and protected.

larly if approached from the right. Repositioning of the Babcock retractor toward the fundic side of the stomach facilitates retraction for this portion of the procedure. The posterior vagus nerve may be encountered in the low left crural dissection. It should be looked for and protected.

A window behind the gastroesophageal junction can generally now be easily created (Fig 8A–29). Attention is returned to the right side of the esophagus where the left-handed instrument is used to retract the esophagus anteriorly. This allows the right hand to perform the dissection behind the esophagus. The posterior vagus nerve should be identified and left on the esophagus. The left crus is identified and the dissection kept caudad to it. There is a tendency to dissect into the mediastinum and left pleura. In the presence of severe esophagitis, transmural inflammation, esophageal shortening and/or a large posterior fat pad, this dissection may be particularly difficult. If unduly difficult, abandon this route of dissection and approach the hiatus from the left side by dividing the short gastric vessels at this point in the procedure rather than later. After completing the posterior dissection, pass a grasper (via the surgeon's left-handed port) behind the esophagus and over the left crus and pull a Penrose drain around the esophagus to be used as an esophageal retractor for the remainder of the procedure.

Fundic Mobilization. Complete fundic mobilization allows construction of a tension-free fundoplication. The gastrosplenic omentum is suspended anteroposteriorly, in a clothesline fashion via both atraumatic grasping forceps and the lesser sac entered approximately one third the distance down the greater curvature of the stomach where the short gastric vessels are longer and easier to expose (Fig 8A–30). Short gastric vessels are sequentially dissected, and divided using ultrasonic shears. An anterior-posterior rather than medial to lateral orientation of the vessels is the preferred, with the exception of those close to the spleen. The dissection includes pancreaticogastric branches posterior to the upper stomach and continues until the right crus and caudate lobe can be seen from the left side. With caution and meticulous dissection, the fundus can be completely mobilized in most patients. The most superior short gastric vessels may be difficult to expose. Occasionally, removal of the liver retractor and placement of a second Babcock forceps through the right anterior axillary port facilitates retraction during division of the short gastric vessels.

Esophageal Mobilization & Crural Closure. The esophagus is mobilized into the posterior mediastinum for several centimeters in order to provide maximal intra-abdominal esophageal length. Posterior and right lateral mobilization is readily accomplished. The anterior and left lateral mobilization must take care not to injure the anterior vagus nerve. Gentle traction on the Penrose drain around the GE junction facilitates exposure. The right and left pleural reflection often come into view and should be avoided. Continue the crural dissection to enlarge the space behind the gastroesophageal junction as much as possible. Following mobilization and an assessment of intraabdominal esophageal length the hiatus is closed in all patients. The esophagus is held anterior and to the left and the crura approximated with two to four interrupted figure of eight 0-Ethibond sutures, starting just above the aortic decussation and working anterior. A large needle (CT1) passed down the left up-

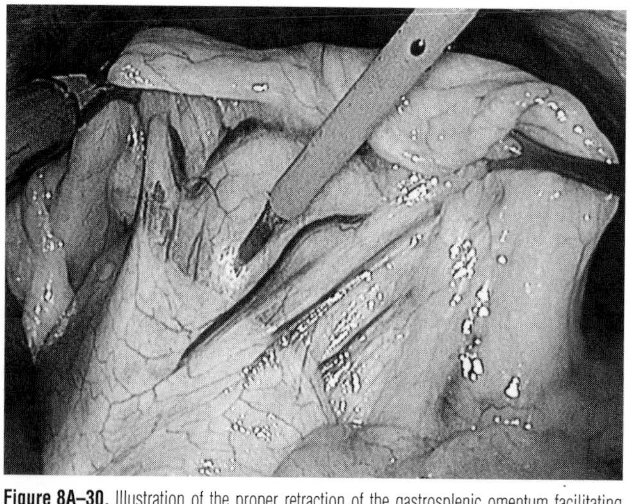

Figure 8A–30. Illustration of the proper retraction of the gastrosplenic omentum facilitating the initial steps in short gastric division. Complete fundic mobilization is continued by retraction of the stomach rightward and the spleen and omentum left and downward. These maneuvers allow opening of the lesser sac and facilitates division of the high short gastric vessels.

per 10-mm port to facilitate a durable crural closure. Because space is limited, it is often necessary to use the surgeon's left-handed (nondominant) instrument as a retractor, facilitating placement of single bites through each crus with the surgeon's right hand. The aorta may be punctured while suturing the left crus. Identification of its anterior surface and often retracting the left crus away from the aorta via the left handed grasper will help avoid inadvertent aortic puncture. Extracorporeal knot tying using a standard knot pusher or a "tie knot" device is common, although tying within the abdomen is perfectly appropriate. More recently we have inspected the crural closure at the completion of the procedure following creation of the fundoplication and removal of the bougie. Doing so will often reveal that the bougie has dilated the hiatal opening such that a final stitch should be placed to further approximate it.

Creation of the Fundoplication. A short loose fundoplication is fashioned with particular attention to the geometry of the wrap. The mid- posterior fundus is grasped and passed left to right behind the esophagus rather than pulling right to left. This assures that the posterior fundus is used for the posterior aspect of the fundoplication. This is accomplished by placing a Babcock clamp through the left lower port, and grasping the mid portion of the posterior fundus (Figure 8A–31). Gently bring the posterior fundus behind the esophagus to the right side with an upward, rightward, and clockwise twisting motion. This maneuver can be difficult particularly for the novice. If so, placement of a 0-silk suture in the mid posterior fundus and grasping it from the right side facilitates brining the posterior fundus around to create the fundoplication. The anterior wall of the fundus is then folded over the esophagus to meet the posterior at about the 10–11 o'clock position above the supporting Penrose drain.

The posterior and anterior fundic lips should be maneuvered (as in a "shoe shine") to allow the fundus to envelope the esophagus without twisting. Laparoscopic visualization has a tendency to exaggerate the size of the posterior opening that has been dissected. Consequently, the space for the passage of the fundus behind the esophagus may be tighter than thought and the fundus relatively ischemic when brought around. If the right lip of the fundoplication has a bluish discoloration, the stomach should be returned to its original position and the posterior dissection enlarged. A 60-French bougie is

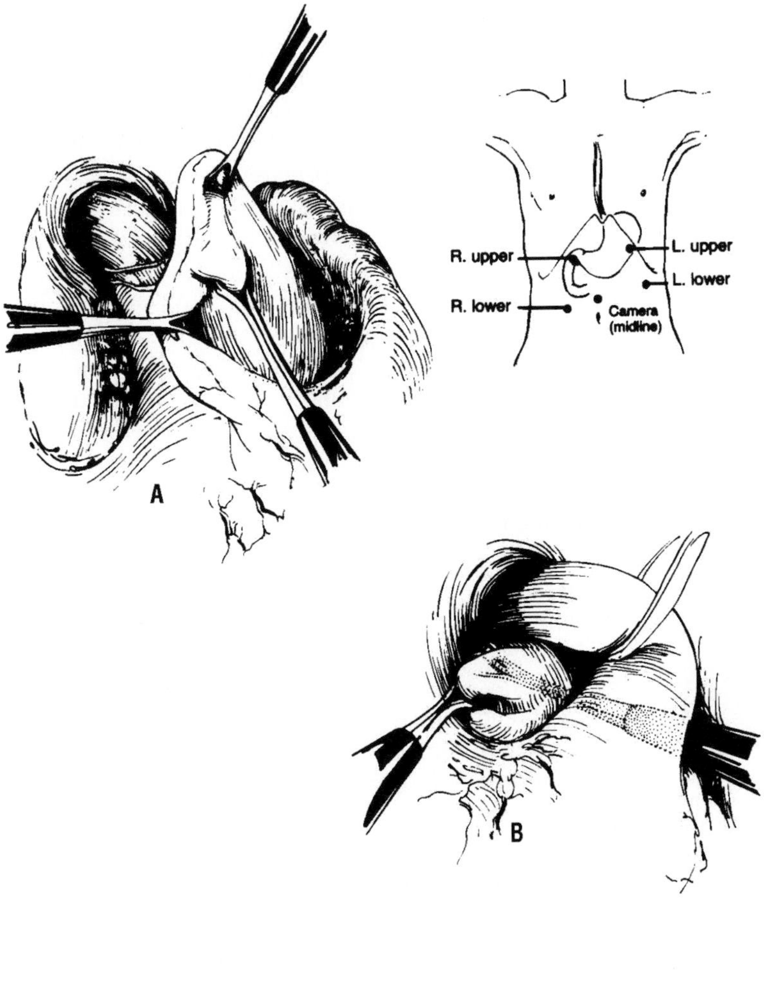

Figure 8A–31. Placement of Babcock on the posterior fundus in preparation for passing it behind the esophagus to create the posterior or right lip of the fundoplication. *Inset:* To achieve the proper angle for passage the Babcock is placed through the left lower trocar. The posterior fundus is passed left to right and grasped from the right via a Babcock through the right upper trocar.

passed to properly size the fundoplication, and the "lips" of the fundoplication sutured utilizing a single U-stitch of 2-0 Prolene buttressed with felt pledgets. The most common error is an attempt to grasp the anterior portion of the stomach to construct the right lip of the fundoplication rather than the posterior fundus. The esophagus should comfortably lie in the untwisted fundus prior to suturing. Finally, two anchoring sutures of 2-0 silk are placed above and below the U-stitch to complete the fundoplication. When finished, the suture line of the fundoplication should be facing in a right anterior direction (Fig 8A–32). The abdomen is then irrigated, hemostasis checked, and the bougie, Penrose drain and any sponges placed into the abdomen removed.

TRANSABDOMINAL OPEN NISSEN FUNDOPLICATION

An open abdominal fundoplication may be the best approach used in the setting of:

1. Multiple previous abdominal procedures.
2. Previous antireflux or hiatal surgery.
3. Large Type III hiatal hernia or intrathoracic stomach.

Excellent exposure of the esophageal hiatus is paramount in performing an open procedure. This can be achieved by utilizing an "upper hand" retractor fit with two blades for the right and left costal margins and a specialized liver retractor constructed by welding a Weinberg retractor to a Balfour handle. This retractor is placed under the liver down to the esophageal hiatus. The operating table is placed in a reverse Trendelenburg position and the retractor is lifted cephalad in a

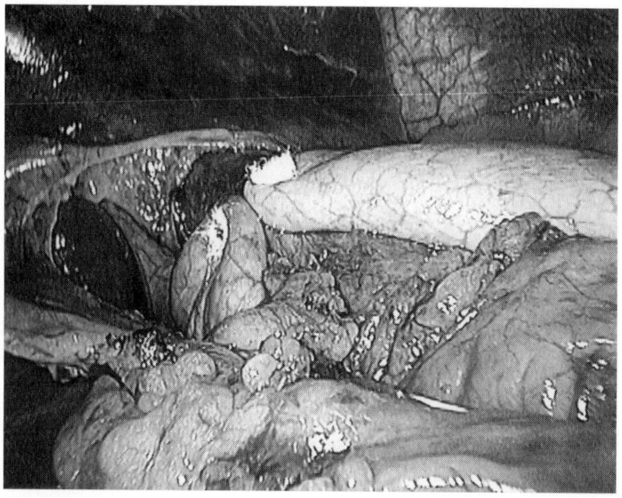

Figure 8A–32. Intraoperative photograph of the completed fundoplication. The fundoplication is sutured in place with a single U-stitch of 2-0 Prolene pledgeted on the outside. A 60 French mercury weighted bougie is passed through the gastroesophageal junction prior to fixation of the wrap to assure a floppy fundoplication. Note the orientation of the fundic wrap slightly to the right.

45° angle and secured to the overhead bar attached to the table. This elevates the anterior chest wall and lifts the liver out of the way. The wound is retracted laterally with a Balfour retractor. Another option is to divide the triangular ligament to mobilize the left lateral segment of the liver which can then be gently folded to the right and held with a deep malleable retractor fixed to a Buchwalter or Gomez retractor system to expose the hiatus This retraction is critical since, without this exposure, careful dissection of the hiatus is difficult, time-consuming, and dangerous.

Similar to the laparoscopic approach, the esophageal hiatus is approached by dividing the gastrohepatic ligament in the area where it is thin and usually transparent. The cephalad portion of the gastrohepatic ligament is divided and the incision carried superiorly over the anterior surface of the esophagus and down the left crus of the esophageal hiatus.

The esophagus is dissected circumferentially within the posterior mediastinum by blunt finger dissection. A soft rubber drain is passed around the esophagus, excluding the posterior or right vagal trunk. While retracting on the rubber drain, the loose fibroareolar tissue within the hiatus is divided to clearly identify the medial surface of the right and left crus.

The procedure continues with mobilization of the gastric fundus by dividing the short gastric vessels. The proximal third of the greater curvature is freed. One can appreciate how these vessels, if not divided, force the surgeon to construct the fundoplication with a portion of the body of the stomach rather than the fundus. The esophageal hiatus is closed by retracting the esophagus to the left, and approximating the right and left crura with interrupted 0-silk sutures. Care is taken not to place the uppermost sutures on the right side in the fascia of the diaphragm, as this will result in a constriction of the hiatus and dysphagia. When complete, the hiatus should freely admit a fingertip adjacent to the esophagus.

Construction of the fundic wrap completes the procedure. The pad of areolar tissue which lies on the anterior surface of the gastroesophageal junction is removed to allow proper identification of the junction and encourage the fusion of the fundic wrap to the esophagus. The freed posterior wall of the fundus is passed behind the esophagus or alternatively pulled between the right vagal trunk and the posterior wall of the esophagus. A 60F bougie is passed by the anesthesiologist into the stomach, and the anterior wall of the fundus is pulled across the anterior wall of the esophagus. This results in enveloping the distal esophagus between the anterior and posterior fundic wall. We prefer a short wrap secured with Teflon pledgets and permanent monofilament sutures. The suture is tied with a single throw to approximate the two lips of the fundic wrap around the esophagus containing the 60F bougie. When drawn together the fundic wrap should be large enough to accept the insertion of the surgeon's index finger alongside the esophagus containing the 60F bougie. If the surgeon is unable to insert his finger or feels tight bands over his finger, the wrap is too tight, and the left end of the horizontal U-stitch must be replaced more laterally and inferiorly on the anterior wall of the fundus. This enlarges the internal diameter of the wrap. If there is excessive space, the wrap is too floppy, and the left or anterior end of the U-stitch must be replaced more medially and superiorly on the anterior wall of the fundus. This reduces the internal diameter of the wrap. When the wrap is of proper size, and the limbs of the U-stitch are tied securely, the bougie is removed and the abdomen is closed.

TRANSTHORACIC NISSEN FUNDOPLICATION

The indications for performing an antireflux procedure by a transthoracic approach are as follows:

1. A patient who has had a extensive transabdominal hiatal surgery. In this situation, a peripheral circumferential incision in the diaphragm is made to provide simultaneous exposure of the upper abdomen. This allows safe dissection of the previous repair from both the abdominal and thoracic sides of the diaphragm.
2. A patient who requires a concomitant esophageal myotomy for diffuse spasm.
3. A patient who has a short esophagus. This is usually associated with a stricture or Barrett's esophagus. In this situation, the thoracic approach is preferred in order to obtain maximum mobilization of the esophagus in order to place the repair without tension below the diaphragm.
4. A patient with a large paraesophageal hiatal hernia that does not reduce below the diaphragm during a roentgenographic barium study in the upright position. This can indicate esophageal shortening and, again, a thoracic approach is preferred for maximum mobilization of the esophagus.
5. A patient who has associated pulmonary pathology. In this situation, the nature of the pulmonary pathology can be evaluated and the proper pulmonary surgery, in addition to the antireflux repair, can be performed.

The hiatus is approached transthoracically through a left posterior lateral thoracotomy incision in the sixth intercostal space; i.e., over the upper border of the seventh rib. For patients who have a failed antireflux repair and are undergoing a second procedure, the seventh intercostal space is preferred; i.e., above the superior border of the eighth rib. This allows better exposure of the abdomen through the diaphragm incision. When necessary, the diaphragm is incised circumferentially 2–3 cm from the chest wall for a distance of approximately 10–15 cm. An adequate fringe of diaphragm must be preserved along the chest wall for reapproximation of the muscle. The operation is made easier if the anesthetic is delivered through a double-lumen endotracheal tube and the left lung is selectively deflated.

The first step in the operation is to mobilize the esophagus from the level of the diaphragm to underneath the aortic arch. Care is taken not to injure the vagal nerves. There are usually two arteries which arise from the proximal descending thoracic aorta and pass over the left lateral surface of the esophagus to the left main stem bronchus. They are the left superior and inferior bronchial arteries. These are ligated individually and represent the cephalad extension of the esophageal mobilization. In addition to these arteries there are two or three esophageal arteries coming directly from the distal descending thoracic aorta to the lower third of the esophagus. They are also ligated and divided. One need not worry about ischemic necrosis of the esophagus with this degree of dissection. There is sufficient blood supply through the intrinsic arterial plexus of the esophagus, fed by the inferior thyroid artery in the neck and branches of the right bronchial artery in the thorax, to maintain the integrity and prevent ischemic necrosis of the muscle. Mobilization up to the aortic arch is usually necessary to place the reconstructed cardia of a shortened esophagus into the abdomen without undue tension. Failure to do this is one of the major causes for subsequent breakdown of a transthoracic repair and return of symptoms. The second step of the operation is to free the cardia from the diaphragm. It is the most difficult portion of the transthoracic approach. To accomplish this, it is *not* necessary to make an incision through the central tendon of the diaphragm or to enlarge the hiatus by dividing the crura. With experience, this portion of the operation can be completed through the hiatus. The dissection is started by gaining access into the abdominal cavity through the phrenoesophageal membrane along the anterior border of the left crus, close to the wall of the stomach, away from the gastric vessels. It can be difficult to find the correct tissue plane, since the pro-peritoneal fat tends to protrude through the incision once the superior leaf of the membrane has been divided. Persistence and dissection above the protruding pro-peritoneal fat will eventually be rewarded with entry into the free peritoneal space. Entry into the abdominal cavity is easier when a hiatal hernia is present.

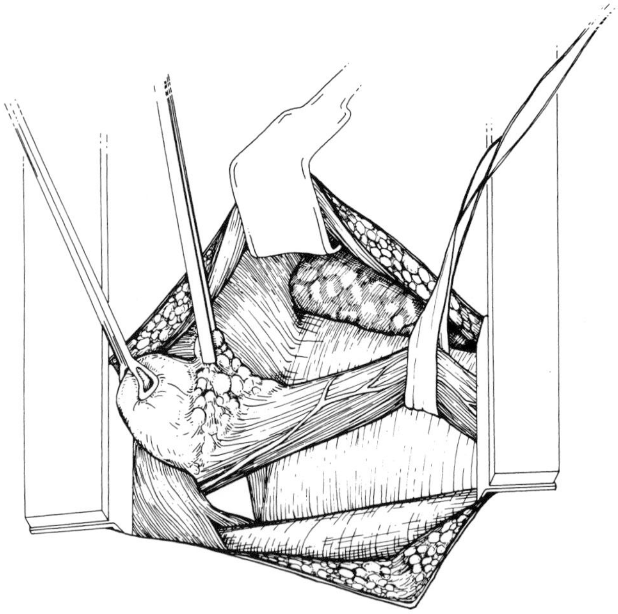

Figure 8A–33. Transthoracic antireflux procedure through a left posterolateral thoracotomy, showing mobilization of the esophagus and freeing of the cardia from the diaphragmatic hiatus. The fundus of the stomach is drawn through the hiatus into the chest with a Babcock clamp. The forceps is on the vascular fat pad at the cardioesophageal junction. (From DeMeester TR. Transthoracic antireflux procedures. In: Nyhus LM, Baker RJ (eds), *Mastery of Surgery.* Boston: Little, Brown; 1984:385.)

The proper stance of the surgeon at the operating table will aid him in the dissection of the hiatus. He should stand adjacent to the patient, facing the head of the table. The left index and middle fingers are placed through the diaphragmatic hiatus into the abdominal cavity with the palm of the hand facing the patient's feet. The surgeon's line of vision is down and backward under his left axilla. With judicial use of the left thumb, index, and middle fingers, the surgeon is able to spread the hiatal tissues and guide the dissection done with the scissors in his right hand. In this position, the left hand is also used to retract the esophagus and protect the vagal trunks. Although the description of this stance sounds somewhat awkward, its use greatly facilitates the most difficult part of the operation. In fact, the stance is quite natural and would be assumed eventually by any surgeon who, on numerous occasions, has experienced the struggle of freeing the cardia from the hiatus through a transthoracic approach.

When all the attachments between the cardia and diaphragmatic hiatus are divided, the fundus and part of the body of the stomach are drawn up through the hiatus into the chest. This requires dividing 4–6 short gastric arteries supplying the proximal stomach. When the stomach is brought up into the chest, the vascular fat pad that lies on the anterior lateral surface of the cardia is excised in a manner similar to that described for the abdominal approach (Fig 8A–33). The third step of the procedure is the placement of the crural sutures used to close the hiatus. To do so the stomach is placed back into the abdomen and the mobilized esophagus is retracted anteriorly to expose the posterior limbs of the right and left crus. Usually there is a decussation of muscle fibers from the right crus around the aorta, but occasionally the aorta lies free within the enlarged hiatus. In either situation, the first crural stitch is placed close to the aorta, taking a generous bite of crural muscle. Traction on this first suture elevates the crura toward the surgeon and facilitates the placement of subsequent crural stitches. Each stitch should incorporate the fascia from the periphery of the central tendon that blends with the muscle fibers of the right crus. Approximately six sutures, placed 1 cm apart, are necessary to approximate the crura adequately and reduce the size of the hiatus. To insert the most anterior crural stitch, it is often necessary to push the esophagus posteriorly against the previously placed sutures and pass a stitch through the right crus, anterior to the esophagus, then bring it posterior to the esophagus and through the left crus. The crural sutures are not tied until the reconstruction of the cardia is complete (Fig 8A–34).

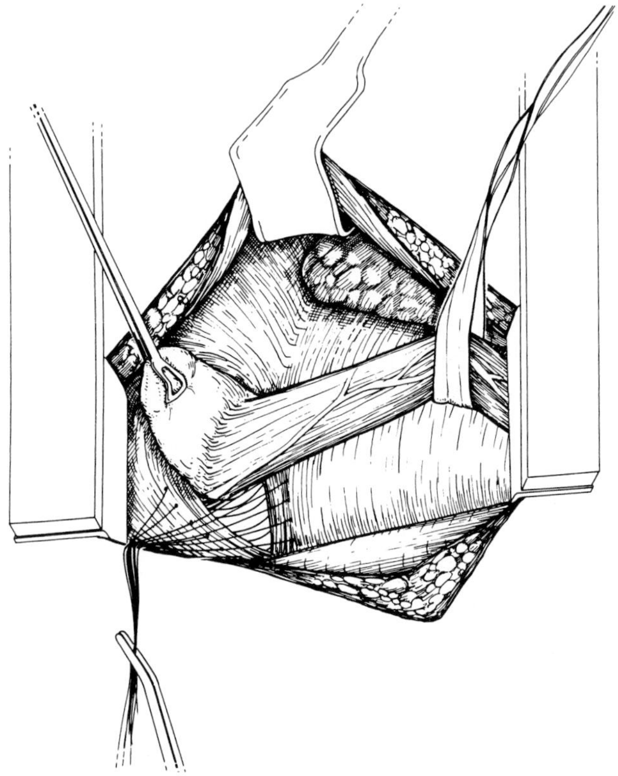

Figure 8A–34. Transthoracic antireflux procedure, showing the vascular fat pad removed and anterior retraction of the esophagus, with placement of the crural sutures for closure of this hiatus posteriorly. (From DeMeester TR. Transthoracic antireflux procedures. In: Nyhus LM, Baker RJ (eds), *Mastery of Surgery.* Boston: Little, Brown; 1984:386.)

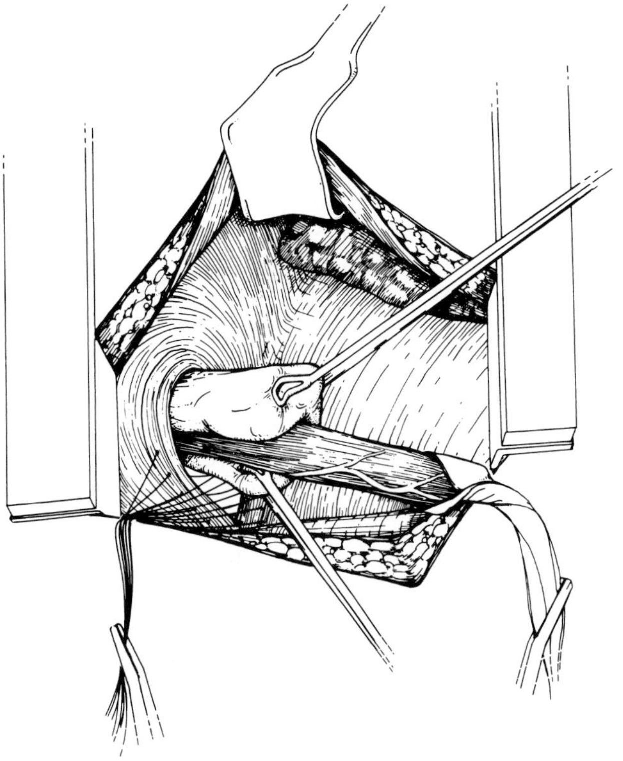

Figure 8A–35. Construction of a Nissen 360° gastric fundic wrap, showing the fundus of the stomach brought up through the hiatus anterior to the esophagus. (From DeMeester TR. Transthoracic antireflux procedures. In: Nyhus LM, Baker RJ (eds), *Mastery of Surgery*. Boston: Little, Brown; 1984:388.)

The fourth step of the operation is to construct the fundoplication. The fundus of the stomach is withdrawn through the hiatus into the chest. The wrapping of the fundus around the distal esophagus is performed in a manner similar to that described for the abdominal approach. As in the abdominal approach, the distal esophagus is invaginated into the stomach by placing the fundus lip between the posterior or right vagal nerve and the esophageal body (Fig 8A–35). A 60F bougie is passed by the anesthesiologist into the stomach to size the wrap (Fig 8A–36). The technique used to secure the wrap is similar to that described in the transabdominal approach.

When complete, the fundoplication is placed into the abdomen by compressing the fundic ball with the hand and manually maneuvering it through the hiatus. Resistance to placing the repair into the abdomen can result from the shoelace obstruction of the previously placed crural sutures. Opening the crural sutures, like loosening the laces of a shoe, relieves the obstruction and aids in placing the reconstructed cardia into the abdomen. Once in the abdomen, the fundoplication should remain there, and a gentle up-and-down motion on the diaphragm should not encourage it to emerge back through the esophageal hiatus into the chest. If the repair remains in the abdomen unaided, the previously placed crural sutures are tied.

If the fundoplication tends to ride up through the hiatus, tension on the repair is too great, usually due to inadequate mobilization of the esophagus. If there has been complete mobilization and the fundoplication still tends to ride up through the hiatus, the branches of the left vagus nerve to the left pulmonary plexus can be divided in an effort to reduce the tension. If, after this maneuver, the tendency to ride up through the hiatus persists, a Collis gastroplasty is done. If a short wrap of 1–2 cm is used and the esophagus has been adequately mobilized, the need for a Collis gastroplasty becomes a serious consideration in less than 10% of the repairs. This, however, will vary depending on how long the referring gastroenterologist persists in treating these patients.

At the completion of the procedure, a nasogastric tube should be able to be passed, without guidance from the surgeon, directly into the stomach to ensure that there has been no angulation of the distal esophagus. A chest tube for drainage of the pleural cavity is properly placed and the chest incision closed.

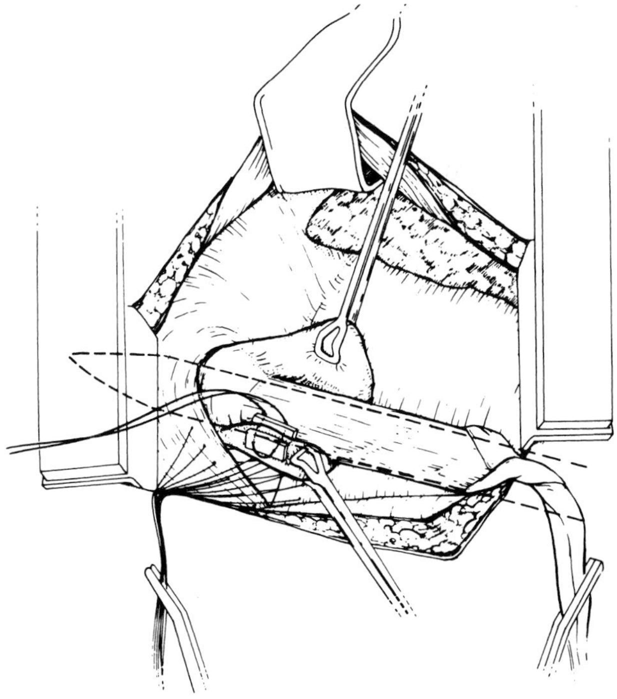

Figure 8A–36. Continued construction of a Nissen 360° gastric wrap, showing placement of the U stitch with the Teflon pledgets in the right lateral lip of the fundic wrap. The esophagus and stomach have been rotated to the right for easier placement of this suture. When the suture has been placed, a 60-F bougie is passed into the stomach to allow accurate sizing of the wrap and to allow identification of the posterior border of the gastroesophageal junction. (From DeMeester TR. Transthoracic antireflux procedures. In: Nyhus LM, Baker RJ (eds), *Mastery of Surgery*. Boston: Little, Brown; 1984:389.)

PARTIAL FUNDOPLICATION

In the presence of altered esophageal motility, where the propulsive force of the esophagus is not sufficient to overcome the outflow obstruction of a complete fundoplication, a partial fundoplication may be indicated. The most common laparoscopic partial fundoplications are a 270 degree posterior fundoplication (modified Toupet from 180 to 270 degrees) and an anterior (Dor) fundoplication. The Belsey Mark IV repair is the prototype of such a partial fundoplication and consists of a 270 degree gastric fundoplication performed through the chest. The dissection of the Belsey Mark IV and the transthoracic Nissen operations are the same, differing only in the technique of constructing the gastric fundoplication (Fig 8A–37).

Historically, partial fundoplications were used rather liberally in patients with esophageal motor disorders. Early results with partial fundoplication were equivalent to Nissen fundoplication with respect to reflux control and associated with less postoperative dysphagia. Most long term outcome studies show however that partial fundoplications are not as durable as Nissen fundoplications, and are associated with significantly higher failure rates.[106,116] Horvath et al reported the long term results of 100 consecutive patients with a modified Toupet procedure for symptomatic gastroesophageal reflux. They found a symptomatic failure rate of 20% and a 51% failure rate with objective testing at 22 months.[116] Multiple studies have shown that postoperative dysphagia is not significantly higher with a short, floppy Nissen fundoplication in patients with altered but not absent esophageal motility.[107]

The laparoscopic approach and dissection is identical to that described for laparoscopic Nissen. To perform a modified Toupet fundoplication the fundus is mobilized posterior to the esophagus as with a Nissen fundoplication. The posterior wall of the fundus on each side of the esophagus is sutured to the esophagus with interrupted 2-0 or 3-0 non absorbable suture approximately 45 degrees to either side of the mid-anterior esophageal wall. A total of 3 interrupted sutures are placed on each side, approximately 1 cm apart, resulting in a 2 cm fundoplication. Care should be taken to position the fundoplication on the esophagus and not onto the stomach. The anterior vagus nerve should be identified and should not be trapped within the suture.

In contrast, the Dor fundoplication is constructed by accentuating the angle of His and folding the fundus over the anterior surface of the esophagus. It is then

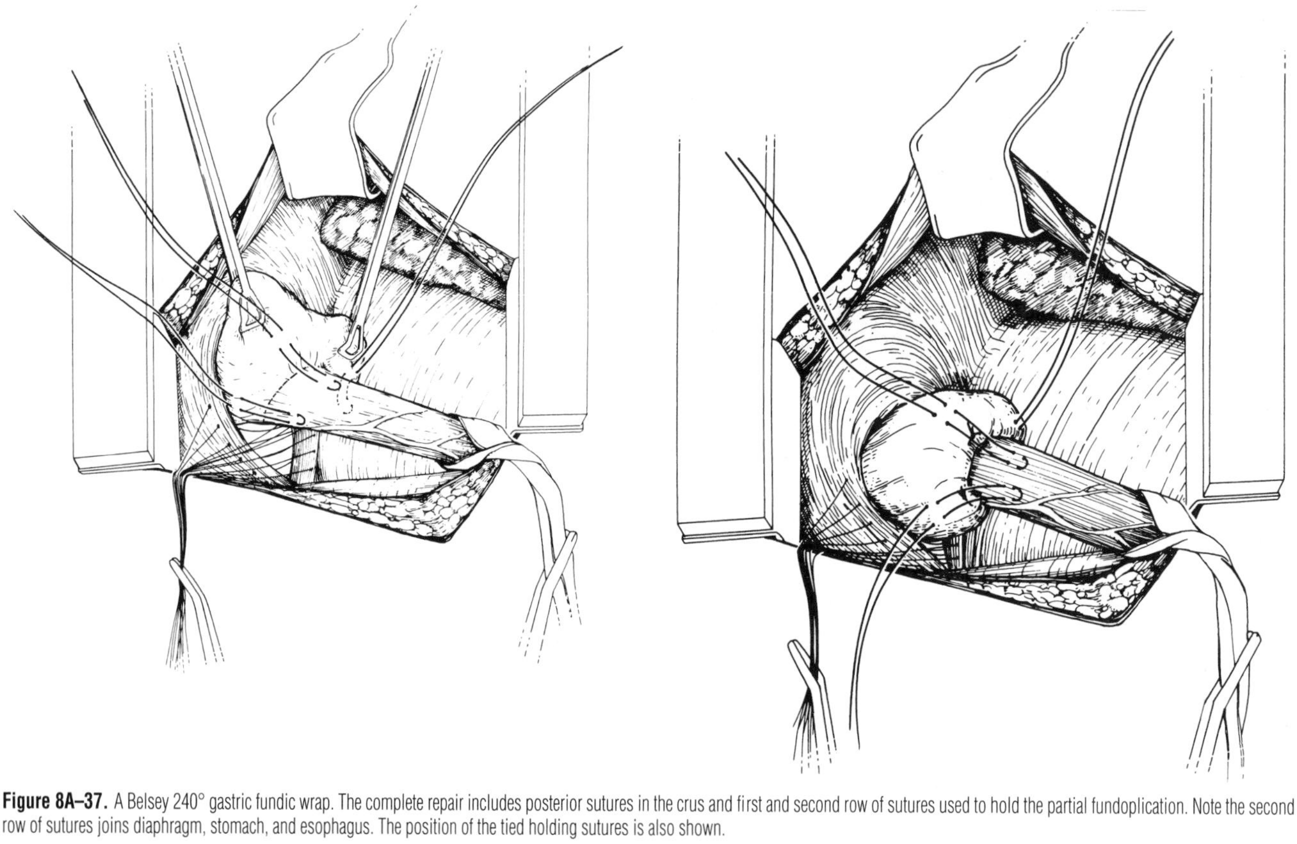

Figure 8A–37. A Belsey 240° gastric fundic wrap. The complete repair includes posterior sutures in the crus and first and second row of sutures used to hold the partial fundoplication. Note the second row of sutures joins diaphragm, stomach, and esophagus. The position of the tied holding sutures is also shown.

fixed to the left crus, left and right esophageal wall, and right crus. It is important to choose the appropriate portion of the fundus such that it will easily reach the right side of the esophagus without tension. The first suture fixes the medial wall of the fundus near the angle of His to the anterior aspect of the left crus (Fig 8A–38). This will pull the fundus closer to the esophagus. Here the fundus can be "tacked" to the left lateral aspect of the esophagus with one 2-0 or 3-0 nonabsorbable sutures. The next suture is placed between the fundus and the left anterior aspect of the hiatus. The fundus is then further folded over the anterior aspect of the hiatus by placing a suture between the fundus and the right anterior aspect of the hiatus. Several (usually 2 to 4) additional sutures are then placed at approximately 1 cm intervals, approximating the fundus of stomach to the right posterolateral wall of the esophagus and the right crus.

▪ COMPLICATIONS OF ANTI-REFLUX SURGERY

Carlson and Frantzides reported on complications and results of primary minimally invasive antireflux operations based on a literature review.[117] 41 papers were included in their analysis, comprising 10,489 procedures. Post-operative complications were found to occur in approximately 8% of patients, with a rate of conversion to an open procedure of about 4%. The most common perioperative complication was early wrap herniation (1.3%), defined as occurring within 48 hours of surgery. This is one complication that may be more common with the laparoscopic than open approach. The explanation for this is unclear but may be related to the opening of tissue planes by the pneumoperitoneum and the reduced tendency for adhesion formation after laparoscopic compared to open surgery. In an attempt to eliminate this complication, most surgeons routinely perform a crural repair.

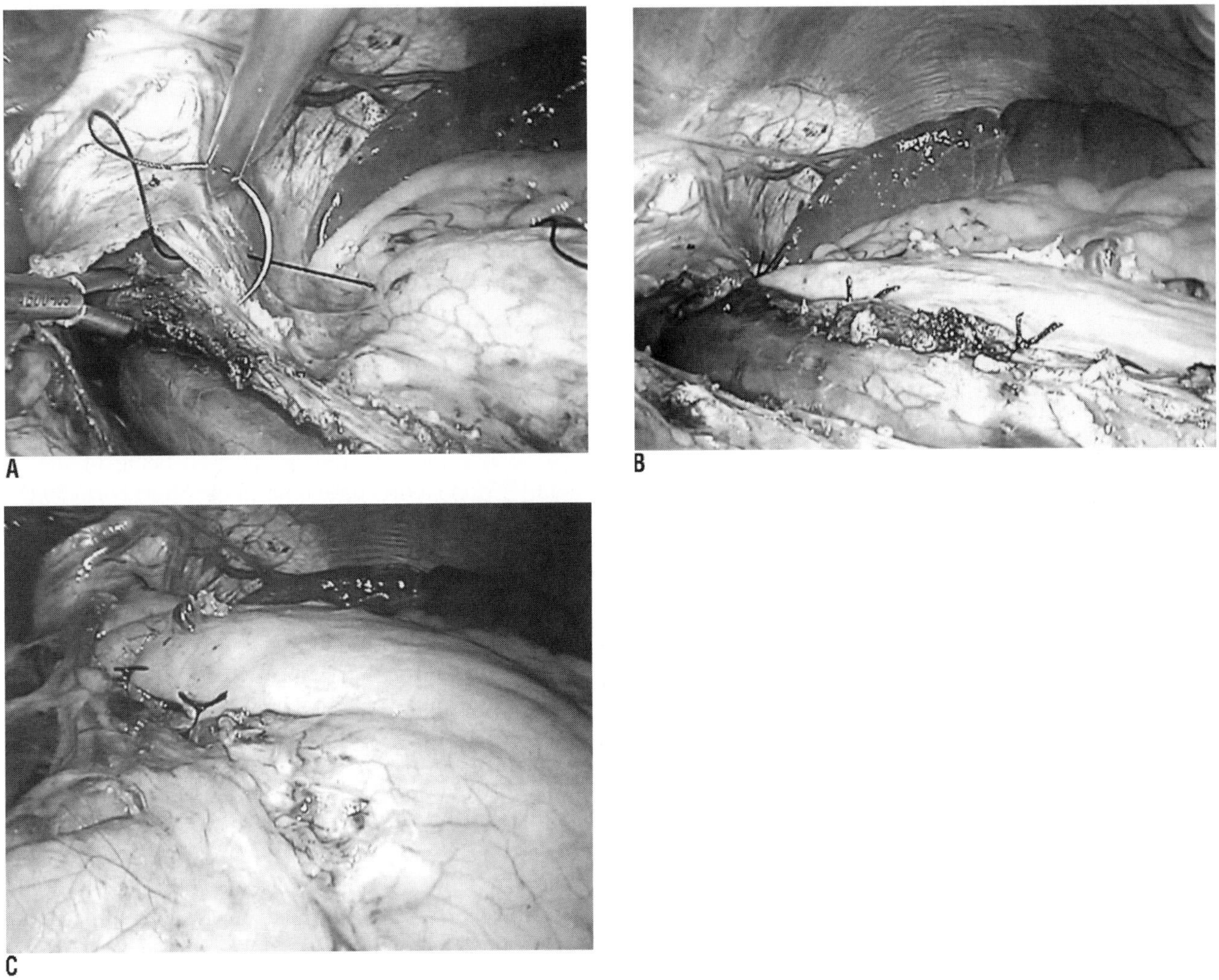

Figure 8A–38. Intraoperative photograph of Dor anterior hemifundoplication. **A.** The angle of His is accentuated and the fundus folder over the anterior esophagus. **B.** Three sutures of 2-0 silk are placed along both right and left anterior esophageal margins with the superior most suture placed through the left and right crural pillars respectively. **C.** The fundus is then folded over the anterior esophagus and the process is repeated on the right side of the esophagus.

Both pneumothorax and pneumomediastinum have been reported. The occurrence of pneumothorax is related to breach of either pleural membrane, usually the left, during the hiatal dissection. Chest drain insertion is usually not required, as accumulated carbon dioxide rapidly dissipates following release of the pneumoperitoneum by a combination of positive pressure ventilation and absorption.

As with any laparoscopic procedure, instrumental perforation of the hollow viscera may occur. Early esophageal perforation may arise during passage of the bougie, during the retroesophageal dissection or during suture pull-through. Late esophageal perforation is related to diathermy injury at the time of mobilization. Gastric perforations are usually related to excessive traction on the fundus for retraction purposes. Recognition of the problem at the time of surgery requires repair which may be performed either laparoscopically or by an open technique.

Hemorrhage during the course of laparoscopic fundoplication usually arises from the short gastric vessels or spleen. Rarer causes include retractor trauma to the liver, injury to the left inferior phrenic vein, an aberrant left hepatic vein or the inferior vena cava. Cardiac tamponade as a result of right ventricular trauma has also been reported. Major vascular injury mandates immediate conversion to an open procedure in order to achieve hemostasis. One complication that has been virtually eliminated since the advent of laparoscopic fundoplication is incidental splenic injury necessitating splenectomy (0.06%), which occurred with a frequency of around 2-5% during the open era. The mortality rate for primary minimally invasive antireflux surgery has fortunately been quite low, reported at 0.08%.

OUTCOMES FOLLOWING ANTIREFLUX SURGERY

Studies of long term outcome following both open and laparoscopic fundoplication document the ability of laparoscopic fundoplication to relieve typical reflux symptoms (heartburn, regurgitation, and dysphagia) in more than 90% of patients at follow-up intervals averaging 2–3 years and 80–90% of patients 5 years or more following surgery.[118–122] This includes evidence-based reviews of antireflux surgery,[123] prospective randomized trials comparing antireflux surgery to PPI therapy[124] and open to laparoscopic fundoplication[125] and analysis of US national trends in utilization and outcomes.[126] Laparoscopic fundoplication results in a significant increase in lower esophageal sphincter pressure and length, generally restoring these values to normal. Postoperative pH studies indicate that more than 90% of patients will normalize their pH tracings. The results of laparoscopic fundoplication compare favorably with those of the "modern" era of open fundoplication. They also indicate the less predictable outcome of atypical reflux symptoms (cough, asthma, laryngitis) after surgery, being relieved in only two-thirds of patients.[127]

The goal of surgical treatment for GERD is to relieve the symptoms of reflux by reestablishing the gastroesophageal barrier. The challenge is to accomplish this without inducing dysphagia or other untoward side effects. Dysphagia, existing prior to surgery, usually improves following laparoscopic fundoplication. Temporary dysphagia is common after surgery and generally resolves within three months. Dysphagia persisting beyond three months has been reported in up to 10% of patients. In our experience, dysphagia, manifest by occasional difficulty swallowing solids, was present in 7% of patients at 3 months, 5% at six months, 2% at 12 months, and in a single patient at twenty four months following surgery.[119] Others have observed a similar improvement in postoperative dysphagia with time. Induced dysphagia is usually mild, does not require dilatation and is temporary. It can be induced by technical misjudgments but this explanation does not hold in all instances. In experienced hands its prevalence should be less than 3% at 1 year. Other side effects common to antireflux surgery include the inability to vomit and increased flatulence. Most patients cannot vomit through an intact wrap, though this is rarely clinically relevant. Hyperflatulence is a common and noticeable problem, likely related to increased air swallowing that is present in most patients with reflux disease.

Quality of life analyses have become an important part of surgical outcome assessment, with both generic and disease-specific questionnaires in use, in an attempt to quantitate quality of life, before and after surgical intervention. In general, these measures relate the effect of disease management to the overall well being of the patient.[128] Most studies have utilized the Short Form 36 (SF-36) instrument, as it is rapidly administered and well-validated. This questionnaire measures twelve different health-related quality of life parameters encompassing mental and physical well-being. Data from Los Angeles indicate significant improvements in scores for the area of bodily pain and in a portion of the general health index.[119] Most other measures were improved but failed to achieve statistical significance. Trus et al.[129] have also analyzed SF-36 scores before and after laparoscopic antireflux surgery. In contrast to our data, scores in all fields were significantly better after surgery. In this study preoperative scores were dramatically lower than were found in our study. Thus, the difference is likely to be secondary to the relatively high scores of our patients prior to surgery (perhaps reflecting good disease control on medical therapy) and to our small sample size. Other investigators have also reported improvement in quality of life following antireflux surgery.[130,131]

REFERENCES

1. Allison PR. Peptic ulcer of the esophagus. *J Thorac Surg* 1946;15:308
2. Allison PR. Reflux esophagitis, sliding hiatus hernia and the anatomy of repair. *Surg Gynecol Obstet* 1951;92:419
3. Allison PR. Hiatus hernia: a 20 year retrospective survey. *Ann Surg* 1973;178:273
4. Boerema I. Gastropexia anterior geniculata for sliding hiatus hernia and cardiospasm. *J Int Coll Surg* 1958;29:533
5. Nissen R. Gastropexy as the lone procedure in the surgical repair of hiatus hernia. *Am J Surg* 1956;92:389
6. Hill LD, Tobias JA. An effective operation for hiatal hernia: an eight year appraisal. *Ann Surg* 1967;166:681
7. Baue AE, Belsey RHR. The treatment of sliding hiatus hernia and reflux esophagitis by the Mark IV technique. *Surgery* 1967;62:396
8. Nissen R. Eine einfache Operation zur Beeinflussung der Reflux oesophagitis. *Schweiz Med Wochenschr* 1956;86:590
9. Nissen R. Gastropexy and 'fundoplication' in surgical treatment of hiatus hernia. *Am Dig Dis* 1961;6:954
10. Negre JB. Hiatus hernia: Post-fundoplication symptoms: do they restrict the success of Nissen fundoplication? *Ann Surg* 1983;198:698
11. Pearson FG, Cooper JD, Patterson GA, et al. Gastroplasty and fundoplication for complex reflux problems. *Ann Surg* 1987;206:473–480
12. Shaker R, Castell DO, Schoenfeld PS, Spechler SJ. Nighttime heartburn is an under appreciated clinical problem that impacts sleep and daytime function; the results of a Gallup survey conducted on behalf of the American Gastroenterologic Association. *Am J Gastroenterol* 2003;98:1487–1493
13. DeMeester TR, O'Sullivan GC, Bermudez G, et al. Esophageal function in patients with angina-type chest pain and normal coronary angiograms. *Ann Surg* 1982; 196:488–498
14. Schofield PM, Bennett DH, Whorwell PJ, et al. Exertional gastroesophageal reflux; a mechanism for symptoms in patients with angina pectoris and normal coronary angiograms. *Br Med J* 1987;294:1459
15. Alban-Davies H, Jones DB, Rhodes J, Newcombe RJ. Angina like esophageal pain; Differentiation from cardiac pain by history. *J Clin Gastroenterol* 1985;7:477
16. Davies HA, Jones DB, Rhodes J. Esophageal angina as the cause of chest pain. *JAMA* 1982;248:2274–2278
17. Nevens F, Janssens J, Piessens J, et al. Prospective study on the prevalence of esophageal chest pain in patients referred on an elective basis to a cardiac unit for suspected myocardial ischemia. *Dig Dis Sci* 1991;36:229–235
18. Pope JH, Aufderheide TP, Ruthazer R, et al. Missed diagnosis of acute cardiac ischemia in the emergency department. *N Engl J Med* 2000;342:1207–1210
19. Harding R, Titchen DA. Chemosensative vagal endings in the esophagus of the cat. *J Physiol* 1975; 247:52P–53P
20. Fass R, Naliboff B, Higa L, et al. Differential effect of long term esophageal acid exposure on mechanosensativity and chemosensativity in Humans. *Gastroenterology* 1998;115:363–1373
21. Peghini PL, Johnston BT, Leite LP, Castell DO. Esophageal acid exposure sensitizes a subset of normal subjects to intraesopahgeal balloon distention. *Eur J Gastroenterol Hepatol* 1996;8:979–983
22. Castell DO, Wood JD, Freiling T, et al. Cerebral electrical potential evoked by balloon distention of the human esophagus. *Gastroenterology* 1990;98:662–666
23. Pehlivanov N, Liu J, Mittal RK. Sustained esophageal contraction; a major correlate of heartburn symptom. *Am J Physiol* 2001;281:G743–G751
24. Kern MK, Birn RM, Jaradeh S, et al. Identification and characterization of cerebral cortical response to esophageal mucosal acid exposure and distention. *Gastroenterology* 1998;115:1353–1362
25. Aziz Q, Anderson JLR, Valind S, et al. Thompson DG. Identification of human brain loci processing esophageal sensation using positron emission tomography. *Gastroenterology* 1997; 113:50–59
26. Polland WS, Bloomfield. Experimental referred pain from the gastrointestinal tract. Part I; the esophagus. *J Clin Inv* 1931;435–452
27. Pace F, Santalucia F, Porro GB. Natural history of gastrooesophageal reflux disease without esophagitis. *Gut* 1991;32: 845–848
28. Ollyo JB, Monnier P, Fontolliet C, et al. The natural history, prevalence and incidence of reflux esophagitis. *Gullet* 1993;3(suppl):3–10
29. Oberg S, Werrner J, Johansson J, et al. Barrett's esophagus; risk factors for progression to dysplasia and adenocarcinoma. *Ann Surg* 2005;242:49–54
30. Bonavina L, Evander A, DeMeester TR, et al. Length of the distal esophageal sphincter and competency of the cardia. *Am J Surg* 1986;151:25–34
31. O'Sullivan GC, DeMeester TR, Joelsson BE, et al. The interaction of the lower esophageal sphincter pressure and length of sphincter in the abdomen as determinants of gastroesophageal competence. *Am J Surg* 1982; 143:40–47
32. Zaninotto G, DeMeester TR, Schwizer W, et al. The lower esophageal sphincter in health and disease. *Am J Surg* 1988;155:104–11
33. Stein HJ, Barlow AP, DeMeester TR, Hinder RA. Complications of gastroesophageal reflux disease: role of the lower esophageal sphincter, esophageal acid and acid/alkaline exposure, and duodenogastric reflux. *Ann Surg* 1992;216:35–43
34. Kuster E, Ros E, Toledo-Pimentel V, et al. Predictive factors of the long term outcome in gastro-oesophageal reflux disease: six year follow up of 107 patients. *Gut* 1994; 35:8–14
35. Stein HJ, Eypasch EP, DeMeester TR, Smyrk TC. Circadian esophageal motor function in patients with gastroesophageal reflux disease. *Surgery*. 1990;108:769–78
36. DeMeester TR, Johnson WE. Outcome of respiratory symptoms after surgical treatment of swallowing disorders. *Sem Resp Crit Care Med* 1995;16:514–19
37. DeMeester TR, Ireland AP. Gastric Pathology as an initiator and potentiator of gastroesophageal reflux disease. *Dis Esoph* 1997;10:1–8

38. Bremner RM, Hoeft SF, Costantini M, et al. Pharyngeal swallowing: the major factor in clearance of esophageal reflux episodes. *Ann Surg* 1993;218:364–70
39. Ismail T, Bancewicz J, Barlow J. Yield pressure, anatomy of the cardia and gastroesophageal reflux. *Br J Surg* 1995;82:943–47
40. Pandolfino JE, Shi G, Trueworthy B, Kahrilas PJ. Esophagogastric junction opening pressure during relaxation distinguishes nonhernia reflux patients, hernia patients and normal subjects. *Gastroenterology* 2003; 125:1018–1024
41. Fletcher J, Wirz A, Young J, et al. Unbuffered highly acidic gastric juice exists at the gastroesophageal junction after a meal. *Gastroenterology* 2001;121:775–783
42. Fletcher J, Wirz A, Henry E, McColl KEL. Studies of acid exposure immediately above the gastroesopahgeal squamocolumnar junction; evidence of short segment reflux. *Gut* 2004;53:168–173
43. Iljima KX, Henry E, Moriya AZ, et al. Dietary nitrate generaties potentially mutagenic concentrations of nitric oxide at the gastroesophageal junction. *Gastroenterology* 2002; 122:1248–1257
44. Joelsson BE, DeMeester TR, Skinner DB, et al. The role of the esophageal body in the antireflux mechanism. *Surgery* 1982;92:417–424
45. DeMeester TR, Lafontaine E, Joelsson BE, et al. The relationship of a hiatal hernia to the function of the body of the esophagus and the gastroesophageal junction. *J Thorac Cardiovasc Surg* 1981;82:547–558
46. Helm JF, Riedel DR, Dodds WJ, et al. Determinants of esophageal acid clearance in normal subjects. *Gastroenterology* 1983;85:607–612
47. Kahrilas PJ, Dodds WJ, Hogan WJ. Effect of peristaltic dysfunction on esophageal volume clearance. *Gastroenterology* 1988;94:73–80
48. Helm JF, Dodds WJ, Pelc LR, et al. Effect of esophageal emptying and saliva on clearance of acid from the esophagus. *N Engl J Med* 1984;310:284–288
49. Helm JF, Dodds WJ, Hogan WJ. Salivary responses to esophageal acid in normal subjects and patients with reflux esophagitis. *Gastroenterology* 1982;93:1393–1397
50. Mittal RK, Lange RC, McCallum RW. Identification and mechanism of delayed esophageal acid clearance in subjects with hiatus hernia. *Gastroenterology* 1987;92:132
51. Sloan S, Kahrilas PJ. Impairment of esophageal emptying with hiatal hernia. *Gastroenterology* 1991;100:596–605
52. Lillimoe KD, Johnson LF, Harmon JW. Role of the components of the gastroduodenal contents in experimental acid esophagitis. *Surgery* 1982;92:276–284
53. Lillimoe KD, Johnson LF, Harmon JW. Alkaline esophagitis: A comparison of the ability of components of gastroduodenal contents to injure the rabbit esophagus. *Gastroenterology* 1983;85:621–628
54. Kauer WKH, Peters JH, DeMeester TR, et al. Mixed reflux of gastric juice is more harmful to the esophagus than gastric juice alone. The need for surgical therapy reemphasized. *Ann Surg* 1995;222:525–533
55. Oh D, Hagen JA, Fein MF, et al. The impact of reflux composition on mucosal injury and esophageal function. *J Gastrointest Surg* 2006;10:787–797
56. Stein HJ, Feussner H, Kauer W, et al. Alkaline gastroesophageal reflux: assessment by ambulatory esophageal aspiration and pH monitoring. *Am J Surg* 1994; 167:163–168
57. Kauer WKH, Burdiles P, Ireland A, et al. Does duodenal juice reflux into the esophagus in patients with complicated GERD? Evaluation of a fiberoptic sensor for bilirubin. *Am J Surg* 1995;169:98
58. El-Serag HB, Sonnenberg A. Comorbid occurrence of laryngeal or pulmonary disease with esophagitis in United States Military Veterans. *Gastroenterology* 1997;113:755–760
59. Sontag SJ, O'Connell S, Khandewal S, et al. Most asthmatics have gastroesophageal reflux with or without bronchodilator therapy. *Gastroenterology* 1990;99:613–20
60. Gastal OL, Castell JA, Castell DO. Frequency and site of gastroesophageal reflux in patients with chest symptoms. *Chest* 1994;106:1793–1796
61. Tuchman DN, Boyle JT, Pack AI, et al. Comparison of airway responses following tracheal or esophageal acidification in the cat. *Gastroenterology* 1984;87:872–881
62. Mansfield LE, Hameister HH, Spaulding HS, et al. The role of the vagus nerve in airway narrowing caused by intraesophageal hydrochloric acid provocation and esophageal distention. *Ann Allergy* 1981;47:431–434
63. Levin TR, Sperling RM, McQuaid KR. Omeprazole improves peak expiratory flow rate and quality of life in asthmatics with gastroesophageal reflux. *Am J Gastroenterol* 1998;93:1060–1063
64. Boeree MJ, Peters FTM, Postma DS, Kleibeuker JH. No effects of high-dose omeprazole in patients with severe airway hyperresponsiveness and symptomatic gastrooesophageal reflux. *Eur Respir J* 1998;11:1070–1074
65. Harding SM, Richter JE, Guzzo MR, et al. Asthma and gastroesophageal reflux: acid suppressive therapy improves asthma outcome. *Am J Med* 1996;100:395–405
66. Sontag SJ, O'Connell S, Khandelwal S, et al. Asthmatics with gastroesophageal reflux; Long term results of a randomized trial of medical and surgical antireflux therapies. *Am J Gastroenterol* 2003;98:987–999
67. Perrin-Fayolle M, Gormand F, Braillon G, et al. Long-term results of surgical treatment for gastroesophageal reflux in asthmatic patients. *Chest* 1989;96:40–45
68. Spechler SJ. The Columnar lined esophagus: history, terminology and clinical issues. *Gastroenterol Clin N Am* 1997; 26:455–466
69. Peters JH, Hagen JA, DeMeester SR. Barrett's Esophagus. *J Gastrointest Surg* 2004;8:1–17
70. Chandrasoma P. Norman Barrett: So close, yet 50 years away from the truth. *J Gastrointest Surg* 1999;3:7–14
71. Campos GMR, DeMeester SR, Peters JH, et al. Predictive factors of Barrett's esophagus; Multivariate analyses of 502 patients with GERD. *Arch Surg* 2001;136:1267–1273
72. Oberg S, Peters JH, DeMeester TR, et al. Inflammation and specialized intestinal metaplasia of cardiac mucosa is a manifestation of gastroesopahgeal reflux disease. *Ann Surg* 1997;226:522–532
73. Katzka DA, Castell DO. Successful elimination of reflux symptoms does not insure adequate control of acid re-

flux in patients with Barrett's esophagus. *Am J Gastroenterol* 1994;89:989–991

74. Ouatu-Lascar R, Triadafilopolous G. Complete elimination of reflux symptoms does not guarantee normalization of intraesophageal acid reflux in patients with Barrett's esophagus. *Am J Gastroenterol* 1998;93:711–716
75. Sampliner RE, Fennerty B, Garewal HS. Reversal of Barrett's esophagus with acid suppression and multipolar electrocoagulation: preliminary results. *Gastrointest Endos* 1996;44:532–535
76. Hofstetter WA, Peters JH, DeMeester TR, et al. Long term outcome of antireflux surgery in patients with Barrett's esophagus. *Ann Surg* 2001;234:532–539
77. Farrell TM, Smith CD, Metreveli RE, et al. Fundoplication provides effective and durable symptom relief in patients with Barrett's esophagus. *Am J Surg* 1999;178: 18–21
78. Oelschlager BK, Barreca M, Chang L, et al. Clinical and pathologic response of Barrett's esophagus to laparoscopic antireflux surgery. *Ann Surg* 2003;238:458–466
79. Overholt BF, Panjehpour M, Halberg DL. Photodynamic therapy for Barrett's esophagus with dysplasia and/or early stage carcinoma; long term results. *Gastrointest Endosc* 2003;58:183–188
80. Pacifico RJ, Wang KK, Wongkeesong LM, et al. Combined endoscopic mucosal resection and photodynamic therapy versus esophagectomy for management of early adenocarcinoma in Barrett's esophagus. *Clin Gastroenterol Hepatol* 2003;1:252–257
81. Peters JH, Clark GWB, Ireland AP, et al. Outcome of adenocarcinoma arising in Barrett's esophagus in endoscopically surveyed and non–surveyed patients. *J Thorac Cardiovasc Surg* 1994;108:813–822
82. Altorki NK, Sunagawa M, Little AG, Skinner DB. High-grade dysplasia in the columnar-lined esophagus. *Am J Surg* 1991;161:99–100
83. Pera M, Trastek VF, Carpenter HA, et al. Barrett's esophagus with high grade dysplasia; an indication for esophagectomy. *Ann Thorac Surg* 1992;54:199–204
84. Ferguson MK, Naunheim KS. Resection for Barrett's mucosa with high-grade dysplasia: implications for prophylactic photodynamic therapy. *J Thorac Cardiovasc Surgery* 1997;114:824–9.
85. Jessurun J, Yardley JH, Giardiello FM, et al. Intracytoplasmic plasma proteins and distended esophageal squamous cells (balloon cells). *Mod Patho* 1988;1(3):175–181
86. Ismail Beigi F, Pope CE. Distribution of histological changes of gastroesophageal reflux in the distal esophagus in man. *Gastroenterology* 1975;66:1109–1113
87. Johnson LF, DeMeester TR, Haggitt RC. Esophageal epithelial response to gastroesophageal reflux: a quantitative study. *Am J Dig Dis* 1978;23:498–509
88. Attwood SEA, Smyrk TC, Barlow AP, et al. The sensitivity and specificity of histologic parameters in the diagnosis of gastroesophageal reflux disease. In: Little AG, Ferguson MK, Skinner DB (eds), *Diseases of the Esophagus, vol II, Benign Diseases.* Mount Kisco, NY: Futura; 1990:73–83
89. Nayar DS, Vaezi MF. Classifications of esophagitis; who needs them. *Gastrointest Endoscopy* 2004;60:253–257
90. Dhiman RK, Saraswat VA, Naik SR. Ambulatory esophageal pH monitoring; technique, interpretations and cilincal indications. *Dig Dis Sciences* 2002;47:241–250
91. Jamieson JR, Stein HJ, DeMeester TR, et al. Ambulatory 24-hour esophageal pH monitoring: normal values, optimal thresholds, specificity, sensitivity, and reproducibility. *Am J Gastroenterol* 1992;87(9):1102–1111
92. Johnson LF, DeMeester TR. Development of 24-hour intraesophageal pH monitoring composite scoring. *J Clin Gastroenterol* 1986;8:52–58
93. Fuchs KH, DeMeester TR, Albertucci M. Specificity and sensitivity of objective diagnosis of gastroesophageal reflux disease. *Surgery* 1987;102:575–580
94. Pandolfino JE, Richter JE, Ours T, et al. Ambulatory esophageal pH monitoring using a wireless system. *Am J Gastroenterol* 2003;98:740–749
95. Tseng D, Rizvi AZ, Fennerty B, et al. Forty-eight hour pH monitoring increases sensitivity in detecting abnormal esophageal acid exposure. *J Gastrointest Surg* 2005;9: 1043–1052
96. Technology Assessment Committee. ASGE technology status evaluation report; wireless esophageal pH monitoring system. 2005;62:485–487
97. Shay SS, Tutuian R, Sifrim D, et al. Twenty-four hour ambulatory simultaneous impedance and pH monitoring; a multicenter report of normal values from 60 healthy volunteers. *Am J Gastroenterol* 2004;99:1037–1043
98. Bredenoord AJ, Weusten BLAM, Timmer R, Smout AJPM. Reproducibility of multichannel imtraluminal electrical impedance monitoring of gastroesopahgeal reflux. *Am J Gastroenterol* 2005;100:265–269
99. Tatuian R, Vela MF, Shay SS, Castell DO. Multichannel intraluminal impedance in esophageal function testing and gastroesophageal reflux monitoring. *J Clin Gastroenterol* 2003;37:206–215
100. Balaji NS, Blom D, DeMeester TR, Peters JH. Redefining gastroesophageal reflux; detection using multichannel intraluminal impedance. *Surgical Endosc* 2003;17:1380–1385
101. American Gastroenterological Association medical position statement; clinical use of esophageal manometry. *Gastroenterology* 2005;128:207–208
102. Pandolfino JE, Ghosh SK, Zhang Q, et al. Quantifying EGJ morphology and relaxation with high resolution manometry; a study of 75 asymptomatic volunteers. *Am J Physiol Gastrointest Liver Physiol* 2006;290:G1033–G1040
103. Campos GM, Peters JH, DeMeester TR, et al. The pattern of esophageal acid exposure in GERD influences the severity of the disease. *Arch Surg* 1999;134:882–888
104. Ritter MP, Peters JH, DeMeester TR, et al. Outcome after laparoscopic fundoplication is not dependent upon a structurally defective lower esophageal sphincter. *J Gastrointest Surg* 1998;2:567–572
105. Campos GMR, Peters JH, DeMeester TR, et al. Multivariate analysis of the factors predicting outcome after Laparoscopic Nissen fundoplication. *J Gastrointest Surg* 1999;3:292–300
106. Bell RC, Hanna P, Mills MR, Bowrey D. Patterns of success and failure with laparoscopic partial fundoplication. *Surg Endosc* 1999;13:1189–1194

107. Patti MG, Robinson T, Galvani C, et al. Total fundoplication is superior to partial fundoplication even when esophageal peristalsis is weak. *J Am Coll Surg* 2004;198: 863–870
108. Horvath KD, Swanstrom LL, Jobe BA. The short esophagus: pathophysiology, incidence, presentation, and treatment in the era of laparoscopic antireflux surgery. *Ann Surg* 2000;232:630–40
109. Terry ML, Vernon A, Hunter JG. Stapled-wedge Collis gastroplasty for the shortened esophagus. *Am J Surg* 2004;188: 195–199
110. Schwizer W, Hinder RA, DeMeester TR. Does delayed gastric emptying contribute to gastroesophageal reflux disease? *Am J Surg* 1989;157:74
111. Lind JF, Duthie HL, Schlegal JR, et al. Motility of the gastric fundus. *Am J Physiol* 1961;201:197
112. Richardson JD, Larson GM, Polk HC. Intrathoracic fundoplication for shortened esophagus: treacherous solution to a challenging problem. *Am J Surg* 1982;143:29
113. DeMeester TR, Bonavina L, Albertucci M. Nissen fundoplication for gastroesophageal reflux disease—evaluation of primary repair in 100 consecutive patients. *Ann Surg* 1986; 204:9
114. Weerts JM, Dallemagne B, Hamoir E, et al. Laparoscopic Nissen fundoplication; detailed analysis of 132 patients. *Surg Laparosc Endosc* 1993;3:359–364
115. Hinder RA, Fillipi CJ. The technique of laparoscopic Nissen fundoplication. *Surg Laparosc Endosc* 1993;3:265–272
116. Horvath KD, Jobe BA, Herron DM, Swanstrom LL. Laparoscopic Toupet is an inadequate procedure for patients with severe reflux disease. *J Gastrointest Surg* 1999; 3:583–591.
117. Carlson MA, Frantzides CT. Complications and results of primary minimally invasive antireflux procedures.a review of 10,735 reported cases. *J Am Coll Surg* 2001;193:429–439
118. Hinder RA, Filipi CJ, Wetscher G, et al. Laparoscopic Nissen fundoplication is an effective treatment for gastroesophageal reflux disease. *Ann Surg* 1994;220:472–81
119. Peters JH, DeMeester TR, Crookes P, et al. The treatment of gastroesophageal reflux disease with laparoscopic Nissen fundoplication. Prospective evaluation of 100 patients with "typical" symptoms. *Ann Surg* 1998; 228:40–50
120. DeMeester TR, Bonavina L, Albertucci M. Nissen fundoplication for gastroesophageal reflux disease—evaluation of primary repair in 100 consecutive patients. *Ann Surg* 1986;204:9–20
121. Hinder RA, Klaus A, Klinger PJ. Five-to eight year outcome of the first lapaoscopic Nissen fundoplications. *J Gastrointest Surg* 2001;5:42–48
122. Granderath FA, Kamolz T, Schweiger et al. Long-term results of laparoscopic antireflux surgery; surgical outcomes and alaysis of failure after 500 laparoscopic antireflux procedures. *Surg Endosc* 2002;16:753–757
123. Catarci M, Gentileschi P, Papi C, et al. Evidence-based appraisal of antireflux fundopplicaion. *Ann Surg* 2004; 239:325–337
124. Lundell L, Miettinen P, Myrvold HE, et al. Continued (5-year) follow-up of a randomized clinical study comparing antireflux surgery and omeprozole in gastroesopahgeal reflux diesease. *J Am Coll Surg* 2001;192:172–181
125. Nilsson G, Wenner J, Larsson S, Johnson F. Randomized clinical trial of laparoscopic versus open fundoplication for gastroesophageal reflux. *Br J Surg* 2004;91:552–559
126. Finlayson SRG, Laycock WS, Birkmeyer JD. National trends in utilization and outcomes of antireflux surgery. *Surg Endosc* 2003;17:864–867
127. So JB, Zeitels SM, Rattner DW. Outcomes of atypical symptoms attributed to gastroesophageal reflux treated by laparoscopic fundoplication. *Surgery* 1998;124:28–32
128. Testa MA, Simonson DC. Assessment of quality-of-life outcomes. *N Engl J Med* 1996;334:835–840
129. Trus TL, Laycock WS, Waring JP, et al. Improvement in quality of life measures following laparoscopic antireflux surgery. *Ann Surg* 1999;229:331–336
130. Glise H, Hallerbäck B, Johansson B. Quality-of-life assessments in evaluation of laparoscopic Rosetti fundoplication. *Surg Endosc* 1995;9:183–189
131. Velonovich V, Vallance SR, Gusz JR, et al. Quality of life scale for gastroesophageal reflux disease. *J Am Coll Surg* 1996;183:217–224

9

Cancer of the Esophagus

Simon Law ▪ *John Wong*

▪ HISTORICAL PERSPECTIVES

One of the earliest descriptions of esophageal cancer was in the second century AD, when Galen described a fleshy obstructing growth in the esophagus, which was responsible for the inability to swallow and led to emaciation and death. In early Chinese literature, a patient who had esophageal cancer was described as "one suffers in autumn, and does not live to see the coming summer." Unfortunately this description of the natural course of the disease is still true for many in modern times. In 1877, Czerny was the first to successfully resect a cervical esophageal cancer and the patient lived for 15 months. Torek in 1913 performed the first successful transthoracic resection.[1] A 67-year old woman had a squamous cell cancer of the mid-esophagus. Through a left thoracotomy, the esophagus was resected. The proximal cervical esophagus was brought out through an incision anterior to the sternocleidomastoid muscle and tunneled subcutaneously along the anterior chest wall, where a cutaneous esophagostomy was fashioned. The patient was fed via a rubber tube connecting the esophagostomy with a gastrostomy. The patient lived for 17 years.

The first successful resection of a thoracic esophageal cancer with reconstruction using the stomach was performed by Ohsawa, a Japanese surgeon in Kyoto, who reported the technique in 18 patients in 1933.[2] In 1946, Ivor Lewis described esophageal resection using a two-phase approach via a right thoracotomy and laparotomy.[3] Tanner independently also described the procedure in 1947.[4]

Although surgical resection has remained the mainstay treatment for esophageal cancer, recent years have seen a proliferation of treatment options, especially with regard to different combinations of chemotherapeutic agents, radiotherapy, and surgery. There has also been a divergence in the epidemiological pattern between Western and Eastern countries, which has made an impact on the management of this disease.

▪ EPIDEMIOLOGY

There is marked geographic variation in the incidence of squamous cell cancer of the esophagus, and to some extent, among different ethic groups within a common area. The disease is especially common in countries of the Asian esophageal cancer belt, which stretches from eastern Turkey and east of the Caspian Sea through northern Iran, northern Afghanistan, and southern areas of the former Soviet Union, such as Turkmenistan, Uzbekistan, and Tajikistan, to northern China and India. High incidences are also found in the Transkei province of South Africa and Kenya. In high-incidence areas, the occurrence of esophageal cancer is 50- to 100-fold higher than in the rest of the world. It is the fourth most common cancer in China.[5] In the southern area of Hebei province, the incidence is as high as 199 cases per 100,000 population. By contrast, esophageal cancer is relatively uncommon in the United States, Canada, and most areas of Europe. The age-adjusted incidence rate in the United States approximates 5 per

100,000 population and there were 13,200 new cases in 2001.[6] In Europe, esophageal cancer represents 5.9% of intestinal malignancies.[7] In some countries such as France, Ireland, Iceland, and the United Kingdom, it represents a higher proportion of gastrointestinal cancers; approximately 10% of gastrointestinal cancers are esophageal in origin. Esophageal cancer most commonly presents in the sixth and seventh decades of life, and the male:female ratio ranges from 1.5:1 to 8:1.

The most striking change in the epidemiological pattern for esophageal cancer in the past two decades has been the shift from squamous cell cancers to adenocarcinomas of the lower esophagus and cardia in the Caucasian populations in Western countries. In the United States, squamous cell cancers predominate in African Americans, but the incidence of this cancer has seen a decline since the mid 1980s, while adenocarcinoma has been rapidly rising in incidence in the white population.[6] The incidence of adenocarcinoma has surpassed squamous cell cancers since 1990.[8] Similar changes have been observed in Europe and Australia among the white population. In Asia, however, esophageal cancers remain predominantly squamous cell in type, and are mostly located in the middle third of the esophagus. There has not been a noticeable rise in the incidence of adenocarcinoma of the esophagus and gastric cardia in published Asian data.[9]

Apart from squamous cell cancers and adenocarcinomas, other tumor types less commonly encountered include mucoepidermoid cancer, adenosquamous cancer,[10] small cell cancer,[11] basaloid squamous tumor,[12] sarcomatoid carcinoma, lymphoma, melanoma,[13] and various subtypes of stromal tumors.[14]

▪ ETIOLOGICAL FACTORS

Various factors associated with the development of esophageal cancer are shown in Table 9–1. Smoking and drinking are independent contributing factors as shown by prospective studies of patients who drink but do not smoke, and conversely of patients who smoke but do not drink.[15]

For squamous cell cancers, in addition to drinking and smoking, dietary and environmental factors are important, especially in Asian countries. Nitrosamines and their precursors (nitrate, nitrite, and secondary amines), such as pickled vegetables, are incriminated.[16] Nutritional depletion of certain micronutrients, particularly vitamins A, C, E, niacin, riboflavin, selenium, molybdenum, manganese, zinc, and magnesium, as well as fresh fruits and vegetables, together with an inadequate protein intake, predisposes the esophageal epithelium to neoplastic transformation. Other dietary risk factors include consumption of hot beverages, opium smoking, chewing betel nuts, and maté drinking in South American countries.

TABLE 9–1. FACTORS ASSOCIATED WITH PATHOGENESIS OF ESOPHAGEAL CANCER

Factor	Squamous Cell Cancer	Adenocarcinoma
Smoking	+++	+
Alcohol consumption	+++	–
Hot beverages	+	–
N-nitroso compounds (e.g., pickled vegetables)	+	–
Betel nut chewing	+	–
Maté drinking	+	–
Deficiencies of green vegetables and vitamins	+	–
Low socioeconomic class	+	–
Fungal toxin or virus	+	–
History of radiation to the mediastinum	+	+
Lye corrosive stricture	+	–
History of aerodigestive malignancy	+++	–
Plummer-Vinson syndrome	+	–
Obesity	–	++
Achalasia	+	–
Gastroesophageal reflux	–	+++
Barrett's esophagus	–	++++

The human papillomaviruses[17] and certain fungi belonging to the genera *Fusarium*, *Alternaria*, *Geotrichum*, *Aspergillus*, *Cladosporium*, and *Penicillium*, are infective agents variably found to be associated with esophageal cancer.

Patients with other aerodigestive malignancies have a particularly high risk of developing squamous cell carcinoma of the esophagus, presumably because of exposure to similar environmental carcinogens and "field cancerization." Using esophageal cancer as the index tumor, multiple primary cancers were found in 9.5% of patients, and 70% were in the aerodigestive tract.[18] The overall incidence of synchronous or metachronous esophageal cancer in patients with primary head and neck cancer is estimated to be 3%.[19]

Diseases that are known to predispose to squamous cell esophageal cancer are few. The risk from achalasia is estimated to be seven- to 33-fold, but symptoms of achalasia are present for an average of 15–20 years before the emergence of cancer.[20] Other diseases include lye corrosive strictures, Plummer-Vinson syndrome, tylosis, and celiac disease.

The reasons accounting for the dramatic rise in incidence of adenocarcinoma in the white population is widely attributed to gastroesophageal reflux disease, obesity, and Barrett's esophagus,[21–23] which are uncommon in Asian populations.[24] Gastroesophageal reflux disease affects up to 44% of the general population in the U.S., and approximately 5–8% will develop Barrett's esophagus,[25] with an estimated annual rate of neoplastic transformation of 0.5%.[26] Epidemiological data suggest a protective role of *Helicobacter pylori* against reflux. The high prevalence of *Helicobacter pylori* infection in Eastern populations may guard against reflux and Barrett's esophagus, and may account for the differences in cancer cell type.[27] However, this association remains controversial.

▪ DIAGNOSIS

EARLY CANCER

Diagnosis of symptomatic esophageal cancer is usually straightforward since most cases are advanced at presentation. Diagnosing the disease at the asymptomatic or early stage is crucial in improving prognosis, although at present this is only possible in the minority of patients. In high-incidence areas such as China, abrasive cytology is used for population screening. Two principal types of samplers have been used: an inflatable balloon developed in China,[28], and an encapsulated sponge sampler developed in Japan.[29] When early-stage cancers are diagnosed by this method, excellent long-term results with 5-year survival rates approaching 90% and 25-year survival rates of 50% can be achieved, comparable to those of the normal population.[30]

Primary endoscopic screening has also been reported in alcoholics and smokers in Japan and France, with prevalence of esophageal cancer reported at 3.3–8.2% of individuals screened.[31] Widespread use of this method is limited by the cost and expertise required. In very-high-incidence areas such as China, endoscopy is being investigated as a screening tool, integrated with early treatment and chemoprevention programs.[32]

Advances in endoscopic methods, such as chromoendoscopy using Lugol's iodine, indigo carmine, methylene blue, and toluidine blue,[33] magnifying endoscopy with instruments that provide magnification of 35–115 times, light-induced fluorescence endoscopy, light-scattering spectroscopy, optical coherence tomography, and confocal laser scanning microscopy are promising techniques to aid early diagnosis.[33,34]

For cancer due to Barrett's esophagus, screening and surveillance for early cancers has been controversial. The American Gastroenterological Association recommends screening endoscopy for patients with chronic reflux symptoms, especially those over 50 years of age, who are most likely to suffer from Barrett's esophagus. Those identified to have Barrett's esophagus should enter surveillance programs carried out using a systematic four-quadrant, 2-cm–interval biopsy protocol with large biopsy forceps.[35] Dysplasia is so far the only reliable indicator of the risk of development of invasive cancer. Endoscopy is performed every 3 years for those with no dysplasia, and yearly for low-grade dysplasia. Diagnosis of high-grade dysplasia implies the need for either therapy (by surgery or endoscopic means), or more intensive surveillance. If the latter is preferred, a four-quadrant, 1-cm–interval protocol is required for diagnosis of early invasive cancer,[36] and endoscopy and biopsy every 3 months is recommended.[35]

The real benefits of these strategies remain unproved. Gastroesophageal reflux is prevalent; approximately 20% of adults have heartburn at least once per week, 5% of whom have Barrett's esophagus, thus a very substantial number of people will require screening. However, the absolute risk of adenocarcinoma is low, even in subgroups of patients with severe reflux symptoms. Moreover, 40% or more of patients with esophageal adenocarcinoma have no prior reflux symptoms and therefore would not be detected through screening programs targeted to those with such symptoms.[22] Most patients with Barrett's esophagus also die from unrelated causes,[37] and the presence of Barrett's esophagus does not change life expectancy or overall survival.[38,39] These arguments together with the high cost of endoscopy militate against general population screening. Although retrospective studies have demonstrated survival benefits in patients with Barrett's esophagus undergoing surveillance,[40] these studies may have been biased because of selection, lead-time, and length bias.[41] There is currently no confirmed evidence proving that screening or surveillance will lead to improved survival in patients with Barrett's esophagus.[34] Computer models based on various assumptions and cost analyses, however, have supported screening and surveillance, albeit at considerable financial outlay.[42]

ADVANCED CANCER

For symptomatic patients, the spectrum of symptoms varies depending on the extent of disease. The duration of symptoms does not necessarily correlate with tumor stage, curability, or resectability. It is important that in localities where the disease is not rare, the threshold for endoscopic examination should be low. Patients with chronic reflux symptoms who develop dysphagia must have the diagnosis of tumor entertained in addition to a reflux stricture. In advanced cases the most common presenting symptom is dysphagia (80–95%), which is progressive in severity. However, many patients delay seeking medical attention until severe dysphagia and weight loss have occurred. Regurgitation is common. In high-grade obstruction, this symptom may be worse at night when the patient lies supine. Fluid regurgitation can lead to bouts of coughing, aspiration, and even chest infection. Odynophagia (retrosternal pain associated with swallowing) is not uncommon. Hoarseness is the result of recurrent laryngeal nerve compression and more commonly affects the left side because of its longer intrathoracic course, and most squamous cell tumors are located in the middle third of the esophagus. Right recurrent laryngeal nerve palsy indicates a proximal tumor, or lymph node metastasis to the apex of the right chest or the neck.

The demographics of patients who suffer from squamous cell cancers and adenocarcinomas are different.[43] Patients with adenocarcinomas tend to be of higher socioeconomic class, and have obesity-related chronic disease such as ischemic heart disease (Table 9–2). Examination of these patients therefore rarely reveals a wasted individual. Patients with squamous cell cancers are blue-collar workers, and general examination may show evidence of weight loss and muscle wasting. Chronic smoking and alcohol intake leads to a higher prevalence of chronic lung disease and liver cirrhosis. The more proximal tumor location more easily predisposes to pneumonia from aspiration or the development of a tracheoesophageal fistula. Lymph nodes in the supraclavicular regions should be sought in all patients.

TABLE 9–2. COMPARISON OF PATIENTS WITH SQUAMOUS CELL CANCERS AND ADENOCARCINOMAS OF THE ESOPHAGUS ASIDE FROM ETIOLOGY: ASIA VERSUS THE WEST

	Asia	West
Cell type	Squamous cell cancer	Adenocarcinoma
Location	Middle and lower esophagus	Lower esophagus and cardia
Comorbid diseases	Pulmonary disease, cirrhosis	Ischemic heart disease
Identifiable premalignant lesions	? Dysplasia	Barrett's esophagus and dysplasia
Screening and surveillance	Balloon cytology, endoscopy (in endemic areas such as China)	Endoscopic surveillance for Barrett's esophagus
Surgical approaches	Predominantly transthoracic, two- and three-field lymphadenectomy	Transthoracic and transhiatal, two-field or minimal lymphadenectomy
Prognosis	Worse?	Better?

■ TUMOR STAGING

Accurate staging serves to provide information for stage-directed therapies and is important for quality control for clinical trials.

The clinical staging system follows the American Joint Committee on Cancer (AJCC) TNM staging system[44] (Table 9–3). The AJCC lymph node station classification is different from that of the Japanese Society for Esophageal Diseases[45] (Fig 9–1). There is no agreed upon preference, but the AJCC system is less complicated. The definitions of the various levels of the esophagus are shown in Figure 9–2A. For adenocarcinomas of the lower esophagus and cardia, Siewert's classification is also used, and the three types have different etiologic and therapeutic implications (Fig 9–2B).[46] Apart from physical examination and simple chest radiography, specific methods used for clinical staging include barium contrast studies, bronchoscopy, CT scanning, percutaneous ultrasound of the cervical lymph nodes with or without fine-needle aspiration (FNA) cytology, endoscopic ultrasound (EUS) with or without FNA, 2-[^{18}F] fluoro-2-deoxy-D-glucose (FDG) positron emission tomography (PET) scanning, and laparoscopy and/or thoracoscopy.

BARIUM CONTRAST STUDY

Typical features on a contrast barium study include mucosal irregularity and shouldering, narrowing of the lumen, and proximal dilatation of the esophagus (Fig 9–3). It gives a longitudinal graphical view of the tumor in relation to other mediastinal structures, especially the trachea and main bronchi. It is a useful guide to the endoscopist, and in addition, it can detect tracheoesophageal fistula. Tortuosity, angulation, axis deviation from the midline, sinus formation, and fistula formation to the bronchial tree are signs indicative of an advanced tumor that has traversed the adventitia and involved the neighboring fixed organs.[47]

BRONCHOSCOPY

Use of the fiberoptic endoscope allows histologic confirmation of the cancer by biopsy or brush cytology. Flexible bronchoscopy is performed to assess tumor involvement of the tracheobronchial tree, especially for tumors in the middle and upper esophagus. Signs of involvement include a widened carina, external compression, tumor infiltration, and fistulization (Fig 9–4). The last two signs contraindicate resection.[48] Gross macroscopic bronchoscopic appearance may not be accurate, and biopsy or brush cytology confirmation is recommended.[49]

TABLE 9–3. STAGING OF ESOPHAGEAL CANCER ACCORDING TO TNM CLASSIFICATION

T—PRIMARY TUMOR
TX: Tumor cannot be assessed
Tis: In-situ carcinoma
T1: Tumor invading the lamina propria or the submucosa, but does not reach the submucosa
T2: Tumor invading into but not beyond the muscularis propria
T3: Tumor invading the adventitia but not the adjacent structures
T4: Tumor invading the adjacent structures

N—REGIONAL LYMPH NODES[a]
NX: Regional nodal status cannot be assessed
N0: No regional lymph node involvement
N1: Regional lymph node involved

M—DISTANT METASTASES
MX: Distant metastases cannot be assessed
M0: No distant metastasis
M1a: Upper thoracic esophagus with metastases to cervical nodes or lower thoracic esophagus with metastases to celiac nodes
M1b: Upper thoracic esophagus with metastases to other nonregional nodes or other distant sites; lower thoracic esophagus with metastases to other nonregional nodes or other distant sites; and middle thoracic esophagus with metastases to cervical, celiac, or other nonregional nodes or other distant sites.

STAGE GROUPINGS

Stage	T	N	M
Stage 0	Tis	N0	M0
Stage I	T1	N0	M0
Stage IIa	T2	N0	M0
	T3	N0	M0
Stage IIb	T1	N1	M0
	T2	N1	M0
Stage III	T3	N1	M0
	T4	N0–N1	M0
Stage IVa	Any T	Any N	M1a
Stage IVb	Any T	Any N	M1b

[a]For cervical esophageal cancer, regional nodes are the cervical nodes. For intrathoracic cancers, the mediastinal and perigastric nodes (excluding the celiac nodes), are considered regional.

COMPUTED TOMOGRAPHY SCAN

The main value of CT scanning in staging of esophageal cancer lies in its ability to detect distant disease, such as that of the liver, lungs, bone, and kidney. When metastasis to the liver is larger than 2 cm, sensitivity is 70–80%, although it drops to approximately 50% when size is less than 1 cm.[50] Solitary lung metastases are rare in patients presenting with esophageal carcinoma,[51] and thus when seen on CT are more likely to be primary lung cancers or benign nodules and should be investigated as such.

CT cannot distinguish the various tumor stages, and its value is for the diagnosis of T4 disease (Fig 9–5). Obliteration of the fat plane between the esophagus and the aorta, trachea and bronchi, and in the pericardium is suggestive of invasion, but the paucity of fat in cachectic patients makes this criterion unreliable. When the area of contact between the esophagus and the aorta extends for more than 90° of the circumference, an 80% accuracy of infiltration was reported,[52] but this is by no means absolute and the accuracy is inferior to that of EUS.

The sensitivity of detecting mediastinal and abdominal nodal involvement is suboptimal with CT scans because only size can be used as a diagnostic criterion. However, normal-sized lymph nodes may contain metastatic deposits and enlargement of lymph nodes may be due to reactive and inflammatory hyperplasia. Recent studies using high-resolution helical CT scanning have demonstrated sensitivities of 11–77% as well as specificities of 71–95% for detection of regional nodal disease.[53,54] Experience with magnetic resonance imaging has shown limitations similar to those of CT scanning.[55]

ENDOSCOPIC ULTRASOUND AND PERCUTANEOUS ULTRASOUND

EUS is the only imaging modality able to distinguish the various layers of the esophageal wall, usually seen as five alternating hyper- and hypoechoic layers (Fig 9–6). The accuracy of EUS for tumor and nodal staging averages 85% and 75%, respectively, compared to 58% and 54% for CT scanning.[56] One problem with EUS is the

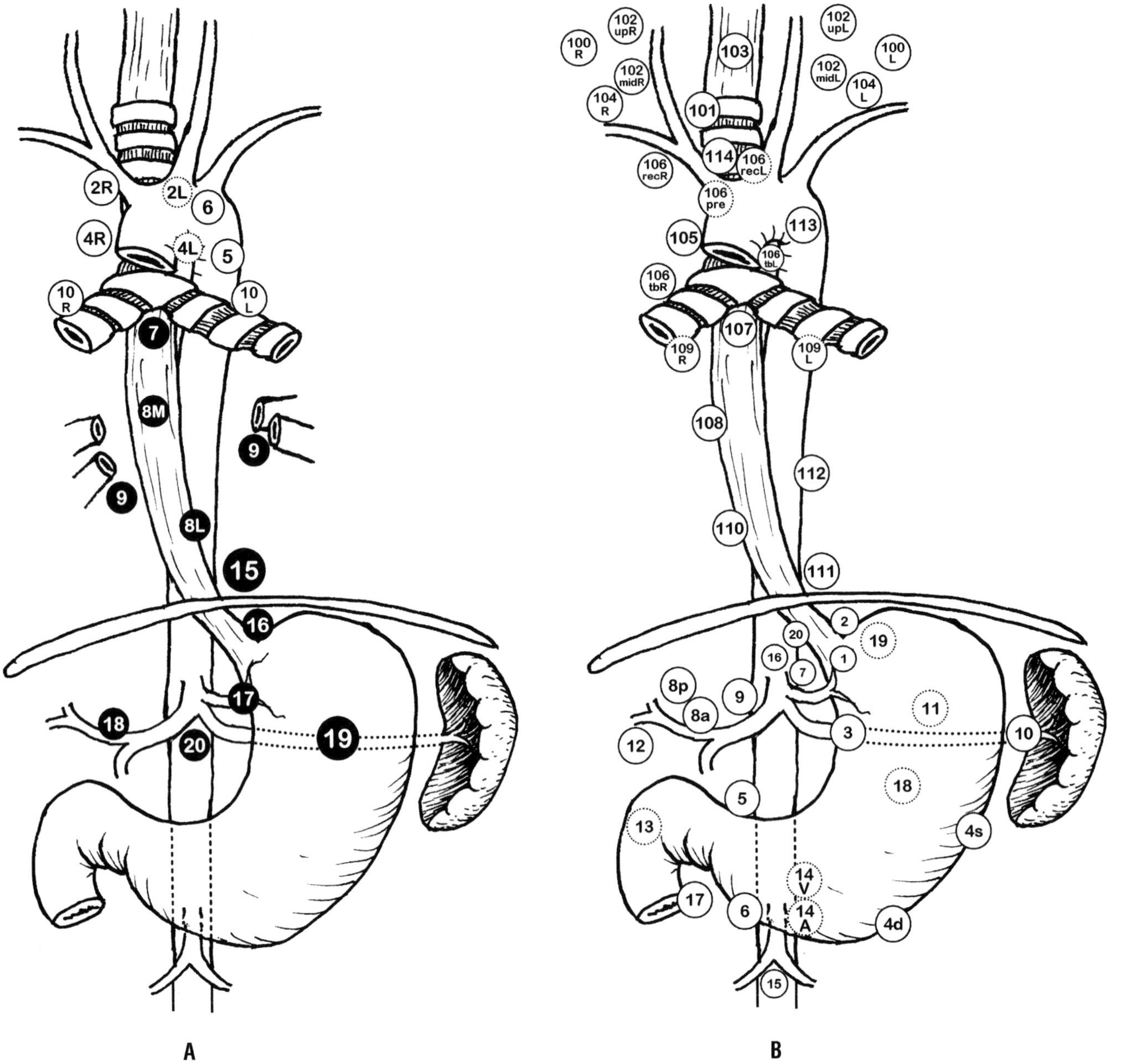

Figure 9–1. A. Lymph node stations according to the AJCC classification. **B.** Lymph node stations according to the Japanese Society for Esophageal Diseases. Much more detailed classification of lymph node number and stations are used in the Japanese system.

non-traversable tumor stricture, which occurs in about one-third of patients.[57,58] Early studies showed that pre-dilatation may result in up to a 25% risk of perforation.[59,60] More recent results suggest that pre-dilatation is safe, and the success rate of complete examination depends on the size of dilatation: 36% for 11–12.8 mm, and 87% for 14–16 mm.[61] An alternative is to use a miniaturized ultrasound catheter probe passed through the working channel of a conventional endoscope.[62]

The use of higher-frequency echo-ultrasound allows fine distinction of early mucosal and submucosal esophageal cancers into intraepithelial cancer (m1), tumor involving the lamina propria (m2), tumor penetrating the lamina muscularis mucosa (m3), and various degrees of submucosal infiltration (sm1–sm3).[63] Such information is of particular importance when endoscopic mucosal resection is a treatment option for early cancers, or for the detection of submucosal invasion, high-grade dysplasia, or carcinoma in situ in Barrett's esophagus.[64]

Echo features of lymph nodes that suggest malignant involvement include echo-poor (hypoechoic) structure,

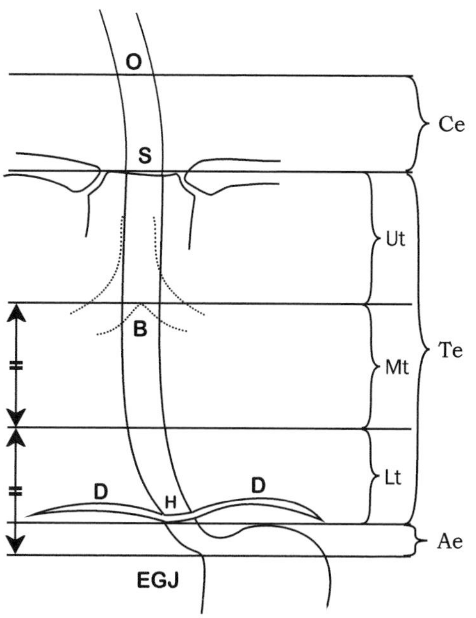

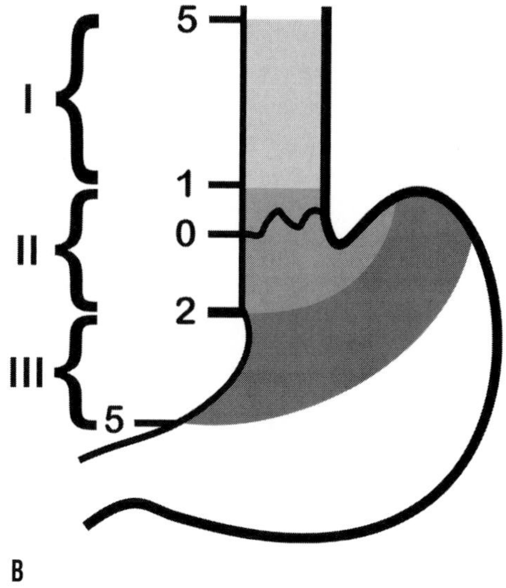

Figure 9–2. A. Description of the different levels of esophageal tumors. Ce, cervical esophagus; Te, thoracic esophagus; Ut, upper third; Mt, middle third; Lt, lower third; Ae, abdominal esophagus; EGJ, esophagogastric junction; O, esophagus; S, sternal notch; B, tracheal bifurcation; D, diaphragm; H, hiatus. **B.** Classification of adenocarcinomas around the gastroesophageal junction. Type I, esophageal; type II, cardiac; type III, subcardiac.

sharply demarcated borders, rounded contour, and size greater than 10 mm, in increasing order of importance.[65] The accuracy of EUS may differ for different lymph node locations, and is related to the limited depth of penetration of EUS (about 3 cm). It is best for detecting paraesophageal nodes, and sensitivity varies inversely with the axial distance of the nodes from the esophageal axis.[66] The ability to perform EUS-guided FNA cytology of suspicious nodes (such as celiac nodes) is another factor that makes EUS superior to CT scanning.[67]

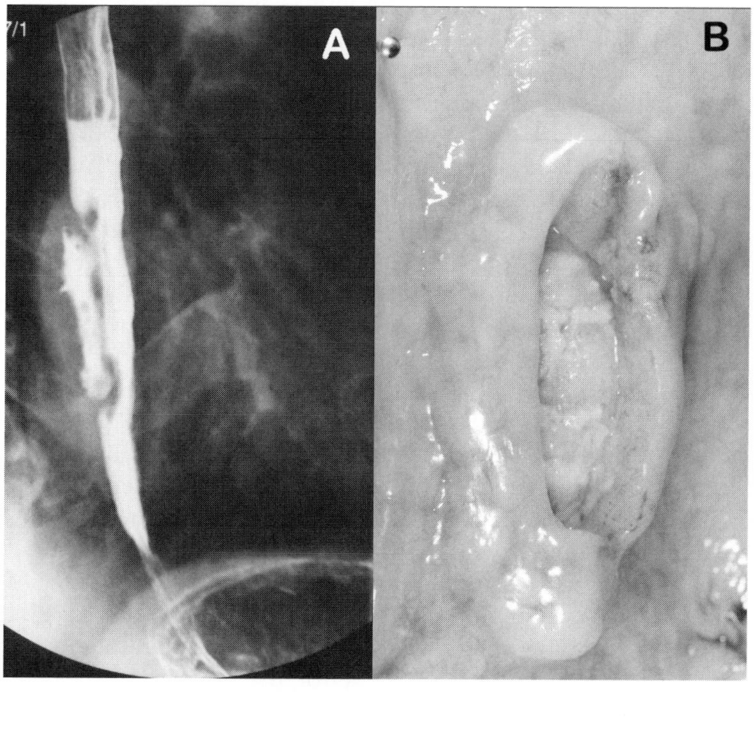

Figure 9–3. A. Barium contrast study showing an ulcerative but localized tumor of the mid-esophagus. **B.** Corresponding surgical specimen.

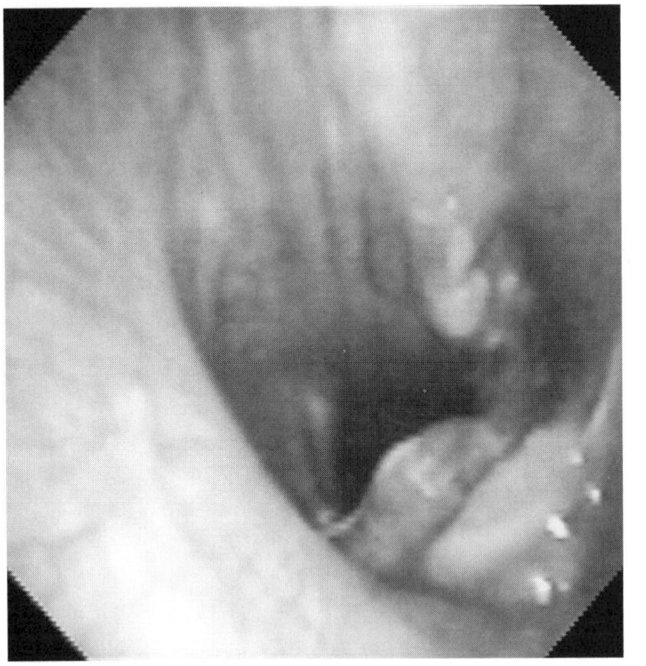

Figure 9–4. Bronchoscopy showing tumor involvement of the trachea, contraindicating resection.

Percutaneous ultrasound is particularly useful for obtaining FNA biopsies of cervical lymph nodes. In one large study of 519 patients, cervical lymph node metastasis was detected in 30.8% of patients (160/519). The sensitivity, specificity, and accuracy of US diagnosis in patients who underwent subsequent cervical lymphadenectomy were 74.5%, 94.1%, and 87.6%, respectively. In those who did not undergo neck dissection, the chance of cervical nodal recurrence was low, at less than 5%.[68]

Information gained by combining preoperative cervical ultrasound and EUS can be highly prognostic. In one study, when the number of metastatic nodes was stratified into subdivisions of 0, 1–3, 4–7, and 8 or more, the number of involved lymph nodes was prognostically similar to the eventual subdivisions as determined by histological diagnosis.[69] However, both percutaneous and endoscopic ultrasound are highly operator-dependent, and their meticulous application is required to produce these results.

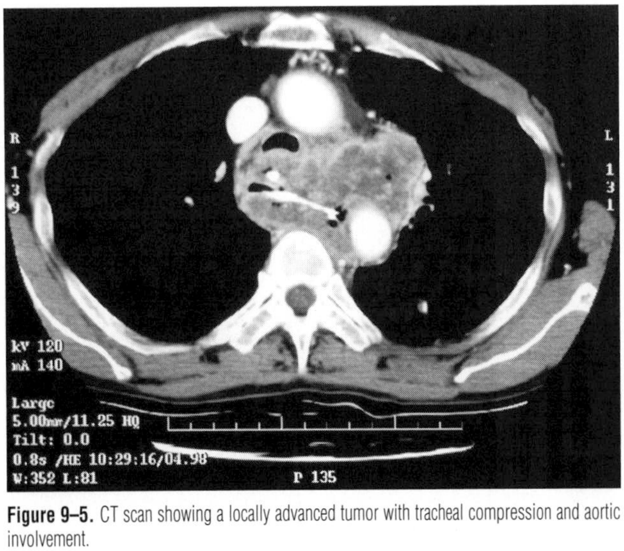

Figure 9–5. CT scan showing a locally advanced tumor with tracheal compression and aortic involvement.

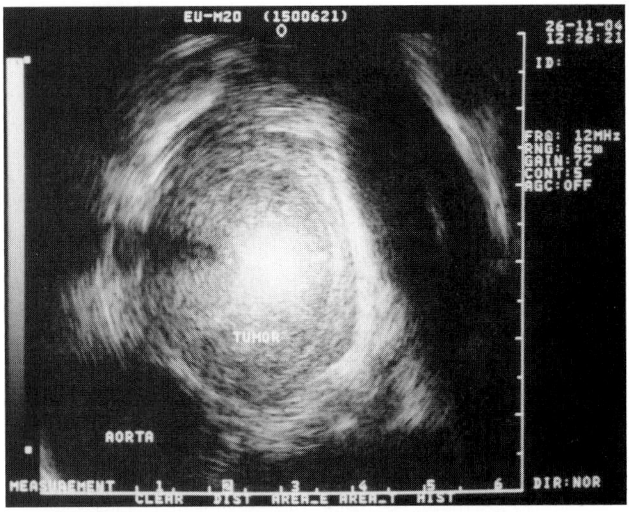

Figure 9–6. EUS examination with a mini-probe showing a tumor involving the full thickness of the esophageal wall. The aorta is not infiltrated.

FDG-POSITRON EMISSION TOMOGRAPHY SCANS

PET scanning is gaining popularity in esophageal cancer staging[70,71] (Fig 9–7). For detection of the primary tumor, the sensitivity of PET scanning ranges from 78–95%, with most false-negative tests occurring in patients with T1 or small T2 tumors.[53,72] PET scan does not provide definition of the esophageal wall and thus has no value in tumor staging. For locoregional nodal metastases, its spatial resolution is also insufficient to separate the primary tumor from juxtatumoral lymph nodes because of interference from the primary tumor, and thus most studies demonstrated poor sensitivity.[72,73] This is especially true for nodes in the middle and lower mediastinum, where most primary tumors are found. In one study, the sensitivities of PET for detecting cervical, upper thoracic, and abdominal nodes were 78%, 82%, 60%, respectively, but were only 38% and 0%, respectively, for the middle and lower mediastinum.[53] Specificity of PET scanning in detecting regional nodes is usually much better, reaching 95–100% in some studies.[72,73] The low rate of false-positive findings is important in preoperative staging.

A recent meta-analysis of 12 publications on PET scanning in esophageal cancer showed that the pooled sensitivity and specificity for the detection of locore-

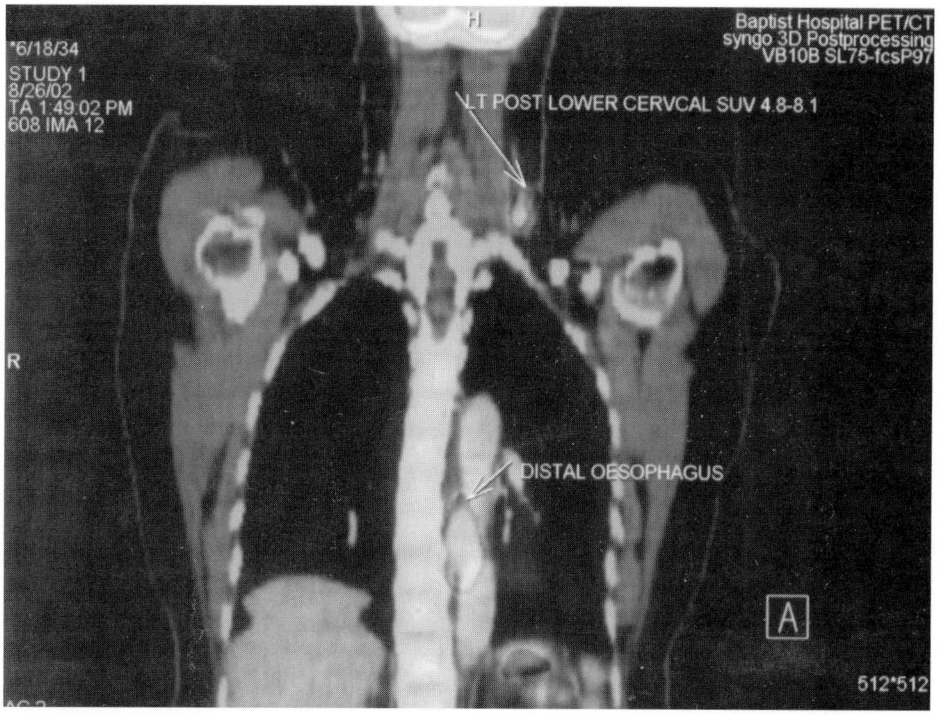

Figure 9–7. PET scan showing a lower-third esophageal cancer with metastasis to cervical lymph nodes. The node has a standard uptake value (SUV) of over 4.8.

gional metastases were 0.51 and 0.84, respectively. For distant metastases the corresponding figures were 0.67 and 0.97. When two studies (out of 11) that had particularly low sensitivities for detection of distant metastases were excluded (probably because they included more early tumors), the pooled sensitivity improved to 0.72 and specificity to 0.95.[74] This study highlights again that the accuracy of PET scanning in detecting locoregional nodes is only moderate; EUS-FNA is superior in this regard. PET is more useful for picking up distant metastases.

THORACOSCOPY AND LAPAROSCOPY

Thoracoscopy and laparoscopy have their advocates. Thoracoscopic staging usually involves a right-sided approach, with opening of the mediastinal pleura from below the subclavian vessels to the inferior pulmonary vein for lymph node sampling. Laparoscopic staging can include celiac lymph node biopsy and the use of laparoscopic ultrasound for detecting liver metastases. One multi-institutional study (CALGB 9380) reported results in 113 patients, and the strategy was shown to be feasible in 73%. Thoracoscopy and laparoscopy identified nodes or metastatic disease missed by CT scan in 50% of patients, by magnetic resonance imaging in 40%, and by EUS in 30%. Although no deaths or major complications occurred, the procedure did involve general anesthesia, single-lung anesethesia, a median operating time of 210 minutes, and a hospital stay of 3 days.[75] For lower-third or gastric cardia cancers, laparoscopy can be of use in diagnosing metastases or identifying unsuspected cirrhosis that may contraindicate resection. Its value is minimal for more proximally located tumors.[76] Given their invasiveness, thoracoscopy and laparoscopy should be reserved for cases in whom positive confirmation of metastatic disease not otherwise obtainable is essential in deciding on treatment.

▪ TREATMENT

STAGE-DIRECTED THERAPY

The information derived from staging methods already described is only useful if stage-directed therapy is used.[77,78] If so, it is important to make three assumptions: (1) that current staging methods have enough accuracy to direct treatment; (2) that segregation of patients into different stages has proven prognostic significance to guide therapy; and (3) most importantly, that patients of different stages can derive benefits from different treatment strategies, such as recruitment into neoadjuvant programs.

These assumptions are intuitive and reasonable, and are obviously true for extreme differences such as those between stage I disease and stage IV diseases with visceral metastases. The stratification of patients into more distinct intermediate stages is difficult, and treatments are not necessarily evidence-based and require further refinement. These assumptions and their drawbacks should be kept in mind when treatments are considered for individual patients.

TREATMENT FOR HIGH-GRADE DYSPLASIA AND EARLY ADENOCARCINOMA

Barrett's high-grade dysplasia, synonymous with intraepithelial cancer, is the last preinvasive stage in the metaplasia-dysplasia-cancer sequence. Options for treatment include intensive surveillance, mucosal ablation, and esophagectomy.

Proponents of endoscopic surveillance claim that such a strategy can diagnose invasive cancer at an early stage and treatment can be delayed until then without adversely affecting prognosis. The high morbidity and mortality rate of esophagectomy is also thought by some to be a deterrent to immediate surgical resection. Opponents of surveillance note that most patients with high-grade dysplasia will have an invasive adenocarcinoma identified in the following 5–10 years: in approximately 25% of patients at 1.5 years, 50% at 3 years, and up to 80% 8 years later.[21] High-grade dysplasia is currently the only reliable marker in preinvasive cancer detection, but interobserver concordance is suboptimal in distinguishing invasive and noninvasive lesions.[79] When esophagectomy is carried out in patients who have high-grade dysplasia, invasive cancer is identified in the surgical specimen in up to 42% of patients, even when patients have been recruited from surveillance programs.[80] Surveillance biopsies are also costly and require frequent endoscopies. The American College of Gastroenterology recommends surveillance biopsy every 3 months.[35] The intense surveillance required of patients with high-grade dysplasia makes this an unattractive option.

Mucosal ablative therapies consist of various techniques for ablating the metaplastic mucosa combined with high-dose acid-suppressive therapy so that normal squamous mucosa will replace the ablated metaplastic mucosa in a pH-neutral environment. Methods include bipolar electrocautery, lasers (Nd:YAG), argon beam, and photodynamic therapy (PDT). PDT, given its ability to treat the entire area of dysplastic mucosa, has special merits. A prospective multicenter trial of 208 patients with Barrett's esophagus and high-grade dysplasia who were randomized to PDT or observation suggested a decrease in the development of high-grade dysplasia and adenocarcinoma after 24 months. Cancer, however, did develop in 13% of patients.[81] While regression of dysplastic mucosa can certainly occur, complications such as stricture (up to 58% in PDT) can develop.[82] It is also difficult to ascertain complete eradication of the dysplastic mucosa; residual metaplastic mucosa beneath the regenerated squamous mucosa can be present (pseudoregression), which makes continual surveillance necessary. Because these methods do not treat nodal disease, accurate pretherapy diagnosis of noninvasiveness is necessary, which is difficult. The lack of the ability to histologically examine the resected specimen makes the diagnosis even more uncertain.

Endoscopic mucosal resection (EMR) can be done for Barrett's esophagus and a histological specimen can be thus obtained. However, up to 30% of patients can develop high-grade dysplasia or neoplasia within 2 years despite EMR.[34] This method requires more evaluation.

Surgical resection is the only method to ensure complete eradication of the dysplastic mucosa, and the frequently unsuspected invasive cancer. In specialized centers, the mortality rate from esophagectomy, especially in this group of patients, is minimal, and excellent long-term survival is reported.[40] Although there are morbidities and functional impairment after esophagectomy, the patients are relieved of the regimen of constant, rigorous endoscopic surveillance. The procedure chosen for high-grade dysplasia or early Barrett's esophagus should aim at eliminating the entire area of the abnormal mucosa, have a low morbidity and mortality rate, result in good long-term quality of life, and cure the disease.

A limited surgical procedure is preferred, provided that any lymph node metastases are resected as well. While the incidence of lymph node metastases is negligible for truly high-grade dysplasia or intramucosal cancers, once the tumor invades into the submucosa, the incidence reaches at least 30%.[21,83] In one study, the incidence of nodal metastases was low in the absence of an endoscopically-visible lesion and when biopsies revealed high-grade dysplasia or intramucosal cancer only, but four of nine patients with an endoscopically-visible lesion had nodal metastases.[21]

Study of lymph node spread from these early Barrett's cancers suggests that nodal spread is preferentially distal. A modified Merendino procedure with limited surgical resection of the distal esophagus and gastroesophageal junction, together with lymphadenectomy of the lower mediastinum and upper abdominal compartment has been advocated, and an isoperistaltic jejunal interposition graft is used to restore intestinal continuity. This procedure combines adequacy of lymph node dissection and improved quality-of-life over other procedures, as the jejunal loop prevents gastroesophageal reflux.[84]

An alternative is a transhiatal esophagectomy with placement of a gastric conduit to the neck. This eliminates the entire Barrett's field and the reconstruction is a single anastomosis. A limited lower mediastinal and upper abdominal lymphadenectomy can also be performed. Another method is to perform vagal-sparing esophageal stripping with colonic interposition. Sparing the vagi eliminates the sequelae of postvagotomy diarrhea and gastric atony. This procedure, however, is very extensive and is unlikely to gain widespread support.[85]

TREATMENT FOR EARLY SQUAMOUS CELL CANCERS

Mucosal lesions can be divided into m1–m3. Intraepithelial cancer or cancer that barely breaks the basement membrane is defined as m1, cancer that is close to or infiltrates the lamina muscularis mucosa is m3, and lesions between these two are m2. In a national survey in Japan, the incidence of lymph node involvement in m1, m2, and m3 tumors were 0%, 3.3%, and 12.2%, respectively. Submucosal lesions can be similarly divided into sm1, sm2, and sm3; the incidence of lymph node involvement was 26.5%, 35.8%, and 45.9%, respectively.[86] For mucosal cancers, 5-year survival rates are 80–100%, and for submucosal cancers 50–65%.[87]

The fine distinction of early cancers into m1–m3 and sm1–sm3 is important because the more superficial lesions are readily amenable to EMR. As implied by the foregoing discussion, m1 and m2 lesions are very suitable for EMR, given the low incidence of lymph node metastases. Sm2 and sm3 tumors should be treated as invasive cancers, with esophagectomy and lymphadenectomy. For m3 and sm1 tumors, indications for EMR are relative because of the fairly frequent nodal metastases. It is also well suited for patients who are not fit for or who refuse surgery. High-frequency EUS (up to 30 MHz) with chromoendoscopy and even magnification endoscopy can aid in selecting patients for EMR.[88]

There are many techniques of EMR but the most commonly performed is perhaps EMR-cap. Using a cap-fitted forward-viewing endoscope, saline is injected into the submucosal layer in order to raise the lesion from the deeper wall layer. The lesion is sucked into the cap and a snare wire which has been prelooped is used to snare the lesion. The strangulated mucosa is cut by blend-current electrocautery. In a series of 250 patients, 72% had absolute indications when EMR was performed for m1–m2 lesions. In these patients, no local or distant metastases occurred during follow-up. The 5-year survival rate was 95%. All those who died within 5 years died of non–cancer-related causes.[89] Complications of EMR include bleeding (which is usually minor), perforation (which can be prevented by adequate submucosal saline injection and can sometimes be treated with hemoclips), and stenosis (which tends to occur when the lesion is large). All these should be rare events.

SURGICAL RESECTION FOR ESOPHAGEAL CANCER

Surgical resection remains the mainstay of treatment for patients with localized esophageal cancer. In dedicated high-volume centers, mortality rates from surgery of 2–3% can be achieved.[43,90–95] It is, however, also true that the overall mortality rate still approximates 10% when nonspecialized hospitals are included in national figures.[96–99]

The results of surgical resection are dependent on many factors, and are mainly related to: (1) selecting appropriate patients for resection and optimizing the patients' physiologic status before surgery; (2) choice of surgical techniques and their proper execution; and (3) enhancing perioperative care.

Patient Selection for Esophagectomy

How disease stage directs treatment has been alluded to in the previous discussion. An R_0 resection, with clear resection margins, should be the aim of surgical resection, since it has been consistently shown to have the best prognosis. The role of obviously palliative resections is limited.

Complete resection rates differ among reports. These rates depend on many factors, including (1) the referral pattern of individual centers; (2) the prevailing treatment philosophy; (3) the availability of alternative therapies; and (4) the potential mortality that the surgeon and patient are prepared to accept. Reported resection rates range from 21% to 70–80%.[93,98,100,101] This wide variation suggests probable pre-referral bias or a higher prevalence of early cancers in those with high resection rates.

In studies that report on improvement of surgical results over time, more stringent patient selection often comes into play, either by excluding high-risk patients, or by treating advanced disease with nonoperative means, such as chemoradiation.[102]

Factors often cited as being predictive of morbidity and mortality after esophagectomy include advanced age,[103–105] poor performance status,[102] nutritional depletion and weight loss,[106] more proximally located tumor,[105] abnormal chest radiograph,[107] poor pulmonary function,[107] cirrhosis,[108] and abnormal cardiac evaluation.[102] Patients suffering from adenocarcinoma and squamous cell cancers also have different risk profiles;

those with squamous cell cancers are more likely to be malnourished, have high alcohol intake, and are smokers and thus have more impairment of pulmonary and hepatic function. On the other hand, patients with adenocarcinomas are more likely to be overweight (up to 50% of patients), and are more at risk from cardiovascular diseases.[109]

Assessing a patient's fitness is often based on surgeon experience and intuition and is not an exact science. Objective scores to assess operative risk and help patient selection have been generated using various statistical methods.[102,107] In one series of studies using a scoring system based on compromised general status and poor cardiac, hepatic, and respiratory function as independent predictors of postoperative death, 30% of patients with otherwise resectable tumors were excluded from surgery. When this was applied in prospective patient selection, it led to a decreased postoperative mortality rate, from 9.4% to 1.6%.[102]

Objective risk scores like this have their practical drawbacks. These scores require a suitably large patient database to generate, and another group of patients for validation before it can be applied clinically. Problems arise when changes in surgical experience and management protocols take place over time, thus the factors derived may become less relevant by the time they are put into clinical decision-making protocols. Scores that are applicable for one institution or population may not be useful at another. It is thus uncertain if patient selection based on a strict mathematical scoring system is better than one based on surgeon and anesthesiologist assessment alone. They are more likely to be complementary to one another.

Technical Aspects of Esophagectomy

There are many important variables in an esophagectomy, such as surgical access, the extent of resection and lymphadenectomy, the type and the method of preparation of the esophageal substitute, the route of reconstruction, and the technique of esophageal anastomosis. Many of these variables are interrelated and could affect immediate morbidity and mortality rates, long-term quality of life, and survival. Tumor location and stage, the patient's risk profile, and the surgeon's preferences and experience are important variables in selecting the surgical procedure. The surgeon should be versatile and well versed in the many techniques available in order to adapt to different clinical situations.

Cervical Esophageal Cancer. In 1960, Ong and Lee first described the procedure of pharyngo-laryngo-esophagectomy (PLE) as a one-stage, three-phase operation which involved cervical, abdominal incisions and a thoracotomy.[110] Tumors involving the hypopharyngeal and upper cervical esophageal region were resected together with the whole esophagus, and the stomach was delivered via the posterior mediastinum to the neck for pharyngogastric anastomosis. A terminal tracheostome was constructed. The thoracotomy was later replaced by transhiatal esophageal mobilization. Thoracoscopic esophageal mobilization has become another and our preferred alternative.[111] PLE is associated with significant morbidity and mortality, partly related to the fact that the procedure is often performed as a last resort for salvage, when no other means of palliation exists.[111] So despite improvement in surgical care, results remain worse compared to patients with intrathoracic cancers. At the authors' institution, of 317 PLEs performed from 1966–1995, the mortality rate decreased from 31% to 9%.[112]

For tumors confined to the proximal portion of the cervical esophagus with sufficient distal margin, free jejunal interposition graft or deltopectoral or pectoralis major myocutaneous flaps are options for reconstruction after resection. The use of a free jejunal graft is advantageous because it avoids mediastinal dissection, though expertise in performing microvascular anastomosis is essential. Graft necrosis, fistula formation, and late graft strictures are specific problems. When compared with gastric pull-up, graft survival and leak rates are similar. Stricture was the most common late complication for free jejunal transfers, whereas reflux was most common in gastric pull-ups, both occurring in approximately 20% of patients.[113] Functional study showed satisfactory swallowing mechanism in all patients.[114] The jejunal graft is also tolerant of postoperative radiotherapy.[115] The need to sacrifice the larynx does make surgical resection an unattractive option and chemoradiation has been used up-front in many series, with surgery reserved for salvage.[116]

Intrathoracic Esophageal Cancer. For tumors in the upper thoracic esophagus, obtaining a sufficient proximal resection margin dictates an anastomosis placed in the neck. For this reason resection is best carried out by a three-phase esophagectomy or the McKeown approach.[117] In this procedure a right thoracotomy is first carried out to mobilize the thoracic esophagus together with lymphadenectomy, and this is followed by abdominal and neck incisions for the mobilization of the esophageal substitute placing the anastomosis in the neck. The split-sternum approach is an alternative, especially for tumors close to the thoracic inlet.[118,119]

The majority of intrathoracic cancers are squamous esophageal cancers located in the middle and lower esophagus, and Barrett's adenocarcinomas in the lower esophagus. The most widely used approach was that described independently by Lewis (1946)[3] and Tanner (1947).[4] The operation begins with an abdominal phase, in which the stomach is prepared; a right thoracotomy and resection of the tumor together with lymphadenectomy follows this. The stomach is then brought up into the chest for anastomosis with the proximal esophagus at the apex of the pleural cavity.

An alternate approach involves a single left thoracotomy incision. Through a left thoracotomy and incision in the diaphragm, both the esophagus and stomach can be mobilized and resection carried out, and the stomach delivered into the chest for anastomosis, either below or above the aortic arch. Proximally the aortic arch does hinder surgical access, making mobilization of the proximal esophagus and subsequent anastomosis difficult. The approach is therefore more suitable for cancer of the cardia or the distal esophagus where an adequate resection margin is obtained below the aortic arch.

A transhiatal approach, whereby the thoracic part of the esophagus is mobilized by blunt and often blind dissection through the enlarged esophageal hiatus, and the mobilized stomach is then delivered to the neck and anastomosed to the cervical esophagus, is advocated especially for distal esophageal tumor or early-stage tumors of other parts of the esophagus.

Abdominal Esophagus and Gastric Cardia Tumors. For cancers that are limited to the abdominal esophagus or gastric cardia cancers, an abdominal–right thoracic approach as in a Lewis-Tanner esophagectomy is one option, with the proximal stomach also resected in order to gain an adequate distal resection margin. A left thoracoabdominal incision through the seventh or eighth rib space also gives excellent exposure of the low mediastinum and upper abdomen. A single left thoracotomy with opening up of the diaphragm is also an option. This gives reasonable exposure to the upper abdomen as well. However, lymphadenectomy towards the hepatoduodenal ligament is hampered. When a thoracotomy is not desired, opening the hiatus widely by splitting the crura laterally and the diaphragm anteriorly can gain access to the low posterior mediastinum, and distal esophagectomy can be performed with the anastomosis performed from the abdomen without the need for a thoracic incision. The anastomosis is made easier with a mechanical stapler. When the proximal stomach is involved by tumor, a total gastrectomy with Roux-en-Y reconstruction is preferred by many.

Transthoracic versus Transhiatal Resection. This continues to be controversial. Proponents of transhiatal resection believe that surgical resection for esophageal cancer is mostly palliative and a cure is a chance phenomenon that is only for those with very early tumors. More thorough lymphadenectomy through a thoracotomy merely improves staging, but does not affect prognosis. The operating time is also shorter and postoperative morbidity is less with the transhiatal approach.[120] Conversely, surgeons who practice transthoracic esophagectomy consider the open approach to be safer, with the ability to dissect under direct vision.[121] A more thorough lymphadenectomy leads to better staging and survival.

Two large meta-analyses concluded that the transthoracic approach probably resulted in higher perioperative morbidity and mortality rates, but long-term survival was no different.[122,123] Four randomized trials were published comparing the two approaches.[124–127] The largest compared 106 patients who underwent transhiatal esophagectomy with 114 patients who had the transthoracic approach for middle- to lower-third/cardia adenocarcinomas. Pulmonary complication rates were 27% in the former group compared to 57% in the later. Ventilation time, ICU, and hospital stay were longer in the transthoracic group. There were no significant differences in in-hospital mortality at 2% and 4%. Significantly more lymph nodes were dissected in the transthoracic group (16 versus 31). There was a trend toward a survival benefit with the transthoracic approach at 5 years: disease-free survival was 27% compared with 39%, and overall survival was 29% compared with 39%.[124]

The location and stage of the primary tumor has bearing on which surgical approach is selected. From a purely safety point of view, transhiatal resection is not suitable for patients with advanced middle- or upper-third tumors, especially in patients with tumors closely related to the tracheobronchial tree and after neoadjuvant radiation therapy; tumor infiltration or fibrosis may obliterate tissue planes and make blind dissection unsafe. As such, its application is more suitable for lower esophageal tumors for which much of the mobilization can be performed under vision. From an oncological standpoint, the philosophy towards lymphadenectomy dictates the surgical approach (see later section on lymphadenectomy).

Minimally Invasive Surgery. Various combinations of minimally invasive approaches including thoracoscopy, laparoscopy, mediastinoscopy, hand-assisted laparoscopy, and open laparotomy and thoracotomy have been explored.[128] The myriad of surgical methods tried implies a lack of consensus on which is superior.

Potentially serious intraoperative complications can occur. These include bleeding from the azygos vein[129] and from intercostal vessel,[130] and injury to the aorta,[131,132] tracheobronchial tree,[133–135] and recurrent laryngeal nerve.[136] The lack of tactile control is probably a contributory factor. On the contrary, the increased magnification and excellent visualization offered by thoracoscopy might in fact help lessen complications. Less blood loss[137] and reduction in transient recurrent laryngeal nerve palsy from 80% to 18% was reported.[138]

For postoperative complications, similar anastomotic leak and respiratory complication rates, but shortened intensive care and hospital stay,[139] or reduction of the incidence of pulmonary complications from 33% to 20%,[138] have been demonstrated by some. Osugi and colleagues experienced longer operation duration, but reduction of vital capacity and performance status was lower for the thoracoscopy group, and the number of retrieved lymph nodes, blood loss, and morbidity were similar.[140,141] When thoracoscopic esophagectomy was selectively applied to patients with elevated risk, similar outcome was obtained compared to those who underwent open thoracotomy, implying a benefit in high-risk patients.[137]

Except for the few studies mentioned, clear advantages of the minimally invasive methods could not be demonstrated, partly because the number of patients studied generally was too small to have enough statistical power to demonstrate a difference. There are also other reasons why benefits are difficult to confirm. With modern analgesic methods such as epidural analgesia, postoperative pain control is less critical a problem.[142] The genesis of cardiopulmonary complications is multifactorial and does not depend solely on the size of the incision. Surgical trauma due to mediastinal dissection is also independent of the incision size. The benefit of smaller port sites compared with open thoracotomy may be offset by the lengthened time of single-lung anesthesia. A learning curve obviously exists for such complicated procedures.[138,143] The duration of the thoracoscopic procedure, blood loss, and the incidence of postoperative pulmonary infection were all less, and the number of mediastinal nodes retrieved was more, in the later half of a group of 80 patients who had thoracoscopic esophagectomy.[143] Most reports to date studied only limited numbers of patients. Only three reports had patient numbers close to or over 100, and each used a different technique.[140,144,145] Thus for most series the full technical potential may not have been realized.

Patient selection is also evident in many series, and in some of these studies most subjects had early-stage disease or high-grade dysplasia in Barrett's esophagus.[145,146] The most important test will be long-term survival by stage-to-stage comparison, but stage migration may be hard to eliminate. Most series do not report on survival data, and in those that do, there is no reported difference compared with historical controls. The place of minimally invasive esophagectomy thus remains controversial without a well-conducted randomized controlled trial.

Extent of Resection: Axial and Lateral Margin. One of the most controversial aspects of treating gastrointestinal malignancies is the appropriate extent of resection, and this debate is exemplified by esophageal cancer. [147]

An R_0 resection is consistently identified as the most important prognostic factor for long-term survival. An R_0 resection results in total removal of the tumor mass (primary and lymph nodes) with clear proximal, distal, and lateral margins. The need to obtain clear axial and lateral margins is less controversial. The propensity of esophageal cancer to spread intramurally and to have multiple separate tumors in the esophagus is well recognized. The prevalence of intraepithelial, subepithelial, or intramural spread was as high as 46% and 54%,[148,149] and multiplicity of tumors was found in around 30% of patients.[149,150] The deeper the wall penetration of the primary tumor, the further away such spread can take place.[148] It is clear that the chance of a histologically positive margin reduces with increasing distance at which the esophagus is transected away from the tumor edge, and that the frequency of anastomotic recurrence is a function of the length of proximal resection margin attained. Taking into account shrinkage of the specimen after resection, as a guide to surgery, an in-situ margin of 10 cm (fresh contracted specimen of approximately 5 cm) should be the goal, to allow a <5% chance of anastomotic recurrence.[151] Intraoperative frozen section is one method to ensure a negative margin. However, a histologically involved resection margin does not necessarily lead to definite anastomotic recurrence, and a negative margin does not preclude anastomotic recurrence. The occurrence of skip lesions or submucosal spread can be missed, even by conscientious pathologists, and so margins may be falsely negative. Extramural recurrence with infiltration back to the anastomosis may also be indistinguishable from true anastomotic recurrence. Patients who have positive histologic margins are those likely to have more advanced disease, and early recurrences at more distant sites may make anastomotic recurrence less relevant. In our study, a positive histologic margin (diagnosed with definitive histology and not with frozen section) occurred in 7.5% of patients who had esophagectomy, and these patients had an anastomotic recurrence rate of 10.3% compared to 4.9% in those with a negative margin. The difference, however, did not reach statistical significance.[151]

Microscopic involvement of the lateral margin (macroscopically clear) results in increased chance of local recurrence and worse survival.[152] Obtaining a clear lateral margin is difficult with esophageal cancer because of its anatomic position and adjacent indispensable structures. Some Western centers advocate the concept of en-bloc resection, which in addition to lymphadenectomy, removes the primary tumor together with the pericardium, thoracic duct, azygos vein, intercostal vessels, and bilateral pleurae overlying the primary tumor and a surrounding cuff of crura (where the primary tumor is abutting) to enhance lateral clearance.[91,153] Obviously this type of resection is less suitable for upper esophageal cancers in close proximity to the trachea. The concept of en-bloc resection is thus more applicable for Western patients, in whom most tumors are adenocarcinomas of the lower esophagus.

Extent of Resection: Lymphadenectomy. For early cancers (m1–m2 tumors involving tissue up to the lamina propria), the prevalence of lymphatic spread is negligible and thus lymph node dissection is not indicated. Instead these are readily treated by EMR. For m3 tumors that have penetrated the lamina muscularis mucosa, and cancers that have infiltrated further into the esophagus (sm1 and deeper), the chance of lymphatic spread increases substantially, and lymphadenectomy is indicated. The optimal extent of lymphadenectomy is controversial. The ability to perform lymphadenectomy is closely related to the surgical approach utilized, and an open transthoracic approach is necessary, unless a limited lower mediastinal dissection is planned. Surgeons who perform transhiatal esophagectomy mostly disregard the benefits of lymph node dissection.[120]

Conventional transthoracic resection usually involves a "standard two-field" lymphadenectomy, which entails removing the nodes and peri-esophageal tissue below the level of the carina, and the lymph node stations around the celiac trifurcation. When superior mediastinal lymph node dissection is performed, it is sometimes known as "extended two-field lymphadenectomy." "Three-field" lymphadenectomy involves additional bilateral cervical lymph node clearance (Figs 9–8, 9–9, and 9–10). While improvement in survival is the ultimate test

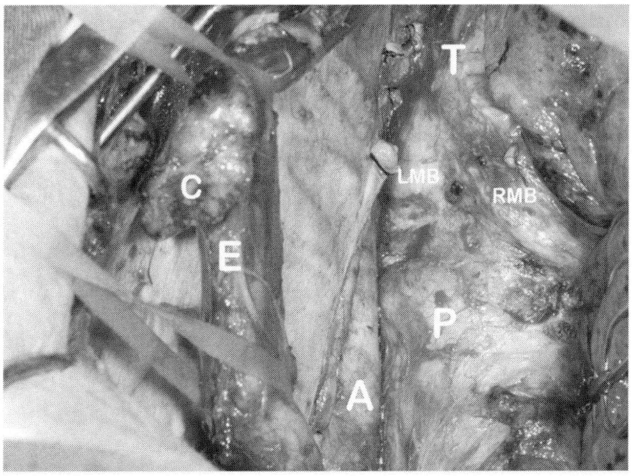

Figure 9–8. Two-field lymphadenectomy with infra-carinal lymph node dissection. T, trachea; RMB, right main bronchus; LMB, left main bronchus; P, pericardium; E, esophagus; A, aorta; C, carinal lymph node.

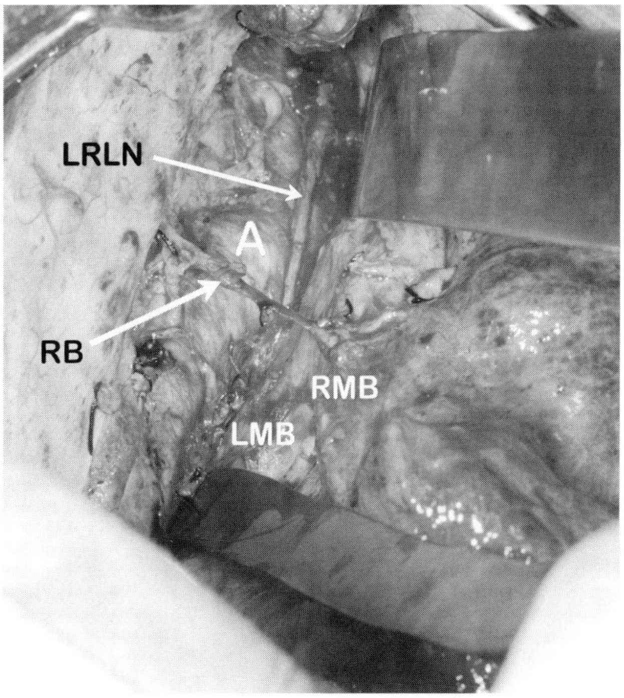

Figure 9–9. Superior mediastinal dissection completed. A large metal retractor is used to retract the trachea anteriorly to expose the left recurrent laryngeal nerve (LRLN). RB, right bronchial artery, which is preserved; A, aortic arch; RMB, right main bronchus; LMB, left main bronchus.

for different philosophies of resection, locoregional recurrence remains an important cause of death and produces symptoms that are difficult to palliate. Ways to achieve local control, if not cure, should be sought, hence the importance of defining the appropriate extent of lymphadenectomy.

The rationale for extensive lymphadenectomy is that lymph node spread occurs widely in esophageal cancer. When preoperative endoscopic injection of technetium-labeled rhenium colloid into the thoracic esophageal wall is performed, radioactivity can be detected to drain via lymphatics to all three fields. However, there is preferential lymphatic flow from the upper and middle esophagus to the neck and upper mediastinum and from the lower esophagus to the abdomen.[154] The overall rate of cervical lymph node metastasis has been documented by three-field lymphadenectomy in Japan and is approximately 30%. In relation to the level of primary tumor, cervical lymph nodes are involved in 60%, 20%, and 12.5% of upper-, middle-, and lower-third tumors, respectively.[155]

For Barrett's adenocarcinomas of the lower esophagus, presumably with less chance of superior mediastinal and cervical lymph node spread, radical lymphadenectomy mostly involves a standard infra-carinal and upper abdominal node dissection. In a detailed study of nodal metastases and recurrence for adenocarcinomas of the lower esophagus after en-bloc esoph-

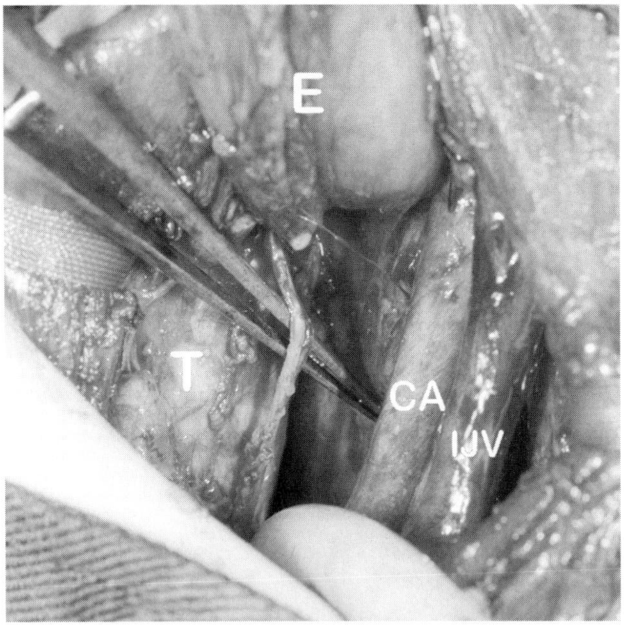

Figure 9–10. Left cervical lymph node dissection completed. A metal forceps is used on the left recurrent laryngeal nerve. T, trachea; CA, carotid artery; IJV, internal jugular vein; E, esophagus.

agectomy, most subsequent nodal recurrences were found outside the limits of dissection in the superior mediastinum or aortopulmonary window, suggesting that the recurrences arose from nodes along the recurrent laryngeal nerve that were not routinely removed.[156] It is claimed that local recurrence can be reduced to an impressive 5% within the field of dissection.[153,156–158] However, in selected centers in the United States and Europe, three-field lymphadenectomy has been tested, which interestingly also yielded similar incidences of positive cervical lymph nodes of around 30%.[92,158]

Removing positive lymph nodes in the neck may not be clinically significant, although it is intuitive that it would be so. In a study of 108 patients who underwent esophagectomy without cervical nodal dissection, 11% of patients developed recurrent disease in the neck, but only 4% had isolated cervical nodal recurrence. The higher incidences of mediastinal recurrence (25%), and systemic organ metastases (26%) further limited the role of additional neck dissection.[159] A very similar study of 176 patients documented comparable results.[160]

Although studies of recurrence pattern in the neck suggest a limited role of neck dissection, it is also realized that the most important group of lymph nodes lies along the recurrent laryngeal nerves, which transgress the thoracic inlet. Reports on recurrence patterns rarely segregate the upper (where no extensive lymphadenectomy is carried out) from the lower mediastinum (where lymph node dissection is usually adequate). When nodes along the recurrent laryngeal nerves from the superior mediastinum are considered together with the cervical nodes as one entity, this "cervico-thoracic" group of nodes are involved in up to 63.4% of proximal-third, 45.2% of middle-third, and 42.0% of lower-third cancers in patients undergoing three-field lymphadenectomy.[155] Thus the value of three-field lymphadenectomy may not lie with the addition of a cervical phase, but may lie in the completeness of the superior mediastinal dissection along the recurrent laryngeal nerves.

A recent review of three-field lymphadenectomy as practiced in Japan showed an overall hospital mortality rate of 4%.[161] Although this very low mortality rate is achieved, most of these results come from experienced and specialized institutions, and such extensive surgery is expected to carry with it more unfavorable outcomes if such procedures are more widely and unselectively applied. The other major criticism of three-field dissection is that the prognostic superiority over conventional resection is only a result of stage migration. While retrospective studies provide evidence for benefits of three-field dissection,[162,163] the more robust evidence of a well-performed randomized controlled trial is lacking.

Only two small randomized trials have been published. The first showed a higher postoperative mortality rate for two-field and a survival advantage for three-field dissection. In the second, 5-year survival rates were not statistically different for three-field (66.2%) and two-field dissection (48%). In both studies the patient groups appeared to be highly selected and not well-matched, and adjuvant therapies were not controlled for.[164,165]

Review of three-field lymphadenectomy indicates a morbidity rate of 44.8%; septic complications were the most common at 26.8%, followed by pulmonary complications at 21.3%. Recurrent laryngeal nerve injury can occur in more than 50% of patients, which predisposes to pulmonary complications and impairs long-term quality of life.[166] Perhaps realizing such an extensive operation carries with it substantial morbidity, and that not all patients could benefit, the recent focus of research in this area is to further refine the indication of extended lymphadenectomy. A survival advantage was demonstrable only for upper- and middle-third cancers by various investigators.[155,167,168] Other poor prognostic factors include: (1) when all three fields have metastatic nodes; (2) when a lower-third tumor has positive cervical nodes; and (3) when five or more lymph nodes are involved. These situations indicate advanced metastatic disease and three-field lymphadenectomy may not be justified.[169] Other suggested strategies include using intraoperative polymerase chain reaction to examine recurrent laryngeal nerve lymph nodes to predict the need for cervical dissection,[170] similarly to the concept of sentinel lymph node metastasis;[171] and taking a two-stage operative approach to select patients suitable for cervical lymphadenectomy.[172] Replacing three-field lymphadenectomy with neoadjuvant, adjuvant, or intraoperative radiotherapy[173] are alternatives, but their roles remain controversial.

Reconstruction after Esophagectomy. The reconstruction phase of an esophagectomy determines to a significant extent the postoperative morbidity and long-term quality of life. The most commonly used conduit is the gastric tube, and of the many configurations attempted, a tailored iso-peristaltic tube based on the greater curvature with preservation of the right gastric and right gastroepiploic vessels is most reliable. A 4-cm gastric tube on the greater curvature gives the best blood supply (Fig 9–11).[174] It can usually reach the neck with ease even after a pharyngo-laryngo-esophagectomy. The simplicity of preparation, adequate length, and robust blood supply make it the first choice as the esophageal substitute.

Disadvantages of the gastric conduit are that patients who had an intrathoracic stomach often experience postprandial discomfort and early satiety related to loss of normal gastric function such as receptive relaxation. Patients may also suffer from acid reflux, possible gastric ulceration, and dysfunctional propulsion.[175] In addition, Barrett's esophagus has been reported to develop in the esophageal remnant,[176] although the clinical relevance of this finding is at present unknown. These are important considerations, though in our experience serious problems are uncommon. Patients who have a low intrathoracic anastomosis tend to have more severe reflux and esophagitis compared with the high intrathoracic or cervical anastomosis. Preserving a longer length of esophagus, on the other hand, theoretically may enhance swallowing function, although no conclusive data are available on this point. Inadequate gastric emptying can also be a problem. A pyloric drainage procedure is not universally practiced. In a randomized trial, 13% of patients who did not have a pyloroplasty had problems with gastric emptying.[177] A one-layer technique was comparable to a two-layer method,[178] and a pyloromyotomy was shown to be as effective as a pyloroplasty.[179] A meta-analysis suggests that a drainage procedure lessens the chance of early postoperative gastric stasis, but long-term function is not affected.[180]

Many other factors contribute to emptying of the intrathoracic gastric conduit. A smaller stomach enhances postoperative emptying.[181] The straighter position of the stomach when delivered to the neck via the orthotopic (posterior mediastinal) or the retrosternal route may make the stomach empty more efficiently compared to one placed in the right pleural cavity, where the angulation at the diaphragmatic hiatus as the stomach continues from the right paravertebral gutter into the abdomen may produce relative obstruction. Rotation of the stomach at the hiatus should be avoided. With a gastric conduit, diet modifications and the use of acid-suppressive and prokinetic drugs such as erythromycin may be useful.[182,183]

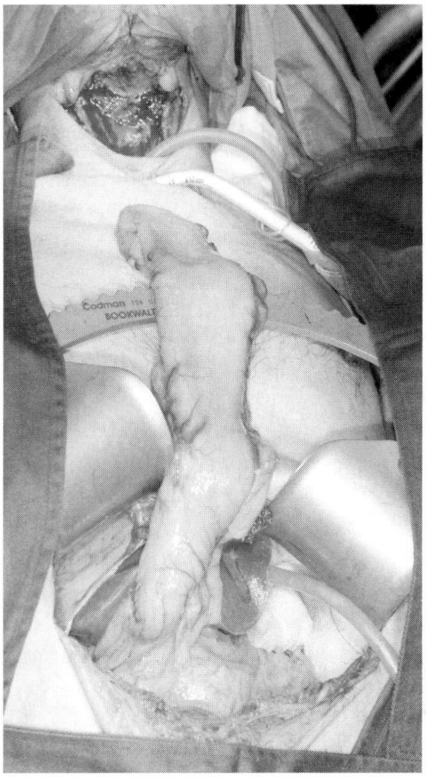

Figure 9–11. Gastric conduit prepared for transposition to the neck for pharyngo-esophagostomy after pharyngo-laryngo-esophagectomy. Ample length is evident.

There are instances when the stomach cannot be used, such as after previous gastric resection, or tumor involvement of a substantial part of the stomach dictating its removal. In these situations use of the colon is preferred. For most, colonic interposition remains an infrequently performed procedure and has the potential for more complications.[184] Bowel preparation is required; mobilization of the loop is more complex; its blood supply is less reliable than that of the gastric conduit; three anastomoses are required; and when the colon becomes ischemic, the choice of alternative conduit is restricted. In our experience, use of a colon loop is associated with more blood loss, a longer operating time, and a higher anastomotic leak rate. Colon ischemia occurs in 1 of 42 patients (2.4%), which compares favorably to a rate of 3–10% reported in the literature.[185]

It has been suggested that a colon conduit is more durable, and the supposed long-term functional benefits of colon interposition make it the preferred esophageal substitute, especially in those with benign disease, and also in patients whose cancer disease stage predicts long survival. A colonic conduit provides good long-term swallowing function and normal oral intake is restored in 65–88% of patients.[186,187] A colonic conduit seems to have active peristalsis, and this is cited as an explanation for its superior function as an esophageal substitute compared with a passive gastric conduit.[188,189] Although peristalsis can be demonstrated immediately following surgery,[190] long-term emptying likely relies on gravity.[191] When the distal stomach is retained in the abdomen after a colon interposition with a colo-gastric anastomosis, the latter provides additional reservoir function.[186]

Unique to the colonic conduit is the risk of redundancy which can manifest years later.[192] Redundancy can cause obstructive symptoms such as dysphagia and regurgitation and correction can be a complex undertaking. Very few cases of revision are reported in the literature, and in our patients only 1 out of 42 patients required a revision of a redundant loop in the neck. In another series of 69 patients with long colonic loops, 10% required anastomotic revision and 25% developed significant colonic redundancy.[193]

The jejunum is used most frequently after distal esophagectomy and total gastrectomy for cancer of the lower esophagus and gastric cardia. A Roux-en-Y configuration seems best, as it prevents bile reflux to the esophagus. A jejunal loop used in a modified Merendino procedure to interpose between the esophagus and proximal stomach after limited resection of the distal esophagus and gastroesophageal junction has also been advocated.[84] Excellent postoperative quality of life and function is claimed. A long jejunal loop is sometimes used to reach the neck, but preparation is tedious and the vasculature may not be reliable, and "supercharge" involving microvascular anastomosis to cervical vessels may be required.[194] A free jejunal graft is used for reconstructing the defect after resection of the pharyngo-esophageal segment in the neck.[115]

The route of reconstruction is in part related to the surgical approach for resection. When a cervical anastomosis is chosen, one must decide whether to place the conduit via the orthotopic, retrosternal, or subcutaneous route. The subcutaneous route is rarely used because it is cosmetically unsightly. The retrosternal route has variably been shown to be associated with increased or similar cardiopulmonary morbidity and mortality rates.[195–197] The retrosternal route is 2–3 cm longer compared to the orthotopic route,[198] but this is rarely of relevance because the esophageal replacement conduit is usually of sufficient length. Some suggest that the tight space at the thoracic inlet in the neck could cause constriction of the conduit, and recommend partial manubrium, clavicular head, and first rib resection[120]; we have found this to be unnecessary. The angulation at the inlet to the retrosternal tunnel from the neck may result in some hold-up sensation during food intake. In addition, the same angulation makes endoscopic bougie dilatation more difficult should it be required for benign or malignant anastomotic strictures. Functionally, although it was shown that there was a higher rate of gastric retention when the retrosternal route was used, quality of life was not adversely affected.[196,199]

When palliative resection is carried out for advanced tumor, recurrent tumor could infiltrate into the conduit placed in the posterior mediastinum. In a retrospective study of 209 patients who had undergone curative resection and orthotopic reconstruction, of 73 patients (35%) who had locoregional tumor recurrence, 46 (22%) had secondary dysphagia as a result. The authors concluded that in 27 patients (13%), dysphagia would likely have been prevented by using a retrosternal reconstruction route.[200] However, the site of the obstruction that produced dysphagia was not clearly stated. The stomach is usually spacious and tumor infiltration will not readily result in dysphagia. Only at the thoracic inlet and in the cervical region, where there is limited space, can tumor involvement lead to obstruction and dysphagia. Using the retrosternal route will eliminate tumor involvement in the posterior mediastinum, but infiltration from tumors in the neck cannot be avoided. The effect of choosing the retrosternal route to reduce secondary dysphagia from recurrent tumor infiltration may therefore be overemphasized. In our own study, only 4 out of 28 patients (14%) developed tumor infiltration into the gastric conduit in the posterior mediastinum. The main symptom was bleeding in two patients and none had dysphagia.[201] It is our policy therefore to use the retrosternal route for reconstruction when resection is palliative, especially when postoperative radiotherapy is planned, or when the reconstructive phase of the operation precedes tumor resection.

PERIOPERATIVE CARE AND POSTOPERATIVE MORBIDITY AND MORTALITY

With adequate preoperative work-up, serious cardiac events like myocardial infarction should be rare. Atrial arrhythmia is common, affecting about 20% of patients. In itself, atrial fibrillation is benign, but it serves as a marker for more serious underlying pulmonary and septic surgical complications.[202] Occurrence of atrial arrhythmia should prompt a thorough search for a more ominous underlying cause.

Pulmonary complications remain the most common and serious form of postoperative morbidity. Most report a major complication rate of about 20%.[97] Pneumonia and respiratory failure occurs in 15.9% of our patients and is responsible for 55% of hospital deaths. Predictive factors include advanced age, supracarinal tumor location, and lengthened operating time. Neoadjuvant therapy did not lead to increased morbidity.[105] Measures to improve respiratory outcome include cessation of smoking preoperatively, chest physiotherapy, avoidance of recurrent laryngeal nerve injury, cautious fluid administration to avoid fluid overload, use of a smaller chest tube,[203] early ambulation, regular bronchoscopy, and early tracheostomy for sputum retention.[204] Epidural analgesia is invaluable in postoperative pain relief and has been shown to improve outcome.[142]

The most common surgical complication after esophagectomy is still anastomotic leak, and the incidence can reach 30%,[205] although in experienced centers leak rates of below 5% can be achieved. Most leaks are probably related to technical faults,[107,206] such as tension between the conduit and the esophageal stump, ischemia of the conduit because of rough handling and poor preparation, and suboptimal technique. The actual method of anastomosis is perhaps less important than its proper application. Stapled anastomosis is popular for intrathoracic anastomosis, while the hand-sewn technique is preferred in the neck. There is no evidence from randomized trials that leak rates differ between stapled and hand-sewn anastomoses, but the circular stapler may give rise to more strictures.[207] Use of the linear stapler has also been advocated in the neck. One group reduced their cervical leak rate from 10–15% using a hand-sewn technique to 2.7% using linear staples with a side-to-side anastomosis.[208] With experience, however, the hand-sewn method is as safe, if not more so, and certainly less expensive. Leak rate was 3% in our patients who had an intrathoracic anastomosis, 35% of whom died, resulting in an overall leak-related mortality of 1% out of all patients who had esophagectomy.[206,209]

The clinical presentation of postoperative anastomotic leak ranges from an asymptomatic radiographic finding to a florid thoracic infection. Early detection of anastomotic leaks is important so that timely intervention can be instituted; sometimes a high index of suspicion is important when other seemingly unrelated complications develop. Treatment principles dictate adequate drainage, whether by radiological, endoscopic, or surgical means. Maintenance of nutritional status is important, preferably via the enteral route, either by a fine-bore nasoduodenal tube placed endoscopically, or by feeding jejunostomy. The mortality of leaks remains high, in spite of recent improvements in perioperative care and intensive care support. Improvements in the management of leak-related sepsis would likely lead to a decrease in morbidity and mortality.

Other surgical complications such as chylothorax and herniation of bowel through the diaphragmatic hiatus are rare, but should be recognized early and both are corrected by surgical re-exploration.

COMBINED MULTIMODAL TREATMENT STRATEGIES

The past decade has seen a proliferation of additional treatments for esophageal cancer. The rationale is based on the suboptimal long-term results of surgery or radiotherapy. Both the spatial and synergistic actions of chemotherapeutic agents and radiotherapy are explored in multimodality treatments. How surgical resection and these new combinations should be integrated into treatment programs is an active area of research.

Neoadjuvant Radiotherapy

Trials of neoadjuvant radiotherapy have failed to show increased resection rate or improved survival compared with surgery alone.[210–215] The European Organization for Research and Treatment of Cancer study suggested improved local disease control but no better long-term outcome.[212] One study, which also involved chemotherapy, suggested a survival advantage imparted by preoperative radiotherapy, but only in the pooled groups of patients receiving radiotherapy.[215] A Cochrane meta-analysis showed that if preoperative radiotherapy regimens do improve survival, then the effect is likely to be modest, with an absolute improvement in 5-year survival of around 3–4%.[216]

Adjuvant Radiotherapy

Postoperative radiotherapy was studied in three randomized trials,[217–219] and all three demonstrated improved local disease control. The largest study published to date randomized 495 patients with intrathoracic squamous cell cancers. Postoperative radiotherapy of 50–60 Gy was given to 220 patients to the entire mediastinum and bilateral supraclavicular fossa. Per protocol, analysis showed no overall difference in 5-year survival, with 31.7% for the surgery-alone group and 41.3% for the radiotherapy group. A benefit in the radiotherapy group was observed in stage III patients; 5-year survival rates were 13.1% and 35.1%, respectively. In patients with node-positive disease, difference in survival was of borderline significance. The chance of mediastinal, cervical lymph node, and anastomotic recurrences was also reduced.[219] Survival benefit was not demonstrated by the other trials. From these studies it seems reasonable to give postoperative radiotherapy to subgroups of patients, especially those who had palliative resections, to enhance local disease control. Suitable meta-analysis should be carried out to further test the statistical validity of the conclusions.

Neoadjuvant Chemotherapy

Eleven randomized trials studied the role of preoperative chemotherapy.[96,215,220–228] The two largest trials were the Intergroup trial and the MRC trial. The first study randomized patients to undergo surgery alone, or to have three cycles of cisplatin and 5-fluorouracil before surgery, and in those who had stable or responsive disease, two additional postoperative courses.[228] Of 440 eligible patients, 213 were assigned to the neoadjuvant group. The median survival was 14.9 months for the chemotherapy group compared with 16.1 months for the surgery-alone group. Two-year survival rates were no different at 35% and 37%, respectively. The MRC trial involved 802 patients and similar preoperative regimens with two courses of cisplatin and 5-fluorouracil.[96] Overall survival was better in the chemotherapy group. Median survival was 16.8 months versus 13.3 months, and 2-year survival rates were 43% and 34%, respectively.

The differences in findings in these two studies are difficult to resolve. There are many differences, including the chemotherapy regimen, distribution of histologic cell types, number of patients undergoing resection, time to resection, type of surgery performed, and number of patients who also had radiotherapy.

A meta-analysis was conducted by the Cochrane group.[229] Altogether 2051 patients were analyzed. Neoadjuvant therapy was found not to alter the rate of resection, rate of complete resection, or postoperative complications. The pooled clinical response was 36%, and pathologically complete response was only 3%. There appears to be a significant survival advantage for chemotherapy. At 3, 4, and 5 years, the increased survival was 21%, 24%, and 44%, respectively, but only reached statistical significance at 5 years. It was estimated that 11 patients needed to be treated to attain one extra survivor at 5 years. It is also worth noting that all trials evaluated patients with squamous cell cancers except the Intergroup and MRC trial. Subgroup analysis did not show any difference between the two cell types.

Adjuvant Chemotherapy

This is the area perhaps least well studied, and trials of pure postoperative chemotherapy are limited. A recent report on 242 patients compared surgical resection with the addition of postoperative cisplatin and 5-fluorouracil.[230] The 5-year disease-free survival rate was significantly different, at 45% with surgery alone and 55% with surgery plus chemotherapy, respectively. The overall 5-year survival rates were not significantly different at 52% and 61%, respectively. The effect was more marked in the subgroup with lymph node metastasis. However, another small French study also using cisplatin and 5-fluorouracil as adjuvant therapy did not show advantage with chemotherapy.[231]

Neoadjuvant Chemoradiation

Several groups have explored chemoradiation as neoadjuvant therapy (Table 9–4).[215,232–238] The radiation dose ranged from 20 Gy to 45.6 Gy. In five trials, only squamous cell cancers were recruited,[215,232,233,235,238] two included mostly adenocarcinomas,[236,237] and one treated adenocarcinomas only.[234] A survival advantage with neoadjuvant chemoradiation over surgery alone was demonstrated only in one trial.[234] Three-year survival rates were 32% and 6% for the preoperative treatment group and surgery-onlygroups, respectively. This trial has been criticized on the grounds of inadequate preoperative staging, unclear surgical procedure, a large number of protocol violations, and because survival in the surgery group was exceptionally poor. In a French study, the chemoradiation group had longer disease-free survival, a longer interval free of local disease, a lower rate of cancer-related deaths, and a higher frequency of curative resection, but overall survival was no different. The postoperative mortality rate was also higher for the treatment group (12.3% versus 3.6%), mainly related to respiratory and septic complications.[235] An Australian trial also could not demonstrate survival advantage with combined treatment.[237] The results from these studies are conflicting and thus inconclusive. Despite this, the use of chemoradiation has increased, and the Patterns of Care studies showed that preoperative chemoradiation therapy increased from 10.4% during 1992–1994, to 26.6% in 1996–1999. Interestingly, trimodal therapy was three times more common in patients with adenocarcinomas compared to those with squamous cell cancers.[239] Notwithstanding the lack of concrete data supporting such regimens, their use is commonplace.

Chemoradiation as Definitive Therapy

The Radiation Therapy Oncology Group trial of chemoradiation versus radiotherapy provided convincing evidence of the superiority of chemoradiation.[32,33,34] The 5-year survival rate reported for the combined therapy group was 26% compared to 0% following radiotherapy (median survival 14 months versus 9 months). Data on recurrence patterns showed that both local and distant disease control were superior with combined treatment. Local persistence of disease and recurrence was 47% compared to 65%. Intensifica-

TABLE 9–4. RANDOMIZED TRIALS ON NEOADJUVANT CHEMORADIATION VERSUS SURGERY ALONE

	No.	Histology	Chemotherapy and Dose of RT (cGy)	CR Rate	Mortality (%)	Median Survival (Months)	3-Year Survival (%)
Nygaard et al.[215]							
S	41	SCC	Cisplatin, bleomycin	NA	13	7.5	9
CRT + S	47		3500		24	7.5	17
Apinop et al.[233]							
S	34	SCC	Cisplatin, fluorouracil	NA	15	7.4	20
CRT + S	35		4000		14	9.7	26
Le Prise et al.[232]							
S	41	SCC	Cisplatin, fluorouracil	12.5[c]	7	10	14
CRT + S	45		2000	8.5	10	19	
Walsh et al.[234]							
S	55	Adeno	Cisplatin, fluorouracil	25%	8	11	6
C + S	58		4500		4	16	32[d]
Bosset et al.[235]							
S	139	SCC	Cisplatin	26%	4	19	34[a]
C + S	143		3700		12.3	19	37
Burmeister et al.[237]							
S	128	SCC (37%)	Cisplatin, fluorouracil	15%	5[b]	22	32[a]
C + S	128	Adeno (62%)	3500	SCC (27%) Adeno (9%)		19	34
Urba et al.[236]							
S	50	SCC (25%)	Cisplatin, vinblastine, fluorouracil	28%	2	17	16
C + S	50	Adeno (75%)	4500		7	17	30
Lee et al.[238]							
S	50	SCC	Cisplatin, fluorouracil	21%	NA	27	51
C + S	51		4560	(43%[c])		28	49 (2-year)

[a]Extrapolate from graphs. [b]Treatment-related mortality. [c]In patients who had resection. [d]$p<0.05$.
C, chemotherapy; CRT, chemoradiotherapy; CR, complete remission; NA, not available; RT, radiotherapy; S, surgery; SCC, squamous cell cancers; Adeno, adenocarcinoma.

tion of radiation dose to beyond 50.4 Gy, whether by external beam,[240] or by brachytherapy,[241] did not yield further advantage, but did increase complication rates.

A recent Cochrane meta-analysis on 13 randomized trials which compared chemoradiation with radiation confirmed the superiority of chemoradiation. Concurrent chemoradiation provides significant overall reduction in mortality at 1 to 2 years, an absolute reduction of death by 7%, reduction of local persistence/recurrence rate by 12%. The downside is a 17% increase in grade 3-4 toxicities. Sequential chemoradiation provides no benefit, perhaps demonstrating the need to maximize the radiosensitizing properties of chemotherapy.[242]

The Role of Surgery

The Radiation Therapy Oncology Group trial suggested that in patients with T1–3,N0–1,M0 disease, a 14–26% 5-year survival rate can be expected. It has been suggested that surgery may be of no additional value to chemoradiation, and should be relegated to use as an adjuvant treatment.

Two clinical trials attempted to examine whether surgical resection was necessary after chemoradiation. A French study[243] was an equivalence trial that treated 455 patients with both squamous cell cancers and adenocarcinomas of stage T3–4,N0–1,M0 with two cycles of 5-fluorouracil, cisplatin, and concurrent radiation (46 Gy at 2 Gy/day, or a split course of 15 Gy on weeks 1 and 3). Only 259 patients who had at least a partial response were randomized to undergo immediate surgery, or to have three more cycles of chemotherapy with 20 Gy at 2 Gy/day or a split course of 15 Gy times two. The death rate within 3 months after starting induction treatment was 9% for the surgery group compared with 1% in the chemoradiation group. Two-year survival rates were no different at 34% and 40%; so were median survival rates, at 17.7 months and 19.3 months for surgical and nonsurgical groups, respectively. However, patients in the surgical arm required stenting (13% versus 27%) and dilatation (22% versus 32%) less often.[243] There was no difference in the long-term quality of life, but the surgery arm had transient deterioration in the immediate postoperative period.[244]

A German multicenter equivalence trial recruited 172 patients with squamous cell cancers (T3–4,N0–1, M0). Three cycles of 5-fluorouracil/leucovorin/etoposide/cisplatin were given followed by chemoradiation (cisplatin/etoposide + 40 Gy). Resection was then performed. This was compared to a control group with the same chemotherapy, followed by definitive chemoradiation (cisplatin/etoposide + >60 Gy). Treatment-related mortality rates were 12.8% in the surgical arm versus 3.5% in the nonsurgical arm. Local tumor control was significantly worse in the nonsurgical arm, but median survival time and 3-year survival rates were no different at 16.4 months and 31.3% (surgical arm) versus 14.9 months and 24.4% (nonsurgical arm). The 3-year survival rate was 32% in nonresponders undergoing complete tumor resection compared to 11% in nonresponders who did not undergo resection.[245] Both studies concluded that surgical resection may not be necessary after chemoradiation therapy.

It may be premature to negate the value of surgical resection. First, chemoradiation is by no means harmless, and surgical resection may not be as morbid as described. Treatment duration of chemoradiation is often long and compliance is problematic. Only 68% of the patients in the RTOG-8501 trial could complete the planned treatment.[246] In the control arm of INT 0123, acute grade 3 and 4 toxicity affected 43% and 26%, and long-term grade 3 and 4 toxicity affected 24% and 13% of patients.[240] Treatment-related mortality was 5–9% as reported by the Intergroup trials.[240,247] In studies that showed a benefit for chemoradiation or questioned the value of surgical resection, the results of the surgical arm were often suboptimal. In the FFCD 9102 trial, death rate within 3 months in the surgical arm was 9% compared to 1% in the nonsurgical arm,[243] and in the German trial again the mortality rates were 12.8% and 3.5%, respectively.[245] The early surgical deaths likely biased the long-term survival results. An unusually poor 6% 3-year survival rate was cited earlier in an Irish study.[234] Comparisons with nonoperative treatments will only be valid when better results from high-volume centers are integrated into clinical trials.

Second, local disease control with chemoradiation alone is less than satisfactory. It can be shown that with increasing extent of lymphadenectomy, better local control is achieved with surgery; by comparison nonoperative chemoradiation has a much higher local persistence/recurrence rate of over 50%.[240] The relief of dysphagia, the main symptom requiring palliation, is much more certain with surgical resection, and the need to treat dysphagia with a stent was twice that in the nonsurgical group in the FFCD 9102 trial.[243]

Third, for the majority of patients treated by chemoradiation, residual disease exists. The pathological complete response rate for most trials is in the region of 25%. Thus it is logical to assume that surgical resection would enhance cure, at least in the remaining 75%. In the German trial, the 3-year survival rate of nonresponding patients who underwent resection was 32% compared with 11% in those who did not.[245] Conversely, the role of surgery is less obvious in those with complete response. However, ascertaining true complete response is difficult, whether by endoscopy, EUS, or CT scans.[248,249] Recent studies using 18-FDG-PET scans showed promise,[72,250] but while PET scan can more reliably distinguish responders and nonresponders, it is not accurate enough to pinpoint the complete pathological responders.[251]

Prediction of Response

Reliable predictors for response to chemoradiation would be useful, since multimodality treatments are toxic, time consuming, and costly. Various markers both in tissue and serum have been explored, such as simple histology,[252] p53, proliferative cell nuclear antigen, epithelial growth factor, Ki-67, cyclin D1, thymidylate synthase, and microvessel density. None are reliable and thus they cannot help clinical decision making.[253] Metabolic imaging with PET scan is promising, with its ability to predict response early in the course of treatment (Fig 9–12).[251] How all of these data should be used requires further study.

It seems that cisplatin and 5-fluorouracil–based chemoradiation therapy has reached its therapeutic limit in treating esophageal cancer. More novel chemotherapeutic agents are being explored, including paclitaxel, docetaxel, the topoisomerase I inhibitor irinotecan (CPT-11), vinorelbine, gemcitabine, herceptin, oxaliplatin, and biomodulators such as interferon.[254] This remains a very active area of research. In addition, advances in techniques in radiation delivery, such as intensity-modulated radiotherapy, may further reduce radiation toxicity.[255]

ENDOSCOPIC PALLIATION

Endoscopic palliative treatments for more advanced tumors include placement of an esophageal prosthesis, laser therapy, intralesional injection of various substances, and photodynamic therapy. The two most commonly employed techniques are insertion of a prosthesis and laser therapy. Insertion of self-expanding metallic stents (SEMS) has become the preferred method in many institutions (Fig 9–13).[256,257] The smaller diameter of the delivery mechanism makes aggressive dilatation of the tumor before insertion un-

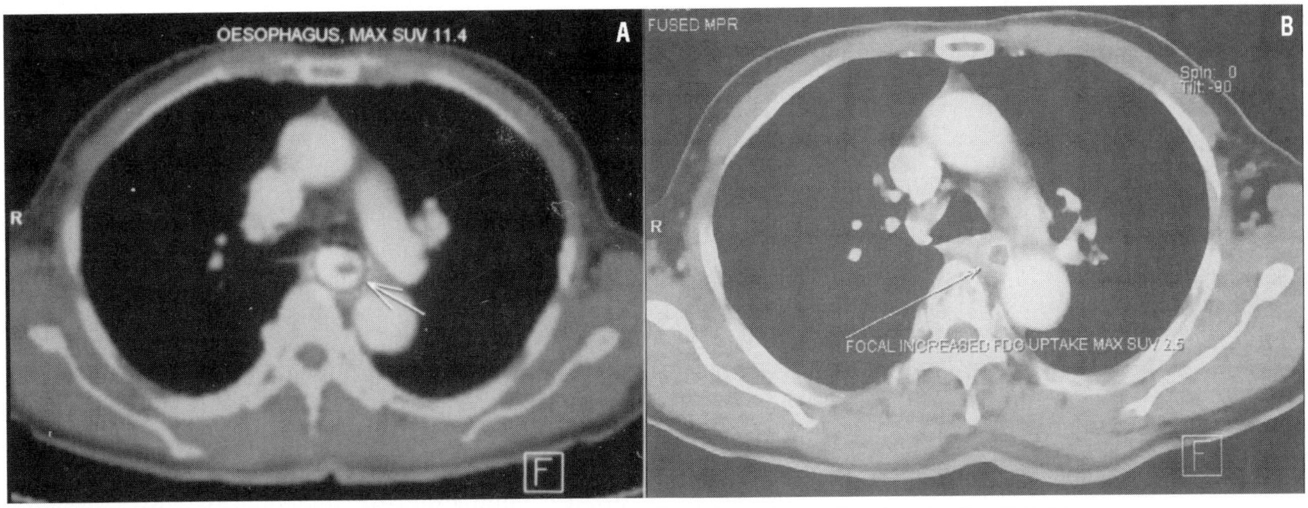

Figure 9–12. A. PET/CT before chemoradiation therapy. **B.** PET/CT after chemoradiation therapy. The standard uptake value of tumor has reduced from 11.4 to 2.5.

necessary. These stents are more flexible than plastic prostheses, and membrane-covered versions have been developed to seal esophagotracheal fistulae and prevent tumor ingrowth. Three randomized trials were reported comparing the use of metallic stents with plastic prostheses. Perforation, pneumonia, bleeding, and migration rates were significantly less with metallic stents. Because of the lower morbidity, metallic stents were also more cost-effective despite their higher initial cost.[258–260] The choice of various metallic stents depends on their individual characteristics in terms of flexibility, tensile force, and degree of shortening on deployment in relation to the site of placement.

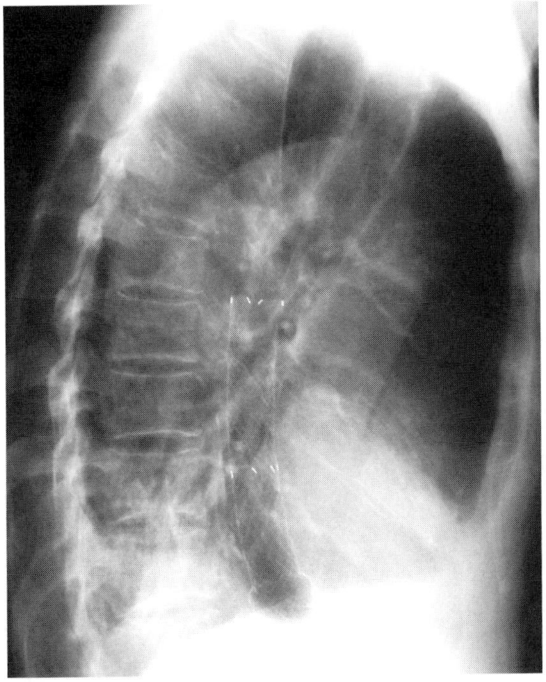

Figure 9–13. A self-expanding metallic stent in-situ.

The main problems with SEMS are stent migration, tumor ingrowth or overgrowth, and if placed across the gastroesophageal junction, they allow acid reflux. Placing uncovered stents across the cardia lessens the chance of migration, and newer stents have been developed with a one-way flap valve to prevent reflux.[261] It has also been shown that apparent tumor ingrowth is actually sometimes granulation tissue or a hyperplastic reaction by the esophageal mucosa.[262] Patency can be achieved again by laser argon beam application, or sometimes via placement of a second stent within the first. Another problem with stent insertion is placement near the upper esophageal sphincter. Foreign body sensation, pain, odynophagia, and airway compression can be troublesome, and demand accurate placement. This is illustrated when recurrent disease is found at the anastomosis or in the esophageal remnant after subtotal esophagectomy. Placement of a SEMS is still possible in these patients and achieves good palliation.[263]

Compared with more conventional methods of palliation such as laser therapy, patients with SEMS spent less time in hospital, and required less frequent re-interventions.[264]

Photodynamic therapy (PDT) is also effective in relieving dysphagia and bleeding from esophageal cancer. The depth of penetration and tumor necrosis after PDT is limited to about 5 mm, and therefore has a low chance of perforation compared to laser therapy, which is more operator-dependent. One study comparing Nd:YAG laser with PDT showed that tumor response and palliation were similar, but PDT was easier and associated with significantly fewer perforations.[265] Disadvantages of PDT include photosensitivity, inability to relieve extrinsic compression, and the costs of specialized equipment. Stricture, especially in combination with radiotherapy and chemotherapy, can occur after PDT.[266]

▪ THE TREATMENT STRATEGY AT THE UNIVERSITY OF HONG KONG

The predominant esophageal cancer treated in our institution is a squamous cell cancer lying within the thoracic cavity. Treatment strategies are based on a patient's disease stage and physical fitness (Fig 9–14). Measures are employed to maximize the chance of an R_0 resection, since this is the single factor that is unequivocally shown to achieve a good prognosis. For tumors that suggest a high likelihood of R_0 resection on preoperative investigation, surgical resection with two-field lymphadenectomy is performed. For patients with tumors that are locally advanced or those with cervical and celiac lymph nodes metastases, upfront chemoradiation is given. Surgical resection is offered when good response is obtained. Patients with obviously incurable disease or those who are not fit for surgical intervention are treated with chemoradiation or stent insertion. A neoadjuvant chemoradiation randomized trial is already closed for accrual, and long-term results are awaited. Study of the benefit of superior mediastinal and cervical lymphadenectomy is ongoing. The results after surgical resection for intrathoracic squamous cell cancers are shown in Figures 9–15 and 9–16.

▪ SUMMARY AND FUTURE PERSPECTIVES

Advances have been made in the management of esophageal cancer; the key is to select the most appropriate combination for individual patients. Surgeons play a central role in directing treatment of this disease by advising on how best to integrate surgical resection with nonoperative programs. Surgeons should aim at improving their results further, so that low mortality rates for resections are used to compare with seemingly safer therapies. The technique and extent of surgical resection may change when more informa-

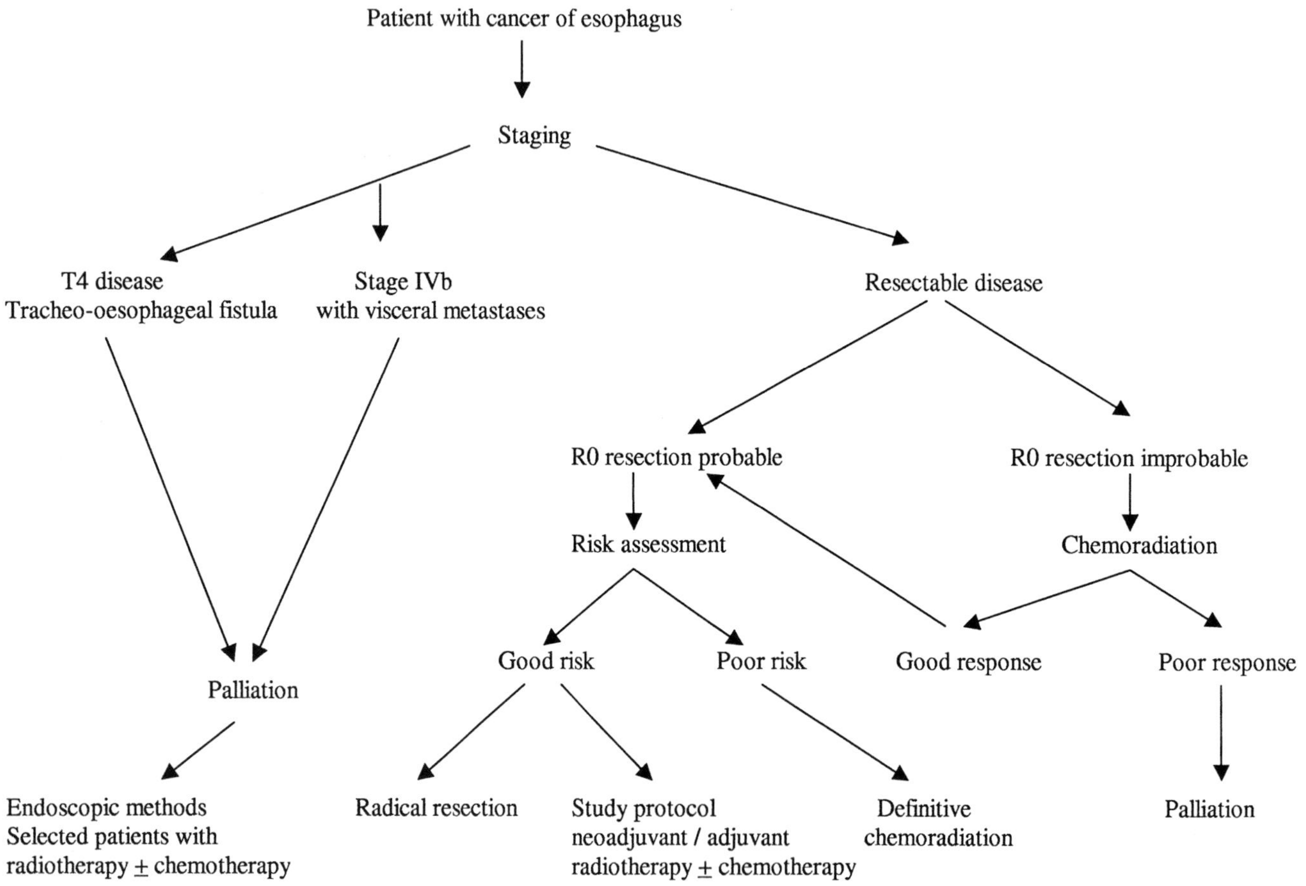

Figure 9–14. The University of Hong Kong Protocol.

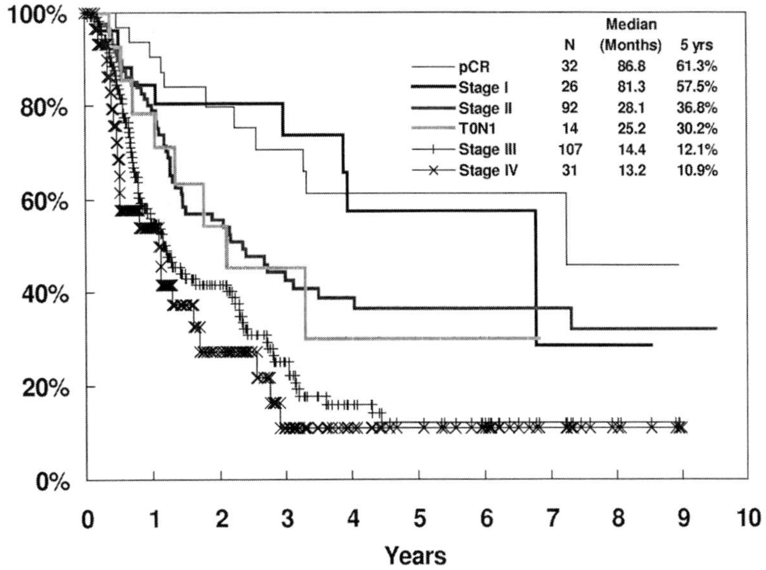

Figure 9–15. Survival curves of patients resected from 1995–2003 by pathological stage. PCR, pathologically-complete response; T0N1, patients who had sterilization of the primary tumor by neoadjuvant therapy but had residual disease in lymph nodes.

tion is made available, and should vary with patients and disease stage. Chemoradiation therapy has made a real impact on current management strategies,[90] but perhaps its overenthusiastic adoption and its presumed benefit have to be balanced against the lack of clear evidence of superiority over surgery.[267] Distant failure remains a major problem, and the search for more effective systemic drugs as well as enhanced ability to predict responders with precision must be therapeutic targets. Management strategies are going to evolve further, with improvements in molecular techniques, imaging methods, and the introduction of more novel tumoricidal agents. The challenge for the future is for us to critically test our strategies in a scientific, unbiased manner, and to explore other innovative treatments.

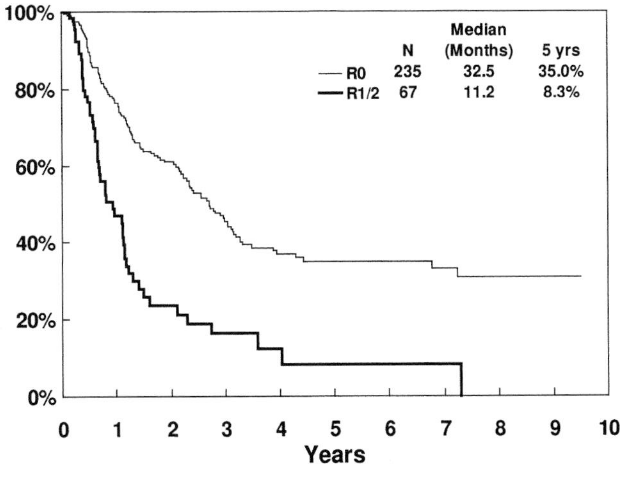

Figure 9–16. Survival curves of patients stratified into R_0 and $R_{1/2}$ resection.

REFERENCES

1. Torek F. The first successful case of resection of the thoracic portion of the esophagus for carcinoma. *Surg Gynecol Obstet* 1913;16:614
2. Ohsawa T. Esophageal surgery. *J Jpn Surg Soc* 1933;34: 1318–1950
3. Lewis I. The surgical treatment of carcinoma of the esophagus with special reference to a new operation for growths of the middle third. *Br J Surg* 1946;34:18
4. Tanner NC. The present position of carcinoma of the esophagus. *Postgrad Med J* 1947;23:109
5. Li L, Lu F, Zhang S. [Analysis of cancer modality and distribution in China from year 1990 through 1992—an epidemiologic study]. *Zhonghua Zhong Liu Za Zhi* 1996; 18:403–407
6. Ries LAG, Eisner MP, Kosary CL, et al. SEER cancer statistics review, 1975–2001. Bethesda, MD: National Cancer Institute; 2004
7. Keighley MR. Gastrointestinal cancers in Europe. *Aliment Pharmacol Ther* 2003;18(Suppl 3):7–30
8. Devesa SS, Blot WJ, Fraumeni-JF J. Changing patterns in the incidence of esophageal and gastric carcinoma in the United States. *Cancer* 1998;83:2049–2053
9. Law S, Wong J. Changing disease burden and management issues for esophageal cancer in the Asia-Pacific region. *J Gastroenterol Hepatol* 2002;17:374–381
10. Fegelman E, Law SY, Fok M, et al. Squamous cell carcinoma of the esophagus with mucin-secreting component. Mucoepidermoid carcinoma. *J Thorac Cardiovasc Surg* 1994;107:62–67

11. Law SY, Fok M, Lam KY, et al. Small cell carcinoma of the esophagus. *Cancer* 1994;73:2894–2899
12. Lam KY, Law S, Luk JM, Wong J. Oesophageal basaloid squamous cell carcinoma: a unique clinicopathological entity with telomerase activity as a prognostic indicator. *J Pathol* 2001;195:435–442
13. Lam KY, Law S, Wong J. Malignant melanoma of the oesophagus: clinicopathological features, lack of p53 expression and steroid receptors and a review of the literature. *Eur J Surg Oncol* 1999;25:168–172
14. Lam KY, Law SY, Chu KM, Ma LT. Gastrointestinal autonomic nerve tumor of the esophagus. A clinicopathologic, immunohistochemical, ultrastructural study of a case and review of the literature. *Cancer* 1996;78:1651–1659
15. Cheng KK, Duffy SW, Day NE, Lam TH. Oesophageal cancer in never-smokers and never-drinkers. *Int J Cancer* 1995;60:820–822
16. Cheng KK, Day NE, Duffy SW, et al. Pickled vegetables in the aetiology of oesophageal cancer in Hong Kong Chinese. *Lancet* 1992;339:1314–1318
17. He D, Zhang DK, Lam KY, et al. Prevalence of HPV infection in esophageal squamous cell carcinoma in Chinese patients and its relationship to the p53 gene mutation. *Int J Cancer* 1997;72:959–964
18. Poon RT, Law SY, Chu KM, Branicki FJ, Wong J. Multiple primary cancers in esophageal squamous cell carcinoma: incidence and implications. *Ann Thorac Surg* 1998;65:1529–1534
19. Shaha AR, Hoover EL, Mitrani M, Marti JR, Krespi YP. Synchronicity, multicentricity, and metachronicity of head and neck cancer. *Head Neck Surg* 1988;10:225–228
20. Ribeiro U, Posner MC, Safatle RA, Reynolds JC. Risk factors for squamous cell carcinoma of the oesophagus [see comments]. *Br J Surg* 1996;83:1174–1185
21. Peters JH, Hagen JA, DeMeester SR. Barrett's esophagus. *J Gastrointest Surg* 2004;8:1–17
22. Lagergren J, Bergstrom R, Lindgren A, Nyren O. Symptomatic gastroesophageal reflux as a risk factor for esophageal adenocarcinoma. *N Engl J Med* 1999;340:825–831
23. Lagergren J, Bergstrom R, Nyren O. Association between body mass and adenocarcinoma of the esophagus and gastric cardia. *Ann Intern Med* 1999;130:883–890
24. Goh KL, Chang CS, Fock KM, et al. Gastro-oesophageal reflux disease in Asia. *J Gastroenterol Hepatol* 2000;15:230–238
25. Romero Y, Cameron AJ, Schaid DJ, et al. Barrett's esophagus: prevalence in symptomatic relatives. *Am J Gastroenterol* 2002;97:1127–1132
26. Shaheen N, Ransohoff DF. Gastroesophageal reflux, Barrett esophagus, and esophageal cancer: scientific review. *JAMA* 2002;287:1972–1981
27. Graham DY. The changing epidemiology of GERD: geography and *Helicobacter pylori*. *Am J Gastroenterol* 2003;98:1462–1470
28. Shu YJ. Cytopathology of the esophagus. An overview of esophageal cytopathology in China. *Acta Cytol* 1983;27:7–16
29. Nabeya K, Hanaoka T, Onozawa K, et al. Early diagnosis of esophageal cancer. *Hepatogastroenterology* 1990;37:368–370
30. Wang GQ, Jiao GG, Chang FB, et al. Long-term results of operation for 420 patients with early squamous cell esophageal carcinoma discovered by screening. *Ann Thorac Surg* 2004;77:1740–1744
31. Ban S, Toyonaga A, Harada H, Ikejiri N, Tanikawa K. Iodine staining for early endoscopic detection of esophageal cancer in alcoholics. *Endoscopy* 1998;30:253–257
32. Dong Z, Tang P, Li L, Wang G. The strategy for esophageal cancer control in high-risk areas of China. *Jpn J Clin Oncol* 2002;32(Suppl):S10–S12
33. Dye C, Waxman I. Interventional endoscopy in the diagnosis and staging of upper gastrointestinal malignancy. *Surg Oncol Clin North Am* 2002;11:305–320
34. Sharma P, McQuaid K, Dent J, et al. A critical review of the diagnosis and management of Barrett's esophagus: the AGA Chicago Workshop. *Gastroenterology* 2004;127:310–330
35. Sampliner RE. Updated guidelines for the diagnosis, surveillance, and therapy of Barrett's esophagus. *Am J Gastroenterol* 2002;97:1888–1895
36. Reid BJ, Blount PL, Feng Z, Levine DS. Optimizing endoscopic biopsy detection of early cancers in Barrett's high-grade dysplasia. *Am J Gastroenterol* 2000;95:3089–3096
37. van der Burgh A, Dees J, Hop WCJ, van Blankenstein M. Oesophgeal cancer is an uncommon cause of death in patients with Barrett's oesophagus. *Gut* 1996;39:5–8
38. Shaheen NJ. Does surveillance endoscopy improve life expectancy in those with Barrett's esophagus? *Gastroenterology* 2001;121:1516–1518
39. Eckardt VF, Kanzler G, Bernhard G. Life expectancy and cancer risk in patients with Barrett's esophagus: a prospective controlled investigation. *Am J Med* 2001;111:33–37
40. Peters JH, Clark GW, Ireland AP, et al. Outcome of adenocarcinoma arising in Barrett's esophagus in endoscopically surveyed and nonsurveyed patients. *J Thorac Cardiovasc Surg* 1994;108:813–21; discussion 821–822
41. Shaheen NJ, Provenzale D, Sandler RS. Upper endoscopy as a screening and surveillance tool in esophageal adenocarcinoma: a review of the evidence. *Am J Gastroenterol* 2002;97:1319–1327
42. Spechler SJ, Barr H. Review article: screening and surveillance of Barrett's oesophagus: what is a cost-effective framework? *Aliment Pharmacol Ther* 2004;19(Suppl 1):49–53
43. Siewert JR, Stein HJ, Feith M, et al. Histologic tumor type is an independent prognostic parameter in esophageal cancer: lessons from more than 1,000 consecutive resections at a single center in the Western world. *Ann Surg* 2001;234:360–367
44. American Joint Committee on Cancer. Esophagus. In: Greene FL (ed). *AJCC Cancer Staging Manual.* New York, NY: Springer; 2002:91–95
45. Japanese Society for Esophageal Diseases. Guidelines for clinical and pathologic studies on carcinoma of the esophagus. Tokyo, Japan: Kanehara & Co, Ltd; 2001

46. Siewert JR, Feith M, Werner M, Stein HJ. Adenocarcinoma of the esophagogastric junction: results of surgical therapy based on anatomical/topographic classification in 1,002 consecutive patients. *Ann Surg* 2000;232:353–361
47. Akiyama H, Kogure T, Itai Y. The esophageal axis and its relationship to the resectability of carcinoma of the esophagus. *Ann Surg* 1972;176:30–36
48. Cheung HC, Siu KF, Wong J. A comparison of flexible and rigid endoscopy in evaluating esophageal cancer patients for surgery. *World J Surg* 1988;12:117–122
49. Riedel M, Stein HJ, Mounyam L, Lembeck R, Siewert JR. Extensive sampling improves preoperative bronchoscopic assessment of airway invasion by supracarinal esophageal cancer: a prospective study in 166 patients. *Chest* 2001;119:1652–1660
50. Rice TW. Clinical staging of esophageal carcinoma. CT, EUS, and PET. *Chest Surg Clin North Am* 2000;10:471–485
51. Margolis ML, Howlett P, Bubanj R. Pulmonary nodules in patients with esophageal carcinoma. *J Clin Gastroenterol* 1998;26:245–248
52. Picus D, Balfe DM, Koehler RE, Roper CL, Owen JW. Computed tomography in the staging of esophageal carcinoma. *Radiology* 1983;146:433–438
53. Kato H, Kuwano H, Nakajima M, et al. Comparison between positron emission tomography and computed tomography in the use of the assessment of esophageal carcinoma. *Cancer* 2002;94:921–928
54. Berger AC, Scott WJ. Noninvasive staging of esophageal carcinoma. *J Surg Res* 2004;117:127–133
55. Lehr L, Rupp N, Siewert JR. Assessment of resectability of esophageal cancer by computed tomography and magnetic resonance imaging. *Surgery* 1988;103:344–350
56. Rosch T. Endosonographic staging of esophageal cancer: a review of literature results. *Gastrointest Endosc Clin N Am* 1995;5:537–547
57. Fok M, Cheng SW, Wong J. Endosonography in patient selection for surgical treatment of esophageal carcinoma. *World J Surg* 1992;16:1098–1103
58. Bumm R. Staging and risk-analysis in esophageal carcinoma. *Dis Esophagus* 1996;9:20–29
59. Vickers J, Alderson D. Influence of luminal obstruction on oesophageal cancer staging using endoscopic ultrasonography. *Br J Surg* 1998;85:999–1001
60. Van Dam J, Rice TW, Catalano MF, Kirby T, Sivak-MV J. High-grade malignant stricture is predictive of esophageal tumor stage. Risks of endosonographic evaluation. *Cancer* 1993;71:2910–2917
61. Wallace MB, Hawes RH, Sahai AV, Van Velse A, Hoffman BJ. Dilation of malignant esophageal stenosis to allow EUS guided fine-needle aspiration: safety and effect on patient management. *Gastrointest Endosc* 2000;51:309–313
62. Hunerbein M, Ghadimi BM, Haensch W, Schlag PM. Transendoscopic ultrasound of esophageal and gastric cancer using miniaturized ultrasound catheter probes. *Gastrointest Endosc* 1998;48:371–375
63. Yanai H, Yoshida T, Harada T, et al. Endoscopic ultrasonography of superficial esophageal cancers using a thin ultrasound probe system equipped with switchable radial and linear scanning modes. *Gastrointest Endosc* 1996;44:578–582
64. Nijhawan PK, Wang KK. Endoscopic mucosal resection for lesions with endoscopic features suggestive of malignancy and high-grade dysplasia within Barrett's esophagus. *Gastrointest Endosc* 2000;52:328–332
65. Catalano MF, Sivak-MV J, Rice T, Gragg LA, Van DJ. Endosonographic features predictive of lymph node metastasis. *Gastrointest Endosc* 1994;40:442–446
66. Chandawarkar RY, Kakegawa T, Fujita H, et al. Endosonography for preoperative staging of specific nodal groups associated with esophageal cancer. *World J Surg* 1996;20:700–702
67. Parmar KS, Zwischenberger JB, Reeves AL, Waxman I. Clinical impact of endoscopic ultrasound-guided fine needle aspiration of celiac axis lymph nodes (M1a disease) in esophageal cancer. *Ann Thorac Surg* 2002;73:916–920
68. Natsugoe S, Yoshinaka H, Shimada M, et al. Assessment of cervical lymph node metastasis in esophageal carcinoma using ultrasonography. *Ann Surg* 1999;229:62–66
69. Natsugoe S, Yoshinaka H, Shimada M, et al. Number of lymph node metastases determined by presurgical ultrasound and endoscopic ultrasound is related to prognosis in patients with esophageal carcinoma. *Ann Surg* 2001;234:613–618
70. Flanagan FL, Dehdashti F, Siegel BA, et al. Staging of esophageal cancer with 18F-fluorodeoxyglucose positron emission tomography. *AJR Am J Roentgenol* 1997;168:417–424
71. Luketich JD, Friedman DM, Weigel TL, et al. Evaluation of distant metastases in esophageal cancer: 100 consecutive positron emission tomography scans. *Ann Thorac Surg* 1999;68:1133–1136
72. Flamen P, Lerut A, Van Cutsem E, et al. Utility of positron emission tomography for the staging of patients with potentially operable esophageal carcinoma. *J Clin Oncol* 2000;18:3202–3210
73. Rasanen JV, Sihvo EI, Knuuti MJ, et al. Prospective analysis of accuracy of positron emission tomography, computed tomography, and endoscopic ultrasonography in staging of adenocarcinoma of the esophagus and the esophagogastric junction. *Ann Surg Oncol* 2003;10:954–960
74. van Westreenen HL, Westerterp M, Bossuyt PM, et al. Systematic review of the staging performance of 18F-fluorodeoxyglucose positron emission tomography in esophageal cancer. *J Clin Oncol* 2004;22:3805–3812
75. Krasna MJ, Reed CE, Nedzwiecki D, et al. CALGB 9380: a prospective trial of the feasibility of thoracoscopy/laparoscopy in staging esophageal cancer. *Ann Thorac Surg* 2001;71:1073–1079
76. Stein HJ, Kraemer SJ, Feussner H, Fink U, Siewert JR. Clinical value of diagnostic laparoscopy with laparoscopic ultrasound in patients with cancer of the esophagus or cardia. *J Gastrointest Surg* 1997;1:167–173
77. Law S, Wong J. Therapeutic options for esophageal cancer. *J Gastroenterol Hepatol* 2004;19:4–12
78. Stein HJ, Brucher BL, Sendler A, Siewert JR. Esophageal cancer: patient evaluation and pre-treatment staging. *Surg Oncol* 2001;10:103–111

79. Ormsby AH, Petras RE, Henricks WH, et al. Observer variation in the diagnosis of superficial oesophageal adenocarcinoma. *Gut* 2002;51:671–676
80. Korst RJ, Altorki NK. High grade dysplasia: surveillance, mucosal ablation, or resection? *World J Surg* 2003;27: 1030–1034
81. Overholt B, Lightdale C, Wang K, et al, on behalf of 23 other investigators. International, multicenter, partially blinded, randomized study of the efficacy of photodynamic therapy (PDT) using porfimer sodium (POR) for the ablation of high-grade dysplasia (HGD) in Barrett's esophagus (BE): results of 24-month follow-up. *Gastroenterology* 2003;124:A20
82. Overholt BF, Panjehpour M. Photodynamic therapy for Barrett's esophagus: clinical update. *Am J Gastroenterol* 1996;91:1719–1723
83. Feith M, Stein HJ, Siewert JR. Pattern of lymphatic spread of Barrett's cancer. *World J Surg* 2003;27:1052–1057
84. Stein HJ, Feith M, von Rahden BH, Siewert JR, Rahden BA. Approach to early Barrett's cancer. *World J Surg* 2003;27:1040–1046
85. Banki F, Mason RJ, DeMeester SR, et al. Vagal-sparing esophagectomy: a more physiologic alternative. *Ann Surg* 2002;236:324–336
86. Kodama M, Kakegawa T. Treatment of superficial cancer of the esophagus: a summary of responses to a questionnaire on superficial cancer of the esophagus in Japan. *Surgery* 1998;123:432–439
87. Holscher AH, Siewert JR. Surgical treatment of early esophageal cancer. *Dig Surg* 1997;14:70–76
88. Inoue H, Sugaya S, Kudo S. Impact of ultrasonography on diagnosis of T1 esophageal cancer as a candidate for endoscopic mucosal resection. *Digestive Endoscopy* 2004; 16(Suppl):S173–S175
89. Inoue H, Fukami N, Yoshida T, Kudo SE. Endoscopic mucosal resection for esophageal and gastric cancers. *J Gastroenterol Hepatol* 2002;17:382–388
90. Law S, Kwong DL, Kwok KF, et al. Improvement in treatment results and long-term survival of patients with esophageal cancer: impact of chemoradiation and change in treatment strategy. *Ann Surg* 2003;238:339–348
91. Hagen JA, DeMeester SR, Peters JH, Chandrasoma P, DeMeester TR. Curative resection for esophageal adenocarcinoma: analysis of 100 en bloc esophagectomies. *Ann Surg* 2001;234:520–530
92. Altorki N, Kent M, Ferrara C, Port J. Three-field lymph node dissection for squamous cell and adenocarcinoma of the esophagus. *Ann Surg* 2002;236:177–183
93. Ando N, Ozawa S, Kitagawa Y, Shinozawa Y, Kitajima M. Improvement in the results of surgical treatment of advanced squamous esophageal carcinoma during 15 consecutive years. *Ann Surg* 2000;232:225–232
94. Birkmeyer JD, Siewers AE, Finlayson EV, et al. Hospital volume and surgical mortality in the United States. *N Engl J Med* 2002;346:1128–1137
95. Birkmeyer JD, Stukel TA, Siewers AE, et al. Surgeon volume and operative mortality in the United States. *N Engl J Med* 2003;349:2117–2127
96. Medical Research Council Oesophageal Cancer Working Party. Surgical resection with or without preoperative chemotherapy in oesophageal cancer: a randomised controlled trial. *Lancet* 2002;359:1727–1733
97. Bailey SH, Bull DA, Harpole DH, et al. Outcomes after esophagectomy: a ten-year prospective cohort. *Ann Thorac Surg* 2003;75:217–222
98. Hospital Authority Hong Kong. Clinical audit on esophagectomy and hepatectomy in Hong Kong. 2002
99. Comprehensive registry of esophageal cancer in Japan (1998, 1999) & long-term results of esophagectomy in Japan (1988–1997). In: Ide H (ed). http://jsed.umin.ac.jp: 2002
100. Pye JK, Crumplin MK, Charles J, et al. One-year survey of carcinoma of the oesophagus and stomach in Wales. *Br J Surg* 2001;88:278–285
101. Bachmann MO, Alderson D, Edwards D, et al. Cohort study in South and West England of the influence of specialization on the management and outcome of patients with oesophageal and gastric cancers. *Br J Surg* 2002;89:914–922
102. Bartels H, Stein HJ, Siewert JR. Preoperative risk analysis and postoperative mortality of oesophagectomy for resectable oesophageal cancer. *Br J Surg* 1998;85:840–844
103. Poon RT, Law SY, Chu KM, Branicki FJ, Wong J. Esophagectomy for carcinoma of the esophagus in the elderly: results of current surgical management. *Ann Surg* 1998; 227:357–364
104. Ellis-FH J, Williamson WA, Heatley GJ. Cancer of the esophagus and cardia: does age influence treatment selection and surgical outcomes? [see comments]. *J Am Coll Surg* 1998;187:345–351
105. Law S, Wong KH, Kwok KF, Chu KM, Wong J. Predictive factors for postoperative pulmonary complications and mortality after esophagectomy for cancer. *Ann Surg* 2004;240:791–800
106. Law SYK, Wong J. Complications: prevention and management. In: Daly JM, Hennessy TPJ, Reynolds JV, (eds). *Management of Upper Gastrointestinal Cancer.* London, England: WB Saunders; 1999:240–262
107. Law SY, Fok M, Wong J. Risk analysis in resection of squamous cell carcinoma of the esophagus. *World J Surg* 1994;18:339–346
108. Ruol A, Rossi M, Baldan N, et al. Esophageal and cardial cancers concomitant with liver cirrhosis: prevalence and treatment results in 273 consecutive cases. Peracchia, A., Bonavina, L., Fumagalli, U., Bona, S., and Chella, B. 183-188. 1996. Bologna, Monduzzi Editore. Recent advances in diseases of the esophagus
109. Bollschweiler E, Schroder W, Holscher AH, Siewert JR. Preoperative risk analysis in patients with adenocarcinoma or squamous cell carcinoma of the oesophagus. *Br J Surg* 2000;87:1106–1110
110. Ong GB, Lee Y. Pharyngogastric anastomosis after oesophago-pharyngectomy for carcinoma of the hypopharynx and cervical oesophagus. *Br J Surg* 1960;48:193–200
111. Law SY, Fok M, Wei WI, et al. Thoracoscopic esophageal mobilization for pharyngolaryngoesophagectomy. *Ann Thorac Surg* 2000;70:418–422

112. Wei WI, Lam LK, Yuen PW, Wong J. Current status of pharyngolaryngo-esophagectomy and pharyngogastric anastomosis. *Head Neck* 1998;20:240–244
113. Schusterman MA, Shestak K, de VE, et al. Reconstruction of the cervical esophagus: free jejunal transfer versus gastric pull-up. *Plast Reconstr Surg* 1990;85:16–21
114. Reece GP, Schusterman MA, Miller MJ, et al. Morbidity and functional outcome of free jejunal transfer reconstruction for circumferential defects of the pharynx and cervical esophagus. *Plast Reconstr Surg* 1995;96:1307–1316
115. Wei WI, Lam LK, Yuen PW, Kwong D, Chan KW. Mucosal changes of the free jejunal graft in response to radiotherapy. *Am J Surg* 1998;175:44–46
116. Burmeister BH, Dickie G, Smithers BM, Hodge R, Morton K. Thirty-four patients with carcinoma of the cervical esophagus treated with chemoradiation therapy. *Arch Otolaryngol Head Neck Surg* 2000;126:205–208
117. McKeown KC. Total three-stage oesophagectomy for cancer of the oesophagus. *Br J Surg* 1976;63:259–262
118. Orringer MB. Partial median sternotomy: anterior approach to the upper thoracic esophagus. *J Thorac Cardiovasc Surg* 1984;87:124–129
119. Moorehead RJ, Paterson I, Wong J. The split-sternum approach to carcinoma of the superior mediastinal esophagus. *Dig Surg* 1989;6:114–117
120. Orringer MB, Marshall B, Iannettoni MD. Transhiatal esophagectomy: clinical experience and refinements. *Ann Surg* 1999;230:392–400
121. Katariya K, Harvey JC, Pina E, Beattie EJ. Complications of transhiatal esophagectomy. *J Surg Oncol* 1994;57:157–163
122. Hulscher JB, Tijssen JG, Obertop H, van Lanschot JJ. Transthoracic versus transhiatal resection for carcinoma of the esophagus: a meta-analysis. *Ann Thorac Surg* 2001; 72:306–313
123. Rindani R, Martin CJ, Cox MR. Transhiatal versus Ivor-Lewis oesophagectomy: is there a difference? *Aust N Z J Surg* 1999;69:187–194
124. Hulscher JB, van Sandick JW, de Boer AG, et al. Extended transthoracic resection compared with limited transhiatal resection for adenocarcinoma of the esophagus. *N Engl J Med* 2002;347:1662–1669
125. Chu KM, Law SY, Fok M, Wong J. A prospective randomized comparison of transhiatal and transthoracic resection for lower-third esophageal carcinoma. *Am J Surg* 1997;174:320–324
126. Goldminc M, Maddern G, Le Prise E, et al. Oesophagectomy by a transhiatal approach or thoracotomy: a prospective randomized trial. *Br J Surg* 1993;80:367–370
127. Jacobi CA, Zieren HU, Muller JM, Pichlmaier H. Surgical therapy of esophageal carcinoma: the influence of surgical approach and esophageal resection on cardiopulmonary function. *Eur J Cardiothorac Surg* 1997;11:32–37
128. Law S, Wong J. Use of minimally invasive oesophagectomy for cancer of the oesophagus. *Lancet Oncol* 2002;3: 215–222
129. Peracchia A, Rosati R, Fumagalli U, Bona S, Chella B. Thoracoscopic dissection of the esophagus for cancer. *Int Surg* 1997;82:1–4
130. Collard JM, Lengele B, Otte JB, Kestens PJ. En bloc and standard esophagectomies by thoracoscopy. *Ann Thorac Surg* 1993;56:675–679
131. McAnena OJ, Rogers J, Williams NS. Right thoracoscopically assisted oesophagectomy for cancer. *Br J Surg* 1994;81:236–238
132. Cuschieri A. Thoracoscopic subtotal oesophagectomy. *Endosc Surg Allied Technol* 1994;2:21–25
133. Bumm R, Feussner H, Bartels H, et al. Radical transhiatal esophagectomy with two-field lymphadenectomy and endodissection for distal esophageal adenocarcinoma. *World J Surg* 1997;21:822–831
134. Kawahara K, Maekawa T, Okabayashi K, et al. Video-assisted thoracoscopic esophagectomy for esophageal cancer. *Surg Endosc* 1999;13:218–223
135. Gossot D, Cattan P, Fritsch S, et al. Can the morbidity of esophagectomy be reduced by the thoracoscopic approach? *Surg Endosc* 1995;9:1113–1115
136. Dexter SP, Martin IG, McMahon MJ. Radical thoracoscopic esophagectomy for cancer. *Surg Endosc* 1996;10: 147–151
137. Law S, Fok M, Chu KM, Wong J. Thoracoscopic esophagectomy for esophageal cancer. *Surgery* 1997;122:8–14
138. Akaishi T, Kaneda I, Higuchi N, et al. Thoracoscopic en bloc total esophagectomy with radical mediastinal lymphadenectomy. *J Thorac Cardiovasc Surg* 1996;112: 1533–1540
139. Nguyen NT, Follette DM, Wolfe BM, et al. Comparison of minimally invasive esophagectomy with transthoracic and transhiatal esophagectomy. *Arch Surg* 2000;135:920–925
140. Osugi H, Takemura M, Higashino M, et al. A comparison of video-assisted thoracoscopic oesophagectomy and radical lymph node dissection for squamous cell cancer of the oesophagus with open operation. *Br J Surg* 2003;90:108–113
141. Taguchi S, Osugi H, Higashino M, et al. Comparison of three-field esophagectomy for esophageal cancer incorporating open or thoracoscopic thoracotomy. *Surg Endosc* 2003;17:1445–1450
142. Tsui SL, Law S, Fok M, et al. Postoperative analgesia reduces mortality and morbidity after esophagectomy. *Am J Surg* 1997;173:472–478
143. Osugi H, Takemura M, Higashino M, et al. Learning curve of video-assisted thoracoscopic esophagectomy and extensive lymphadenectomy for squamous cell cancer of the thoracic esophagus and results. *Surg Endosc* 2003;17:515–519
144. Smithers BM, Gotley DC, McEwan D, et al. Thoracoscopic mobilization of the esophagus. A 6 year experience. *Surg Endosc* 2001;15:176–182
145. Luketich JD, Alvelo-Rivera M, Buenaventura PO, et al. Minimally invasive esophagectomy: outcomes in 222 patients. *Ann Surg* 2003;238:486–494
146. Nguyen NT, Roberts P, Follette DM, Rivers R, Wolfe BM. Thoracoscopic and laparoscopic esophagectomy for benign and malignant disease: lessons learned from 46 consecutive procedures. *J Am Coll Surg* 2003;197:902–913

147. Law S, Wong J. Two-field dissection is enough for esophageal cancer. *Dis Esophagus* 2001;14:98–103
148. Tsutsui S, Kuwano H, Watanabe M, Kitamura M, Sugimachi K. Resection margin for squamous cell carcinoma of the esophagus. *Ann Surg* 1995;222:193–202
149. Lam KY, Ma LT, Wong J. Measurement of extent of spread of oesophageal squamous carcinoma by serial sectioning. *J Clin Pathol* 1996;49:124–129
150. Pesko P, Rakic S, Milicevic M, Bulajic P, Gerzic Z. Prevalence and clinicopathologic features of multiple squamous cell carcinoma of the esophagus. *Cancer* 1994;73: 2687–2690
151. Law S, Arcilla C, Chu KM, Wong J. The significance of histologically infiltrated resection margin after esophagectomy for esophageal cancer. *Am J Surg* 1998;176: 286–290
152. Dexter SP, Sue-Ling H, McMahon MJ, et al. Circumferential resection margin involvement: an independent predictor of survival following surgery for oesophageal cancer. *Gut* 2001;48:667–670
153. Altorki N, Skinner D. Should en bloc esophagectomy be the standard of care for esophageal carcinoma? *Ann Surg* 2001;234:581–587
154. Ianabe G, Baba M, Kuroshima K, et al. [Clinical evaluation of the esophageal lymph flow system based on RI uptake of dissected regional lymph nodes following lymphoscintigraphy]. *Nippon Geka Gakkai Zasshi* 1986;87: 315–323
155. Akiyama H, Tsurumaru M, Udagawa H, Kajiyama Y. Radical lymph node dissection for cancer of the thoracic esophagus. *Ann Surg* 1994;220:364–372
156. Clark GW, Peters JH, Ireland AP, et al. Nodal metastasis and sites of recurrence after en bloc esophagectomy for adenocarcinoma. *Ann Thorac Surg* 1994;58:646–653
157. Hagen JA, Peters JH, DeMeester TR. Superiority of extended en bloc esophagogastrectomy for carcinoma of the lower esophagus and cardia. *J Thorac Cardiovasc Surg* 1993;106:850–858
158. Lerut T, Coosemans W, De Leyn P, et al. Reflections on three field lymphadenectomy in carcinoma of the esophagus and gastroesophageal junction. *Hepatogastroenterology* 1999;46:717–725
159. Law SY, Fok M, Wong J. Pattern of recurrence after oesophageal resection for cancer: clinical implications. *Br J Surg* 1996;83:107–111
160. Dresner SM, Wayman J, Shenfine J, et al. Pattern of recurrence following subtotal oesophagectomy with two field lymphadenectomy. *Br J Surg* 2000;87:362–373
161. Tachibana M, Kinugasa S, Yoshimura H, Dhar DK, Nagasue N. Extended esophagectomy with 3-field lymph node dissection for esophageal cancer. *Arch Surg* 2003; 138:1383–1389
162. Udagawa H, Akiyama H. Surgical treatment of esophageal cancer: Tokyo experience of the three-field technique. *Dis Esophagus* 2001;14:110–114
163. Isono K, Sato H, Nakayama K. Results of a nationwide study on the three fields of lymph node dissection in esophageal cancer. *Oncology* 1991;48:411–420
164. Kato H, Watanabe H, Tachmimori Y, Iizuka T. Evaluation of neck lymph node dissection for thoracic esophageal carcinoma. *Ann Thorac Surg* 1991;51:931–935
165. Nishihira T, Hirayama K, Mori S. A prospective randomized trial of extended cervical and superior mediastinal lymphadenectomy for carcinoma of the thoracic esophagus. *Am J Surg* 1998;175:47–51
166. Baba M, Aikou T, Natsugoe S, et al. Quality of life following esophagectomy with three-field lymphadenectomy for carcinoma, focusing on its relationship to vocal cord palsy. *Dis Esophagus* 1998;11:28–34
167. Fujita H, Kakegawa T, Yamana H, et al. Mortality and morbidity rates, postoperative course, quality of life, and prognosis after extended radical lymphadenectomy for esophageal cancer. Comparison of three-field lymphadenectomy with two-field lymphadenectomy. *Ann Surg* 1995;222:654–662
168. Baba M, Aikou T, Yoshinaka H, et al. Long term results of subtotal esophagectomy with three-field lymphadenectomy for carcinoma of the thoracic esophagus. *Ann Thorac Surg* 1994;219:310–316
169. Nishimaki T, Suzuki T, Suzuki S, Kuwabara S, Hatakeyama K. Outcomes of extended radical esophagectomy for thoracic esophageal cancer. *J Am Coll Surg* 1998;186:306–312
170. Yoshioka S, Fujiwara Y, Sugita Y, et al. Real-time rapid reverse transcriptase-polymerase chain reaction for intraoperative diagnosis of lymph node micrometastasis: clinical application for cervical lymph node dissection in esophageal cancers. *Surgery* 2002;132:34–40
171. Kitagawa Y, Fujii H, Mukai M, et al. [The validity of the sentinel node concept in gastrointestinal cancers]. *Nippon Geka Gakkai Zasshi* 2000;101:315–319
172. Noguchi T, Wada S, Takeno S, et al. Two-step three-field lymph node dissection is beneficial for thoracic esophageal carcinoma. *Dis Esophagus* 2004;17:27–31
173. Hosokawa M, Shirato H, Ohara M, et al. Intraoperative radiation therapy to the upper mediastinum and nerve-sparing three-field lymphadenectomy followed by external beam radiotherapy for patients with thoracic esophageal carcinoma. *Cancer* 1999;86:6–13
174. Liebermann-Meffert DMI, Meier R, Siewert JR. Vascular anatomy of the gastric tube used for esophageal reconstruction. *Ann Thorac Surg* 1992;54:1110–1115
175. Cerfolio RJ, Allen MS, Deschamps C, Trastek VF, Pairolero PC. Esophageal replacement by colon interposition. *Ann Thorac Surg* 1995;59:1382–1384
176. O'Riordan JM, Tucker ON, Byrne PJ et al. Factors influencing the development of Barrett's epithelium in the esophageal remnant postesophagectomy. *Am J Gastroenterol* 2004;99:205–211
177. Fok M, Cheng SW, Wong J. Pyloroplasty versus no drainage in gastric replacement of the esophagus. *Am J Surg* 1991;162:447–452
178. Lee YM, Law S, Chu KM, Wong J. Pyloroplasty in gastric replacement of the esophagus after esophagectomy: one-layer or two-layer technique? *Dis Esophagus* 2000;13: 203–206

179. Law S, Cheung MC, Fok M, Chu KM, Wong J. Pyloroplasty and pyloromyotomy in gastric replacement of the esophagus after esophagectomy: a randomized controlled trial. *J Am Coll Surg* 1997;184:630–636
180. Urschel JD, Blewett CJ, Young JE, Miller JD, Bennett WF. Pyloric drainage (pyloroplasty) or no drainage in gastric reconstruction after esophagectomy: a meta-analysis of randomized controlled trials. *Dig Surg* 2002; 19:160–164
181. Bemelman WA, Taat CW, Slors JFM, van Lanschot JJB, Obertop H. Delayed postoperative emptying after esophageal resection is dependent on the size of the gastric substitute. *J Am Coll Surg* 1995;180:461–464
182. Nakabayashi T, Mochiki E, Garcia M, et al. Gastropyloric motor activity and the effects of erythromycin given orally after esophagectomy. *Am J Surg* 2002;183:317–323
183. Gutschow CA, Collard JM, Romagnoli R, et al. Bile exposure of the denervated stomach as an esophageal substitute. *Ann Thorac Surg* 2001;71:1786–1791
184. Furst H, Huttl TP, Lohe F, Schildberg FW. German experience with colon interposition grafting as an esophageal substitute. *Dis Esophagus* 2001;14:131–134
185. Davis PA, Law S, Wong J. Colonic interposition after esophagectomy for cancer. *Arch Surg* 2003;138:303–308
186. DeMeester TR, Johansson KE, Franze I, et al. Indications, surgical technique, and long-term functional results of colon interposition or bypass. *Ann Surg* 1988; 208:460–474
187. Thomas P, Fuentes P, Giudicelli R, Reboud E. Colon interposition for esophageal replacement: current indications and long-term function. *Ann Thorac Surg* 1997;64: 757–764
188. Moreno-Osset E, Tomas-Ridocci M, Paris F, et al. Motor activity of esophageal substitute (stomach, jejunal, and colon segments). *Ann Thorac Surg* 1986;41:515–519
189. Paris F, Tomas-Ridocci M, Galan G, et al. The colon as oesophageal substitute in non-malignant disease. Long-term clinical results and functional studies. *Eur J Cardiothorac Surg* 1991;5:474–478
190. Myers JC, Mathew G, Watson DI, Jamieson GG. Peristalsis in an interposed colonic segment immediately following total oesophagogastrectomy. *Aust N Z J Surg* 1998;68:278–280
191. Isolauri J, Koskinen MO, Markkula H. Radionuclide transit in patients with colon interposition. *J Thorac Cardiovasc Surg* 1987;94:521–525
192. Urschel JD. Does the interponat affect outcome after esophagectomy for cancer? *Dis Esophagus* 2001;14:124–130
193. Jeyasingham K, Lerut T, Belsey RH. Revisional surgery after colon interposition for benign oesophageal disease. *Dis Esophagus* 1999;12:7–9
194. Ascioti AJ, Hofstetter WL, Miller MJ, et al. Long-segment, supercharged, pedicled jejunal flap for total esophageal reconstruction. *J Thorac Cardiovasc Surg* 2005;130:1391–1398
195. Bartels H, Thorban S, Siewert JR. Anterior versus posterior reconstruction after transhiatal oesophagectomy: a randomized controlled trial. *Br J Surg* 1993;80:1141–1144
196. Gawad KA, Hosch SB, Bumann D, et al. How important is the route of reconstruction after esophagectomy: a prospective randomized study. *Am J Gastroenterol* 1999; 94:1490–1496
197. van Lanschot JJ, van Blankenstein M, Oei HY, Tilanus HW. Randomized comparison of prevertebral and retrosternal gastric tube reconstruction after resection of oesophageal carcinoma. *Br J Surg* 1999;86:102–108
198. Ngan SYK, Wong J. Lengths of different routes for esophageal replacement. *J Thorac Cardiovasc Surg* 1986; 91:790–792
199. van Lanschot JJ, Hop WC, Voormolen MH, et al. Quality of palliation and possible benefit of extra-anatomic reconstruction in recurrent dysphagia after resection of carcinoma of the esophagus. *J Am Coll Surg* 1994;179:705–713
200. van Lanschot JJ, Tilanus HW, Voormolen MH, van Deelen RA. Recurrence pattern of oesophageal carcinoma after limited resection does not support wide local excision with extensive lymph node dissection. *Br J Surg* 1994;81:1320–1323
201. Wong AC, Law S, Wong J. Influence of the route of reconstruction on morbidity, mortality and local recurrence after esophagectomy for cancer. *Dig Surg* 2003;20:209–214
202. Murthy SC, Law S, Whooley BP, et al. Atrial fibrillation after esophagectomy is a marker for postoperative morbidity and mortality. *J Thorac Cardiovasc Surg* 2003;126: 1162–1167
203. Law S, Boey JP, Kwok KF, et al. Pleural drainage after transthoracic esophagectomy: experience with a vacuum system. *Dis Esophagus* 2004;17:81–86
204. Whooley BP, Law S, Murthy SC, Alexandrou A, Wong J. Analysis of reduced death and complication rates after esophageal resection. *Ann Surg* 2001;233:338–344
205. Hsu HK, Hsu WH, Huang MH. Prospective study of using fibrin glue to prevent leak from esophagogastric anastomosis. *J Surg Assoc ROC* 1992;25:1248–1252
206. Whooley BP, Law S, Alexandrou A, Murthy SC, Wong J. Critical appraisal of the significance of intrathoracic anastomotic leakage after esophagectomy for cancer. *Am J Surg* 2001;181:198–203
207. Law S, Fok M, Chu KM, Wong J. Comparison of hand-sewn and stapled esophagogastric anastomosis after esophageal resection for cancer: a prospective randomized controlled trial. *Ann Surg* 1997;226:169–173
208. Orringer MB, Marshall B, Iannettoni MD. Eliminating the cervical esophagogastric anastomotic leak with a side-to-side stapled anastomosis. *J Thorac Cardiovasc Surg* 2000;119:277–288
209. Lorentz T, Fok M, Wong J. Anastomotic leakage after resection and bypass for esophageal cancer: lessons learned from the past. *World J Surg* 1989;13:472–477
210. Launois B, Delarue D, Campion JP, Kerbaol M. Preoperative radiotherapy for carcinoma of the esophagus. *Surg Gynecol Obstet* 1981;153:690–692
211. Fok M, McShane J, Law SY, Wong J. A prospective randomized study on radiotherapy and surgery in the treatment of oesophageal carcinoma. Symposium on oesophageal carcinoma in the Asian-Pacific rim. *Asian J Surg* 1994;17:223–229

212. Gignoux M, Roussel A, Paillot B, et al. The value of preoperative radiotherapy in esophageal cancer: results of a study of the E.O.R.T.C. *World J Surg* 1987;11:426–432
213. Wang M, Gu XZ, Yin WB, et al. Randomized clinical trial on the combination of preoperative irradiation and surgery in the treatment of esophageal carcinoma: report on 206 patients. *Int J Radiat Oncol Biol Phys* 1989;16: 325–327
214. Arnott SJ, Duncan W, Kerr GR, et al. Low dose preoperative radiotherapy for carcinoma of the oesophagus: results of a randomized clinical trial. *Radiother Oncol* 1992; 24:108–113
215. Nygaard K, Hagen S, Hansen HS, et al. Pre-operative radiotherapy prolongs survival in operable esophageal carcinoma: a randomized, multicenter study of pre-operative radiotherapy and chemotherapy. The second Scandinavian trial in esophageal cancer. *World J Surg* 1992;16:1104–1109
216. Arnott SJ, Duncan W, Gignoux M, et al (Oesophageal Cancer Collaborative Group). Preoperative radiotherapy for esophageal carcinoma (Cochrane Review). In: *The Cochrane Library.* Chichester, UK: John Wiley & Sons, 2004.
217. Ténière P, Hay J-M, Fingerhut A, Fagniez P-L. Postoperative radiation therapy does not increase survival after curative resection for squamous cell carcinoma of the middle and lower esophagus as shown by a multicenter controlled trial. *Surg Gynecol Obstet* 1991;173:123–130
218. Fok M, Sham JS, Choy D, Cheng SW, Wong J. Postoperative radiotherapy for carcinoma of the esophagus: a prospective, randomized controlled study. *Surgery* 1993;113:138–147
219. Xiao ZF, Yang ZY, Liang J, et al. Value of radiotherapy after radical surgery for esophageal carcinoma: a report of 495 patients. *Ann Thorac Surg* 2003;75:331–336
220. Law S, Fok M, Chow S, Chu KM, Wong J. Preoperative chemotherapy versus surgical therapy alone for squamous cell carcinoma of the esophagus: a prospective randomized trial. *J Thorac Cardiovasc Surg* 1997;114:210–217
221. Roth JA, Pass HI, Flanagan MM, et al. Randomized clinical trial of preoperative and postoperative adjuvant chemotherapy with cisplatin, vindesine, and bleomycin for carcinoma of the esophagus. *J Thorac Cardiovasc Surg* 1988;96:242–248
222. Schlag PM. Randomized trial of preoperative chemotherapy for squamous cell cancer of the esophagus. *Arch Surg* 1992;127:1446–1450
223. Kok TC, van Lanschot JJ, Siersema PD, et al. Neoadjuvant chemotherapy compared with surgery in esophageal squamous cell cancer. *Can J Gastroenterol* 1998; 12(Suppl B):297
224. Wang C, Ding T, Chang L. [A randomized clinical study of preoperative chemotherapy for esophageal carcinoma]. *Zhonghua Zhong Liu Za Zhi* 2001;23:254–255
225. Maipang T, Vasinanukorn P, Petpichetchian C, et al. Induction chemotherapy in the treatment of patients with carcinoma of the esophagus. *J Surg Oncol* 1994;56:191–197
226. Baba M, Natsugoe S, Shimada M, et al. Prospective evaluation of preoperative chemotherapy in resectable squamous cell carcinoma of the thoracic esophagus. *Dis Esophagus* 2000;13:136–141
227. Ancona E, Ruol A, Santi S, et al. Only pathologic complete response to neoadjuvant chemotherapy improves significantly the long term survival of patients with resectable esophageal squamous cell carcinoma: final report of a randomized, controlled trial of preoperative chemotherapy versus surgery alone. *Cancer* 2001;91: 2165–2174
228. Kelsen DP, Ginsberg R, Pajak TF, et al. Chemotherapy followed by surgery compared with surgery alone for localized esophageal cancer. *N Engl J Med* 1998;339:1979–1984
229. Malthaner R, Fenlon D. Preoperative chemotherapy for resectable thoracic esophageal cancer (Cochrane Review). In: *The Cochrane Library.* Chichester, UK: John Wiley & Sons; 2004
230. Ando N, Iizuka T, Ide H, et al. Surgery plus chemotherapy compared with surgery alone for localized squamous cell carcinoma of the thoracic esophagus: a Japan Clinical Oncology Group Study—JCOG9204. *J Clin Oncol* 2003;21:4592–4596
231. Pouliquen X, Levard H, Hay JM, et al. 5-Fluorouracil and cisplatin therapy after palliative surgical resection of squamous cell carcinoma of the esophagus. A multicenter randomized trial. French Associations for Surgical Research. *Ann Surg* 1996;223:127–133
232. Le Prise E, Etienne PL, Meunier B, et al. A randomized study of chemotherapy, radiation therapy, and surgery versus surgery for localized squamous cell carcinoma of the esophagus. *Cancer* 1994;73:1779–1784
233. Apinop C, Puttisak P, Preecha N. A prospective study of combined therapy in esophageal cancer. *Hepatogastroenterology* 1994;41:391–393
234. Walsh TN, Noonan N, Hollywood D, et al. A comparison of multimodal therapy and surgery for esophageal adenocarcinoma. *N Engl J Med* 1996;335:462–467
235. Bosset JF, Gignoux M, Triboulet JP, et al. Chemoradiotherapy followed by surgery compared with surgery alone in squamous-cell cancer of the esophagus. *N Engl J Med* 1997;337:161–167
236. Urba SG, Orringer MB, Turrisi A, et al. Randomized trial of preoperative chemoradiation versus surgery alone in patients with locoregional esophageal carcinoma. *J Clin Oncol* 2001;19:305–313
237. Burmeister BH, Smithers BM, Gebski V, et al. Surgery alone versus chemoradiotherapy followed by surgery for resectable cancer of the oesophagus: a randomised controlled phase III trial. *Lancet Oncol* 2005; 6:659–668
238. Lee JL, Park SI, Kim SB, et al. A single institutional phase III trial of preoperative chemotherapy with hyperfractionation radiotherapy plus surgery versus surgery alone for resectable esophageal squamous cell carcinoma. *Ann Oncol* 2004;15:947–954
239. Suntharalingam M, Moughan J, Coia LR, et al. The national practice for patients receiving radiation therapy for carcinoma of the esophagus: results of the 1996–1999 Patterns of Care Study. *Int J Radiat Oncol Biol Phys* 2003;56:981–987
240. Minsky BD, Pajak TF, Ginsberg RJ, et al. INT 0123 (Radiation Therapy Oncology Group 94-05) phase III trial of combined-modality therapy for esophageal cancer:

high-dose versus standard-dose radiation therapy. *J Clin Oncol* 2002;20:1167–1174

241. Gaspar LE, Winter K, Kocha WI, et al. A phase I/II study of external beam radiation, brachytherapy, and concurrent chemotherapy for patients with localized carcinoma of the esophagus (Radiation Therapy Oncology Group Study 9207): final report. *Cancer* 2000;88:988–995
242. Wong R, Malthaner R. Combined chemotherapy and radiotherapy (without surgery) compared with radiotherapy alone in localized carcinoma of the esophagus (Cochrane Review). In: *The Cochane Library*. Chichester, UK: John Wiley & Sons; 2004:CD002092
243. Bedenne L, Michel P, Bouche O, et al. Randomized phase III trial in locally advanced esophageal cancer: radiochemotherapy followed by surgery versus radiochemotherapy alone (FFCD 9102). *Proc Am Soc Clin Oncol* 2002;21:130a
244. Bennetain F, Bedenne L, Michel P, et al. Definitive results of a comparative longitudinal quality of life study using the Spitzer index in the randomized multicentric phase III trial FFCD 9102 (surgery vs radiochemotherapy in patients with locally advanced esophageal cancer). *Proc Am Soc Clin Oncol* 2003;22:250(abst 1002)
245. Stahl M, Stuschke M, Lehmann N, et al. Chemoradiation with and without surgery in patients with locally advanced squamous cell carcinoma of the esophagus. *J Clin Oncol* 2005;23:2310–2317
246. Cooper JS, Guo MD, Herskovic A, et al. Chemoradiotherapy of locally advanced esophageal cancer: long-term follow-up of a prospective randomized trial (RTOG 85-01). Radiation Therapy Oncology Group. *JAMA* 1999;281:1623–1627
247. Minsky BD, Neuberg D, Kelsen DP, et al. Final report of Intergroup Trial 0122 (ECOG PE-289, RTOG 90-12): Phase II trial of neoadjuvant chemotherapy plus concurrent chemotherapy and high-dose radiation for squamous cell carcinoma of the esophagus. *Int J Radiat Oncol Biol Phys* 1999;43:517–523
248. Jones DR, Parker LAJ, Detterbeck FC, Egan TM. Inadequacy of computed tomography in assessing patients with esophageal carcinoma after induction chemoradiotherapy. *Cancer* 1999;85:1026–1032
249. Zuccaro G, Rice TW, Goldblum J, et al. Endoscopic ultrasound cannot determine suitability for esophagectomy after aggressive chemoradiotherapy for esophageal cancer. *Am J Gastroenterol* 1999;94:906–912
250. Weber WA, Ott K, Becker K, et al. Prediction of response to preoperative chemotherapy in adenocarcinomas of the esophagogastric junction by metabolic imaging. *J Clin Oncol* 2001;19:3058–3065
251. Wieder HA, Brucher BL, Zimmermann F, et al. Time course of tumor metabolic activity during chemoradiotherapy of esophageal squamous cell carcinoma and response to treatment. *J Clin Oncol* 2004;22:900–908
252. Lam KY, Law S, Ma LT, Ong SK, Wong J. Pre-operative chemotherapy for squamous cell carcinoma of the oesophagus: do histological assessment and p53 overexpression predict chemo-responsiveness? *Eur J Cancer* 1997;33:1221–1225
253. Walsh TN, Grannell M, Mansoor S. Predictive factors for success of neo-adjuvant therapy in upper gastrointestinal cancer. *J Gastroenterol Hepatol* 2002;17(Suppl):S172–S175
254. Law S, Wong J. New adjuvant therapies for esophageal cancer. *Adv Surg* 2001;35:271–295
255. Nutting CM, Bedford JL, Cosgrove VP, et al. A comparison of conformal and intensity-modulated techniques for oesophageal radiotherapy. *Radiother Oncol* 2001;61:157–163
256. Baron TH. Expandable metal stents for the treatment of cancerous obstruction of the gastrointestinal tract. *N Engl J Med* 2001;344:1681–1687
257. Ramirez FC, Dennert B, Zierer ST, Sanowski RA. Esophageal self-expandable metallic stents—indications, practice, techniques, and complications: results of a national survey. *Gastrointest Endosc* 1997;45:360–364
258. Knyrim K, Wagner HJ, Bethge N, Keymling M, Vakil N. A controlled trial of an expansile metal stent for palliation of esophageal obstruction due to inoperable cancer. *N Engl J Med* 1993;329:1302–1307
259. De Palma G, Di Matteo E, Romano G, et al. Plastic prosthesis versus expandable metal stents for palliation of inoperable esophageal thoracic carcinoma: a controlled prospective study. *Gastrointest Endosc* 1996;43:478–482
260. Siersema PD, Hop WCJ, Dees J, Tilanus HW, van Blankenstein M. Coated self-expanding metal stents versus latex prostheses for esophagogastric cancer with special reference to prior radiation and chemotherapy: a controlled, prospective study. *Gastrointest Endosc* 1998;47:113–120
261. Kocher M, Dlouhy M, Neoral C, et al. Esophageal stent with antireflux valve for tumors involving the cardia: work in progress. *J Vasc Intervent Radiol* 1998;9:1007–1010
262. Mayoral W, Fleischer D, Salcedo J, et al. Nonmalignant obstruction is a common problem with metal stents in the treatment of esophageal cancer. *Gastrointest Endosc* 2000;51:556–559
263. Law S, Tung PH, Chu KM, Wong J. Self-expanding metallic stents for palliation of recurrent malignant esophageal obstruction after subtotal esophagectomy for cancer. *Gastrointest Endosc* 1999;50:427–436
264. Nicholson DA, Haycox A, Kay CL, et al. The cost effectiveness of metal oesophageal stenting in malignant disease compared with conventional therapy. *Clin Radiol* 1999;54:212–215
265. Lightdale CJ, Heier SK, Marcon NE, et al. Photodynamic therapy with porfimer sodium versus thermal ablation therapy with Nd:YAG laser for palliation of esophageal cancer: a multicenter randomized trial. *Gastrointest Endosc* 1995;42:507–512
266. Litle VR, Luketich JD, Christie NA, et al. Photodynamic therapy as palliation for esophageal cancer: experience in 215 patients. *Ann Thorac Surg* 2003;76:1687–1692
267. Law S. Chemoradiotherapy—Panacea for esophageal cancer? Commentary for "Chemoradiotherapy" of locally advanced esophageal cancer. Long-term follow-up of a prospective randomized trial (RTOG 85-01). *JAMA Southeast Asia* 1999;15:9–11

10

Surgical Procedures to Resect and Replace the Esophagus

Philip A. Linden ▪ *David J. Sugarbaker*

Billroth and Czerny described the first esophageal resections in the 1870s, and they consisted of resections of the cervical esophagus without reconstruction. In 1913, Torek described the first transthoracic esophageal resection.[1] He employed a left thoracotomy to resect the esophagus, but did not attempt reconstruction. Instead, a cervical esophagostomy and abdominal gastrostomy were performed. A 3-foot-long external rubber tube was used to connect the ostomies, and it allowed the patient to eat for 17 more years (Fig 10–1).

Ivor Lewis is credited with popularizing transthoracic resection of the esophagus. Initially, he performed the procedure in two stages, first mobilizing the stomach via laparotomy, and several days later resecting the intrathoracic esophagus and reconstructing with the stomach. In 1962, McKeown described a tri-incisional approach. McKeown used a right thoracotomy to mobilize the esophagus. The patient was then repositioned in the supine position, the gastric conduit was mobilized by laparotomy and the anastomosis was performed in the neck.[2] In the past 10 years, total endoscopic approaches for esophageal resection have been developed.[3,4]

▪ NEOADJUVANT TREATMENT

Surgery is recommended for all esophageal cancer patients without metastatic disease who are fit enough for surgery. Nonetheless, the long-term results of surgery alone for esophageal cancer are disappointing. Five-year survival for stage I cancers (T1,N0) is 51%, for stage IIA cancers (T2,T3,N0) is 38%, for stage IIB cancers (T1,T2,N1) is 16%, and for stage III cancers (T3,N1 or T4) is 13%.[5] Preoperative chemoradiation has been proposed as a means of improving long-term survival. Eight randomized trials have been performed employing preoperative chemoradiation. Although the two largest randomized trials of preoperative chemoradiation followed by surgery compared to surgery alone showed no difference in survival,[6,7] two smaller randomized trials have been used to support the use of preoperative chemoradiation. Urba and colleagues looked at 100 total patients randomized to preoperative chemoradiation or surgery alone.[8] Median survival was about 18 months in both groups, although there was a trend toward improved survival at 3 years (30% versus 16%; not statistically significant). Walsh and associates randomized 113 patients, and at 3 years 32% of those receiving preoperative chemoradiation were alive versus 6% of those undergoing surgery alone.[9] Most of the studies to date have been small and have included a variety of stages, and there have been few pre-enrollment staging studies (see Chapter 9).

Recently, the long-term results of a prospective randomized intergroup trial, CALGB 9781 have become available. Patients with stages 1–3 esophageal cancer were randomized to surgery alone or to preoperative cisplatin and 5-FU with concurrent radiation (50.4 Gy) followed by surgery. Poor accrual (most likely due to referring physician bias) resulted in premature closure of the study with 56 patients.

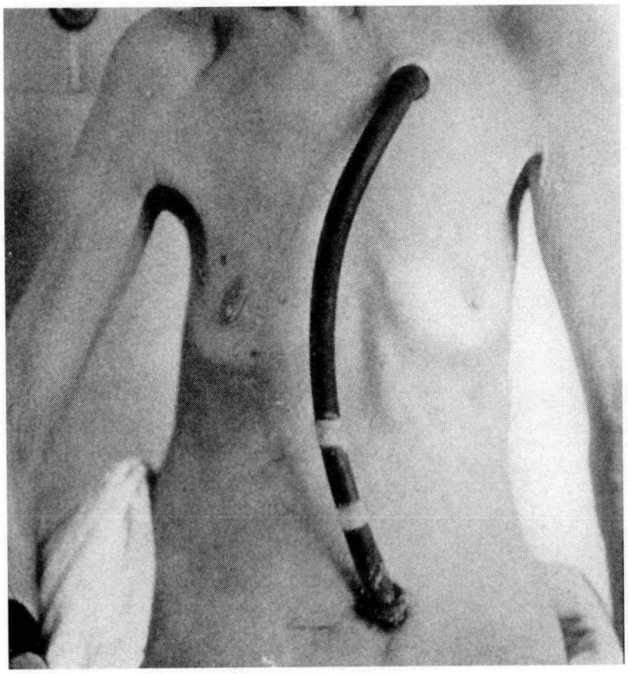

A

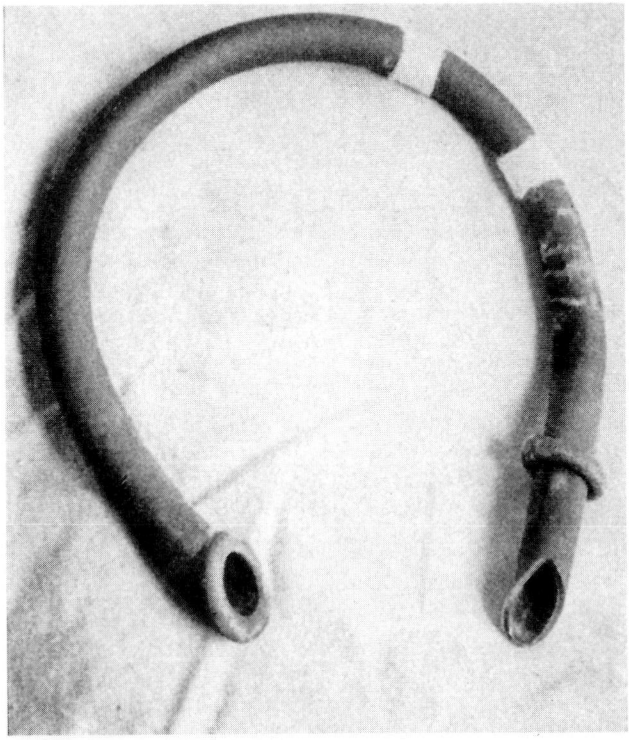

B

Figure 10–1. A. Depiction of Torek's first patient after esophageal resection. The rubber tube connected the lower end of the esophagus with a gastrostomy. The patient lived 17 years after the surgery and died at age 80. **B.** Removable rubber tube conduit with beveled ends. (Reproduced, with permission, from Torek F. The operative treatment of carcinoma of the esophagus. *Ann Surg* 1915;61:385.)

Nonetheless, with median follow up now at 6 years, five-year survival was 39% for the trimodality group vs. 16% for the surgery alone group. Median survival was 4.5 years for the trimodality group vs. 1.8 years for the surgery alone group (p=.02). The dramatic and statistically significant results from this most recent randomized trial provide a strong argument in favor of preoperative chemoradiation in appropriately selected patients.[10]

▪ STAGING

It is important to recognize those patients with stage IV disease, because the mean survival in these patients is less than 6 months. In the past, palliative esophagectomy was often thought necessary to restore swallowing and oral nutrition. With recent advances in photodynamic therapy and expandable endoscopic stents it is unusual that anyone would require esophageal replacement to re-establish swallowing ability. Hence, stage IV patients should be spared the perioperative mortality, morbidity, and recovery time associated with esophagectomy. The appropriate use of neoadjuvant treatment requires accurate staging. Patients with nodal involvement, invasion through the esophagus, or possibly even invasion into the muscularis often undergo preoperative chemoradiation, while patients with simple mucosal involvement generally proceed directly to surgery.

The main staging modalities available today are computed tomography (CT) scan, positron emission tomography (PET) scan, and endoscopic ultrasound (EUS). CT scans are used mainly for detecting distant metastases in the lungs, liver, or other remote sites, including the brain. CT scan may be useful for excluding T4 tumors if a fat plane can be demonstrated between the adjacent structure and the esophagus. Such staging is often not possible if the patient is severely cachectic or if there are no natural fat planes, such as that between the trachea and esophagus. In regard to nodal status, CT is not as sensitive or as accurate as EUS.

PET scan seems to be superior to CT scan for detecting distant metastatic disease. In a series of 91 patients, CT scan had a sensitivity of 46%, a specificity of 74%, and an overall accuracy of 73%. In contrast, PET scan had a sensitivity of 69%, specificity of 93%, and overall accuracy of 84%. All metastases that were missed by PET were less than 1 cm in size.[4] Other studies have shown similar results.[11,12] In addition, PET scan may aid in the diagnosis of primary tumor where it may be difficult to perform biopsy because of obstruction. Conversely, a certain percentage of nonbulky tumors of the esophagus may be PET-negative.

EUS gives detailed images of the esophageal wall and nearby structures (Fig 10–2). Accurate identification of the layers of the esophageal wall is possible. Muscle layers tend to be hypoechoic. The first hyperechoic layer and second hypoechoic layer correspond to the mucosa and muscularis mucosa. The third hyperechoic layer is submucosa. The fourth hypoechoic layer is the muscularis propria, and the fifth hyperechoic layer is the outside of the esophagus. Tumor infiltration of the wall disrupts the normal layered appearance, and extent of penetration is usually clearly visible. EUS has an overall accuracy of 80–90% in ascertaining T status. The differentiation between T1 and T2 is most difficult. In addition, biopsy of deeper layers of tumor not accessible by traditional grasping forceps is possible. It should be noted that EUS is not accurate in defining post-neoadjuvant treatment T status because of fibrosis induced by the chemoradiation.

Nodal status is determined by examining four characteristics. Malignant nodes tend to be round and hypoechoic. They have discrete borders and are larger than 1 cm in size. Nodes that meet such criteria have a 90% chance of being malignant. Fine-needle aspiration (FNA) further increases the accuracy in determining nodal status. If the tumor is from a node, then the cytopathologist should be able to identify lymphoid tissue in the specimen. False-positives can result with FNA if the needle passes through the primary tumor. The accuracy of EUS in N status staging is between 70% and 80%. EUS is 10–15% more accurate than CT scan.[13]

Recent developments in EUS and PET scanning have lessened the enthusiasm for pre-resection operative staging of esophageal cancer patients. Operative staging involving laparoscopy and thoracoscopy is more invasive, but may be superior to EUS. Luketich and associates studied 26 patients and detected N1 disease in a considerable number of patients staged N0 by EUS.[14] It should be noted, however, that the sensitivity of EUS in this series was only 60%, considerably lower than that described in other series. In addition, 15% of patients with no radiographic metastatic disease were found to have liver metastases by laparoscopic staging. The average cost of surgical staging was $20,000–$25,000 versus $2000 for EUS.

A common algorithm used in staging patients includes endoscopy for primary diagnosis, CT scanning with PET to evaluate for metastatic disease, and EUS if the patient is an operative candidate and neoadjuvant therapy is considered. In cases of esophageal obstruction, where EUS scanning is known to be less accurate, the incidence of lymph node metastasis is very high (90%) and neoadjuvant therapy should be considered (see Chapter 9).

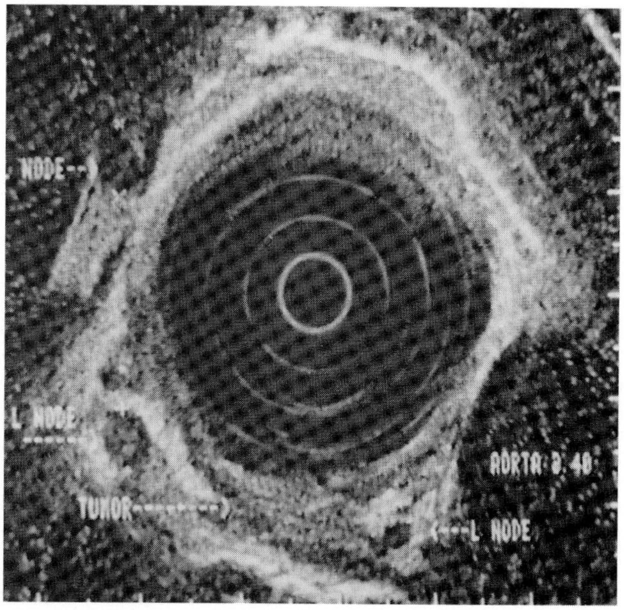

Figure 10–2. Endoesophageal ultrasound image of an adenocarcinoma of the esophagus (T3) and multiple lymph nodes suspicious for metastatic disease (N1). (Reproduced, with permission, from Van Dam J. Endosonographic evaluation of the patient with esophageal carcinoma. *Chest Surg Clin North Am* 1994;4:269–284.)

▪ APPROACH TO THE CERVICAL LESION

The treatment of a cancer of the cervical esophagus is challenging and requires a multidisciplinary approach involving an otorhinolaryngologist, a thoracic surgeon, and occasionally a plastic surgeon. Frequently, radiation will be required preoperatively to maximize margins and spare the larynx, if possible. The neck incision is made along the anterior border of the sternocleidomastoid muscle and can be extended across the midline if additional exposure is needed. If the tumor is fixed to the spine or neck vessels, then the procedure is aborted and palliative radiotherapy is considered. If the larynx is involved, it is removed en bloc with the upper esophagus along with the upper paraesophageal nodes bilaterally. A radical neck dissection is not routinely performed. The dissection spares the jugular vein, sternocleidomastoid muscles, and spinal accessory nerves. The trachea is transected, leaving enough length to allow construction of a permanent end tracheostomy. The endotracheal tube is inserted into the distal trachea and the hypopharynx is divided sharply.

By this point, a separate midline abdominal incision will have been performed, and blunt dissection is begun on the esophagus from the abdomen. A two-team approach should be considered with one team at the neck, while the other prepares the gastric conduit. The gastric conduit is elevated to the neck with traction and the gastroesophageal junction is divided. The pharyngogastrostomy anastomosis is performed using a single-layer, interrupted hand-sewn anastomosis with a nonabsorbable suture. The cervical tracheostomy is performed above the sternal notch. If too much trachea has been resected to allow for this, then manubrial resection will permit placement of the end tracheostomy lower in the midline.

▪ STRATEGY FOR LESIONS BELOW THE THORACIC INLET

Lesions below the thoracic inlet can be divided according to their location in the upper esophagus (below the thoracic inlet but above the carina), mid-esophagus (between the carina and inferior pulmonary vein), or lower esophagus (below the inferior pulmonary vein). While we favor the tri-incisional approach for all malignant lesions (for reasons to be discussed later), lesions in the upper thoracic esophagus generally must be approached with this technique to ensure adequate proximal margins. If the lesion is in the mid-thoracic esophagus, then either the tri-incisional approach or the Ivor Lewis approach may be adequate. Lower esophageal tumors can be resected with either of these two approaches, or additionally with a transhiatal approach or left thoracotomy and distal esophagectomy. With any resection, accommodation must be made for additional resection with reconstruction if frozen margins are involved with tumor.

TRANSHIATAL VERSUS TRANSTHORACIC TECHNIQUES

Numerous retrospective analyses have been performed comparing the transhiatal to the transthoracic (mainly Ivor Lewis) approach. These are summarized in two meta-analyses. Rindani and associates reviewed 44 trials involving either Ivor Lewis or transhiatal esophagectomy that were published in the English language between 1986 and 1996.[15] Overall, the incidence of bleeding, cardiac complications, or pneumonia was no different between the two groups. Differences were seen in the anastomotic leak rate (16% transhiatal versus 10% Ivor Lewis), stricture rate (28% transhiatal versus 16% Ivor Lewis), and incidence of recurrent nerve injury (11% transhiatal versus 5% Ivor Lewis). Mortality was higher after the Ivor Lewis approach (9.5%) than the transhiatal approach (6.3%). Long-term survival was about 25% with either technique. Hulscher and colleagues also performed a meta-analysis of 50 studies published between 1990 and 1999 involving transthoracic and transhiatal resection.[16] Cardiac complications (20% versus 7%), anastomotic leakage (24% versus 7%), and vocal cord paralysis (10% versus 4%) were higher in the transhiatal group as opposed to the transthoracic group. Pulmonary complications (19% versus 13%), in-hospital mortality (9% versus 6%), and operative time (5 hours versus 4.2 hours) were higher in the transthoracic group. Overall long-term survival was similar between the two groups (23% for transthoracic and 21.7% for transhiatal resections). These reviews are retrospective and nonrandomized, and caution should therefore be used in applying these findings to individual institutions and patients.

Three prospective, randomized trials have been performed comparing transhiatal to transthoracic resection. The first was published in 1993 by Goldminc and associates.[17] Sixty-seven patients under the age of 70 with squamous cell cancer were randomized to Ivor Lewis resection or transhiatal resection. Operative time was longer (6 hours versus 4 hours) in the Ivor Lewis group. There was no difference in the incidence of pneumonia (20%), anastomotic leak, recurrent nerve injury, bleeding, perioperative mortality, or length of hospital stay. For those patients with nodal disease, however, none of the transhiatal patients were alive at 18 months, while 30% of the transthoracic patients were alive at 18 months.

Chu and coworkers randomized 39 patients with lower-third esophageal cancers to either Ivor Lewis or transhiatal resection.[18] Limitations of the study were small sample size, short follow-up (mean 15 months), and patient exclusions. Patients undergoing neoadjuvant therapy or those with forced expiratory volume in 1 second <70% of expected were excluded. There were no perioperative deaths in either group. Intraoperative hypotension occurred in 60% of transhiatal patients but only 5% of transthoracic patients. There was no difference in blood loss, pneumonia, or recurrent nerve injury. The mean proximal margin was 3 cm longer in the transhiatal group. No significant difference was seen in tumor recurrence or survival during the brief follow-up period.

The most recent study comparing transhiatal resection to transthoracic, tri-incisional en bloc resection for distal adenocarcinoma of the esophagus or cardia was performed in the Netherlands. One hundred six patients were randomized to transhiatal resection and 114 patients to transthoracic resection. In-hospital mortality was 2–4% in each group. Chyle leak was higher in the transthoracic resection group (10% versus 2%).

Respiratory complications including atelectasis and pneumonia were higher in the transthoracic group (57% versus 27%). Although statistical significance was not reached, 39% of the transthoracic group was alive at 5 years, while only 29% of the transhiatal group survived 5 years.[19]

Meta-analyses show that the incidence of bleeding, ischemic cardiac events, and length of stay are not necessarily different between the transthoracic and transhiatal approaches. Placement of the anastomosis in the cervical position appears to increase the risk of recurrent laryngeal nerve injury, anastomotic leak, and stricture. The mortality rate from an anastomotic leak, however, is less than that of a leak in the chest. The transthoracic approach increases operative time and in-hospital mortality.

The randomized trials show no statistically significant difference in survival, but they are small, and trends toward improved survival are observed in patients undergoing transthoracic dissection. No difference in mortality, blood loss, or incidence of pneumonia was detected. It should also be noted that unlike the meta-analyses, the randomized trials showed no difference in recurrent nerve injury or anastomotic leak. This is a testament to the importance of experience and volume in preventing these complications. Wong and associates noted intraoperative hypotension in 60% of transhiatal dissections, but in only 5% of transthoracic dissections.[20] This finding confirms every surgeon's experience with transhiatal resection. While some may argue that transhiatal dissection may be less taxing on an elderly or debilitated patient (either because of shorter operative time or avoidance of a thoracotomy), the operation may be more taxing to a patient with severe cardiac valvular or atherosclerotic disease who cannot tolerate fluctuations in blood pressure. In these patients, transthoracic esophagectomy is safer.

▪ SURGICAL APPROACHES TO LESIONS BELOW THE THORACIC INLET

TRI-INCISIONAL ESOPHAGECTOMY (MCKEOWN TECHNIQUE)

The tri-incisional technique of esophageal resection combines the most attractive aspects of the Ivor Lewis and transhiatal approaches. It allows for dissection of the intrathoracic esophagus under direct vision with complete nodal resection, and brings the anastomosis to the neck, allowing for maximal proximal margins and minimizing the risk of an intrathoracic leak.

Under general anesthesia, bronchoscopy is performed to rule out tracheal or bronchial (most commonly left main bronchial) involvement with tumor. Esophagogastroduodenoscopy is performed to localize the tumor and rule out disease of the stomach or duodenum. The patient is then reintubated with a double-lumen endotracheal tube and placed in the left lateral decubitus position. A right posterolateral thoracotomy incision is made large enough, approximately 10 cm in length, to introduce the surgeon's hand (Fig 10–3). The serratus muscle is spared. Division of the intercostal muscles anteriorly and posteriorly often permits adequate rib spreading without the need to remove a small portion, or shingle, of a rib. The chest is entered through the fifth or sixth interspace depending on the location of the tumor. The inferior pulmonary ligament is divided using electrocautery and the lung is retracted anteriorly.

Dissection of the esophagus begins at a point away from tumor and any associated scarring, and the esophagus is encircled with a Penrose drain. Traction on the Penrose drain allows for cautery dissection encompassing all adjacent nodes. Arterial branches directly off the aorta are clipped or ligated. The settings on the electrocautery should be low when cauterizing near the trachea. The azygos vein is typically divided, although this is not always necessary (Fig 10–4). At this level, the vagus nerves are identified. Dissection cranial to this level involves the vagus nerves; the vagus nerves are peeled off and away from the esophagus to avoid injury to the recurrent vagus branches.

Dissection between the trachea and esophagus must be done with care and with low cautery dissection to avoid injury to the membranous trachea. Much of the dissection high in the chest can be done bluntly (Fig 10–5). The cranial aspect of the dissection is complete when one's fingers reach easily above the first rib. The Penrose drain is knotted and passed into the lower neck with the knot against the vertebral body for later retrieval during the neck phase of the dissection (Fig 10–6).

Another Penrose drain is used to gain traction on the lower esophagus and dissection continues caudally. All tissue between the pericardium, aorta, and azygos vein is dissected and incorporated into the specimen. No effort is made to resect the thoracic duct, although it is sometimes injured. For tumors near the gastroesophageal junction, a rim of diaphragm is incorporated into the specimen. The knotted Penrose drain is placed in the abdomen for later retrieval (Fig 10–7). At this point, careful inspection is made for hemostasis and injury to the thoracic duct. Often, injury to the thoracic duct is evident when slightly cloudy or crystallized fluid is seen pooling in the region of the duct. If an injury to the duct is seen it should be closed with a pledgeted fine suture such

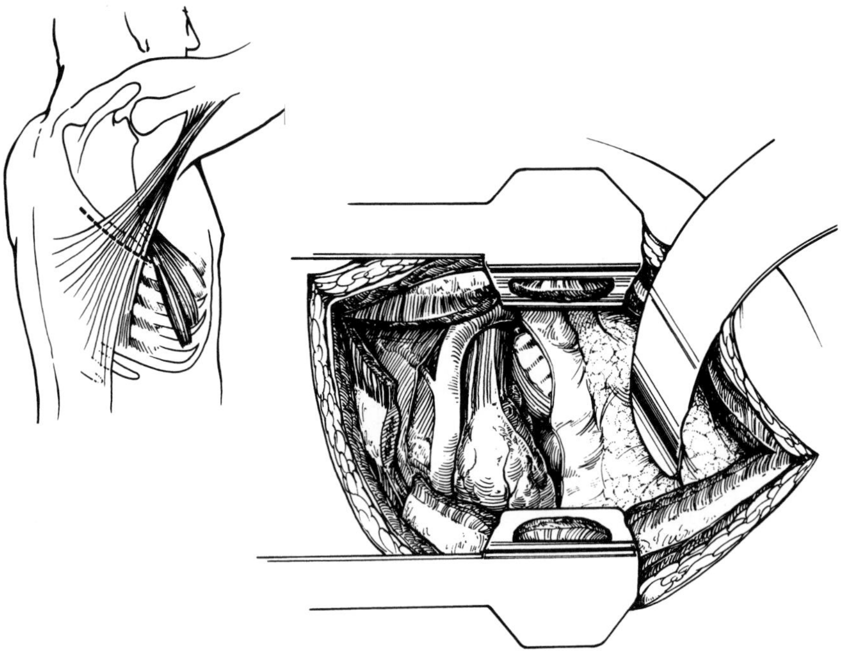

Figure 10–3. The right chest has been entered through the fifth interspace. A piece of the posterior sixth rib has been "shingled" to aid in exposure. The lung is retracted anteromedially and the mediastinal pleura has been incised posteriorly to expose the esophageal tumor. *Inset:* The patient is placed in the left lateral decubitus position. The *dotted line* marks the skin incision for a right posterolateral thoracotomy. The latissimus muscle is divided as caudally as possible and the serratus muscle is spared and reflected medially.

as 5-0 Prolene. Mass ligature of the duct as it enters the chest is then performed by encompassing all tissue between the spine, aorta, and azygos vein at the level of the hiatus with a 0 silk suture. A 28F straight chest tube is inserted via a separate stab incision and directed to the apex of the chest. An additional hole in the tube can be made to facilitate dependent fluid drainage. The ribs are reapproximated with #2 Vicryl sutures. The latissimus layer is closed using a running 0 Vicryl suture. A subdermal layer is closed with 2-0 Vicryl and the skin is closed in subcuticular fashion.

The patient is placed in the supine position and is reintubated with a single-lumen tube. A roll is placed under the back to permit neck extension, and the head is turned to the right. A midline laparotomy is performed from the umbilicus to the xiphoid. Exploration of the abdomen should include a careful palpation of the liver and inspection of the serosal surfaces for tumor implants. Palpation of the GE junction and proximal stomach should be performed to rule out gastric spread of tumor. The left lobe of the liver is mobilized and retracted to the right. The Penrose drain left from the chest dissection is used for retraction of the GE junction (Fig 10–8). The gastroepiploic artery is identified and palpated. The pulse should be easily palpable provided the patient has a physiologic blood pressure. Staying at least 2 cm away from the gastroepiploic artery, the lesser sac is entered. Dissection continues cranially on the stomach along the greater curvature. Dissection may be performed by dividing tissue and ligating with 2-0 silk ties, or by use of an ultrasonic scalpel. The stomach is retracted medially, and the omentum laterally. The artery itself should not be grasped or used for retraction. The gastroepiploic arcade ends near the point where the short gastric arteries begin. A pack placed behind the spleen often aids in exposure of the short gastric vessels (Fig 10–9). The short gastric vessels can be ligated, double clipped, or divided with an ultrasonic scalpel. Large vessels should be tied. Care should be taken not to incorporate stomach wall in the ligature, as this may result in delayed necrosis of stomach wall and a postoperative intrathoracic leak. Dissection on the greater curvature proceeds to the hiatus, and is complete when the Penrose drain is reached.

Proximal dissection on the greater curvature of the stomach proceeds in likewise fashion. The gastroepiploic artery migrates farther from the stomach as one dissects toward the pylorus, and care must be taken not to injure the vessel. The gastrohepatic ligament is divided with cautery up to the GE junction. The stomach is lifted anteriorly, and thin adhesions between the stomach and pancreas are divided with cautery. The left gastric vessels are approached from behind the stomach (Fig 10–10). The vessels are skeletonized, and lymph nodes are swept up onto the specimen.

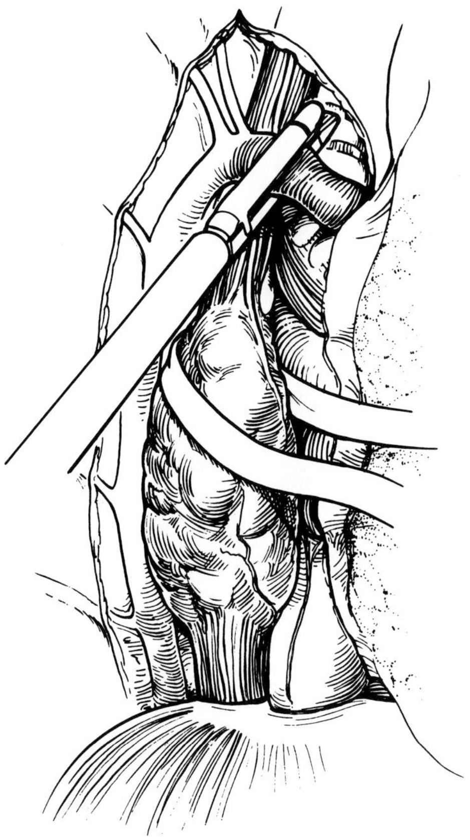

Figure 10–4. The esophagus has been isolated circumferentially at a point superior to the tumor and encircled with a Penrose drain. An endostapling device is used to divide the azygos vein near its caval connection.

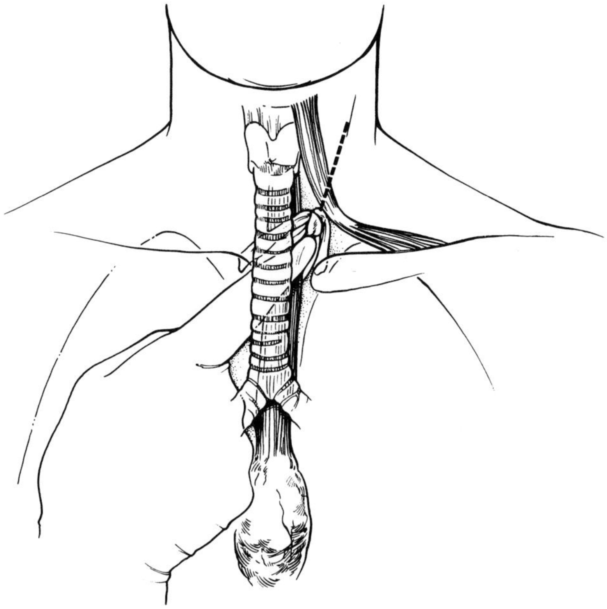

Figure 10–6. The knotted Penrose drain is pushed up through the thoracic inlet and left to lie beneath the omohyoid muscle on the left side of the neck.

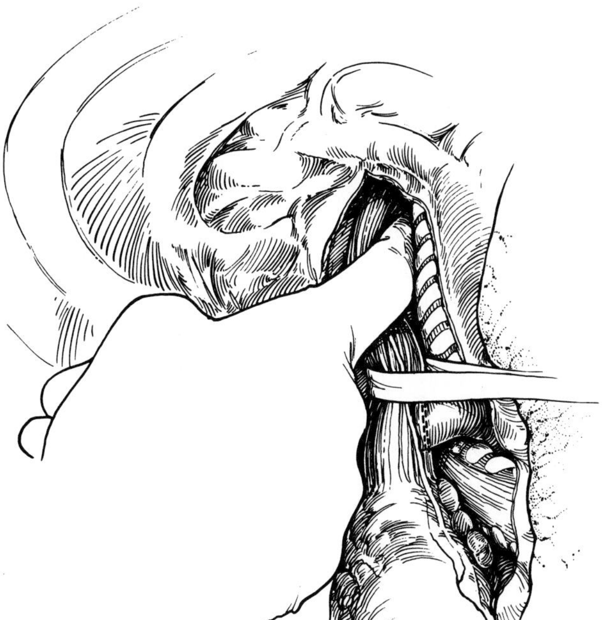

Figure 10–5. With countertraction applied to the Penrose drain encircling the esophagus above the tumor, blunt finger dissection is used to develop the tracheoesophageal plane to and above the thoracic inlet.

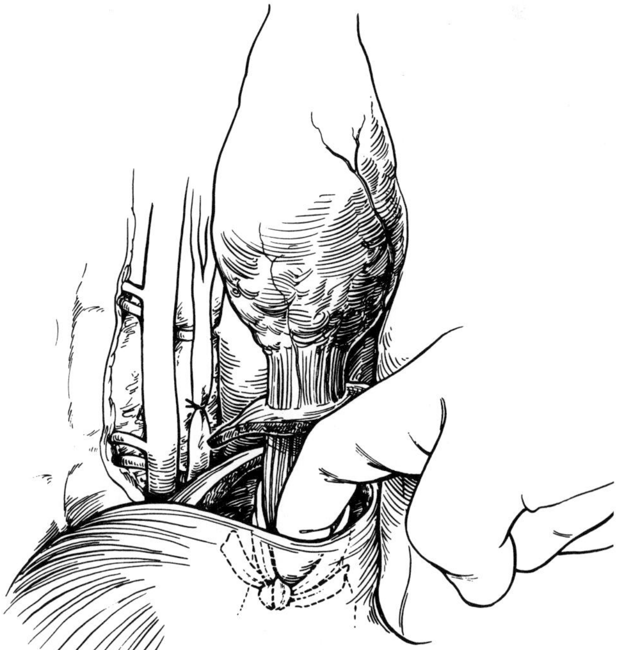

Figure 10–7. The lower Penrose drain is pushed down onto the gastroesophageal junction below the diaphragm. The thoracic duct is shown ligated and a rim of the diaphragmatic hiatus encircles the lower esophagus.

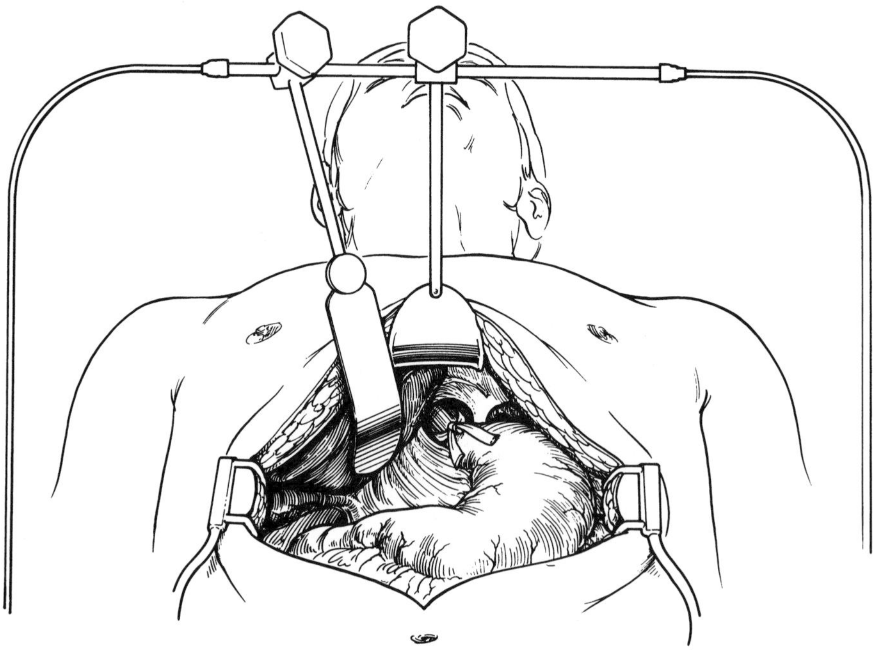

Figure 10–8. Exposure achieved by upper midline laparotomy. The large Balfour retractor is on the lateral abdominal walls and the upper hand retractor reflects the liver to the right exposing the hiatus and lower Penrose drain around the GE junction.

The vessels are clamped with a vascular endoscopic 30-mm stapler. The gastroepiploic pulse should be palpated at this time to ensure that the celiac axis itself has not been clamped, and the stapler is then fired. The duodenum is then mobilized using a Kocher maneuver, bringing it to the midline (Fig 10–11). A pyloromyotomy or pyloroplasty may be performed with equivalent efficacy in aiding gastric emptying. If a pyloroplasty is performed, it is best to close it in a single layer with interrupted (3-0 silk) sutures. A leak is exceedingly rare.

A neck incision is then made 6 cm in length along the anterior border of the left sternocleidomastoid muscle starting at the sternal notch. Deep to the platysma, dissection proceeds medial to the sternocleidomastoid muscle and carotid sheath, and lateral to the thyroid. The omohyoid can be divided with cautery (Fig 10–12). Blunt dissection is then used to approach the vertebral bodies (Fig 10–13). Lying along the vertebral body, the Penrose drain is grasped and brought out into the neck wound with the encircled esophagus. Proximally, the esophagus can be gently mobilized. The nasogastric tube is removed, and the esophagus is divided with a GIA 75-mm stapler (Fig 10–14). A #2 silk suture is attached to the proximal margin and the specimen is drawn out into the abdomen (Fig 10–15). The cervical end of this tie is fastened to a clamp.

The gastric tube is then constructed by resecting the GE junction and the lesser curvature of the stomach down to the crow's foot of veins with a series of thick tissue 75-mm GIA staplers (Fig 10–16). A narrow gastric tube is believed to aid in emptying; however, a diameter of less than 5–6 cm may compromise conduit perfusion. The right gastric artery along the lesser curvature can be divided in order to allow

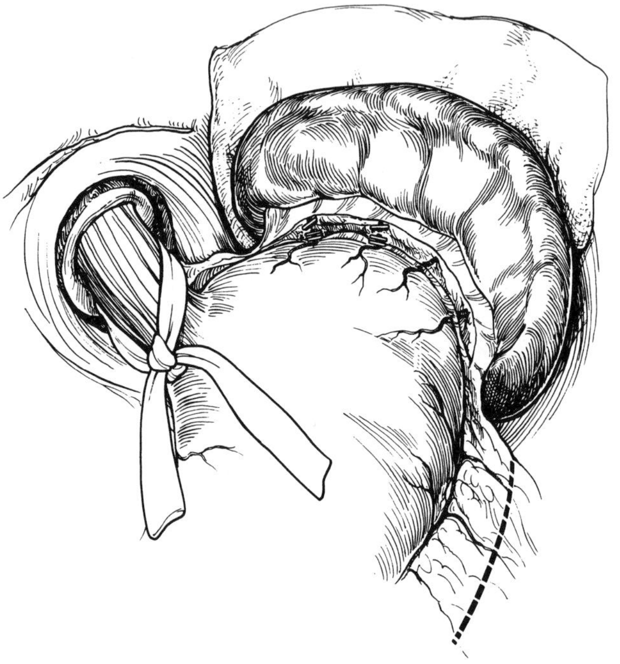

Figure 10–9. Gastric mobilization is begun at the superior greater curvature near the hiatus. A rolled Miculitz pad is placed behind the spleen to aid in exposure. The short gastric vessels between the spleen and the stomach are divided and the transition zone between the left and right gastroepiploic arteries is identified. Mobilization proceeds at least 2 cm away from the right gastroepiploic arcade (*dotted line*).

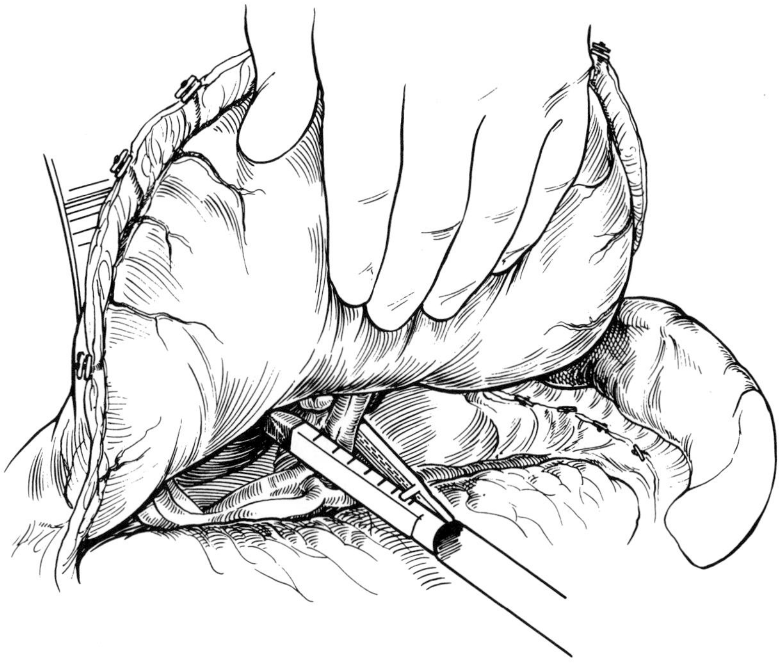

Figure 10–10. After the greater curvature is mobilized, the stomach is reflected superiorly and to the right, exposing the left gastric artery and coronary vein. These are ligated and divided with an endostapler, near their origin, from the celiac axis.

elongation of the conduit (Fig 10–17). The specimen is removed and frozen sections are performed on the margins. Inspection for hemostasis is made of the gastric bed. The esophageal hiatus should admit four fingers. One ampule of IV glucagons is administered to ensure relaxation and lengthening of the gastric conduit. The silk tie that traverses the mediastinum is then attached to the valved end of a Foley catheter with a 30-cc balloon (Fig 10–18). An endoscopic camera bag is secured around the 30-cc balloon (Fig 10–19). The conduit is advanced into the bag, ensuring appropriate orientation. Suction is applied to the bag via the Foley catheter, and the conduit is drawn up into the neck incision (Fig 10–20). The assistant

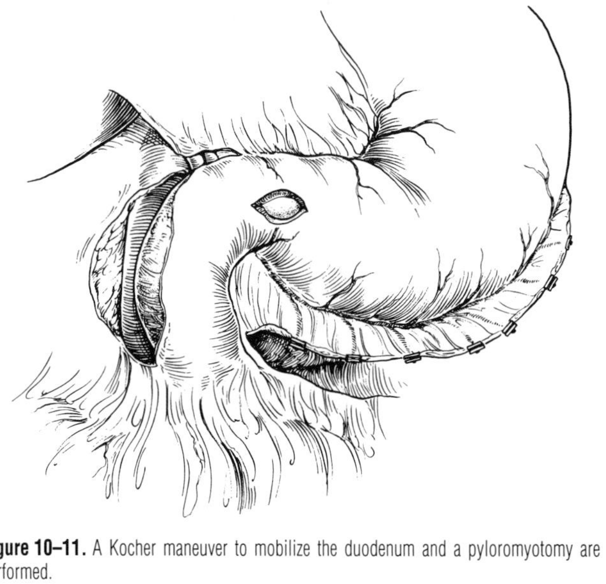

Figure 10–11. A Kocher maneuver to mobilize the duodenum and a pyloromyotomy are performed.

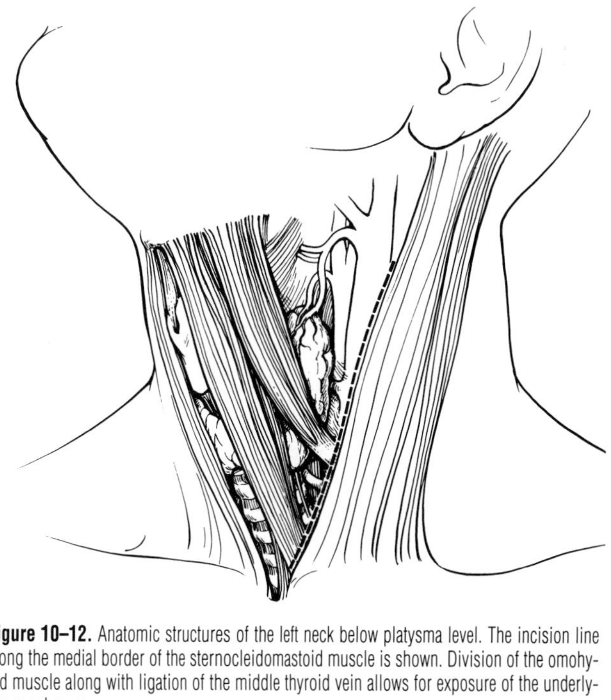

Figure 10–12. Anatomic structures of the left neck below platysma level. The incision line along the medial border of the sternocleidomastoid muscle is shown. Division of the omohyoid muscle along with ligation of the middle thyroid vein allows for exposure of the underlying esophagus.

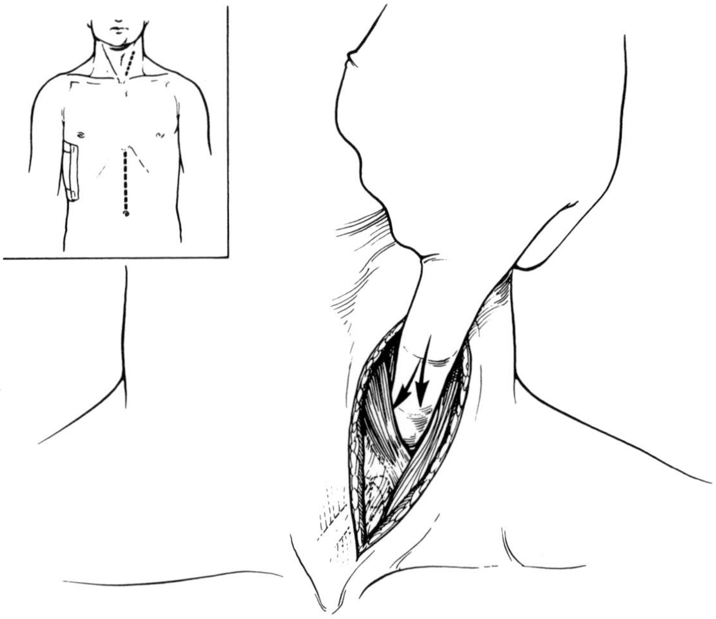

Figure 10–13. Left cervical incision with the sternocleidomastoid muscle reflected laterally. Finger dissection beneath the omohyoid muscle develops a plane to the knotted Penrose drain. *Inset:* The patient is placed supine for the neck and abdominal incisions (*outlined*).

must actively guide the conduit through the hiatus. At the end, the pylorus should sit at the hiatus.

The neck anastomosis can be hand sewn using interrupted full-thickness 3-0 silk sutures (Fig 10–21). The anastomosis may also be stapled in side-to-side, functional end-to-end fashion. A portion of the esophageal staple line is removed, an enterotomy is created on the posterior aspect of the gastric tube, and a linear GIA 75-mm stapler is inserted to create the anastomosis (Fig 10–22). An additional fire of an endoscopic 30-mm stapler may be used to gain additional length on the anastomosis. The enterotomy is usually closed with a TA 30 or 60 stapler after guiding the nasogastric tube down toward the hiatus. Hybrid anastomosis has been described with the back wall of the anastomosis created using a 30-mm stapler and the anterior wall closed with sutures. A soft drain should be placed posterior to the anastomosis and the platysma and skin are closed separately. It is wise to use an interrupted closure, as this will allow for reopening of a portion of the wound should a cervical leak develop. Before closing the abdomen, a J-tube should be inserted at a

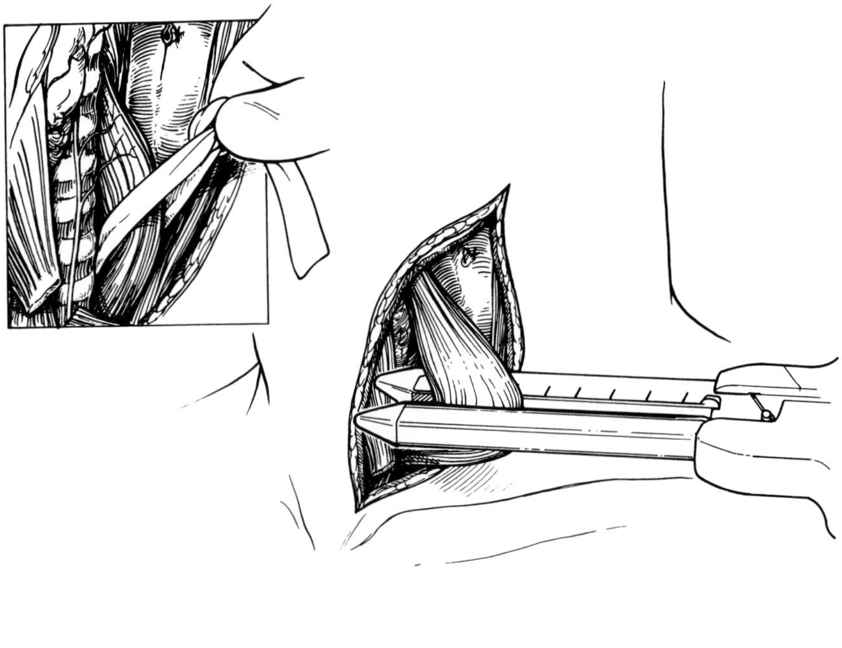

Figure 10–14. A GIA stapler is used to divide the cervical esophagus. Note the ligated middle thyroid vein and divided omohyoid muscle. *Inset:* Traction is placed on the Penrose drain around the cervical esophagus.

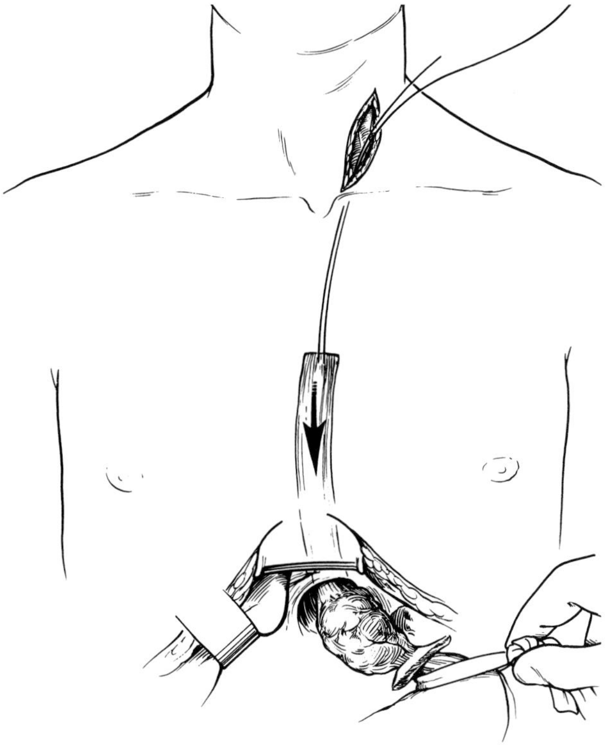

Figure 10–15. The specimen is removed through the abdominal incision with a long heavy silk suture attached to the end of the esophagus.

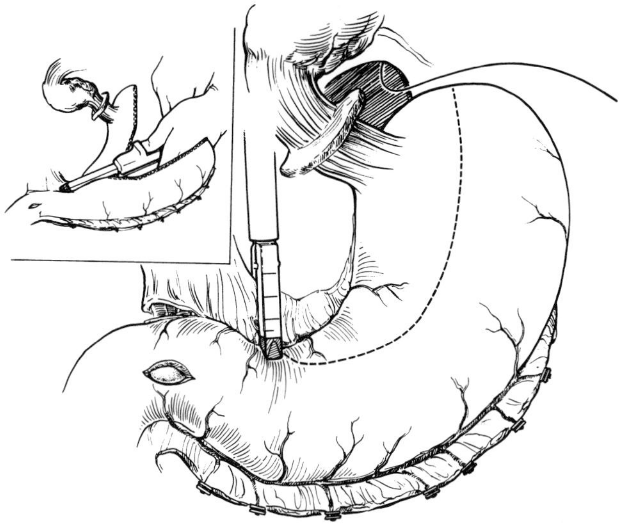

Figure 10–17. The right gastric artery and lesser omentum are divided with an endostapling device. *Inset:* A GIA stapler divides the stomach along the lesser curvature, creating the gastric conduit.

point approximately 40 cm distal to the ligament of Treitz. The fascia is closed using a #2 running monofilament suture and the skin is closed with staples.

IVOR LEWIS TECHNIQUE

The patient is placed in the supine position. Bronchoscopy to rule out tracheobronchial invasion and esopha-

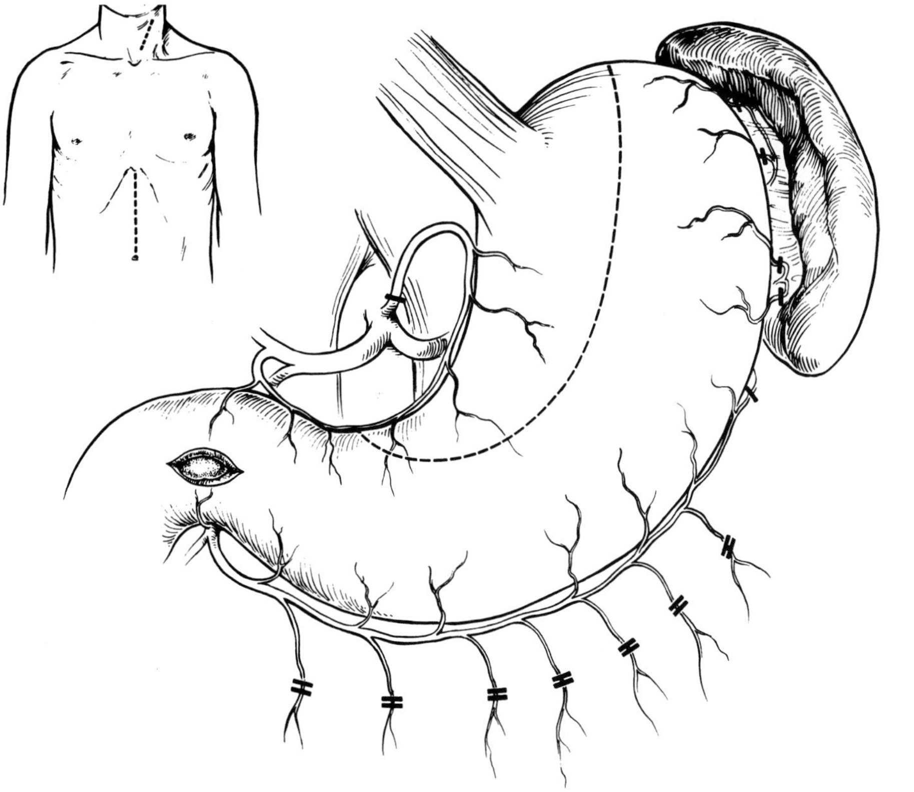

Figure 10–16. The stomach is mobilized as a pedicle based on the right gastroepiploic vessels. *Inset:* Incisions illustrated.

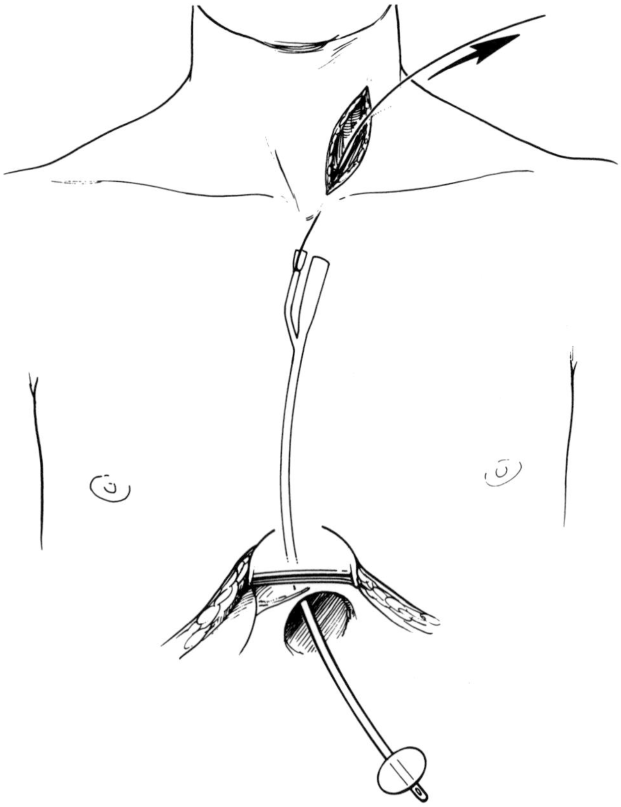

Figure 10–18. The heavy silk is tied to the port of a 30-cc balloon Foley catheter and is pulled up partially through the neck incision.

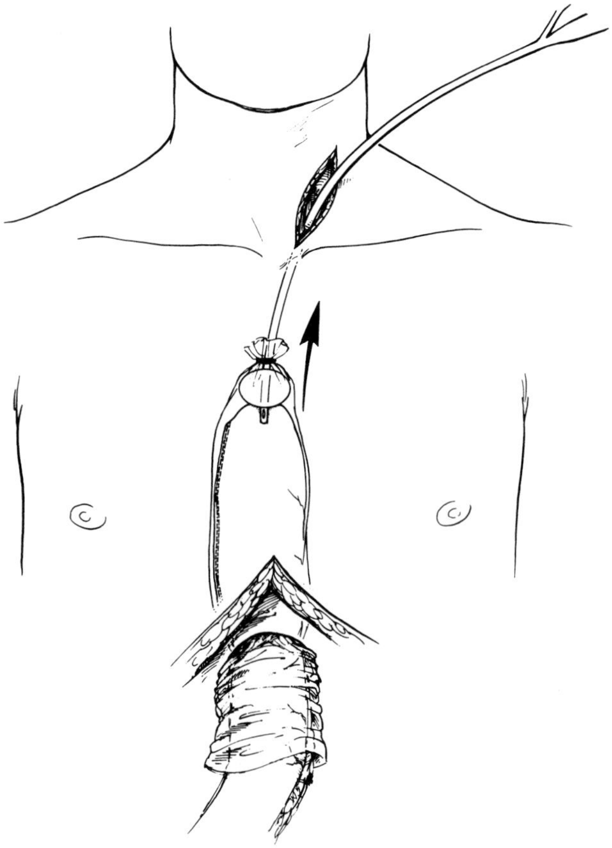

Figure 10–20. The gastric conduit is atraumatically pulled through the posterior mediastinum into the cervical wound.

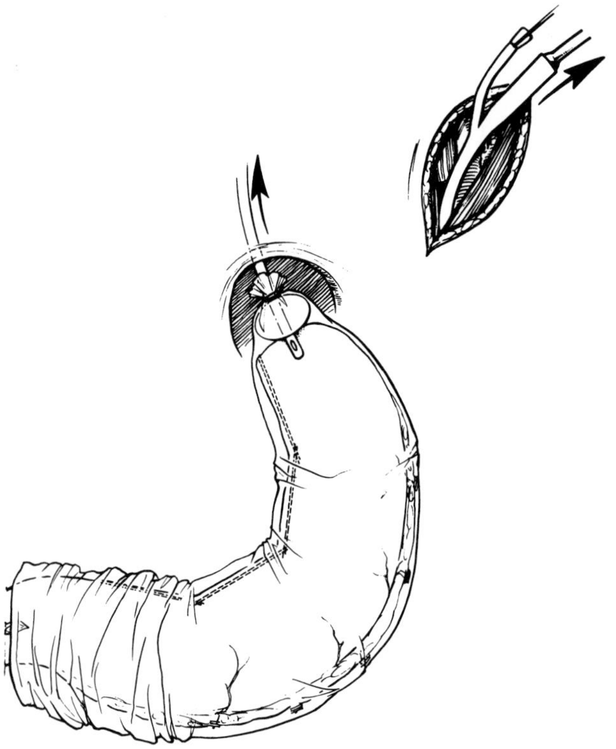

Figure 10–19. An arthroscopy camera bag is tied around the Foley catheter balloon and the gastric conduit is placed in the folded-up arthroscopy bag ensuring the proper axial orientation. *Inset:* A Yankauer suction is attached to the Foley catheter to collapse the bag around the neoesophagus.

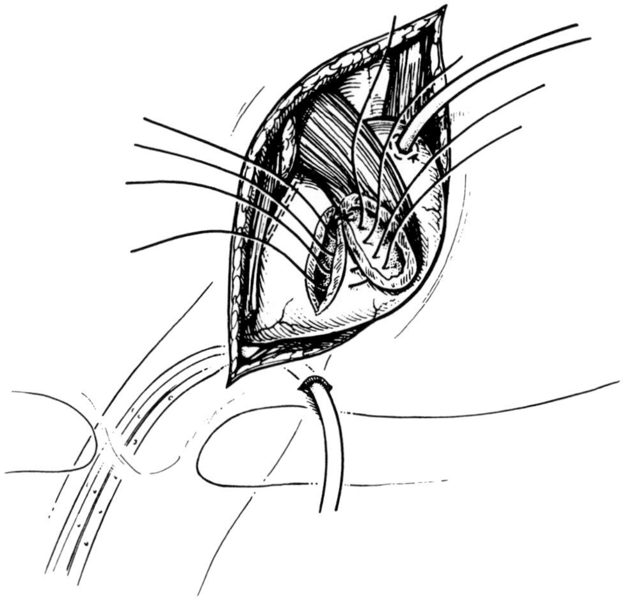

Figure 10–21. The esophagogastric anastomosis is performed with a single layer of full-thickness interrupted nonabsorbable sutures. The Silastic sump drain is shown emanating from the fundus of the gastric conduit. A Jackson-Pratt drain is shown positioned alongside the gastric conduit inferiorly and exiting from a separate stab wound above the clavicle.

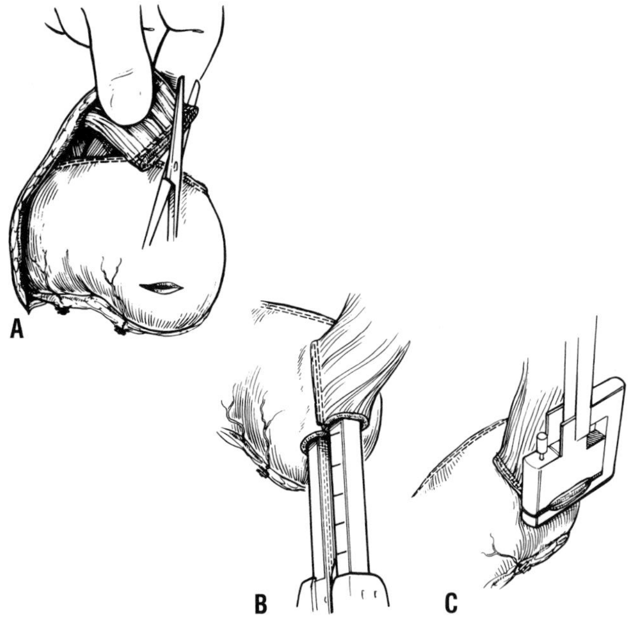

Figure 10–22. A. and **B.** The stapled functional end-to-end anastomosis is performed using the GIA stapler to approximate the side of the esophagus to the anterior wall of the stomach. **C.** The TA linear stapler is then used to close the defect between the two free walls.

goscopy to confirm the location of the tumor are performed. An upper midline incision is made from the umbilicus to the xiphoid. The abdominal phase of this operation is identical to the previously described tri-incisional technique. If the stomach does not need to reach to the neck, then the right gastric artery may be preserved. Enlargement of the hiatus and dissection of the lower esophagus are more easily performed through the abdomen than through a high thoracotomy incision. The stomach is advanced as far into the chest as possible, and a J-tube is placed before closing the abdomen.

A double-lumen endotracheal tube is placed and the patient is re-positioned in the left lateral decubitus position. A right posterolateral thoracotomy is performed, and the chest is entered through the fourth or fifth interspace. A rib is often shingled, allowing for greater spreading of the ribs without fracture. The azygos vein is divided and the intrathoracic esophagus is dissected. All lymphatic tissue is included with the esophagus. Because a gross margin of 5 cm, and ideally 10 cm, is desired, the anastomosis is usually performed high in the chest at or above the level of the azygos vein. The proximal esophagus is dissected only several centimeters above the proposed level of transection to preserve its blood supply. The mobilized stomach is pulled up into the chest. The GE junction and lesser curvature of the stomach are resected using a GIA stapler. The specimen is left attached to the esophagus to facilitate a hand-sewn anastomosis. The anastomosis can be constructed using an EEA stapler or hand-sewn technique. If an EEA stapler is used, a large 33 size should be selected to lessen the incidence of postoperative stricture. If a hand-sewn anastomosis is chosen, a double-layer technique is advisable (Fig 10–23). In 1942, Churchill and Sweet described a method of double-layer anastomosis that is still often used today.[21,22] A point on the gastric tube at least 2 cm away from the staple line is chosen for the anastomosis. A circle of stomach serosa 2 cm in diameter is scored and the underlying gastric vessels are ligated with 4-0 silk sutures. The back outer layer of the anastomosis is constructed with interrupted 4-0 silk horizontal mattress sutures. These are placed 4 mm away from the serosal edge. Full-thickness stomach and esophageal wall are used. The esophagus is opened with a sharp instrument and the inner layer is constructed with interrupted suture incorporating esophageal mucosa and full-thickness

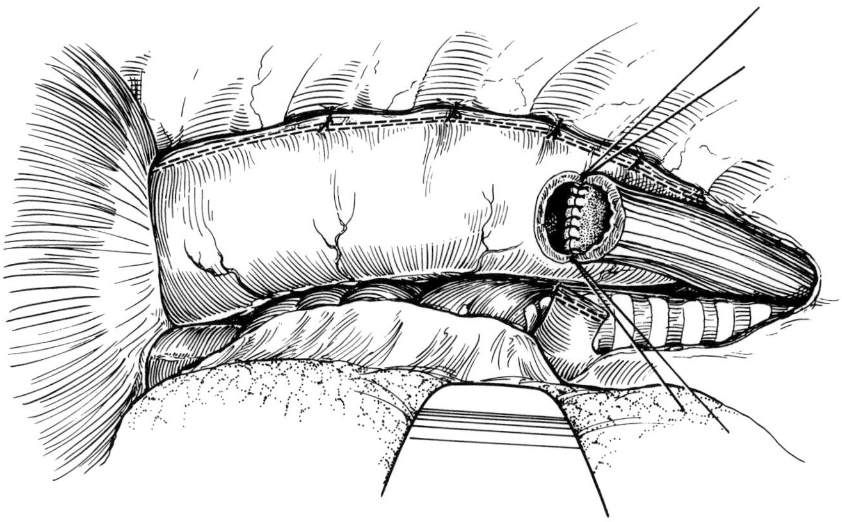

Figure 10–23. View through a right thoracotomy incision showing an esophagogastric end-to-side anastomosis in the apical right chest. Note the tacking sutures from stomach to the posterior chest wall to avoid torsion.

stomach edge. The nasogastric tube is passed after completion of the posterior wall. A continuous Connell suture may also be used. The anterior outer layer anastomosis is constructed with 4-0 silk horizontal mattress sutures. The anastomosis should be wrapped or buttressed with omentum. At all times, atraumatic handling of mucosal edges and tying of sutures without crushing of tissues is advised. Some surgeons advise tacking the edge of the stomach wall to mediastinal tissue or paravertebral fascia to decrease tension on the anastomosis, although it is not clear if this is necessary.

A 28F straight chest tube is placed into the apex of the chest via a separate stab incision. The chest is closed with interrupted #2 Vicryl paracostal sutures, followed by a 0 Vicryl running latissimus layer, a 2-0 Vicryl running subdermal layer, and a 3-0 Vicryl subcuticular layer. Postoperative toilet bronchoscopy should be performed.

TRANSHIATAL TECHNIQUE

Considerations

We believe that a tri-incisional approach gives better exposure to the thoracic esophagus, allowing for a safer and wider resection and better lymphadenectomy. As discussed, there may be survival advantages to the radical resection permitted by the transthoracic technique, although trials to date have not shown a statistically significant survival advantage using this approach. In cases in which the thoracic esophagus is not involved with tumor (either high-grade dysplasia or a laryngeal tumor involving the proximal esophagus), the transhiatal technique may be performed with equivalent oncological efficacy. The approach to the benign mega-esophagus, as seen in achalasia, is also more easily performed through the chest.

Technique

The patient is placed in the supine position with the head rotated 45 degrees to the right. The abdominal phase of the operation is performed in identical fashion to that described in the tri-incisional section above. An upper hand retractor is useful in elevating the sternum and costal margin. The phrenoesophageal ligament is divided using cautery and the lower esophagus is encircled with a 1" wide Penrose drain. If the operation is being performed for a tumor at the GE junction, it is wise to include a rim of diaphragm with the specimen. The phrenic vein must first be identified and ligated. This will also enlarge the window for dissection of the intrathoracic esophagus. The hiatus is dilated to allow entry of the surgeon's hand. Arterial branches from the aorta are clipped on the aortic side and divided using cautery. Thin hand-held malleable retractors are used to retract either side of the pleura during the dissection. Dissection under direct vision is usually possible up to the level of the inferior pulmonary veins.

At this point, an incision is made in the left neck along the anterior border of the sternocleidomastoid muscle starting at the sternal notch and extending 6–8 cm. The platysma is divided. The sternocleidomastoid muscle and carotid sheath are retracted laterally. The omohyoid is often divided. The middle thyroid vein is ligated and divided. A retractor may be used but must not rest on the recurrent nerve in the tracheoesophageal groove. The esophagus is palpated anterior to the spine and posterior to the trachea. Sharp dissection is carried out immediately on the esophagus, separating the esophagus from the membranous trachea and recurrent nerve. The esophagus is looped with a 1" Penrose drain.

Blunt dissection of the posterior plane of the esophagus is performed first. From the abdomen, the surgeon's hand is placed in between the spine and esophagus with the palmar aspect of the fingertips immediately against the esophagus (Fig 10–24). This is performed in conjunction with raising the esophagus anteriorly with the aid of the Penrose drain. An identical maneuver is performed through the cervical incision. When sufficient dissection has been done from either side, both hands are introduced simultaneously and an attempt is made to touch fingertips. Intervening loose areolar tissue must then be torn, uniting the fingertips. If the surgeon's fingertips will not reach from the neck, then a sponge stick can be used. While the surgeon's hand is behind the heart, there must be constant communication between the surgeon and the anesthesiologist. Hypotension often results from compression of the left atrium and impairment of left ventricular filling. It is wise to have the arterial line tracing and numbers in direct view of the surgeon; the surgeon's eyes should be on these numbers as he performs the blind dissection with his fingers.

Dissection anterior to the esophagus is then performed in nearly identical fashion. The palmar aspect of the hand is again kept directly against the esophagus (Fig 10–25). As dissection approaches the carina from below, the surgeon will note an increase in the tenacity of the anterior attachments to the esophagus. Dissection must be gentler in this area. A gentle side-to-side motion of the fingertips will also separate the trachea from esophagus. Eventually the fingertips from both hands are united. Once the anterior and posterior dissection has been completed, the lateral attachments are then divided. From the neck incision, as much blunt dissection of the lateral attachments as possible is performed under direct vision. Next the surgeon's hand is introduced anterior to the esophagus with the

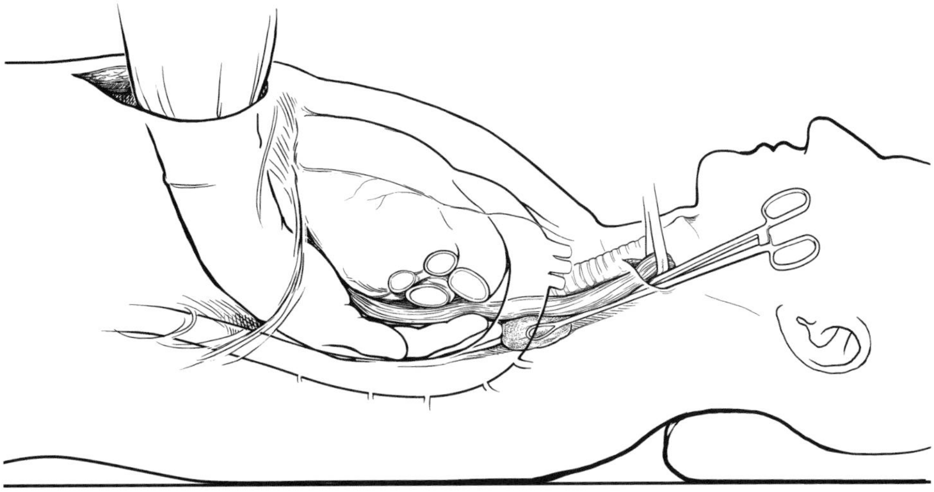

Figure 10–24. Lateral view of the blunt dissection posterior to the esophagus in the chest. A sponge stick is used, as it may be difficult to insert one's hand completely through the cervical incision. (Redrawn, with permission, from Orringer MB, Sloan H. Esophagectomy without thoracotomy. *J Thorac Cardiovasc Surg* 1978;76:643.)

palmar aspect of the hand facing the esophagus. The hand is inserted until the first and second fingers are above the level of dissection of the lateral attachments. These attachments are pressed against the spine, and using a raking motion the surgeon pulls his hand back toward the abdomen, releasing the lateral attachments (Fig 10–26). Care must be taken in the region of the azygos vein and its branches.

The remainder of the operation, including the anastomosis, is identical to that of the tri-incisional technique. After removing the specimen, it is wise to pack the mediastinum with a lap pad (without compressing the heart) to facilitate hemostasis. Prior to drawing the conduit into the neck, a final inspection is made for hemostasis and for entry into either pleural space. If either pleural space is entered, a chest tube should be placed.

LEFT THORACOABDOMINAL APPROACH

Considerations

Limited resection of the distal esophagus via left thoracotomy is almost always a compromise procedure. Only the distal esophagus is readily accessible via the left chest, as the aortic arch obscures much of the upper esophagus. A tumor that extends more proximally than 30 cm should not be approached through the left, as a difficult dissection behind the aortic arch will be required. In addition, placement of the esophagogastric anastomosis low in the left chest can be associated with severe GE reflux. This approach is best reserved for a GE junction cancer that involves a significant portion of the proximal stomach and when there is concern that the residual stomach may be of insufficient length to reach the neck.

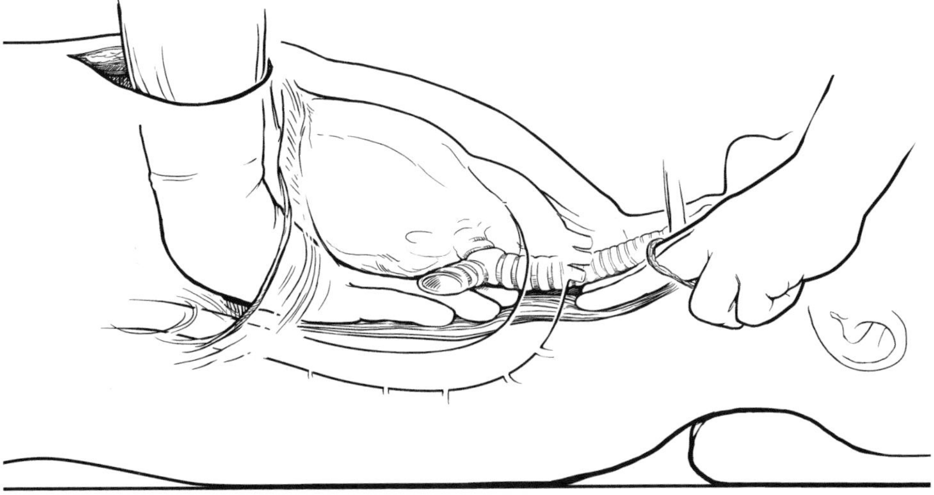

Figure 10–25. Anterior blunt dissection of the esophagus in the chest. Dissection must be gentle and deliberate around the level of the carina to avoid tracheal as well as azygos vein injury. (Redrawn, with permission, from Orringer MB. Transhiatal esophagectomy without thoracotomy. In: Cohn LH. *Modern Techniques in Cardiothoracic Surgery.* Mt. Kisco, NY: Futura Publishing; 1983.)

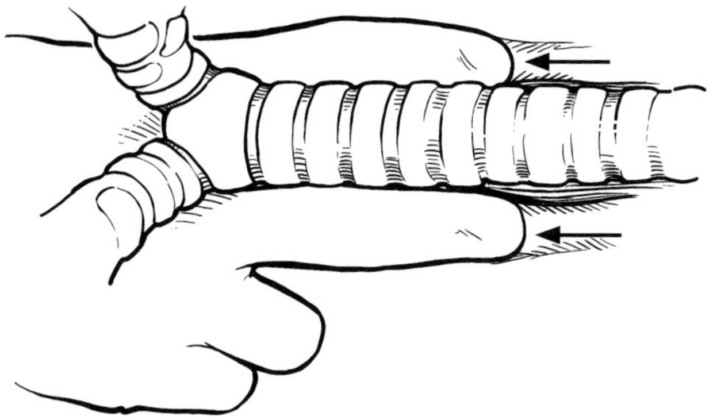

Figure 10–26. The esophagus has been freed from the trachea and the lateral attachments are avulsed from a cranial to caudal direction. (Redrawn, with permission, from Orringer MB. Transhiatal esophagectomy without thoracotomy. In: Cohn LH. *Modern Techniques in Cardiothoracic Surgery.* Mt. Kisco, NY: Futura Publishing; 1983.)

A variety of incisions or a combination of left thoracic and abdominal incisions can be utilized for this approach. An upper midline laparotomy can be extended across the costal margin. This is the least versatile approach and its use is limited to instances in which use of the esophagus is unexpected, as with proximal extension of a gastric tumor. A second approach involves placing the patient in full right lateral decubitus position and taking the diaphragm down in radial fashion 2–3 cm from the chest wall to gain exposure to the abdomen. This approach permits good exposure to the upper abdomen, although exposure of the pylorus and duodenum may be difficult.

Technique

The most versatile thoracoabdominal approach involves positioning the patient in the right lateral decubitus position with the hips rotated posteriorly 45 degrees. A left sixth interspace thoracotomy is performed beginning at the tip of the scapula and extending across the costal margin toward the abdominal midline. The latissimus is divided and the serratus is spared. The costal margin is divided with a rib cutter. The left lung is deflated. The diaphragm is incised circumferentially 2–3 cm away from the chest wall (Fig 10–27). Doing so avoids injury to the radial branches of the phrenic nerve. The abdomen is explored for metastatic disease. Cautery is used to divide the inferior pulmonary ligament. The mediastinal pleura overlying the esophagus is incised and the esophagus is encircled in the lower chest including all tissue from the aorta to the pericardium. The esophagus is dissected proximally behind the inferior pulmonary vein. A proximal gross in-situ margin of 10 cm is ideal, though lesser margins, if confirmed negative by frozen section, may be adequate. A point of division of the proximal esophagus is identified and mobilization above this point is minimized to preserve blood supply to the anastomosis. At the hiatus, a 2-cm cuff of diaphragm is included around the esophagus at the hiatus. The thoracic duct should be located at this level and ligated.

The incision permits excellent exposure of the short gastric vessels, which are ligated starting at the hiatus. Care is taken along the greater curvature, where the short gastric vessels end and the right gastroepiploic vessel begins. The right gastroepiploic artery is preserved. The gastrohepatic ligament is divided. The left gastric artery is identified and all celiac lymph nodes are swept up onto the specimen. The stomach is retracted anteriorly and the left gastric artery is divided with a vascular endoscopic stapler. The gastric tube is constructed by sequential fires of GIA staplers starting at the fundus and extending down to the crow's foot of veins. Six centimeters of distal margin is desirable. A Kocher maneuver and pyloroplasty or pyloromyotomy are performed and the tube is passed through the enlarged hiatus into the chest. The anastomosis is typically constructed inferior to the aortic arch and may be hand-sewn as described in the previous section or stapled.

If needed, the dissection can be carried to the neck with this incision with some difficulty. The proximal

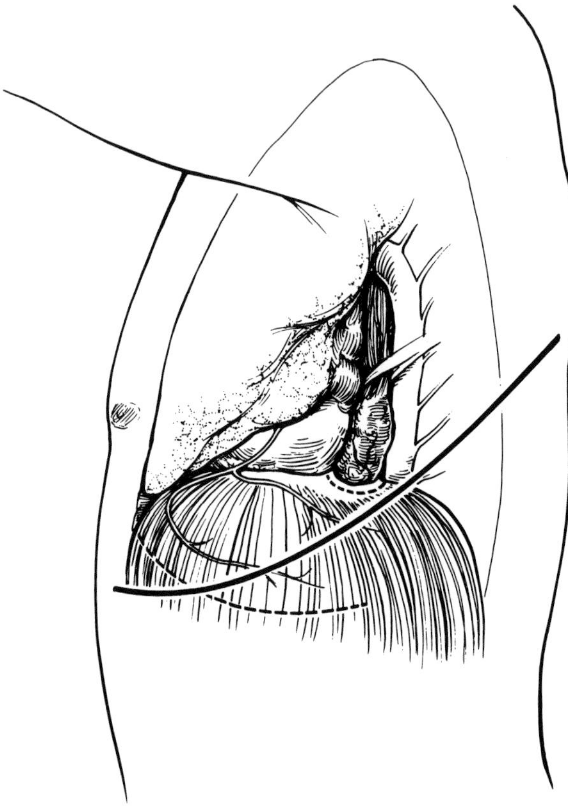

Figure 10–27. Left thoracoabdominal approach; *dotted lines* delineate the circumferential diaphragmatic incision as well as the hiatal margin incision. A Penrose drain encircles the esophagus above the tumor.

esophagus can be dissected bluntly under the aortic arch, and provided the neck has been prepped into the field, a left cervical incision is made as in the tri-incisional technique and the conduit pulled into the neck. Closure begins with careful re-approximation of the diaphragm with interrupted horizontal mattress 0 silk sutures followed by solid reapproximation of the costal margin with figure-of-eight wire or heavy nonabsorbable suture such as #1 Prolene. Some surgeons prefer not to divide the costal margin, and, instead, perform all intra-abdominal work through the divided diaphragm.

▪ ALTERNATE METHODS OF RECONSTRUCTION: COLON AND JEJUNUM

COLONIC INTERPOSITION

The stomach is the preferred organ for esophageal replacement because of its blood supply, the resistance of these vessels to atherosclerotic disease, the need for a single anastomosis, and the ability of the stomach to reach the neck without difficulty. Prior gastric surgery, scarring from peptic ulcer disease, or involvement with tumor may preclude use of the stomach as a conduit. In this instance, colon interposition may be employed. The left colon is preferred over the right colon for several reasons. Its diameter more closely resembles that of the esophagus, its vascular supply has less variation, and greater length can be obtained. Unfortunately, atherosclerotic disease most commonly affects the inferior mesenteric artery, and the left colon is often more affected by diverticular disease than the right.

Preoperative preparation includes colonoscopy or barium enema to ensure normal anatomy and the absence of any intrinsic colonic disease. Patients over age 40 or any patients with atherosclerotic risk factors should undergo mesenteric angiography. Significant vascular disease of the conduit vessel would preclude its use as a conduit. A complete bowel prep and oral antibiotics are necessary prior to operation.

Left Colon

After completion of the thoracic phase of the operation, the patient is placed in the supine position and a midline laparotomy is performed. After a careful search for metastatic disease, the left colon is mobilized by dividing the white line of Toldt and by dividing the attachments to the spleen and omentum. The colon is freed proximal to the hepatic flexure. A careful inspection is made of the vascular supply including the marginal artery of Drummond (Fig 10–28). A pulse should be palpable in the left colonic artery as well as the marginal artery. The middle colic artery supplying the hepatic flexure is clamped with a soft bulldog clamp and its perfusion is inspected for 10 minutes.

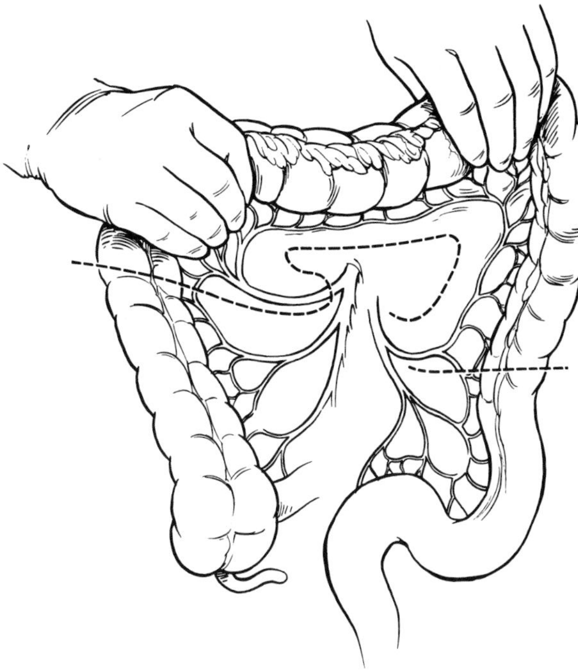

Figure 10–28. The mobilized colon is elevated and the arterial supply and venous drainage are examined. The arterial and venous ligation sites and the mesenteric incision lines are illustrated for an isoperistaltic conduit based on a left colic artery supply.

Prior to conduit isolation, the GE junction is isolated and the cardia and lesser curvature are dissected with division of the phrenoesophageal ligament and the gastrohepatic ligament. The stomach is divided using a GIA stapler. A pyloric drainage procedure is performed. The length of colon needed is estimated by placing an umbilical tie along the proposed route of colonic interposition. This tie is placed alongside the colon and the length of required colon is determined.

After ensuring adequate blood supply to the conduit, the marginal artery is ligated distal to both branches of the left colic artery. The middle colic artery is divided near its origin. The mesentery is scored and divided between clamps. The colon is divided with GIA staplers and the conduit is packed in moist gauze. The colocolonic anastomosis is most easily stapled in side-to-side functional end-to-end fashion. The mesenteric defect is closed with a running suture to avoid internal herniation. The esophagus is identified in the neck and the esophagectomy is completed as previously described in the tri-incisional esophagectomy section.

The colon can be brought to the neck via either the anterior mediastinum (substernal) or the in-situ route (bed of the resected esophagus). The in-situ route is preferred, as it provides the shortest route to the neck (Fig 10–29). In instances of prior infection or scarring

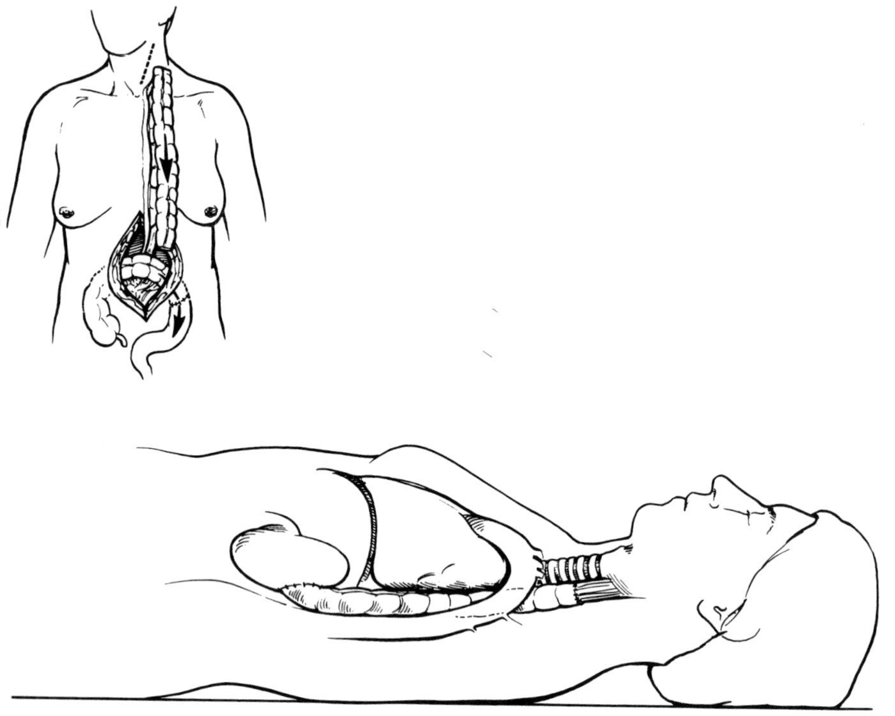

Figure 10–29. Lateral view of the colonic conduit in the posterior mediastinal esophageal bed. Cervical esophagocolonic and posterior cologastric anastomoses are shown. *Inset:* Neck incision marked and left colon conduit mobilized on the anterior chest wall, based on the marginal artery pedicle of left colonic artery and placed in isoperistaltic position.

(as seen with gastric conduit necrosis or leak), the in-situ route may be scarred and unusable. The substernal route may then be used with resection of the manubrium required to prevent acute angulation and possible obstruction in the neck. The colon is oriented in isoperistaltic position and drawn to the neck in an endoscopic camera bag as described previously. The proximal anastomosis is most easily performed using a single layer interrupted technique with fine 4-0 silk sutures. An EEA or functional end-to-end stapled anastomosis is also acceptable. The nasogastric tube is guided through prior to completion of the anastomosis. The cologastric anastomosis is then performed onto the posterior aspect of the stomach. The easiest method of anastomosis employs a size 33 EEA stapler. The handle is placed through an anterior gastrotomy and creates the anastomosis in the posterior wall of the stomach. The gastrotomy is then closed with a TA stapler. The nasogastric tube must be guided through the anastomosis into the stomach. Any excess length in the conduit should be pulled into the abdomen; if it remains in the chest, obstruction may result. The colon is sutured to the left crus of the diaphragm at the hiatus using seromuscular sutures in a two-thirds circumferential fashion in order to prevent herniation of abdominal contents into the chest.

Right Colon

There are numerous conditions that may make the left colon unsuitable as a conduit, including extensive diverticular disease, stricture from ischemia or infection, atherosclerotic occlusion of the inferior mesenteric artery, or splenic vein thrombosis and thrombosis of the inferior mesenteric vein. In these instances the right colon may be used as a conduit to reach the neck. The right colon is mobilized by lysis of its retroperitoneal attachments. The length of colon needed is estimated with an umbilical tape as described previously. The greater omentum is removed from the hepatic flexure and proximal half of the transverse colon. Its mesentery is transilluminated revealing the ileocolic, right colic, middle colic, and marginal arteries. The ileocolic and right colic arteries are clamped in preparation for division of these vessels and mobilization of the conduit based on the middle colic artery. If perfusion appears adequate, these vessels are ligated. The peritoneum overlying the base of the mesentery is scored, and the remainder of the mesentery is divided between clamps and ligated. The proximal and distal ends of the conduit are divided with a linear cutting stapler. Some incorporate the ileocecal valve and distal ileum in the conduit because the diameter of the ileum closely approximates that of the esophagus. Others prefer not to use distal ileum in the anastomosis, as the valve may contribute to dysphagia.

The colocolonic anastomosis is performed with staplers. The right colon conduit is then rotated in clockwise fashion (as the surgeon looks into the abdomen) in preparation for isoperistaltic transfer into the chest. As stated previously, the preferred route is via the esophageal bed. This route is often unavailable for use in colon transposition, as one of the most common indications is a failed gastric conduit placed in the esophageal bed. The retrosternal route is most often used. The diaphragm is bluntly detached from its inferior sternal attachments and blunt dissection with the hand is performed to enlarge the tract. Division of cartilaginous attachments behind the manubrium is also necessary. The conduit is drawn into the neck via a plastic endoscopy bag as described previously. If the thoracic inlet is thought to be too constricting, then the head of the clavicle, manubrium, and anterior aspect of the first rib may be resected. The proximal and distal anastomoses are performed as described for left colon conduits. The conduit may also be passed to the neck via the transpleural or subcutaneous route (with great cosmetic deformity).

JEJUNAL INTERPOSITION

Jejunal interposition may be applied as a free graft, pedicled graft, or Roux-en-Y replacement. Jejunum is often the third choice (after stomach and colon) for esophageal replacement, since it cannot replace the entire esophagus to the neck, but can be used to replace a portion of the distal or proximal esophagus. When distal esophagectomy is necessary for peptic stricture, jejunum or colon interposition is preferred, as both conduits are relatively resistant to reflux. The isoperistaltic conduits are believed to have a lower incidence of recurrent reflux than the simple gastric pull up procedure. Free jejunal grafts are used in limited reconstructions of the cervical esophagus. Patients undergoing jejunal interposition should receive preoperative antibiotics. Although a mechanical bowel preparation is not needed, it should be used if it is possible that colon may be needed.

Roux-en-Y Replacement

Roux-en-Y replacement is most commonly used after total gastrectomy and distal esophagectomy (Fig 10–30). Unlike stomach, it will not reliably reach to the cervical esophagus. The jejunum is divided approximately 20–30 cm beyond the ligament of Treitz. The jejunum and its mesentery are held up and its arcade is transilluminated. The proposed point of division is identified, as are the mesenteric vessels to be divided. The first few arcades are not divided to preserve blood flow to the native jejunum. Up to 60 cm of jejunum can be mobilized using this technique. The mesentery is scored and these vessels are clamped near their origin from the superior mesenteric artery with soft bulldog clamps. The conduit is observed for about 10 minutes for evidence of ischemia.

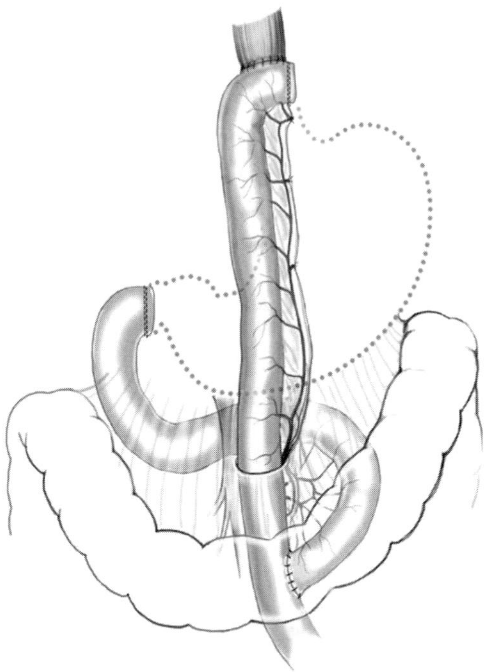

Figure 10–30. Roux-en-Y jejunal replacement of the distal esophagus.

The vessels are then ligated and divided. A hole is made in the transverse mesocolon to the left of the middle colic artery, just large enough to pass the jejunum and its mesentery. For replacement after total gastrectomy, the proximal anastomosis is made to the very distal esophagus in the upper abdomen. If resection of the distal esophagus is required, the incision is usually extended across the costal margin to the sixth or seventh interspace. If additional length is needed on the conduit, the next vessel in the arcade is identified, test clamped, and then divided. The anastomosis can be performed by stapled or hand-sewn technique. The stapled anastomosis is most easily performed with an EEA stapler. The largest EEA stapler possible should be used for the anastomosis. The distal esophagus may first be dilated with a lubricated metal dilator. A full thickness 2-0 Prolene suture is used to create a purse-string in the distal esophagus. The shaft may be introduced by opening the stapled end of the jejunum. It can then be passed out the side of the jejunum and united with the anvil. Care must be taken not to occlude the ongoing lumen of the jejunum with the stapler. Two full-thickness anastomotic doughnuts should be verified. After removing the stapler, the jejunal end is closed with a TA 60 stapler. A hand-sewn anastomosis in one or two layers can also be performed. The jejunum is tacked to the hiatus at several points using interrupted silk sutures. This prevents herniation of abdominal contents into the chest and limits tension on the esophagojejunal anastomosis. Likewise, defects in the colonic mesentery should be closed to prevent an internal hernia. The distal anastomosis can be hand-sewn or more rapidly performed with a side-to-side functional end-to-end stapled anastomosis.

Pedicled Jejunal Interposition

Pedicled jejunal interposition is most often used to replace a strictured distal esophagus (Fig 10–31). A left thoracoabdominal incision is employed with a left seventh interspace incision extended across the costal margin and rectus muscle. The jejunum is transilluminated and an appropriate length of jejunum is selected, beginning 20 cm beyond the ligament of Treitz. A single large vessel is chosen as the conduit feeder vessel. The jejunum is transected proximally and distally using a GIA stapler, and the mesentery is divided down each side toward the feeder vessel (Fig 10–32A). The jejunum is reconnected using a side-to-side functional end-to-end stapled anastomosis (Fig 10–32B). The pedicled jejunum is tunneled through the colonic mesocolon and brought up to the left chest through an enlarged hiatus. (Figure 10–33) The proximal anastomosis can be constructed with an EEA stapler (usually 28 cm in size, but a larger anastomosis may be more resistant to postoperative stricture). The jejunogastric anastomosis is easily performed using an EEA stapler (inserting the handle through a separate gastrotomy). A two-layered hand-sewn anastomosis may also be used.

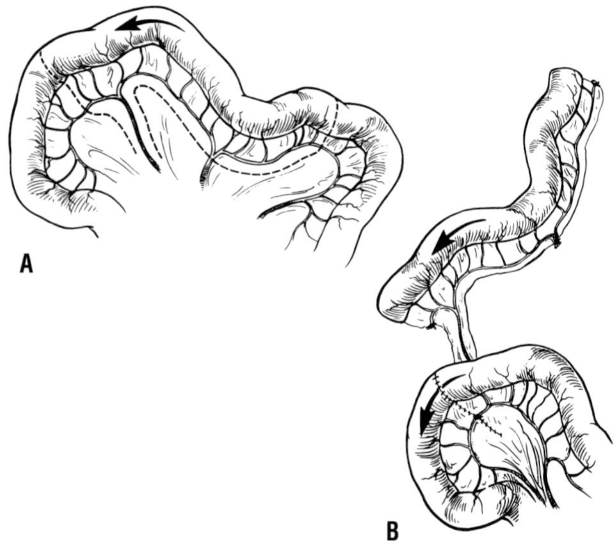

Figure 10–32. A. The jejunum is prepared in an isoperistaltic fashion (*arrows*) based on a distal mesenteric branch and proximal marginal arcade. The *dotted line* illustrates the line of resection of mesentery and the division of vessels. **B.** After dividing the mesentery and preserving the pedicle, jejunal continuity is restored and the mesenteric defect closed.

Free Jejunal Transfer

Free jejunal transfer is needed if the pedicle is not of sufficient length, such as in replacement of a portion of the cervical esophagus for benign disease. It is not clear

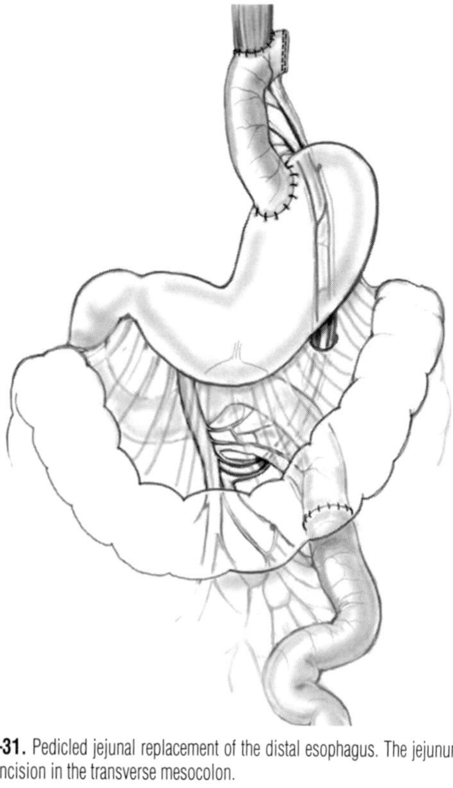

Figure 10–31. Pedicled jejunal replacement of the distal esophagus. The jejunum is brought through an incision in the transverse mesocolon.

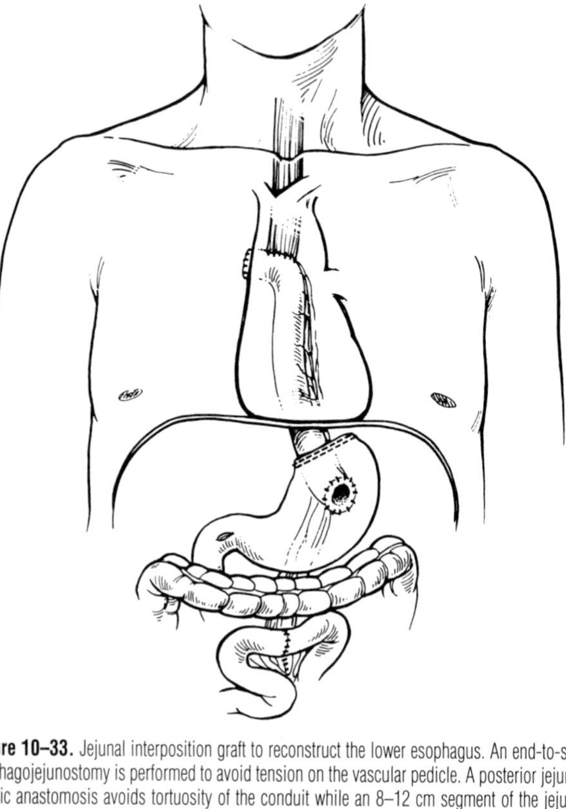

Figure 10–33. Jejunal interposition graft to reconstruct the lower esophagus. An end-to-side esophagojejunostomy is performed to avoid tension on the vascular pedicle. A posterior jejunogastric anastomosis avoids tortuosity of the conduit while an 8–12 cm segment of the jejunal graft situated below the hiatus aids in the control of reflux.

whether use of a free jejunal transfer is preferable to total esophagectomy and gastric pull-up. The use of jejunum does carry a lower incidence of postoperative reflux, and avoids dissection of the thoracic esophagus; however, there is increased risk of graft ischemia and gangrene. Two anastomoses are required and there is an increased risk of anastomotic leak. As with a pedicled jejunal graft, a short segment of jejunum is chosen for harvest. A left cervical incision is made, and the esophagus as well as the carotid artery and jugular vein are isolated. A dominant feeder vessel in the jejunal segment is identified and divided with a scalpel. The artery and vein are flushed with heparinized saline. The proximal anastomosis is constructed first and is performed with a two-layer end-to-side hand-sewn anastomosis. An operating microscope is then used to perform the arterial and venous anastomosis to the carotid artery and jugular vein with 9-0 or 10-0 Prolene suture. The distal anastomosis is then performed in fashion identical to the proximal anastomosis (Fig 10–34). Typically, a meshed skin graft is placed over the conduit for continuous postoperative monitoring. A feeding jejunostomy tube is placed as with every case of esophageal replacement.

▪ COMPLICATIONS AND HOW TO AVOID THEM

ANASTOMOTIC LEAK

The incidence of anastomotic leak is higher following cervical anastomosis (10–15%) than intrathoracic anastomosis (5–10%).[15,22,23] The incidence of leak is believed to be higher in the cervical position for several reasons. First, increased length is needed and this may place increased tension on the anastomosis. The tip of the stomach, which is used in the cervical anastomosis, may have a more tenuous blood supply, as it is farther from the gastroepiploic artery. Additionally, venous engorgement due to a tight thoracic inlet may impair blood supply. A recent analysis of anastomotic leaks found that albumin level below 3 g/dL, positive margins, and cervical anastomosis were risk factors for anastomotic leak following esophagectomy.[24] A randomized comparison of hand-sewn versus stapled anastomosis in 102 patients undergoing Ivor Lewis esophagectomy did not show any significant difference in the incidence of anastomotic leak. The incidence was 5% after a single-layer monofilament anastomosis and 2% after a stapled anastomosis.[25] The incidence of leak following hand-sewn anastomosis is more operator-dependent, and those who perform few of these procedures may wish to use a stapled technique.

Anastomotic leak following Ivor Lewis esophagectomy is a feared complication that in the past was associated with a 50% mortality rate. Centers that routinely employ this technique have refined their techniques resulting in very low leak rates in the 2% range. Early detection and aggressive management can reduce the high mortality rate usually associated with this complication. Unexplained fever, elevated white cell count, respiratory failure, delirium, hypotension, or low urine output may signal the onset of an intrathoracic leak. Confirmation is usually possible by Gastrografin swallow or instillation of contrast through the nasogastric tube. Immediate intervention is required, and attempts at direct repair with muscle flap reinforcement and wide drainage are often successful. Patients who are un-

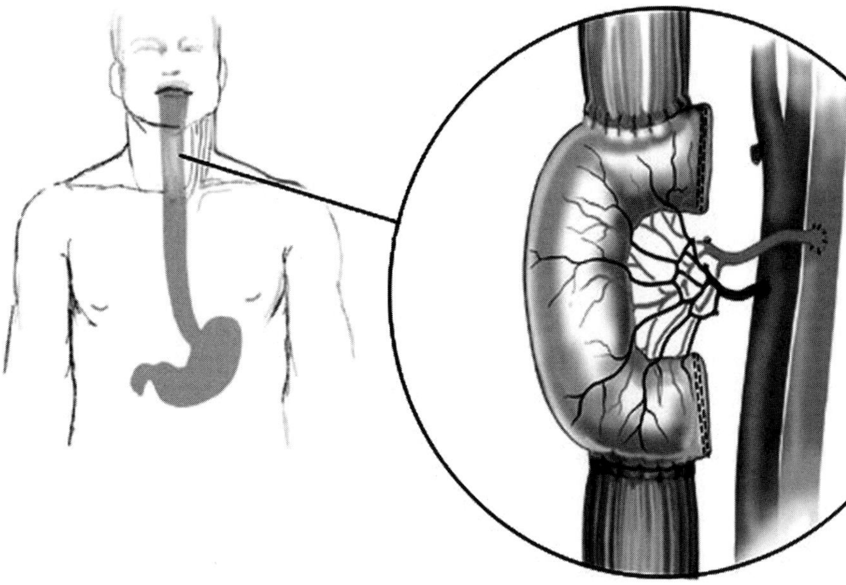

Figure 10–34. Free jejunal graft used as a cervical esophageal replacement. It is typically covered with a meshed skin graft so that conduit health can be observed postoperatively.

stable or severely ill should be diverted with a spit fistula, and either excluded at the hiatus, or have the conduit closed and returned to the abdomen. In rare instances, a clinically silent, small, contained leak that is not adjacent to vital structures such as the trachea or aorta may be observed and treated with strict NPO status and enteral feeds.

Although leak is more common following cervical anastomosis, it is rarely life-threatening. Occasionally a cervical anastomosis may leak into the chest, and must be treated like an intrathoracic leak. Initially, mortality from a cervical leak was estimated at 20%, though recent series have shown that the mortality is much lower.[26] Cervical anastomotic leak is usually signaled by fever, erythema, and fluctuance in the neck incision. Opening of the neck incision and probing down to the prevertebral fascia (with placement of a drain) is usually all that is needed. Patients can be allowed clear liquids by mouth and may be fed via jejunostomy tube until the leak is sealed. Barium swallow following esophagectomy may miss 10% of cervical leaks. Giving patients purple grape juice to drink and observing the drain during swallow may detect leaks missed by barium swallow.

ANASTOMOTIC STRICTURE

The same risk factors that predispose to anastomotic leak also predispose one to stricture. Indeed, it is very common to present with stricture following treatment for an anastomotic leak. Retrospective meta-analyses have shown that the incidence of stricture is higher after cervical reconstruction (28%) than after Ivor Lewis reconstruction (16%).[18] The definition of stricture is not precise, and is usually determined by the need for intervention (i.e., dilatation). As some surgeons are more aggressive than others with regard to dilatation, this value may be misleading. A retrospective analysis of transhiatal esophagectomy patients revealed that the use of a stapled anastomosis, anastomotic leak, and the presence of cardiac disease were the only risk factors associated with the development of stricture.[27] Other studies have mentioned intraoperative blood loss and poor conduit vascularization as risk factors. A unifying theme in anastomotic stricture (other than mechanical stapler issues) is impaired blood supply to the region of anastomosis. In an effort to avoid ischemia, it is wise not to place the anastomosis too close to the tip of the gastric conduit. Careful handling of the gastroepiploic artery, ensuring systemic oxygen delivery, and avoidance of congestion all are important in avoiding anastomotic leak and stricture.

Mechanical factors may also contribute to development of stricture, especially when an EEA stapled anastomosis is performed. In a randomized evaluation of the EEA stapler for Ivor Lewis anastomosis, the incidence of stricture was found to be 40% with a stapled anastomosis versus 9% with a hand-sewn anastomosis. When a small (25-mm) EEA stapler was used, the incidence of stricture was 43% as opposed to a 12.5% incidence with a 29-mm stapler, and no strictures seen with a 33-mm stapler.[25]

Postoperative strictures may nearly always be managed by bougie dilation. Often repeat dilations are needed. In the above-mentioned study of strictures following Ivor Lewis esophagectomy, 53% of patients needed one dilatation, 20% required two, 12% required three, and 8% required four. No patient was treated with reoperation. In Honkoop and associates' study of anastomotic stricture following transhiatal esophagectomy, the average patient required three dilations to achieve normal swallowing. Perforations occurred in two of the 519 patients requiring dilation.[27]

RECURRENT LARYNGEAL NERVE INJURY

The clearest risk factor for recurrent nerve injury is cervical anastomosis. In a retrospective analysis, the incidence of recurrent nerve injury with a cervical anastomosis was double (11%) that for intrathoracic anastomosis (5%).[15] The recurrent nerve can be injured at any point, from its "recurrence" from the vagus nerve (around the subclavian artery on the right and around the aortic arch on the left), to its course in the tracheoesophageal groove, to its insertion into the larynx. Although an Ivor Lewis resection should not touch the recurrent nerve, traction or cautery injury to the vagus nerve may cause injury to the recurrent nerve.

A left neck incision is often used to approach the cervical esophagus. The right recurrent nerve is farther from the esophagus than the left, and it is easier to avoid the right nerve from a left neck incision than it is to avoid the left nerve from a right neck incision. During neck dissection, it is important to stay immediately against the esophagus in order to avoid injury to the nerve. In a review of tri-incisional esophagectomy by Swanson and colleagues, refinements in technique resulted in a reduction of recurrent nerve injury from 14% to 7%.[28] In the Brigham and Women's Hospital technique, the vagus nerves are divided at the level of the azygos vein, and cranial dissection of the esophagus proceeds within the nerves. A Penrose drain is used to surround the esophagus and is positioned in the neck for later retrieval during the cervical phase of the operation to ensure isolation of the esophagus inside the recurrent nerves.

Early recognition and aggressive treatment is necessary to minimize respiratory complications from recurrent nerve injury. Recurrent nerve injury prevents cord apposition, making an effective cough impossible and interfering with protective reflexes involved in swallowing. Hoarseness is present with recurrent nerve injury, but may be present after any intubation. Loss of effective cough is another hallmark of recurrent nerve injury, but may not be present immediately following extubation, since there may be swelling of the cords after use of a double-lumen tube, a prolonged operation, and large fluid shifts. Effective cough may be lost between 24 and 48 hours after extubation as cord swelling decreases. Any patient with hoarseness and ineffective cough should undergo fiberoptic laryngoscopy. Immediate injection of the affected cord with gelfoam will allow an effective cough and clearance of secretions.

RESPIRATORY COMPLICATIONS

In early series, anastomotic leak and infection were the most common cause of death following esophagectomy. In modern series, the most common cause of death is respiratory failure. The incidence of pneumonia following esophagectomy ranges from 2–57%.[19,23] The assumption that the incidence of pneumonia is higher with transthoracic esophagectomy than transhiatal esophagectomy has not been definitively borne out by the literature. A large meta-analysis by Rindani and coworkers showed no difference in incidence of pneumonia between the two techniques.[15] Two randomized trials, one by Goldminc and associates and one by Chu and colleagues, also showed no difference in the incidence of pneumonia.[17,18] A more recent, larger randomized trial comparing tri-incisional, en bloc esophagectomy with transhiatal esophagectomy did show a higher incidence of combined atelectasis and pneumonia in the tri-incisional group (57%) versus the transhiatal group (27%). The unexpectedly high incidence of pulmonary complications in the transthoracic group should be questioned, as reported rates are typically around 20–35%.[13,14]

A variety of modifications and maneuvers can be employed to limit the incidence of pulmonary complications. All efforts must be made to spare injury to the recurrent nerve, and if injured, aggressive intervention including cord medialization is necessary. Efforts at limiting pain associated with thoracotomy, including a limited muscle-sparing thoracotomy, are helpful. The use of thoracic epidurals has been shown to decrease the incidence of pulmonary complications in thoracotomy patients. Early ambulation and aggressive pulmonary toilet are necessary. It has yet to be determined whether avoidance of thoracotomy by totally thoracoscopic dissection of the esophagus will decrease the incidence of respiratory complications.

BLEEDING

Bleeding following esophagectomy occurs about 5% of the time regardless of the technique used. Meta-analyses have shown that estimates of blood loss are slightly higher with the transthoracic group as opposed to the transhiatal group.[16] Preoperatively, antiplatelet agents should be stopped well in advance of surgery. Low-dose subcutaneous heparin or low-dose low-molecular-weight heparin should not increase the incidence of perioperative bleeding. Intraoperatively, arterial branches from the aorta to the esophagus should be clipped whenever possible. If blunt dissection is used, staying immediately against the esophagus should help avoid larger arteries, as the esophageal arterioles tend to form a fine plexus of vessels approximately 1–2 cm away from the wall of the esophagus. A notorious site of bleeding during the transhiatal dissection is the azygos vein or one of its branches. This bleeding usually occurs at about the level of the carina, and as always, extra care should be taken at this level. A common site of bleeding after any thoracotomy is the chest wall itself, including intercostal vessels; these should be inspected after removing the retractor.

CHYLE LEAK

The thoracic duct enters the chest through the aortic hiatus and lies between the spine, azygos vein, and aorta at the level of the diaphragm. At approximately the T6 level, it crosses to the left side and eventually empties into the left subclavian vein. The incidence of chyle leak following esophagectomy ranges from 2–10% and is at greatest risk during en bloc resection. If the thoracic duct is taken during en bloc dissection, then the duct is ligated at the hiatus and inspected for leak. It is wise to inspect the area of the thoracic duct at the end of any transthoracic dissection of the esophagus. Often, clear fluid (in the unfed patient) can be seen welling up in the area and may lead one to a laceration of the thoracic duct. In such instances, the leak should be repaired directly with pledgeted 4-0 Prolene sutures. Prophylactic ligation of the thoracic duct following esophagectomy is advocated by many. In this maneuver, all tissue between the aorta, spine, and azygos vein at the level of the hiatus is ligated with a large (0 or #1) ligature.

The diagnosis of a thoracic duct leak should be suspected if chest tube output remains high (>800 mL per day) in a patient despite a normal volume status. Definitive diagnosis may be difficult, because chyle is not milky unless the patient has been fed fats. Fluid should be sent for Gram's stain, triglyceride level, cell count, and cholesterol level. A triglyceride level greater than 1 mmol/L is strongly suggestive of a chyle leak, as is a lymphocyte count greater than 90%. If chylomicrons can be confirmed by electrophoresis, then the diagnosis can also be established. A good bedside test involves feeding the patient cream enterally 200–300 mL over 2 hours and observing for a change in character of chest tube effluent, from serous to milky white.

Chyle leak following esophagectomy must be repaired. These patients are recovering from major surgery and most are malnourished. The loss of protein and lymphocytes associated with a chyle leak may be associated with infections and may interfere with healing. Once the diagnosis is confirmed, or even if it is strongly suspected, patients should be brought to the operating room and the thoracotomy incision reopened. The patient is given enteral cream 1 hour before the procedure to help locate the leak. The defect is repaired with a pledgeted 4-0 or 5-0 Prolene suture. A careful inspection for other leaks should be performed before closure, and mass ligation of the duct at the hiatus should be considered as well.

CT-guided noninvasive methods have been proposed for repairing chyle leaks. The cisterna chyli can sometimes be located under CT guidance, cannulated, and injected with either coils or glue. In a published trial of 42 patients (including 9 post-esophagectomy patients), the thoracic duct could be embolized in 26, and 16 of these cases were cured.[28,29]

IMPAIRED CONDUIT EMPTYING

Numerous factors affect conduit emptying post-esophagectomy. These include vagotomy, drainage through the pylorus, width of the conduit, redundancy and/or kinking of the conduit, and postoperative swelling. Studies objectively looking at conduit emptying following esophagectomy give conflicting results as to the effect of pyloroplasty on gastric conduit emptying time. A prospective trial studied 200 patients and randomized half to pyloroplasty and half to no pyloroplasty following Ivor Lewis esophagectomy.[30] The average daily postoperative nasogastric drainage was no different between the two groups. Thirteen patients who did not undergo pyloroplasty had symptoms from delayed gastric emptying, and two died of aspiration pneumonia. There were no complications from the pyloroplasty procedure. Six months after the procedure, gastric emptying was 6 minutes in the pyloroplasty group versus 24 minutes in the group without pyloroplasty. These patients had more symptoms attributable to delayed emptying as well. The same group conducted a randomized trial of pyloroplasty versus pyloromyotomy and found both to be equally effective and safe.

Width of the gastric conduit may also affect emptying. A gastric tube has been shown to have a lower incidence of symptoms related to poor gastric emptying (3%) than either patients with whole stomach (38%) or distal two-thirds stomach (14%) acting as conduit.[31] A conduit diameter of 5–6 cm is probably ideal. Excess conduit length or angulation may also impair emptying, and excess colon conduit length or angulation is known to cause immediate or delayed problems with emptying.

LOCAL RECURRENCE

Direct invasion into periesophageal tissue, regional lymph nodal disease, and recurrence at the remaining margins of stomach or esophagus may all contribute to local recurrence. Clearance of the radial margins is best addressed by en-bloc dissection. Unfortunately, most analyses of en-bloc resections fail to include an analysis of local recurrence, instead focusing on survival. Discussion of adequate margin length must make note of whether the margin is an in-situ margin, resected margin, or fixed and resected margin. It is estimated that after fixation, the margin length is only 50% of the in-situ margin.[32] Perhaps the most detailed analysis of adequate margin length was performed by Tam and Wong et al. In their analysis of squamous cell carcinoma patients, in-situ proximal margin was measured and patients were observed for anastomotic recurrence.[33] If the proximal margin was less than 2 cm (only four patients) then the risk of recurrence was 25%. If the margin was between 2 and 6 cm then the risk was about 15%, if the margin was between 6 and 10 cm the risk was about 8%, and if the margin was greater than 10 cm no recurrence was seen. Clearly, a 10-cm margin can only be obtained for tumors of the middle and lower esophagus, unless one agrees to sacrifice the larynx. It is useful to know, however, that if one can obtain a 2-cm gross proximal margin, then the risk of recurrence will be 15% or lower. This certainly justifies leaving the larynx intact in such tumors. Intraoperative frozen section should be considered routine in establishing a clear margin. The optimal distal margin is unclear but authors have stated that an adequate margin following resection of GE junction adenocarcinoma is 6 cm.[34]

■ CONCLUSION

Esophagectomy has the potential to be an extremely morbid operation. The combination of a long operation that traverses the neck, chest, and abdomen and a nutritionally deficient patient may result in mortality exceeding 10% and morbidity exceeding 50%. Careful patient selection, preoperative preparation, and choice of operation, as well as meticulous surgical technique, excellent anesthetic and intensive care, and aggressive management of postoperative complications limit the morbidity of this operation.

REFERENCES

1. Torek F. The operative treatment of carcinoma of the esophagus. *Ann Surg* 1915;61:385
2. McKeown K. Total three-stage oesphagectomy for cancer of the oesophagus. *Br J Surg* 1976;63:259
3. Swanstrom L, Hansen P. Laparoscopic total esophagectomy. *Arch Surg* 1997;132:943–949
4. Nguyen N, Schauer P, Luketich J. Combined laparoscopic and thoracoscopic approach to esophagectomy. *J Am Coll Surg* 1999;188:328–332
5. Ellis FH Jr, Watkins E Jr, Krasna MJ, et al. Staging of carcinoma of the esophagus and cardia: a comparison of different staging criteria. *J Surg Oncol* 1993;52:231–235
6. Burmeister B, Smithers B, Fitzgerald L, et al. A randomized phase III trial of preoperative chemoradiation followed by surgery versus surgery alone for localized resectable cancer of the esophagus. *Prog Proc Am Soc Clin Oncol* 2002;21:130A
7. Bosset JF, Gignoux M, Triboulet JP, et al. Chemoradiotherapy followed by surgery compared to surgery alone in squamous-cell cancer of the esophagus. *N Engl J Med* 1997;337:161–167
8. Urba SG, Orringer MB, Turrisi A, et al. Randomized trial of preoperative chemoradiation versus surgery alone in patients with locoregional esophageal carcinoma. *J Clin Oncol* 2001;19:305–313
9. Walsh TN, Noonan N, Hollywood D, et al. A comparison of multimodal therapy and surgery for esophageal adenocarcinoma. *N Engl J Med* 1996;335:462–467
10. Tepper JE, Krasna M, Niedzwiecki D et al. Superiority of trimodality therapy to surgery alone in esophageal cancer: Results of CALGB 9781. J Clin Oncol 2006 ASCO Annual Meeting Proceedings Part I;24(182): Abstract #4012
11. Flanagan FL, Dehdashti F, Siegel BA, et al. Staging of esophageal cancer with 18-fluorodeoxyglucose positron emission tomography. *Am J Roentgenol* 1997;168:417–424
12. Block M, Patterson G, Sundaresan R, et al. Improvement in staging of esophageal cancer: 100 consecutive positron emission tomography scans. *Ann Thorac Surg* 1999;68:1133
13. Saltzman J. Endoscopic and other staging techniques. *Semin Thorac Cardiovasc Surg* 2003;15:180–186
14. Luketich JD, Schauer P, Landreneau R, et al. Minimally invasive surgical staging is superior to endoscopic ultrasound in detecting lymph node metastases in esophageal cancer. *J Thorac Cardiovasc Surg* 1997;114:817–821; discussion 821–823
15. Rindani R, Martin C, Cox M. Transhiatal versus Ivor-Lewis oesophagectomy: is there a difference? *Aust N Z J Surg* 1999;69:187–194
16. Hulscher J, Tijssen J, Lanschot J. Transthoracic versus transhiatal resection for carcinoma of the esophagus: A meta-analysis. *Ann Thorac Surg* 2001;72:306–313
17. Goldminc M, Maddern G, Le Prise E, et al. Oesophagectomy by a transhiatal approach or thoracotomy: a prospective randomized trial. *Br J Surg* 1993;80:367–376
18. Chu KM, Law SY, Fok M, et al. A prospective randomized comparison of transhiatal and transthoracic resection for lower-third esophageal carcinoma. *Am J Surg* 1997;174:320–324
19. Hulscher J, Van Sandick J, Van Lanschot J. Extended transthoracic resection compared with limited transhiatal resection for adenocarcinoma of the esophagus. *N Engl J Med* 2002;347:1662–1669
20. Wong J. Esophageal resection for cancer: the rationale of current practice. *Am J Surg* 1987;153:18–24
21. Churchill E, Sweet R. Transthoracic resection of tumors of the stomach and esophagus. *Ann Surg* 1942; 115:897
22. Mathisen DJ, Grillo HC, Wilkins EW Jr, Moncure AC, Hilgenberg AD. Transthoracic esophagectomy: a safe approach to carcinoma of the esophagus. *Ann Thorac Surg* 1988;45:137
23. Orringer M, Marshall B, Iannettoni M. Transhiatal esophagectomy: Clinical experience and refinements. *Ann Surg* 1999;230:392–403
24. Patil P, Patel S, Desai P. Cancer of the esophagus: esophagogastric anastomotic leak—a retrospective study of predisposing factors. *J Surg Oncol* 1992;49:163–167
25. Law S, Fok M, Chu KM, Wong J. Comparison of hand-sewn and stapled esophagogastric anastomosis after esophageal resection for cancer. A prospective randomized controlled trial. *Ann Surg* 1997;226:169–173
26. Urschel J. Esophagogastrostomy anastomotic leaks complicating esophagectomy: A review. *Am J Surg* 1995;169: 634–639
27. Honkoop P, Siersema PD, Tilanus HW, et al. Benign anastomotic strictures after transhiatal esophagectomy and cervical esophagogastrostomy: Risk factors and management. *J Thorac Cardiovasc Surg* 1996;111:1141–1146
28. Swanson SJ, Batirel HF, Bueno R, et al. Transthoracic esophagectomy with radical mediastinal and abdominal lymph node dissection and cervical esophagogastrostomy for esophageal carcinoma. *Ann Thorac Surg* 2001; 72:1918–1925
29. Cope C, Kaiser L. Management of unremitting chylothorax by percutaneous embolization and blockage of retroperitoneal lymphatic vessels in 42 patients. *J Vasc Intervent Radiol* 2002;13:1139–1148
30. Fok M, Cheng S, Wong J. Pyloroplasty versus no drainage in gastric replacement of the esophagus. *Am J Surg* 1991;162:447–452

31. Bemelman W, Taat C, Slors F. Delayed postoperative emptying after esophageal resection is dependent on the size of the gastric substitute. *J Am Coll Surg* 1995;180:461–464
32. Siu K, Cheung H, Wong J. Shrinkage of the esophagus after resection for carcinoma. *Ann Surg* 1986;203:173–176
33. Tam PC, Siu KF, Cheung HC, et al. Local recurrences after subtotal esophagectomy for squamous cell carcinoma. *Ann Surg* 1987;205:189–194
34. Papachristou D. Histologically positive esophageal margin in the surgical treatment of gastric cancer. *Am J Surg* 1980;139:711

section IV

STOMACH AND DUODENUM

11

Benign Gastric Disorders

Michael W. Mulholland ■ *Diane M. Simeone*

■ *HELICOBACTER PYLORI* INFECTION

In 1984, Marshall and Warren published a seminal paper entitled "Unidentified curved bacilli in the stomach of patients with gastritis and peptic ulceration."[1] These investigators identified a spiral-shaped flagellated organism associated with peptic ulcers. Originally referred to as *Campylobacter pyloridis*, the organism is now known as *Helicobacter pylori*. The proposal that peptic ulcer disease might have an infectious etiology revolutionized the practice of gastroenterology and provided important insights into diseases ranging from gastritis to gastric adenocarcinoma.

Helicobacter pylori (*H. pylori*) is a gram-negative spiral organism that currently infects more than half of the people in the world. The prevalence of *H. pylori* infection varies among populations and is strongly correlated with socioeconomic conditions. In a number of developing countries, *H. pylori* infection affects more than 80% of middle-aged adults. Infection rates are lower in industrialized countries. Epidemiological data indicate that the prevalence of infection in the United States has been declining since the second half of the 19th century, decreases corresponding to improved sanitation. Nonetheless, *H. pylori* infection is predicted to remain endemic in the U.S. for the next century.

Human beings are the only reservoir for *H. pylori*. Infection is presumed to occur by oral ingestion of the bacterium. Direct transmission from person to person occurs via saliva and feces, and infection also occurs through contact with contaminated water. In developing countries, most individuals are infected during childhood. Family members are at increased risk of infection. A number of occupations also show increased rates of *H. pylori* infestation, notably health care workers. Infection with *H. pylori* is a chronic disease and does not resolve spontaneously without specific treatment.

The gastric contents are normally nearly sterile as a consequence of the acidic luminal environment and the effects of gastric emptying. *H. pylori* has adapted to this hostile ecological environment and displays a number of features that permit its entry into the surface mucus layer, attachment to gastric epithelial cells, evasion of immune responses, and persistent colonization.

Because of its important role in disease pathogenesis, the organism has been intensively studied. The *H. pylori* genome encodes approximately 1500 proteins and contains 1.65 million base pairs. *H. pylori* expresses a number of novel proteins including urease. Urease hydrolyzes urea to carbon dioxide and ammonia. Ammonia acts as a neutralizing agent for hydrochloric acid and permits the bacterium to survive in an acidic microenvironment. Motility is also central for colonization, and the organism contains a flagellum, which permits the organism to move through mucus and approach the epithelial surface. The *H. pylori* genome also encodes a number of bacterial surface adhesins. These outer membrane proteins bind to the Lewis B blood group antigen. Mucosal adhesion is essential to bacterial pathogenesis and persistent infestation.

Most *H. pylori* strains express a 95-kd exotoxin, vacuolating cytotoxin. This toxin becomes inserted into the epithelial cell outer membrane and forms an anion-selective, voltage-dependent channel. Bicarbonate and organic ions are released through this channel, potentially providing the bacterium with nutrient substrate. The exotoxin is also incorporated into the host mitochondrial membrane. The VacA exotoxin causes the release of cytochrome c from mitochondria and induces apoptosis. This exotoxin is not essential for human colonization, and there is extensive variability in bacterial expression of VacA. A number of observations suggest that some VacA gene variants are associated with more severe disease.

The bacterium also produces a nontoxigenic high-molecular-weight protein encoded by the *cagA* gene. The cagA protein is translocated into the host epithelial cell. Within the epithelial cell, cagA is phosphorylated and binds to a tyrosine phosphatase. This binding is associated with inflammatory phenomena including production of interleukin-8. The cagA gene product serves as a pathogenicity phenotype marker.

TABLE 11–1. MEDIATORS OF *HELICOBACTER PYLORI*–INDUCED INJURY

TOXINS
VacA
cagA
IMMUNE RESPONSE
Elaboration of cytokines
Recruitment of inflammatory cells
Production of immunoglobulins
ACID SECRETION
Initial hypochlorhydria
Long-term hyperchlorhydria
Elevated serum gastrin
Reduced somatostatin expression
Increased gastric N-methylhistamine
BICARBONATE SECRETION
Reduced duodenal secretion of bicarbonate

(Reproduced, with permission, from Kaufman GL. Duodenal ulcer disease: treatment by surgery, antibiotics, or both. *Adv Surg* 2000;34:121–135.)

HOST RESPONSE TO *H. PYLORI*

H. pylori infestation is followed by continuous gastric inflammation in virtually all individuals. Worldwide, *H. pylori*–induced gastritis is the most common form, comprising 80–90% of all types of gastritis. Complete healing of infected mucosa is extremely rare, with rates of 0.4% per year in the absence of active treatment. For most individuals, this persistence means that *H. pylori* infestation causes gastritis which is lifelong.

The initial inflammatory response is characterized by recruitment of neutrophils, followed sequentially by T and B lymphocytes, plasma cells, and macrophages. *H. pylori* infection is not invasive of the gastric mucosa, and the host immune response is triggered by the attachment of bacteria to surface epithelial cells. The resultant chronic gastric inflammation in affected individuals is characterized by enhanced expression of interleukin-1β, interleukin-2, interleukin-6, interleukin-8, and tumor necrosis factor-α (Table 11–1). These interleukins serve as potent chemoattractants and as activators of neutrophils. A sustained systemic and mucosal immune response is also noted. The resulting antibody response does not lead to eradication of *H. pylori*, but does cause sustained tissue damage. Some individuals infected with *H. pylori* develop autoantibodies directed against gastric parietal cells. This autoimmunity correlates with subsequent atrophy of gastric mucosa.

H. pylori infestation is accompanied by an abnormal T-cell response. Immature T-helper cells can differentiate into two functional subtypes. Th1 cells are characterized by the secretion of interleukin-2 and interferon-γ. Th2 cells secrete interleukins-4, -5, and -10. In response to extracellular pathogens, Th2 cells stimulate T cells. Intracellular pathogens cause induction of Th1 cells. *H. pylori* infection is noninvasive and a Th2-cell response would be expected. However, *H. pylori* gastric infection induces mainly a Th1 phenotype. The Th1 response is associated with the production of cytokines that promote gastric inflammation, whereas Th2 cytokines would be expected to be cytoprotective. This abnormal response may be partially responsible for the long-term persistence of *H. pylori* infestation.

DIAGNOSIS

H. pylori infection can be diagnosed by both invasive and noninvasive means. Noninvasive methods include the urea breath test, serology, and detection of antigen in stool samples. The urea breath test is based on production of urease by *H. pylori* in the gastric mucosa. C^{14}-labeled urea is ingested and C^{14}-labeled CO_2 is produced and excreted in the breath. This test has a sensitivity and specificity of greater than 90% and indicates ongoing infection. The urea breath test is useful for initial diagnosis of infection and for follow-up after eradication therapy.

Because *H. pylori* induces a strong immunologic response, serological testing is useful. *H. pylori* serology is widely used for epidemiologic studies and for the diagnosis of *H. pylori* infection in patients before treatment. Sensitivity and specificity are greater than 90% for serology, comparable with those of the urea breath test. Because *H. pylori*–induced serology does not return to normal after bacterial eradication, this test is not reliable in monitoring therapy.

H. pylori infection can also be diagnosed on the basis of biopsies in patients undergoing upper endoscopic examination. Individuals more than 50 years of age, or those with significant symptoms including gastrointestinal bleeding, anemia, and weight loss, should undergo endoscopic diagnosis. During endoscopy, antral biopsies can be obtained and the organism cultured in agar containing both urea and a pH-sensitive colorimetric agent. *H. pylori* hydrolysis of urea causes a diagnostic change in color. The sensitivity of this test varies from 80–100% and specificity exceeds 90%. The test is associated with false-negative results in patients with active or recurrent bleeding and in those taking antibiotics or antisecretory compounds. Biopsy also permits histologic examination with visualization of the organism. Culture of *H. pylori* is not routine and is usually reserved for recurrent infection and for antibiotic sensitivity testing when second-line therapy has failed.

TREATMENT

Complete eradication of *H. pylori* infection is the goal of treatment, and recurrence of disease signifies reinfection in most circumstances. An enormous worldwide experience has developed relating to *H. pylori* eradication. More than 2000 articles report the results of antibiotic trials, and a large number of summary articles and meta-analyses are available.

It is important to note that none of the therapeutic regimens reported to date cure *H. pylori* infection in 100% of patients. To be effective, antimicrobial drugs must be combined with gastric acid secretion inhibitors or bismuth salts. Cure rates of 80–85% are achieved using combination therapy, usually proton pump inhibitors, ranitidine, or bismuth citrate with two antibiotics. The most common antibiotics used are clarithromycin, amoxicillin, and metronidazole or tinidazole. A combination of two drugs is more effective than one antibiotic alone, as there seems to be synergistic response. Treatment duration does not strongly influence outcome.

Metronidazole has been a mainstay of *H. pylori* treatment. With use, nitroimidazole resistance has increased over time. In developing countries, resistance rates are currently reported to be 80–90%; in most developed countries the resistance rates are much lower at 10–50%. Current evidence indicates that eradication therapy with a proton pump inhibitor, metronidazole, and amoxicillin decreases the prevalence of metronidazole-resistant *H. pylori* strains. The prevalence of clarithromycin-resistant strains varies greatly from country to country, with the highest rates reported in southern Europe. In this region, clarithromycin resistance now approximates 15%. This rate is predicted to rise over the next several years with increasing use of macrolide antibiotics. In patients failing therapy, culture of *H. pylori* from gastric mucosa is possible for resistance testing.

■ NON-ULCERATIVE DYSPEPSIA

Dyspepsia is a very common symptom complex which is characterized by pain and discomfort centered in the upper abdomen. Dyspepsia is among the most common disorders encountered by primary care physicians and gastroenterologists in the United States and Western countries. It is estimated that approximately 25% of the population will experience dyspepsia and that this problem accounts for 5% of visits to primary care providers.

Dyspepsia is characterized by symptoms which are focused in the upper abdomen. Symptoms may include heartburn, but a symptom complex limited to this complaint suggests gastroesophageal reflux disease and excludes the diagnosis of dyspepsia. Non-ulcerative dyspepsia is considered when no anatomic or biochemical abnormality is discovered that explains the patient's symptoms. This common disorder is not associated with increased morbidity or mortality. However, it is generally long lasting and responsible for impaired quality of life. Investigation of non-ulcerative dyspepsia and its treatment represents a large economic burden. Optimal treatment is controversial.

Since the description of *Helicobacter pylori* as a cause of gastritis, its association with non-ulcerative dyspepsia has been disputed. *H. pylori* infestation is always associated with histologic gastritis, absent in cases of non-ulcerative dyspepsia. A large number of studies have reported the efficacy of therapy for *H. pylori* infection on symptoms of non-ulcerative dyspepsia. A number of prospective randomized trials have been performed; analysis of these trials does not support the use of *H. pylori* eradication therapy in the treatment of non-ulcerative dyspepsia.[2–4] For surgeons, the importance of non-ulcerative dyspepsia relates to its place in the differential diagnosis of epigastric pain. There is no role for surgery for the treatment of this disorder.

■ PEPTIC ULCER DISEASE

EPIDEMIOLOGY

Peptic ulcer disease is a major public health problem in the United States and a source of substantial health care expenditure.[5] Each year, approximately 300,000 cases of peptic ulcer are diagnosed, and several million people receive treatment for ulcer symptoms. Overall, peptic ulcer mortality and hospitalization rates have declined for the past two decades, and surgeons are now treating a cohort of older patients with frequent comorbidity and ulcer disease of greater chronicity. Mortality attributed to complications of peptic ulcer disease is low relative to cardiovascular disorders or cancer; ulcer disease is a contributing cause of death in 10,000 cases annually.

The surgical treatment of peptic ulcer has changed dramatically, with the virtual elimination of elective operations for ulcer disease. Operative therapy is now used only for emergent treatment of complicated disease. Antibiotics have become primary anti-ulcer therapy with the realization that in most cases, peptic ulceration is an infectious disease. A wide variety of antisecretory drugs are available for clinical practice. Endoscopic and surgical therapies are frequently integrated in the care of individual patients.

PATHOPHYSIOLOGY

The pathogenesis of peptic ulceration is multifactorial, but increasingly understood to be a consequence of *H. pylori* infection. Before the recognition of the role of *H. pylori*, ulcer disease was conceived as an imbalance between acid and pepsin secretion and mucosal defense, with the balance shifted toward peptic injury and disease. In groups of patients, increases in acid secretion are well-documented, and although gastric acid is crucial in the development of ulcers, an acquired defect in mucosal defense exists to tip the balance away from health. Mucosal infestation with *H. pylori* is the factor that contributes to ulceration in most patients.

Helicobacter pylori

The relationship between *H. pylori* infection and ulceration is overwhelmingly strong; multiple observations establish *H. pylori* as a factor in the pathogenesis of duodenal ulceration.[6–10] Most of the evidence is inferential. A causal relationship between human *H. pylori* infection and peptic ulceration has not been tested directly because the organism is difficult to eradicate with certainty. For this reason, intentional exposure of humans to the organism to establish Koch's postulates is not justified. An effective vaccine has not yet been developed.

Observations that support *H. pylori* as a factor in the pathogenesis of human duodenal ulceration include:

1. *H. pylori* infection is invariably followed by the development of chronic gastritis and the organism is the primary cause of chronic active gastritis worldwide. The infectious response to *H. pylori* is characterized by nonerosive inflammation of the gastric mucosa. Antral gastritis is present histologically in patients with duodenal ulcer, and *H. pylori* can be isolated from gastric mucosa of ulcer patients.
2. *H. pylori* binds only to gastric-type epithelium. Gastric metaplasia of the duodenal bulb is a nonspecific response to damage, which develops after infestation of the gastric mucosa. Antral gastritis with *H. pylori* is preceded by active chronic duodenitis. Metaplastic gastric epithelium is colonized by *H. pylori* from gastric sources. Gastric metaplasia is extremely common in duodenal epithelium surrounding areas of ulceration.
3. Eradication of *H. pylori* with antibiotics that have no effect on acid secretion leads to ulcer healing.
4. Therapy of peptic ulceration with bismuth compounds, which eradicate *H. pylori*, is associated with reduced rates of ulcer relapse relative to acid suppression therapy.
5. Relapse of duodenal ulcer after eradication of *H. pylori* is preceded by reinfection of the gastric mucosa by the organism.

However, infection by *H. pylori* alone does not cause peptic ulceration in most individuals, suggesting the existence of other pathogenetic factors. Half of patients evaluated for dyspepsia have histologic evidence of bacterial infection. In developed countries, one-fifth of healthy volunteers harbor the bacteria, and the incidence of bacterial infestation increases with age in the healthy, asymptomatic population. The occurrence of peptic ulcers in only a fraction of individuals who harbor the organism suggests that other factors must also act to induce ulceration.

Gastric Acid Secretion

Abnormalities of gastric acid secretion in patients with peptic ulceration have been recognized for more than 50 years. The formation of duodenal ulcers clearly depends on gastric secretion of acid and pepsin. This association is symbolized by the dictum "no acid–no ulcer." *H. pylori* infection is now known to secondarily induce alterations in gastric acid secretion as a prerequisite for ulcer development, and a more complete and accurate statement might be "no acid and no *H. pylori*–no ulcer."

Patients with duodenal ulceration have increased gastric acid-secretory capacity relative to normals. Maximal acid output in normal men is approximately 20 mEq/h in response to intravenous histamine stimulation. Patients with duodenal ulcer secrete an average of approximately 40 mEq/h upon maximal stimulation. The increase in acid-secretory capacity in patients with duodenal ulceration has been postulated to be secondary to increased parietal cell mass in the acid-secreting gastric mucosa. Overlap in acid-secretory capacity exists between ulcer patients and normal individuals and the values for most ulcer patients fall within the normal range.

Patients with duodenal ulcer demonstrate a larger and more prolonged acid-secretory response to an ingested meal than do normal subjects. As with histamine-stimulated acid output, overlap in meal responses between patients with duodenal ulcer and normal subjects exists. Disturbances in gastric motility parallel meal-stimulated acid-secretory abnormalities. Duodenal ulcer patients have accelerated emptying of liquid gastric contents after a meal, and duodenal acidification fails to slow emptying appropriately. In these circumstances, the duodenal mucosa can be exposed to a low pH for prolonged periods relative to normal subjects.

Fasting acid secretion is elevated in patients with duodenal ulceration. Basal secretion is measured by nocturnal collection of gastric secretions. Basal acid secretion in patients with duodenal ulcer correlates with circulating concentrations of vagally-released gastrointestinal peptides, suggesting that increased vagal nerve activity is a contributing mechanism. Sham feeding, which is vagally mediated, does not increase acid output above basal secretion in duodenal ulcer patients.[12]

Many of the secretory abnormalities are a long-term consequence of *H. pylori* infection.[11] The first, acute phase of *H. pylori* infection is accompanied by marked decrease in gastric acid secretion. Initial acute antral infection is followed by fundic inflammation. Inflammation of the fundic mucosa is associated with local production of a number of cytokines, including interleukin (IL)-1β, IL-6, IL-8, and tumor necrosis factor-α (TNF-α). IL-1β potently inhibits gastric acid secretion.[13] The acute and transient reduction in gastric acid secretion is believed to facilitate further gastric colonization with *H. pylori*. Hypochlorhydria resolves despite continued infection of *H. pylori* and is replaced by a state of chronically increased acid secretion.

Abnormalities in acid secretion and parietal cell mass that were documented prior to the identification of *Helicobacter pylori* now appear to be a consequence of *H. pylori*–induced hypergastrinemia. Individuals that are infested with *H. pylori* demonstrate increased basal circulating gastrin levels, augmented gastrin responses to meal stimulation, and increased sensitivity to intravenous gastrin-releasing peptide. Antibiotic treatments that cause eradication of *H. pylori* infection are followed over several weeks by return of serum gastrin levels to normal. Gastric mucosal inflammatory cells and epithelial cells are induced by *H. pylori* infection to secrete cytokines such as IL-8, interferon-γ, and TNF-α. These cytokines act as gastric secretagogues, releasing gastrin from canine gastrin cells in vitro.

Acid secretory responses are, in turn, correlated with circulating serum gastrin levels. While basal and peak acid outputs are increased in patients with duodenal ulcer, following eradication of *H. pylori*, basal acid output returns to normal within 4 weeks, and peak acid output declines to the normal range by 6 months.[14] Maximal acid output indirectly reflects parietal cell mass; the return to normal levels suggests that *H. pylori* infection increases parietal cell mass. *H. pylori* produces N-histamine methyltransferase. This enzyme produces N-methylhistamine, an abnormal analogue of histamine that can also act as a gastric acid secretory stimulant.

Somatostatin is an inhibitory peptide produced by distinctive endocrine cells in the gastric mucosa. Somatostatin inhibits the release of gastrin from antral gastric cells and counters the acid-stimulatory actions of gastrin on fundic parietal cells. The concentration of somatostatin in gastric mucosa and the presence of somatostatin-producing cells in the antrum are diminished in *H. pylori*–infected patients. Alterations in somatostatin physiology appear to be causally related to *H. pylori* infection; antibiotic treatment is followed by increases in numbers of somatostatin cells and in expression of mucosal somatostatin mRNA.[15] By removing the inhibitory effects of somatostatin on gastrin release, altered mucosal somatostatin metabolism may contribute to hypergastrinemia in *H. pylori*–infected patients. Somatostatin release is suppressed by N-methylhistamine.

Mucosal Defense

In health, the duodenal mucosa is resistant to potentially injurious effects of luminal acid and pepsin. Because many patients with peptic ulceration secrete normal amounts of acid and pepsin, abnormalities of mucosal function have been invoked as contributing factors to peptic injury. In support of this concept, several agents that are used to treat peptic ulceration are cytoprotective. Cytoprotective agents inhibit mucosal injury at concentrations lower than threshold doses which suppress acid secretion.[16] The ability of such agents to heal ulcers suggests that abnormalities in mucosal defense, in addition to abnormalities in acid secretion, cause ulceration. Most cytoprotective agents act via mucosally secreted bicarbonate or on mucosal prostaglandin production.

Gastric and duodenal epithelial cells secrete mucus and bicarbonate, creating a pH gradient within the mucus layer. Immediately adjacent to the epithelial cell surface, pH is significantly higher than in the highly acidic lumen. Abnormalities in local bicarbonate secretion could result in exposure of surface epithelial cells to the peptic activity of gastric secretions at low pH. Groups of patients with duodenal ulceration have significantly lower basal bicarbonate secretion in the proximal duodenum than normal subjects. In addition, in response to a physiologically relevant challenge of hydrochloric acid instilled into the duodenal bulb, stimulated bicarbonate output was decreased to approximately 40% of the normal response.[17] Abnormalities in duodenal bicarbonate secretion normalize after eradication of *H. pylori* in affected individuals.

Prostaglandins and synthetic prostaglandin analogues exhibit cytoprotective effects, accelerate ulcer healing, and decrease acid secretion. Decreased mucosal prostaglandin production has also been proposed to contribute to the development of duodenal ulcer.[18,19] In subjects with active duodenal ulceration, gastric mucosal production of prostaglandin E_2 and other prostanoids is diminished. Ulcer healing is followed by increased prostanoid synthesis within gastric mucosa. In the duodenal mucosa, locally produced prostaglandins stimulate mucosal bicarbonate secretion, and duodenal bicarbonate secretion in response to prostaglandin E_2 is suppressed in patients with duodenal ulcer.

Other Environmental Factors

Substantial evidence implicates cigarette smoking as an additive risk factor in the development of duodenal ulcers. Smokers appear to have an increased risk of developing *H. pylori* infection relative to nonsmokers. Cigarette smoking impairs ulcer healing and increases the risk of recurrent ulceration. Continued smoking blunts the effectiveness of active ulcer therapy. Cigarette smoking increases both the probability that surgery will be required and the risks of operative therapy. When *H. pylori* is eradicated in smokers, they appear to have no greater risk of peptic ulceration than nonsmokers.[20,21] This observation suggests that smoking is probably not an independent risk factor for ulcer disease, but acts by increasing the harmful effects of bacterial infection. Cessation of smoking is a key goal of anti-ulcer therapy.

Nonsteroidal anti-inflammatory drugs (NSAIDs) are a major risk factor for the development of acute ulceration, and for hemorrhagic complications of ulceration. NSAIDs produce a variety of lesions, ranging from superficial mucosal erosions to deeper ulcerations. While the mucosal injury caused by NSAIDs is more common in the stomach than in the duodenum, ulcer complications occur with equal frequency in these two sites. *H. pylori* and NSAID use independently increase the risk of peptic ulcer and ulcer bleeding. These agents also act synergistically. In the duodenum, it appears likely that invasive *H. pylori*–associated ulcers are compounded by the direct injurious effects of NSAIDs.

The injurious actions of NSAIDs are secondary to systemic suppression of prostaglandin production. Numerous experimental models have demonstrated that NSAIDs injure the gastroduodenal mucosa. Ulcers resembling those occurring in humans can be produced by administration of NSAIDs to animals, and NSAID-associated gastric ulcers can be prevented by the coadministration of prostaglandin analogues. Ulcers associated with NSAIDs heal rapidly when the drug is withdrawn, corresponding temporally to reversal of antiprostaglandin effects.

None of the currently available NSAIDs are free of the hazard of gastroduodenal ulceration.[19] Clinically significant ulceration of the stomach and duodenum is estimated to occur at a rate of 2–4% per patient-year. The risks of long-term NSAID use are increased by *H. pylori* infection and cigarette smoking. The incidence of NSAID-related ulcer complications is highest in older patients, as is attendant mortality rate. Peptic ulcer disease is rare in individuals that are *H. pylori*–negative and that do not receive NSAID medications.[22]

DIAGNOSIS

Duodenal ulceration is characterized by epigastric pain. The pain is usually localized to the upper abdomen without radiation and is described as burning, stabbing, or gnawing. In the absence of complications such as perforation or penetration into the head of the pancreas, referral of pain to extra-abdominal sites is not common. Many patients report that pain is worsened by fasting. Ingestion of antacids usually provides prompt relief. In uncomplicated cases, physical examination is usually normal.

The differential diagnosis includes a variety of diseases originating in the epigastrium and upper gastrointestinal tract. Common disorders to be distinguished include non-ulcer dyspepsia, gastritis, gastric neoplasia, cholelithiasis and related diseases of the biliary system, neoplastic lesions of the liver, and both inflammatory and neoplastic disorders of the pancreas. In dyspeptic patients, especially those over 50 years of age, the most important differential diagnoses are peptic ulceration and gastric cancer.

The evaluation of patients with suspected peptic ulceration usually involves endoscopic examination of the esophagus, stomach and duodenum. In most circumstances, contrast radiography is not the preferred initial diagnostic method; endoscopy has become the standard to which other modalities are compared. Endoscopy eliminates the need for radiation, is safe, is tolerated by elderly patients, and permits both visual inspection and biopsy of the esophagus, stomach, and duodenum. In controlled trials, endoscopy was both more sensitive (92% versus 54%) and more specific

(100% versus 91%) than radiographic examination.[23] Endoscopy must be utilized with discretion because of the potential for perforation (approximately 1 per 5000 cases) and cost.

Endoscopically, duodenal ulceration is characterized by lesions that are erosive to the intestinal wall. When viewed endoscopically, peptic ulcers have a typical appearance, with edges that are usually sharply demarcated. The ulcer consists of the exposed underlying submucosa. With chronic ulcers, the base is usually clean and smooth. Acute ulcers and ulcers with recent hemorrhage may demonstrate clot, eschar, or adherent exudate. The surrounding duodenal mucosa may be friable, but marked inflammation is uncommon. The most frequent site for peptic ulceration is the first portion of the duodenum, with the second portion less frequently involved. Peptic ulceration of the third or fourth portions of the duodenum is distinctly unusual; occurrence of ulcers in these locations raises the possibility of gastrinoma. Peptic ulcers in the pyloric channel or the prepyloric area are similar in appearance to duodenal ulcers. Endoscopic demonstration of a duodenal ulcer does not require duodenal biopsy, but should prompt mucosal biopsy of the gastric antrum to demonstrate the presence of *H. pylori* and guide subsequent therapy.

Contrast radiographs demonstrate retention of contrast within the ulcer. When viewed tangentially, the ulcer projects beyond the level of the duodenal mucosa. Distortion of the duodenal bulb by spasm or scarring is a secondary sign of current or previous ulceration.

DRUG TREATMENT

In the absence of treatment, eradication of *H. pylori* infection is very rare, occurring in less than 0.5% per patient-year. Current treatment of peptic ulcer in *H. pylori*–positive patients involves a combination of an antisecretory drug, usually a proton pump inhibitor, with antibiotics. A large number of drug regimens have been described. The most widely used treatment protocols combine a proton pump inhibitor, usually omeprazole, with two antibiotics, usually clarithromycin and metronidazole or amoxicillin.[24,25] A combination of antibiotics is more effective than a single antibiotic in almost all series. *H. pylori* eradication rates of greater than 90% have been reported. After eradication of *H. pylori,* ulcer recurrence rates essentially equal rates of reinfection. In developed countries, reinfection rates of less than 10% at 5 years have been reported. Elimination of *H. pylori* improves quality of life, as measured by symptoms, drug prescriptions, physician visits, and days of lost employment.

Histamine-Receptor Antagonists

Histamine is a major gastric acid secretagogue. Histamine is released by cells in the fundic mucosa and diffuses to mucosal parietal cells. Histamine is released in response to a number of physiologic stimuli and blockade of histamine receptors inhibits all forms of stimulated acid secretion in humans. All clinically useful gastric histamine-receptor antagonists are of the H_2 type. Parietal cell histamine receptors are classified as H_2 receptors because they are blocked by agents such as cimetidine.

H_2-receptor antagonists produce reversible inhibition of acid secretion by binding competitively to parietal cell H_2 receptors. The agents are both effective and safe. When endoscopy is used to evaluate healing, 70% of patients are ulcer free within 4 weeks of therapy. By 8 weeks, approximately 90% of patients are symptom free and without endoscopic evidence of ulceration. Most studies of maintenance therapy have used single nocturnal doses of H_2-receptor antagonists; ulcer recurrence during maintenance therapy occurs in approximately 15% of patients.

H_2-receptor blockers do not affect underlying ulcer disease. If H_2-receptor antagonists are discontinued, ulceration recurs in more than half of patients within 1 year. With current understanding of *H. pylori* in ulcer pathogenesis, the role of H_2-receptor antagonists has changed from primary therapy. These agents are now substitutes for proton pump inhibitors in conjunction with antibiotic treatment.

Proton Pump Inhibitors

Acid secretion by the gastric parietal cells is due to the active transport of hydrogen ions from parietal cells into the gastric lumen. Omeprazole is a member of a family of compounds that selectively block the parietal cell proton pump. Omeprazole binds to membrane-bound H^+-K^+-adenosine triphosphatase of the parietal cell. If enough omeprazole is administered to occupy all parietal cell binding sites, complete suppression of acid secretion can be achieved. Omeprazole, at 20–30 mg, causes nearly complete inhibition of stimulated gastric acid secretion within 6 hours. The agent has a long half-life, such that at 24 hours after drug administration, 60–70% reduction in acid secretion persists.

Repeated daily dosing with omeprazole results in additive inhibition of gastric acid secretion and decreased intragastric degradation of the drug. Acid suppression is maximal after approximately 3 days. Controlled studies have demonstrated significant inhibition of peak acid output, marked relief of epigastric pain, and decreased use of supplemental antacids during omeprazole therapy of peptic ulceration. Direct comparisons of omeprazole with H_2-receptor antagonists have favored omeprazole in terms of pain relief and rate of ulcer healing.

Sucralfate

Sucralfate is an aluminum salt of sulfated sucrose. When sucralfate contacts gastric acid, the agent polymerizes and adheres to the gastroduodenal mucosa. The drug has almost no buffering capacity, and is believed to provide a protective barrier, binding bile salts and inhibiting the actions of pepsin. Sucralfate stimulates the production of mucus, increases mucosal prostaglandin E_2 production, and increases duodenal bicarbonate secretion. Sucralfate binds epidermal growth factor and may increase epithelial proliferation at the ulcer margin. The drug has no systemic absorption.

Antacids

Antacids are a time-honored treatment for peptic ulceration, but the availability of compounds that effectively and more conveniently suppress acid production has greatly reduced the use of antacid therapy. Nonetheless, intensive treatment of acute ulcers with antacids (approximately 1000 mEq of buffering capacity) heals ulcers in 78% of patients at 4 weeks.[26] The need for frequent dosing is unacceptable to many patients, and a significant proportion of patients have diarrhea on such a regimen.

Bismuth Compounds

A number of bismuth compounds have antimicrobial activity. Useful antibiotic regimens may be based on a bismuth compound (colloidal bismuth subsalicylate or colloidal bismuth subcitrate) plus metronidazole, used alone or in combination with amoxicillin or tetracycline. Bismuth compounds act intraluminally to achieve gastric concentrations above the minimum inhibitory concentration for 90% of *H. pylori* isolates.

■ OPERATIVE TREATMENT OF ULCER DISEASE

The realization that peptic ulceration is an infectious disease has fundamentally altered the role of surgery in ulcer treatment.[27,28] Indications for operative intervention have changed over the past 15 years as a consequence, with the virtual elimination of elective operations.[29] Operative intervention is now reserved for the treatment of complicated ulcer disease. Three complications are most common and constitute contemporary indications for peptic ulcer surgery—hemorrhage, perforation, and obstruction. Evolving indications have been reflected in changed forms of operative therapy and in surgical training experience.[30,31]

The first goal of current surgical therapy is treatment of anatomic complications, such as pyloric stenosis or perforation. The second major goal should be patient safety in the acute setting, combined with freedom from undesirable chronic side effects. The third goal in contemporary surgical treatment of complicated ulcer disease should be alteration of the ulcer diathesis so that ulcer healing is achieved and recurrence is minimized. To achieve these goals, the gastric surgeon can combine therapy through endoscopic, radiologic, or operative means, the appropriate choice depending on the clinical circumstances.

OPERATIVE PROCEDURES

There is currently no indication for surgical treatment of uncomplicated ulcer disease. A number of operative procedures have been developed to treat peptic ulcer, but have been used with decreasing frequency in the past decade. Operative treatment of gastric outlet obstruction has decreased by approximately 50%. The majority of surgical patients are currently treated emergently for the complications of bleeding or perforation.

Truncal vagotomy and drainage, truncal vagotomy and antrectomy, and proximal gastric vagotomy, have been most widely utilized in the operative treatment of peptic ulcer disease. However, surgical therapy of complicated peptic ulcer disease is directed increasingly at correction of the immediate problem without gastric denervation. The underlying cause of the ulcer diathesis may then be addressed after recovery from surgery by antibiotic therapy directed at *H. pylori*. This approach is applicable to most patients with peptic ulcer undergoing emergent operation and reflects a greatly diminished role for vagotomy in the future. The role of vagotomy in clinical surgery diminished significantly in the 1990s. In 1998, only 7000 vagotomies were performed in the United States, among more than 41 million operative procedures.[28]

Transection of both vagal trunks at the esophageal hiatus, termed truncal vagotomy, denervates the acid-producing fundus of the stomach. The procedure also denervates the remainder of the vagally supplied viscera, including the liver and biliary tree, pancreas, small bowel, and colon to the mid-transverse portion. Because denervation impedes normal pyloric coordination and impairs gastric emptying, truncal vagotomy is usually combined with a procedure to eliminate pyloric sphincteric function. Usually, gastric drainage is ensured by performance of a pyloroplasty. Several methods of pyloroplasty have been developed, referred to eponymously. The Heineke-Mikulicz pyloroplasty consists of a longitudinal incision of the pyloric sphincter extending into the antrum and the duodenum. The incision is closed transversely, eliminating sphincteric closure and increasing the lumen of the pyloric channel.

Truncal vagotomy can be combined with resection of the gastric antrum to further reduce acid secretion by removing antral sources of gastrin. The limits of antral resection are defined by external landmarks. The stomach is divided proximally along a line from a point above the incisura angularis to a point along the greater curvature midway from the pylorus to the gastroesophageal junction. Reconstruction via a gastroduodenostomy is termed a Billroth I procedure. A Billroth II procedure uses a gastrojejunostomy to restore gastrointestinal continuity.

Proximal gastric vagotomy, also termed highly selective vagotomy, differs from truncal vagotomy in that only the nerve fibers to the acid-secreting fundic mucosa are transected (Fig 11–1). The hepatic and celiac divisions are not divided, and vagal nerve fibers to the antrum and pylorus remain intact. The operation has also been called parietal cell vagotomy to emphasize the intended functional consequence.

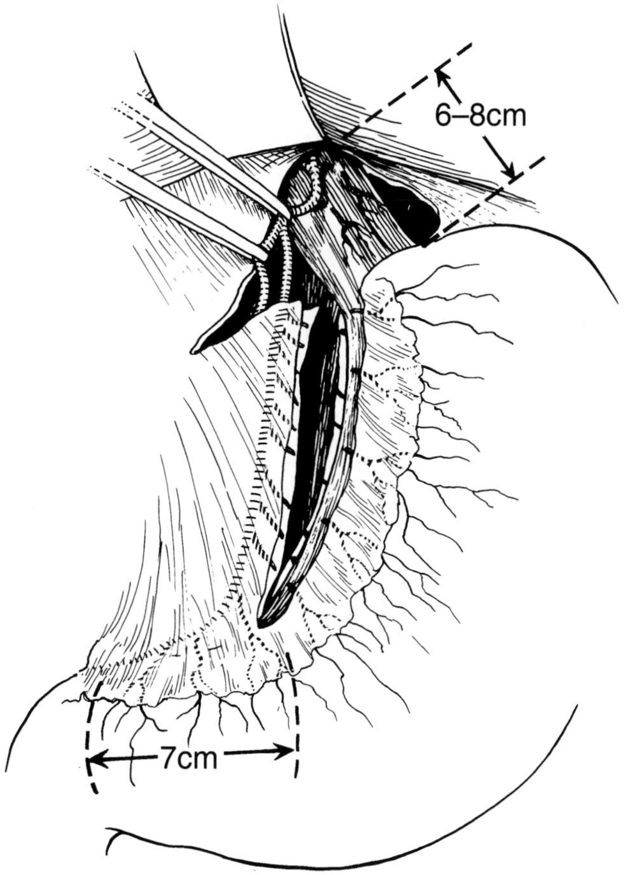

Figure 11–1. Technique of proximal gastric vagotomy. The distal 6 cm of the esophagus is skeletonized. Denervation spares the antrum and pylorus by stopping 7 cm proximal to the pylorus. *(Redrawn from Griffith CA. Selective gastric vagotomy. In: Nyhus LM, Wastell C (eds). Surgery of the Stomach and Duodenum, 3rd ed. Boston, MA: Little, Brown; 1977:275. After Gloege)*

POSTOPERATIVE ALTERATIONS

Division of vagal nerve fibers alters gastric acid secretion by reducing cholinergic stimulation of parietal cells. Vagal denervation also decreases parietal cell responsiveness to gastrin and histamine. Basal acid secretion is diminished by approximately 80% in the immediate postoperative period. Basal acid secretion remains unchanged long term. The maximal acid output in response to secretagogues such as pentagastrin is reduced by approximately 70%. After 1 year, pentagastrin-stimulated maximal acid output increases to 50% of prevagotomy values but remains at this level on subsequent testing. Acid secretion due to meal stimulation is reduced by 60–70% relative to normal subjects. The inclusion of antrectomy to truncal vagotomy further reduces acid secretion. Maximal acid output is reduced by 85% relative to values recorded before antrectomy.

Both forms of vagotomy cause postoperative hypergastrinemia. Fasting gastrin values are increased to approximately twice preoperative levels. Postprandial gastrin response is exaggerated. Hypergastrinemia is due to decreased luminal acid, with loss of feedback inhibition of gastrin release. Chronic hypergastrinemia is caused by mucosal gastrin cell hyperplasia in addition to loss of inhibitory feedback. When antrectomy is performed, circulating gastrin levels are decreased. Basal gastrin values are reduced by approximately half and postprandial gastrin levels by two-thirds.

Operations that involve vagotomy affect gastric emptying. Both truncal vagotomy and proximal gastric denervation abolish vagally-mediated receptive relaxation. Receptive relaxation allows the ingestion of a meal with no increase in intragastric pressure; the process involves a vagal reflex arc. After vagotomy, the intragastric pressure rise is greater for any given volume ingested, and the gastroduodenal pressure gradient higher than in normal subjects. As a result, emptying of liquids, which depends on the gastroduodenal pressure gradient, is accelerated. Because nerve fibers to the antrum and pylorus are preserved with proximal gastric vagotomy, the function of the distal stomach to mix solid food is preserved, and emptying of solids is nearly normal. Truncal vagotomy affects the motor activity of the distal stomach, and solid and liquid emptying rates are usually increased when truncal vagotomy is accompanied by pyloroplasty.

The surgical literature regarding peptic ulcer operations, developed in an era of elective procedures, is of high quality, though dated. A number of prospective randomized trials have compared surgical options in terms of postoperative symptoms, including dumping, diarrhea, weight loss, and disturbance of lifestyle. Dumping is defined by a postprandial symptom complex of abdominal discomfort, weakness, and vasomotor symptoms of sweating and dizziness. Dumping occurs transiently in 10–15% of patients after truncal vagotomy and antrectomy and is persistent in 1–2%. Dumping is present initially in 10% of patients undergoing truncal vagotomy and pyloroplasty, and remains in approximately 1%. Permanent symptoms of dumping are unusual after proximal gastric vagotomy. The incidence of diarrhea, presumably caused by denervation of the pylorus and small bowel and by elimination of pyloric function, parallels the incidence of dumping when truncal vagotomy is performed. Persistent and disabling diarrhea is present in less than 1% of patients after proximal gastric vagotomy.

Proximal gastric vagotomy is a safe operation. The procedure has a reported operative mortality rate of less than 0.05%, lower than the reported mortality for any other gastric procedure for peptic ulcer. Truncal vagotomy and pyloroplasty has an accepted mortality rate of 0.5–0.8%, whereas mortality after truncal vagotomy and antrectomy approximates 1.5%. These statistics require an important caveat; almost all large series report the results of elective operations on patients with peptic ulceration and may not accurately reflect expected results when similar procedures are performed emergently.

The largest surgical series examining ulcer recurrence rates were reported at a time before the pathogenic role of *H. pylori* was appreciated. With appropriate use of antibiotics directed against *H. pylori*, ulcer recurrence rates are currently expected to be much lower. Although recurrence rates (without *H. pylori* treatment) as low as 5% have been reported, a more generally representative figure is 10%. This rate is similar to that of reinfection with *H. pylori* after successful eradication. Ulcer recurrence rates after proximal gastric vagotomy can be adversely affected by the inclusion of prepyloric and pyloric channel ulcers. Proximal gastric vagotomy is significantly less effective when used to treat ulcers in this position than when used for duodenal ulceration.

ULCER HEMORRHAGE

Hemorrhage continues to be a major source of morbidity in patients with peptic ulceration. Bleeding is the leading cause of death associated with peptic ulcer. The incidence of hemorrhage has not changed since the introduction of H_2-receptor antagonists.[28] The lifetime risk of hemorrhage for patients with duodenal ulcer who do not undergo specific therapy approximates 35%. Hemorrhage usually occurs during the initial episode of ulceration or during relapse; patients who have bled previously have a higher risk of bleeding again. Patients with recurrent bleeding and elderly patients are at greatest risk of death.[29,30]

The contemporary risk of mortality from bleeding peptic ulcer is surprisingly high, approximating 10–20%. When surgery is necessary, operative risk is increased in patients that have shock at admission, recurrent bleeding, delay in operative intervention, or comorbid illnesses. Surgical delay leads to recurrent hypovolemia, and subsequently multisystem organ failure.

Upper gastrointestinal endoscopy is the appropriate initial diagnostic test, following resuscitation, when hemorrhage from duodenal ulceration is suspected. Endoscopy identifies the site and source of bleeding in over 90% of patients. An ulcer should be accepted as the bleeding source only if it exhibits a stigmata of active or recent hemorrhage (Table 11–2). Active hemorrhage is defined by an arterial jet, active oozing, or oozing beneath an adherent clot. Signs of recent hemorrhage include adherent clot without oozing, adherent slough in the ulcer base, or visible vessel in the ulcer. The predictive power of these findings to accurately predict recurrent hemorrhage has been extensively validated. Up to 30% of patients who have stigmata of recent hemorrhage experience rebleeding, and most of the patients who bleed recurrently require emergency treatment. The signs are not sufficiently accurate, nor are rebleeding rates high enough, to be indications for surgery. Endoscopic stigmata indicate that aggressive therapy is needed and close follow-up mandatory. The occurrence of hypovolemic shock, rebleeding during hospitalization, and a posteroinferior location of the ulcer are clinical features that are associated with increased risk of recurrent bleeding. Acute reduction of acid secretion by H_2-receptor antagonists or proton pump inhibitors is not sufficient to prevent recurrent hemorrhage.[31]

The ability to visualize bleeding duodenal ulcers endoscopically permits endoscopic treatment. Methods of

TABLE 11–2. ULCER STIGMATA AND REBLEEDING IN PEPTIC ULCERS

	Prevalence (%)	Rebleeding (%)
Active arterial bleeding	12	88
Nonbleeding visible vessel	22	50
Nonbleeding flat clot	10	33
Oozing	14	10
Nonbleeding flat spots	10	7
Clean ulcer base	32	3

(Reproduced, with permission, from Machiado G. Thermal probes alone or with epinephrine for the endoscopic haemostasis of ulcer haemorrhage. *Baillières Clin Gastroenterol* 2000;14:442–458.)

TABLE 11–3. FAILURE RATES FOR ENDOSCOPIC HEMOSTASIS

Rebleed (%)	Urgent Surgery (%)	Mortality (%)
0–40%	0–32%	0–16%

(Reproduced, with permission, from Lundell L. Upper gastrointestinal hemorrhage—surgical aspects. *Dig Dis* 2003;21:16–18.)

endoscopic therapy include thermal coagulation by bipolar electrocoagulation or direct application of heat through a heater probe.[32] Injection of epinephrine into the base of the bleeding ulcer is also an established method to control ulcer hemorrhage.

Both reduced rebleeding rates and avoidance of operation have been demonstrated for endoscopic hemostasis.[32,33] Proof of efficacy for endoscopic treatment of hemorrhage is complicated by the 70% rate of spontaneous, sometimes temporary, cessation of bleeding without intervention (Table 11–3). In addition to endoscopic stigmata, hemodynamic instability, continuing transfusion requirements, red stool or hematemesis, age older than 60 years, and medical comorbidity are clinical features that mandate endoscopic therapy. Rebleeding during hospitalization and the endoscopic findings of visible vessel, oozing, or bleeding associated with an adherent clot are also indications for endoscopic hemostasis. Ulcers with clean bases and no stigmata of recent hemorrhage require no treatment.

Failure of endoscopic treatment is usually due to inaccessibility of the ulcer because of pyloric scarring, rapid active bleeding, or an obscuring clot. Patients treated endoscopically should be observed closely for further hemorrhage. Those who rebleed within 72 hours of initial endoscopic control may be successfully retreated without increased risk of mortality.[33]

The efficacy of endoscopy diagnosis and therapy is dependent upon timing. Early endoscopy correctly classifies patients as low-risk for recurrent hemorrhage and permits safe avoidance of hospitalization. Early endoscopy also benefits high-risk patients by directing specific, active hemostatic therapy. Patients with early endoscopy have been demonstrated to have fewer episodes of rebleeding, lower rates of operation, less resource consumption, and shorter hospitalizations.[34]

Operative intervention is indicated for the following:

- Massive hemorrhage leading to shock or cardiovascular instability
- Prolonged blood loss requiring continuing transfusion
- Recurrent bleeding during medical therapy or after endoscopic therapy
- Recurrent hemorrhage requiring hospitalization

The need for emergency intervention significantly increases surgical risks, and not surprisingly, mortality

TABLE 11–4. REBLEEDING RATES BY PROCEDURE FOR BLEEDING PEPTIC ULCER

Ulcer Suture or Excision	Truncal Vagotomy and Pyloroplasty	Truncal Vagotomy and Antrectomy
10–30%	0–30%	0–10%

(Reproduced, with permission, from Legrand MJ, Jacquet N. Surgical approach in severe bleeding peptic ulcer. *Acta Gastroenterol Belg* 1996;59:240–244.)

is increased 10-fold. Emergent operative therapy should consist of duodenotomy with direct suture ligation of the bleeding vessel in the ulcer base (Tables 11–4 and 11–5). Postoperatively, patients should receive antibiotics directed against *H. pylori.* This treatment approach is based on the observation, in medically-treated patients, that peptic ulcer hemorrhage recurs in 20% of patients when *H. pylori* is not eradicated, while rebleeding is reduced to 3% in patients that receive *H. pylori* antibiotic therapy.[35–37] This recommendation is an extrapolation; the studies that support this practice were not designed to evaluate postoperative hemorrhage (Table 11–6).

■ PERFORATION

The lifetime risk for perforation in patients with duodenal ulceration not receiving therapy approximates 10%, while ulcer perforation is unusual if initial ulcer healing has been achieved. Duodenal ulcer perforation is followed by sudden and severe epigastric pain. The pain is caused by contact of the peritoneum with highly caustic gastric secretions. Pain is often instantaneous and remains constant. Radiation to the right scapular region is common with right subphrenic collection of gastric contents. If gastric contents travel caudally through the paracolic gutter, pain may be sensed in the lower abdomen. Peritoneal irritation is usually intense, and causes most patients to avoid movement.

Physical examination reveals fever, diminished bowel sounds, rigidity of the abdominal musculature, and guarding. Upright abdominal radiographs demonstrate pneumoperitoneum in 80% of cases. If free intraperitoneal air is not present, computed tomography of the abdomen is very sensitive for demonstrating perforation.

TABLE 11–5. MORTALITY RATES BY PROCEDURE FOR BLEEDING PEPTIC ULCER

Ulcer Suture or Excision	Truncal Vagotomy and Pyloroplasty	Truncal Vagotomy and Antrectomy
26%	10–45%	0–30%

(Reproduced, with permission, from Legrand MJ, Jacquet N. Surgical approach in severe bleeding peptic ulcer. *Acta Gastroenterol Belg* 1996;59:240–244.)

TABLE 11–6. ERADICATION OF *H. PYLORI* AND ULCER REBLEEDING

TREATMENT GROUP		
No. Patients	Eradication Rate (%)	Rebleeding (%)
133	83	6
CONTROL GROUP		
No. Patients	Eradication Rate (%)	Rebleeding (%)
129	4	28

(Reproduced, with permission, from Sharma VK, et al. *Helicobacter pylori* eradication is superior to ulcer healing with or without maintenance therapy to prevent further ulcer haemorrhage. *Ailment Pharmacol Ther* 2001;15:1939–1947.)

Occasional reports have described nonoperative treatment of this complication, but this approach is not consistent with contemporary therapy. Perforation is a strong indication for surgery in most circumstances. Laparotomy or laparoscopy affords the opportunity to relieve intraperitoneal contamination and to close the perforation.

The results of surgical treatment of duodenal perforation in the era preceding the recognition of *H. pylori* are instructive. Signs of preexisting duodenal ulceration, in terms of history of prior symptoms and anatomic evidence of duodenal scarring, should be sought, but a lack of antecedent symptoms is not protective. Patients without antecedent symptoms are at substantial risk for recurrent ulceration. By 5–6 years, symptomatic ulcer recurrence in patients with acute ulcer perforation is similar to that for patients with chronic disease. Before the role of *H. pylori* was appreciated, simple omental closure of duodenal perforation did not provide satisfactory long-term results; up to 80% of patients so treated had recurrent ulceration and 10% experienced reperforation. It is now known that four-fifths of all patients with perforation have *H. pylori* infestation and therefore are at risk of recurrent disease.

The mortality of emergent ulcer operations is most clearly correlated with the existence of preoperative shock, coexisting medical illness, and presence of perforation for more than 48 hours.[38] For patients that receive prompt surgical attention, the operation can be performed with safety. Proximal gastric vagotomy with omental patch closure of the perforation is one option in this circumstance. This procedure has been shown to be both safe and effective in preventing ulcer relapse. Incorporation of the site of perforation as part of a pyloroplasty or resection of the perforation during antrectomy can also be combined with truncal vagotomy. The performance of these operations has declined significantly, however, with the focus on *H. pylori* as the cause of most ulcer recurrences.

Several investigators advocate omental patch closure alone with postoperative anti–*H. pylori* therapy.[39–44] Omental patching can often be accomplished laparoscopically. This approach rests upon three assumptions: (1) that most perforated duodenal ulcers are caused by *H. pylori*; (2) that the duodenal perforation is small enough that secure closure can be obtained; and (3) that further surgical therapy will be obviated by the effects of postoperative antibiotic therapy. Minimally invasive approaches are becoming standard practice.

▪ OBSTRUCTION

Gastric outlet obstruction can develop either acutely or chronically in patients with duodenal ulcer disease. Acute obstruction, due to edema and inflammation, is associated with ulcers in the pyloric channel and the first portion of the duodenum. Pyloric obstruction causes recurrent vomiting and dehydration. Hypochloremic alkalosis, due to loss of hydrochloric acid in gastric secretions, is distinctive of gastric obstruction. Hypokalemia may develop as a secondary renal compensation for alkalosis. Acute gastric outlet obstruction is treated by nasogastric suction, rehydration, and intravenous administration of antisecretory agents. Acute obstruction due to pyloric inflammation resolves with supportive measures within 72 hours.

Repeated episodes of ulceration can lead to pyloric scarring and a fixed stenosis with chronic gastric outlet obstruction. In cases of recurrent duodenal ulceration, the lifetime risk of chronic pyloric stenosis approximates 10%.

Initial investigation begins with upper gastrointestinal endoscopy to confirm the site of obstruction and to exclude neoplasm. Endoscopic hydrostatic balloon dilatation of pyloric stenosis can also be attempted; approximately 85% of pyloric stenoses are anatomically amenable to balloon dilatation.[45] Most treated patients note immediate symptomatic improvement, but only 40% have sustained improvement by 3 months after balloon dilatation. Recurrent symptoms are presumed due to residual scarring in the pyloric channel. In most cases, operative correction is required. Operative correction should include treatment of the underlying ulcer disease and relief of the anatomic abnormality. Truncal vagotomy with antrectomy and truncal vagotomy with drainage have both been used with success in this circumstance.

▪ GASTRIC ULCER DISEASE

DIAGNOSIS

Benign gastric ulcers occur at one-third the frequency of benign duodenal ulceration in the United States. Gastric ulcer is more common in men than women and occurs in a patient cohort approximately 10 years older than that of duodenal ulceration. In symptomatic patients, upper gastrointestinal endoscopy is the preferred method for diagnosing gastric ulceration. The visual appearance of benign and malignant gastric ulcers may be identical and differentiation may be made only by biopsy. Benign gastric ulcers appear smooth and flat and are often covered by a gray, fibrous exudate. The margin is often raised and erythematous. The ulcer margin is friable and may bleed with manipulation. All gastric ulcers should undergo multiple biopsies, obtained from the perimeter of the lesion. The addition of endoscopic brushings to biopsy increases diagnostic accuracy to approximately 95%.

Although benign gastric ulcers may occur in any location in the stomach, more than half are located along the lesser curvature proximal to the incisura angularis. Fewer than 10% of benign ulcers are located on the greater curvature. Virtually all gastric ulcers lay within 2 cm of the histologic transition between fundic and antral mucosa.

Similar to duodenal ulceration, *H. pylori* infection is key to the pathogenesis of benign gastric ulcers. Antibiotic treatment regimens useful for duodenal ulcer have also been employed for benign gastric ulceration. The response of gastric ulcers to antibiotic therapy is equivalent to that of duodenal ulcers. Recurrence of gastric ulcers after *H. pylori* eradication is equal to the rate of reinfection.

In addition to *H. pylori* infection, alterations in gastric motility have been demonstrated in some patients with benign gastric ulcers. Motility defects include delayed gastric emptying, abnormal pyloric sphincter function, prolonged high-amplitude gastric contractions, duodenogastric reflux, and alterations in the gastric migrating motor complex. These alterations have not been definitively demonstrated to be pathogenic, and their relevance to gastric ulceration is unsettled. A definite association between chronic NSAID use and benign gastric ulceration has been recognized. As with duodenal ulceration, cigarette smoking is associated with development of gastric ulceration, and continued smoking impairs medical therapy. Gastric and duodenal ulcers may occur in patients that receive hepatic artery chemotherapy if improper placement of the catheter permits perfusion of gastric and duodenal mucosa. A variety of agents, including 5-fluorouracil, cisplatin, doxorubicin, and mitomycin C, have been implicated.

THERAPY

The primary therapy for benign gastric ulceration is antibiotic treatment of *H. pylori* infection using treatment protocols similar to those for duodenal ulceration. Antibiotic response rates are similar. Cessation of NSAID therapy is required for many patients. Operative treatment is reserved for complications of gastric ulcer, including hemorrhage and perforation. Unlike duodenal ulcer, failure of a recurrent ulcer to respond to medical therapy may be an indication for operation, usually because nonhealing raises concerns about the inability to exclude malignant disease.

For benign gastric ulcers, the elective operation of choice is usually a distal gastrectomy with either gastroduodenal (Billroth I) or gastrojejunal (Billroth II) anastomosis. The ulcer should be excised with the gastrectomy specimen (Fig 11–2). Performed electively, operative mortality approximates 2–3%, and ulcer recurrence rates are less than 5%. Inclusion of vagotomy does not improve recurrence rates. The occurrence of a benign ulcer near the gastroesophageal junction represents a difficult surgical problem. The ulcer may be excised via a distal gastrectomy with an extension along the lesser curvature and reconstruction with gastrojejunostomy. Emergency treatment of hemorrhage or perforation requires ulcer excision. Distal gastrectomy, including the site of perforation or bleeding, is usually the procedure of choice. Operative mortality rates average 10–20% in the presence of hemorrhage or perforation.

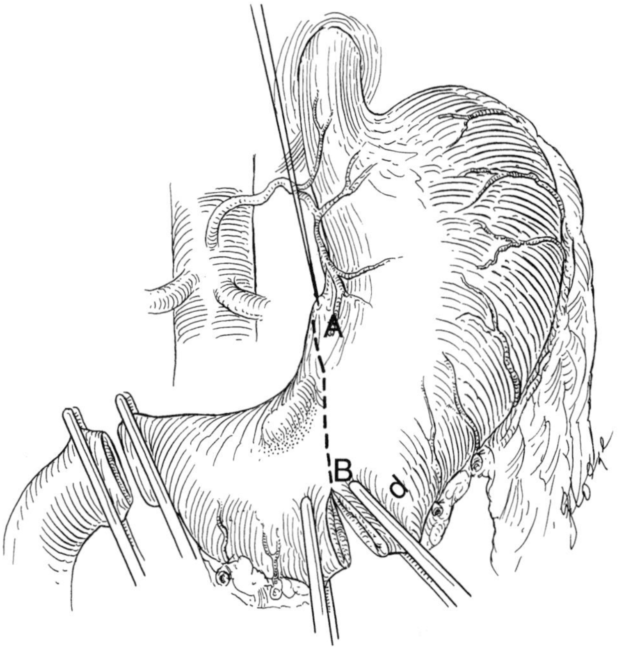

Figure 11–2. Points of transection for distal gastrectomy performed to resect a gastric ulcer along the lesser curvature. d, the approximate diameter of the duodenum.

▪ POSTGASTRECTOMY SYNDROMES

A number of syndromes have been described after gastric operations performed for peptic ulceration or gastric neoplasm. The occurrence of disabling postoperative symptoms is uncommon, 1–3% of cases, and unpredictable. The two most common postgastrectomy syndromes are dumping and alkaline reflux gastritis.

DUMPING

Dumping is defined as a postoperative clinical syndrome with gastrointestinal and vasomotor symptoms. The cause of dumping is uncertain but is likely related to unregulated entry of ingested food into the proximal small bowel following vagotomy and resection or division of the pyloric sphincter. Early dumping symptoms occur within 1 hour of ingestion of a meal and include nausea, epigastric discomfort, tremulousness, and sometimes dizziness or syncope. Late dumping symptoms follow a meal by 1–3 hours. Late symptoms also include reactive hypoglycemia.

Most patients that undergo vagotomy or gastrectomy do not experience dumping symptoms postoperatively. For patients that experience mild dumping symptoms in the early postoperative period, dietary alterations and time bring improvement in all but approximately 1%. For those that remain persistently symptomatic, the long-acting somatostatin analogue, octreotide, improves dumping symptoms when administered subcutaneously before a meal.[46] The effects of somatostatin on the vasomotor symptoms of dumping are postulated to be due to effects of the compound on splanchnic vessels that prevent vasodilatation. Octreotide also inhibits the release of vasoactive peptides from the gut and slows intestinal transit, effects that may alleviate dumping symptoms. Octreotide administration before meal ingestion has been shown to prevent changes in pulse, systolic blood pressure, and red blood cell volume.

ALKALINE REFLUX GASTRITIS

Alkaline reflux gastritis is a postoperative syndrome characterized by postprandial epigastric pain associated with nausea and vomiting. Endoscopic examination reveals reflux of bile into the stomach, and biopsy demonstrates histologic evidence of gastritis. These findings occur transiently in up to one-fifth of patients after truncal vagotomy and pyloroplasty or gastrectomy, but are persistent in only 1–2% of patients.

Alkaline reflux gastritis is a diagnosis of exclusion. The differential diagnosis of postoperative epigastric pain includes recurrent ulceration, calculous biliary disease, pancreatic inflammation, afferent loop obstruction, and esophagitis. Upper endoscopic examination is essential to exclude recurrent ulcer. The gastric mucosa appears inflamed, friable, and edematous. Gastric inflammation is often uneven and nonulcerative. Histologic examination shows glandular atrophy, mucosal and submucosal edema, and the presence of acute and chronic inflammatory cells in the lamina propria. Intestinal metaplasia may be present.

Postoperative alkaline reflux gastritis is resistant to medical treatment. Antacids, proton pump inhibitors, and dietary manipulations have not been definitively demonstrated to be beneficial. The most effective treatment for persistent alkaline reflux gastritis is operative diversion of intestinal contents from contact with the gastric mucosa. This solution usually requires conversion of a Billroth I or II gastrectomy to a Roux-en-Y gastrojejunostomy with an intestinal limb of 50–60 cm (Fig 11–3). The length of the Roux limb prevents reflux of intestinal contents. This procedure is very effective in eliminating bilious vomiting. However, persistent pain is reported in up to 30% of patients, and 20% of patients develop postoperative delayed gastric emptying.

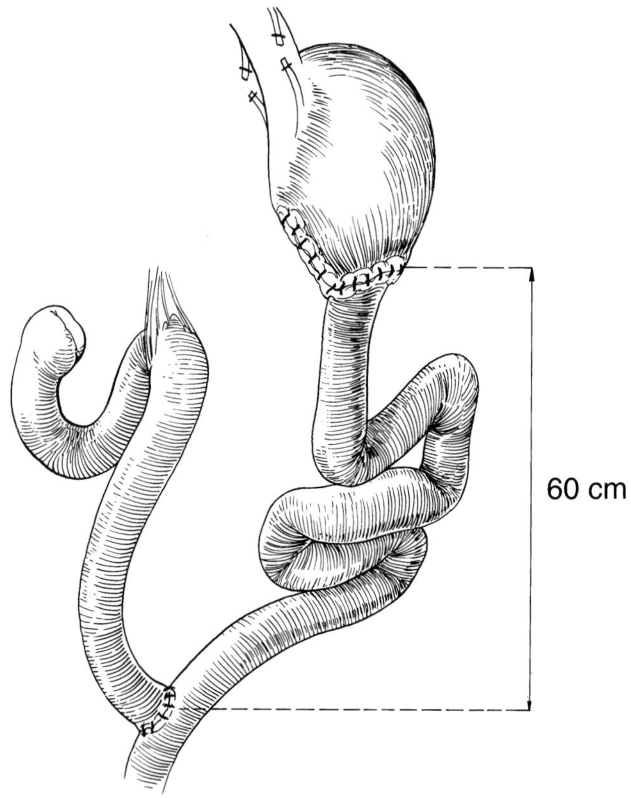

Figure 11–3. Roux-en-Y gastrojejunostomy used to treat alkaline reflux gastritis. (Redrawn from Schwartz SI, Ellis H. *Maingot's Abdominal Operations*, 9th ed. Stamford, CT: Appleton & Lange; 1989:716.)

■ STRESS ULCER DISEASE

Gastritis and gastric ulceration can be induced by physiologic stress. Usually occurring in hospitalized patients with critical illness, stress gastritis can be demonstrated endoscopically in the majority of patients recovering from shock. While occult bleeding in this population is common, clinically significant hemorrhage defined by the need for blood transfusion, hypotension, or alteration in other vital signs occurs in only 0.5–5% of patients. The incidence of clinically significant stress-related bleeding has decreased in the past several decades with the improved understanding of pathogenesis and with widespread adoption of prophylactic treatment protocols. In four recent surgical series comprising more than 28,000 patients, the incidence of clinically significant stress ulceration was 0.4%.[47] In another series of 16,612 hospitalized patients, the incidence of overt stress bleeding was only 0.1%.[48] In a review of patients admitted to both surgical and medical intensive care units, the incidence of clinically significant and endoscopically proven stress ulceration was 0.17%.[49]

Major trauma, especially if accompanied by hypotension, sepsis, respiratory failure, hemorrhage, or multiple injuries, predisposes to acute stress gastritis (Table 11–7). Acute stress gastritis is also common after thermal injury with greater than 35% total body surface area burned. A form of gastritis similar to that following trauma may complicate central nervous system injury or intracranial hypertension. When viewed endoscopically, multiple ulcerations are observed in the proximal, acid-secreting portion of the stomach. Fewer lesions are found in the antrum, and only rare ulcerations in the duodenum.

The major complication of stress gastritis is hemorrhage. Patients with coagulopathy and those requiring mechanical ventilation are at increased risk of hemorrhage. Patients without these two risk factors have been reported to have an overall risk of hemorrhage of only 0.1%, while those with both demonstrate clinically significant bleeding in 3.7% of cases. Respiratory failure is defined as greater than 48 hours on a mechanical ventilator. Coagulopathy is defined as platelet count less than 50,000 per mm^3, an International Normalized Ratio greater than 1.5, or partial thromboplastin time greater than 2 times control.

TABLE 11–7. RISK FACTORS FOR STRESS ULCER BLEEDING

Respiratory failure
Coagulopathy
Hypotension
Sepsis
Hepatic failure
Renal failure
Steroids
Injury Severity Score > 16
Spinal cord injury
Age >55 years

Admission to an intensive care unit by itself does not place patients at risk for hemorrhage, and patients undergoing major gastrointestinal surgery do not have an increased risk of stress-related bleeding in the absence of complications. Increased patient age, emergency surgery, need for reoperation, and the occurrence of hypotension are risk factors for postoperative gastric bleeding. The occurrence of sepsis and respiratory failure are also risk factors. Multiple regression analysis has shown that mechanic ventilation and coagulopathy impart the greatest risk.

The pathogenesis of stress gastritis has been the subject of intensive investigation. Experimental studies suggest that the central event underlying the development of stress gastritis is mucosal ischemia. In clinical practice, most patients who develop stress gastritis have survived an episode of sepsis, hemorrhage, or shock. In animal studies, depletion of high-energy phosphate compounds such as adenosine triphosphate predisposes to the development of stress gastritis. Luminal gastric acid secretion is not the cause of stress gastritis, but is a required concurrent condition. A decline in epithelial energy charge permits proton back-diffusion into the mucosa; the resultant decrease in mucosal pH initiates cellular damage.

The diagnosis of stress ulceration requires endoscopic examination. Acute mucosal ulcerations may be observed as early as 12 hours post-insult; lesions appear as multiple shallow areas of erythema and friability, accompanied by focal hemorrhage. Histologically, the lesions consist of coagulation necrosis of the superficial endothelium with infiltration of leukocytes into the lamina propria. Signs of chronicity, such as fibrosis and scarring, are absent. With resolution of injury or sepsis, healing is accomplished by mucosal restitution and regeneration.

Because hemorrhage does not occur in all patients, studies that use bloody nasogastric discharge as a sign of stress gastritis underestimate the true incidence in critically ill patients. In one endoscopically-controlled study, 100% of patients with life-threatening injuries had evidence of gastric erosions by 24 hours. A high prevalence of gastric erosions is also noted in burn patients, while gastrointestinal hemorrhage occurs in only 25–50% of patients with burn wound infection. Barium contrast examinations have no role in the diagnosis of stress gastritis and interfere with endoscopic examination.

It is important to distinguish stress ulceration from other causes of postoperative hemorrhage. Several recent studies have demonstrated that duodenal ulcer-

TABLE 11–8. RISK FACTOR FOR RESPIRATORY INFECTION IN VENTILATED PATIENTS

Supine position
Nasogastric tube
Continuous enteral feeding
Alkaline enteral feeding

(Reproduced, with permission, from Tryba M. Role of acid suppressants in intensive care medicine. *Best Pract Res Clin Gastroenterol* 2001;15:447–461.)

ation and gastric ulcers are common in postoperative patients. In one series, sources of clinically significant bleeding included duodenal ulcer in 26%, gastric ulcer in 13%, esophagitis in 18%, and esophageal varices in 7%. Similar results have been reported in other series, emphasizing the need for specific diagnosis obtained by endoscopy.

Aspiration of gastric contents into the lungs occurs in more than half of mechanically ventilated intensive care unit patients that are positioned supine (Table 11–8). Nosocomial pneumonia is the most common infection noted in mechanically ventilated patients. Prophylaxis against stress ulceration has been postulated to cause bacterial colonization of the stomach and has been linked to the pathogenesis of pneumonia in treated populations (Table 11–9).

Gastric bacterial colonization occurs from both oral and enteric sources and occurs after 12–24 hours of gastric acid suppression. A recent meta-analysis has demonstrated a trend toward increased risk of pneumonia with H_2-receptor antagonist prophylaxis relative to no prophylaxis. Sucralfate was associated with lower instances of nosocomial pneumonia. Despite the trend toward lower pneumonia rates with sucralfate, no significant difference in overall mortality or duration of intensive care unit care has been demonstrated.

PROPHYLAXIS

Because gastric acidity is a required condition for stress ulcer development, prophylaxis focuses on control of gastric luminal pH. Effective stress ulcer prophylaxis requires that intragastric pH be maintained above 3.5. A number of high-quality prospective studies have demonstrated that administration of H_2-receptor antagonists are as effective as antacids for prophylaxis of stress gastritis. Continuous-infusion H_2-receptor antagonist therapy appears to be equally effective relative to intermittent dosing with H_2 blockers or antacids. Proton pump inhibitors have also been shown to be effective as stress ulcer prophylaxis.[50]

TABLE 11–9. RISK OF PNEUMONIA WITH STRESS ULCER PROPHYLAXIS

Comparison	Odds Ratio
Sucralfate vs. pH-altering drugs	0.63
Sucralfate vs. antacids	0.55
Sucralfate vs. H_2 antagonists	0.69

(Reproduced, with permission, from Tryba M. Role of acid suppressants in intensive care medicine. *Best Pract Res Clin Gastroenterol* 2001;15:447–461.)

Although it has no buffering capacity, sucralfate has demonstrated efficacy as prophylactic treatment for stress gastritis. Sucralfate is not absorbed in the gastrointestinal tract and has no antisecretory activity. The agent binds to exposed collagen in areas of epithelial erosions, but the mechanism of action of sucralfate is incompletely understood. A lower rate of pneumonia has been observed in patients receiving sucralfate relative to prophylactic H_2-receptor antagonist therapy. When stress gastritis causes gastrointestinal bleeding, endoscopic therapy is used as first-line treatment. Endoscopic examination is diagnostic and permits application of electrocautery or heater probe hemostasis.

▪ UPPER GASTROINTESTINAL BLEEDING

Acute upper gastrointestinal (GI) hemorrhages are frequent medical events occurring at a rate of approximately 50 cases per 100,000 persons per year. Acute GI hemorrhage still has a significant associated mortality, approximating 10%. Although urgent esophagogastroduodenoscopy has been used for the past 20 years for the diagnosis and management of acute upper GI hemorrhage, the mortality rate has not substantially declined since the introduction of endoscopic intervention. Patients with acute upper GI hemorrhage are increasingly at advanced age and have preexisting medical comorbidities. Currently, more than one-fourth of patients admitted with acute upper GI hemorrhage in the United States are older than 80 years. It is estimated that acute GI hemorrhage imparts more than $2.5 billion of health care costs in the United States annually.

Endoscopy has become the preferred method for diagnosis in patients with acute upper GI bleeding. This method is informative in most patients, correctly identifying the site and source of bleeding in 90% of cases. While the efficacy of upper endoscopy has been established for diagnosing acute upper gastrointestinal tract hemorrhage, optimal timing has been controversial. The majority of existing studies support the claim that early endoscopy is both safe and effective for all risk groups.

For low-risk patients, the current evidence demonstrates that early endoscopy promotes safe patient disposition. In many instances, these patients can avoid hospitalization with a very low risk of recurrent bleeding. For high-risk patients, there is benefit of early endoscopy for outcomes including transfusion requirements, rebleeding rate, and the need for emergency surgery. Early endoscopy directs therapy and significantly reduces length of hospitalization relative to delayed endoscopy without evidence of cost shifting to the outpatient setting. In this sense, early endoscopy provides prompt diagnosis and assists in decision making regarding clinical triage and subsequent management. Current evidence does not demonstrate, however, that early endoscopy decreases overall mortality. There is no evidence that the practice of early endoscopic intervention results in patient harm.

Based on current information, gastroduodenal ulceration accounts for approximately 40% of cases of acute upper gastrointestinal hemorrhage. Other diagnoses, in decreasing frequency, include acute gastritis, esophageal variceal bleeding, esophagitis, duodenitis, Mallory-Weiss tears, and upper gastrointestinal tract malignancies.

Initial treatment of upper gastrointestinal tract hemorrhage begins with intravascular repletion. Hemodynamic monitoring is crucial. Most patients should be initially treated in an intensive care unit setting. Rationale exists for use of agents that inhibit acid secretion in upper gastrointestinal tract hemorrhage. It is theoretically attractive that reduction in gastric acidity would diminish bleeding or its recurrence. Numerous trials have examined the efficacy of H_2-receptor antagonists in patients with bleeding peptic ulcers. These trials have not demonstrated consistent therapeutic benefit either individually or when examined by meta-analysis. Sixteen prospective trials have also examined the use of proton pump inhibitors in the setting of acute ulcer bleeding. Only 7 of these 16 trials have demonstrated a statistically significant benefit in terms of rebleeding or need for urgent surgical intervention. None of the trials have shown a reduction in mortality. Over half (9 of 16) of the studies did not demonstrate reduction in any of the primary outcomes which included rebleeding, surgery, or mortality.

In addition to providing diagnostic information, aggressive endoscopy also presents an opportunity for therapeutic intervention. Relative to medical therapy alone, patients with stigmata of active bleeding, visible vessels, and nonbleeding adherent clots benefit from endoscopic ulcer hemostasis. The major modalities employed include bipolar electrocautery probes, heater probes, and epinephrine injection.

Patients with hemorrhage from peptic ulceration experience arterial bleeding, as the ulcer erodes into branches of the pancreaticoduodenal arcade. The endoscopic "visible vessel" represents a pseudoaneurysm, an organized clot covering a side hole in an artery. The mean diameter of involved arteries underlying gastric ulcers is reported to be 0.7 mm. The mean arterial diameter of fatal duodenal ulcer hemorrhage has been reported at 1.0 mm. Contact probes control hemorrhage from these large vessels by coaptive coagulation. The stiff probe is used to initially compress the artery, interrupting arterial blood flow. Subsequent application of energy causes coaptive coagulation. Proteins are coagulated above 60°C. Both heater probes and bipolar probes can weld arteries as large as 2.5 mm in diameter. Vessel compression is important. Vessel erosion and worsened bleeding may result when arteries larger than 0.5 mm in diameter are treated by methods that do not involve compression.

Mechanisms by which epinephrine injections cause ulcer hemostasis have been examined experimentally. Epinephrine causes intense vasoconstriction, platelet aggregation, and vessel sclerosis. These combined effects permit permanent control of arterial hemorrhage in most patients. Absolute alcohol has also been used for injection therapy with good results.

Potential complications of endoscopic therapy include bowel perforation and incitement of active bleeding from a nonbleeding vessel. The rate of perforation is low, and has been reported to approximate 0.7%. New bleeding is induced by therapy in less than 1% of patients.

Under selective circumstances, repeated attempts at endoscopic therapy may also be employed. In a prospective randomized trial, investigators evaluated whether emergency surgery or repeated endoscopic therapy resulted in better outcomes for patients with severe ulcer hemorrhage. Endoscopic therapy consisted of a combination of epinephrine injection and heater probe application. Definitive hemostasis was significantly higher in surgically treated patients (93% versus 73%), but the complication rate was significantly higher in the surgery group (36%) relative to the endoscopy group (15%).

Acute therapy of variceal bleeding may also be directed endoscopically. Major approaches have included variceal injection with sclerosants and band ligation. Because of efficacy and safety, endoscopic variceal ligation has largely replaced sclerotherapy as the endoscopic method of choice for acute variceal hemorrhage.[51] This method has also been employed for secondary prevention of esophageal variceal hemorrhage. Prospective randomized trials indicate that prophylactic variceal ligation decreases the risk of first variceal bleeding relative to no treatment or to treatment with propranolol. In addition, ligation decreases the risk of recurrent bleeding and associated mortality relative to no treatment. In this circumstance, however, relative to propranolol therapy, ligation does not improve mortality.

In patients with acute peptic ulcer as a cause for upper gastrointestinal hemorrhage, *H. pylori* is a common etiology. After initial control of hemorrhage, eradication of infection should be a treatment imperative. Because eradication of *H. pylori* eliminates ulcer recurrence, it is logical to assume that it would also decrease the rate of recurrent ulcer bleeding. Randomized trials demonstrate that recurrent hemorrhage usually occurs in patients who have persistent or recurrent *H. pylori* infection. Without antibiotic treatment recurrent hemorrhage occurs in as many as 20% of patients. The risk of recurrent hemorrhage can be reduced to approximately 3% in individuals treated with an effective antibiotic regimen after hemorrhage.

REFERENCES

1. Marshall BJ, Warren JR. Unidentified curved bacilli in the stomach of patients with gastritis and peptic ulceration. *Lancet* 1984;1:1311–1315
2. Lassen AT, Pedersen FM, Bytzer P, et al. *Helicobacter pylori* test-and-eradicate versus prompt endoscopy for management of dyspeptic patients: a randomized trial. *Lancet* 2000;356:455–460
3. Moayyedi P, Soo S, Deeks J, et al. Eradication of *Helicobacter pylori* for non-ulcer dyspepsia [review]. *The Cochrane Library* 2004;2
4. Laine L, Schoenfeld P, Fennerty MB. Therapy for *Helicobacter pylori* in patients with nonulcer dyspepsia. *Ann Intern Med* 2001;134:361–369
5. Logan RPH, Hirschl AM. Epidemiology of *Helicobacter pylori* infection. *Curr Opin Gastroenterol* 1996;12:1–5
6. National Institutes of Health. *Helicobacter pylori* in peptic ulcer disease. *NIH Consensus Statement* 1994;12:1–18
7. Suerbaum S, Michetti P. *Helicobacter pylori* infection. *N Engl J Med* 2002;347:1175–1186
8. Kokoska ER, Kauffman GL Jr. *Helicobacter pylori* and the gastroduodenal mucosa. *Surgery* 2001;130:13–16
9. Blaser MJ. *Helicobacter* are indigenous to the human stomach: duodenal ulceration is due to changes in gastric microecology in the modern era. *Gut* 1998;43:721–727
10. Atherton JC. The clinical relevance of strain types of *Helicobacter pylori.* Gut 1997;40:701–703
11. Hatz R, Schildberg FW. *Helicobacter pylori* infections—are these diseases relevant for surgical treatment? *Arch Surg* 2003;385:75–83
12. Morris A, Nicholson G. Ingestion of *Campylobacter pyloridis* causes gastritis and raised fasting gastric pH. *Am J Gastroenterol* 1987;82:192–199
13. Crabtree JE, Farmery SM, Lindley IJD, et al. Cag A/cytotoxic strains of *Helicobacter pylori* and interleukin-8 in gastric epithelial cell lines. *J Clin Pathol* 1994;47:945–950
14. Peterson WL, Barnett CC, Evans DJ, et al. Acid secretion and serum gastrin in normal subjects and patients with duodenal ulcer: the role of *Helicobacter pylori. Am J Gastroenterol* 1993;88:2038–2043
15. Queiroz DM, Mendez EN, Rocha GA, et al. Effect of *Helicobacter pylori* eradication on antral gastrin- and somatostatin-immunoreactive cell density and gastrin and somatostatin concentrations. *Scand J Gastroenterol* 1993;28:858–864
16. Cryer B. Mucosal defense and repair. *Gastroenterol Clin North Am* 2001;30:877–894
17. Isenberg JI, Selling JA, Hogan DL, et al. Impaired proximal duodenal mucosal bicarbonate secretion in patients with duodenal ulcer. *N Engl J Med* 1987;316:374
18. Bukhave K, Rask-Madsen J, Hogan DL, et al. Proximal duodenal prostaglandin E2 release and mucosal bicarbonate secretion are altered in patients with duodenal ulcer. *Gastroenterology* 1990;99:951
19. Peskar BM, Maricic N, Gretzer B, et al. Role of cyclooxygenase-2 in gastric mucosal defense. *Life Sci* 2001;69: 2993–3003
20. Parasher G, Eastwood GL. Smoking and peptic ulcer in the *Helicobacter pylori* era. *Eur J Gastroenterol Hepatol* 2000; 12:843–853
21. Sontag S, Graham DY, Belsito A, et al. Cimetidine, cigarette smoking, and recurrence of duodenal ulcer. *N Engl J Med* 1984;311:689
22. Huang JQ, Sridhar S, Hunt RH. Role of *Helicobacter pylori* infection and non-steroidal anti-inflammatory drugs in peptic-ulcer disease: a meta-analysis. *Lancet* 2002;359:14–22
23. Hopkins RJ, Girardi LS, Turney EA. Relationship between *Helicobacter pylori* eradication and reduced duodenal and gastric ulcer recurrence: a review. *Gastroenterology* 1996;110:1244–1252
24. Laheij RJR, Van Rossum LGM, Jansen JBMJ, et al. Evaluation of treatment regimens to cure *Helicobacter pylori* infection—a meta-analysis. *Aliment Pharmacol Ther* 1999; 13:857–864
25. Houben MHMG, Van De Beek D, Hensen EF, et al. A systematic review of *Helicobacter pylori* eradication therapy—the impact of antimicrobial resistance on eradication rates. *Aliment Pharmacol Ther* 1999;13:1047–1055
26. Berstad A, Weberg R. Antacids in the treatment of gastroduodenal ulcer. *Scand J Gastroenterol* 1986;21:385
27. Johnson AG. Proximal gastric vagotomy: does it have a place in the future management of peptic ulcer? *World J Surg* 2000;24:259–263
28. Kleeff J, Friess H, Büchler MW. How *Helicobacter pylori* changed the life of surgeons. *Dig Surg* 2003;20:93–102
29. Millat B, Fingerhut A, Borie F. Surgical treatment of complicated duodenal ulcers: controlled trials. *World J Surg* 2000;24:299–306
30. Espat NJ, Ong ES, Helton WS, et al. 1990–2001 U.S. General Surgery chief resident operative experience: analysis of paradigm shift. *J Gastrointest Surg* 2004;8:471–477
31. Bustamante M, Stollman N. The efficacy of proton-pump inhibitors in acute ulcer bleeding. A qualitative review. *J Clin Gastroenterol* 2000;30:7–13
32. Machicado GA, Jensen DM. Thermal probes alone or with epinephrine for the endoscopic haemostasis of ulcer haemorrhage. *Baillieres Clin Gastroenterol* 2000;14:443–458
33. Hepworth CC, Swain CP. Mechanical endoscopic methods of haemostasis for bleeding peptic ulcers: a review. *Baillieres Clin Gastroenterol* 2000;14:467–476

34. Spiegel BMR, Vakil NB, Ofman JJ. Endoscopy for acute nonvariceal upper gastrointestinal tract hemorrhage: is sooner better? *Arch Intern Med* 2001;161:1393–1404
35. Gisbert JP, Khorrami S, Carballo F, et al. H. pylori eradication therapy vs. antisecretory non-eradication therapy (with or without long-term maintenance antisecretory therapy) for the prevention of recurrent bleeding from peptic ulcer. *The Cochrane Library* 2004;2
36. Sharma VK, Sahai AV, Corder FA, et al. Helicobacter pylori eradication is superior to ulcer healing with or without maintenance therapy to prevent further ulcer haemorrhage. *Ailment Pharmacol Ther* 2001;15:1939–1947
37. Leivonen MK, Haglund CH, Nordling SFA. *Helicobacter pylori* infection after partial gastrectomy for peptic ulcer and its role in relapsing disease. *Eur J Gastroenterol Hepatol* 1997;9:369–374
38. Boey J, Wong J, Ong GB. A prospective study of operative risk factors in perforated duodenal ulcers. *Ann Surg* 1982;195:265
39. Matsuda M, Nishiyama M, Hanai T, et al. Laparoscopic omental patch repair for perforated peptic ulcer. *Ann Surg* 1995;221:236–240
40. Lau W-Y, Leung K-L, Kwong K-H, et al. A randomized study comparing laparoscopic versus open repair of perforated peptic ulcer using suture or sutureless technique. *Ann Surg* 1996;224:131–138
41. Dubois F. New surgical strategy for gastroduodenal ulcer: laparoscopic approach. *World J Surg* 2000;24:270–276
42. Lagoo S, McMahon RL, Kakihara M, et al. The sixth decision regarding perforated duodenal ulcer. *JSLS* 2002; 6:359–368
43. Donovan AJ, Berne TV, Donovan JA. Perforated duodenal ulcer: an alternative therapeutic plan. *Arch Surg* 1998;133:1166–1171
44. Matsuda M, Nishiyama M, Hanai T, et al. Laparoscopic omental patch repair for perforated peptic ulcer. *Ann Surg* 1995;221:236–240
45. Hogan RB, Hamilton JK, Polter DE. Preliminary experience with hydrostatic balloon dilation of gastric outlet obstruction. *Gastrointest Endosc* 1986;32:71
46. Lamers CBHW, Bijlstra AM, Harris AG. Octreotide, a long-acting somatostatin analog, in the management of postoperative dumping syndrome. *Dig Dis Sci* 1993;38:359
47. Hiramoto JS, Terdiman JP, Norton JA. Evidence-based analysis: postoperative gastric bleeding: etiology and prevention. *Surg Oncol* 2003;12:9–19
48. Wijdicks EF, Fulgham JR, Batts KP. Gastrointestinal bleeding in stroke. *Stroke* 1994;25:2146–2148
49. Pimental M, Roberts DE, Bernstein CN, et al. Clinically significant gastrointestinal bleeding in critically ill patients in an era of prophylaxis. *Am J Gastroenterol* 2000; 95:2801–2806
50. Yang Y, Lewis JD. Prevention and treatment of stress ulcers in critically ill patients. *Semin Gastrointest Dis* 2003;14:11–19
51. Imperiale TF, Chalasani N. A meta-analysis of endoscopic variceal ligation for primary prophylaxis of esophageal variceal bleeding. *Hepatology* 2001;33:802–807

12

Ulcer Complications

Timothy J. Broderick ■ Jeffrey B. Matthews

■ BACKGROUND

Recognition of the roles that *Helicobacter pylori* (*H. pylori*) and nonsteroidal anti-inflammatory drugs (NSAIDs) play in peptic ulcer disease has revolutionized the care of patients who suffer from gastroduodenal ulcer. Research over the last decade confirmed that *H. pylori* infection and NSAID use are highly associated with peptic ulcer disease.[1–4] Recent data suggest that more than 99% of all duodenal ulcers and 96% of all gastric ulcers are associated with either *H. pylori* infection or NSAID use.[5] Medical therapy has become significantly more effective with eradication of *H. pylori*, improved antisecretory medicines (histamine-2 receptor antagonists and proton pump inhibitors), and introduction of NSAIDs that have less effect on mucosal integrity. Endoscopic diagnosis and therapy also have improved in the last decade.

Better understanding of the pathogenesis and improvement in the treatment of peptic ulcer disease have decreased the incidence of intractable ulcer disease that requires surgical intervention dramatically.[6,7] While medical advances have translated into fewer elective ulcer operations, ulcer disease continues to exact a heavy personal and financial toll. Currently, the personal toll of ulcer disease is seen mainly in the complications of perforation and bleeding. The incidence of and morbidity and mortality from perforation and hemorrhage have remained essentially unchanged over the preceding decade.[6,7]

The financial cost incurred by treatment of peptic ulcer disease is staggering. It was estimated recently that peptic ulcer disease costs approximately $3.1 billion dollars annually in the United States.[8] While research supports antibiotic eradication of *H. pylori* and the use of proton pump inhibitors in the treatment of peptic ulcer disease, the cost of management continues to escalate, with the increase driven primarily by the expense of antisecretory drugs.[9,10] For example, while only a portion of proton pump inhibitors are prescribed for peptic ulcer disease, sales of these agents totaled more than $10 billion in the United States in 2001.[9,11]

■ EVOLUTION IN PEPTIC ULCER DISEASE TREATMENT

HELICOBACTER PYLORI

H. pylori eradication represents a paradigm shift in the treatment of peptic ulcer disease.[1,12] *H. pylori* is found in the mucus layer of the surface epithelium and the crypts of gastric glands in nearly all patients with duodenal ulcer and the majority of patients with gastric ulcer.[12] *H. pylori* infection is diagnosed easily via urea breath test, serology, or antigen stool assay. The diagnosis also can be made with analysis of endoscopic antral biopsies via urease test, histology, culture, or polymerase chain reaction (PCR). While the contribution of *H. pylori* to specific complications of ulcer disease is still debated, the vast majority of patients who suffer a complication of peptic ulcer disease are *H. pylori*–positive or take NSAIDs.[2] Further studies are needed to determine the exact prevalence of this bacteria in complicated peptic ulcer disease. *H. pylori* treatment should reflect evidence-based guidelines as well as patterns of local bacterial resistance. Eradication should be confirmed after completion of treatment. The crucial role that *H. pylori* plays in peptic ulcer disease is emphasized by the decrease in ulcer recurrence by over 90% with its eradication.[13–16]

The pathophysiology of *H. pylori* infection is not completely understood. Putative mechanisms by which *H. pylori* promotes ulcer formation include stimulation of gastrin release, inhibition of somatostatin release, interruption of inhibitory vagal reflexes, and inhibition of gastroduodenal bicarbonate secretion.[12] As discussed throughout this chapter, *H. pylori* eradication has decreased the need for elective surgery significantly and also has changed the selection of which procedures are performed commonly in the urgent setting in the treatment of ulcer complications. Additional investigation is needed to determine the optimal combination of medical, endoscopic, and surgical therapy in the treatment of peptic ulcer disease.

NONSTEROIDAL ANTI-INFLAMMATORY DRUGS

Recent research has confirmed the association of NSAIDs with peptic ulcer disease.[2,3] Amelioration of the gastrointestinal complications related to these agents can be achieved through patient counseling to limit or stop medication use, prescription of additional agents to minimize the gastrointestinal side effects (such as antibiotics in *H. pylori*–positive patients, prostaglandins, and antisecretory medicines), and prescription of NSAIDs with minimal gastrointestinal side effects to patients at risk of developing gastrointestinal complications.

In the last decade, cyclooxygenase-2 (COX-2)–selective NSAIDs have been introduced that are associated with markedly fewer gastrointestinal complications and peptic ulcer disease. For example, a recent study of lumiracoxib showed a three- to fourfold reduction in ulcer complications compared with other NSAIDs in the treatment of patients with osteoarthritis.[17] Unfortunately, selective NSAIDs cost significantly more than nonselective agents, with sales of selective drugs totaling billions of dollars in the United States annually. Recently, an increased rate of serious cardiovascular events has prompted withdraw of one of the most commonly prescribed selective inhibitors. In the long term, refinement of NSAIDs and improved treatment protocols should further reduce the incidence of peptic ulcer disease and its complications.

SURGICAL INDICATION AND PROCEDURE SELECTION

Surgical treatment of peptic ulcer disease has evolved from elective surgery for medically refractory ulcer disease to urgent surgery in the treatment of perforation or hemorrhage.[6,7,18,19] Classically, complications of peptic ulcer disease requiring surgery included intractability, obstruction, perforation, and hemorrhage. With more effective medical therapy, elective operations to treat intractable peptic ulcer disease have become very uncommon.[6,7,19] Currently, gastric resection for malignancy, gastric surgery in the treatment of morbid obesity, and fundoplication in the management of gastroesophageal reflux disease represent the most frequent indications for elective gastric surgery.[20–24] Perforated or bleeding ulcers remain a relatively common indication for urgent surgery.[6,7,19] Gastric outlet obstruction for peptic ulcer disease is a less common indication for elective gastric surgery.[25]

▪ COMPLICATIONS OF PEPTIC ULCER DISEASE

Epidemiological data suggest that the incidence of ulcer complications has remained stable or has increased slightly over the last decade. For example, elective operations for peptic ulcer disease decreased from 157 to 17 operations per 100,000 inhabitants between 1987 and 1999 in Finland.[7,19] The annual incidence of emergency surgery increased concomitantly from 52 to 70 operations per 100,000 inhabitants. During this period, the annual hospital admission rate nearly doubled to 687 admissions per 100,000 inhabitants primarily owing to bleeding from gastric ulcer in elderly women. The overall surgical mortality rate remained 8%. While emergency surgery remained constant, elective surgery for peptic ulcer disease now is infrequent in Finland.

Interestingly, local procedures such as suture duodenorrhaphy and gastrorrhaphy were applied in 25% of operations for peptic ulcer disease in 1987 and were applied in 90% of operations for peptic ulcer disease surgery in 1999. Other procedures, specifically parietal cell vagotomy, are now performed quite infrequently in Finland. Additional studies from the United Kingdom demonstrated that most surgeons there no longer perform any form of vagotomy for peptic ulcer complications.[26,27]

A recent study from the United States suggests that surgical treatment of peptic ulcer disease has evolved similarly.[28] Within a large tertiary-care hospital, the number of operations performed for peptic ulcers decreased annually from 24 to 11 per 100,000 inhabitants. Seventy-seven percent of all cases were done urgently, and the most common indication was perforated ulcer. Over the last two decades, the 30-day mortality rate of

13% remained unchanged. Despite a decrease in surgical volume, there was an increase in the proportion of urgent operations performed.

Clearly, the indication for and selection of operations for peptic ulcer disease have evolved in the last decade secondary to improvements in medical therapy. The majority of surgeons now select the simplest and quickest operation that will address the ulcer complication while minimizing the postoperative gastrointestinal side effects. The decrease in ulcer recurrence provided by definitive acid-reduction surgery has been replaced by *H. pylori* eradication, tailored NSAID drug therapy, and proton pump inhibitor therapy.[19,26,27,68] The recommended operative procedures in complicated peptic ulcer disease are summarized in Table 12–1. The rationale for these recommendations is explained in detail in the remainder of this chapter.

INTRACTABILITY

Incidence

As mentioned previously, surgical treatment of peptic ulcer disease has evolved from elective surgery for medically refractory ulcer disease to urgent surgery in the treatment of perforation or hemorrhage. Elective surgical treatment of intractable peptic ulcer has virtually disappeared over the last decade.[108]

Diagnosis

Diagnosis begins with a thorough history and physical examination. Chronic ulcer disease often is associated with midepigastric pain. Detailed questioning about the pain can help to differentiate intractable ulcer disease from pain associated with other diseases such as symptomatic cholelithiasis. The patient should be questioned regarding the clinical course of his or her peptic ulcer disease and the success of prior treatment. Specific questions should be asked about compliance with previously recommended therapy, including *H. pylori* eradication, limitation of NSAID use, maintenance antisecretory medication therapy, smoking cessation, and limitation of alcohol intake. A family history of intractable ulcer disease and multiple endocrine neoplasia should be explored. The patient also should be asked about the complications of peptic ulcer disease, including perforation and bleeding.

The history and physical is complemented by a directed laboratory examination that includes a complete blood count, comprehensive metabolic profile, and serum gastrin determination. In most cases of intractable ulcer disease, the laboratory examination is normal, but chronic anemia can be present. Although the history and physical examination can narrow the differential diagnosis, an upper gastrointestinal barium series or endoscopy is necessary to diagnose an intractable gastroduodenal ulcer accurately. Endoscopic biopsy can provide tissue and thereby direct therapy for persistent *H. pylori* infection or malignancy.

TABLE 12–1. RECOMMENDED OPERATIVE PROCEDURES IN COMPLICATED PEPTIC ULCER DISEASE

Complication	Location	Operation
Intractability	DU bulb	PGV
	GU I	Distal gastrectomy
	GU II + III	Distal gastrectomy
	GU IV	Subtotal gastrectomy
Perforation	DU anterior bulb	Lap or open closure/onlay
	GU II	Excision/closure or distal gastrectomy
Bleeding	DU posterior bulb	Oversew
	GU I	Distal gastrectomy
	GU II + III	Excision/closure or distal gastrectomy
	GU IV	Subtotal gastrectomy
Obstruction	DU bulb	Distal gastrectomy
	GU III	Distal gastrectomy

Treatment

Surgical. *Intractable Duodenal Ulcer.* Proximal gastric vagotomy is recommended for elective use in the very unusual patient with intractable symptoms of peptic ulcer despite maximal medical treatment. A patient with persistent duodenal ulcer in the absence of *H. pylori* infection that requires continued treatment with NSAIDs is also an indication for elective definitive surgical treatment through proximal gastric vagotomy. Proximal gastric vagotomy results are technique-dependent, and elective surgical patients should be referred to a center with expertise in performing this operation.[26]

This procedure has been called a variety of names, e.g., *highly selective vagotomy, superselective vagotomy,* and *parietal cell vagotomy.* We prefer *proximal gastric* or *highly selective vagotomy.* While some minor technical details are debated, the basic procedure is well described.[29–34] A drainage procedure is not necessary and has been shown to be detrimental to the clinical results.[31,35] The procedure can be performed open or laparoscopically.

In the proximal gastric vagotomy, the surgeon spares the "crow's foot" of the vagi that innervate the pylorus and antrum. The crow's foot is the distal branch of the nerve of Latarjet (the gastric vagi distal to the hepatic and celiac divisions). By preserving the crow's foot, innervation of the last 6 cm of the stomach immediately proximal to the pylorus is preserved. In the proximal gastric vagotomy, the surgeon denervates the distal esophagus and proximal stomach by dividing the anterior and posterior vagal branches that innervate the distal 6 cm of the esophagus, the gastric fundus, and gastric body. The denervation is accomplished by division of the vagi and vessels of the anterior and posterior leaflets of the gastrohepatic ligament. The deserosalized lesser curve is closed subsequently with interrupted sutures. Proximal gastric vagotomy and other standard forms of vagotomy are illustrated schematically in Figure 12–1.[36]

Intractable Gastric Ulcer. Gastric ulcer is a heterogeneous disorder. The relationship between the anatomic location and pathophysiology of gastric ulcer that was described originally by Johnson is illustrated in Figure 12–2.[37]

Type I, or primary, ulcers typically are located on the lesser curvature at the junction of the fundic and antral regions of the stomach, occur in older patients, and are associated with gastric acid hyposecretion. Type II, or combined, gastric and duodenal ulcers are lesser-curvature lesions that occur in association with active or quiescent duodenal ulcer disease. Type III ulcers are prepyloric lesions. Type II and III ulcers occur in younger patients with high acid secretory rates, and their management is similar to the management of duodenal ulcer. Up to 30% of gastric ulcers are associated with duodenal ulcers. Type IV ulcers are juxtaesophageal ulcers that are situated high on the lesser curvature near the gastroesophageal junction and probably are variants of type I ulcers. They are discussed separately in this chapter because of the technical difficulty associated with surgical treatment of these lesions.

Recent analysis of the risk factors associated with the development of different types of gastric ulcer support the heterogeneity of gastric ulcer pathogenesis.[38] Among all gastric ulcer subsets, cigarette smoking, NSAID use, and *H. pylori* infection are independent ulcer risk factors. Smoking and NSAID use are associated with type I ulceration. In type II and III gastric ulcers, smoking, NSAID use, and *H. pylori* infection are identified as risk factors. *H. pylori* infection is associated most strongly with gastroduodenal ulcer in type II ulceration, and NSAID use is associated most often with type III ulceration. NSAID use markedly raised the likelihood of multiple gastric ulcers. Patients with all types of gastric ulcer should be advised to limit use of these agents as much as possible, to stop smoking, and to take proton pump inhibitors and antibiotics to eradicate *H. pylori*.

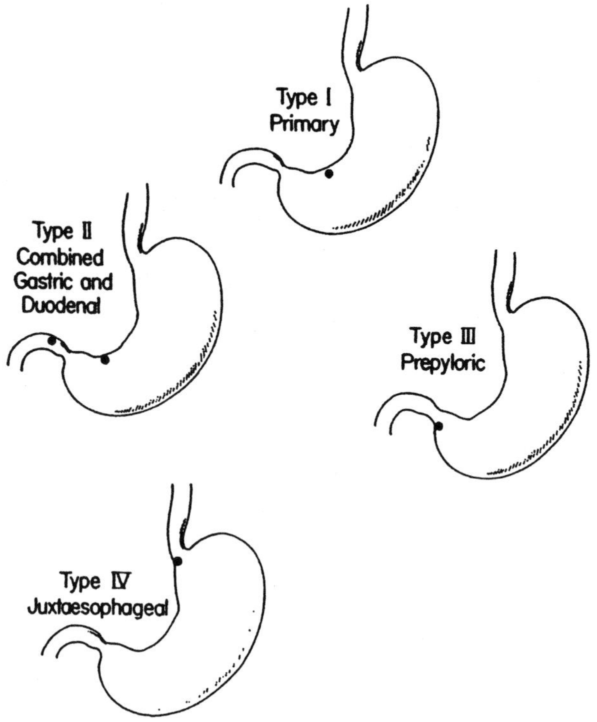

Figure 12–2. Types of gastric ulcers. (Reprinted from Peptic ulcer surgery. In: Sleisenger MH, Fordtran JS (eds). *Gastrointestinal Disease: Pathophysiology, Diagnosis, Management.* Philadelphia: Saunders, 1993:719, with permission from Elsevier.)

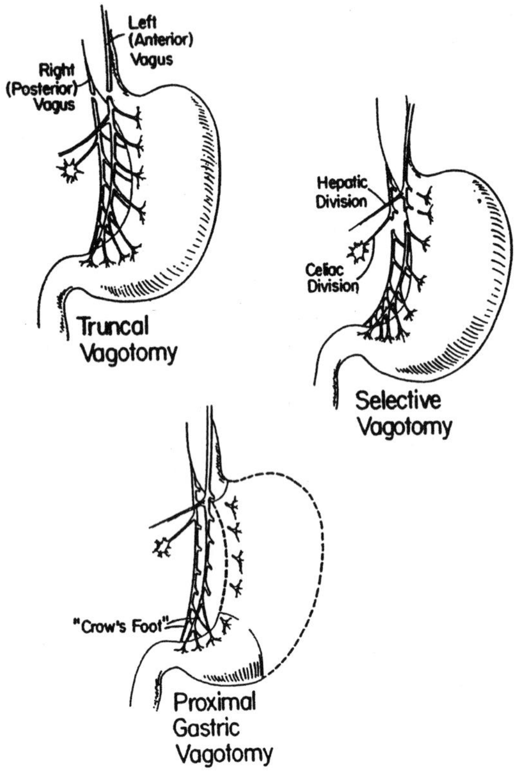

Figure 12–1. Schematic representation of the three standard forms of vagotomy. (Reprinted from Peptic ulcer surgery. In: Sleisenger MH, Fordtran JS (eds). *Gastrointestinal Disease: Pathophysiology, Diagnosis, Management.* Philadelphia: Saunders, 1993:717, with permission from Elsevier.)

Recommendations regarding surgical treatment of intractable gastric ulcer are best discussed within the context of this classification system. In type I ulcers, the pathogenesis is not clearly understood, and like gastric cancer, they often occur at the junction of antral and fundic mucosa. Therefore, surgical recommendations include excision of the ulcer. At this point on the lesser curve, wedge excision often is difficult, and minimal additional dissection is required to perform a formal distal gastrectomy. Therefore, a partial gastrectomy is recommended unless the patient is unable to tolerate a resection because of comorbid disease or intraoperative instability. If the patient is unstable, the ulcer should be excised and closed. A vagotomy is not recommended for type I gastric ulcers.

H. pylori and acid hypersecretion are associated with type II and type III gastric ulcers, and treatment should parallel treatment recommended for duodenal ulcers. There is no consensus regarding surgical treatment of these ulcers. Because of the concern for malignancy in gastric ulcer, excision of these gastric ulcers is recommended. The anatomy and inflammation found at operation dictate procedure selection. Excision with primary closure is acceptable when technically feasible. When simple closure would narrow the gastric outlet or multiple ulcers are present, a distal gastrectomy is recommended. When significant duodenal inflammation would make a distal gastrectomy technically challenging, gastric ulcer excision with a vagotomy and pyloroplasty is suggested.

Juxtaesophageal ulcers likely represent a variant of type I ulcers that are described primarily because of the technical difficulty associated with their excision. Postoperative morbidity and mortality are increased with juxtaesophageal ulcer location.[39] Excision is complicated by large-diameter ulcers, significant surrounding inflammation, and location near the gastroesophageal junction. Operative procedures used to treat such ulcers are illustrated in Figure 12–3.[40]

Ulcer excision with primary closure usually is not feasible because of the proximal lesser-curve location of these ulcers. Subtotal gastrectomy is recommended when the ulcer can be excised without restricting the esophageal lumen. Another alternative is the Pauchet procedure—a distal gastrectomy with a sleevelike extension along the lesser curvature to incorporate the ulcer. A Roux-en-Y may be helpful in reconstruction after a high subtotal gastrectomy. The Kelling-Madlener procedure, in which the ulcer is biopsied and a distal gastrectomy is performed, is not recommended because of the risk of recurrent symptoms and of missing malignant disease.[41] Truncal vagotomy plus antrectomy or pylorplasty with ulcer excision has been used in the past, but the addition of vagotomy in the current era is

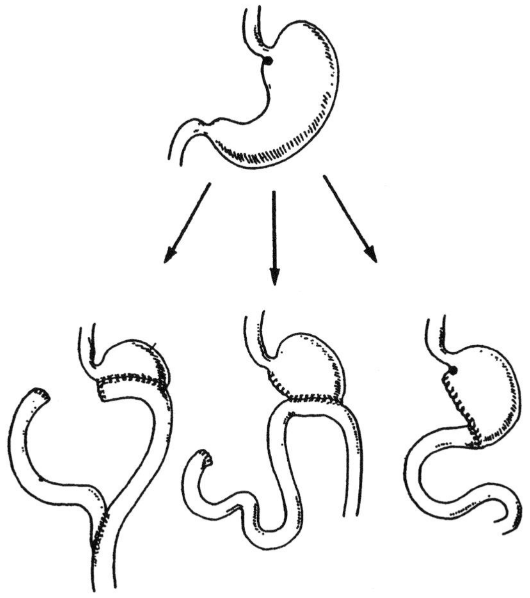

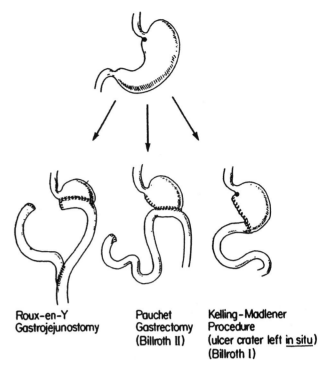

Figure 12–3. Surgical procedures used in juxtaesophageal gastric ulcer. (Reprinted from Peptic ulcer surgery. In: Sleisenger MH, Fordtran JS (ed). *Gastrointestinal Disease: Pathophysiology, Diagnosis, Management.* Philadelphia: Saunders, 1993:720, with permission from Elsevier.)

of questionable value. As a general rule, proximal gastric resection that includes the gastroesophageal junction should be avoided.

PERFORATION

Incidence

In general, the incidences of emergency surgery, hospital admission, and mortality for perforated peptic ulcer have remained stable through the last two decades. In older patients, admission rates for duodenal ulcer perforation increased and gastric ulcer perforation decreased in the last decade. Duodenal perforation currently accounts for approximately 75% of peptic perforation. Of note, the mortality rate for perforated ulcer is higher in the elderly and is higher after gastric than after duodenal perforation. In a recent study, a postoperative mortality rate of 19% in perforated peptic ulcer patients increased to 41% among the elderly.[42]

Factors such as concomitant diseases, shock on admission, delayed surgery (>24 hours), resectional surgery, and postoperative abdominal and wound infections have been associated with increased morbidity and mortality in perforated ulcer patients.[43–46] For decades, delay in operative treatment has remained a primary determinant of morbidity, mortality, and cost. A recent study suggests that a positive peritoneal fungal culture is common and is a significant risk factor for adverse outcome in patients with a perforated peptic ulcer.[47] A positive peritoneal fungal culture has been associated with a higher incidence of surgical-site infection, a longer hospital stay, and a significantly higher mortality rate.

The mean prevalence of *H. pylori* infection in patients with perforated peptic ulcer is approximately 60% compared with 90–100% in uncomplicated ulcer disease. However, if NSAID use is excluded, the prevalence of infection is similar to that found in patients with nonperforated ulcer disease at 90%.[107] In addition to *H. pylori* and NSAID use, smoking and alcohol consumption are also associated with perforated peptic ulcer.

Diagnosis

Diagnosis begins with a thorough history and physical examination. The history and physical examination are complemented by a directed laboratory examination that includes a complete blood count, comprehensive metabolic profile, coagulation profile, and amylase determination. In patients who present with a clinical picture worrisome for shock, an arterial blood gas analysis and lactate level may provide additional information concerning the degree of physiologic compromise and help to guide resuscitation. A type and screen should be sent to the blood bank prior to operation. Early after perforation, laboratory tests usually are normal, with the exception of leukocytosis and possibly mild hyperamylasemia. Later, additional abnormalities suggestive of a systemic inflammatory response syndrome develop, such as decreased renal function and hypoxia.

The selection of radiologic examinations is determined by the clinical presentation. If severe diffuse peritonitis is present, suggesting an acute surgical abdomen, no imaging is necessary prior to exploration. If the diagnosis and need for operation are less clear, it is appropriate to begin with plain abdominal radiography. The acute abdominal series includes an upright chest (if tolerated), supine abdominal, and upright or left lateral decubitus abdominal films. Free air indicating a perforated viscus is present in 70% of patients with perforated peptic ulcer, and therefore, its absence cannot be taken as evidence against the diagnosis (Fig. 12–4).

If free air is not present and the abdominal series is otherwise unremarkable, the diagnosis can be made with either a computed tomographic (CT) scan of the abdomen and pelvis or a Gastrografin upper gastrointestinal series. CT scan provides more information and is the preferred diagnostic test if the differential diagnosis remains wide. While an upper gastrointestinal series can be of help in establishing the diagnosis, it is used more frequently to delineate anatomy and confirm a contained perforation, especially if nonoperative management of the perforated ulcer is being considered.

While the diagnosis is easily made in many patients, it can be surprisingly difficult to diagnose a perforated peptic ulcer in some patients. Difficulty and delay in diagnosis are seen in patients who are young, elderly, obese, immunocompromised, and in the immediate postoperative period. Early diagnosis of a perforated ulcer in patients with altered mental status from mental illness, spinal cord injury, or substance abuse requires a high index of suspicion and liberal use of diagnostic tests.

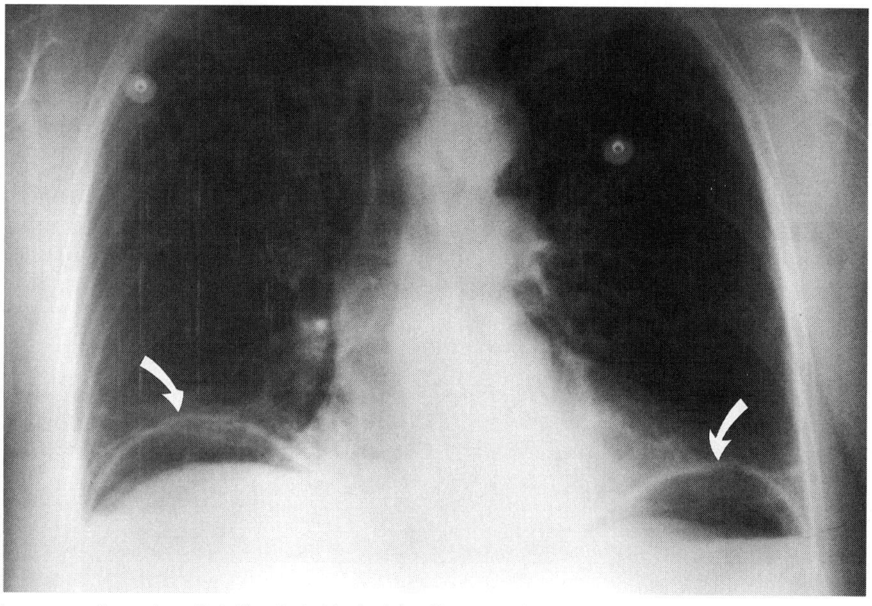

Figure 12–4. Chest x-ray showing pneumoperitoneum in a patient with perforated duodenal ulcer. The arrows point to free intra-abdominal air beneath the right and left hemidiaphragms.

Treatment

Treatment begins with insertion of a sump nasogastric tube to decompress the gastrointestinal tract and limit additional peritoneal soilage. A Foley catheter is inserted to monitor urine output and direct resuscitation. The patient is resuscitated aggressively by administration of intravenous crystalloid. Intravenous broad-spectrum antibiotics are also administered. Invasive hemodynamic monitors (e.g., central venous, arterial, and pulmonary artery catheters) are inserted as clinical status and comorbid medical conditions dictate. Associated medical illnesses such as coronary artery disease should be treated quickly and effectively so as to minimize complications. Since morbidity and mortality are associated with delay in operation, it is important to avoid prolonged preoperative resuscitation and to proceed to the operating room as quickly as possible. Informed consent should include the local procedure and more extensive procedures that could be necessary. These procedures include acid-reduction procedures, resection, and feeding tubes required for postoperative nutritional support.

Medical. *Conservative.* In patients who do not have generalized peritonitis, hemodynamic instability, or free peritoneal perforation on a Gastrografin upper gastrointestinal study, nonoperative management can be considered. In conservative management, the patient is observed closely through serial physical and laboratory examinations while being treated with nasogastric suction, intravenous acid secretion suppression, and intravenous broad-spectrum antibiotics. Patients in whom the diagnosis is uncertain or in whom the abdominal examination is not reliable are not good candidates for conservative management. As such, the subsets of patients who were mentioned earlier who represent a diagnostic challenge should not be included. In the largest published series of patients with perforated duodenal ulcer who were managed conservatively, patients who were 70 years of age and older were much more likely to require operative therapy and had a higher mortality rate.[48] If at any time during conservative management the patient deteriorates, an operation is indicated. Conservatively managed patients often develop intra-abdominal abscesses, especially in the subhepatic or subdiaphragmatic locations, and these abscesses usually can be managed percutaneously. Retrospective and prospective, randomized studies suggest that conservative management is effective in properly selected patients.[48–53]

Surgical. *Minimally Invasive Surgery.* Over the last decade, much has been published regarding the minimally invasive approach to peptic ulcer disease. While essentially all the procedures used to treat peptic ulcer disease have been performed laparoscopically, the more complicated procedures are challenging laparoscopic procedures even in the elective setting. Fortunately, open management of peptic ulcer disease has evolved such that most surgeons currently perform simple closure in perforated duodenal ulcer and do not routinely add complex acid-reduction procedures. Simple closure translates well from the open to the laparoscopic approach for surgeons with advanced laparoscopic skills.

Most surgeons agree that diagnosis of perforated ulcer is readily apparent with the laparoscope in the majority of cases. Laparoscopic surgery has not been as widely used as expected in perforated ulcer secondary to concerns regarding the technical challenge of two-handed manipulation and intracorporeal suturing of indurated and friable tissue. Recent studies have confirmed the appropriateness of the laparoscopic approach to perforated peptic ulcer in appropriately selected patients.[54–61] As described below, laparoscopic duodenal ulcer closure with omental patch combined with postoperative *H. pylori* eradication and proton pump inhibitor therapy has been shown to be technically feasible and associated with low morbidity and mortality and an appropriately low rate of ulcer recurrence.

Perforated Duodenal Ulcer. The most frequently performed operation for a perforated duodenal ulcer is simple closure with an omental onlay reinforcement or patch. The operation usually is performed through an upper midline incision. After clearing the peritoneal cavity of purulent and/or bilious fluid, visual inspection and palpation direct the surgeon to the site of perforation. The point of perforation usually is recognized easily in the proximal anterior duodenum. If not apparent, exploration of the remainder of the duodenum, the anterior and posterior gastric walls, and the jejunum is undertaken.

In the *H. pylori* era, a perforated duodenal ulcer is closed routinely with interrupted sutures. Omentum is laid over the closure and secured with the ends of the previously placed sutures. Additional sutures can be placed as necessary to plicate the omentum about the closure (Fig. 12–5).

When combined with postoperative *H. pylori* eradication, the morbidity, mortality, and ulcer recurrence rate after closure and omental onlay have been shown to be acceptably low.[62–64] This current practice is in marked contrast to the prior recommendation suggesting the addition of a concomitant acid-reduction procedure to ulcer closure.

Since there is no significant alteration in gastrointestinal anatomy with ulcer closure, patients suffer no postvagotomy or postgastrectomy side effects after this procedure. Ulcer closure without a concomitant acid-

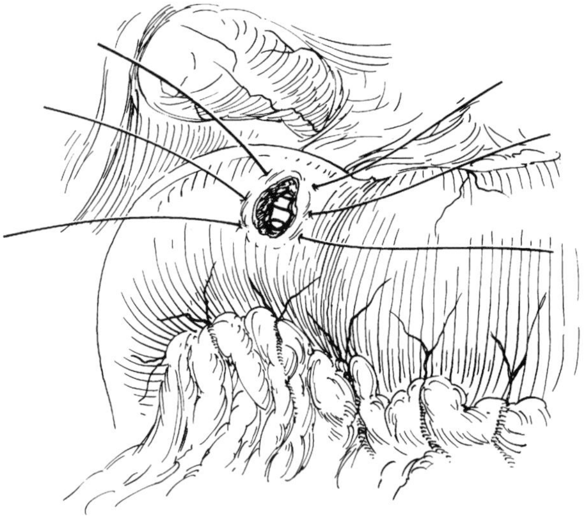

Figure 12–5. Perforated duodenal ulcer closure with omental onlay patch. The omentum is secured with the sutures that are used to primarily close the ulcer.

reduction procedure is especially indicated with generalized peritonitis, shock, perforation for more than 24 hours, or if the patient has not had significant symptoms for 3 months before perforation.

While many methods of postoperative duodenal decompression have been described, a transpyloric nasogastric sump tube is the simplest method. While some surgeons place a closed suction drain in the subhepatic space, strong data do not exist to support this practice.[65] Insertion of a nasoenteric or jejunal feeding tube should be considered, especially in patients with evidence of chronic malnutrition or in whom a prolonged postoperative course is expected. A retrograde duodenal drain and jejunal feeding tube also can be placed in the proximal jejunum to decompress the duodenum if the closure appears tenuous. If duodenal induration or edema precludes closure of the defect, then use of an omental or jejunal serosal patch can be helpful. In the unusual circumstances of a large ulcer and significant inflammation, duodenal drainage and pyloric exclusion as described for use in the treatment of traumatic duodenal injuries can be helpful. A combination of gastrostomy, duodenostomy, and jejunostomy tubes then would be indicated. Alternatively, a lateral duodenal fistula can be prevented by a Roux-en-Y jejunal "patch" sutured over the defect with a transjejunal drain that extends from the duodenum through the jejunal "patch" and exits via a Witzel closure several centimeters downstream in the jejunal limb.

Postoperatively, patients should be treated with antisecretory medications and antibiotics to eradicate *H. pylori.* There are a number of effective regimens for such eradication.[66,67] Treatment should be started during the immediate postoperative period, and elimination should be confirmed at the conclusion of therapy. Eradication of *H. pylori* after ulcer closure has been shown to decrease ulcer recurrence significantly in patients with *H. pylori*–associated perforated ulcers.[62] Antifungal therapy is indicated in patients with a positive peritoneal fungal culture or a high Mannheim Peritonitis Index score that suggests that prophylactic antifungal therapy could be of benefit.[47] (The Mannheim Peritonitis Index uses clinical information obtained during initial evaluation and laparotomy to classify the severity of peritonitis and thereby provide prognostic information that could help to direct surgical therapy.) We routinely study the patient with a Gastrografin and barium swallow in the week following closure prior to removal of the nasogastric tube and resumption of diet.

Laparoscopic closure of perforated duodenal ulcer is a simple and safe procedure. While initial reports of laparoscopic closure of perforated duodenal ulcer demonstrated little difference in comparison with open duodenal ulcer closure, recent data demonstrate that the approach is safe and maintains the benefits of the minimally invasive approach.[54,56–61] Specifically, laparoscopic closure of perforated duodenal ulcers has been associated with shorter operating time, less postoperative pain, a shorter postoperative hospital stay, and earlier return to normal daily activities than the conventional open repair.

Patients with shock on admission or symptoms for more than 24 hours more often require conversion to an open operation. The Acute Physiology and Chronic Health Evaluation (APACHE) II score may be a useful tool for stratifying patients with perforated peptic ulcer into various risk groups, and a high score has been associated with an increased likelihood of leak after laparoscopic repair.[55] Patients in shock, with delayed presentation, or with a high APACHE II score are better served by expeditious open closure of the ulcer.

The laparoscopic procedure performed is interrupted suture closure of the perforated ulcer with omental onlay patch. After closure, the peritoneum is cleaned through saline lavage and aspiration. An intraluminal endoscope can be used as necessary to help identify the site of perforation, guide the repair, and pull omentum into the perforation.[61] Fibrin glue application also has been used to facilitate closure.[57] Laparoscopic ulcer closure compares favorably with open ulcer closure with regard to operative time, morbidity, and mortality. When followed by treatment for *H. pylori,* ulcer recurrence rate is low. Further study of its long-term effectiveness and comparability with existing therapy is still needed.

In patients with bleeding or perforated duodenal ulcers, proximal gastric vagotomy has been used in conjunction with suturing the vessel or patching the perforation. Patients with a perforated ulcer who are appropriate candidates for proximal gastric vagotomy and ulcer closure do well. However, the benefit of proximal gastric vagotomy over closure and antibiotic therapy has not been demonstrated. Fewer surgeons doing emergency peptic ulcer surgery have experience with proximal gastric vagotomy, so simple suture followed by medical treatment is recommended as the safest option.

Perforated Gastric Ulcer. Perforated gastric ulcer has a higher mortality rate than perforated duodenal ulcer. In most series, the mortality rate of perforated gastric ulcer is 15–20%. Clinical condition and comorbid disease dictate which surgical procedure should be chosen to address a perforated gastric ulcer. Surgical options include simple closure with biopsy, excision and closure, and resection. Most perforated gastric ulcers are prepyloric. Prepyloric and pyloric ulcers are best treated with distal gastric resection because this avoids the 15% incidence of postoperative gastric obstruction seen with simple closure and also allows histologic assessment.[69] If a gastric ulcer is difficult to include in a resection, generous biopsies should be taken to exclude malignancy, and the ulcer is closed or patched primarily with omentum.

Perforated gastric ulcers can pose a diagnostic challenge in a few clinical situations. Posterior gastric ulcer perforation is characterized by the insidious onset of upper abdominal pain and delayed presentation.[70] When a retroperitoneal collection is noted on diagnostic imaging or laparotomy, posterior perforation of peptic ulcer should be actively excluded. Diagnosis of perforated gastric ulcer in morbidly obese patients who have undergone gastric bypass surgery also can be difficult.[71] Since the bypassed stomach is not readily available for endoscopic or radiographic evaluation and obesity can obscure signs of perforation, diagnosis and treatment of peptic ulcer disease and its complications in the gastric bypass patient can be quite difficult. A high index of suspicion regarding marginal and remnant gastric ulceration in these patients is important.

BLEEDING

Incidence

Bleeding ulcers not associated with *H. pylori* or NSAIDs are uncommon. Recent data demonstrate that a negative biopsy urease test is unreliable for exclusion of *H. pylori* infection during the acute phase of ulcer bleeding and that approximately 4% of bleeding peptic ulcers are not associated with *H. pylori* or NSAIDs.[72] Approximately one-half of patients with peptic ulcer bleeding use NSAIDs.

The risk of developing bleeding ulcer with corticosteroid use is debated. While data suggest that an independent causal association between steroid use and bleeding gastroduodenal ulcer does not exist, concomitant use of NSAIDS and steroids raises the risk of ulcer hemorrhage 10-fold.[73–75] The Medicaid database suggests that steroids have a low ulcer risk associated with their use at 2.8 events per 10,000 patient-months of exposure. Data suggest an adverse role for alcohol and smoking in the long-term survival of peptic ulcer disease with bleeding.[76]

The incidence of peptic ulcer hemorrhage decreased over the last decade. For example, in the Netherlands, the incidence was 62 per 100,000 persons in 1993 and 48 per 100,000 persons in 2000.[77] Interestingly, despite changing treatment patterns during the 1990s, the mortality rates from gastrointestinal bleeding have been relatively stable.[77,78] The incidence remained stable for both duodenal and gastric ulcer bleeding but was higher among patients of more advanced age. Bleeding from peptic ulcer disease occurs most often in the sixth decade of life. Epidemiological data suggest that the incidence of emergency surgery has not changed over the last decade despite major improvements in endoscopic treatment.[79] Similarly, rebleeding rates (~15–22%) and mortality (~14–15%) in the modern endoscopic era remain unchanged.[77]

Ulcer bleeding remains a frequent cause of upper gastrointestinal bleeding and has been estimated to account for approximately 40–46% of such bleeds.[77] However, a recent study from the United States suggested that the percentage of patients with peptic ulcer as the source of upper gastrointestinal bleeding is decreasing.[80] A review of endoscopic data from 7822 patients with upper gastrointestinal bleeding from December 1999 until April 2001 in the national Clinical Outcome Research Initiative database demonstrated that peptic ulcers were the source of upper gastrointestinal bleeding in 20% of patients, and a nonbleeding visible vessel was present in only 7% of the ulcers.

Increasing age, presence of shock on presentation, severe comorbidity, and rebleeding are associated with higher mortality in bleeding ulcer.[77] The cause of death usually is multiple-system-organ failure and not exsanguinating hemorrhage. Elderly patients with hemorrhagic gastric ulcer have higher incidences of severe ulcer disease and concomitant medical problems.[81,82] While initial endoscopic diagnosis and therapy of hemorrhagic peptic ulcer disease in the elderly are agreed on, debate exists regarding the advisability of early surgical intervention in elderly patients who have stopped bleeding.[79,83–88]

Critically ill patients who bleed while in the hospital have similar sources of bleeding and rates of endoscopically directed therapy as patients admitted to the hospital with bleeding.[89] The mortality rate is very high in patients with bleeding that develops in the hospital primarily as the result of significant systemic disease.

Diagnosis

Clinical signs and symptoms of peptic ulcer bleeding vary according to amount of bleeding, rate of bleeding, and the comorbid illnesses of the patient. The diagnosis usually is suggested by hematemesis, melena, or hematochezia. Hematemesis can vary from minimal to massive. Melena can result from the introduction of even a small amount of blood into the upper gastrointestinal tract. When associated with peptic ulcer bleeding, hematochezia generally signifies bleeding of over 1 L of blood.

Diagnosis begins with a thorough history and physical examination. Specific questions regarding NSAID use, past *H. pylori* treatment, recent antisecretory medication use, anticoagulant use, coagulopathy, and bleeding should be asked. For example, upper gastrointestinal bleeding in a patient with a past history of peptic ulcer bleeding is secondary to recurrent peptic ulcer bleeding in 75% of patients. Recent vigorous retching suggests a Mallory-Weiss tear. A history of prior variceal bleeding and evidence of liver failure suggest variceal bleeding as the etiology. A history of sodium warfarin (Coumadin) use for the treatment of atrial fibrillation suggests iatrogenic coagulopathy.

The history and physical examination are complemented by a directed laboratory examination that includes a complete blood count, comprehensive metabolic profile, coagulation profile, and blood type and cross-match. In patients who present with a clinical picture worrisome for shock, an arterial blood gas determination and a lactate level will help to assess the degree of physiologic compromise and guide resuscitation. With mild bleeding, laboratory tests usually are normal. In more severe bleeding, anemia, coagulopathy, and abnormalities suggestive of hemorrhagic shock can be present.

Although the history and physical examination can narrow the differential diagnosis, endoscopy is necessary for accurate diagnosis and treatment of gastrointestinal bleeding. Generally, endoscopy establishes the source of bleeding and thereby directs medical and surgical therapy. During resuscitation, urgent upper endoscopy should be performed to aid in diagnosis, provide therapy, and guide further medical and surgical treatment. Initial findings on upper endoscopy also have prognostic value.[90–93] A flat, clean-based ulcer is associated with a lower rate of recurrent bleeding and mortality. Active bleeding, fresh clot in the ulcer base, a visible vessel, and a large ulcer are associated with higher rates of rebleeding and mortality. As described below, endoscopic findings and therapeutic success determine the need for operation, as well as the operative approach.

Treatment

Medical. Multidisciplinary, evidence-based care of patients with upper gastrointestinal hemorrhage in a unit that specializes in gastrointestinal bleeding has been associated with a lower mortality rate.[94] Inadequate resuscitation is a common error made by those inexperienced in the management of these patients' hemorrhages.[95] The initial Rockall score is predictive of mortality in patients with peptic ulcer bleeding, and the complete Rockall score is predictive of peptic ulcer rebleeding.[90,94,96]

To provide cost-effective, quality care to patients with peptic ulcer bleeding, it is important to determine the clinical significance of the bleeding. The amount and rate, as well as the patient's comorbid conditions, may have therapeutic implications. Physiologic compromise is assessed initially through physical examination. In the absence of underlying cardiovascular disease, tachycardia and orthostatic hypotension indicate mild to moderate blood loss, whereas hypotension suggests moderate to severe blood loss of greater than 25% of circulating blood volume.

The location and severity of bleeding are assessed further by insertion of a nasogastric sump tube. The presence of blood in the nasogastric tube confirms an upper gastrointestinal source; the absence of blood suggests a lower gastrointestinal source of bleeding only when the aspirate is bilious. The nasogastric tube also can be helpful in monitoring ongoing bleeding and in the detection of recurrent bleeding. Gastric decompression may help to prevent aspiration in the obtunded patient. The presence or absence of blood in the nasogastric aspirate helps to guide selection of upper endoscopy or colonoscopy as the initial endoscopic procedure.

Outpatient management is safe for patients with nonvariceal upper gastrointestinal bleeding who are at low risk of recurrent bleeding and death. Selected patients with bleeding peptic ulcer can be managed safely as outpatients after endoscopic therapy. Criteria used to identify such patients include ulcer size less than 15 mm in diameter, absence of hypovolemia, no associated severe disease, and appropriate family support.[92] This policy conserves health care resources without compromising standards of care.

Severe gastrointestinal bleeding requires early intensive resuscitation to decrease mortality. Resuscitation begins with insertion of large-bore intravenous catheters for the administration of crystalloid and blood products. Resuscitation should be focused on rapid correction of hemodynamics, return of hemoglobin to a near-normal level (>10 g/dL), and correction of the underlying coagulopathy. A Foley catheter should be inserted to monitor urine output and guide resuscitation. Central venous, arterial, and pulmonary artery catheters are used as necessary to assess ongoing blood loss and resuscitation. Associated medical illnesses such as coronary artery disease should be treated quickly and effectively so as to minimize complications, but use of NSAIDs and anticoagulants should be limited.

An intravenous proton pump inhibitor should be administered. Proton pump inhibitors have been shown to be more effective than an intravenous histamine-2 receptor antagonist or placebo in reducing the rate of rebleeding in patients with bleeding peptic ulcer.[97,98] While proton pump inhibitors are superior to histamine antagonists in preventing rebleeding and in reducing the need for surgery in patients with gastrointestinal bleeding, they do not appear to reduce mortality.[99] Of note, about 5% of patients with peptic ulcer bleeding respond poorly to standard doses of intravenous omeprazole, as evidenced by a mean intragastric pH of less than 6 despite therapy.[100] Standard treatment should be modified in these patients because the rebleeding rate is significantly higher. Somatostatin has not been shown to be of benefit in patients with bleeding peptic ulcers in controlled clinical trials.

Not enough data have accumulated to prove the superiority of intravenous proton pump inhibitors to intravenous histamine-2 receptor antagonists for prophylaxis of clinically important stress ulcer bleeding.[97] A recent meta-analysis demonstrated that omeprazole, famotidine, or sucralfate prophylaxis did not affect the already very low incidence of clinically important stress-related bleeding in high-risk surgical intensive-care-unit patients.[101] Furthermore, the data suggested that medications increasing gastric pH also could increase the risk for nosocomial pneumonia. Further clinical investigation of stress ulcer prophylaxis is necessary.

Endoscopic. Endoscopy is useful in the diagnosis and treatment of gastrointestinal bleeding. Endoscopy establishes the source of bleeding in over 90% of upper gastrointestinal bleeding and thereby directs medical and surgical therapy. Mallory-Weiss tears, variceal sources, gastritis, and peptic ulcer bleeding usually can be differentiated by upper endoscopy. As mentioned previously, endoscopy can help to select peptic ulcer disease patients for early discharge and outpatient management. The endoscopic appearance of the ulcer has prognostic value. A flat, clean-based ulcer is less likely to rebleed than an ulcer that is actively bleeding, has fresh clot in its base, contains a visible vessel, or is of large diameter. Rebleeding is associated with an increase mortality rate and often is used as an indication for operative treatment.

Currently, combination therapy with epinephrine injection and bicap or heater probe therapy is employed most commonly in the United States.[102,103] Other techniques, such as endoscopic band ligation, have shown promise in selected populations (such as patients with small-sized, nonfibrotic acute peptic ulcer bleeding).[104] In one study, combination endoscopic treatment of ulcers with an adherent clot was associated with a significant reduction in recurrent ulcer hemorrhage compared with medical therapy alone.[102] However, combination therapy did not reduce the need for ulcer surgery or 30-day mortality significantly. Other recent studies instead suggest that endoscopic therapy may decrease the need for surgery and the mortality.[93,105] Larger randomized, prospective studies are needed to delineate the optimal combination of endoscopic and surgical therapy in patients with acute peptic ulcer bleeding.

After endoscopic treatment of bleeding peptic ulcers, a high-dose infusion of omeprazole substantially reduces the risk of recurrent bleeding.[98] The combination of endoscopic therapy and omeprazole infusion is superior to omeprazole infusion alone for preventing recurrent bleeding from ulcers with nonbleeding visible vessels and adherent clots.[93] In patients who had endoscopically confirmed bleeding peptic ulcer with stigmata of acute bleeding, visible vessels, or adherent clot, a scheduled repeat endoscopy with appropriate therapy 16–24 hours after initial endoscopic hemostasis reduced the number of cases of recurrent bleeding.[106] In general, if a patient develops recurrent bleeding, a second therapeutic endoscopy is performed.[83,84,87] Additional endoscopies to control recurrent bleeding are not indicated routinely.

The concern regarding malignancy in gastric ulcer has prompted follow-up endoscopy in many patients. Recent data suggest that the endoscopic impression correlates with the histologic diagnosis even in a geographic region of intermediate gastric cancer incidence.[109] Endoscopic follow-up studies may be restricted to cases of uncertain or malignant endoscopic impression.

Surgical. The optimal surgical management of patients with bleeding peptic ulcer is debated. Most surgeons agree that patients with profusely bleeding peptic ulcer associated with hemodynamic instability require aggressive resuscitation, endotracheal intubation to protect their airway, and emergent exploration to control the hemorrhage. However, the necessity and timing of surgical intervention to prevent or treat recurrent bleeding are less clear.[79,85,87] Some surgeons offer elderly patients with comorbid disease and an ulcer with stigmata worrisome for recurrent bleeding a semielective surgical therapy as soon as the initial bleeding stops spontaneously or is controlled endoscopically.[84,88,91] The role of angiographic embolization in the control of recurrent or intractable hemorrhage remains unclear. Further investigation is required to delineate the optimal medical, endoscopic, and surgical treatment of acute peptic ulcer bleeding.

Bleeding Duodenal Ulcer. The patient is approached through an upper midline incision. A longitudinal duodenotomy is performed to identify the ulcer, which is usually located in the posterior duodenal bulb. As necessary, the duodenotomy is extended proximally across the pylorus or distally beyond the first portion of the duodenum to find the ulcer. The bleeding is controlled with digital pressure and suture ligation. Figure-of-eight sutures are applied at the cephalad and caudad margins of the ulcer to ligate the gastroduodenal artery. A U stitch is placed in the ulcer base to occlude pancreatic branches from the gastroduodenal artery. The technique suggested for suture control of ulcer bleeding is illustrated in Figure 12–6.

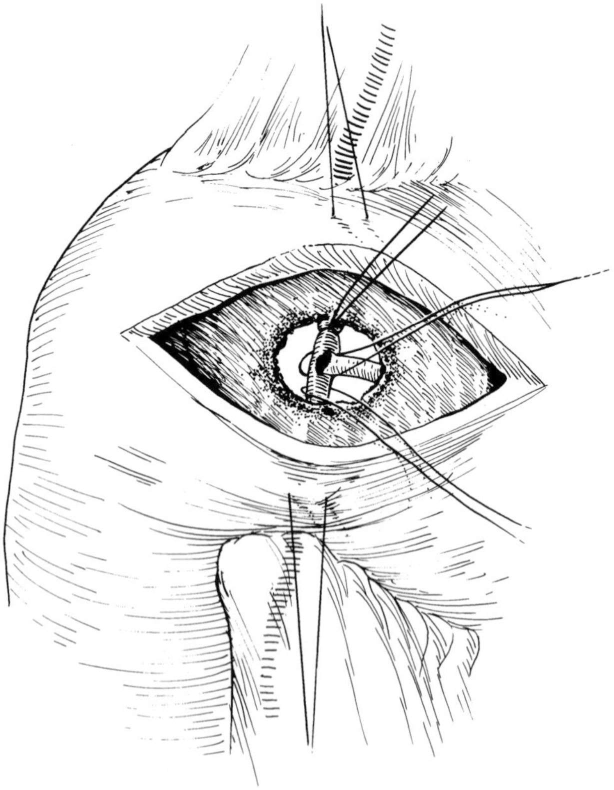

Figure 12–6. Technique of suture control of bleeding duodenal ulcer. Through a longitudinal pyloric incision, figure-of-eight sutures are placed at the cephalad and caudad aspects of the ulcer deep enough to occlude the gastroduodenal artery.

After hemostasis is obtained, the duodenal bulb and prepyloric stomach are examined for additional ulcers. As necessary, the duodenotomy is extended to control bleeding from additional ulcers. A small duodenotomy is closed primarily, and longer duodenotomies are closed via a Heineke-Mikulicz or a Finney pyloroplasty.[110]

In the past, the addition of a truncal vagotomy had been recommended to decrease recurrent bleeding. As described earlier, surgeons are less likely to add vagotomy to pyloroplasty in the *H. pylori* era. While a vagotomy is not recommended, further study of the natural history of bleeding duodenal ulcer is required to validate this recommendation. In the past, many surgeons favored the aggressive addition of a truncal vagotomy and antrectomy to oversewing a duodenal ulcer in the hope of further decreasing the incidence of recurrent bleeding and ulceration. Studies of vagotomy and antrectomy without *H. pylori* treatment suggest that the morbidity and mortality of antrectomy are equal to those of pyloroplasty, and that antrectomy decreases the incidence of recurrent bleeding.[111] Regardless of which procedure is performed, patients with bleeding duodenal ulcer likely will have a lower rebleeding rate if *H. pylori* is eradicated than if they are treated with surgery alone. NSAID use also should be limited.

Bleeding Gastric Ulcer. Surgical treatment of bleeding gastric ulcer is determined by the clinical status of the patient, as well as by gastric ulcer type. In general, the recommended surgical treatment of a bleeding gastric ulcer mirrors the surgical treatment described previously for intractable gastric ulcers.

In type I ulcers, the pathogenesis is not clearly understood, and surgical recommendations include excision of the ulcer. A partial gastrectomy is recommended unless the patient is unstable, in which case the ulcer should be excised and closed. In extreme instability, the ulcer is biopsied and oversewn, and the gastrotomy is closed.

Vagotomy and pyloroplasty have been recommended previously in high-risk patients requiring urgent operation. However, the functional outcome of vagotomy and pyloroplasty is worse than the outcome of vagotomy and distal gastrectomy. In addition, the lesser-curve ulcer should be excised, and this makes vagotomy and pyloroplasty less attractive. Since the duodenal dissection usually is easy in patients who do not have duodenal ulceration, distal gastrectomy is recommended over vagotomy and pyloroplasty.

There is no consensus regarding the surgical treatment of type II and type III bleeding ulcers. Secondary to the concern for malignancy in gastric ulcer, excision of these is recommended. The anatomy, inflammation, and patient condition at operation dictate procedure selection. Excision with primary closure is acceptable when technically feasible. When simple closure would narrow the gastric outlet or multiple ulcers are present, a distal gastrectomy is recommended. When significant duodenal inflammation would make a distal gastrectomy technically challenging, gastric ulcer excision with a vagotomy and pyloroplasty is used. When combined with gastric ulcer excision, proximal gastric vagotomy is less appealing and has been associated with a high recurrence rate. Evidence suggests that patients with bleeding ulcers associated with critical illness are best served by a relatively aggressive surgical approach.[79] Postoperatively, patients should have *H. pylori* infection eradicated and avoid the use of NSAIDs.

OBSTRUCTION

Incidence

In peptic ulcer disease, gastric outlet obstruction is less common than perforation or bleeding. Obstruction from a duodenal ulcer is the most common cause of gastric outlet obstruction and occurs in approximately 2% of patients with chronic duodenal ulcer. Gastric outlet obstruction related to peptic ulcer disease has continued to decrease over the last decade. While prepyloric, pyloric, and duodenal ulcers previously caused up to 80% of gastric outlet obstructions, it is likely that the percentage caused by ulcer disease has decreased significantly, although this decrease has not been confirmed. Malignancy and chronic pancreatitis continue to cause gastric outlet obstruction and must be considered in all patients who present with a clinical picture suggestive of gastric outlet obstruction.

Risk factors for the development of peptic gastric outlet obstruction are similar to those for other complications of ulcer disease and include NSAID use and *H. pylori* infection.

Diagnosis

Patients with peptic gastric outlet obstruction usually present with a history of ulcer disease and years of worsening symptoms. The patients describe progressively worsening early satiety and vomiting. The early satiety can result in weight loss and cachexia if untreated. The presence of cachexia without vomiting should raise the suspicion of malignancy. Vomiting from pyloric obstruction often begins intermittently and occurs later in the day. In more severe chronic obstruction, vomiting of foul-smelling, nonbilious liquid and partially digested food occurs multiple times during the day. Severe vomiting results in dehydration and classic electrolyte and acid-base abnormalities.

Diagnosis begins with a physical examination. On examination, the patient usually is thin, and the chronically dilated, fluid-filled stomach often can be detected as a succession splash heard with movement of the abdomen.

Laboratory evaluation is helpful in making the diagnosis. An elevated hematocrit on a complete blood count reveals dehydration. A renal profile demonstrates dehydration as well as a severe hypokalemic, hypochloremic metabolic alkalosis. A comprehensive metabolic profile reveals hypoalbuminemia related to malnutrition in more advanced disease. On urinalysis, the urine is concentrated and paradoxically acidotic. It seems counterintuitive that the kidney secretes acid when gastric losses of acid are high. However, in gastric outlet obstruction associated with severe chronic dehydration, the kidney exchanges H^+ for Na^+ in an attempt to maintain extracellular fluid volume.

The diagnosis is confirmed with a barium upper gastrointestinal series and upper endoscopy. The upper gastrointestinal series demonstrates an atonic, dilated, fluid-filled stomach. The details of gastric anatomy may be difficult to discern secondary to flocculation of the barium. Gastric emptying is delayed, but a small amount of barium eventually passes through the pylorus to demonstrate a narrow, scarred duodenum. Upper endoscopy is important to exclude malignancy. A dilated stomach filled with fluid and partially digested food is seen. The examination can be compromised secondary to retained fluid and food . The pylorus usually is narrowed to the point that the scope cannot be passed into the duodenum. Multiple biopsies and brushings should be taken to evaluate for malignancy. Of historical interest, the saline load test to quantify gastric emptying is of little clinical value in the modern era.[112]

Treatment

Medical. Treatment begins with insertion of a sump nasogastric tube to decompress the stomach and prevent aspiration. The patient should be resuscitated with intravenous normal saline. The electrolyte abnormalities should be corrected by intravenous potassium chloride administration. Treatment of severe hypokalemia should be done in a monitored setting because of potential cardiac dysrhythmias. The metabolic alkalosis usually resolves with saline resuscitation and potassium repletion. However, in some cases it is necessary to administer dilute hydrochloric acid to correct the acid-base abnormalities. Intravenous proton pump inhibitors help to limit acid and fluid loss from the nasogastric tube. A Foley catheter should be inserted to monitor urine output and guide resuscitation.

After the electrolyte and acid-base abnormalities have begun to normalize, nutritional support with total parenteral nutrition should be started. Total parenteral nutrition usually is started within the first few days of admission and continues until enteral nutrition can provide adequate nutrition. In some cases, after the inflammation and edema partially resolve, a small nasoenteric feeding tube can be passed through the pylorus under fluoroscopic or endoscopic guidance to provide enteral nutrition until gastric emptying normalizes.

H. pylori should be eradicated, and NSAID use should be limited as much as possible. Fortunately, experience has shown that many cases of gastric outlet obstruction will resolve with such treatment. While recurrent gastric outlet obstruction has been a significant problem in the past, anecdotal clinical experience suggests that improved medical treatment of peptic ulcer disease has decreased recurrent peptic gastric outlet obstruction. However, in a number of cases, obstruction is associated with significant irreversible cicatrix formation, and nonoperative management will not provide lasting resolution.

Endoscopic. While endoscopy is recognized as a valuable diagnostic aid, the role of therapeutic endoscopy in peptic gastric outlet obstruction is less clear. As mentioned previously, endoscopic-guided nasoenteric feeding tube placement can be helpful in selected patients. Endoscopic balloon dilation is associated with little morbidity. A recent small case series suggests that balloon dilation in conjunction with medical treatment could be of benefit in peptic obstruction.[113] With 2-year follow-up, a good response was seen in the majority of patients. Further study of the long-term effectiveness of dilation of peptic obstruction is required.

Surgical. Surgical treatment of peptic gastric outlet obstruction has been required less frequently over the last decade. In the unusual patient who requires surgical therapy, most surgeons prefer to decompress the stomach preoperatively with a nasogastric tube for a period of at least a week. While gastric decompression is an integral part of the medical therapy that helps most outlet obstructions resolve, decompression also probably helps to restore gastric muscular tone and decreases the duration of postoperative delayed gastric emptying. Stagnant gastric contents should be removed preoperatively through sump suction, saline irrigation, and endoscopy. Some surgeons recommend irrigation of the stomach with dilute antibiotic solution the evening prior to surgery to decrease wound infections related to bacterial overgrowth in the chronically obstructed stomach. Prophylactic perioperative intravenous antibiotics should be administered as appropriate for gastrointestinal surgery. Ideally, the patient should receive preoperative nutritional support until he or she has a positive nitrogen balance.

The recommended operation is vagotomy and antrectomy with insertion of a feeding jejunostomy tube to provide postoperative enteral nutritional support. In cases of severe inflammation that preclude safe resection of the duodenum, vagotomy and gastrojejunostomy are recommended. A prolonged preoperative period of obstruction suggests that a gastrostomy tube could help to decompress the stomach and avoid the need for prolonged use of a nasogastric tube in the postoperative period.

The etiology of postoperative delayed gastric emptying is unclear, but gastric emptying usually returns to normal in approximately a week. If gastric emptying has not returned to normal after a week, a barium upper gastrointestinal study should be obtained to evaluate for mechanical obstruction. The study usually shows no evidence of such obstruction, and supportive therapy is provided while waiting for return of motility. Promotility agents have not been shown to be of benefit, but proton pump inhibitors help to decrease gastric secretion and fluid loss. Chronic gastric outlet obstruction can be associated with delayed gastric emptying that lasts for weeks to months. Enteral nutrition should be provided through the feeding jejunostomy tube until adequate oral intake is confirmed. While waiting for the return of gastric emptying, selected patients can be managed as outpatients after the supportive care has reached a minimal level.

Recent data suggest that the morbidity and mortality of elective surgical treatment of intractable gastric outlet obstruction have decreased. Interestingly, in one small series, *H. pylori* infection was present in a minority of patients with peptic gastric outlet obstruction who required surgical intervention. Endoscopic balloon dilation was used in a number of these patients without success. The operative morbidity was low, and mortality was zero. Importantly, patient satisfaction was high.[25] Further investigation is required to determine the optimal combination and timing of medical, endoscopic, and surgical treatment in peptic gastric outlet obstruction.

▪ RECURRENT ULCER DISEASE

POSTOPERATIVE

Incidence

Recurrent postoperative ulceration after peptic ulcer surgery has become an increasingly uncommon problem in the last decade. Primary treatment with *H. pylori* eradication, NSAIDs with fewer gastrointestinal side effects, and proton pump inhibitors have decreased the incidence of peptic surgery, as well as the need for acid-reduction procedures such as vagotomy and gastrectomy. Despite less aggressive surgical procedures, postoperative recurrence rates are low secondary to improved medical treatment in the postoperative period.

The contribution of incomplete vagotomy, inadequate gastric resection (specifically, retained gastric antrum after gastrojejunal reconstruction), and gastrinoma in the development of recurrent ulcer disease requires further study in the *H. pylori* era. Since the incidence of acid-reduction surgery has decreased and the incidence of gastrinoma has remained stable, it is likely that the percentage of postoperative patients with gastrinoma will increase from the 2% previously described. Gastrinoma is described in more detail below. As mentioned previously, the diagnosis and treatment of ulcer disease after gastric bypass surgery represent increasingly common and challenging postoperative problems.

Diagnosis

The clinical presentation of recurrent ulcer disease is often confused with other postoperative conditions. Pain and hemorrhage are the most common symptoms of postoperative recurrent ulceration, each occurring in about 40% of patients.[115] Obstruction is the presenting symptom in approximately 10% of patients. Rarely, recurrent ulceration presents as a free perforation or as a gastrojejunocolic fistula, as evidenced by diarrhea and weight loss.

Diagnosis begins with a thorough history and physical examination. The patient should be asked and the medical record should be reviewed regarding the initial operative indication and the procedure performed. Furthermore, past treatment of *H. pylori*, use of NSAIDs and antisecretory agents, smoking, alcohol consumption, and a family history of multiple endocrine neoplasia should be explored. Surreptitious use of aspirin or other NSAIDs is probably the most common cause or recurrent ulceration. Laboratory evaluation includes a complete blood count to detect anemia, comprehensive metabolic profile to detect dehydration, a coagulation profile to detect coagulopathy in the presence of bleeding, and a gastrin level. Gastrin levels of greater than 1000 pg/mL are diagnostic of a gastrinoma, and normal levels below 100 pg/mL exclude this diagnosis.[116] Moderate hypergastrinemia should be evaluated further with a secretin stimulation test. An increase in gastrin secretion greater than 100 pg/mL with secretin administration suggests gastrinoma.

Prior vagotomy, G-cell hyperplasia, and retained gastric antrum are not associated with a significant increase in gastrin levels with secretin administration. Protein meal–stimulated gastrin levels above 300 pg/mL suggest G-cell hyperplasia or retained gastric antrum in patients who have had a prior gastrectomy. Measurement of postoperative acid secretory function and sham feeding to evaluate the completeness of vagotomy are necessary infrequently and have little clinical relevance in the modern era.

Upper gastrointestinal barium study and upper endoscopy are useful in the evaluation of recurrent postoperative ulcer. Barium studies help to delineate postoperative anatomy and functional abnormalities. Barium studies are less sensitive and specific for recurrent ulcer disease than endoscopy.[117–118] Upper endoscopy can help to make the diagnosis of recurrent ulcer disease, as well as localize the ulcer. Biopsies are taken to assess for the presence of *H. pylori* and malignancy. Malignant ulceration is more common in gastric ulcers and is surprisingly uncommon in duodenal or jejunal ulcers.

Treatment

The management of patients with recurrent ulcer disease after acid-reducing operations consists of antibiotics directed at *H. pylori* if present, limitation of NSAID use, treatment with an antisecretory medication, smoking cessation, and limitation of alcohol intake. Ulcer disease refractory to such treatment is unusual. If the ulcer persists for more than 3 months despite eradication of *H. pylori* and maintenance antisecretory therapy or the ulcer is associated with perforation, bleeding, or obstruction, operation is indicated. Although little data exist regarding therapeutic endoscopy in the treatment of complicated postoperative recurrent ulcer, endoscopic control of bleeding and dilation of the obstruction have been employed in this setting.

The choice of operation for recurrent postoperative ulcer depends on the indication for initial operation, the operation performed, the etiology of the recurrence, and patient comorbidity.[119] Since these ulcers have recurred despite prior peptic ulcer disease surgery and maximal medical therapy, surgery should be appropriately aggressive. A few general rules are helpful in selection of the operation. Persistent ulcers are worrisome for malignant disease and should be resected. Gastric resection should be performed for a recurrent peptic ulcer after initial procedures that did not include a resection. Truncal vagotomy should be included. For recurrences related to gastrinoma, the operative procedure is detailed below. Table 12–2 lists the recommended operative procedures for recurrent ulcers that develop after acid-reduction surgery.

Operation for recurrent ulcer after local procedures such as perforation closure or oversewn bleeding should include ulcer resection, truncal vagotomy, and gastrectomy (at least antrectomy). Operation after prior gastrectomy should include truncal vagotomy and resection of retained antrum if present. After prior vagotomy and pyloroplasty, operation should include another vagot-

TABLE 12–2. RECOMMENDED OPERATIVE PROCEDURES FOR RECURRENT POSTOPERATIVE ULCERS

Initial Operation	Recommended Operation
Local procedure	Truncal vagotomy and antrectomy
Gastrectomy	Truncal vagotomy and resection of retained antrum if present
Vagotomy and pyloroplasty	Re-vagotomy and antrectomy
Vagotomy and antrectomy	Re-vagotomy and resection of retained antrum if present
Proximal gastric vagotomy	Truncal vagotomy and antrectomy
Subtotal gastrectomy	Truncal vagotomy and resection of retained antrum if present

omy and antrectomy. Operation after prior vagotomy and antrectomy should include resection of retained antrum if present and another vagotomy. Operation after prior subtotal gastrectomy includes resection of retained antrum if present and truncal vagotomy. The recommendation for recurrence after proximal gastric vagotomy is debatable but includes truncal vagotomy and antrectomy.[114] Of note, functional results after reoperative surgery are not as good as functional results after primary surgery, with good to excellent results achieved in only 60–70% of patients.[115,120–122] Fortunately, even in the pre–*H. pylori* era, second recurrences were unusual and developed in fewer than 10% of patients managed by gastric resection.[122]

ZOLLINGER-ELLISON SYNDROME

Zollinger and Ellison first described a syndrome of severe peptic ulcer disease and hypersecretion of gastric acid that was associated with an islet cell tumor of the pancreas.[123] Subsequently, the postulated hormone was identified as gastrin, and these tumors were called *gastrinomas*.[124]

Incidence

Gastrinomas are uncommon, with an annual incidence of 1 in 2.5 million people. They occur sporadically, but approximately 20% of patients who develop gastrinomas have multiple endocrine neoplasia type I. Approximately 60% of sporadic gastrinomas are malignant, 35% are adenomas, and 5% are islet cell hyperplasia. Metastasis and invasion establish the diagnosis of malignancy rather than histology. Ninety percent of primary tumors are located within the pancreas or duodenum within the gastrinoma triangle. The triangle is defined by the cystic duct, the junction of the neck and body of the pancreas, and the junction of the second and third portions of the duodenum. The gastrinoma triangle is illustrated in Figure 12–7.

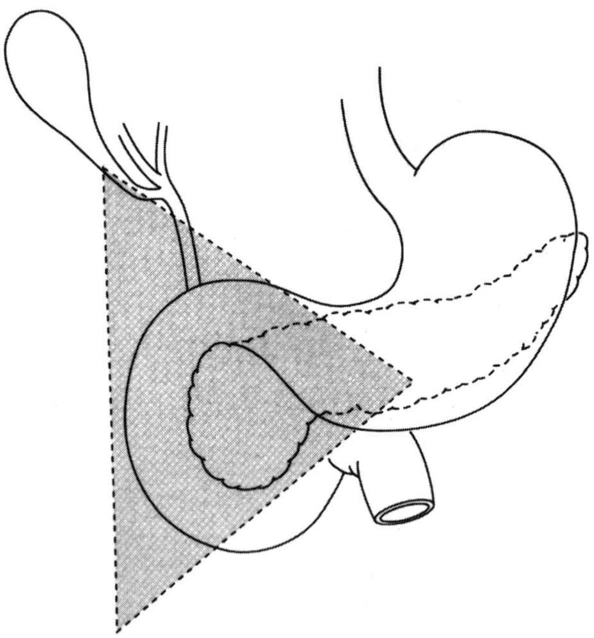

Figure 12–7. The gastrinoma triangle in which approximately 90% of gastrinomas are found. (From Stabile BE, Morrow DJ, Passaro E. The gastrinoma triangle: Operative implications. Am J Surg 1984;147:26.)

Approximately 60% of gastrinomas metastasize, usually to the liver and/or peripancreatic lymph nodes. The magnitude of fasting serum gastrin level at presentation is associated with the size and site of tumor and the presence of hepatic metastases, factors that are each significant independent predictors of outcome.[125] Liver metastases are associated with decreased survival. Surgery is indicated potentially to cure the patient or to control the malignant disease and prolong survival.[126] The most favorable outcomes are observed in patients with benign functional tumors and in those with completely resected malignant tumors.

Diagnosis

Abdominal pain and diarrhea are the most common symptoms and are present in approximately three-quarters of patients. Heartburn is present in nearly half, and gastrointestinal bleeding is present in a quarter. It is unusual for patients to present with a single symptom—pain and diarrhea are the most common combination and occur in half of patients.[127] Patients with multiple endocrine neoplasia type I present less frequently with abdominal pain and more frequently with symptoms related to nephrolithiasis related to their hyperparathyroidism.[127,128] The extent and location of the gastrinoma have minimal effects on clinical presentation.[127] The presence of weight loss, especially with abdominal pain, diarrhea, or heartburn, is an important clue suggesting the presence of gastrinoma.

In the era of widespread use of potent antisecretory medicines, small series and anecdotal experience suggest that patients present with less severe symptoms and fewer complications. Large clinical series suggest that there has been no change in the time to diagnosis, frequency of presenting symptoms, or frequency of peptic complications in gastrinoma in the last decade.[127] Data suggest that the stage of disease at presentation and 5-year cure rate for malignant gastrinoma may have been slightly worsened by widespread use of antisecretory medicines.[129] Antisecretory therapy has decreased the need for acid-reduction surgery, and fewer patients now present with gastrinoma after having undergone prior gastric surgery.[127]

A mean delay to diagnosis of over 5 years suggests that gastrinoma is difficult to identify. In one series, the correct diagnosis of gastrinoma was made by the referring physician in only 3% of patients.[127] Diagnosis begins with a thorough history and physical examination. The presence of abdominal pain, diarrhea, heartburn, gastrointestinal bleeding, and weight loss should be ascertained. A family history of ulcer disease and multiple endocrine neoplasia, including hyperparathyroidism, should be explored. Laboratory evaluation includes complete blood count to evaluate for anemia, a complete metabolic profile to evaluate for hypercalcemia, and a serum gastrin level. As mentioned previously, a gastrin level greater than 1000 pg/mL is diagnostic of gastrinoma, and a level below 100 pg/mL excludes this diagnosis. Moderately elevated levels should be evaluated further with a secretin stimulation test. A marked stimulation of gastrin secretion (>100 pg/mL) on secretin administration strongly favors the diagnosis of gastrinoma.[130]

Other diagnostic modalities include ultrasound, computed tomography, magnetic resonance imaging, upper endoscopy, endoscopic ultrasound, somatostatin receptor scintigraphy, and selective secretin or calcium arteriography. The referring physician usually has performed an ultrasound or CT scan of the abdomen as part of the initial evaluation of the gastrointestinal complaints. These tests often are unsuccessful in locating the primary tumor but can detect metastatic liver disease. Upper endoscopy also is ordered commonly prior to referral. If the endoscopist has a high index of suspicion regarding gastrinoma, prominent gastric body folds likely will be noted because they are present in over 90% of patients with Zollinger-Ellison syndrome. Esophageal stricture and duodenal or pyloric scarring occur in fewer than 10% of patients.

Localization studies, especially somatostatin receptor scintigraphy, are indicated to identify the site and extent of disease. Somatostatin receptor scintigraphy is the best preoperative localization study and identifies the site of gastrinoma in up to 93% of patients.[131,132] If not performed previously, an abdominal CT scan or magnetic resonance imaging should be done to evaluate for metastatic disease.[133] If scintigraphic localization is unsuccessful, endoscopic ultrasound should be performed in attempt to localize the gastrinoma.[131,133–136]

Administration of secretin or calcium via selective angiography also has been used.[137] Under angiographic control, secretin or calcium gluconate is injected selectively into the arteries supplying the pancreas and duodenum. An intravenous gastrin level is drawn after each injection, and the gastrin level is elevated with injection of the artery that supplies the gastrinoma. The gastrinoma thereby is localized by vascular distribution.

Small primary tumors often are not found preoperatively.[132] With recent advances in operative technique and technology, gastrinoma can be located in up to 98% of patients.[139] Intraoperative palpation, intraluminal endoscopic duodenal transillumination, ultrasound, and duodenotomy are used routinely.

Treatment

Medical. Gastrinoma treatment has evolved considerably in the last 20 years. Effective antisecretory therapy has changed the consequences of gastrinoma from those of acid hypersecretion to a disease characterized by tumor growth and spread. While symptoms can be controlled using proton pump inhibitors and somatostatin analogues, cure is possible only with resection.

While medical therapy can control acid hypersecretion in virtually every patient, the role of adjuvant therapy for gastrinoma remains limited.[140] A recent study suggests that octreotide is helpful in the treatment of progressive malignant gastrinoma.[141] In patients in whom chemotherapy with dimethyltrizenoimidazole carboxamide was not effective, subcutaneous administration of octreotide was useful in controlling the growth of the liver metastases and in stabilizing serum gastrin in approximately 50% of patients. The inhibition of growth response was long lasting and was associated with a low incidence of serious side effects. Additional studies involving larger numbers of patients will be needed to determine whether there is a convincing effect on survival.

Surgical. Surgery will cure approximately one-third of patients with sporadic gastrinoma.[142] Surgery provides symptomatic improvement in the majority of patients; it also provides short-term palliation in patients with nonresectable disease.[143]

Most experts agree that all sporadic cases of localized gastrinoma should be excised.[144] In addition, debulking of metastatic tumor may improve symptoms and survival even when cure is not possible.[145–146] However, there is controversy as to the surgical approach for gastrinoma found in the setting of multiple endocrine neoplasia.[147] Some surgeons suggest that gastrinoma in these patients should be excised when the tumors exceed 2.5 cm in diameter.[148] This tumor size has been associated with a higher likelihood of hepatic metastases and decreased survival. Recent studies suggest that surgical resection should be performed in patients with multiple endocrine neoplasia even in the presence of advanced disease.[145,146] Despite previous studies of these patients demonstrating decreased survival rates, these recent series suggested that those with advanced tumor who underwent surgical resection had the same survival as patients with limited disease or those without identifiable tumor. Some surgeons advocate nonoperative management of patients with multiple endocrine neoplasia and gastrinoma because it is unclear whether surgical intervention offers survival or disease-free benefit in this population.[148]

Operation in sporadic gastrinoma begins with exploration of the gastrinoma triangle. Dissection of lymph nodes in this region is important because lymph node primaries and metastases are common.[149,150] If the gastrinoma is not found, a duodenotomy should be performed to search for duodenal primary tumors.[139] Extraduodenal, extrapancreatic, and extranodal gastrinomas are encountered in 5% of patients who undergo exploration with curative intent. If no gastrinoma is found in the usual locations, other ectopic sites should be examined carefully. Reported sites include liver, common bile duct, jejunum, omentum, pylorus, and ovary.[138] Resection of these ectopic tumors can be curative. Gastrinomas not found at operation are likely to be small duodenal gastrinomas, but blind resection is not indicated.[151] Intraoperative gastrin measurement can confirm complete resection or suggest the need for additional exploration. Normalization of hypergastrinemia during surgery signifies removal of all gastrin-secreting tumors.[152] A parietal cell vagotomy can be considered in the event of residual tumor.

For patients with hepatic metastasis, initial expectant observation and medical management of symptoms are appropriate in view of the indolent course of the disease. Hepatic arterial embolization is the preferred mode of palliation for pain and hormonal symptoms.[153] The role of other minimally invasive techniques in surgery of gastrinoma has not been established. Isolated cases of the successful use of laparoscopic radiofrequency ablation of solitary hepatic gastrinoma metastasis suggest that the role of minimally invasive surgery in gastrinoma will continue to evolve.[154]

A curative hepatic resection may be possible in selected patients.[155,156] Aggressive surgery, including pancreatectomy, pancreaticoduodenectomy, and liver resection, can be performed by experienced surgeons with acceptable morbidity and mortality rates in patients with advanced neuroendocrine tumors.[155] Although survival rates following surgery are excellent, most patients will develop recurrent tumor. Postoperative evaluation should include a secretin test because it is the most sensitive method to document cure and detect tumor recurrence.

Molecular diagnosis in gastrinoma includes mutational analysis for frequently involved exons of the gene *menin* on chromosome 11 in multiple endocrine neoplasia.[157,158] In sporadic gastrinoma, recent research suggests that chromosome 1 defects, aneuploidy, and mismatch repair defects are important features of gastrinomas.[159] Chromosomal loss of heterogeneity (X in female patients and 1q in all patients) and high frequent allelic loss at 1q31-32 as well as 1q21-23 have been shown to be common in gastrinoma specimens, and their presence is a potentially useful molecular prognostic factor for aggressive growth that could be useful clinically.[160,161] In addition to prognostic significance, HER-2/neu levels in gastrinoma could help to identify patients who might benefit from trastuzumab treatment.[162]

▪ CONCLUSION

Recognition of the roles that *H. pylori* and NSAIDs play in peptic ulcer disease has revolutionized the care of patients who suffer from gastroduodenal ulcer. While better understanding and treatment of peptic ulcer disease have translated into fewer elective operations, the incidence of urgent operations required to treat complications of peptic ulcer has remained stable over the last decade. *H. pylori* eradication also has changed the selection of procedures that are performed commonly in the treatment of ulcer complications. Most surgeons now select the simplest and quickest operation that will address the ulcer complication while minimizing the postoperative gastrointestinal side effects. The decrease in ulcer recurrence provided by definitive acid-reduction surgery such as vagotomy has been replaced by *H. pylori* eradication, tailored NSAID drug therapy, and proton pump inhibitor therapy. Additional investigation is needed to determine the optimal combination of medical, endoscopic, and surgical therapy to treat complicated peptic ulcer disease in the modern era.

REFERENCES

1. NIH Consensus Development Panel. *Helicobacter pylori* in peptic ulcer disease. *JAMA* 1994;272:65–69

2. Huang JQ, Sridhar S, Hunt RH. Role of *Helicobacter pylori* infection and nonsteroidal anti-inflammatory drugs in peptic-ulcer disease: A meta-analysis. *Lancet* 2002;359:14–22
3. Hawkey CJ, Naesdal J, Wilson I, et al. Relative contribution of mucosal injury and *Helicobacter pylori* in the development of gastroduodenal lesions in patients taking nonsteroidal anti-inflammatory drugs. *Gut* 2002;51:336–343
4. Garcia Rodriguez LA, Hernandez-Diaz S. Risk of uncomplicated peptic ulcer among users of aspirin and nonaspirin nonsteroidal anti-inflammatory drugs. *Am J Epidemiol* 2004;159:23–31
5. Arroyo MT, Forne M, de Argila CM, et al. The prevalence of peptic ulcer not related to *Helicobacter pylori* or nonsteroidal anti-inflammatory drug use is negligible in southern Europe. *Helicobacter* 2004;9:249–254
6. Schwesinger WH, Page CP, Sirinek KR, et al. Operations for peptic ulcer disease: Paradigm lost. *J Gastrointest Surg* 2001;5:438–443
7. Paimela H, Paimela L, Myllykangas-Luosujarvi R, et al. Current features of peptic ulcer disease in Finland: Incidence of surgery, hospital admissions and mortality for the disease during the past 25 years. *Scand J Gastroenterol* 2002;37:399–403
8. Sandler RS, Everhart JE, Donowitz M, et al. The burden of selected digestive diseases in the United States. *Gastroenterology* 2002;122:1500–1511
9. Chan J, Hui RL, Szpakowski JL. Prescribing proton pump inhibitors for initial treatment of acid-related gastrointestinal diseases in a managed care population. *Am J Manag Care* 2004;10:433–441
10. Erstad BL. The cost of enhanced acid suppression. *Pharmacotherapy* 2003;23:94–100S
11. Agency for Healthcare Research and Quality. http://www.ahrq.gov
12. Graham DY, Go MF. *Helicobacter pylori:* Current status. *Gastroenteremology* 1993;105:279–282
13. Miwa H, Sakaki N, Sugano K, et al. Recurrent peptic ulcers in patients following successful *Helicobacter pylori* eradication: A multicenter study of 4940 patients. *Helicobacter* 2004;9:9–16
14. Graham DY, Lew GM, Klein PD, et al. Effect of treatment of *Helicobacter pyloric* infection on the long-term recurrence of gastric and duodenal ulcer: A randomized, controlled study. *Ann Intern Med* 1992;116:705–708
15. Hentschel E, Brandstatter G, Dragosics B, et al. Effect of ranitidine and amoxicillin plus metronidazole on the eradication of *Helicobacter pylori* and the recurrence of duodenal ulcer. *N Engl J Med* 1993;328:308–312
16. Forbes GM, Glaser ME, Cullen DJ, et al. Duodenal ulcer treated with *Helicobacter pylori* eradication: Seven-year follow-up. *Lancet* 1994;343:258–260
17. Schnitzer TJ, Burmester GR, Mysler E, et al. Comparison of lumiracoxib with naproxen and ibuprofen in the Therapeutic Arthritis Research and Gastrointestinal Event Trial (TARGET) reduction in ulcer complications: Randomized, controlled trial. *Lancet* 2004;364:665–674
18. Kleeff J, Friess H, Buchler MW. How *Helicobacter pylori* changed the life of surgeons. *Dig Surg* 2003;20:93–102
19. Paimela H, Oksala NK, Kivilaakso E. Surgery for peptic ulcer today: A study on the incidence, methods and mortality in surgery for peptic ulcer in Finland between 1987 and 1999. *Dig Surg* 2004;21:185–191
20. Hundahl SA, Phillips JL, Menck HR. The National Center Data Base Report on poor survival of U.S. gastric carcinoma patients treated with gastrectomy: Fifth Edition American Joint Committee on Cancer Staging, proximal disease, and the "different disease" hypothesis. *Cancer* 2000;88:921–932
21. Livingston EH. Procedure incidence and in-hospital complication rates of bariatric surgery in the United States. *Am J Surg* 2004;188:105–110
22. Pope GD, Birkmeyer JD, Finlayson SR. National trends in utilization and in-hospital outcomes of bariatric surgery. *J Gastrointest Surg* 2002;6:855–860
23. Finlayson SR, Laycock WS, Birkmeyer JD. National trends in utilization and outcomes of antireflux surgery. *Surg Endosc* 2003;17:864–867
24. Espat NJ, Ong ES, Helton WS, et al. 1990–2001 US general surgery chief residence gastric surgery operative experience: Analysis of paradigm shift. *J Gastrointest Surg* 2004;8:471–478
25. Gibson JB, Behrman SW, Fabian TC, et al. Gastric outlet obstruction resulting from peptic ulcer disease requiring surgical intervention is infrequently associated with *Helicobacter pylori* infection. *J Am Coll Surg* 2000;191:32–37
26. Johnson AG. Proximal gastric vagotomy: Does it have a place in the future management of peptic ulcer? *World J Surg* 2000;24:259–263
27. Gilliam AD, Speake WJ, Lobo DN, et al. Current practice of emergency vagotomy and *Helicobacter pylori* eradication for complicated peptic ulcer in the United Kingdom. *Br J Surg* 2003;90:88–90
28. Towfigh S, Chandler C, Hines OJ, et al. Outcomes from peptic ulcer surgery have not benefited from advances in medical therapy. *Am Surg* 2002;68:385–389
29. Johnston D, Wilkinson A. Selective vagotomy with innervated antrum without drainage for duodenal ulcer. *Br J Surg* 1969;56:626
30. Amdrup E, Jensen H. Selective vagotomy of the parietal cell mass preserving innervation of the undrained antrum. *Gastroenterology* 1970;59:522
31. Holle F. New method for surgical treatment of gastroduodenal ulceration. In: Harkins HN, Nyhus LM (eds). *Surgery of the Stomach and Duodenum*, 2nd ed. Boston: Little, Brown; 1969:629
32. Jordan PL. A prospective study of parietal cell vagotomy and selective vagotomy-antrectomy for treatment of duodenal ulcer. *Ann Surg* 1976;183:619
33. Hallenbeck GA, Gleysteen JJ, Aldrete JS, et al. Proximal gastric vagotomy: Effects of two operative techniques on clinical and gastric secretory results. *Ann Surg* 1976;184:435
34. Herrington JL, Davidson J, Shumway SJ. Proximal gastric vagotomy: Follow-up of 109 patients for 6–13 years. *Ann Surg* 1986;204:108
35. Wastell C, Colin J, Wilson T, et al. Prospectively randomized trial of proximal gastric vagotomy either with or

without pyloroplasty in treatment of uncomplicated duodenal ulcer. *Br Med J* 1977;2:851
36. Sleisenger MH, Fordtran JS (eds). *Gastrointestinal Disease: Pathophysiology, Diagnosis, Management.* Philadelphia: Saunders, 1993:717
37. Johnston HD. Gastric ulcer: Classification, blood group characteristics, secretion patterns and pathogenesis. *Ann Surg* 1965;162:996
38. Chen MH, Wu MS, Lee WC, et al. A multiple logistic regression analysis of risk factors in different subtypes of gastric ulcer. *Hepatogastroenterology* 2002;49:589–592
39. Welch CE, Burke JF. Gastric ulcer reappraisal. *Surgery* 1969;65:708
40. Sleisenger MH, Fordtran JS (eds). *Gastrointestinal Disease: Pathophysiology, Diagnosis, Management.* Philadelphia: Saunders, 1993:720.
41. Greenall MJ, Lenhart T. Vagotomy or gastrectomy for elective treatment of benign gastric ulceration? *Dig Dis Sci* 1985;30:353
42. Uccheddu A, Floris G, Altana ML, et al. Surgery for perforated peptic ulcer in the elderly: Evaluation of factors influencing prognosis. *Hepatogastroenterology* 2003;50: 1956–1958
43. Noguiera C, Silva AS, Santos JN, et al. Perforated peptic ulcer: Main factors of morbidity and mortality. *World J Surg* 2003;27:782–787
44. Hermansson M, Stael von Holstein C, Zilling T. Surgical approach and prognostic factors after peptic ulcer perforation. *Eur J Surg* 1999;165:566–572
45. Testini M, Portincasa P, Piccinni G, et al. Significant factors associated with fatal outcome in emergency open surgery for perforated peptic ulcer. *World J Gastroenterol* 2003;9:2338–2340
46. Svanes C. Trends in perforated peptic ulcer: Incidence, etiology, treatment, and prognosis. *World J Surg* 2000;24: 277–283
47. Shan YS, Hsu HP, Hsieh YH, et al. Significance of intraoperative peritoneal culture of fungus in perforated peptic ulcer. *Br J Surg* 2003;90:1215–1219
48. Crofts TJ, Park KG, Steele RJ, et al. A randomized trial of nonoperative treatment for perforated peptic ulcer. *New Eng J Med* 1989;320:970–973
49. Berne TV, Donovan AJ. Nonoperative treatment of perforated duodenal ulcer. *Arch Surg* 1989;124:830–832
50. Keane TE, Dillon B, Afdhal HH, et al. Conservative management of peforated duodenal ulcer. *Br J Surg* 1988;75:583–584
51. Donovan AJ, Berne TV, Donovan JA. Perforated duodenal ulcer: An alternative therapeutic plan. *Arch Surg* 1998;133:1166–1171
52. Marshall C, Ramaswamy P, Bergin FG, et al. Evaluation of a protocol for the nonoperative management of perforated peptic ulcer. *Br J Surg* 1999;86:131–134
53. Crofts TJ, Park KG, Steele RJ, et al. A randomized trial of nonoperative treatment for perforated peptic ulcer. *N Engl J Med* 1989;320:970–973
54. Katkhouda N, Mavor E, Mason RJ, et al. Laparoscopic repair of perforated duodenal ulcers: Outcome and efficacy in 30 consecutive patients. *Arch Surg* 1999;134:845–848
55. Lee FY, Leung KL, Lai PB, et al. Selection of patients for laparoscopic repair of perforated peptic ulcer. *Br J Surg* 2001;88:133–136
56. Bergamaschi R, Marvik R, Johnsen G, et al. Open vs laparoscopic repair of perforated peptic ulcer. *Surg Endosc* 1999;13:679–682
57. Khoursheed M, Fuad M, Safar H, et al. Laparoscopic closure of perforated duodenal ulcer. *Surg Endosc* 2000; 14:56–58
58. Arnaud JP, Tuech JJ, Bergamaschi R, et al. Laparoscopic suture closure of perforated duodenal peptic ulcer. *Surg Laparosc Endosc Percutan Tech* 2002;12:145–147
59. Siu WT, Leong HT, Law BK, et al. Laparoscopic repair for perforated peptic ulcer: A randomized, controlled trial. *Ann Surg* 2002;235:313–319
60. Siu WT, Chau CH, Law BK, et al. Routine use of laparoscopic repair for perforated peptic ulcer. *Br J Surg* 2004; 91:481–484
61. Malkov IS, Zaynutdinov AM, Veliyev NA, et al. Laparoscopic and endoscopic management of perforated duodenal ulcers. *J Am Coll Surg* 2004;198:352–355
62. Ng EK, Lam YH, Sung JJ, et al. Eradication of *Helicobacter pylori* prevents recurrence of ulcer after simple closure of duodenal ulcer perforation: Randomized, controlled trial. *Ann Surg* 2000;231:153–158
63. Gisbert JP, Pajares JM. *Helicobacter pylori* infection and perforated peptic ulcer prevalence of the infection and role of antimicrobial treatment. *Helicobacter* 2003;8:159–167
64. Kate V, Ananthakrishnan N, Badrinath S. Effect of *Helicobacter pylori* eradication on the ulcer recurrence rate after simple closure of perforated duodenal ulcer: Retrospective and prospective, randomized, controlled studies. *Br J Surg* 2001;88:1054–1058
65. Pai D, Sharma A, Kanungo R, et al. Role of abdominal drains in perforated duodenal ulcer patients: A prospective, controlled study. *Aust N Z J Surg* 1999;69: 210–213
66. McMahon BJ, Hennessy TW, Bensler JM, et al. The relationship among previous antimicrobial use, antimicrobial resistance, and treatment outcomes for *Helicobacter pylori* infections. *Ann Intern Med* 2003;139:463–469
67. Duck WM, Sobel J, Pruckler JM, et al. Antimicrobial resistance incidence and risk factors among *Helicobacter pylori*–infected persons, United States. *Emerg Infect Dis* 2004;10:1088–1094
68. Millat B, Fingerhut A, Borie F. Surgical treatment of complicated duodenal ulcers: Controlled trials. *World J Surg* 2000;24:299–306
69. McGee GS, Sawyers JL. Perforated gastric ulcers: A plea for management by primary gastric resection. *Arch Surg* 1987;122:555
70. Wong CH, Chow PK, Ong HS, et al. Posterior perforation of peptic ulcers: Presentation and outcome of an uncommon surgical emergency. *Surgery* 2004;135:321–325
71. Papasavas PK, Yeaney WW, Caushaj PF, et al. Perforation in the bypassed stomach following laparoscopic Roux-en-Y gastric bypass. *Obes Surg* 2003;13:797–799

72. Chan HL, Wu JC, Chan FK, et al. Is non–*Helicobacter pylori,* non-NSAID peptic ulcer a common cause of upper GI bleeding? A prospective study of 977 patients. *Gastrointest Endosc* 2001;53:438–442
73. Guslandi M, Tittobello A. Steroid ulcers: a myth revisited. *Br Med J* 1992;304:655–656
74. Piper JM, Ray WA, Daugherty JR, et al. Corticosteroid use and peptic ulcer disease: Role of nonsteroidal anti-inflammatory drugs. *Ann Intern Med* 1991;114:735–740
75. Carson JL, Strom BL, Schinnar R, et al. The low risk of upper gastrointestinal bleeding in patients dispensed corticosteroids. *Am J Med* 1991;91:223–228
76. Duggan JM, Zinsmeister AR, Kelly KA, et al. Long-term survival among patients operated upon for peptic ulcer disease. *J Gastroenterol Hepatol* 1999;14:1074–1082
77. van Leerdam ME, Vreeburg EM, Rauws EA, et al. Acute upper GI bleeding: Did anything change? Time trend analysis of incidence and outcome of acute upper GI bleeding between 1993–1994 and 2000. *Am J Gastroenterol* 2003;98:1494–1499
78. Lewis JD, Bilker WB, Brensinger C, et al. Hospitalization and mortality rates from peptic ulcer disease and GI bleeding in the 1990s: Relationship to sales of nonsteroidal anti-inflammatory drugs and acid suppression medications. *Am J Gastroenterol* 2002;97:2540–2549
79. Ohmann C, Imhof M, Roher HD. Trends in peptic ulcer bleeding and surgical treatment. *World J Surg* 2000;24: 284–293
80. Boonpongmanee S, Fleischer DE, Pezzullo JC, et al. The frequency of peptic ulcer as a cause of upper-GI bleeding is exaggerated. *Gastrointest Endosc* 2004;59:788–794
81. Yamaguchi Y, Yamato T, Katsumi N, et al. Endoscopic treatment of hemorrhagic gastric ulcer in patients aged 80 years or more. *Hepatogastroenterology* 2001;48:1195–1198
82. Fowler SF, Khoubian JF, Mathiasen RA, et al. Peptic ulcers in the elderly is a surgical disease. *Am J Surg* 2001; 182:733–737
83. Imhof M, Ohmann C, Roher HD, et al. Endoscopic versus operative treatment in high-risk ulcer bleeding patients: Results of a randomized study. *Langenbecks Arch Surg* 2003;387:327–336
84. Schoenberg MH. Surgical therapy for peptic ulcer and nonvariceal bleeding. *Langenbecks Arch Surg* 2001;386: 98–103
85. Barkun A, Bardou M, Marshall JK, et al. Consensus recommendations for managing patients with nonvariceal upper gastrointestinal bleeding. *Ann Intern Med* 2003; 139:843–857
86. Monig SP, Lubke T, Baldus SE, et al. Early elective surgery for bleeding ulcer in the posterior duodenal bulb: Own results and review of the literature. *Hepatogastroenterology* 2002;49:416–418
87. Ohmann C, Imhof M, Roher HD. Trends in peptic ulcer bleeding and surgical treatment. *World J Surg* 2000;24: 284–293
88. Imhof M, Schroders C, Ohmann C, et al. Impact of early operation on the mortality from bleeding peptic ulcer: Ten years' experience. *Dig Surg* 1998;15:308–314
89. Lewis JD, Shin EJ, Metz DC. Characterization of gastrointestinal bleeding in severely ill-hospitalized patients. *Crit Care Med* 2000;28:46–50
90. Church NI, Palmer KR. Ulcers and nonvariceal bleeding. *Endoscopy* 2003;35:22–26
91. Monig SP, Lubke T, Baldus SE, et al. Early elective surgery for bleeding ulcer in the posterior duodenal bulb: Own results and review of the literature. *Hepatogastroenterology* 2002;49:416–418
92. Brullet E, Campo R, Calvet X, et al. A randomized study of the safety of outpatient care for patients with bleeding peptic ulcer treated by endoscopic injection. *Gastrointest Endosc* 2004;60:15–21
93. Sung JJ, Chan FK, Lau JY, et al. The effect of endoscopic therapy in patients receiving omeprazole for bleeding ulcers with nonbleeding visible vessels or adherent clots: A randomized comparison. *Ann Intern Med* 2003; 139:237–243
94. Sanders DS, Perry MJ, Jones SG, et al. Effectiveness of an upper-gastrointestinal hemorrhage unit: A prospective analysis of 900 consecutive cases using the Rockall score as a method of risk standardization. *Eur J Gastroenterol Hepatol* 2004;16:487–494
95. Baradarian R, Ramdhaney S, Chapalamadugu R, et al. Early intensive resuscitation of patients with upper gastrointestinal bleeding decreasing mortality. *Am J Gastroenterol* 2004;99:619–622
96. Sanders DS, Carter MJ, Goodchap RJ, et al. Prospective validation of the Rockall risk scoring system for upper GI hemorrhage in subgroups of patients with varices and peptic ulcers. *Am J Gastroenterol* 2002;97:630–635
97. Cash BD. Evidence-based medicine as it applies to acid suppression in the hospitalized patient. *Crit Care Med* 2002;30:S373–378
98. Lau JY, Sung JJ, Lee KK, et al. Effect of intravenous omeprazole on recurrent bleeding after endoscopic treatment of bleeding peptic ulcers. *N Engl J Med* 2000;343: 310–316
99. Zed PJ, Loewen PS, Slavik RS, et al. Meta-analysis of proton pump inhibitors in treatment of bleeding peptic ulcers. *Ann Pharmacother* 2001;35:1528–1534
100. Hsieh YH, Lin HJ, Tseng GY, et al. Poor responders to intravenous omeprazole in patients with peptic ulcer bleeding. *Hepatogastroenterology* 2004;51:316–319
101. Kantorova I, Svoboda P, Scheer P, et al. Stress ulcer prophylaxis in critically ill patients: A randomized, controlled trial. *Hepatogastroenterology* 2004;51:757–761
102. Bini EJ, Cohen J. Endoscopic treatment compared with medical therapy for the prevention of recurrent ulcer hemorrhage in patients with adherent clots. *Gastrointest Endosc* 2003;58:707–714
103. Blocksom JM, Tokioka S, Sugawa C. Current therapy for nonvariceal upper gastrointestinal bleeding. *Surg Endosc* 2004;18:186–192
104. Park CH, Lee WS, Joo YE, et al. Endoscopic band ligation for control of acute peptic ulcer bleeding. *Endoscopy* 2004;36:79–82
105. Thomopoulos KC, Vagenas KA, Vagianos CE, et al. Changes in etiology and clinical outcome of acute up-

per gastrointestinal bleeding during the last 15 years. *Eur J Gastroenterol Hepatol* 2004;16:177–182
106. Chiu PW, Lam CY, Lee SW, et al. Effect of scheduled second therapeutic endoscopy on peptic ulcer rebleeding: A prospective, randomized trial. *Gut* 2003;52:1403–1407
107. Gisbert JP, Legido J, Garcia-Sanz I, et al. *Helicobacter pylori* and perforated peptic ulcer prevalence of the infection and role of nonsteroidal and anti-inflammatory drugs. *Dig Liver Dis* 2004;36:116–120
108. Bardhan KD, Nayyar AK, Royston C. History in our lifetime: The changing nature of refractory duodenal ulcer in the era of histamine H_2 receptor antagonists. *Dig Liver Dis* 2003;35:529–536
109. Bustamante M, Devesa F, Borghol A, et al. Accuracy of the initial endoscopic diagnosis in the discrimination of gastric ulcers: Is endoscopic follow-up study always needed? *J Clin Gastroenterol* 2002;35:25–28
110. Knight CD, van Heerden JA, Kelly KA. Proximal gastric vagotomy: update. *Ann Surg* 1983;197:22
111. Millat B, Hay JM, Valleur P, et al. Emergency surgical treatment for bleeding duodenal ulcer: Oversewing plus vagotomy versus gastric resection, a controlled, randomized trial. French Associations for Surgical Research. *World J Surg* 1993;17:568–573
112. Dubois A, Price SF, Castell DO. Gastric retention in peptic ulcer disease: A reappraisal. *Am J Dig Dis* 1978;23: 993–997
113. Kochhar R, Sethy PK, Nagi B, et al. Endoscopic balloon dilatation of benign gastric outlet obstruction. *J Gastroenterol Hepatol* 2004;19:418–422
114. Hoffman J, Meisner S, Jensen HE. Antrectomy for recurrent ulcer after parietal cell vagotomy. *Br J Surg* 1983; 70:120
115. Schirmer BD, Meyers WC, Hanks JB, et al. Marginal ulcer: A difficult surgical problem. *Ann Surg* 1982;195:653
116. McGuigan JE, Wolfe MM. Secretin injection test in the diagnosis of gastrinoma. *Gastroenterology* 1980;79:1324
117. Ott DJ, Munitz HA, Gelfand DW, et al. The sensitivity of radiography of the postoperative stomach. *Radiology* 1982;144:741
118. Mosiman F, Donovan IA, Alexander-Wiliams J. Pitfalls in the diagnosis of recurrent ulceration after surgery for peptic ulcer disease. *J Clin Gastroenterol* 1985;7:133
119. Turnage RH, Sarosi G, Cryer B, et al: Evaluation and management of patients with recurrent peptic ulcer disease after acid-reducing operations: A systematic review. *J Gastrointest Surg* 2003;7:606–626
120. Stabile BE, Passaro E. Recurrent peptic ulcer. *Gastroenterology* 1976;70:124
121. Koo J, Lam SK, Ong GB. Cimetidine versus surgery for recurrent ulcer after gastric surgery. *Ann Surg* 1982;195:406
122. Hoffman J, Shokouh-Amiri H, Klarskov P, et al. Gastrectomy for recurrent ulcer after vagotomy: 5 to 19 year follow-up. *Surgery* 1986;99:517
123. Zollinger RM, Ellison EH. Primary peptic ulcerations of the jejunum associated with islet cell tumors of the pancreas. *Ann Surg* 1955;142:709–723
124. Gregory RA, Grossman MI, Tracy HJ, et al. Nature of the gastric secretagogue in Zollinger-Ellison tumors. *Lancet* 1967;2:543–544
125. Berger AC, Gibril F, Venzon DJ, et al. Prognostic value of initial fasting serum gastrin levels in patients with Zollinger-Ellison syndrome. *J Clin Oncol* 2001;19:3051–3057
126. Norton JA: Gastrinoma: Advances in localization and treatment. *Surg Oncol Clin North Am* 1998;7:845–861
127. Roy PF, Venzon DJ, Shojamanesh H, et al. Zollinger-Ellison syndrome: Clinical presentation in 261 patients. *Medicine* 2000;79:379–411
128. Gibril F, Schumann M, Pace A, et al. Multiple endocrine neoplasia type I and Zollinger-Ellison syndrome: A prospective study of 107 cases and comparison with 1009 cases from the literature. *Medicine* 2004;83:43–83
129. Ellison EC, Sparks J. Zollinger-Ellison syndrome in the era of effective acid suppression: Are we unknowingly growing tumors? *Am J Surg* 2003;186:245–248
130. Wada M, Komoto I, Doi R, et al. Intravenous calcium injection test is a novel complementary procedure in differential diagnosis for gastrinoma. *World J Surg* 2002;26: 1291–1296
131. Proye C, Malvaux P, Pattou F, et al. Noninvasive imaging of insulinomas and gastrinomas with endoscopic ultrasonography and somatostatin receptor scintigraphy. *Surgery* 1998;124:1134–1143
132. Alexander HR, Fraker DL, Norton JA, et al. Prospective study of somatostatin receptor scintigraphy and its effect on operative outcome in patients with Zollinger-Ellison syndrome. *Ann Surg* 1998;228:228–238
133. Zimmer T, Scherubl H, Faiss S, et al. Endoscopic ultrasonography of neuroendocrine tumors. *Digestion* 2000; 1:45–50
134. Gauger PG, Scheiman JM, Wamsteker EJ, et al. Role of endoscopic ultrasonography in screening and treatment of pancreatic endocrine tumors in asymptomatic patients with multiple endocrine neoplasia type I. *Br J Surg* 2003;90:748–754
135. Anderson MA, Carpenter S, Thompson NW, et al. Endoscopic ultrasound is highly accurate and directs management in patients with neuroendocrine tumors of the pancreas. *Am J Gastroenterol* 2000;95:2271–2277
136. Bansal R, Tierney W, Carpenter S, et al. Cost-effectiveness of EUS for preoperative localization of pancreatic endocrine tumors. *Gastrointest Endosc* 1999;49:19–25
137. Turner JJ, Wren AM, Jackson JE, et al. Localization of gastrinomas by selective intra-arterial calcium injection. *Clin Endocrinol (Oxf)* 2002;57:821–825
138. Wu PC, Alexander HR, Bartlett DL, et al. A prospective analysis of the frequency, location, and curability of ectopic (nonpancreaticoduodenal, nonnodal) gastrinoma. *Surgery* 1997;122:1176–1182
139. Norton JA, Alexander HR, Fraker DL, et al. Does the use of routine duodenotomy (DUODX) affect rate of cure, development of liver metastases, or survival in patients with Zollinger-Ellison syndrome? *Ann Surg* 2004; 239:617–625
140. Saijo F, Naito H, Funayama Y, et al. Octreotide in control of multiple liver metastases from gastrinoma. *J Gastroenterol* 2003;38:905–908
141. Shojamanesh H, Gibril F, Louie A, et al. Prospective study of the antitumor efficacy of long-term octreotide

treatment in patients with progressive metastatic gastrinoma. *Cancer* 2002;94:331–343

142. Norton JA, Jensen RT. Current surgical management of Zollinger-Ellison syndrome (ZES) in patients without multiple endocrine neoplasia-type I (MEN1). *Surg Oncol* 2003;12:145–151
143. Phan GQ, Yeo CJ, Hruban RH, et al. Surgical experience with pancreatic and peripancreatic neuroendocrine tumors: Review of 125 patients. *J Gastrointest Surg* 1998;2:472–482
144. Norton JA, Fraker DL, Alexander HR, et al. Surgery to cure the Zollinger-Ellison syndrome. *N Engl J Med* 1999; 341:635–644
145. Norton JA, Alexander HR, Fraker DL, et al. Comparison of surgical results in patients with advanced and limited disease with multiple endocrine neoplasia type I and Zollinger-Ellison syndrome. *Ann Surg* 2001;234: 495–505
146. Norton JA, Kivlen M, Li M, et al. Morbidity and mortality of aggressive resection in patients with advanced neuroendocrine tumors. *Arch Surg* 2003;138:859–866
147. Norton JA, Jensen RT. Resolved and unresolved controversies in the surgical management of patients with Zollinger-Ellison syndrome. *Ann Surg* 2004;240:757–773
148. Li ML, Norton JA. Gastrinoma. *Curr Treat Options Oncol* 2001;2:337–346
149. Zogakis TG, Gibril F, Libutti SK, et al. Management and outcome of patients with sporadic gastrinoma arising in the duodenum. *Ann Surg* 2003;238:42–48
150. Norton JA, Alexander HR, Fraker DL, et al. Possible primary lymph node gastrinoma: occurrence, natural history, and predictive factors: A prospective study. *Ann Surg* 2003;237:650–657
151. Jordan PH Jr. A personal experience with pancreatic and duodenal neuroendocrine tumors. *J Am Coll Surg* 1999;189:470–482
152. Proye C, Pattou F, Carnaille B, et al. Intraoperative gastrin measurements during surgical management of patients with gastrinomas: Experience with 20 cases. *World J Surg* 1998;22:643–649
153. Azimuddin K, Chamberlain RS. The surgical management of pancreatic neuroendocrine tumors. *Surg Clin North Am* 2001;81:511–525
154. Deol ZK, Frezza E, DeJong S, et al. Solitary hepatic gastrinoma treated with laparoscopic radiofrequency ablation. *JSLS* 2003;7:285–289
155. Norton JA, Warren RS, Kelly MG, et al. Aggressive surgery for metastatic liver neuroendocrine tumors. *Surgery* 2003;134:1057–1063
156. Okuzawa A, Kobayashi S, Sakamoto K, et al. Metastatic gastrinoma to the liver 20 years after primary resection. *J Gastroenterol* 2000;35:717–720
157. Glascock MJ, Carty SE. Multiple endocrine neoplasia type I: Fresh perspective on clinical features and penetrance. *Surg Oncol* 2002;11:143–150
158. Plockinger U, Wiedenmann B. Neuroendocrine tumors of the gastroenteropancreatic system: The role of early diagnosis, genetic testing and preventive surgery. *Dig Dis* 2002;20:49–60
159. Yu F, Jensen RT, Lubensky IA, et al. Survey of genetic alterations in gastrinomas. *Cancer Res* 2000;60:5536–5542
160. Chen YJ, Vortmeyer A, Zhuang Z, et al. X-chromosome loss of heterozygosity frequently occurs in gastrinomas and is correlated with aggressive tumor growth. *Cancer* 2004;100:1379–1387
161. Chen YJ, Vortmeyer A, Zhuang Z, et al. Loss of heterozygosity of chromosome 1q in gastrinomas: Occurrence and prognostic significance. *Cancer Res* 2003;63:817–823
162. Goebel SU, Iwamoto M, Raffeld M, et al. *Her-2/neu* expression and gene amplification in gastrinomas: Correlations with tumor biology, growth, and aggressiveness. *Cancer Res* 2002;62:3702–3710

13

Stomach and Duodenum: Operative Procedures

Subroto Paul ■ *David I. Soybel* ■ *Michael J. Zinner*

■ HISTORICAL PERSPECTIVE

The earliest recorded operations on the stomach were performed for penetrating injuries.[1] In the late 1800s, experimental studies in the surgical laboratories of Billroth confirmed the feasibility of removing the pylorus, a concept developed by Michaelis in the early part of that century. In 1881, Rydygier performed the first successful pylorectomy, and in 1884 he performed the first gastroenterostomy. Both of these operations were performed for benign peptic ulcer disease. In 1881, Billroth performed the first successful pylorectomy for malignancy. In this case, the duodenum was anastomosed to the lesser curvature of the stomach and the greater curvature was oversewn. The patient initially did well, but died from disseminated abdominal carcinomatosis 4 months later. In 1885, Billroth performed a resection of a large pyloric carcinoma, using an anterior gastrojejunostomy for the reconstruction. In subsequent years, Billroth, his students, and others devised several approaches to gastroduodenal and gastrojejunal reconstruction,[2,3] some of which will be detailed below. Following popularization of gastrojejunostomy for reconstruction after gastric resection or palliation of unresectable gastric malignancy, surgeons were confronted with early complications such as bleeding, anastomotic leak, intestinal obstruction, and late complications such as stomal ulceration, bilious vomiting, afferent and efferent limb obstructions, and dumping.[4,5] At present, these problems remain unsolved.

Pyloroplasty was initially devised by Heineke for treatment of congenital hypertrophic pyloric stenosis, and the results were poor. Jaboulay's side-to-side anastomosis of the distal greater curvature and duodenum in 1892, and the Faience extension of this anastomosis to include the pylorus itself were subsequently refined by Kocher. Kocher improved the technical ease of the operation by including a mobilization of the duodenum from its lateral peritoneal attachments. The first pyloromyotomy was performed for this lesion in 1912 by Ramstedt.

In the early part of the 20th century, a dramatic rise was observed in the incidence of duodenal ulceration. A period of intense clinical and laboratory investigation from 1920–1940 led to the recognition that surgically performed vagotomy could reduce gastric acidity under resting conditions and in response to luminal and humoral stimuli. The use of vagotomy for patients with complications of ulcer disease was pioneered by Latarget, who reported 24 such cases in 1922. Latarget himself recognized that vagotomy might lead to delayed gastric emptying and had added a drainage procedure, gastrojejunostomy. Confusion regarding the role of delayed gastric emptying in the pathogenesis of peptic ulcers, however, led many surgeons away from vagotomy and drainage as a treatment for recurrent peptic ulceration. It remained for Dragstedt and his colleagues at the University of Chicago to resurrect this concept in the 1940s.[6] Subsequently, Farmer and Smithwick and others introduced the combination of truncal vagotomy and hemigastrectomy, an operation that also removed the gastrin-producing antral mucosa.[2] In the 1950s, Harkins' group in Seattle began to evaluate forms of vagotomy that left intact the celiac and hepatic branches (proximal selective vagotomy), along with or in combination with the preservation of vagal motor branches to the antrum (highly selective vagotomy, HSV, or parietal cell vagotomy).[7,8] These modifications arose from an appreciation of the contributions of antral motility to proper digestion, as well as improved understanding of specific postvagotomy complications such as dumping and diarrhea. The popularization of HSV is largely attributable to the efforts of Johnston, Goligher, Amdrup, and others, who in the 1960s and 1970s demonstrated the feasibility of obtaining ulcer recurrence rates as low as those of conventional truncal vagotomy (TV) without the incidence of dumping and diarrhea that was associated with TV with drainage or gastrectomy.[9,10] It is worth noting that surgeons have done more than develop new and interesting operative approaches to acid peptic disease. They played a major role in advancing current concepts of pathophysiology in ulcer disease and recurrence, and in understanding the physiological consequences of ulcer treatments, both medical and surgical.

▪ VAGOTOMY

Even though the increasing use of medications that inhibit gastric acid secretion, such as proton pump inhibitors, have made elective antisecretory operations essentially nonexistent, they remain part of the surgeon's armamentarium in dealing with patients who remain refractory to maximal medical therapy for ulcer disease, and in some selected cases for patients with ulcer perforation and bleeding. Hence, to understand the importance of the technical details in the execution of antisecretory operations, it is necessary to fully appreciate the anatomy of the vagus nerve and the gastric microvasculature, as well as the physiology of acid secretion, mucosal barrier function, and gastric motility, which are expanded upon below.

TESTS OF VAGAL CONTROL OF ACID SECRETION

Historically, vagal control of acid secretion has been assessed by measuring acid secretion in response to various stimuli. Acid secretion can be measured directly by the placement of a tube into the stomach, through which gastric juice is aspirated and the titratable acidity is measured by adding known quantities of 0.1 N NaOH. Gastric output is measured at baseline and after stimulation with pentagastrin or sham feeding. Measurements of gastric acid output pre– and post–vagotomy operations can be measured to assess the efficacy of vagotomy.[11,12] Acid secretion also can be assessed semiquantitatively, using pH sensitive dyes such as Congo red, that coat the mucosa and turn color when acid is being secreted from the gastric glands.[13] Although the former analytic methods permit accurate and quantitative assays of secretory capacity before and after the operation, the latter colorimetric methods can provide relatively rapid means of assessing secretory capacity of the stomach during the operation itself. These tests are rarely used today with the increasing use of medications that inhibit gastric acid secretion such as proton pump inhibitors and the consequent rarity of performing elective anti-ulcer gastric acid–reducing operations.

VAGAL REGULATION OF GASTRIC MOTILITY AND EMPTYING

As stated by Professor David Johnson in a previous edition of this book, "... Only when one fully understands the physiologic rationale of highly selective vagotomy will be one sufficiently motivated to do it well." This statement was made not in reference to the innervation of parietal cells that secrete HCl, but to the neural regulation of gastric motor function and emptying. The vagus dominates the motor activity of the normally functioning stomach in three ways. First, it mediates receptive relaxation and gastric accommodation; that is, the relaxation of the gastric fundus when intraluminal pressures in the proximal esophagus and stomach are increased by the presence of chyme. Second, the vagus mediates increases in antral myoelectrical activity that result from distention of the proximal stomach by chyme. Third, the vagus appears to mediate coordination of pyloric emptying with antral myoelectrical activity, in response to changes in proximal gastric motor activity, and perhaps in response to changes in composition and pH of duodenal content.[14]

It should be recognized that while truncal or selective vagotomy interrupts the vagal pathways to the antrum and pylorus, all three forms of vagotomy (truncal, selective, and highly selective) abolish receptive relaxation and gastric accommodation. It has been claimed that in the absence of pyloric scarring or stenosis, that vagotomy only temporarily impairs gastric emptying. This rationale has been used to justify combinations of selective and relatively nonselective approaches, such as a posterior truncal and anterior highly selective (or anterior seromyotomy) vagotomy. Such arguments become important in thinking about the feasibility of laparoscopic approaches to the vagus and the need for, and choice of, drainage procedures. Nevertheless, caution is advisable in recommending mixtures of approach or dispensing with drainage procedures after truncal or selective vagotomy. The assumptions that antral/pyloric coordination will return after truncal vagotomy or that gastric emptying after pyloromyotomy is as good as that after pyloroplasty are currently being tested, but have been disputed.[15] In addition, the full spectrum of complications following such mixtures of approach remains relatively uncharacterized and has not been studied in properly controlled trials.[16–18] It remains the surgeon's primary responsibility to ensure that the quality of care provided by newer laparoscopic approaches is comparable to that which has already been achieved with conventional surgical approaches.

OPEN APPROACHES TO THE VAGUS

Patient Position, Incisions, and Exposure

To perform a complete vagotomy, access to the upper part of the stomach and lower esophagus is crucial. It is helpful for the operating surgeon, standing on the patient's right, to wear a headlight. When access to the duodenum is required, as in a gastrectomy, excellent exposure is available through a chevron incision. However, in most patients, both thin and obese, a midline incision carried up along the xiphoid will be adequate. In the obese, extension of the incision below the umbilicus facilitates exposure. Placing the patient in reverse Trendelenburg position is helpful. A nasogastric (NG) tube is placed with its tip at the most dependent portion of the greater curvature. The NG tube helps to keep the position of the esophagus in mind. A self-retaining retractor is required. We use a Bookwalter retractor that provides excellent accessories for securing wide exposure to the upper abdomen, and by means of well-placed Mikulicz pads, for holding the small bowel and transverse colon in the lower abdomen (Fig 13–1). Some surgeons advocate routine mobilization of the left lobe of the liver by dividing the left triangular ligament. This mobilization is not always necessary, and when the lobe is floppy, can impede exposure. If this maneuver is performed, the lateral segment of the left lobe is held upward and to the right by a Richardson or Herrington-type retractor accessory. Care must be taken to place sponges or a pack between the retractor attachment and liver, and not to put much tension on the liver. Otherwise, fracture of the liver parenchyma and bleeding will result.

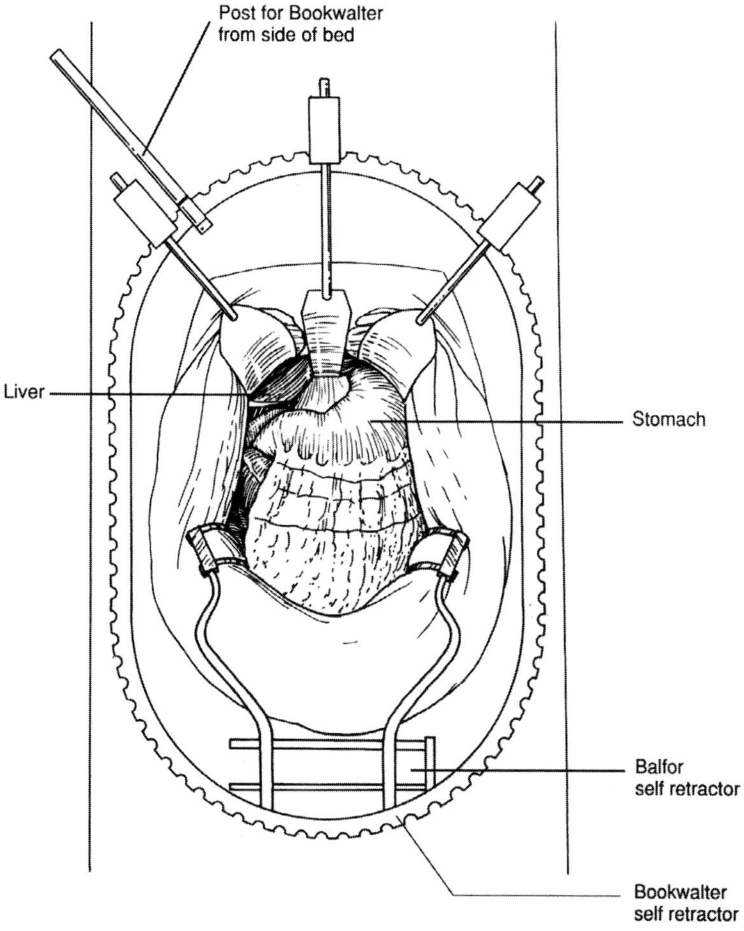

Figure 13–1. The use of the Bookwalter retractor for exposure of the upper abdomen.

Truncal Vagotomy

Truncal vagotomy (TV) is performed in conjunction with some form of drainage procedure. In the elective setting, it is used in conjunction with antrectomy for definitive management of refractory symptoms of duodenal ulcer, pyloric channel ulcer (gastric ulcer type III), or gastric ulcers combined with duodenal (Dragstedt) ulcers. In the current era of highly effective antisecretory therapies such as omeprazole, and anti-*Helicobacter* antibiotics, the main indication for TV and antrectomy is in the setting of pyloric outlet obstruction with a long-standing history of ulcer symptoms or complications such as bleeding and perforation. TV and pyloroplasty is reserved for emergency operations for complications such as bleeding or perforation. Occasionally, TV plus gastroenterostomy will be an appropriate compromise when the duodenum is too scarred to permit safe antrectomy and duodenal closure. The anatomy of the vagal trunks and nerves of Latarget is shown in Figures 13–2 and 13–3.

Using a Mikulicz pad or carefully applied Babcock clamps, the assistant places downward traction on the greater curvature of the stomach, thereby placing traction on the gastroesophageal junction and lower esophagus. The first step is to incise the peritoneal covering of the gastroesophageal junction. The peritoneum is opened horizontally, from the angle at the lesser curvature to the cardiac notch at the greater curvature. The surgeon's thumb and right index finger are used in a blunt dissection to encircle the esophagus. When teaching this maneuver, it is not uncommon for the trainee to confuse the right crus of the diaphragm with the esophagus itself or even the posterior vagal trunk. Extra time spent at this juncture to correctly identify all structures is part of the teaching aspect of the operation. A Penrose drain is passed around the junction in order to place more effective downward traction on the gastroesophageal junction. When encircling the esophagus, the surgeon stays wide of the esophagus in order to prevent inadvertent entry into the lumen and to include the vagal trunks. In the course of this maneuver, the posterior vagal trunk usually will be palpated as a taut cord.

A single anterior vagal trunk is usually identified in the anterior midportion of the esophagus, 2–4 cm above the gastroesophageal junction (Fig 13–4). At this level, however, it is not uncommon for vagal fibers to be distributed among two or three smaller cords. These cords are palpable as much as they are visible and can be separated from surrounding esophageal muscle fibers using a nerve hook. These trunks are individually lifted up and 2- to 4-cm segments of each are separated from surrounding tissues. A medium-sized clip is applied at the most superior end, and a clamp is applied inferiorly. The 2-cm length of nerve is resected and a clip is applied below the clamp; small bleeders are cauterized precisely. If it has not been done, the esophagus should be more widely mobilized for a distance of 4–5 cm above the gastroesophageal junction. Smaller, individual vagal fibers that ramify from the main trunks toward the lesser curvature and the cardiac notch then can be identified and cut or cauterized. The "criminal nerve" of Grassi, dis-

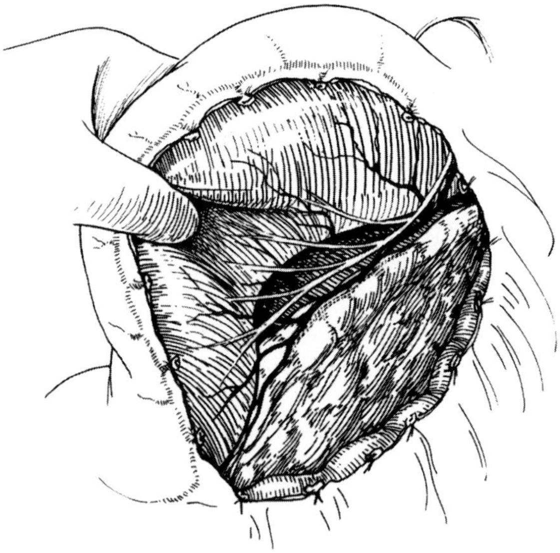

Figure 13–3. The posterior wall of the stomach and posterior nerve of the Latarget are shown. The terminal Y fork of the nerve is preserved and all of the branches to the stomach are divided, leaving about 5 cm of the distal portion of the stomach innervated. (Redrawn, with permission, from Johnston D. Vagotomy. In: Schwartz SI, Ellis H [eds]. *Maingot's Abdominal Operations*, 8th ed. Norwalk, CT: Appleton-Century-Crofts; 1982. After R.N. Lane.)

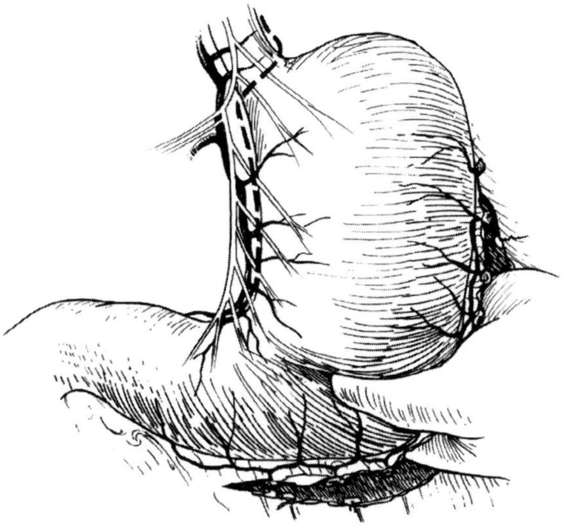

Figure 13–2. The distribution of the anterior vagus nerve is shown. The *dotted line* indicates the line of dissection. Note that it goes around the incisura to within about 6 cm of the pylorus. The gastrocolic omentum has been partially divided to permit access to the posterior nerve of Latarget and to allow the stomach to be grasped and used as a retractor. Note that the gastroepiploic arteries are carefully preserved. (Redrawn, with permission, from Johnston D. Vagotomy. In: Schwartz SI, Ellis H [eds]. *Maingot's Abdominal Operations*, 8th ed. Norwalk, CT: Appleton-Century-Crofts; 1982. After R.N. Lane.)

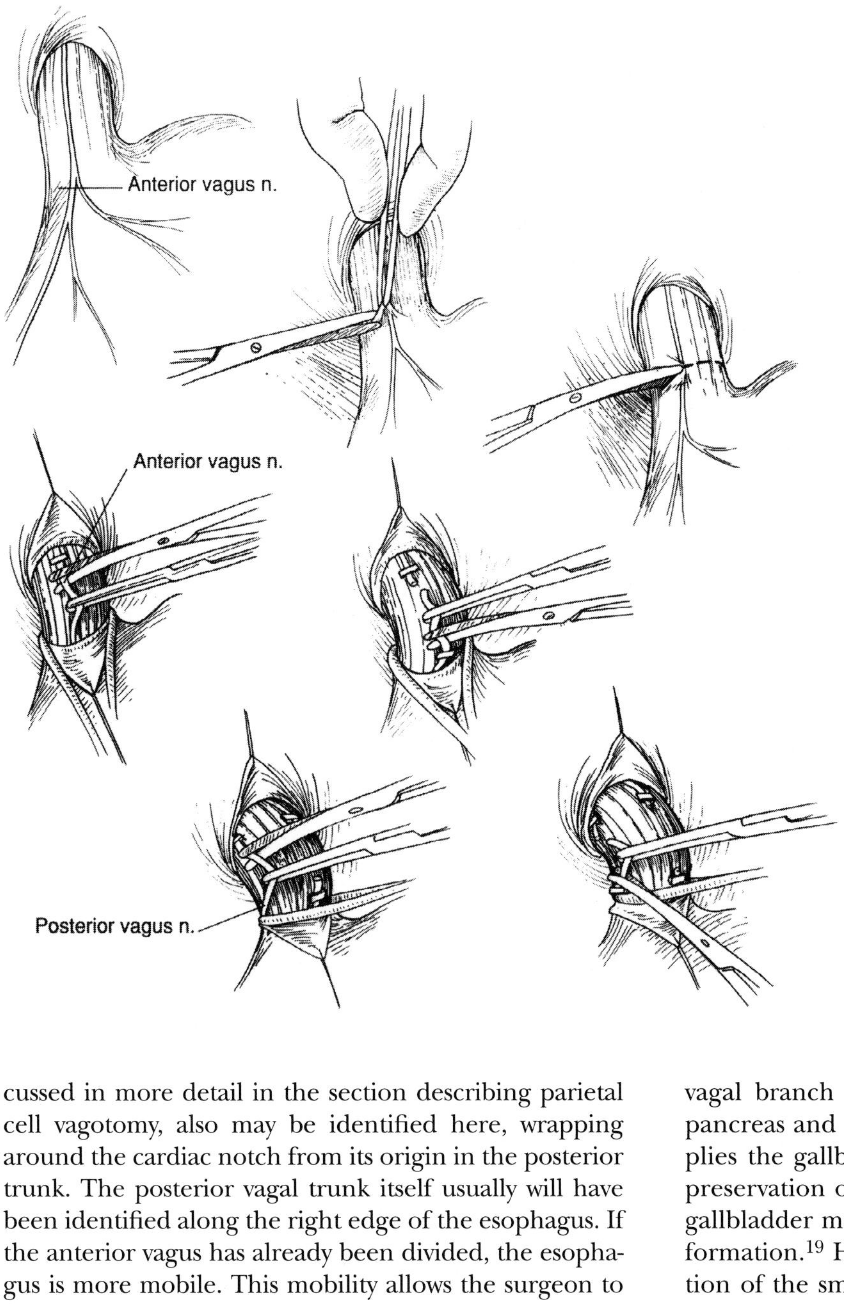

Figure 13–4. Division at both vagus nerves. (Redrawn, with permission, from Zinner MJ. *Atlas at Gastric Surgery.* New York, NY: Churchill Livingstone; 1992. After Gloege.)

cussed in more detail in the section describing parietal cell vagotomy, also may be identified here, wrapping around the cardiac notch from its origin in the posterior trunk. The posterior vagal trunk itself usually will have been identified along the right edge of the esophagus. If the anterior vagus has already been divided, the esophagus is more mobile. This mobility allows the surgeon to place downward traction on the gastroesophageal junction, which causes the posterior vagus to "bowstring" and make it easier to identify. A 2- to 4-cm segment is separated from surrounding tissues, its margins marked with clips, and resected. Major branches of the anterior vagus and the posterior vagal trunk should be sent to pathology for examination in frozen section. Care should be taken to note the results of the pathologist's frozen section diagnosis in the dictated operative note.

Selective Vagotomy

Selective vagotomy (SV) is not commonly practiced in the United States, but has found favor with European surgeons, who prefer not to cut the posteriorly derived vagal branch that innervates the small intestine and pancreas and anteriorly derived vagal branch that supplies the gallbladder and liver. There is evidence that preservation of such branches can avoid alterations in gallbladder motility that might lead to stasis and stone formation.[19] However, it is not clear whether preservation of the small intestinal and pancreatic nerves protects against some symptoms of the dumping syndrome.[16,20–22] SV involves interruption of both nerves of Latarget and therefore does not avoid the need for a drainage procedure. Thus the main indication for SV may be in patients undergoing elective antrectomy with vagotomy for refractory ulcer symptoms or obstruction.

Exposure to the vagus, gastroesophageal junction, and esophagus are obtained in the same way that the surgeon would perform TV. Anteriorly, the nerve of Latarget is identified by following the anterior vagal trunk as it descends from the esophagus to the lesser curvature of the stomach. Frequently, the descending branch of the left gastric artery is in close proximity to the site where the hepatic/gallbladder branches take off toward the liver in the gastrohepatic (lesser) omentum. A segment of the nerve of Latarget is severed between clips and sent for examination on frozen section. The most expeditious way to perform this maneuver is to cross-clamp the portion of the lesser omentum that contains the artery and nerve, ligating and dividing these structures together (Fig 13–5). The dissection continues upward along the lesser curvature, gastroesophageal junction, and esophagus. Division and ligation of blood vessels and nerves in this bundle avoids the hepatic/gallbladder branches and denervates the cardia, as was described for TV. This dissection opens up the plane for dissection and ligation of the posterior nerve of Latarget.

Highly Selective Vagotomy

Generally accepted indications for highly selective vagotomy (HSV) include: elective management of intractable symptoms of duodenal ulcer disease, emergency treatment for perforated duodenal ulcer, and emergency treatment of perforated gastric ulcer when the ulcer is to be excised in a wedge rather than resected in continuity with the distal stomach. HSV also has been advocated for management of bleeding gastric or duodenal ulcers, but this has not been widely practiced. Finally, there is published experience in pyloric outlet obstruction using HSV in combination with finger or endoscopic balloon dilatation,[22,23] but long-term persistence or recurrence rates of obstructing symptoms are not known.

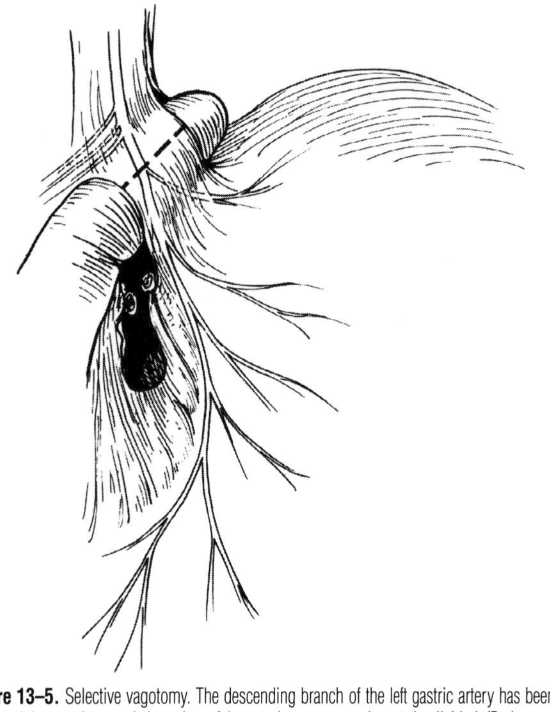

Figure 13–5. Selective vagotomy. The descending branch of the left gastric artery has been divided and the anterior gastric branches of the anterior vagus are about to be divided. (Redrawn, with permission, from Griffith CA. Selective gastric vagotomy. In: Nyhes LM, Wastell C [eds]. *Surgery of the Stomach and Duodenum,* 3rd ed. Boston, MA: Little, Brown; 1977:275. After Gloege.)

A number of variations of the technique have been described and will not all be reviewed here. However, it is worth cataloging the decisions that the surgeon must make in preparing for and performing this operation. The first decision is whether to use Congo red dye for intraoperative testing of the completeness of vagotomy. It may be difficult, and sometimes contraindicated, to perform endoscopy in the setting of acute bleeding or perforation. If the test is to be used, the endoscopic equipment and reagents should be assembled in the operating room before the operation begins. Conceptually then, the operation is divided into four phases: (1) exposure and gastric mobilization; (2) dissection of the anterior leaf of the lesser omentum; (3) dissection of the posterior leaf of the lesser omentum; and (4) dissection of vagal fibers traveling to the stomach along the distal esophagus.

Exposure and Gastric Mobilization. Exposure of the vagus nerves, esophagus, and gastroesophageal junction is obtained as described above. A wide-bore (18F) NG tube should be placed by the anesthesia team. A number of authors have emphasized the importance of the stomach as a retractor in this operation. We recommend mobilization of the distal part of gastrocolic omentum. The dissection should be carried outside the gastroepiploic arcade, in order to avoid loss of any blood supply to the greater curvature. Congenital adhesions between the stomach and peritoneum overlying the pancreas are divided sharply. The goal of this dissection is to obtain sufficient mobility of the stomach so that it can be rotated upward and to the patient's right, thus permitting visualization of the posterior leaf of the lesser omentum and the posterior nerve of Latarget through the lesser sac. The nerve can be seen running close to the descending branch of the left gastric artery. Vagal fibers can be seen running transversely toward the lesser curvature.

Dissection of the Anterior Leaf of the Lesser Omentum. The anterior leaf of the lesser omentum now is dissected. The next decision point is to define the distal margin of the dissection of the branches of the nerve of Latarget (Fig 13–6). An important landmark is the incisura angularis. The "crow's foot" is the neurovascular bundle that innervates the junction of the corpus and antrum, and has three characteristic branches from which its name derives. These nerves contain motor branches to the antrum and secretory branches to the oxyntic mucosa. Thus, leaving this bundle intact makes the antisecretory operation less complete, but fully severing it may lead to disturbances in gastric emptying. Two approaches for defining the distal margin of the dissection have been advocated. First, one may arbitrarily be-

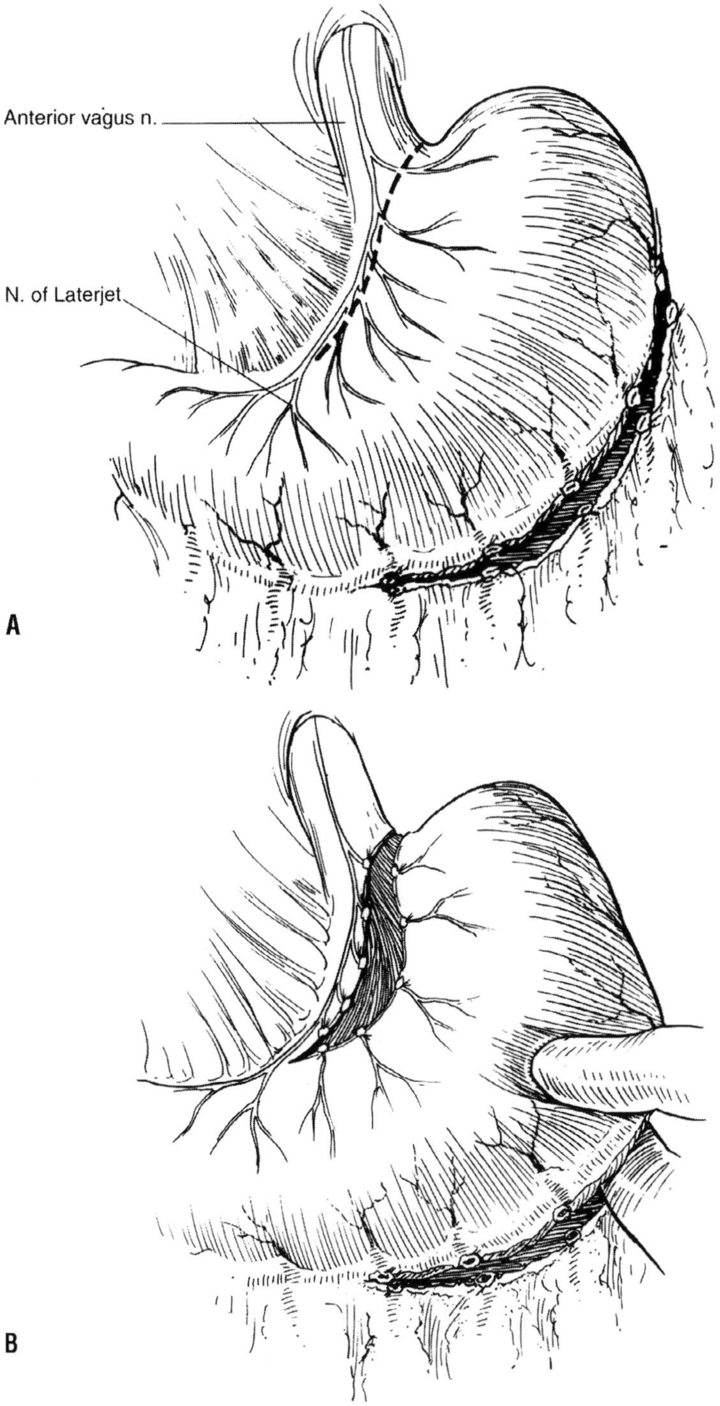

Figure 13–6. Highly selective vagotomy. **A.** Planned line of dissection of the anterior leaf of the gastrohepatic ligament. **B.** The dissection is carried out, beginning just proximal to the crow's foot and extending upward, to the left of the gastroesophageal unction. (Redrawn, with permission, from Zinner MJ. *Atlas of Gastric Surgery.* New York, NY: Churchill Livingstone; 1992. After Gloege.)

gin the dissection at a predetermined point 6–7 cm proximal to the pylorus, a distance that usually corresponds to the most proximal of the three branches of the crow's foot. Alternatively, one may identify this most proximal branch and begin the dissection there. It is helpful to begin the dissection a few centimeters proximal to the agreed upon distal margin, since strong traction during subsequent parts of the operation may cause traction injury on the antral motor branches and vessels that accompany them. These last few centimeters are dealt with last.

The assistant provides downward and leftward traction on the greater curvature, thus placing tension on the anterior nerve of Latarget as it runs along the lesser curvature. The hepatic fibers usually are visualized without difficulty in the upper part of the lesser omentum. It is helpful to "score" the serosa of the lesser curvature, from the incisura to the cardia, and then transversely across the gastroesophageal junction. The incision is performed with dissecting scissors or a no. 15 knife, not electrocautery. This maneuver widens the gap between the nerve and the gastric wall. Individual vessels run transversely from the lesser omentum onto the lesser curvature. These structures are ligated in continuity with 3-0 silk ligatures before division. (We avoid the use of hemostats in this dissection.) This part of the operation is performed gently and should not cause blood loss. The dissection proceeds along the lesser curvature until the gastroesophageal junction is reached. The left anterior aspect of the esophagus is now uncovered, and for the moment, the dissection stops.

Dissection of the Posterior Leaf of the Lesser Omentum. The posterior leaf of the lesser omentum then is dissected. Care should be taken in setting up exposure for this part of the operation. In one approach, the stomach is rotated upward and to the patient's right. Alternatively, the posterior leaf can be reached by working through the anterior leaf as illustrated in Figure 13–7. Using the thumbs and fingers, the gastroesophageal junction is "rolled" counterclockwise so that the posterior wall moves to the right and the anterior wall moves to the left. The nerve branches and their accompanying vessels then are ligated in continuity and divided. The dissection should not be carried to less than 6 cm from the pylorus. To avoid the main left gastric vessels, this approach to the dissection should be carried about two-thirds of the distance along the lesser curvature. After reaching the left gastric vessels, the surgeon returns to the anterior approach, ligating and dividing the remainder of the posterior leaf through the window in the anterior leaf.

Dissection of the Distal Esophagus. The goal of this dissection is to clear the distal esophagus of all nerve fibers for a distance of approximately 5 cm above the gastroesophageal junction. The importance of this part of the dissection is well documented.[24] It should be noted that the prior dissection of the lesser omentum has allowed the main vagal trunks to move upward and to the patient's right, thereby minimizing the risk of damaging the main trunks in this part of the dissection. Nevertheless, the operative technique requires that this dissection stay close to the lesser curvature and esophagus. Any dissection toward the tissues to the right (i.e., toward the main vagal trunks) should be avoided.

This part of the procedure begins with the dissection of the left side of the esophagus (Fig 13–8). Denuding the surface can be performed gently, using a finger or "peanut" dissector to isolate the adventitia that contains nerves, vessels, and lymphatics. This dissection is where the "criminal nerve" of Grassi is likely to be encountered. Tissues are ligated in continuity and divided. This dissection should also clear 2 or 3 cm of the cardia, just distal to the gastroesophageal junction, and small fibers running to the greater curvature will be divided here. It is usually not necessary to divide any of the short gastric arteries.

The anterior aspect of the esophagus is now cleared of vagal fibers (Fig 13–9). Gentle traction and lifting of the fibers will isolate them for division between ligatures or by cautery. We prefer ligation in continuity with fine (4-0 or 5-0) silk to avoid injury to the esophageal muscle. The posterior aspect is now re-exposed with downward traction of the gastroesophageal junction and a counterclockwise rotation of the distal esophagus. Working through the window of the anterior leaflet, the upward branches of the left gastric artery are visualized as they pass to the cardia and the gastroesophageal junction. They are ligated in continuity and divided. The dissection continues upward along the cardia and gastroesophageal junction, until it is possible to encircle the lower esophagus with a Penrose drain. Downward traction on the gastroesophageal junction is provided by this drain, and additional nerve fibers are seen in the adventitia. Smaller fibers are cauterized while held away from the esophageal muscularis, whereas larger ones are ligated with clips or fine silk and divided. Throughout this dissection, the positions of the nerves of Latarget and the main trunks should be checked.

The final part of the operation involves completion of the distal dissection to the crow's foot and checks for hemostasis. A number of authors have in the past suggested that reperitonealization of the lesser curvature be performed. The rationale for this maneuver is that the devascularization that is part of HSV may lead to small areas of necrosis of the gastric wall and localized perforations. Such leaks have been reported in about 0.2% of patients.[25] Also, it has been argued that reperitonealization might impede re-establishment of vagal nerve connections to the gastric wall.[26] The reperitonealization would thus protect against such leaks. The repertionealization can be performed by inversion of the serosa of the lesser curvature with running or continuous 3-0 Maxon or Prolene suture. Alternatively, a vascularized pedicle of omentum can be used to cover the deserosalized lesser curvature. Bleeding complications have been reported with this latter method, but it minimizes tension within the gastric wall.

Reoperative Approaches to the Vagus Nerves

Approximately two-thirds of patients with duodenal or pyloric channel ulcer recurrence after an initial anti-

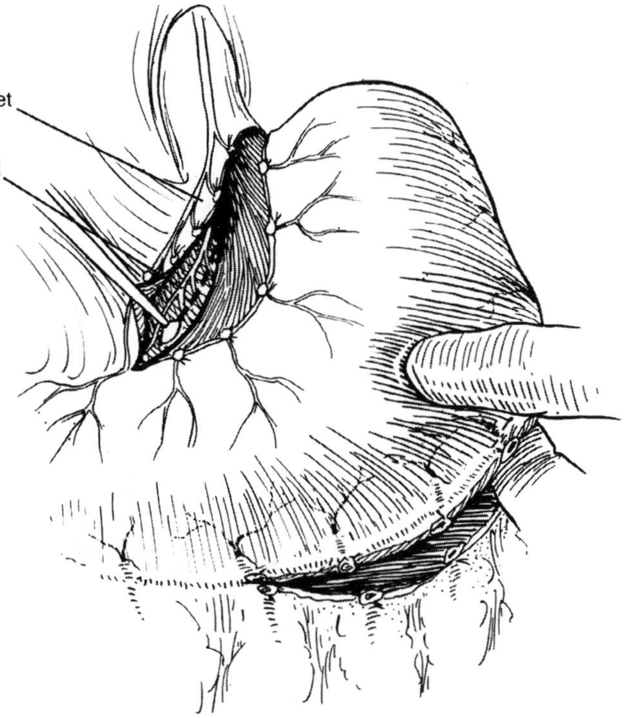

A

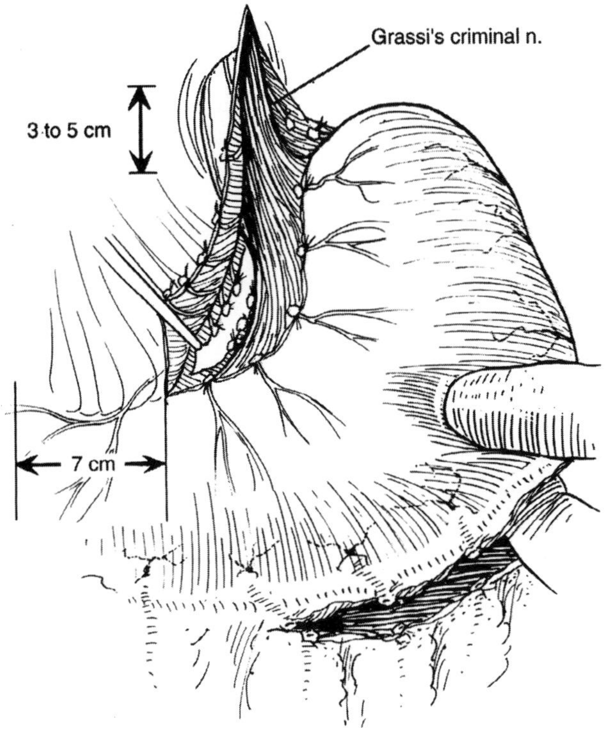

B

Figure 13–7. Parietal cell vagotomy. **A.** The line of dissection of the posterior leaf of the gastrohepatic ligament is illustrated. **B.** The dissection is carried out through the window created by prior dissection of the anterior leaf. (Redrawn, with permission, from Zinner MJ. *Atlas of Gastric Surgery.* New York, NY: Churchill Livingstone; 1992. After R.N. Lane.)

secretory operation (TV, SV, or HSV) have evidence of intact vagal innervation.[11,27] Although many such recurrences are amenable to medical regimens, a small fraction ultimately may be considered for reoperation, especially if surgery is required to control an acute complication such as bleeding or perforation following a period of ulcer-related symptoms. Prior surgery will have made the standard approaches to the lesser curvature and gastroesophageal junction hazardous, which is often caused by dense adhesions to a previously mobilized left lobe of the liver. Thus, two approaches to the vagus, both nonselective, may be considered for com-

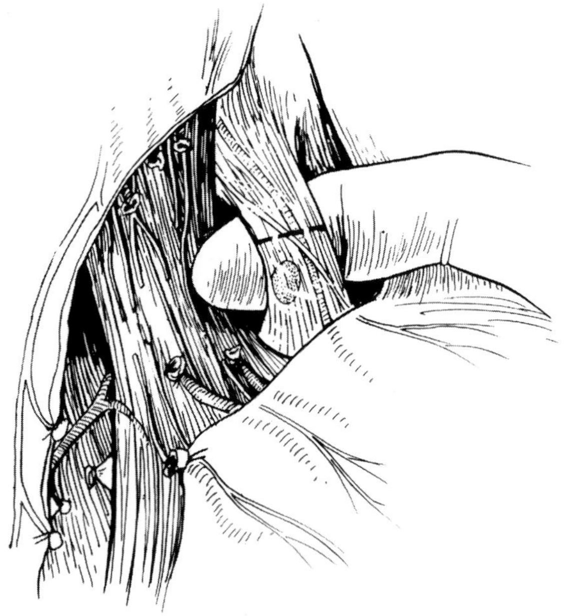

Figure 13–8. The serosa has been cut to the left of the esophagus, and fatty areolar tissue to the left of the esophagus, containing nerve fibers, blood vessels, and lymphatics is hooked up by the right index finger.The angle of His and the adjacent esophagus with a 2–3 cm portion of the fundus of the stomach are thoroughly cleaned. In this way, small nerve fibers running to the proximal 3 cm portion of fundus ("criminal nerves of Grassi") are eliminated. (Redrawn, with permission, from Johnston D. Vagotomy. In: Schwartz SI, Ellis H [eds]. *Maingot's Abdominal Operations.* Norwalk, CT: Appleton-Century-Crofts; 1982. After R.N. Lane.)

pletion of the failed vagotomy, especially if it was performed in conjunction with antrectomy. It should be stressed that when such a reoperation is contemplated, especially in a nonemergent setting, it is prudent to obtain some form of acid secretion profile to document the hypersecretory state. Also, because of the nonselective nature of the completion vagotomy, an antrectomy or drainage procedure must be performed.

In the setting in which standard access is difficult due to prior surgery, Barroso and associates have utilized a transabdominal suprahepatic approach to the vagi.[28] A high midline incision is used, with mechanical retraction to elevate the subcostal margin. A 18F NG tube is placed. The triangular, left coronary, and falciform ligaments and adhesions are divided, permitting downward retraction of the left lobe. Using the NG tube, the esophagus and hiatus are located. The esophagus and vagi are dissected at the level of the diaphragm at the hiatus and incised anteriorly for a distance of 3–5 cm, exposing the esophagus at the lower mediastinum. The trunks are easily identified and ligated in the unoperated area of the lower thoracic esophagus. The hiatus is closed with interrupted nonabsorbable sutures.

A transthoracic approach to this region has also been used,[29] and with the advent of thoracoscopy, may become increasingly attractive for this limited set of patients. The operation is performed through the left chest, entered via the eighth intercostal space. A NG tube is positioned with its tip in the stomach. After division of the inferior pulmonary ligament, the base of the left lung is retracted upward and laterally. The mediastinal pleura overlying the esophagus is incised for a distance of 8 cm. The esophagus is then mobilized and encircled with a Penrose drain. Vessel loops are used to retract individual vagal trunks as they are identified. The supradiaphragmatic anterior vagus nerve may have multiple branches above the level of the diaphragm, but rarely are there multiple branches at a level 4 cm above the diaphragm.[30] In contrast, the posterior vagus has multiple branches above the level of the diaphragm, but is a single trunk at this level more than 90% of the time (Fig 13–10). Thus, the best opportunity for a complete vagotomy lies 4 cm above the diaphragm for the posterior trunk. A circumferential dissection of the 6 cm of esophagus just above the diaphragm is carried out, with technique similar to that performed during the HSV. Tube thoracostomy is required for 2–3 days postoperatively.

▪ DRAINAGE PROCEDURES

In the context of bilateral truncal or selective vagotomies, the purpose of a drainage procedure is to preserve the pylorus but bypass or render it ineffective. The options for drainage include (1) gastroenterostomy; (2) pyloric dilatation; (3) pyloromyotomy; and (4) pyloroplasty. Gen-

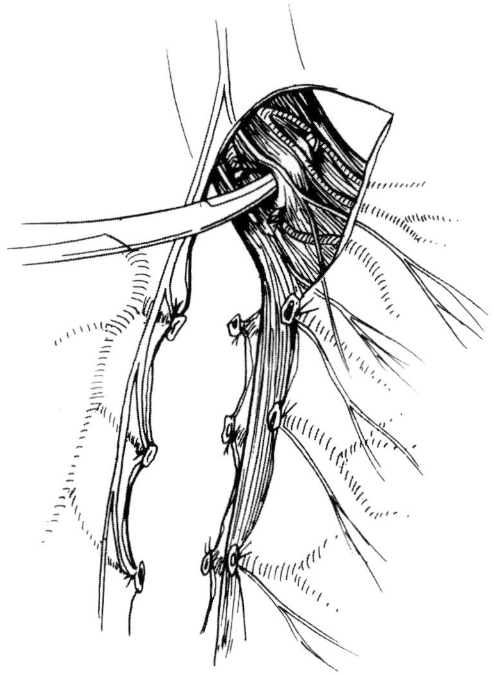

Figure 13–9. Anterior gastric branches of the anterior vagal trunk running downward on the anterior surface of the esophagus are gently lifted with a hemostat and either ligated or clipped before being divided, or destroyed with diathermy. (Redrawn, with permission, from Johnston D. Vagotomy. In: Schwartz SI, Ellis H [eds]. *Maingot's Abdominal Operations,* 8th ed. Norwalk, CT: Appleton-Century-Crofts; 1982. After R.N. Lane.)

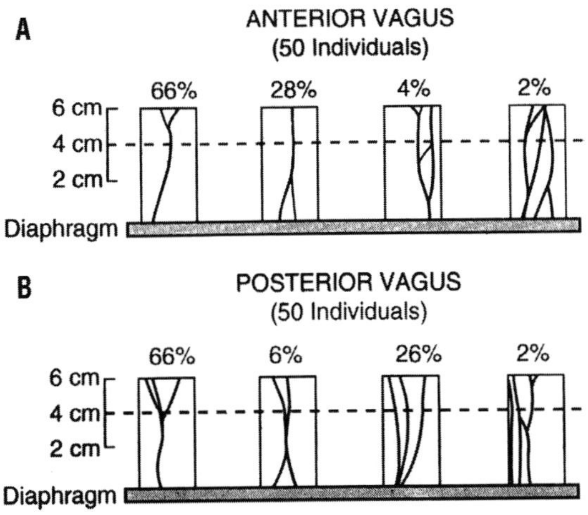

Figure 13–10. Anatomy of the anterior **(A)** and posterior **(B)** vagus nerves above the diaphragm in 50 cadavers. Incidence of each anatomic group is indicated by percentage. (Redrawn, with permission, from Jackson RG. Anatomy of the vagus nerve in the region of the lower esophagus and stomach. Anat Rec 1949;103:1.)

erally, these techniques are used when TV or SV is performed, but they also may be used with HSV in order to treat obstruction resulting from peptic acid scarring. We will discuss techniques for performing gastrojejunostomy in the subsequent discussion ofgastric resection.

▪ PYLORIC DILATATION

In open procedures, the simplest technique reported for performing pyloric dilatation is to perform a small gastrotomy, approximately 3–4 cm in length, proximal to the pylorus. A finger is introduced through the pylorus, forcing it to widen. The gastrotomy then is used with a single layer of 3-0 silk interrupted sutures. A second technique, advocated for use in laparoscopic cases, is to use a balloon. The balloon, 15 mm in length, may be positioned endoscopically and inflated to 45 psi for 10 minutes. Other dilators are available for positioning over a wire and inflation to higher pressures, which may prevent pyloric spasm. Advocates of pyloric dilatation after laparoscopic TV or SV have suggested that a drainage procedure is not required as often as previously thought, or may only be necessary in the early postoperative phase and not permanently.[31,32] Thus, it is argued, dilatation can be repeated postoperatively and in the outpatient setting. Most surgeons, however, subscribe to the need for some form of formal drainage procedure after SV or TV.

▪ PYLOROMYOTOMY

Pyloromyotomy is performed using the same techniques as those described in the setting of hypertrophic pyloric stenosis in the infant (Fig 13–11). An incision is made to score the anterior surface of the stomach from 1–2 cm proximal to 1 cm distal to the pyloric ring. The separation of pyloric muscles is accomplished mainly with a fine-tip hemostat and the knife. Cautery is avoided and only used in the muscularis, not the submucosa. When this procedure is performed in the setting of esophagogastrectomy, the pylorus is usually soft and unscarred. In the setting of chronic duodenal ulcer disease, the pylorus is often scarred and it is difficult to perform the gentle, meticulous dissection of muscle layers that is required, and at the same time, to avoid entering the mucosa. Laparoscopic versions of this procedure also have been advocated in the setting of laparoscopic TV or SV.[33]

▪ PYLOROPLASTY

The most expeditiously performed pyloroplasty is the Heineke-Mikulicz procedure (Fig 13–12). This is difficult to perform if the pyloric region is very scarred. The operation usually is performed in the setting of emergency surgery for bleeding or perforation of a gastric or duodenal ulcer. A vagotomy is performed, usually after bleeding has been controlled. If the indication is a bleeding or perforated duodenal or pyloric channel ulcer, the incision for pyloroplasty may include the ulcer or be used to gain access to the ulcer. The incision is thus the planned pyloroplasty incision.

It is not always necessary to perform a Kocher maneuver; however, duodenal mobilization is usually helpful in relieving any tension on the intended suture line. Unless the duodenal bulb is unusually mobile, we recommend this as the initial step. In this maneuver, the peritoneum along the right border of the duodenum is incised from the lateral border of the common bile duct to the junction of the second and third portions of the duodenum. After duodenal mobilization, 3-0 silk stay sutures are placed untied, superior and inferior to the site of the intended incision, which then is made on the anterior surface in a longitudinal direction, using electrocautery, from 2 cm distal to the pyloric muscle to 3 cm proximal to the pylorus. The closure of the pyloroplasty is performed vertically, in order to minimize narrowing of the lumen. The Gambee stitch (see Fig 13–12) is a single-layer inverting suture used in this setting. The suture, usually performed with 3-0 or 2-0 silk, begins on the outside and (1) is placed full thickness (serosa to mucosa) on the same side; (2) is brought, on the same side, back through the mucosa to the submucosa; (3) is carried through the submucosa to the mucosa on the opposite side; and (4) is brought full thickness from mucosa to serosa on that side. When the pylorus is scarred and the tissues inflexible, it is often helpful to tie the sutures after they have been placed, rather than as they are being placed. The stay sutures

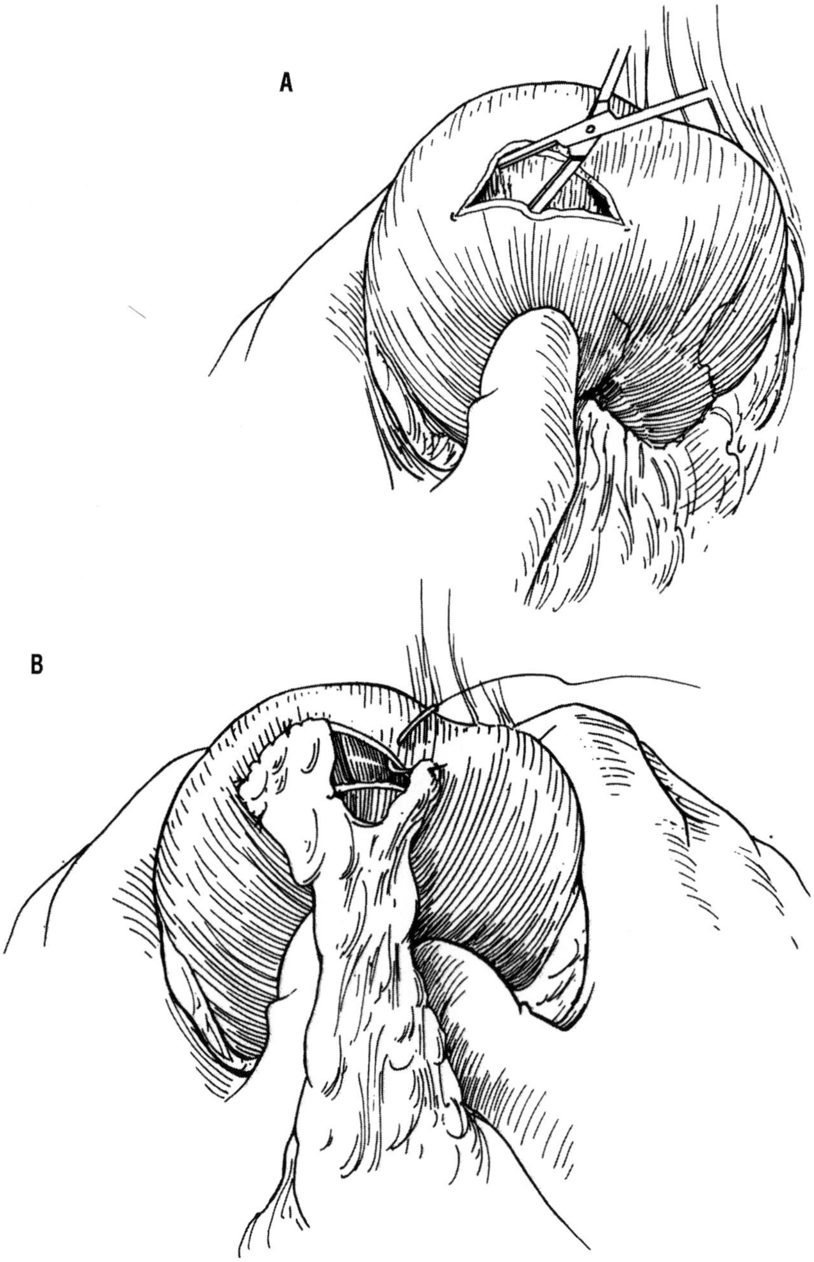

Figure 13–11. Pyloromyotomy. **A.** Dissection of seromuscular layers, avoiding entry into bowel. **B.** An omental patch is used to cover the dissected area. (Redrawn, with permission, from Welch CE. *Surgery of the Stomach and Duodenum.* Chicago, IL: Year Book Medical; 1973.)

then are removed, after completion of the pyloroplasty. A tongue of vascularized omentum may be brought up to cover the closure and it is sutured to the gut wall with 3-0 Vicryl sutures.

The Finney pyloroplasty can be used when scarring has involved the pylorus and duodenal bulb and would not permit a tension-free, patulous Heineke-Mikulicz pyloroplasty. The Finney pyloroplasty is in essence a side-to-side gastroduodenostomy (Fig 13–13). When beginning this operation, dense adhesions often are encountered surrounding the pylorus and duodenal bulb. These must be lysed systematically. The Kocher maneuver then is performed, carrying the mobilization distally. Complete mobility of the duodenum and freedom from surrounding adhesions are essential to this operation.

A 2-0 silk stay suture is placed on the upper anterior surface of the pyloric ring. Another stay suture is placed on the greater curvature of the stomach approximately 10 cm proximal to the pylorus, and a third stay suture is placed approximately 10 cm distal to the pylorus. Traction cranially on the pyloric suture and caudally on the other two sutures brings the anterior surfaces on the stomach and duodenum into apposition. The apposed surfaces are sutured together using interrupted 3-0 silk Lembert seromuscular sutures. Using electrocautery an inverted U-shaped incision is made

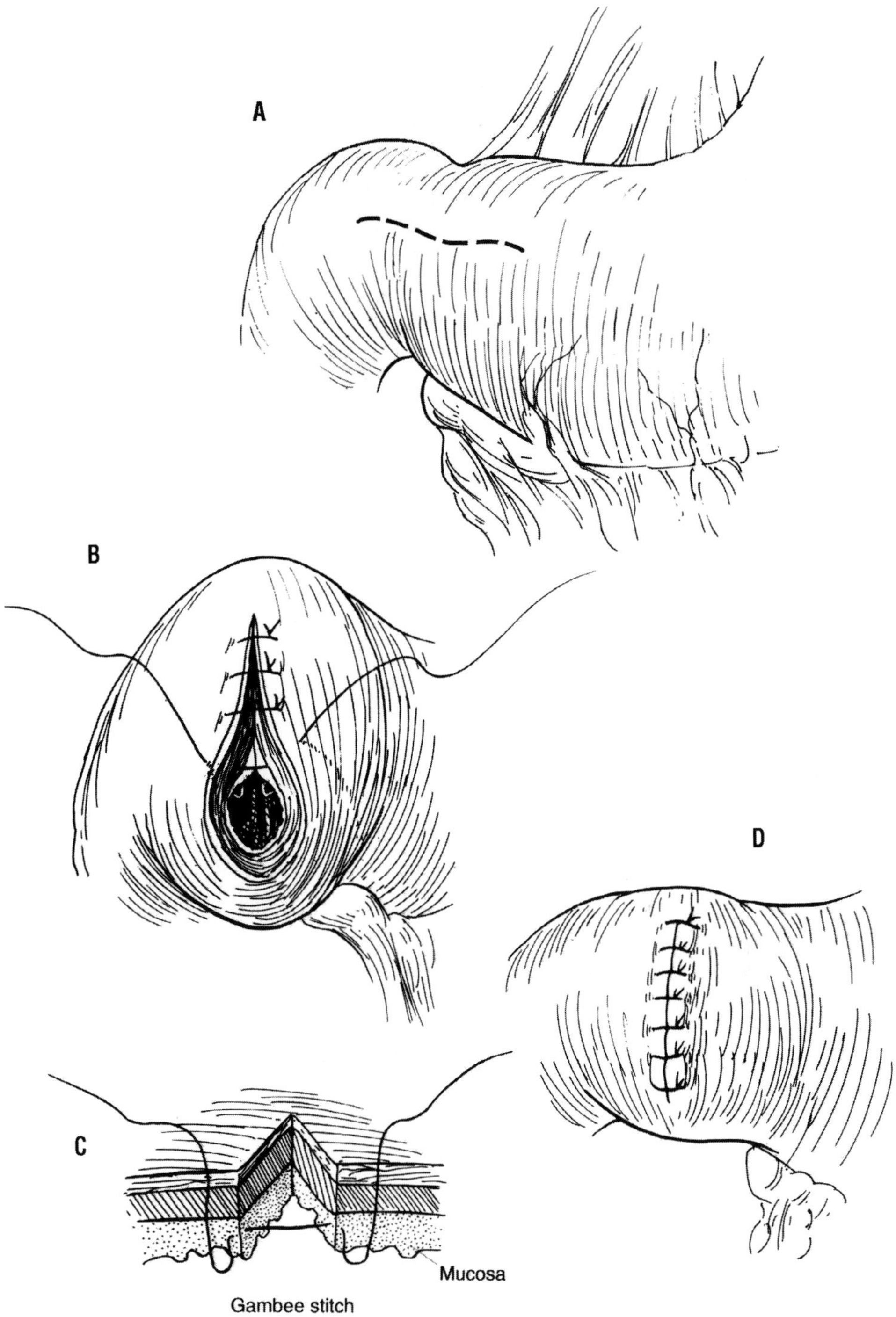

Figure 13–12. Heinecke-Mikulicz pyloroplasty. **A.** Full-thickness incision extends from 2 cm proximal to 1–2 cm distal to the pyloric ring. **B.** The incision is closed vertically. **C.** Illustration of Gambee stitch. **D.** Finished pyloroplasty. (Redrawn, with permission, from Zinner MJ. *Atlas of Gastric Surgery.* New York, NY: Churchill Livingstone; 1992. After Gloege.)

beginning on the gastric side just distal to the traction suture, traveling longitudinally through the pylorus, then distally to a point just proximal to the traction suture. If the ulcer is present on the anterior surface of the duodenal bulb, it is excised. The posterior inner layer between the stomach and the duodenum then is sutured closed with a continuous over-and-over 3-0 Vicryl or chromic catgut suture. This closure is begun at the superior edge, is carried caudally, and then converted into a Connell inverting technique as the suture is brought around the inferior edge to begin closing the anterior portion of the inner layer. The anterior outer layer then is closed using interrupted 3-0 Lambert sutures. Some surgeons use 3-0 Maxon or PDS su-

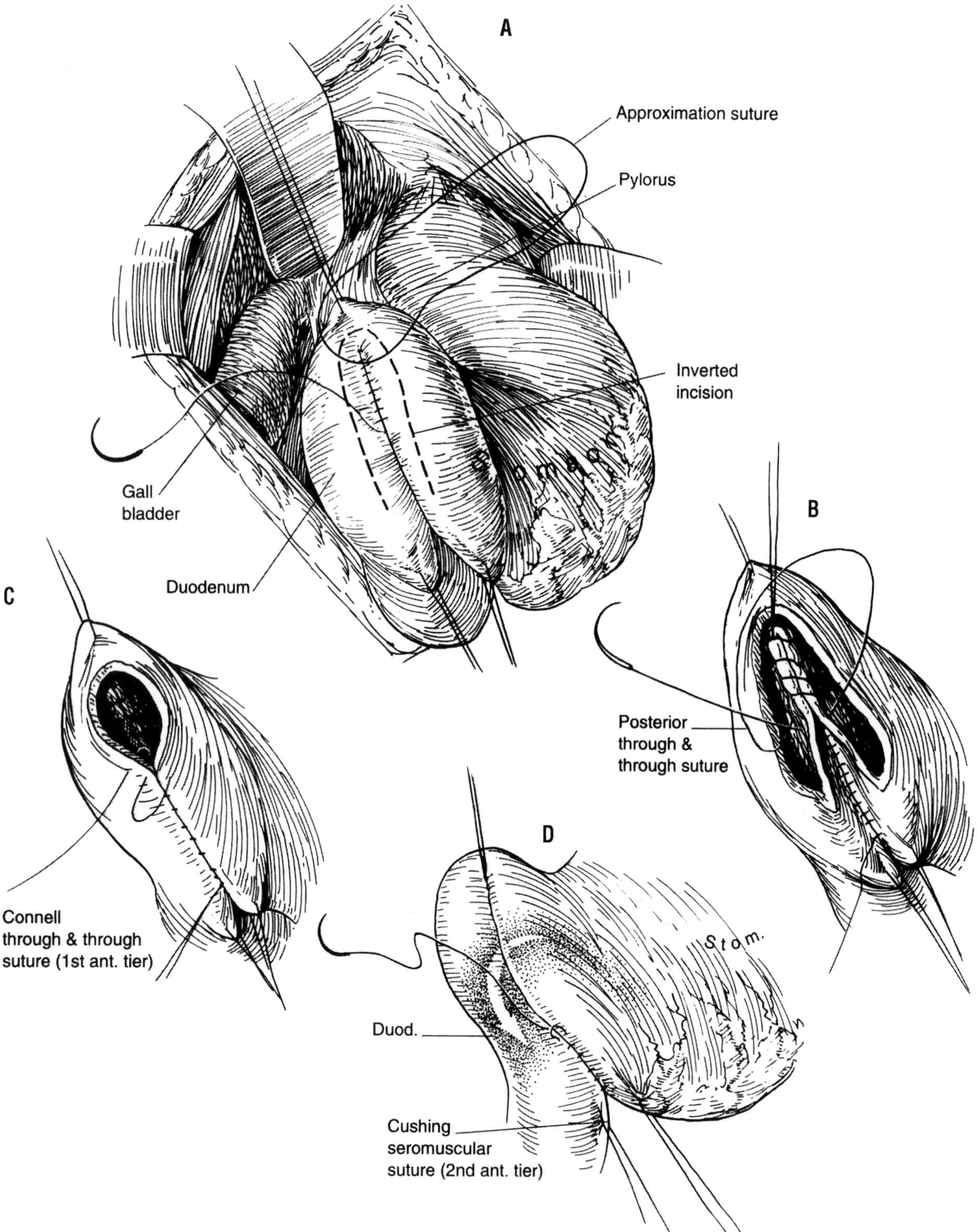

Figure 13–13. Finney U-shaped pyloroplasty. **A.** The distal stomach and proximal duodenum are aligned with traction strands and their adjacent walls approximated with a Cushing suture; the inverted U-shaped incision into the lumens of the stomach and duodenum is indicated. **B.** Suture of the posterior septum of the stomach and duodenum. **C.** The first anterior tier of sutures (Connell) is placed. **D.** The operation is completed with a reinforcing tier of Cushing sutures. (Redrawn, with permission, from Zuidema GD [ed]. *Shackelford's Surgery of the Alimentary Tract,* Vol. II, 3rd ed. Philadelphia, PA: WB Saunders; 1991.)

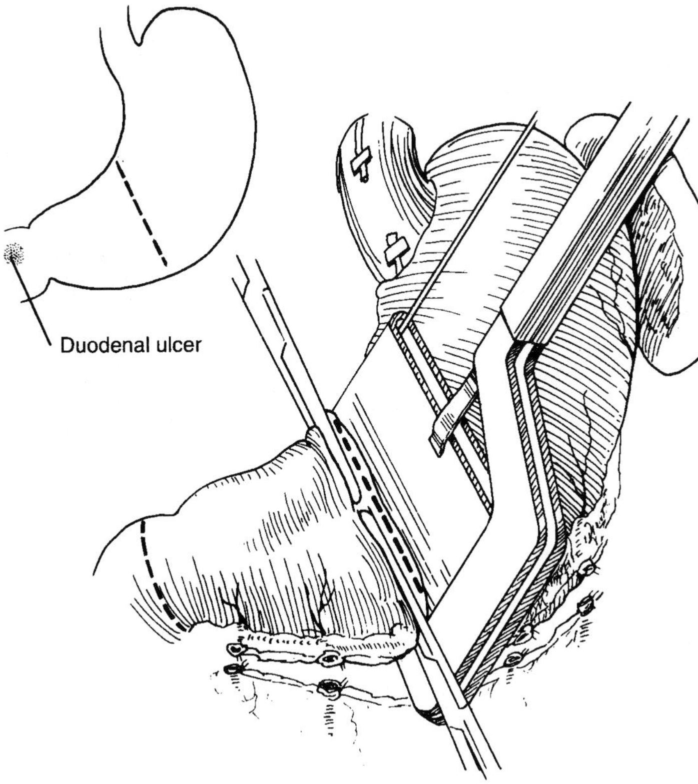

Figure 13–18. Billroth I operation. Division of stomach beyond the incisura. The gastric 90 stapler facilitates this maneuver. Note the truncal vagotomy has already been performed. (Redrawn, with permission, from Zinner MJ. *Atlas of Gastric Surgery.* New York, NY: Churchill Livingstone; 1992. After Gloege.)

stump. Careful attention should be given to mobilizing the duodenal stump and obtaining a secure tension-free closure. If the duodenum is relatively free of scar or inflammation, this presents no problem and the TA-55 stapler may be used for closure as described above. If heavily scarred, dissection of the duodenum and performance of the antrectomy may be abandoned in favor of a safer vagotomy and gastroenterostomy.

If one is committed to the antrectomy and scarring prevents mobilization of the pylorus and duodenal bulb, one may rarely find a need to perform a Bancroft procedure, in which the most distal portion of the pyloric channel and antrum are left in situ after resection of the more proximal antrum (Fig 13–23). The mucosa of the retained segment is stripped,[38] removing all gastrin-secreting tissue that could cause a retained antrum syndrome. In the classic approach for this procedure, the greater and lesser curvatures are mobilized without dissecting too far into the tissues surrounding the pylorus. About 7–8 cm from the pylorus, the seromuscular coat of the antrum is incised circumferentially down to the level of the submucosa. Using sharp dissection, the muscle coat is separated from underlying mucosa. This dissection can be facilitated by submucosal injection of 1: 100,000 epinephrine solution, as has been described for the mucosal proctectomy in ileal pouch–anal anastomosis procedures.[39] When the pyloric channel opening is reached, a fine purse-string absorbable suture (3-0 chromic catgut or Vicryl) picks up small bites of submucosa at the pyloric ring. Transfixion and ligation of the mucosa is tempting, but should be avoided, as this would lead to mucosal ischemia and subsequent perforation. A small margin of mucosa is left to be invaginated into the pylorus as the purse-string is gently closed and tied. The proximal margins of the seromuscular cuff are excised, leaving just enough to close over the purse-string. Omentum is used to cover this closure, if possible.

One other important circumstance to be prepared for is the closure of the duodenum distal to a posteriorly perforated or deeply penetrating ulcer. In this setting, the ulcer crater is left in situ (Fig 13–24). In other settings, the anterior wall of the duodenum can be sutured to the ulcer base, with care being taken to suture ligate any exposed vessels. The suture line can be protected by a vascularized tongue of omentum.

Position of the Jejunal Loop: Antecolic or Retrocolic. The second decision in performing a B-II reconstruction is whether to bring the loop of jejunum behind (retro) or in front of (ante) the transverse colon. In performing the gastrectomy for benign disease, there is no clear evidence that this makes any difference and we prefer the retrocolic position. For malignant disease, it has generally been held that the retrocolic position may be predis-

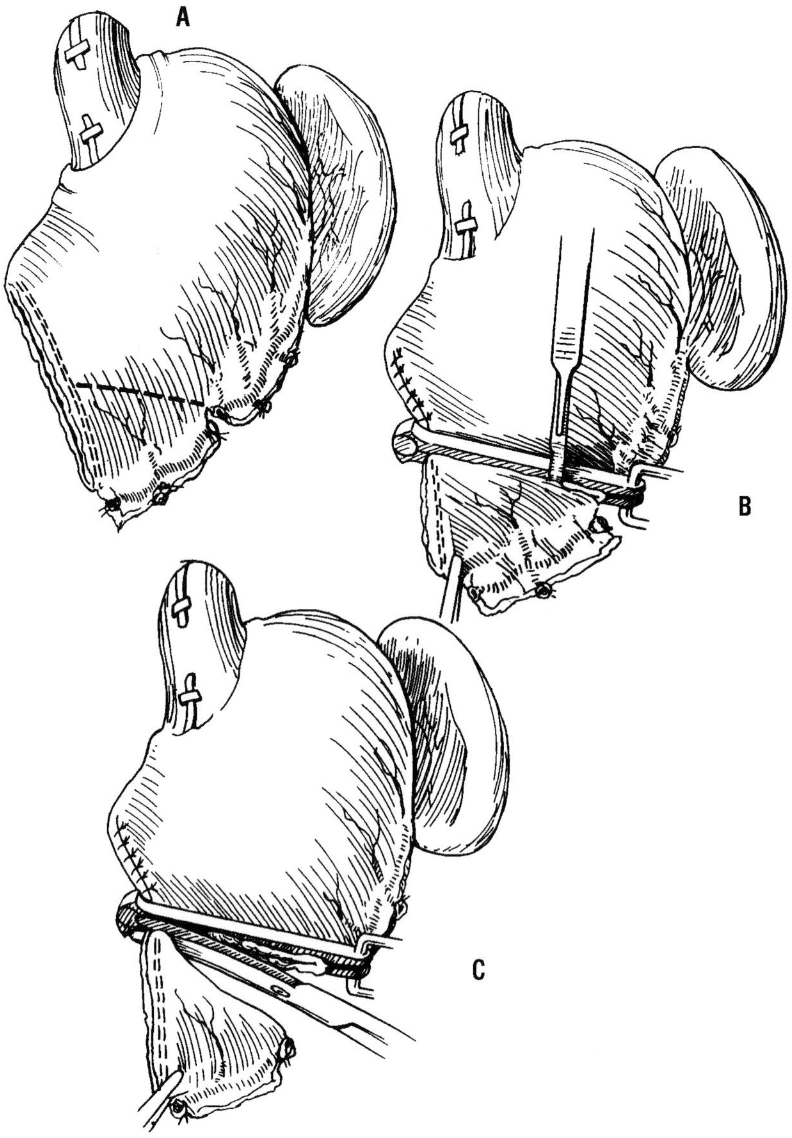

Figure 13–19. Billroth I operation. Division of the lower portion of the suture line. (Redrawn, with permission, from Zinner MJ. *Atlas of Gastric Surgery.* New York, NY: Churchill Livingstone; 1992. After Gloege.)

posed to obstruction owing to enlargement of lymph nodes or serosal implants in the transverse mesocolon. Whether or not this predisposition exists, positioning the jejunal limb in front of the colon requires a somewhat longer mesentery. As long as the anastomosis will not be under tension, the antecolic position will permit emptying as effective as that through a retrocolic anastomosis. If a retrocolic position is chosen, the window in the transverse mesocolon should be wide enough to permit both the afferent and efferent limbs of the jejunum to slide comfortably through. When this window is closed following construction of the anastomosis, it is preferable to tack the mesentery above, on the gastric side, rather than on the jejunal side. This will prevent kinking and obstruction of the jejunal limbs and positions the anastomosis below the mesentery.

Length of the Afferent Limb. The third decision is the choice of the segment of jejunum used for the anastomosis. In general, the segment should be as close to the ligament of Treitz as possible and still reach the stomach without tension. This generally leaves 10–20 cm of the proximal jejunum as the afferent limb. The shorter this length, the less likely the possibility of an afferent limb syndrome developing. The incidence of other complications such as alkaline reflux gastritis, dumping, or postvagotomy diarrhea should not be influenced by the length of the afferent limb.

Anastomotic Position on the Stomach and Technique. Figure 13–25 schematically illustrates a number of described variations on the B-II reconstruction. We will describe one handsewn and one stapled technique for anastomosis. As shown in Figure 13–26, a portion of the gastric

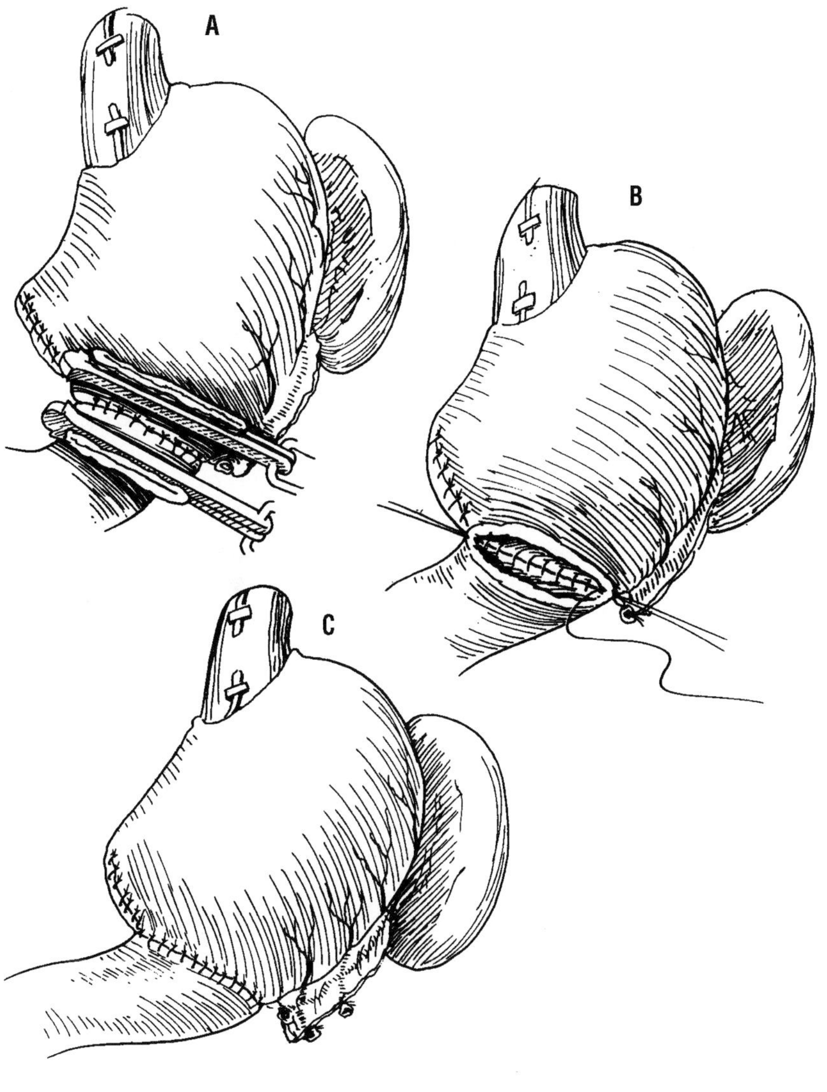

Figure 13–20. Billroth I operation. The construction of the gastroduodenostomy is performed end to end in two layers. (Redrawn, with permission, from Zinner MJ. *Atlas of Gastric Surgery.* New York, NY: Churchill Livingstone; 1992. After Gloege.)

staple line is excised with electrocautery, taking a small wedge of stomach behind the staple line. The superior portion of the staple line can be reinforced with 3-0 silk Lembert sutures at this time or can be reinforced later by tacking the afferent limb of jejunum, just beyond the anastomosis, to the gastric wall. The proximal jejunal limb is brought, untwisted, through a window in the transverse mesocolon (Fig 13–27). Traction seromuscular sutures (2-0 or 3-0 silk) are placed at both corners of the anastomosis. The gastrojejunal anastomosis is performed in two layers (Fig 13–28), between the most caudal part of the stomach and the jejunal limb. The outer layer is comprised of 3-0 silk Lembert seromuscular sutures. The inner layer is performed in the posterior row by running two 3-0 Vicryl sutures in opposite directions around the corners and then in Connell fashion for the anterior row. Placement of the anastomosis on the posterior gastric wall, about 2–3 cm from the gastric staple line, also will provide a suitably dependent position for drainage of gastric contents. The window in the transverse mesocolon is closed, as illustrated in Fig 13–29.

Figures 13–30 and 13–31 illustrate the technique for stapled gastroenterostomy. As before, the jejunal limb is placed in the retrocolic position. Traction sutures are placed on the gastric wall posterior to the anastomosis, bringing the jejunal limb into apposition. The 55-mm GIA stapler is fired after its two limbs are placed through a small gastrotomy and small enterotomy, respectively. The open end of the anastomosis is then closed with a TA-55 stapler. It should be noted that these staple lines, especially from the TA-55, are difficult to reinforce without undue tension. The blood supply of the gastric and intestinal walls are ample and reinforcement with Lembert sutures generally is not necessary.

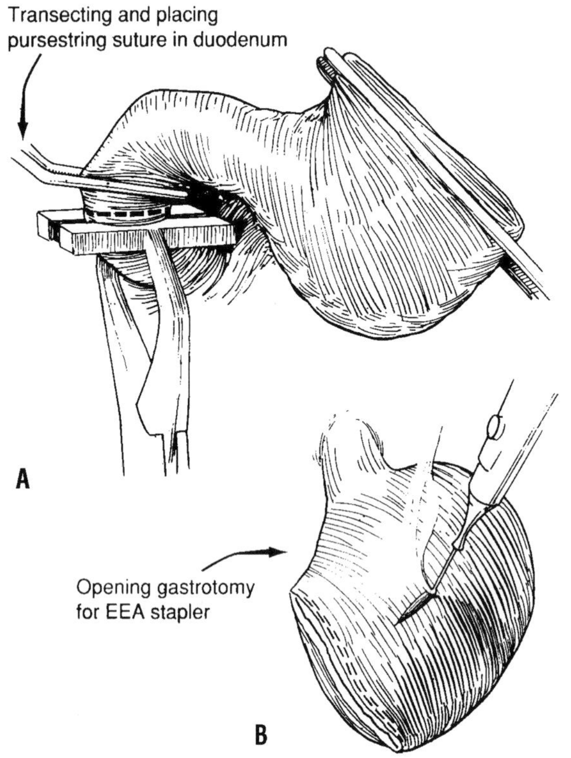

Figure 13–21. A. A Dennis clamp can be placed across the proximal duodenum, and the purse-string device can be placed at the selected site of duodenal division. **B.** A gastrotomy is made with the cautery on the anterior surface of the stomach, carefully avoiding large vascular arcades. This should be done at least 3 cm proximal to the row of staples. The gastrotomy should be large enough to accommodate the end-to-end stapling device easily. (Redrawn, with permission, from Siegler HF. Gastric resection: Billroth I. In: Sabiston DC Jr [ed]. *Atlas of General Surgery.* Philadelphia, PA: WB Saunders; 1994. After R. Gordon.)

SUBTOTAL AND TOTAL GASTRIC RESECTIONS

The main indications for subtotal (70–80%) gastric resection are carcinoma of the antrum or pylorus or primary gastric lymphoma. However, in cases of ulcers that lie very proximal on the lesser curvature, the proximity to the gastroesophageal junction prevents excision without significant narrowing of the gastric inlet. Similarly, the main indication for total gastric resection is a bulky carcinoma of the body or distal fundus, and rarely, otherwise unmanageable symptoms of an unresectable gastrinoma. Indications for near-total (>90%) gastric resection include the uncommon settings of the Roux stasis syndrome and gastroparesis unresponsive to medical management, as well as carcinoma or lymphoma of the body of the stomach. The approaches for subtotal and near total gastrectomy will be discussed only briefly, focusing on issues of exposure and techniques for resection of the stomach itself and reconstruction. The principles of resection for gastric carcinoma will be presented subsequently in conjunction with the discussion of radical total gastrectomy for carcinoma.

Subtotal and Near-Total Gastric Resections

In principal, a subtotal gastrectomy is simply an extended antrectomy or hemigastrectomy. A few technical issues are worth noting. First, the exposure provided by midline incision is usually not as adequate as

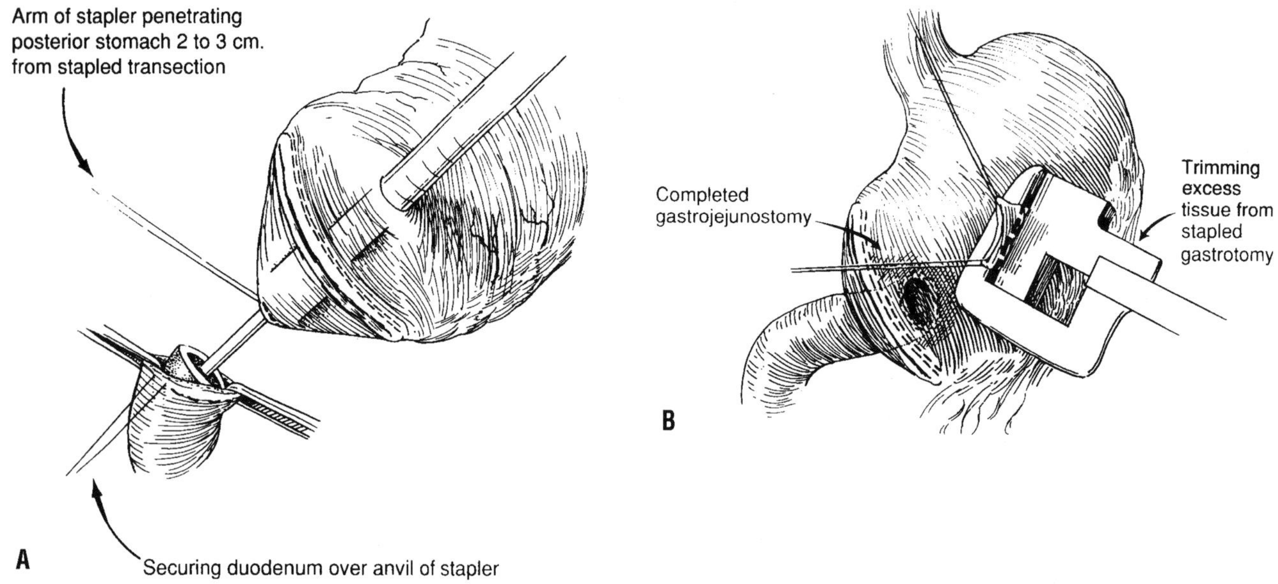

Figure 13–22. A. The gastrotomy edges should be grasped with two Babcock clamps and the end-to-end stapling device, minus the anvil, should be passed into the lumen of the stomach. The center rod should be gently pressed against the posterior wall of the stomach approximately 4 cm from the gastric line, and cautery should be used to permit passage of the rod through the posterior wall of the stomach. A purse-string suture will ensure that the stomach does not tear at the site of center rod penetration. The selected anvil size should be applied, and the open end of the duodenum should be grasped with Allis clamps. The duodenal wall should be gently pulled over the anvil, and the purse-string suture should be snugly tied around the center rod. **B.** The cartridge and the anvil should then be approximated, being certain that no extraneous tissues are caught between the anvil and the circular cartridge. The instrument should be fired, and the anastomosis should then be carefully observed by direct visualization to ensure that hemostasis is adequate. The surgeon should then remove the anvil and check the circular tissue from both the duodenum and the stomach to be certain that the tissue doughnuts are intact. If the doughnuts are defective, external Lambert sutures will need to be applied to secure a complete anastomosis. The gastrotomy is closed by grasping each end with Allis clamps and incorporating the entire thickness of the stomach wall through the jaws of the 55-mm stapler. (Redrawn, with permission, from Siegler HF. Gastric resection: Billroth I. In: Sabiston DC Jr [ed]. *Atlas of General Surgery.* Philadelphia, PA: WB Saunders; 1994. After R. Gordon.)

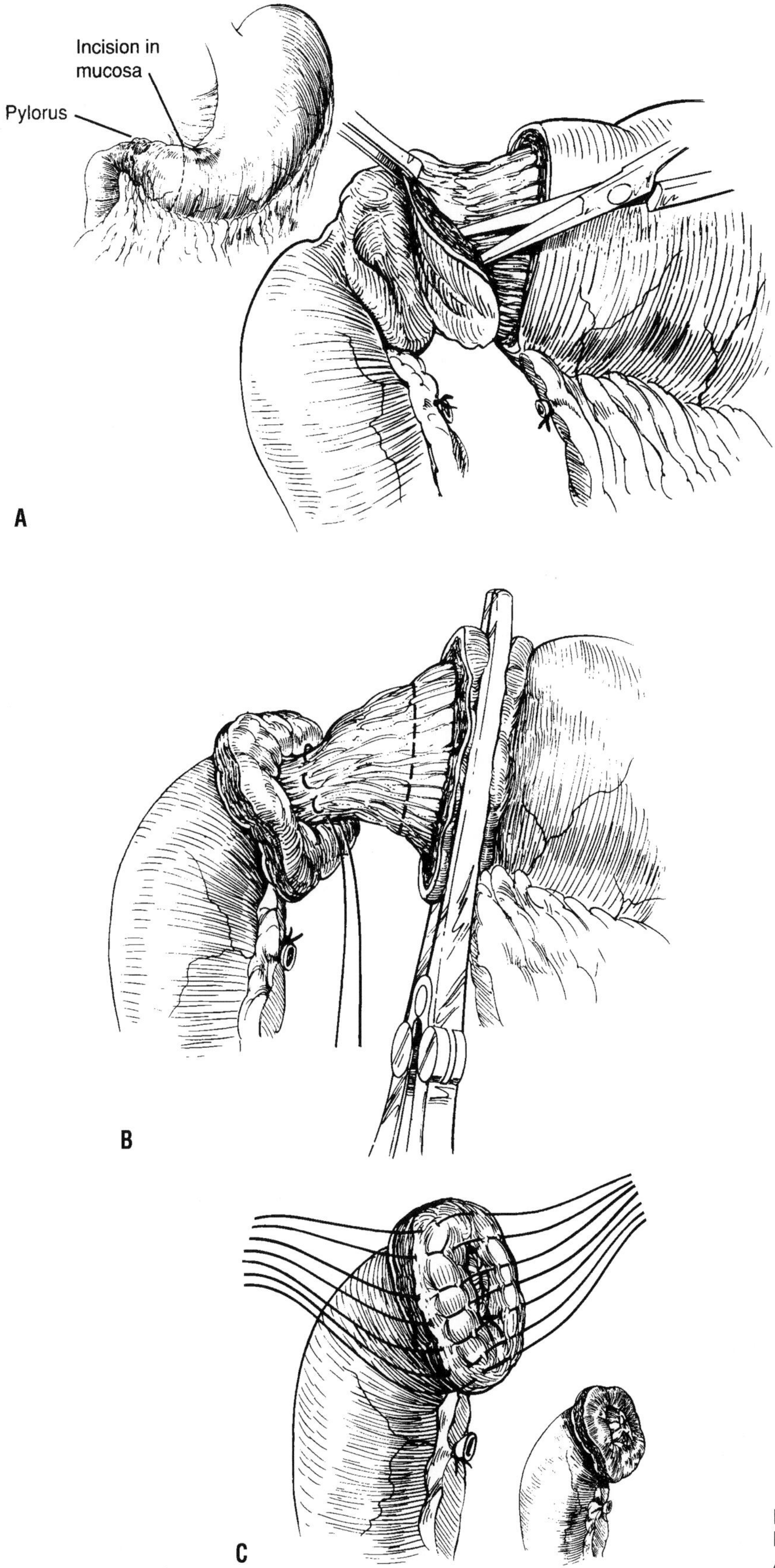

Figure 13–23. Bancroft procedure. (Redrawn, with permission, from Kirkham JS. Partial and total gastrectomy. In: Schwartz SI, Ellis H. *Maingot's Abdominal Operations.* Norwalk, CT: AppletonCentury-Crofts; 1982.)

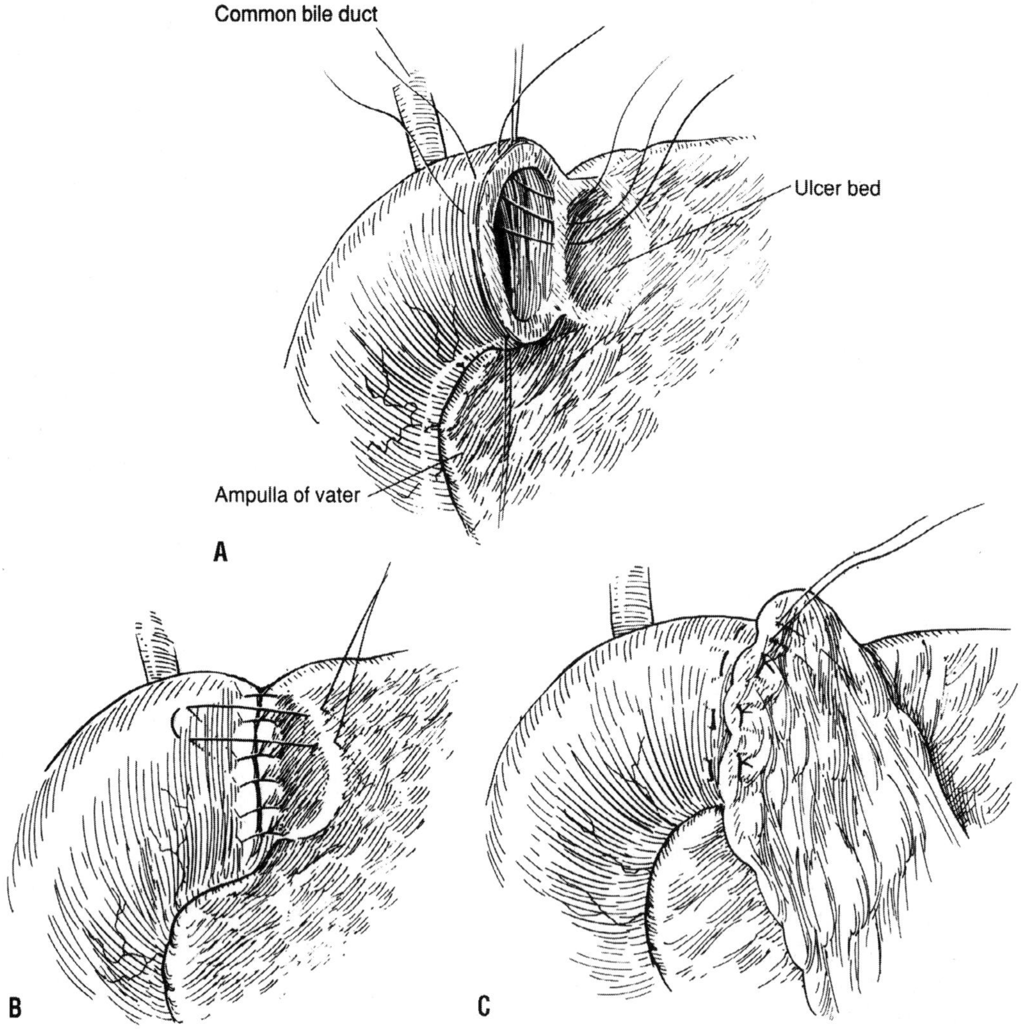

Figure 13–24. Closure of a chronic, ulcer-scarred duodenal stump. (Redrawn, with permission, from Zinner MJ. *Atlas of Gastric Surgery.* New York, NY: Churchill Livingstone; 1992. After Gloege.)

that provided by a chevron incision. Second, the left gastric artery always is ligated and divided in this dissection, and once the level of gastric transection has been determined, the branches of the left gastroepiploic artery and short gastric arteries are ligated in continuity and divided up to this predetermined level. Third, in opting for a near-total gastric resection, a 1- to 2-cm cuff of gastric wall is left behind and is the margin for the anastomosis. For this operation, it is desirable to preserve the uppermost one or two short gastric vessels, in order to ensure the adequacy of the blood supply for the gastric side of the anastomosis.

Fourth, a greater extent of lymph node dissection has shown in some series, both Japanese and Western series, to improve survival for gastric cancer after resection although with increased morbidity.[40–43] Earlier Western studies had not found a benefit,[44] but newer studies seem to confirm Japanese findings of improved survival.[40–43] Extended lymphadenectomy (D2 resection) involves dissection and removal of the perigastric lymph nodes, as well as those of the celiac axis, and the hepatoduodenal ligament.[42,43] Skeletonization of the celiac artery and its branches (left gastric artery, common hepatic artery, and splenic artery) is required to achieve adequate lymphadenectomy if it is desired. However, further studies are needed before it can be routinely recommended outside of highly specialized centers with surgeons who have specific expertise in this dissection. Finally, although it is often possible to reconstruct with a standard gastrojejunostomy, we prefer a Roux-en-Y reconstruction since this minimizes tension on the suture line, and theoretically reduces the risk of anastomotic obstruction by persistence or recurrence of tumor.

Total Gastrectomy for Carcinoma

The goals of total gastrectomy for carcinoma are (1) clear margins on both esophageal and duodenal sides; (2) re-

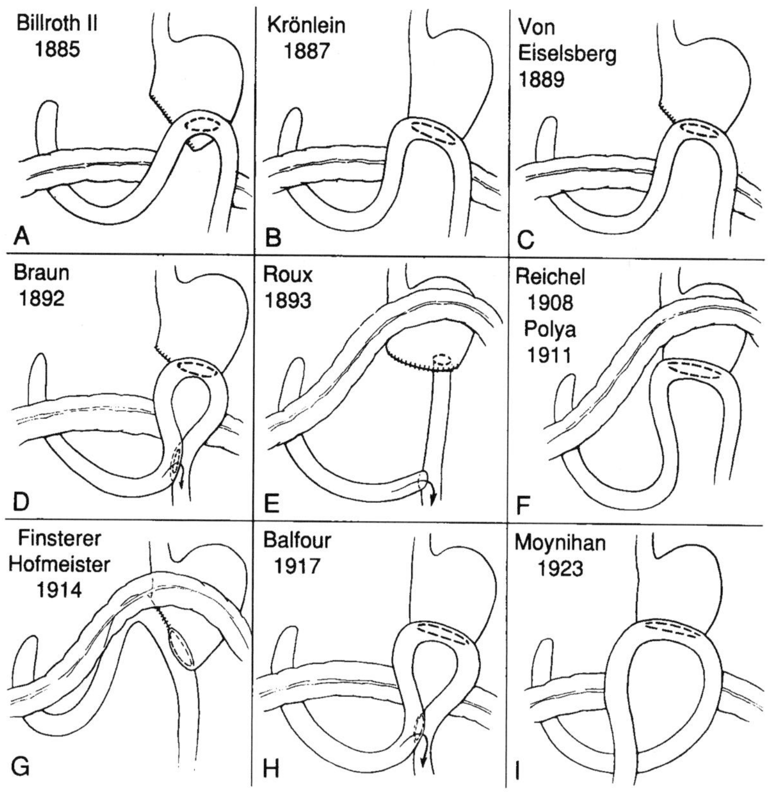

Figure 13–25. Billroth II operation and some of its modifications.

moval of local and regional lymph node–bearing tissues, including those surrounding the right and left gastric arteries, right gastroepiploic artery, and short gastric arteries; (3) removal of the omentum en bloc with the stomach; and (4) removal of the lymphatic tissues overlying the pancreatic capsule. Extended lymph node dissection (D2 resection) can be done here as described in the prior section.[40–43] However, as before, its potential survival benefit as shown in some studies must be weighed against its increased morbidity. After total gastric resection, we favor a Roux-en-Y reconstruction with a direct esophagoenterostomy rather than a jejunal pouch, al-

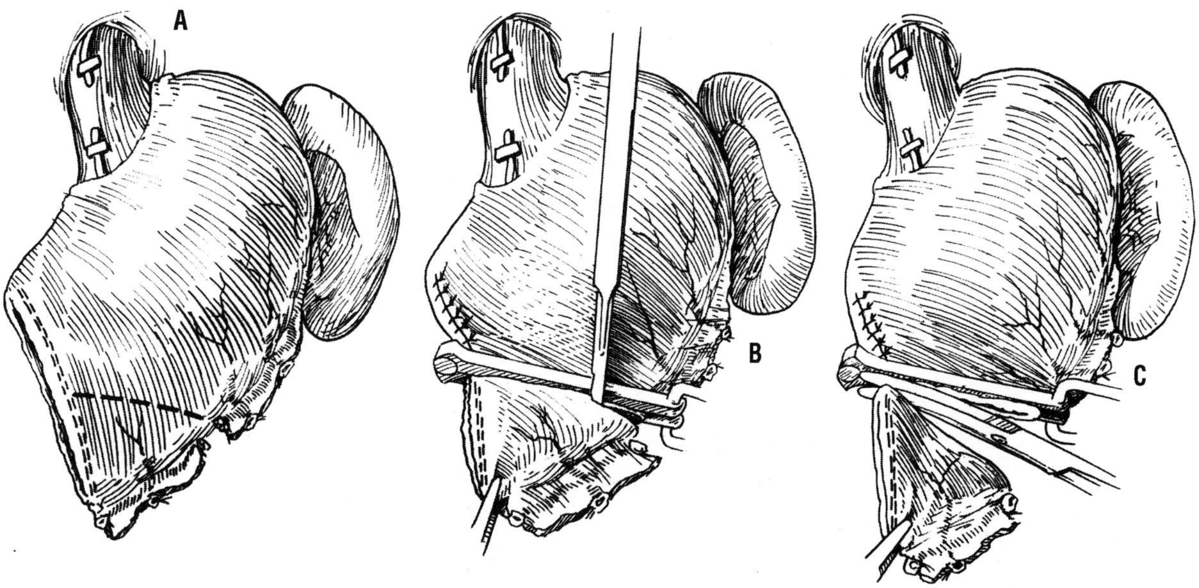

Figure 13–26. Billroth II operation. The antrum is resected as in a Billroth I operation. The distal portion of the resection line is excised. (Redrawn, with permission, from Zinner MJ. *Atlas of Gastric Surgery.* New York, NY: Churchill Livingstone; 1992. After Gloege.)

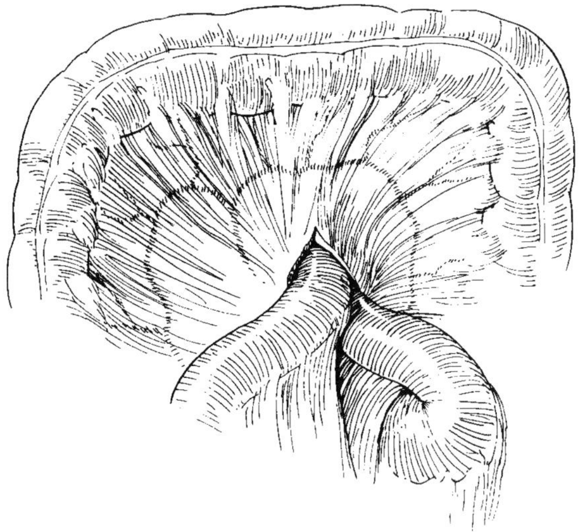

Figure 13–27. Billroth II operation. The jejunal segment, located 10–20 cm beyond the ligament of Treitz, is brought through a window in the retrocolic mesentery. (Redrawn, with permission, from Zinner MJ. *Atlas of Gastric Surgery.* New York, NY: Churchill Livingstone; 1992. After Gloege.)

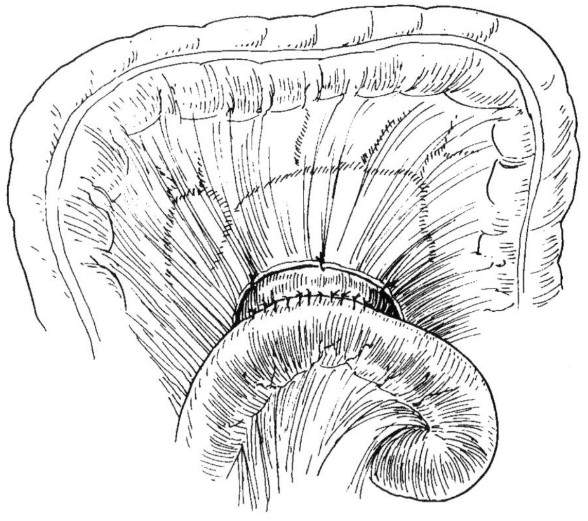

Figure 13–29. Billroth II operation. The retrocolic window in the mesentery is closed in order to avoid herniation of other viscera. The mesentery is linked to gastric wall, positioning the anastomosis below the closure. (Redrawn, with permission, from Zinner MJ. *Atlas of Gastric Surgery.* New York, NY: Churchill Livingstone; 1992. After Gloege.)

though the techniques for both forms of reconstruction will be described.

Figure 13–32 illustrates the en bloc resection. Generally, an upper midline or chevron incision will provide good exposure. A thoracoabdominal incision (Fig 13–33) is rarely necessary, but can provide better exposure when the patient's habitus suggests a deep hiatus. This latter incision also should be considered when preoperative endoscopy suggests that the tumor is close enough to the cardia so that the distal thoracic portion of the esophagus might be included with the resection. If this latter approach is chosen, the abdominal portion of the incision is performed first, in order to assess resectability. The patient is placed in a left thoracotomy position. The incision is carried from the line of the eighth rib obliquely toward the umbilicus. If resection appears feasible, the incision is extended over the eighth rib to the posterior angle. Occasionally, the seventh rib will provide better exposure. A separate rib retractor for the chest, and a self-retaining retractor without a ring for the abdominal portion, provide the best retraction. The diaphragm is divided toward the hiatus, but the muscle does not always have to be divided completely. Thus it may be possible to spare the neurovascular bundle. Significant bleeding is encountered and requires suture ligation with 2-0 or 0-0 Vicryl.

In the abdominal approach, the Bookwalter retractor is used. Extra care in positioning retractors on the left lobe of the liver, diaphragm, and small intestine, for optimal exposure of the hiatus is time well spent. The dissection is begun by dividing the omentum

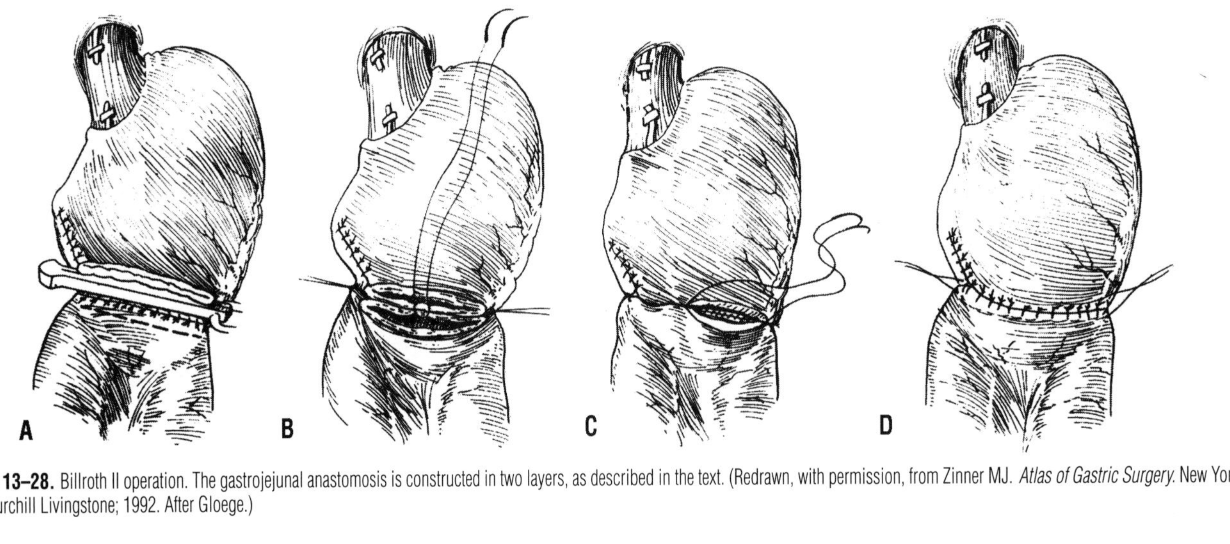

Figure 13–28. Billroth II operation. The gastrojejunal anastomosis is constructed in two layers, as described in the text. (Redrawn, with permission, from Zinner MJ. *Atlas of Gastric Surgery.* New York, NY: Churchill Livingstone; 1992. After Gloege.)

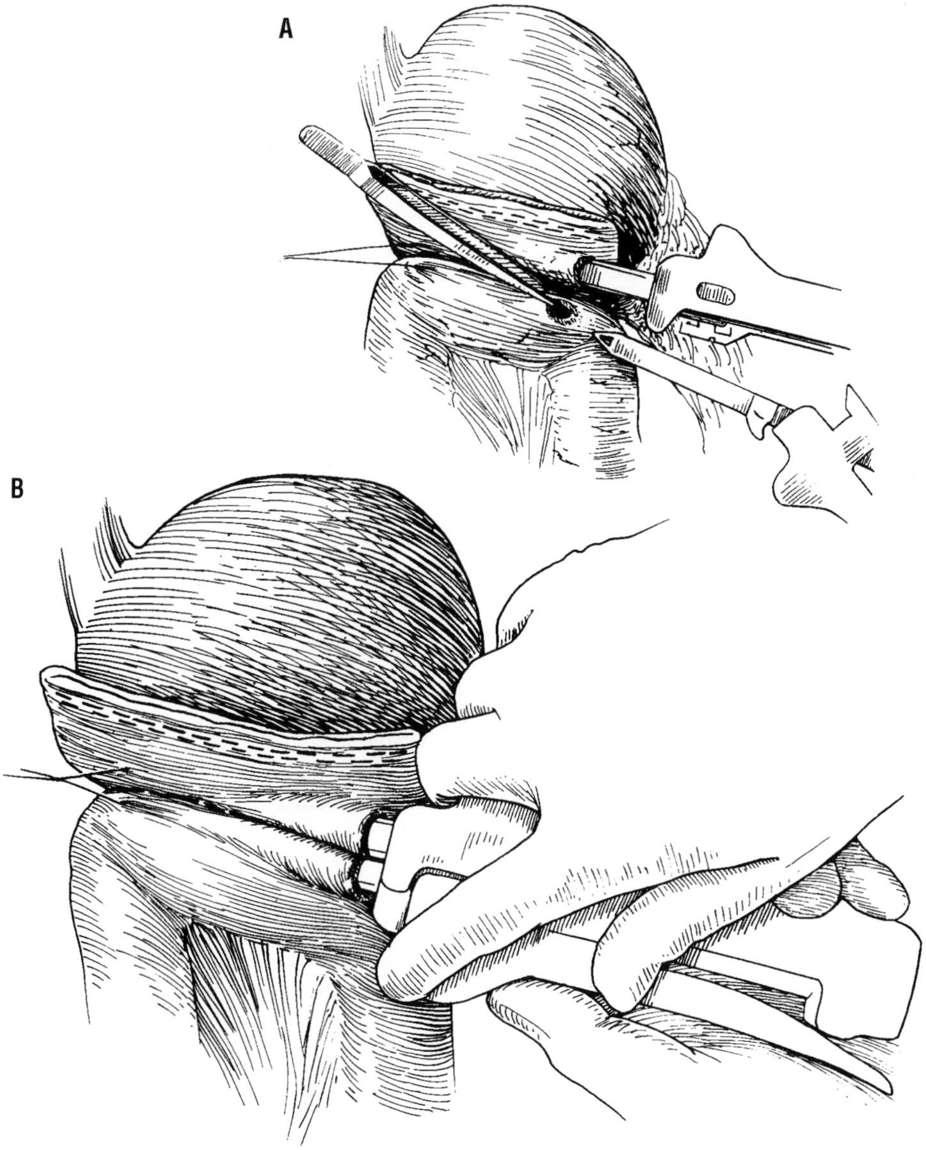

Figure 13–30. Stapling technique for Billroth II gastrojejunostomy. (After W. Baker.)

from the transverse colon (Fig 13–34). This relatively avascular plane can be separated using the electrocautery. Deviation from this plane will injure the colon or require tedious ligation and division of omental blood vessels. The lesser sac is then entered, allowing assessment of the retroperitoneum, with regard to local tumor extension and lymph node involvement. The distal portion of the gastrectomy is then performed. The origin of the right gastric artery at the common hepatic artery is identified, ligated in continuity with 2-0 silk ligatures, and divided.

Lymphatic-bearing tissues are swept toward the gastric side. The right gastroepiploic artery is identified, usually by palpation, and traced as far to the right as possible. It is usually possible to trace the artery to its origin at the gastroduodenal artery, which is similarly ligated in continuity and divided. Using the electrocautery, the lesser omentum is incised near the liver and its tissues are swept toward the lesser curvature, from the duodenum to the esophagus. Any small vessels are ligated with 3-0 ligatures. The dissection is carried onto the peritoneal surface of the esophagus. The duodenum may then be divided using the GIA stapler or a TA-55 stapler that is fired twice, once on the duodenum and once directly on the pylorus. The duodenum is divided just distal to the pyloric ring (Fig 13–35).

With the distal portion of the stomach divided, full access to the left gastric artery is obtained posteriorly through the lesser sac. This approach optimizes visualization of the celiac axis and its branches. With the assistant retracting the stomach upward and anteriorly, a number of congenital adhesions between the

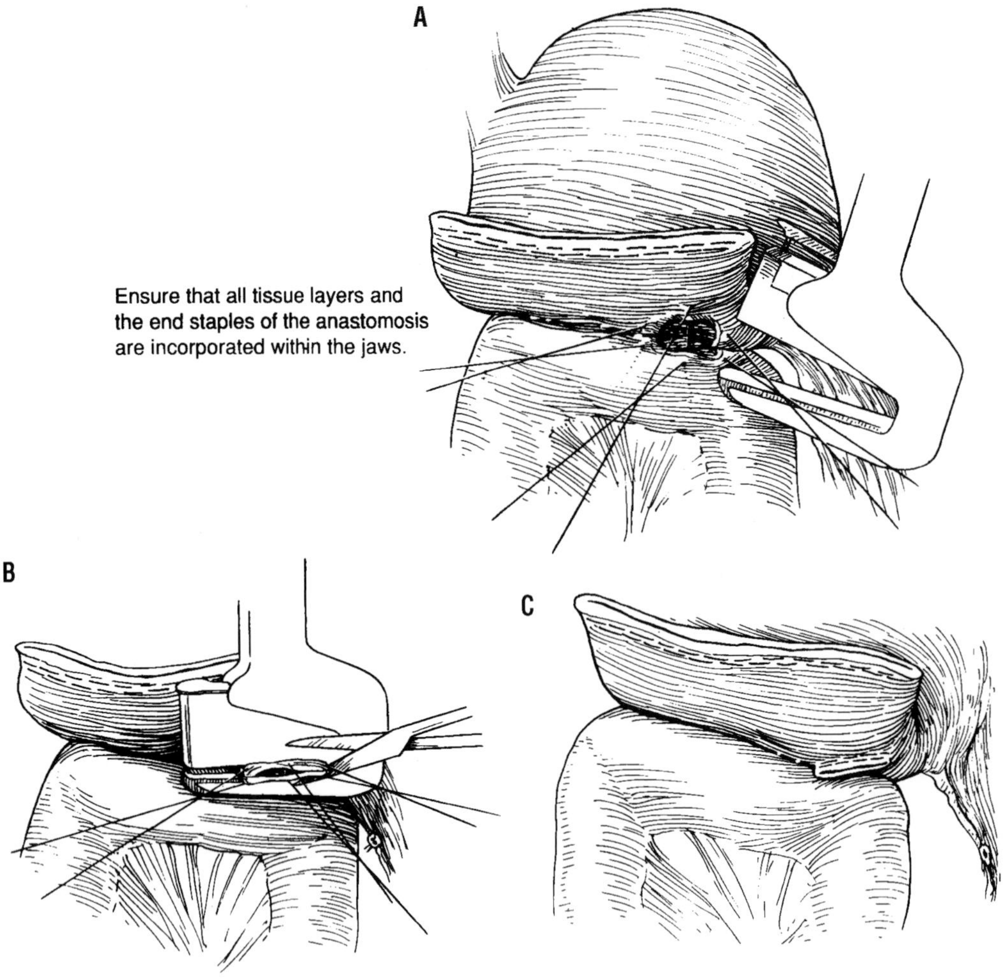
A
Ensure that all tissue layers and
the end staples of the anastomosis
are incorporated within the jaws.
B
C

Figure 13–31. A. Billroth II operation. **B** and **C.** The transverse stapler is used to close the common opening over the gastrojejunal anastomosis. (After W. Baker.)

posterior gastric wall and the peritoneum overlying the pancreas are observed (Fig 13–36). If tumor is invading this plane, a decision must be made regarding inclusion of the body and tail of the pancreas in the specimen. In our view, the arguments for this radical approach are weak. However, the plane made by the peritoneum overlying the pancreas is a natural plane and there may be sense in taking this peritoneum with the en bloc specimen. This layer can be dissected off the anterior face of the pancreas and swept gently to the front toward the left gastric vessels and splenic hilum. If a curative resection appears to be feasible, but would require removal of the body and/or tail of the pancreas, we do not see this as a contraindication to resection. The origin of the left gastric artery is then identified at the celiac axis, ligated in continuity using 2-0 silk, and divided (Fig 13–37). The stump of the artery is suture-ligated as well. From the celiac axis side, the tissue surrounding the artery contains lymphatics and is swept toward the lesser curvature. When the tumor is located in the more proximal body and corpus, the case for inclusion of the spleen with the en bloc specimen has not been persuasive.[45–47] Inclusion of the spleen is indicated if there are obvious tumor-bearing nodes or if there is direct invasion of the splenic hilum. Through the lesser sac, the tail of the pancreas is identified. The splenic artery and vein are separated, suture ligated, and divided individually. At this point, the short gastric vessels are then part of the en bloc specimen and are not dissected or divided.

The posterior aspect of the esophagus then comes into view as the stomach and spleen are lifted upward. Posteriorly, the front of peritoneal tissue can be dissected bluntly until the superior border of the pancreas is reached. The peritoneum is continuous with the peritoneum investing the gastric side of the gastroesophageal junction. If this layer has not been included with the dissection, the peritoneum must be divided here, exposing the gastroesophageal junction posteriorly. Figure 13–38 demonstrates the stomach completely mobilized except for its attachment to the

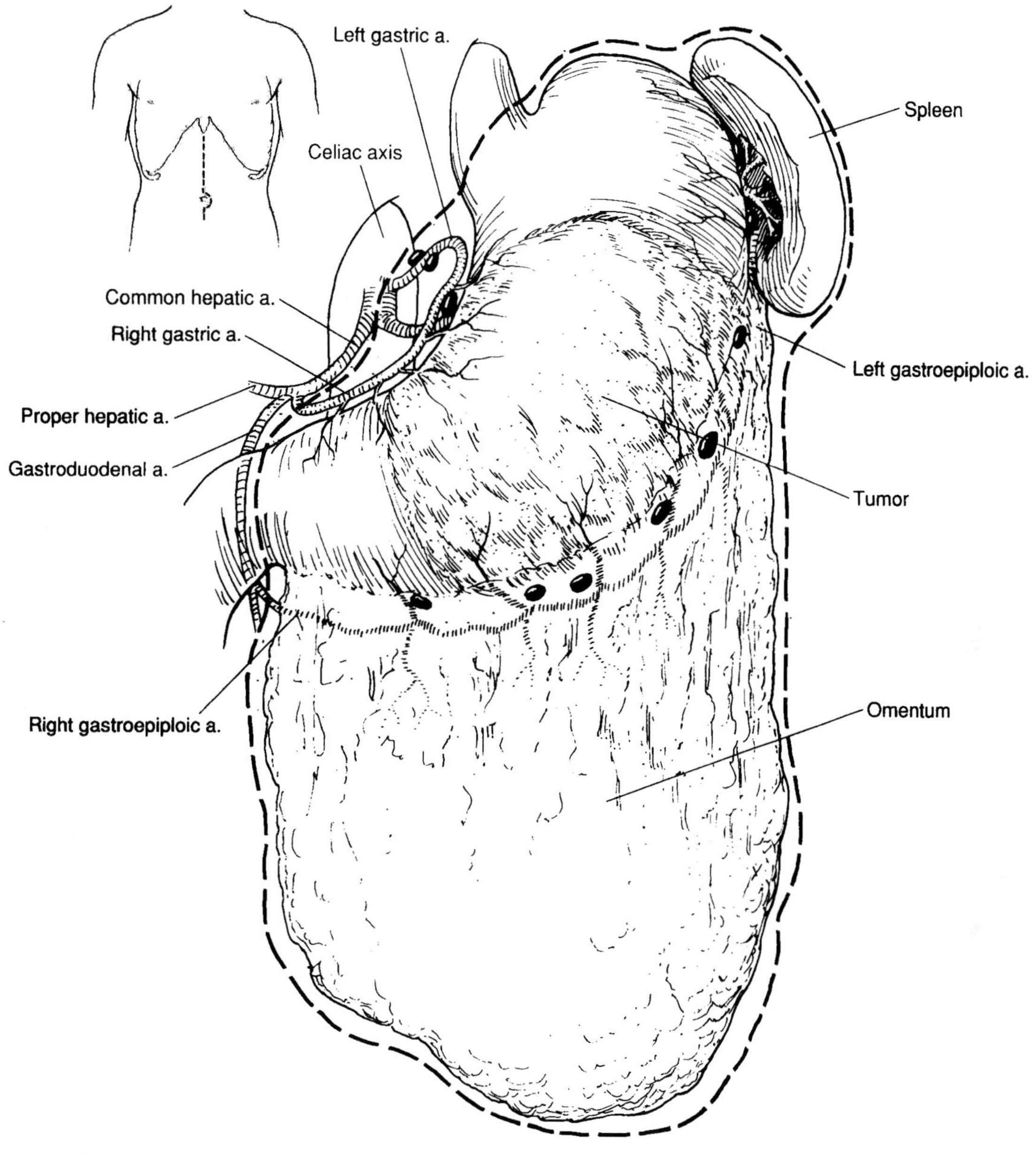

Figure 13–32. Anatomy relevant to resections for gastric carcinoma. (Redrawn from Zinner MJ. *Atlas of Gastric Surgery.* New York, NY: Churchill Livingstone; 1992. After Gloege.)

esophagus. A noncrushing clamp is placed on the mobilized esophagus and the specimen is resected. To minimize spillage of luminal contents, a second clamp is placed on the gastric side or the TA-55 stapler may be fired below the line of resection and above the gastroesophageal junction.

Our preferred technique for reconstruction is a simple Roux-en-Y, with an end-to-side esophagojejunal anastomosis with the Roux limb. Using the GIA stapler, a section of jejunum is divided 10–15 cm beyond the ligament of Treitz (Fig 13–39). The Roux limb is brought antecolic up to the esophagus. An enteroenterostomy is constructed between the jejunum on the duodenal side of the Y and the jejunum, 40–45 cm distal to the Roux limb staple line (Fig 13–40). The enteroenteral anastomosis can be performed using hand-sewn two-layer technique or stapling technique. The esophagojejunal anastomosis is performed using interrupted 3-0 silk sutures for both the inner and outer layers, as shown in Figure 13–41. The completed reconstruction is shown in Figure 13–42. This figure emphasizes the antecolic position of the anastomosis when the operation is performed for malignant disease. Areas of potential internal herniation in the mesentery are closed with absorbable 3-0 sutures.

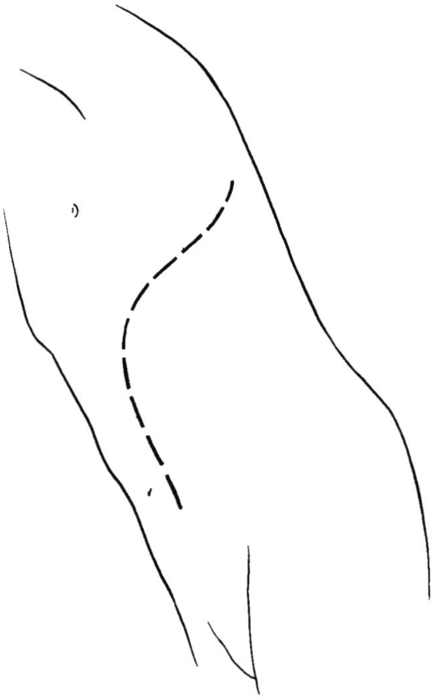

Figure 13–33. Thoracodominal incision for radical total gastrectomy for carcinoma of the stomach. The incision is carried along the seventh or the eighth interspace.

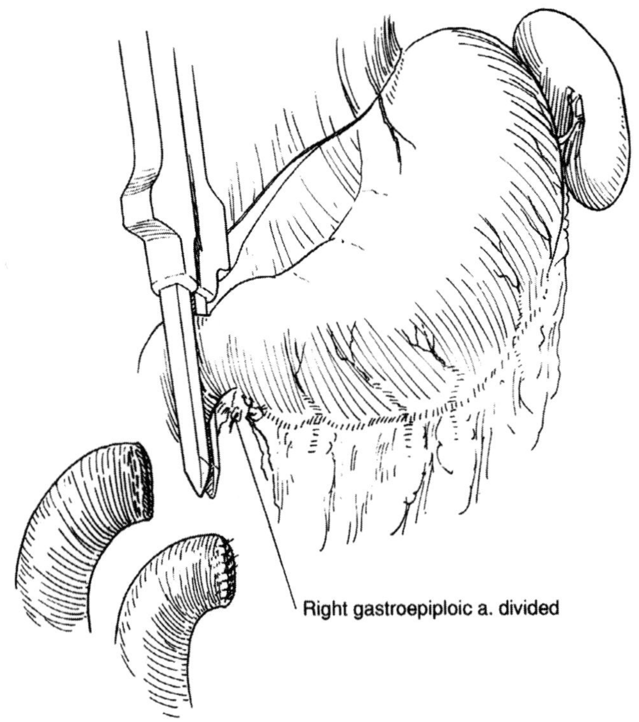

Figure 13–35. Resection for gastric carcinoma. The duodenum is divided beyond the pylorus. Either the linear cutter or transverse stapling instruments are appropriate. If feasible, the duodenal staple line is reinforced using 3-0 silk Lambert sutures. (Redrawn, with permission, from Zinner MJ. *Atlas of Gastric Surgery.* New York, NY: Churchill Livingstone; 1992. After Gloege.)

A jejunal pouch (Hunt-Lawrence pouch) also may be constructed, with the idea of anastomosing the esophagus in end-to-side fashion with the antimesenteric border of the pouch.[48–50] The technique is illustrated in Figures 13–43 through 13–45 and can be performed expeditiously using surgical staplers. The pouch is constructed with the goal of providing a reservoir function. Alternatively, a number of surgeons expressed a preference for leaving an island of undivided intestine at the bend in the pouch. This should theoretically optimize the blood supply to the anastomosis. The circular stapler can be passed through the open

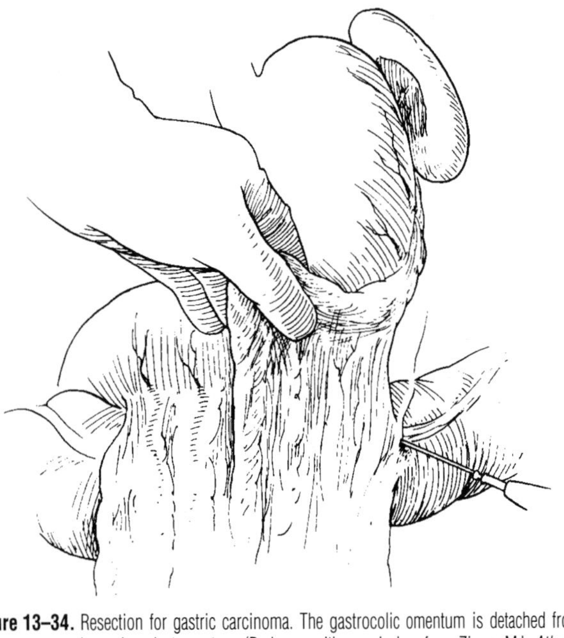

Figure 13–34. Resection for gastric carcinoma. The gastrocolic omentum is detached from the transverse colon using electrocautery. (Redrawn, with permission, from Zinner MJ. *Atlas of Gastric Surgery.* New York, NY: Churchill Livingstone; 1992. After Gloege.)

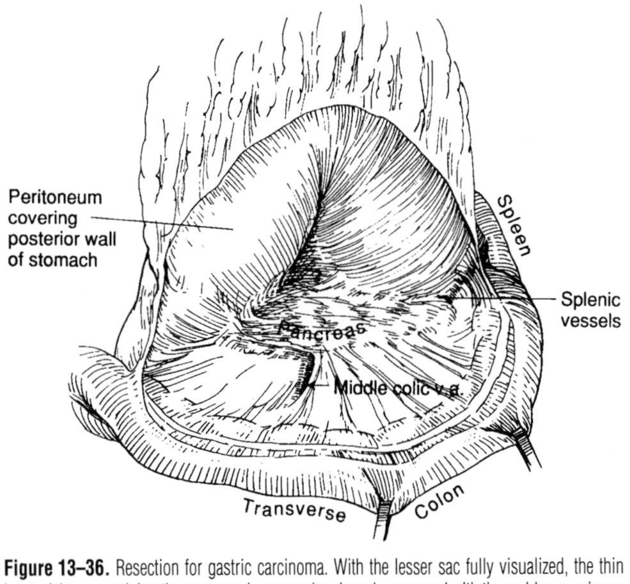

Figure 13–36. Resection for gastric carcinoma. With the lesser sac fully visualized, the thin layer of tissue overlying the pancreas is exposed and can be removed with the en bloc specimen. (Redrawn, with permission, from Zinner MJ. *Atlas of Gastric Surgery.* New York, NY: Churchill Livingstone; 1992. After Gloege.)

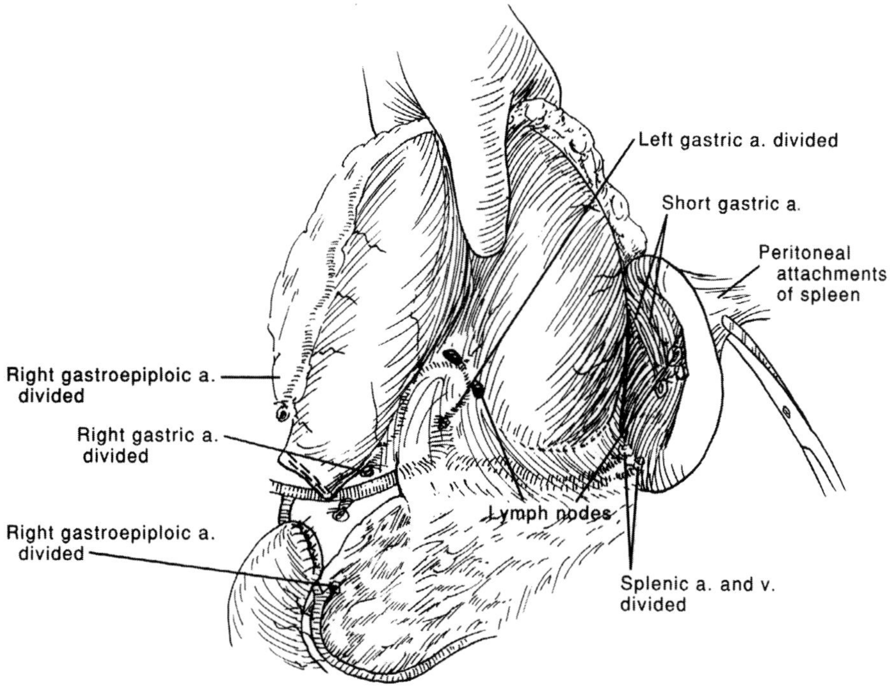

Figure 13–37. Resection for gastric carcinoma. Exposure of the left gastric artery through the lesser sac. (Redrawn, with permission, from Zinner MJ. *Atlas of Gastric Surgery.* New York, NY: Churchill Livingstone; 1992. After Gloege.)

end of the Roux limb in order to perform the end-esophagus to side-jejunum anastomosis. The linear stapler then can be fired in such a way as to leave the island of undivided intestine. One important point is that the pouch can be made too long, giving rise to stasis and ineffective clearance of food from the pouch into the intestine. The pouch should not be more than 15 cm in length.

LAPAROSCOPIC APPROACHES

Laparascopic Approaches to the Vagus Nerve

As noted above, the advent of laparoscopic approaches has led surgeons to reconsider traditional approaches to peptic ulcer disease. The advantages of minimally invasive approaches revolve largely around the minimal postoperative discomfort and rapid recovery, with a potential benefit in reduced cost of surgery versus the cost of long-term medication.[51,52] At the same time, rapid advances have occurred in our understanding of the role of *Helicobacter pylori* and mucosal growth, and angiogenetic factors in ulcer healing and recurrence. In addition, limitations in access and suturing techniques have increased the difficulty of access to the lesser sac and of performing drainage procedures. These considerations have led surgeons to question the rationale for drainage procedures whenever truncal vagotomy has been performed. A number of approaches have evolved to address these difficulties and have been given credibility in the laparoscopic experience. One such approach has been to combine truncal vagotomy with pyloric dilatation or seromyotomy. Another has been to combine a posterior truncal vagotomy with an anterior highly selective vagotomy or with an anterior seromyotomy. The important elements of the laparoscopic approach to the vagi are discussed here.

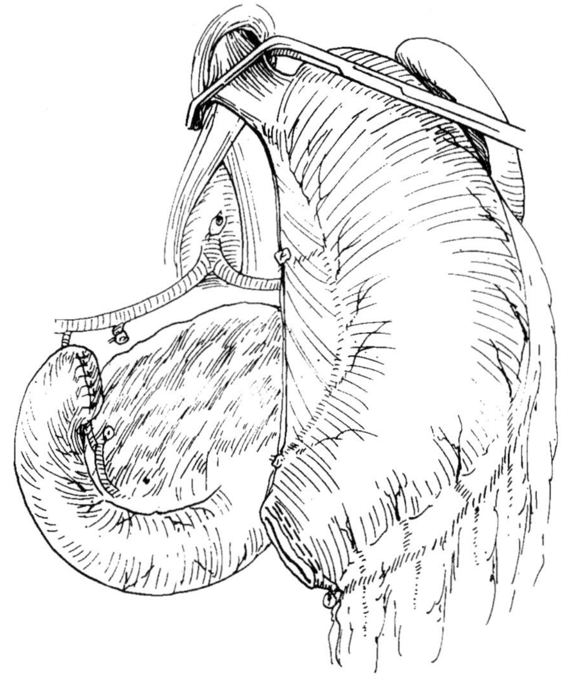

Figure 13–38. Gastric resection for carcinoma. The esophagus is transected just above the gastroesophageal junction. (Redrawn, with permission, from Zinner MJ. *Atlas of Gastric Surgery.* New York, NY: Churchill Livingstone; 1992. After Gloege.)

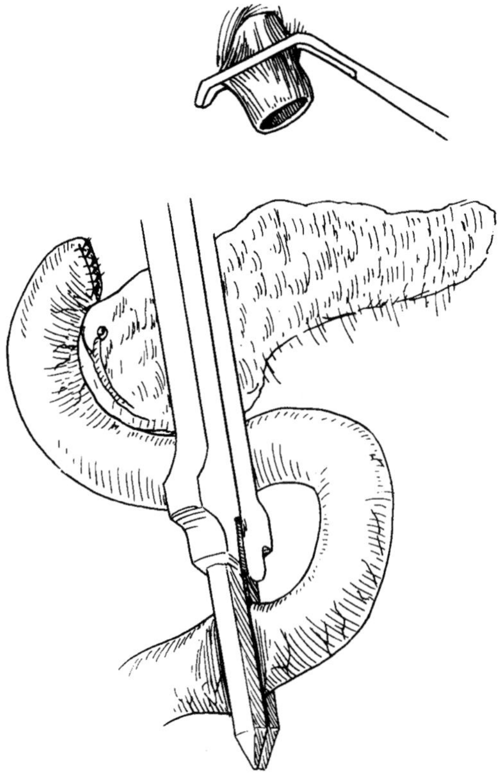

Figure 13–39. Gastric insert for carcinoma. Construction of Roux-en-Y limb begins with division of the jejunum beyond the ligament of Treitz. (Redrawn, with permission, from Zinner MJ. *Atlas of Gastric Surgery.* New York, NY: Churchill Livingstone; 1992. After Gloege.)

Patient Position and Port Placement

The patient is placed on the operating room table with legs in stirrups and apart (Fig 13–46). Video monitors are placed on either side at the head; often the surgeon works best when standing between the legs, with the camera operator on the right and the first assistant on the patient's left. The scrub nurse/technician and instrument table are placed at the patient's right foot. A large esophageal tube or even a gastroscope is placed in the stomach to facilitate visualization of the distal esophagus. Frequent aspiration of the gastric contents is crucial to maintain total collapse of the stomach and the best visualization. We recommend an open technique to gain access to the peritoneum, insufflating to a pressure of 14 mm Hg. Five ports are placed in the following locations: (1) a 12-mm laparoscope port at the superior edge of the umbilicus or placed 5 cm above and lateral to the left of midline; (2) a 5-mm irrigation/suction and dissection port in the subxiphoid position, just to the right of midline; (3) a 10-mm port for retraction and grasping forceps midway between the umbilicus and xiphoid, to the right of the rectus, and possibly as far as the midclavicular line; (4) a 10-mm port for grasping forceps midway between the umbilicus and xiphoid, almost to the anterior axillary line on the left; and (5) a 12-mm operating port just lateral to the rectus 3 cm above the umbilicus. A number of surgeons prefer the angled 30° laparoscope for this operation.

Laparoscopic Truncal Vagotomy

The left lobe of the liver is retracted using a probe placed via the subxiphoid port or the 10-mm fan retractor placed via the higher right-side port (Fig 13–47). Visualization is improved when tissues from the hiatus are dissected away from the esophagus and lesser curvature (Figs 13–48 and 13–49). One can encounter a coronary hepatic vein or accessory hepatic artery in this dissection. These do not always need to be sacrificed. The right crus of the diaphragm usually is seen here and can be retracted with one of the blades of the liver retractor (Fig 13–50). A Babcock clamp or other atraumatic grasper is used to retract the anterior greater curvature (distal to the cardia) to the patient's left. A hook coagulator or dissecting forceps is used to incise the lesser omentum, entering the lesser sac just above the take-off of the hepatic branch of the anterior vagus nerve. A plane is developed between the right crus and the esophagus and continued posteriorly. Continued dissection along the wall of the esophagus reveals the posterior trunk, which is ligated between clips and divided (Fig 13–51). The excised nerve segment is sent for frozen-section examination. The next step is identification of the anterior vagal trunk(s). The phrenoesophageal membrane usually has been entered and incision is extended toward the left, first by scoring the membrane with scissors and then bluntly pushing away the membrane with a cotton dissector. The visualization of major anterior trunks is often easier in the laparoscopic approach, owing to magnification and excellent video optics. These branches also are ligated and divided between clips (Fig 13–52), with frozen-section confirmation of the nerve segment. Smaller anterior branches are identified and cauterized after being held away from the esophageal wall. It is possible to dissect tissues on either side of the esophagus for a distance of 5–6 cm, thereby ensuring division of any nerve branches to the lesser curvature and cardia. The main difficulty can occur in visualizing the angle of His and possibly missing major vagal branches, including the "criminal nerve." With the use of a traction forceps placed through the subxiphoid port and a cotton dissector placed via the left grasping forceps, it is possible to expose the left edge of the gastroesophageal junction and cauterize or clip any branches.

Anterior Proximal Vagotomy or Seromyotomy

A laparoscopic dissection of the posterior leaf is feasible.[53] However, the combination of posterior truncal vagotomy and an anterior selective operation is appealing, since it avoids the difficult maneuver of work-

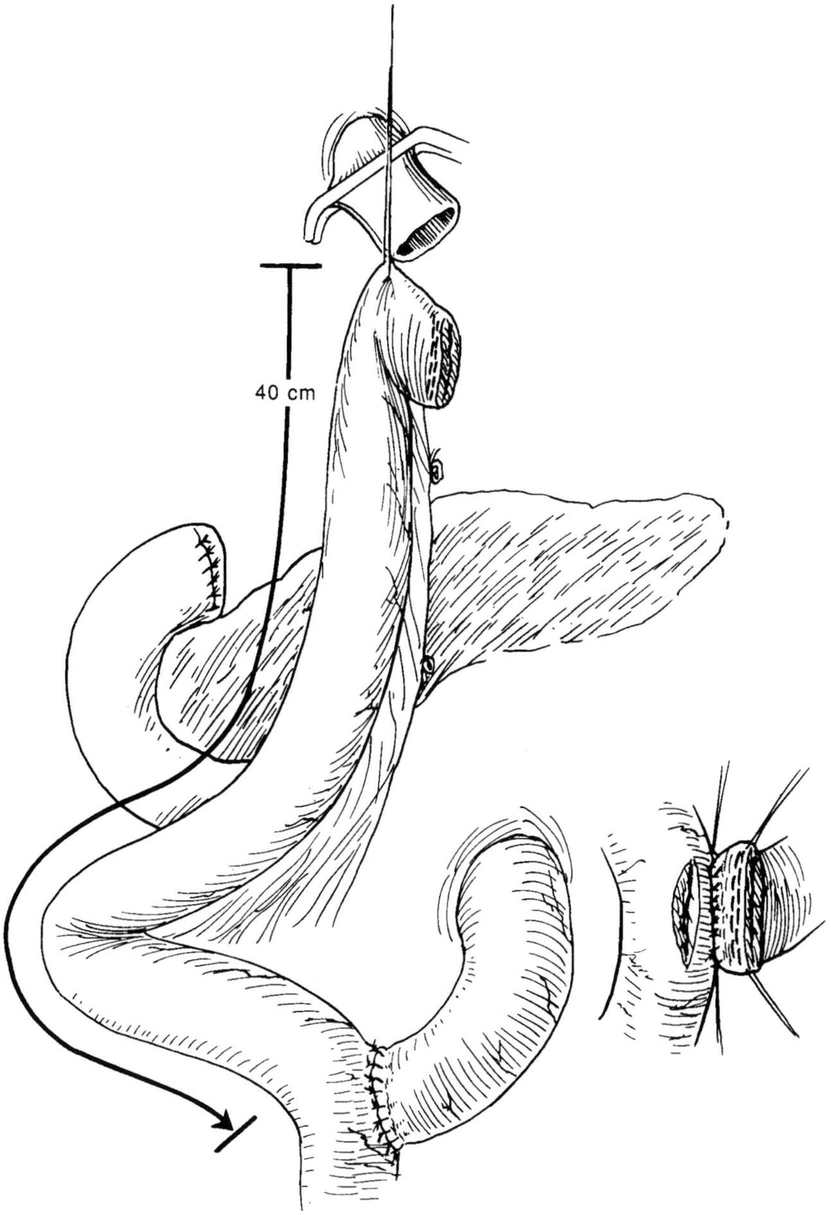

Figure 13–40. Construction of Roux-en-Y anastomosis. The enteroenterostomy is performed in two layers. The length of the Roux limb measures 40 cm. (Redrawn, with permission, from Zinner MJ. *Atlas of Gastric Surgery.* New York, NY: Churchill Livingstone; 1992. After Gloege.)

ing through the lesser sac in order to visualize the posterior lesser omentum and nerves accompanying the ascending left gastric artery branches. For highly selective vagotomy, dissection is begun at the crow's foot, approximately 6 cm from the pylorus. Retraction of the greater curvature is performed using a Babcock clamp (Fig 13–53). With the magnification available through the scope, the proximal branch of the crow's foot is often, but not always, relatively easy to identify. The anterior leaf of the lesser omentum is approached by dividing and ligating the neurovascular bundle between clips. Electrocautery is used sparingly, and preferably not at all. The serosa overlying the gastroesophageal junction is scored as in the open procedure. Dissection of the distal 5 cm of esophagus and cardiac branches is carried out as described above for truncal vagotomy.

The goal of an anterior seromyotomy, as described originally by Taylor and others, is to sever the neurovascular bundles dividing the serosa and muscularis that transmit these nerves to the mucosa.[54–56] The anterior surface of the stomach is retracted and placed on stretch using the right and left grasping ports. The outline of the seromyotomy is scored using a coagulator hook or spatula, on the anterior surface of the stomach, 1 cm from the visible border of the lesser curvature. Moving caudad and parallel to the lesser curvature, a line is traced from the gastroesophageal

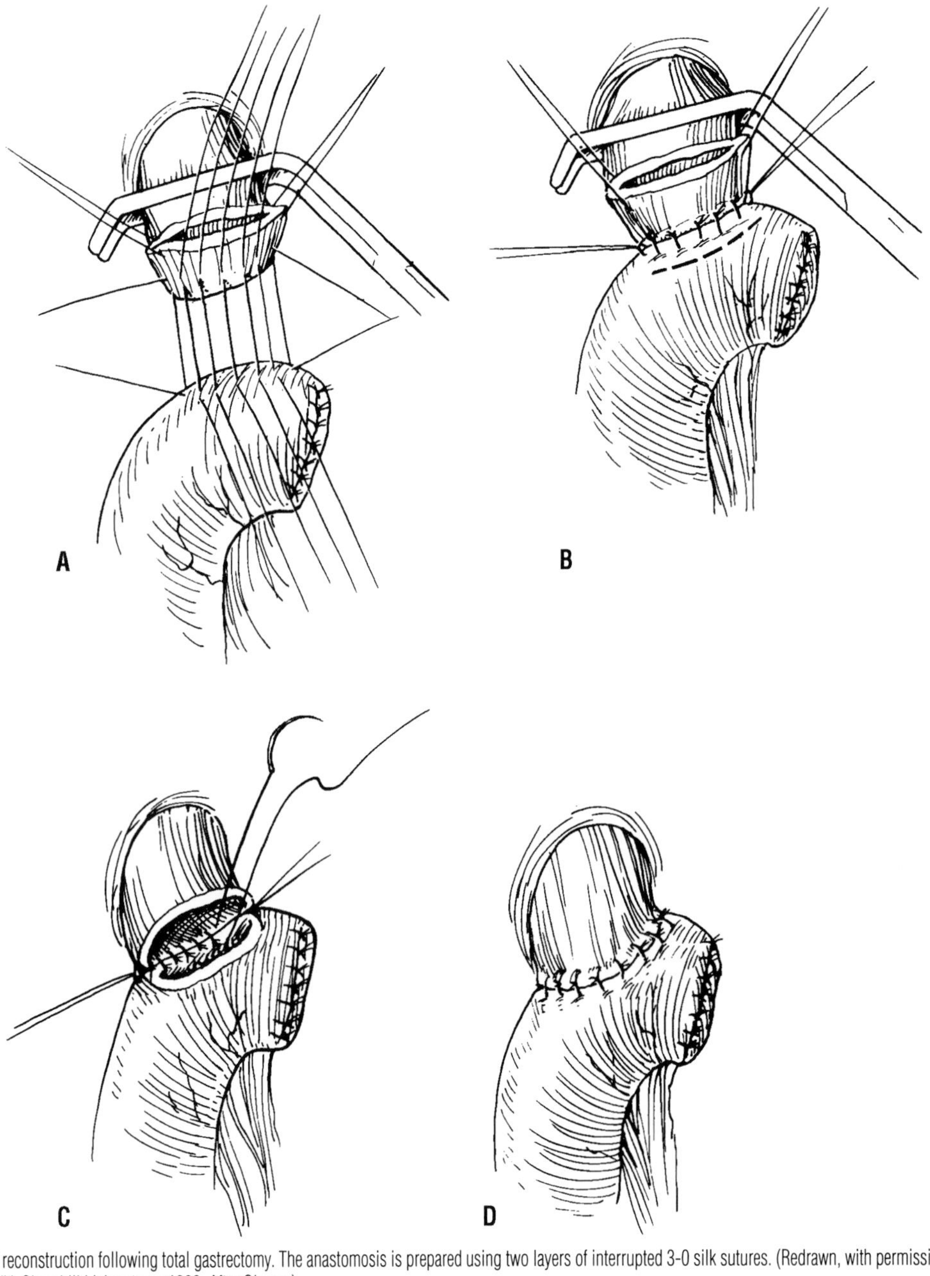

Figure 13–41. Roux-en-Y reconstruction following total gastrectomy. The anastomosis is prepared using two layers of interrupted 3-0 silk sutures. (Redrawn, with permission, from Zinner MJ. *Atlas of Gastric Surgery.* New York, NY: Churchill Livingstone; 1992. After Gloege.)

junction to the first branch of the crow's foot, or arbitrarily 6 cm from the pylorus. The hook coagulator is most suitable for performing the seromyotomy, using monopolar current for electrocoagulation. The hook cuts through successive layers of gastric wall, of the serosa, outer oblique muscle fibers, middle longitudinal fibers, and inner circular fibers. The two grasping ports then are used to place traction on the two edges of the gastric wall, exposing the deep circular fibers that may split as much from traction as from cautery. The darker submuscosa/mucosa layer pops through the muscularis. This layer is inspected for any evidence of full-thickness cautery injury or perforation. With a complete seromyotomy, the gap between the cut edges should be about 6–8 mm. Alternatively, a laparoscopic surgical stapling device can be used for creation of a modified seromyotomy.[56]

A number of decent-sized vessels may be encountered in the dissection. Prolonged cauterization may provide hemostasis but risks a full-thickness burn and subsequent perforation. The hook can be used to isolate these vessels and lift them for clipping in continuity. Recent advances in the design of needle holders may make it possible to suture these vessels in continu-

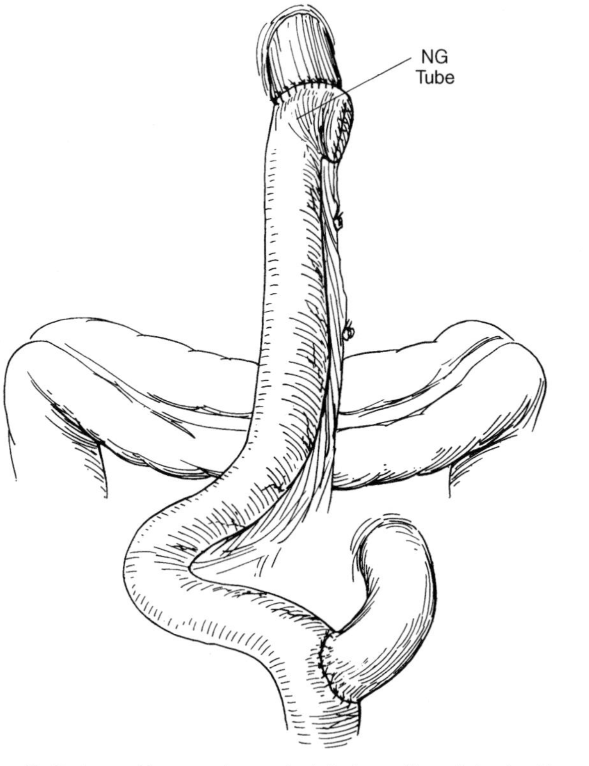

Figure 13–42. Roux-en-Y reconstruction completed. (Redrawn, with permission, from Zinner MJ. *Atlas of Gastric Surgery.* New York, NY: Churchill Livingstone; 1992. After Gloege.)

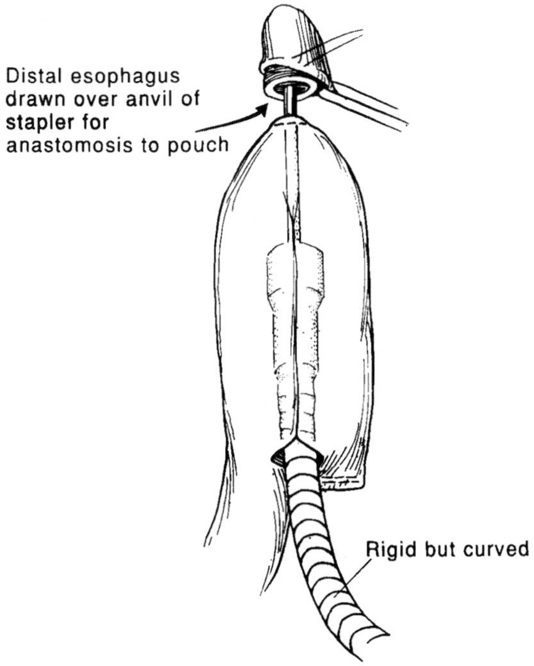

Figure 13–44. Total gastrectomy. The circular stapler is positioned via the enterotomies. The center rod is pushed through the antimesenteric border of the jejunum using cautery to prevent tearing. (Redrawn, with permission, from Siegler HF. Total gastrectomy: stapler. In Sabiston DC Jr [ed]. *Atlas of General Surgery.* Philadelphia, PA: WB Saunders; 1994.)

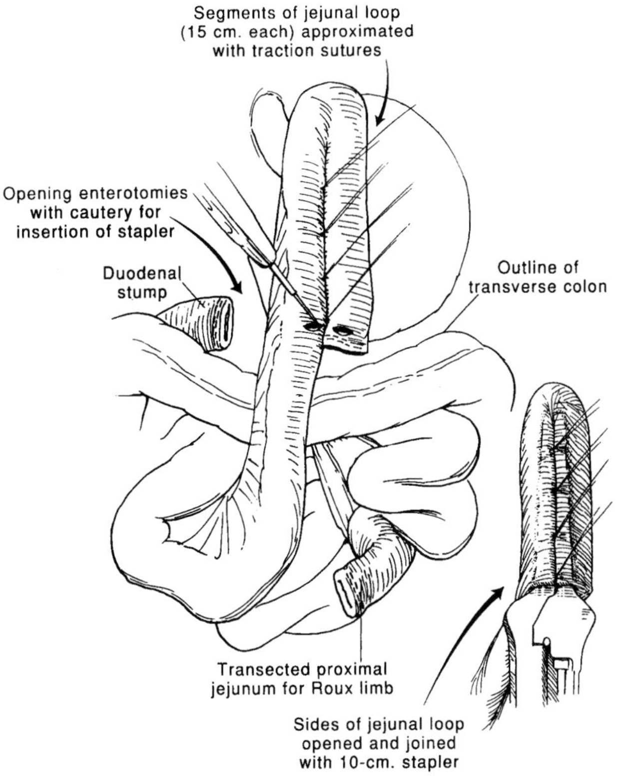

Figure 13–43. Total gastrectomy with jejeunal pouch reconstruction.

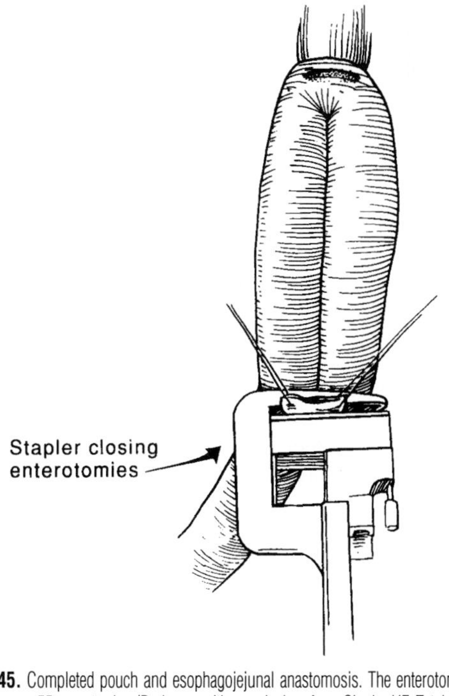

Figure 13–45. Completed pouch and esophagojejunal anastomosis. The enterotomy is closed with the transverse 55-mm stapler. (Redrawn, with permission, from Siegler HF. Total gastrectomy: stapler. In: Sabiston DC Jr [ed]. *Atlas of General Surgery.* Philadelphia, PA: WB Saunders; 1994.)

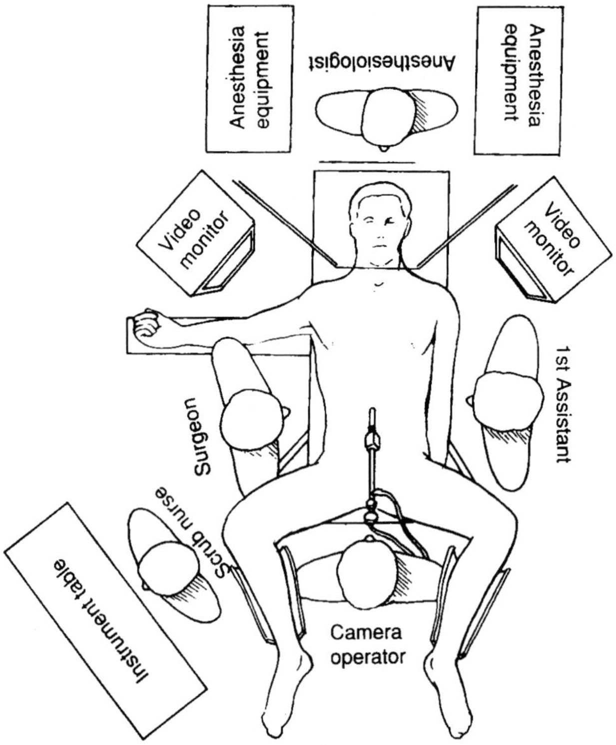

Figure 13–46. Set up for laparoscopically-assisted vagotomy. (Redrawn, with permission, from Bailey RW, Zucker KA, Flowers JL. Vagotomy. In: Ballantyne GH [ed]. *Laparoscopic Surgery.* Philadelphia, PA: WB Saunders; 1994.)

ity before division by scissors. Surgical stapling devices can be used for this purpose, as well as newer devices such as the harmonic scalpel, which utilizes ultrasonic energy for coagulating vessels, or the electrothermal bipolar coagulator device (LigaSure Vessel Sealing System, Valleylab, Boulder, CO). After creation of the seromyotomy, the integrity of the mucosa should be verified by moderate expansion of the stomach using the NG tube for insufflation. Some authors use methylene blue solution (1 vial per 200 mL), placed intragastrically, for this maneuver. The seromyotomy then is closed using a continuous suturing technique. A tongue of omentum may be mobilized and secured over the seromyotomy as a patch, secured with sutures placed through either edge of the seromyotomy.

Laparoscopic Approaches to the Gastric Resection

The patient is positioned the same way as for laparoscopic antisecretory surgery, with the patient supine with legs in stirrups and apart as shown in Figure 13–46. Port placement is similar with five ports placed in the following locations: (1) a 12-mm laparoscope port at the superior edge of the umbilicus or placed 5 cm above and lateral to the left of midline; (2) a 5-mm irrigation/suction and dissection port in the subxiphoid position, just to the right of midline; (3) a 10-mm port for retraction and grasping forceps midway between

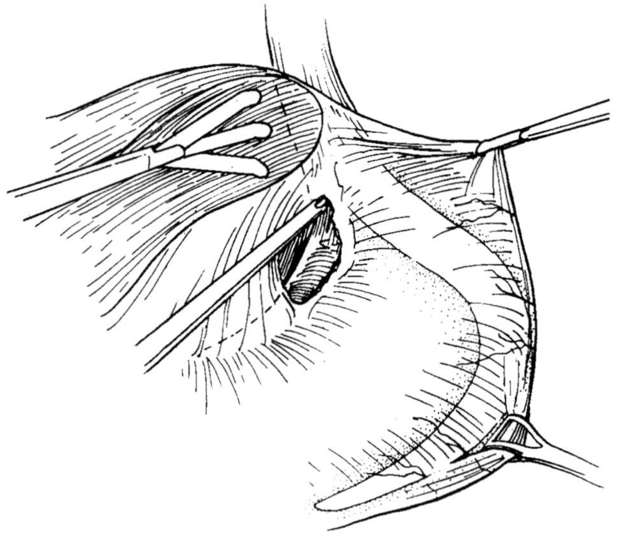

Figure 13–47. Laparoscopic view of the hiatus.

the umbilicus and xiphoid, to the right of the rectus and possibly as far as the midclavicular line; (4) a 10-mm port for grasping forceps midway between the umbilicus and xiphoid, almost to the anterior axillary line on the left; and (5) a 12-mm operating port just lateral to the rectus 3 cm above the umbilicus. A angled 30° laparoscope is useful for gastric resections, as it allows improved visualization of the stomach from multiple perspectives. If resections high in the lesser curvature are planned, retraction of the left lobe of the liver using a probe placed via the subxiphoid port or the 10-mm fan retractor placed via the higher right-side port (see Fig 13–47) is useful as described for laparoscopic truncal vagotomy.

Wedge resections of benign but symptomatic masses on the greater curvature can be done by grasping the greater curvature with a Babcock or other atraumatic grasper and use of a laparoscopic stapling device to resect the involved portion of stomach. Occasionally intraoperative endoscopic confirmation of the position of intraluminal masses not readily apparent intraoperatively is useful. Wedge resections on the lesser curvature are more difficult due to the presence of the left lobe of the liver, which usually needs to be retracted, and the proximity of the esophagus and vagus nerves. However, with careful attention to the gastroesophageal junction, wedge resections of the lesser curvature can be done. If the vagus nerve or its major branches are sacrificed in lesser curvature resections, a laparoscopic or endoscopic drainage procedure is recommended (endoscopic pyloric dilatation or laparoscopic pyloric seromyotomy).

Both laparoscopic subtotal and total gastrectomy have been described.[36,57–61] Only laparoscopic subtotal gastrectomy will be described here, as laparoscopic total

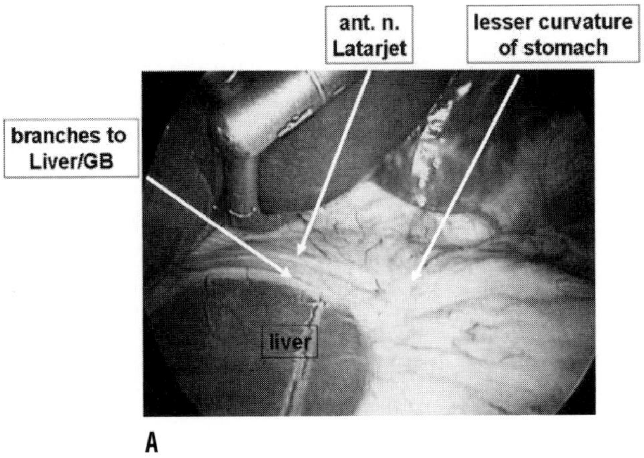

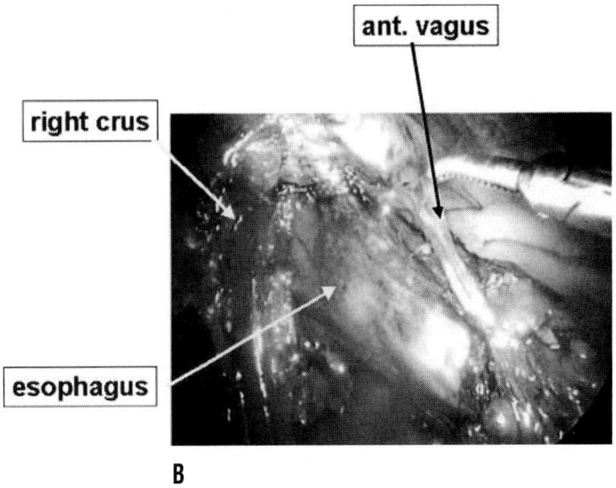

Figure 13–48. Laparoscopic view of the anterior vagus nerve. **A.** Before dissection. **B.** After dissection.

gastrectomy is rarely performed and is only done at specialized centers. Port placement is similar to that for wedge resections and antisecretory procedures. Gastric mobilization, resection, and reconstruction are done in a similar fashion to that of the open procedures. After entry into the abdominal cavity and port placement, the left lobe of the liver is mobilized and retracted laterally with a fan retractor or probe through the subxiphoid port if the lesser curvature cannot be adequately visualized or if extensive dissection of the lesser curvature is required. The stomach is grasped with a laparoscopic Babcock clamp and the distal stomach is mobilized by incising the gastrocolic ligament, which is taken bluntly if the plane is avascular and with the harmonic scalpel or electrothermal bipolar coagulator device if small vessels are encountered. The dissection is carried distally along the greater curvature, dividing the small branches of the gastroepiploic artery to the gastric wall similarly with the harmonic scalpel or electrothermal bipolar coagulator device. Others have used endoscopic vascular staplers to take much of gastrocolic omentum and its vessels. Once the proximal portion of the gastric dissection is reached, the stomach is divided with laparoscopic staplers at our institution (2.5-mm stapler load on U.S. Surgical, Norwalk, CT; or Ethicon, Somerville, New Jersey laparoscopic staplers). The gastric resection is then completed by division of the distal stomach at or just past the pylorus with a laparoscopic stapler. Reconstruction is completed as a B-II gastrojejunal anastomosis. Babcock clamps are used to locate the jejunum at the ligament of

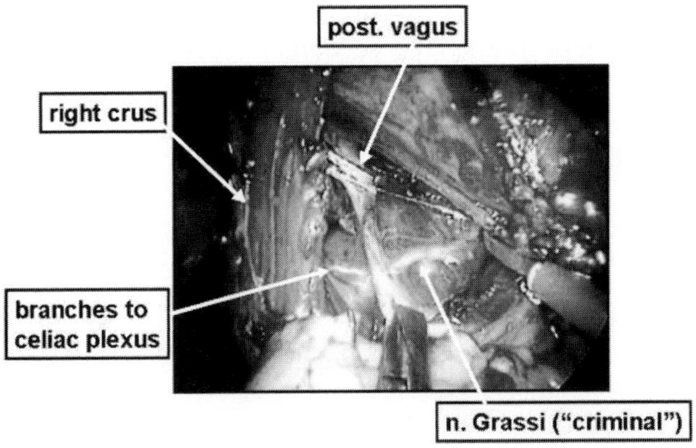

Figure 13–49. Laparoscopically-assisted vagotomy. The gastrohepatic ligament is dissected anteriorly without injury to the vagus nerves. (Redrawn, with permission, from Katkhouda N, Mouiel J. Laparoscopic treatment of peptic ulcer disease. In: Brooks DC [ed]. *Current Techniques in Laparoscopy.* Philadelphia, PA: Current Medicine; 1994.)

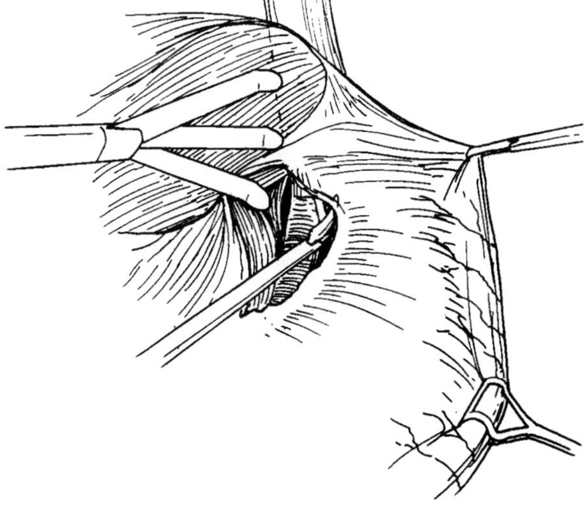

Figure 13–50. Laparoscopically-assisted vagotomy. The crus of the diaphragm is retracted to the patient's right. The anterior vagal trunk is exposed at the gastroesophageal junction. (Redrawn, with permission, from Katkhouda N, Mouiel J. Laparoscopic treatment of peptic ulcer disease. In: Brooks DC [ed]. *Current Techniques in Laparoscopy.* Philadelphia, PA: Current Medicine; 1994.)

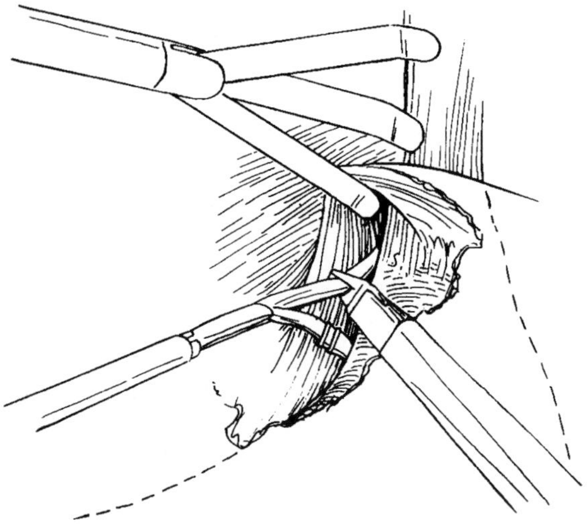

Figure 13–51. Laparoscopically assisted vagotomy. The posterior trunk is ligated between clips and divided. (Redrawn, with permission, from Katkhouda N, Mouiel J. Laparoscopic treatment of peptic ulcer disease. In: Brooks DC [ed]. *Current Techniques in Laparoscopy.* Philadelphia, PA: Current Medicine; 1994.)

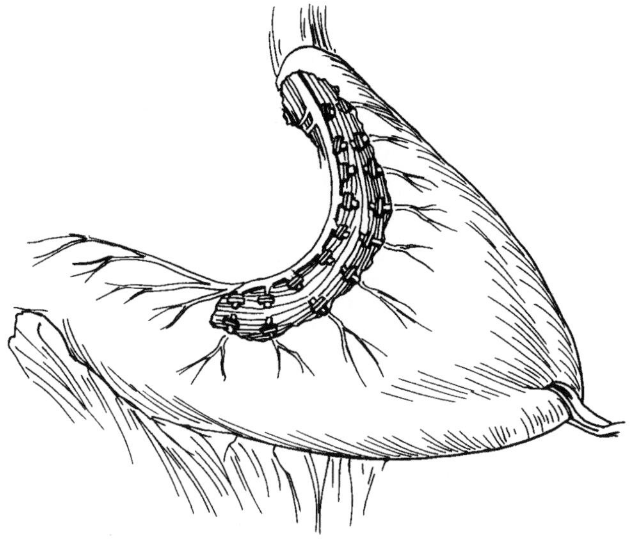

Figure 13–53. Laparoscopically-assisted parietal cell vagotomy. Dissection of the anterior leaf of the gastrohepatic ligament. (Redrawn, with permission, from Katkhouda N, Mouiel J. Laparoscopic treatment of peptic ulcer disease. In: Brooks DC [ed]. Current Techniques in Laparoscopy. Philadelphia, PA: Current Medicine; 1994.)

Treitz and bring a freely mobile portion of jejunum typically 20–30 cm distal to the ligament of Treitz up to the proximal gastric remnant in an antecolic or retrocolic fashion through an avascular window in the transverse colon mesentery. The gastric remnant and jejunum are aligned together, being careful not to twist the jejunal mesentery, and then secured to each other at the proximal and distal suture lines by interrupted 3-0 Vicryl sutures placed either with an Endostitch (Endostitch, Auto Suture Company, Norwalk, CT) or with a laparoscopic needle driver. After the gastric and jejunal limbs are aligned, Bovie cautery is used to place enterotomies in the proximal gastric remnant and jejunum. A laparoscopic stapler is placed into the gastric and jejunal limbs and then deployed to form the anastomotic staple line.

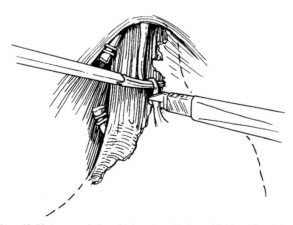

Figure 13–52. Laparoscopically-assisted vagotomy. Ligation and division of the anterior vagus between clips. (Redrawn, with permission, from Katkhouda N, Mouiel J. Laparoscopic treatment of peptic ulcer disease. In: Brooks DC [ed]. *Current Techniques in Laparoscopy.* Philadelphia, PA: Current Medicine; 1994.)

The proximal portion of the anastomosis is then closed using a laparoscopic stapler or sutured closed using an Endostitch device or with a laparoscopic needle driver. The mesenteric defect in the transverse colon is then closed if a retrocolic anastomosis was done.

One of the concerns with laparoscopic subtotal gastrectomy, especially for those done in patients with gastric cancer, is if an adequate lymphadenectomy is being performed. One approach being investigated for use is sentinel node mapping as has been used for breast cancer.[62,63] All nodes that are identified as sentinel nodes at the time of laparoscopy are resected with the hopes of performing a complete lymphadenectomy of affected nodes. However, this is controversial and more studies are needed before it can be widely recommended. It is also unclear how this influences survival in light of the some studies showing improved survival with extended lymphadenectomy (D2 resection).

REFERENCES

1. Finney J. The development of surgery of the stomach with special reference paid to the part played by American surgeons. *Ann Surg* 1929;90:829
2. Herrington J. Historical aspects of gastric surgery. In: Scott H, Sawyers J (eds). *Surgery of the Stomach, Duodenum, and Small Intestine,* 2nd ed. Boston, MA: Blackwell Scientific; 1992:1–28
3. Absolon KB. The surgical school of Theodor Billroth. *Surgery* 1961;50:697–715
4. Mikulicz-Radecki J. Small contributions to the surgery of the intestinal tract. *Trans Am Surg Assoc* 1903;21:124

5. Stabile BE, Passaro E Jr. Duodenal ulcer: a disease in evolution. *Curr Probl Surg* 1984;21:1–79
6. Waisbren SJ, Modlin IM, Lester R. Dragstedt and his role in the evolution of therapeutic vagotomy in the United States. *Am J Surg* 1994;167:344–359
7. Harkins HN, Schmitz EJ, Harper HP et al. A combined physiologic operation for peptic ulcer (partial distal gastrectomy, vagotomy and gastroduodenostomy); a preliminary report. *West J Surg Obstet Gynecol* 1953;61:316–319
8. Griffith CA, Harkins HN. Partial gastric vagotomy: an experimental study. *Gastroenterology* 1957;32:96–102
9. Johnston D, Wilkinson A. Selective vagotomy with innervated antrum without drainage procedure for duodenal ulcer. *Br J Surg* 1969;56:626
10. Goligher JC, Hill GL, Kenny TE, Nutter E. Proximal gastric vagotomy without drainage for duodenal ulcer: results after 5–8 years. *Br J Surg* 1978;65:145–151
11. Feldman M, Richardson CT, Fordtran JS. Experience with sham feeding as a test for vagotomy. *Gastroenterology* 1980;79:792–795
12. Thirlby RC. Studies of gastric secretion. In: Scott H, Sawyers J (eds). *Surgery of the Stomach, Duodenum, and Small Intestine*, 2nd ed. Boston, MA: Blackwell Scientific; 1992:124–143
13. Andrus CM. St. Louis University Department of Surgery, St. Louis, MO. (Personal communication)
14. Mayer EA. The physiology of gastric storage and emptying. In: Johnston LR (ed). *Physiology of the Gastrointestinal Tract.* New York, NY: Raven; 1994:929–976
15. Johnston D. Vagotomy. In: Schwartz SI (ed). *Maingot's Abdominal Operations*, 8th ed. Norwalk, CT: Appleton-Crofts; 1985:797–820
16. Morris DL, Harrison JD, Jorgensen JO, Perkins AC, Stanley J. Posterior truncal vagotomy and stapling of the anterior stomach wall in 30 patients with duodenal ulcer: acid inhibition, gastric emptying, and endoscopic dye spraying. Prospects for endoscopic vagotomy. *Surg Laparosc Endosc* 1993;3:375–380
17. Fich A, Neri M, Camilleri M, Kelly KA, Phillips SF. Stasis syndromes following gastric surgery: clinical and motility features of 60 symptomatic patients. *J Clin Gastroenterol* 1990;12:505–512
18. Paimela H, Hallikainen D, Ahonen J et al. The prognostic significance of radiologically determined gastric emptying time before proximal gastric vagotomy. *Acta Chir Scand* 1986;152:611–615
19. Pechlivanides G, Xynos E, Chrysos E et al. Gallbladder emptying after antiulcer gastric surgery. *Am J Surg* 1994; 168:335–339
20. Saik RP, Greenburg AG, Peskin GW. Pros and cons of parietal cell versus truncal vagotomy. *Am J Surg* 1984;148:93–98
21. Cheadle WG, Baker PR, Cuschieri A. Pyloric reconstruction for severe vasomotor dumping after vagotomy and pyloroplasty. *Ann Surg* 1985;202:568–572
22. Rossi RL, Dial PF, Georgi B, Braasch JW, Shea JA. A five to ten year follow-up study of parietal cell vagotomy. *Surg Gynecol Obstet* 1986;162:301-306
23. Wang CS, Tzen KY, Chen PC, Chen MF. Effects of highly selective vagotomy and additional procedures on gastric emptying in patients with obstructing duodenal ulcer. *World J Surg* 1994;18:131–137; discussion 137–138
24. Hallenbeck GA, Gleysteen JJ, Aldrete JS, Slaughter RL. Proximal gastric vagotomy: effects of two operative techniques on clinical and gastric secretory results. *Ann Surg* 1976;184:435–442
25. Johnston D. Operative mortality and postoperative morbidity of highly selective vagotomy. *Br Med J* 1975;4:545–547
26. Grassi G. Highly selective vagotomy with intraoperative acid secretive test of completeness of vagal section. *Surg Gynecol Obstet* 1975;140:259–264
27. Butterfield DJ, Whitfield PF, Hobsley M. Changes in gastric secretion with time after vagotomy and the relationship to recurrent duodenal ulcer. *Gut* 1982;23:1055–1059
28. Barroso FL, Caltabiano A, Ornellas A. Transabdominal suprahepatic approach to repeat vagotomy after proximal gastric vagotomy. *Surg Gynecol Obstet* 1990;171:167–168
29. Thirlby RC, Feldman M. Transthoracic vagotomy for postoperative peptic ulcer. Effects on basal, sham feeding- and pentagastrin-stimulated acid secretion, and on clinical outcome. *Ann Surg* 1985;201:648–655
30. Jackson RG. Anatomy of vagus nerves in the region of the lower esophagus and stomach. *Anat Rec* 1949;103:1
31. Bemelman WA, Brummelkamp WH, Bartelsman JF. Endoscopic balloon dilation of the pylorus after esophagogastrostomy without a drainage procedure. *Surg Gynecol Obstet* 1990;170:424–426
32. McDermott EW, Murphy JJ. Laparoscopic truncal vagotomy without drainage. *Br J Surg* 1993;80:236
33. Pietrafitta JJ, Schultz LS, Graber JN, Hickok DF. Laser laparoscopic vagotomy and pyloromyotomy. *Gastrointest Endosc* 1991;37:338–343
34. Clancy TV, Moore PM, Ramshaw DG, Kays CR. Laparoscopic excision of a benign gastric tumor. *J Laparoendosc Surg* 1994;4:277–280
35. Llorente J. Laparoscopic gastric resection for gastric leiomyoma. *Surg Endosc* 1994;8:887–889
36. Huscher CG, Anastasi A, Crafa F, Recher A, Lirici MM. Laparoscopic gastric resections. *Semin Laparosc Surg* 2000;7:26–54
37. Donahue PE, Nyhus LM. Surgical excision of gastric ulcers near the gastroesophageal junction. *Surg Gynecol Obstet* 1982;155:85–88
38. Bancroft FW. A modification of the Devine operation of pyloric exclusion for duodenal ulcer. *Am J Surg* 1932;16:223
39. Becker JM, Kelly KA, Haddad AC, Zinsmeister AR. Proximal gastric vagotomy and mucosal antrectomy: a possible operative approach to duodenal ulcer. *Surgery* 1983; 94:58–64
40. Degiuli M, Sasako M, Ponti A, Calvo F. Survival results of a multicentre phase II study to evaluate D2 gastrectomy for gastric cancer. *Br J Cancer* 2004;90:1727–1732
41. Degiuli M, Sasako M, Calgaro M et al. Morbidity and mortality after D1 and D2 gastrectomy for cancer: interim analysis of the Italian Gastric Cancer Study Group (IGCSG) randomised surgical trial. *Eur J Surg Oncol* 2004;30:303–308

42. Collard JM, Malaise J, Mabrut JY, Kestens PJ. Skeletonizing en-bloc gastrectomy for adenocarcinoma in Caucasian patients. *Gastric Cancer* 2003;6:210–216
43. Roukos DH, Lorenz M, Encke A. Evidence of survival benefit of extended (D2) lymphadenectomy in western patients with gastric cancer based on a new concept: a prospective long-term follow-up study. *Surgery* 1998;123: 573–578
44. Wanebo HJ, Kennedy BJ, Chmiel J et al. Cancer of the stomach. A patient care study by the American College of Surgeons. *Ann Surg* 1993;218:583–592
45. Robertson CS, Chung SC, Woods SD et al. A prospective randomized trial comparing R1 subtotal gastrectomy with R3 total gastrectomy for antral cancer. *Ann Surg* 1994;220:176–182
46. Brady MS, Rogatko A, Dent LL, Shiu MH. Effect of splenectomy on morbidity and survival following curative gastrectomy for carcinoma. *Arch Surg* 1991;126:359–364
47. Adachi Y, Kamakura T, Mori M, Maehara Y, Sugimachi K. Role of lymph node dissection and splenectomy in node-positive gastric carcinoma. *Surgery* 1994;116:837–841
48. Lehnert T, Buhl K. Techniques of reconstruction after total gastrectomy for cancer. *Br J Surg* 2004;91:528–539
49. Barone RM. Reconstruction after total gastrectomy: construction of a Hunt-Lawrence pouch using Auto Suture staples. *Am J Surg* 1979;137:578–584
50. Gioffre' Florio MA, Bartolotta M, Miceli JC et al. Simple versus double jejunal pouch for reconstruction after total gastrectomy. *Am J Surg* 2000;180:24–28
51. Oddsdottir M, Soybel D. Peptic ulcer disease. In: Ballantyne G (ed). *Laparoscopic Surgery*. Philadelphia, PA: WB Saunders; 1994:137
52. Millat B, Fingerhut A, Borie F. Surgical treatment of complicated duodenal ulcers: controlled trials. *World J Surg* 2000;24:299–306
53. Dallemagne B, Weerts JM, Jehaes C, Markiewicz S, Lombard R. Laparoscopic highly selective vagotomy. *Br J Surg* 1994;81:554–556
54. Taylor TV, Lythgoe JP, McFarland JB et al. Anterior lesser curve seromyotomy and posterior truncal vagotomy versus truncal vagotomy and pyloroplasty in the treatment of chronic duodenal ulcer. *Br J Surg* 1990;77: 1007–1009
55. Katkhouda N, Heimbucher J, Mouiel J. Laparoscopic posterior truncal vagotomy and anterior seromyotomy. *Semin Laparosc Surg* 1994;1:154–160
56. Petrakis I, Vassilakis SJ, Chalkiadakis G. Anterior lesser curve seromyotomy using a stapling device and posterior truncal vagotomy for the treatment of chronic duodenal ulcer: long term results. *J Am Coll Surg* 1999; 188:623–628
57. Kitano S, Shiraishi N. Current status of laparoscopic gastrectomy for cancer in Japan. *Surg Endosc* 2004;18:182–185
58. Adrales GL, Gandsas A, Mastrangelo MJ Jr, Schwartz R. An introduction to laparoscopic gastric resection. *Curr Surg* 2003;60:385–389
59. Shimizu S, Noshiro H, Nagai E, Uchiyama A, Tanaka M. Laparoscopic gastric surgery in a Japanese institution: analysis of the initial 100 procedures. *J Am Coll Surg* 2003;197:372–378
60. Uyama I, Sugioka A, Fujita J et al. Laparoscopic total gastrectomy with distal pancreatosplenectomy and D2 lymphadenectomy for advanced gastric cancer. *Gastric Cancer* 1999;2:230–234
61. Kim YW, Han HS, Fleischer GD. Hand-assisted laparoscopic total gastrectomy. *Surg Laparosc Endosc Percutan Tech* 2003;13:26–30
62. Kitagawa Y, Fujii H, Mukai M et al. Intraoperative lymphatic mapping and sentinel lymph node sampling in esophageal and gastric cancer. *Surg Oncol Clin N Am* 2002;11:293–304
63. Kitagawa Y, Ohgami M, Fujii H et al. Laparoscopic detection of sentinel lymph nodes in gastrointestinal cancer: a novel and minimally invasive approach. *Ann Surg Oncol* 2001;8:86S–89S

14

Gastric Adenocarcinoma

Murray F. Brennan

▪ INCIDENCE AND PREVALENCE

The incidence of gastric adenocarcinoma has fallen in the Western world in the last four decades. However, gastric cancer continues to be seen in much of the rest of the world, and the mortality rate continues to be high. Age-standardized incidence of gastric adenocarcinoma varies from less than 10 per 100,000 population to in excess of 80 per 100,000[1] (Fig 14–1). Age-adjusted death rates vary from 5 per 100,000 in the United States to 35 per 100,000 in Russia (Fig 14–2).

Improved survival rates in Japan initially led to the suggestion that the biology of gastric cancer differed according to the country of residence. This has not been supported by any known biologic observations. It is correct that the site of gastric cancer varies by country, with antral (distal) cancer the major site-specific type in Asia, whereas proximal gastric cancer has begun to predominate in Europe and the United States.

This increasing incidence of proximal gastric cancers is particularly of the gastroesophageal (GE) junction. In my own institution, the prevalence of proximal gastric cancer has changed since my colleagues and I initiated our prospective database in 1985 (Fig 14–3) to where proximal gastric cancer is more common than distal or antral gastric cancer in 2004.

The stage of disease at the time of diagnosis appears to be the predominant factor in predicting outcome accurately. Overall survival is highly correlated with the stage at presentation. In countries where there is a high degree of advanced gastric cancer, mortality remains high.

Unfortunately, accurate staging is poorly applied outside specialized units. In the National Cancer Data Base (NCDB), only 46% of patients were staged by the American Joint Committee on Cancer (AJCC) system in 1985–1986, although some improvement in staging was obtained by 1991, when 77% were staged by the AJCC system.[2]

The accuracy of staging is highly questionable because survival figures reported by national registries such as the NCDB even for early-stage disease (e.g., 5-year survival of 43% for stage I disease, 37% for stage II)[2] when compared with similar survival figures for patients treated in specialized units (stage I, 75–90%; stage II, 40–50%)[3] are so disparate as to suggest gross understaging in many national registries.

Much of the improved overall survival is associated with early-stage diagnosis. Surveillance programs in Asia have increased the number of patients diagnosed with early gastric cancer and are a major factor in the improved survival rates.

In the United States, increases have been found in the prevalence of early gastric cancer, with my own data showing an increasing incidence of T1 and T2 lesions and a corresponding decrease in T3 and T4 lesions (Fig 14–4). While early gastric cancer is common in Japan, advanced gastric cancer is the norm in the West. Nevertheless, progressively in the United States, early gastric cancer is becoming more common. In my own prospective database, earlier-stage gastric cancer as defined by N0 curatively resected patients has gone from 36% in 1985–1986 to 58% in 2000–2004 (Table 14–1) with a corresponding decrease in N2 disease.

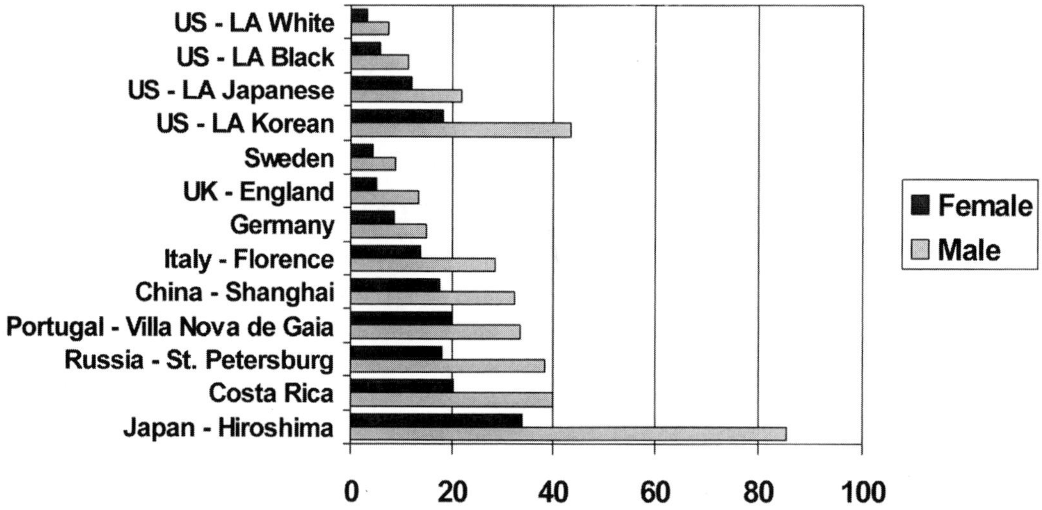

Figure 14–1. Age-standardized incidence per 100,000 population in gastric adenocarcinoma in selected populations. Data from Parkin DM, Whelan SL, Ferlay J, et al (eds). *Cancer Incidence in Five Continents,* Vol VIII. Lyon, France: International Agency for Research on Cancer; 2002.

Age distribution of gastric adenocarcinoma for patients undergoing R_0 resection is shown in Figure 14–5, emphasizing that gastric cancer remains a disease predominantly of the seventh and eighth decades but can occur at any age.

Familial gastric cancer has been identified and associated with mutations in the *E-cadherin* gene, the most famous family of which appears to be the Bonapartes. Inherited or familial gastric cancer [hereditary diffuse gastric cancer (HDGC)] should be searched for in patients with gastric cancer identified before age 40. Prophylactic gastrectomy has been performed in these familial kindreds with almost uniform findings of multifocal pathologic adenocarcinoma in the resected specimen.[4,5] The finding of an *e-cadherin* mutation results in a lifetime risk of gastric cancer of 60–90%.

HDGC is a fascinating entity that is being identified increasingly. This entity provides a challenge to surgeons because total gastrectomy appears curative since most of the multiple lesions (as many as 300–400 per specimen) are of an early stage. Significant issues arise as to risks of any preemptive operations, particularly one as significant as total gastrectomy performed at a young age. No data are available as to the consequences of 40 years without a stomach! Surveillance has been suggested as an alternative to prophylactic gastrectomy using a chromoendoscopic approach in these families.[6] Other familial associations of the development of gas-

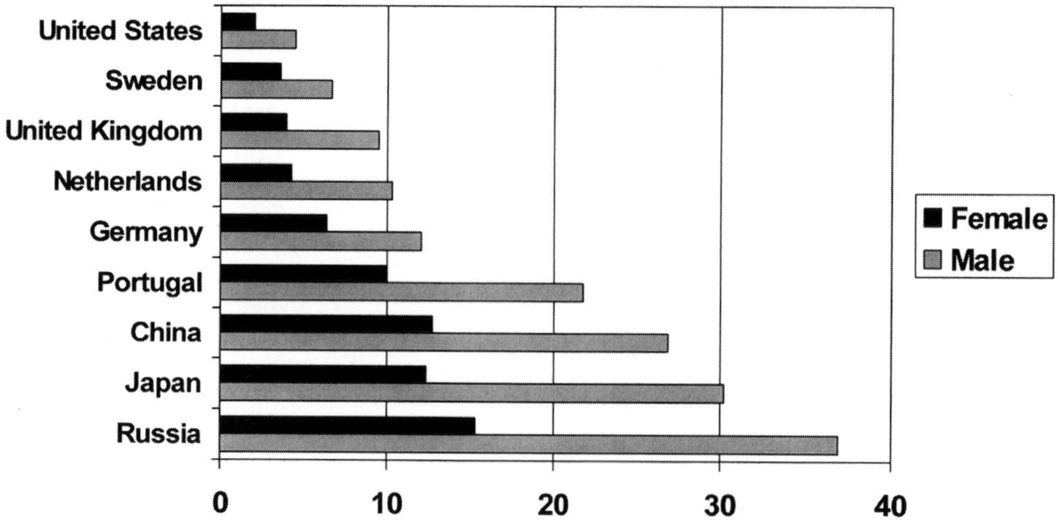

Figure 14–2. Age-adjusted deaths per 100,000 population in gastric adenocarcinoma in selected populations, 1994–1997. Data from Greenlee RT, Murray T, Bolden S, Wingo PH. Cancer Statistic, 2000. *CA Cancer J Clin* 2000;50:7–33.

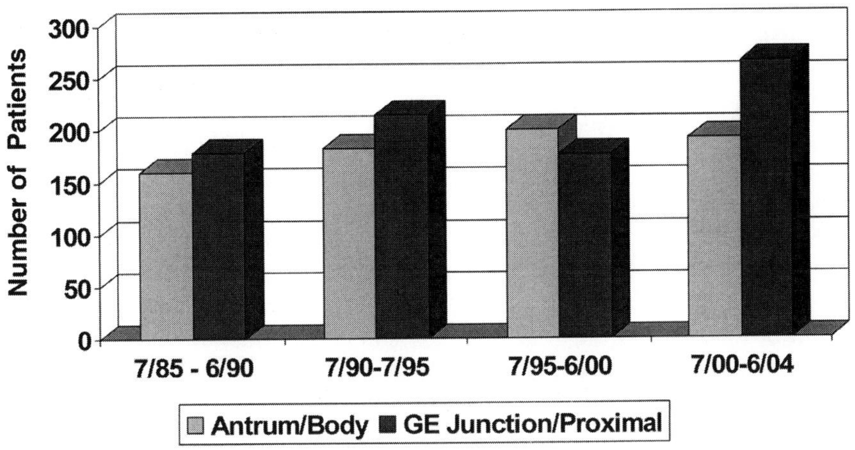

Figure 14–3. Gastric adenocarcinoma—primary admissions by site and yearly intervals. Memorial Sloan-Kettering Cancer Center, 7/1985–7/2004 ($n = 1571$).

tric cancer include those related to hereditary nonpolyposis colon cancer (HNPCC).

Helicobacter pylori appears to correlate with the presence of the intestinal-type gastric cancer and is thought to be a contributing factor to gastric carcinogenesis, now defined by the World Health Organization (WHO) as a class 1 carcinogen.[7] But since *H. pylori* are present in 80% of patients in developing countries, the presence of such bacteria is of limited value in detection, and the majority of infected patients have chronic gastritis.

Other factors associated with an increased incidence include poorly prepared (raw) food, tobacco use, low vitamin A and C intake, and high nitrate intake.

▪ DIAGNOSIS

The primary diagnosis of gastric adenocarcinoma is made by upper gastrointestinal endoscopy with or without endoscopic ultrasound. Histologic diagnosis is confirmed by biopsy. Upper gastrointestinal barium imaging remains only of historical interest in the West.

▪ PREOPERATIVE EVALUATION

Once the diagnosis of gastric adenocarcinoma has been established, then evaluation of the extent of disease is required. The extent of local disease can be evaluated by upper gastrointestinal endoscopy and, where endoscopic ultrasound is performed, delineation of the T and N stage defined, although the N-stage findings are based predominantly on size greater than 1 cm, an imprecise determinant. The early claims for high correlation of endoscopic ultrasound (EUS) T and N stage with pathologic stage have been questioned recently. Our early studies of EUS showed a very high concordance with pathologic T stage, with accuracy of from 70–90% for both T and N stage.[8,9] More recent analyses, with routine application of EUS without selectivity[10] of 296 patients

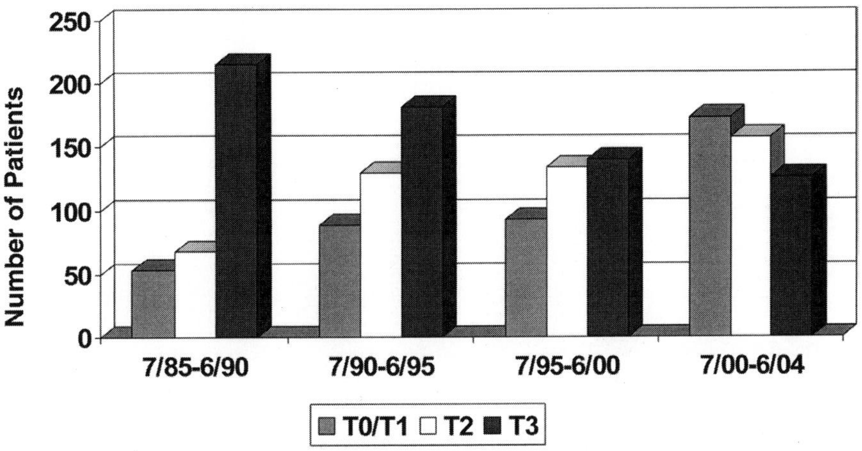

Figure 14–4. Gastric adenocarcinoma by T stage by interval showing increasing early-stage disease with time. Memorial Sloan-Kettering Cancer Center, 7/1985–7/2004 ($n = 1558$).

TABLE 14–1. GASTRIC ADENOCARCINOMA BY N STAGE, MEMORIAL SLOAN-KETTERING CANCER CENTER, JULY 1, 1985 TO JUNE 30, 2004

	N0	N1	N2
1985–1986, $n = 325$	118 (36%)	136 (42%)	71 (22%)
1990–1994, $n = 451$	199 (44%)	179 (39%)	73 (16%)
1995–1999, $n = 415$	217 (52%)	152 (37%)	46 (11%)
2000–2004, $n = 326$	192 (58%)	89 (27%)	45 (14%)

undergoing EUS followed by R_0 resection, suggested an accuracy for T stage of 57% and for N stage of 50%. Thirty-two percent were overstaged by T and 25% by N. Concordance for T3 lesions was greater than 70%, an important issue when EUS is used to define patients for investigational neoadjuvant strategies. In the latter series, EUS serosal extension was still a powerful indicator of poor outcome. EUS T stage is particularly unreliable in patients who have undergone preoperative chemoradiotherapy or when local ulceration is extensive.

On rare occasions, when identified, small amounts of ascitic fluid identified by EUS can be aspirated, and metastatic lesions identified in the left lateral segment of the liver can be biopsied. If there is a suspicion of a locally advanced lesion, i.e., a T3 or T4 lesion, then CT scanning is appropriate. The majority of patients with T3 disease show extensive wall thickening with or without accompanying nodal disease. I have reserved laparoscopy for patients with advanced disease, finding little benefit for detecting unsuspected metastatic disease in T1 and early T2 lesions, where metastatic disease is rare. In the absence of findings of wall thickening or nodal enlargement by CT scan, laparoscopy is of limited value in finding more advanced disease.[11]

The patient then must be evaluated for the suitability of the proposed procedure. If the lesion is a proximal GE junction lesion, then consideration has to be made as to whether or not the patient will require a thoracotomy. Many patients with GE junction lesions (Siewert types II and III) can be operated on with a subdiaphragmatic approach or transhiatal resection, but where the potential for a thoracotomy exists, then consideration must be made as to the adequacy of pulmonary function because many patients are prior or current cigarette smokers. While bleeding is not frequent in the majority of gastric cancer patients, attention to the adequacy of red cell mass is appropriate. Conventional cardiovascular evaluation is limited to electrocardiogram (ECG) unless there is known cardiovascular disease. Preoperative antibiotics are not used uniformly unless there has been prolonged gastric outlet obstruction or there is a suggestion of colonic involvement.

Questions that need resolution include the extent of gastric resection, the extent of lymphadenectomy, the type of reconstruction, the value of perioperative nutritional support, and the role of pre- and postoperative radiation and chemotherapy.

■ OPERATIVE MANAGEMENT

The first successful gastric resection was described in 1881 by Billroth, who at the time of the procedure performed the first lymphadenectomy, although the patient died of gastric cancer 14 months later.

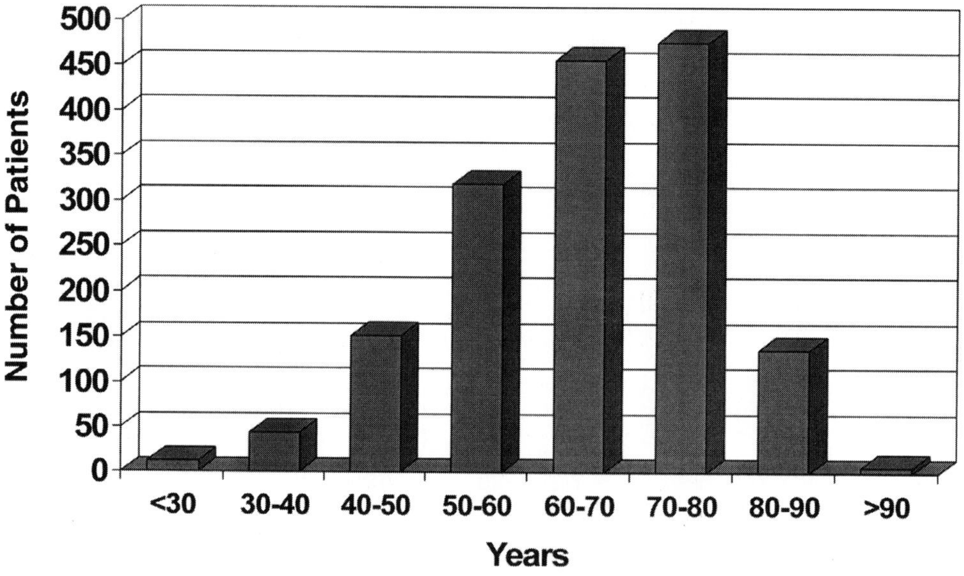

Figure 14–5. Age distribution for R_0 resected gastric adenocarcinoma. Memorial Sloan-Kettering Cancer Center 7/1/1985–6/30/2004 ($n = 1600$).

EXTENT OF GASTRIC RESECTION

There is no evidence that an extended gastric resection above and beyond complete clearance of the primary tumor improves survival; i.e., total gastrectomy does not improve survival over distal or proximal gastrectomy, provided that the tumor is removed completely with negative transection margins (R_0 resection). This has been confirmed in a number of randomized trials. The extent of the gastrectomy therefore is site-dependent and focuses on complete removal of the gastric carcinoma with preferably a 4- to 5-cm margin from the gross edge of the tumor. Clearly, anatomic limitations influence this margin because in antral lesions close to or involving the pylorus, only a limited portion of the duodenum can be removed. In similar fashion, a lesser extent of uninvolved esophageal margin may be acceptable provided complete histologic resection is possible.

In patients with a distal lesion, a distal subtotal gastrectomy is performed essentially regardless of T stage. For proximal gastric cancers and true GE junction cancers (Siewert types II and III), I have liberally used subdiaphragmatic proximal gastrectomy with esophagogastrectomy, whereas others prefer total gastrectomy for any lesion not in the antrum. For midbody or more extensive lesions, total gastrectomy is required, whereas for more distal lesions, a subtotal gastrectomy is the preferred approach. It is important to emphasize that in most studies there is an increase in morbidity and mortality when total gastrectomy is performed over distal subtotal gastrectomy. Since long-term survival is not improved by the more extensive resection, this is a further factor in favor of subtotal resection, provided that an R_0 resection can be obtained.

Proximal resections, however, appear to have similar perioperative morbidity and mortality to total gastrectomy.

Extended organ resection is reserved for patients with apparently node-negative T4 lesions, in which complete resection requires resection of the invaded portions of the diaphragm, pancreas, spleen, adrenal gland, or colon. In my institution, these patients usually are pretreated with chemotherapy (see below).

USE OF PREOPERATIVE CHEMORADIATION THERAPY

For patients with T3–4 lesions without metastatic disease, a number of trials use preoperative chemotherapy with or without radiation therapy. Despite several trials of this approach, there are no data to prove conclusively that this approach has survival benefit. In most experienced centers, a number of patients have a significant histologic response, and operative morbidity does not seem to be increased. Given the relatively poor outcome of advanced T3 and T4 lesions and the ability to characterize those patients by endoscopic ultrasound (at least those with advanced T3 disease accompanied by prelaparotomy laparoscopy), such an approach remains justified, although it should take place under a clinical-trial scenario.

USE OF LAPAROSCOPY

I have used laparoscopy liberally in patients with defined T3 and greater lesions because of the 20–30% incidence[12] of radiologically unsuspected metastatic disease. At the time of laparoscopy, I perform peritoneal lavage for cytology. Patients with cytologically positive washings in the absence of visible M1 disease have a similar outcome to patients with defined M1 disease.[12] In obviously advanced disease where laparoscopy is only designed to confirm metastatic disease, this can be done as an outpatient procedure. More commonly, however, for the suspected T3–4 lesion where the patient is a candidate for resection, laparoscopy is performed as the initial part of the procedure, and if advanced local disease is found, a neoadjuvant chemotherapy protocol is performed. For less advanced disease (T1–2), I proceed directly to the definitive procedure, usually without laparoscopy.

▪ OPERATIVE PROCEDURES

ENDOSCOPIC SUBMUCOSAL RESECTION

Risk factors that determine lymph node metastasis are based predominately on extent of primary tumor invasion. For mucosal cancers, approximately 3% will be expected to have positive lymph nodes and selectively justify the use of an endoscopic submucosal resection (ESMR). Patients with submucosal cancer, where the risk of nodal positivity can reach 20%, would be better considered for limited laparoscopic resections or limited open operations. Lymph node metastasis in both these situations is associated with larger tumor size, undifferentiated histology, and the presence of histologic lymphatic or blood vessel invasion. As a working rule, lymph node metastases are rare if the tumor is less than 2 cm in diameter and well differentiated regardless of the depth of mucosal invasion.

In the main, minimally invasive procedures have tended to be performed in the United States by gastroenterologists rather than surgeons, and the technique is well described elsewhere. Given the increasing incidence of early gastric cancers, such approaches can be expected to increase; however, in the West, they remain the province of specialized centers.

LAPAROSCOPIC RESECTION

Laparoscopic resection is being used increasingly for early-stage cancer. This is performed essentially by an extragastric approach after appropriate tattooing of the lesion endoscopically so as to ensure the ability to identify the lesion and the adequacy of the resection. The procedure can be prolonged, and it is essential that clear margins be obtained. Progressively more advanced procedures such as distal gastrectomy are being performed with the laparoscopic hand-assisted approach using a minilaparotomy. The relative benefits of these are questionable, with some small decrease in hospital stay but at the cost of prolonged operative time. For the present time, both would be considered investigational and confined to the hands of a few. Because of the high incidence of early gastric cancer in Japan and the increasing incidence of early gastric cancer in this country, laparoscopic and endoscopic procedures can be expected to increase. The laparoscopic and laparoscopic-assisted gastrectomy, except for wedge resection for small lesions, is essentially the same procedure as that of the open approach done by an alternate method. Accurate visualization and extended lymph node dissection can be performed as described for open operations (see below) with a limited incision for removal of the specimen and extracorporeal anastomosis. In Europe and North America, the laparoscopic approach is more favored for benign lesions such as benign leiomyomas or early-stage gastrointestinal stromal tumors.[13]

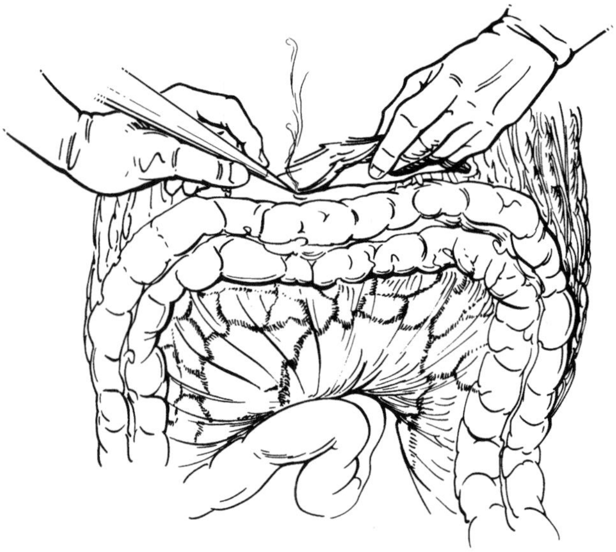

Figure 14–6. Detachment of the greater omentum from the colon through the avascular plane using the cautery.

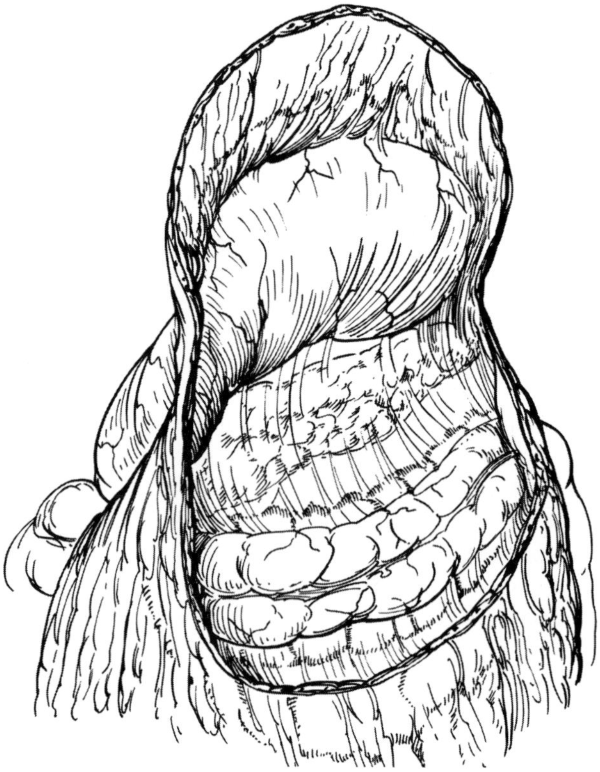

Figure 14–7. The anterior layer of the mesocolon is sharply dissected from the mesocolonic vessels in an avascular plane.

DISTAL SUBTOTAL GASTRECTOMY

Following laparoscopy, the patient is explored through a midline incision, although some prefer a bilateral subcostal incision. An assessment for metastasis is made, and the lesion is identified, usually by palpation. I prefer to start with the inferior dissection, taking the omentum from the colon through the avascular plane using the cautery (Fig 14–6), and the anterior layer of the mesocolon is sharply dissected from the mesocolonic vessels in an avascular plane (Fig 14–7). This procedure is readily accomplished in the thin patient but can be difficult in the very obese patient, in whom the small omental vessels are not so readily identified and preserved. At the base of the mesocolon, the pancreatic capsule is incised, and the capsule is dissected from the anterior surface of the pancreas (Fig 14–8). While removal of the pancreatic capsule is a standard approach, the value of the capsular dissection is unproven and may result in minor pancreatic leaks. Increasingly, I leave the pancreatic capsule intact. As the mobilization continues, the right epiploic vessels are divided under direct control. Once the superior border of the pancreas is identified, then the proximal splenic artery nodes can be dissected after identification of the splenic artery and elevation of all the nodal tissue along the splenic artery. This dissection can be delayed until the portal dissection is begun. The splenic hilus is

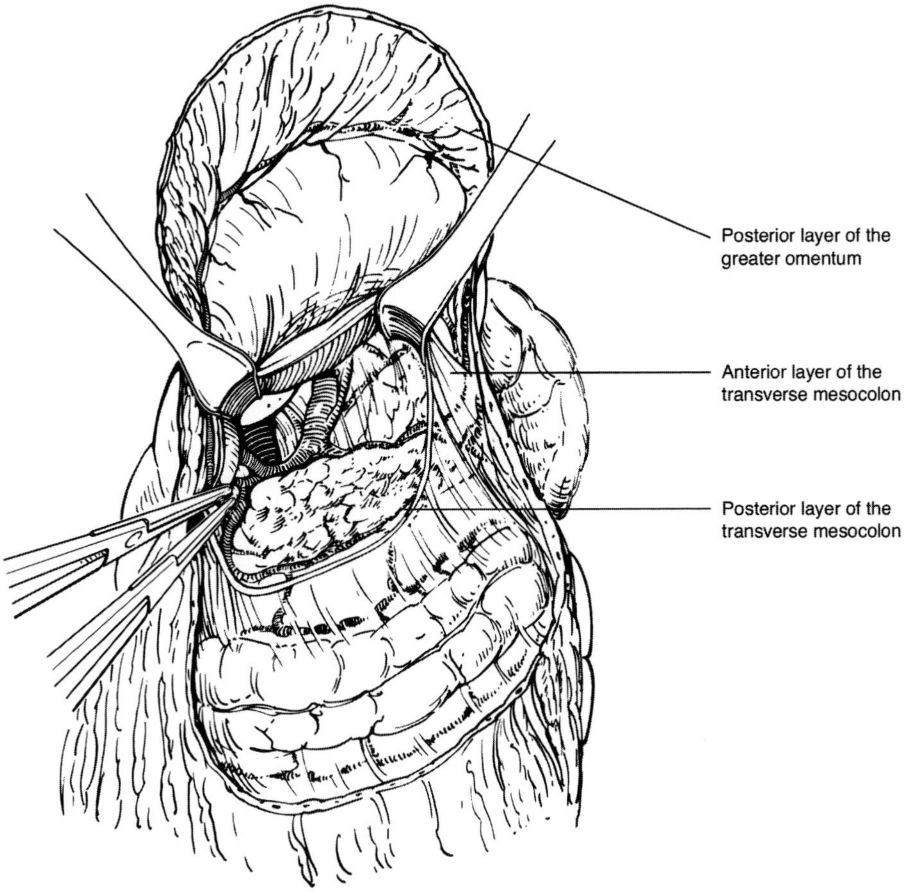

Figure 14–8. Careful ligation of the gastroepiploic vessels is essential to avoid annoying hemorrhage.

only rarely dissected completely in most Western centers. The splenic artery dissection, especially in obese patients, is achieved more easily once the duodenum has been divided. The duodenum is either isolated between straight clamps (Fig 14–9) or divided with the GIA stapler (Fig 14–10). I prefer to oversew the divided duodenum with interrupted absorbable monofilament sutures (Fig 14–11), although this may not be essential. If there is to be an oversewn closure, then there must be adequate mobilized duodenum from the pancreas to ensure invagination without damage to the pancreas.

The porta hepatis is dissected by coming down the left side of the left hepatic artery, dissecting the left side of the portal vein and the node-bearing tissue in that area and then taking the dissection back along the common hepatic artery to the celiac axis and base of the aorta. At this site, the crus of the right diaphragm is cleared, and the left gastric artery origin similarly is cleared of any node-bearing tissue, which is removed with the specimen. The left lateral segment needs to be mobilized by taking down the falciform ligament to gain better access to the esophageal hiatus and the right crus.

The nodal tissue inferior to the common hepatic artery, superior to the pancreas, and in front of the portal vein is cleared from the gastroduodenal artery back to the origin of the splenic artery, and the proximal splenic artery nodes are taken, if not already mobilized

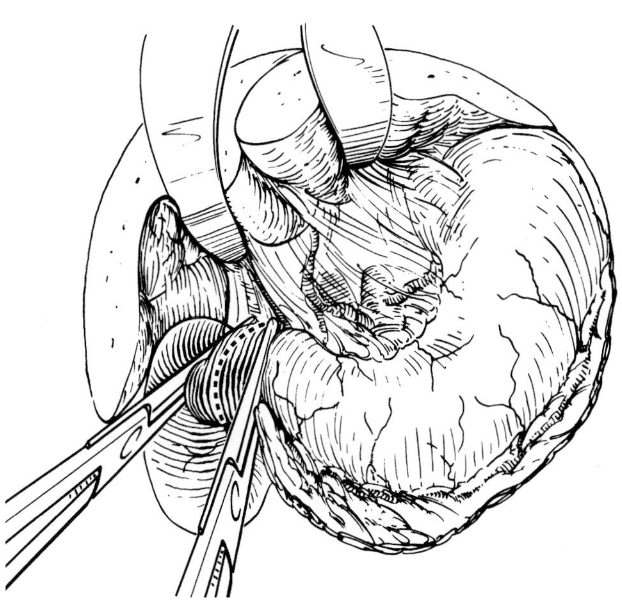

Figure 14–9. The duodenum is divided carefully with the scalpel between straight clamps.

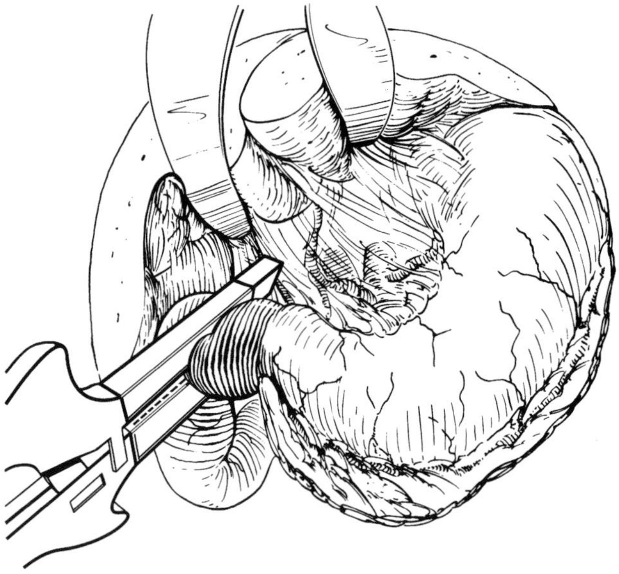

Figure 14–10. The duodenum can be divided using the GIA stapler if a Billroth I anastomosis is not planned.

with the gastric specimen. The left gastric artery is divided close to its origin (Fig 14–12), and the crus of the diaphragm on the right is cleared further back to the esophageal hiatus. The right paracardial nodes then are reflected down from the proximal stomach, taking care not to devascularize the lesser curvature (Fig 14–13). That portion of the omentum not to be removed with the specimen is detached at the greater curvature, taking care to preserve the distal short gastric vessels, and the remaining omentum is retained with the specimen. I prefer to divide the stomach with straight and curved Kocher clamps, completing the division with the GIA stapler, coming high on the lesser curvature at or close to the GE junction (Fig 14–14).

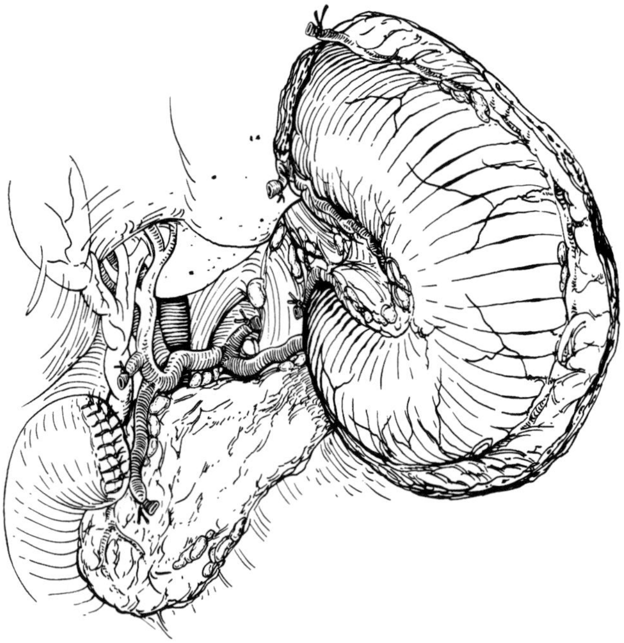

Figure 14–12. The left gastric artery is divided close to its origin, with the perivessel lymph nodes reflected with the stomach.

Multiple different approaches to this transection can be made, with some preferring to divide the stomach completely with the stapler. However, it is quite simple to reconstruct if the lateral aspect of the stomach is divided between the straight and curved Kocher clamps (see Fig 14–14), allowing the orifice for the gastrojejunal anastomosis. The stapled suture line can be over-

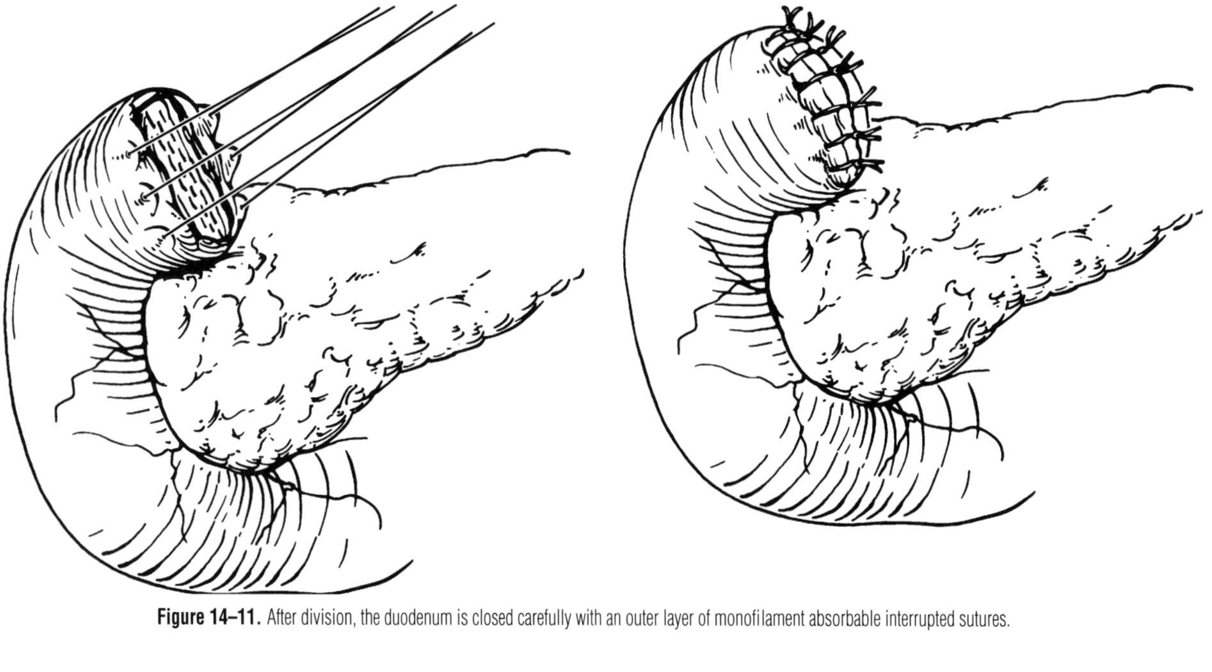

Figure 14–11. After division, the duodenum is closed carefully with an outer layer of monofilament absorbable interrupted sutures.

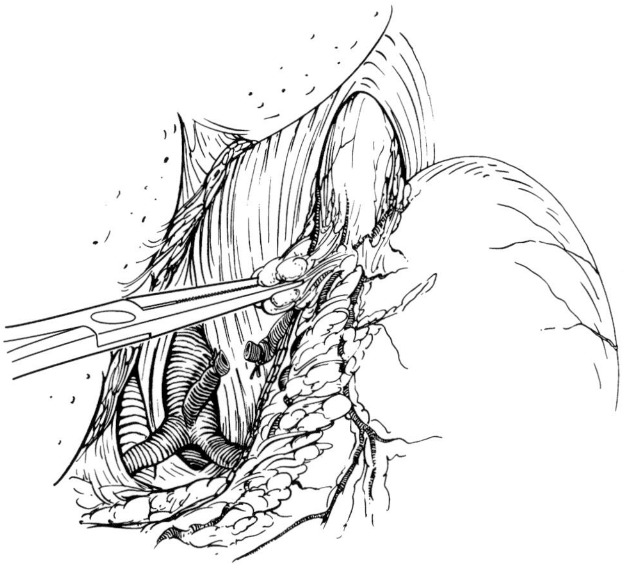

Figure 14–13. The paracardial and periesophageal lymph nodes are dissected and reflected inferiorly with the specimen.

sewn, but this is not essential. If a Billroth I anastomosis is to be performed, then the division of the duodenum (see Fig 14–9) should be done with straight clamps to allow reanastomosis. If a Billroth II anastomosis is to be performed, then the gastrojejunal anastomosis usually is performed in an antecolic fashion with running 3-0 PDS sutures (Fig 14–15). If the stomach has been divided completely by the GIA stapler, then a posterior gastrojejunostomy is performed by rotating the stomach remnant upward and forward, being sure that the anastomosis is well clear of the staple line so as not to develop an avascular bridge. In most patients, a routine enteroenterostomy is not performed but can be performed at the surgeon's preference. In addition, in early-stage disease, some consideration is given to a Roux-en-Y reconstruction in an effort to avoid postoperative reflux with concomitant distal enteroenterostomy.

TOTAL GASTRECTOMY

In a total gastrectomy, the dissection proceeds in a similar fashion. Early mobilization of the left lateral segment of the liver will be necessary to evaluate the extent of a more proximal lesion. However, once the right side of the esophagus is isolated, then the esophagus can be encircled, and the left paracardial nodes and the paraesophageal nodes can be reflected inferiorly with the specimen (Fig 14–16). In this situation, the short gastric vessels need to be divided, and I prefer to divide these close to the spleen. The left crus is skeletonized, and the left adrenal gland is identified commonly. I prefer to transect the stomach with the placement of a proximal Satinsky vascular clamp, which allows ready stabilization of the esophagus (Fig 14–17). In proximal lesions, a frozen section of the esophageal margin is performed. In locally invasive extensive proximal lesions, the mucosal margin can be benign, but extraesophageal extension can be found in the periserosal tissues. Once this specimen is removed, the jejunal loop is isolated and divided with the GIA stapler (Fig 14–18). The small in-

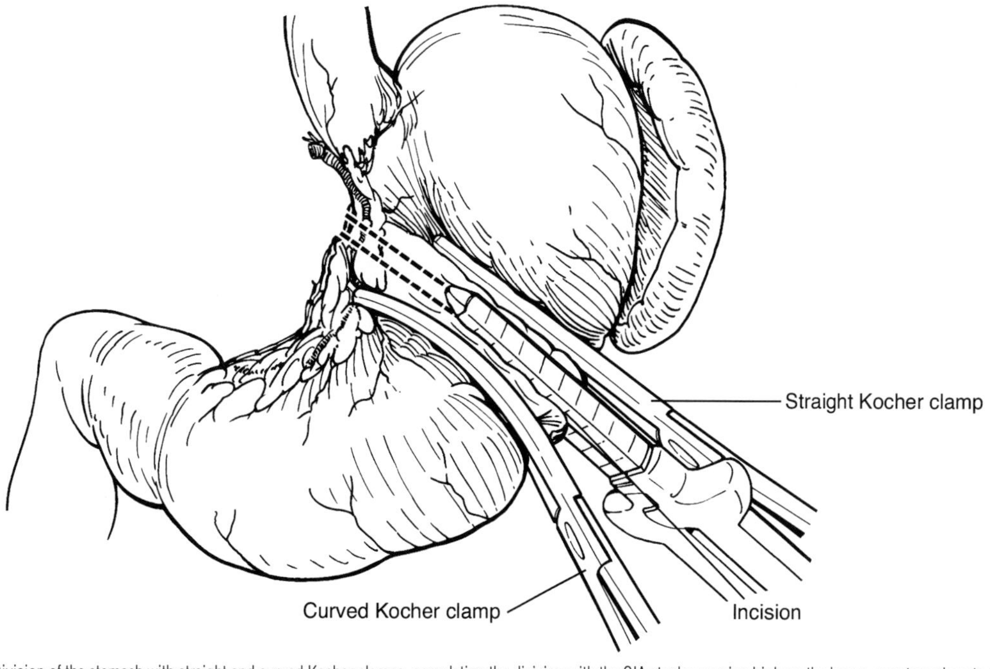

Figure 14–14. Division of the stomach with straight and curved Kocher clamps, completing the division with the GIA stapler, coming high on the lesser curvature close to the GE junction.

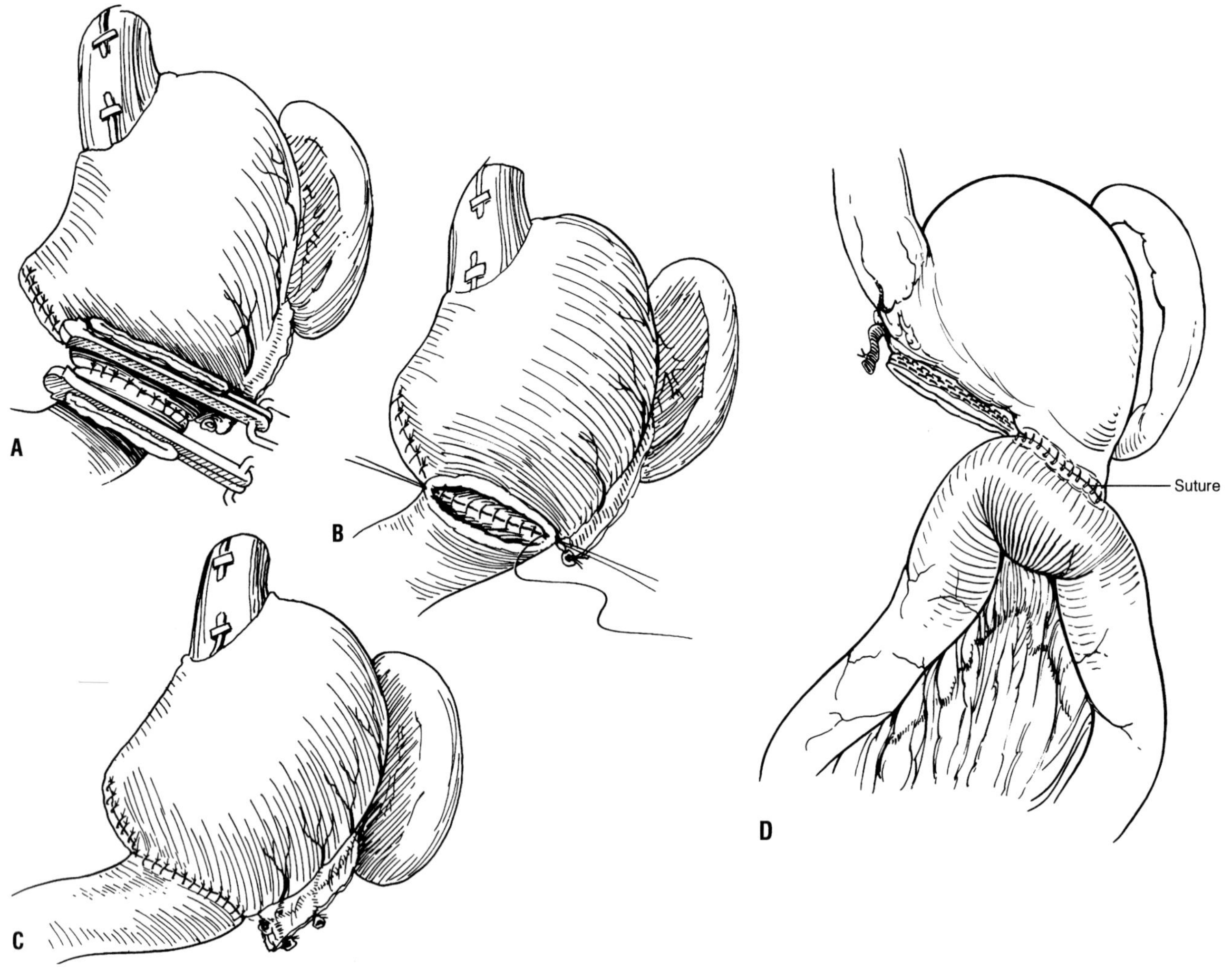

Figure 14–15. For a Billroth II anastomosis, a gastrojejunal anastomosis is performed with two layers of running absorbable monofilament sutures.

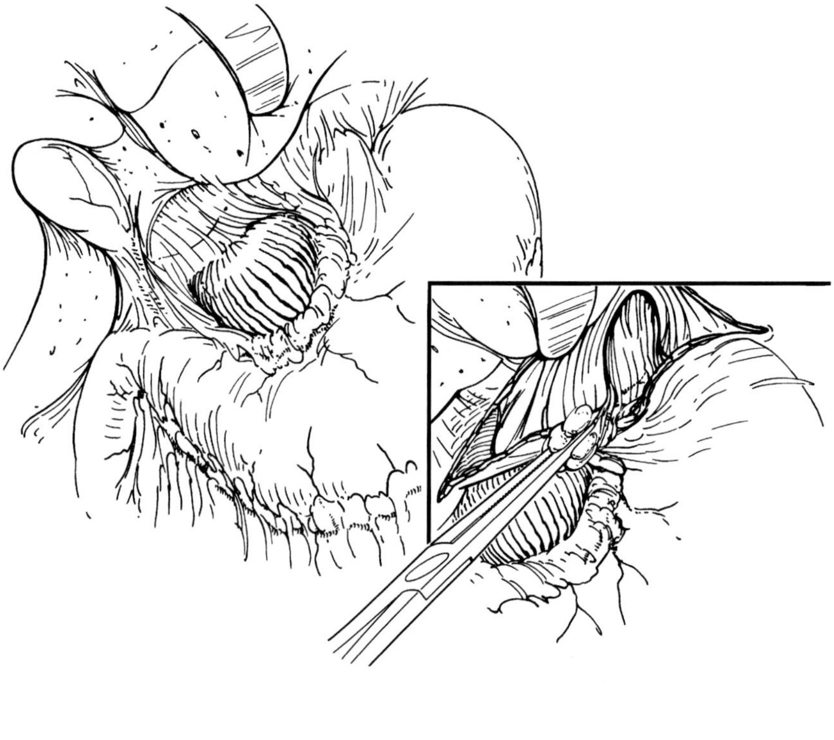

Figure 14–16. Mobilization of the esophageal hiatus is completed by detaching the peritoneal reflection from the diaphragm.

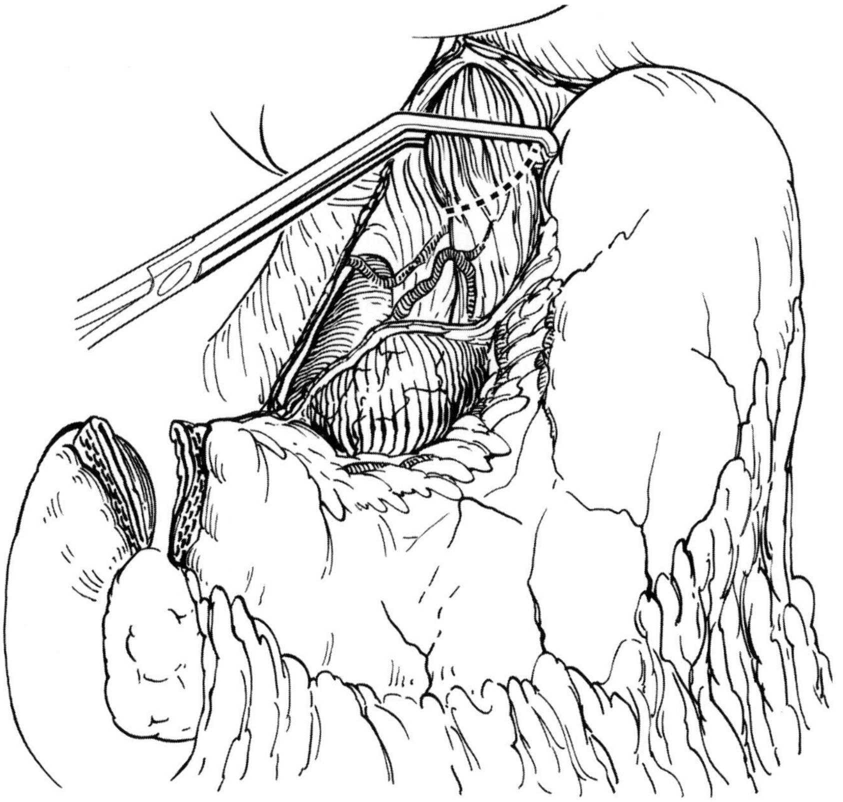

Figure 14–17. The esophagus is divided sharply by knife or scissors, usually stabilized by a noncrushing vascular clamp.

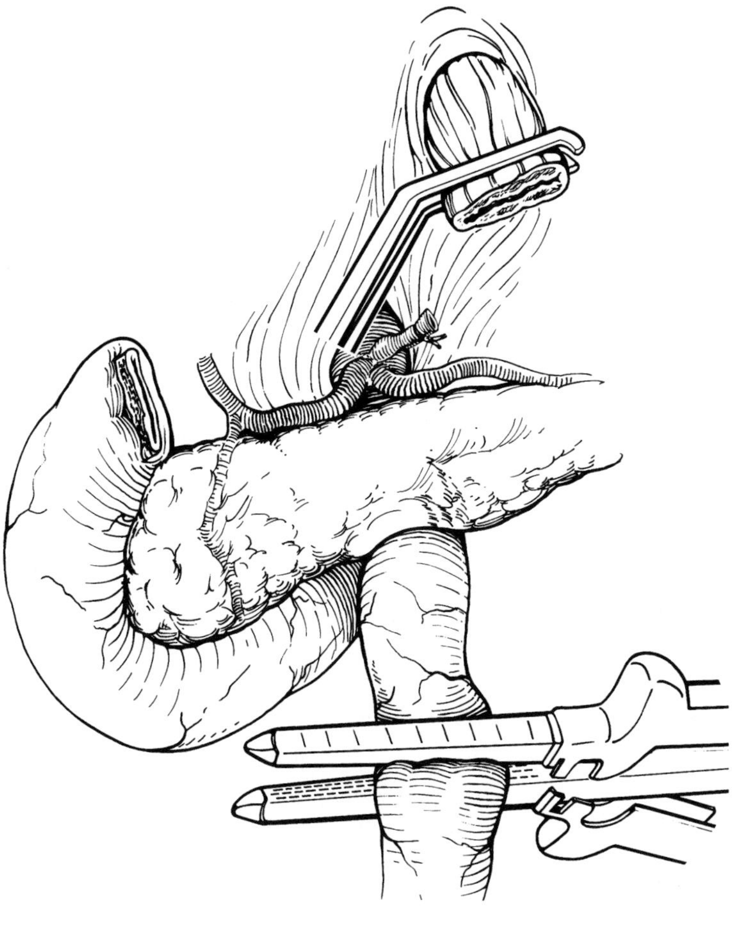

Figure 14–18. The small intestine is divided with a GIA stapler 60 to 70 cm distally.

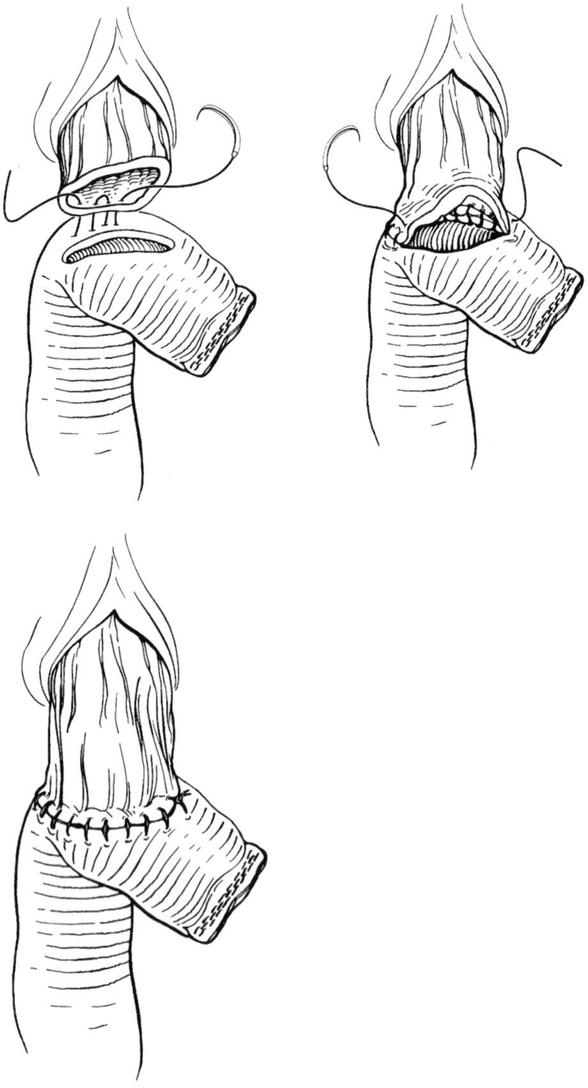

Figure 14–19. Standard end-to-side reconstruction using monofilament absorbable sutures in a single continuous layer.

testine for the Roux-en-Y anastomosis is divided with the stapler. Attention should be paid to ensure adequate vascularity of the limb, and some require careful transillumination to be sure that the arterial arcade is maintained without subsequent tension. The reconstruction can be performed by a direct end of esophagus to jejunum anastomosis (Figs 14–19 and 14–20). It is helpful in the sutured anastomosis to place a single stabilizing suture in the posterior aspect of the esophagus, suturing the posterior aspect to the posterior surface of the jejunum, which stabilizes and aligns the appropriate reconstruction. I then begin in the midline posteriorly with a running over-and-over suture tied anteriorly. An alternative reconstruction uses the EEA stapler (Figs 14–21 and 14–22).

Reconstruction with the EEA stapler requires (see Fig 14–21A) the placement of a purse-string suture, which now can be performed with a purse-string applicator instrument. The head of the stapler (see Fig 14–21B) is placed in the esophagus and the purse string tied. The anvil of the stapler is placed through the divided bowel end to allow closure and firing (see Fig 14–21B). The open bowel limb can be closed by a stapler once two adequate "donuts" have been obtained (see Fig 14–21D).

An alternative approach providing an end-to-end stapled anastomosis is shown in Figure 14–22. This requires a more distal enterostomy site in the small bowel loop, with the prior standard proximal purse string on the esophagus. This can be more difficult, requiring a much greater length of passage of the bulky stapler through the small bowel, with some risk of mucosal laceration. Most patients readily take a 28F stapler, but many prefer the smaller 25F instrument to allow ease of passage through the small intestine.

CREATION OF A POUCH

Much debate is held about the creation of a pouch to increase capacity. In most patients, this is probably not necessary, although when the prognosis is expected to be very good, e.g., in a total gastrectomy for an early

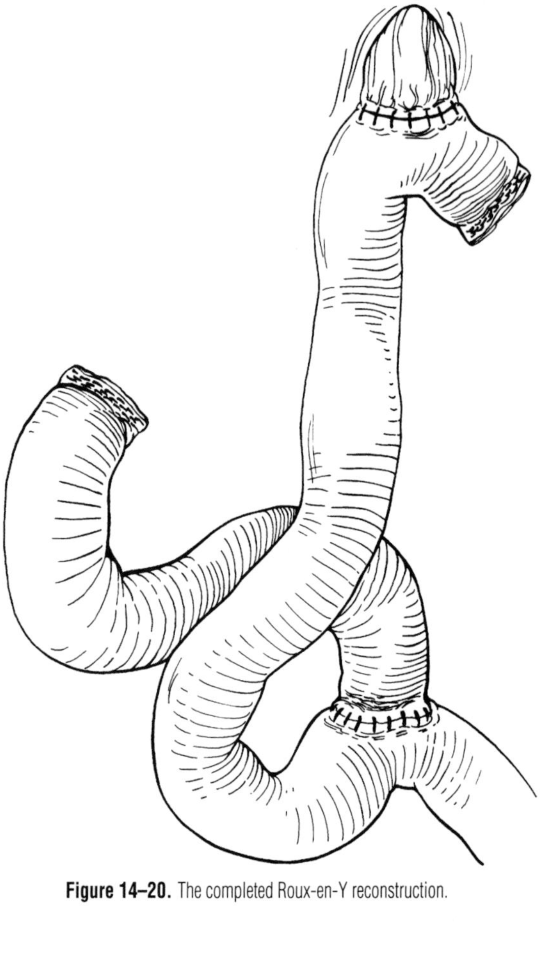

Figure 14–20. The completed Roux-en-Y reconstruction.

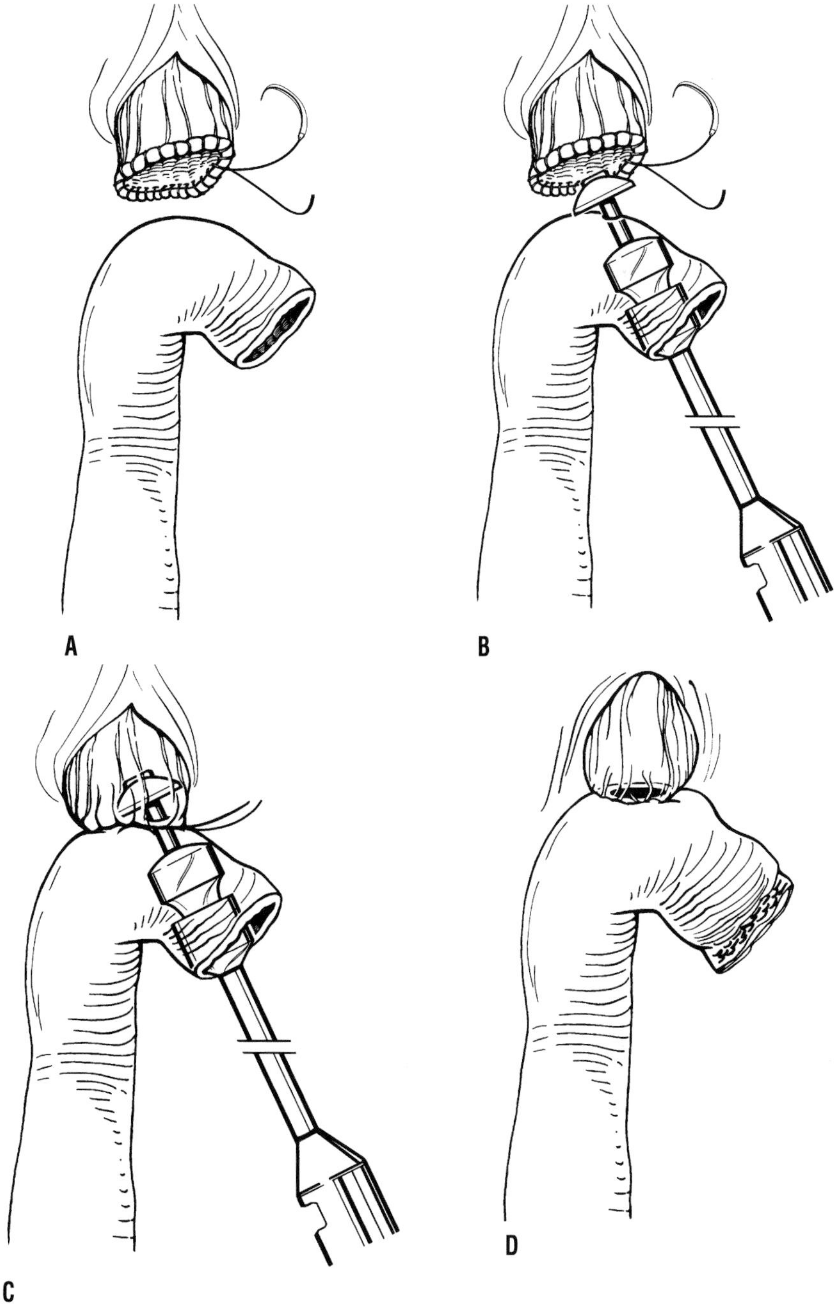

Figure 14–21. Reconstruction using the EEA stapler. **A.** Placement of a full-thickness running suture or using a purse-string applicator. **B.** Placement of the EEA stapler through the divided loop. **C.** Closer of the stapler. **D.** Staple line.

gastric cancer with extensive metaplasia or familial gastric cancer, a simple pouch as outlined in Figure 14–23 can be used. I prefer to make this pouch by two passages of the GIA stapler, and then I perform the esophagojejunal anastomosis. This is technically simple because the pouch can be made in the field. If the anastomosis is made first, then it is sometimes awkward to create the pouch more distally. Multiple other options for pouch formation are available, and these are outlined in Figures 14–24 and 14–25.

DETERMINATION OF PROXIMAL MARGIN FROZEN SECTION

I reserve the proximal margin frozen section for situations where the procedure would be changed should the margin prove positive. My colleagues and I have shown previously that in patients with advanced disease, i.e., greater than five nodes positive, a positive microscopic margin, provided that the gross margin is negative, has not had an impact on survival.[14] Often the positive margin is not the mucosal margin but is the ex-

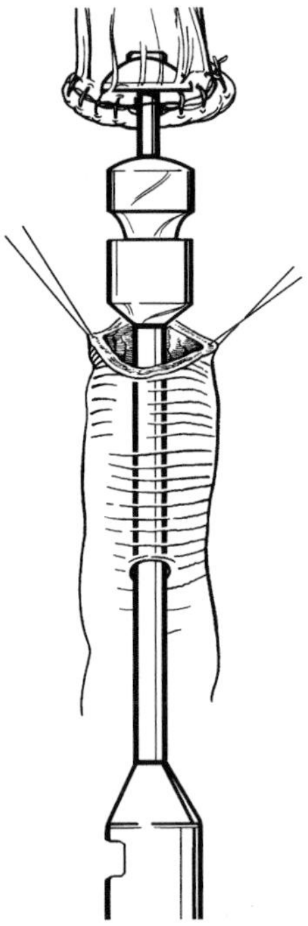

Figure 14–22. Alternative reconstruction with the EEA stapler using a separate enterotomy and end-to-end anastomosis.

tensive perigastric infiltration of the soft tissues outside the mucosa and into the musculature of the esophagus of advanced lesions. In the situation, where the margin is positive but the lesion early, with the absence of proven nodal disease, it may be necessary to convert the procedure to a thoracoabdominal incision or the standard Ivor-Lewis approach (see Chapter 9).

PROXIMAL GASTRECTOMY

Proximal gastrectomy is an operation that has been viewed with some cynicism historically, based mainly on the concept that with any intrathoracic anastomosis, alkaline reflux is a problem. However, in my experience, proximal gastrectomy is an adequate operation, particularly if done subdiaphragmatically. I have not encountered the problems of reflux that have been suggested previously. However, many patients may be asymptomatic but have evidence of alkaline reflux esophagitis or gastritis on routine endoscopy. As a cancer operation, proximal gastrectomy is receiving increasing support in various parts of the world. My colleagues and I have previously published[15] the results of a comparison between proximal gastrectomy and total gastrectomy for patients with proximal gastric adenocarcinoma. No difference in survival was found, as would be expected between proximal gastrectomy and total gastrectomy. This is consistent with other randomized trials where the extent of gastrectomy is not a factor in outcome. I believe that proximal gastrectomy is an operation that is of value for patients with proximal gastric (cardia) and localized GE junction lesions (Siewert types II and

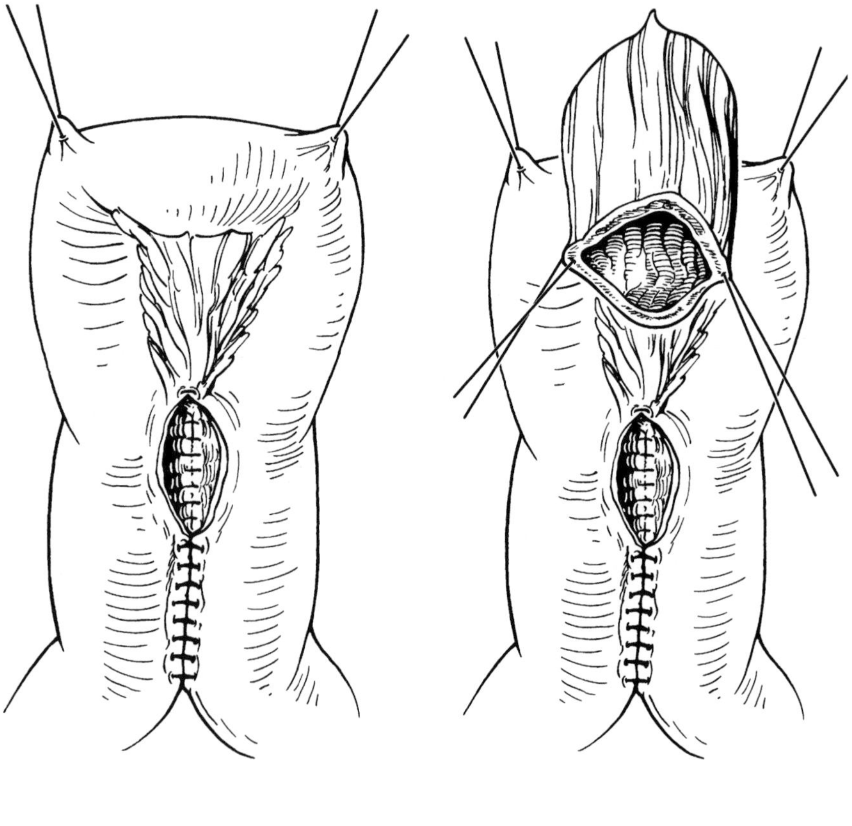

Figure 14–23. The creation of a pouch is rarely necessary but can be simply performed using a GIA stapler to approximate two loops.

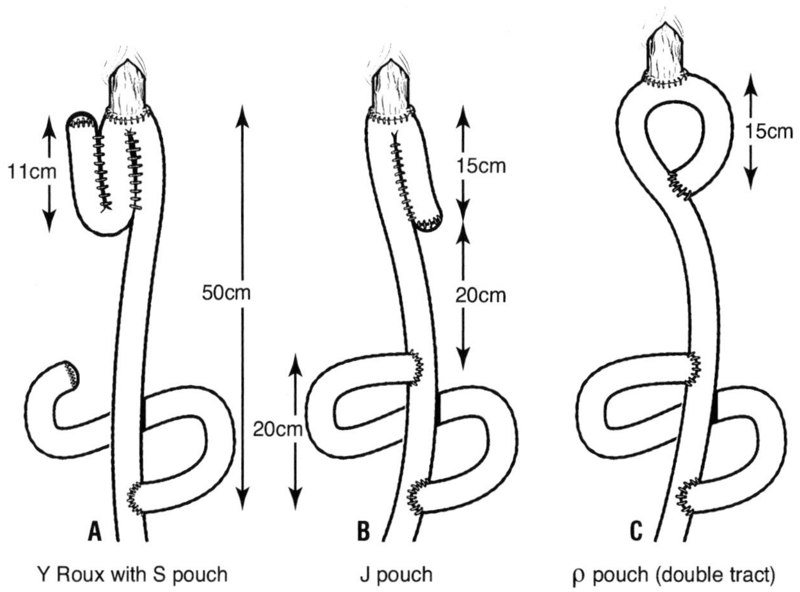

Figure 14–24. A. S-pouch reconstruction with Roux-en-Y drainage of duodenum. **B.** J-pouch with proximal and distal drainage of duodenum into efferent loop. **C.** ρ-pouch reconstruction with proximal and distal drainage of duodenum into efferent loop. Esophagojejunostomy to free limb of 2 × 15 cm jejunal loop.

III). Many still prefer total gastrectomy for all proximal lesions.[16] Consideration prior to the procedure must be given to whether it is likely that the chest will need to be entered if the lesion extends over a significant portion of the esophagus.

Technique of Proximal Gastrectomy

With accurate preoperative staging, this usually can be determined ahead of time, and I prefer an approach by a simple midline incision. The left lateral segment of the liver is taken down and retracted, the esophageal hiatus is identified, and the soft tissue around the diaphragmatic hiatus is incised. The extent of the lesion is appreciated rapidly, and on occasion, local invasion into the crura of the diaphragm may need crural resection. The retroperitoneal attachments to the diaphragm on the left side then are incised, coming down toward the anterior surface of the left adrenal gland. Once the esophagus is mobilized, it can be retracted upward and forward, and a decision can be made as to the extent of resection required.

For cardiac lesions that are locally extensive, the spleen is mobilized and taken with the specimen. In more localized lesions, the short gastric vessels are taken close to the splenic hilum to enable greater mobilization. On the right side, the right crus is cleared, and all tissue is taken back to the celiac axis origin. The section then is carried forward along the anterior surface of the celiac axis to identify the left gastric artery.

Depending on the extent of the lesion, the nodal dissection can be focused on just the left gastric vessels and the proximal celiac axis or can be extended more distally. In the majority of patients, all lymph nodes along the lesser curvature can be dissected readily and reflected back toward the proximal gastrectomy with the specimen. Care must be taken not to devascularize the lesser curvature. An appropriate distal site on the greater curvature is identified, and the stomach is divided with two passages of the GIA-60 or TA stapler. This can be done in an oblique fashion so as to create a relative tube of the distal stomach (Fig 14–26). Dissection continues back into the diaphragmatic hiatus, and I prefer to divide the esophagus below a soft Satinsky clamp. Where appropriate, frozen-section

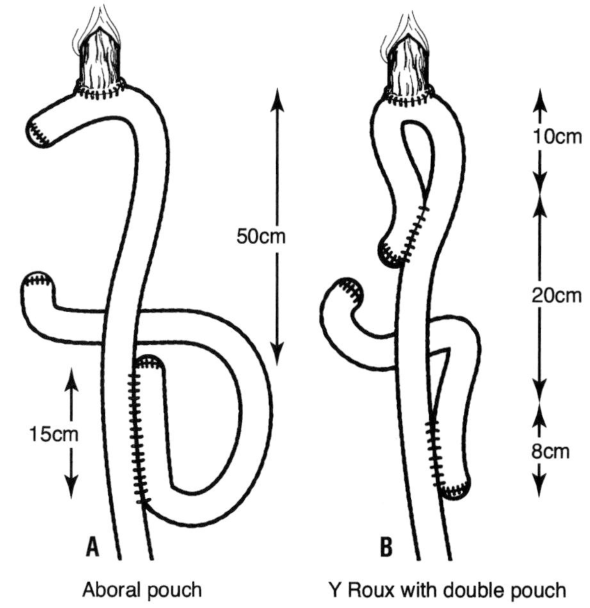

Figure 14–25. A. Distal-pouch reconstruction without preservation of duodenal transit; formation of one large 15-cm pouch by extension of the Roux anastomosis. **B.** Double-pouch reconstruction without preservation of duodenal transit; proximal 10-cm pouch with free jejunal limb and small (8-cm) distal pouch at extended Roux anastomosis.

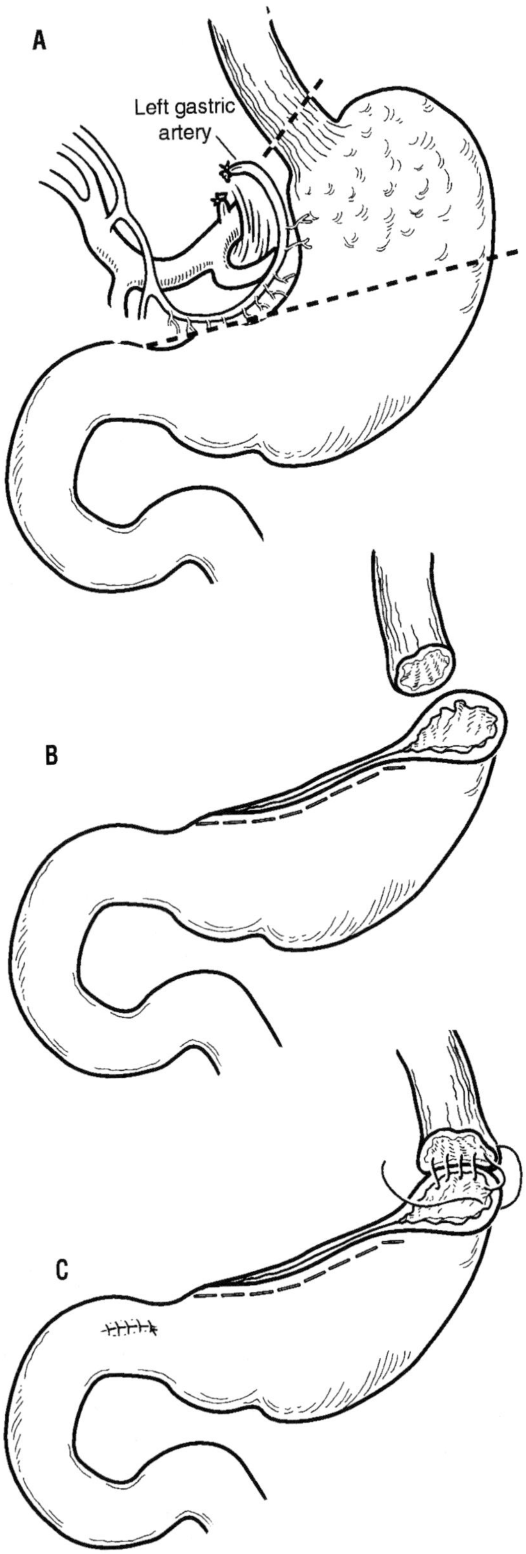

Figure 14–26. A. The esophagus is divided, the node-bearing tissue on the lesser curvature of the stomach is dissected from the crus back to the celiac artery origin, and the left gastric artery is divided. The greater curvature and proximal nodes are included with the specimen. The stomach is divided with the stapler. **B, C.** The reconstruction is done in simple fashion by dividing the transected suture line at the greater-curvature apex and performing a simple end-to-end running anastomosis with 3-0 PDS sutures; best secured with a posterior stay suture at the initiation, a pyloroplasty is performed.

margins are taken (see above), and further resection of the esophagus is performed if the margin is inadequate. It is clear that microscopic positive margins are of limited significance in patients with extensive multinodal disease.[14] As the specimen is removed, the reconstruction can be done in simple fashion by dividing the transected suture line at the greater-curvature apex and performing a simple end-to-end running anastomosis with running 3-0 PDS sutures best secured with a posterior stay suture at the initiation (Fig 14–26). Conversely, a second incision can be made in the anterior surface of the stomach, stay sutures can be applied posteriorly, and the esophagus can be sewn directly into the anterior surface of the stomach (Fig 14–27). It is important to recognize when the latter procedure is performed that the distal stomach performs a partial posterior wrap to the intra-abdominal esophagus. All other aspects of the resection remain as for other procedures. Alternately, a transgastric end-to-end anastomosis can be made with a stapler. The extent of the nodal dissection is determined by the site of the tumor and the expected nodal draining areas. A simple pyloroplasty or pyloromyotomy is performed.

EXTENT OF LYMPH NODE DISSECTION

The extent of lymph node involvement can be predicted by the site of the primary lesion (Fig 14–28). The extent of the node dissection then can be standarized to that approach, as described earlier. Progressively, rather than characterizing individual nodal stations, as has been

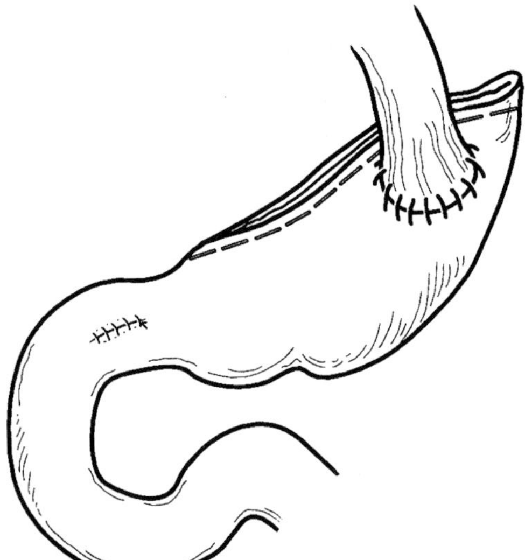

Figure 14–27. A second incision can be made in the anterior surface of the stomach, stay sutures are applied posteriorly, and the esophagus is sewn directly into the anterior surface of the stomach.

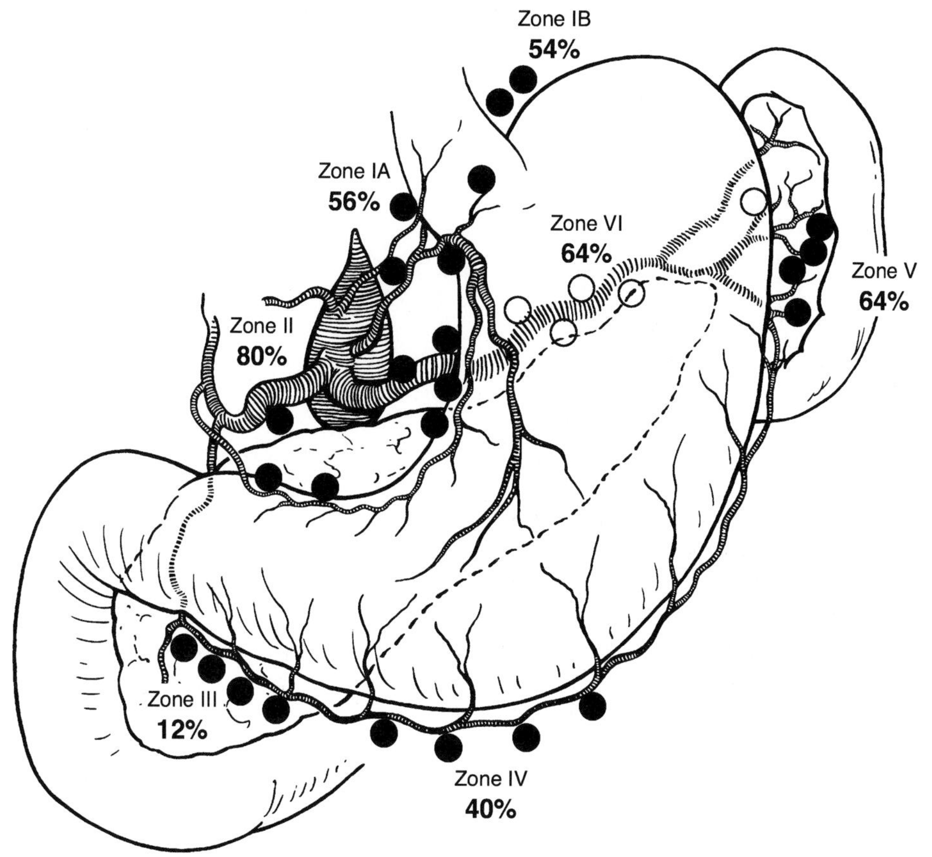

Figure 14–28. Proximal gastric cancer node-bearing areas.

done based on extensive studies by the Japanese, it has become imperative that at least 15 lymph nodes be sampled to give adequate staging. With 15 nodes sampled, accurate N staging can be obtained: with N1, one to five nodes positive; with N2, six to 15 nodes positive; with N3, greater than 15 nodes positive. Clear differences in outcome can be based solely on the number of negative nodes identified, which in essence affirms the accuracy of the extent of actual nodal involvement. The accuracy of this approach has been established by comparative studies between the site of the positive nodes and the number of positive nodes (Fig 14–29).

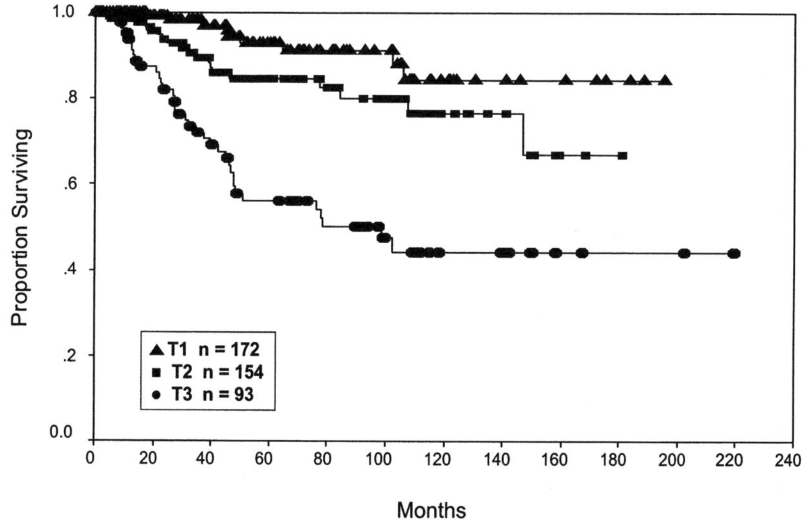

Figure 14–29. Gastric adenocarcinoma survival for N0 by T stage with more than 15 nodes sampled (staging by number of nodes positive). Memorial Sloan-Kettering Cancer Center, 7/1/1985–6/30/2004 ($n = 419$).

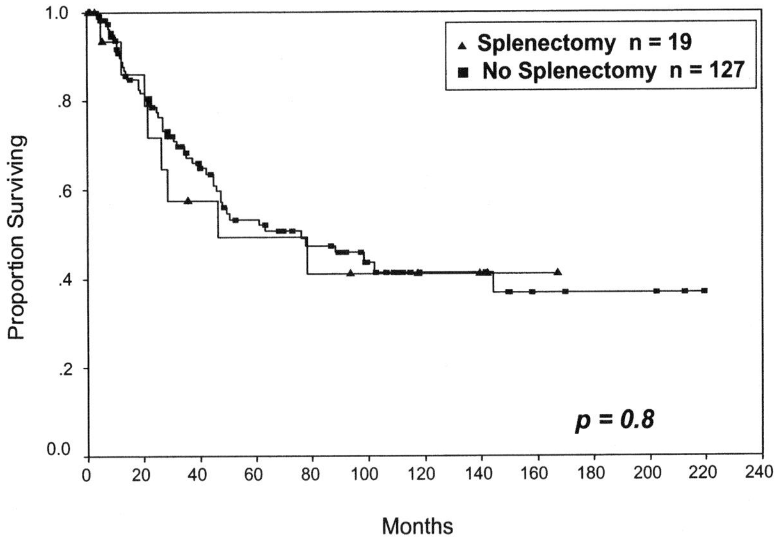

Figure 14–30. Gastric adenocarcinoma R_0-resected survival in T3N0 stage—influence of splenectomy. Memorial Sloan-Kettering Cancer Center, 7/1/1985–6/30/2004 ($n = 146$).

EXTENDED GASTRIC RESECTIONS

It is now clear that anything less than an R_0 resection does not translate into significant survival benefit for the patient with gastric cancer. Consistent with this approach is whether or not more extended resections, which would allow an R_0 resection, can improve survival. The most common organs resected in extended resections are the spleen and pancreas. These almost invariably occur in patients with large legions, more extensive T stage, and a higher incidence of advanced nodal disease.

The relevance of splenic resection has been debated widely, with most authors suggesting that splenectomy is associated with a poorer outcome. Certainly in the Dutch randomized trial, morbidity in patients with splenectomy was 32.7% and mortality 12.7% compared to patients who did not have splenectomy, in whom morbidity and mortality were 10.8% and 4.8%, respectively. In my own experience, however, when one corrects for nodal status, the survival of T3N0 patients is not altered by splenectomy (Fig 14–30). Five-year survival for patients with R_0 resections for T3N1 lesions was 34% in the absence of splenectomy and 23% for patients with splenectomy (Fig 14–31).

Standard resections for T3 and T4 disease are accompanied by a 27% survival when an additional organ resection is required.[17] However, if an R_0 resection can be achieved, then the outcome depends solely on the extent of the T stage and N stage. Extended operations therefore can be encouraged when an R_0 resection results, and morbidity is low.

Patterns of postoperative care vary widely between institutions. I rarely use nasogastric suction for more

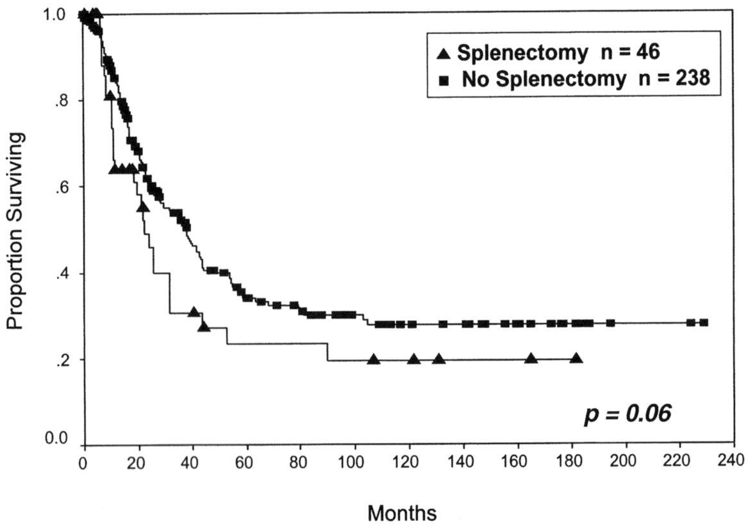

Figure 14–31. Gastric adenocarcinoma R_0-resected survival in T3N1 stage—influence of splenectomy. Memorial Sloan-Kettering Cancer Center, 7/1/1985–6/30/2004 ($n = 284$).

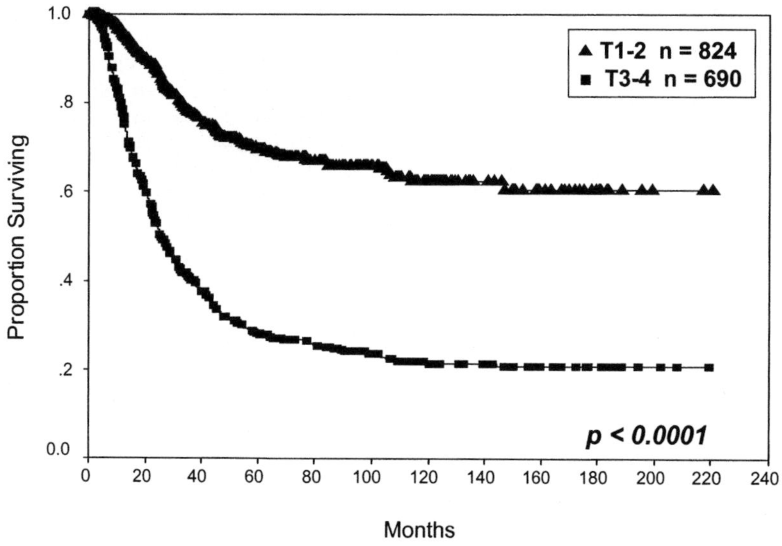

Figure 14–32. Survival by T classification and resections for primary gastric adenocarcinoma. Memorial Sloan-Kettering Cancer Center, 7/1/1985–6/30/2004 ($n = 1514$).

than 24 hours, whereas others deem it mandatory.[18] In the absence of benefit, I do not use intraperitoneal drains.[19] The routine application of postoperative nutritional support has not been shown to be beneficial in randomized trials.[20,21] Postgastrectomy deficiency states have been defined, with weight loss common initially and then stabilizing at a less than preoperative level. Vitamin B_{12}, folate, and iron supplementation is required for patients following total gastrectomy.

Operative mortality and morbidity, as with other major operations, are volume-dependent.[22] Results in high-volume centers by high-volume surgeons are clearly better than in low-volume centers, with operative mortality being decreased fourfold.[23]

■ SURGICAL RESULTS

Survival is the ultimate absolute outcome measure, but Western society rarely has matched the results of those seen in Japan. More recently, however, in specialized centers, results have begun to parallel those seen in Japan.

Dominant factors in outcome are T stage, N stage, presence or absence of complications, and histologic grade. When examined by T stage, the results show a clear differentiation between T1–2 and T3–4 lesions (Fig 14–32) and N stage (Fig 14–33). As mentioned previously, the extent of gastric resection has not been shown to influence outcome, so where infradiaphragmatic proximal gastric resection can be performed, it can be justified.[15] It is important

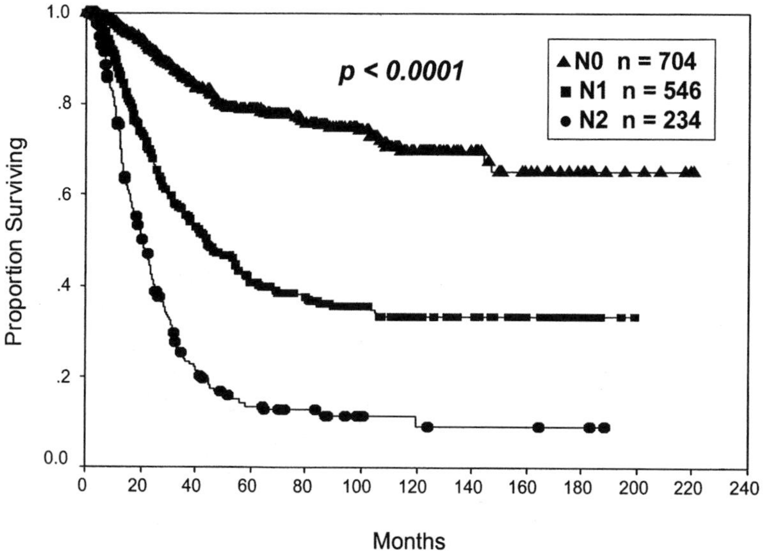

Figure 14–33. Survival by N classification and resections for primary gastric adenocarcinoma. Memorial Sloan-Kettering Cancer Center, 7/1/1985–6/30/2004 ($n = 1484$).

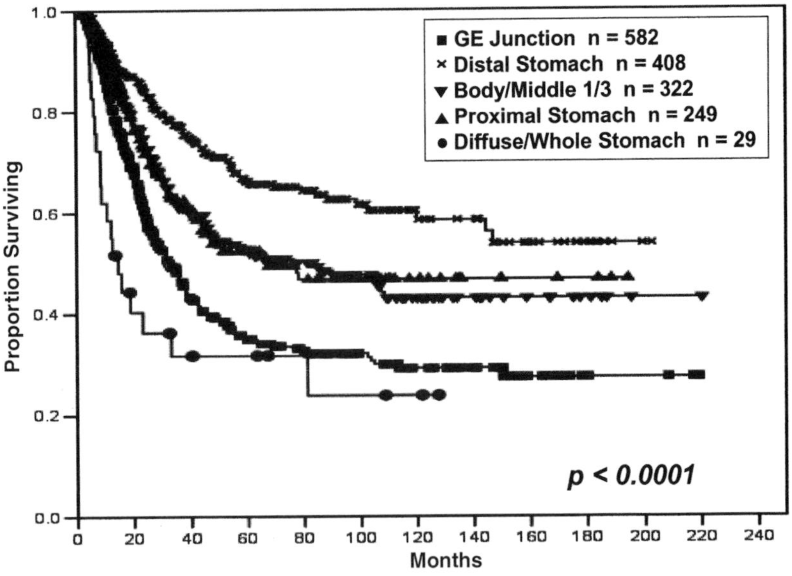

Figure 14–34. Survival by site. R_0 resections for primary gastric adenocarcinoma includes all patients with any node dissection. Memorial Sloan-Kettering Cancer Center, 7/1/1985–6/30/2004 ($n = 1590$).

that I emphasize that site appears to be a variable in outcome that is not readily explained by either extent of the lesion or extent of the operative procedure (Fig 14–34).

SURVIVAL VERSUS STAGE

It is important to emphasize that there is a relationship between depth of invasion (T stage) and nodal involvement (N stage). Advancing T stage predicts increasing N stage.

Historically, nodal staging relied on the Japanese Research Study Group for Gastric Cancer (JRSGC), with American (AJCC) and international (UICC) staging being similar. However, the JRSGC required diligent attention to identifying specific nodal testing in relation to the primary tumor site. This was well accepted and performed in Japan but rarely followed in most Western centers.

The latest staging system for the UICC and AJCC relies on the number of involved regional nodes as opposed to the specific location of such involved nodes. This approach has several obvious advantages for surgeon, patient, and pathologist. The most obvious advantage is simplicity and thereby adherence to such an approach.

As a consequence of more diligent attempts to identify at least 15 lymph nodes, stage migration can occur; i.e., with more diligent dissection and identification of involved lymph nodes, patients are placed in a higher stage than they would be if fewer nodes were removed, identified, and examined. This is a major factor in the apparent improved survival of Japanese patients over their Western counterparts. In the Dutch Gastric Cancer Trial, the performance of a D_2 dissection resulted in 30% stage migration. When such attempts are made to appropriately stage Western patients, survival rates begin to approximate those of the Japanese.

One factor rarely commented on is the relative differences in body mass index (BMI) in different countries.[24] A recent Japanese analysis[25] has shown that only 7% of their patients were obese as defined by Western standards. With a more restrictive definition, obesity was associated with increase infection, blood loss, and length of hospital stay but no difference in long-term survival.

Other factors influencing survival include age,[26] where patients under age 65 had a mortality of 3.5% and a 5-year survival of 62% and patients over age 80 had a 15.2% mortality and 22% 5-year survival. When I look at my own data, the mortality for patients younger than age 65 was 5%; ages 65–75, 2%; and over age 75, 8%.

The influence of surgical volume on outcome has been studied. My colleagues and I showed that low surgical volume and low hospital volume were strongly associated with increased mortality.[22] For gastric cancer in New York State, this has been examined,[23] with operative mortality in low-volume hospitals 11.16% compared with high-volume hospitals at 2.85%, a risk-adjusted rate increase of 7.1.

With the advent of nomograms, multiple factors in addition to T and N stage can be evaluated for individual patient undergoing an R_0 resection. This provides a useful tool for the practicing clinician to predict outcome.[27] Such nomograms developed from my data set now have been validated by other national and international[28] databases.

REFERENCES

1. Parkin DM, Whelan SL, Ferlay J, et al (eds). *Cancer Incidence in Five Continents,* Vol VIII. Lyon, France: International Agency for Research on Cancer; 2002

2. Lawrence W Jr, Menck HR, Steele G Jr, et al. The National Cancer Data Base report on gastric cancer. *Cancer* 1995;75:1734–1744
3. Schwarz RE, Karpeh MS, Brennan MF. Surgical management of gastric cancer: The Western experience. In: Hennessy PJ, Daly JM, Reynolds JV (eds). *Management of Upper Gastrointestinal Cancer.* New York: Harcourt Brace; 1999:84–107
4. Charlton A, Blair V, Shaw D, et al. Hereditary diffuse gastric cancer: Predominance of multiple foci of signet ring cell carcinoma in distal stomach and transitional zone. *Gut* 2004;53:814–820
5. Guilford P, Hopkins J, Harraway J, et al. *E-cadherin* germline mutations in familial gastric cancer. *Nature* 1998; 392:402–405
6. Shaw D, Blair V, Martin IG. Chromoendoscopic surveillance in a Maori kindred genotypically predisposed to hereditary diffuse gastric cancer: An alternative to prophylactic gastrectomy. *Gastrointest Endosc* 2003;57: AB158
7. Forman D. *Helicobacter pylori* and gastric cancer. *Scand J Gastroenterol Suppl* 1996;215:48–51
8. Tio TL, Schouwink MH, Cikot RJ, et al. Preoperative TNM classification of gastric carcinoma by endosonography in comparison with the pathological TNM system: A prospective study of 72 cases. *Hepatogastroenterology* 1989;36:51–56
9. Botet JF, Lightdale CJ, Zauber AG, et al. Preoperative staging of gastric cancer: Comparison of endoscopic US and dynamic CT. *Radiology* 1991;181:426–432
10. Bentrem D, Gerdes H, Brennan MF, et al. Clinical correlation of endoscopic ultrasound with pathologic stage and outcome in patients undergoing curative resection for gastric cancer. *Ann Surg Oncol* (submitted)
11. Sarela AI, Turnbull AD, Coit DG, et al. Accurate lymph node staging is of greater prognostic importance than subclassification of the T2 category for gastric adenocarcinoma. *Ann Surg Oncol* 2003;10:783–791
12. Burke EC, Karpeh MS, Conlon KC, et al. Laparoscopy in the management of gastric adenocarcinoma. *Ann Surg* 1997;225:262–267
13. Cuschieri A. Laparoscopic gastric resection. *Surg Clin North Am* 2000;80:1269–1284
14. Kim SH, Karpeh MS, Klimstra DS, et al. Effect of microscopic resection line disease on gastric cancer survival. *J Gastrointest Surg* 1999;3:24–33
15. Harrison LE, Karpeh MS, Brennan MF. Proximal gastric cancers resected via a transabdominal-only approach: Results and comparisons to distal adenocarcinoma of the stomach. *Ann Surg* 1997;225:678–685
16. Ito H, Clancy TE, Osteen RT, et al. Adenocarcinoma of the gastric cardia: What is the optimal surgical approach? *J Am Coll Surg* 2004;199:880–886
17. Martin RCG, Jaques DP, Brennan MF, et al. Extended local resection for advanced gastric cancer: Increased survival versus increased morbidity. *Ann Surg* 2002;236: 159–165
18. Doglietto GB, Papa V, Tortorelli AP, et al. Nasojejunal tube placement after total gastrectomy: A multicenter prospective, randomized trial. *Arch Surg* 2004;139:1309–1313
19. Conlon KC, Labow D. Leung D, et al. Prospective, randomized clinical trial of the value of intraperitoneal drainage after pancreatic resection. *Ann Surg* 2001;234: 487–494
20. Heslin MJ, Latkany L, Leung D, et al. A prospective, randomized trial of early enteral feeding after resection of upper GI malignancy. *Ann Surg* 1997;226:567–580
21. Brennan MF, Pisters PWT, Posner MC, et al. A prospective, randomized trial of total parenteral nutrition following major pancreatic resection for malignancy. *Ann Surg* 1994;22:436–444
22. Begg CB, Cramer LD, Hoskins WJ, et al. Impact of hospital volume on operative mortality for major cancer surgery. *JAMA* 1998;280:1747–1751
23. Hannan EL, Radzyner M, Rubin D, et al. The influence of hospital and surgeon volume on in-hospital mortality for colectomy, gastrectomy and lung lobectomy in patients with cancer. *Surgery* 2002;131:6–15
24. Noguchi Y, Yoshikawa T, Tsuburaya A, et al. Is gastric cancer different between Japan and the United States? A comparison of patient survival among three institutions. *Cancer* 2000;89:2237–2246
25. Kodera Y, Ito S, Yamamura Y, et al. Obesity and outcome of distal gastrectomy with D2 lymphadenectomy for carcinoma. *Hepatogastroenterology* 2004;51:1225–1228
26. Kranenbarg EK, van de Velde CJ. Gastric cancer in the elderly. *Eur J Surg Oncol* 1998;24:384–390
27. Karpeh MS, Leon L, Klimstra D, et al. Lymph node staging in gastric cancer: Is location more important than number? An analysis of 1038 patients. *Ann Surgery* 2000; 232:362–371
28. Peeters KCMJ, Kattan MW, Hartgrink HH, et al. Validation of a nomogram for predicting disease-specific survival following a R_0 resection for gastric cancer. *Cancer* 2005;103:702–707

15

Gastrointestinal Stromal Tumors

Monica M. Bertagnolli

Gastrointestinal stromal tumors (GIST) are rare malignancies. Although they are the most common sarcoma of the gastrointestinal (GI) tract, they represent only 0.2% of all GI tumors, with an annual incidence in the United States of 14.5 per million persons.[1,2] GIST have recently been the subject of considerable clinical and experimental interest, because of the identification of their activating signal (oncogenic mutation of the c-kit receptor) and the development of a therapeutic agent that suppresses tumor growth by inhibiting this signal (imatinib mesylate). The current management of these malignancies represents a proof of the principle that specific inhibition of tumor-associated receptor tyrosine kinase activity can produce effective cancer treatment. The advent of effective chemotherapy for GIST has altered, but not diminished, the role of surgery for this disease. This chapter reviews the biology of these fascinating mesenchymal tumors, and describes the new challenges in clinical management of GIST in the post-imatinib era.

■ PATHOLOGIC FEATURES

The term GIST was first employed in 1983 by Mazur and Clark to describe nonepithelial tumors of the GI tract that lacked the ultrastructural features of smooth muscle cells as well as the immunohistochemical characteristics of Schwann cells.[3] GIST exhibit heterogeneous histologic features, and are most often composed of long fascicles of bland spindle cells with pale to eosinophilic cytoplasm and rare nuclear pleomorphism. GIST occasionally exhibit epithelioid characteristics, including sheets of round- to oval-shaped cells with abundant eosinophilic cytoplasm and nuclear atypia (Fig 15–1). Based upon their histologic and immunohistochemical features, GIST are thought to arise from the interstitial cells of Cajal (ICC), which are components of the intestinal autonomic nervous system that serve as pacemakers regulating intestinal peristalsis.[4] Until recently, similarities in histology led to misclassification of many GIST as leiomyomas, leiomyosarcomas, or GI tumors of nerve cell origin (Fig 15–1).[5]

In 1998, Hirota and colleagues demonstrated gain-of-function mutations of the KIT proto-oncogene in the vast majority of GIST.[6] KIT is a receptor tyrosine kinase that is activated when bound to a ligand known as steel factor or stem cell factor.[7] KIT is important in the development and maintenance of components of hematopoiesis, gametogenesis, and intestinal pacemaker cells.[8–10] Oncogenic mutations of KIT have been identified in neoplasms corresponding to these functions, including mast cell tumors, myelofibrosis, chronic myelogenous leukemia, germ cell tumors, and GIST.[10] GIST are now identified by the near universal expression of the CD117 antigen (~95%), part of the KIT receptor, in the appropriate histopathologic context (Fig 15–2). CD117 expression is characteristic of most GIST, but not of other gastrointestinal smooth muscle tumors, which are more likely to express high levels of desmin and smooth muscle actin[1,10] (Fig 15–1). The application of CD117 staining as a diagnostic criterion for GIST has altered our understanding of the prevalence of this disease. In a population-based review of patients diagnosed with GIST prior to 2000, in-

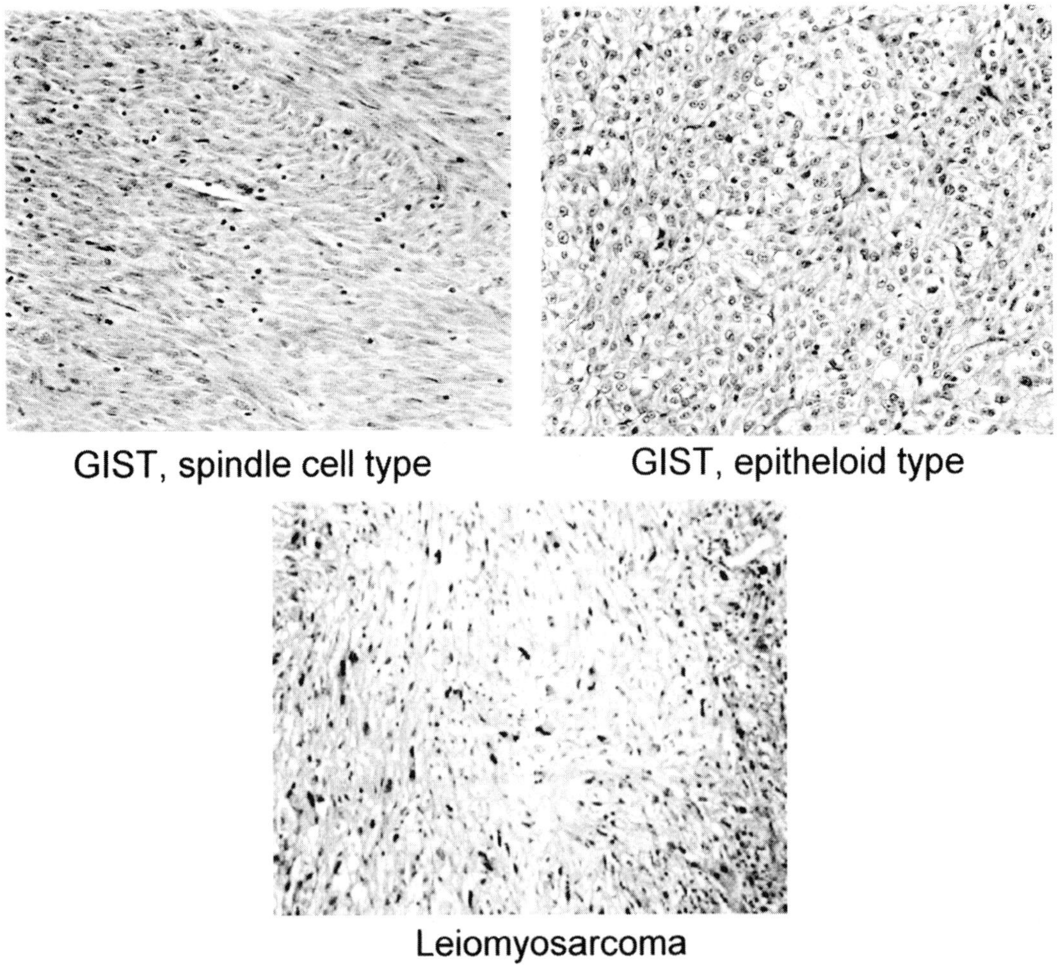

Figure 15–1. GIST histology. Staining of tumor paraffin sections with hematoxylin and eosin (H&E) reveals two patterns of GIST histology: spindle cell, and epithelioid. A comparison of the spindle cell variant of GIST and a leiomyosarcoma specimen demonstrates similarities between the two tumors by standard H&E examination. (Photos courtesy of Dr. J. Hornick, Brigham and Women's Hospital.)

vestigators in Sweden found that two thirds of these tumors had been misclassified as leiomyomas, leiomyoblastomas, or leiomyosarcomas, and only 28% were correctly identified as GIST (Table 15–1).[5]

In a small proportion of GIST, estimated at 5–10%, KIT staining may be faint or truly negative.[11,12] In these cases, a diagnosis of GIST can often be confirmed by mutational analysis of KIT, which reveals mutations of exon 11 in approximately 68% of cases and of exon 9 in 11% of GIST[13] (Fig 15–3). A small percentage of GIST (0.6–4.0%) contain mutations of KIT exons 13 or 17. Approximately 7% of GIST have gain-of-function mutations in the PDGFRA tyrosine kinase receptor.[14] Finally, a few GIST show no detectable KIT or PDGFRA mutations. Tumor progression studies suggest that, in most cases, mutation of KIT or PDGFRA is the earliest alteration in a series of genetic losses leading to GIST formation. Animal models and studies of familial GIST kindreds suggest that mutation of KIT or PDGFRA alone is not sufficient for tumor formation, although this condition does produce ICC hyperplasia.[15]

A few specific genotype-phenotype correlations have been identified for GIST. Interestingly, approximately 95% of GIST harboring exon 9 KIT mutations are of small bowel origin.[16] The transition from ICC hyperplasia to low-risk GIST is often accompanied by 14q deletion, and additional loss of 22q is frequently observed in high-risk or metastatic GIST.[15] The clinical behavior of a GIST also depends to a certain degree upon KIT or PDGFRA genotype. For example, a higher percentage of GIST with aggressive behavior contain mutations of KIT exon 9.[15]

Examination of KIT-mutant GIST has led to identification of several components of signaling downstream of the activated kinase. These include phosphorylation of the GRB and PI_3K binding sites of KIT, as well as activation of mitogen-activated protein (MAP) kinase and Akt.[14,17] Inhibitor studies also suggest activation of mammalian target of rapamycin (mTOR) signaling.[18] Studies of this type provide potential new targets of drug therapy for GIST.

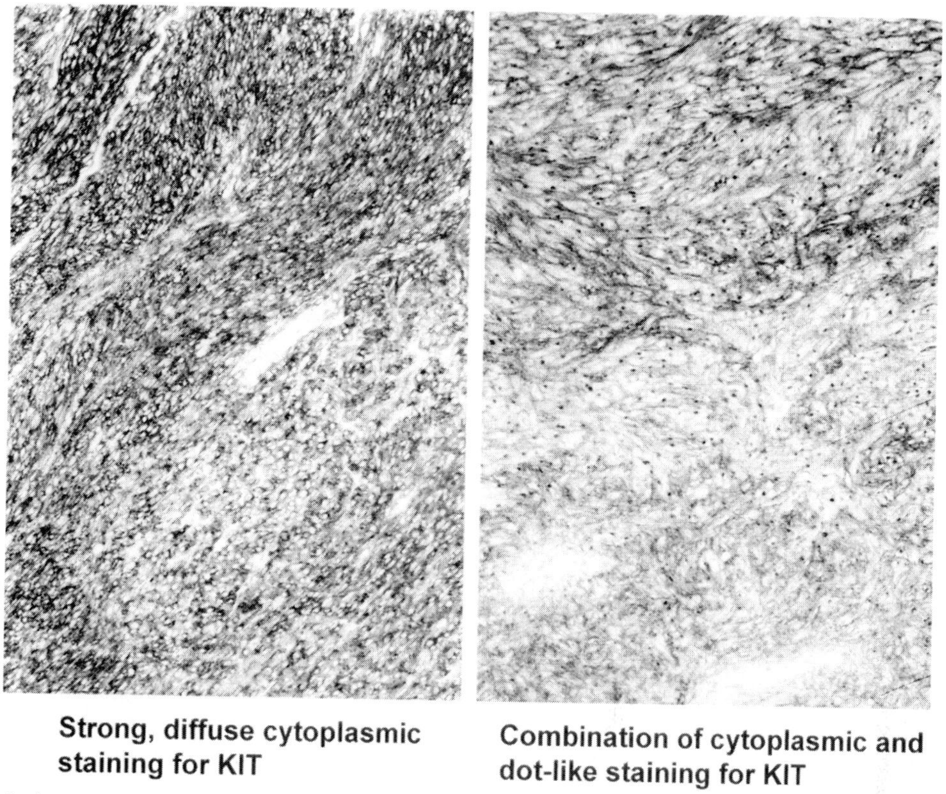

Strong, diffuse cytoplasmic staining for KIT
Combination of cytoplasmic and dot-like staining for KIT

Figure 15–2. Immunohistochemistry to detect c-KIT expression. Immunohistochemistry to detect expression of KIT (CD117) is present in approximately 95% of GIST and varies among tumors from predominantly cytoplasmic (left), to perinuclear and dot-like (bottom, right). Variable expression within a given tumor also occurs (right). (Photos courtesy of Dr. J. Hornick, Brigham and Women's Hospital.)

▪ CLINICAL PRESENTATION

Primary GIST can arise throughout the GI tract, but are most common in the stomach (40–70%), followed by small bowel (20–40%) and colorectum (5–15%), and are rarely found in the esophagus (<5%).[11] GIST usually present in patients from 40 to 60 years of age, although they have been diagnosed in children younger than age 10 years. They are equally common in men and women, and occur in all racial and ethnic groups. A very few GIST are familial, caused by an activating germline mutation of KIT. Most of these kindreds have mutations of the KIT juxtamembrane region (exon 11), and the phenotype often includes hyperpigmentation of the skin and diffuse hyperplasia of the intestinal myenteric plexus.[15] A recent report also described a kindred with GIST in which a germline mutation of PDGFRA was identified as the causative factor.[19] Carney triad is the association of paragangliomas, pulmonary chondromas, and gastric lesions that were classified as leiomyosarcomas in the initial report of this condition in seven unrelated young women.[20] Carney triad occurs predominantly in females, and affected individuals are generally diagnosed with tumors before age 30 years. The gastric tumors characteristic of this syndrome are now thought to represent multifocal GIST, based upon their morphology and the presence of KIT immunohistochemical staining. Mutational analyses, however, have failed to document the presence of activating KIT or PDGFRA mutations in patients with Carney triad.[21] A newly recognized syndrome involves the autosomal dominant transmission of a condition associated with multifocal GIST and multiple functional paragangliomas. The genetic defect responsible for this syndrome is unknown.[22] A small subset of patients with neurofibromatosis type 1 (NF1) also have multifocal GIST.[23] In the past, these tu-

TABLE 15–1. DIFFERENTIAL DIAGNOSIS OF SUBMUCOSAL TUMORS OF THE INTESTINE

Gastrointestinal stromal tumor
Leiomyoma
Leiomyosarcoma
Schwannoma
Malignant peripheral nerve sheath tumor
Solitary fibrous tumor
Inflammatory myofibroblastic tumor
Desmoid tumor (fibromatosis)
Metastatic melanoma

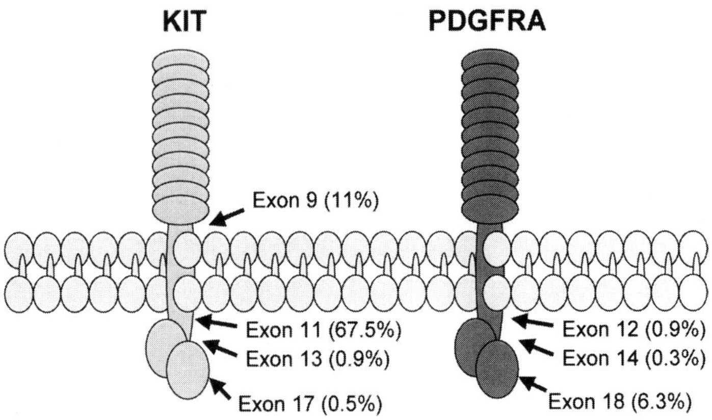

Figure 15–3. KIT and PDGFRA mutations in GIST. KIT and PDGFRA mutations in GIST produce constitutive ligand-independent receptor activation. Response to tyrosine kinase inhibitors correlates with the location of the activating mutation, with best response in patients whose tumors contain mutations in KIT exon 11.[35]

mors, which are present in approximately 7% of individuals with NF1, were frequently misclassified as leiomyomas or autonomic nerve tumors.

Many GIST are asymptomatic, discovered upon imaging or at laparotomy for other reasons. Patients with advanced disease may present with a mass lesion or vague abdominal pain, although tumors can grow to a large size before producing symptoms (Fig 15–4). GIST can be highly vascular, and bleeding is one of the more common presenting symptoms. These tumors are typically soft and friable, and can cause life-threatening hemorrhage by erosion into the intestinal lumen. Additionally, tumor rupture with intraperitoneal bleeding can occur, and this complication carries a high risk of dissemination by peritoneal seeding of the tumor. Obstruction of the GI tract is occasionally a presenting condition, and can lead to perforation. Between 15–50% of GIST present with overtly metastatic disease,[11,24] with the most common metastatic sites being liver and peritoneum. The pattern of metastatic spread is almost entirely intraabdominal, with less than 5% of patients demonstrating pulmonary metastases. GIST almost never metastasize to regional lymph nodes; however they can invade adjacent organs, the common sites being intestine, liver, or bladder. Diffuse peritoneal spread is not uncommon, and may involve innumerable small tumor nodules essentially replacing the omentum, studding the diaphragmatic surface, or covering the serosal surfaces of the bowel (Fig 15–4). In these cases, tumor-associated ascites is typical. It is not unusual to encounter tumor nodules in abdominal incisions, as a lesion that has metastasized to the peritoneum of the anterior abdominal wall can grow through the weakened tissue of a previous incision. Large, necrotic tumors occasionally form fistulas with bowel, the biliary tree, or the skin. In this setting, intratumoral abscesses or enterocutaneous fistulae can occur.

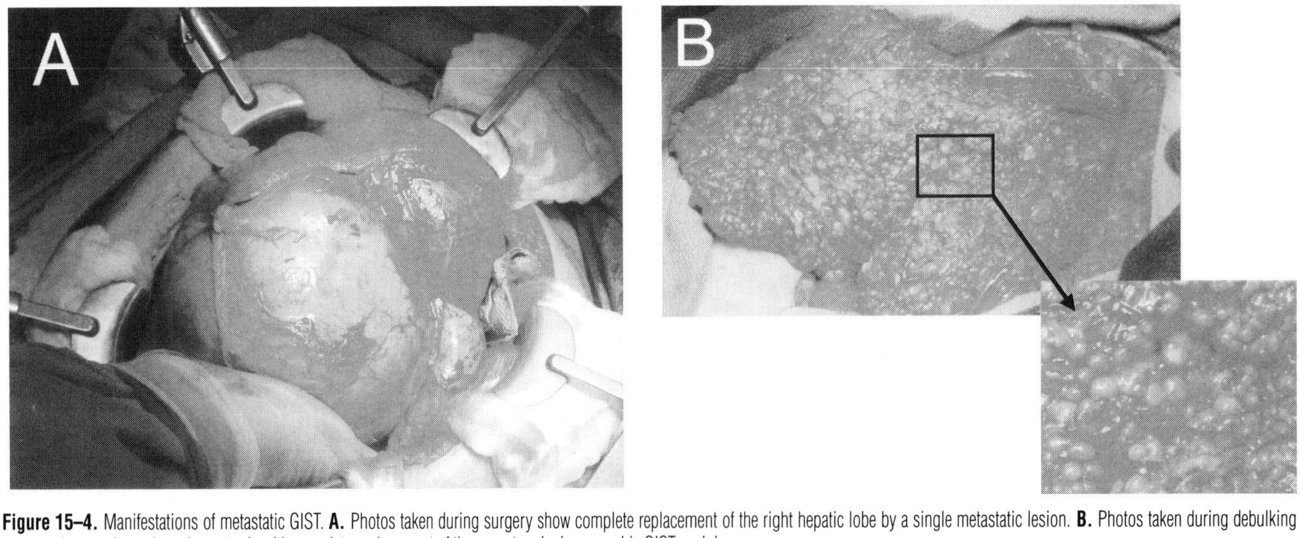

Figure 15–4. Manifestations of metastatic GIST. **A.** Photos taken during surgery show complete replacement of the right hepatic lobe by a single metastatic lesion. **B.** Photos taken during debulking surgery show peritoneal carcinomatosis with complete replacement of the omentum by innumerable GIST nodules.

■ IMAGING AND DIAGNOSTIC STUDIES

The endoscopic appearance of a primary GIST is that of a submucosal lesion, with or without ulceration, present in the upper or lower GI tract. These lesions are visually indistinguishable from other GI tumors of smooth muscle origin (Fig 15–5). Because of their submucosal location, fine-needle aspiration (FNA) or core biopsy with endoscopic ultrasound guidance is commonly required to obtain tissue for diagnosis.[25] CT scans are critical to determine the anatomic extent of a GIST and to assist with operative planning. The CT findings vary with the size of the lesions (Fig 15–6). Ghanem and colleagues[26] recently reported that small GIST have sharp margins, an intraluminal growth pattern, and are of homogenous density on both unenhanced and contrast-enhanced scans. In contrast, larger lesions have irregular margins, extraluminal growth patterns, and inhomogeneous density. Radiographic signs corresponding to aggressive malignant GIST include calcification, ulceration, necrosis, cystic areas, fistula formation, metastasis, ascites, and signs of infiltration of local tissues. Unfortunately, CT is unable to differentiate between inflammatory adhesions and malignant involvement of adjoining organs. It is also unlikely to identify any peritoneal metastasis smaller than 2 cm in diameter.

Positron emission tomography (PET) is a useful adjunct to CT for evaluating GIST, particularly as a means of assessing response to chemotherapy. Metabolically active GIST accumulate 18-fluorodeoxyglucose (^{18}FDG), and blockade of the KIT receptor results in a rapid suppression of this activity. Functional blockade of KIT activation is produced by specific inhibitors of KIT tyrosine kinase activity, such as imatinib mesylate. This orally administered drug is widely used for treatment of advanced GIST. Sequential scans prior to and following imatinib mesylate therapy reliably and rapidly indicate the responsiveness or resistance of the tumor to therapy. There is a strong correlation between early decreases in FDG-PET uptake and symptomatic improvement, both of which can occur as early as a week after starting therapy (Fig 15-7). In one study, FDG-PET uptake at 8 days after starting imatinib therapy showed a partial response in 57%, while 17% had stable disease and 24% progressed.[27] Evidence of early metabolic response by FDG-PET correlated with significant progression free survival, suggesting that this imaging can be used to guide decisions regarding systemic therapy very early in the course of treatment. As a result of these data, PET scanning to assess imatinib response is generally recommended to guide therapeutic dosing or timing of surgery, with a baseline pretreatment scan followed by a repeat scan after 2 to 4 weeks of drug therapy.

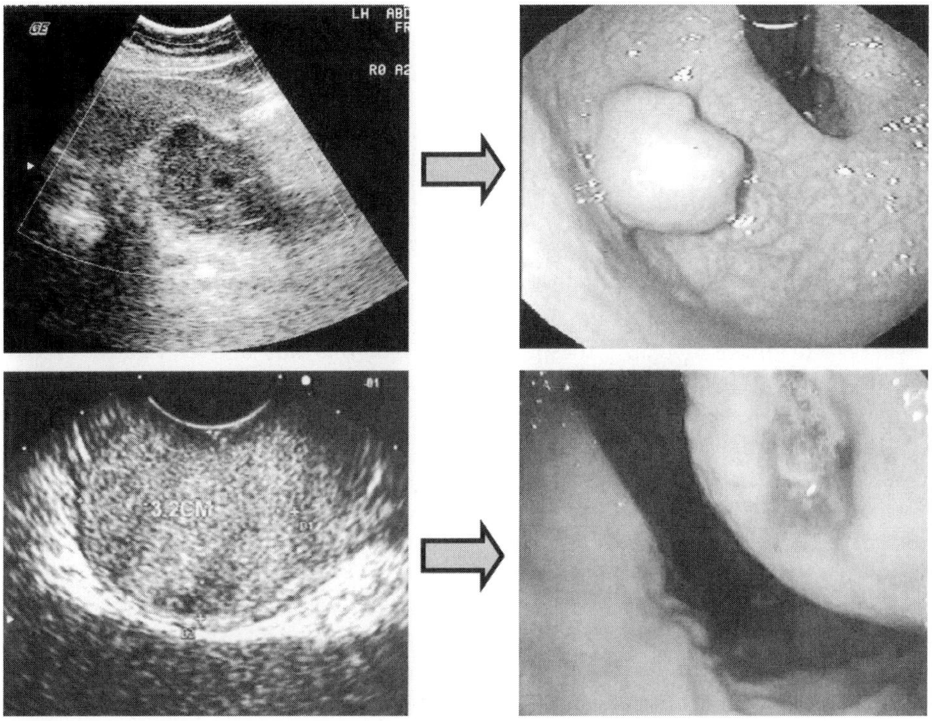

Figure 15–5. Endoscopic examination of primary gastric GIST. GIST commonly present as submucosal tumors in the wall of the GI tract. Central necrosis of high-risk tumors or erosion into blood vessels can produce local inflammation or significant GI bleeding (bottom, right). (Courtesy of Dr. W. Brugge, Massachusetts General Hospital.)

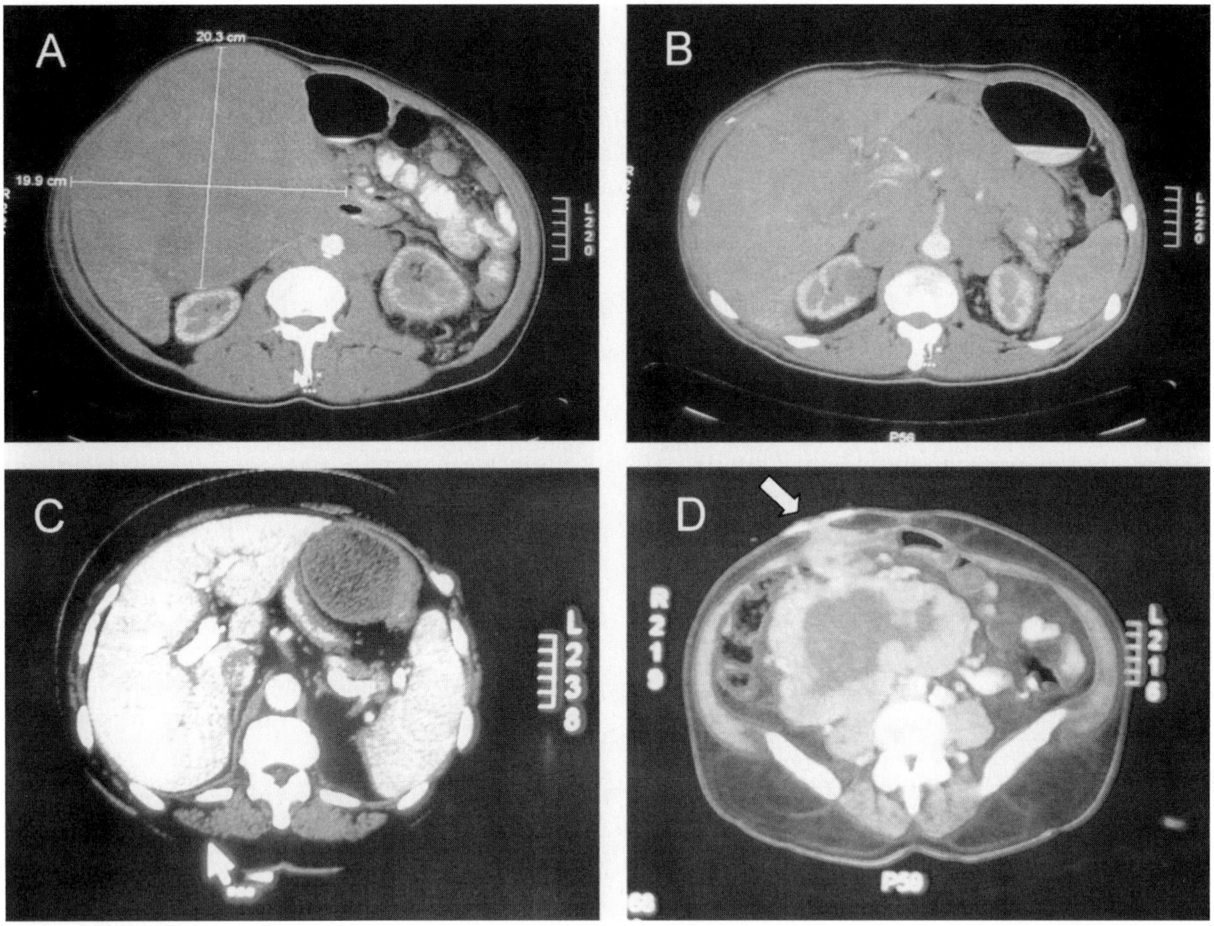

Figure 15–6. CT characteristics of GIST. Various manifestations of GIST include: **A.** large heterogeneous primary tumor; **B.** hepatic metastases with diffuse mesenteric disease; **C.** cystic lesion; and **D.** large necrotic GIST with enterocutaneous fistula.

■ PROGNOSTIC FEATURES

GIST exhibit a wide spectrum of clinical behavior. Small lesions may remain stable for years, although some lesions rapidly progress to widely metastatic disease. At the time of diagnosis of a primary tumor, features associated with a poor prognosis include large size (>5 cm) and increased mitotic activity.[1] In some studies, location of the tumor in the small bowel indicated a worse outcome.[1,28] Large retrospective studies from the pre-imatinib era showed that the 5-year disease specific survival following resection of a primary GIST larger than 10 cm was approximately 20%, versus 60% for tumors less than 5 cm in size.[29] Although tumors giving rise to metastases are generally >5 cm in diameter and have a high mitotic rate (>10 mitoses per high powered field), up to 20% of small GIST (<5 cm) exhibit metastatic behavior.[30] Additionally, lesions <2 cm and those with low mitotic rates occasionally demonstrate metastases.[1] It is difficult to label a particular GIST as either benign or malignant based upon histology alone. The recognition that all GIST have some malignant potential has now led to their classification as either low-, intermediate-, or high-risk based upon tumor size and mitotic count (Table 15–2).[1] This risk stratification was assembled by consensus during a National Institute of Health/National Cancer Institute-sponsored workshop in 2001.[1]

Correlations between KIT or PDGFRA mutational status and clinical outcome following resection of localized disease are an active area of investigation. In a report of 275 patients with resected localized primary tumors, the frequency of *KIT* exon 11 mutations in the low-risk category was 87%.[15] KIT exon 9 mutations were found in 17% of the high-risk tumors, but only 3.0% and 2.5% of the intermediate- and low-risk tumors, respectively. These data suggest that GIST arising from KIT exon 9 mutations may be more aggressive than those bearing exon 11 mutations. The relationship between surgical outcome and the presence of PDGFRA and WT KIT mutations has not been established for localized, resectable disease.

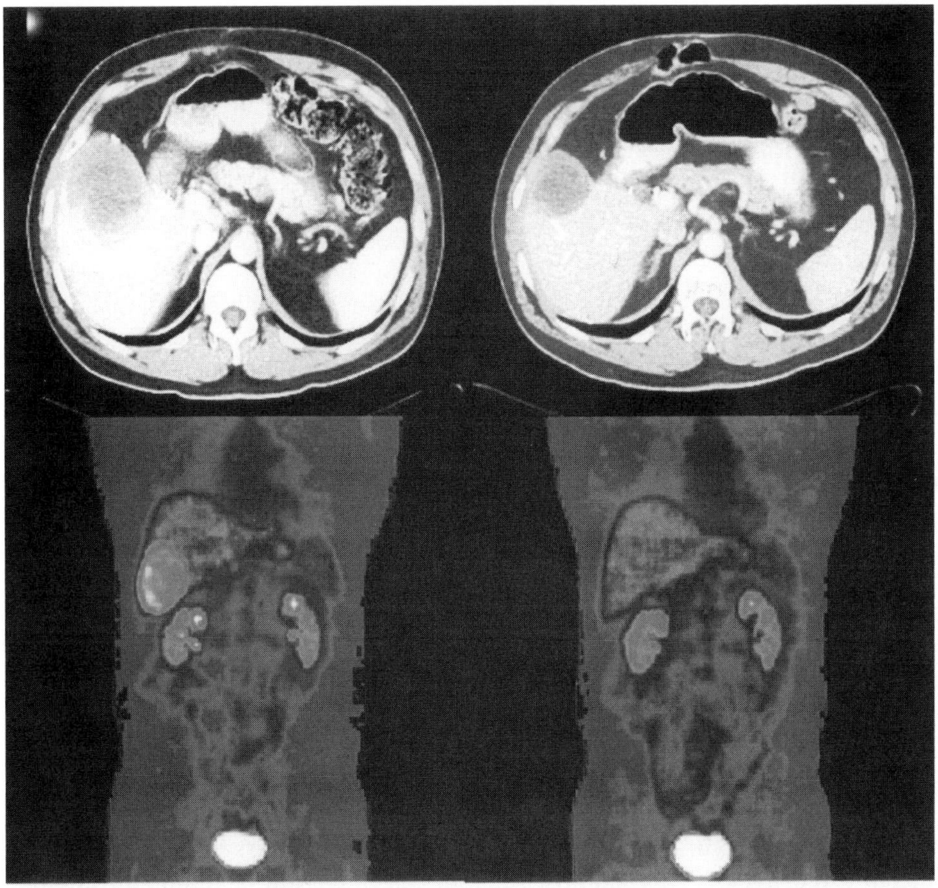

Figure 15–7. Early imatinib response indicated by ^{18}FDG-PET. Tumors responding to imatinib exhibit a marked decrease in ^{18}FDG-PET activity that is discernible within days to weeks following initiation of therapy. (Courtesy of Drs. A. van den Abbeele and G. Demetri, Dana Farber Cancer Institute.)

▪ RADIATION AND CHEMOTHERAPY OF GIST

Prior to 2001, traditional cytotoxic chemotherapy had little to offer in the management of GIST. Standard sarcoma regimens, such as those employing adriamycin and ifosfamide, achieved marginal benefit in patients with metastatic disease, and had no role in adjuvant therapy. Nonstandard regimens, such as those using intraperitoneal mitoxantrone and chemoembolization, also achieved marginal, if any, benefit. A dramatic change in the treatment of GIST occurred following the recognition that activated KIT provided the driving force for GIST growth. Under physiological conditions, binding of ligand to KIT causes dimerization of the receptor, leading to phosphorylation of intracellular proteins and transmission of a signal resulting in cell growth. Oncogenic mutations of KIT result in receptor dimerization and constitutive activation of the kinase.[6] This discovery led to the development of therapeutic agents that are relatively specific inhibitors of KIT kinase activity.

Imatinib mesylate, known commercially as Gleevec in the United States and Glivec in other countries, is a small molecule originally developed to treat chronic myelogenous leukemia (CML). In CML, tumor-promoting activity of the *BCR-ABL* fusion gene product is inhibited by imatinib, and more than 85% of patients with chronic-phase CML achieve a complete hematologic response. This orally administered drug also inhibits KIT and PDGFRA protein tyrosine kinases.[31,32] Imatinib suppresses KIT activity by lodging in an ATP-binding pocket that forms upon receptor dimerization. Unable to bind ATP, the source of the phosphate group required for phosphorylation, the kinase is rendered inactive (Fig 15–8).

TABLE 15–2. CLASSIFICATION OF PRIMARY GASTROINTESTINAL STROMAL TUMORS BY RISK OF METASTASIS[1]

Risk Category	Size	Mitotic Count
Very Low	<2 cm	<5 per 50 HPFs*
Low	2–5 cm	<5 per 50 HPFs
Intermediate	<5 cm	6–10 per 50 HPFs
	5–10 cm	<5 per 50 HPFs
High	>5 cm	>5 per 50 HPFs
	>10 cm	Any mitotic rate
	Any size	>10 per 50 HPFs

*HPF, high powered field.

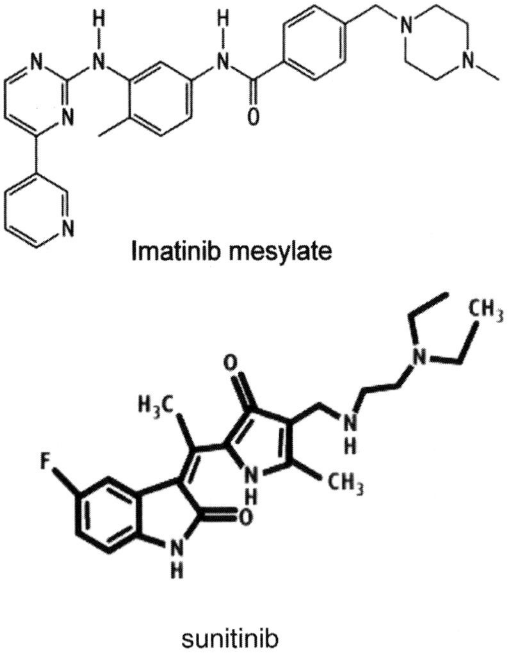

Figure 15–8. Chemical structures of imatinib mesylate (Gleevec) and sunitinib (Sutent).

Imatinib was first studied in a patient with liver metastases from GIST in March 2000. This patient experienced a dramatic antitumor response, with resolution of all cancer-related symptoms in a few weeks.[33] The first multicenter trial conducted in patients with metastatic GIST, reported in 2001, documented partial responses in 54%, stable disease in 28%, and disease progression in 14%, with a minimum follow-up of 6 months.[34] After additional studies confirming this result, imatinib was approved in Europe and the United States for use in patients with advanced or metastatic GIST. The optimal dose of imatinib therapy remains to be determined. Phase III studies comparing daily doses of 400 versus 800 mg have been completed in both the United States and Europe; however further follow-up will be required to detect any clinical differences between these dose levels. The toxicities of imatinib, which include edema, nausea, muscle cramps, diarrhea, headache, dermatitis, fatigue, anemia, and neutropenia are dose-related. Fortunately, most side effects (>70%) are mild to moderate in severity and often resolve with continuing therapy.

The location of KIT mutation correlates with response to imatinib therapy. In 121 patients studied by Heinrich and associates from the United States-Finland study, patients whose disease harbored an exon 11 mutation had a response rate of 72%, while only 32% of patients with exon 9 KIT mutants and 12% of wild type KIT patients responded to imatinib.[35] In a study of 117 patients treated with imatinib for metastatic GIST, the median event-free survival for patients whose tumors had mutations of exon 11 was 22.5 months, compared to 6.6 months for patients with mutations in exon 9. The poorest response occurred in patients with no detectable KIT or PDGFRA mutation. These individuals had a median event-free survival of only 2.7 months.[35]

Radiation has a very limited role in the management of GIST.[33] Because of their intra-abdominal location, radiation therapy is associated with considerable toxicity to surrounding organs. The advent of effective chemotherapy has limited the role of radiation therapy for GIST to rare situations where symptom palliation can be achieved by localized tumor shrinkage.

▪ SURGICAL MANAGEMENT OF LOCALIZED PRIMARY DISEASE

Surgery remains the standard therapy for all resectable nonmetastatic tumors. Figure 15–9 shows a summary of clinical management for primary GIST. The reported resectability rate for localized primary GIST is 70–80%.[24,29,30] The importance of clear resection margins cannot be overemphasized. Tumor rupture or any other violation of the tumor pseudocapsule is associated with an increased risk of recurrence, including a risk of dissemination of tumor throughout the peritoneum. If the lesion involves adjacent organs, en bloc resection is considered essential to avoid tumor spillage. This also includes resection of any associated inflammatory adhesions, as these adhesions frequently contain tumor cells. Although endoscopic resection of small lesions has been reported, it remains controversial because of the risk of incomplete margins and the possibility of tumor spillage during manipulation of these lesions that are sometimes very friable.[33,36]

The 5-year overall survival rates following complete resection of localized GIST ranges from 40–55%.[29,33,37,38] In a review of patients treated prior to imatinib approval, Singer and associates[39] reported a 5-year recurrence free survival of 76 ± 9% for patients undergoing an R0 resection with clear surgical margins, compared to 15 ± 8% in patients with grossly or microscopically positive margins ($p = 0.0001$). The optimum width of margin has not been determined. Because GIST generally do not exhibit an infiltrative pattern of spread, modest margins of approximately 1 cm are a standard goal. Because lymph node metastases are extremely uncommon, regional lymphadenectomy is not recommended. Intraoperative incisional biopsy prior to resection should be avoided, because it risks tumor spillage.[40] This adverse factor does not

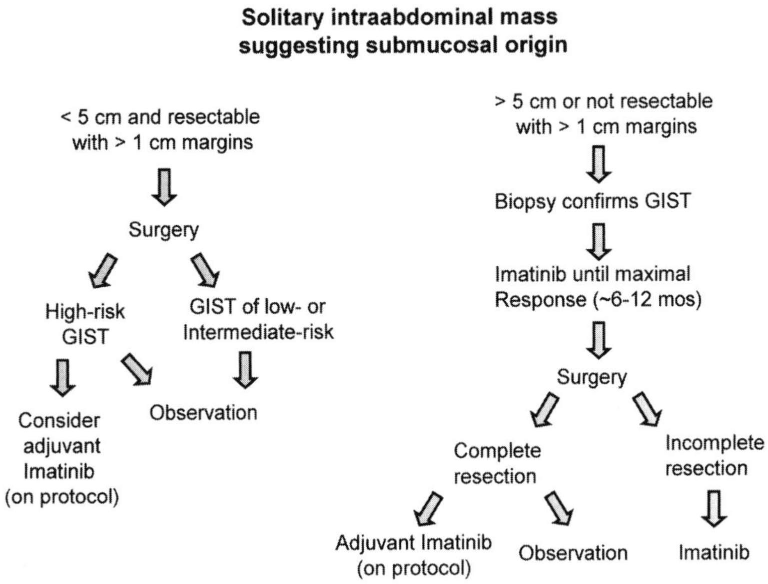

Figure 15–9. Management of primary localized GIST.

appear to apply to percutaneous biopsy techniques employing either thin- or core-needles, as instances of needle tract seeding or dissemination following these procedures have not been observed (C. Fletcher, personal communication).

Controversy exists concerning which GIST, if any, can be followed without intervention. It has been common practice to consider that smaller tumors (<1 cm), particularly in the esophagus and stomach, may be followed without resection with evaluations at 6-month intervals. However, the recognition that even small GIST can exhibit aggressive behavior leads most surgeons to recommend excision of all tumors in patients who are acceptable operative candidates.

▪ POSTSURGICAL FOLLOW-UP

The typical sites of tumor recurrence following resection of a GIST with curative intent are the local resection bed, the liver, and the peritoneum. Pulmonary metastases are uncommon. In general, the time to recurrence reflects the original growth pattern of the tumor, and recurrences as early as 3 months following resection have been observed. Most centers use abdominal/pelvic CT scanning for posttreatment follow-up, with PET scanning or MRI reserved for clarification of equivocal CT findings. Because more recurrences occur within the first 5 years after surgery, imaging intervals of 3 to 6 months are standard for patients in the first 5 years of posttreatment follow-up, with annual evaluation thereafter. At present there are no specific serum-based markers for the detection of recurrent GIST.

▪ ADJUVANT THERAPY

For patients with localized GIST treated with surgery alone, the reported recurrence rate at 5 years varies considerably, with recurrent disease developing in 2–15% of those with low-risk and 70–90% of those with high-risk primary tumors.[5,30,41] In the absence of adjuvant therapy, approximately 50% of patients receiving potentially curative surgery will develop either locally recurrent or metastatic disease within 5 years, yielding 5-year survival rates of 40–55%.[29,33,37,38] The effectiveness of imatinib in managing metastatic disease has led to combined modality treatment of high-risk localized tumors. This practice is supported by anecdotal reports suggesting that postoperative administration of imatinib improves disease control. In a small series of patients treated with imatinib after resection of GIST with positive margins, Bumming and associates reported a recurrence-free interval of 7 to 13 months.[42] The American College of Surgeons Clinical Oncology Group (ACOSOG) is currently sponsoring two adjuvant trials of imatinib following GIST resection with curative intent. In one pilot study, ACOSOG Z9000, patients with high-risk primary tumors (>10 cm in size, intraperitoneal tumor rupture or hemorrhage, or multifocal (<5) primary tumors) are treated with imatinib for 1 year after complete gross resection. Results from this open-label study will be evaluated as overall survival compared to historical controls. A second larger trial, ACOSOG Z9001, is a randomized, double-blind study comparing imatinib to placebo for 1 year in patients with fully resected, nonmetastatic primary GIST tumors larger than 3 cm in size. No preliminary data are yet available from either of these trials.

■ USE OF IMATINIB IN UNRESECTABLE PRIMARY DISEASE

The success of imatinib in managing metastatic disease led to its use as a means of improving the resectability of technically inoperable primary tumors. Although no series have yet been published, anecdotal reports indicate that this is an excellent approach that can reduce tumor size to the extent that surgery with curative intent is often possible.[43] This approach is also warranted when surgery with curative intent cannot be undertaken without significant loss of function. An example of this is the presence of a primary GIST of the rectum for which reduction in tumor volume could allow sphincter preservation. Objective responses to imatinib are evident in 30–40% of patients after 7 months and 50–60% after 9 months of treatment.[34] Surgery is performed when tumor size has decreased to the point at which resection is technically possible, and/or when successive CT scans show no further tumor shrinkage. Generally, this occurs from 9 to 12 months following initiation of chemotherapy. Following surgery, these high-risk patients are routinely maintained on imatinib indefinitely, as long as drug-related toxicity is minimal.

■ MANAGEMENT OF METASTATIC DISEASE

At present, all unresectable, recurrent, and metastatic GIST are considered for therapy with imatinib. In this setting, the standard of care is life-long imatinib use, or treatment at least until significant, generalized disease progression occurs.[44] Although initial disease response is occasionally rapid, the median time to an objective response is approximately three months.[35] Complete responses are rarely seen. The short-term prognosis is relatively good for patients who achieve even partial responses with imatinib. The 2-year survival for these individuals is approximately 85–90%.[45] Patients whose disease remains stable during imatinib treatment also benefit, with an overall survival comparable to those who achieve a partial response.[46] Patients who continue to have generalized disease progression have a median survival of 38 weeks, which is similar to that of untreated disease.[46]

Patients with metastatic GIST who respond to chemotherapy can experience an excellent quality of life. Upon initiation of therapy, patients with widespread, symptomatic disease often demonstrate a rapid improvement in performance status that corresponds to the decreased tumor metabolism visualized by PET. Because imatinib produces relatively few side effects, this suppressive therapy generally allows patients to remain fully functional. This is sometimes the case even in the setting of a relatively large burden of stable disease.

Figure 15–10 shows a summary of clinical management of previously untreated metastatic GIST.

■ PRIMARY AND ACQUIRED RESISTANCE TO CHEMOTHERAPY

GIST harboring mutations in KIT exon 9 or containing wild-type KIT tend to respond poorly to imatinib. The same is true for GIST associated with mutation of PDGFRA.[35] GIST that express little or no KIT by immunohistochemistry are often PDGFRA-mutant tumors. Absence of KIT staining, however, is not always associated with imatinib resistance, as some tumors with low or absent expression of KIT by IHC have mutations in exon 11 and respond favorably to imatinib treatment.[11]

Although imatinib produces dramatic antitumor responses in most GIST patients, for patients with widespread metastatic disease, its effects are not permanent. Imatinib leads to death of many tumor cells, achieving disease regression or stability for months to years. Unfortunately, the quiescent tumor cells can develop new mutations of KIT that alter the ATP-binding site in a way that no longer provides access for imatinib blockade. Disease progression typically occurs from 18 to 24 months after initiation of imatinib therapy.[34]

Clues to the nature of acquired imatinib resistance come from studies of patients treated with imatinib for CML. In many CML patients, initial imatinib response is followed by disease progression. These individuals often have secondary mutations in the ABL domain of the Philadelphia chromosome, and these mutations can be found at low levels before the emergence of clinical drug resistance. It is unclear whether these additional mutations are newly acquired, or whether they represent the outgrowth of cells present prior to imatinib treatment. Amplification of the BCR-ABL oncogene is also identified in a subset of patients with imatinib-resistant CML.[47–49] Preliminary studies of GIST suggest that acquisition of a second point mutation in KIT or PDGFRA confers imatinib resistance.[50] Increased kinase activity resulting from genomic amplification of KIT has also been observed. Some resistant clones in patients with GIST show loss of KIT staining by IHC, suggesting activation of an alternate activation pathway.[51]

■ CHARACTERIZING DISEASE RESPONSE AND PROGRESSION

As previously mentioned, PET scanning can be used to rapidly assess changes in tumor metabolism that reflect effective disease suppression by imatinib. In contrast, changes seen on CT scan may take months to become apparent.[52] A substantial degree of hetero-

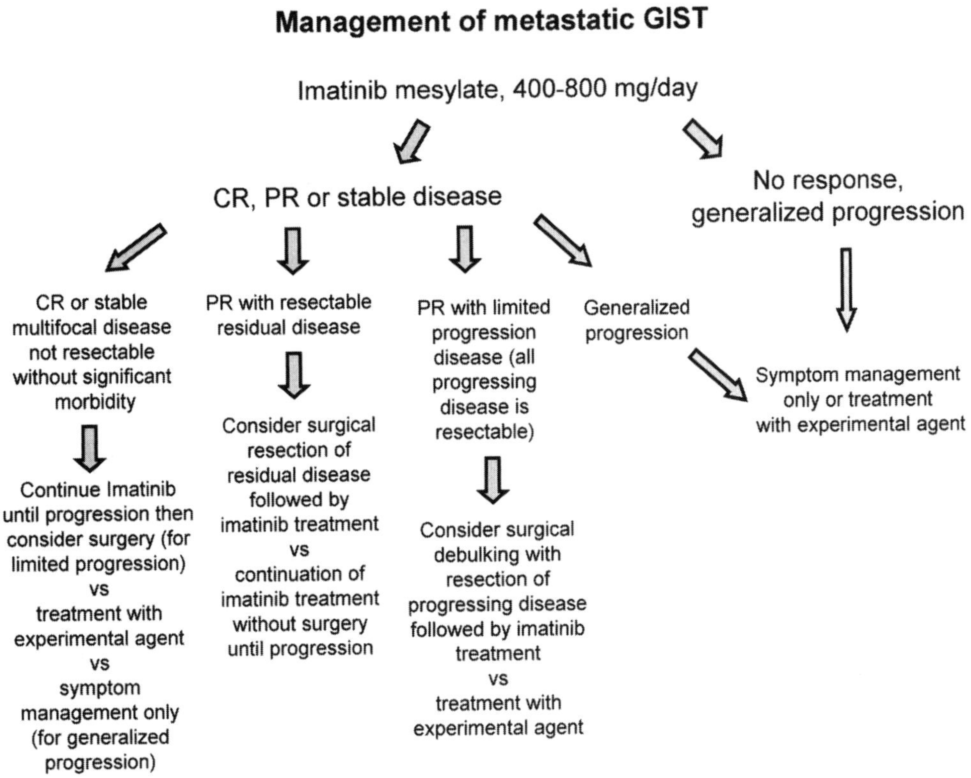
Management of metastatic GIST
Imatinib mesylate, 400-800 mg/day
CR, PR or stable disease
No response, generalized progression
CR or stable multifocal disease not resectable without significant morbidity
PR with resectable residual disease
PR with limited progression disease (all progressing disease is resectable)
Generalized progression
Symptom management only or treatment with experimental agent
Continue Imatinib until progression then consider surgery (for limited progression) vs treatment with experimental agent vs symptom management only (for generalized progression)
Consider surgical resection of residual disease followed by imatinib treatment vs continuation of imatinib treatment without surgery until progression
Consider surgical debulking with resection of progressing disease followed by imatinib treatment vs treatment with experimental agent

Figure 15–10. Management of metastatic GIST.

geneity of response among different metastatic sites is common (Fig 15–11). Responding lesions can shrink in size and, when palpable, become noticeably softer. In addition to tumor shrinkage, evidence of disease response can be visualized in the form of qualitative changes in the character of tumor sites. Treatment response is often evident in the form of cystic transformation of lesions, a change that is most easily detected in the liver. Occasionally, quiescent disease appears as completely homogeneous, fluid-filled structures on CT. Despite their benign appearance, the thin walls of these cystic structures invariably contain active tumor cells. The development of acquired drug resistance within these lesions can

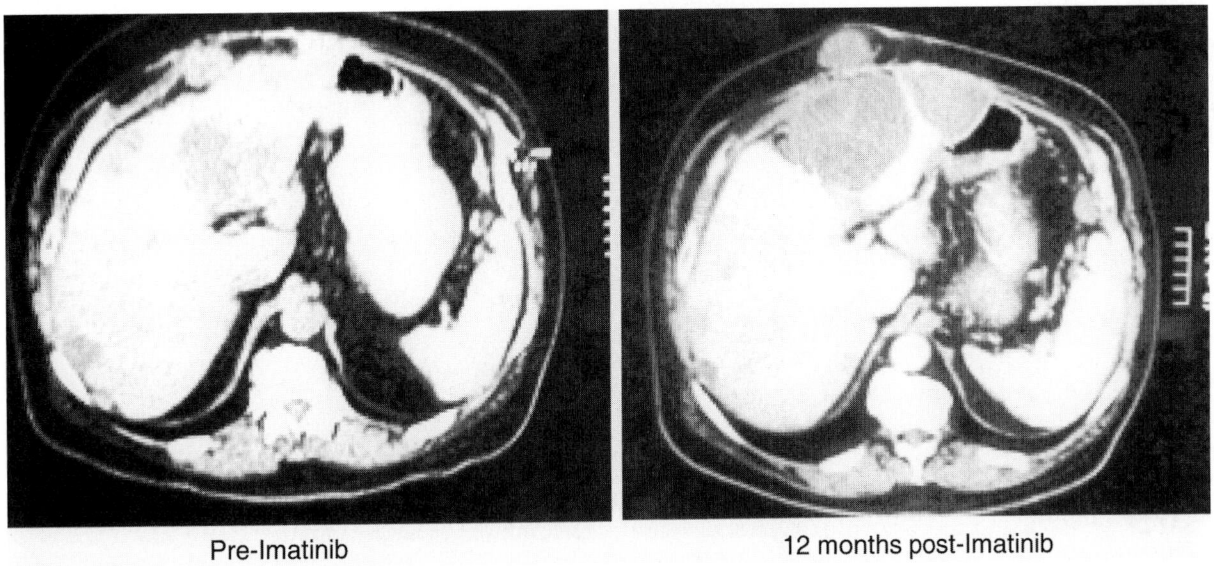
Pre-Imatinib
12 months post-Imatinib

Figure 15–11. Changes in tumor character during imatinib response. While some responding tumors shrink and eventually disappear during imatinib treatment, others, like that shown here, undergo cystic degeneration, sometimes even enlarging slightly without tumor progression.

sometimes be seen as new solid masses arising within these cysts (Fig 15–12).

The pattern of disease progression varies among different patients, reflecting the clonal evolution of metastatic GIST. Some patients experience generalized progressive disease, similar to that seen with primary drug resistance. Once this clinical picture develops, these individuals have a poor prognosis, with a median survival of only approximately 38 weeks.[46] A common type of progression, at least initially, is of a more limited nature, characterized by drug responsiveness or growth stability in most metastatic tumor deposits, with progressive growth in isolated lesions. It appears likely that continued drug therapy alters the natural history of this "limited progression" disease. For example, rapid generalized growth of tumor has been observed upon discontinuation of drug therapy in this setting, indicating that patients benefit from suppression of sensitive tumor clones when limited disease progression occurs.[53]

▪ ROLE OF SURGERY IN MANAGEMENT OF RECURRENT OR METASTATIC DISEASE

Surgery has an important role in the palliation of patients with incurable GIST. Large lesions that produce significant symptoms such as pain or early satiety should be considered for surgical therapy even if the symptomatic lesion is incompletely resectable or occurs in the presence of metastatic disease.[33] GIST can also result in GI or intraperitoneal bleeding, and can disrupt the intestinal wall to the extent that a tumor-associated fistula or abscess occurs. These complications can develop during chemotherapy in patients with stable or responding disease, and in this setting, surgery can improve quality of life and likely has a significant impact upon survival. In rare instances, patients with metastatic GIST will exhibit primary drug resistance, yet demonstrate an indolent course of disease progression. In these cases, which are more common in younger patients, surgical debulking can provide long-term palliation.

In theory, surgical resection following imatinib therapy may be curative in some patients with limited disease recurrence. By removing clones of disease that have acquired drug resistance, surgical debulking may also prolong survival in patients with metastatic disease, as long as remaining disease remains responsive to imatinib. For selected patients, radiofrequency ablation may be the optimal approach to disease control. Unfortunately, like surgical resection, ablative techniques have little to offer in the setting of generalized disease progression, as they are unlikely to alter the course of disease unless they can help a patient achieve disease stability.[54]

▪ NEW THERAPIES FOR MANAGEMENT OF PRIMARY AND SECONDARY DRUG RESISTANCE

A number of different agents are currently under investigation in clinical trials to determine their utility as second-line drugs for the management of imatinib-resistant GIST. These agents have been selected based

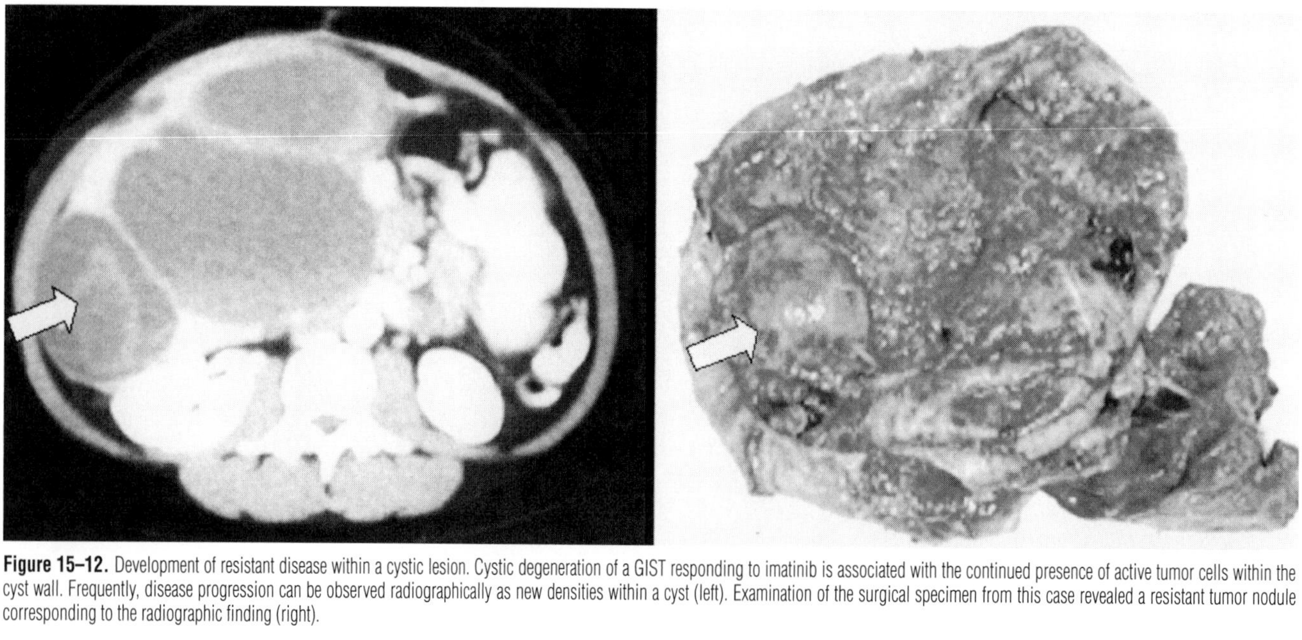

Figure 15–12. Development of resistant disease within a cystic lesion. Cystic degeneration of a GIST responding to imatinib is associated with the continued presence of active tumor cells within the cyst wall. Frequently, disease progression can be observed radiographically as new densities within a cyst (left). Examination of the surgical specimen from this case revealed a resistant tumor nodule corresponding to the radiographic finding (right).

upon their ability to disrupt KIT tyrosine kinase activity, or to inhibit targets that are downstream of KIT or PDGFRA. At least one of these, sunitinib, has shown some efficacy in phase II studies. Sunitinib (Fig 15–8) is a tyrosine kinase inhibitor with activity against KIT, PDGFR, FLT3, and VEGFR.[55] In a study of 92 GIST patients whose tumors exhibited primary or acquired imatinib resistance, treatment with sunitinib achieved an objective response rate of 8%, with disease stabilization in 58%.[55] A recently completed phase III study confirmed the efficacy of sunitinib in imatinib-refractory disease, and this agent has been approved by the FDA for this indication.[56]

▪ SUMMARY

In response to the dramatic change in GIST treatment following the introduction of imatinib therapy, the National Comprehensive Cancer Network (NCCN) issued a set of updated guidelines for GIST management. These guidelines, first presented in March 2004, emphasize the importance of a multidisciplinary approach to management of patients with GIST. These guidelines can be accessed on the following web site:

www.nccn.org/professionals/physician_gls/PDF/sarcoma.pdf

Although imatinib has had a profound impact on the course of disease, many patients with advanced GIST ultimately fail chemotherapy. In addition, questions concerning the optimal use of chemotherapy in the adjuvant setting remain unanswered. In the near term, therefore, it is important for patients with these rare tumors to be referred to specialty centers where they can be offered participation in clinical trials.

REFERENCES

1. Fletcher CD, Berman JJ, Corless C, et al. Diagnosis of gastrointestinal stromal tumors: A consensus approach. *Hum Pathol* 2002;33:459–465
2. Jemal A, Murray T, Ward E, et al. Cancer statistics. *CA Cancer J Clin* 2005;55:10–30
3. Mazur MT, Clark HB. Gastric stromal tumors: Reappraisal of histogenesis. *Am J Surg Path* 19837:507–519
4. Kindblom LG, Remotti HE, Aldenborg F, et al. Gastrointestinal pacemaker cell tumor (GIPACT): Gastrointestinal stromal tumors show phenotypic characteristics of the interstitial cells of Cajal. *Am J Pathol* 1998; 152:1259–1269
5. Nilsson B, Bumming P, Meis-Kindblom JM, et al. Gastrointestinal stromal tumors: The incidence, prevalence, clinical course, and prognostication in the pre-imatinib mesylate era. *Cancer* 2005;103:821–829
6. Hirota S, Isozaki K, Moriyama Y, et al. Gain-of-function mutations of c-kit in human gastrointestinal stromal tumors. *Science* 1998;279:577–580
7. Fleischman RA. From white spots to stem cells: The role of the Kit receptor in mammalian development. *Trends Genet* 1993;9:285–290
8. Ward SM, Burns AJ, Torihashi S, et al. Mutation of the proto-oncogene c-kit blocks development of interstitial cells and electrical rhythmicity in murine intestine. *J Physiol* 1994;480:91–97
9. Tian Q, Frierson HFJ, Krystal GW, et al. Activating c-kit gene mutations in human germ cell tumors. *Am J Pathol* 1999;154:1643–1647
10. Rubin BP, Singer S, Tsao C, et al. KIT activation is a ubiquitous feature of gastrointestinal stromal tumors. *Cancer Res* 2001;61:8118–8121
11. Bauer S, Corless CL, Heinrich MC, et al. Response to imatinib mesylate of a gastrointestinal stromal tumor with very low expression of KIT. *Cancer Chemother Pharmacol* 2003;51:261–265
12. Medeiros F, Corless CL, Duensing A, et al. KIT-negative gastrointestinal stromal tumors: proof of concept and therapeutic implications. *Am J Surg Pathol* 2004;28:889–894
13. Heinrich MC, Rubin BP, Longley BJ, et al. Biology and genetic aspects of gastrointestinal stromal tumors: KIT activation and cytogenetic alterations. *Hum Pathol* 2002; 33:484–495
14. Heinrich MC, Corless CL, Duensing A, et al. PDGFRA activating mutations in gastrointestinal stromal tumors. *Science* 2003;299:708–710
15. Corless CL, Fletcher JA, Heinrich MC. Biology of gastrointestinal stromal tumors. *J Clin Oncol* 2004;22:3813–3825
16. Lasota J, Wozniak A, Sarlomo-Rikala M, et al. Mutations in exons 9 and 13 of KIT gene are rare events in gastrointestinal stromal tumors. A study of 200 cases. *Am J Pathol* 2000;157:1091–1095
17. Hirota S, Ohashi A, Nishida T, et al. Gain-of-function mutations of platelet-derived growth factor receptor alpha gene in gastrointestinal stromal tumors. *Gastroenterology* 2003;125:660–667
18. Maki RG. Gastrointestinal Stromal Tumors Respond to Tyrosine Kinase-targeted Therapy. *Curr Treat Options Gastroen* 2004;7:13–17
19. Chompret A, Kannengiesser C, Barrois M, et al. PDGFRA germline mutation in a family with multiple cases of gastrointestinal stromal tumor. *Gastroenterology* 2004; 126:318–321
20. Carney JA. Gastric stromal sarcoma, pulmonary chondroma, and extra-adrenal paraganglioma (Carney Triad): Natural history, adrenocortical component, and possible familial occurrence. *Mayo Clin Proc* 1999;74: 543–552
21. Amieux PS. Getting the GIST of the Carney Triad: growth factors, rare tumors, and cellular respiration. *Pediatr Dev Pathol* 2004;7:306–308
22. Boccon-Gibod L, Boman F, Boudjemaa S, et al. Separate occurrence of extra-adrenal paraganglioma and gas-

trointestinal stromal tumor in monozygotic twins: probable familial Carney syndrome. *Pediatr Dev Pathol* 2004;7: 380–384
23. Kinoshita K, Hirota S, Isozaki K, et al. Absence of c-kit gene mutations in gastrointestinal stromal tumours from neurofibromatosis type 1 patients. *J Pathol* 2004; 202:80–85
24. Roberts PJ, Eisenberg B. Clinical presentation of gastrointestinal stromal tumors and treatment of operable disease. *Eur J Cancer* 2002;38:S37–S38
25. Rader AE, Avery A, Wait CL, et al. Fine-needle aspiration biopsy diagnosis of gastrointestinal stromal tumors using morphology, immunocytochemistry, and mutational analysis of c-kit. *Cancer* 2001;93:269–275
26. Ghanem N, Altehoefer C, Furtwangler A, et al. Computed tomography in gastrointestinal stromal tumors. *Eur Radiol* 2003;13:1669–1678
27. Stroobants S, Goeminne J, Seegers M, et al. 18FDG-Positron emission tomography for the early prediction of response in advanced soft tissue sarcoma treated with imatinib mesylate (Glivec). *Eur J Cancer* 2003;39:2012–2020
28. Miettinen M, El-Rifai W, Sobin LH, et al. Evaluation of malignancy and prognosis of gastrointestinal stromal tumors: a review. *Hum Pathol* 2002;33:478–483
29. DeMatteo RP, Lewis JL, Leung D, et al. Two hundred gastrointestinal stromal tumors: Recurrence patterns and prognostic factors for survival. *Ann Surg* 2000;231:51–58
30. Rossi CR, Mocellin S, Mencarelli R, et al. Gastrointestinal stromal tumors: from a surgical to a molecular approach. *Int J Cancer* 2003;107:171–176
31. Buchdunger E, Cioffi CL, Law N, et al. Abl protein-tyrosine kinase inhibitor STI571 inhibits in vitro signal transduction mediated by c-kit and platelet-derived growth factor receptors. *J Pharmacol Exp Ther* 2000;295: 139–145
32. Buchdunger E, Zimmermann J, Mett H, et al. Inhibition of the Abl protein-tyrosine kinase in vitro and in vivo by a 2-phenylaminopyrimidine derivative. *Cancer Res* 1996; 56:100–104
33. Joensuu H, Fletcher C, Dimitrijevic S, et al. Management of malignant gastrointestinal stromal tumours. *Lancet Oncol* 2002;3:655–664
34. Demetri GD, von Mehren M, Blanke CD, et al. Efficacy and safety of imatinib mesylate in advanced gastrointestinal stromal tumors. *N Engl J Med* 2002;347:472–480
35. Heinrich MC, Corless CL, Demetri GD, et al. Kinase mutations and imatinib response in patients with metastatic gastrointestinal stromal tumor. *J Clin Oncol* 2003; 21:4342–4349
36. Davila RE, Faigelm DO. GI stromal tumors. *Gastrointest Endosc* 2003;58:80–88
37. Crosby JA, Catton CN, Davis A, et al. Malignant gastrointestinal stromal tumors of the small intestine: a review of 50 cases from a prospective database. *Ann Surg Oncol* 2001;8:50–59
38. Pierie JP, Choudry U, Muzikansky A, et al. The effect of surgery and grade on outcome of gastrointestinal stromal tumors. *Arch Surg* 2001;136:383–389
39. Singer S, Rubin BP, Lux ML, et al. Prognostic value of KIT mutation type, mitotic activity, and histologic subtype in gastrointestinal stromal tumors. *J Clin Oncol* 2002;20:3898–3905
40. Dematteo RP, Maki RG, Antonescu C, et al. Targeted molecular therapy for cancer: the application of STI571 to gastrointestinal stromal tumor. *Curr Probl Surg* 2003; 40:144–193
41. Demetri GD. Identification and treatment of chemoresistant inoperable or metastatic GIST: experience with the selective tyrosine kinase inhibitor imatinib mesylate (STI571). *Eur J Cancer* 2003;38:S52–S59
42. Bumming P, Andersson J, Meis-Kindblom JM, et al. Neoadjuvant, adjuvant and palliative treatment of gastrointestinal stromal tumours (GIST) with imatinib: a centre-based study of 17 patients. *Br J Cancer* 2003;89: 460–464
43. Wu PC, Langerman A, Ryan CW, et al. Surgical treatment of gastrointestinal stromal tumors in the imatinib (STI-571) era. *Surgery* 2003;134:656–665
44. Demetri GD, Delaney T. NCCN Sarcoma Practice Guidelines Panel. *Cancer Control* 2001;8:94–101
45. Rankin C, Von Mehren M, Blanke C, et al. Dose effect of imatinib (IM) in patients with metastasis GIST — Phase III Sarcoma Group Study S0033. *J Clin Oncol* 2004;22:9005
46. Blanke CD, Joensuu H, Demetri GD, et al. Outcome of advanced gastrointestinal stromal tumor (GIST) patients treated with imatinib mesylate: Four-year follow-up of a phase II randomized trial. *Amer Soc Clin Oncol* 2006 Gastrointestinal Cancers Symposium (abstract 7). http://www.asco.org/portal/site/ASCO/menuitem.34d60f5624ba07fd506fe310ee37a01d/?abstractID=226&confID=41&index=y&vmview-abst_detail_view
47. Branford S, Rudzki Z, Walsh S, et al. High frequency of point mutations clustered within the adenosine triphosphate-binding region of BCR/ABL in patients with chronic myeloid leukemia or Ph-positive acute lymphoblastic leukemia who develop imatinib (STI571) resistance. *Blood* 2002;99:3472–3475
48. Roche-Lestienne C, Soenen-Cornu V, Grardel-Duflos N, et al. Several types of mutations of the Abl gene can be found in chronic myeloid leukemia patients resistant to STI571, and they can pre-exist to the onset of treatment. *Blood* 2002;100:1014–1018
49. Gorre ME, Mohammed M, Ellwood K, et al. Clinical resistance to STI-571 cancer therapy caused by BCR-ABL gene mutation or amplification. *Science* 2001;293:876–880
50. Tamborini E, Bonadiman L, Greco A, et al. A new mutation in the KIT ATP pocket causes acquired resistance to imatinib in a gastrointestinal stromal tumor patient. *Gastroenterology* 2004;127(1):294–299
51. Fletcher JA, Corless CL, Dimitrijevic S, et al. Mechanisms of resistance to imatinib mesylate (IM) in advanced gastrointestinal stromal tumor (GIST). *Proc Am Soc Clin Oncol* 2003;22:815
52. Vanel D, Albiter M, Shapeero L, et al. Role of computed tomography in the follow-up of hepatic and peritoneal metastases of GIST under imatinib mesylate treatment: a prospective study of 54 patients. *Eur J Radiol* 2005;54:118–123

53. Le Cesne A, Perol D, Ray-Coquard I, et al. Interruption of imatinib (IM) in GIST patients with advanced disease: Updated results of the prospective French Sarcoma Group randomized phase III trial on survival and quality of life. *J Clin Oncol* 2005;23:823s
54. Dileo P, Randhawa R, VanSonnenberg E, et al. Safety and efficacy of percutaneous radio-frequency ablation (RFA) in patients with metastatic gastrointestinal stromal tumor with clonal evolution of lesions refractory to imatinib mesylate. *J Clin Oncol* 2004;22:9024
55. Demetri GD, Desai J, Fletcher JA, et al. SU11248, a multi-targeted tyrosine kinase inhibitor, can overcome imatinib resistance caused by diverse genomic mechanisms in patients with metastatic gastrointestinal stromal tumor. *J Clin Oncol* 2004;22:3001
56. Demetri GD, van Oosterom AT, Blackstein M, et al. Phase III multicenter, randomized, double-blind, placebo-controlled trial of SU11248 in patients following failure of imatinib for metastatic GIST. *Proc Am Soc Clin Oncol* 2005;23:4000a

16

Morbid Obesity and Operations for Morbid Obesity

Danny O. Jacobs ▪ *Malcolm K. Robinson*

Obesity is a very serious health problem. The excess morbidity or mortality attributable to obesity or obesity-related diseases exceeds that of tobacco and alcohol.[1] The prevalence of obesity has increased dramatically over the past three decades. Health problems related to obesity represent a significant cost to society from lost wages and increased costs. The financial impact is such that the obesity epidemic consumes approximately 6% of all health care expenditures.[2] It is estimated that as many as 300,000 patients may die annually from obesity or obesity-related diseases and over $100 billion are spent yearly on obesity-related health care problems.[3]

The advent of modern bariatric surgery is increasingly recognized as an important therapeutic option for many patients with clinically significant obesity. The increased prevalence of obesity in the United States and Europe is associated with a dramatic increase in the number of gastrointestinal operations that are performed to treat the condition. For example, the number of bariatric procedures has increased more than sixfold over the past decade. The development of new and innovative minimally invasive operations to treat morbid obesity has certainly contributed to the increase in the number of bariatric procedures that are being performed. This chapter will briefly review key aspects of obesity, including its epidemiology, pathogenesis, health effects, medical treatment, the rationale for surgical intervention, perioperative management, outcomes and complications.

▪ ASSESSING SEVERITY

The body mass index (BMI), which is calculated by dividing the weight in kilograms by the height in meters squared, is commonly used to define, describe, and screen for obesity. As such, it does not account for potentially important factors such as body frame or lean body mass. However, in adults, a normal body mass index measures between 18.5 and 24.9. The BMI is closely, but not necessarily precisely, related to body fat content. As one might suspect, its error varies according to the demographic characteristics of the population in question. For example, the relationship between BMI and obesity (and therefore between obesity and outcome) in children is not as well established. Furthermore, in the United States the association between obesity and mortality appears to be weaker for African Americans as compared with Anglo Americans.[2] Although the BMI's accuracy, and therefore its validity, may vary in some patient populations according to their demographic characteristics, including ethnicity and perhaps age, the body mass index has proven to be a clinically relevant measure of obesity that can be linked to health outcomes. The BMI associated with the lowest risk of death is within the normal range for most men and lies within the normal to overweight range for most women.[2] A few studies suggest that the mortality risk of obesity decreases with aging.

It is important to note that not every obese patient has an elevated risk of an adverse medical outcome. For example, a significant proportion of overweight or obese patients are not resistant to insulin. Because the risk of significant medical comorbidities (e.g., type II or adult-onset diabetes, hypertension, and coronary artery disease) is significantly less in patients who do not manifest clinical sequelae of insulin resistance, an important objective should be to identify those obese patients who have the greatest risk of excess morbidity or mortality (i.e., those who have the "metabolic syndrome"). These are also patients who may benefit the most from significant weight loss.

Abdominal obesity is more predictive of the presence of metabolic risk factors (e.g., insulin resistance) than is an elevated BMI alone.[4] Waist circumference and the waist:hip ratio, used in conjunction with the BMI, may more accurately identify patients with central adiposity who are at risk for significant medical comorbidities, including cardiovascular disease.[2] Waist circumference is more closely correlated with visceral obesity in African Americans. Population survey data indicate that a waist circumference exceeding 98 cm in men and 87 cm in women (after adjusting for age, menopausal status, smoking history, alcohol consumption, education, and income as appropriate) can help identify patients who have an increased risk for cardiovascular disease. Other risk factors include: (1) elevated fasting triglycerides (>150 mg/dL); (2) elevated high-density lipoprotein cholesterol; (3) hypertension (blood pressure >130/85 mm Hg); and (4) hyperglycemia (fasting plasma glucose levels >110 mg/dL). The presence of any three of these risk factors identifies patients who have the metabolic syndrome.

The National Heart, Lung and Blood Institute guidelines define patients with body mass indices between 25 and 29.9 kg/m^2 body surface area as overweight (Table 16–1). Those with BMIs exceeding 30 kg/m^2 are classified as obese. Medical obesity is further subclassified into three categories: class 1 obesity for patients with body mass indices between 30 and 34.9 kg/m^2, class 2 obesity for BMIs between 35 and 39.9, and class 3 obesity for patients with BMIs that exceed 40 kg/m^2.[5] In 1991, the National Institutes of Health defined morbidly obese patients as those with BMIs of 35 kg/m^2 or greater who had significant obesity-related conditions, or those with BMIs 40 kg/m^2 or greater in the absence of medical comorbidities.[6] Superobesity is a term that is occasionally used to identify patients who have BMIs equal to 50 kg/m^2 or greater. The National Institutes of Health definitions are similar to those of the World Health Organization.

■ EPIDEMIOLOGY

Over the past four decades, the prevalence of obesity has increased worldwide and dramatically in the United States (Fig 16–1).

TABLE 16–1. THE RELATIONSHIP BETWEEN BODY MASS INDEX (BMI) AND WEIGHT CLASSIFICATION

BMI <18.5	Underweight
BMI 18.5–24.9	Normal
BMI 25.0–29.9	Overweight
BMI 30.0–34.9	Obesity class 1
BMI 35.0–39.9	Obesity class 2
BMI >40.0	Obesity class 3

In the United States, obesity has reached epidemic proportions. In 1994, the National Health and Nutrition Examination Survey revealed that approximately 35% of adults in the U.S. were overweight or obese.[7] Although the rate of increase in the prevalence of obesity is more dramatic in the U.S., the adult population in Europe is also becoming more obese.[8,9] Similar trends are also reported in other industrialized countries.

In the 1990s, approximately 55% of the adults in U.S. were overweight. Of these, at least half were obese according to their body mass indices.[10,11] Obesity is more common among the poor and some minorities—for example, African-American women appear to be disproportionately affected.[12,13] Among the latter, the prevalence of obesity was approximately 20% of the population in the mid-1990s and appears to be continuing to increase.

Therefore, more people than ever are at least 100 pounds overweight, and thereby have clinically severe obesity. Between 1986 and 2000, the prevalence of adults in the United States with a BMI of at least 40 kg/m^2 body surface areas increased from approximately 1 in 200 to 1 in 50, while the prevalence of severe obesity (as defined by the presence of a BMI >50 kg/m^2 sur-

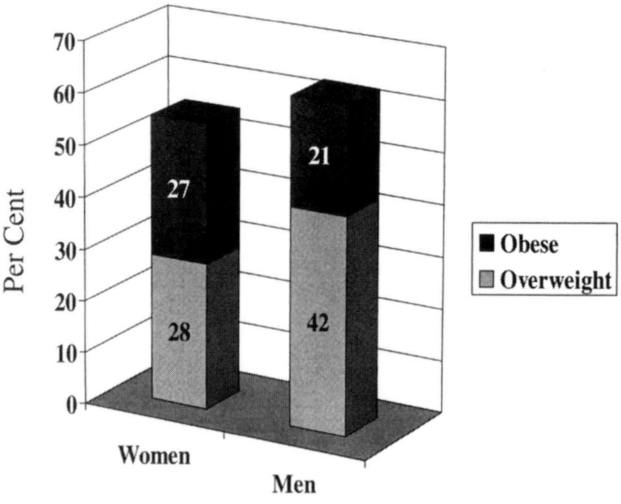

Figure 16–1. Prevalence of overweight and obese adults 25 years or older in the United States. (Adapted, with permission, from Must A, Spadano J, Coakly EH et al. The disease burden associated with overweight and obesity. *JAMA* 1999;282:1523–1529.)

face area) increased fivefold.[8,14] In the U.S., the age-adjusted prevalence of obesity increased by 33% between 1999 and 2000, and the prevalence of extreme or superobesity (see above) increased by 62% over the same time period.[15] In 2002, 30–34% of the adult population in the U.S. had a BMI between 25 and 29.9, and approximately 27% were obese, with a BMI over 30 kg/m^2. Thus the prevalence of obesity has increased by more than 75% since 1980.

These disturbing trends are also evident among young adults and children. For example, among people aged 12–19 years of age, the prevalence of obesity has increased by nearly 50% according to the Centers for Disease Control and Prevention.[16] The prevalence of children who are overweight has at least doubled (Fig 16–2).[17] Recent reviews show that at least 20% of children between the ages of 6 and 17 are overweight as defined by a BMI that is equal to or greater than the 85th percentile.[18] Half of these patients have BMIs greater than or equal to the 95th percentile for their age.

▪ ETIOLOGY

Storage of consumed energy as triglycerides within adipose tissue is a normal physiological process. It is teleologically appropriate to suppose that such a storage process would provide a survival advantage to the host during times of starvation or increased energy demands because the consumption of adipose tissue via hydrolysis releases fatty acids that can used as an energy source by many tissues. It is also logical to reason that starvation, rather than obesity, constituted the greater survival threat for most of human history. Such pressure likely resulted in the evolution of a phenotype that was energy efficient and fat retentive.[11] Thus from a geneticist's point of view, what was once advantageous as humans evolved from an environment characterized by high energy demands but relatively low food availability to the current environment in many industrialized countries in which high-density foods are much more readily available and physical demands are significantly reduced, now favors the development of morbid obesity.[11] Of these factors, the decline in physical activity may be the most important factor influencing the increasing prevalence of obesity in Westernized societies.[19] The changes that have been witnessed over the past decades most likely have occurred as energy expenditure has declined due to less physical activity, while food intake has remained the same or increased.

Energy balance is regulated by the balance between food intake and energy expenditure. The properties of the major macronutrients consumed by humans have substantially different core properties (e.g., caloric content and energy density), that predict their effect on energy intake in most instances (Table 16–2). A macronutrient's thermic effect, otherwise known as nutrient-induced thermogenesis, is the energy cost to the body of absorbing, processing, and storing an orally ingested food. As the table illustrates, fat has a very high energy density and storage capacity, is subject to less autoregulation, suppresses appetite somewhat less than other macronutrients in general, and requires the least amount of energy for it to be metabolized. For these reasons, the importance of fat intake as a determinant of weight gain should be apparent—especially as compared with protein or carbohydrate.

The major determinants of energy expenditure are the resting metabolic rate (which is the amount of energy needed to maintain the body's core functions at rest), the energy required to process the food consumed (which is the nutrient-induced thermogenesis described above), and the energy consumed by physical activity. The latter is the most variable component of the daily energy expenditure and may vary greatly. Nevertheless, it is very difficult to lose substantial

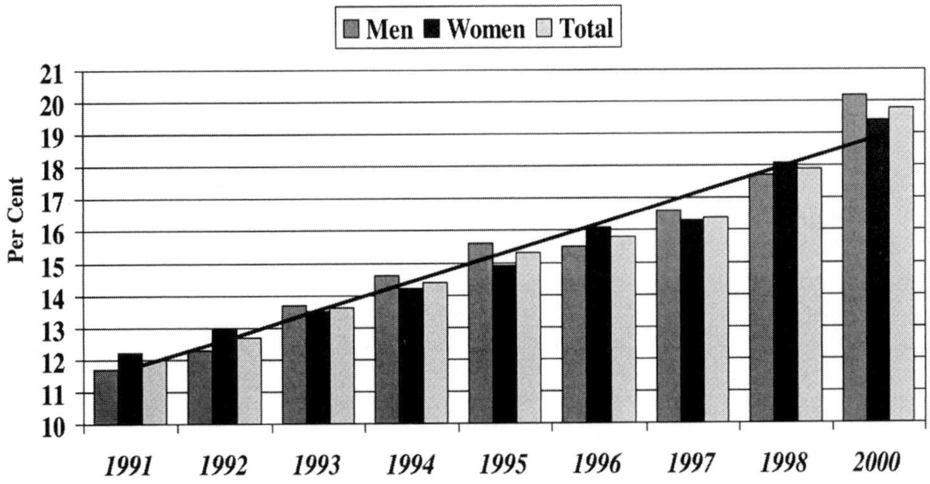

Figure 16–2. Prevalence of obesity among adults 18 years and older in the United States. (Modified, with permission, from Mokdad AH, Serdula MK, Dietz WH et al. The spread of the obesity epidemic in the United States: 1991–1998. *JAMA* 1999;282:1519–1522.)

TABLE 16–2. NUTRITIONAL AND METABOLIC PROPERTIES OF THE COMMON MACRONUTRIENTS

Properties	Fat	Protein	Carbohydrate	Alcohol
Kcal/g	9	4	4	7
Energy density	High	Low	Low	High
Nutrient-induced thermogenesis (percent of energy content)	2–3%	25–30%	6–8%	15–20%
Storage capacity	High	None	Low	None
Autoregulation	Poor	Good	Good	Poor
Ability to suppress hunger	Low	High	High	May stimulate hunger

Reproduced, with permission, from Labib M. The investigation and management of obesity. *J Clin Pathol* 2003; 56:17–25.

amounts of weight from physical activity alone. For example, a typical adult who weighs 75 kilograms consumes approximately 100 kcal for each mile walked at a comfortable pace. He or she would need to walk approximately 70 miles just to burn a single kilogram of body fat (each kilogram of body fat contains approximately 2000 kcal). Such levels of activity are extremely difficult for healthy, normal-weight adults to perform, and would be an extraordinary, if not impossible, task for those who are significantly overweight and unfit. There are also behavioral factors that may vary genetically, including the preference for fat in the diet, metabolic adaptations to food restriction, tolerance for physical activity, and the frequency of meals.[11] Many Americans consume between 500 and 1000 more calories per day than are needed to maintain a stable and safe body weight. This level of excess caloric intake is sufficient to cause weight gain of a pound per week or more on average.

Neural, metabolic, and endocrine signals passed between the central nervous system and peripheral sites in the body vary according to changes in energy balance. A complex neural network in the hypothalamus regulates the body's metabolic responses to starvation and feeding by stimulating or inhibiting appetite, and by modulating changes in energy expenditure—including physical activity. Changes in satiety may not only modify food intake but also help to regulate long-term changes in body weight. Finally, it should be noted that we are just beginning to understand the effects of various metabolites, besides fatty acids or triglycerides, that are released by adipose tissue during starvation. These metabolites include various cytokines and prostaglandins that may help regulate energy balance, and others that may influence carbohydrate metabolism such as resistin and fibronectin.[20] Unlike rodents, humans have very little adipose tissue that is metabolically active—the so called "brown fat." However, there may be some uncoupling proteins active in human adipose tissue that can help dissipate energy and may play an important role in energy regulation. Overall, energy balance and total caloric intake appear to be governed by neuropeptide effects in and around the hypothalamus.

Nutrient ingestion into the stomach or proximal intestine elicits hormonal signals that release neuropeptides, which in turn alter body metabolism. Hormones known to be important in these processes include pleptin, ghrelin, which is normally associated with appetite stimulation (i.e., is orexigenic), and those which are normally anorexic such as insulin and cholecystokinin. Many hormonal signals and their effect on obesity are just beginning to be elucidated.

One such hormone is leptin. It is worthy of a brief review because it is a good example for some of the fundamental principles of neurohormonal signaling between the periphery and the central nervous system, although its relevance to the efficacious treatment of most morbidly obese patients has been disappointing thus far. Leptin is a cytokinelike polypeptide hormone that is known to influence long-term changes in satiety. It is produced predominantly by adipose tissue and its circulating levels are proportional to the amount of fat stored as adipose tissue.[21] Its effects on food intake are governed by its effects on receptors within the arcuate nucleus of the hypothalamus. There it induces the production of α-melanocyte stimulating hormone (α-MSH) from propiomelanocortin. α-MSH then binds with melanocortin 4 receptors within hypothalamic nuclei and inhibits food intake. Leptin also decreases the production of appetite-inducing neuropeptides such as neuropeptide Y.[20] Although many obese patients appear to be leptin resistant, the relationship between leptin resistance and obesity is not well understood.

Humans born with homozygous loss of function mutations of the leptin gene (and who, therefore cannot produce leptin) eventually develop morbid obesity. These unfortunate individuals continuously seek food and eat much more than normal. Such monogenic causes of obesity are extremely rare. Other phenotypical manifestations including adrenal insufficiency, changes in hair color, and impaired fertility are commonly observed. The Prader-Willi syndrome is a well-recognized disorder characterized by childhood-onset upper body obesity, short stature, mental retardation, and hypogonadism. In general, when such syndromes are identified, they most often include alterations in the leptin-hypothalamic feedback loop (i.e., of important signal precursors such as propiomelanocortin, the leptin gene, and the leptin receptor).[19] Melanocortin 4 receptor mutations have also been described but are extremely rare.[22]

Ghrelin, which was only discovered in 1999, is a growth hormone secretagogue that is synthesized predominantly by the stomach. Its levels rise just before meals and with short-term food restriction, or prolonged starvation in general and may be an important orexigenic (i.e., appetite-stimulating) signal. Ghrelin levels normally fall rapidly after meals. Like leptin, ghrelin metabolism may be dysregulated in obese subjects. Obesity is associated with decreased circulating ghrelin levels. After gastric bypass surgery, ghrelin levels fall but do not increase as expected before meals.[21] Low levels of ghrelin and its metabolic dysregulation may be at least partially responsible for the sustained weight loss after surgical procedures that resect and/or bypass a significant portion of the stomach.

In rodent models, the genes responsible for changes in body fatness appear to most often involve the regulation of food intake. Similarly, in humans most of the genes identified in commonly recognized monogenetic syndromes are involved in the regulation of food intake. However, as suggested earlier, although a number of genetic syndromes have been identified with obesity as dominant feature, susceptibility to obesity in humans is most likely polygenic in origin.[20] Surveys indicate that between 25% and 70% of a person's average body weight is controlled by genetic factors.[19,23] These data show that BMI is closely correlated among first-degree relatives. Adoption studies have confirmed genetic contributions to observed variations in body fatness and the BMI as well.[24] Binge eating disorders appear to be highly inheritable.

We do not yet know if a limited number of genes will ultimately be found that modulate obesity in adults. The overwhelming majority of obese humans who will present for surgical evaluation, however, will not have mutations of any neurohormonal pathways that are known to be able to induce or predispose to obesity.

▪ HEALTH EFFECTS OF OBESITY AND WEIGHT LOSS

Many epidemiological studies show that obesity has an effect on public health that is equivalent to or greater than the effect of cigarette smoking, physical inactivity, or high cholesterol levels.[25] Overall, mortality is significantly and dramatically elevated for the obese and severely obese.[11] The relationship between overweight and obesity and the frequency of medical conditions such as type II diabetes, hypertension, and osteoarthritis are well recognized. Table 16–3 displays a list of the medical conditions to which the clinically obese are predisposed.[11,19] In general, obesity increases the risk of mortality at any age, although this effect is strongest until the age of 50. For example, a woman who is a nonsmoker with a BMI >32 kg/m^2 has a relative risk of death from cardiovascular disease or cancer that may be up to two to four times greater than that of a woman who is otherwise comparable but with a BMI <19 kg/m[19,26] (Fig 16–3).

TABLE 16–3. SOME MEDICAL CONDITIONS ASSOCIATED WITH OR AGGRAVATED BY OBESITY

Type II adult-onset diabetes mellitus
Gastroesophageal reflux
Coronary artery disease
Cerebrovascular accident
Congestive heart failure
Hypertension
Dyslipidemia
Cholelithiasis and gallbladder disease
Osteoarthritis and degenerative joint disease
Sleep apnea
Cancer (inluding esophageal, stomach, liver, pancreatic, kidney, non-Hodgkin's lymphoma, multiple myeloma, prostate, ovarian, uterine, gallbladder, and colon malignancies)
Menstrual abnormalities
Impaired fertility and increased risk of adverse outcomes after pregnancy
Stress incontinence

The pathogenesis of many of the pathological manifestations of obesity is certainly related to the metabolic sequelae of insulin resistance, but other mechanisms are poorly understood.[27] Some data suggest that hypertension and other abnormalities detected in patients who are severely obese are secondary to increased intra-abdominal pressure and activation of the renninangiotensin-aldosterone system.[28]

Overall, the risk of excess morbidity appears to increase concordantly with an increase in the BMI. The risk appears to be greatest for cardiovascular disease and for colon, uterine, breast, and ovarian malignancies.[28] In the U.S., although the risk for mortality and morbidity appears to vary somewhat according to ethnicity, the underlying relationship remains valid. The greater the obesity, the more likely is a patient to develop hypertension or adult-onset type II diabetes. This combination is more frequently observed in elderly patients. Population studies suggest that up to 75% of cases of simple hypertension can be directly attributed to excess weight or obesity.[18] African Americans in general are more likely to be hypertensive and severely obese, but are less likely to be diabetic. Severely obese subjects are also more likely to suffer from obesity-related hypoventilation and obstructive sleep apnea and venous stasis disease.[29] Women are more likely to have urinary incontinence and pseudotumor cerebri, as well as problems with menstruation and fertility.

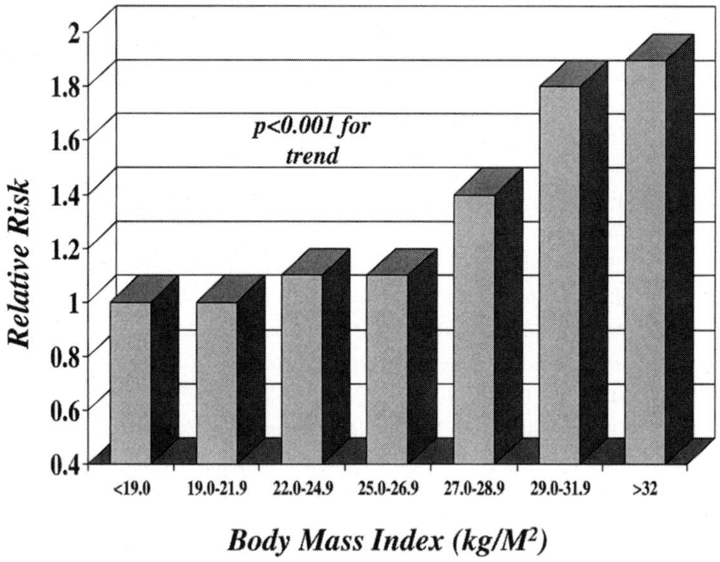

Figure 16–3. The relationship between body mass index and the relative risk of death in non-smoking women. (Reproduced, with permission, from Manson J, Willett W, Stampfer M. Body weight and mortality among women. *N Engl J Med* 1995; 333:677–685.)

Morbidity from obesity is increased in the presence of preexisting coronary artery or peripheral artery disease, type II diabetes, hypertension, smoking, elevated low-density or decreased high-density lipoprotein levels, increased fasting blood sugar concentrations, and in patients with a family history of early-onset heart disease.

When considering population studies describing the relationship between obesity and the risk of developing cancer, it is important to realize that in countries with a very high prevalence of obesity, only a small incremental increase in mortality is required to demonstrate that a very large patient population could be adversely affected.[27] Calle and colleagues followed more than 400,000 men and women to evaluate the relationship between BMI and death from cancer.[30] They then calculated the proportion of all deaths that could be attributed to excess body weight (i.e., for patients who were either overweight or obese). Members of their cohorts with BMIs >40 kg/m^2 had death rates from cancer that were 52% higher in men and 62% higher in women compared with their normal-weight counterparts. In both men and women, increased BMI was positively correlated with higher rates of death from cancers of the esophagus, colon and rectum, liver, gallbladder, pancreas, and kidney, as well as for non-Hodgkin's lymphoma and multiple myeloma. Less strong associations were noted for the relationship between stomach and prostate cancer in men, and breast, uterine, ovarian, and cervical cancer in women. The authors concluded that excess body weight could account for as much as 14% of all deaths from cancer in men and 20% of deaths in women.

Similar observations have been made regarding cardiovascular risks associated with significant obesity.[31] Overweight women have a 50% greater risk of heart failure compared to women with normal BMIs. The risk is twofold higher in obese females. Obese men have a 90% greater risk of heart failure. Overall, approximately 11% of all heart failure cases in men and 14% in women can be attributed to obesity alone.

Others have described the increased risk of adverse outcomes obese patients experience after many operations. For example, the presence of morbid obesity is associated with an increased risk of death after heart transplantation.[32] Studies of the effects of obesity on mortality risk after liver transplantation have been less conclusive, perhaps because patients with preexisting cardiac disease are typically excluded from consideration. However, the perioperative complication rate is higher for patients with BMIs >31 kg/m^2, although the long-term survival rate is similar to that of normal controls.[33] Obesity also increases the risk of an adverse outcome after renal transplantation, although some of this morbidity may be due to the cardiovascular disease that develops in these patients.[34]

▪ MANAGEMENT OF THE OBESE PATIENT

MEDICAL THERAPY

Although much research effort is being expended to develop more effective medical therapies to treat obesity, the treatments available to date are unsatisfactory for many patients. Most patients will eventually regain most or all of the weight that is lost by dieting. Despite this observation, the American public spends significant dollars on prescription medicine to treat obesity. Over $32 million were spent in 1999 alone.[17]

Medical treatment of obesity has been the subject of several comprehensive reviews. Two of the most recent publications will be reviewed here.[2,17] One was a systematic review of Medline and The Cochrane Library for published studies of treatments and their efficacy for obesity in adults.[2] The modern era for drug treatment of obesity began in the early 1990s after studies were published by Weintraub and colleagues that showed that fenfluramine and phentermine given in combination with behavioral modification could sustain weight loss in some patients for an extended period of time. Although this drug combination was eventually withdrawn from the market because of its association with the development of pulmonary hypertension and valvular heart disease, Weintraub's approach heralded a change in the medical community, where obesity increasingly came to be recognized as a chronic disease process that warranted sustained medical attention and treatment.

Medical treatments for obesity have evolved over the past several decades as new drugs have been developed and introduced to the market. Medications that are approved for use for weight loss in the United States can be broadly categorized as those that decrease food intake by suppressing appetite or increasing satiety, and those that decrease nutrient absorption. Appetite suppressants are believed to work by increasing the availability of neurotransmitters such as norepinephrine, serotonin, and dopamine, which suppress appetite. Sibutramine works by inhibiting the uptake of these neurotransmitters. This drug may also stimulate thermogenesis, although this effect is modest and constitutes only 3–5% of the average person's resting metabolic rate. Randomized controlled trials indicate that the average patient will lose approximately 3–4 kg over 8–52 weeks of treatment. All subjects regained weight after treatment was discontinued.

Orlistat (Xenical) and sibutramine are the only FDA-approved medications to treat obesity. Orlistat reduces nutrient absorption by binding to gastrointestinal lipase and prevents the hydrolysis of dietary fat into absorbable free fatty acids and monoacylglycerols. Patients who are treated with orlistat excrete about a third of the dietary fat that they consume in their stools and can be expected to lose about 9% of their baseline weight on average. Randomized controlled trials also indicate that patients treated with orlistat tend to regain all of the weight that was lost when treatment is ended.

Thus, pharmacotherapy typically induces relatively small amounts of weight loss, in the range of 3–5 kg over 6 months. Similar outcomes are to be expected from behavioral counseling. Although long-term medical therapy can decrease the likelihood of a given patient regaining the lost weight, long-term data on the safety and efficacy of using any medication is sparse. As of 2002, there were no long-term randomized controlled trials demonstrating that prescription weight loss medications were safe or efficacious in children less than 16 years of age.[17]

Other medications with different mechanisms of action are being evaluated in clinical trials, including bupropion, which has been shown to be associated with small amounts of weight loss in patients who were being treated for depression; topiramate, which can reduce food intake; and metformin, which has been shown to inhibit hepatic glucose production and increase sensitivity to insulin.[17] It should be noted that the utility of prescription medication in concert with surgical procedures to treat morbid obesity has not been sufficiently investigated.

Despite the lack of durable success with medical therapy in many obese patients, the relationship between weight loss and reduction of much, if not all, of the risk of excess morbidity and mortality is well established. Loss of as little as 5–10% of pretreatment weight improves blood glucose control in type II diabetes, hypertension, and cardiovascular disease.[19] Loss of 10 kg of body weight is associated with a 20–25% decrease in mortality from all causes, including 30–50% reductions in deaths related to diabetes and cancer.[19]

For these reasons and others that will become apparent, the currently accepted approach is to combine caloric restriction with exercise and behavioral modification as the initial treatment recommendation for most overweight or obese patients. Diet modification, exercise, and behavioral modifications should be the cornerstones of every treatment plan. The National Institutes of Health has published guidelines on the identification and treatment of obesity, including medical therapy, in adults. These guidelines are available online at http://www.nhlbi.nih.gov/guidelines/obesity/Ob_home.htm (Table 16–4). Many patients can be expected to lose between 5% and 10% of the starting body weight over 4–6 months, and this may be sufficient to improve their health by reducing obesity-related comorbidities.[17] Medical treatment of obesity is appropriate therapy for patients who fail these more conservative approaches and who have a BMI of at least 27 kg/m^2 body surface area and obesity-related medical conditions (e.g., hypertension, dyslipidemia, coronary artery disease, adult-onset diabetes mellitus, or sleep apnea), or 30 kg/m^2 or higher in the absence of comorbidities.[17] Initial treatment failure is defined as when a patient fails to lose at least 10% of his or her initial body weight or at least 0.5 kg per week over a 6-month period. Medical therapy is continued as long as it is effective or until unacceptable side effects occur. Patients who fail lifestyle manage-

TABLE 16–4. GUIDELINES FOR THE TREATMENT OF OVERWEIGHT AND OBESE INDIVIDUALS

BMI (kg/m^2)	Health Risk	Risk with Comorbidities	Treatment
<25	Minimal	Low	Healthy eating, exercise, and lifestyle changes
25–26.9	Low	Moderate	
27–29.9	Moderate	High	All of the above plus low-calorie diet
30–34.9	High	Very high	All of the above plus pharmacotherapy or very low calorie diet
35–39.9	Very high	Extremely high	
>40	Extremely high	Extremely high	All of the above plus bariatric surgery

ment, behavioral modification, and pharmacotherapy, and who have significant obesity are candidates for surgical intervention.[35]

SURGICAL TREATMENT

The National Institutes of Health has concluded that surgical therapy offers the best long-term chance of successfully treating morbid obesity for most patients.[6] Bariatric surgery should be offered to appropriate patients with BMIs of 40 kg/m^2 or greater (or between 35 and 40 kg/m^2 if any of the previously described significant medical comorbidities are present) who have failed medical treatment, nutritional treatment, lifestyle changes, behavioral modification, or other conservative therapies. Candidates for surgical therapy must be willing and able to comply with postoperative dietary recommendations, exercise, and follow-up requirements. Patients who have ongoing drug or alcohol dependency, who are unstable or otherwise unfit psychiatrically, or who are unable to undergo general anesthesia should not undergo bariatric surgery (Table 16–5).

The technology evaluation center of the Blue Cross and Blue Shield Association recently concluded that "surgery improves health outcomes for most patients with morbid obesity as compared with nonsurgical treatment."[36] In all instances, the best care for morbidly obese patients provides unfettered access to, and evaluation by, a multidisciplinary team comprised of nutritionists, physical or exercise therapists, surgeons, medical specialists, and psychiatrists. Nutritional evaluation and education are critically important components of preoperative preparation. Psychiatric evaluation helps to prepare patients for operation and their postoperative recuperation, and also helps to identify patients with eating disorders, severe depression, psychosis, or other mood disturbances that could adversely affect outcome. Psychiatric evaluation also helps some patients cope more effectively with various stressors that may surface in their interpersonal relationships after surgery.

It is also likely that centers of excellence where a large number of procedures are performed each year by experienced surgeons who devote a significant portion of their practices to bariatric surgery, those that have organized and supervised patient support groups, and those with a comprehensive system for documenting and following patients and their outcomes will provide the highest quality and safest treatment and will achieve the best overall results.

Selection criteria for surgical treatment of obesity are summarized in Table 16–6.

Preoperative Preparation

In all cases, the mortality rate for patients with severe obesity is two to three times higher perioperatively than it is for normal-weight subjects. Because many obese patients will have cardiovascular disease (including hypertension, congestive heart failure, and ischemic heart disease), a careful preoperative work-up is mandatory.[37] All patients should have an electrocardiogram performed preoperatively. Those with significant cardiac disease should be evaluated by a cardiologist. Some patients, especially those with a prior history of treatment with fenfluramine and phentermine, should undergo echocardiography. Stress testing and even cardiac catheterization may be indicated for intermediate- or high-risk patients. The signs and symptoms of obstructive sleep apnea are highly variable and can be difficult to interpret.

TABLE 16–5. MAJOR CONCLUSIONS OF THE 1991 NIH CONSENSUS CONFERENCE ON THE SURGICAL TREATMENT OF MORBID OBESITY

Surgical treatment is the only way to obtain consistent, durable weight loss for most morbidly obese patients
Surgical treatment is indicated for patients with:
BMIs of 40 kg/m^2 or greater
BMIs of 35–40 kg/m^2 with obesity-related comorbidities
When medical, nutritional, and behavioral therapies are ineffective

TABLE 16–6. SELECTION CRITERIA FOR SURGICAL TREATMENT OF OBESITY

BMI >40 or BMI between 35 and 40 in individuals with high-risk comorbid conditions or severe lifestyle limitations for greater than 5 years
Absence of secondary cause of morbid obesity
Ability and willingness to cooperate with long-term follow-up
Acceptable operative risk
Not yet uniformly recommenced for children or adolescents (less than 18 years of age), or patients over the age of 60

Many patients with this disease may not be noted to snore loudly and may not have daytime hypersomnolence. For these reasons, some centers refer all morbidly obese patients who are being evaluated for surgical treatment for polysomnographic evaluation at a sleep center. Patients who are diagnosed with significant sleep apnea require treatment with continuous positive airway pressure and are at risk for acute upper airway obstruction and significant cardiac arrhythmias postoperatively. Obesity hypoventilation syndrome may also be present in many obese patients. The syndrome is defined by the presence of significant hypoxemia with arterial partial pressure of oxygen less than 55 mm Hg, and hypercarbia with a partial pressure of carbon dioxide greater than 47 mm Hg. Patients with sleep apnea, the obesity hypoventilation syndrome, or any other significant airway or parenchymal lung disease should be evaluated by a pulmonologist preoperatively. Finally, many patients with severe gastroesophageal reflux, dysphagia, nausea, vomiting, abdominal pain, or a prior history of gastric or intestinal surgery may require formal evaluation of the gastrointestinal tract including barium swallow, upper gastrointestinal series, esophagogastroduodenoscopy, esophageal manometry, and pH testing and computed tomography of the abdomen with and without contrast. Preoperative laboratory evaluation will typically include hemoglobin, hematocrit, and platelet count measurements, along with assessment of electrolyte levels, BUN, creatine, blood glucose, and liver function. In women, Pap smears and pregnancy testing should be performed routinely. Hemoglobin A_{1c} measurements are appropriate for patients with adult-onset diabetes mellitus. Posteroanterior and lateral radiographs of the chest should also be evaluated routinely.

Obesity likely increases the risk of postoperative wound infections. For this reason antibiotic prophylaxis is indicated according to the likelihood of wound contamination and the type of procedure planned. The rate of wound infection after laparoscopic gastric bypass appears to be reduced by at least 75% compared with open gastric bypass surgery.[37]

As mentioned previously, obese patients have an increased risk (approximately 3%) of developing deep venous thrombosis. The risk of pulmonary embolism is estimated to be approximately 1%. Deep venous thrombosis prophylaxis is considered the standard of care, though there is some disagreement as to how this should be accomplished. Two approaches are described; 5000 units of unfractionated heparin may be administered subcutaneously pre- and postoperatively to reduce the risk of deep venous thrombosis.[37] Alternatively, low-molecular-weight heparin therapy at a typical dose of 40 mg administered twice daily may also be effective, although the maximally effective dose has not been clearly established.[37]

Intraoperative Management

Morbidly obese patients can be extremely difficult to manage intraoperatively.[37] Partnering with an anesthesiologist who is knowledgeable about the metabolic and physiological changes induced by obesity is extremely important to provide high-quality, safe patient care.

Positioning also requires careful attention and is important to help prevent pressure sores and nerve injury. The brachial plexus and sciatic nerve may be particularly susceptible to injury due to excessive stretch. The lateral femoral cutaneous nerve and the ulnar nerve are also susceptible to traction injury. For severely obese patients with BMIs >60 kg/m^2, those with severe cardiopulmonary disease, or for patients in whom measurements from standard noninvasive sphygmomanometers are unreliable, invasive arterial monitoring is recommended. Central venous cannulation and pressure measurements may also be needed in patients who have poor peripheral access. A Foley catheter is recommended to assess volume status, although the effects of carbon dioxide pneumoperitoneum may make urine output an unreliable indicator of overall volume status in patients who have undergone laparoscopic procedures.[37] Surgeons must remember that pressure-induced rhabdomyolysis is a rare but potentially lethal complication that has been described in morbidly obese patients.

Postoperative Management

Close observation postoperatively is imperative for morbidly obese patients who undergo bariatric surgical procedures. High-risk patients should be admitted to an intermediate "step-down" or intensive care unit postoperatively. Respiratory complications, most commonly atelectasis, may occur, especially in patients who have undergone open surgical procedures. Patients who have their operations performed laparoscopically may experience less pain and less pulmonary compromise. All patients should be encouraged to ambulate as quickly as possible after operation, ideally on the first postoperative day. The use of incentive spirometry should be encouraged. If epidural anesthesia is not employed or is otherwise unsuccessful, patient-controlled analgesia should be used. Some surgeons administer ketorolac in the postoperative period to improve pain control, especially in patients with degenerative joint disease or osteoarthritis. In many major centers, a Gastrografin swallow is obtained routinely on the first or second postoperative day (followed by the instillation of barium if needed), especially if a gastric bypass is performed laparoscopically, to help rule out the presence of an anastomotic leak.[38] Other surgeons use a selective approach to performing radiographic evaluations based on intraoperative findings, the course and conduct of the operation, and postoperative signs or symptoms, especially respiratory decompensation. Many experts also perform esophagogastroduodenoscopy once gastric bypass is completed to check the integrity of the gastrojejunal anastomosis, especially if the operation has been performed laparoscopically. Thereafter, patients are allowed to resume oral intake beginning first with clear liquids. Dietary progression varies greatly by center and according to surgeon preference. The key is to reinvolve the expert dietitian to help guide the patient about food choices and to address any food intolerances that may develop or that may have been identified preoperatively. In general, patients need to be encouraged to hydrate themselves adequately since weight loss can be associated with significant water loss. Food and liquids should be consumed separately. Hyperosmolar, dense foods should be avoided—especially by patients who have undergone gastric bypass procedures. In general, low-residue, high-protein, low-carbohydate diets are the best tolerated and such foods are introduced gradually. Supplementary calcium, multivitamins, and trace elements should begin immediately and should be continued indefinitely. Women should take at least 1 g of calcium (as gluconate or carbonate) daily. Bone density measurements by x-ray absorptiometry are recommended beginning approximately 1 year after surgery for women. Additional calcium supplementation may be required to prevent or treat bone demineralization.

The Operations

Historical Perspective and Overview. Historically, the rationale for the surgical treatment of obesity has been based on three fundamental goals: (1) reducing caloric absorption by bypassing portions of the stomach and small bowel; (2) reducing gastric capacity via banding, stapling, or transection; or (3) performing operations that induce malabsorption and restrict food intake. Much of the latest research described earlier suggests that this classification scheme may be too simplistic. The mechanisms of action of many of the bariatric surgical procedures may involve more than rerouting or restriction of food intake, and include alterations of metabolic pathways and other signaling processes that may modulate appetite and dietary intake. For example, gastrointestinal hormone secretion and feedback may be substantially modified after gastric bypass or biliopancreatic diversion, but not by operations such as the laparoscopic banding procedure or the vertical-banded gastroplasty.

Although the mechanisms of action of the various operations that are used to treat morbid obesity are the subject of ongoing research and are being refined, a useful paradigm is to categorize bariatric procedures as restrictive, malabsorptive, or a combination of both[39] (Table 16–7). The so-called restrictive procedures can certainly limit the amount of some foods that can be ingested and can induce a sense of fullness. Malabsorptive procedures alter normal nutrient digestion and absorption. Over the years, many different bariatric operations have been described. Only the major variants will be discussed. Although the indications for each operation may vary somewhat according to the patient population for which it is best suited, and the outcomes may differ somewhat between centers, each modern procedure may have a place in the surgeon's armamentarium. Ideally, the expert bariatric surgeon should be capable of performing each operation or should be part of a team that together provides the complete range of services including the care of patients who require reoperation.

The jejunoileal bypass was one of the earliest operations developed to treat morbid obesity. This operation induced substantial weight loss by surgically rerouting the intestine and cause extreme malabsorption.[40] In this operation, the proximal jejunum is divided 35 cm from the ligament of Treitz and then is anastomosed to the distal ileum approximately 10 cm from the ileocecal valve. A very long excluded "blind loop" of intestine is created through which no food or biliopancreatic secretions flowed. This segment drains into the small intestine or colon to avoid closed-loop obstruction. Most patients suffered severe diarrhea, electrolyte imbalances, vitamin deficiencies, and severe end-organ dysfunction such that their risk of mortality was substantially and unacceptably increased.[41]

Restrictive procedures include the various gastroplasties as well as the gastric banding procedures. To perform the vertical banded gastroplasty, a small gastric pouch was created near the gastroesophageal junction with a narrowed outlet. The gastric pouch, however, originally remained in continuity with the remaining stomach. The adjustable gastric banding procedures

TABLE 16–7. MAJOR TYPES OF BARIATRIC SURGICAL PROCEDURES

Malabsorptive
Jejunoileal and jejunocolic bypasses (no longer recommended)
Restrictive
Vertical banded gastroplasty
Adjustable silicone gastric banding
Mostly restrictive
Short-limb (50–100 cm) Roux-en-Y gastric bypass
Long-limb (150 cm) Roux-en-Y gastric bypass
Mostly malabsorptive
Biliopancreatic diversion with or without duodenal switch

were designed to be performed laparoscopically and position an adjustable inflatable bandlike device near the gastric cardia to limit oral intake. Of course, the adjustable gastric band can also be positioned using a traditional open approach to the abdomen.

The first gastric bypass operation to treat morbid obesity was described by Mason and Ho in 1969. Their procedure connected a small horizontally divided gastric pouch to a loop gastrojejunostomy.[42] As such, it was thought to combine elements of restriction as well as mild malabsorption. Over the years the operation has been extensively modified to include, in various iterations, reinforced staple lines, vertically-oriented gastric pouches, Roux-en-Y reconstructions with gastrojejunostomy to minimize the risk of bile reflux gastritis, divided gastric pouches to minimize the risk of staple-line disruption with reinforcement to decrease the risk of gastric leakage, as well as banding of the pouch outlet.

The Roux-en-Y gastric bypass procedures were designed to combine limitation of oral intake, accomplished by restricting the size of the stomach pouch, with some malabsorption and appetite suppression by construction of the Roux limb and gastrojejunostomy. The creation of the gastrojejunostomy would inhibit intake of hyperosmolar or densely caloric foods while bypassing the distal stomach and duodenum. The reported lengths of the Roux-en-Y and afferent biliopancreatic limbs vary. Most surgeons now construct a Roux limb that is between 50 (short) and 150 cm (long) in length (usually at least 100 cm), and an afferent limb that is between 50 and 75 cm in length.

The biliopancreatic diversion was introduced by Scopinaro and others.[43] Like the jejunoileal bypass, this operation disrupts intestinal absorptive capacity by short-circuiting a portion of the small intestine. However, it has not been associated with the severe complications described in patients who had jejunoileal bypasses performed. A likely explanation is that there are no defunctionalized limbs that are created.[37]

Gastric bypass procedures and biliopancreatic diversion operations, with or without duodenal switch, account for approximately 80% of the bariatric procedures that are performed in the U.S. and Canada.[44] Between 1998 and 2002, the number of bariatric operations performed in the U.S. increased dramatically.[45,46] Laparoscopic restrictive procedures are more commonly performed in Europe, where its overall outcomes appear to be superior to the outcomes reported from most centers in North America. This disparity has been attributed to the presence of more favorable dietary habits among the Europeans, and their lower average body mass indices, as well as to surgeon experience.[44] All of the modern procedures can be performed laparoscopically or open with acceptable mortality risks.

Vertical Banded Gastroplasty. *Open Approach.* Edward Mason also described the first vertical banded gastroplasty in 1982 (Fig 16–4).[47] Access to the peritoneal cavity is accomplished via a vertical midline incision precisely dividing the linea alba. Such an approach facilitates optimal wound closure.

In his original description, Mason inserted a 32F Ewald tube transorally into the stomach. A large caliber nasogastric tube is equally useful in our opinion and may be less traumatic. Otherwise, the procedure has changed very little since it was originally described.

The esophagus is encircled with a Penrose drain at the level of the esophageal hiatus and gastroesophageal junction using a combination of blunt and sharp dissection. Exposure to the posterior wall of the stomach is obtained by opening the lesser or greater omentum to access the lesser sac. The authors prefer dividing the gastrocolic ligament to access the lesser sac. Blunt dissection posteriorly proceeds at the angle of His facilitated by blunt dissection with the index and middle fingers of the right hand. A no. 2 Prolene suture or its equivalent is grasped between the fingertips and pulled posterior to the stomach to exit the lesser sac along the greater curvature of the stomach where the gastrocolic ligament was divided.

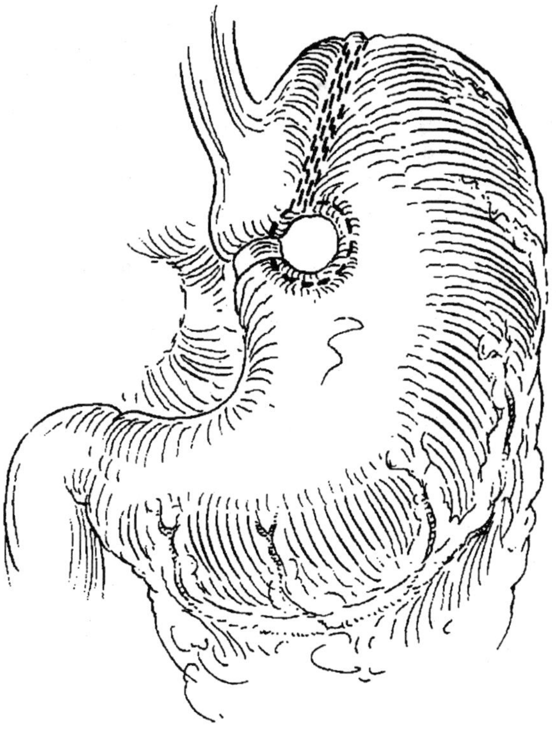

Figure 16–4. The original vertical banded gastroplasty. (Redrawn, with permission, from Sugerman HJ, Starkey JV, Birkenhauer R. A randomized prospective trial of gastric bypass versus vertical banded gastroplasty for morbid obesity and their effects on sweets versus nonsweets eaters. *Ann Surg* 1987;205:613.)

The lesser curvature of the stomach is the dissected free of its mesentery 10–15 cm below the gastroesophageal junction. The anterior and posterior walls of the stomach are punctured 3 cm from the lesser curvature of the stomach with a right angle clamp that is used to grasp a no. 22 filiform and follower. The anvil of a no. 25 circular stapler is fitted in the follower which allows it to be easily passed sequentially through the posterior and anterior walls of the stomach. The stapler post is mated to the anvil and fired to create a window in the proximal stomach. Care must be taken to be sure not to capture the nasogastric tube. The Prolene suture is passed from posterior to anterior through the gastric window and tied to a no. 32 chest tube, the end of which is fashioned to fit the TA-90B surgical stapler (Tyco). The Prolene suture is used to guide the chest tube and heavy duty surgical stapler in place and create a line of four rows of 90-mm staples. We reinforce the staple line with a figure-of-eight seromuscular stitch along the greater curvature of the stomach. Other surgeons may use the linear cutting stapler to create the pouch. This technique creates a pouch that is approximately 50 mL in volume. A strip of polypropylene mesh measuring approximately 7 × 1.5 cm is marked to 5.0-cm circumference and is secured around the gastric outlet by securing the mesh to itself with 3-0 polypropylene suture.

Laparoscopic Approach. Five or six ports are inserted into the upper abdomen for access. Pneumoperitoneum is established using a Veress needle and the patient is placed in a steep reverse Trendelenburg position. Dissection begins on the lesser curvature of the stomach approximately 6–15 cm below the gastroesophageal junction. The peritoneal attachments lateral to the angle of His are also incised. The lesser curvature of the stomach is dissected free from its mesentery and the lesser sac is entered by dividing the gastrocolic ligament. In this manner, the anterior and posterior walls of the stomach are freed. A 12- to 16-F nasogastric tube is inserted transorally and grasped with a laparoscopic Babcock clamp. Next, a 21-mm diameter circular stapler is introduced via one of the 15-mm port sites in the upper abdomen. The stapler's post is used to puncture both walls of the stomach, mated with the anvil, and fired. A 60-mm stapler is inserted into the gastrotomy and fired along the nasogastric tube toward the angle of His (again taking care not to include it in the staple line) separating the gastric pouch from the residual stomach. As with the open procedure a strip of polypropylene mesh is sewn to itself with nonabsorbable suture to create an outlet with a 5-cm circumference. All staple lines are carefully inspected for continuity and hemostasis and are reinforced as needed.

Vertical banded gastroplasties are easier to perform than gastric bypasses, are associated with less morbidity, and require less operative time to perform, but induce less weight loss on average. Patients may modify their eating habits to consume more sweets or ingest liquids with high caloric content.[48]

Adjustable Gastric Banding. The Food and Drug Administration approved a laparoscopic band for use in the United States in 2001. The band can be placed using an open or laparoscopic approach (Fig 16–5). The theoretical advantage of the band is that the amount of restriction to foods, especially solids, can be increased or decreased to facilitate optimal weight loss of the patient.

Open Approach.[49,50] The patient is placed in a supine position and a midline incision is performed to enter the upper abdomen. Self-retaining retractors are ideal to allow full access to the operative field. The gastrohepatic ligament is opened approximately 2 cm below the gastroesophageal junction at the level of the right diaphragmatic crus close to the lesser curvature of the stomach. This is described as the "pars flaccida" technique. Blunt dissection is used to create a retrogastric tunnel running from the lesser curvature of the stomach toward the esophagus. The gastrophrenic ligament is opened very close to the greater curvature of the stomach approximately 1–1.5 cm distal to the gastroesophageal junction above the short gastric vessels. The inflatable band is then passed behind the stomach. A

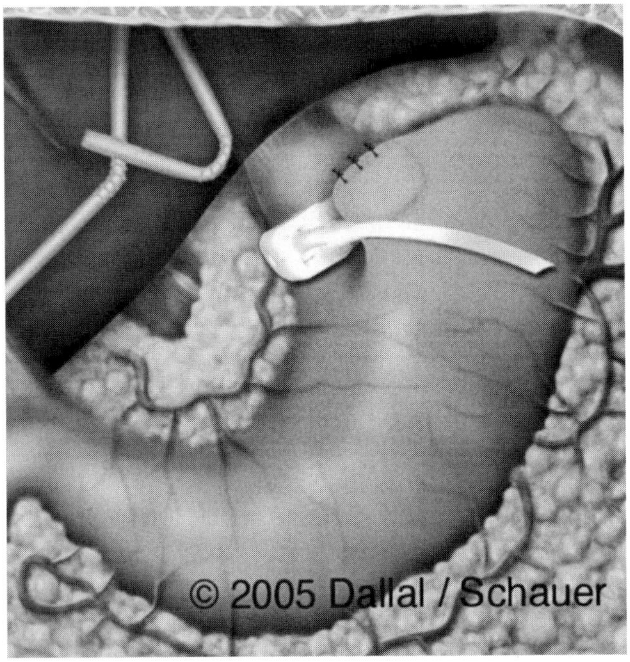

Figure 16–5. Adjustable silicone gastric band. (Reproduced, with permission, from http://asbs.org/html/patients/banding.html. Accessed 12/13/05.)

calibration tube that has a 15-mm balloon and pressure sensor at its distal end is used to facilitate positioning. The band is prefabricated to secure to itself via a buckle. The end of the silicone tubing that attaches to the band is brought out to the upper abdomen via a separate puncture site and is secured to the port. The port is typically positioned in the upper abdomen and secured to the anterior rectus sheath. It is important that it is located so it is easily accessible without radiographic guidance so that saline can easily be instilled or withdrawn to adjust the band as needed.

Laparoscopic Approach. The patient is placed in a modified lithotomy position. Typically, pneumoperitoneum is established via cutdown directly opening the fascia of the anterior abdomen above or below the umbilicus, or by introducing the Veress needle in the same area or in the subcostal region of the upper abdomen. Five 10- to 12-mm trocars are placed in the upper abdomen. A sixth trocar is sometimes needed to insert a retractor to suspend the liver away from the operative field when the left lobe is hypertrophied. A calibration tube is introduced transorally into the stomach and 25 mL of saline is instilled into the balloon that is then seated against the gastroesophageal junction using gentle traction. Next, a retrogastric tunnel is created in line with the equator of the balloon. The dissection should continue close to the gastric wall taking care to avoid entering the lesser sac. The surgeon must be mindful of the possibility that the left hepatic artery could be aberrant and course directly within the operative field.

The retrogastric tunnel should exit the posterior gastric space anterior and superior to the short gastric vessels. Once the crus of the left diaphragm is reached, the lap band is introduced through a 15-mm port in the upper abdomen. With the calibration balloon still inflated, the band is positioned and locked. Three or four seromuscular gastrogastric nonabsorbable sutures are placed to secure the band in place. The tubing used to inflate the band is then tunneled from the abdomen via one of the access sites to the port that is typically seated in the upper abdomen overlying the rectus fascia. Many surgeons are now leaving the band deflated for 10–12 weeks because this is believed to reduce the risk of band slippage.[51,52] More recently, surgeons have emphasized the importance of minimal posterior dissection to create a tiny virtual pouch just inferior to the Belsey fat pad, and have taken care to ensure that the band's closing mechanism is rotated to the left.

Clear liquids are allowed on the first postoperative day after a Gastrografin swallow is obtained to confirm the band's position and patency. Most patients are discharged by the second postoperative day and are maintained on a liquid diet for 4 weeks. Band adjustment is typically performed initially with fluoroscopic guidance after 10–12 weeks. Patients are then followed carefully and the band is adjusted according to the weight loss and food tolerance. Band adjustments may be necessary every 4–6 weeks during the first year.

Roux-en-Y Gastric Bypass. *Open Approach.*[53] An upper midline incision is used to access the peritoneal cavity. Opening the linea alba at the midline facilitates wound closure. The abdominal wall is carefully inspected to detect associated umbilical or epigastric hernias that may be present in up to 30% of patients. Self-retaining retractors are used to facilitate exposure of the operative field. The current recommendation is to create a very small gastric pouch based on the cardia of the stomach. The gastrohepatic ligament is opened and the surgeon passes his or her left hand posterior to the stomach and upwards to expose the left aspect of the gastroesophageal junction. The right hand courses anteriorly to facilitate exposure of the angle of His by elevating Belsey's fat pad. Blunt dissection is used to divide the avascular connective tissue found in this region. Silastic tubes of at least 20F diameter are passed to the retrogastric tunnel and then are redirected to be directly adjacent to the lesser curvature of the stomach to avoid injury to the neurovascular pedicle in this region when the stomach is divided. Two 90-mm linear staplers are guided into place around the gastric cardia using the Silastic tubes. The staples are fired and the cardia between the two staple lines is transected. Alternatively, the 90-mm stapler can be fired a third time without dividing the stomach. The jejunum is then transected approximately 50–100 cm distal to the ligament of Treitz, where the branching of the vessels allows an excellent arterial and venous mesenteric blood supply and typically provide sufficient laxity to mobilize the Roux limb without difficulty. The Roux limb is then coursed through the mesentery of the transverse colon anterior to the stomach. The opening in the transverse mesocolon is created just to the left of the middle colic vessels through an avascular space. This routing is preferred if a stapled gastrojejunostomy will be created. In addition, should reconstruction be necessary, dissection can be more easily performed. The Roux limb can also be brought anterior to the colon, but usually necessitates freeing an additional 5- or 10-cm length of jejunum, even if an opening is created through the omentum.

The gastrojejunostomy can be created using an EEA mechanical stapler. The circular anvil head is placed in the proximal pouch and secured with a 2-0 polypropylene suture so as to occlude the entry point. The post of the circular stapler is exposed through the antimesenteric wall of the Roux-en-Y limb at its most superior portion and mated with the anvil, taking care to exclude any excess fatty tissue and fired. The donuts are inspected. Most surgeons reinforce the anastomosis with several seromuscular sutures. The end of the Roux limb is closed using a linear stapler. Patency of the anastomosis is tested by instilling methylene blue into the gastric pouch under slight pressure. There are three mesenteric defects that must be closed. The first is located near the enteroenterostomy and the second occurs where the Roux-en-Y limb passes through the transverse mesocolon. Care is taken to be sure that no redundant jejunum lies in the lesser sac. The Roux limb is sutured to the transverse mesocolon after any redundancy is eliminated, but avoiding excessive tension on the gastrojejunal anastomosis. Peterson's space is located posterior to the Roux limb below the transverse colon and anterior to the posterior peritoneum (Fig 16–6).

An alternative approach to performing an open gastric bypass is as follows. Access to the abdominal cavity is accomplished through a vertical midline incision as previously described. With experience, the length of the incision can be minimized, often to as small as 5 or 6 inches. Minimizing the length of the incision may minimize postoperative pain and other morbidity. Infiltrating the wound with 0.5% bupivacaine with epinephrine may also minimize postoperative discomfort in patients who are not receiving epidural anesthesia. In this method, the first part of the operation proceeds as if a vertical banded gastroplasty would be performed as described previously. A marking pen is used to measure 15 cm vertically down from the gastroesophageal junction and 3 cm from the lesser curvature after the esophagus is encircled at the level of the gastroesophageal junction with a wide Penrose drain. The lesser sac is entered via the gastrocolic ligament. The anterior and posterior walls of the stomach are punctured and a no. 22 filiform with follower is used to seat the anvil of a no. 25 circular stapler coursing anteriorly. It is mated with the post and fired, creating a circular gastrotomy. The right or left hand is used to bluntly free the avascular tissue along the greater curvature of the stomach at the angle of His superior to the short gastric vessels. A no. 2 polypropylene stitch is grasped between the fingertips, and ultimately brought out through the gastrotomy. It is tied to a no. 32 Silastic chest tube and then used to position the 90-mm linear stapler that is fired to place four rows of heavy duty titanium staples. The staple line is reinforced at its superior apex with a figure-of-eight polypropylene suture. At this point, if the patient is stable and the operation has proceeded uneventfully, a Roux-en-Y reconstruction can be performed by dividing the gastric outlet. This is done using the 30-mm linear stapler to occlude the gastric outlet of the newly created, vertically-oriented gastric pouch at the level of the gastrotomy. The pouch is opened just above the 30-mm staple line using electrocautery. The Roux limb is created as previous described, but is coursed in a retrocolic and retrogastric fashion to the lesser curvature side of the stomach, where an end-to-side gastrojejunal anastomosis is created using a running double-armed 3-0 polypropylene suturing technique (Fig 16–7). The potential spaces where hernias can occur are closed as previously described.

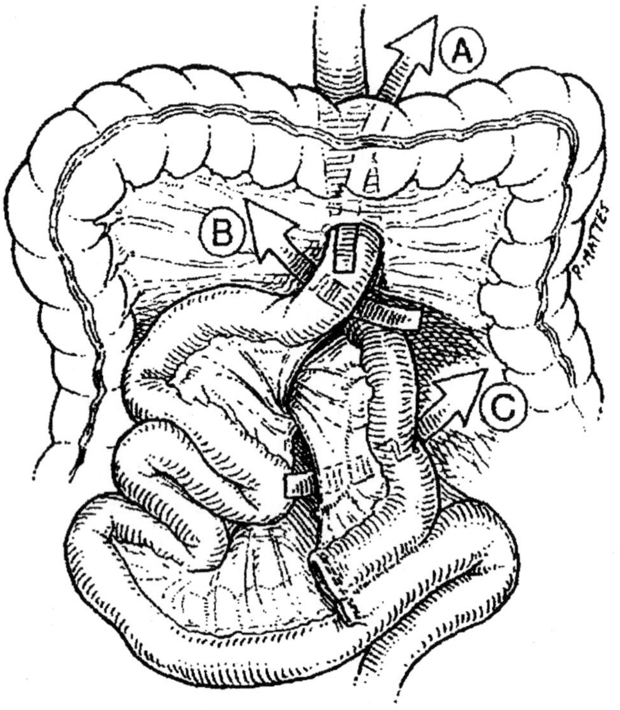

Figure 16–6. Depiction of mesenteric spaces where internal herniation may occur. **A.** Transverse mesocolon. **B.** Peterson's hernia, represented by the infracolic space posterior to the mesentery of the Roux limb and anterior to the posterior peritoneum. **C.** Jejunomesenteric hernia potential space near the jejunojejunostomy. (Reproduced, with permission, from Sarr MG. Open roux-en-y gastric bypass: indications and technique. *J Gastroint Surg* 2004;8:390–392.)

Laparoscopic Approach.[54,38] The laparoscopic Roux-en-Y gastric bypass was first described by Wittgrove and colleagues in 1994.[55] A six-port technique is commonly used. After carbon dioxide pneumoperitoneum is established by inserting a Veress needle in the left subcostal region, a 12-mm trocar is inserted. Additional trocars are usually placed in the left supraumbilical area (12 mm) in the subxiphoid position (5 mm). This allows a transabdominal liver retractor to be inserted to retract the left lateral segment of the liver. Five- and ten-millimeter trocars are typically placed in the right upper abdomen and are used by the operating surgeon. Another 5-mm trocar is inserted in the patient's left upper abdomen for the assistant to use. The gastrohepatic ligament is opened using an ultrasonic dissector to expose the lesser sac. The lesser curvature is

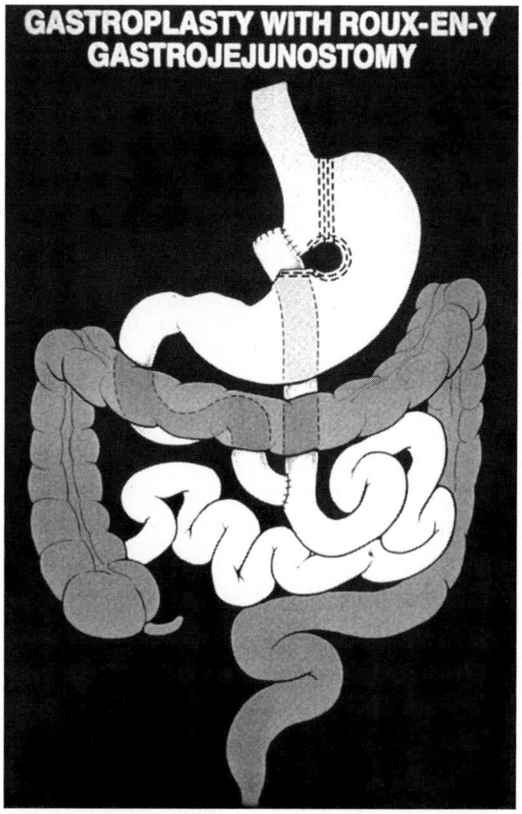

Figure 16–7. Vertical gastroplasty with Roux-en-Y reconstruction in a form that is most often used with the open approach.

freed approximately 10 cm distal to the gastroesophageal junction. The stomach is then serially transected using a linear cutting stapler angling toward the gastroesophageal fat pad. These are typically done with a 60-mm cartridge and 3.5-mm staples. The residual stomach may be calibrated to the size of a 15-mL balloon seated against the gastroesophageal junction. If the Roux limb is to be passed in a retrocolic and retrogastric fashion, a soft latex-free rubber drain may be positioned in the lesser sac to facilitate identification of the correct plane. Dissection through the transverse mesocolon in an avascular plane allows the drain to be identified. Alternatively the transverse mesocolon may be opened inferiorly, laterally and superior to the ligament of Treitz, and the Roux limb passed directly into the lesser sac and grasped above the transverse mesocolon.

An appropriate length of small bowel is then identified 30–100 cm distal to the ligament of Treitz and divided using the 60-mm linear cutting stapler; 2.5-mm staples are recommended for use for this. A portion of the mesentery is also divided to facilitate construction of the enteroenterostomy. This can be accomplished using either another vascular staple load or the ultrasonic dissector. The Roux limb is constructed with a length of 50–100 cm for the standard proximal bypass, or 150 cm if a long-limb reconstruction will be used, measured from the point where the small bowel was resected. Seromuscular stay sutures placed in the jejunal limbs may facilitate construction of the side-to-side jejunojejunostomy. Enterotomies are created in the small bowel using the ultrasonic dissector. The 60-mm linear cutting stapler with 2.5-mm staples are used to create the anastomosis and the enterotomies are carefully closed to avoid narrowing. The mesenteric defects are closed using running absorbable suture.

The linear stapling device is also used to create the gastrojejunostomy. An enterostomy and gastrotomy are made using the harmonic dissector. A 45-mm linear stapler with 3.5-mm staples is used for the anastomosis. The insertion sites are closed with another application of the stapler and the gastrojejunal anastomosis is reinforced using nonabsorbable 2-0 suture material.

Alternatively, upper endoscopy may be performed to create a circular gastrojejunostomy. A transabdominal cannula is used to introduce a wire into the lumen of the gastric pouch. The wire is grasped using a gastroscope and attached to the anvil of a 21- or 25-mm circular stapler. The anvil is then passed down the esophagus to the stomach, where electrocautery may be needed to expose its end. A left-sided access site is enlarged to admit the end of the circular stapler that is passed through the open end of the Roux limb, mated with the anvil, and fired. The end of the Roux limb is closed with a linear stapler.

The integrity of the gastrojejunal anastomosis is tested by insufflation of air instilled via a nasogastric tube or the gastroscope. Methylene blue can also be instilled via the nasogastric tube to check for anastomotic leaks. The fascia is closed at the large port sites (>5 mm) using absorbable sutures.

Biliopancreatic Diversion with and without Duodenal Switch. Scopinaro and Papadia described the first biliopancreatic diversion procedure[43] to treat morbid obesity, although DeMeester and colleagues had introduced the procedure in 1987 as a treatment for bile reflux gastritis and to minimize morbidity in patients who had undergone distal gastrectomies with Billroth I reconstruction (Figs 16–8 and 16–9).[56] Scopinaro and Papadia combined a partial gastrectomy with closure of the duodenal stump and created a distal Roux-en-Y gastrojeunostomy to contain ingested food. The alimentary limb is coursed through the mesentery of the transverse colon. The biliopancreatic limb connected the proximal small bowel to the ileum 50 cm from the ileocecal valve. The proce-

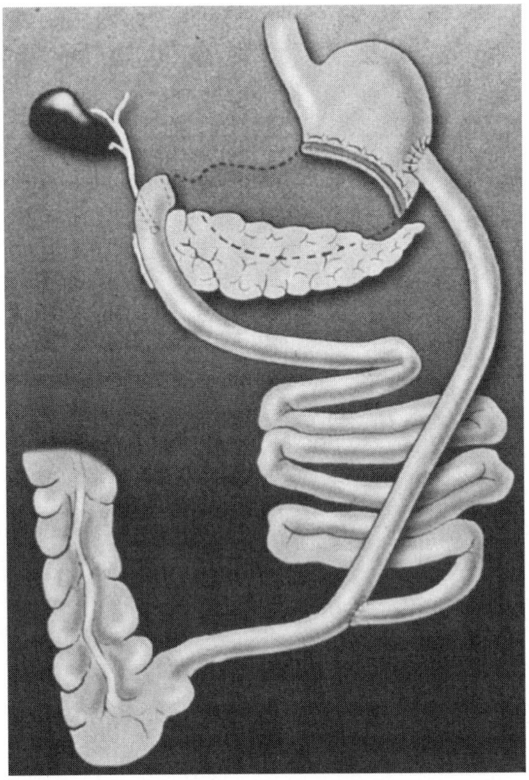

Figure 16–8. Biliopancreatic diversion procedure before the gallbladder is removed. The common channel's length is most often 100 cm.

dure was later modified to decrease the volume of the residual stomach to approximately 200–400 mL. Later modifications were introduced by Hess[57] and Marceau[58] so that a sleeve gastrectomy was performed by resecting the lesser curvature of the residual stomach. The intent was to enhance feelings of satiety in the first few months of recovery.

Presently, the biliopancreatic diversion consists of the following key elements. A subtotal gastrectomy is performed leaving a gastric remnant between 200 and 400 mL in size. A smaller pouch is recommended for superobese patients. A Roux-en-Y gastrojejunal anastomosis is created 100 cm from the ileocecal valve, and the distal small bowel is anastomosed to the gastric pouch. This alimentary limb typically measures about 250 cm and is approximately one-third of the total length of small intestine. A cholecystectomy should be performed because of the high risk of postoperative cholelithiasis in these patients. The operation has been successfully performed laparoscopically but is performed in an open fashion most often.

The duodenal switch modification was introduced in an effort to minimize the risk of dumping syndrome and marginal ulceration by preserving the antrum, pylorus, and duodenum. A sleeve resection of the greater curvature of the stomach is performed to leave a residual capacity of 150–200 mL. As before, the ileum is divided approximately 250 cm proximal to the ileocecal valve and anastomosed to the duodenum distal to the pylorus. The biliopancreatic limb is anastomosed to the ileum 100 cm from the ileocecal valve.

A Gastrografin swallow is typically obtained on the second or third postoperative day to help exclude the presence of anastomotic leak or stenosis. If this test is negative, a clear liquid diet is begun.

POSTOPERATIVE COMPLICATIONS

Early and late complications after bariatric surgical procedures have been the subject of an excellent recent comprehensive review, elements of which are summarized below.[39]

Early Complications

The most serious early complications are anastomotic leak and pulmonary embolus. Anastomotic leaks can

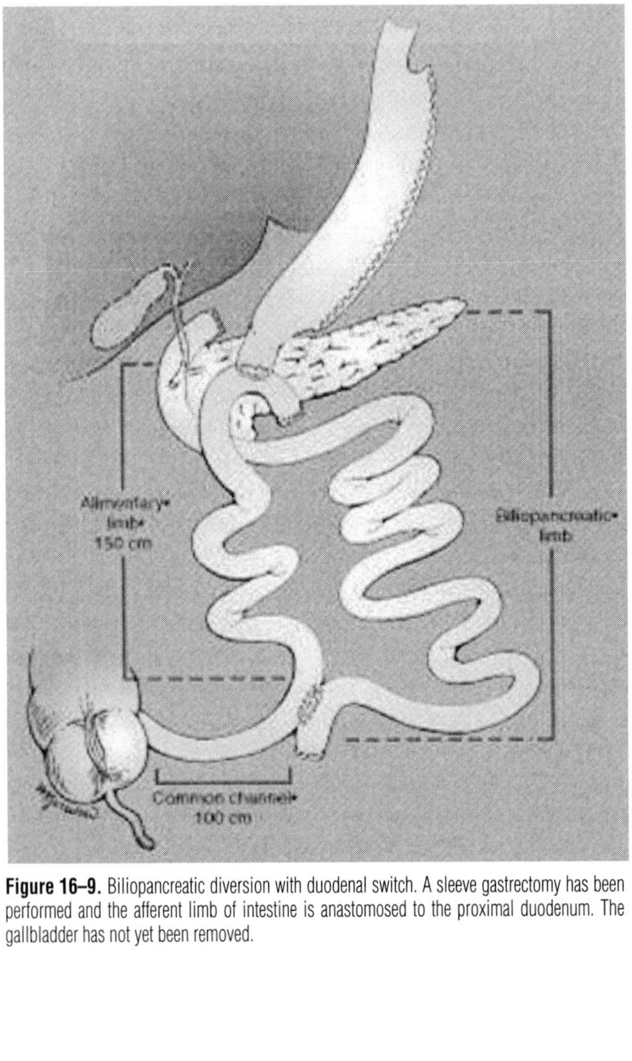

Figure 16–9. Biliopancreatic diversion with duodenal switch. A sleeve gastrectomy has been performed and the afferent limb of intestine is anastomosed to the proximal duodenum. The gallbladder has not yet been removed.

occur at any of the sites where the GI tract is entered or reconstructed, although it most commonly occurs at the gastrojejunostomy. Leakage has been described at the gastrotomy site used in the vertical banded gastroplasty. Peritonitis secondary to anastomotic leakage is the most common cause of death after bariatric surgery. The initial signs and symptoms may be minimal. Patients with unexplained tachycardia, dyspnea, restlessness, or oxygen desaturation should be evaluated carefully because these may be early warning signs of an anastomotic disruption. Depending on the procedure that was performed, Gastrografin x-rays of the upper GI tract or abdominal computed tomography scanning may be indicated. A high index of suspicion is warranted and emergent re-exploration may be indicated in patients with otherwise unexplained septic physiology.

Although obstruction of the Roux-en-Y limb is rare after gastric bypass surgery (<1%), it may cause acute distention of the gastric remnant. These patients will often complain of severe bloating and persistent hiccups. Plain films of the abdomen may show dilatation of the remnant stomach. Emergent reoperation may be necessary, although percutaneous decompression has been described and may be successful. Internal hernias and adhesion formation are also rare causes of intestinal obstruction. Obstruction of the gastric pouch outlet in patients who have undergone vertical banded gastroplasty has been described and may be due to edema or other technical errors when it occurs early in the postoperative period.

Pulmonary complications may be observed even in patients who have their procedures performed laparoscopically. These complications include pneumonia and atelectasis. Pulmonary embolism is the second most frequent cause of death, with an incidence of approximately 1%.

Besides wound infections that usually become immediately evident, other wound complications are usually detected within 1 month of surgery, with a reported frequency of between 20% and 30% after open procedures and 5% or less after laparoscopic procedures. Most wound complications occur within 1 month of operation.

Late Complications

Vomiting. Vomiting is a common complaint after bariatric surgery and may be severe in up to 30% of patients. Careful evaluation is warranted. Causes include noncompliance, inadequate chewing, obstruction of the stoma or anastomosis, food impaction, internal herniation, and partial bowel obstruction secondary to adhesion formation. Other less frequent causes include gastroesophageal reflux, food intolerance (especially to red meat), overfilling of the gastric pouch, marginal ulceration, medication side effects, and cholelithiasis.

Patients who are not losing at least 1 pound per week on average for the first 6 months to a year after operation may be ingesting large quantities of food or drinking, especially immediately after eating. They should be encouraged to drink between meals to minimize the risk of overdistention of the gastric pouch. They should also be encouraged to chew their food very well and to eat slowly, over a period of at least 20 minutes, and to make sure that their meal volume is less than 60 mL at each sitting. Patients should also be instructed to discontinue eating before discomfort ensues and to avoid red or other stringy meats.

Patients who gradually develop intolerance to both solids and liquids may have developed stomal stenosis. Stomal stenosis occurs after Roux-en-Y gastric bypass or vertical banded gastroplasty with a reported incidence between 4% and 20%. The sudden onset of vomiting and epigastric pain may herald acute obstruction secondary to a bezoar or food impaction. Emergency esophagogastroscopy may be required and can be used to extract the obstructing material. Patients typically present within 6 months of initial operation and complain of a gradual onset of intolerance to solids or liquids, epigastric pain, and vomiting. An upper GI series is most often performed initially, although endoscopy is the diagnostic procedure of choice because it is more sensitive and allows for therapeutic intervention. Dilatation is recommended based on symptoms and the presence of a stoma diameter of less than 15 mm. Repeated dilatations may be required to achieve the optimum result. Patients who fail to respond satisfactorily after three balloon treatments may require surgical intervention. Obstruction at the jejunojejunal anastomosis is a less common cause of vomiting that most often requires operative correction.

Prolonged vomiting can cause significant malnutrition and thiamine deficiency, especially in the absence of sufficient carbohydrate intake. Patients who are thiamine deficient can develop significant neurological deficits, including Wernicke's encephalopathy. Parenteral multivitamin and thiamine supplementation may be required.

Diarrhea. There are many causes of diarrhea including alterations in bowel frequency and consistency caused by the operations. Patients who undergo biliopancreatic diversion typically have between four and six bowel movements per day on average that may be steatorrheic. Patients who experience diarrhea after Roux-en-Y gastric bypass may have dumping associated with the ingestion of hyperosmolar food substances. Other possibilities include lactose intolerance or food sensitivities, bacterial overgrowth, and infection.

Gatroesophageal Reflux. Gastroesophageal reflux is frequently observed after vertical banded gastroplasty or silicone adjustable gastric banding. Reflux may be exaggerated by pouch overfilling secondary to excessive food intake, vagal nerve injury, stomal stricture, or alterations in gastric motility. Diagnostic evaluation of these patients may require upper endoscopy, esophageal manometry, and 24-hour esophageal pH monitoring if the symptoms are severe and not controlled by medication. Some patients will need to have their gastroplasties reversed or their gastric bands removed. In this instance, conversion to a Roux-en-Y gastric bypass may be indicated, especially if weight loss has been unsatisfactory.

Strictures are treated symptomatically and with serial dilatation. Up to three treatments may be required to elicit a satisfactory result.

Cholelithiasis. The rapid weight loss associated with bariatric surgery increases the likelihood of gallstone formation in the immediate perioperative period. As many as 36% of patients may develop sludge or cholelithiasis within 6 months of gastric bypass operations and at least half of them will be symptomatic.

If the gallbladder is diseased, it should be removed at the time of operation. Intraoperative ultrasonography may facilitate decision making. Some surgeons remove the gallbladder routinely even if no disease is evident. Cholecystectomy is routinely performed when patients undergo biliopancreatic diversion. Other surgeons will leave a normal gallbladder in place and treat with bile salt binders (ursodiol, 600 mg per day in divided doses) for 6 months to 1 year after operation. Patients who take ursodiol have an incidence of new gallstone formation that is equivalent to that of normal control subjects.

Access to the common bile duct can be difficult in patients who have undergone gastric bypass. Magnetic resonance cholangiopancreatography can be used to assess the biliary tree noninvasively. When choledocholithiasis is demonstrated, endoscopic retrograde cholangiopancreatography can be performed after the bypass and the stomach is accessed percutaneously.

Stomal Ulceration. Stomal ulceration is more common after gastric bypass procedures in which the distal stomach is not transected. The reported incidence is less than 8%. Endoscopy is the preferred diagnostic test and biopsies should be performed to help rule out the presence of *Helicobacter pylori*. Patients with large gastric pouches or who have suffered staple line disruption have the greatest risk. Prophylaxis is key. Patients are treated with proton pump inhibitors during the immediate postoperative period. Many centers continue such treatment through discharge and the first several months of recovery until meal intake normalizes.

Upper Gastrointestinal Bleeding. Upper gastrointestinal bleeding is rare. Possible causes include bleeding at the gastrojejunal anastomosis, at the gastric pouch staple line, from sources within or near the gastric remnant such as stomal ulceration, or at the jejunojejunal anastomosis. Endoscopy can readily identify and treat many sources of bleeding. Occasionally, angiography may be required to identify the causes of hemorrhage. Access to the bypassed stomach may be obtained percutaneously or may require operative exposure. The risk of cancer forming in the bypassed stomach is minimal.

Dumping Syndrome. Patients who experience the dumping syndrome are often noncompliant with the recommended diet. Typical symptoms include diarrhea, abdominal colic, nausea, and vomiting, as well as systemic effects of hypotension, tachycardia, lightheadedness, flushing, and syncope, and are believed to be caused by exposure of the proximal small bowel to hyperosmolar foods or liquids. The dumping syndrome most commonly occurs after Roux-en-Y gastric bypass; patients who undergo surgical gastroplasty should not have dumping and it is rarely seen after biliopancreatic diversion with duodenal switch.

Complications of Gastric Banding. Gastric banding procedures are technically less complicated than laparoscopic gastric bypass or the biliopancreatic diversion. It may be a better choice for high-risk patients, including the elderly, but also may be more appropriate for children or for treating patients who have relatively lower body mass indices. Complications of the gastric banding procedures include intractable vomiting, esophageal injury, band slippage or erosion, pouch dilatation, esophageal dilatation, gastroesophageal reflux, outlet stenosis, and failure to lose weight. The reoperation rate for complications is prohibitive in many published studies from centers in the U.S., ranging from 15–20% to as high as 40%. More recently published studies show more promising results.

Complications after Biliopancreatic Diversion. The duodenal switch version may reduce the risk of stomal ulceration and the dumping syndrome. However, both the biliopancreatic diversion and the biliopancreatic diversion with duodenal switch are associated with an increased risk of nutritional and metabolic complications, including protein-calorie malnutrition, calcium depletion, and fat-soluble vitamin and other micronutrient deficiencies. The risk of bone demineralization is minimized by the appropriate use of oral supplements. Indeed, all patients who undergo bariatric surgery should receive oral vitamin and trace mineral supplementation indefinitely in the absence of significant organ dysfunction.

Vitamin and Mineral Deficiencies. Patients should be tested for micronutrient deficiencies routinely after bariatric surgery and testing may be required indefinitely.

Iron deficiency anemia is common in patients after Roux-en-Y gastric bypass with an incidence that is reported to be as high as 50%. Its etiology is multifactorial, including reduced absorption of dietary iron in association with the achlorhydria that is induced by gastric partitioning. Iron absorption is also inhibited by histamine blockers and proton pump inhibitors that are commonly prescribed after surgery. Furthermore, iron absorption occurs predominantly in the duodenum which is bypassed. Lastly, the intake of iron-rich foods is significantly diminished in most patients. As mentioned previously, multivitamin and trace metal supplementation should be routinely prescribed for all patients after any bariatric surgical procedure. Additional iron supplementation may be needed if iron deficiency anemia is recognized.

Vitamin B_{12} and Folate. Patients who undergo Roux-en-Y gastric bypass or biliopancreatic diversion may also develop vitamin B_{12} deficiency. The mechanisms of action include achlorhydria, suboptimal vitamin consumption, and a reduced production of intrinsic factor, which is required for normal absorption of vitamin B_{12} to occur in the distal ileum. The likelihood of significant deficiency is reduced in patients who receive vitamin supplements.

Folate deficiency may also occur after gastric bypass secondary to reduced secretion of hydrochloric acid. Folate deficiency is also seen and in association with decreased vitamin B_{12} absorption. Vitamin B_{12} is needed for the conversion of inactive folate to active folate. Reduced food intake may also play an important role.

Fat-Soluble Vitamins. Patients who have undergone long-limb Roux-en-Y gastric bypasses or biliopancreatic diversion may have significant steatorrhea and an associated loss of the fat-soluble vitamins A, D, and K. Vitamin D is important for normal calcium homeostasis and bone mineralization. Daily supplementation may be required. Bone mineralization studies should probably be performed in most women who have undergone bariatric surgery procedures after their weight loss has stabilized.

Thiamine. Thiamine is normally absorbed in the proximal small bowel. Oral supplementation is mandatory, because it can not be synthesized by humans. As alluded to previously, thiamine deficiency can result in the Wernicke-Korsakoff syndrome, characterized by ophthalmoplegia, ataxia, and alterations in mental status, and can ultimately result in confusion, coma, and death if thiamine is not replaced. Patients with nausea and vomiting are at increased risk. When thiamine deficiency is suspected, it can be administered intravenously or intramuscularly as needed.

Calcium. Calcium is normally absorbed in the duodenum. Thus patients who have undergone Roux-en-Y gastric bypasses or biliopancreatic diversion (see above) have the greatest risk of developing calcium deficiency. Long-term consequences include osteoporosis and therefore routine calcium supplementation is recommended postoperatively at doses of 1500–2000 mg per day taken in divided doses.

■ CONCLUSION

This chapter has reviewed important elements of the pathogenesis of obesity and the impact of operative intervention with the hope of providing a useful reference for surgeons and surgical trainees. We will likely witness great progress over the next decade in our understanding of the effects of medical and surgical approaches and the development of even more effective treatment options.

REFERENCES

1. Sturm R. The effects of obesity, smoking and drinking on medical problems and cost. Obesity outranks both smoking and drinking in its deleterious effects of health and health costs. *Health Aff* 2002;21:245–253
2. McTigue KM, Harris R, Hemphill B et al. Screening and interventions for obesity in adults: summary of the evidence for the U.S. preventive services task force. *Ann Intern Med* 2003;139:933–949
3. Fernandez AZ, DeMaria EJ, Tichansky DD et al. Multivariate analysis of risk factors for death following gastric bypass for treatment of morbid obesity. *Ann Surg* 2004; 239:698–703
4. Grundy SM, Hansen B, Smith SC et al. Clinical management of metabolic syndrome. *Circulation* 2004;109:551–556
5. Pi-Sunyer FX. NHLBI obesity education initiative expert panel on the identification, evaluation, and treatment of overweight and obesity in adults—the evidence report. *Obes Res* 1998;6(Suppl 2):51s–209s
6. NIH Consensus Conference. Gastrointestinal surgery for severe obesity: Consensus Development Panel. *Ann Intern Med* 1991;115:695–962

7. Kuczmarski RJ, Flegal MM, Campbell S, Johnson DL. Increasing prevalence of overweight among US adults. The National Health and Nutrition Examination Survey, 1960–1991. *JAMA* 1994;272:205–211
8. Mokdad AH, Serdula MK, Dietz WH et al. The spread of the obesity epidemic in the United States: 1991–1998. *JAMA* 1999;282:1519–1522
9. Mokdad AH, Ford ES, Bowman BA et al. Prevalence of obesity, diabetes and obesity-related risk factors. *JAMA* 2001;289:76–79
10. Must A, Spadano J, Coakly EH et al. The disease burden associated with overweight and obesity. *JAMA* 1999;282: 1523–1529
11. Devlin MJ, Yanovski SZ, Wilson GT. Obesity: what mental health professionals need to know. *Am J Psychiatry* 2000;157:854–866
12. Flegal KM, Kuczmarski RJ, Johnson CL. Overweight and obesity in the United States: prevalence and trends, 1960–1994. *Int J Obes Relat Metab Disord* 1998;22:39–47
13. Leigh JP, Fries JF, Hubert HB. Gender and race differences in the correlation between body mass and education in the 1971–1975 NHANES I. *J Epidemiol Comm Health* 1992;46:191–196
14. Sturm R. Increases in clinically severe obesity in the United States. *Arch Intern Med* 2003;163:2146–2148
15. Flegal KM, Carroll MD, Ogden CL, Johnson CL. Prevalence and trends in obesity among US adults, 1999–2000. *JAMA* 2002;288:1723–1727
16. Steinbrook R. Surgery for severe obesity. *N Engl J Med* 2004;350:1075–1079
17. Yanovski SZ, Yanovski JA. Obesity. *N Engl J Med* 2002; 346:591–602
18. Krauss RM, Winston M, Fletcher BJ, Gundy SM. Obesity: impact on cardiovascular disease. *Circulation* 1998;98: 1472–1476
19. Labib M. The investigation and management of obesity. *J Clin Pathol* 2003;56:17–25
20. Clément K, Ferré P. Genetics and the pathophysiology of obesity. *Pediatr Res* 2003;53:721–725
21. Flier JS, Maratos-Flier E. The stomach speaks—ghrelin and weight regulation. *N Engl J Med* 2002;346:1662–1663
22. James F, Habener JF. Defective melanocortin 4 receptors in hyperphagia and morbid obesity. *N Engl J Med* 2003;348:1160–1163
23. Maes HH, Neale MC, Eaves LJ. Genetic and environmental factors in relative body weight and human adiposity. *Behav Genet* 1997;27:325–351
24. Poirier P, Després J-P. Waist circumference, visceral obesity, and cardiovascular risk. *J Cardiopulm Rehabil* 2003; 23:161–169
25. Donahue M, Fuster V, Califf RM. Introduction: cardiologists should target obesity. *Am Heart J* 2001;142:1088–1090
26. Manson J, Willett W, Stampfer M. Body weight and mortality among women. *N Engl J Med* 1995;333:677–685
27. Adami H-O, Trichopoulos D. Obesity and mortality from cancer. *N Engl J Med* 2003;348:1623–1624
28. Sugerman HJ, Wolfe LG, Sica DA, Clore JC. Diabetes and hypertension in severe obesity and effects of gastric bypass induced weight loss. *Ann Surg* 2003;237:751–758
29. Sugerman HJ, Sugerman EL, Wolfe L et al. Risks and benefits of gastric bypass in morbidly obese patients with severe venous stasis disease. *Ann Surg* 2001;234:41–46
30. Calle EE, Rodriguez C, Walker-Thurmond K, Thun MJ. Overweight, obesity, and mortality from cancer in a prospectively studied cohort of U.S. adults. *N Engl J Med* 2003;248:1625–1638
31. Kenchaiah S, Evans JC, Levy D et al. Obesity and the risk of heart failure. *N Engl J Med* 2002;347:305–313
32. Lietz K, John R, Burke EA. Pre-transplant cachexia and morbid obesity are predictors of increased mortality after heart transplantation. *Transplantation* 2001;72:277–284
33. Nair S, Cohen DB, Cohen MP, Tan H. Post-operative morbidity, mortality, costs and long-term survival in severely obese patients undergoing orthotopic liver transplantation. *Am J Gastroenterol* 2001;96:842–851
34. Johnson DW, Isbel NM, Brown AM et al. The effect of obesity on renal transplant outcomes. *Transplantation* 2002;74:600–601
35. Weigle DS. Pharmacological therapy of obesity: past, present and future. *J Clin Endocrinol Metab* 2003;88: 2462–2469
36. Blue Cross and Blue Shield Association Technology Evaluation Center. Special Report: the relationship between weight loss and changes in morbidity following bariatric surgery for morbid obesity. September 2003. http://www.bcbs.com/tec/vol18/18-09.html Accessed December 15, 2004
37. Abir F, Bell R. Assessment and management of the obese patient. *Crit Care Med* 2004;32(Suppl):S87–S91
38. Schauer PR, Ikramuddin S, Gourash W et al. Outcomes after laparoscopic roux-en-y gastric bypass for morbid obesity. *Ann Surg* 2000;232:515–529
39. Ukleja A, Stone RL. Medical and gastroenterologic management of the post-bariatric surgery patient. *J Clin Gastroenterol* 2004;38:312–321
40. Payne JH, Dewind LT, Commons RR. Metabolic observations in patients with jejunocolic shunts. *Am J Surg* 1963; 105:273–289
41. Livingston EH. Obesity and its surgical management. *Am J Surg* 2002;184:103–113
42. Mason EE, Ho C. Gastric bypass. *Ann Surg* 1969;170: 329–335
43. Scopinaro N, Papadia F. Malabsoprtive procedures. In: Schein M, Wise L (eds). *Controversies in Surgery,* Vol 4. New York, NY: Springer; 2001:353–360
44. Morino M, Toppino N, Bonnet G, del Genio G. Laparoscopic adjustable silicone gastric banding versus vertical banded gastroplasty in morbidly obese patients. *Ann Surg* 2003;238:835–842
45. Nguyen NT. Open vs. laparoscopic procedures in bariatric surgery. *J Gastrointest Surg* 2004;8:393–395
46. Nguyen NT. The relationship between hospital volume and outcome in bariatric surgery at academic medical centers. *Ann Surg* 2004;240:586–594

47. Mason EE. Vertical banded gastroplasty for obesity. *Arch Surg* 1982;117:701–706
48. Brolin RL, Robertson LB, Kenler HA. Weight loss and dietary intake after vertical banded gastroplasty and Roux-en-Y gastric bypass. *Ann Surg* 1994;220: 782–789
49. O'Brien PE, Brown WA. Prospective study of a laparoscopically placed, adjustable gastric band in the treatment of morbid obesity. *Br J Surg* 1999;86:113–118
50. de Wit LT, Mathus-Vliegen L, Hey C et al. Open versus laparoscopic adjustable silicone gastric banding. *Ann Surg* 1999;230:800–807
51. Ceelen W, Walder J, Cardon A et al. Surgical treatment of severe obesity with a low-pressure adjustable gastric band. *Ann Surg* 2003;237:10–16
52. DeMaria EJ, Sugerman HJ, Meador JG et al. High failure rate after laparoscopic adjustable silicone gastric banding for treatment of morbid obesity. *Ann Surg* 2001;233:809–818
53. Sarr MG. Open roux-en-y gastric bypass: indications and technique. *J Gastrointest Surg* 2004;8:390–392
54. DeMaria EJ, Sugerman HJ, Kellum JM et al. Results of 281 consecutive total laparoscopic roux-en-y gastric bypasses to treat morbid obesity. *Ann Surg* 2002;235:640–647
55. Wittgrove AC, Clark W. Laparoscopic gastric bypass, Roux-en-Y: Preliminary results of five cases. *Obes Surg* 1994;4:353–357
56. Pories WJ. Diabetes: the evolution of a new paradigm. *Ann Surg* 2004;239:12–13
57. Hess D. Biliopancreatic diversion with a duodenal switch procedure. *Obes Surg* 1994;4:106
58. Marceau P, Biron S, Bourgue R-A et al. Biliopancreatic diversion with a new type of gastrectomy. *Obes Surg* 1993; 3:29–35

Section V

SMALL INTESTINE AND COLON

17

Bowel Obstruction

Scott G. Houghton ▪ *Antonio Ramos De la Medina* ▪ *Michael G. Sarr*

Bowel obstruction was recognized, described, and treated by Hippocrates. Indeed, the earliest recorded operation as treatment was performed by Praxagoras circa 350 BC, when he created an enterocutaneous fistula to relieve the obstruction of a segment of bowel.

Bowel obstruction remains one of the most common intra-abdominal problems faced by general surgeons in their practice. Whether caused by hernia, neoplasm, adhesions, or related to biochemical disturbances, intestinal obstruction of either the small or large bowel continues to be a major cause of morbidity and mortality. Its early recognition and aggressive treatment in patients of all ages, including neonates, can prevent irreversible ischemia and transmural necrosis, thereby decreasing mortality and long-term morbidity. Despite many recent advances in our diagnostic and treatment armamentarium, intestinal obstruction will continue to occur. The aim of this chapter is to review the etiologies, pathogenesis, diagnosis, and management in the current era.

▪ DEFINITION

Bowel obstruction occurs when the normal propulsion and passage of intestinal contents does not occur. This obstruction can involve only the small intestine (small bowel obstruction), the large intestine (large bowel obstruction), or via systemic alterations, involving both the small and large intestine (generalized ileus). The "obstruction" can involve a mechanical obstruction or, in contrast, may be related to ineffective motility without any physical obstruction, so-called functional obstruction, "pseudo-obstruction," or ileus. Intestinal obstruction can also be classified according to etiopathogenesis (mechanical or functional obstruction), time of presentation, and duration of obstruction (acute or chronic obstruction), the extent of obstruction (partial or complete), and the type of obstruction (simple, closed-loop, or strangulation obstruction). The latter two fall into the category of "complicated" obstruction.

MECHANICAL BOWEL OBSTRUCTION

This term is used to define intestinal obstruction caused by a physical blockage of the intestinal lumen. This blockage may be intrinsic or extrinsic to the wall of the intestine or on occasion may occur secondary to luminal obstruction arising from the intraluminal contents (e.g., an intraluminal gallstone) (Table 17–1). Partial obstruction occurs when the intestinal lumen is narrowed but still allows the transit of some intestinal content aborally. On the other hand, complete obstruction implies that the lumen is totally obstructed, and none of the intestinal contents can move distally. Complete obstruction carries a markedly increased risk of strangulation (vascular compromise). Complete intestinal obstruction can be categorized as simple obstruction, closed-loop obstruction, or strangulation obstruction. Simple obstruction implies an obstruction without any vascular compromise; with simple obstruction, it is possible to decompress the intestine proxi-

TABLE 17–1. MECHANICAL BOWEL OBSTRUCTION

Lesions Extrinsic to the Intestinal Wall	Lesions Intrinsic to the Intestinal Wall
ADHESIONS	CONGENITAL
Postoperative	Intestinal atresia
Congenital	Meckel's diverticulum
Postinflammatory	Duplications/cysts
HERNIA	INFLAMMATORY
External abdominal wall (congenital or acquired)	Crohn's disease
Internal	Eosinophilic granuloma
Incisional	INFECTIONS
CONGENITAL	Tuberculosis
Annular pancreas	Actinomycosis
Malrotation	Complicated diverticulitis
Omphalomesenteric duct remnant	NEOPLASTIC
NEOPLASTIC	Primary neoplasms
Carcinomatosis	Metastatic neoplasms
Extraintestinal neoplasm	Appendicitis
INFLAMMATORY	MISCELLANEOUS
Intra-abdominal abscess	Intussusception
"Starch" peritonitis	Endometriosis
MISCELLANEOUS	Radiation enteropathy/stricture
Volvulus	Intramural hematoma
Gossypiboma	Ischemic stricture
Superior mesenteric artery syndrome	INTRALUMINAL/OBTURATOR OBSTRUCTION
	Gallstone
	Enterolith
	Phytobezoar
	Parasite infestation
	Swallowed foreign body

Adapted, with permission, from Tito WA, Sarr MG. Intestinal obstruction. In: Zuidema GD (ed). Surgery of the Alimentary Tract. Philadelphia, PA: WB Saunders; 1996:375–416.

mally. Closed-loop obstruction occurs when both ends of the involved intestinal segment are obstructed (e.g., volvulus) with a consequent increase in intraluminal pressure secondary to increased intestinal secretion and accumulation of fluid in the involved intestinal segment; a closed-loop obstruction, however, results in a much higher risk of vascular compromise and irreversible intestinal ischemia. Finally, strangulation occurs when the blood supply to the affected segment is compromised. The strangulation is either reversible (i.e., the viability of the bowel is maintained with relief of the obstruction), or irreversible when the vascular obstruction has caused irreversible ischemia of the bowel that will progress to transmural necrosis whether or not the strangulation is relieved.

FUNCTIONAL BOWEL OBSTRUCTION

When the obstruction is secondary to factors that cause either paralysis or dysmotility of intestinal peristalsis that prevents coordinated aboral transit of luminal contents, the obstruction is called a functional or pseudo-obstruction (Table 17–2). With functional obstruction, no physical site of mechanical obstruction is present. Postoperative ileus is the most common form of functional bowel obstruction, since it is present to some extent after most intra-abdominal operative procedures. A transient ileus may also develop in response to various types of extra-abdominal medical and surgical conditions. In addition to these forms of ileus that occur in response to local or systemic stimuli, there is a group of rare, progressive, chronic, idiopathic gastrointestinal pseudo-obstructions that are related either to hereditary or acquired visceral myopathies, visceral neuropathies, or a poorly understood disruption of myoneural coordination of organized contractile activity.

Postoperative ileus represents the most common cause of delayed hospital discharge after abdominal operations. The duration of postoperative ileus tends to correlate with the degree of surgical trauma as well as the type of operation, and might even be considered a "physiologic" response. Patients operated on for radiation enteropathy, chronic obstruction, or severe perito-

TABLE 17–2. FUNCTIONAL BOWEL OBSTRUCTION, ILEUS, AND PSEUDO-OBSTRUCTION

Intra-Abdominal Causes	Extra-Abdominal Causes
INTRAPERITONEAL PROBLEMS	THORACIC PROBLEMS
Peritonitis	Myocardial infarction
Intra-abdominal abscess	Congestive heart failure
Postoperative (physiologic)	Pneumonia
Chemical:	Thoracic trauma
Gastric juice	METABOLIC ABNORMALITIES
Bile	Electrolyte imbalance
Blood	Sepsis
Autoimmune:	Lead poisoning
Serositis	Porphyria
Vasculitis	Hyperglycemia/ketoacidosis
Intestinal ischemia:	Hypothyroidism
Arterial or venous	Hypoparathyroidism
Sickle-cell disease	Uremia
RETROPERITONEAL PROBLEMS	MEDICINES
Urolithiasis	Opiates
Pyelonephritis	Anticholinergics
Metastasis	Alpha-adrenergic agonists
Pancreatitis	Antihistamines
Retroperitoneal trauma/hematoma	Catecholamines
	MISCELLANEOUS
	Spinal cord injury
	Pelvic fracture
	Head trauma
	Chemotherapy
	Radiation therapy
	Renal transplantation

Modified, with permission, from Helton WS, Fisichella P. Intestinal obstruction. In: *ACS Surgery Principles and Practice.* New York, NY: WebMD Professional Publishing; 2004.

nitis are susceptible to a more prolonged postoperative ileus; with radiation enteropathy, the ileus is probably related to radiation-induced damage to neuromuscular coordination in the irradiated segments. Different anatomic segments of the gastrointestinal tract also recover at different rates after manipulation and trauma. The small bowel generally recovers effective motor function within several hours after the operation; indeed, contractile activity in the small intestine remains present even during a celiotomy. In contrast, the stomach may take 24–48 hours to regain normal motor activity, while the colon recovers in about 3–5 days postoperatively; neither of these organs show spontaneous contractions or respond to manual compression with visible contraction (as does the small intestine) during a celiotomy.[1] It is important to differentiate postoperative ileus both from an early postoperative mechanical bowel obstruction and from postoperative "paralytic" ileus in which there is a prolonged inhibition of coordinated bowel activity that can take days or even weeks to resolve. This distinction may be important, because paralytic or generalized ileus usually is secondary to or caused by different pathophysiologic mechanisms.[2]

EARLY POSTOPERATIVE (MECHANICAL) BOWEL OBSTRUCTION

Bowel obstruction occurring within the first 6 weeks postoperatively is classified as an early postoperative bowel obstruction. This type of obstruction can be considered a distinct clinical entity with a unique pathophysiology that should be differentiated from classic mechanical bowel obstruction and from postoperative ileus. Acute adhesions are the responsible cause in over 90% of the episodes of early postoperative obstruction that require surgical management. Other causes include internal herniation, intra-abdominal abscess, intramural intestinal hematoma, and anastomotic edema or leak. The special circumstance of the patient who has recently undergone an operation may make early postoperative bowel obstruction quite difficult or impossible to differentiate from postoperative ileus. Nausea, vomiting, abdominal distention, and obstipation are themselves relatively common findings in the early postoperative period. Initially, the symptoms of early postoperative mechanical obstruction tend to be vague, and patients are often labeled as having postoperative ileus. The abdominal exam is seldom helpful because of pain secondary to the recent incision or the use of narcotic analgesics masking the underlying pain picture. Imaging studies may also be difficult to interpret, since early postoperative bowel obstruction and ileus can manifest with similar findings on plain abdominal radiographs. Contrast studies and CT can help to differentiate between patients that need only conservative management and those that may need operative intervention by identifying the presence or absence of either a focal site of obstruction or the presence of dilated proximal with decompressed distal small bowel; the latter defines a mechanical etiology.[3]

▪ EPIDEMIOLOGY

There are wide variations in the frequency and etiology of bowel obstruction throughout the world depending on ethnicity, age group, dietary habits, and geographic location, among other factors. Both the etiology and frequency of bowel obstruction changed dramatically during the 1900s. During the first third of the 20th century, the most common cause of bowel obstruction was incarcerated hernia. The widespread growth of therapeutic intra-abdominal surgery in the second half of the 20th century led to an increase in the frequency of postoperative adhesive obstruction and a decrease in the relative frequency of obstruction secondary to hernias. This decrease in the frequency of obstruction secondary to incarcerated hernias is due to the early diagnosis and surgical management of most abdominal wall hernias, especially in industrialized countries. Bowel obstruction in Third World nations manifests as with different clinical picture resembling that found in the early 20th century in Western societies. In the future, wider application of minimal access laparoscopic approaches may decrease the frequency of bowel obstruction secondary to postoperative adhesions,[4] but this putative trend has yet to be confirmed.

There is a slightly higher frequency of bowel obstruction in women due to the fact that obstetric, gynecologic, and other pelvic surgical procedures are important etiologies for the development of postoperative adhesions.

About 80% of bowel obstructions occur in the small intestine; the other 20% occur in the colon. Colorectal cancer is responsible for 60–70% of all large bowel obstructions, while diverticulitis and volvulus account for the majority of the remaining 30%. Although possible, abdominal wall hernias rarely cause a true, isolated large bowel obstruction, while adhesions, unlike for small bowel obstruction, represent an exceedingly uncommon cause of a large bowel obstruction. In contrast, small bowel obstruction in most advanced Western societies is caused most commonly by adhesions, neoplasms, or abdominal wall hernias.

The costs incurred and the resources expended in the treatment of intestinal obstruction represent a significant burden on the national health care system for any country. One study estimated that bowel obstruction accounted for over one million days of inpatient care and $1.33 billion dollars in health care expenditures in the United States in 1994. Indeed, it has been estimated that 1% of all hospitalizations, 3% of emergency surgical admissions to general hospitals, and 4% of major celiotomies (about 250,000) are secondary to bowel obstruction or procedures requiring adhesiolysis.[5] Another study showed that between 12% and 17% of patients who have undergone a total colectomy are admitted for small bowel obstruction within 2 years of their index operation, while approximately 3% will require an operation to treat an established small bowel obstruction.

The overall mortality and morbidity of bowel obstruction is substantial. Mortality rates range from up to 3% for simple obstructions to as much as 30% when there is vascular compromise or perforation of the obstructed bowel, depending on the clinical setting and other related or unrelated comorbidities. In addition, bowel obstruction is frequently a recurrent problem, adding to the overall morbidity of an operation or successful nonoperative management. Recurrence rates vary according to method of management (conservative or operative). Future intestinal obstruction will recur in about 12% of patients after primary conservative treatment and in between 8% and 32% of patients after operative management for adhesive bowel obstruction.

▪ PATHOPHYSIOLOGY

Luminal obstruction results in prominent alterations of the normal intestinal physiology. Despite the many changes noted, the pathophysiology of bowel obstruction remains incompletely understood. Bowel distension, decreased absorption, intraluminal hypersecretion, and alterations in motility are found universally, yet the mechanisms responsible for these pathophysiologic derangements are not clear. Neural and hormonal control mechanisms, endogenous bacterial flora, and the innate immunity of the gut are also disrupted.

The older classic literature addressing the pathophysiology of bowel obstruction maintains that a decrease in blood flow is responsible for most of the pathophysiologic changes. More recent experimental work, however, suggests that many of the pathophysiologic changes that occur with bowel obstruction are in part related to the increases in blood flow seen during the early phases of bowel obstruction in association with an intramural inflammatory reaction. Indeed, strong evidence suggests that this inflammatory reaction plays a key role in the pathophysiology of the intestinal response to obstruction. Recent data show that mucosal production of reactive oxygen species may be one important mediator of some changes seen in simple mechanical bowel obstruction.[6]

DISTENTION, ABSORPTION, AND SECRETION

Bowel distension represents a characteristic, fundamental, and constant physiologic derangement present in mechanical bowel obstruction. The mechanism underlying the intestinal distention has also not been elucidated fully. Most of the gas distending the small bowel in the early phases of obstruction accumulates from swallowed air. As would be expected, intraluminal gas consists of approximately 75% nitrogen in the obstructed bowel. Other sources of gas arise from the fermentation of sugars, production of carbon dioxide by interaction of gastric acid and bicarbonates in pancreatic and biliary secretions, and diffusion of oxygen and carbon dioxide from the blood. Dilatation and inflammation of the bowel wall may cause activated neutrophils and macrophages to accumulate within the muscular layer of the bowel wall, inhibiting or causing damage to secretory and motor processes by release of reactive proteolytic enzymes, cytokines, and other locally active substances. This inflammatory response leads to an increase in the local release of nitric oxide, itself a potent inhibitor of smooth-muscle tone, further aggravating the intestinal dilatation and inhibition of contractile activity. The amount and activity of nitric oxide synthase, the enzyme that synthesizes nitric oxide, correlates with the severity of intestinal dilatation. Experimental data also support the presence of a close relationship between distension and the intramural production of reactive oxygen metabolites which modulate not only gut motility but also gut permeability.

During the first 12 hours of an obstruction of the small bowel, water and electrolytes accumulate within the lumen secondary to a decrease in net absorption. By 24 hours, intraluminal water and electrolytes accumulate more rapidly secondary to a further decrease in absorptive flux and a concomitant increase in net intestinal secretion (secretory flux) apparently secondary to mucosal injury and increased permeability; intraluminal leakage of plasma, electrolytes, and extracellular fluid occurs. Whether associated neural or systemic humoral/hormonal mechanisms also aggravate this upregulation of unidirectional secretory flux remains likely but poorly investigated.

Intraluminal bacteria-derived toxins, bile acids, prostaglandins, vasoactive intestinal polypeptide, and mucosa-derived oxygen free radicals accumulate and all exacerbate this fluid secretion into the lumen of the obstructed bowel. The decrease in the absorptive capacity and increase in secretion leads to important fluid losses which can lead to dehydration if not recognized and treated. Although the intestinal wall distal to the obstruction maintains relatively normal function, the inability of the luminal content to reach the unobstructed small bowel and colonic absorptive surface is an important component of the overall dehydration.

INTESTINAL MOTILITY

In the early phase of bowel obstruction, intestinal contractile activity increases in an attempt to propel intraluminal contents past the obstruction. Later in the course of the bowel obstruction, the contractile activity diminishes, probably secondary to intestinal wall hypoxia and the exaggerated intramural inflammation; however, the exact mechanisms have not been adequately described. Some investigators[7] have suggested that the alterations in intestinal motility are secondary to a disruption of the normal autonomic parasympathetic (vagal) and sympathetic splanchnic innervation.

The splanchnic innervation has been the focus of extensive research, and especially so in the pathogenesis of ileus. Chemical sympathectomy has been successful in ameliorating the ileus in several experimental models of ileus. Other approaches have focused on blocking the neural inhibitory mechanisms affecting enteric neuromuscular coordination. Still other experimental approaches have been designed to prevent or inhibit the inflammatory response that accompanies the "physiologic" (postoperative) response to celiotomy or the abnormal inflammatory response accompanying generalized ileus.

CIRCULATORY CHANGES

Ischemia of the bowel wall can occur by several different mechanisms. Extrinsic compression of the mesenteric arcades by adhesions, fibrosis, a mass, or a hernia defect; an axial twist of the mesentery; local chronic serosal-based pressure on a segment of the bowel wall (e.g., a fibrous band); or progressive distention in the presence of a closed-loop bowel obstruction can all cause vascular compromise or strangulation. The worry about vascular compromise is more acute in large bowel obstruction, because about 40% of people have a competent ileocecal valve, which functionally leads to a form of closed-loop obstruction.

Progressive distention of the bowel lumen with a concomitant increase in intraluminal pressure results in increased transmural pressure on capillary blood flow within the wall of the bowel. For simple (non–closed loop) obstruction, this scenario rarely occurs, because the obstructed distended bowel can decompress proximally. In contrast, the possibility of intestinal wall ischemia is a very real concern in large bowel obstruction, when the ileocecal valve is competent and the distended colon cannot decompress retrograde into the small bowel. The resultant bowel wall ischemia may eventually lead to compromise of blood flow by exceeding venous pressure. This scenario is most common in the ascending colon where the luminal diameter is the greatest and (by Laplace's law) the wall tension (and ischemia) is also the greatest. This potential phenomenon actually makes large bowel obstruction more of a surgical emergency than small bowel obstruction. This type of bowel wall ischemia leads to further disruption of intestinal absorption with a relative increase in net secretion, an unregulated increase in mucosal permeability, and intramural production of reactive oxygen species by activated resident and recruited leukocytes, causing peroxidation of the lipid components of the cellular membrane, release of cytokines and other inflammatory mediators, and systemic toxicity. With strangulation, there can also be blood loss into the infarcted bowel, which together with the preexistent fluid loss leads to further hemodynamic instability, which exacerbates the already compromised blood flow of the intestinal wall.

MICROBIOLOGY AND BACTERIAL TRANSLOCATION

The upper small intestine contains resident and transient flora consisting mainly of gram-positive facultative organisms in small concentrations, usually $<10^6$ colonies/mL. More distally, the bacterial count increases in concentration to about 10^8 colonies/mL in the distal ileum, and the flora changes to primarily coliforms and anaerobic organisms. However, in the presence of obstruction, a rapid proliferation of bacterial organisms occurs proximal to the point of obstruction, consisting predominantly of fecal-type organisms. These fecal flora proliferate in direct proportion to duration of obstruction, reaching a plateau of 10^9–10^{10} colonies/mL after 12–48 hours of an established obstruction. The bowel distal to the obstruction tends to maintain its usual bacterial flora until a generalized ileus sets in, and then even here, bacterial proliferation occurs. Bacterial toxins have an important role in the mucosal response to bowel obstruction. Experiments in germ-free dogs with a mechanical bowel obstruction have shown that intraluminal accumulation of fluid and net electrolytes does not occur and net absorption continues.

In persistent bowel obstruction, experiments in rodents showed that bacterial translocation can occur secondary to impairment of the barrier function of the intestinal mucosa. This disruption of the mucosal barrier begins to occur early after the onset of bowel obstruction. The endoplasmic reticulum dilates as early as 4 hours after onset of bowel obstruction. Mitochondrial edema, focal epithelial necrosis, intracellular swelling, and degenerative lesions in the nucleus of epithelial cells (apoptosis) have been demonstrated after 6–12 hours of obstruction in these experimental models.[8] Reduction of perfusion of the intestinal wall further compromises the mucosal defenses. When the mechanical integrity of the mucosa is lost, luminal bacteria invade the submucosa and enter the systemic circulation via the portal venous and lymphatic systems. Several bacterial substances can be retrieved from peritoneal fluid and lymphatic channels even in the absence of perforation. In rodents, bacteria can be cultured from the spleen, liver, and mesenteric lymph nodes, indicative of a marked increase in bacterial translocation.

The very elegant studies demonstrating bacterial translocation in the rodent led to erroneous assumptions about similar bacterial "translocation" in humans. However, documentation of true bacterial translocation in humans is notably lacking, and true bacterial translocation in man seems unlikely. Several studies that tried to document the presence of bacteria in intra-abdominal lymph nodes, spleen, liver, and even lymphatics have been unsuccessful in reproducing the results noted in the animal models. In contrast, more recent work has shown that lipopolysaccharide and other inflammatory mediators, but not bacteria, can be recovered from the mesenteric lymphatics. The eventual drainage of these vasoactive substances into the systemic circulation may lead both to the systemic manifestations of sepsis and further disruption of the mucosal barrier function.

The importance of this change in the intraluminal bacteriology in simple intestinal obstruction is that the risk of infective complications is increased markedly, and especially so if an intestinal resection is required or if an inadvertent enterotomy is made with intraperitoneal spillage of "obstructed" enteric contents. In contrast, with strangulation obstruction, it is clear that a myriad of local and systemic alterations, such as systemic entry of bacterial products, activation of immunocompetent cells, release of cytokines, and increased formation of reactive oxygen intermediates, can promote the systemic inflammatory response syndrome and can progress to multiple organ dysfunction.

▪ ETIOLOGY

ADHESIONS

Adhesions may be defined as abnormal connective tissue attachments between tissue surfaces. Adhesions can be congenital or acquired (postinflammatory and postoperative). Congenital or inflammatory adhesions are infrequent causes of bowel obstruction, except in selected circumstances such as malrotation or persistent urachus, among others. Postoperative adhesions are the leading cause of small bowel obstruction in Western societies and are responsible for 40–80% of bowel obstructions seen in most hospital surgical services. This wide variation in incidence of adhesive obstruction varies with different referral patterns, community settings, racial cultures, and countries.

Some element of adhesion formation is nearly universal after celiotomy and starts as early as the first postoperative hours.[9] Much of the pathogenesis of adhesion formation remains unknown. Experts agree that it is a surface event associated with some form of peritoneal injury. The inciting trauma triggers an inflammatory response leading to activation of the complement and coagulation cascades, along with exudation of fibrinogen-rich fluid; the full establishment of this response is present 5–7 days after the peritoneal trauma of a celiotomy.[10] Recent findings have identified the presence of sensory nerve fibers in human peritoneal adhesions, suggesting that these structures may even be capable of conducting pain.[11]

Peritoneal healing appears to differ from the response in skin, where re-epithelialization occurs from the periphery inwards. In the peritoneum, surgical or traumatic defects are re-peritonealized by implantation of mesothelial cells in multiple areas of the defect. This mesothelialization takes place quite rapidly and is often complete by 2–5 days after the injury, depending on local conditions.[12]

Normal peritoneal healing is a complex, interrelated, programmed inflammatory process. The initial response involves the influx of polymorphonuclear leukocytes and lymphocytes within fibrin strands. During the next 24–36 hours, numerous macrophages have infiltrated the wounded area, recruited by various chemokines. By 48 hours, a fibrin scaffold overlying the defect has been established, covered by macrophages and a few mesothelial cells which then coalesce to fully mesothelialize the defect over the next 2–4 days. The underlying fibrin scaffold is populated by fibroblasts and other mesenchymal cells that begin to lay down a basement membrane, so that by 8–10 days, a single layer of mesothelial cells resting on a continuous basement membrane is established; the underlying reactive matrix and inflammatory cells then regress.

Adhesion formation can be considered a pathologic process as opposed to the above described process. It appears that adhesions form in response to the initial fibrin gel matrix combined with the local microenvironment. This fibrin gel matrix consists of numerous types of cells, including the initial leukocytes, but also other humorally active cells such as platelets, mast cells, and erythrocytes, as well as surgical debris and possibly bacteria. The resultant spectrum between mesothelial healing versus adhesion formation varies among individuals and is dependent on many other conditions, such as inflammation, infection, devitalized tissue, and foreign bodies as well.

If the fibrin gel allows apposition of adjacent surfaces, a band or bridge may form (i.e., an adhesion). This process of adhesion formation also is a dynamic process, consisting predominantly of macrophages early on, but by 2–4 days, larger strands of fibrin and fibroblasts begin to appear. By 5 days, distinct bundles of collagen are apparent, and fibroblasts begin to form a syncytium within the matrix. These cells thereafter predominate, and eventually the fibrin matrix and cellular elements are replaced by a vascularized, granulation-type tissue containing macrophages, fibroblasts, giant cells, and a rich vascular supply. Eventually the surface of the adhesions are covered by a mesothelial layer, but only after formation of the underlying fibrous scar leading to surface opposition and transperitoneal bands.

The type of surgical procedure is also an important factor in determining the risk of future adhesive bowel obstruction. The operations most frequently associated with adhesive bowel obstruction are those involving the structures in the inframesocolic compartment, and especially the pelvic region, such as colonic, rectal, and gynecologic procedures. Adhesive bowel obstruction may occur at any time postoperatively after a celiotomy, with reports ranging as early as within the first postoperative month to more than 8 decades after the index operation. A study by Menzies and Ellis[13] found that about 20% of adhesive bowel obstructions occur within 30 days after the initial celiotomy, about 20% occur between 1 and 12 months postoperatively, another 20% tend to occur between 1 and 5 years postoperatively, and the remainder (~30%) occur after 5 years. A Norwegian study of patients requiring an operation for adhesive bowel obstruction found that most episodes of recurrent bowel obstruction occurred within 5 years after the previous episode, but the risk was still present more than 20 years after a prior episode, reaching an incidence as great as 29% at 25 years.[14] Therefore, a common predisposition to adhesive obstruction is the presence of a prior episode of adhesive obstruction. Numerous attempts to decrease or prevent the development of postoperative adhesions have been reported and will be discussed below.

HERNIA

Incarceration of the bowel in congenital abdominal wall hernias (umbilical, epigastric, inguinal, femoral, spigelian, obturator, sciatic, lumbar, and perineal), internal hernias, or postoperative hernias (incisional, ostomy-related, or mesenteric defects after intestinal resection) are the second most common cause of bowel obstruction in most series. Hernias as an etiology are more common in males than in females, primarily because of the predominance of inguinal hernias in men.

Approximately 5% of external hernias will require emergency operation if they are not repaired electively. The presence of acute incarceration should prompt emergent surgical management, since 10–15% of incarcerated hernias contain necrotic bowel at exploration (Figs 17–1 and 17–2); chronically incarcerated hernias can develop strangulation, but most chronically incarcerated hernias can be managed electively.

MALIGNANT BOWEL OBSTRUCTION

Primary intra-abdominal neoplasms are a common cause of both large and small bowel obstruction. Colorectal, gastric, small bowel, and ovarian neoplasms are among the most frequent causes of malignant bowel obstruction. Because bowel obstruction is often a terminal event in many of these patients and the recurrence and morbidity are high, decisions about management need to be individualized by carefully weighing risks, benefits, and life expectancy. The study by Mucha[15] on bowel obstruction from the Mayo Clinic showed that 50% of patients undergoing operation for malignant bowel obstruction died within 6 months. Palliative operative management, however, may be indicated in many patients. Patients in whom abdominal exploration is not possible or desirable may benefit from placement of a percutaneous endoscopic gastrostomy or tube pharyngostomy[16] to help relieve symptoms. Hospital stay tends to be longer for bowel obstruction secondary to intra-abdominal malignancy than for other causes of bowel obstruction.

Metastatic cancer can also cause bowel obstruction. The most common form of obstructing metastatic lesion is peritoneal carcinomatosis, but melanoma and carcinoma of the breast, kidney, or lung

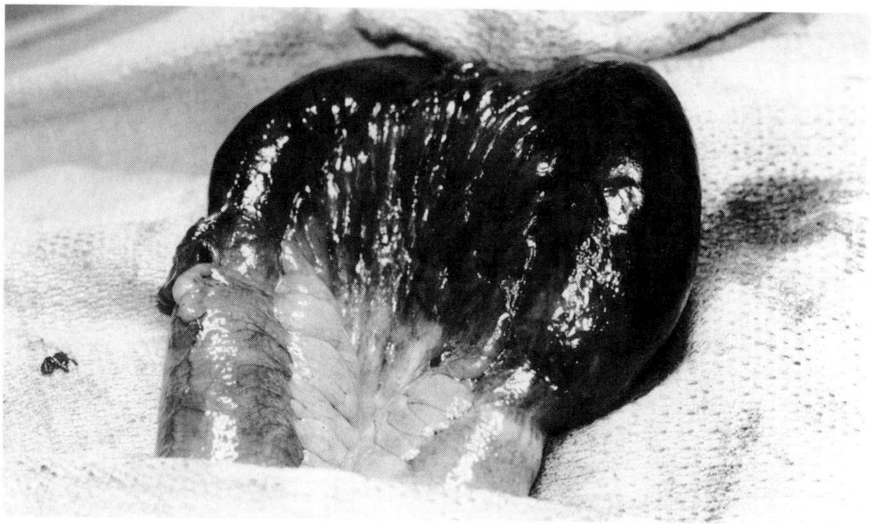

Figure 17–1. Gangrenous bowel from an irreversible, strangulated, incarcerated inguinal hernia.

can also cause intraperitoneal metastases that can obstruct the bowel (Fig 17–3).

GRANULOMATOUS DISEASES AND CROHN'S DISEASE

Crohn's disease is a chronic, transmural, inflammatory disease of the gastrointestinal tract that may affect any part of the alimentary tract from the mouth to the anus. Crohn's disease is responsible for about 5% of cases of small bowel obstruction, the cause of which is usually secondary to the inflammatory process or to stricture formation. Other granulomatous diseases causing obstruction, such as tuberculosis and actinomycosis, are much less common in most Western countries, but in Third World countries and especially where AIDS and HIV infection are endemic, intra-abdominal tuberculosis must be entertained in the diagnosis of intestinal obstruction.

INTUSSUSCEPTION

Intussusception is a relatively frequent cause of bowel obstruction in infancy (the first 2 years of life) but accounts for only 2% of bowel obstruction in the adult population.[17] The median age of presentation in adults with intussusception is the sixth to seventh decade. The etiology of intussusception differs greatly between adult and pediatric patients. In the vast majority of adult intussusceptions, there is a demonstrable inflammatory lesion or a neoplasm that is malignant in almost 50% of patients. Although rare in the Western Hemisphere, intussusception is the most common cause of bowel obstruction in central Africa, for reasons as yet not fully explained.

VOLVULUS

Volvulus represents an axial twist of the bowel and its mesentery and is an infrequent cause of small or large bowel obstruction in the Western Hemisphere (Figs

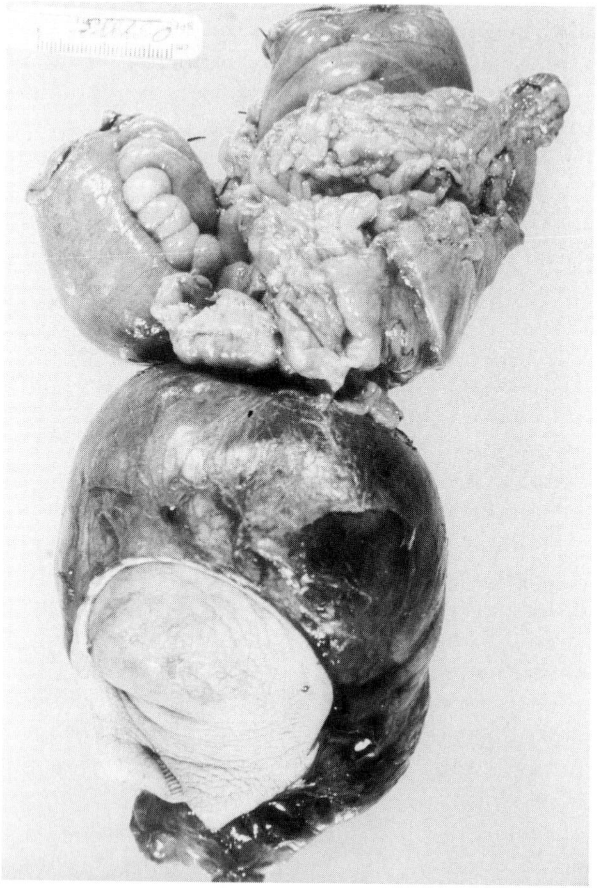

Figure 17–2. Umbilical hernia. Operative en bloc resection of hernia sac, umbilical skin, and irreversible strangulation obstruction.

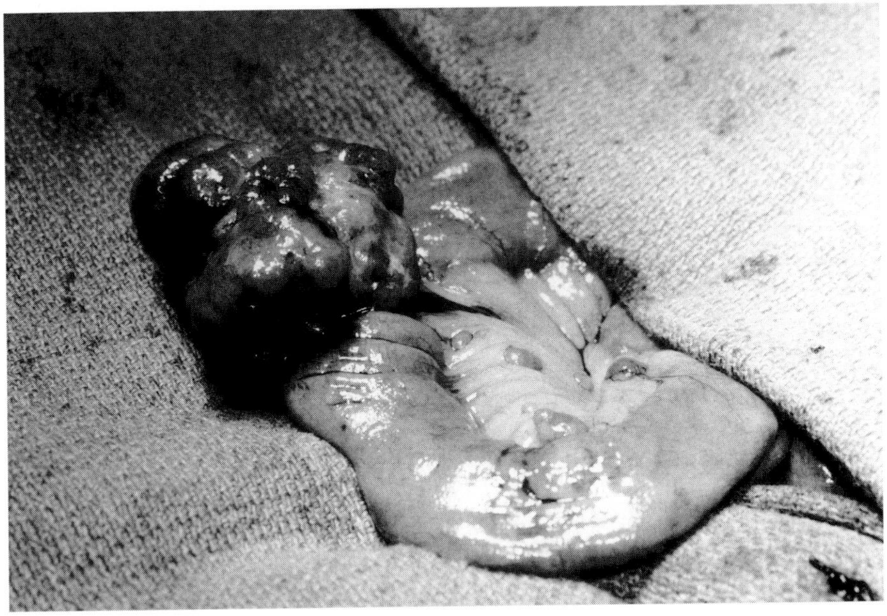

Figure 17–3. Renal cell carcinoma metastatic to small intestine.

17–4 and 17–5). When present, volvulus is more frequently encountered in the geriatric population, in individuals with a long history of constipation, or in institutionalized or neurologically impaired or psychiatric patients. Colonic volvulus represents about 1–4% of all bowel obstructions and about 10–15% of all large bowel obstructions. The volvulated segment has to be relatively mobile to allow the degree of freedom necessary to permit an axial twist of the mesentery. Either the affected segment has an especially long, narrow mesentery (e.g., malrotation or cecal volvulus) and/or a lack of bowel wall fixation (floppy cecum syndrome) or one aspect of the affected segment is fixed, around which the contiguous segment can twist (e.g., a deep fibrous band fixing the other end of the segment).

Other variables may also play a role in the etiology of volvulus. In the Bolivian and Peruvian Andes at more than 10,000 feet above sea level, sigmoid volvulus represents 79% of all bowel obstructions. The high altitude appears to play a role in the high incidence in this population.

Overall, sigmoid volvulus accounts for 75% of all patients with volvulus. In contrast, cecal volvulus is responsible for the majority of the remaining 25% of bowel volvulae in the United States and is the most common cause of large bowel obstruction in pregnancy. A somewhat unique, though less common form of cecal volvulus is the "cecal bascule" which occurs when the true anatomic cecum (i.e., that part of the ascending colon which lies caudal to the entrance of the ileocecal valve) flops anteriorly over onto the ascending colon, obstructing the lumen. This form of cecal volvulus may be intermittent, recurrent, and more difficult to diagnose.

Primary volvulus of the small intestine is extremely rare in the United States, but is quite prevalent in central Africa, India, and the Middle East. Speculation about etiology has been related to abrupt dietary changes that occur during the religious holiday when the people celebrating Ramadan fast during the day and then consume a large meal after dark. Some investigators, however, maintain that this racial group has an exceedingly long, floppy mesentery that permits generous mobility of the small bowel.

OTHER CAUSES

Other causes of bowel obstruction include the following: congenital lesions such as Meckel's diverticula, duplication cysts, intestinal malrotation, annular pancreas, and omphalomesenteric duct remnant; infections such as appendicitis and complicated diverticulitis; inflammatory conditions like starch peritonitis, intra-abdominal abscess, and localized perforations; intraluminal obstruction from stricture, gallstones, phytobezoar, swallowed foreign body, and parasitic infestation; posttraumatic lesions like mesenteric or intramural hematomas; and miscellaneous extraluminal conditions such as radiation enteropathy (Figs 17–6 and 17–7), endometriosis, and superior mesenteric artery syndrome.

■ DIAGNOSIS

The diagnosis of bowel obstruction is suspected clinically based on the presence of classic signs and symptoms and

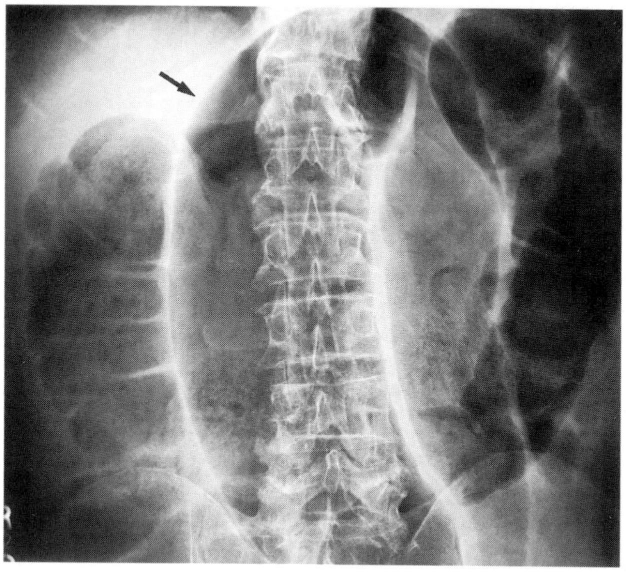

A

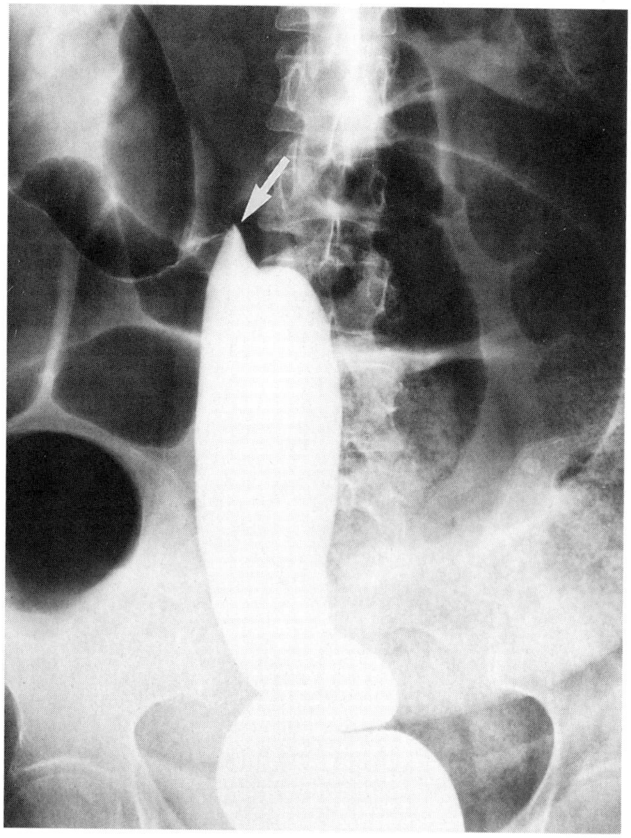

B

Figure 17–4. Sigmoid volvulus. **A.** Supine abdominal radiograph showing the dilated, volvulated segment of redundant sigmoid colon pointing toward the right upper quadrant; *arrows* show the space between the sigmoid and hepatic and splenic flexures. **B.** Contrast enema in sigmoid volvulus showing cut off at distal site of volvulated sigmoid having a "bird-beak" appearance.

then confirmed by some form of imaging test, such as abdominal radiography or more recently by computed tomography. The etiology can often be pinpointed by careful history-taking complemented with imaging studies.

HISTORY AND PHYSICAL EXAMINATION

The classic clinical picture of a patient suffering from bowel obstruction includes crampy abdominal pain, distention, acute obstipation, nausea, and vomiting. Usually the abdominal pain and then distention precede the appearance of nausea and vomiting by several hours. The more proximal the obstruction, the earlier and more prominent are the symptoms of nausea and vomiting while distension is usually less. Vomiting is relatively uncommon in colonic obstruction until its later stages. The abrupt onset of symptoms makes an acute obstructive cause more likely. The location and character of pain may be helpful in differentiating mechanical bowel obstruction and ileus. The former usually presents as severe, crampy pain localized to the midabdomen, while the latter tends to have a more diffuse and mild pain, often without the waves of colic.

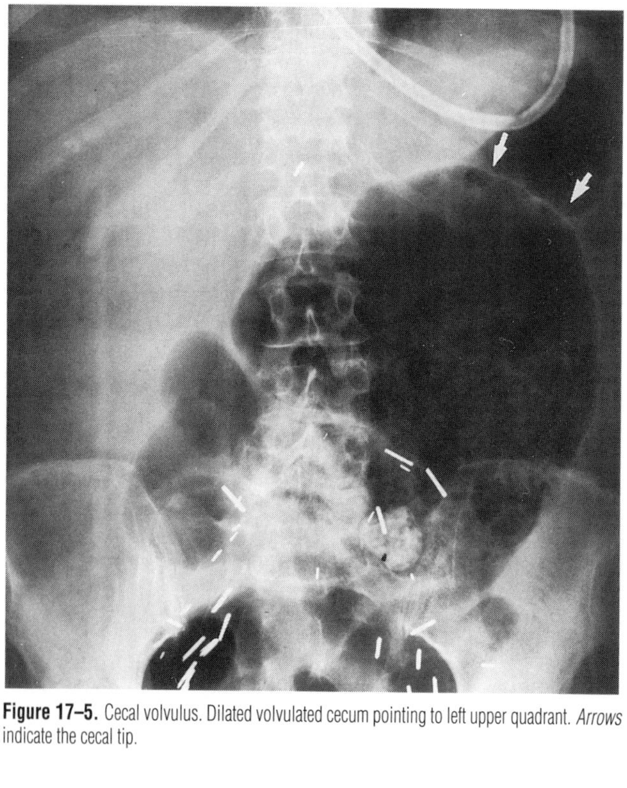

Figure 17–5. Cecal volvulus. Dilated volvulated cecum pointing to left upper quadrant. *Arrows* indicate the cecal tip.

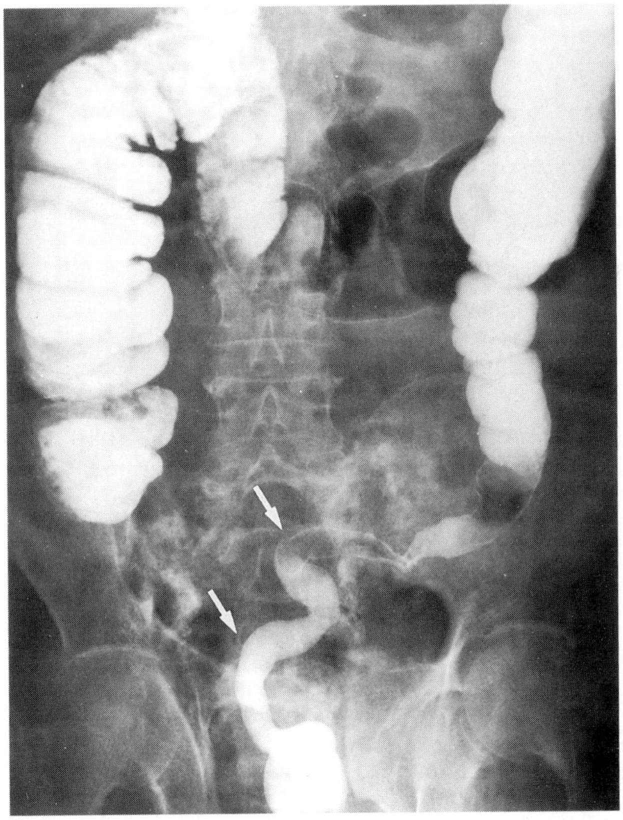

Figure 17–6. Radiation changes in distal colon/rectum (*arrows*).

Characteristically, with mechanical small bowel obstruction, the pain is usually described as visceral, poorly localized, and crampy with recurrent paroxysms occurring in short (30 seconds to 2 minutes) crescendo/decrescendo episodes. In contrast, in mechanical large bowel obstruction, the episodes are usually spaced farther apart in time and tend to last longer (minutes rather than seconds) compared to small bowel obstruction. Classically, the presence of constant or a localized pain has been regarded as a sign of strangulation, although several studies have shown that these findings are neither specific nor sensitive for the detection of strangulation.

It is of utmost importance to obtain a complete medical history. The past medical history of the patient may be key in making both the diagnosis and establishing the cause. It is especially important to inquire about previous events of bowel obstruction, recent and distant abdominal operations, current medications, a history of chronic constipation, recent changes in the caliber of stools, a history of cancer and its stage at presentation and related treatments (surgery, chemotherapy, or radiation therapy), and a history of Crohn's disease.

A thorough physical examination is mandatory and should include assessment of vital signs and hydration status, abdominal inspection, auscultation, palpation, a search for potential hernia defects, and a rectal exam (palpation and test for occult blood). One must look closely for previous surgical incisions, including inguinal incisions for previous "extraperitoneal" herniorrhaphies (recurrent hernias are common). Some consideration should be given to the possibility of internal hernias or those not associated with an obvious external "bulge," such as obturator or femoral hernias.

Tachycardia, hypotension, and oliguria are signs of advanced dehydration that should be corrected aggressively while continuing with further evaluation. Fever may be associated with an infectious cause or with strangulation. Auscultation can determine the presence, frequency, and quality of the "obstructed" bowel sounds. Mechanical bowel obstruction presents with an increase in the frequency of bowel sounds, but more specifically the high-pitched metallic "rushes" and "groans" followed by the metallic tinkling sounds of "water dripping into a large hollow container," indicative of dilated bowel with an air-fluid interface. In contrast, functional bowel obstruction lacks the rushes and groans, but continues to have the metallic tinkling indicative of dilated bowel. Sometimes functional obstruction (ileus) may present with the absence of bowel sounds. In both mechanical and functional bowel obstruction, a succussion splash is usually present (dilated stomach or markedly dilated small bowel filled with an air-fluid interface); the presence of a succussion splash is not normal in a patient who has not eaten or ingested liquids in the previous 1–2 hours and should be

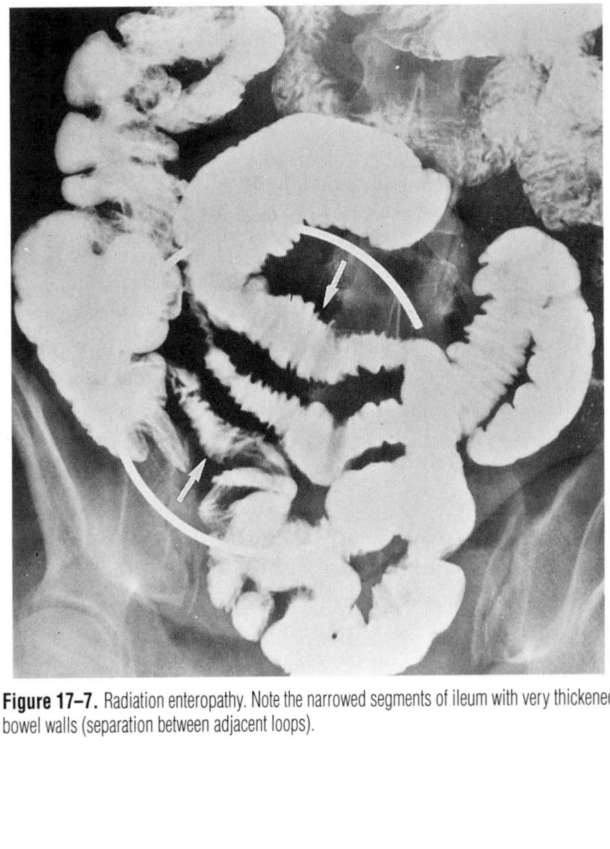

Figure 17–7. Radiation enteropathy. Note the narrowed segments of ileum with very thickened bowel walls (separation between adjacent loops).

regarded as an important but often underappreciated sign of bowel obstruction (unless the patient just recently vomited his or her gastric contents).

Abdominal palpation can reveal the presence of peritoneal signs such as rebound, localized tenderness, and involuntary guarding that herald vascular compromise or perforation. The presence of these findings cannot be ignored. Abdominal masses should be sought and noted. A meticulous search for inguinal and femoral hernias is essential, since they can easily be overlooked. The rectal exam should rule out fecal impaction and should look for occult or macroscopic blood.

LABORATORY

Laboratory data, although nondiagnostic, may be helpful in determining the condition of the patient and guides the resuscitation. A complete blood cell count and differential, electrolyte panel, blood urea nitrogen, creatinine, and urinalysis should be obtained to evaluate fluid and electrolyte imbalance and to rule out sepsis. Arterial blood pH, serum lactate concentrations, and amylase and lactic dehydrogenase activity are useful (but not sensitive) tests in the evaluation of bowel obstruction, especially when trying to rule out bowel necrosis. Others have suggested that serum concentrations of phosphate, intestinal fatty acid binding protein, and isoforms of creatine phosphokinase (isoform B) may identify the presence of intestinal cell necrosis; however, the specificity and especially the sensitivity are not accurate enough to base a management decision solely on these values.

RADIOLOGIC FINDINGS

Flat and Upright Abdominal Radiographs

An upright chest x-ray combined with supine and upright abdominal radiographs should be the initial imaging studies in the diagnostic work-up of the patient with suspected bowel obstruction. The chest x-ray is helpful to detect extra-abdominal conditions that may present with a clinical picture similar to bowel obstruction (e.g., pneumonic process) and the presence of subdiaphragmatic free air indicative of a perforated viscus. The typical findings of small bowel obstruction on abdominal films are dilated loops of small intestine with air-fluid levels (Fig 17–8). The gaseous pattern often helps to determine the type and location of the obstruction. Proximal bowel obstruction can present with little if any intestinal dilation, because the length of obstructed bowel may be short, and it may readily decompress proximally back into the stomach. In contrast, distal bowel obstruction usually has multiple loops of distended small intestine

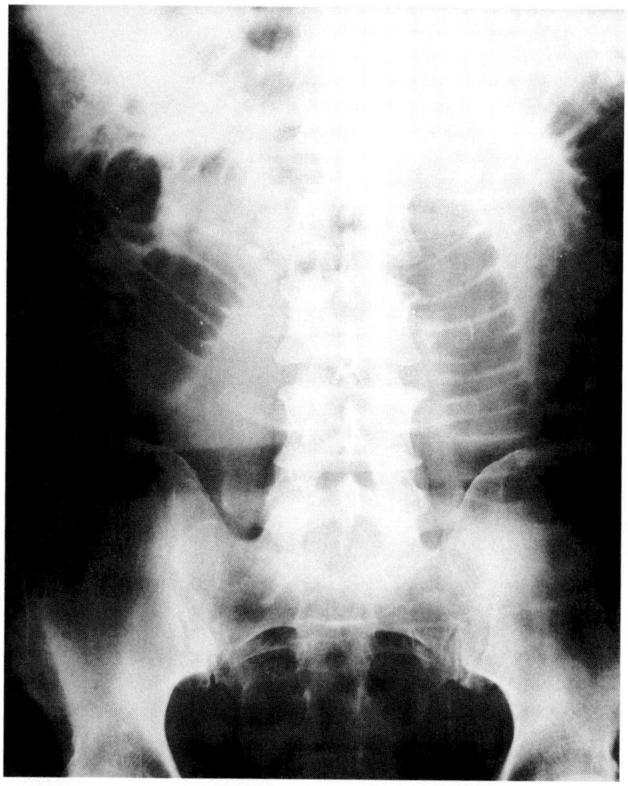

Figure 17–8. Supine abdominal radiograph showing an incomplete small intestinal obstruction. Note the dilated loops of small bowel.

(Figs 17–9 and 17–10) and/or large intestine; proximal decompression into the stomach is less common because of the well-recognized relative "obstruction" to jejunoduodenal reflux of enteric contents exerted by the duodenojejunal junction. The small intestine is considered dilated if loops of bowel measure more than 3 cm in diameter. Measurements for the large bowel vary among different anatomic segments, with a relative threshold of 9 cm in diameter for the proximal colon and 5 cm for the sigmoid colon. There are no really good parameters of colonic dilatation, especially in patients with preexistent symptoms or complaints of constipation, because chronic enlargement of the colonic diameter is often present in these patients and may represent their normal baseline luminal diameter.

It is extremely important to differentiate the gas patterns of small and large intestinal distention. Dilated loops of small intestine tend to lay in the central portion of the abdomen and are recognized by the presence of the valvulae conniventes or plicae circulares that traverse the full diameter of the bowel (see Fig 17–8). Dilated segments of large intestine are usually visualized in the periphery of abdominal films and are identified by the presence of haustral markings that only partially traverse the bowel wall. When the bowel becomes markedly dilated from a subacute or chronic obstruction, it may be impossible to differentiate large from small bowel. All

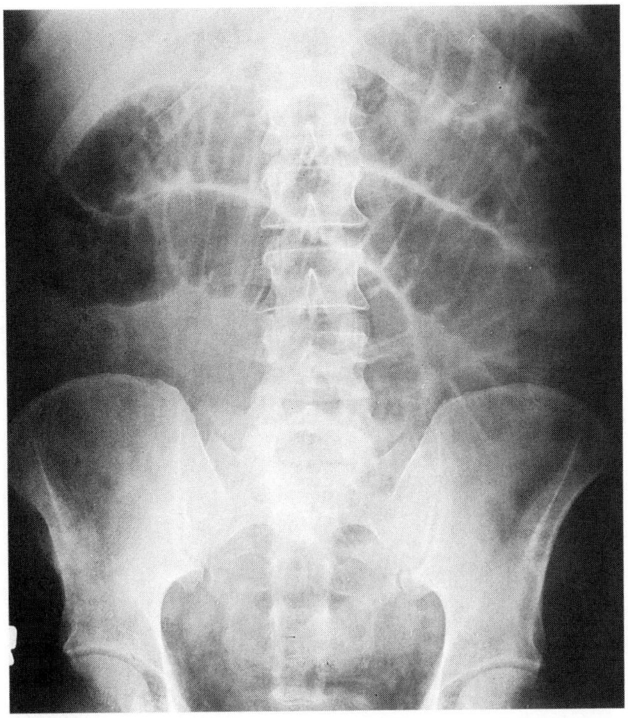

A

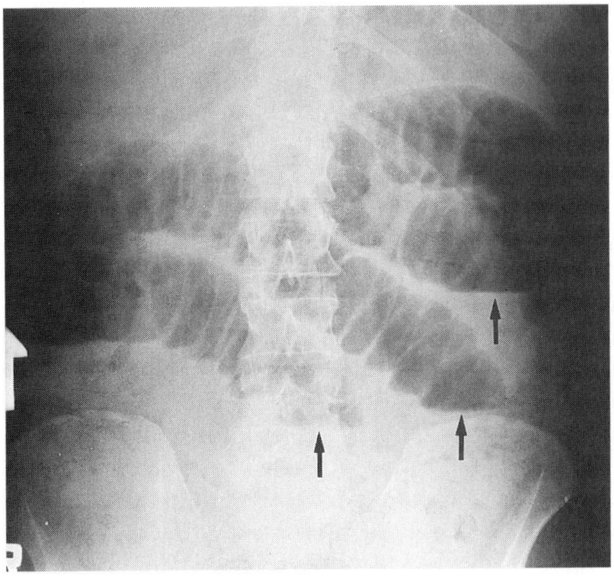

B

Figure 17–9. Complete small bowel obstruction. **A.** Supine abdominal radiograph shows multiple loops of dilated small bowel with colonic gas. **B.** Upright radiograph shows multiple air-fluid levels in the small intestine (*arrows*).

this discussion about differentiation of large from small bowel obstruction is not just academic, because a complete large bowel obstruction in the presence of a competent ileocecal valve is a surgical emergency, while a complete small bowel obstruction is a more subacute emergency (unless related to an acutely incarcerated hernia) and is more subject to the classic adage, "The sun should never rise and set on a (complete) small bowel obstruction."

The cause of the bowel obstruction can often be determined by the findings on plain abdominal films. The presence of pneumobilia in the absence of instrumentation of the biliary tree strongly suggests the diagnosis of gallstone ileus. Cecal and sigmoid volvulae usually produce pathognomonic images on abdominal films. Plain abdominal films can be diagnostic in 50–80% of patients. Closed-loop obstruction carries the greatest risk for strangulation and is also more difficult to diagnose with plain abdominal films, because the obstructed (at both ends) loop may contain very little gas and be completely filled with liquid, thus making it hard to recognize on the film. This lack of an air-fluid level can lead to delayed recognition (and management) with an increase in morbidity and mortality.

Contrast Studies

The indications for prograde or retrograde intraluminal radiologic contrast studies in bowel obstruction are controversial. The use of contrast is helpful when the diagnosis is uncertain in patients with a nonresolving partial small bowel obstruction and to differentiate between partial and complete bowel obstruction. These intraluminal contrast studies can also identify the specific site

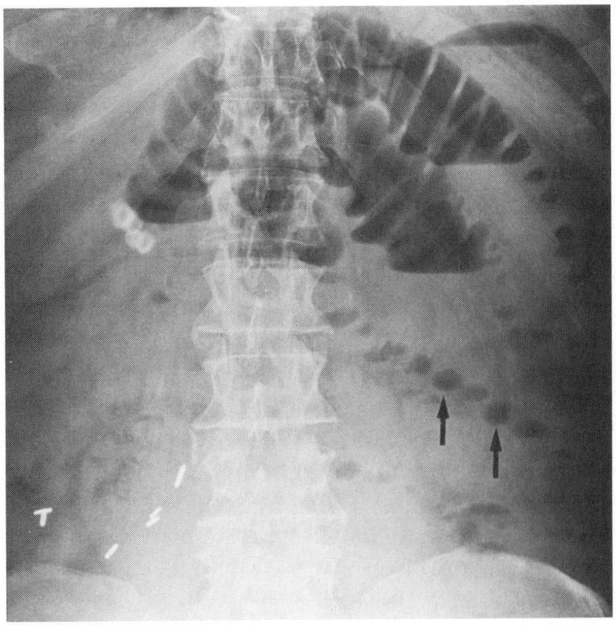

Figure 17–10. Small bowel obstruction with fluid-filled loops of small bowel in left lower quadrant (*arrows*).

and often the cause of the obstruction. A retrograde contrast study (barium enema) can be useful in the patient with suspected large bowel obstruction (Fig 17–11) or in those with a clinical and radiologic picture of a distal small bowel obstruction but with no history of abdominal operations or evidence of an external hernia.

The contrast agent of choice has often been a matter of intense debate. Some groups prefer dilute barium, since it allows a better visualization of mucosal detail, while others advocate the use of water-soluble contrast due to a potential therapeutic effect and the fear of a barium impaction. Water-soluble, hyperosmotic solutions, which tend to draw fluid into the intestinal lumen, are believed to decrease intestinal wall edema, and thereby increase contractile activity, allegedly promoting transit of intraluminal contents distally. Exactly how an earlier resolution of the obstruction occurs is unknown, but may involve more mobility of the distended loops which allows them to detort or to "flop over" and thereby unobstruct. Others have suggested that the contractile activity may increase the propulsive force which itself may allow resolution of the obstruction, also by decompressing a dilated obstructed bowel.

A study by Assalia and associates in 1994 found that patients receiving Gastrografin had a much shorter time to their first bowel movement (6.2 hours versus 23.3 hours), a lower rate of operative treatment (10% versus 21%), and shorter mean hospital stay (2.2 days versus 4.4 days) when compared to those patients who did not receive the water-soluble contrast.[18] In 2002, Choi and coworkers[19] reported a prospective randomized study that showed that the therapeutic use of Gastrografin not only has a role in determining the need for eventual operative management of patients with a presumed small bowel obstruction, but its use appeared to reduce the need for an operation by 74%. On the other hand, Feigin and associates could not confirm any benefit of the use of water-soluble contrast in patients with small bowel obstruction.[20]

The use of both types of contrast agent has risks. In patients with large bowel obstruction, barium within the lumen of the colon proximal to the site of obstruction can become inspissated and itself cause a complete obstruction; in contrast, inspissation of barium is not of concern in small bowel obstruction, because the lumen of the obstructed small intestine is filled with fluid. However, should the patient require a small bowel resection, should an inadvertent enterotomy be made, or should there be an intestinal perforation with intraperitoneal extravasation of the luminal barium contrast, the risk of infective complications and barium peritonitis is a very real concern. Gastrografin and other water-soluble agents are relatively safe even if extravasation occurs, but other potential complications have been reported. Pulmonary aspiration of these agents is more troublesome than that of barium, and in the presence of a distal small bowel obstruction, progressive dilution of the water-soluble agent often precludes any useful data concerning site and/or cause of the obstruction. Most surgeons would agree that contrast studies are contraindicated in patients with a clear diagnosis of complete bowel obstruction and when strangulation or perforation is suspected.

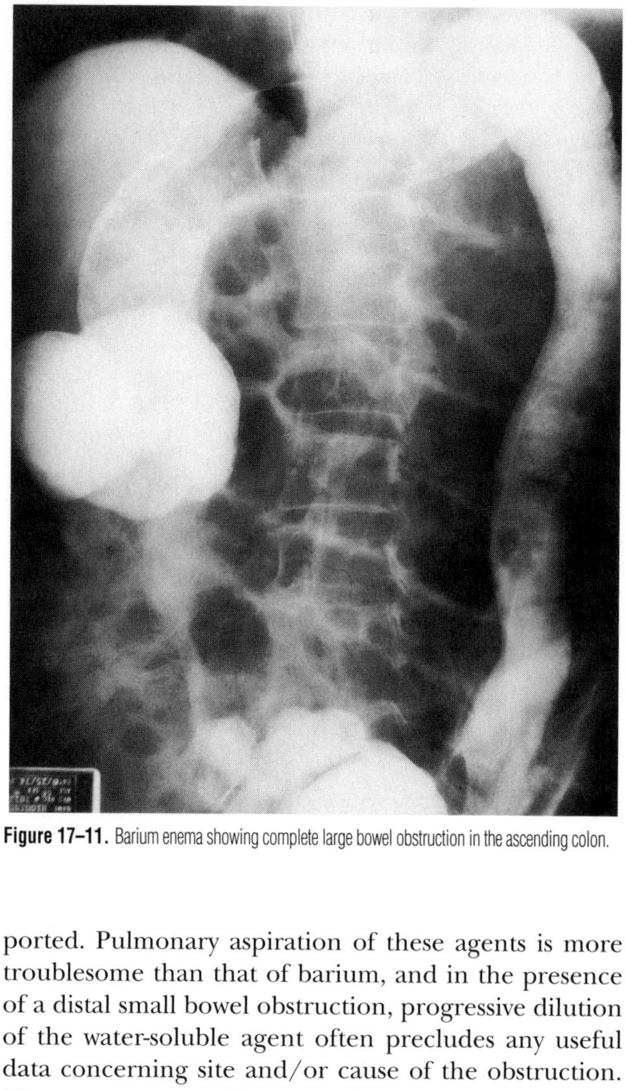

Figure 17–11. Barium enema showing complete large bowel obstruction in the ascending colon.

Computed Tomography

Recently, computed tomography (CT) has become a valuable tool in the diagnosis of bowel obstruction, especially when abdominal films are nonspecific and fail to provide an accurate diagnosis or when strangulation is suspected. The advantages of CT have led to a marked increase in its use, especially because CT allows imaging of structures other than just mucosal detail, which may outline both the site as well as the etiology of the obstruction. With its sensitivity of 93%, specificity of up to 100%, and accuracy of 94% in diagnosing small bowel obstruction, CT has replaced the typical small bowel contrast studies in many centers.

CT findings diagnostic of bowel obstruction include intestinal loops greater than 25 mm in diameter and a transition zone between dilated and collapsed bowel loops. Another advantage of CT is the ability to visualize the entire intra-abdominal compartment as well as defects in the abdominal wall. In addition, because CT can demonstrate changes in the intestinal wall and associated mesentery, as well as showing enhancement or lack thereof by the intravenously administered contrast, some evidence about the severity of the local vascular changes and the presence or absence of strangulation may also be available.

Ultrasonography

Although ultrasonography (US) has been disregarded by many clinicians, in experienced hands, US is more sensitive and specific than plain abdominal films for the diagnosis of bowel obstruction. One should always bear in mind that US is very much operator-dependent, and the accuracy may be quite variable. The diagnosis of small bowel obstruction is made when the intestinal loops measure more that 25 mm in diameter and the distal ileum is found to be collapsed. The etiology can sometimes be determined, but US is less accurate than CT, except in cases of intraluminal obstructions. The reported specificity is 82%, sensitivity is 95%, and overall accuracy is 81%, but the reader should be cautioned that the figures reported in the literature come from centers with extensive experience and interest in the use of US. The authors doubt that similar accuracy can be obtained in most practices or even in most large medical centers. The sensitivity and specificity are not, however, as great as for CT. Abdominal US has been reported to be useful for the early recognition of strangulation in several Japanese and European studies[21,22]; however, experience and reliability are questionable.

DETECTION OF ISCHEMIA

The primary concern in the patient with an intestinal obstruction is the possibility of ischemia. Clinical judgment and laboratory findings have been notoriously unreliable for early detection of intestinal vascular compromise. Acidosis, leukocytosis with left shift, and increased serum amylase activity and lactate concentration may indicate strangulation, and while abnormalities of these parameters may prove sensitive markers of strangulation, they generally lack specificity and useful positive or negative predictive value. Abdominal US and pulsed Doppler US have been reported to be useful in identifying patients with strangulation. Ogata and associates reported that an akinetic dilated loop observed on real-time US has a high sensitivity (90%) and specificity (93%) for the recognition of strangulation; the positive predictive value was 73%. The presence of peritoneal fluid was also sensitive for strangulation.[23] Further studies of the usefulness of US are needed.

■ MANAGEMENT

SMALL BOWEL OBSTRUCTION

The initial management of patients with small bowel obstruction should focus on aggressive fluid resuscitation, potentially on decompression of the obstructed bowel, and on prevention of aspiration. These steps are the same for all patients, whether they will be managed operatively or undergo a trial of nonoperative management. Blood should be sampled for serum electrolyte concentrations, cross-match, and when necessary, arterial blood gas analysis. Steps should also be taken to correct metabolic or electrolyte imbalances, which may be severe. Specifically, in patients who have experienced prolonged vomiting, potassium (and chloride) should be measured and replaced appropriately. The patient should also be considered for possible operative therapy.

The most important initial step in management is vigorous fluid resuscitation. Patients with small bowel obstruction often present with profound volume losses and may require large amounts of isotonic crystalloid solutions such as normal saline or lactated Ringer's solution, usually with additional potassium. Resuscitation should be guided by urine output, provided the patient is hemodynamically stable and has normal renal function. Patients who are hemodynamically unstable or have impaired cardiac, pulmonary, or renal function may require hemodynamic monitoring of central venous or pulmonary arterial pressure to evaluate their volume status. Colloid solutions such as 5% albumin or hetastarch have little or no role in the resuscitation of patients with a small bowel obstruction. Broad-spectrum antibiotics should be given to patients requiring an operation, but have no defined utility in those patients initially managed nonoperatively.

Most surgeons believe that nasogastric decompression is important to prevent further intestinal distention from swallowed air. In addition, nasogastric decompression also prevents aspiration during vomiting and on induction of general anesthesia. Symptomatically, decompression helps relieve abdominal distension and can improve ventilation in patients with respiratory compromise.

Some authors have advocated nasointestinal "long tube" intubation over nasogastric "short tube" intubation. The rationale behind this theory is that a long tube placed distal to the pylorus promotes more complete intestinal decompression, allowing the now decompressed bowel increased mobility and more opportunities to become unobstructed. Success rates of up to 90% have been reported in some series of patients treated with a long nasointestinal tube.[24] However, most prospective and retrospective studies have failed to demonstrate the superiority of nasointestinal versus nasogastric intubation,[24,25] making the added expense of fluoroscopic or endoscopic placement of a nasointestinal tube unwarranted. Some groups have also recommended intestinal splinting with these long nasointestinal tubes (an intraluminal Noble plication) to prevent kinking in the postoperative period.[24] Based on the literature, the authors believe that a functioning nasogastric tube is the best therapeutic approach and that a nasointestinal tube has not been shown to add benefit to the treatment of patients with small bowel obstruction. One might imagine a situation in which a nasogastric tube fails to relieve a massive small bowel dilatation (because of incomplete intestinogastric reflux); in this situation, placement of a nasointestinal tube distal to the ligament of Treitz may provide symptomatic benefit.

Nonoperative Management

Only patients with uncomplicated small bowel obstruction should be considered for a trial of nonoperative management. Nonoperative management of small bowel obstruction is reported to be successful in 62–85% of patients treated by this approach.[26–30] The rate of success is likely influenced by patient selection, type of bowel obstruction (complete versus partial, or recurrent, among others), etiology (e.g., adhesions, hernia, or neoplasm), the surgeon's threshold for conversion to operative management, and practice differences related to suspected ischemia. Patients successfully managed nonoperatively require shorter hospital stays[26,27] and do not experience the morbidity or convalescence necessitated by an operation. Few studies have compared the long-term outcomes of patients with a small bowel obstruction treated nonoperatively versus operatively. One such study reported by Landercasper and colleagues[31] found a recurrence rate of 29% in patients managed surgically versus a recurrence rate of 53% for patients managed nonoperatively, with over 4 years of follow-up. While the recurrence rates may be greater with nonoperative management, the authors point out that about half of the patients managed nonoperatively did not develop a recurrent small bowel obstruction.

Contraindications to nonoperative management include suspected ischemia, large bowel obstruction, closed-loop obstruction, strangulated hernia, and perforation. In an attempt to define which patients with an uncomplicated small bowel obstruction can be successfully treated nonoperatively, Chen and colleagues[30] used an orally administered, water-soluble contrast agent (Urografin) to study 116 patients with small bowel obstruction. The presence of contrast material within the colonic lumen within 8 hours of oral administration had an accuracy of 93% for predicting which patients would benefit from nonoperative therapy. In their study, only 19% of patients with a small bowel transit time of more than 8 hours had resolution of their obstruction with nonoperative treatment. However, one of the criteria for conversion to operative treatment was the failure of contrast to reach the colon within 8 hours. Therefore the 81% failure rate of patients without contrast reaching their colon 8 hours after administration may be artificially high based on study design.

A relative contraindication to nonoperative management is complete small bowel obstruction. In a prospective study by Fleshner and associates,[26] all patients with an uncomplicated small bowel obstruction underwent a trial of nonoperative management. They were able to successfully manage 45% of patients with a complete obstruction nonoperatively, while 66% of patients with a partial obstruction were successfully managed nonoperatively. These investigators, however, did not describe the incidence of intestinal ischemia at operation based on the presence or absence of complete versus partial obstruction. These investigators reported a 0% mortality rate in their study, which led them to conclude that a trial of nonoperative management is safe in patients without signs and symptoms of bowel strangulation or ischemia at presentation. Another study by Fevang and colleagues[27] reported a 42% success rate in managing patients with a complete small bowel obstruction nonoperatively. When they compared complete and partial obstructions managed nonoperatively, there was a higher rate of bowel strangulation (10% versus 4%) and need for resection (14% versus 8%) in the group with complete obstruction at the time of operation for treatment failure. This group noted a mortality rate of 6% in patients with a complete obstruction initially managed nonoperatively versus a 0% mortality rate for patients with a partial obstruction initially managed nonoperatively. Other groups have also noted a higher rate of ischemic bowel coupled with a lower success rate in those patients with a complete obstruction managed nonoperatively.[25,32] These studies and the unreliability of clinical acumen to reliably recognize strangulation obstruction have led many surgeons to favor early operation for all patients with a complete small bowel obstruction.[29] If nonoperative management is attempted in a patient with complete obstruction, the decision should be made with the understanding that there is a definite risk of overlooking an underlying strangulation obstruction,[32] and thus there should be a low threshold for operative intervention.

When patients with a small bowel obstruction are initially managed nonoperatively, several treatment principles need to be considered. Adequate proximal decompression is important to allow the bowel an opportunity to become unobstructed. This concept is accomplished by maintaining a functioning nasogastric tube. If patients become progressively more distended or develop vomiting, tube placement should be evaluated with an abdominal radiograph and tube function confirmed by bedside evaluation. If the tube is noted on radiograph to be out of position, it should be repositioned and imaged again for proper placement. Upon evaluation, the tube should be properly connected to the suction apparatus, it should be sumping properly (if the tube has a sump port), and checked for patency by flushing and aspirating water through the suction lumen.

Patients managed nonoperatively require aggressive resuscitation and realistic replacement of daily losses with an appropriate crystalloid solution and electrolyte replacement as necessary. Fluid replacement should take into consideration the volume and electrolyte content of the output of the nasogastric tube, urinary output, and insensible losses. Electrolytes should be monitored frequently and corrected as necessary.

When to Convert to Operative Management

If a patient being treated nonoperatively develops evidence of a complicated obstruction, operative intervention is indicated. Signs and symptoms suggestive of a complicated obstruction include fever, tachycardia, leukocytosis, localized tenderness, continuous abdominal pain, and peritonitis. The presence of any three of the following signs—continuous pain, tachycardia, leukocytosis, peritoneal signs, and fever—has an 82% predictive value for strangulation obstruction.[32] Similarly, the presence of any four of the above signs has a near 100% predictive value for strangulation obstruction. Patients who develop free air or signs of a closed-loop obstruction on abdominal radiograph require operative exploration. If evidence of ischemia, strangulation, or vascular compromise is noted on CT, such as pneumatosis intestinalis, bowel wall thickening, portal venous gas, generalized ascites, or nonenhancement of the bowel wall, then operative intervention is usually indicated.[29]

The timing of conversion to operative management in a patient with a small bowel obstruction who is not improving with nonoperative management is more controversial. Some surgeons advocate surgical intervention in any patient who fails to show improvement within 48 hours of initiating therapy.[25,28] Others advocate a more liberal use of nonoperative therapy, citing a mean time to successful resolution of up to 4.6 days.[26] The authors feel that nonoperative management can be continued longer than 48 hours with the understanding that delaying inevitable operative treatment will result in a longer overall hospital stay, increased costs, and place the patient at increased risk for perioperative morbidity. It is important for the surgeon to remember that nonoperative management always carries a calculated risk of overlooking an underlying complicated obstruction.[32]

Operative Management

Once the decision has been made to pursue operative management, steps should be taken to prevent peri- and postoperative complications. Preoperative preparation includes assessing and addressing the medical fitness of the patient, and as time allows, taking steps to optimize the patient's medical status. Consideration should be given to the administration of beta-blockers to patients with cardiovascular comorbidities.[33] Special consideration should be given to ensuring that the patient has been resuscitated adequately, appropriate antibiotics have been given, and any electrolyte abnormalities have been addressed. A nasogastric tube should already be in place to decrease the risk of aspiration during the induction of anesthesia.

Several decisions must be made with regard to operative planning to provide the safest operation that will afford the best outcome for each individual patient. The choice of operative approach and incision is important to allow the surgeon adequate exposure and visibility. A laparoscopic approach should at least be considered in some patients.[34] When an obstruction develops in the early postoperative period, the original incision should be reopened provided extensive adhesions were not present originally. However, in patients without a history of operation or in those remote from their original operation, a midline celiotomy affords the best exposure to all four quadrants of the abdomen. For example, patients with upper oblique, transverse, or subcostal type incisions may have pelvic adhesions that are difficult to address from the upper abdomen.

Once within the abdominal cavity, the first step is to identify the site and cause of obstruction. If the point of obstruction is not obvious, decompressed bowel distal to the obstruction can be identified and followed proximally to the point of obstruction. Care should be taken when handling the obstructed bowel at or near the point of obstruction when acutely obstructed, if it is fixed at an apparent site of obstruction, or if it is ischemic. This region is at high risk for strangulation and infarction, making it more likely to rupture with spillage of bacteria-laden enteric contents into the abdomen. The dilated bowel proximal to the offending obstruction is often very thin-walled and at increased risk for perforation. After the offending obstruction has been corrected, a thorough exploration of all four quadrants should always be undertaken to ensure that all intestinal injuries are repaired, nonviable segments are resected, and a second site of obstruction is not overlooked. Sometimes obstructing bands traversing a sizeable part of the peritoneum can affect more than one loop of bowel. When a small bowel resection is necessary, intestinal continuity of the small bowel can generally be accomplished with a primary anastomosis unless there is generalized peritonitis and the edges of the remnant bowel are of questionable viability.

Abdominal closure may be difficult to achieve when the small bowel is massively dilated. In these cases, intraoperative intestinal decompression will facilitate closure. Techniques described for intraoperative decompression include manual retrograde decompression into the stomach (with careful handling of the obstructed bowel), passage of a long nasointestinal tube, and performance of a controlled enterotomy with passage of a decompressing tube; the latter technique is strongly discouraged except under very select circumstances. Manual retrograde decompression of luminal contents around the ligament of Treitz, through the pylorus, and into the stomach allows them to be aspirated through the nasogastric tube by the anesthetist.[15] This maneuver is the safest and quickest technique, because it allows closure of the abdominal wall while avoiding an enterotomy and excessive manipulation of the bowel. When decompressing the bowel, care must be taken to handle the inflamed and distended bowel gently, as experimental studies have demonstrated an increased rate of bacteremia after extensive manipulation of obstructed bowel.[35] Although intraoperative decompression has not been shown to decrease the rate of postoperative complications or speed return of bowel function, it certainly does make the closure easier, faster, and safer.

Nonviable bowel needs to be identified and resected. Resection should be undertaken with caution, especially in patients with a limited length of bowel from a previous resection or those with large sections of ischemia. Adjuncts for determining bowel viability include the use of Doppler ultrasonography and intravenous fluorescein. These tests are relatively subjective, should be used with caution, and are only adjuncts to sound clinical judgment. In patients who will be left with less than two-thirds of their original bowel length after resection, consideration may be given to performing end ostomies or a second look procedure 12–24 hours later, particularly if the viability of the ends to be anastomosed is in question.

In patients with malignant small bowel obstruction or if the offending obstruction is unable to be released or it is deemed unsafe to attempt to dissect out the point of obstruction, intestinal bypass can be performed. Bypass relieves the obstruction while reestablishing intestinal continuity and preventing a closed-loop obstruction. However, the advisability of a bypass procedure should be considered. For instance, in the presence of carcinomatosis, a bypass may prove fastest and safest, since patient survival will be short. In contrast, patients with certain chronic inflammatory diseases will remain at risk for ongoing problems (e.g., Crohn's disease or tuberculosis) related to the inflammation and may be served better by resection than simple bypass.

The surgeon should at least consider an initial laparoscopic minimal access approach in patients with uncomplicated small bowel obstruction. Laparoscopy is known to cause fewer adhesions than laparotomy,[36] and in that regard may be superior to laparotomy for the treatment of adhesive small bowel obstruction. Several studies have shown laparoscopy to be a safe and effective means of access for treatment of small bowel obstruction.[34,37–39] When successful, a laparoscopic approach decreases the duration of hospital stay[34,38,39] and the complication rate.[38,39] Patients successfully treated laparoscopically appear to have more rapid return of bowel function.[38,39] However, these reports showing a large benefit to laparoscopic treatment for small bowel obstruction need to be interpreted carefully. Many series compare patients successfully treated laparoscopically to those who failed initial laparoscopic treatment. Those patients unable to be treated laparoscopically likely had more extensive adhesions or complicated pathology possibly requiring resection. Surgical intervention in these patients would be more involved and complex whether done open or laparoscopically. One would expect these patients to have longer hospital stays, higher complication rates, and slower return of bowel function independent of the method of abdominal access. In addition, the skill and confidence level of the surgeon should weigh in the decision to approach the obstruction laparoscopically. First, if the surgeon lacks skill in using moderately advanced laparoscopic techniques, an open operation may be a better choice. Similarly, if the patient is known to have a frozen abdomen or is found to have multiple dense adhesions at the time of insertion of the laparoscope, conversion to an open procedure is wise. It should not be necessary to point out that the initial access for creating the pneumoperitoneum in a patient with a small bowel obstruction should be a fully open approach under total visual control.

Recurrent Small Bowel Obstruction

Although the results of individual studies vary, between 4% and 34% of patients, depending on the clinical scenario, will experience a recurrent small bowel obstruction, regardless of management modality.[5,14,28,29,31,40,41] This wide range of recurrence rates likely results from variations both in the duration and quality of follow-up between studies as well as the etiology of the original bowel obstruction. Recurrent obstruction is more common in patients with multiple adhesions, matted adhesions, previous admissions for small bowel obstruction, and previous pelvic, colonic, and rectal surgery.[5,31]

In the past, numerous attempts have been made by surgeons to control the formation of adhesions in an effort to prevent future mechanical obstruction. A simple technique to prevent adherence of the bowel to the undersurface of the fascial incision is to interpose the omentum between the bowel and the incision. Theoretically, when adhesions form after omental interposition, they will involve the omentum and not the underlying bowel. Other more intricate techniques such as the Noble plication and the Childs-Phillips transmesenteric plication have been described. These procedures involve the suturing of adjacent loops of small bowel into an orderly pattern in an attempt to permanently plicate the bowel in a position that will not allow mechanical obstruction.[40] Although initial reports were encouraging, the Noble and Childs-Phillips procedures have multiple complications and are of historical interest only. The problems associated with plication procedures include prolonged operative times and high rates of enterocutaneous and entero-enteric fistula, abdominal abscess, and wound infection; moreover, the rate of recurrent obstruction is as high as 19%, questioning their efficacy.

Another method used to prevent mechanical obstruction of the small bowel is intraluminal "stenting" or "splinting" of the bowel with a long intestinal tube[40] (Fig 17–12). White, whose method involved suture plication of the small bowel over a tube, initially proposed intestinal stenting for the prevention of recurrent small bowel obstruction.[40] Baker described the use of a more rigid, balloon-tipped tube and did not suture the loops of bowel together.[40] Baker's technique involved the creation of a tube jejunostomy with passage of a "Baker" tube through the small bowel into the proximal colon. The tube was left in place as a stent for at least 10 days to allow for adhesion formation and simultaneous decompression of the affected bowel. The most frequent complications experienced by patients after Baker's procedure were related to the proximal jejunostomy, including intra-abdominal leak, intra-abdominal abscess, persistent enterocutaneous fistula, and obstruction at the jejunostomy site. Patients treated with this technique occasionally required reoperation for problems stemming from their jejunostomy. In an attempt to avoid the problems with the jejunostomy, others have placed the Baker tube retrograde into the jejunoileum via a cecostomy or even nasointestinally. Another tube used similarly via the nasointestinal route

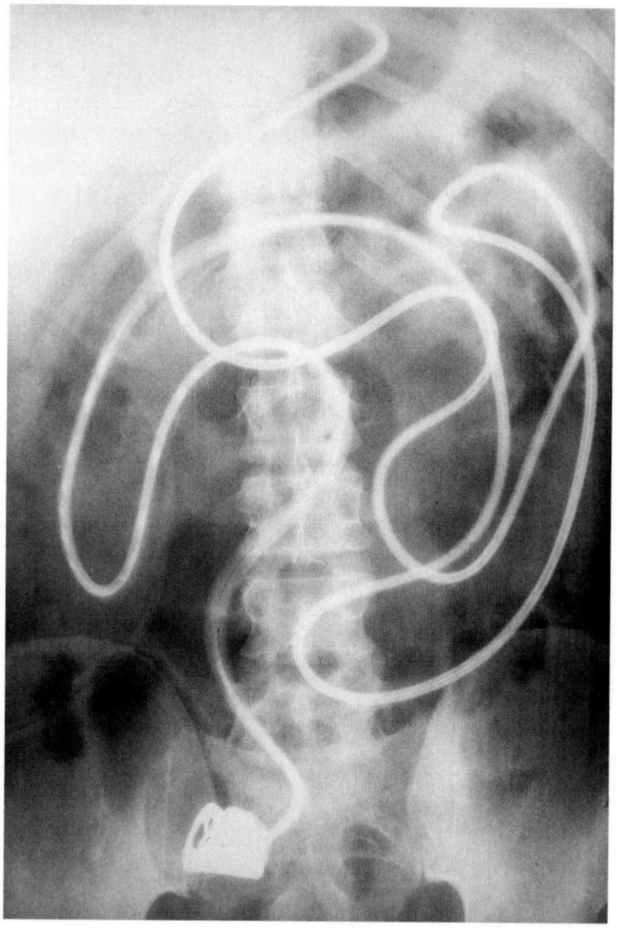

Figure 17–12. Abdominal radiograph showing distal passage of a long nasointestinal decompression tube into the small bowel distal to the ligament of Treitz.

has been the Lennard tube; however, it is much more rigid (designed so to aid passage through the duodenal C loop) and has not been as well-tolerated. The real question is whether the concept of an intraluminal stent is a valid one and how long the tube should be left in place to assure the appropriate maturation of the "friendly" intestino-intestinal adhesions. No prospective, randomized studies exist examining the best method of bowel plication and are unlikely to be done given the relative infrequency with which these methods are employed.

Occasionally patients will fall into a cycle of recurrent small bowel obstruction requiring frequent adhesiolysis. Others may have developed dense adhesions throughout the abdomen related to multiple previous celiotomies or peritonitis unrelated to bowel obstruction. When these patients develop a bowel obstruction, surgical intervention can be quite challenging technically. Operative intervention in this setting is associated with a high rate of iatrogenic bowel injury and serosal injury during the dissection, on occasion culminating in fistula formation. Patients having had multiple previous obstructions are less likely to develop bowel ischemia related to adhesions because of the relative lack of mobility of the bowel. For these reasons it may be advisable to attempt nonoperative therapy a bit more liberally in patients with multiple recurrences, provided there are no absolute indications for operative intervention (as described above). Patience of the treating surgeon and patient alike is also important, because these patients may require weeks of total parenteral nutritional support before the obstruction resolves.

In some patients it will become evident during the course of the operation that complete or adequate adhesiolysis is not possible. This situation is especially common when celiotomy is deemed necessary or performed too soon after a previous intra-abdominal procedure (see section below on early postoperative obstruction). This situation is especially common when the previous operation involved extensive adhesiolysis. In such situations, it may be important to control any bowel injuries present and conclude the operation to prevent further bowel injury and its potential sequelae. This approach has been used by the senior author five times in 25 years of practice. This "conservative" approach may allow the acute inflammatory process to resolve or regress (often 3–6 months); should the obstruction not resolve by 6 months, the plan should be to reoperate at a time when the adhesions have matured, allowing a more controllable and safer adhesiolysis. In some situations, the mature decision might be to provide proximal diversion with a proximal enterostomy if the obstruction has no chance for resolution (e.g., due to malignancy or radiation), or if a more distal bowel repair is tenuous, or to place a tube gastrostomy for diversion and patient comfort. Pushing on in a futile attempt to complete the adhesiolysis puts the patient at risk for further serious bowel injury, devascularization injury necessitating resection of otherwise normal bowel, and/or subsequent enterocutaneous fistulization.

Adhesion Prevention

Over the last 100 years, multiple approaches have been employed in an attempt to prevent the formation of unwanted postoperative adhesions. These include, among others, cow cecum, shark peritoneum, and fish bladder, and multiple fluids, mechanical barriers, and gels.[41] The concept of separating injured surfaces to prevent adhesions is a very attractive one. The formation of fibrin bridges (and thus adhesions) may be preventable by separating injured surfaces in the postoperative interval during the critical period of healing and mesothelialization by application of an absorbable "biofilm." Estimates of the minimum amount of time necessary for an impermeable or semipermeable barrier to prevent adhesion formation appears to be about 36 hours. Some authors have placed a Silastic® sheet between two injured peritoneal surfaces; when left in place for 36 hours, no adhesions formed thereafter.[12] Others have postulated that separating the surfaces at risk for the first 5–7 days until full mesothelialization occurs would seem to be most effective. However, the barrier should not incite its own inflammatory response and should not reduce fibrinolytic activity or suppress access to oxygen. The ideal product, therefore, should be bioabsorbable (preferably via a process such as hydrolysis), last only about 5–7 days, be easy to apply, and be interposed between all injured surfaces. Similarly, it cannot itself cause a foreign body reaction or impair either the normal wound healing process of an intestinal anastomosis or the fascial closure or mesothelial cell migration and proliferation. These ideal requirements are quite lofty. The most effective method to date has been the application of a sheet of bioresorbable, hyaluronate membrane; this approach has been shown to decrease the formation of adhesions at the site of application.[42,43] Although it is unknown, it is unlikely that this method will result in decreased adhesion formation at sites other than at the site of application. It is also important to remember that these studies have shown hyaluronate barriers to decrease the rate of postoperative adhesion formation, not postoperative bowel obstructions. Data from the Adhesion Study Group suggest hyaluronate barriers may modestly decrease the relative risk of developing an adhesive bowel obstruction among patients undergoing resection (personal communication).

Initial concerns were raised over the safety of hyaluronate barriers. Interest centered on worry about an increased risk of postoperative abscess, pulmonary embolism, fistula formation, peritonitis, and anastomotic leak. Concerns over the safety of hyaluronate membranes stemmed from initial studies on the impact of hyaluronate membranes on adhesion formation, as well as complications related to a gel preparation of hyaluronate cross-linked with iron, which has been withdrawn from the market. A subsequent prospective, randomized, controlled trial showed that hyaluronate barriers did not increase the risk of intra-abdominal abscess or pulmonary embolism.[43] However, in a post-hoc subgroup analysis of 289 patients in whom the hyaluronate membrane was wrapped around a fresh anastomosis, the rates of leak, fistula formation, peritonitis, abscess, and sepsis were increased. This observation suggests that "adhesions" or at least the access of the intraperitoneal microenvironment play an important role in the normal healing of bowel anastomoses. Indeed, peritoneal fluid contains multiple growth factors that may promote certain aspects of wound healing. Therefore, future attempts to prevent adhesions using materials such as more fluid-type gels and liquids that can more completely interpose between surfaces at risk need to bear in mind that not all adhesions are bad. For instance, use of sea snake venom, a potent protease with intense fibrinolytic activity, effectively prevented all adhesions, but in doing so also prevented healing of the surgical wound and any other wounds as well. Also, any surface coating agent that prevents contact of the peritoneal fluid and even the omentum, both of which contain certain growth factors that promote sealing and healing of anastomoses or areas of peritoneal trauma, may actually be detrimental to outcome. Based on these studies and assumptions, the use of hyaluronate membranes in elective abdominal surgery decreases the amount of postoperative adhesions and may decrease the rate of mechanical obstruction, although their routine use may not be warranted and awaits further study.

Other materials are being developed that someday may move to the forefront of adhesion prevention. These include gel and liquid preparations such as hyaluronic acid and carboxymethylcellulose, hydrogel, fibrin sealant, and protein polymers. Other adhesion barriers include oxidized regenerated cellulose (ORC). ORC has been well studied and does help prevent adhesion formation, but its use requires a blood-free field which at times is not practical to achieve. The use of ORC, like hyaluronate membranes, has not been shown to decrease the incidence of adhesive small bowel obstruction.[44]

Early Postoperative Small Bowel Obstruction

Early postoperative small bowel obstruction is a relatively uncommon problem, but one encountered in every practice performing abdominal operations. The definition of an "early" obstruction is not consistent in the surgical literature; multiple time frames have been used to define early postoperative obstruction, including up to 30 days postoperatively, within 6 weeks postoperatively, and those episodes occurring during the same hospitalization after a celiotomy. For the purposes of this chapter, we will consider early intestinal obstructions as those occurring within 6 weeks of operation; obstructions occurring after 6 weeks are managed similarly to other bowel obstructions.

It is often difficult, if not impossible, to distinguish early obstruction from postoperative ileus, but fortunately the management is usually quite similar. Patients with suspected early mechanical small bowel obstruction should be managed initially by nasogastric decompression, fluid resuscitation, and correction of any electrolyte abnormalities. After a thorough physical examination and the decision that emergent intervention is not indicated, a search for the cause of obstruction should be undertaken. CT can be helpful in determining the etiology of an obstruction caused by external bowel compression. Some such causes may be amenable to percutaneous correction, including fluid collections, abscesses, and hematomas. CT may be able to detect those causes of obstruction that will likely require surgical intervention such as internal hernia, fascial dehiscence, and uncontrolled anastomotic leak. CT can also aid in the detection of areas of ischemia.

Generally, two categories of patients with early postoperative small bowel obstructions have been recognized.[29] The first category includes those in whom the obstruction becomes evident within 10 days of surgery. Conservative management is advised as long as signs and symptoms of ischemia and strangulation obstruction are not present and other remediable causes have been excluded. Patients within this time frame are not at a substantially increased risk of bowel-related complications after celiotomy. It is important to rule out correctable causes of external compression and reverse any electrolyte abnormalities, especially if ileus is also suspected. Strangulation obstruction, although rare, can occur in this group of patients and a high index of suspicion must always be maintained; the etiology of a strangulation obstruction in this group is almost never related to adhesions, but rather to some surgical misadventure, such as internal hernia, an overlooked segment of ischemia at the original celiotomy, bowel entrapped in the fascial closure, or an overlooked abdominal wall hernia.

The second category of patients is those presenting between 10 days and 6 weeks after surgery.[29] Conservative management is strongly advised whenever possible for patients in this category as well. The risk of iatrogenic bowel complications during and after reoperation so early after celiotomy increases dramatically in this group secondary to the dense adhesions present during this period after abdominal operation. The time period from 7–10 days up until 6–12 weeks postoperatively represents the window when the greatest inflammatory reaction is present intraperitoneally. The developing adhesions are highly vascularized, friable, and very immature. If the patient had no or very minimal adhesions at the time of celiotomy, reoperation is warranted. However, in a small, unpredictable group of patients without any previous adhesions, and reliably so in those with dense adhesions that had required substantial adhesiolysis at the time of celiotomy, an acute inflammatory reaction involving the peritoneal surface may agglutinate adjacent loops of bowel, often involving the omentum and mesenteric surfaces.

Operations performed during this period have a much higher rate of iatrogenic injury and subsequent fistula formation. Those patients not responding to conservative management during this period should be placed on parenteral nutrition until the obstruction resolves or they are more than 6–12 weeks out from their last celiotomy. At this time, the decision to reoperate is made based on several considerations. First, if the patient had relatively few adhesions at the time of celiotomy, re-exploration at 6 weeks to 3 months postoperatively may be warranted. In contrast, in those patients who required an extensive adhesiolysis at the time of original celiotomy, many experienced surgeons wait for a full 6 months prior to reoperation for several reasons: (1) by 6 months, the adhesions are reliably less vascular and more mature; (2) reoperation prior to 3 months may reveal a frozen abdomen in which the obstruction may be unable to be dissected free safely; and (3) about half the time, the obstruction will resolve as the adhesions mature (see section above on recurrent small bowel obstruction).

Radiation Enteropathy

The management of radiation enteropathy is often difficult and frustrating. The clinical presentation can be quite diverse with recurrent intermittent small bowel obstruction, a true chronic persistent partial small bowel obstruction, or chronic diarrhea/malabsorption. Surgical management is often extremely challenging secondary to dense adhesions present after radiation. These patients also tend to develop recurrent areas of enteropathy (progression of disease) in bowel that appeared normal previously, because this ischemic disease is an ongoing chronic process. The need for surgical correction with a resection and anastomosis has been reported to have a mortality rate as high as 21% in some series.[40] Patients with radiation enteropathy also have a high rate of anastomotic leak and fistulization after operation because of the compromised vascular supply to the bowel. These effects are magnified in patients with atherosclerosis, hyperlipidemia, or type 2 diabetes. For these reasons, a cautious, conservative approach to the patient with radiation enteropathy is warranted whenever possible.

When surgical management is necessary, the surgeon must decide between resection, bypass of the affected segment, or adhesiolysis. As mentioned above, resection has been reported to have a high mortality rate and a 36% incidence of leak after primary anastomosis.[40] In the same study, bypass of the affected segment had a 10% mortality rate and 6% leak rate. However, surgeons advocating aggressive resection back to healthy bowel have reported leak rates between 0% and 8% when confounding conditions (abscess, fistula, necrosis, or recurrent cancer) were absent; this aggressive approach may require an extensive resection.

Most surgeons approach the treatment of radiation enteropathy selectively. In those patients with recurrent cancer and radiation enteropathy, treatment should consist of palliative bypass of the diseased segment with creation of an anastomosis in visibly normal tissue. If the obstructive process is localized, wide resection back to healthy, non-irradiated tissue (if possible) and primary anastomosis is acceptable. Usually this means anastomosis from small bowel to ascending colon, because the terminal ileum has usually been involved in the radiation field. While ideally, resection of the entire involved small bowel is optimal, the surgeon must consider the extent of the resection necessary as well as the anatomic segment involved. Usually, the involved small intestine is the ileum; major resection back to reliably normal, non-irradiated small bowel may require a total or subtotal ileectomy which carries its own complications, and a decision will need to be made concerning preservation of mildly involved but functional ileum if the only alternative is complete resection. In contrast, if the bowel is severely involved and nonfunctional, resection (despite its side effects) may be the best option. When the affected area contains dense adhesions or is stuck deep within the pelvis, bypass may be a better choice for avoiding potential iatrogenic injury to the bowel, bladder, pelvic organs, and ureters; however, if there is a localized abscess or associated septic process, this is not a good option, just as with Crohn's disease, because the ischemic, inflammatory process will continue. Attempts at complete lysis of adhesions alone without resection are controversial due to the risk of traumatizing the intestine with potential fistula formation. For the patient with advanced disease years after irradiation, adhesiolysis may not be a good option, especially if the bowel is matted and agglutinated together. In contrast, in the case of isolated adhesive bands and the patient early (<2 years) after irradiation, lysis alone may be warranted; much of the decision needs to be based on the quality of the involved bowel and the site of obstruction. If the bowel is thickened, woody, and strictured, resection or bypass is best.

Carcinomatosis and Malignant Obstruction

Bowel obstruction in the setting of carcinomatosis often represents the terminal phase of the malignant disease. Surgical management is purely palliative and needs to be applied selectively. In the case of limited life expectancy and malignant cachexia, nonoperative palliative measures are advised, as surgical intervention would be cruel and unnecessary. However, other patients with a good performance status may have a long life expectancy, and in this case surgical bypass with the idea of permitting renewed oral intake may be indicated. Patients and their families should be counseled that the relief of their obstruction will not affect disease progression but can improve quality of life. In addition, the surgeon should remember that up to one-third of bowel obstructions presenting in the setting of carcinomatosis are due to adhesions and not to malignant obstruction.[28] Therefore, a short trial of conservative therapy with rehydration and nasogastric decompression is usually advisable, although many (possibly most) patients with carcinomatosis will fail this intervention.

An initial minimal access, laparoscopic approach should be at least entertained in patients with a malignant obstruction, provided the access to the peritoneal cavity is safe. The least invasive approach is best for these patients, and if palliation can be achieved laparoscopically, the patient would benefit substantially with decreased pain, possibly a shorter convalescence, and decreased duration of hospital stay, all of which are important considerations in the palliative care of patients with a limited life expectancy.

Upon exploration, multiple scenarios may be encountered. Some patients will have an isolated area of adhesions and require only adhesiolysis. Others will have a solitary metastasis causing either intra- or extraluminal obstruction that can be corrected with a limited resection or bypass. If multiple areas of adhesions are present or the affected area is adherent to the abdominal wall or intra-abdominal structures, bypass of the involved segment will provide symptom relief and the fewest opportunities for complication. One should consider placement of a tube gastrostomy if there is any question of the success of the operation, if impending obstruction seems imminent, or if relief of the obstruction is not possible. In the event of re-obstruction, a tube gastrostomy can be used to decompress the stomach and avoid the discomfort associated with a nasogastric tube. The decision to place a palliative decompressive tube gastrostomy is more difficult in the presence of ascites. In this situation, a better option would be a tube pharyngostomy.[16]

▪ LARGE BOWEL OBSTRUCTION

Virtually all patients with complete acute large bowel obstruction require prompt surgical intervention and should not undergo a trial of nonoperative management. Acute complete large bowel obstruction in a patient with a competent ileocecal valve is a true surgical emergency because of the high risk of perforation. Once the diagnosis has been made, surgical exploration should be undertaken as soon as possible after appropriate resuscitation. Prior to exploration, the same principles apply for large bowel obstruction as for small bowel obstruction. Volume losses may be substantial, and patients should be resuscitated aggressively with an isotonic crystalloid solution. Electrolyte and acid-base abnormalities should be corrected. Nasogastric decompression is also important in patients with a large bowel obstruction to decrease the amount of air and gastric contents delivered to the bowel. About 50% of colonic gas is from swallowed air. Nasogastric decompression will help relieve intraluminal pressure, prevent further dilation of the proximal bowel, and possibly decrease the risk of perforation. A bladder catheter should be inserted to help guide resuscitation and as preparation for the operating room. As with small bowel obstruction, invasive monitoring may be necessary depending on the hemodynamic status of the patient. Antibiotics targeted at both skin and colonic flora should be administered. If time permits, patients with large bowel obstructions should have several possible stoma sites marked by a stoma therapist before being taken to the operating room to help ensure appropriate placement of the stoma device. It can be notoriously difficult to select a satisfactory site in the operating room with the patient supine and anesthetized, especially if the patient is obese or has redundant abdominal wall skin.

Exploration in patients with large bowel obstructions is best performed through a low midline incision. The role of initial laparoscopic exploration for large bowel obstruction is much less well defined; however, there are situations in which laparoscopic management might be beneficial. An example is a patient with an obstructing rectal cancer. Initial laparoscopic exploration could be used to determine the extent of disease and to perform a diverting loop ileostomy or proximal loop colostomy. This approach might allow mechanical bowel preparation and early resection with primary anastomosis. Similarly, some of these patients may be best managed initially with neoadjuvant therapy with the definitive resection performed at a later time.

For most patients, however, an open exploration is best. Patients with large bowel obstructions should be placed in the lithotomy or modified lithotomy position if access to the anus is anticipated. Once inside the abdominal cavity, the surgeon should proceed with exploration of all four quadrants as well as examination of the liver, omentum, and retroperitoneal lymph nodes for any suspicious lesions.[45] Obstructing lesions of the cecum and ascending colon should be resected via right hemicolectomy, usually with a primary anastomosis. Lesions in the transverse colon should be managed with an extended right hemicolectomy and again, with a primary anastomosis. Proximal diversion with an end ileostomy is not necessary in all patients; however, proximal diversion should be considered when there is any concern about bowel viability, if the patient is unstable, or in the case of substantial peritoneal contamination or peritonitis.

The management of obstructing lesions in the descending and sigmoid colon is more controversial. Intraoperative "on-the-table" bowel preparation can be performed when the surgeon and the operating room team are experienced and comfortable with this technique. Intraoperative bowel preparation allows for segmental resection and primary anastomosis of the involved colon provided the remnant bowel to be reanastomosed is healthy and neither too edematous nor too dilated; this approach has an acceptable leak rate of around 5%. Primary anastomosis should not, however, be carried out in the setting of fecal contamination, peritonitis, hemodynamic instability, or possible ischemia of the remaining colonic segments. Many surgeons prefer a more classic approach with a Hartmann's procedure of segmental resection of the affected colon, an end colostomy, and a blind distal pouch or mucous fistula. An end colostomy at the time of operation is safe and may decrease the incidence of perioperative complications compared to an on-the-table bowel preparation with primary anastomosis. However, patients undergoing end colostomy will require another procedure to reestablish intestinal continuity and will thus be subject to the complications associated with a second procedure[45]; this consideration should be weighed in the decision about therapy. A diverting loop ileostomy can be added to a primary anastomosis if there is any question of anastomotic integrity; the surgeon should remember that if the fecal load in the proximal colon has not been evacuated, the colonic anastomosis is still at risk for anastomotic leakage. The loop ileostomy will require takedown at a later time, but it is a less morbid operation than the celiotomy required after a Hartmann's procedure. Another option for left-sided lesions is subtotal colectomy and primary ileosigmoidostomy or ileorectostomy. This approach may be advisable when there is concern about possible cecal perforation, when there are multiple serosal tears in the colon,[45] or if the patient had a previous colonic cancer and the current obstruction is from a new colonic carcinoma.

In the case of obstructing rectal cancers, a different approach may be necessary. Primary resection is usually contraindicated in this situation secondary to an unacceptably high risk of leak with any primary anastomosis below the peritoneal reflection, and the technical difficulty of a future delayed primary colorectal or coloanal anastomosis after a Hartmann-type resection, since the blind end will be below the peritoneal reflection.[45] In contrast, if the patient is not a candidate for restoration of intestinal continuity, primary resection with end colostomy may be an acceptable approach. Usually, however, the surgical objectives in the case of an obstructing rectal cancer are a diversion to prevent perforation and allow bowel decompression, and preparation for later resection and possible sphincter-saving restoration of coloanal continuity. Proximal colonic diversion can be accomplished, preferably using a diverting sigmoid or transverse loop colostomy and mucous fistula. While proximal diversion can be accomplished with a loop ileostomy or an end ileostomy with distal mucous fistula, this type of diversion may not fully decompress the colon if the ileocecal valve is competent and mechanical preparation of the colon is quite difficult. Thus, diversion via ileostomy is usually discouraged. After discharge, patients with localized disease can undergo neoadjuvant therapy with definitive surgical resection after completing the chemoradiation.

Consideration should be given to an initial laparoscopic exploration in patients with obstructing or near obstructing lesions of the large bowel,[45,46] and especially if proximal diversion alone is anticipated. Laparoscopic exploration has several advantages over exploratory celiotomy for obstructing colonic lesions, including shorter hospital stays, early return of bowel function, earlier initiation of neoadjuvant therapy, and the potential to provide a diagnosis when the cause of obstruction is not known preoperatively.[45,46] Another advantage of laparoscopic exploration is the ability to detect peritoneal and metastatic disease not identified preoperatively. Because long-term survival and prognosis are dismal, palliative diversion can be established without subjecting the patient to a full celiotomy[45,47]; the advisability of resection of the primary lesion can then be discussed electively. Laparoscopy is particularly useful in patients with obstructing rectal cancers, because most of these patients should be diverted and undergo neoadjuvant therapy prior to definitive resection with primary anastomosis if feasible.[45,46] Finally, laparoscopic resection of colorectal cancers is a safe alternative to open resection with good quality of life and shorter hospital stays.[47]

Another option to consider in the early management of the patient with an obstructing lesion in the large bowel is the use of a self-expanding intraluminal metal stent (SEMS) to allow immediate colonic decompression (Fig 17–13) and the ability to perform elective mechanical bowel preparation.[48] The use of SEMS is becoming widely available and it can be a useful tool for the surgeon managing a large bowel obstruction. In experienced hands, a SEMS can be placed successfully in about 90% of patients with low complication rates.[48] A SEMS can avoid the need for urgent or emergent operation by intraluminally decompressing the distended proximal colon and allowing distal passage of stool. This approach converts an otherwise emergent operation into an elective operation. A SEMS is also useful when palliating patients who might not tolerate surgi-

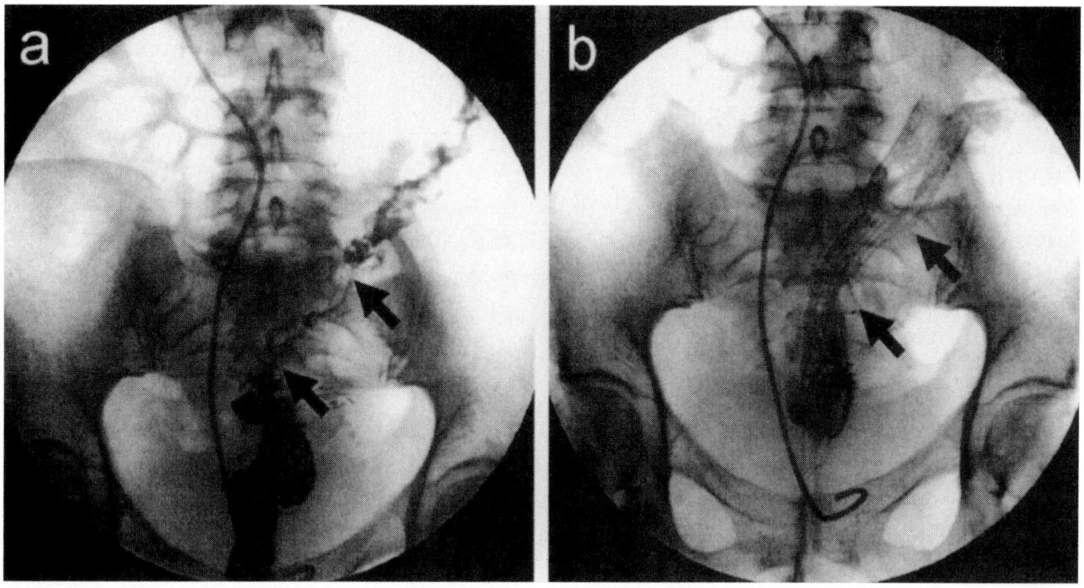

Figure 17–13. A. Obstructing rectal cancer (*arrows*). **B.** Intraluminal self-expanding metal stent restores luminal patency. (Reproduced, with permission, from Hünerbein M, Krause M, Moesta KT, Rau B, Schlag PM. Palliation of malignant rectal obstruction with self-expanding metal stents. Surgery 2005;137:42–47.)

cal diversion or those with unresectable disease and a limited survival. Successfully placed stents provide time for medical conditions to be identified and optimized, as well as a thorough mechanical bowel preparation to be performed.[48] These steps can decrease the morbidity and mortality associated with an emergent operation, as well as increasing the rate of an eventual one-stage operation with primary anastomosis. With a locally advanced obstructing rectal cancer, after placement of a SEMS, the patient can undergo neoadjuvant therapy followed by surgical resection, again increasing the chances for a successful one-stage operation.[49]

■ ILEUS

Postoperative ileus is usually differentiated from early small bowel obstruction by the presence of dilated small and large bowel (Fig 17–14). Currently, the treatment of ileus involves supportive measures only. Nasogastric decompression is important to prevent further intestinal distension from swallowed air and secretions as well as to decrease the risk of vomiting and subsequent aspiration. Patients with an ileus can sequester a substantial volume in the dilated bowel, causing intravascular volume depletion; therefore these patients require diligent fluid and electrolyte replacement. Most importantly, the underlying cause of ileus needs to be addressed. Aggressive treatment of sepsis, electrolyte abnormalities, and associated intra-abdominal processes will hasten the return of bowel function. Ileus is almost always self-resolving and results in very few long-term sequelae.

Early postoperative ileus (in the first 3–5 days) after abdominal operation has been called a "physiologic" ileus by some. It is well known that the stomach, small bowel, and large bowel recover normal motor activity at different rates after operative trauma and anesthesia. Within a few hours of operation, the small bowel returns to normal motor activity. The stomach recovers normal motor activity and emptying characteristics in 24–48 hours, while the large bowel takes 3–5 days to recover coordinated propulsive function.[1] It is therefore felt that early postoperative ileus is predominantly a colonic problem.

Because early postoperative ileus may prolong hospitalization after an otherwise innocuous celiotomy, a

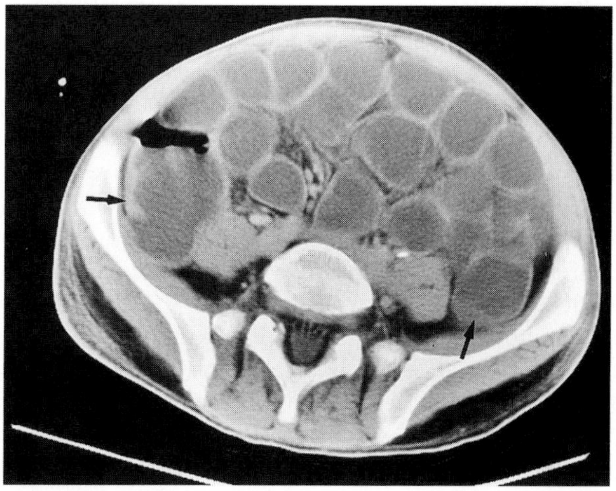

Figure 17–14. Ileus. CT of multiple loops of dilated, fluid-filled loops of small and large bowel (*arrows* point to the ascending and descending colon).

wide range of therapies have been tried to decrease the rate and impact of early postoperative ileus. These approaches have included physiologic-based therapies, such as blockade of sympathetic input and stimulation of the parasympathetic system, perioperative fluid restriction,[50] and more novel approaches such as gum chewing. Parasympathetic stimulation has been marginally effective in some patients, but overall the results with these agents have been disappointing. Similarly, results of central sympathetic blockade with ganglionic blocking agents have also been discouraging, demonstrating no difference in resolution of ileus. Other interventions that have been claimed to result in a shorter time to return of bowel function include prolonged, segmental epidural anesthesia[51] and transcutaneous nerve stimulation. Both interventions are cumbersome to employ and have a poorly defined, small risk:benefit ratio. Other pharmacological agents that have shown promise in the past include intravenous erythromycin and cisapride. However, neither has been used routinely in clinical practice, and the latter has been withdrawn from the market.

During the last decade, models of postoperative ileus have been proposed that focus on other aspects of the physiology of ileus. Inflammation within the wall of the bowel has been shown to play an important role in postoperative ileus in animal models and may be a target of future therapies.[52] In animal models, opioid receptor stimulation results in slower return of bowel function, even in nonabdominal surgery. This animal work has led to human trials of opioid antagonists for treatment of early postoperative ileus.[53,54] Alvimopan, a peripherally acting mu opioid-receptor antagonist, appears to decrease the time to recovery of bowel function after major abdominal operations and to accelerate hospital discharge by 20 hours compared to placebo.[55,56] These and future therapies may decrease the morbidity and cost associated with abdominal surgery, allowing shorter hospital stays and less patient discomfort.

In contrast to the more universal early postoperative ileus which is of limited duration, a generalized, adynamic ileus is much less common but may persist for many days to weeks in some patients. Most investigators believe this motor problem to be a systemic disorder involving a dysregulation of neuromotor coordination of the entire gut. Obviously, every attempt should be made to correct electrolyte disorders (especially sodium, chloride, and magnesium), treat any site of sepsis, and exclude a mechanical cause of potential obstruction. Despite addressing all correctable abnormalities, on occasion the ileus can persist and can be a very vexing problem for both patient and physician, requiring prolonged gastric decompression and intravenous nutritional support. Studies of pharmacological parasympathetic stimulation with parenteral neostigmine (on occasion with a concomitant sympatholytic agent) have been successful (see the section below on acute colonic pseudo-obstruction). This treatment should be given in a monitored setting.

ACUTE COLONIC PSEUDO-OBSTRUCTION

Acute pseudo-obstruction of the colon is often suspected based both on abdominal radiography and the clinical setting, but it remains a diagnosis of exclusion. It is imperative that a mechanical obstruction be excluded before proceeding with nonoperative or pharmacological treatment. When peritonitis or perforation is present or ischemia is suspected, the patient requires semi-emergent operative intervention, but only after appropriate resuscitation. Exclusion of a mechanical obstruction can be accomplished via either a careful, complete (and potentially therapeutic) colonoscopy minimizing air insufflation, or by demonstrating free retrograde flow of contrast without obstruction to the cecum on water-soluble enema;[57] a barium solution should not be used. These water-soluble contrast enemas can also be therapeutic; some patients achieve decompression after contrast instillation because of stimulation of defecation. Initial management of pseudo-obstruction is the same as that for small bowel obstruction and includes placement of a nasogastric tube, nothing by mouth, rehydration, correction of electrolyte abnormalities, and if possible, discontinuation of narcotics.[57]

The decision to pursue colonic decompression is based in part on the cecal diameter as determined by abdominal radiographs (Fig 17–15), on symptomatology, and on the duration of obstruction. In general, the maximum accepted safe cecal diameter is 12 cm; above this diameter, the risk of perforation increases substantially. When the cecum is less than 12 cm in diameter and the patient is not distressed, initial treatment should be continued, as immediate decompression is not necessary.[45,57] If at any time during therapy the patient develops peritonitis or signs of ischemia, emergent surgical therapy is indicated.

When the cecal diameter exceeds 12 cm or the patient has a significant amount of abdominal discomfort, decompression is indicated.[57] The two methods of colonic decompression include intravenous neostigmine and colonoscopic decompression.[57,58] Neostigmine is the first line of treatment in the patient without contraindications.[57] Neostigmine has been shown to be effective for treatment of acute colonic pseudo-obstruction, achieving success in about 90% of patients.[57,58] However, neostigmine should only be administered with

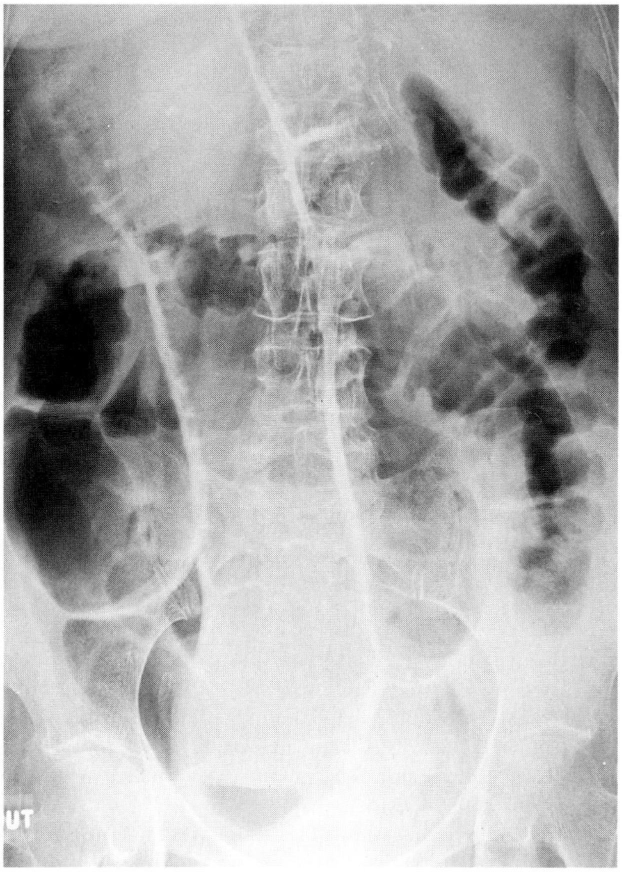

Figure 17–15. Acute colonic pseudo-obstruction, with a markedly dilated proximal colon; endoscopy confirmed no distal obstruction.

cardiac monitoring. Atropine and emergency airway equipment should be available in case severe bradycardia or respiratory compromise develop, which are potential side effects of neostigmine administration.[57] The initial dose of neostigmine is 2 mg intravenously. If one 2-mg dose of neostigmine is unsuccessful, a second dose may be administered.

Colonoscopic decompression, once the first line of therapy for acute colonic pseudo-obstruction, is now considered the second-line treatment for patients with uncomplicated pseudo-obstruction. Colonoscopic decompression is indicated in those patients with contraindications to neostigmine administration or those who have failed neostigmine therapy.[57] Another role for colonoscopy is to exclude a source of mechanical obstruction, in which case it may be both diagnostic and therapeutic. A long, large-diameter colonic tube can be placed at the time of colonoscopy, and although controversial, may aid in further decompression in those patients with refractory pseudo-obstruction.[57] Most surgeons, however, do not place a long colonic tube at the time of first colonoscopic decompression, but do leave a tube should the patient require another colonoscopic decompression for recurrent obstruction. When a colonic tube is deemed necessary, the tube is left within the dilated segment, not just in the rectum.

Success must be confirmed by a decrease in the cecal diameter on posttherapy abdominal radiograph[57,58] and by a notable decrease in abdominal girth. Serial exams and abdominal films must continue to ensure that the pseudo-obstruction does not recur or persist. If the cecal diameter is unchanged after colonoscopic decompression, then another treatment modality should be pursued and/or the diagnosis of pseudo-obstruction revisited and the diagnosis of mechanical obstruction re-entertained.

Operative intervention is indicated when signs and symptoms of perforation or ischemia are present or when conservative measures have failed.[57] In the presence of ischemia or when splitting of the teniae coli is evident, resection of the involved segment, usually the cecum and ascending colon, is warranted. Primary anastomosis can often be performed without a bowel preparation on the right side of the colon,[57] as long as the residual tissues and medical condition of the patient are favorable.

When surgical intervention is necessary after failed medical therapy and no evidence of ischemia exists, some authors recommend a surgical cecostomy tube be placed.[57,59] The tube placed should have a large diameter (>32F) and be flushed frequently to prevent obstruction with stool, which can be quite problematic.[57,59,60] Cecostomy tubes have been associated traditionally with a high incidence of leakage, but recent series have reported a low rate of leakage and a minor complication rate of 23–45%.[59,60] Most complications were wound-related or tube-related, with wound infection being the most commonly reported problem.[59,60] One technique employed to decrease the leakage rate is placement of an intervening wrap or tunnel of omentum between the cecum and the abdominal wall.[57] Other options for patients without evidence of perforation or ischemia include percutaneous and endoscopic cecostomy. Endoscopic cecostomy can be done at the time of colonoscopy and has been shown to be safe in experienced hands for the treatment of colonic motility disorders.[61]

REFERENCES

1. Woods JH, Erickson LW, Condon RE et al. Postoperative ileus: a colonic problem? *Surgery* 1978;84:527–533
2. Baig MK, Wexner SD. Postoperative ileus: A review. *Dis Colon Rectum* 2004;47:516–526
3. Sajja SB, Schein M. Early postoperative small bowel obstruction. *Br J Surg* 2004;91:683–691

4. Duepree HJ, Senagore AJ, Delaney CP et al. Does means of access affect the incidence of small bowel obstruction and ventral hernia after bowel resection? Laparoscopy versus laparotomy. *J Am Coll Surg* 2003;197:177–181
5. Miller G, Boman J, Shrier I et al. Natural history of patients with adhesive small bowel obstruction. *Br J Surg* 2000;87:1240–1247
6. Lu RH, Chang TM, Yen MH et al. Involvement of superoxide anion in the pathogenesis of simple mechanical intestinal obstruction. *J Surg Res* 2003;115:184–190
7. Miedema BW, Johnson JO. Methods for decreasing postoperative gut dysmotility. *Lancet Oncol* 2003;4:365–372
8. Kabaroudis A, Papaziogas B, Koutelidakis I et al. Disruption of the small-intestine mucosal barrier after intestinal occlusion: a study with light and electron microscopy. *J Invest Surg* 2003;16:23–28
9. Hellebrekers BW, Trimbos-Kemper GC, Bakkum EA et al. Short-term effect of surgical trauma on rat peritoneal fibrinolytic activity and its role in adhesion formation. *Thromb Haemost* 2000;84:876–881
10. Wilson MS, Ellis H, Menzies D et al. A review of the management of small bowel obstruction. Members of the Surgical and Clinical Adhesions Research Study (SCAR). *Ann R Coll Surg Engl* 1999;81:320–328
11. Sulaiman H, Gabella G, Davis C et al. Presence and distribution of sensory nerve fibers in human peritoneal adhesions. *Ann Surg* 2001;234:256–261
12. di Zerega GS, Campeau JD. Peritoneal repair and postsurgical adhesion formation. *Hum Reprod Update* 2001;7: 547–555
13. Menzies D, Ellis H. Intestinal obstruction from adhesions—how big is the problem? *Ann R Coll Surg Engl* 1990;73:60–63
14. Fevang BS, Fevang J, Lie SA et al. Long-term prognosis after operation for adhesive small bowel obstruction. *Ann Surg* 2004;240:193–201
15. Mucha P Jr. Small intestinal obstruction. *Surg Clin North Am* 1987;67:597–620
16. Kendrick ML, Sarr MG. Prolonged gastrointestinal decompression of the inoperable abdomen: the forgotten tube pharyngostomy. *J Am Coll Surg* 2000;191:221–223
17. Begos DG, Sander A, Modlin IM. The diagnosis and management of adult intussusception. *Am J Surg* 1997; 173:88–94
18. Assalia A, Schein M, Kopelman D et al. Therapeutic effect of oral Gastrografin in adhesive, partial small-bowel obstruction: a prospective randomized trial. *Surgery* 1994;115:433–437
19. Choi HK, Chu KW, Law WL. Therapeutic value of Gastrografin in adhesive small bowel obstruction after unsuccessful conservative treatment: a prospective randomized trial. *Ann Surg* 2002;236:1-6
20. Feigin E, Seror D, Szold A et al. Water-soluble contrast material has no therapeutic effect on postoperative small-bowel obstruction: results of a prospective, randomized clinical trial. *Am J Surg* 1996;171:227–229
21. Okada T, Yoshida H, Iwai J et al. Pulsed Doppler sonography for the diagnosis of strangulation in small bowel obstruction. *J Pediatr Surg* 2001;36:430–435
22. Cozza S, Ferrari FS, Stefani P et al. Ileal occlusion with strangulation: importance of ultrasonography findings of the dilated loop with intraluminal fluid-fluid resulting from sedimentation. *Radiol Med (Torino)* 1996;92:394–397
23. Ogata M, Imai S, Hosotani R et al. Abdominal ultrasonography for the diagnosis of strangulation in small bowel obstruction. *Br J Surg* 1994;81:421–424
24. Gowen GF. Long tube decompression is successful in 90% of patients with adhesive small bowel obstruction. *Am J Surg* 2003;185:512-515
25. Brolin RE. The role of gastrointestinal tube decompression in the treatment of mechanical intestinal obstruction. *Am Surg* 1983;49:131–137
26. Fleshner PR, Siegman MG, Slater GI et al. A prospective, randomized trial of short versus long tubes in adhesive small-bowel obstruction. *Am J Surg* 1995;170:366–370
27. Fevang BT, Jensen D, Svanes K et al. Early operation or conservative management of patients with small bowel obstruction? *Eur J Surg* 2002;168:475–481
28. Pickleman J. Small bowel obstruction. In: Zinner MJ, Schwartz SI, Ellis H (eds). *Maingot's Abdominal Operations,* 10th ed. New York, NY: McGraw-Hill; 1997:1159–1172
29. Baerga-Varela Y. Small bowel obstruction. In: Kelly KA, Sarr MG, Hinder RA (eds). *Mayo Clinic Gastrointestinal Surgery,* 1st ed. Philadelphia, PA: Saunders; 2004:421–437
30. Chen SC, Chang KJ, Lee PH et al. Oral Urografin in postoperative small bowel obstruction. *World J Surg* 1999;23:1051-1054
31. Landercasper J, Cogbill TH, Merry WH et al. Long-term outcome after hospitalization for small bowel obstruction. *Arch Surg* 1993;128:765–771
32. Sarr MG, Bulkley GB, Zuidema GD. Preoperative recognition of intestinal strangulation obstruction: Prospective evaluation of diagnostic capability. *Am J Surg* 1983; 145:176–181
33. Fleisher LA, Eagle KA. Lowering cardiac risk in noncardiac surgery. *N Engl J Med* 2001;345:1677–1682
34. Luque-de Leon E, Metzger A, Tsiotos GG et al. Laparoscopic management of small bowel obstruction: Indications and outcome. *J Gastrointest Surg* 1998;2:132–140
35. Merrett ND, Jorgenson J, Schwartz P et al. Bacteremia associated with operative decompression of a small bowel obstruction. *J Am Coll Surg* 1994;179:33–37
36. Polymeneas G, Theodosopoulos T, Stamatiedis A et al. A comparative study of postoperative adhesion formation after laparoscopic vs. open cholecystectomy. *Surg Endosc* 2001;15:41–43
37. Suzuki K, Umehara Y, Kimura T. Elective laparoscopy for small bowel obstruction. *Surg Laparosc Endosc Percutan Tech* 2003;13:254–256
38. Strickland P, Lourie DJ, Suddleson EA et al. Is laparoscopy safe and effective for treatment of acute small-bowel obstruction? *Surg Endosc* 1999;13:695–698
39. Wullstein C, Gross E. Laparoscopic compared with conventional treatment of acute adhesive small bowel obstruction. *Br J Surg* 2003;90:1147–1151
40. Tito WA, Sarr MG. Intestinal obstruction. In: Zuidema GD (ed). *Shackelford's Surgery of the Alimentary Tract,* 4th ed. Philadelphia, PA: Saunders; 1996:375–416

41. Becker JM, Stucchi AF. Intra-abdominal adhesion prevention: are we getting any closer? *Ann Surg* 2004;240:202–204
42. Becker JM, Dayton MT, Fazio VW et al. Prevention of postoperative abdominal adhesions by a sodium hyaluronate-based bioresorbable membrane: a prospective, randomized, double-blind multicenter study. *J Am Coll Surg* 1996;183:297–306
43. Beck DE, Cohen Z, Fleshman JW et al. A prospective, randomized, multicenter, controlled study of the safety of Seprafilm adhesion barrier in abdominopelvic surgery of the intestine. *Dis Colon Rectum* 2003;46:1310–1319
44. Al-Jaroudi D, Tulandi T. Adhesion prevention in gynecologic surgery. *Obstet Gynecol Surv* 2004;59:360–367
45. Hughes SJ. Large bowel obstruction. In: Bland KI (ed). *The Practice of General Surgery,* 1st ed. Philadelphia, PA: Saunders; 2002:473–477
46. Koea JB, Guillem JG, Conlon KC et al. Role of laparoscopy in the initial multimodality management of patients with near-obstructing rectal cancer. *J Gastrointest Surg* 2000;4:105–108
47. Clinical Outcomes of Surgical Therapy Group. A comparison of laparoscopically assisted and open colectomy for colon cancer. *N Engl J Med* 2004;350:2050–2059
48. Baron TH, Kozarek RA. Endoscopic stenting of colonic tumours. *Best Pract Res Clin Gastroenterol* 2004;18:209–229
49. Alder DG, Young-Fadok TM, Smyrk T et al. Preoperative chemoradiation therapy after placement of a self-expanding metal stent in a patient with an obstructing rectal cancer: clinical and pathologic findings. *Gastrointest Endosc* 2002;55:435–437
50. Lobo DN, Bostock KA, Neal KR et al. Effect of salt and water balance on recovery of gastrointestinal function after elective colon resection: a randomized controlled trial. *Lancet* 2002;359:1812–1818
51. Jorgensen H, Wetterslev J, Moiniche S et al. Epidural local anesthetics versus opioid-based analgesic regimens on postoperative gastrointestinal paralysis, PONV, and pain after abdominal surgery. *Cochrane Database Syst Rev* 2000;4:CD001893
52. Schwarz NT, Kalff JC, Turler A et al. Selective jejunal manipulation causes postoperative pan-enteric inflammation and dysmotility. *Gastroenterology* 2004;126:159–169
53. Taguchi N, Sharma N, Saleem RM et al. Selective postoperative inhibition of gastrointestinal opioid receptors. *N Engl J Med* 2001;345:935–940
54. Bauer AJ, Beckxstaens GE. Mechanisms of postoperative ileus. *Neurogastroenterology* 2004;16(Suppl 2):54–60
55. Delaney CP. Clinical perspective on postoperative ileus and the effect of opiates. *Neurogastroenterology* 2004; 16(Suppl 2):61–66
56. Wolff BG, Michelassi F, Gerkin TM et al. Alvimopan, a novel, peripherally acting μ opioid antagonist: results of a multicenter, randomized, double-blind, placebo-controlled, phase III trial of major abdominal surgery and postoperative ileus. *Ann Surg* 2004;240:728-735
57. Suggs WJ, Young-Fadok TM. Pseudo-obstruction of the colon. In: Bland KI (ed). *The Practice of General Surgery,* 1st ed. Philadelphia, PA: Saunders; 2002:499–502
58. Paran H, Silverberg D, Mayo A et al. Treatment of acute colonic pseudo-obstruction with neostigmine. *J Am Coll Surg* 2000;190:315–318
59. Benacci JC, Wolff BG. Cecostomy. Therapeutic indications and results. *Dis Colon Rectum* 1995;38:530–534
60. Perrier G, Peillon C, Leberge N et al. Cecostomy is a useful surgical procedure: study of 113 colonic obstructions caused by cancer. *Dis Colon Rectum* 2000;43:50–54
61. Ramage JI, Baron TH. Percutaneous endoscopic cecostomy: a case series. *Gastrointest Endosc* 2003;57:752–755

18

Diverticular Disease of the Colon

Angus J. M. Watson ▪ *Frank A. Frizelle*

Colonic diverticula are the most common structural abnormality of the bowel. However, they are not true diverticula in that they do not contain all layers of the colonic wall, but rather are false diverticula because they are acquired herniations of mucosa through the muscle wall. In Western countries the prevalence of diverticular disease has increased during the last century.[1] This rise probably reflects both an increase in detection and an aging population. Diverticular disease is currently one of the five most costly gastrointestinal disorders affecting the United States population.[2,3] Until 30 years ago, the proportion of patients requiring surgery or dying from diverticular disease was decreasing[4]; however, during the last 20 years the rates of hospital admission and surgical intervention have increased, while inpatient and population mortality rates have remained unchanged.[5]

Colonic diverticuli affect less than 10% of people in their fifth decade of life, increasing to around 50–66% in their ninth decade.[6] The management of the complications of diverticular disease is challenging and good outcome relies on timely intervention.

▪ HISTORY

Diverticular disease was initially described by Littre in 1700 as saccular outpouchings of the colon.[7] Cruveilhier is credited with the first clear and detailed description of the pathogenesis of diverticulitis and complicated diverticular disease.[8] In 1899 Graser introduced the term "peridiverticulitis" and suggested that diverticula were caused by herniation of colonic mucosa through areas of penetration of the vasa recta. This is now well established as the pathogenesis of colonic diverticulosis.[9] In contrast, the mechanism for diverticulitis was not identified until 1904 by Beer.[10] He proposed that impacted fecal matter at the neck of the diverticulum caused inflammation and subsequent abscess and fistula formation.

Moynihan reported a case of peridiverticulitis in 1907 and underlined the difficulties in distinguishing diverticular disease from malignancy.[11] Telling and Gruner's classic paper describing complex diverticular disease was not published until 1917.[12] At this time the prevalence and pathophysiology of diverticular disease were well recognized, as were the complications including acute diverticulitis, abscess, fistula, perforation, and obstruction.

The development of radiological imaging of the large intestine was important in establishing a diagnosis and documenting the extent of diverticular disease.[13] De Quervain (1914) and Case (1914, 1929) were the first to demonstrate colonic diverticula with x-rays.[14–16]

▪ ETIOLOGY

Diverticular disease is a disease of Western populations. A number of studies have shown an increase in incidence over the last 30 years.[1,5] Migrant studies likewise confirm increases in incidence when populations move to a Western country. There is a widely held view that fiber content of food is important, and the high intraluminal pressure associated with low-fiber diets precipitated by colonic compartmentalization causes an unsustainable increase in tension within the bowel wall. This is compounded by the hyperelastosis and altered collagen structure seen in the colon due to aging.[17,18] Both mechanisms ultimately lead to a loss of bowel wall integrity and the formation of diverticula. Exercise and a reduction in the intraluminal pressure associated with a high-fiber diet may be protective.[19]

High intraluminal pressures are generated because of colonic motility. Colonic motility is complex and not easily studied. The most common motor patterns are tonic segmenting and rhythmic contraction. Tonic segmentation creates stationary narrow rings that appear as haustral markings. Their purpose is to slow the fecal stream and to permit water absorption and electrolyte exchange. Infrequent propulsive peristaltic contractions move fecal matter in a caudal direction; these occur around six times a day.[20]

The alteration in pressure caused by these movements has been implicated in the pathogenesis of colonic diverticulosis. Several groups have studied colonic motility with intraluminal manometry in humans and animals. Most of the studies agree that there is increased phasic pressure activity, but this relates more to the presence of symptoms rather than diverticula. However, the results are heterogenous, principally because of methodological differences, in particular relating to bowel preparation and pressure sensors.[21] It may therefore be unreasonable to draw firm conclusions from these investigations.[22]

More generalized alterations in colonic motility have been implicated in the pathogenesis of colonic diverticular disease. In vitro and in vivo studies, however, are conflicting, with some demonstrating an absence of slow-wave activity (favoring nonpropagating contractile activity), and some demonstrating unimpaired or increased slow-wave activity.[23–25] Other workers have demonstrated an increase in fast-wave activity, which persists after resectional surgery.[26] The exact relevance of these myoelectric changes remains uncertain.

Diverticulosis is a Western disease that has a striking geographic distribution. The disease is rare in rural Africa and Asia with the highest prevalence seen in the U.S., Europe, and Australia.[27] Within a single country the disease incidence can vary depending on ethnicity.[28] Urbanization can also increase diverticular disease incidence, possibly attributed to a dietary change.[29–31] The incidence of complicated diverticular disease also seems to be increasing.[32]

Diverticular disease in Asian patients is often right-sided. The reasons for this variation are unknown; however, it has been suggested that both diet and elastin/collagen differences may play a role.[33]

▪ MORPHOLOGIC FEATURES

Colonic diverticula are false diverticula. The muscular colonic wall is comprised of both longitudinal and circular layers. The circular layer of the muscularis propria forms a continuous sheet of muscle throughout the large bowel. The longitudinal layer forms three discrete condensations called taeniae; one of these is adjacent to the mesentery the other two are antimesenteric. The taeniae coalesce to form an enveloping muscular layer in the rectum. Much of the colonic wall is therefore devoid of longitudinal muscle and it is in these areas that diverticula form. Herniations of muscularis mucosa occur between the taeniae along the arteries that penetrate the muscle wall en route to the submucosa and mucosa (Fig 18–1).

Many studies have demonstrated a change in the histological structure of the muscularis propria in diverticular disease. In a classic study, Whiteway and Morson found the muscle cells to be normal with no evidence of hyperplasia or hypertrophy, but both layers were thickened. They demonstrated excessive amounts of elastin in the taeniae but not in the circular muscle.[34] Repeated intermittent distension of the colon can result in increased synthesis of connective tissue components.[35] It may be that the Western diet with its lower fecal load only intermittently distends the bowel wall and encourages elastin deposition.

The importance of collagen and elastin types in the colonic wall is increasingly being recognized. Elastin deposition, termed "elastosis," explains the contracted and thickened appearance of the diverticula-affected colon. The taeniae shorten and because of fascial linkage between the longitudinal and circular muscles, the colonic wall looks like a concertina. Thickened circular muscle folds project into the lumen causing a decrease in caliber. The mesocolon is also foreshortened, possibly as a result of chronic inflammation. Other studies have suggested the type of collagen may be important.[36] One study has shown that in the bowel sections of patients with diverticulitis, there were decreased levels of mature collagen type I and increased levels of collagen type III with a resulting lower collagen I:III ratio. The expression of matrix metalloproteinase 1 was reduced significantly in the diverticulitis group.[36] These findings support the theory of structural changes in the colonic wall as one of the predisposing pathogenic factors for the development of diverticuli[36] (Figs 18–2A and 18–2B).

▪ PRESENTATION

Given the high incidence of diverticulosis, it is surprising that clinical manifestations are relatively infrequent.

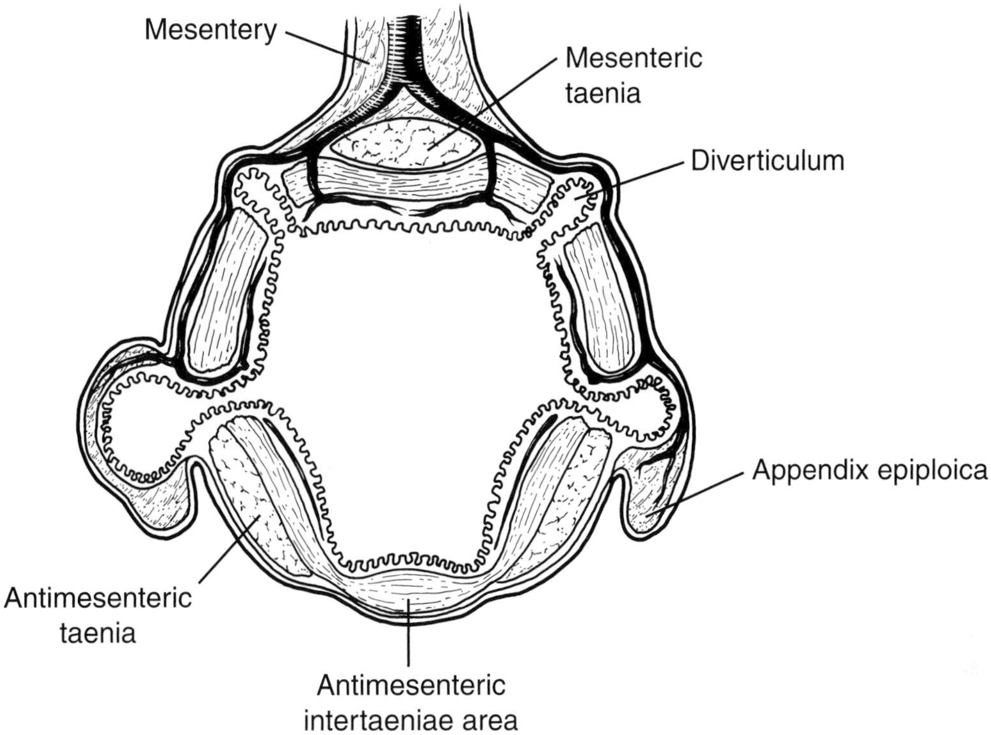

Figure 18–1. Diagrammatic representation of the relationship of diverticula and blood vessels to the taeniae coli.

Many patients are unaware that they have colonic diverticula until they develop acute symptoms. Typically an acute attack begins with lower abdominal pain which then localizes to the left iliac fossa. An inflamed sigmoid colon can lie against the dome of the bladder or the cecum, mimicking a urinary tract infection or appendicitis. Fever, tachycardia, and a leukocytosis accompany the acute attack. The inflammatory response starts at the site of a blocked diverticulum and bacterial proliferation leads eventually to abscess formation. Minor episodes may be self-limiting but an abscess can develop and then rupture into the abdomen causing a purulent peritonitis. More rarely feculent peritonitis occurs when a diverticulum ruptures freely into the peritoneum.

Physical examination will often reveal peritonitis localized to the left iliac fossa; a palpable mass is not un-

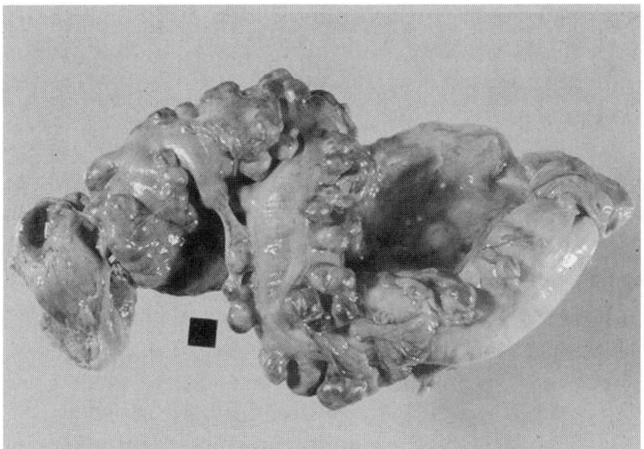

A

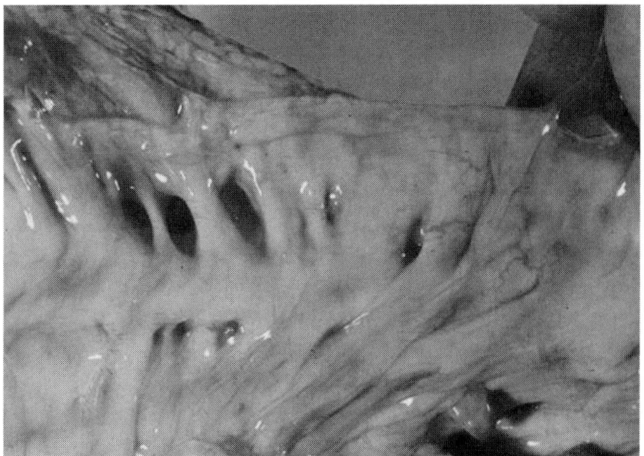

B

Figure 18–2. A, B. Pathological specimen showing numerous diverticula within the sigmoid colon.

common. In the absence of complications these patients are best managed conservatively. Generalized rigidity suggests purulent or fecal peritonitis, and in this situation there is no benefit from wasting time for further investigation. Once fully resuscitated, an emergency laparotomy and an appropriate colonic resection should be performed.

Often diverticular disease presents in a more indolent manner with nagging left iliac fossa pain, abdominal distension, and a change in bowel habits. In the course of investigations to exclude colon cancer, diverticular disease may be discovered by barium enema or colonoscopy (Fig 18–3). In the majority of these patients dietary modification and verbal advice will suffice. A small number of patients who continue to have symptoms despite long periods of medical management may benefit from surgery in the absence of other specific complications of the disease.

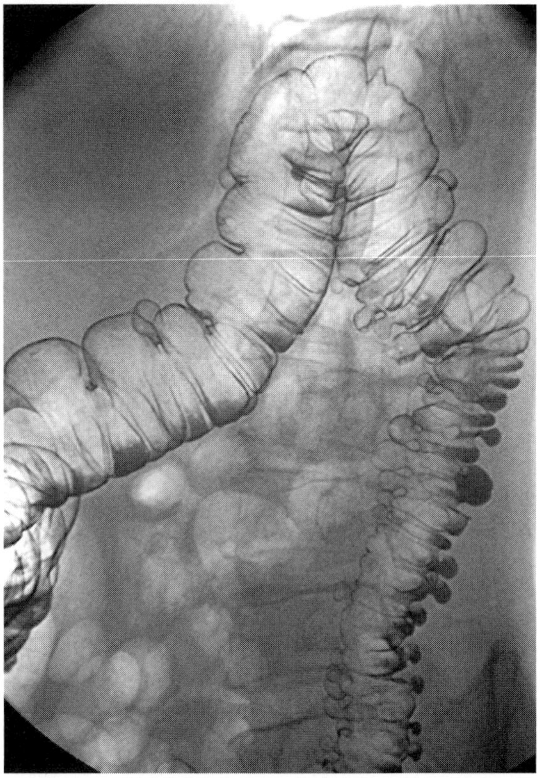

Figure 18–3. Double contrast barium enema of the colon. Note how the diverticula protrude beyond the normal line of the colonic wall, some filled with air (*white*) and others with barium (*black*).

COMPLICATIONS

Fistula

An inflamed segment of sigmoid colon can adhere to a number of intra-abdominal structures or to the abdominal wall. A fistula may arise spontaneously as a result of the inflammatory condition itself or as a result of surgical intervention. Diverticular fistulas can drain either internally or externally.

Colocutaneous. Occasionally a paracolic diverticular abscess will discharge spontaneously through the abdominal wall causing a colocutaneous fistula. More often a fistula will result from incision and drainage of a pointing paracolic abscess or from a drain placed under radiological control. A fistula can arise from a leaking colonic anastomosis in patients who have undergone resection for diverticular disease.

Colovesical. This is the most common fistula associated with diverticular disease. It is more common in males because in females the uterus is interposed between the bladder and the colon. A relatively mobile sigmoid colon becomes adherent to the dome of the bladder and a communication develops. Patients present with recurrent urinary sepsis, urgency, frequency, and pneumaturia. Cystoscopy sometimes identifies an area of inflamed transitional epithelium but is more useful to exclude bladder cancer. A double contrast enema provides a useful map of the anatomy and in some cases can confirm the presence of a fistula. Caution should be exercised when using barium in an acute situation to avoid peritoneal contamination (Figs 18–4A and 18–4B).

Coloenteric. Small bowel can become adherent to an inflamed diverticulum-affected colon. Fistulas form when an abscess discharges through the small bowel wall. This may be asymptomatic.

Colovaginal. This is a particularly debilitating fistula. The patient may pass flatus and feces through the vagina and suffer recurrent vaginal infections. Colovaginal fistulas are more likely to occur if a hysterectomy has been performed. Barium studies of both the bowel and the vagina can confirm the diagnosis; an examination of the vagina is mandatory to exclude a gynecological malignancy.

Single-stage operative resection with primary anastomosis and repair of the contiguous organ can be performed in most circumstances.[37] Interposition of the pediclized greater omentum between the anastomosis and the site of the fistula is a useful adjunct in preventing recurrent fistula formation.

Bleeding

Severe hemorrhage from diverticular disease is rare (5%).[38,39] However, distinguishing diverticular bleeding from other causes can be a diagnostic challenge, particularly because diverticular disease is so prevalent.[40,41] In elderly patients, angiodysplasia is the most common co-

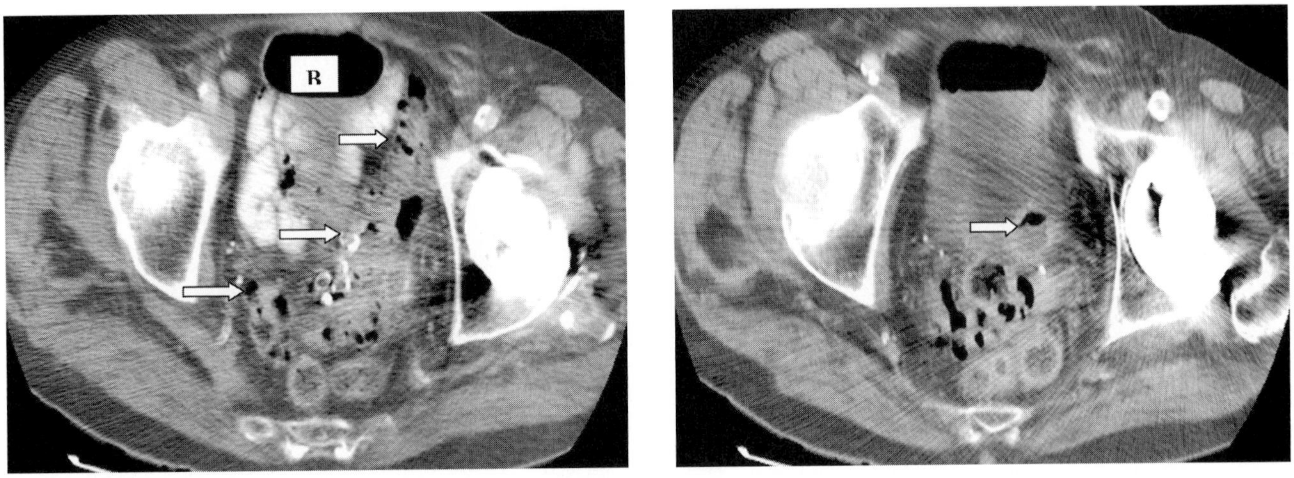

A B

Figure 18–4. Enhanced transverse CT scan through the pelvis. **A.** Arrows are pointing at several diverticula. Note also the fluid level in the bladder (**B**). (There is an artifact from a left total hip replacement.) The image shows a diverticular abscess adjacent to the bladder causing a colovesical fistula.

lonic cause for rectal bleeding. Taken together, bleeding from angiodysplasia and diverticuli accounts for 90% of cases of severe lower intestinal hemorrhage.

Diverticular hemorrhage presents with the passage of bright or dark red blood per rectum and may be associated with left iliac fossa pain. Most diverticular bleeding occurs from left-sided diverticuli except in patients of Asian ethnic origin, in whom it is more common to find the bleeding occurring on the right side.[42] Colonoscopy should be performed to confirm the diagnosis and exclude malignancy. Identifying the site of colonic bleeding can be difficult, as a combination of poor bowel preparation in the emergency setting and the retrograde passage of blood into the more proximal bowel can obscure endoscopic visualization. However, if a bleeding point is identified, then a variety of endoscopic treatment options are available.[43] In these circumstances a radiolabeled red blood cell scan can be invaluable in locating the source of the hemorrhage. Scintigraphy is noninvasive and sensitive to bleeding rates as low as 0.1 mL/min, but only gives information on the anatomic site of bleeding, not its cause.[44]

Most diverticular hemorrhage ceases spontaneously (70–80%) with rebleeding rates of 22–38%.[38,39,45] For those patients who have recurrent or severe hemorrhage, mesenteric angiography is advisable. Angiography has sensitivity for lower gastrointestinal hemorrhage at a rate of 0.5 mL/min.[46] Visualization should include both the superior and inferior mesenteric arteries (Figs 18–5A and 18–5B). This allows surgery to be tailored so that half the colon may be resected rather than doing a blind subtotal colectomy. If a bleeding point is not demonstrated then an intraoperative colonoscopic examination can be a useful adjunct when the abdomen is open and the operating surgeon can guide the colonoscope to the cecum. In patients who are unfit for surgery, embolization of bleeding colonic lesions can be performed. In experienced hands, this is a highly effective method of hemorrhage control; however, the risk of colonic wall infarction cannot be discounted.[47]

Obstruction

Diverticular disease causes colonic obstruction through either luminal stenosis or extrinsic compression from an abscess (Fig 18–6). Small bowel obstruction can occur if a loop of small bowel becomes adherent to the inflamed sigmoid colon. The diagnosis is usually apparent from the patient's history. Radiological confirmation either by contrast enema or by CT with oral/rectal contrast should be obtained. Direct visualization and histological exclusion of malignancy is mandatory.

Management of colonic obstruction in this setting depends on the mode of presentation and the medical fitness of the patient. An insidious onset is characterized by pain, increasing constipation, and the passage of ribbon-like stools. However, the majority of patients will present acutely with a classic large bowel obstruction. The surgical options include a Hartmann's resection and resection with primary anastomosis or rarely with a diverting loop ostomy. In those patients deemed unfit for surgery, the endoscopic or fluoroscopic deployment of a colon stent is a useful alternative procedure with a high clinical success rate.[48]

Abscess

Abscess formation is the most common complication of acute diverticulitis. It occurs when the center of the

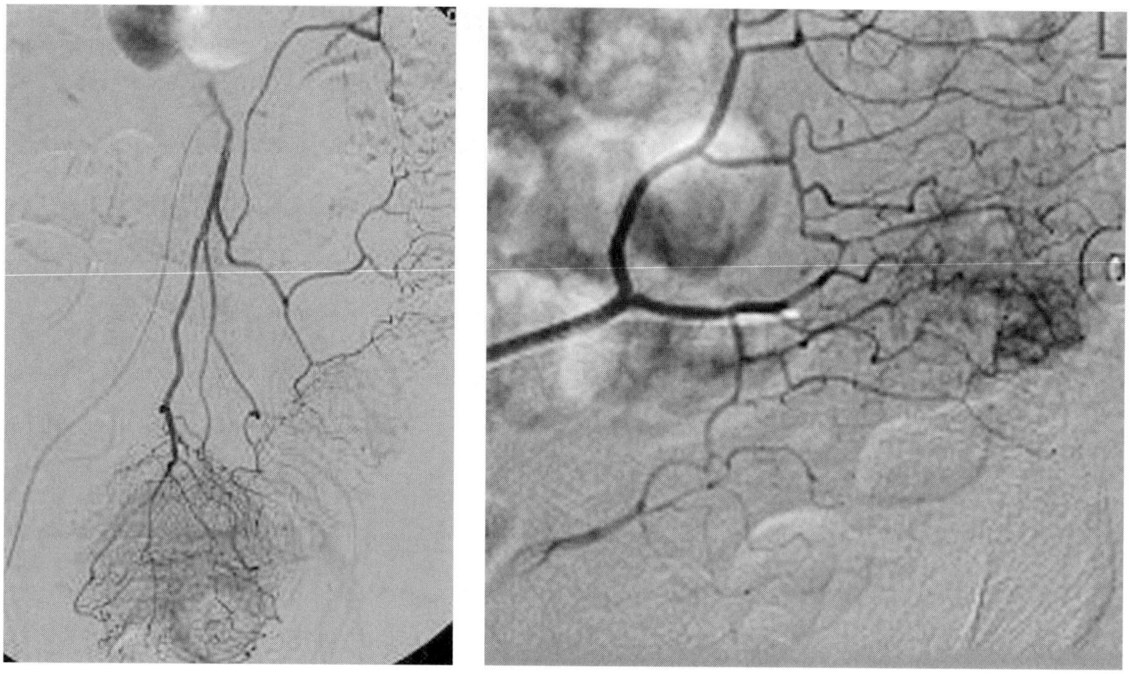

A B

Figure 18–5. A, B. Mesenteric angiogram demonstrating the inferior mesenteric artery with bleeding into the sigmoid colon.

inflammatory mass or phlegmon becomes necrotic (Fig 18–7). The patient presents with worsening abdominal pain, undulating fever, a leukocytosis, and raised inflammatory markers. A mass is often palpable in the left iliac fossa and may also be felt during vaginal or rectal examination. The most common site for a diverticular abscess is in the sigmoid mesocolon, although a variety of unusual presentations have been described.[49] A significant number of abscesses are detected radiologically on CT or ultrasound scanning. Most small (<5 cm) pericolic abscesses can be treated medically with bowel rest and antibiotics.[50] CT- or ultrasound-guided drainage is indicated for larger or unresolving abscesses. Drainage may eliminate the need for a two-stage procedure with interval colostomy, instead allowing temporary abscess decompression and subsequent observational management or single-stage resection.[51,52]

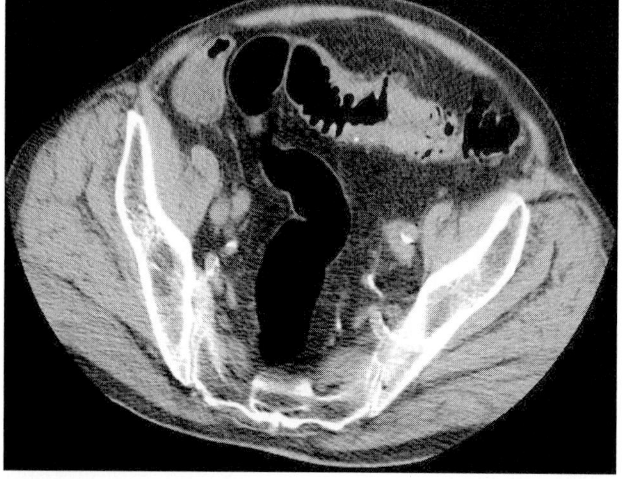

Figure 18–6. Computed tomography pneumocolon image of sigmoid diverticular disease with a thickened and stenotic colon wall.

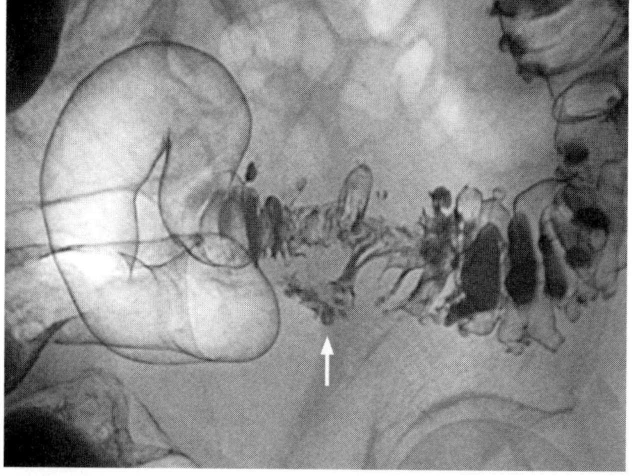

Figure 18–7. Double contrast barium enema of the sigmoid colon demonstrating diverticular disease and contrast flowing into a contained abscess cavity (*arrow*).

Giant Colonic Diverticulum

Giant colonic diverticulum (GCD) was first described in 1946 by Bonvin and Bonte[53] in the French literature. The first radiological description was by Hughes and Greene[54] in the American literature in 1953. Various names have been used to describe GCD including solitary air cyst, giant air cyst, giant gas cyst, encysted pneumatocele, colonic pneumocyst, and giant diverticulum. The variety of names highlights the fact that there has been no clear definition or a single accepted name for these poorly defined lesions which present as large gas filled cysts attached to the colon (diverticulum). GCD are rare clinical entities with just over 100 cases reported. The age at presentation is comparable to that of patients with conventional diverticular disease. Abdominal pain is the most common symptom, affecting 70% of patients, while 10% are asymptomatic. The most common physical finding is an abdominal mass, affecting 60% of patients, while 4% have normal physical examinations. Plain abdominal radiology is usually diagnostic of GCD. Treatment is recommended early, preferably soon after presentation, because of the high complication rate. Surgical treatment may either require a diverticulectomy or segmental resection and the outcome is usually good.[55]

Cancer

There is little evidence to support an association of diverticular disease and colorectal cancer; however, recently a population-based, case-control study from Sweden identified a causal association between sigmoid diverticulitis and a long-term increased risk of left-sided colon cancer.[56]

■ INVESTIGATIONS

The spiral CT scan has changed the investigation of acute diverticular disease (Fig 18–8). Although it is debatable whether CT alters disease management in minor diverticular disease, it is invaluable in excluding other causes of abdominal pain and documenting the extent of extraluminal disease. In circumstances in which access to CT is limited, a water-soluble contrast study may show mucosal thickening, edema, irregularity, and occasional extravasation of contrast. Sensitivity is high.[57] Any free perforation is usually contained in an abscess cavity. Contrast enemas are particularly useful for demonstrating the presence and course of an enteric fistula. Barium should be avoided in the emergency setting, as the consequences of barium-induced peritonitis are catastrophic.

The real advantage that CT scanning affords, in addition to confirmation of the diagnosis, is to direct the treatment of complicated diverticular disease.[58–60] Radiologically-guided drainage of diverticular abscesses is a useful adjunct to medical management, and can, if successful, avoid the requirement for emergency surgery.

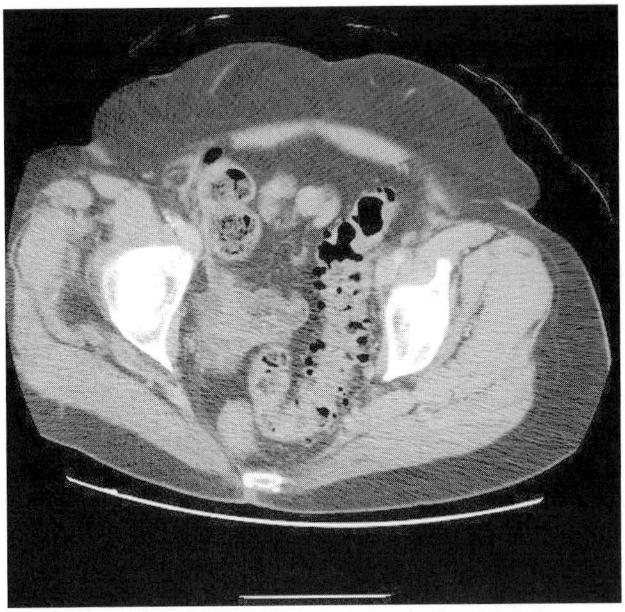

Figure 18–8. Computed tomography image of a diverticular loop of sigmoid colon.

The role of ultrasound scanning in patients suspected of having diverticular disease has been confined to the treatment and follow-up of diverticular abscess. It is highly operator-dependent, but it can be used to insert drains and to measure the response of the abscess to drainage.

■ CLASSIFICATION OF DIVERTICULITIS

The Hinchey classification is a useful grading system for diverticulitis.[61]

Stage I	Diverticulitis with associated pericolic abscess
Stage II	Diverticulitis associated with distant abscess (retroperitoneal or pelvic)
Stage III	Diverticulitis associated with purulent peritonitis
Stage IV	Diverticulitis associated with fecal peritonitis

Its usefulness is related to the direction the classification gives for initial treatment; with stages I and II being suitably managed with drainage and antibiotics and stages III and IV usually requiring surgery.

■ MANAGEMENT

The majority of patients with acute diverticular disease can be managed conservatively. In the absence of complications, most patients will respond to a targeted course of antimicrobial therapy. The decision to operate should be made at a senior level, as the actual number of patients who require resectional surgery for diverticular disease is small.[62] The increasing use of interventional radiology and laparoscopic surgery has impacted on how diverticular disease is currently managed. This is coupled with a drive to perform resectional surgery with a primary anastomosis in patients presenting with acute complicated diverticulitis.

ELECTIVE SURGERY

Surgery in this setting should be reserved for patients who are medically fit with several proven attacks of acute diverticulitis or who have ongoing sequelae from complicated diverticular disease. Even then, caution should be exercised, as a significant minority of patients whose principal symptom is chronic pain will continue to be symptomatic after resectional surgery.[63] This possibility should be explained to patients during their preoperative work-up.

Elective resection has generally been offered to patients who have suffered two attacks of acute diverticulitis in a short period of time. However, there is a lack of good prospective data comparing surgical intervention with conservative management in this situation. Risk-reducing measures in elective surgery include weight control, routine administration of prophylactic preoperative antibiotics, and preoperative optimization of the respiratory status of the patient with chronic pulmonary disease.[64] Attempts have been made to stratify the management of diverticular disease by pathological and radiological means.[65,66] Patients characterized as having a mild attack of diverticulitis had a 14% risk of having a recurrent episode, whereas severe forms had a risk of 39%. Ultimately the wide spectrum of disease encountered makes dogmatic statements about intervention unreliable and sound clinical judgement is still required to decide when to intervene.

Indications for operative intervention are different in two patient subgroups: those under the age of 40 years and the immunocompromised. Data on young patients with diverticular disease are mainly retrospective. The prevalence of colonic diverticula has been estimated at between 6% and 9% in the general population 40 years of age or younger,[67,68] with a male preponderance (62–100%).[68–71] Patients in this age group are thought to have a more malignant course and an aggressive policy of surgical resection has been proposed.[72] Between 29% and 55% of younger patients will be readmitted to the hospital with acute diverticulitis following their initial presentation, with the majority of these subsequently undergoing elective or emergency surgery.[73–75] However, it is unclear whether there is an advantage to operating after the initial acute attack. If such a policy is to be pursued, it will inevitably mean that a number of patients who do not require surgery will undergo colonic resection.

It is uncertain whether patients who are chronically immune-suppressed are more at risk of developing diverticular disease. It is thought that patients who have long-term uremia have a higher incidence of diverticulosis, possibly due to chronic constipation and generalized tissue weakness. Patients with polycystic kidney disease have a very high incidence of colonic diverticular disease.[76] Several groups have reported that immunocompromised patients with acute diverticulitis have a more complicated course compared to nonimmunosuppressed patients.[77–79] Patients who are recipients of renal transplants have a high mortality rate from acute complicated diverticular disease. In some centers routine colonic screening of patients awaiting renal allografts is performed.[80]

There is limited evidence that the cessation of smoking and stopping nonsteroidal anti-inflammatory drugs will reduce the rate of recurrent attacks of diverticulitis, as will the long-term administration of a poorly absorbed antibiotic.[81–85]

EMERGENT ACUTE DIVERTICULITIS WITH LOCALIZED PERITONITIS

Patients with acute diverticulitis present with localized left iliac fossa peritonitis, fever, tachycardia, and a leukocytosis. Tenderness can spread to the hypogastrium and even to the right iliac fossa. Generalized peritonitis is highly suspicious for a free diverticular perforation. Patients should be rehydrated with an intravenous infusion; in septic patients a urinary catheter is invaluable for assessing an adequate hourly urine output. Other supportive measures including oxygen therapy, adequate opioid analgesia, and antimicrobial therapy should be instituted.

Early oral feeding may commence when tolerated and a switch to oral antibiotics can be made with signs of resolution of inflammation. In the majority of patients, this conservative therapy will lead to the resolution of symptoms. On discharge from hospital, the patient should have their large bowel visualized with a double-contrast barium enema or colonoscopy to rule out a colonic malignancy.

EMERGENT ACUTE DIVERTICULITIS WITH GENERALIZED PERITONITIS

When either an abscess or a diverticulum ruptures into the peritoneal cavity, widespread bacterial contamination ensues with resultant generalized peritonitis. Surgery is principally directed at controlling peritoneal sepsis and should be tailored to each situation. A conservative approach can be taken with elderly and medically unfit patients who are unlikely to survive surgical intervention. The combined use of appropriate antibiotic therapy and regular review is surprisingly successful in this cohort, even in the presence of a pneumoperitoneum.

In patients who are fit for surgery, a period of vigorous resuscitation and antibiotic therapy is still warranted. Even in the face of advanced peritoneal signs a number of patients will respond to these measures and avoid the requirement for surgery. Serial clinical observation is of greatest benefit when pursuing this course. If there is no sustained improvement in 24 hours, then the patient should be offered surgery.

There is little place for nonresectional surgery in the emergent situation. The aim of surgery is clear: to remove the source of sepsis and to toilet the abdominal cavity. Resection of the affected colon is associated with a lower morbidity and mortality compared with nonresection procedures, which rely on drainage and proximal colostomy.[86] Occasionally, during diagnostic laparoscopy for the assessment of the acute abdomen, an inflamed segment of sigmoid colon is visualized. If there is no evidence of perforation and minimal peritoneal contamination, it is reasonable to thoroughly lavage the abdominal cavity and adopt a nonresectional approach relying on systemic antibiotics. This avoids unnecessary resectional surgery and its associated morbidity and mortality, as well as stoma formation. The need for a second laparotomy for reanastomosis is similarly avoided.[87]

The amount of resected tissue depends on the extent of the diverticular disease. At the time of the initial acute surgery, the inflamed bowel needs to be resected. The extent of this resection depends on whether a primary anastomosis is being undertaken or a Hartmann's procedure is being performed. When bowel continuity is restored after a Hartmann's procedure, all visible left-sided colonic diverticula should be removed; this will usually require a left hemicolectomy with mobilization of the splenic flexure. The anastomosis should be to the upper rectum, not the distal sigmoid colon.

The decision of whether to undertake an anastomosis in the acute setting is dependent on a number of criteria: the frailty of the patient, the degree of contamination and sepsis, the preparedness of the bowel, and the experience of the surgeon. Hartmann's procedure entails resection of the sigmoid colon with formation of end colostomy and is the safest option when conditions do not favor primary anastomosis. However, this form of surgery is not without its own complications. A considerable minority of patients will never have their stoma closed.[88] There is definite morbidity and mortality related to restoration of continuity, and occasionally there are complications related to rectal stump dehiscence.[89]

Primary anastomosis can be performed in the emergency setting but only if conditions are wholly favorable.[90–91] Performing anastomoses in the presence of gross purulent or fecal contamination is controversial and should only be performed by experienced hands. The requirement for bowel preparation for left-sided anastomosis is equally controversial, but a recent study has cast doubt on the need for bowel preparation.[92]

LAPAROSCOPIC SURGERY FOR DIVERTICULAR DISEASE

The widespread acceptance of laparoscopic surgery has led to its use in both benign and malignant colorectal disease. Laparoscopic colonic resection of diverticular disease is challenging and is being increasingly utilized by specialist centers with good results.[93] Published studies comparing laparoscopic and open resection of left-sided colonic diverticular disease have demonstrated benefits in terms of shorter hospital stay and convalescence.[94,95] However, publication bias is likely to promote laparoscopic resection more favorably, and the true morbidity, cost, and conversion rates may differ from figures published in the medical literature. In over 1100 patients reported over the last 5 years, the postoperative complication rates range from 7.3–21%. Conversion rates range between 4% and 14%, operating time from 141 to 300 minutes, and return of bowel activity takes between 2 and 2.9 days.[94] A recent analysis of the cost of laparoscopic surgery compared with open surgery demonstrated that the total cost of the laparoscopic approach was significantly less ($3458 versus $4321; $p<0.05$).[84] Clearly this may have economic ramifications for the future.

▪ SUMMARY

The prevalence of diverticular disease has increased and is continuing to do so in Western countries. The management of diverticular disease is becoming an increasing financial burden to health systems with limited resources. There is little evidence that a change in lifestyle measures can reduce the prevalence of diverticular disease. Fortunately colonic diverticula are usually asymptomatic.

The acute management of diverticulitis is usually conservative with antibiotics and bowel rest, with few patients needing emergency operations. Abscesses can be adequately treated with percutaneous drainage. When an operation is required the quality of the surgery appears to be more important than whether the operation is undertaken open or laparoscopically. In the acute setting the affected segment of colon should be resected. Following resection the distal anastomosis should be to the rectum, not the sigmoid colon. The place of elective resection is uncertain. There is support for the concept of elective operation after two attacks in patients who are otherwise well; however, to date the data to support such management is inadequate. The wide spectrum of disease encountered makes dogmatic statements about intervention unreliable and sound clinical judgement is still required to decide when to intervene.

REFERENCES

1. Hughes LE. Postmortem survey of diverticular disease of the colon. Diverticulosis and diverticulitis. *Gut* 1969; 10:336–344
2. American Gastroenterological Association. *The Burden of Gastrointestinal Diseases.* Bethesda, MD: American Gastroenterological Association; 2001
3. Papagrigoriadis S, Debrah S, Koreli A et al. Impact of diverticular disease on hospital costs and activity. *Colorectal Dis* 2004;6:81–84
4. Kyle J, Davidson AI. The changing pattern of hospital admissions for diverticular disease of the colon. *Br J Surg* 1975;62:537–541
5. Kang JY, Hoare J, Tinto A et al. Diverticular disease of the colon on the rise: a study of hospital admissions in England between 1989/1990 and 1999/2000. *Aliment Pharmacol Ther* 2003;17:1189–1195
6. Parks TG. Natural history of diverticular disease of the colon. *Clin Gastroenterol* 1975;4:53–69
7. Littre A. 1700. Cited by: Finney JM. Diverticulitis and its surgical management. *Proc Interstate Post-Grad Med Assembly North Am* 1928;55:57–65
8. Cruveilhier J. *Traite d'Anatomie Pathologique Generale,* Vol. 1. Paris: Bailliere; 1849
9. Graser E. Das falsche Darmdivertikel. *Arch Klin Chir* 1899;59:638–647
10. Beer E. Some pathological and clinical aspects of acquired (false) diverticula of the intestine. *Am J Med Sci* 1904;128:135–145
11. Moynihan BFA. The mimicry of malignant disease in the large intestine. *Edinb Med J* 1907;21:228
12. Telling WH, Gruner OC. Acquired diverticula, diverticulitis, and peridiverticulitis of the large intestine. *Br J Surg* 1917;4:468–530
13. Spriggs EI, Marxer OA. Multiple diverticula of the colon. *Lancet* 1927;1:1067
14. De Quervain F. Zur diagnose der erworbenen dickdarmdivertikel und der sigmoiditis diverticularis. *Dtsch Z Chir* 1914;128:67
15. Case JT. The roentgen demonstration of multiple diverticula of the colon. *Am J Roentgenol* 1914;2:654
16. Case JT. The roentgen study of colonic diverticula. *Am J Roentgenol* 1929;21:207
17. Whiteway J, Morson BC. Elastosis in diverticular disease of the sigmoid colon. *Gut* 1985;26:258–266
18. Wess L, Eastwood MA, Wess TJ et al. Cross linkage of collagen is increased in colonic diverticulosis. *Gut* 1995; 37:91–94
19. Aldoori WH, Giovannucci EL, Rimm EB et al. Prospective study of physical activity and the risk of symptomatic diverticular disease in men. *Gut* 1995;36:276–282
20. Bassotti G, Germani U, Morelli A. Human colonic motility: physiological aspects. *Int J Colorectal Dis* 1995;10:173–180
21. Parks TG, Connell AM. Motility studies in diverticular disease of the colon. *Gut* 1969;10:534–542
22. Simpson J, Scholefield JH, Spiller RC. Pathogenesis of colonic diverticula. *Br J Surg* 2002;89:546–554
23. Huizinga JD, Waterfall WE, Stern HS. Abnormal response to cholinergic stimulation in the circular muscle layer of the human colon in diverticular disease. *Scand J Gastroenterol* 1999;34:683–688
24. Katschinski M, Lederer P, Ellermann A et al. Myoelectric and manometric patterns of human rectosigmoid colon in irritable bowel syndrome and diverticulosis. *Scand J Gastroenterol* 1990;25:761–768
25. Taylor I, Duthie HL, Smallwood R. Proceedings of the Fourth International Symposium on Gastrointestinal Motility. Vancouver, BC, Canada: Mitchell Press; 1974
26. Parks TG. Rectal and colonic studies after resection of the sigmoid for diverticular disease. *Gut* 1970;11:121–125
27. Painter NS, Burkitt DP. Diverticular disease of the colon: a deficiency disease of Western civilisation. *BMJ* 1971;2:450–454
28. Kyle J, Adesola A, Tinckler L et al. Incidence of diverticulitis. *Scand J Gastroenterol* 1967;2:77–80
29. Lee YS. Diverticular disease of the large bowel in Singapore: an autopsy survey. *Dis Colon Rectum* 1986;29: 330–335
30. Walker AR, Segal I. Epidemiology of noninfective intestinal disease in various ethnic groups in South Africa. *Isr J Med Sci* 1979;15:309–313
31. Ogunbiyi OA. Diverticular disease of the colon in Ibadan, Nigeria. *Afr J Med Sci* 1989;18:241–244
32. Makela J, Kiviniemi H, Laitinen S. Prevalence of perforated sigmoid diverticulitis is increasing. *Dis Colon Rectum* 2002;45:955–961
33. Wong SK, Ho YH, Leong AP, Seow-Choen F. Clinical behavior of complicated right-sided and left-sided diverticulosis. *Dis Colon Rectum* 1997;40:344–348
34. Whiteway J, Morson BC. Elastosis in diverticular disease of the sigmoid colon. *Gut* 1985;26:258–266
35. Leung DYM, Glagov S, Mathews MB. Cyclic stretching stimulates synthesis of matrix components of arterial smooth muscle cells in vivo. *Science* 1976;191:475–477
36. Stumpf M, Cao W, Klinge U et al. Increased distribution of collagen type III and reduced expression of matrix metalloproteinase 1 in patients with diverticular disease. *Int J Colorectal Dis* 2001;16:271–275

37. Stefansson T, Ekbom A, Sparen P et al. Association between sigmoid diverticulitis and left-sided colon cancer; a nested, population-based, case control study. *Scand J Gastroenterol* 2004;39:743–747
38. McGuire HH Jr, Haynes BW Jr. Massive hemorrhage of diverticulosis of the colon: guidelines for therapy based on bleeding patterns observed in fifty cases. *Ann Surg* 1972;175:847–855
39. Zuckerman GR, Prakash C. Acute lower intestinal bleeding: part II—etiology, therapy, and outcomes. *Gastrointest Endosc* 1999;49:228–238
40. Peura DA, Lanza FL, Gostout CJ et al. The American College of Gastroenterology bleeding registry: preliminary findings. *Am J Gastroenterol* 1997;92:924–928
41. Longstreth GF. Epidemiology and outcome of patients hospitalized with acute lower gastrointestinal hemorrhage: a population-based study. *Am J Gastroenterol* 1997; 92:419–424
42. Wong SK, Ho YH, Leong AP et al. Clinical behavior of complicated right sided and left sided diverticulosis. *Dis Colon Rectum* 1997;40:344–348
43. Alavi A, Ring EJ. Localization of gastrointestinal bleeding: superiority of 99mTc sulfur colloid compared with angiography. *Am J Roentgenol* 1981;137:741–748
44. McGuire HH Jr. Bleeding colonic diverticula: a reappraisal of natural history and management. *Ann Surg* 1994;220:653–656
45. Potter GD, Sellin JH. Lower gastrointestinal bleeding. *Gastroenterol Clin North Am* 1988;17:341–356
46. Jensen DM, Machicado GA, Jutabha R et al. Urgent colonoscopy for the diagnosis and treatment of severe diverticular hemorrhage. *N Engl J Med* 2000;342:78–82
47. Gordon RL, Ahl KL, Kerlan RK et al. Selective arterial embolization for the control of lower gastrointestinal bleeding. *Am J Surg* 1997;174:24–28
48. Watson AJM, Shanmugam V, Mackay I et al. Outcomes after placement of colorectal stents. *Colorectal Dis* 2005; 7:70–73
49. Ravo B, Khan SA, Ger R et al. Unusual extraperitoneal presentations of diverticulitis. *Am J Gastroenterol* 1985;80: 346–351
50. Wong WD, Wexner SD, Lowry A et al. Practice parameters for the treatment of sigmoid diverticulitis: supporting documentation. *Dis Colon Rectum* 2000;43:290–297
51. Schechter S, Eisenstat TE, Oliver GC et al. Computerised tomographic scan-guided drainage of intra-abdominal abscesses: preoperative and postoperative modalities in colon and rectal surgery. *Dis Colon Rectum* 1994; 37:984–988
52. Stabile BE, Puccio E, van Sonnenberg E et al. Preoperative percutaneous drainage of diverticular abscesses. *Dis Colon Rectum* 1988;31:591–596
53. Bonvin P, Bonte G. Diverticules geants du sigmoide. *Arch Mal Appar Dig Mal Nutr* 1946;35:353
54. Hughes WL, Greene RC. Solitary air cyst of peritoneal cavity. *Arch Surg* 1953;67:931–936
55. Choong CK, Frizelle FA. Giant colonic diverticulum: report of four cases and review of the literature. *Dis Colon Rectum* 1998;41:1178–1185; discussion 1185–1186
56. Stefansson T, Ekbom A, Sparen P et al. Association between sigmoid diverticulitis and left-sided colon cancer; a nested, population-based, case control study. *Scand J Gastroenterol* 2004;39:743–747
57. Smith TR, Cho KC, Morehouse HT et al. Comparison of computed tomography and contrast enema evaluation of diverticulitis. *Dis Colon Rectum* 1990;33:1–6
58. Eggesbo HB, Jacobsen T, Kolmannskog F et al. Diagnosis of acute left sided colonic diverticulitis by three radiological modalities. *Acta Radiol* 1998;39:315–321
59. Brengman ML, Otchy DP. Timing of computed tomography in acute diverticulitis. *Dis Colon Rectum* 1998;41: 1023–1028
60. Poletti PA, Platon A, Rutschmann O et al. Acute left colonic diverticulitis: can CT findings be used to predict recurrence? *Am J Roentgenol* 2004;182:1159–1165
61. Hinchey EJ, Schaal PG, Richards GK. Treatment of perforated diverticular disease. *Adv Surg* 1978;12:85–109
62. Tudor RG, Farmakis N, Keighley MRB. National audit of complicated diverticular disease: analysis of index cases. *Br J Surg* 1994;81:733–735
63. Munson KD, Hensien MA, Jacob LN et al. Diverticulitis: a comprehensive follow up. *Dis Colon Rectum* 1996;39: 318–322
64. Pessaux P, Muscari F, Ouellet JF et al. Risk factors for mortality and morbidity after elective sigmoid resection for diverticulitis: prospective multicenter multivariate analysis of 582 patients. *World J Surg* 2004;28: 92–96
65. Killingback M, Barron PE, Dent OF. Elective surgery for diverticular disease: an audit of surgical pathology and treatment. *ANZ J Surg* 2004;74:530–536
66. Ambrosetti P, Becker C, Terrier F. Colonic diverticulitis: impact on imaging on surgical management—a prospective study of 542 patients. *Eur Radiol* 2002;12:1145–1149
67. Acosta JA, Grebenc ML, Doberneck RC et al. Colonic diverticular disease I patients 40 years old or younger. *Am Surg* 1992;58:605–607
68. Freischlag J, Bennion RS, Thompson JE. Complications of diverticular disease of the colon in young people. *Dis Colon Rectum* 1986;29:639–643
69. Schauer PR, Ramos R, Ghiatas AA et al. Virulent diverticular disease in young obese men. *Am J Surg* 1992;164: 443–448
70. Marinella MA, Mustafa M. Acute diverticulitis in patients 40 years of age and younger. *Am J Emerg Med* 2000; 18:140–142
71. Ouriel K, Schwartz SI. Diverticular disease in the young patient. *Surg Gynecol Obstet* 1983;156:1–5
72. Simonwitz D, Paloyan D. Diverticular disease of the colon in patients under 40 years of age. *Am J Gastroenterol* 1977;67:69–72
73. Chodak GW, Rangel DM, Passaro E. Colonic diverticulosis in patients under 40: need for earlier diagnosis. *Am J Surg* 1981;141:699–702
74. Ambrosetti P, Robert JH, Witzig JA et al. Acute left colonic diverticulitis in young patients. *J Am Coll Surg* 1994; 179:156–160

75. Tudor RG, Farmakis N, Keighley MRB. National audit of complicated diverticular disease: analysis of index cases. *Br J Surg* 1994;81:733–735
76. Scheff RT, Zuckerman GM, Harter H et al. Diverticular disease in patients with chronic renal failure due to polycystic kidney disease. *Ann Intern Med* 1980;92:202–204
77. Church JM, Fazio VW, Braun WE et al. Perforation of the colon in renal homograft recipients. A report of cases and a review of the literature. *Ann Surg* 1986;203:69–76
78. Myers WC, Harris N, Stein S et al. Alimentary tract complications after renal transplantation. *Ann Surg* 1979; 190:535–542
79. Sawyer OI, Garvin PJ, Codd JE et al. Colorectal complications of renal allograft transplantation. *Arch Surg* 1978;113:84–86
80. McCune TR, Nylander WA, Van Buren DH et al. Colonic screening prior to renal transplantation and its impact on post-transplant colonic complications. *Clin Transplant* 1992;6:91–96
81. Campbell KC, Steele RJ. Non-steroidal anti-inflammatory drugs and complicated diverticular disease: a case control study. *Br J Surg* 1991;78:190–191
82. Papi C, Ciaco A, Koch M, Capurso L. Efficacy of rifaximin in the treatment of symptomatic diverticular disease of the colon. A multicentre double-blind placebo controlled trial. *Aliment Pharmacol Ther* 1995;9:33–39
83. Papagrigoriadis S, Macey L, Bourantas N et al. Smoking may be associated with complications in diverticular disease. *Br J Surg* 1999;86:923–926
84. Latella G, Pimpo MT, Sottili S et al. Rifaximin improves symptoms of acquired uncomplicated diverticular disease of the colon. *Int J Colorectal Dis* 2003;18:55–62
85. Morris CR, Harvey IM, Stebbings WSL et al. Anti-inflammatory drugs, analgesics and the risk of perforated colonic diverticular disease. *Br J Surg* 2003;90:1267–1272
86. Krukowski ZH, Matheson NA. Emergency surgery for diverticular disease complicated by generalised and faecal peritonitis. *Br Med J* 1985;290:1490–1492
87. Krukowski ZH. In: Phillips, Robin KS (eds). *Diverticular Disease in Colorectal Disease: A Companion to Specialist Surgical Practice.* London, England: WB Saunders; 2001
88. Wigmore SJ, Duthie IE, Young EM et al. Restoration of intestinal continuity following Hartmann's procedure: the Lothian experience 1987–1992. *Br J Surg* 1995;82: 27–30
89. Khoury DA, Beck DE, Opelka FG et al. Colostomy closure. *Dis Colon Rectum* 1996;39:605–609
90. Biondo S, Perea MT, Rague JM et al. One-stage procedure in non-elective surgery for diverticular disease complications. *Colorectal Dis* 2001;3:42–45
91. Gooszen AW, Tollenaar RAE, Geelkerken RH et al. Prospective study of primary anastomosis following sigmoid resection for suspected acute complicated diverticular disease. *Br J Surg* 2001;88:693–697
92. Slim K, Vicaut E, Panis Y et al. Meta-analysis of randomised clinical trials of colorectal surgery with or without mechanical bowel preparation. *Br J Surg* 2004;91: 1125–1130
93. Gonzalez R, Smith CD, Mattar SG et al. Laparoscopic vs open resection for the treatment of diverticular disease. *Surg Endosc* 2004;18:276–280
94. Senagore AJ, Duepree HJ, Delaney CP et al. Cost structure of laparoscopic and open sigmoid colectomy for diverticular disease. Similarities and differences. *Dis Colon Rectum* 2002;45:485–490
95. Schwander O, Farke S, Fischer F et al. Laparoscopic colectomy for recurrent and complicated diverticulitis: a prospective study of 396 patients. *Langenbecks Arch Surg* 2004;389:97–103

19

Crohn's Disease

Fabrizio Michelassi ■ *Roger D. Hurst* ■ *Alessandro Fichera*

Crohn's disease is a chronic inflammatory condition of the gastrointestinal tract that can give rise to strictures, inflammatory masses, fistulas, abscesses, hemorrhage, and cancer. This disease commonly affects the small bowel, colon, rectum, or anus. Less commonly, it can also involve the stomach, esophagus, and mouth. Often the disease will simultaneously affect multiple areas of the gastrointestinal tract.

The cause of Crohn's disease is not known and there is no curative treatment. Current medical and surgical treatment is effective at controlling the disease but even with optimal treatment, recurrences and relapses are frequent. The combined approach of optimal medical treatment with timely and strategic surgical intervention offers the most effective management to patients affected by Crohn's disease. Crohn's disease, however, can be particularly challenging, as the disease has a myriad of manifestations and potential complications. Additionally, the course of the disease and its response to therapy can be difficult to predict. To add to the overall complexity, there are many therapeutic options that must be tailored to each individual patient and to each site of involvement to achieve optimal outcomes.

■ HISTORY

Crohn's disease was fully recognized as a specific pathological entity in 1932 when Crohn, Ginsberg, and Oppenheimer first identified regional enteritis as a unique clinical entity.[1] In retrospect, case descriptions of what appeared to be Crohn's disease date back to at least 1612, when Fabry reported on the death of a boy experiencing severe abdominal pain.[2] Autopsy revealed a contracted ulcerated cecum and ileum with complete bowel obstruction. In 1761, Morgagni described a case of an inflamed ileum with perforation and thickened mesentery in a young man with a history of diarrhea and fever.[3,4]

It is unclear how common Crohn's disease might have been prior to 1932, as it is likely that cases of Crohn's disease occurring in an era of limited abdominal surgery may have been mistaken for other processes such as tumor or intestinal tuberculosis. In 1913, Sir Kennedy Dalziel of Glasgow, Scotland, reported in the *British Medical Journal* on 13 patients and provided what is now recognized as a classical clinical and pathologic description of Crohn's disease.[5] Although not often cited, Dalziel's description predates the one by Crohn, Ginsberg, and Oppenheimer, and some have argued that the disease should be known by the eponym "Dalziel-Crohn's disease."

After the report by Crohn, Ginsberg, and Oppenheimer, increased awareness of the disease led to a marked increase in reported cases in the 1930s through the 1950s. The general public's awareness of the disease increased when in 1956, one of the most famous figures of the 20th century, President Dwight Eisenhower, was diagnosed with Crohn's disease at the terminal ileum. That same year, President Eisenhower underwent intestinal bypass surgery with the small intestine proximal to the area of disease anastomosed to the transverse colon.[6] Following this operation, he remained relatively free of symptoms for the remainder of his life.[7]

Early on in the surgical management of Crohn's disease, optimal surgical management remained disputed. Initially, many thought that the disease was one of both the bowel and the mesentery, and much like malignancies, wide excision with radical dissection of the mesentery was the best way to provide for the optimal long-term outcome.[8] It was also appreciated that diversion of the fecal stream was effective at decreasing active inflammation and ameliorating symptoms. Frequently performed in the 1940s and 1950s, bypass operations are now only rarely undertaken for Crohn's disease.[9–11] Additionally, a greater understanding of the clinical course of Crohn's disease has led to more conservative resections, as it is appreciated that wide surgical margins of normal tissue and radical resection of the mesentery are not necessary to avoid early recurrence of disease.

In spite of the increased attention given to Crohn's disease of the ileum, Crohn's colitis was not widely recognized as a form of Crohn's disease until 1960 when Lockhart-Mummery and Morson firmly established the pathologic criteria for distinguishing Crohn's disease from idiopathic ulcerative colitis.[12]

■ EPIDEMIOLOGY

After the original description of Crohn's disease in 1932, the number of reported cases increased greatly. Today it is estimated that the incidence of Crohn's disease in the United States is approximately four new cases per year for every 100,000 persons. The disease is chronic and patients live for many years with the ailment, thus the prevalence is much higher and is reported to be between 80 and 150 cases per 100,000.[13,14] The incidence of Crohn's disease increased rapidly from 1930 to at least the 1980s, but the incidence of new cases now appears to have stabilized.

The United States, Canada, and Europe have the highest incidence of Crohn's disease. It is much less common in Asia, South America, and Japan. Crohn's disease is believed to be uncommon in Africa, but accurate data regarding the incidence of inflammatory bowel disease in this region of the world are lacking. The peak age for contracting Crohn's disease is between 15 and 25. As such, Crohn's disease typically affects young adults, yet the disease can occur at almost any age. It should be noted, however, that Crohn's disease is very rare in children under the age of 6.[15]

In the U.S., the incidence of Crohn's disease is highest among Caucasians, low among blacks, and lowest among Hispanics and Asians. Crohn's disease is three to four times more common among ethnic Jews than non-Jewish whites. It also appears to be slightly more common in women than in men, although a slight male predominance has been reported in some populations.[16]

Familial clusters of disease are not uncommon, with a six- to tenfold increase in the risk of Crohn's disease in first-degree relatives of those affected by Crohn's disease or its sister ailment, ulcerative colitis. Although familial aggregations are common, the distribution within families does not indicate a pattern of simple mendelian inheritance.

■ ETIOLOGY

The etiology of Crohn's disease is not known. Many possible causes have been the subject of both speculation and investigation.[4] Basic science research into the molecular biology of Crohn's disease has begun to give some better insight into the genetics of this condition, but much regarding the ultimate causes of Crohn's disease remains unclear.

It is known that Crohn's disease is an altered immune response that results in inflammation and destruction of intestinal tissues. It is not clear if this altered immune response is the result of a primary dysfunction in the gut-related immune system or whether an unknown pathological trigger induces an otherwise normal immune system to overreact. Most believe that Crohn's disease occurs in individuals with a genetic predisposition and that development of the disease is dependent upon exposure to environmental triggers that start the pathological sequence that ultimately manifests as Crohn's disease.

To date, no specific primary defect in the systemic or mucosal immune system has been identified. Studies of intestinal transport mechanisms have demonstrated an increase in intestinal permeability in both Crohn's disease patients and their symptom-free first-degree relatives.[17–21] This has led some to speculate that Crohn's disease is the result of an altered mucosal barrier function that allows abnormal interactions to take place between the multitude of antigenic substrates normally found in the gut lumen and the immunocompetent tissue of the submucosa.

As indicated by the observed familial aggregations and variability of risks among differing ethnic and racial groups, a genetic predisposition is very likely to have a major role in the etiology of Crohn's disease. The distribution of Crohn's disease within family aggregates is complex and defies classification with simple mendelian transmission of disease. Genetic linkage studies have identified susceptibility to Crohn's to the *CARD15/NOD2* gene mapped to chromosome 16q12.[22,23] CARD15 is a gene product related to innate immunity and it is preferentially expressed to Paneth cells of the ileum.[24,25] While the *CARD15/NOD2* gene has been linked to susceptibility to Crohn's disease, the known mutations of CARD15 are neither necessary nor sufficient to contract the disease. Hence, it appears that the genetic relationship of *CARD15/NOD2* to Crohn's disease is complex and still poorly understood.

The suspicion that infectious agents may play a role, either directly as a primary cause of Crohn's disease, or indirectly as a trigger to stimulate a defective immune system, has generated much attention. This hypothesis has always found strength in the identification of non-caseating granulomas as the characteristic histopathologic lesion found in Crohn's specimens, and in the isolation of *Mycobacterium paratuberculosis* from resected Crohn's disease specimens. This finding has been far from consistent, and even sensitive preliminary chain reaction studies have been unable to provide definitive evidence for the presence of *Mycobacterium paratuberculosis*-specific DNA in Crohn's-affected segments of the bowel. Other infectious agents have been studied and have been shown not to be causative agents for Crohn's disease. These include measles virus, non-pylori *Helicobacter* species, *Pseudomonas*, and *Listeria monocytogenes*.[26] To date, no single infectious agent has been consistently associated with Crohn's disease.

Although diet modification can ameliorate the symptoms of Crohn's disease, no dietary factor has been identified as a cause of Crohn's disease. Smoking, however, has been associated with the development of Crohn's disease, with smokers having a substantially higher risk for contracting Crohn's disease than nonsmokers.[27–30] Additionally, smoking is known to exacerbate existing Crohn's disease and can accelerate the recurrence of disease after resection.[31,32] The component of cigarette smoke that is responsible for these deleterious effects on the clinical course of Crohn's disease is not known.

▪ PATHOLOGY

Histopathologic examination of Crohn's disease typically demonstrates transmural inflammation characterized by multiple lymphoid aggregates in a thickened submucosa. Lymphoid aggregates may extend beyond the mucosa and can be found within the muscularis propria.[33] The presence of well-formed lymphoid aggregates in an edematous fibrotic submucosa is a classic histological feature of the disease. Another sentinel microscopic feature of Crohn's disease is the presence of non-caseating granulomas. Non-caseating granulomas are a valuable diagnostic feature of Crohn's disease, but they are seen in only 50% of resected specimens and are rarely seen on endoscopic biopsies. Additionally the presence of granulomas does not correlate with disease activity, as areas of active inflammation are no more likely to contain granulomas than areas of quiescent disease.[34]

The earliest gross manifestations of Crohn's disease are the development of small mucosal ulcerations call aphthous ulcers.[33] Aphthous ulcers appear as red spots or focal mucosal depressions and they typically occur directly over submucosal lymphoid aggregates. As the inflammation progresses, the aphthous ulcers enlarge and become stellate. The enlarging ulcerations then coalesce to form longitudinal mucosal ulcerations. In Crohn's disease of the small bowel, these linear ulcerations always occur along the mesenteric aspect of the bowel lumen. Further progression leads to a serpiginous network of linear ulcerations that surround islands of edematous mucosa producing the classic "cobblestone" appearance. Mucosal ulcerations may penetrate through the submucosa to form intramural channels that can bore deeply into the bowel wall and create sinuses, abscesses, or fistulas.

The inflammation process progresses to extend through all layers of the bowel wall. The inflammation of Crohn's disease also involves the mesentery and regional lymph nodes such that the mesentery may become massively thickened. With early acute intestinal inflammation, the bowel wall is hyperemic and boggy. As the inflammation becomes chronic, fibrotic scarring develops and the bowel wall becomes thickened and leathery in texture.

▪ CLINICAL PRESENTATION OF CROHN'S DISEASE

The clinical presentation and symptoms of Crohn's disease vary greatly depending on the segment of intestine involved[35] and the predominant features of the disease: stricturing, perforating, or inflammatory. In the next few paragraphs the influence of disease pattern and location will be described.

PATTERNS OF DISEASE

Crohn's disease can be categorized into three general manifestations: stricturing disease, perforating disease, and inflammatory disease.[36] These three classes do not represent truly distinct forms of the disease; rather they are terms that are used to describe the predominant gross manifestation of the disease.[37] It is typical for more than one pattern to occur in the same patient or even the same segment of intestine; even so, one pattern tends to predominate in most cases. It is generally the predominant pattern of disease that determines the clinical presentation and affects the therapeutic options.

Stricturing Disease

Chronic inflammation of Crohn's disease results in the development of fibrotic scar tissue that constricts the intestinal lumen with cicatricial strictures often referred to as "fibrostenotic lesions." Patients with a stricturing pattern of disease generally develop partial or complete intestinal obstruction, and hence their symptoms are primarily obstructive in nature. Being the result of scar tissue, fibrostenotic strictures are not reversible with medical therapy. Once fibrostenotic areas become symptomatic, significant improvement rarely occurs and surgical intervention is often required.

Perforating Disease

Perforating Crohn's disease is characterized by the development of sinus tracts, fistulae, and abscesses. Penetrating sinus tracts develop from deep mucosal ulcerations. These sinus tracts penetrate through the muscularis propria and give rise to abscesses or to fistulas if they penetrate into surrounding structures. The term "perforating" disease can be misleading, as free perforation with spillage of intestinal contents into the abdominal cavity is not a common phenomenon with Crohn's disease. Inflammatory response around the advancing sinus tract typically results in adhesion to surrounding structures. The sinus usually bores through the area of adhesion such that abscess formation or fistulization to other structures occurs much more often than free perforation into the abdominal cavity. Typically, perforating disease is accompanied by a degree of stricture formation, but the fistula or abscess generated by the perforating component of the disease dominates the clinical picture.

Inflammatory Pattern

The inflammatory pattern of Crohn's disease is characterized by mucosal ulceration and bowel wall thickening. The edema that results from inflammation can lead to an adynamic segment of intestine and luminal narrowing. This pattern often gives rise to obstructive symptoms in the small intestine and diarrhea in the colon. Of the three patterns of disease, the inflammatory pattern is much more likely to respond to medical therapy.

LOCATION OF DISEASE

Crohn's disease is a panintestinal condition which may affect any area from the mouth to the anus. The most commonly affected location is the terminal ileum and one-fifth of all patients have more than one intestinal segment affected simultaneously.

Gastroduodenal and Esophageal Crohn's Disease

Crohn's disease of the upper gastrointestinal tract gives rise to symptoms of nausea, vomiting, dysphagia, or odynophagia.[38] Oral Crohn's disease usually manifests with aphthous ulcers in the hard palate that may cause discomfort, especially during mastication. Esophageal Crohn's disease is uncommon in both children and adults, but it is believed to be more frequent in children than in adult patients.[39] Esophageal involvement with Crohn's disease may be asymptomatic or may give rise to dysphagia or odynophagia. Esophageal Crohn's disease is associated with Crohn's disease elsewhere within the gastrointestinal tract, as disease isolated to the esophagus is almost never seen. Symptomatic Crohn's disease of the stomach and duodenum is more common than disease of the esophagus, yet both locations are the least frequently involved by Crohn's. The symptoms are usually related to the obstructive nature of the disease with delayed gastric emptying, a sense of postprandial gastric fullness, nausea, and vomiting.

Crohn's Disease of the Small Intestine

Abdominal pain is the predominant symptom of small bowel Crohn's disease, as it occurs in 90% of cases.[35] Abdominal pain may be the result of obstructive or septic complications. Pain related to partial obstruction is mostly postprandial and crampy in nature; pain from septic complications is typically steady and associated with fevers. Other common symptoms and findings include anorexia and weight loss. Weight loss is usually related to food avoidance, but in severe cases weight loss may be the result of malabsorption. With disease of the small intestine, patients may develop a palpable mass, usually located in the right lower quadrant, related to an abscess or phlegmon in perforating disease or a thickened loop of intestine in obstructive disease. Evidence of fistulization to the skin, urinary bladder, or vagina may also be elicited with an accurate history and physical exam.

Crohn's Colitis

Crohn's involvement of the colon typically results in diarrhea that may or may not be bloody. Acute flares of Crohn's colitis are often associated with fever and abdominal pain that is often exacerbated by bowel movements. Stricturing of the colon with more advanced disease can give rise to colonic obstruction. Like Crohn's disease of the small intestine, Crohn's colitis can give rise to abscess formation and fistulas. Toxic megacolon can occur with Crohn's disease, but this severe complication is rare and less frequently seen than in ulcerative colitis.[40]

Perineal Crohn's Disease

Crohn's disease frequently affects the anal crypts and gives rise to perianal fistulas, abscesses, and anal strictures. Perineal Crohn's disease is also associated with hypertrophic perianal skin tags, fissures, and perineal scarring. Approximately 40% of patients will develop perineal manifestations of Crohn's disease.[41,42] Anal Crohn's disease is almost always associated with Crohn's disease present elsewhere in the GI tract, although perianal disease can be the initial symptomatic manifestation of Crohn's disease.

Extraintestinal Crohn's Disease

In addition to the inflammation of the gastrointestinal tract, a variety of extraintestinal manifestations can occur in Crohn's disease. These include ocular, dermatological, hepatobiliary, and joint disorders.[43,44] Such extraintestinal manifestations occur in a minority of patients, but when present, they produce symptoms that can be more severe than those of the primary intestinal disease. Ocular manifestations of Crohn's disease include uveitis and episcleritis.[45] Cutaneous manifestations of Crohn's disease include erythema nodosum and pyoderma gangrenosum. Joint disorders such as ankylosing spondylitis, sacroiliitis, and seronegative polyarteritis can occur. Patients with Crohn's disease are also at risk for the development of primary sclerosing cholangitis. However, the risk for primary sclerosing cholangitis is much less in Crohn's disease patients than in patients who suffer from ulcerative colitis.

Peripheral polyarteritis, episcleritis, uveitis, and erythema nodosum typically correlate with the activity of intestinal Crohn's disease. These particular extraintestinal manifestations typically regress with complete surgical resection of the affected segment of intestine or with successful medical control of the intestinal inflammation. Pyoderma gangrenosum may also improve with treatment of primary intestinal disease, but available clinical data on this particular issue have not always been consistent. The clinical course of ankylosing spondylitis and primary sclerosing cholangitis tend to be independent of the level of disease activity within the intestine. Ankylosing spondylitis and primary sclerosing cholangitis do not improve with surgical resection of the Crohn's-affected bowel.

▪ DIAGNOSIS

The onset of Crohn's disease is often insidious and many patients will experience some symptoms for months or even years before the diagnosis is made. The diagnosis of Crohn's disease is typically made by a thorough history and physical examination along with intestinal radiography and endoscopy. There is no specific laboratory test that is diagnostic for Crohn's disease. Advanced imaging studies such as CT scan or MRI can assess or detect some of the complications and manifestations of Crohn's disease,[46] but they are generally not useful in making the initial diagnosis of Crohn's disease.[47]

HISTORY AND PHYSICAL EXAMINATION

The symptoms of Crohn's disease are dependent upon the location of the involved segment, the pattern and the severity of disease, and the associated complications. As noted above, in most cases, the onset of disease is gradual with the most common complaints being intermittent abdominal pain, bloating, diarrhea, nausea, vomiting, weight loss, and fever.[48] Patients may also have symptoms related to complications of the disease including abdominal masses, pneumaturia, perianal pain and swelling, or skin rash. In some cases the onset of symptoms can be more sudden, with patients relating a history reminiscent of acute appendicitis. In these cases, pain in the right lower quadrant may have been present only for a few hours or days. However, a brief history of symptoms such as this is atypical.

In patients suspected of having Crohn's disease, a complete physical exam should include a thorough abdominal assessment. In cases of ileal Crohn's disease, tenderness is typically present in the right lower quadrant and occasionally a palpable mass is present. The oral cavity should be examined for the presence of aphthous ulcers. The perianal area should be examined for the presence of fistulas, abscesses, or enlarged skin tags. A digital rectal examination should assess for the presence of anal strictures, fissures, and rectal mucosal ulcerations. The skin in the extremities should be examined for erythema nodosum and pyoderma gangrenosum.

SMALL BOWEL RADIOGRAPHY

Upper intestinal contrast studies, either small bowel follow-through or enteroclysis, are the best means for assessing the small bowel for Crohn's disease.[49–52] The radiographic abnormalities of small bowel Crohn's disease are often distinctive[53] (Fig 19–1). With early Crohn's disease, mucosal granulations with ulceration and nodularity can be identified. Thickening of the mucosal folds and edema of the bowel wall itself can be demonstrated as the disease progresses. With more advanced disease, cobblestoning becomes radiographically apparent. Small

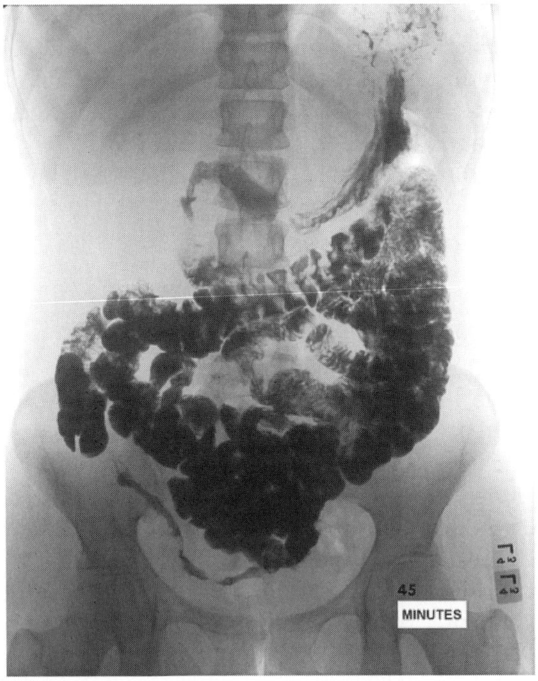

Figure 19–1. Small bowel radiograph demonstrating Crohn's disease of the terminal ileum. (Reprinted, with permission, from the University of Chicago General Surgery Archives.)

bowel contrast studies can also provide information regarding enlargement of the mesentery, as well as formation of an inflammatory mass or abscess. Such findings are demonstrated by a general mass effect separating and displacing contrast-filled loops of small intestine (see Fig 19–1; Fig 19–2). Small bowel contrast studies can demonstrate some of the complications of Crohn's disease, including high-grade strictures and fistulas. It is important to note, however, that small bowel radiography may not identify all such lesions. For instance, many enteric fistulas including ileosigmoid and ileovesical fistulas are not typically demonstrated on contrast radiography.[54,55] Thus the absence of radiographic evidence for fistulization does not exclude this possibility. Additionally, small bowel studies may not demonstrate all the areas of disease with significant strictures.[56] While small bowel radiographs may underestimate the extent of complicated Crohn's disease, small bowel studies performed by an experienced gastrointestinal radiologist are very effective as a diagnostic tool for the disease. Besides their diagnostic utility, small bowel radiographs can also help in assessing the extent of the disease by identifying the location and length of involved and uninvolved intestine, and by recognizing whether the disease is continuous or discontinuous with skip lesions separated by areas of normal intestine (Fig 19–3). Experienced radiologists can also assess areas of luminal narrowing and determine if they are the result of acute inflammatory swelling or are the result of fibrostenotic scar tissue. Such a distinction provides valuable information regarding the value of medical therapy versus early surgical intervention, as inflammatory stenoses are likely to respond to medical therapy while fibrotic strictures are best treated with surgery.

COLONOSCOPY

Colonoscopy allows for inspection of mucosal disease and provides an opportunity for a biopsy for histologic evaluation. In many cases the terminal ileum can be entered and evaluated. Characteristic colonoscopic features of Crohn's disease include aphthous ulcers, longitudinal ulcerations, skip lesions often with rectal sparing, pseudopolyps, and strictures.[53]

CAPSULE ENDOSCOPY

Capsule endoscopy is a new tool in the diagnosis and evaluation of Crohn's disease.[57,58] With this study, a small camera constructed within a capsule-size casing is swallowed and images from the camera are transmitted to a small electronic receiver worn by the patient. The image from the capsule endoscopy can detect subtle mucosal lesions that may not be apparent on small bowel x-rays. The value of capsule endoscopy in the diagnosis of Crohn's disease is yet to be fully established.

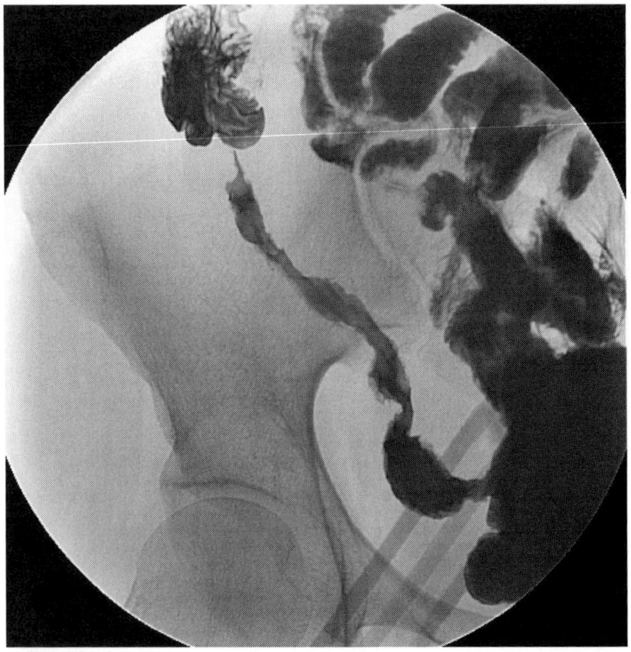

Figure 19–2. Small bowel radiograph demonstrating Crohn's disease of the terminal ileum with high-grade strictures and ulcerations. (Reprinted, with permission, from the University of Chicago General Surgery Archives.)

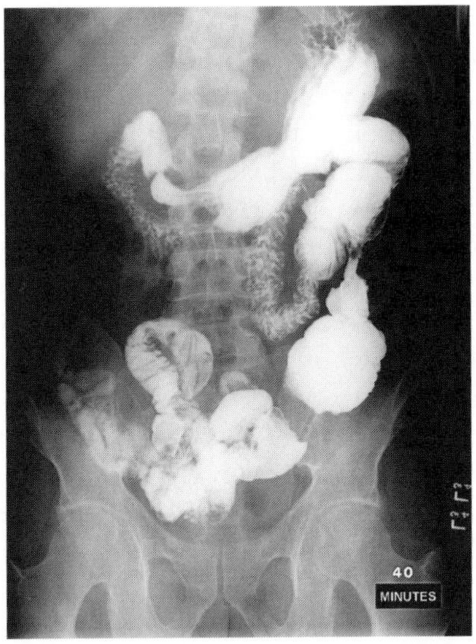

Figure 19–3. Small bowel radiograph demonstrating Crohn's disease with strictures in the jejunum. (Reprinted, with permission, from the University of Chicago General Surgery Archives.)

This diagnostic study should be reserved for those cases in which there is a substantial diagnostic uncertainty. All patients with suspected Crohn's disease should undergo a small bowel contrast study to exclude stricture formation prior to the capsule endoscopy, as the capsule may fail to pass through areas of narrowing and result in intestinal obstruction.

COMPUTED TOMOGRAPHY

Computed tomography (CT) findings of uncomplicated Crohn's disease are nonspecific and routine CT is not necessary for the diagnosis of Crohn's disease. CT, however, is very useful in identifying the complications associated with Crohn's disease.[59,60] Specifically, CT can readily identify thickened and dilated intestinal loops, inflammatory masses, or abscesses. CT scan can also demonstrate hydronephrosis resulting from retroperitoneal fibrosis and ureteral narrowing. CT scans are often the most sensitive indicator for the presence of an enterovesical fistula as identified by the presence of air within the urinary bladder.

▪ DIFFERENTIAL DIAGNOSIS

The differential diagnosis for small bowel Crohn's disease includes irritable bowel syndrome, acute appendicitis, intestinal ischemia, pelvic inflammatory disease, endometriosis, and gynecological malignancies. Other disorders that are within the differential diagnosis include radiation enteritis, *Yersinia* infections, intestinal injury from nonsteroidal anti-inflammatory agents, intestinal tuberculosis, and small bowel tumors.

Among the most important ailments to consider are small bowel malignancy and intestinal tuberculosis. In cases in whom small bowel malignancy is suspected, resection should be undertaken to make certain the diagnosis. The exclusion of intestinal tuberculosis can be difficult, as the inflammation and stricturing of the terminal ileum can occur in a manner that closely mimics Crohn's disease. The patient should be assessed for exposure to tuberculosis and screened for tuberculosis with a purified protein derivative skin test. Chest radiography should also be considered. Even when the diagnosis of Crohn's disease is certain, patients who coincidentally are found to also have latent tuberculosis should be treated in accordance with American Thoracic Society guidelines prior to the initiation of immunosuppressive therapy for management of their Crohn's disease.[61]

Intestinal injury from nonsteroidal anti-inflammatory drugs (NSAIDs) can result in focal enteritis with ulceration and stricture formation.[62,63] These manifestations can be very difficult to distinguish from Crohn's disease of the small bowel. This rare side effect from the very commonly used NSAIDs often requires resection or biopsy to confirm the diagnosis.

For Crohn's disease of the colon, the differential diagnosis includes ulcerative colitis, infectious colitis, collagenous colitis, ischemic colitis, diverticular disease, Behçet's disease, colonic neoplasm, solitary rectal ulcer syndrome, and NSAID colopathy.

The entity that is most difficult to discern from Crohn's colitis is ulcerative colitis. The diagnosis of ulcerative colitis cannot be made with absolute certainty, as it is possible for Crohn's disease of the colon to reproduce all the features of ulcerative colitis. It is only when features appear that are unique to Crohn's disease that the diagnosis of Crohn's disease can be made. Such distinguishing features of Crohn's disease include small bowel involvement, perianal disease, skip lesions, transmural inflammation, fistulas, abscesses, and noncaseating granulomas. After a complete history and physical exam complemented by appropriate radiological, endoscopic, and humoral studies, Crohn's and ulcerative colitis can be distinguished with a high degree of confidence in as many as 85–90% of cases; yet in the remaining 10–15% of cases, the differential diagnosis will remain indeterminate. This has major bearing on the surgical options available for such patients.

▪ MEDICAL MANAGEMENT

The goal of medical treatment of Crohn's disease is to provide long-lasting symptomatic relief while avoiding excessive morbidity. Crohn's disease cannot be cured by medical treatment but it may afford long periods of disease control and avoidance of surgical intervention. Thus it is important that the surgeon have an understanding of the basics of medical therapy for Crohn's disease. Selecting the optimal medical treatment for each individual requires experience and special expertise because of the variable course of the disease, the myriad of different clinical presentations and associated complications, and the desire to optimize medical treatment for each clinical situation.

CORTICOSTEROIDS

Corticosteroids are the most effective agents for controlling acute exacerbations of Crohn's disease, but their use is limited due to the risk of serious side effects. The majority of patients with active small bowel Crohn's disease will experience clinical remission with a short course of oral prednisone given in a dose between 0.25 and 0.5 mg/kg/day.[64] For patients unable to take oral medications, methylprednisolone can be administered in the adult at doses of 40–60 mg given as a daily infusion.[65] Common side effects from corticosteroids include diabetes, osteoporosis, cataracts, osteonecrosis, myopathy, psychosis, opportunistic infections, and adrenal suppression. The risks for these side effects are related to both the dose and the duration of steroid therapy.

5-AMINOSALICYLIC ACID

The aminosalicylates as a group of medications include sulfasalazine and 5-aminosalicylic acid (5-ASA) derivatives. The exact mechanism of action for these agents is not clear, but 5-ASA is thought to function through various pathways.[69] 5-ASA compounds inhibit leukotriene production by inhibition of 5-lipooxygenase activity. 5-ASA also inhibits the production of interleukin-1 and tumor necrosis factor (TNF). 5-ASA compounds are weak inhibitors of cyclooxygenase activity and it is unlikely that they act through the inhibition of prostaglandin production. Aminosalicylates are effective in the treatment of mild to moderate Crohn's disease. 5-ASA given in a controlled-release preparation is also effective as maintenance therapy to prevent recurrence after a flare of disease has been effectively managed either medically or surgically.[70–73]

Aminosalicylates come in a variety of preparations, each designed to deliver the drug in a topical fashion to the affected segments of intestine.[74] For instance, Asacol is 5-aminosalicylic acid contained within a pH-dependent resin designed to release the drug in the terminal ileum and colon where the pH is typically >7.0. Pentasa is 5-aminosalicylic acid contained within ethylcellulose-coated microgranules designed to slowly release the active compound throughout the entire small bowel and colon. Colazal is 5-aminosalicylic acid bound to an inert carrier by an AZO bond. This bond is broken by bacterial enzymes found within the colon, releasing the active 5-ASA compound to the colonic mucosa.

It is important to emphasize that mesalamine and its derivatives should not be confused with acetylsalicylic acid (aspirin) and other NSAIDs. Unlike 5-ASA compounds, classic NSAIDs are powerful inhibitors of cyclooxygenase (COX)-1 and COX-2. Many clinicians have had concerns that NSAIDs may exacerbate Crohn's disease.[75–77] Although the basis of these concerns has been challenged,[78–80] it is recommended that patients with Crohn's disease avoid NSAIDs and use alternative medications when appropriate.

IMMUNOMODULATORS (AZATHIOPRINE AND 6-MERCAPTOPURINE)

Azathioprine and 6-mercaptopurine (6-MP) are immunosuppressive agents that inhibit cytotoxic T-cell and natural killer cell function. These agents are effective in treating mild to moderate Crohn's disease.[64,81] Azathioprine given at 2.0–2.5 mg/kg/day or 6-MP in doses of 1.0–1.5 mg/kg/day will result in a 50–60% response rate in patients with active Crohn's disease.[65,82] Both 6-MP and azathioprine are also effective in maintaining remission following surgery or successful medical management.[71]

INFLIXIMAB

Infliximab is a chimeric mouse-human monoclonal antibody to TNF. TNF is a proinflammatory cytokine that is believed to be important in the pathophysiology of Crohn's disease. Infliximab binds to both free and membrane-bound TNF and prevents TNF from binding to its cell surface receptors.[69] Clinical trials have demonstrated an 80% response rate with a single dose of infliximab.[83,84] It is important to note that the doses and dosing intervals of infliximab must be individualized, but a typical regimen would include 5 mg/kg of infliximab given IV at weeks zero, two, and six, with a dose of 5 mg/kg every 8 weeks thereafter.

OTHER MEDICAL THERAPIES

Other agents that are used with varying success in the treatment of Crohn's disease include methotrexate, metronidazole, cyclosporine, tacrolimus, and thalidomide. With the exception of metronidazole, each one of these agents requires a complete and sophisticated knowledge of appropriate dosing, side effects and therapeutic efficacy, which is beyond the scope of this chapter. Metronidazole is indicated in the maintenance therapy of chronic perineal septic complications and in the treatment of bacterial overgrowth associated with chronic obstructive disease of the small bowel. Long-term side effects include peripheral paresthesias, which are usually transient if the drug is discontinued as soon as they are experienced.

▪ SURGICAL TREATMENT OF CROHN'S DISEASE

Similarly to medical treatment, the goal of surgical treatment of Crohn's disease is to provide long-lasting symptomatic relief while avoiding excessive morbidity. Crohn's disease cannot be cured by surgical therapy and thus surgery, like medical treatment, should be considered palliative. Complete extirpation of disease should not be the primary goal of surgery, as this does not produce cure and is frequently counterproductive. Rather, treatment of complications and palliation of symptoms while avoiding excessive loss of intestine should be the main aims of surgical treatment.

To avoid excessive loss of intestine, nonresectional techniques such as strictureplasty may be required. Additionally, optimal surgical therapy may require leaving behind segments of the intestinal tract affected by mild but asymptomatic disease with resection of only the areas of severe and symptomatic Crohn's disease. The best surgical strategy for each patient with Crohn's disease takes into account the indications for surgical treatment and the natural history of the disease, with its high risk for recurrence and the need for repeated surgeries.

INDICATIONS FOR SURGERY

Failure of Medical Treatment

The failure to respond to medical treatment or the inability to tolerate effective therapy are the most common indications for surgical treatment of Crohn's disease.[85] Some patients may respond to the initial medical therapy only to rapidly relapse with tapering of the medical treatment. For example, some patients respond well to steroid therapy, but become steroid-dependent as tapering of the steroid dose results in recurrent symptoms. Due to the severe complications that are virtually inevitable with prolonged steroid treatment, surgery is warranted if the patient cannot be weaned from systemic steroids within 3–6 months. The occurrence of complications related to the medical treatment or the progression of disease while on maximal medical treatment represent additional indications for surgical treatment.

Intestinal Obstruction

Partial or complete intestinal obstruction is a common indication for operation for Crohn's disease.[86] The clinical presentation of chronic partial small bowel obstruction is much more typical than complete obstruction. Patients with chronic partial small bowel obstruction due to Crohn's disease may experience postprandial cramps, abdominal distension, borborygmi, and weight loss. To avoid symptoms, many patients will restrict their diets to soft foods or even liquids. If partial obstruction from Crohn's disease is primarily due to acute inflammation and bowel wall thickening, then initial medical therapy is warranted. If, however, the obstructive symptoms are due to high-grade fibrostenotic lesions, then medical treatment will not reverse these lesions and surgery is indicated.

When complete intestinal obstruction occurs, initial conservative treatment with nasogastric decompression and intravenous hydration is warranted.[34,87] Intravenous steroids are also administered. This allows for decompression of acutely distended and edematous bowel, and in most cases, for resolution of the complete obstruction. Resolution of the complete obstruction should not lead the physician to attempt treating the patient with medical treatment. Patients with complete obstruction who respond well to initial conservative therapy are at high risk for persistent or recurrent symptoms of obstruction and are best managed with surgery once adequate decompression is achieved. The surgery can be performed under elective and safer conditions after appropriate bowel preparation.

Fistulas

Intestinal fistulas occur in one-third of Crohn's disease patients.[54] Intestinal fistulas, however, are the primary indication for surgery in only a minority of patients. Thus the presence of an intestinal fistula is not in and of itself an indication for surgery.[88,89] In general, intestinal fistulas are the primary indication for surgical treatment if they connect with the genitourinary tract, or if their drainage is cause for personal embarrassment and discomfort (enterocutaneous and enterovaginal fistulas), or if they create a bypass of such magnitude as to cause intestinal malabsorption.

Fistulas between the ileum and the urinary bladder often result in recurrent urinary tract infections including pyelonephritis. While it is not mandatory to operate on all cases of enterovesical fistulas, surgery is warranted to avoid deterioration of renal function with recurrent infections or if symptoms persist in spite of appropriate medical therapy.

Enterocutaneous fistulas and enterovaginal fistulas often cause physical discomfort and personal embarrassment. A trial of medical therapy may be elected for enterocutaneous and enterovaginal fistulas, but most such cases will require surgery.[90,91]

Occasionally, an enteroenteric fistula can result in significant symptoms. Fistulas that result in functional bypass of a major intestinal segment can result in malabsorption or diarrhea. These fistulas need to be addressed surgically.

Abscesses and Inflammatory Masses

Intra-abdominal abscesses and inflammatory masses occur less frequently than fistulae but are more often an indication for operative intervention.[92] Small abscesses seen on CT may warrant a trial of treatment with antibiotics, but almost all intra-abdominal abscesses will require drainage. In a vast majority of cases, Crohn's abscesses can be drained percutaneously with CT or ultrasound guidance.[93–95] The rare large intra-loop abscesses may require open surgical drainage. Often in such cases the abscess can be completely extirpated with the resection of the diseased segment of intestine.

Crohn's abscesses usually originate from a severely diseased segment of bowel. A Crohn's abscess that has been drained percutaneously is very likely to recur or result in an enterocutaneous fistula, and surgical resection is often advised even after successful drainage.[95] Inflammatory masses indicate severe disease and often harbor an unrecognized abscess.[92] Thus, inflammatory masses that do not readily respond to antibiotic treatment should be considered for surgical treatment.

Perforation

Free perforation is a rare complication of Crohn's disease occurring in only about 1% of cases.[96] When this complication occurs, it is an obvious indication for urgent operation. The diagnosis of free perforation is made by detecting a sudden change in the patient's symptoms along with the development of the physical findings of peritonitis or the identification of free intraperitoneal air as demonstrated on plain x-rays or CT scans. The use of immunosuppressants and glucocorticosteroids can blunt many of the physical findings of acute perforation, therefore the index of suspicion for perforation must be higher in immunocompromised patients who complain of worsening symptoms or show early signs of sepsis. Most patients, however, will demonstrate classic signs of peritonitis with rebound, rigidity, guarding, and loss of bowel sounds.

Hemorrhage

Hemorrhage is an uncommon complication from Crohn's disease. Massive gastrointestinal hemorrhage is rare and occurs more frequently from Crohn's colitis than in small bowel Crohn's disease.[97] Hemorrhage from small bowel Crohn's disease tends to be indolent with episodic or chronic bleeding requiring intermittent transfusions, but rarely requires emergent surgery. Localization of the site of bleeding is accomplished by angiography in the presence of brisk bleeding; otherwise colonoscopy can be attempted preoperatively to localize a source of lower gastrointestinal hemorrhage. Intraoperative localization can be aided by enteroscopy or colonoscopy.

When severe hemorrhage occurs in Crohn's disease, it is usually due to erosion of a single vessel by a deep ulcer or fissure. Recurrent bleeding in an area of small bowel disease is a common phenomenon and it has been argued that even after control of hemorrhage from small bowel Crohn's disease with conservative management, elective resection of the areas of Crohn's disease should be undertaken to prevent recurrent bleeding.

Patients with Crohn's disease are also at risk for bleeding from peptic ulcer disease. This is particularly true for patients receiving corticosteroid therapy. For this reason, Crohn's disease patients who develop gastrointestinal bleeding should undergo an upper endoscopy to rule out gastric or duodenal ulcers.

Cancer or Suspicion of Cancer

The diagnosis of Crohn's disease increases the risk of adenocarcinoma of the colon and small intestine.[98] The diagnosis of adenocarcinoma of the small bowel is difficult because symptoms and radiographic findings of small bowel malignancy can be similar to those of the underlying Crohn's disease. Male patients and patients with long-standing disease appear to be at increased risk for small bowel adenocarcinoma.[98] Defunctionalized segments of bowel also seem to be at particular risk for malignancy.[99] For this reason, bypass surgery should be avoided for Crohn's disease of the small intestine and defunctionalized rectal stumps should either be restored to their function or excised.

Adenocarcinoma of the small intestine should be suspected in any patient with long-standing disease whose symptoms of obstruction progress after a lengthy quiescent period. Surveillance for colonic malignancies can be undertaken by colonoscopy with random mucosal biopsy. If dysplasia is encountered, then resection of the areas of Crohn's disease should be considered.[100,101] Areas of stricture formation within the colon should be closely examined and biopsied. Strictures that are too narrow to allow passage of the colonoscope or cannot be adequately assessed colonoscopically should be resected.

Growth Retardation

Growth retardation occurs in a quarter of children affected by Crohn's disease. Although steroid treatment may delay growth in children, the major cause of growth retardation in Crohn's disease patients is due to the malnutrition associated with active intestinal disease.[102]

PREOPERATIVE PREPARATION AND EVALUATION

A complete assessment of the gastrointestinal tract is required prior to surgery. Full delineation of the extent of disease and associated complications is necessary to plan for the optimal surgical strategies.

Assessment of the small intestine requires either a small bowel follow-through or an enteroclysis study. The colon and rectum is best evaluated by colonoscopy. Barium enema studies can also be used to evaluate for colonic disease, particularly in cases in which strictures do not allow passage of the colonoscope. If the patient has had a previous resection of the ileocecal valve, a contrast enema can be a useful means of evaluating the ileocolonic anastomosis and the preanastomotic segment for recurrent disease. If an abscess or inflammatory mass is suspected, a CT scan of the abdomen and pelvis with both oral and IV contrast should be obtained. In cases in whom urgent surgery is required, a full evaluation of the gastrointestinal tract prior to surgery may not be feasible. In these cases, evaluation of disease must be accomplished intraoperatively and both the patient and the surgeon must be prepared for a wide variety of surgical possibilities.

As with preparation for any major operation, metabolic derangements must be treated prior to surgery. Fluid and electrolyte abnormalities must be corrected. Patients with profound anemia need to be transfused and coagulopathies must be addressed. Patients with cardiovascular or pulmonary disease should have the condition stabilized and their functional capacity optimized prior to operation. Most patients with Crohn's disease will not require preoperative parenteral nutrition, as most suffer from only a minor degree of malnutrition. There are rare cases, however, in which the nutritional status of the patient has been so severely compromised that they benefit from several weeks of bowel rest, hyperalimentation, and ongoing medical treatment before operation.

The absolute need for mechanical bowel preparation is controversial.[104–106] Traditionally mechanical bowel preparations have been an unquestioned standard to lessen the risks of sepsis and to allow for a safe anastomosis. Recently these advantages have been challenged.[104,105] Even so, it is common practice for patients undergoing intestinal resection for Crohn's disease to undergo a complete mechanical bowel preparation with either polyethylene glycol or sodium phosphate. Should the patient be unable to tolerate oral preparations, then enemas can be utilized. Prophylactic broad-spectrum antibiotics are administered perioperatively[107] and stress dose steroids must be given to patients suspected of hypothalamic-pituitary-adrenal suppression. If feasible, well-contained intra-abdominal abscesses should be drained percutaneously prior to surgery. If an abdominal stoma is contemplated, then the optimal site for the stoma location should be marked preoperatively. In cases in whom preoperative CT scan suggests significant inflammation in proximity to the ureters, then preoperative ureteral stenting can be helpful.

Some have suggested that to improve the safety of surgery for Crohn's disease anti-inflammatory Crohn's medication should be either lowered or discontinued prior to elective surgery. Recent studies, however, have shown that preoperative use of steroids and antimetabolites do not appear to affect the perioperative morbidity, and hence discontinuation of these medications is not likely to result in significant benefit. Methotrexate, on the other hand, is one medication that may be worth discontinuing at least 2 weeks prior to surgery. Laboratory studies have shown decreased wound healing with methotrexate,[108] and clinical data to evaluate the safety of methotrexate in patients undergoing bowel resection with anastomosis are lacking.

SURGICAL OPTIONS

Intestinal Resection

Intestinal resection with anastomosis or stoma formation is the most common surgical procedure performed for the treatment of Crohn's disease. Most cases of Crohn's disease require only limited resections that are generally well tolerated and do not place these patients at risk for short bowel syndrome. Cumulative clinical data including randomized studies have indicated that resection of Crohn's disease need only encompass the grossly apparent disease, as wider resections do not improve the outcome after surgery.[109–112] Microscopic resection margins that are grossly normal but demonstrate microscopic evidence for Crohn's activity do not result in early recurrence or other complications. Hence, intraoperative frozen section of the resection margins is not necessary.[113]

The extent of mesenteric dissection does not affect the long-term results either, hence the mesentery can be divided at the most advantageous level. Division of the thickened mesentery of small bowel Crohn's disease can be the most challenging aspect of the procedure. Identification and isolation of individual mesenteric vessels is not feasible with a thickened Crohn's mesentery. Although many approaches to this problem have been described, a common technique is to apply overlapping clamps on either side of the intended line of transection. The mesentery is then divided between the clamps and the tissue contained within the clamps is suture ligated (Fig 19–4). In severe cases, additional hemostatic mattress sutures may need to be applied to the mesentery to control bleeding. The use of tissue welding devices such as the LigaSure device can be useful for sealing vessels within the thickened mesentery. Even with these devices, mattress sutures in the mesentery are commonly needed for complete hemostasis. In spite of the difficulty dealing with the thickened and often hyperemic mesentery, resection can be performed with a low risk for postoperative hemorrhage, and the risk for hemorrhage requiring re-exploration has been reported to be less than 0.5%.[85]

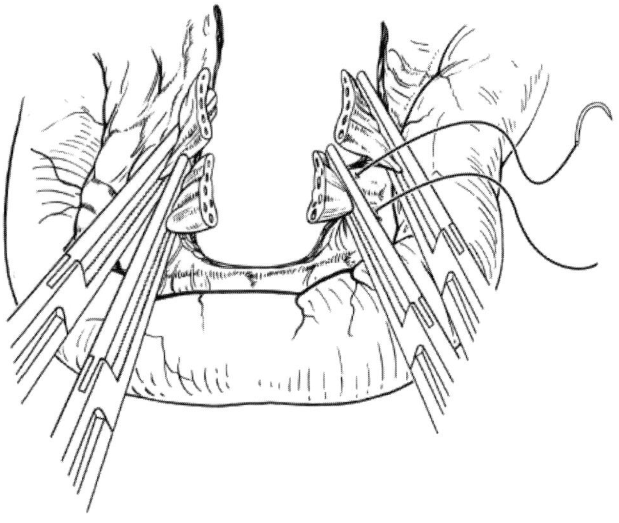

Figure 19–4. Technique for division of thickened Crohn's mesentery.

Anastomosis

There is no overriding consensus regarding the optimal technique for intestinal anastomosis in Crohn's disease.[70,114–118] It is well established that recurrent Crohn's disease after resection of terminal ileal disease is most likely to occur at the ileocolonic anastomosis or at the preanastomotic ileum. It has been proposed that large caliber anastomoses require a longer period to stricture down to a critical diameter that becomes symptomatic. The argument is made that a longer side-to-side anastomosis may be beneficial over an end-to-end or end-to-side anastomosis.[117] To date, however, clinical data do not indicate a benefit for one particular intestinal configuration over another.[116] Intestinal anastomosis for Crohn's disease cases can be fashioned with a stapling device or may be hand sutured. When performed under selective conditions, resection with primary anastomosis for Crohn's disease can be performed with a high degree of safety, and small bowel anastomotic dehiscence rates can be kept under 1%.[85] In the presence of sepsis, severe scarring, or malnutrition, it may be wise to protect the anastomosis with a proximal loop stoma or to forego the anastomosis altogether and bring out an end stoma at the point of resection.

Stoma Formation

Permanent stomas are required for the surgical treatment of Crohn's proctitis and are occasionally required for the management of severe, unrelenting perianal disease. Temporary stomas are much more common and are typically employed as a means of protecting a distal anastomosis or when an anastomosis is not advisable.

If an ileostomy or colostomy is contemplated, selection of the optimal placement of the stoma should be determined preoperatively.[119] Proper stoma location is critical to achieve a satisfactory stoma. It is preferable to locate the ileostomy over the left or right rectus abdominis muscle on a flat area away from deep skin folds and bony prominences.[120] The surface of the abdomen must be evaluated in both the sitting and standing positions, as this will often demonstrate skin folds and creases not evident in the supine position. Attention must be paid to determining the level of the patient's belt line and every effort is made to place the stoma below it. Once the optimal position of the stoma has been identified, it is marked in a manner that will remain visible at the time of surgery.

Complications related to intestinal stomas are common. They include peristomal hernia, prolapse, and stricture. Peristomal hernia is the most common ostomy-related complication. It can be anticipated that approximately 25% of patients with a permanent stoma will require surgical revision of their ostomy to deal with one or more of these complications.[121]

Bypass Procedures

Bypass procedures became popular in the 1940s and 1950s once physicians and surgeons realized that aggressive enterectomies did not reduce the incidence of recurrence and were fraught with the development of short gut syndrome. Initially conceived to bypass an area of stricture or obstruction, the use of bypass procedures was eventually extended to Crohn's disease complicated by septic complications. Increased experience with bypass procedures revealed that persistence of disease put patients at risk of persistent sepsis, and eventually neoplastic transformation. Because of these complications, bypass procedures were supplanted by limited intestinal resection as the main surgical option in the late 1960s in all intestinal districts except the duodenum, where a simple side-to-side retrocolic gastrojejunostomy adequately relieves the obstructive symptoms. With increased experience and confidence in the performance of strictureplasty, duodenal disease is nowadays more and more commonly handled with strictureplasties.

Strictureplasty

Strictureplasty techniques have gained popularity as a safe and effective means of treating stricturing Crohn's disease of the small intestine without resorting to lengthy resections. Strictureplasties are best employed when resection would otherwise result in loss of a lengthy segment of bowel and thus place the patient at risk for short bowel syndrome. This would include cases with long segments of stricturing disease and patients with multiple prior resections. They are also indicated when they offer a simpler alternative to resection, such as in short recurrent disease at a previous ileocolic or enteroenteric anastomosis.

It is generally accepted that the advantage conferred by a strictureplasty over a resection in the preservation of intestinal absorptive capacity is mainly due to the sparing of normal areas in between strictures which would be otherwise sacrificed. Although this is true, there is increased evidence that the acuity of the disease decreases at the site of the strictureplasty and the disease becomes quiescent.[122] Whether this correlates with a simultaneous restoration of absorptive function has not yet been established.

The most commonly performed strictureplasty is the Heinecke-Mikulicz strictureplasty.[123–125] The Heinecke-Mikulicz is named after the pyloroplasty technique from which this procedure is derived. With the Heinecke-Mikulicz strictureplasty, a longitudinal incision is made along the antimesenteric border of the stricture (Fig 19–5). This incision should extend for 1–2 cm into the normal elastic bowel on either side of the stricture. Once the enterotomy is made, the area of the stricture should be closely examined. If there is any concern that the stricture may harbor a malignancy, a biopsy with frozen section must be obtained. Complete hemostasis should be obtained with precise application of electrocautery. The longitudinal enterotomy of the Heinecke-Mikulicz strictureplasty is then closed in a transverse fashion. The closure can be accomplished with either single- or double-layered sutures. The Heinecke-Mikulicz stricture technique is appropriate for short segment strictures of 2–3 cm in length.

The Finney strictureplasty, also named for the pyloroplasty technique from which this approach is derived, can be used for strictures up to 15 cm in length.[123] With the Finney strictureplasty technique, the strictured segment is folded onto itself in a U-shape[126] (Fig 19–6). A row of seromuscular sutures is placed between the two arms of the U and a longitudinal U-shaped enterotomy is then made paralleling the row of sutures. The mucosal surface is examined and biopsies are taken as necessary. Hemostasis is obtained with electrocautery. Full-thickness sutures are then placed beginning at the posterior wall of the apex of the strictureplasty and then continued down to approximate the proximal and distal ends of the enterotomy. This full-thickness suture line is then continued anteriorly to close the strictureplasty. To complete the procedure, a row of seromuscular Lembert sutures is placed anteriorly. In essence, the Finney is a short side-to-side functional anastomosis. A very long Finney strictureplasty may result in a functional bypass with a large lateral diverticulum. This diverticulum, in theory, could be at risk for bacterial overgrowth and the blind loop syndrome. Fortunately, this theoretical concern has not been observed in clinical practice.

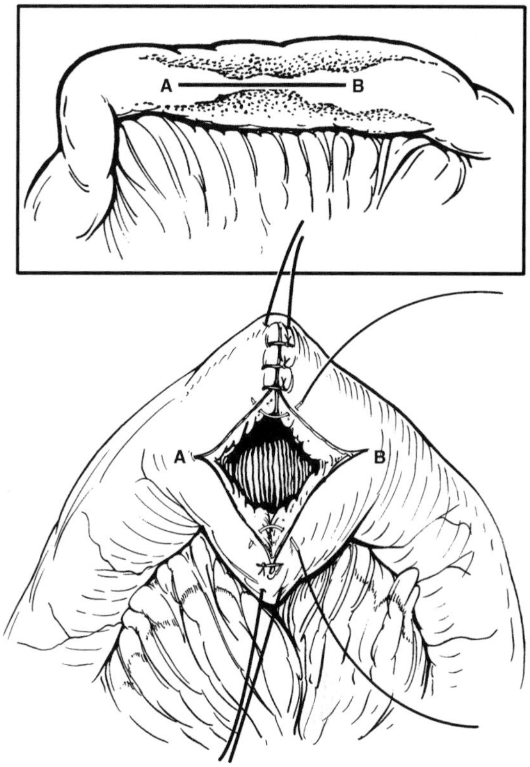

Figure 19–5. Heineke-Mikulicz strictureplasty.

The purpose of the strictureplasty is to preserve intestinal length that otherwise would be sacrificed with resection. Those cases with long segments of stricturing disease are the ones in which nonresectional methods should be aggressively pursued. To manage such cases, multiple strictureplasties are typically required. In general, however, repeated Heinecke-Mikulicz or Finney strictureplasties should be separated from each other by at least 5 cm. Otherwise the result can be a bulky and relatively unyield-

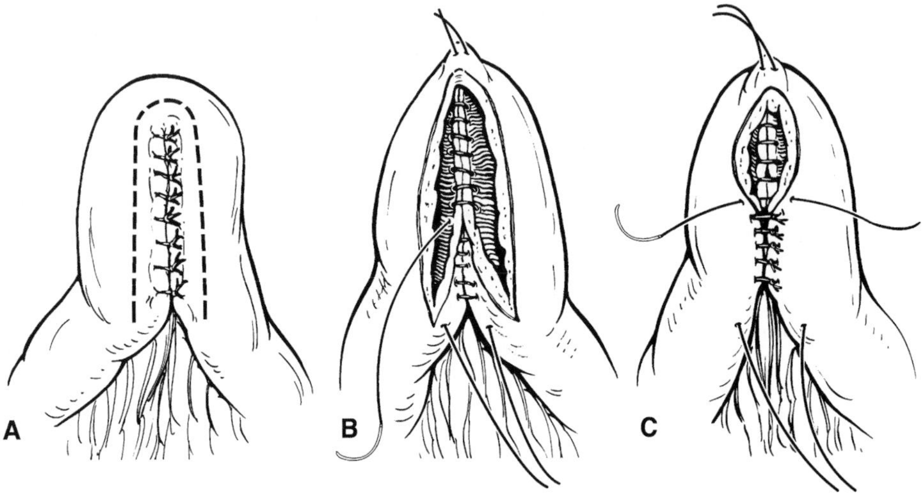

Figure 19–6. Finney strictureplasty.

ing segment of intestine with considerable tension placed on each suture line.

Patients with long segment stricturing disease and multiple strictures grouped close together are best managed with an isoperistaltic side-to-side strictureplasty.[127] With this technique, the segment of stricturing disease is divided at its midpoint. The proximal and distal ends are then drawn onto each other in a side-to-side fashion (Fig 19–7). Division of some of the mesenteric vascular arcades facilitates the positioning of the two limbs over each other. The proximal and distal loops are then sutured together with a layer of interrupted seromuscular sutures. A longitudinal enterotomy is then made along both of the loops (Fig 19–8). The intestinal ends are spatulated to provide a smoothly tailored fit to the ultimate closure of the strictureplasty. Again, this is the time to examine the mucosal surface of the intestine to detect potential areas of neoplastic transformation and control bleeding. The outer suture line is reinforced with an interior row of either interrupted or running full-thickness sutures. This inner suture line is continued anteriorly. The anterior closure is then reinforced with an outer layer of interrupted seromuscular sutures to complete the strictureplasty (Fig 19–9).

Originally described in 1996, this procedure has been utilized with increasing frequency. The isoperistaltic side-to-side strictureplasty is recognized as an effective means of treating extensive small bowel Crohn's disease and provides the best option for those cases that would otherwise require extensive intestinal resection with loss of significant length of small bowel.[122,125,128,129]

Unlike resection, diseased segments are retained with strictureplasty and suture lines are placed in Crohn's-affected tissue. This has been a cause of concern regarding the risk of intestinal suture line dehiscence, long-term recurrences, and risk for malignancy. The ongoing and now substantial clinical experience with these techniques has allayed these concerns.[130] In appropriately selected patients, perioperative morbidity from strictureplasty appears to be similar to that of resection and primary anastomosis. Specifically, intestinal suture line dehiscence appears to be uncommon with any of the described strictureplasty techniques.[131,132] The most common postoperative complication directly related to strictureplasty is hemorrhage from the strictureplasty site. This has been reported to occur in up to 9% of cases. Fortunately, the gastrointestinal hemorrhage following strictureplasty is typically minor and can be managed conservatively with transfusions alone. Rarely, more persistent bleeding may require intra-arterial infusion of vasopressin, but the need for reoperation to control hemorrhage after strictureplasty is very rare. It is by now also well established that strictureplasty techniques provide excellent long-term symptomatic relief which is comparable to resections with

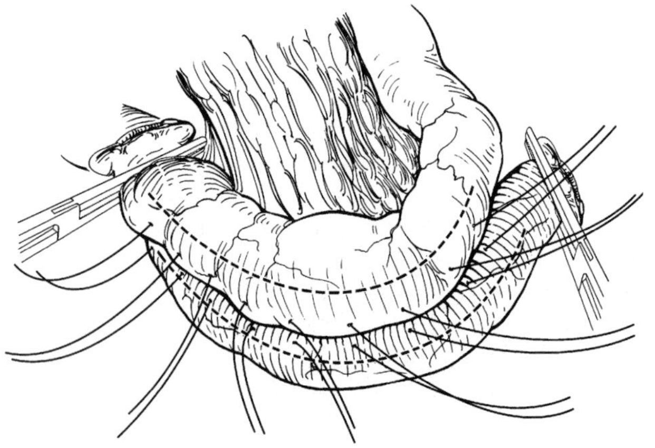

Figure 19–7. Isoperistaltic side-to-side strictureplasty. The segment of intestine affected by Crohn's strictures is divided and the two limbs are drawn onto each other.

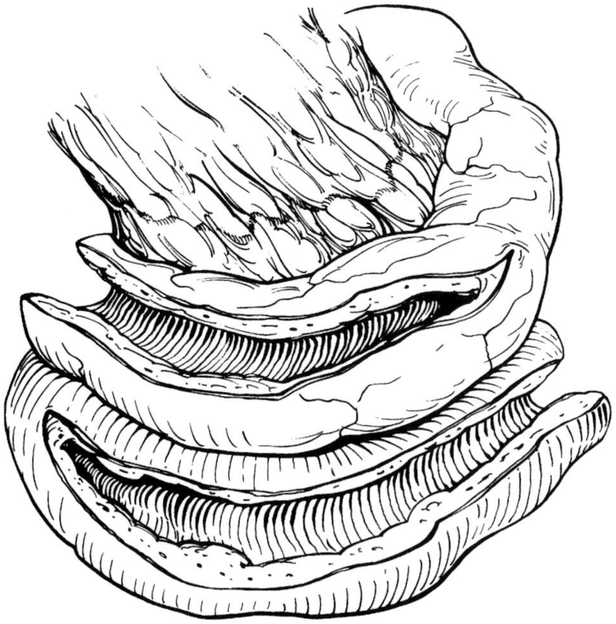

Figure 19–8. Isoperistaltic side-to-side strictureplasty. Longitudinal enterotomies are made along the antimesenteric borders of the two limbs.

anastomosis. Although there are no controlled studies directly comparing strictureplasty to resection, multiple reports of the observed symptomatic recurrence rates after strictureplasty compare well with published recurrence rates after resection and anastomosis.[125,132,133]

Epidemiological studies have shown an increased risk for small bowel adenocarcinoma in Crohn's disease patients.[100] This risk is increased in patients with long-standing disease. It is not known if strictureplasty by virtue of its retention of diseased tissue increases this risk. At the time of the writing of this chapter, there have been only two reported cases of an adenocarcinoma developing at a site of previous small bowel strictureplasty, and it is thus believed that the risk of malignancy after strictureplasty is low.[134,135]

LAPAROSCOPY

Over the past two decades, laparoscopy has been dramatically changing all aspects of gastrointestinal surgery. Specifically in colon and rectal surgery, laparoscopy has been widely used in benign disease,[136,137] including inflammatory bowel disease, and more recently in colon cancer.[138] Several single-institution small reports suggest that not only is laparoscopic surgery for Crohn's disease feasible and safe, but also it reduces length of hospitalization and recovery, and allows for a smaller wound, with an overall reduction in morbidity.[139–152]

Most Crohn's disease patients are well suited for laparoscopy. They are usually young, otherwise healthy, and interested in undergoing an operation that involves minimal scarring, since they are facing the risk of multiple major abdominal operations in their lifetime. On the other hand, Crohn's disease represents a difficult arena even for the experienced open colorectal surgeon. Many of the unique features of Crohn's disease, such as the intense inflammation and thickened mesentery, enteric fistula, inflammatory masses or abscesses, and the multiplicity of areas of intestinal involvement, have deterred many surgeons from even considering a laparoscopic approach.

Two prospective controlled studies have shown several advantages of the laparoscopic-assisted approach over the conventional approach.[139,141] Bemelman and colleagues compared 48 open ileocolic resections with 30 laparoscopic-assisted resections. This study showed similarly low morbidity rates in both groups, but a shorter hospital stay and improved cosmetic results in favor of the laparoscopic group.[141] Alabaz and associates compared 48 open ileocolic resections with 26 laparoscopic-assisted resections. The patients in the laparoscopic group returned to work more quickly, had better cosmetic results, and were more likely to have improved postoperative quality of life.[139] A prospective randomized trial comparing open and laparoscopic-assisted resections in 60 patients undergoing elective ileocecectomy for Crohn's disease not complicated by abscess formation or complex fistula showed a faster postoperative recovery of respiratory function (measured as recovery of 80% of forced respiratory volume and forced vital capacity), shorter abdominal incisions, and longer performance time in the laparoscopic-assisted group. These differences were all statistically significant. With limited follow-up,

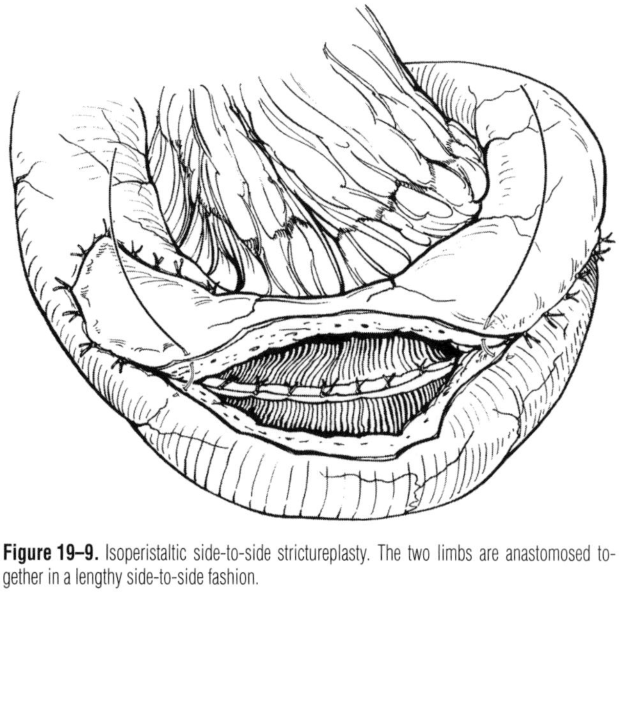

Figure 19–9. Isoperistaltic side-to-side strictureplasty. The two limbs are anastomosed together in a lengthy side-to-side fashion.

there was no difference in recurrence rate.[147] This paper demonstrated that in experienced hands, morbidity from the laparoscopic approach compares favorably with that of a conventional open approach. Obviously these results need to be confirmed by larger series with longer follow-up.

The indications for laparoscopic surgery for Crohn's disease should not differ from conventional open surgery as described before. Contraindications to a laparoscopic approach include patients who are critically ill and unable to tolerate the pneumoperitoneum due to hypotension or hypercarbia, patients with extensive intra-abdominal sepsis (abscess, free perforation, or complex fistula), and difficulty in identifying the anatomy (previous surgery, obesity, or adhesions). The same variety of surgical procedures described earlier can be performed laparoscopically.

After induction of general anesthesia, the patient is placed on the operating table in the modified lithotomy position. Rectal irrigation with diluted iodine solution is performed, especially in patients with involvement of the rectum and sigmoid colon. An epidural catheter is usually inserted at the time of surgery. The sympathetic blockade achieved with epidural administration of local anesthetics and opioids prevents bowel distension, hence facilitating exploration of the gastrointestinal tract and handling of the bowel. Depending on the procedure planned, four or five trocars are utilized, with the camera placed at the level of the umbilicus.

Every operation for Crohn's disease, whether open or laparoscopic, should start with a complete examination of the entire gastrointestinal tract starting from the ligament of Treitz. The patient is placed in the reverse Trendelenburg position and right lateral decubitus with the assistant standing on the patient's left side retracting the transverse colon into the upper quadrants and the surgeon between the patient's legs, tracing the intestine from the ligament of Treitz all the way to the ileocolic pedicle. This maneuver is facilitated by progressively rotating the patient from the reverse Trendelenburg to a full Trendelenburg position and left lateral decubitus. In the presence of skip areas of involvement from Crohn's disease, these are marked intracorporeally with sutures in order to facilitate retrieval of the diseased segments when the specimen is exteriorized.

Laparoscopic-assisted ileocolic resection is the most commonly performed laparoscopic procedure for Crohn's disease. For laparoscopic ileocolectomy, a four-trocar technique is utilized (Fig 19–10). Five-millimeter trocars can be used exclusively, as a 5-mm 30° camera offers the same resolution as larger ones and the vascular pedicles can be divided intracorporeally with 5-mm

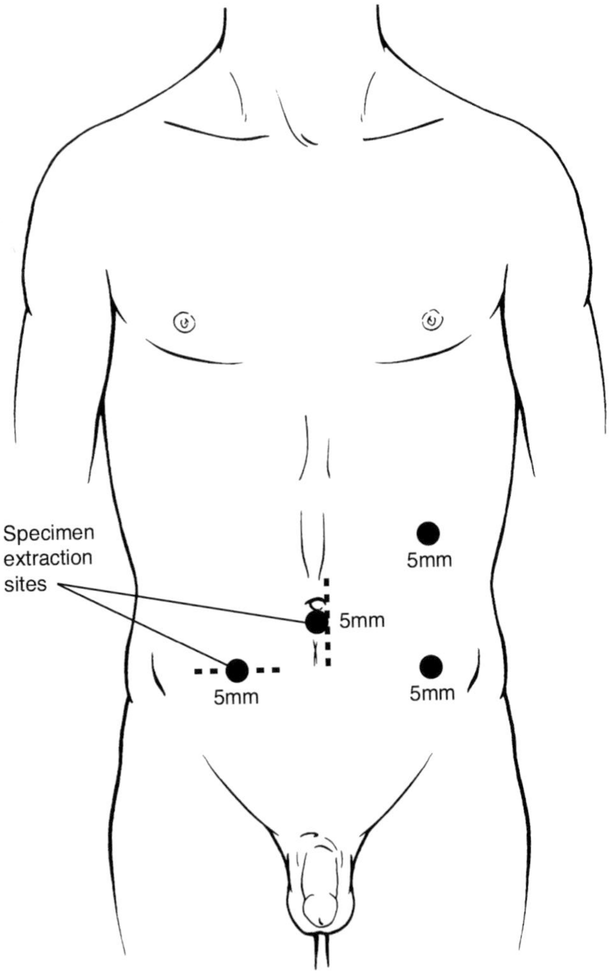

Figure 19–10. Port site locations for laparoscopic ileocecectomy.

instruments. After the bowel has been evaluated in its entirety as previously described, the assistant, standing between the patient's legs using the right lower quadrant trocar site, places the ileocolic pedicle under tension (Fig 19–11). The surgeon on the patient's left side dissects and divides it (Fig 19–12). Once this is accomplished, a medial-to-lateral submesenteric mobilization of the ascending colon all the way to the hepatic flexure is completed (Fig 19–13). The assistant between the legs is in charge of lifting the colon to allow clear visualization of the submesenteric plane. When the submesenteric mobilization is completed, the lateral colonic peritoneal reflection is divided all the way to the hepatic flexure (Fig 19–14). The terminal ileum is completely mobilized by dividing the peritoneum at the level of the pelvic rim to allow a tension-free anastomosis through a small incision. It is often necessary to completely mobilize the hepatic flexure without dividing the right branch of the ileocolic vessels in order to facilitate exteriorization of the specimen (Fig 19–15). It

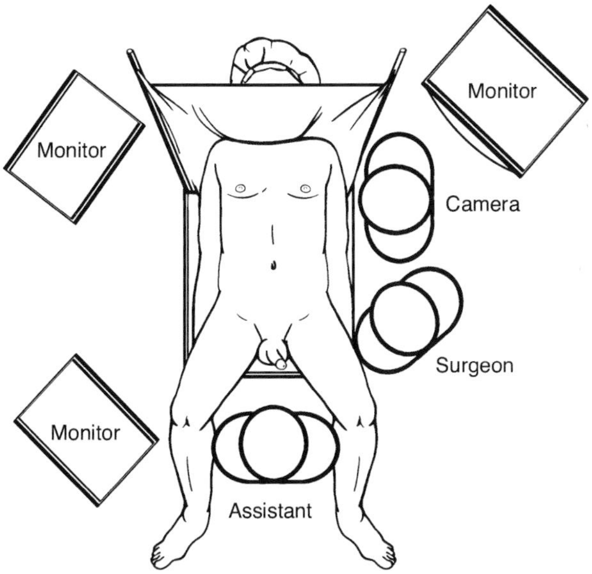

Figure 19–11. Optimal position of the surgeons and assistants for laparoscopic ileocecectomy.

is imperative to make sure that the mobilization is adequate before evacuating the pneumoperitoneum and making an incision to avoid a difficult anastomosis through a small incision or the need for a larger incision to exteriorize the specimen.

Once the ileum, cecum, and ascending colon are fully mobilized, the instruments are removed. With the pneumoperitoneum still in place, the umbilical port site or the right lower quadrant port site is enlarged. The pneumoperitoneum is evacuated and the specimen is exteriorized. The ileocolonic resection is then completed by dividing the remainder of the mesentery and the bowel extracorporeally. An anastomosis is then constructed in a standard fashion.

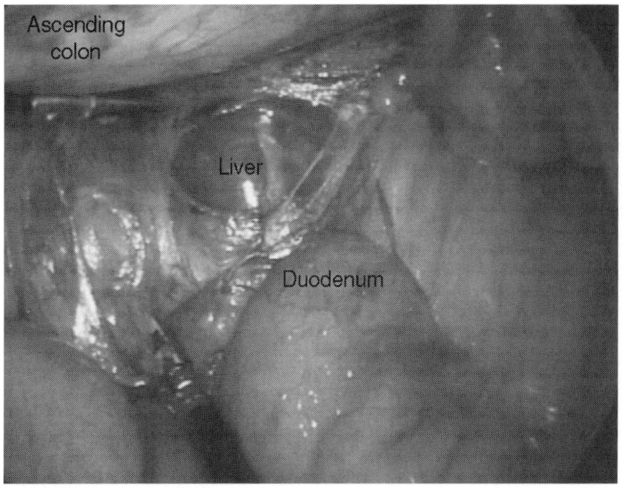

Figure 19–13. Submesenteric mobilization of the ascending colon and hepatic flexure with exposure of the duodenum. (Reprinted, with permission, from the University of Chicago General Surgery Archives.)

▪ MANAGEMENT OF COMPLICATED CROHN'S DISEASE

CROHN'S DISEASE OF THE DUODENUM

Primary Crohn's disease of the duodenum almost always manifests with stricturing disease that can be managed by strictureplasty or with bypass procedures (Fig 19–16). Fortunately, resection of the duodenum for Crohn's disease is almost never required.[153–155] Perforating Crohn's disease almost never affects the duodenum. When the duodenum is involved with Crohn's fistulas, it is always the result of disease within a distal segment (typically the terminal ileum or neoterminal ileum) that fistulizes into an otherwise normal duodenum.[156] Yet, Crohn's disease of the duode-

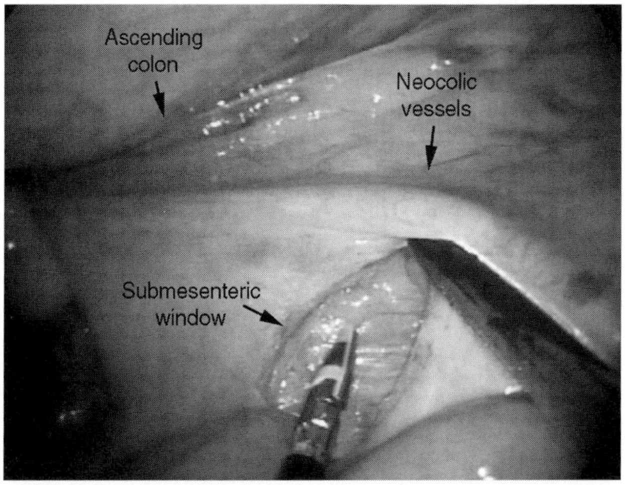

Figure 19–12. Laparoscopic isolation of the ileocolic vessels. (Reprinted, with permission, from the University of Chicago General Surgery Archives.)

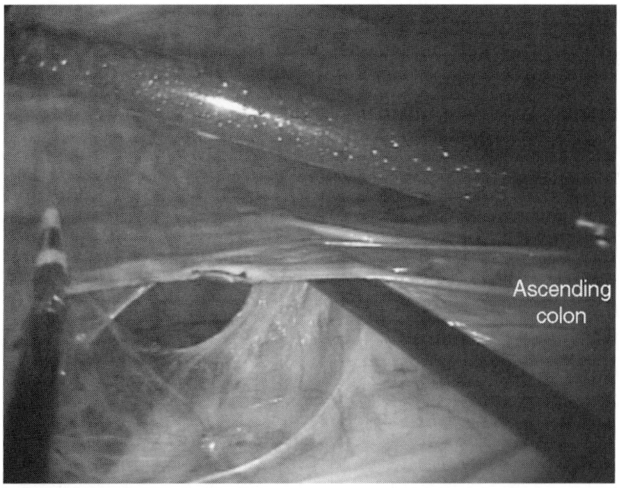

Figure 19–14. Division of the lateral peritoneal attachments to the ascending colon. (Reprinted, with permission, from the University of Chicago General Surgery Archives.)

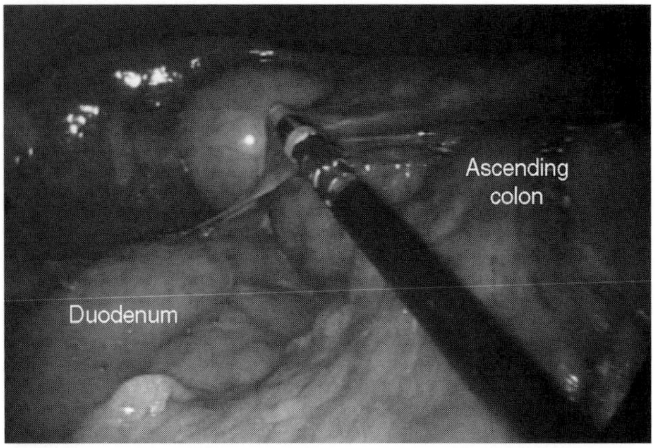

Figure 19–15. Final mobilization of the hepatic flexure. (Reprinted, with permission, from the University of Chicago General Surgery Archives.)

num can offer a particularly challenging problem due to the retroperitoneal location of the organ and its intimate proximity with the pancreas.

Stricturing disease of the duodenum is often focal and many cases can be managed with a Heinecke-Mikulicz strictureplasty.[157] In order to safely accomplish a strictureplasty, the duodenum must be fully mobilized with a generous Kocher maneuver. Strictureplasties can be safely performed in the first, second, and proximal third portion of the duodenum. Strictures of the last portion of the duodenum are better handled with a Finney strictureplasty constructed by creating an enteroenterostomy between the fourth portion of the duodenum and the first loop of the jejunum.

If the duodenal stricture is lengthy or the tissues around the stricture are too rigid or unyielding, then a strictureplasty should not be performed and an intestinal bypass procedure should be undertaken. The most common bypass procedure performed for duodenal Crohn's disease is a simple side-to-side retrocolic gastrojejunostomy.[113] This procedure effectively relieves the symptoms of duodenal obstruction related to Crohn's strictures, but carries a high risk for stomal ulcerations. To lessen the likelihood of ulcerations forming at the anastomosis, it has been recommended that a vagotomy be performed along with the gastrojejunostomy.[113] Because of the concerns of vagotomy-related diarrhea, a highly selective vagotomy is preferred over a truncal vagotomy. If the stricturing Crohn's disease is limited to the third or fourth portions of the duodenum, then a Roux-en-Y duodenojejunostomy to the proximal duodenum is preferred over a gastrojejunostomy.[156] The Roux-en-Y duodenojejunostomy has the advantage of bypassing strictures and eliminates the concern regarding acid-induced marginal ulceration and the need for vagotomy.

As noted above, when the duodenum is involved with a Crohn's fistula, it is almost always the case that the diseased segment is located distal in the GI tract and the duodenum itself is otherwise free of active Crohn's disease.[156] Most of these duodenal fistulas are small in caliber and asymptomatic, but larger fistulas may shunt the duodenal contents to the distal small bowel such that malabsorption and diarrhea result. In the majority of cases, duodenoenteric fistulas are identified with preoperative small bowel radiography; however, many are discovered only at the time of surgery.[158] With complex fistulizing disease involving an inflammatory mass, great care at the time of surgery should be undertaken to limit the size of the duodenal defect resulting from the resection of the fistula. Most duodenal fistulas are located away from the juncture of the duodenal wall at the head of the pancreas, and thus these fistulas can be managed by resection of the primary Crohn's disease with primary closure of the duodenal defect. Larger fistulas or fistulas that are involved with a large degree of inflammation may result in a sizable duodenal defect. Such large defects may require closure with a Roux-en-Y duodenojejunostomy or with a jejunal serosal patch.[158,159] As noted above, duodenal resections are almost never necessary for Crohn's disease and they should be considered the surgical option of last resort.

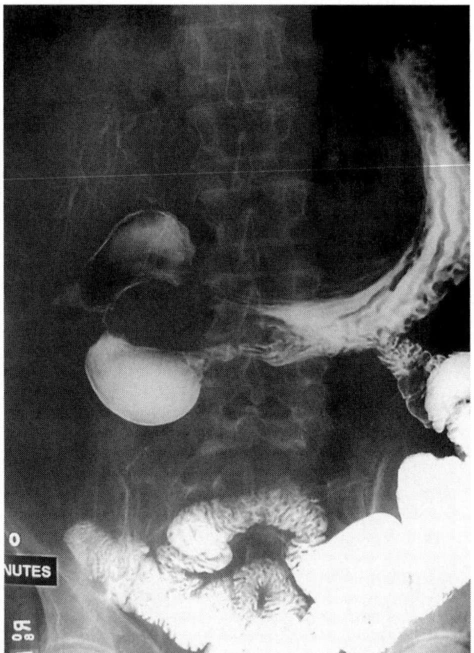

Figure 19–16. Upper GI study demonstrating Crohn's strictures of the duodenum. Contrast seen within the biliary ducts is due to deformity and incompetence of the ampullary sphincter secondary to the Crohn's disease. (Reprinted, with permission, from the University of Chicago General Surgery Archives.)

CROHN'S DISEASE OF THE SMALL BOWEL

Complete Intestinal Obstruction

Complete small intestinal obstruction resulting from Crohn's disease only rarely requires urgent surgical intervention, as the vascular supply to the intestinal loop is never compromised and almost all cases of complete or high-grade partial small bowel obstruction from Crohn's disease respond to conservative management. Such patients should be treated with nasogastric decompression, intravenous hydration, and steroid therapy.[113] This program allows for resolution of the acute episode of obstruction in a vast majority of cases. Unfortunately, most patients whose Crohn's disease is severe enough to experience an episode of complete or high-grade partial obstruction are at high risk for recurrent episodes and persistent symptoms. For this reason, elective surgery should be considered once the episode of complete obstruction has resolved. The advantage of this approach is that surgery can be performed under safer conditions when the obstruction has resolved, the bowel is not distended or edematous, and an appropriate bowel preparation has been performed. If the obstruction fails to respond to appropriate conservative treatment, then surgery is required. In these situations, the surgeon needs to have a high index of suspicion for small bowel cancer as the cause of the obstruction, as obstructions from cancers do not respond to bowel decompression and steroid treatment.

Ileosigmoid Fistulas

Ileosigmoid fistula is a common complication of perforating Crohn's disease of the terminal ileum. Typically, the inflamed terminal ileum adheres to the sigmoid colon that is otherwise normal and free of primary involvement of Crohn's disease. Most ileosigmoid fistulas are small and do not produce any symptoms. Asymptomatic ileosigmoid fistulas do not in and of themselves require operative management. On the other hand, large ileosigmoid fistulas can result in bypass of the intestinal contents from the terminal ileum to the distal colon and thus give rise to debilitating diarrhea (Fig 19–17). Such symptomatic fistulas often fail to respond to medical therapy and should be managed surgically.

More than half of the ileosigmoid fistulas from Crohn's disease are not recognized prior to surgery.[160] For this reason, the surgeon should be prepared to deal with this complication in any case of Crohn's disease that involves the terminal ileum. Ileosigmoid fistulas can be managed by simple division of the fistulous adhesion and resection of the ileal disease. The defect in the sigmoid colon is then débrided and simple closure is undertaken. Seventy-five percent of ileosigmoid fistulas can be managed in this manner.[55,160] The remainder require resection of the sigmoid colon. Sigmoid colon resection is necessary when primary closure of the fistula is at risk for poor healing. This is the case when either the sigmoid is also involved in Crohn's disease, when the fistulous opening is particularly large, or when there is extensive fibrosis extending along the sigmoid colon. Also, fistulous tracts that enter the sigmoid colon in proximity to the mesentery can be difficult to close and often require resection and primary anastomosis.

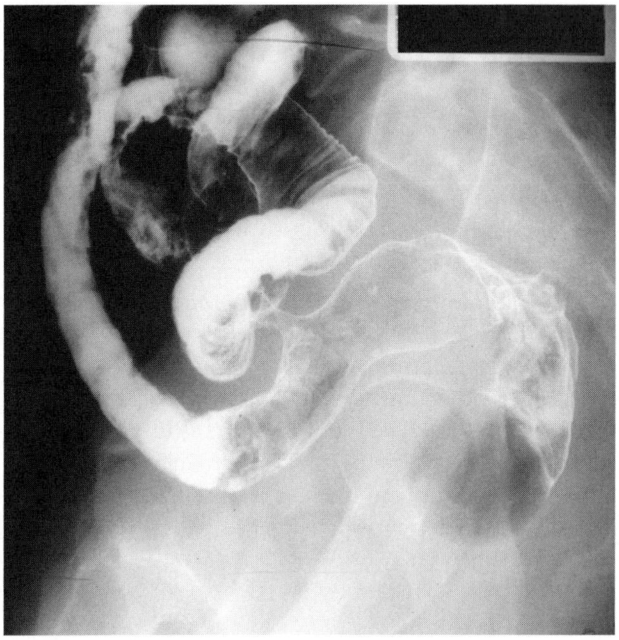

Figure 19–17. Contrast enema demonstrating large ileosigmoid fistula. (Reprinted, with permission, from the University of Chicago General Surgery Archives.)

Ileovesical Fistula

Ileovesical fistulae occur in approximately 5% of Crohn's disease patients.[85] Hematuria and fecaluria are virtually diagnostic of ileovesical fistula but these symptoms are absent in one-third of cases.[161] Small bowel x-rays, cystograms, and cystoscopy often do not detect the fistula. Air within the bladder, as noted on CT scan, is often the best indirect evidence for the presence of an enterovesical fistula. An ileovesical fistula is an indicator of complex fistulizing disease, as most ileovesical fistulas occur along with other enteric fistulae. For example, as many as 60% of patients with an ileovesical fistula will also have an ileosigmoid fistula.[55]

The necessity for surgery for ileovesical fistula is controversial. Many patients with ileovesical fistulae can be managed medically for extended periods of time without significant complications. Healing rates with medical treatment are not clearly defined, but are probably low and most patients with ileovesical fistulae will ultimately come to surgery. Surgery is indicated when recurring urinary infections occur, particularly pyelonephritis, with concomitant potential for worsening of renal function.

Surgical treatment of ileovesical fistulae requires resection of the ileal disease with closure of the bladder defect. Most ileovesical fistulas involve the dome of the bladder, and thus débridement and primary closure can be accomplished without risk of injury to the trigone. Decompression of the bladder with an indwelling Foley catheter should be continued postoperatively until the bladder is confidently healed without leaks. A cystogram taken on postoperative day five is a convenient means for confirming the seal of the bladder repair and the safety of removing the Foley catheter.

Abscess

Intra-abdominal abscesses that result from Crohn's disease tend to follow an indolent course with modest fever, abdominal pain, and leukocytosis. Rapidly progressive and overwhelming sepsis is not typical for the clinical course of Crohn's disease–related abscesses. In fact, in up to one-third of intra-abdominal Crohn's abscesses preoperative clinical signs of localized infection are absent and the abscesses are discovered only at the time of operation. When an abscess is suspected or an abdominal mass is palpated, a CT scan should be obtained, as 50% of tender intra-abdominal masses will harbor an abscess collection within.[92] The CT scan can detect most chronic abscesses and can also delineate the size and location of the abscess as well as the relationship of the abscess to critical structures such as the ureters, duodenum, and the inferior vena cava (Fig 19–18).

Most abscesses with Crohn's disease are in fact very small collections that are contained within the area of diseased intestine and its mesentery. In the case of small intraloop or intramesenteric abscesses, resection of the defective segment and its mesentery often extirpates the abscess such that drains are not necessary and primary anastomosis can be performed without risk.

Large abscesses related to Crohn's disease are best managed with CT-guided percutaneous drainage.[94] Percutaneous drainage is often very effective at controlling the sepsis and healing the abscess cavity.[93] With percutaneous drainage of a Crohn's disease abscess, an enterocutaneous fistula often occurs, as the abscess typically connects to a deeply penetrating sinus emanating from a segment of Crohn's-affected intestine. Percutaneous drainage then completes the fistulous tract from the intestine through the sinus to the abscess cavity and out the drain. Such a fistula may

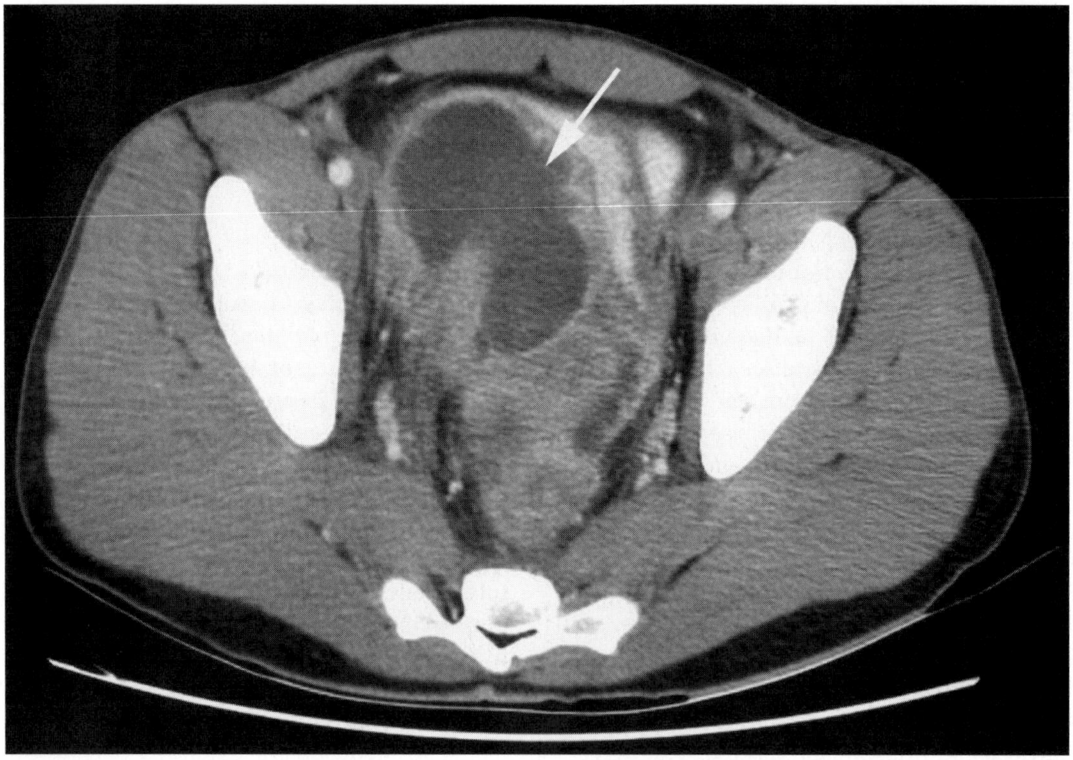

Figure 19–18. CT scan of the pelvis demonstrating large Crohn's abscess. (Reprinted, with permission, from the University of Chicago General Surgery Archives.)

spontaneously close or it may persist and the intestine may continue to be a source of sepsis. With successful drainage of the abscess, the sepsis often clears well enough that it can be tempting to try to manage the disease without subsequent surgery. Published clinical data on the optimal approach to such patients are unfortunately lacking. Even so, in the absence of Crohn's symptoms, initial nonoperative management after successful percutaneous drainage can be undertaken in carefully selected patients.[95] On the other hand, if drainage through the fistula continues, surgical resection of the affected segment of intestine becomes necessary.

Perforation

Free perforation is a surprisingly uncommon phenomenon because the chronic progressive inflammation of Crohn's disease normally leads to adhesions with adjacent structures. Most perforations from Crohn's disease occur in the ileum and are usually proximal to a stenotic lesion.[96,113] The diagnosis of free perforation is made by detecting a sudden change in the patient's symptoms along with the development of the physical findings of peritonitis or the identification of free intra-peritoneal air as demonstrated on plain x-rays or CT scans. Free perforation is an absolute indication for emergent laparotomy with resection of the diseased segment and exteriorization of the proximal bowel as an end-ileostomy. Primary closure of the perforation should never be attempted, as sutures will not be able to approximate the edges of the perforated, edematous, and diseased bowel in a satisfactory and tension-free way. The distal bowel end can be exteriorized as a mucous fistula or closed as a defunctionalized pouch, depending on the degree of peritoneal contamination. In the presence of free perforation, creation of a primary anastomosis even with a proximal protecting loop ileostomy carries a high risk of anastomotic breakdown and should be avoided.

Hemorrhage

Hemorrhage from small bowel Crohn's disease is managed by resection of the diseased portion of intestine. For patients with multiple skip areas of Crohn's disease, small bowel angiography may be attempted to localize the exact site of bleeding.[97] Localization with angiography may be unsuccessful if the bleeding is episodic or insufficiently brisk to be identified with angiography. In those cases in whom small bowel hemorrhage stops spontaneously, the risk for rebleeding is high. Thus elective resection of active Crohn's disease after the first episode of hemorrhage should be considered.

CROHN'S DISEASE OF THE COLON

The optimal management of Crohn's disease of the colon is dependent on the distribution and the location of the disease (Fig 19–19).

Cecal Disease

Colonic disease limited to the cecum is almost always associated with terminal ileal disease. The terminal ileitis is the predominant component of the ileocecal disease. Terminal ileal disease with extension into the cecum behaves much like disease limited to the terminal ileum. For this pattern of disease, surgical resection should encompass the margins of gross disease with an anastomosis between the neoterminal ileum and the proximal ascending colon. Recurrence of disease at the anastomosis or at the preanastomotic ileum is common but the risk for recurrent disease within the distal colon or the rectum is low. This pattern of disease does not imply a predisposition to more extensive colonic disease.

Right-Sided Colitis

Disease involving the entire right colon can occur alone but more typically occurs along with disease of the terminal ileum. Extensive involvement of the right colon as a form of ileocolonic disease is less common than the ileocecal pattern. Surgical treatment involves a standard right hemicolectomy to encompass the gross limits of the disease. An anastomosis between the ileum

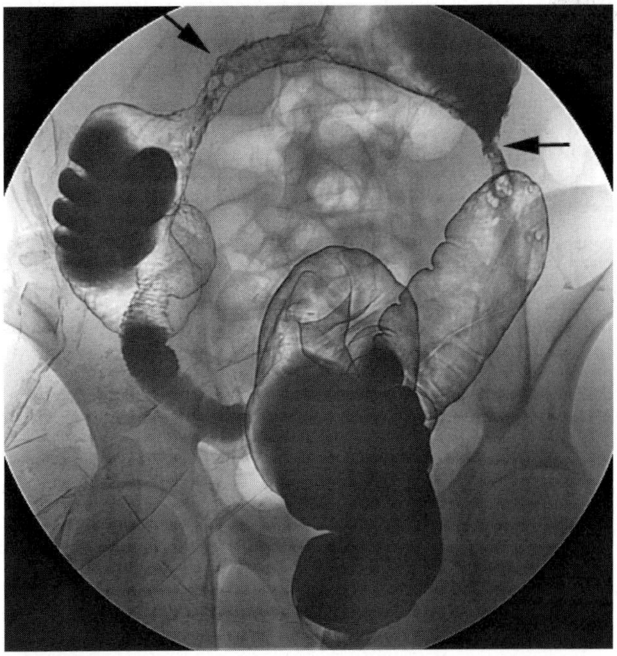

Figure 19–19. Contrast enema demonstrating severe Crohn's colitis with multiple high-grade strictures. (Reprinted, with permission, from the University of Chicago General Surgery Archives.)

and the transverse colon is then fashioned. With a standard right hemicolectomy, the anastomosis may rest in proximity to the duodenum. Recurrent disease at the preanastomotic ileum may thus secondarily involve the duodenum. This phenomenon can place the patient at risk for substantial morbidity should inflammatory encasement of the duodenum or fistulization into the duodenum occur. For this reason it is advantageous to protect the duodenum by interposing omentum between the duodenum and the ileocolonic anastomosis.

Extensive Colitis with Rectal Sparing

Extensive colitis with sparing of the rectum occurs in approximately 20% of individuals suffering from Crohn's colitis. In such cases, the rectum should be closely examined endoscopically and should the rectum be truly free of disease, then a total abdominal colectomy with ileorectal anastomosis can be performed when fecal continence is adequate and the patient does not have extensive perineal septic complications. This procedure often results in good long-term function and enables many patients to avoid an ileostomy. Older patients or patients who have undergone an extensive small bowel resection may experience frequent and loose stools to the point that incontinence may develop after an ileorectal anastomosis. Additionally, recurrent disease within the rectum can result in significant deterioration of bowel function requiring further medical or even surgical intervention. Up to 50% of patients who undergo an ileorectal anastomosis for colonic Crohn's disease will ultimately require a proctectomy with permanent ileostomy due to poor bowel function with incontinence or due to recurrence of disease in the rectum.[162]

Proctocolitis

Surgical management of extensive involvement of the colon and rectum requires total proctocolectomy with permanent ileostomy in almost all cases. In most instances, a total proctocolectomy can be performed in a single step. The presence of severe perianal disease, however, may require that the procedure be performed in two stages. At the first stage, the intra-abdominal colon and majority of the rectum are removed and a short rectal stump is created at the level of the levator muscles. At the same time, perineal abscesses are drained and fistulas are laid open. This first step removes the diseased colon and rectum without creating a perineal wound that may be difficult to heal in the presence of active perineal sepsis. Once the perineal sepsis is cleared and the perineum is healed, the short anorectal stump can be removed through a perineal approach. At this second stage, primary closure of the perineum can be accomplished without the high risk of persistent perineal wounds.

Restorative procedures such as an ileal pouch–anal anastomosis or continent ileostomy have traditionally not been offered to patients who have Crohn's colitis because of the recurrent nature of the disease. Even so, some of these procedures have been performed in patients whose diagnosis of Crohn's disease was not known or suspected at the time of surgery. Various reports indicate that recurrence of Crohn's disease within the pouch is common and removal of the pouch is often necessary. On the other hand, those patients who do not suffer from recurrent disease generally do well and typically experience good pouch function.

While it is commonly accepted that restorative proctocolectomy with J-pouch ileoanal anastomosis should not be undertaken for Crohn's colitis, there is a specific pattern of Crohn's disease that appears to be at low risk for problems with recurrence after an ileoanal anastomosis.[163,164] In cases in whom Crohn's disease is limited to the colon and rectum without any history of small bowel involvement and without any perineal manifestations, the risk for pouch failure after ileoanal anastomosis appears to be low, and such patients can be considered for the ileoanal procedure. This particular pattern of Crohn's disease, however, is rare, as most patients with Crohn's proctocolitis will have some degree of small bowel involvement or perineal manifestations and thus would not be considered candidates for the ileoanal procedure.

Proctitis

Crohn's inflammation limited to the rectum is unusual. Surgical management of Crohn's proctitis mandates proctectomy with permanent stoma. The need for resection of the normal proximal colon is controversial. Abdominoperineal resection with end sigmoid colostomy has been associated in some reports with a high risk for stomal complications and recurrent disease in the proximal intestine when compared to total proctocolectomy with end ileostomy. For these reasons, total proctocolectomy with ileostomy has been recommended for Crohn's disease limited to the rectum and distal colon. This more extensive resection may be of greater value in younger patients who have no history of small bowel Crohn's disease, as it appears that colorectal Crohn's disease without small bowel involvement is unlikely to result in recurrence within the small bowel once a proctocolectomy is performed.[40] If the patient has undergone a prior resection for small bowel Crohn's disease, they may be at risk for high output from the ileostomy, and therefore these patients may benefit from the preservation of colonic absorptive capacity. Preservation of the colonic absorptive capacity may be beneficial also in the elderly patient. Thus these patients may be better managed with a proctectomy and end sigmoid colostomy.

Proctectomy for Crohn's disease does not require a wide excision of perirectal tissue. To avoid injury to pelvic sympathetic and parasympathetic nerves, the dissection should be undertaken close to the rectal wall. In the absence of significant perianal disease, the perineal dissection is best carried out along the plane between the internal and external sphincters.[165] This intersphincteric dissection allows for a perineal closure that is associated with fewer complications and better healing than wider dissections that encompass the entire sphincter mechanism. In some patients, fistula from the perianal Crohn's disease can traverse the intersphincteric plane and a wider dissection is required in order to encompass the diseased tissue. In the presence of significant perianal disease a staged approach, as described above, can be utilized as an option. Occasionally, however, because of extensive rectal disease, closure of the rectal stump may be technically challenging or not feasible, forcing the surgeon to proceed with a proctectomy in the face of perianal sepsis. These dissections may need to be carried out widely and extensive loss of perianal skin and subcutaneous tissue may occur. The resultant defects are often too large for primary closure and closure may require advanced tissue transfer techniques such as gluteal flaps, gracilis flaps, or myocutaneous rectus abdominis pedicle flaps. These closures may have to be staged as well in the presence of perineal sepsis. Large open perineal wounds may be managed temporarily or definitively with the assistance of the vacuum assisted closure device. This device allows for rapid contracture of the wound and facilitates healing.

Segmental Colitis

The optimal management of segmental colitis is dependent primarily upon the location of the disease, and secondarily upon the presence and severity of concurrent perineal complications, the degree of fecal continence, and the natural history of the disease in the residual colon. Segmental involvement of the right colon should be managed by simple right hemicolectomy with ileotransverse anastomosis. For segmental disease involving the transverse colon, an extended right hemicolectomy is generally preferred over a segmental transverse colectomy. Such an approach may have a lower risk of recurrence compared to a segmental resection of the transverse colon. Additionally, the extended right hemicolectomy avoids a colocolonic anastomosis that is associated with a higher risk for anastomotic leak.

For disease in the descending or sigmoid colon, the appropriate surgery is more controversial. Presence and severity of concurrent perineal complications, the degree of fecal continence, and the natural history of the disease in the residual colon all play a role in deciding on the approach for each individual patient. Studies have indicated that segmental colonic resection with colocolonic anastomosis or even colonic strictureplasty can be performed with overall good results.[166,167] However, such a strategy may be at risk for early disease recurrence within the colon.[40] Even if the risk for recurrence is higher with segmental resection, the benefits of preserving the absorptive capacity in appropriately selected cases may outweigh the higher risk of recurrence.

Perianal Disease

The perianal manifestations of Crohn's disease include abscesses, fistulas, fissures, anal stenosis, and hypertrophic skin tags.[168,169] Perianal Crohn's disease originates from inflammation within the anal crypts. This inflammation gives rise to sepsis and to fistulization (Fig 19–20). Perianal Crohn's disease is common and occurs in one-third of the patients who suffer from intestinal Crohn's disease.[42] Perianal Crohn's disease is usually associated with active or quiescent disease elsewhere within the gastrointestinal tract. It is controversial as to whether the activity of perianal Crohn's disease parallels the activity of the intestinal disease. There is also controversy over whether medical or surgical control of the intestinal disease can ameliorate the perianal manifestations. Unlike idiopathic perianal abscesses and fistula-in-ano that occur in patients without Crohn's disease, perianal Crohn's disease tends to be recurrent, complex, and sometimes progressive.

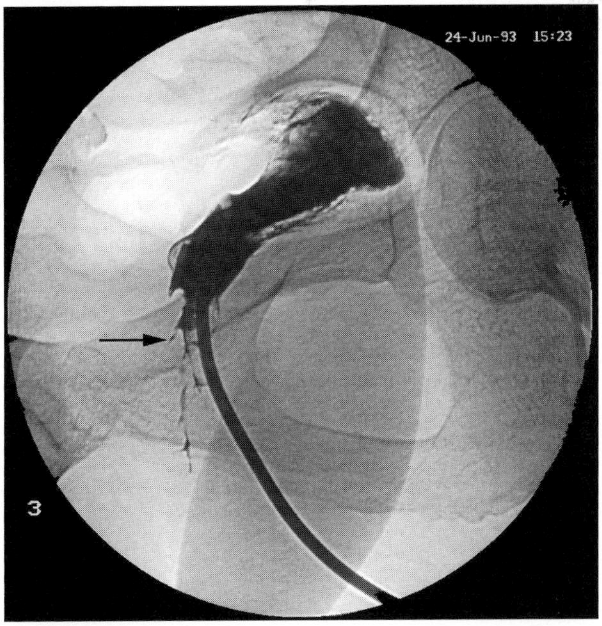

Figure 19–20. Dynamic proctogram demonstrating Crohn's fistula-in-ano. (Reprinted, with permission, from the University of Chicago General Surgery Archives.)

Surgical incision and drainage is required to manage perianal abscesses (Fig 19–21). Attempts at treating purulent collections with antibiotics alone are invariably unsuccessful. With surgical drainage of the abscess the incision should be placed close to the anal margin. The cavity may be packed with ribbon gauze or drained with a 10–16F mushroom catheter. If at the time of drainage of the suppuration a fistula tract can be identified, then a loose seton may be placed to ensure adequate drainage.

Uncomplicated submucosal or intersphincteric fistulas are best treated with an initial trial of either metronidazole or ciprofloxacin. These antibiotics are moderately effective in promoting healing of Crohn's fistulas and are associated with a low risk of complication.[170,171] If a low-lying submucosal or intersphincteric fistula fails to heal with antibiotic treatment, then a surgical fistulotomy can be performed. These low-lying fistulas typically heal well after fistulotomy and the risk of incontinence is low.

Surgical fistulotomies and cutting setons should not be used for suprasphincteric fistulas and should also be avoided for most transsphincteric fistulas. For complex fistulas, the risk for surgical complications is higher and more aggressive medical therapy is warranted before surgery is recommended. Medical treatment for extensive Crohn's fistulas includes the use of 6-mercaptopurine, azathioprine, and cyclosporine. Probably the most effective agent at promoting healing of perianal fistulas related to Crohn's disease is infliximab. With infliximab treatment, healing of complex perianal fistulas is seen in 60% of cases.[172,173] Recurrence of the fistula after infliximab, however, may be high. Additionally, persistent stasis or sepsis within the fistula tract can impede effective healing with medical treatment. To provide for adequate drainage throughout the fistula tract, many patients may benefit from placement of setons. The use of setons with infliximab therapy can improve the overall effectiveness of infliximab.[174] Typically the seton is placed prior to the initiation of infliximab therapy and then it is removed after the second or third dose.

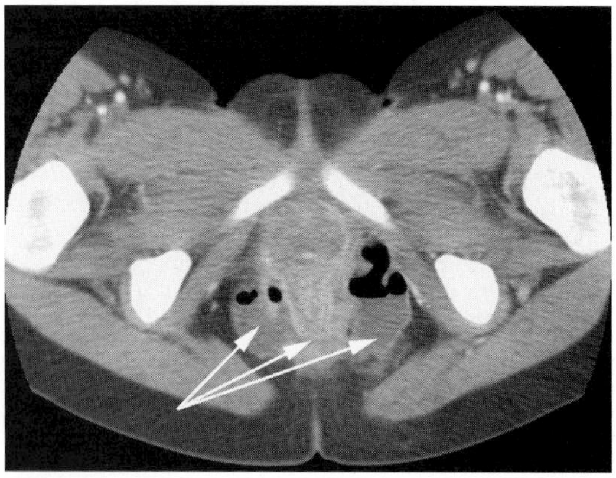

Figure 19–21. CT scan demonstrating a large perirectal abscess secondary to Crohn's disease. (Reprinted, with permission, from the University of Chicago General Surgery Archives.)

Fibrin glue has been used for the treatment of Crohn's disease–related fistulas, but reported experience is limited. Success rates with this approach are low but given the low risk of complications, an attempt at fibrin glue may be worthwhile in selected cases.[175,176]

Closure of the internal opening of the fistula with a rectal advancement flap can be considered in cases of Crohn's disease.[177] With this approach, an incision is made at the dentate line and an advancement flap of mucosa and muscularis is undermined and drawn down over the internal opening of the fistula. The advancement flap is then sutured into position with absorbable sutures. Rectal advancement flaps for Crohn's disease have a low risk for anal incontinence, but are associated with a high failure rate. Rectal advancement flaps are not appropriate in cases in whom the rectal mucosa is involved with Crohn's disease. In severe cases of perianal disease that do not respond to aggressive medical and surgical therapy, fecal diversion with a stoma may be necessary. Diversion of the fecal stream typically results in significant relief of local inflammation and can assist in the healing of perianal fistulas. Proctectomy is indicated when perianal disease is unrelenting or when damage to the sphincters results in debilitating incontinence.

RECURRENT DISEASE

Crohn's disease carries a high risk for recurrence after surgery. The actual incidence of recurrent disease depends on the defining parameters of recurrence. For example, histological evidence for recurrence can be seen in many patients within days of surgical resection.[178] Endoscopic evidence for recurrent Crohn's disease can be seen in over 80% of patients within 3 years.[179] Most cases of histological or endoscopically detected recurrences, however, do not go on to produce symptoms of Crohn's disease. For this reason, histological or endoscopic evidence of recurrent disease may be used as an end point in investigative studies, but are not typically used as a guide for clinical management.[180]

The development of symptoms related to recurrent Crohn's disease activity is the most commonly applied definition of disease recurrence, as it is the recurrence of symptoms that has the most relevance to the patient. The onset of symptoms of recurrent Crohn's disease is often insidious and the severity of symptoms varies greatly. To create a reproducible standard for recurrence of Crohn's disease symptoms, the Crohn's Disease Activity Index (CDAI) can be applied as a means of measuring recurrent disease.[181,182] A CDAI of greater than 150 is generally accepted as defining clinical recurrence. Once symptoms suggestive of recurrent disease occur, it is still necessary to carry out radiological and endoscopic tests to confirm that the symptoms are in fact related to Crohn's.

The clearest end point as a definition of recurrence is the need for reoperation. Dates of surgery are readily documented even in a retrospective fashion. While reoperation is the most precise definition of recurrence, even this standard does not allow for accurate and reproducible comparisons between series, as some centers may submit patients to surgery earlier than other centers.

Reported crude and cumulative recurrence rates vary greatly. Symptomatic or clinical recurrence occurs in about 60% of patients at 5 years and recurrences increase with time such that at 20 years clinical recurrence can occur in between 75% and 95% of cases.[35,183,184] Reports of surgical recurrence rates range from 10–30% at 5 years, 20–45% at 10 years, and 50–70% at 20 years.[63,86,183–187] Some interesting observations regarding the pattern of recurrent disease have been made. Recurrent Crohn's disease is most likely to occur in proximity to the location of the previously resected intestinal segment, typically at the anastomosis and pre-anastomotic bowel.[86] This is particularly true for terminal ileal disease. Additionally, the length of small bowel involved with recurrent disease parallels the length of disease originally resected.[188,189] Short segment disease tends to recur over a short segment of the pre-anastomotic bowel, and lengthy disease typically is followed by lengthy recurrence. Also, to a lesser degree of concordance, stenotic disease tends to recur as stenotic disease and perforating disease tends to recur as perforating disease.[189]

While many factors that may influence the risk of recurrence have been studied, the cumulative literature has validated very few as true risk factors. The data are conflicting for most of the proposed predictors of recurrent Crohn's disease. Much of the clinical data examining potential risk factors are confounded by poorly defined end points and improper study design. There is, however, general consensus that cigarette smoking has a significant effect on the clinical course of Crohn's disease.[30] Smoking not only exacerbates existing Crohn's disease, but also has been identified as a risk factor for the development of Crohn's.[27,28,30] What is so striking about the effect of cigarettes on Crohn's disease is that smoking has the opposite effect on what is thought to be a very similar disease, ulcerative colitis.[29] While smoking exacerbates Crohn's disease, it seems to lessen the activity of ulcerative colitis.

The mechanism by which smoking results in exacerbation of Crohn's disease is not known. Smoking is an independent risk factor for endoscopic, symptomatic, and surgical recurrence.[31,32] The risk from smoking appeared to be dose-related with heavy smokers being at higher risk. This effect is reversible, as smokers who quit smoking prior to surgery can lower their risk of recurrence to a level similar to that of nonsmokers. Because of the harmful effects on the clinical course of Crohn's disease combined with the many other clearly established health hazards caused by cigarette smoking, all patients with Crohn's disease should be strongly counseled to quit smoking.

There is concern that NSAIDs may exacerbate the activity of both ulcerative colitis and Crohn's disease.[63,76] Although there are no studies that have examined the specific issue of NSAIDs and the risks for postoperative recurrence of Crohn's disease, the currently available data certainly warrant some caution and patients with Crohn's disease should be advised to avoid nonsteroidal anti-inflammatory drugs.

▪ POSTOPERATIVE MAINTENANCE THERAPY

The risk for recurrent disease can be lessened with postoperative maintenance therapy. The most common agents employed for postoperative suppression of disease are controlled-release 5-aminosalicylic acid (5-ASA; Pentasa) and 6-mercaptopurine (6-MP).[71–73] Maintenance with 5-ASA is associated with few side effects, but up to sixteen pills have to be taken daily. 6-Mercaptopurine is less expensive and is taken on a once-daily basis. Additionally, 6-MP may be more effective in diminishing the risk of recurrence.[71] 6-MP, however, is associated with potential bone marrow suppression, so that patients on 6-MP maintenance must be followed with periodic blood cell counts. The effect of these agents on the natural course of Crohn's disease is not dramatic and many patients will go on to develop recurrence while on maintenance therapy. The largest benefit demonstrated with 6-MP in a multicenter trial showed a decrease of symptomatic recurrence from 77% with placebo to 50% with 6-MP.[71] The option for maintenance therapy should be considered for Crohn's disease patients, but the decision for such therapy must be individualized for each patient.

REFERENCES

1. Crohn BB, Ginsberg L, Oppenheimer GD. Regional ileitis: a pathological and clinical entity. *JAMA* 1932;99: 1323–1329
2. Fielding JF. Crohn's disease and Dalziel's syndrome. A history. *J Clin Gastroenterol* 1988;10:279–285
3. Morgagni G. *The Seats and Causes of Disease Investigated by Anatomy.* Mount Kisco, NY: Futura Publishing; 1769
4. Kirsner JB. Etiologic concepts of inflammatory bowel disease; past, present, and future. In: Michelassi F, Milsom JW (eds). *Operative Strategies in Inflammatory Bowel Disease.* New York, NY: Springer-Verlag; 1999:3–20

5. Dalziel TK. Chronic intestinal enteritis. *BMJ* 1913;2:1068–1070
6. Heaton LD, Ravdin IS, Blades B, Whelan TJ. President Eisenhower's operation for regional enteritis: a footnote to history. *Ann Surg* 1964;159:661–666
7. Hughes CW, Baugh JH, Mologne LA et al. A review of the late General Eisenhower's operations: epilog to a footnote to history. *Ann Surg* 1971;173:793–799
8. Bergman L, Krause U. Crohn's disease. A long-term study of the clinical course in 186 patients. *Scand J Gastroenterol* 1977;12:937–944
9. Koudahl G, Kristensen M, Lenz K. Bypass compared with resection for ileal Crohn's disease. *Scand J Gastroenterol* 1974;9:203–206
10. Homan WP, Dineen P. Comparison of the results of resection, bypass, and bypass with exclusion for ileocecal Crohn's disease. *Ann Surg* 1978;187:530–535
11. Alexander-Williams J, Fielding JF, Cooke WT. A comparison of results of excision and bypass for ileal Crohn's disease. *Gut* 1972;13:973–975
12. Lockhart-Mummery H, Morson B. Crohn's disease (regional enteritis) of the large intestine and its distinction from ulcerative colitis. *Gut* 1960;1:87–105
13. Loftus EV Jr. Clinical epidemiology of inflammatory bowel disease: Incidence, prevalence, and environmental influences. *Gastroenterology* 2004;126:1504–1517
14. Sandler RS, Glenn ME. Epidemiology of inflammatory bowel disease. In: Kirsner JB (ed). *Inflammatory Bowel Disease*, 5th ed. Philadelphia, PA: WB Saunders; 2000:89–112
15. Ekbom A. The epidemiology of IBD: a lot of data but little knowledge. How shall we proceed? *Inflamm Bowel Dis* 2004;10(Suppl 1):S32–S34
16. Leong RW, Lau JY, Sung JJ. The epidemiology and phenotype of Crohn's disease in the Chinese population. *Inflamm Bowel Dis* 2004;10:646–651
17. Hollander D, Vadheim CM, Brettholz E et al. Increased intestinal permeability in patients with Crohn's disease and their relatives. A possible etiologic factor. *Ann Intern Med* 1986;105:883–885
18. Wyatt J, Vogelsang H, Hubl W et al. Intestinal permeability and the prediction of relapse in Crohn's disease. *Lancet* 1993;341:1437–1439
19. Wyatt J, Oberhuber G, Pongratz S et al. Increased gastric and intestinal permeability in patients with Crohn's disease. *Am J Gastroenterol* 1997;92:1891–1896
20. Puspok A, Oberhuber G, Wyatt J et al. Gastroduodenal permeability in Crohn's disease. *Eur J Clin Invest* 1998;28:67–71
21. May GR, Sutherland LR, Meddings JB. Is small intestinal permeability really increased in relatives of patients with Crohn's disease? *Gastroenterology* 1993;104:1627–1632
22. Cho JH. Advances in the genetics of inflammatory bowel disease. *Curr Gastroenterol Rep* 2004;6:467–473
23. Cho JH. Significant role of genetics in IBD: the NOD2 gene. *Rev Gastroenterol Disord* 2003;3(Suppl 1):S18–S22
24. Gasche C, Grundtner P. Genotypes and phenotypes in Crohn's disease: do they help in clinical management? *Gut* 2005;54:162–167
25. Grimm MC, Pavli P. NOD2 mutations and Crohn's disease: are Paneth cells and their antimicrobial peptides the link? *Gut* 2004;53:1558–1560
26. Sartor R. Microbial influences in inflammatory bowel diseases: role in pathogenesis and clinical implications. In: Sartor R, Sandborn W (eds). *Kirsner's Inflammatory Bowel Diseases*. New York, NY: Saunders; 2004:120–137
27. Thomas GA, Rhodes J, Green JT. Inflammatory bowel disease and smoking—a review. *Am J Gastroenterol* 1998;93:144–149
28. Cosnes J, Carbonnel F, Beaugerie L et al. Effects of cigarette smoking on the long-term course of Crohn's disease. *Gastroenterology* 1996;110:424–431
29. Rhodes J, Thomas GA. Smoking: good or bad for inflammatory bowel disease? *Gastroenterology* 1994;106:807–810
30. Birrenbach T, Bocker U. Inflammatory bowel disease and smoking: a review of epidemiology, pathophysiology, and therapeutic implications. *Inflamm Bowel Dis* 2004;10:848–859
31. Kane SV, Flicker M, Katz-Nelson F. Tobacco use is associated with accelerated clinical recurrence of Crohn's disease after surgically induced remission. *J Clin Gastroenterol* 2005;39:32–35
32. Cottone M, Rosselli M, Orlando A et al. Smoking habits and recurrence in Crohn's disease. *Gastroenterology* 1994;106:643–648
33. Kleer CG, Appelman HD. Surgical pathology of Crohn's disease. *Surg Clin North Am* 2001;81:13–30, vii
34. Block GE, Michelassi F, Tanaka M et al. Crohn's disease. *Curr Probl Surg* 1993;30:173–265
35. Mekhjian HS, Switz DM, Melnyk CS et al. Clinical features and natural history of Crohn's disease. *Gastroenterology* 1979;77(4 Pt 2):898–906
36. Gasche C, Scholmerich J, Brynskov J et al. A simple classification of Crohn's disease: report of the Working Party for the World Congresses of Gastroenterology, Vienna 1998. *Inflamm Bowel Dis* 2000;6:8–15
37. Steinhart AH, Girgrah N, McLeod RS. Reliability of a Crohn's disease clinical classification scheme based on disease behavior. *Inflamm Bowel Dis* 1998;4:228–234
38. Yamamoto T, Allan RN, Keighley MR. An audit of gastroduodenal Crohn disease: clinicopathologic features and management. *Scand J Gastroenterol* 1999;34:1019–1024
39. Decker GA, Loftus EV Jr, Pasha TM et al. Crohn's disease of the esophagus: clinical features and outcomes. *Inflamm Bowel Dis* 2001;7:113–119
40. Hurst RD, Melis M, Michelassi F. Surgery for Crohn's colitis. In: Bayless TM, Hanauer SB (eds). *Advanced Therapy of Inflammatory Bowel Disease*. Hamilton, Ontario, Canada: BC Decker; 2001:495–500
41. Rankin GB, Watts HD, Melnyk CS et al. National Cooperative Crohn's Disease Study: extraintestinal manifestations and perianal complications. *Gastroenterology* 1979;77(4 Pt 2):914–920
42. Michelassi F, Melis M, Rubin M et al. Surgical treatment of anorectal complications in Crohn's disease. *Surgery* 2000;128:597–603
43. Isaacs K. Extra-intestinal manifestations. In: Bayless TM, Hanauer SB (eds). *Advanced Therapy of Inflammatory*

Bowel Disease. Hamilton, Ontario, Canada: BC Decker; 2001:267–270
44. Loftus EV Jr. Management of extraintestinal manifestations and other complications of inflammatory bowel disease. *Curr Gastroenterol Rep* 2004;6:506–513
45. Mintz R, Feller ER, Bahr RL et al. Ocular manifestations of inflammatory bowel disease. *Inflamm Bowel Dis* 2004; 10:135–139
46. Schreyer AG, Seitz J, Feuerbach S et al. Modern imaging using computed tomography and magnetic resonance imaging for inflammatory bowel disease (IBD) AU1. *Inflamm Bowel Dis* 2004;10:45–54
47. Orel SG, Rubesin SE, Jones B et al. Computed tomography vs. barium studies in the acutely symptomatic patient with Crohn disease. *J Comput Assist Tomogr* 1987;11: 1009–1016
48. Munkholm P, Binder V. Clinical features and natural history of Crohn's disease. In: Sartor R, Sandborn WJ (eds). *Kirshner's Inflammatory Bowel Diseases,* 6th ed. New York, NY: Saunders; 2004:289–300
49. Nolan DJ. The radiological appearances of small intestinal Crohn's disease with the enteroclysis technique. *Acta Gastroenterol Belg* 1987;50:513–518
50. Chernish SM, Maglinte DD, O'Connor K. Evaluation of the small intestine by enteroclysis for Crohn's disease. *Am J Gastroenterol* 1992;87:696–701
51. Bernstein CN, Boult IF, Greenberg HM et al. A prospective randomized comparison between small bowel enteroclysis and small bowel follow-through in Crohn's disease. *Gastroenterology* 1997;113:390–398
52. Cirillo LC, Camera L, Della Noce M et al. Accuracy of enteroclysis in Crohn's disease of the small bowel: a retrospective study. *Eur Radiol* 2000;10:1894–1898
53. Rutgeerts P, Vantrappen G, Geboes K. Endoscopy in inflammatory bowel disease. *Scand J Gastroenterol Suppl* 1989;170:12–15; discussion 6–9
54. Michelassi F, Stella M, Balestracci T et al. Incidence, diagnosis, and treatment of enteric and colorectal fistulae in patients with Crohn's disease. *Ann Surg* 1993;218: 660–666
55. Schraut WH, Chapman C, Abraham VS. Operative treatment of Crohn's ileocolitis complicated by ileosigmoid and ileovesical fistulae. *Ann Surg* 1988;207:48–51
56. Otterson MF, Lundeen SJ, Spinelli KS et al. Radiographic underestimation of small bowel stricturing Crohn's disease: a comparison with surgical findings. *Surgery* 2004;136:854–860
57. Kornbluth A, Legnani P, Lewis BS. Video capsule endoscopy in inflammatory bowel disease: past, present, and future. *Inflamm Bowel Dis* 2004;10:278–285
58. Voderholzer WA, Beinhoelzl J, Rogalla P et al. Small bowel involvement in Crohn's disease: a prospective comparison of wireless capsule endoscopy and computed tomography enteroclysis. *Gut* 2005;54:369–373
59. Fishman EK, Wolf EJ, Jones B et al. CT evaluation of Crohn's disease: effect on patient management. *AJR Am J Roentgenol* 1987;148:537–540
60. Zalis M, Singh AK. Imaging of inflammatory bowel disease: CT and MR. *Dig Dis* 2004;22:56–62
61. American Thoracic Society. Targeted tuberculin testing and treatment of latent tuberculosis infection. *MMWR Recomm Rep* 2000;49(RR-6):1–51
62. Bjarnason I, Zanelli G, Smith T et al. Nonsteroidal anti-inflammatory drug-induced intestinal inflammation in humans. *Gastroenterology* 1987;93:480–489
63. Gibson GR, Whitacre EB, Ricotti CA. Colitis induced by nonsteroidal anti-inflammatory drugs. Report of four cases and review of the literature. *Arch Intern Med* 1992; 152:625–632
64. Summers RW, Switz DM, Sessions JT Jr et al. National Cooperative Crohn's Disease Study: results of drug treatment. *Gastroenterology* 1979;77(4 Pt 2):847–869
65. Hanauer SB, Stein RB. Medical therapy. In: Michelassi F, Milsom JW (eds). *Operative Strategies in Inflammatory Bowel Disease.* New York, NY: Springer-Verlag; 1999:138–149
66. Edsbacker S, Andersson T. Pharmacokinetics of budesonide (Entocort EC) capsules for Crohn's disease. *Clin Pharmacokinet* 2004;43:803–821
67. Hofer KN. Oral budesonide in the management of Crohn's disease. *Ann Pharmacother* 2003;37:1457–1464
68. Lichtenstein GR, Hanauer SB, Kane SV et al. Crohn's is not a 6-week disease: lifelong management of mild to moderate Crohn's disease. *Inflamm Bowel Dis* 2004; 10(Suppl 2):S2–S10
69. Mahadevan U, Sandborn WJ. Clinical pharmacology of inflammatory bowel disease. In: Sartor R, Sandborn WJ (eds). *Kirshner's Inflammatory Bowel Diseases,* 6th ed. New York, NY: Saunders; 2004:484–502
70. Caprilli R, Corrao G, Taddei G et al. Prognostic factors for postoperative recurrence of Crohn's disease. Gruppo Italiano per lo Studio del Colon e del Retto (GISC). *Dis Colon Rectum* 1996;39:335–341
71. Hanauer SB, Korelitz BI, Rutgeerts P et al. Postoperative maintenance of Crohn's disease remission with 6-mercaptopurine, mesalamine, or placebo: a 2-year trial. *Gastroenterology* 2004;127:723–729
72. Lochs H, Mayer M, Fleig WE et al. Prophylaxis of postoperative relapse in Crohn's disease with mesalamine: European Cooperative Crohn's Disease Study VI. *Gastroenterology* 2000;118:264–273
73. McLeod RS, Wolff BG, Steinhart AH et al. Prophylactic mesalamine treatment decreases postoperative recurrence of Crohn's disease. *Gastroenterology* 1995;109:404–413
74. Harrell LE, Hanauer SB. Mesalamine derivatives in the treatment of Crohn's disease. *Gastroenterol Clin North Am* 2004;33:303–317, ix–x
75. Bjarnason I, Peters TJ. Intestinal permeability, non-steroidal anti-inflammatory drug enteropathy and inflammatory bowel disease: an overview. *Gut* 1989;30(Spec No):22–28
76. Kaufmann HJ, Taubin HL. Nonsteroidal anti-inflammatory drugs activate quiescent inflammatory bowel disease. *Ann Intern Med* 1987;107:513–516
77. Felder JB, Korelitz BI, Rajapakse R et al. Effects of nonsteroidal antiinflammatory drugs on inflammatory bowel disease: a case-control study. *Am J Gastroenterol* 2000;95:1949–1954
78. Bonner GF, Walczak M, Kitchen L et al. Tolerance of nonsteroidal antiinflammatory drugs in patients with in-

flammatory bowel disease. *Am J Gastroenterol* 2000;95: 1946–1948
79. Bonner GF, Fakhri A, Vennamaneni SR. A long-term cohort study of nonsteroidal anti-inflammatory drug use and disease activity in outpatients with inflammatory bowel disease. *Inflamm Bowel Dis* 2004;10:751–757
80. Forrest K, Symmons D, Foster P. Systematic review: is ingestion of paracetamol or non-steroidal anti-inflammatory drugs associated with exacerbations of inflammatory bowel disease? *Aliment Pharmacol Ther* 2004;20: 1035–1043
81. Choi PM, Targan SR. Immunomodulator therapy in inflammatory bowel disease. *Dig Dis Sci* 1994;39:1885–1892
82. Pearson DC, May GR, Fick GH, Sutherland LR. Azathioprine and 6-mercaptopurine in Crohn disease. A meta-analysis. *Ann Intern Med* 1995;123:132–142
83. Targan SR, Hanauer SB, van Deventer SJ et al. A short-term study of chimeric monoclonal antibody cA2 to tumor necrosis factor alpha for Crohn's disease. Crohn's Disease cA2 Study Group. *N Engl J Med* 1997;337:1029–1035
84. van Dullemen HM, van Deventer SJ, Hommes DW et al. Treatment of Crohn's disease with anti-tumor necrosis factor chimeric monoclonal antibody (cA2). *Gastroenterology* 1995;109:129–135
85. Hurst RD, Molinari M, Chung TP et al. Prospective study of the features, indications, and surgical treatment in 513 consecutive patients affected by Crohn's disease. *Surgery* 1997;122:661–667; discussion 7–8
86. Michelassi F, Balestracci T, Chappell R et al. Primary and recurrent Crohn's disease. Experience with 1379 patients. *Ann Surg* 1991;214:230–238; discussion 8–40
87. Cheung O, Regueiro MD. Inflammatory bowel disease emergencies. *Gastroenterol Clin North Am* 2003;32:1269–1288
88. Broe PJ, Bayless TM, Cameron JL. Crohn's disease: are enteroenteral fistulas an indication for surgery? *Surgery* 1982;91:249–253
89. Glass RE, Ritchie JK, Lennard-Jones JE et al. Internal fistulas in Crohn's disease. *Dis Colon Rectum* 1985;28:557–561
90. Hawker PC, Givel JC, Keighley MR et al. Management of enterocutaneous fistulae in Crohn's disease. *Gut* 1983; 24:284–287
91. Heyen F, Winslet MC, Andrews H et al. Vaginal fistulas in Crohn's disease. *Dis Colon Rectum* 1989;32:379–383
92. Michelassi F, Finco C, Balestracci T, et al. Incidence, diagnosis and treatment of abdominal abscesses in Crohn's patients. *Research in Surgery* 1996;8:35–39
93. Bernini A, Spencer MP, Wong WD et al. Computed tomography-guided percutaneous abscess drainage in intestinal disease: factors associated with outcome. *Dis Colon Rectum* 1997;40:1009–1013
94. Doemeny JM, Burke DR, Meranze SG. Percutaneous drainage of abscesses in patients with Crohn's disease. *Gastrointest Radiol* 1988;13:237–241
95. Gervais DA, Hahn PF, O'Neill MJ et al. Percutaneous abscess drainage in Crohn disease: technical success and short- and long-term outcomes during 14 years. *Radiology* 2002;222:645–651
96. Greenstein AJ, Sachar DB, Mann D et al. Spontaneous free perforation and perforated abscess in 30 patients with Crohn's disease. *Ann Surg* 1987;205:72–76
97. Robert JR, Sachar DB, Greenstein AJ. Severe gastrointestinal hemorrhage in Crohn's disease. *Ann Surg* 1991;213:207–211
98. Ribeiro MB, Greenstein AJ, Heimann TM et al. Adenocarcinoma of the small intestine in Crohn's disease. *Surg Gynecol Obstet* 1991;173:343–349
99. Greenstein AJ, Sachar D, Pucillo A et al. Cancer in Crohn's disease after diversionary surgery. A report of seven carcinomas occurring in excluded bowel. *Am J Surg* 1978;135:86–90
100. Bernstein D, Rogers A. Malignancy in Crohn's disease. *Am J Gastroenterol* 1996;91:434–440
101. Korelitz BI, Lauwers GY, Sommers SC. Rectal mucosal dysplasia in Crohn's disease. *Gut* 1990;31:1382–1386
102. Kelts DG, Grand RJ, Shen G et al. Nutritional basis of growth failure in children and adolescents with Crohn's disease. *Gastroenterology* 1979;76:720–727
103. Werlin SL. Growth failure in Crohn's disease: an approach to treatment. *JPEN J Parenter Enteral Nutr* 1981;5: 250–253
104. Bucher P, Mermillod B, Gervaz P et al. Mechanical bowel preparation for elective colorectal surgery: a meta-analysis. *Arch Surg* 2004;139:1359–1364; discussion 65
105. Wille-Jorgensen P, Guenaga KF, Castro AA et al. Clinical value of preoperative mechanical bowel cleansing in elective colorectal surgery: a systematic review. *Dis Colon Rectum* 2003;46:1013–1020
106. Bucher P, Gervaz P, Soravia C et al. Randomized clinical trial of mechanical bowel preparation versus no preparation before elective left-sided colorectal surgery. *Br J Surg* 2005;92:409–414
107. Song F, Glenny AM. Antimicrobial prophylaxis in colorectal surgery: a systematic review of randomized controlled trials. *Br J Surg* 1998;85:1232–1241
108. Calnan J, Davies A. The effect of methotrexate (amethopterin) on wound healing: an experimental study. *Br J Cancer* 1965;19:505–512
109. Fazio VW, Marchetti F, Church M et al. Effect of resection margins on the recurrence of Crohn's disease in the small bowel. A randomized controlled trial. *Ann Surg* 1996;224:563–571; discussion 71–73
110. Kotanagi H, Kramer K, Fazio VW et al. Do microscopic abnormalities at resection margins correlate with increased anastomotic recurrence in Crohn's disease? Retrospective analysis of 100 cases. *Dis Colon Rectum* 1991;34:909–916
111. Pennington L, Hamilton SR, Bayless TM et al. Surgical management of Crohn's disease. Influence of disease at margin of resection. *Ann Surg* 1980;192:311–318
112. Speranza V, Simi M, Leardi S, Del Papa M. Recurrence of Crohn's disease after resection. Are there any risk factors? *J Clin Gastroenterol* 1986;8:640–646
113. Aufses AH Jr. The surgery of granulomatous inflammatory bowel disease. *Curr Probl Surg* 1983;20:755–826
114. Cameron JL, Hamilton SR, Coleman J et al. Patterns of ileal recurrence in Crohn's disease. A prospective ran-

domized study. *Ann Surg* 1992;215:546–551; discussion 51–52
115. Scott NA, Sue-Ling HM, Hughes LE. Anastomotic configuration does not affect recurrence of Crohn's disease after ileocolonic resection. *Int J Colorectal Dis* 1995;10:67–69
116. Scarpa M, Angriman I, Barollo M et al. Role of stapled and hand-sewn anastomoses in recurrence of Crohn's disease. *Hepatogastroenterology* 2004;51:1053–1057
117. Munoz-Juarez M, Yamamoto T, Wolff BG et al. Wide-lumen stapled anastomosis vs. conventional end-to-end anastomosis in the treatment of Crohn's disease. *Dis Colon Rectum* 2001;44:20–25; discussion 5–6
118. Tersigni R, Alessandroni L, Barreca M et al. Does stapled functional end-to-end anastomosis affect recurrence of Crohn's disease after ileocolonic resection? *Hepatogastroenterology* 2003;50:1422–1425
119. Bass EM, Del Pino A, Tan A et al. Does preoperative stoma marking and education by the enterostomal therapist affect outcome? *Dis Colon Rectum* 1997;40: 440–442
120. Erwin-Toth P, Barrett P. Stoma site marking: a primer. *Ostomy Wound Manage* 1997;43:18–22, 4–5
121. Ritchie JK. Ileostomy and excisional surgery for chronic inflammatory disease of the colon: a survey of one hospital region. *Gut* 1971;12:528–540
122. Michelassi F, Upadhyay GA. Side-to-side isoperistaltic strictureplasty in the treatment of extensive Crohn's disease. *J Surg Res* 2004;117:71–78
123. Milsom JW. Strictureplasty and mechanical dilation in strictured Crohn's disease. In: Michelassi F, Milsom JW (eds). *Operative Strategies in Inflammatory Bowel Disease.* New York, NY: Springer-Verlag; 1999:259–267
124. Fazio VW, Galandiuk S, Jagelman DG et al. Strictureplasty in Crohn's disease. *Ann Surg* 1989;210:621–625
125. Roy P, Kumar D. Strictureplasty. *Br J Surg* 2004;91:1428–1437
126. Sharif H, Alexander-Williams J. The role of strictureplasty in Crohn's disease. *Int Surg* 1992;77:15–18
127. Michelassi F. Side-to-side isoperistaltic strictureplasty for multiple Crohn's strictures. *Dis Colon Rectum* 1996;39: 345–349
128. Tonelli F, Fedi M, Paroli GM et al. Indications and results of side-to-side isoperistaltic strictureplasty in Crohn's disease. *Dis Colon Rectum* 2004;47:494–501
129. Sampietro GM, Cristaldi M, Maconi G et al. A prospective, longitudinal study of nonconventional strictureplasty in Crohn's disease. *J Am Coll Surg* 2004;199:8–20
130. Tichansky D, Cagir B, Yoo E et al. Strictureplasty for Crohn's disease: meta-analysis. *Dis Colon Rectum* 2000;43: 911–919
131. Fazio VW, Tjandra JJ, Lavery IC et al. Long-term follow-up of strictureplasty in Crohn's disease. *Dis Colon Rectum* 1993;36:355–361
132. Hurst RD, Michelassi F. Strictureplasty for Crohn's disease: techniques and long-term results. *World J Surg* 1998;22:359–363
133. Spencer MP, Nelson H, Wolff BG et al. Strictureplasty for obstructive Crohn's disease: the Mayo experience. *Mayo Clin Proc* 1994;69:33–36
134. Jaskowiak NT, Michelassi F. Adenocarcinoma at a strictureplasty site in Crohn's disease: report of a case. *Dis Colon Rectum* 2001;44:284–287
135. Marchetti F, Fazio VW, Ozuner G. Adenocarcinoma arising from a strictureplasty site in Crohn's disease. Report of a case. *Dis Colon Rectum* 1996;39:1315–1321
136. Mavrantonis C, Wexner SD, Nogueras JJ et al. Current attitudes in laparoscopic colorectal surgery. *Surg Endosc* 2002;16:1152–1157
137. Talac R, Nelson H. Laparoscopic colon and rectal surgery. *Surg Oncol Clin North Am* 2000;9:1–12, v
138. Clinical Outcomes of Surgical Therapy Study Group. A comparison of laparoscopically assisted and open colectomy for colon cancer. *N Engl J Med* 2004;350: 2050–2059
139. Alabaz O, Iroatulam AJ et al. Comparison of laparoscopically assisted and conventional ileocolic resection for Crohn's disease. *Eur J Surg* 2000;166:213–217
140. Bauer JJ, Harris MT, Grumbach NM et al. Laparoscopic-assisted intestinal resection for Crohn's disease. Which patients are good candidates? *J Clin Gastroenterol* 1996; 23:44–46
141. Bemelman WA, Slors JF, Dunker MS et al. Laparoscopic-assisted vs. open ileocolic resection for Crohn's disease. A comparative study. *Surg Endosc* 2000;14:721–725
142. Benoist S, Panis Y, Beaufour A et al. Laparoscopic ileocecal resection in Crohn's disease: a case-matched comparison with open resection. *Surg Endosc* 2003;17:814–818
143. Canin-Endres J, Salky B, Gattorno F et al. Laparoscopically assisted intestinal resection in 88 patients with Crohn's disease. *Surg Endosc* 1999;13:595–599
144. Diamond IR, Langer JC. Laparoscopic-assisted versus open ileocolic resection for adolescent Crohn disease. *J Pediatr Gastroenterol Nutr* 2001;33:543–547
145. Duepree HJ, Senagore AJ, Delaney CP et al. Advantages of laparoscopic resection for ileocecal Crohn's disease. *Dis Colon Rectum* 2002;45:605–610
146. Kishi D, Nezu R, Ito T et al. Laparoscopic-assisted surgery for Crohn's disease: reduced surgical stress following ileocolectomy. *Surg Today* 2000;30:219–222
147. Milsom JW, Hammerhofer KA, Bohm B et al. Prospective, randomized trial comparing laparoscopic vs. conventional surgery for refractory ileocolic Crohn's disease. *Dis Colon Rectum* 2001;44:1–8; discussion 9
148. Msika S, Iannelli A, Deroide G et al. Can laparoscopy reduce hospital stay in the treatment of Crohn's disease? *Dis Colon Rectum* 2001;44:1661-1666
149. Reissman P, Salky BA, Pfeifer J et al. Laparoscopic surgery in the management of inflammatory bowel disease. *Am J Surg* 1996;171:47–50; discussion 51
150. Tabet J, Hong D, Kim CW et al. Laparoscopic versus open bowel resection for Crohn's disease. *Can J Gastroenterol* 2001;15:237–242
151. Watanabe M, Ohgami M, Teramoto T et al. Laparoscopic ileocecal resection for Crohn's disease associated with intestinal stenosis and ileorectal fistula. *Surg Today* 1999;29:446–448
152. Wu JS, Birnbaum EH, Kodner IJ et al. Laparoscopic-assisted ileocolic resections in patients with Crohn's dis-

ease: are abscesses, phlegmons, or recurrent disease contraindications? *Surgery* 1997;122:682–688; discussion 8–9
153. Marshak RH, Maklansky D, Kurzban JD et al. Crohn's disease of the stomach and duodenum. *Am J Gastroenterol* 1982;77:340–341
154. Fitzgibbons TJ, Green G, Silberman H et al. Management of Crohn's disease involving the duodenum, including duodenal cutaneous fistula. *Arch Surg* 1980;115: 1022–1028
155. Harold KL, Kelly KA. Duodenal Crohn disease. *Probl Gen Surg* 1999;16:50–57
156. Poggioli G, Stocchi L, Laureti S et al. Duodenal involvement of Crohn's disease: three different clinicopathologic patterns. *Dis Colon Rectum* 1997;40:179–183
157. Schoetz D. Gastroduodenal Crohn's disease. In: Michelassi F et al (eds). *Operative Strategies in Inflammatory Bowel Disease.* New York, NY: Springer-Verlag; 1999:389–393
158. Lee KK, Schraut WH. Diagnosis and treatment of duodenoenteric fistulas complicating Crohn's disease. *Arch Surg* 1989;124:712–715
159. Pichney LS, Fantry GT, Graham SM. Gastrocolic and duodenocolic fistulas in Crohn's disease. *J Clin Gastroenterol* 1992;15:205–211
160. Block GE, Schraut WH. The operative treatment of Crohn's enteritis complicated by ileosigmoid fistula. *Ann Surg* 1982;196:356–360
161. Gruner JS, Sehon JK, Johnson LW. Diagnosis and management of enterovesical fistulas in patients with Crohn's disease. *Am Surg* 2002;68:714–719
162. Lefton HB, Farmer RG, Fazio V. Ileorectal anastomosis for Crohn's disease of the colon. *Gastroenterology* 1975; 69:612–617
163. Panis Y, Poupard B, Nemeth J et al. Ileal pouch/anal anastomosis for Crohn's disease. *Lancet* 1996;347:854–857
164. Regimbeau JM, Panis Y, Pocard M et al. Long-term results of ileal pouch-anal anastomosis for colorectal Crohn's disease. *Dis Colon Rectum* 2001;44:769–778
165. Berry AR, de Campos R, Lee EC. Perineal and pelvic morbidity following perimuscular excision of the rectum for inflammatory bowel disease. *Br J Surg* 1986;73: 675–677
166. Allan A, Andrews H, Hilton CJ et al. Segmental colonic resection is an appropriate operation for short skip lesions due to Crohn's disease in the colon. *World J Surg* 1989;13:611–614; discussion 5–6
167. Sanfey H, Bayless TM, Cameron JL. Crohn's disease of the colon. Is there a role for limited resection? *Am J Surg* 1984;147:38–42
168. Sandborn WJ, Fazio VW, Feagan BG et al. AGA technical review on perianal Crohn's disease. *Gastroenterology* 2003;125:1508–1530
169. Homan WP, Tang C, Thorgjarnarson B. Anal lesions complicating Crohn disease. *Arch Surg* 1976;111:1333–1335
170. Bernstein LH, Frank MS, Brandt LJ et al. Healing of perineal Crohn's disease with metronidazole. *Gastroenterology* 1980;79:599
171. Turunen U, Farkkila M, Seppala K. Long-term treatment of perianal or fistulous Crohn's disease with ciprofloxacin. *Scand J Gastroenterology Suppl* 1989;24:144
172. Present DH, Rutgeerts P, Targan S et al. Infliximab for the treatment of fistulas in patients with Crohn's disease. *N Engl J Med* 1999;340:1398–1405
173. Ardizzone S, Maconi G, Colombo E et al. Perianal fistulae following infliximab treatment: clinical and endosonographic outcome. *Inflamm Bowel Dis* 2004;10:91–96
174. Regueiro M, Mardini H. Treatment of perianal fistulizing Crohn's disease with infliximab alone or as an adjunct to exam under anesthesia with seton placement. *Inflamm Bowel Dis* 2003;9:98–103
175. Loungnarath R, Dietz DW, Mutch MG et al. Fibrin glue treatment of complex anal fistulas has low success rate. *Dis Colon Rectum* 2004;47:432–436
176. Zmora O, Mizrahi N, Rotholtz N et al. Fibrin glue sealing in the treatment of perineal fistulas. *Dis Colon Rectum* 2003;46:584–589
177. Kodner IJ, Mazor A, Shemesh EI et al. Endorectal advancement flap repair of rectovaginal and other complicated anorectal fistulas. *Surgery* 1993;114:682–689
178. D'Haens GR, Geboes K, Peeters M et al. Early lesions of recurrent Crohn's disease caused by infusion of intestinal contents in excluded ileum. *Gastroenterology* 1998; 114:262–267
179. Rutgeerts P, Geboes K, Vantrappen G et al. Predictability of the postoperative course of Crohn's disease. *Gastroenterology* 1990;99:956–963
180. McLeod RS, Wolff BG, Steinhart AH et al. Risk and significance of endoscopic/radiological evidence of recurrent Crohn's disease. *Gastroenterology* 1997;113:1823–1827
181. Best WR, Becktel JM, Singleton JW et al. Development of a Crohn's disease activity index. National Cooperative Crohn's Disease Study. *Gastroenterology* 1976;70:439–444
182. Best WR, Becktel JM, Singleton JW. Rederived values of the eight coefficients of the Crohn's Disease Activity Index (CDAI). *Gastroenterology* 1979;77(4 Pt 2):843–846
183. Greenstein AJ, Sachar DB, Pasternack BS et al. Reoperation and recurrence in Crohn's colitis and ileocolitis: Crude and cumulative rates. *N Engl J Med* 1975;293:685–690
184. Mekhjian HS, Switz DM, Watts HD et al. National Cooperative Crohn's Disease Study: factors determining recurrence of Crohn's disease after surgery. *Gastroenterology* 1979;77(4 Pt 2):907–913
185. Borley NR, Mortensen NJ, Jewell DP. Preventing postoperative recurrence of Crohn's disease. *Br J Surg* 1997;84: 1493–1502
186. Post S, Herfarth C, Bohm E et al. The impact of disease pattern, surgical management, and individual surgeons on the risk for relaparotomy for recurrent Crohn's disease. *Ann Surg* 1996;223:253–260
187. Chardavoyne R, Flint GW, Pollack S et al. Factors affecting recurrence following resection for Crohn's disease. *Dis Colon Rectum* 1986;29:495–502
188. D'Haens G, Baert F, Gasparaitis A et al. Length and type of recurrent ileitis after ileal resection correlate with presurgical features in Crohn's disease. *Inflamm Bowel Dis* 1997;3:249–253
189. D'Haens GR, Gasparaitis AE, Hanauer SB. Duration of recurrent ileitis after ileocolonic resection correlates with presurgical extent of Crohn's disease. *Gut* 1995;36:715–717

20

Ulcerative Colitis

James M. Becker ■ *Arthur F. Stucchi*

Ulcerative colitis, one of the two primary forms of idiopathic inflammatory bowel disease (IBD), is a chronic disease that specifically affects the mucosa of the rectum and colon. Although the etiology of this recurring inflammatory disorder remains essentially unknown, there have been significant advances in identifying likely genetic and environmental factors that contribute to its pathogenesis. The clinical course of the disease typically manifests with remissions and exacerbations characterized by rectal bleeding and diarrhea. Since ulcerative colitis most commonly affects patients in their youth or early middle age, the disease can have serious long-term local and systemic consequences. There is no specific medical therapy that is curative. Although medical therapy can ameliorate the inflammatory process and control most symptomatic flares, it provides no definitive treatment for the disease. Proctocolectomy or total removal of the colon and rectum provides the only complete cure; however, innovative surgical alternatives have eliminated the need for a permanent ileostomy.

The capability to distinguish ulcerative colitis from other forms of inflammatory bowel diseases, especially Crohn's colitis, has important therapeutic and surgical implications. Although improved diagnostic techniques using specific serologic markers are making the differential diagnosis more reliable, uncertainty remains in more than 10% of patients presenting with colitis alone.[1] However, new data collected from epidemiological, genetic, and clinical studies have greatly facilitated our understanding of the natural progression of this disease, as well as the pathological manifestations that distinguish them from one another. Many of these advances are providing the rationale for efficacious therapeutic options; however, optimal medical treatment will not be achieved until the multifactorial etiology of ulcerative colitis is more clearly understood.

Although Hippocrates described diarrheal diseases that were colitislike well before 360 BC, it was not until the late 1800s that ulcerative colitis was distinguished clinically from common infectious enteritis. Ulcerative colitis has now been recognized as a distinct disease entity for nearly 150 years. The first medical account of colitis by Sir Samuel Wilks of London in 1859 described a 42-year-old woman who died after several months of diarrhea and fever. Postmortem examination revealed a transmural ulcerative inflammation of the colon and terminal ileum that while originally designated as "simple ulcerative colitis," may in fact have been Crohn's disease. A subsequent case report in 1875, again by Wilks and Walter Moxon, that described ulceration and inflammation of the entire colon in a young woman who had succumbed to severe bloody diarrhea, was more likely the first detailed account of ulcerative colitis.[2] Despite our long knowledge of the existence of ulcerative colitis, a clear understanding of the factors that underlie its pathogenesis continues to elude investigators.

From a surgical perspective, after Burrill Crohn's landmark description of regional enteritis in the 1930s, distinguishing between ulcerative colitis and Crohn's disease of the large intestine appeared to be relatively uncomplicated. Although the two diseases initially appeared to have distinct pathologic features, a marked overlap is now appreciated not only pathologically, but also in anatomic distribution. The fact remains that the diagnosis is indeterminate in more than 10% of patients,[1] which can have significant therapeutic implications because the surgical approaches to ulcerative colitis and Crohn's disease are inherently quite different. As will be discussed further, the more recent surgical alternatives for ulcerative colitis are generally contraindicated in patients with Crohn's disease.

▪ EPIDEMIOLOGY

Ulcerative colitis poses many challenges to the epidemiologist since the incidence of the disease is low and it is rarely fatal, its clinical presentation can be variable and often insidious, the interval between the initiating event and the diagnosis can be decades, and there are no universal diagnostic criteria.[3] Despite these limitations, epidemiological studies can provide invaluable insight into numerous potential etiologic factors.

In the United States, IBD afflicts about 2–6% of the population, or up to about 1.5 million individuals. Interestingly, while the incidence of ulcerative colitis has risen only slightly in recent years, there has been a noteworthy rise in the incidence of Crohn's disease in the United States since the late 1940s. Of particular note was the sharp increase in the incidence of Crohn's disease over a 20-year period from about 1960 to 1980, which was not mirrored by a similar rise in ulcerative colitis. As a result, the annual incidence of Crohn's disease is nearly equal to that of ulcerative colitis.

Although the incidence of new cases of ulcerative colitis diagnosed each year, as well as the prevalence of individuals with ulcerative colitis varies greatly within populations and throughout the world, no racial, ethnic, or socioeconomic population is spared. Worldwide, the variation in the incidence of ulcerative colitis may serve as a valuable etiological clue. It appears that there is a distinct north-to-south gradient in risk, with the greatest incidence and prevalence occurring in countries of the northern hemisphere such as the United Kingdom, Norway, Sweden, Canada, and the United States,[4] where the annual incidence of ulcerative colitis is about 6–12 per 100,000. In more southern countries such as Australia, South Africa, and the countries of southern Europe, the annual incidence of ulcerative colitis is about 2–8 per 100,000. The incidence in Asia and South America is considerably lower.[4] These trends suggest that the incidence of ulcerative colitis is highest in developed or urban regions of the world and lowest is in developing regions; however, it appears that the incidence rates of ulcerative colitis may be leveling off in the developed countries and starting to increase in the developing nations.

Epidemiological studies have also shown that the incidence of ulcerative colitis among Jewish populations is two to four times higher than that in non-Jewish populations, while the age-adjusted incidence rate for white males is about twice that of non-white males, and the rate for non-white women is actually higher than that for white women.[3]

Although the age of onset of ulcerative colitis is bimodal and it typically occurs between the ages of 15 and 40 years and again after age 60, the disease can present at any age from infancy to the elderly. In fact, nearly 5% of new cases reportedly occur after age 60. Throughout the age range, males and females are affected about equally. The mortality rate from ulcerative colitis has steadily declined worldwide, especially in the U.S., not only as a result of improved medical therapy, but also due to earlier surgical intervention.

GENETICS

In contrast to Crohn's disease, where the *NOD2/CARD15* gene has been associated with genetic susceptibility,[5] no specific gene has yet been linked to ulcerative colitis. Despite this, there is convincing evidence that genetic factors do contribute to susceptibility.[6] Familial studies have shown an increased risk among family members of patients with ulcerative colitis, particularly among first-degree relatives. Although Crohn's disease and ulcerative colitis can occur within the same family, there is an 80–90% concordance for the same disease category within the same family.[3] In twin studies, concordance for disease type and localization has been observed. In genetically isolated groups such as the Ashkenazi Jews, there is a considerably higher prevalence, again implicating an unidentified genetic link.[7] Geographic as well as racial differences can influence the occurrence of the disease, and there is no conclusive evidence regarding the genetic versus the environmental determination of familial patterns. In addition to the likely contribution of genetics to the susceptibility of developing ulcerative colitis, there is a strong possibility that genetics also plays some role in susceptibility to extraintestinal complications of ulcerative colitis such as ankylosing spondylitis, sacroiliitis, peripheral arthropathies, erythema nodosum, and uveitis.[8]

ENVIRONMENT

There are several environmental factors that may provide some insight into the susceptibility to ulcerative colitis.[9] These environmental factors, including smoking, diet, drugs, geographical and socioeconomic status, stress, microbial agents, and appendectomy are now considered fundamental components of the pathogenesis of ulcerative colitis and may underlie the growing incidence worldwide. Epidemiological, clinical, and experimental data support the involvement of each of these factors in predisposing, triggering, or modulating the course of the disease. For example, pathogenic bacteria have long been thought to play a role in triggering ulcerative colitis; however, recent evidence suggests that nonpathogenic commensal bacteria are sufficient to induce colitis in a susceptible individual.[10] Although no bacterial strains that are specific to ulcerative colitis have been identified, bacteria are still strongly implicated since experimental colitis does not develop in animals that are born and maintained in germ-free environments. Interestingly, cigarette smoking continues to play a protective role against the development of ulcerative colitis.[11] Smokers are less likely to develop ulcerative colitis and ex-smokers are more likely to develop extensive or severe colitis. Smoking is also protective against the development of extraintestinal manifestations and postoperative complications associated with ulcerative colitis. Whether transdermal nicotine therapy offers any advantage over standard medical therapy in inducing remission remains unclear.[12] Another consistent epidemiological clue to the pathogenesis of ulcerative colitis is the observation that appendectomy, particularly at a younger age, reduces the probability of developing ulcerative colitis.[13] Interestingly, appendectomy and smoking appear to be additive in protecting against the development of ulcerative colitis.

▪ PATHOPHYSIOLOGY

Although our understanding of the role of familial and genetic factors in the etiology of ulcerative colitis has increased considerably, the pathogenesis of ulcerative colitis remains poorly understood due to complex environmental or extrinsic factors that can significantly influence susceptibility. As mentioned, ulcerative colitis is a chronic inflammatory disease characterized by recurring episodes of intestinal inflammation followed by partial healing. These repetitious inflammatory cycles eventually lead to chronically disrupted bowel function. The clinical manifestations of this pathological process are the result of a series of overlapping interactions between extrinsic environmental factors, genetic intrinsic factors, and mucosal barrier function. Although a single etiological factor has yet to be identified, strong evidence suggests that the disease is perpetuated by a sustained mucosal inflammatory response that the host is unable to downregulate. The failure to attenuate this response enhances the recruitment and activation of numerous immune and inflammatory cells, and coupled with the release of proinflammatory mediators, perpetuates inflammation and facilitates damage to intestinal tissues.

Recent research has focused on the role of the mucosal immune system in the pathogenesis of ulcerative colitis. Immune-mediated inflammatory events include the dysregulation of humoral and cell-mediated immunity and enhanced reactivity against intestinal bacterial antigens. It is currently thought that loss of tolerance against indigenous enteric flora is the fundamental event in the pathogenesis of ulcerative colitis.[10,14] The intestinal mucosa is continually exposed to an immense environmental challenge. Optimal mucosal tolerance lies in the tight regulation of an intricate network of mucosal immune and nonimmune cells, which is orchestrated by a finely tuned network of autocrine and paracrine mediators. Chronic dysregulation of mucosal immunity can initiate an uncontrolled inflammatory response and may be an underlying immunopathological mechanism of ulcerative colitis.

Immunoregulatory and proinflammatory cytokines also play key roles in the modulation of intestinal inflammation. Cytokines can have paracrine and autocrine as well as endocrine functions that mediate both local and systemic manifestations of intestinal inflammation. Proinflammatory cytokines such as interleukin (IL)-1β, IL-6, IL-8, and tumor necrosis factor-α, and prostaglandins such as prostaglandin E_2 and leukotriene B_4 also have been implicated in exacerbating mucosal inflammation, while IL-4 and IL-10 play a pivotal role in suppressing intestinal inflammation as well as initiating repair and healing mechanisms. While the roles of these immunoregulatory and proinflammatory cytokines have yet to be completely defined, it appears that ulcerative colitis is mediated by a Th2-like cytokine pattern.

PATHOLOGY

On gross inspection, the colonic mucosa appears swollen and congested even in mild cases (Fig 20–1A). As the disease progresses, the mucosa begin to erode leaving only small islands of mucosa that resemble polyps but are actually pseudopolyps. The mucosal erosions often coalesce to form linear ulcers and superficial fissures that undermine the remaining mucosa, which becomes friable and erythematous with reduced haustral folds (Fig 20–1B). The recurrent nature of the disease frequently leaves healed granular superficial ulcers superimposed on a friable and thickened mucosa with increased vascularity. This appearance sharply contrasts with the transmural inflammatory changes found in Crohn's disease of the colon, in which all layers of the

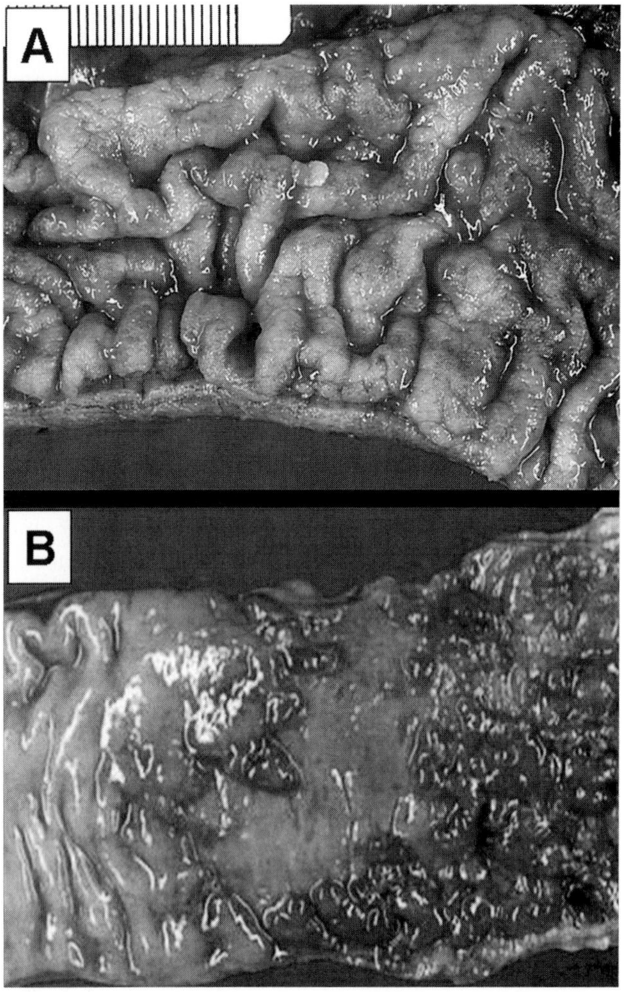

Figure 20–1. Gross pathologic specimens from patients with ulcerative colitis. **A.** Resected rectosigmoid from a patient with mildly active disease showing swollen, congested, and ulcerated mucosa. **B.** Severe ulcerative colitis. Mucosal ulceration and inflammation is characteristically diffuse and uninterrupted, often extending from the rectum proximally. Chronic ulcerative colitis is frequently associated with the appearance of small pseudopolyps, which represent areas of regenerating mucosa among diffuse mucosal destruction. While the risk of colon cancer is higher in patients with ulcerative colitis, pseudopolyps themselves have no malignant potential.

colonic wall may be involved in a granulomatous inflammatory process (Table 20–1).

Histologically, the typical early lesion consists of an infiltration of inflammatory cells, primarily polymorphonuclear leukocytes, into the crypts at the base of the mucosa, forming crypt abscesses. As the lesions progress, there is a coalescence of crypt abscesses and desquamation of overlying cells to form an ulcer. This cryptitis is associated with undermining of adjacent, relatively normal mucosa, which becomes edematous and assumes a polypoid configuration as it becomes isolated between adjacent ulcers. A whole mount section of a colon from a patient with severe disease shows these broad-based undermined ulcers (Fig 20–2A). The absence of fibrosis and the lack of transmural inflammation in part rule out Crohn's disease. Collagen and granulation tissue often occupy the areas of ulceration, which extend down to, but rarely through, the muscularis. On higher magnification, an ulcer edge is shown overhanging inflamed mucosa (Fig 20–2B). Although ulcerative colitis is generally confined to the mucosa and submucosa, in the most severe forms of the dis-

TABLE 20–1. PATHOLOGIC, CLINICAL, ENDOSCOPIC, AND RADIOGRAPHIC FEATURES OF ULCERATIVE COLITIS AND CROHN'S DISEASE

	Ulcerative Colitis	Crohn's Disease
PATHOLOGIC FEATURES		
Transmural inflammation	Uncommon	Common
Granulomas	No	Common
Fissures	Rare	Common
Fibrosis	Occasional	Common
CLINICAL FEATURES		
Location	Colon only	Anywhere in the alimentary tract
Anatomic distribution	Continuous, beginning distally	Asymmetrical skip lesions
Rectal involvement	>90%	Occasionally
Diarrhea/gross bleeding	Severe, often bloody with mucus	Less severe, infrequent bleeding
Abdominal pain	Yes	Occasionally
Perianal fistulas	Rare	Common
Abdominal mass (palpable)	Rare	Common
Strictures and obstructions	Uncommon	Common
Fistulas and perforations	Rare	Common
Extraintestinal manifestations	Common	Common
Recurrence after surgery	If retained rectal mucosa	Yes
P-ANCA-positive	Frequently	Rarely
ASCA-positive	Rarely	Frequently
ENDOSCOPIC FEATURES		
Mucosal involvement	Contiguous	Discontinuous
Discrete ulcers (aphthous)	Rare	Common
Surrounding mucosa	Abnormal	Relatively normal
Longitudinal ulcers	Rare	Common
Cobblestoning	No	In severe cases
Rectal involvement	>90%	Sparing common
Mucosal friability	Common	Uncommon
Vascular pattern	Distorted	Normal
RADIOGRAPHIC FEATURES		
Small bowel abnormalities	No	Yes
Terminal ileum abnormalities	Rare	Yes
Segmental colitis	No	Yes
Asymmetric colitis	No	Yes
Stricturing	Occasionally	Frequently

ASCA, anti-*Saccharomyces cerevisiae* mannan antibodies; P-ANCA, perinuclear antineutrophilic cytoplasmic antibody.

Adapted, with permission, from Forcione DG, Sands BE. Differential diagnosis of inflammatory bowel disease. In: Sartor RB, Sandborn WJ (eds). *Kirsner's Inflammatory Bowel Diseases,* 6th ed. Philadelphia, PA: WB Saunders; 2004; Dayton MT, Trundel JL. Colon, rectum and anus. In: Friedman S, Blumberg RS. *Essentials of Surgery,* 3rd ed. Baltimore, MD; Lippincott Williams & Wilkins; 1999; Inflammatory bowel disease. In: Kasper DL et al (eds). *Harrison's Principles of Internal Medicine,* 16th ed. New York, NY: McGraw-Hill, 2005; Becker JM, Stucchi AF. Ulcerative colitis. In: Greenfield LJ et al (eds). *Surgery: Scientific Principles and Practice,* 3rd ed. Baltimore MD: Lippincott Williams & Wilkins; 2001.

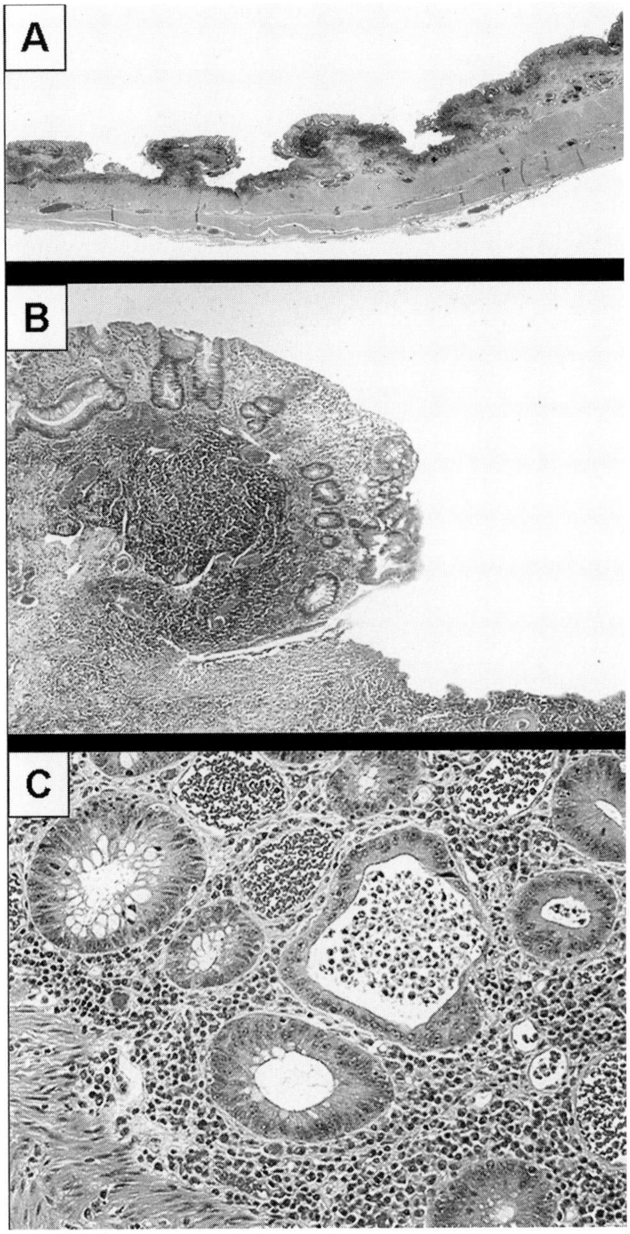

Figure 20–2. Microscopic features of ulcerative colitis. **A.** Typical hematoxylin-eosin (H&E)–stained whole mount section of a colon from a patient with severe ulcerative colitis showing broad-based undermined ulcers. Inflammation is limited to the mucosa with no evidence of transmural inflammation or fibrosis, and that might be indicative of Crohn's disease. **B.** A higher-magnification H&E-stained histological section of an ulcer edge showing overhanging inflamed mucosa. **C.** High-magnification H&E-stained section of inflamed mucosa showing diffuse acute and chronic inflammation with architectural distortion and destruction of some glands, loss of goblet cells and depletion of mucin from the remaining goblet cells, crypt abscesses, and basal plasmacytosis. The glands show hyperchromatic nuclei with inflammatory atypia.

ease, such as fulminant colitis or toxic megacolon, the disease process may extend to the deeper muscular layers of the colon and even to the serosa. For example, we have noted that colectomy specimens from some patients with severe chronic active colitis contain superficial fissuring-type ulcers that extend into the inner half of the muscularis propria of the colon.[15] Aside from the fissures, the pathological features of these colons appear typical of ulcerative colitis. These ulcers appear as knifelike, vertically oriented defects lined by actively inflamed granulation tissue and are often associated with marked chronic inflammation in the vicinity of the ulcer. Although deep fissuring ulcers are normally associated with Crohn's disease, some pathologists believe that superficial fissuring ulcers may be seen in severe cases of ulcerative colitis as well. This type of presentation can certainly complicate the differential diagnosis. Rarely, crypt abscesses (Fig 20–2C) penetrate the muscularis propria, often extending along a blood vessel, eventually leading to perforation.

CLINICAL FEATURES

Patients with a relatively mild episode of ulcerative colitis typically present with bloody diarrhea, abdominal pain, and fever (see Table 20–1). Although the disease may be initially limited to the rectosigmoid, it eventually progresses proximally in most cases. A smaller percentage (25%) present with a moderate attack in which bloody diarrhea is the major symptom. In a small number of patients (15%), ulcerative colitis can present rapidly with a fulminating course. These patients develop the relatively sudden onset of frequent, bloody bowel movements, high fever, weight loss, and diffuse abdominal tenderness.

Physical findings are generally associated with the duration, extent, and severity of disease. Weight loss and pallor usually accompany acute flares, along with detectable alterations in numerous metabolic functions. During active periods, the abdomen, especially in proximity to the colon, is tender to palpation. Acute attacks or fulminating forms of the disease can present much like an acute surgical abdomen, with accompanying fever and decreased bowel sounds. In patients with toxic megacolon, abdominal distention may be identified.

Extraintestinal manifestations of ulcerative colitis are observed in a number of organ systems.[8] Thus, careful examination of the skin, oral cavity and tongue, joints, and eyes can be a vital component of the initial diagnosis because the presence of extraintestinal disease suggests that IBD is the likely cause of the underlying diarrheal illness. Many extraintestinal manifestations of ulcerative colitis are closely related to disease activity and respond to therapy with steroids, immunosuppressive agents, or surgical treatment.[16] Liver and biliary tract disorders also commonly afflict patients with ulcerative colitis. Up to 80% of patients, especially those with pancolitis, show some hepatic involvement. Sclerosing cholangitis, one of the most difficult extraintestinal complications associated with ulcerative colitis, is observed in 1–4% of patients. Although some patients respond to colectomy, most show progression of their hepatic disease even after colon resection. Patients with progressive liver failure ultimately require liver transplantation. Affected patients are also at greater risk of developing carcinoma of the bile duct, although this may also develop de novo in patients with ulcerative colitis.

▪ DIAGNOSIS

ENDOSCOPY

There are no specific laboratory, radiographic, or histologic tests that definitively establish the diagnosis of ulcerative colitis; thus the final diagnosis is generally one of exclusion. However, endoscopy with biopsy can play an integral role in the diagnosis, management, and surveillance of ulcerative colitis.[17] Endoscopy can be very valuable in establishing the final diagnosis, excluding other potential etiologies in patients presenting with bloody diarrhea, delineating the extent and activity of mucosal inflammation, and obtaining mucosal biopsies for histologic evaluation. For the surgeon, endoscopy can be particularly useful in differentiating ulcerative colitis from Crohn's colitis, which can have a significant impact on surgical decisions and on the management of disease-related complications. Major distinguishing clinical characteristics of ulcerative colitis and Crohn's disease are shown in Table 20–1.

Since ulcerative colitis involves the rectum in 90–95% of cases, flexible sigmoidoscopy is the first step in diagnosis. Mild cases may only show a loss of normal vascular pattern, a granular texture, and microhemorrhages when the friable mucosa is touched or wiped (Fig 20–3A). When the disease is moderately active, the mucosa becomes more grossly pitted, and spontaneous bleeding is often present (Fig 20–3B). In severe cases, there is macroulceration and profuse bleeding usually accompanied by a purulent exudate (Fig 20–3C). Chronic ulcerative colitis is frequently associated with the appearance of small pseudopolyps, which represent areas of regenerating mucosa in the midst of diffuse mucosal destruction. The use of flexible sigmoidoscopy as well as other imaging modalities has greatly improved diagnostic accuracy and patient acceptability. Colonoscopy may be useful in determining the extent and activity of the disease, particularly in patients in whom the diagnosis is unclear or cancer is suspected.

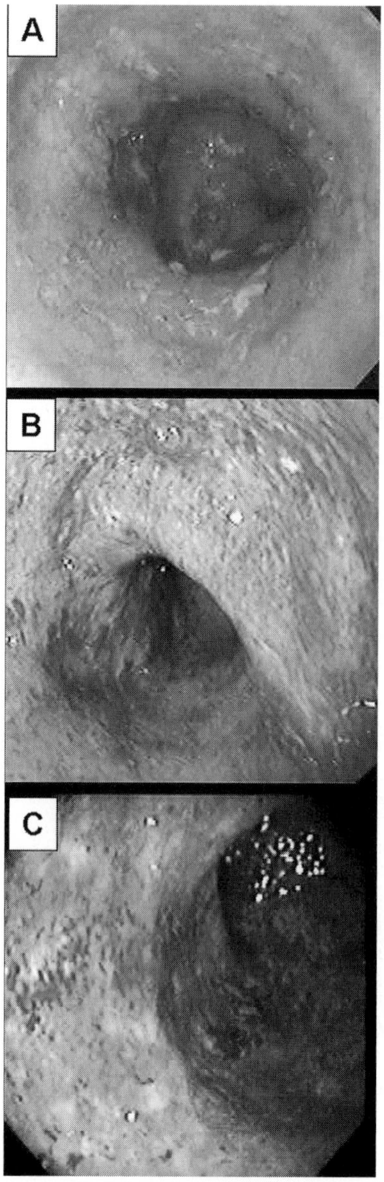

Figure 20–3. Endoscopic views of the sigmoid colon during active ulcerative colitis. **A.** Endoscopic appearance of the rectum in a patient with mild ulcerative colitis, showing mucosal granularity, diffuse erythema, and loss of the normal vascular pattern. The mucosa is friable and often bleeds on contact. **B.** Endoscopic appearance of the rectum in a patient with moderate ulcerative colitis, with pitted mucosa and spontaneous hemorrhage. The mucosa is diffusely erythematous, edematous, and granular, with areas of submucosal hemorrhage. A mucopurulent exudate is evident. **C.** Severe ulcerative colitis showing extensive ulceration with irregular, inflamed, ulcerated mucosa and a patchy exudate.

RADIOGRAPHIC STUDIES

In patients presenting with fulminant or severe ulcerative colitis, a plain abdominal radiograph may be useful initially, especially since more invasive imaging techniques can have serious risks. An abdominal film may demonstrate colonic dilation or toxic megacolon in 3–5% of patients. Although this dilation is most frequently observed in the transverse colon (Fig 20–4A), it can occur anywhere in the colon (Fig 20–4B). A plain radiograph is also useful for detecting free air within the peritoneal cavity, indicating a potential perforation of the diseased colon.

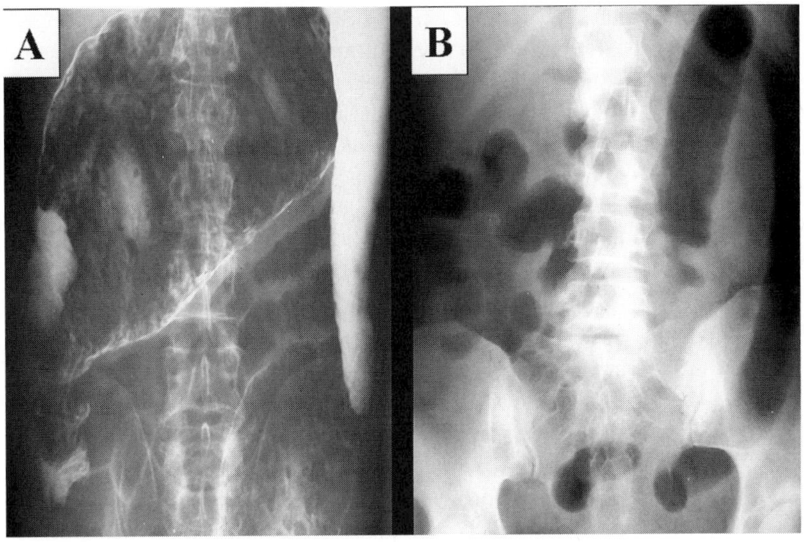

Figure 20–4. Radiographic appearance of toxic megacolon in severe ulcerative colitis. **A.** A single supine film of the abdomen shows marked distension and dilation of the transverse colon in a patient with toxic megacolon. Some distension of the small bowel is also evident. **B.** Air contrast showing severe dilation of the descending colon indicating toxic megacolon.

A lower GI series or barium enema examination of the colon is useful in most patients, although potentially dangerous in those with toxic megacolon. As ulcerative colitis develops, mucosal granularity and microhemorrhages produce a diffusely reticulated pattern, on which are superimposed countless punctate collections of contrast material lodged in microulcerations (Fig 20–5A). More mild cases of acute ulcerative colitis may be manifested by a diffusely granular appearance, which can also be seen in more detail on air-contrast barium enema. In more advanced cases, the colon develops irregular margins with spiculated and undermining collar-button ulcers that can be observed on full-column barium enema (Fig 20–5B). End-stage or "burned-out" ulcerative colitis is characterized by shortening of the colon, loss of normal redundancy in the sigmoid region and at the splenic and hepatic flexures, disappearance of the haustral pattern, a featureless mucosa, absence of discrete ulceration, and narrowed caliber of the bowel (Fig 20–6).

▪ MEDICAL MANAGEMENT

Surgeons are now becoming involved in the management of potential surgical candidates much earlier in the course of their disease, so a general understanding of the medical management of the various presentations and stages of ulcerative colitis is required. Medical therapy for ulcerative colitis is not curative. It is primarily intended to control the patient's symptoms or manage their underlying inflammatory process in order to induce remission. Once the diagnosis of ulcerative colitis has been established, the decision

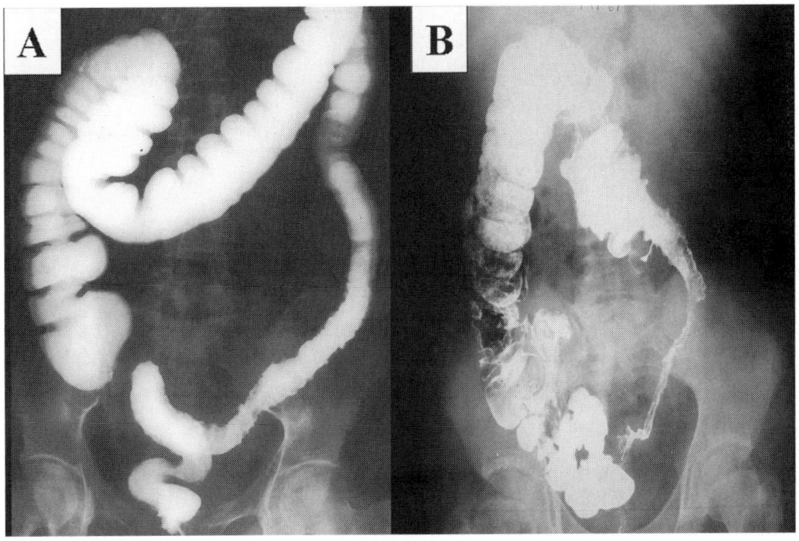

Figure 20–5. Radiographic appearance of active ulcerative colitis. **A.** Single-contrast barium enema showing the typical jagged and ulcerative appearance of the mucosa with characteristic collar-button or undermining ulcers. **B.** Radiographic appearance of severe ulcerative colitis. Single-contrast barium enema showing continuous involvement of the colon from the rectum proximally to the transverse colon along with a large ulcer tract in the transverse colon. The colon is shortened considerably, indicating the chronicity of the inflammation. In general, barium enema and colonoscopy should be avoided in fulminant ulcerative colitis because of the possibility of precipitating toxic megacolon.

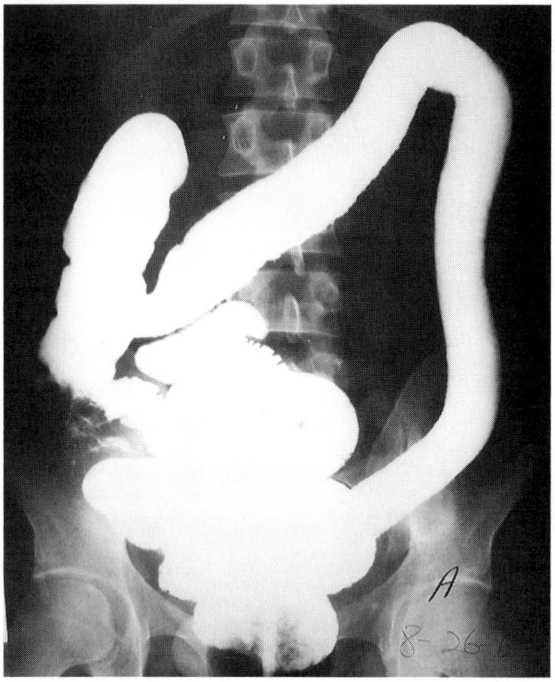

Figure 20–6. Radiographic appearance of ulcerative colitis. Single-contrast barium enema showing chronic ulcerative colitis characterized by shortening and straightening of the colon with loss of haustrations, resulting in the appearance of a featureless tube. No ulcerations are seen.

regarding the implementation of medical therapy depends on the severity of symptoms, the patient's clinical history, and on their endoscopic and radiographic studies. The optimal treatment plan, which may eventually include surgery, is often devised with input from the patient as well as their gastroenterologist and surgeon. Although adherence to individualized treatment plans can result in better long-term outcomes, a significant percentage of patients will eventually become refractory to even the most aggressive treatment regimens or experience other complications that require surgical intervention.[18]

The choice of agents commonly used to induce remission in patients with ulcerative colitis depends on both the extent and severity of the disease and its anatomic location, and can include oral and topical regimens alone or in combination.[19] Drugs commonly used in the treatment of various stages of ulcerative colitis include sulfasalazine and its aminosalicylate analogues, corticosteroids, immunomodulators, suppressive antimetabolites, anti-tumor necrosis factor-α biologics including infliximab, and in some cases antibiotics (Table 20–2). Symptomatic antidiarrheals and antispasmodic agents can also be used in combination therapy as needed.

Sulfasalazine has been a mainstay in the management of mild to moderate disease since the early 1950s and induces remission in up to 80% of patients, particularly with dosages higher than 3 g/d. However, at these higher dosages, the incidence of intolerable side effects increases, largely due to the sulfapyridine moiety. Sulfasalazine consists of the antibacterial sulfapyridine linked to 5-aminosalicylate (5-ASA). The 5-ASA moiety, which is released when the compound is cleaved by enteric bacteria generally in the colon, is responsible for the drug's potent anti-inflammatory effects. The dose-limiting side effects associated with sulfasalazine led to the development of sulfa-free aminosalicylates that could be administered orally or topically without adverse side effects. The 5-ASA agents are now the treatment of choice for mild to moderate disease. They can be administered orally for extensive disease, topically for distal disease, or in combination.[19] Clinical improvement or remission can be attained in nearly 90% of patients, including the majority of those previously intolerant to sulfasalazine. Other common therapeutic modalities for mild to moderate distal ulcerative colitis are oral or topical corticosteroids.

Patients with moderate to severe disease often require more aggressive therapy, usually with the introduction of

TABLE 20–2. MEDICAL MANAGEMENT OF ULCERATIVE COLITIS

- ACTIVE DISEASE
  - Mild–moderate disease
    - Distal colon
      - Sulfasalazine or 5-ASA (oral or topical) or in combination
      - Topical corticosteroid
    - Extensive colitis
      - Sulfasalazine or oral 5-ASA
  - Moderate–severe disease
    - Distal colon
      - Topical or oral 5-ASA (or in combination with sulfasalazine)
      - Oral sulfasalazine
      - Topical or oral corticosteroids
    - Extensive colitis
      - Oral sulfasalazine or 5-ASA
      - Oral corticosteroids
      - Infliximab
  - Severe–fulminant disease
    - Distal or extensive colitis
      - Intravenous corticosteroids
      - Intravenous cyclosporine
- MAINTENANCE THERAPY
  - Distal colitis
    - Sulfasalazine or 5-ASA (oral or topical)
    - Azathioprine or 6-mercaptopurine
  - Extensive colitis
    - Sulfasalazine or oral 5-ASA
    - Azathioprine or 6-mercaptopurine

5-ASA, 5-aminosalicylic acid.

Adapted, with permission, from Hanauer SB. Medical therapy for ulcerative colitis. In: Sartor RB, Sanborn WJ (eds). *Kirsner's Inflammatory Bowel Diseases,* 6th ed. Philadelphia, PA: WB Saunders; 2004; Sands BE. Therapy of inflammatory bowel disease. *Gastroenterology* 2000; 118: S68-S82; Hanauer SB, Present DH. The state of the are in the medical management of inflammatory bowel disease. *Rev Gastroenterol Discord* 2003; 3:81-92; Hanauer SB, Sparrow M. Therapy of ulcerative colitis. *Curr Opin Gastroenterol* 2004; 20:345-350.

oral corticosteroids, and in some chronic cases, systemic therapy. Initially, many of these patients can be managed with oral sulfasalazine or oral and topical 5-ASA, frequently in combination, or with topical corticosteroids. However, if they do not respond or become refractory to this regimen, oral or intravenous corticosteroids are introduced depending on the severity of the flare-up. Because of their potentially serious adverse effects, corticosteroids should be tapered after several weeks if the patient's clinical symptoms and sigmoidoscopic findings improve. Patients must be monitored carefully for the long-term adverse sequelae of corticosteroids, including hypertension, hyperglycemia, cataracts, osteoporosis, and osteomalacia.

A number of immunosuppressive agents have been used for the management of moderate to severe ulcerative colitis, including azathioprine and its metabolite, 6-mercaptopurine (6-MP). Since these immunosuppressive agents do not produce a clinical response for several months, they have no role in treatment of acute flare-ups. Cyclosporine, which has a more rapid onset of action, can be administered intravenously for severe, steroid-refractory ulcerative colitis; however, patients must be monitored closely for nephropathies and infectious complications. As mentioned, anti-tumor necrosis factor-α biologics such as infliximab are also used to treat moderate to severe disease.

Patients with a flare-up of severe ulcerative colitis or with intractable, severe symptoms or complications should be hospitalized. Although intravenous corticosteroids or cyclosporine are currently recommended as the treatments of choice for these patients, therapy is often guided by expert opinion and experience.[19] Depending on the extent and duration, these patients can often require supplemental nutritional support, with either intravenous hyperalimentation or total parenteral nutrition. Although total parenteral nutrition plays no role in ameliorating the inflammatory response, it does provide nutritional maintenance and repletion during the treatment phase. During an acute episode of severe colitis, narcotic pain medications and antidiarrheals should be avoided to prevent provocation of toxic megacolon. Once the patient has responded clinically, oral steroids can be started while parenteral steroids are tapered. For patients that fail to respond to this medical therapy or experience intolerable complications, an urgent colectomy is generally indicated.

For those patients that respond favorably to medical therapy and achieve complete remission, ongoing treatment is usually required to maintain the clinical benefits. As with the initial treatment regimen, maintenance therapy is often individualized in coordination with the patient's medical team. Patients with mild to moderate disease can often be maintained on the same drug and dosage except for high-dose sulfasalazine. Patients can often be titrated to a lower dose and frequency for maintenance to reduce side effects. Topical therapy may also be used to maintain remission in patients with left-sided disease, particularly when this regimen was used previously. In some cases, oral and topical combinations provide the best results for long-term maintenance. Since corticosteroids are generally ineffective for maintenance therapy, patients can be tapered and switched to 5-ASA, azathioprine, or 6-MP. A small number of patients will be refractory to induction or will relapse soon after maintenance therapy has begun. Total colectomy remains the final option for these patients.

▪ SURGICAL MANAGEMENT

INDICATIONS FOR SURGERY

Recent reports estimate that up to 40% of the patients with ulcerative colitis will eventually undergo total proctocolectomy, in part due to the chronicity of the disease and the tendency for relapse, as well as the significant risk for malignant degeneration.[20,21] The indications for surgery can vary widely, and have very different implications for the timing of surgery as well as the choice of operative procedure. At times, surgical treatment is absolutely necessary, such as when life-threatening emergencies arise. However, at other times, when medical therapy is failing or the risk of malignancy is rising, the decision to operate can be elective and is usually mutually agreed upon by the gastroenterologist, the surgeon, and the patient. Thus the indications for surgery can be divided into two categories: emergency and elective operations (Table 20–3).

SURGICAL EMERGENCIES

Although emergency complications of ulcerative colitis are rare, they can be life-threatening and often require immediate surgical intervention for patient survival. Several indications that may potentially require emergency surgery include: fulminant colitis unresponsive to IV corticosteroids; toxic megacolon with impending perforation; massive unrelenting hemorrhage; colonic perforation; and acute colonic obstruction from stricture.[22,23] These complications can parallel the clinical course of the disease and respond to aggressive medical therapy, but most often they result in total proctocolectomy. The primary goal of emergency surgery is to remove nearly the entire diseased colon in order to allow the patient's clinical condition to improve. Despite the

TABLE 20–3. INDICATIONS FOR EMERGENCY AND ELECTIVE SURGERY IN ULCERATIVE COLITIS

SURGICAL EMERGENCIES
Fulminant colitis unresponsive to IV corticosteroids
Toxic megacolon with impending perforation
Massive unrelenting hemorrhage
Colonic perforation
Total obstruction from stricture
Acute intractable colitis
ELECTIVE SURGERY
Intractability or failure of maximal medical therapy
Mucosal dysplasia
Intolerable side effects of medications
Stricture formation without obstruction
Dysplasia-associated lesion or mass (DALM)
Malignancy of the colon or rectum
Anorectal complications
Extraintestinal manifestations
Growth retardation, primarily in children and adolescents

Adapted, with permission, from Fichera A, Michelassi F. Indications for surgery: A surgeon's opinion. In: Sartor RB, Sanburn WJ (eds). *Kirsner's Inflammatory Bowel Diseases,* 6th ed. New York, NY: WB Saunders; 2004: 602-613; Cima RR, Pemberton JH. Surgical indications and procedures in ulcerative colitis. *Curr Treat Options Gastroenterol* 2004; 7:181-190; Cima RR, Pemberton JH. Surgical indications and procedures in ulcerative colitis. In: Sartor RB, Sanburn WJ (eds). *Kirsner's Inflammatory Bowel Diseases,* 6th ed. New York, NY: WB Saunders; 2004: 602-613.

urgency of these situations, emergency operations are intended for life-threatening complications and are not a definitive surgical treatment. Therefore, it is a vitally important consideration for the surgeon to perform an operation that will not compromise a subsequent restorative procedure.

Fulminant Colitis

The clinical course of ulcerative colitis is one of a chronic inflammatory state characterized by sporadic symptomatic flares. However, in a small percentage of patients, the initial presentation can be of a fulminant nature.[24] Fulminant colitis is characterized by the rapid onset of severe symptoms including bloody diarrhea, severe abdominal pain, and dehydration. These patients are often extremely ill, generally anemic and tachycardic, and present with a high fever. They can require immediate and aggressive medical therapy that can include high-dose intravenous steroids, fluid resuscitation, correction of electrolyte abnormalities, and in some cases, blood transfusions. If severe colonic distention is present, nasogastric tube decompression may be required. Approximately 10% of ulcerative colitis patients initially present with fulminant colitis;[22] however, if the patient's history is not known or if the diagnosis of ulcerative colitis is unclear, flexible sigmoidoscopy of the rectum and sigmoid colon should be performed as soon as possible. The gastroenterologist and the surgeon should closely monitor the patient's condition for 24–48 hours and, if there is no improvement or conditions worsen, surgical treatment is recommended. If there is any indication of perforation or peritonitis, the patient should be operated upon immediately.

Toxic Megacolon

Toxic megacolon is a rare but devastating complication occurring in up to 2.5% of patients with ulcerative colitis.[25] Acute toxic megacolon may be the initial presentation of the disease or represent a flare-up in a patient with chronic disease.[22] As mentioned above, usually an isolated segment of the transverse or the left colon (see Fig 20–4) is dilated more than 5.5 cm; however, the entire colon can be involved. Because of the associated high morbidity and mortality, early recognition and aggressive, often surgical management is of vital importance. Medical therapy for toxic megacolon is similar to that of fulminant colitis and includes intravenous fluid and electrolyte resuscitation, nasogastric suction, broad-spectrum antibiotics, and total parenteral nutrition to improve nutritional status.[25] Although the therapeutic role of high-dose steroids in toxic megacolon is controversial, most patients presenting with a severe attack of ulcerative colitis are most likely undergoing steroid therapy and thus need stress doses of corticosteroids to avert adrenal crisis. The medical and surgical teams must also monitor these patients very closely, and if there is no substantial clinical improvement after 24–36 hours of aggressive medical therapy or if there is evidence of perforation, emergency surgery is indicated. Any delay in performing surgery significantly increases the risk of perforation, which raises mortality from under 5% to nearly 30%.[22] Although prompt and aggressive medical therapy can postpone emergency surgery, nearly 50% of these patients will require total proctocolectomy within a year. This observation suggests that more conservative surgery is appropriate in the acute setting. With the popularity of anal sphincter–sparing procedures, the surgeon should always weigh the possibility of the need for later surgery for restoration of continence. Specifically, leaving the rectum intact allows its use for subsequent mucosal proctectomy and ileoanal anastomosis.

Historically, operations such as Turnbull's blow-hole colostomy with loop ileostomy[26] are rarely used because of improved medical care during emergencies and better surgical options. However, the blow-hole colostomy-ileostomy procedure may still be indicated for select patients with toxic megacolon, large bowel obstruction, severe *Clostridium difficile* colitis, adult Hirschsprung's disease, and pancreatitis with obstructing pseudocysts. The procedure may also act as a bridge to a more definitive operation for toxic patients with benign disease and palliates those with malignant obstructions and metastasis.[27]

Massive Unrelenting Hemorrhage

Massive unrelenting hemorrhage severe enough to result in hemodynamic instability is also a rare surgical complication of ulcerative colitis, occurring in less than 1% of patients and accounting for about 10% of urgent colectomies. Initial treatment should consist of aggressive fluid, electrolyte and blood-product resuscitation. If the hemorrhage is continuous but the patient is hemodynamically stable, a 2–3 day course of high-dose steroids may be tried prior to surgical intervention. However, in most cases prompt surgical intervention is indicated, but only after other causes of bleeding such as gastric or duodenal ulcers are ruled out. Uncontrollable hemorrhage from the entire colorectal mucosa may be the one clear indication for emergency proctocolectomy. If possible, the rectum should be spared for later mucosal proctectomy with ileoanal anastomosis, realizing that about 12% of patients will have continued hemorrhage from the retained rectal segment.

Acute Perforation

Although acute colonic perforation occurs infrequently in the absence of toxic megacolon, the incidence is usually directly related to both the severity of the initial episode and extent of the disease. Although the overall incidence of perforation during a first attack is less than 4%, if the attack is severe, the incidence rises to about 10%. If the patient has pancolitis, the perforation rate can rise to 15%; if the pancolitis is associated with a clinically severe attack, the perforation rate rises to nearly 20%. Perforation may not always be directly associated with the underlying ulcerative colitis, and other causes such as gastric or duodenal ulcers from steroid use or even Crohn's disease might be other causes of perforation. However, since perforation is the most lethal complication of ulcerative colitis, there is no role for medical therapy, and the patient should undergo surgery immediately. Although free colon perforation occurs much more frequently in the presence of toxic megacolon than in its absence, it is important to remember that toxic megacolon is not a prerequisite for the development of perforation. In the presence of colonic perforation, the operation should be definitive without being overly aggressive. As discussed below, abdominal colectomy with ileostomy and Hartmann closure of the rectum is the procedure of choice.

Obstructions

Complete obstructions caused by benign strictures occur in 11% of patients, with 34% of the strictures occurring in the rectum. Strictures are usually the result of submucosal fibrosis and occasionally mucosal hyperplasia. Although they do not usually cause acute obstruction, the lesions must be differentiated from carcinoma by biopsy or excision, and particular attention should be given to ruling out Crohn's disease. Strictures caused by carcinoma are less common than those caused by benign disease and are more prone to perforate. Many surgeons now believe that any colonic stricture that causes obstructive symptoms, even if it appears benign on endoscopy, should be treated surgically.[24]

ELECTIVE SURGERY

Many patients with chronic ulcerative colitis are choosing to undergo elective proctocolectomy much earlier in the course of their disease,[28] now that there are restorative procedures that offer low complication rates and excellent outcomes. The patient usually decides on elective surgery in consultation with their gastroenterologist and surgeon, and although ulcerative colitis is a chronic disease, the indications for elective surgery may occur early in the course of a patient's disease or may take place after years of fairly mild disease. The major indications to elect surgical treatment of ulcerative colitis are: intractability or failure of maximal medical therapy to control symptoms; mucosal dysplasia; intolerable side effects of medications; stricture formation without obstruction; dysplasia-associated lesion or mass (DALM); malignancy of the colon or rectum; anorectal complications; extraintestinal manifestations; and growth retardation, primarily in children and adolescents (see Table 20–3).

Intractable Disease

The failure of medical management as indicated by chronic physical disability and physiologic dysfunction is by far the most common indication for elective surgery in chronic ulcerative colitis. Intractability can be characterized as the severe and persistent impairment of a patient's quality of life, created by the underlying disease or the therapy. Since intractability is clinically defined, it can occur in patients with either acute or chronic disease. Acutely, intractability generally refers to the inability to control a patient's symptoms despite maximal medical therapy. Conversely, in the chronic state, intractability refers either to the inability to taper medications without relapse, especially steroids, to a tolerable maintenance dose, or to the development of severe drug-related side effects.[24] There are numerous elective operations for medically intractable ulcerative colitis which are discussed below.

Dysplasia, Malignancy of the Colon or Rectum, or Cancer Prophylaxis

Patients with ulcerative colitis are clearly at an increased risk for the development of dysplasia and colorectal cancer.[29] Most surgeons agree that significant dysplasia, suspected cancer, or frank malignancy are clear indications for colectomy. Despite the fact that colorectal cancer complicating ulcerative colitis only accounts for approximately 2% of all cases of colorectal cancer in the general population, it is considered a serious complication and accounts for approximately 15% of all deaths associated with inflammatory bowel diseases.[29] Ulcerative colitis increases the risk of colon cancer by approximately 0.5–1.0% annually after 10 years. Early age at diagnosis, and increased duration and extent of disease appear to increase the risk substantially.[30] Thus, by the time the patient has had the disease for 20 years, the risk of colon cancer may be as high as 20%, rising to over 30% in patients who have had even quiescent disease for longer than 35 years. This increased risk clearly emphasizes the importance of performing complete colonoscopies with numerous biopsies from the entire colon and rectum at regular intervals in order to detect mucosal dysplasia and to identify possible candidates for prophylactic colectomy.[31] Although the question of timing of surgery for cancer prophylaxis remains controversial, there are few patients in whom this is the sole indication for operation. The role of rectal or colonic biopsy in directing the timing of colectomy also remains controversial. Patients with long-standing colitis, unequivocal high-grade dysplasia, or a DALM are candidates for colectomy.

Dysplasia in ulcerative colitis may be classified as flat or elevated (DALM). Patients with flat high-grade dysplasia are generally candidates for colectomy.[32] Since dysplasia is an unreliable marker for the detection of synchronous carcinoma, some surgeons now advocate that even low-grade dysplasia, if verified by an experienced IBD pathologist, is an indication for colectomy. Dysplasia of any grade increases the probability of coexistent cancer and even low-grade dysplasia has a high positive predictive value.[33] Since advanced cancer has been found in association with dysplastic changes of any grade, confirmed dysplasia of any grade is now an indication for colectomy.[33] The presence of carcinoma is not a contraindication to mucosal proctectomy with ileoanal anastomosis, unless the tumor is found to be of an advanced stage or is located within the rectum. Mucosal proctectomy with ileoanal anastomosis is contraindicated for rectal tumors located in the middle and lower thirds of the rectum. In these patients, a standard proctocolectomy and permanent Brooke ileostomy is recommended. Since these tumors are prone to local recurrence, subsequent radiation therapy may be required which contributes to very poor function. In contrast, patients with tumors located in the upper third of the rectum may safely undergo mucosal proctectomy with ileoanal anastomosis, except in cases in which the tumor is large or advanced, when proctocolectomy with Brooke ileostomy is a safer option. If there is uncertainty about the stage of the tumor at the time of the initial operation, subtotal colectomy with ileostomy and Hartmann closure of the rectum can be performed. This operation would allow subsequent conversion to ileoanal anastomosis if the patient remains disease-free.

Patients with relatively early stage colon cancers have several options including mucosal proctectomy with ileoanal anastomosis or continent or Brooke ileostomy, as discussed below. Colon cancers that have metastasized to the liver should be treated with proctocolectomy with Brooke ileostomy or abdominal colectomy and ileorectal anastomosis, as discussed below. Proctocolectomy and Brooke ileostomy is a safer option than mucosal proctectomy with ileoanal anastomosis in patients presenting with lymph node–positive tumors unless the patient is averse to a permanent stoma.

Extraintestinal Manifestations

Other than for extreme growth and development retardation in children and adolescents, extraintestinal manifestations and complications of ulcerative colitis seldom provide the sole indication for surgical management. However, in come cases colectomy can bring dramatic benefits to children with ulcerative colitis. Joint-, eye-, and skin-associated extraintestinal manifestations often respond to colectomy; however, other more serious manifestations such as ankylosing spondylitis and liver dysfunction or failure may remain unresponsive. The progression of primary sclerosing cholangitis (PSC), a chronic cholestatic syndrome characterized by fibrosing inflammation in the intra- and extrahepatic bile ducts, appears to bear no relation to the presence or absence of the colon or to the degree of the inflammatory process within the diseased mucosa. The epidemiology of PSC and its relationship to ulcerative colitis has become much clearer recently.[16] In fact, ulcerative colitis patients with PSC may represent a distinct subset of IBD patients in which colorectal cancer develops in a significant fraction and overall survival is worse.[34] Therefore, patients with this rare complication require careful and more frequent surveillance prior to colectomy.

Another extraintestinal manifestation of ulcerative colitis that occasionally emerges as a potential surgical indication is progressively destructive pyoderma gangrenosum, which generally resolves in approximately 50% of patients following colectomy. A rare but more urgent extracolonic indication for colectomy is massive hemolytic anemia, usually Coombs test positive, that is unresponsive to steroid and immunosuppressive therapy. Under these circumstances, colectomy is generally accompanied by splenectomy.

Other indications for elective surgery for ulcerative colitis can include anorectal complications, which are more common than generally appreciated and can occasionally confound the differential diagnosis between Crohn's colitis and ulcerative colitis. Most rectal symptoms occur within the first year of onset of symptoms, and in part correlate with the severity of disease. Overall, up to 18% of patients with ulcerative colitis develop perirectal or ischiorectal abscesses and associated anal fistulas that require surgical intervention.

The most common extraintestinal manifestations that present as an emergency include thromboembolic events, ocular complications, and hepatobiliary disease.[23] Hence, for most patients with ulcerative colitis, a colectomy is performed when the disease enters an intractable, chronic phase and becomes a physical and social burden. Again, with sphincter-sparing operations available for patients with ulcerative colitis, it is vitally important to avoid standard proctectomy whenever possible.

SURGICAL APPROACHES

Historical

Although sigmoid colostomy was the first documented surgical procedure for ulcerative colitis, it was not until the 1940s that it became clear that the only definitively curative treatment of chronic ulcerative colitis required total proctocolectomy, or as a compromise, subtotal abdominal colectomy with ileostomy. However, the ileostomy was fraught with technical problems from the outset, including the optimal location of the ostomy site, surgical construction and attachment techniques, and leakproof collection pouches and skin barriers, that all contributed to a high complication rate and patient dissatisfaction. It was not until the early 1950s that Brooke[35] in the U.K. and Crile and Turnbull[36] in the U.S. proposed that the ileal stoma could be immediately matured to the skin with primary mucocutaneous suturing. This innovative procedure, coined the Brooke ileostomy, when performed following a proctocolectomy, rapidly emerged as the procedure of choice for ulcerative colitis and finally offered patients a curative operation with a reasonably manageable outcome. This operation, as described below, is still performed for certain indications. Despite this early advance, patients still remained incontinent, which continued to motivate surgeons to develop techniques for restoring fecal continence following removal of the colon and rectum.

Perhaps the earliest attempt to promote a more functional and continent alternative to a permanent ileostomy was proposed by Stanley Aylett of the U.K., who in the early 1950s began performing a subtotal colectomy and ileorectal anastomosis for ulcerative colitis.[37] Despite the fact that diseased mucosa remaining in the rectal segment clearly increased the risk of persistent symptoms and cancer of the rectum, he performed nearly 400 such procedures through the mid-1970s, with relatively satisfactory functional outcome and a low cancer rate.[38] This operation, as described below, is still performed for certain indications.

Other unique techniques have been proposed for the restoration of continence after colectomy. The continent ileostomy, or Kock pouch, proposed by Nils Kock[39] in the late 1960s, is still used today for some indications, as described below. Although this operation was technically difficult, it offered patients an option for a totally curative single-stage operation that was free of cancer risk and left the patient continent. Despite multiple technical revisions to the procedure, drawbacks included high reoperation and complication rates and the possibility for ileal pouch inflammation. These deficiencies led surgeons to seek even more functional alternatives.

In the early 1970s, the development of anal sphincter–sparing operations, as described below, completely changed the course of surgical management of ulcerative colitis. Patients could now be offered a low-risk operation, the ileal pouch–anal anastomosis (IPAA) or the ileoanal "pull-through" that provided an excellent functional outcome and high patient satisfaction.

SURGICAL OPTIONS

As long as our understanding of the etiology of ulcerative colitis remains essentially unknown and medical therapy is not curative, surgery will continue to play a central role in the management of these patients. Despite significant advances in medical therapy, the fact remains that surgery will be required in up to 40% of these patients at some stage of their disease. Significant advances in the surgical management of ulcerative colitis have been made in the past 50 years. Although restorative proctocolectomy has evolved as the procedure of choice, there are a number of surgical options to choose from depending on the patient's medical circumstance or preference and the surgeon's experience (Table 20–4). Although there is some degree of morbidity associated with every option, functional results for the most part are generally good and patient satisfaction is high.

Proctocolectomy and Ileostomy

Since ulcerative colitis is essentially cured once the colon and rectum are removed, a single-stage total proc-

TABLE 20–4. SURGICAL OPTIONS FOR THE EMERGENCY AND ELECTIVE MANAGEMENT OF ULCERATIVE COLITIS

Procedure	Indications	Contraindications	Advantages	Disadvantages
SURGICAL EMERGENCIES				
Subtotal colectomy with end ileostomy	Life-threatening emergencies	Massive hemorrhage from colon and rectum	Allows option for IPAA; low risk	Requires second operation; may develop rectal recurrence of disease
Proctocolectomy with end ileostomy	Life-threatening emergencies	Severely toxic or unstable patient	Definitive treatment	No option for IPAA; moderate risk for perineal nerve damage
Blow-hole colostomy with end ileostomy	Life-threatening emergencies	Rarely, if ever, indicated	Short, simple decompression procedure	Diseased colon and rectum retained
ELECTIVE PROCEDURES				
Total proctocolectomy with Brooke ileostomy	Patients wanting to avoid risks of IPAA; elderly; poor sphincter function; rectal cancer	Patient aversion to permanent ileostomy; obesity; life-threatening emergencies	Eliminates all disease-bearing mucosa; single operation	Potential for nerve injury in the perineal and pelvic dissection; permanent ileostomy; delayed perineal wound healing; mechanical problems with stoma; high risk of SBO
Subtotal colectomy with ileorectal anastomosis	No rectal involvement; avoid permanent stoma and IPAA; young women of childbearing age to preserve fertility	Poor sphincter tone or dysfunction; active rectal or perianal disease; colonic or rectal dysplasia; or frank cancer	One-stage operation; complete continence with good function; low risk of pelvic nerve injury; eliminates stoma.	30% Recurrence rate requiring conversion to ileostomy; risk of rectal cancer requiring lifelong surveillance
Total proctocolectomy with Kock pouch	Alternative to conventional ileostomy for patients desiring to preserve continence; poor sphincter tone; low rectal cancer; failed IPAA; conversion from ileostomy	Possibility of Crohn's disease; previous resection of small bowel; patients over 60 years old; obesity; coexisting medical illness	Avoids ileostomy; patients remain continent; good quality of live; improved body image over ileostomy	High reoperation rate (35%) due to nipple valve dysfunction or failure; high fistula rate; pouchitis
Total colectomy, mucosal proctectomy and hand-sewn IPAA with temporary diverting loop ileostomy (two-stage operation)	Procedure of choice for ulcerative colitis; colonic dysplasia or cancer; indeterminate colitis	Poor resting tone or anal sphincter dysfunction; low rectal cancers	Completely restorative; mucosectomy eliminates all disease-bearing mucosa; no disease recurrence; no cancer risk; good function, continence, and quality of life.	Two-stage procedure; potential for nerve injury in the perineal and pelvic dissection; reduced fertility in females; mucosectomy and hand-sewn IPAA are technically demanding and difficult to learn; septic complications; pouchitis
Total proctocolectomy without mucosectomy and stapled IPAA with temporary diverting loop ileostomy (two-stage operation)	Procedure of choice for ulcerative colitis, colonic dysplasia, cancer, or indeterminate colitis	Poor resting tone or anal sphincter dysfunction; low rectal cancers	Completely restorative; technically easier and faster than mucosectomy with hand-sewn IPAA; good function and continence; good quality of life	Two-stage procedure; potential for nerve injury in the perineal and pelvic dissection; risk of disease recurrence and rectal cancer from retained mucosa requiring lifelong surveillance; reduced fertility in females; pouchitis.
Laparoscopic total proctocolectomy with or without mucosectomy and IPAA	Procedure of choice for UC, colonic dysplasia or cancer; indeterminate colitis; young age	Poor resting tone or anal sphincter dysfunction; low rectal cancers; obesity	Completely restorative; good function and continence; good quality of life; better cosmesis; reduced postoperative ileus and pain; fewer psychological complications	Prolonged operative time and expense; potential for nerve injury in the perineal and pelvic dissection; risk of rectal cancer from retained mucosa requiring lifelong surveillance; reduced fertility in females; pouchitis.

IPAA, ileal pouch-anal anastomosis; SBO, small bowel obstruction; UC, ulcerative colitis.

Adapted, with permission, from Fazio VW. Inflammatory bowel disease of the colon. In: Zinner MJ, Schwartz SI, Ellis H (eds). *Maingot's Abdominal Operations,* 10th ed. New York, NY: McGraw-Hill; 1997:1249-1279; Cima RR, Pemberton JH. Surgical indications and procedures in ulcerative colitis. *Curr Treat Options Gastroenterol* 2004; 7:181-190; Cima RR, Pemberton JH. Surgical management of ulcerative colitis. In: Sartor RB, Sandborn WJ (eds). *Kirsner's Inflammatory Bowel Diseases,* 6th ed. New York, NY: WB Saunders; 2004:602-613.

tocolectomy with permanent ileostomy has historically been the procedure of choice, especially in elective situations.[40] Though this procedure eliminates all diseased tissue and the risk of malignant transformation, and requires a single operation providing patients with a predictable functional result, it remains poorly accepted by patients and their physicians and is usually performed only after other operations have failed or under special circumstances. The reluctance to undergo this operation is primarily associated with the permanent abdominal ileostomy, which is required after a standard proctocolectomy. Although use of a Brooke ileostomy (Fig 20–7) facilitates the immediate maturation of the stoma and eliminates many of the functional problems previously associated with a permanent ileostomy, patients receiving even the most carefully constructed ileostomies are incontinent and must continuously wear an external collecting device.

Significant postoperative complications are also associated with this operation. A 20% overall morbidity rate is reported for elective, 30% for urgent, and 40% for emergency proctocolectomy. The risks are primarily hemorrhage, contamination, sepsis, and neural injury. Up to 25% of patients require stoma revision and experience perineal wound problems after a standard abdominal perineal proctectomy. Fifteen to twenty percent of patients experience small bowel obstruction at some point in the postoperative period. Of major concern are bladder and sexual dysfunction associated with parasympathetic nerve injury. Impotence is reported to occur in to up to 5% of male patients after proctectomy.

Despite the fact that the majority of patients with a Brooke ileostomy eventually adjust to the stoma, nearly half experience some level of appliance-related problems including skin irritation or excoriation, discomfort, leakage and odor, or just the time, effort, and financial burden of caring for an ileostomy. Perhaps more central than these problems are the significant psychological and psychosocial implications of a permanent ileostomy, particularly for young and physically active patients. It was for these reasons that surgeons sought alternatives to total proctocolectomy and ileostomy.

Subtotal Colectomy and Ileorectal Anastomosis

Subtotal colectomy and ileorectal anastomosis (Fig 20–8), has been utilized in the surgical treatment of ulcerative colitis for over 50 years.[37] An ileorectal anastomosis eliminates the need for an abdominal stoma and since the pelvic autonomic nerves are not disturbed, the risk for impotence and bladder dysfunction are very low. Although abdominal colectomy with ileorectal anastomosis is a less extensive procedure that usually leaves the patient with full continence, it is not performed extensively except under certain circumstances (see Table 20–4) because it is not curative. Mucosal inflammation can persist in the retained rectum and there is an ongoing risk of malignancy that increases with time. Approximately 20% of patients require subsequent proctectomy for uncontrollable proctitis or poor function. Even in the absence of disease recurrence or malignancy, function in the early postoperative period can be poor, averaging four or five stools per 24 hours. Ileorectal anastomosis can also be associated with a number of postoperative complications, including small bowel obstruction in up to 20% of patients. In addition, there is the potential for leakage of the anastomosis between the ileum and the disease-bearing rectum. Subtotal colectomy with ileorectal anastomosis is clearly a compromise operation, except for specific indications, and is obviously contraindicated in patients with anal sphincter dysfunction, severe

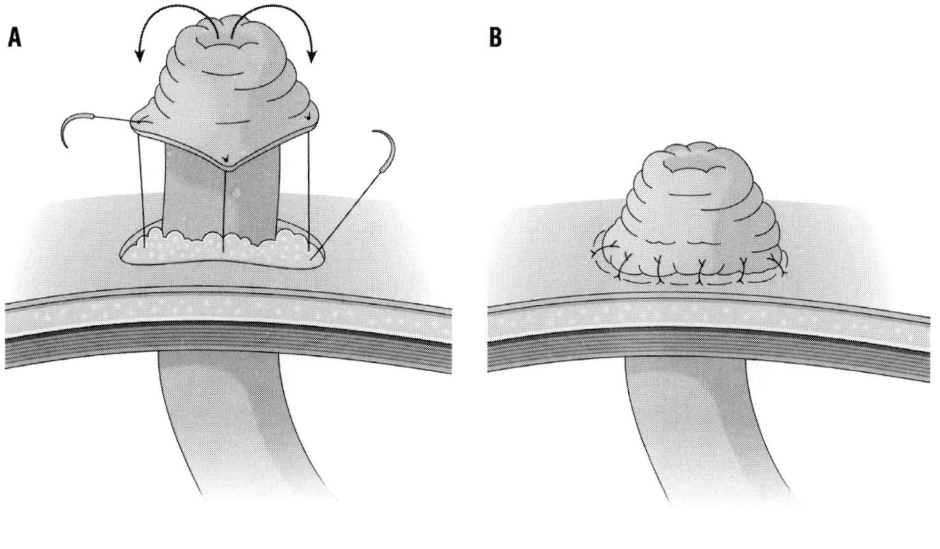

Figure 20–7. Construction of an end ileostomy. **A.** The terminal ileum is brought 5 cm through an abdominal wall defect, everted, **(B)** and sutured to the more proximal ileal seromuscularis and the dermis to mature the ileostomy. (Reproduced, with permission, from Becker JM, Stucchi AF. Inflammatory bowel disease. In: Becker JM, Stucchi AF [eds]. *Essentials of Surgery.* Philadelphia, PA: WB Saunders; 2006:240–256.)

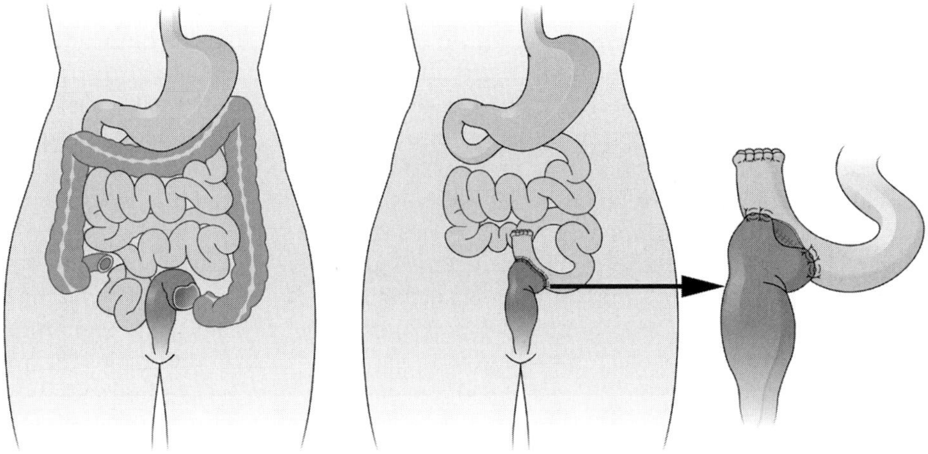

Figure 20–8. Ileorectal anastomosis after abdominal colectomy. This represents a nondefinitive operation for selected patients with chronic ulcerative colitis. (Reproduced, with permission, from Becker JM, Stucchi AF. Inflammatory bowel disease. In: Becker JM, Stucchi AF [eds]. *Essentials of Surgery*. Philadelphia, PA: WB Saunders; 2006:240–256.)

rectal disease, rectal dysplasia, or malignancy. With the availability and success of the definitive mucosal proctectomy and ileoanal anastomosis, ileorectal anastomosis is indicated in very few patients. As discussed below, with the recent concern over infertility in young women following IPAA, subtotal colectomy with or without ileorectal anastomoses became more popular in this patient population.

Continent Ileostomy

Patient dissatisfaction due to mechanical and functional problems with the ileostomy and the associated incontinence has motivated surgeons to seek alternatives to preserving continence. Early attempts at continence, such as the continent ileostomy or Kock pouch, however, were fraught with technical complications.[39] Kock first constructed the continent ileostomy entirely of terminal ileum with an ileal pouch that served as a reservoir for stool and an ileal conduit connecting the pouch to a cutaneous stoma (Fig 20–9). Despite poor functional results, patients undergoing total proctocolectomy could, for the first time, be offered an option for continence. The operation was later modified to include an intestinal nipple valve between the pouch and the stoma.

Typically, 45–50 cm of terminal ileum is required to surgically construct the pouch and the nipple valve. The proximal 30–35 cm is fashioned into a pouch; whereas intussuscepting the outflow tract from the pouch and then securing it with sutures or staples forms the nipple valve. The ileal reservoir is sutured to the peritoneum and fascia, and the efferent limb is externalized through the abdominal wall as a flush stoma. Passing a soft plastic tube through the nipple valve via

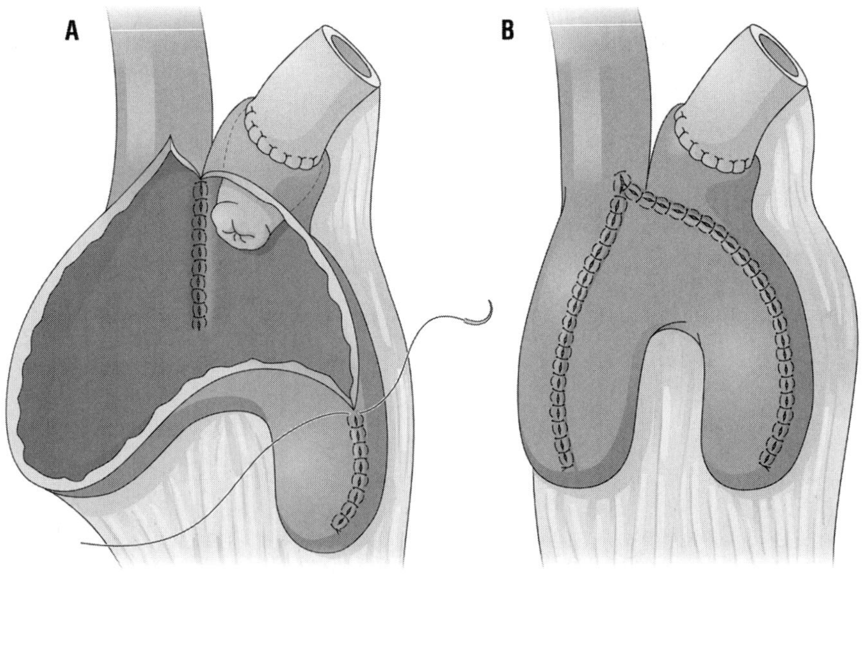

Figure 20–9. The continent ileostomy or Kock pouch consists of an ileal reservoir and nipple valve constructed by **(A)** intussuscepting the efferent limb and fixing it in place with sutures or staples. **B.** The pouch itself is then closed with sutures. This provides a continent internal intestinal reservoir that the patient can drain by intubating the pouch through the flush cutaneous stoma several times throughout the day. (Reproduced, with permission, from Becker JM, Stucchi AF. Inflammatory bowel disease. In: Becker JM, Stucchi AF [eds]. *Essentials of Surgery*. Philadelphia, PA: WB Saunders; 2006:240–256.)

the stoma can then empty the ileal pouch. The significance of this operation for its time was that patients could finally be offered an operation that was curative and did not require the use of an external appliance.

The continent ileostomy has been associated with a number of complications, the most significant being related to dislodgment of the nipple valve, which results in fecal incontinence and difficulty in intubating and emptying the pouch. Nipple valve failure requiring revision reportedly occurs in up to 60% of patients and approximately 20% of patients will experience small bowel obstruction, primarily due to adhesions.[41] The risk of bladder dysfunction, impotence, and perineal wound problems are similar to those of standard proctocolectomy and ileostomy. Several dysfunction syndromes associated directly with the continent ileostomy include stagnant loop syndrome, enteritis, nonspecific ileitis, and pouchitis. Clinically these patients often present with diarrhea, fat and vitamin B_{12} malabsorption, bacterial overgrowth, and mucosal inflammation of the pouch and incontinence. Patients may also develop fistulae between the pouch and the skin or other enteric organs. Crohn's disease is a clear contraindication to performing this operation.

Although the continent ileostomy has clear theoretical advantages over the Brooke ileostomy, especially with respect to continence, its high rate of functional complications has restricted its clinical utility. The continent ileostomy may be useful in patients who have already undergone total proctocolectomy and ileostomy, and after careful counseling, wish to undergo a continence-restoring procedure. This operation also remains an option for patients who wish to remain continent but are either not candidates for or have failed IPAA,[42] or who for other reasons prefer a permanent ileostomy. In major centers that offer all surgical alternatives to patients with ulcerative colitis, the Kock pouch has limited clinical usefulness and few such pouches are currently being constructed despite recent reports of satisfactory long-term function in more than two-thirds of patients for up to 30 years.[41] Although surgical revisions may be needed to restore proper function, the continent ileostomy appears to have good durability. In a more recent study, patients reported adequate function, high satisfaction, and a health-related quality of life similar to that of the general population.[43]

TOTAL PROCTOCOLECTOMY WITH ILEAL POUCH–ANAL ANASTOMOSIS

As mentioned, until about 25 years ago, proctocolectomy with a Brooke ileostomy was the only viable surgical option that surgeons could offer patients with ulcerative colitis requiring colectomy. Even though this procedure eliminated all diseased tissue and the subsequent risk of malignant transformation, patients and their physicians were averse to this option because it required a permanent abdominal ileostomy. It is for this reason that surgeons sought alternatives to total proctocolectomy and ileostomy that could provide the patient with continence and acceptable function. While the options discussed above were being performed, many surgeons were developing more innovative, functional, and acceptable procedures.

Although the first ileoanal anastomosis was reportedly performed by Nissen in Germany in the early 1930s,[44] it was the pioneering efforts of two surgeons, Mark Ravitch and David Sabiston, who more than half a century ago proposed the novel concept of restorative proctocolectomy with anal sphincter preservation.[45] Instead of ablating the entire rectum, anus, and anal sphincter as occurs during a standard proctocolectomy, they purported that since ulcerative colitis is a mucosal disease, the disease-bearing rectal mucosa could be dissected completely down to the dentate line of the anus, and in theory preserve the rectal muscular cuff and the anal sphincter apparatus. The subsequent extension of the terminal ileum into the pelvis endorectally, and suturing it circumferentially to the anus in an end-to-end fashion would re-establish the continuity of the intestinal tract (Fig 20–10). This novel surgical advance incorporated a number of potential advantages including preservation of parasympathetic innervation to the bladder and genitalia, elimination of the abdominal perineal proctectomy, and if performed carefully, preservation of the anorectal sphincter. Most importantly, the permanent abdominal ileostomy was eliminated and continence was maintained. Early on, poor func-

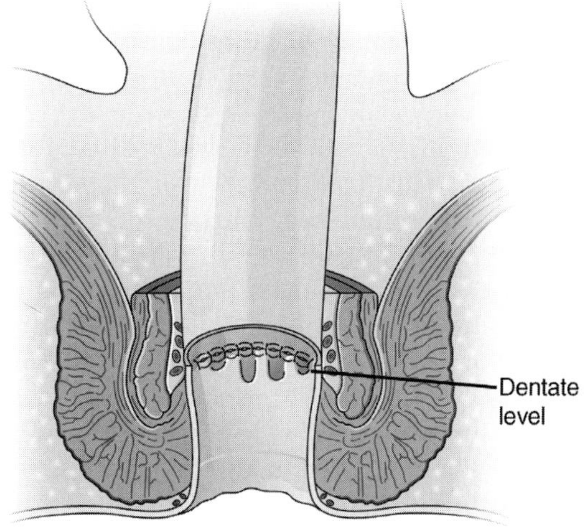

Figure 20–10. End-to-end ileoanal anastomosis after colectomy, mucosal proctectomy, and endorectal ileoanal pull-through. (Reproduced, with permission, from Becker JM, Stucchi AF. Inflammatory bowel disease. In: Becker JM, Stucchi AF [eds]. *Essentials of Surgery.* Philadelphia, PA: WB Saunders; 2006:240–256.)

tional results forced the operation to be largely abandoned, due in part to an inadequate understanding of anal sphincter physiology at the time. The pioneering efforts of these surgeons, however, set the stage for what has become the definitive procedure for patients seeking surgical intervention for ulcerative colitis.

Although a few surgeons continued to experiment with the ileoanal anastomosis procedure throughout the 1950s and 1960s, there were no more human trials until the late 1970s when Martin, LeCoultre, and Schubert reported on a cohort of 17 patients with ulcerative colitis in whom they successfully performed a total colectomy and mucosal proctectomy and straight ileoanal anastomosis.[46] Despite significant postoperative complications and high stool frequency, others who performed them concluded that ileoanal anastomosis is a viable alternative for patients requiring proctocolectomy.[47,48] However, it was the physiologic studies of Heppell and associates in 1982 that showed an inverse relationship between ileal compliance and stool frequency in patients after an end-to-end or straight ileoanal anastomosis.[49] These studies led to perhaps the most significant technical refinement in the evolution of the IPAA procedure, which was the surgical construction of an ileal pouch or reservoir proximal to the ileoanal anastomosis. Increasing the capacity for storage greatly improved function, reduced stool frequency, and led to increased patient satisfaction.

Although the above reports are historically relevant to the revitalization of the ileoanal anastomosis procedure, it was probably the reports by Parks and Nicholls[50] and Utsunomiya and colleagues[51] that motivated the resurgence of the modern ileal pouch–anal anastomosis procedure. They independently developed and were among the first to successfully utilize an ileal reservoir or pelvic pouch proximal to the ileoanal anastomosis to improve the functional outcome following total colectomy and mucosal proctectomy. Subsequent follow-up studies comparing functional outcomes between the straight ileoanal anastomosis and the ileal pouch–anal anastomosis concluded that inclusion of the ileal pouch significantly improved continence, function, quality of life,[52] and overall clinical outcome, due primarily to the increased distensibility of the neorectum.[53]

Since the addition of the ileal pouch, there has been a dramatic increase in the use of restorative proctocolectomy, especially as surgeons became more familiar with the technical aspects of the procedure. Despite the controversies surrounding methodological issues such as mucosectomy, stapled versus hand-sewn anastomoses, diverting loop ileostomy, pouch configurations, and staged procedures, most surgeons agree that restorative proctocolectomy with IPAA is the definitive operation for the surgical treatment of patients with ulcerative colitis. This procedure is also the choice for patients with familial adenomatous polyposis and more recently in select patients with hereditary nonpolyposis colorectal cancer.[54] Although this procedure is generally contraindicated for patients with Crohn's disease, there are reports of acceptable long-term outcomes in select patients.[55]

Patient Selection

Although strict adherence to careful patient selection has always been a guiding principle for success with IPAA, the selection process has become less stringent as surgeons have become more familiar with the technical aspects. However, there still remain established factors associated with improved outcomes.

Until recently, age was not a significant consideration since most ulcerative colitis patients requiring surgery were relatively young. However, as older and even elderly patients were being referred for surgical intervention, surgeons needed to evaluate the impact of age on long-term functional outcome. Initially, IPAA was not recommended for elderly patients, especially in light of studies that showed that functional outcomes were poor in patients who were older than 45 years at the time of surgery.[56] Surprisingly, there were no patients older than 65 years of age in this study on which to base these recommendations. However, Tan and associates[57] evaluated the outcomes in patients from age 50 years to beyond 70 years and found that there were no significant differences in major complications or functional outcomes when patients over 65 were compared with younger patients. Thus, as we and others have shown, IPAA is not contraindicated in healthy older patients, as long as sphincter tone is good.

Preoperative anal sphincter function is perhaps one of the more important predictors of postoperative functional outcome. Anorectal manometry is routinely used at this center to establish preoperative sphincter tone. IPAA is generally contraindicated in patients found to have poor preoperative resting pressures; however, we find that most patients, even into their sixth and seventh decades, meet the minimum acceptable criteria. This raises the confidence of both the patient and surgeon that the outcome will be acceptable. It is also imperative when proposing IPAA that the patient fully understands the physiology as well as the operative procedure and has reasonable expectations regarding the long-term outcome.

One final consideration in patient selection pertains to offering IPAA to women of childbearing age. While young women who have undergone proctocolectomy with Brooke or continent ileostomy can anticipate a normal pregnancy and delivery, IPAA appears to reduce fertility.[58] However, those who do become pregnant are at no increased risk for complications either during pregnancy or after delivery. Furthermore, ileal pouch function and the incidence of long-term complications following pregnancy appears unaffected.[59] Thus, until more definitive studies further evaluate fertility in women considering IPAA, surgeons should inform their patients of the possibility of decreased fertility.

Operative Techniques

At most major centers, the operation is typically performed in two stages. The first stage consists of abdominal colectomy, mucosal proctectomy, endorectal IPAA, and diverting loop ileostomy. Approximately 8 weeks after the initial operation, the second stage is performed in which the loop ileostomy is closed.

As part of the patient's preoperative work-up, anal manometry is performed to assure that the patient has adequate anal sphincter tone. Sufficient preoperative resting pressure is perhaps one of the more important aspects to postoperative continence and satisfactory function. Just prior to surgery, flexible sigmoidoscopy is performed to confirm the final diagnosis and to assess the status of the inflammation in the sigmoid colon and rectum. In patients experiencing active disease, steroid or salicylate treatment can be accelerated in the immediate preoperative period. Patients also undergo a thorough bowel preparation on the day before surgery.

At many major centers, two teams of surgeons work together to perform a multi-part operation that entails a total colectomy, the removal of the rectum with or without mucosal proctectomy, the construction of the ileal pouch, and finally the ileoanal anastomosis. Once the patient is fully anesthetized, they are carefully placed on the operating table in lithotomy position (Fig 20–11), which facilitates access to the abdomen and the perineum simultaneously. One team then accesses the abdomen through a midline vertical incision and performs a standard colectomy as follows: After the colon is freed from its peritoneal attachments, the transverse colon is carefully dissected away from the greater omentum. While some surgeons prefer to leave the omentum intact, we and others generally perform an omentectomy, primarily to reduce the significant intra-abdominal adhesions that form following this procedure.[60] Once the entire colon is completely free, the terminal ileum is transected approximately 1–2 cm proximal to the ileocecal valve with a linear stapler. The mesentery of the colon is divided at a suitable distance from the bowel wall (Fig 20–12), taking care not to compromise the terminal arcade of the superior mesenteric artery supplying the terminal ileum, since this will soon be the major blood supply to the ileal pouch. The ileocolic artery is divided to facilitate mobility of the pouch. The remaining colonic mesentery is serially clamped, divided, and ligated and the colon is removed.

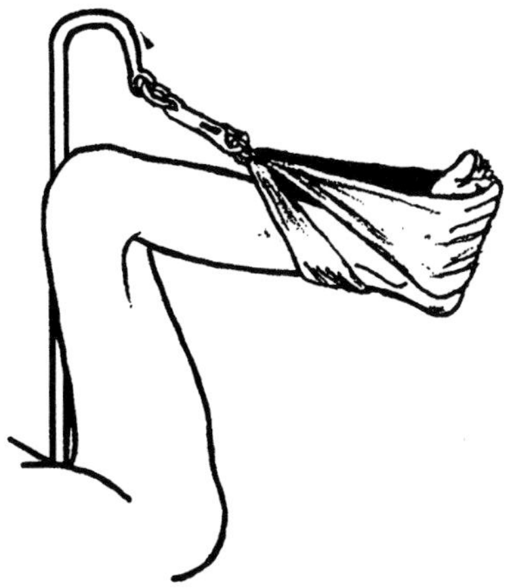

Figure 20–11. The patient is placed on the operating table in the lithotomy position. (Reprinted, with permission, from Paschal CR, Strzelecki LR. Lithotomy positioning devices. *AORN J* 1992;55:1011.)

To facilitate access to the pelvis for the dissection of the rectum and the mucosal proctectomy, if performed, most surgeons prefer that the patient be placed in the Trendelenburg position. The proximal rectum is then mobilized and transected above the levator ani sling, meticulously avoiding the pelvic nerves that lie in this plane. At this center, the rectal team simultaneously performs the transperineal rectal mucosal dissection as described below. However, at other centers, 1.5–2.0 cm of rectal mucosa proximal to the dentate line is left intact in preparation for a double-stapled ileal pouch–anal anastomosis, as discussed further below. Exposure of the anal canal and rectal mucosa is facilitated by the Lone Star retractor (Fig 20–13). Once the submucosa of the anal canal is infiltrated with a dilute (1:200,000) solution of epinephrine, a circumferential incision is completed at the dentate line with a needle-tip electrocautery leaving the anal sphincter intact. The rectal mucosa is then circumferentially dissected away from the anal sphincter and the rectal muscularis (Fig 20–14). Although the largely blunt dissection is facilitated by electrocautery or harmonic scalpel primarily for hemostasis, optimum functional results requires that meticulous care be taken in identifying and preserving maximum anorectal smooth muscle during mucosectomy.

After the proximal rectum is removed and the distal rectal mucosectomy is performed, the next step involves the construction of the ileal pouch from the remaining terminal ileum. In order to ensure that the newly constructed ileal pouch will extend down into the anal canal, the mesentery must be sufficiently mobilized, in most cases to just below the pancreas. A number of pouch configurations have been utilized including the J-pouch,[51] S-pouch,[61] W-pouch,[62] and lateral side-to-side

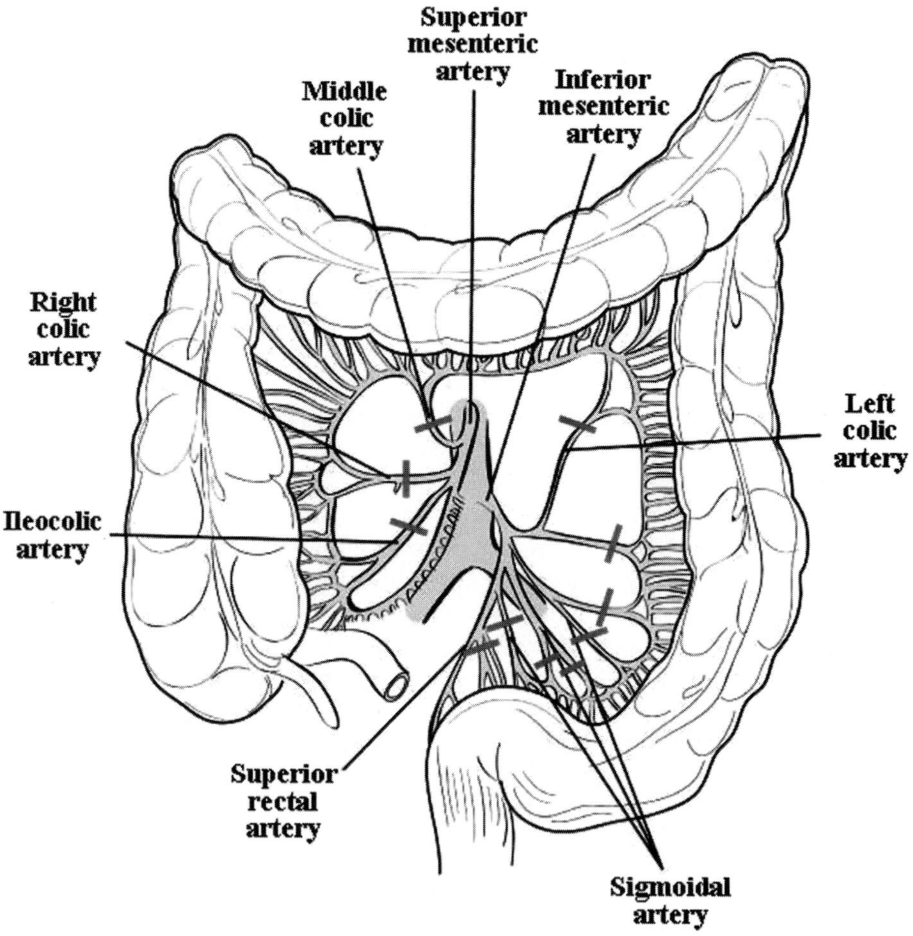

Figure 20–12. Arterial blood supply to the colon showing mesenteric divisions. (Reproduced, with permission, from Schwartz SI, Shires GT, Spencer FC [eds.]: Principles of Surgery, 5th ed. New York: McGraw-Hill, 1989, p 1226.)

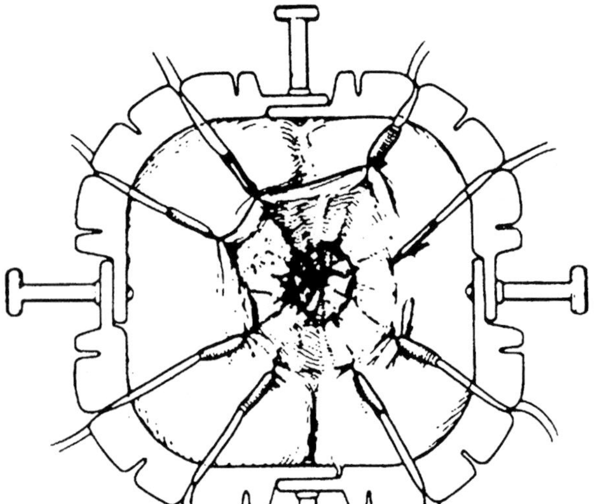

Figure 20–13. The Lone Star retractor (Lone Star Medical Products, Houston, TX) used to facilitate the transanal mucosal proctectomy. (Reproduced, with permission, from Sagar PM, Pemberton JH. Role of the ileal pouch procedure-pouch construction, and the ileoanal anastomosis. In: Allen RN et al [eds]. *Inflammatory Bowel Diseases*, 3rd ed. New York, NY: Churchill Livingstone; 1997:781–791.)

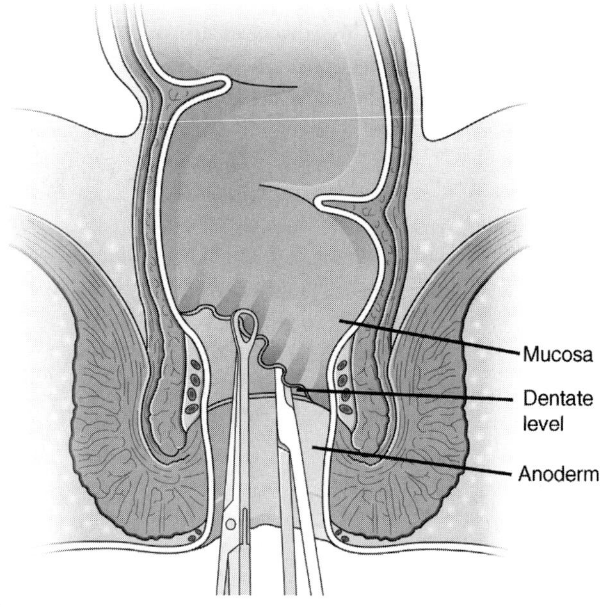

Figure 20–14. Transanal mucosal proctectomy. A circumferential incision is made at the dentate line, and the rectal mucosa is carefully dissected away from the anal sphincter and the rectal muscularis. (Reproduced, with permission, from Becker JM, Stucchi AF. Inflammatory bowel disease. In: Becker JM, Stucchi AF [eds]. *Essentials of Surgery*. Philadelphia, PA: WB Saunders; 2006:240–256.)

isoperistaltic pouch,[63] with varying degrees of success (Fig 20–15). However, the most common configuration used at major centers around the world, including this center, is the ileal J-pouch (Fig 20–16). Technically, ileal J-pouches are faster and less tedious to create, use considerably less ileum, and have similar or better functional results than other pouch configurations.

Approximately 15 cm of the stapled off terminal ileum is folded back onto itself into the shape of a J. This distal or efferent limb of the J is secured to the afferent limb of the small bowel with several interrupted sutures. The ileal J-pouch, approximately 15 cm in length, is then formed using two firings of a 75-mm mechanical stapler applied sequentially through an enterotomy in the apex of the pouch (Fig 20–17). Electrocautery is used to create the enterotomy at the apex of the loop of terminal ileum. The forks of a 75-mm intestinal anastomosing stapler (PROXIMATE Linear Cutter, Ethicon, Johnson & Johnson Health Care Systems, Piscataway, NJ) are passed into the ileal limbs, and the instrument is fired. This is repeated while the limbs are telescoped onto the stapler, until a 15-cm side-to-side anastomosis is completed. The apical enterotomy is closed with a simple 2-0 polypropylene purse-string stitch. The newly constructed pouch is then filled with a saline solution via a catheter to measure pouch volume at a fixed intraluminal pressure of 10 cm of H_2O to assess leakage of the staple lines. The capacity of the pouch should be approximately 200–300 mL. Prior to beginning the final pouch-anal anastomotic step, it is important to confirm that the newly constructed ileal pouch extends into the anal canal without tension. To allow adequate mobility of the terminal ileum, especially in large or obese patients, the ileal branch of the ileocolic artery must be ligated and divided and the superior mesenteric artery must be mobilized to where it arises from below the pancreas.

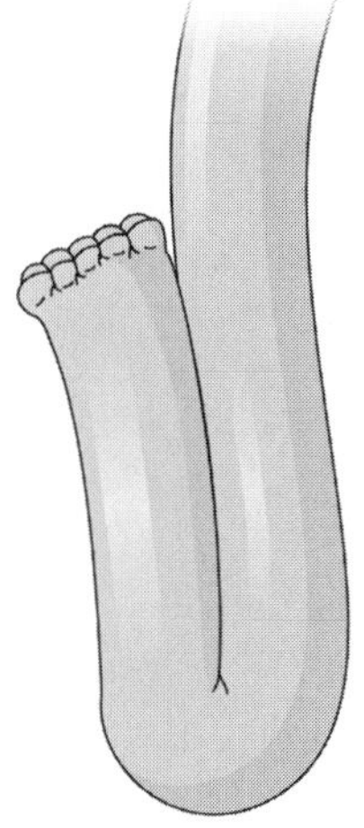

Figure 20–16. Ileal J pouch configuration in patients undergoing ileal pouch–anal anastomosis. (Reproduced, with permission, from Becker JM, Stucchi AF. Inflammatory bowel disease. In: Becker JM, Stucchi AF [eds]. *Essentials of Surgery.* Philadelphia, PA: WB Saunders; 2006:240–256.)

The final step in completing this phase of the operation is to anastomose the newly constructed ileal pouch to the anus or the pouch-anal anastomosis. The two surgical techniques currently used for performing this procedure, the hand-sewn method with mucosal proctectomy used at this center and the double-stapled method without mucosectomy, remain an issue of significant controversy among surgeons, as discussed below. The ileal pouch is extended endorectally into the anal canal and down to the level of the dentate line, making sure that the ileal mesentery proximal to the pouch is not twisted. The apex of the pouch is fixed to the anal sphincter in four quadrants with 2-0 polyglycolic acid sutures and opened. The apex of the pouch is sutured circumferentially to the dentate line with interrupted 3-0 polyglycolic acid sutures to complete a side-to-end ileal pouch–anal anastomosis (Fig 20–18).

As mentioned, the surgical alternative in completing the pouch-anal anastomosis is to secure the distal apex

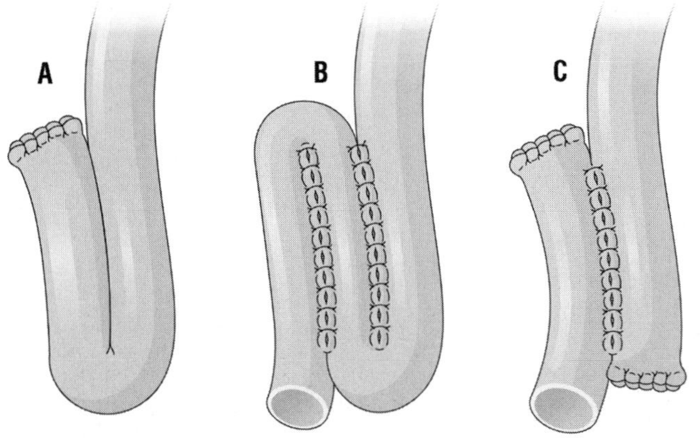

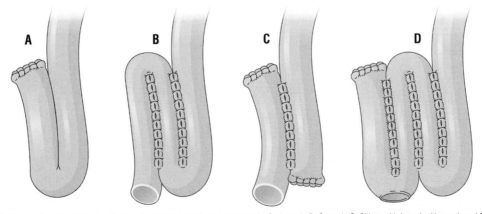

Figure 20–15. Options for ileal pouch configurations in patients undergoing ileal pouch–anal anastomosis. **A.** J-pouch, **B.** S-pouch, **C.** Side-to-side isoperistaltic pouch, and **D.** W-pouch. (Reproduced, with permission, from Becker JM, Stucchi AF. Inflammatory bowel disease. In: Becker JM, Stucchi AF [eds]. *Essentials of Surgery.* Philadelphia, PA: WB Saunders; 2006:240–256.)

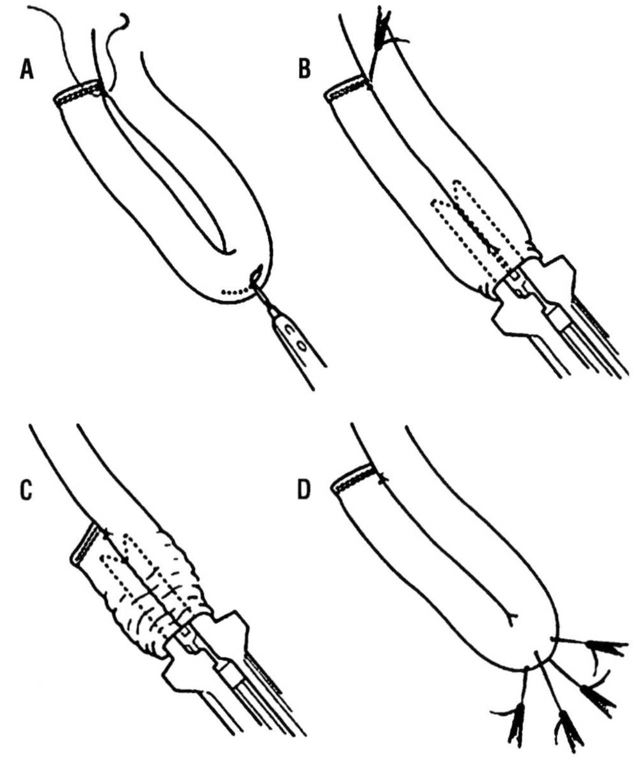

Figure 20–17. Construction of the ileal J-pouch. The ileal pouch is constructed by dividing the common wall of the afferent and efferent limbs of the distal ileum by means of multiple firings of a linear cutting stapler as follows. **A.** An electrocautery is used to create an enterotomy at the apex of the 15-cm loop of terminal ileum. **B.** The forks of a 75-mm intestinal anastomosing stapler are pressed into the intestinal limbs, and the instrument is fired. **C.** This is repeated while the limbs are telescoped onto the stapler, until a 15-cm side-to-side anastomosis is completed. **D.** The apical enterotomy is closed with a simple purse-string stitch. (Reproduced, with permission, from Becker JM, Stucchi AF. Ulcerative colitis. In: Greenfield LJ et al [eds]. *Surgery Scientific Principles and Practice*, 3rd ed. Philadelphia, PA: Lippincott Williams & Wilkins; 2001:1070–1089.)

of the ileal pouch to the anal canal by the double-stapled technique without performing a prior rectal mucosectomy. First, the distal rectum is closed with a TA-30 linear stapler and is divided near the pelvic floor, but leaving the anal transition zone largely intact. The anastomotic technique requires the use of a circular end-to-end anastomosis or EEA stapler. The anvil is affixed to the apex of the newly created ileal pouch with a purse-string suture. After the head of the EEA stapler is advanced into the anal canal, the connection pin is located next to the staple line at the site where the rectum was previously divided at the floor of the pelvis. The anvil of the stapler within the pouch is then brought down into the pelvis and carefully aligned and fit onto the pre-fixed pin of the stapler. The stapler is then fired to secure the pouch to the anus (Fig 20–19). The same principles apply, as above, in assuring that there is no tension on the pouch prior to completing the anastomosis.

With the most technically demanding phase of the operation completed, the patient is taken out of the lithotomy position. The abdominal cavity is thoroughly rinsed several times with an antibiotic-containing saline solution. Gloves and instruments are replaced, and the abdomen is re-draped. A closed suction drain is then placed at the rear of the pouch and exteriorized through the left abdominal wall. In the majority of patients, including those operated on at this center, a temporary loop ileostomy is constructed in the right lower abdomen to divert the fecal stream from the pouch while the staple lines and the anastomosis heal. However, whether a diverting ileostomy is actually required is another of the major controversies regarding the technical aspects of the IPAA, as discussed below. To construct the diverting loop ileostomy, a mobile loop of ileum approximately 40 cm proximal from the top of the efferent limb of the ileal pouch is brought out through the abdominal wall in a previously marked ostomy site and suspended over an ostomy rod. The midline fascia and skin are closed, the ileal loop is opened, and the loop ileostomy is matured with interrupted 4-0 polyglycolate acid sutures (Fig 20–20).

Adhesion Prevention

One final and very important consideration for the surgeon prior to closing the midline abdominal incision pertains to intra-abdominal adhesions. Principles of adhesion prevention during any abdominal operation include gentle handling of tissues, meticulous control of bleeding, avoidance of foreign materials, excision of necrotic tissue, minimization of ischemia and desicca-

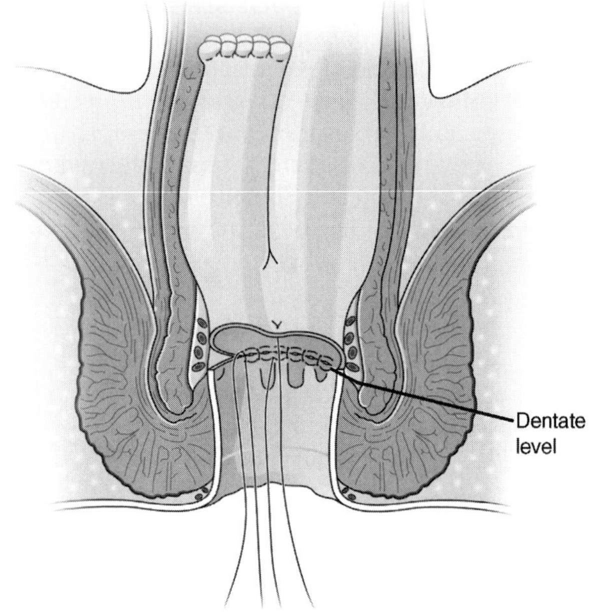

Figure 20–18. Creating the ileal J-pouch–anal anastomosis. The ileal J-pouch is secured to the sphincter in each quadrant with a suture. The purse-string stitch closing the enterotomy is cut to allow the apex of the pouch to open. An anastomosis is then created between the apex of the pouch and the anoderm with interrupted absorbable sutures. (Reproduced, with permission, from Becker JM, Stucchi AF. Inflammatory bowel disease. In: Becker JM, Stucchi AF [eds]. *Essentials of Surgery*. Philadelphia, PA: WB Saunders; 2006:240–256.)

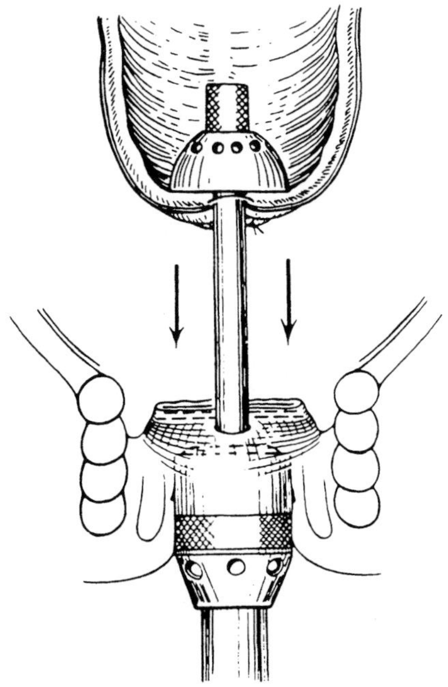

Figure 20–19. Double-staple technique for ileal pouch–anal anastomosis using an end-to-end anastomosing (EEA) stapler. After the pouch is constructed, the head of an EEA stapler is secured in the apex of the pouch and connected to the pin of the stapler, which was placed upward through the anus. (Reproduced, with permission, from Sagar PM, Pemberton JH. Role of the ileal pouch procedure–pouch construction, and the ileoanal anastomosis. In: Allan RN et al [eds]. *Inflammatory Bowel Diseases*, 3rd ed. New York, NY: Churchill Livingstone; 1997:781–791.)

tion, and prevention of infection. Despite adhering to those principles, adhesions occur after IPAA with very high incidence. A recent study showed that up to 94% of patients develop primary abdominal adhesions following IPAA.[60] Abdominal adhesions are associated with a range of adverse sequelae including difficult and dangerous reoperations, infertility, and chronic abdominal and pelvic pain; however, the most serious and life-threatening sequela is adhesive small bowel obstruction (ASBO).[64] At the Cleveland Clinic and the Mayo Clinic, the reported incidence of ASBO was 25% of 1,500 patients and 15% of 1,193 patients, respectively, following IPAA. At both centers, approximately 30% required reoperation. In nearly 750 such operations at this center, the incidence of ASBO is approximately 17% with 6% requiring surgical intervention. Lysis of adhesions for ASBO can lead to inadvertent enterotomy, prolonged operative times, increased clinical workload, and high financial costs, all of which are important adhesion-related problems that need to be addressed. A recent study showed that not only have a significant percentage of patients undergoing adhesiolysis for ASBO experienced recurrent ASBO, but many have endured years of adhesion-related abdominal and pelvic pain.[65]

At the present time, there are a limited number of options for surgeons to reliably and effectively prevent adhesion formation. A prospective, randomized clinical trial showed that the bioresorbable physical barrier Seprafilm® (Genzyme Corporation, Cambridge, MA), composed of carboxymethylcellulose and hyaluronic acid, significantly reduced adhesions after IPAA.[60] While other physical barriers are in use and under development, it is unclear whether physical barriers can provide protection in areas other than the site of application, especially in a complex abdominal and pelvic operation like the IPAA. Our own studies have shown that a midline laparotomy initiates a generalized inflammatory response in the peritoneum that can initiate adhesion formation at uninjured peritoneal sites distant from the midline incision.[66] Barrier agents will likely decrease adhesion formation, particularly when used in conjunction with meticulous surgical technique, thorough hemostasis, and careful tissue handling, and perhaps novel biological agents.

Post-IPAA

Approximately 4 weeks after the IPAA is completed, a barium radiographic study is performed to assess the integrity of the ileal pouch and the ileoanal anastomo-

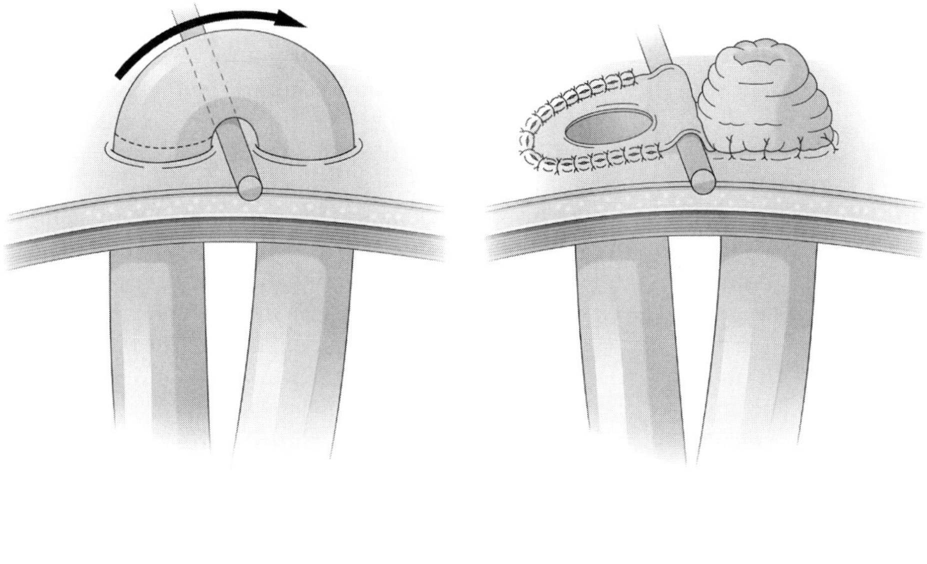

Figure 20–20. A loop ileostomy is constructed 40 cm proximal to the ileal pouch and matured over a rod. (Reproduced, with permission, from Becker JM, Stucchi AF. Inflammatory bowel disease. In: Becker JM, Stucchi AF [eds]. *Essentials of Surgery*. Philadelphia, PA: WB Saunders; 2006:240–256.)

sis. Anastomotic or pouch leaks, such as the one shown (Fig 20–21), can lead to serious septic complications and are a significant cause of morbidity, poor function, and pouch failure.

Approximately 8 weeks after the IPAA is completed, anal manometry is repeated to ensure that the anal sphincter muscles have retained full function. The volume of the ileal pouch is also measured. Pending the satisfactory outcome of these tests, the loop ileostomy is then closed using a stapling technique, which has greatly simplified this operation (Fig 20–22). A transverse elliptical incision is made in the skin around the site of the loop ileostomy. The loop is then dissected free from the subcutaneous tissue and the fascia. The afferent and efferent limbs are divided with a stapling device. A side-to-side functional end-to-end anastomosis is then created between the two limbs with a 75-mm anastomosing stapler. The enterotomy is closed with a 60-mm linear stapler. The anastomosed loops of ileum are then placed back into the peritoneal cavity, and the fascia, subcutaneous tissue, and skin are closed. The standard protocol at this center requires that patients are followed at approximately 1 month, 3 months, 6 months, and 12 months after closure of the loop ileostomy and then are seen at yearly intervals for follow-up. Anorectal manometry is repeated at 1 year. Unless subsequent long-term complications such as pouchitis arise, patients generally undergo flexible fiberoptic pouchoscopy with surveillance biopsies of the ileal pouch approximately every 5 years.

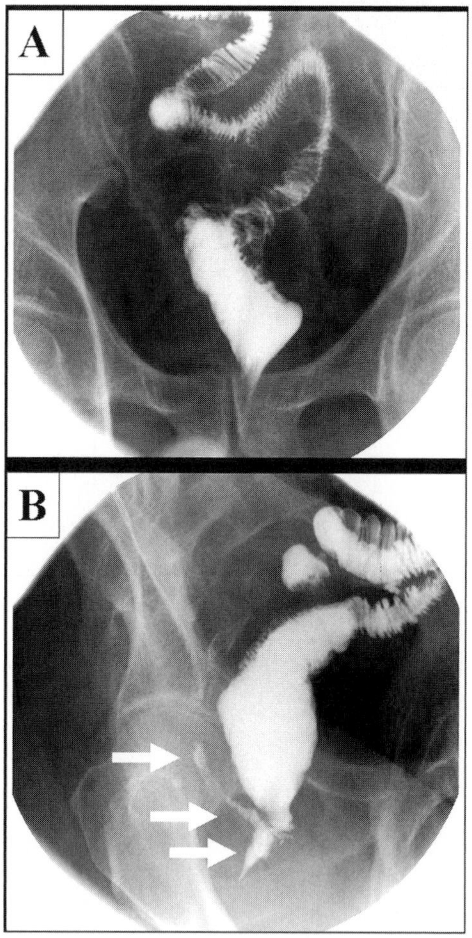

Figure 20–21. A barium radiograph of the ileal J-pouch taken 4 weeks after ileal pouch–anal anastomosis. **A.** Normal pouch showing no apparent leaks. **B.** Pouch with pouch-anal anastomotic leak showing contrast material leaking into the pelvis

SURGICAL CONTROVERSIES

Ever since IPAA became the most common surgical option offered to patients requiring colectomy for ulcerative colitis, controversy has surrounded a number of aspects of the operation. Although a number of small procedural issues are often debated, perhaps the foremost controversies regarding the procedure involve the rectal mucosal resection, the choice of ileoanal anastomotic technique, pouch configuration, and the requirement for a diverting loop ileostomy.[21]

Mucosectomy and Anastomotic Technique

Mucosal proctectomy and hand-sewn IPAA versus a double-stapled IPAA to the intact anal transition zone has been a significant technical controversy among surgeons performing this operation. The disagreement arises over two main issues: the increased risk of ongoing proctitis and rectal cancer if a mucosal proctectomy is not performed, and the purportedly technical and functional advantages of the double-stapled technique. Even though the patient's clinical condition and mitigating complications may play some role, the choice of anastomotic technique generally depends on the surgeon's preference and experience.

Since mucosal proctectomy removes the columnar epithelial layer from the anal transition zone, the subsequent risk of mucosal inflammation, dysplasia, or cancer is presumably eliminated. Despite this benefit, dissection of the rectal mucosa can be tedious, time-consuming, technically demanding, and is not without risk. Damage to underlying smooth muscle layers and prolonged retraction of the anal sphincter muscles has been shown to compromise functional outcomes and impair rectal sensation.[67] Although residual rectal mucosa has been detected in patients following mucosal proctectomy, there have been only isolated reports of associated rectal cancers. Mucosectomy is absolutely indicated in patients with ulcerative colitis who have dysplasia or cancer in the rectum or in patients undergoing IPAA for familial adenomatous polyposis (FAP). From a sagittal view, the ileal pouch can be seen anastomosed to the anus at the dentate line following mucosectomy (Fig 20–23).

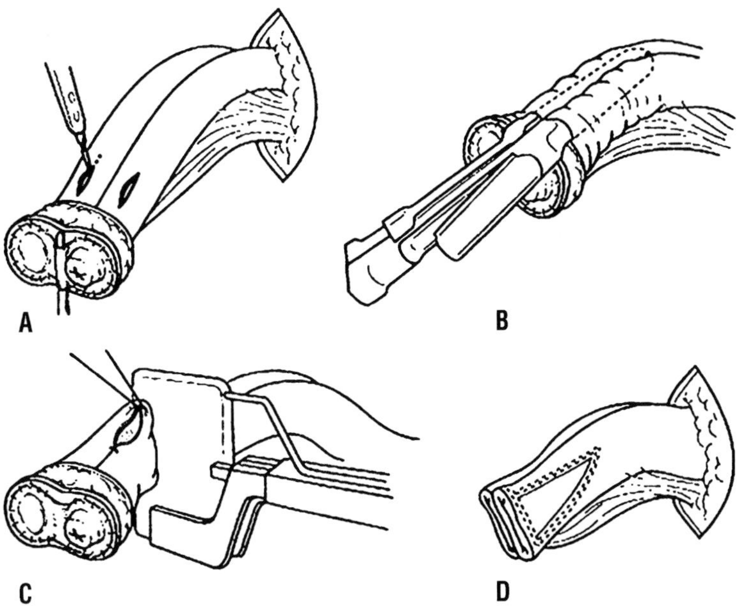

Figure 20–22. Closure of loop ileostomy. **A.** A transverse elliptical incision is made around the stoma, and the limbs are dissected free. **B.** The antimesenteric surfaces of the limb are tacked together, and the jaws of an anastomosing stapler are passed through enterotomies and down into the lumen of each of the intestinal limbs. The stapler is then fired to create a side-to-side anastomosis between the afferent and efferent ileal limbs. **C.** A linear stapler is placed and fired below the former stoma and below the edges of the enterotomy. The stoma and distal limbs are amputated, and the stapler is released. **D.** The anastomosis is dropped back into the peritoneal cavity, and the peritoneum, fascia, and skin are closed. Alternatively, the stoma can be fully excised and a standard side-to-side functional end-to-end stapled anastomosis can be performed. (Reproduced, with permission, from Becker JM, Stucchi AF. Ulcerative colitis. In: Greenfield LJ et al [eds]. *Surgery Scientific Principles and Practice*, 3rd ed. Philadelphia, PA: Lippincott Williams & Wilkins; 2001:1070–1089.)

A number of centers that perform IPAA have now advocated an alternative approach to the pouch-anal anastomosis that eliminates the mucosal proctectomy. As noted above, the distal rectum is stapled and divided near the pelvic floor, leaving the anal transition zone largely intact. The ileal pouch is then stapled to the top of the anal canal with a transanally placed circular stapler. Since ulcerative colitis is a mucosal disease, the obvious objective of surgical therapy is to remove all or as much of the diseased mucosa as possible, thereby eliminating the subsequent risk of disease recurrence and cancer. This very point has probably been the major controversy ever since the technique was introduced in the early 1980s.[68] Since the double-stapled technique does not involve a mucosal proctectomy, this raises concerns regarding the risk of developing cancer in the retained mucosa of the anal transitional zone. IPAA is a technically difficult and very demanding procedure with the mucosal proctectomy and the pouch-anal anastomosis perhaps requiring the most experience. The ease of use has made the double-stapled anastomosis a widely used technique, especially in light of a recent study showing it is significantly faster and easier to learn than the hand-sewn technique.[69] In addition, pundits claim that preserving the distal internal anal sphincter muscle and anal transitional zone contribute to significant functional advantages over the mucosectomy, including increased anal resting pressure, preservation of the rectoanal inhibitory reflex, improved continence, and fewer septic complications.[70] Even though a number of trials have supported this supposition,[71–73] nearly as many have concluded otherwise, showing that a double-stapled IPAA conferred no improvement in stool frequency or continence compared to hand-sewn IPAA.[74–76] All these studies demonstrated that both operations are safe and result in rapid and profound improvement in quality of life. The obvious concern is that by leaving disease-bearing mucosa in the anal canal, patients are exposed to a lifelong risk of malignant transformation that will require careful annual postoperative surveillance.[77] In addition, inflammation of the retained mucosa in the anal transition zone, sometimes referred to as cuffitis, can mimic other postoperative complications such as pouchitis and confound treatment.[78]

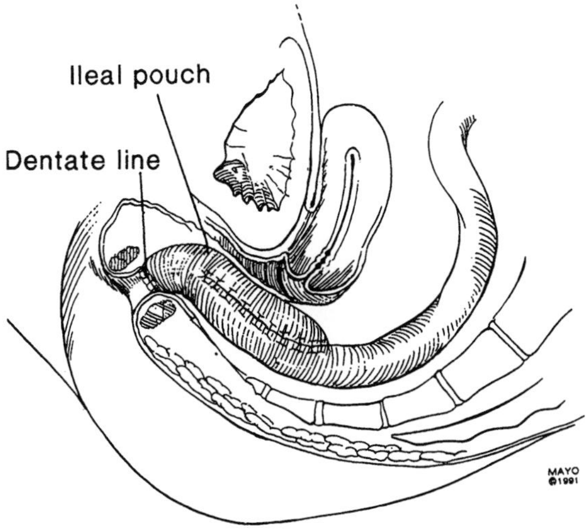

Figure 20–23. A sagittal view of the ileal pouch–anal anastomosis with mucosectomy. (Reproduced, with permission, from Kelly KA. Anal sphincter-saving operations for chronic ulcerative colitis. *Am J Surg* 1992;163:5–11.)

Figure 20–24 represents a sagittal view of the ileal pouch showing the double-stapled anastomosis to the anus above the dentate line with 1.5–4 cm of disease-bearing rectal mucosa remaining. Therefore, at the present time, the best available evidence suggests that there are risks and benefits to both pouch-anal anastomotic techniques, and these must be carefully weighed by the surgeon given each patient's medical circumstances, disease, and ability to comply with careful follow-up (Table 20–5).

Diverting Loop Ileostomy

A significant addition to the IPAA procedure was the construction of a temporary loop ileostomy allowing diversion of the fecal stream during the early weeks of ileal pouch and ileoanal anastomotic healing. Temporary diversion significantly reduces the potential for leakage from the ileal pouch or ileoanal anastomosis, thereby reducing the risk of pelvic sepsis and anastomotic dehiscence, both serious complications associated with significant morbidity and pouch failure. As mentioned above, at most major centers, including this one, the operation is typically performed in two stages. The first stage consists of colectomy with or without mucosal proctectomy, endorectal IPAA, and diverting loop ileostomy. Approximately 8 weeks after the initial operation the second stage is performed in which the loop ileostomy is closed as described above. In the larger series, it appears that most experienced surgeons at major centers prefer to use a temporary ileostomy to divert the fecal stream.[56,79] However, surgeons that routinely use a single-stage procedure without an ileostomy have not reported an increased risk of pelvic sepsis in their patients.[80,81] Analysis of a series of more than 1,000 patients comparing those who had undergone diversion and those who had not

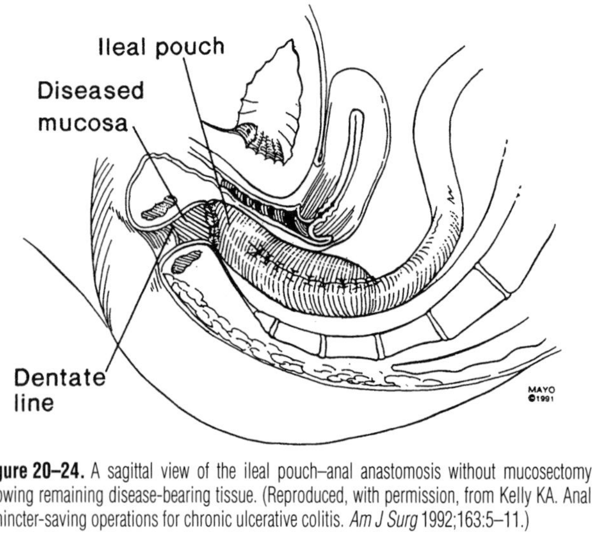

Figure 20–24. A sagittal view of the ileal pouch–anal anastomosis without mucosectomy showing remaining disease-bearing tissue. (Reproduced, with permission, from Kelly KA. Anal sphincter-saving operations for chronic ulcerative colitis. *Am J Surg* 1992;163:5–11.)

TABLE 20–5. ADVANTAGES AND DISADVANTAGES OF A DOUBLE-STAPLED ANASTOMOSIS VERSUS MUCOSAL PROCTECTOMY WITH HAND SEWN ANASTOMOSIS

	Double-Stapled Anastomosis	Mucosal Protectomy with Hand-Sewn Anastomosis
Easy-to-learn technique	Yes	No
Technical ease of use	Yes	No
Preserves anal transition zone	Yes	No
Improved function	?	No
Decreases septic complications	?	?
Increases dysplasia risk	Yes	No
Increases cancer risk	Yes	No
Cuffitis	Yes	No

Adapted, with permission, from Larson DW, Pemberton JH. Current concepts and controversies in surgery for IBD. *Gastroenterology* 2004; 126:1611-1619.

found no differences in complication rates and functional outcomes.[77] It also appears that eliminating this procedure may reduce the mechanical and functional complications and the patient dissatisfaction associated with even a temporary ileostomy.[82] Despite evidence to support these stoma-related complications,[83] there are sufficient studies showing that pelvic sepsis after IPAA is associated with significant complications including pouch failure[84] and an increased risk of death.[85] Therefore, despite the arguments that since the single-stage procedure alleviates the need for a second operation to reverse the loop ileostomy, the hospital stays are shorter and the costs are lower, most experienced surgeons advocate that a diverting ileostomy should remain an essential element of IPAA.

Timing of Surgery

As mentioned earlier, total colectomy offers the only curative treatment for ulcerative colitis. Despite new and highly effective medical therapies, up to 40% of patients will ultimately undergo surgery due to the refractory nature of their disease or the increased risk of malignancy. Medical therapy does not decrease the markedly elevated risk of colorectal cancer associated with chronic ulcerative colitis. Since patients are generally quite young when first diagnosed, the overall financial burden, loss of productivity and the risks associated with decades of medical therapy can be significant.[86–88] The overall morbidity, cost, and disability of medical therapy for ulcerative colitis is rarely compared with surgical therapy. Interestingly, a study by Sher and associates,[89] showed that medical treatment was associated with a significantly higher overall morbidity (65%) than surgical therapy (15%). Aggressive medical therapy may be significantly less cost effective than early surgical intervention, and in fact, delaying surgery until complications arise increases morbidity significantly. Given these potential drawbacks, many surgeons are now advocating earlier surgical intervention as a reasonable alternative to prolonged medical management.[28] When performed by an experienced surgeon, the complication rate is very low, the functional results are excellent, and the majority of patients report a high degree of satisfaction and a quality of life comparable with that of normal healthy patients.[90] Many medically-treated patients often report significant limitations in social activity, even if in remission. In contrast, patients that undergo early surgical treatment are able to resume normal functioning, and enjoy healthy lives with an excellent quality of life.[91]

Despite this reasoning, others argue that colectomy is only rarely required and early surgical intervention is not necessary even for uncontrolled disease.[92] Furthermore, it is argued that the majority of patients can be maintained in long-term remission with 5-ASA and in those who relapse, azathioprine or 6-MP can usually be used to achieve and maintain remission in most patients.[93] Opponents to early or urgent surgery for ulcerative colitis also argue that medical treatment for conditions that may require immediate surgery such as fulminant disease, toxic megacolon, and unremitting colitis can now be managed more conservatively and effectively with aggressive medical therapy. Finally, it is concluded that given that surgical therapy is associated with substantial morbidity and mortality, the preferred treatment should be nonsurgical except for high-grade dysplasia or cancer, imminent perforation despite maximal treatment, or chronic active disease despite maximal treatment.[92]

Indeterminate Colitis

Indeterminate colitis refers to the approximately 10% of IBD patients in whom a definitive diagnosis of ulcerative colitis or Crohn's disease cannot be made at colonoscopy, in colonic biopsies, or in the colectomy specimen. Typically, these patients present with clinical, pathological, and histological features of both ulcerative colitis and Crohn's disease.[94] This presentation can be a particular challenge for the surgeon and has been somewhat controversial with regard to the surgical option offered to the patient whose diagnosis is unclear. From a surgical standpoint, every attempt to differentiate ulcerative colitis from Crohn's disease should be made preoperatively since this can play a significant role in the options presented to the patient. The gastroenterologist, pathologist, and surgeon should carefully review all clinical, endoscopic, radiographic and pathological records. The final diagnosis may be aided by serologic markers such perinuclear antineutrophilic cytoplasmic autoantibodies (P-ANCA) and anti-*Saccharomyces cerevisiae* mannan antibodies (ASCA) for ulcerative colitis and Crohn's disease, respectively.[95] However, these serology tests are not definitively diagnostic by themselves. If the diagnosis is seriously in question, colectomy with a Hartmann's closure of the rectum and a Brooke ileostomy will leave the surgical option for future reconstructive surgery. Although there are varying opinions on this issue, some surgeons feel that if there is any evidence to suggest Crohn's disease, then a proctocolectomy with Brooke ileostomy should be performed and both IPAA and Kock pouch are contraindicated. However, several series have recently shown that most patients with indeterminate colitis that undergo IPAA experience functional outcomes and failure rates similar to those of patients with ulcerative colitis.[96] Since it was recently shown that most patients with indeterminate colitis most likely have ulcerative colitis,[94] many surgeons now feel that they can safely offer these patients IPAA with the expectation of a reasonably good outcome.[97]

Crohn's Disease

Until recently, the general consensus among surgeons was that IPAA was strictly contraindicated in patients diagnosed preoperatively with Crohn's disease. The high risk of recurrent disease, especially Crohn's of the ileal pouch, frequently leads to years of poor function and high morbidity that eventually necessitates pouch excision. Therefore, total proctocolectomy with a permanent Brooke ileostomy was thought to be the only option for these patients. However, there have been reports of acceptable long-term functional outcomes in select Crohn's colitis patients who have undergone IPAA. Although the pouch failure rate is higher in these patients than in patients with ulcerative colitis, acceptable long-term results can be achieved in 55–90% of these patients as long as there were no anoperineal or ileal manifestations of Crohn's disease prior to IPAA.[55] Similarly, other reports have demonstrated good long-term results and low rates of Crohn's disease–related complications and pouch excision up to 10 years after IPAA for colorectal Crohn's disease.[98] A recent report further showed that a subset of Crohn's colitis patients with no evidence of anal or small bowel involvement had favorable outcomes after IPAA.[99] Although many surgeons still do not advocate elective IPAA for patients with Crohn's colitis, the fact that many patients with a secondary diagnosis of Crohn's disease after IPAA have good outcomes and quality of life[100] has prompted some surgeons to offer IPAA to select young patients averse to the prospect of permanent ileostomy if they meet strict preoperative criteria.

LAPAROSCOPIC PROCTOCOLECTOMY WITH ILEAL POUCH–ANAL ANASTOMOSIS

Laparoscopic techniques were first used to perform total proctocolectomy with ileostomy in patients with severe ulcerative colitis in the early 1990s.[101] Since then, this field has advanced rapidly and restorative proctocolectomy is increasingly being performed using laparoscopic and minimally invasive surgical techniques. In most series, laparoscopically-assisted techniques require only a small periumbilical or suprapubic incision of 4 cm or less for vascular dissection of the colon and ileal pouch formation while the remainder of the procedure is usually performed entirely laparoscopically.

Although the ideal candidates for laparoscopic total proctocolectomy are generally young, nonobese, asymptomatic patients with benign colonic or rectal disease, similar indications and contraindications for restorative proctocolectomy apply (see Table 20–4). In these patients, recovery is rapid with minimal lifestyle disruption and reduced apprehension of surgery. However, the functional outcome and quality of life in patients having undergone laparoscopic-assisted IPAA is no different from those that undergo conventional IPAA.[102] In these patients, cosmesis is the most important advantage after laparoscopic surgery. Moreover, since large intraoperative fluid losses and prolonged postoperative ileus are significantly reduced, the length of hospitalization is typically shorter.[103] Also, younger patients do not have to endure the psychological implications of a large abdominal incision.

In brief, after initial medial transection of the three main vascular pedicles, the colon is dissected free laterally towards the ileum. The rectum is mobilized down to the pelvic floor. Through a Pfannenstiel incision, the bowel is extracted and the ileal J-pouch is constructed. The anastomosis is typically completed using a double-stapling technique; however, hand-sewn anastomoses have been reported after transanal rectal mucosectomy. In the hands of a skilled surgeon, laparoscopic restorative proctocolectomy for ulcerative colitis is technically feasible, safe, and effective.[104] Interestingly, similar technical controversies still surround the use of a single-stage laparoscopic-assisted restorative proctocolectomy without diverting ileostomy.[105]

More recently, trials are ongoing comparing the potential applicability, short- and long-term clinical outcomes, inflammatory responses, and overall costs of hand-assisted laparoscopic colectomy versus conventional laparoscopic colectomy.[106,107] Hand-assisted laparoscopic surgery can be a useful adjunct to conventional laparoscopic techniques, especially when difficult situations arise. Although it is a potentially faster and safer procedure with less need to convert to open surgery, hand-assisted techniques do require a small laparotomy which is expanded and compressed throughout the procedure subjecting the intra-abdominal viscera to more intense manipulations.[108] Since these factors can contribute to additional surgical trauma, it is not clear whether hand-assisted procedures actually maintain the true minimally invasive characteristics of laparoscopic surgery. However, a number of studies have now concluded that hand-assisted procedures simplify complicated intraoperative situations and reduce the need for conversion to an open procedure[109] while maintaining the low morbidity rates of conventional laparoscopic techniques.[110] Since hand-assisted laparoscopic colectomy is thought to facilitate colonic mobilization while maintaining the minimally invasive benefits of laparoscopic surgery, surgeons have begun to investigate the efficacy of hand-assisted laparoscopic approaches compared with conventional laparoscopic methods in patients undergoing restorative proctocolectomy. Recent studies have now concluded that compared with conventional laparoscopic restorative proctocolectomy, the hand-assisted method results in a significant reduction in operative time without detriment to bowel function, length of stay, or patient outcome.[111] Despite the continued success of laparoscopic proctocolectomy with IPAA at some centers,[112] many surgeons now feel that the hand-assisted approach to restorative proctocolectomy is expected to replace conventional laparoscopic methods as the preferred laparoscopic approach for this technically challenging procedure.[111,113] However, neither of these minimally invasive approaches appears to reduce the need for a protective ileostomy.[114] These minimally invasive procedures also appear to contribute to a reduction in intra-abdominal adhesion formation,[115] which has been a significant cause of morbidity after IPAA.[60]

OUTCOMES AFTER IPAA

Most large series now conclude that restorative proctocolectomy with IPAA is a very safe procedure. Long-term follow-up of these patients has demonstrated that the functional results are durable for more than 15 years and patient satisfaction remains high.[116–118] In the author's own experience with nearly 750 patients in whom IPAA was performed using mucosal proctectomy and a hand-sewn ileoanal anastomosis over a 25-year period at three major institutions, nearly 90% of those operations were performed in patients with ulcerative colitis and the remainder performed in patients with FAP or a genetic variant (Table 20–6). The mean age is 36 years (range 11–76), and has been slowly increasing as we have become more confident about offering the

TABLE 20–6. ILEAL POUCH–ANAL ANASTOMOSIS PATIENT PROFILE

Study period:	August 1982 to June 2006
Total number of patients:	741
Diagnosis	
Chronic ulcerative colitis	660 (89%)
Familial adenomatous polyposis	81 (11%)
Age	
Mean	36 years
Range	11-76 years
Male:Female ratio	412:329

operation to older patients. There has also been a trend towards earlier surgical intervention as gastroenterologists and surgeons realize the substantial benefits to the patient. The majority of patients with ulcerative colitis report a significant improvement in their quality of life after having undergone IPAA,[118–120] which further supports the concept of surgical treatment much earlier in the course of the disease. In addition, we and others[116] have had excellent results in older patients and now feel confident in offering the operation to patients older than 65 years of age as long as they meet the preoperative anal manometric standards.

In our series, as in most, poor stool consistency, increased stool frequency, and nocturnal leakage are some of the more common postoperative complaints. Late follow-up data from the larger series have demonstrated that the number of bowel movements is in the range of four to nine daily, with an average of six per day. Nocturnal bowel movements occur one to two times nightly, with a mean of slightly more than one. Nocturnal seepage of stool or staining is observed in 20% of patients in the early postoperative period, but by 1 year, it is infrequently observed. Overall, mean 24-hour and nocturnal stool frequencies average five or six bowel movements per 24 hours and 0.5 bowel movements at night in the late follow-up period. In an effort to control stool output, patients can be placed on antidiarrheals such as loperamide with supplementary fiber in the form of cellulose or psyllium mucilloid. In addition, patients are counseled to consume a high-fiber diet that is low in simple sugars, and in some cases to include a high-fat nocturnal snack in their dietary regimen.

IPAA also remains an excellent option for most patients requiring colectomy for FAP, Gardner's syndrome, and in selected patients with hereditary nonpolyposis colon cancer. In our series, the overall outcome, morbidity, and functional results in patients who have received IPAA for indications other than ulcerative colitis have been significantly better when compared to those patients who have received the operation for ulcerative colitis. Patients who have undergone IPAA for FAP have significantly fewer bowel movements per 24 hours than those operated on for ulcerative colitis, which averages about six bowel movements per day at 12 months after ileostomy closure.

Complications

Although the severity and frequency of short- and long-term complications related to IPAA have decreased significantly since its inception, especially as surgeons become more technically adept with the operation, there can be significant morbidity associated with IPAA. Perioperative complications can occur with IPAA as they can with any major abdominal operation, but there are some unique complications associated with IPAA. Short-term complications or those that occur within 30 days of surgery include pelvic sepsis and abscesses primarily due to anastomotic or pouch leakage. Long-term complications including small bowel obstruction, anastomotic strictures, fistulas, sexual dysfunction, pouchitis, and adhesions have also been well documented. We recently performed a meta-analysis of more than 18 major studies from around the world in which complications and outcomes after IPAA were reported in over 8,300 patients (Fig 20–25).[117] Interestingly, in reviewing the world's literature, those series that reported complication rates and outcomes stratified by year showed

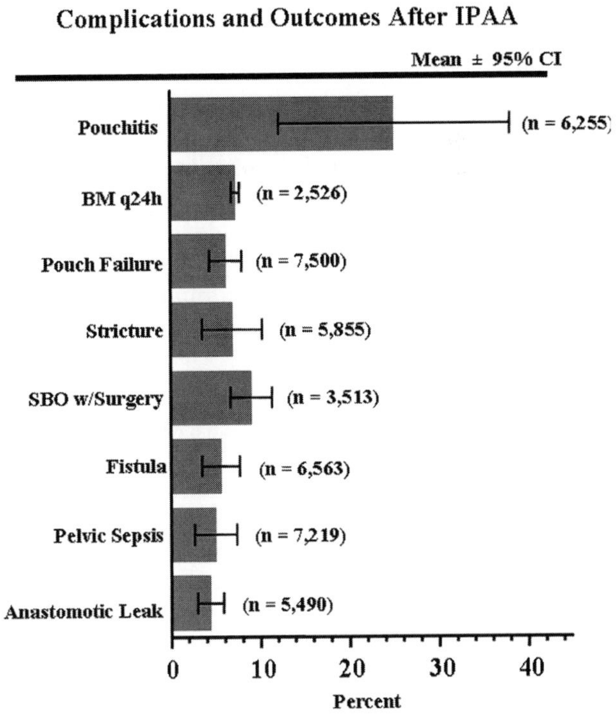

Figure 20–25. Results of a meta-analysis of over 8,300 patients from 18 major studies showing the major complications and outcomes after ileal pouch–anal anastomosis. (Reproduced, with permission, from Lehrmann J, Stucchi AF, LaMorte WW, Herren T, Becker JM. Complications and outcomes after ileal pouch-anal anastomosis: A meta-analysis of more than 8300 patients. *Gastroenterology* 2003;124:A814.)

significantly fewer complications, and improvements in function and quality of life in patients who had received the operation more recently when compared to patients who had received the operation in the earlier years. This finding undoubtedly can be attributed to surgeon experience. One long-term complication that does not show signs of improvement is ASBO requiring reoperation, clearly suggesting the need for more effective adhesion prevention measures. These reports also demonstrated that, despite the fact that patients experience between four and seven bowel movements per day and high rates of pouchitis (discussed below), the patient satisfaction rate and quality-of-life indices were very high (Table 20–7).

In our own series, the postoperative morbidity and complication rate after IPAA in the 570 patients for whom we have reliable follow-up data (Table 20–8) are comparable to those reported from other major centers.[116,118] Single-surgeon experience with IPAA contributes significantly to the low mortality and morbidity rates that can be achieved with this operation if it is performed frequently, carefully, and with a standard operative technique. No operative deaths have occurred in our series, and the overall operative morbidity after IPAA is about 10%. The major operative morbidity is small bowel obstruction, and although lower than the reported incidence, it is likely due to the high rate of adhesion formation associated with IPAA.[60]

Pouch Failure

Pouch failure is a significant long-term complication of IPAA. Although excision of the ileal pouch with construction of a conventional Brooke ileostomy has typically been the procedure of choice after unsuccessful salvage surgery, alternatives include conversion to a Kock pouch or continent ileostomy in patients wishing to remain continent.[42] There are a number of risk factors that were recently shown to be independent predictors of pouch failure including patient diagnosis, prior anal pathology, abnormal anal manometry, pouch-perineal or pouch-vaginal fistulae, pelvic sepsis, anastomotic stricture, and dehiscence.[121]

The pouch failure rate in our series necessitating conversion to permanent Brooke ileostomy is approximately 2%, as compared to the pooled estimate of 6.2% we found when we surveyed the literature.[117] This is due not only to the fact that increased experience decreases the risk of postoperative and pouch-related complications, but also to our continued efforts to salvage failed pouches. Approximately 60% of the failed pouches in our series were successfully salvaged, thus avoiding permanent ileostomy.[122] These results suggest that a continued effort to salvage failed pouches, including the use of total reconstruction, is a viable alternative to permanent ileostomy.

TABLE 20–7. SUMMARY OF OUTCOMES AFTER IPAA FOR ULCERATIVE COLITIS OF 18 MAJOR SERIES

Outcome	Mean (%)	Range
Diagnosis of ulcerative colitis	88.5	84–96
Mortality	1.7	0–9[a]
Pelvic sepsis	5.4	2.3–12[a]
Pouch failure	6.2	1.2–25[a]
Bowel movements	7.3	4.7–7.8[a]
Pouchitis	25.1	22–59[a]
Satisfaction/quality of life	88.0	75–97[a]

[a]More recent series; total number of patients in 18 series was 8,316. Reproduced, with permission, from Lehrman J, Stucchi AF, LaMorte WW, Herren T, Becker JM. Complications and outcomes after ileal pouch-anal anastomosis: A meta-analysis of more than 8300 patients. *Gastroenterology* 2003; 124:A814.

TABLE 20-8. COMPLICATIONS ASSOCIATED WITH ILEAL POUCH-ANAL ANASTOMOSIS

Complications	Percent (Number of Patients)
Perineal complications	1.9% (11)
Small bowel obstruction	17% (97)
SBO requiring operation	6.7% (38)
Pelvic abscess	6.7% (38)
Diverting loop ileostomy re-established	4.7% (27)
Failed pouch w/conversion to Brooke ileostomy	2.0% (12)
Crohn's disease	0.9% (5)
Sinus tract	1.0% (6)
Other	0.1% (1)
	Total 570

Crohn's Disease

The occurrence of Crohn's disease of the ileal pouch often results in severe morbidity and a significant risk of pouch excision. Strong predictors of Crohn's disease in IPAA patients include complex perianal or pouch fistulae, ileitis proximal to the pouch, or afferent limb ulcers.[123] Until recently, gastroenterologists and surgeons could offer these patients little in the way of new or more effective medical therapy. However, the advent of biological therapies for Crohn's disease has made a significant impact on the nonsurgical treatment of these patients. Infliximab and other similar anti–tumor necrosis factor-α strategies have revolutionized the medical treatment of Crohn's disease.[124] In patients refractory to conventional therapies, infliximab has been used successfully to treat Crohn's disease of the ileoanal pouch[125] and in both the short- and long-term treatment of IPAA patients who subsequently develop other Crohn's disease–related complications.[126] Hence, as discussed below, IPAA patients that present with Crohn's disease–like symptoms may benefit from a trial of infliximab or other similar biologics before considering any surgical options.

Pouchitis

Pouchitis is a nonspecific, idiopathic inflammation of the ileal pouch and remains the most common and significant late, long-term complication that in some cases overshadows the benefits of IPAA (see Fig 20–25). Pouchitis occurs only in patients having undergone IPAA for ulcerative colitis and is rarely documented in FAP patients. Since pouchitis reportedly occurs in more than 50% of ulcerative colitis patients,[127] surgeons should be familiar with the diagnosis, treatment, and follow-up.

Patients with pouchitis can present with any number of colitis-like symptoms including increased stool frequency, watery diarrhea, fecal urgency, incontinence, rectal bleeding, abdominal cramping, fever, and malaise. When repeated episodes or chronic clinical symptoms of this nature persist, the diagnosis should be confirmed by flexible ileal pouchoscopy. Endoscopically, the mucosal surface of a normal pouch glistens and has a velvety appearance indicative of normal villi. In sharp contrast, an inflamed ileal pouch appears erythematous, edematous, hyperemic, and granular. The mucosa is often friable, may bleed on contact, and a mucous exudate is often visible. Mucosal and submucosal hemorrhaging and superficial, focal ulceration are also present in more severe cases (Fig 20–26). Occasionally ulcerations may be found along any of the staple or suture lines within the pouch; however, these are generally not associated with more diffuse pouch inflammation. While these mucosal changes may be irregular and not uniform throughout the pouch, the functional integrity of the entire pouch can be affected, in some severe cases including the ileum just proximal to the pouch. There may also be a clear line of distinction between the unaffected proximal ileum and the inflamed pouch. Endoscopic appearance alone, however, does not always correlate well with the overall clinical presentation.

When examining the ileal pouch endoscopically, the anatomic location of the mucosal inflammation can be an important diagnostic consideration. Although pouchitis typically presents in the distal portion of the pouch, factors such as pouch configuration, severity, and chronicity can affect the distribution of the inflammation. Inflammation can extend proximally in the more severe and chronic cases; however, this can also be indicative of Crohn's disease. If this anatomic presentation persists following therapy, further diagnostic evaluation should be considered. Inflammation occurring distal to the pouch in the area of the anal transition zone may indicate that original rectal mucosa still remains and ulcerative colitis has persisted or recurred. Although this generally occurs in patients who have undergone a double-stapled ileal pouch–anal anastomosis, any inflammation found between the dentate line and the distal apex of the pouch is suspect and must be biopsied.

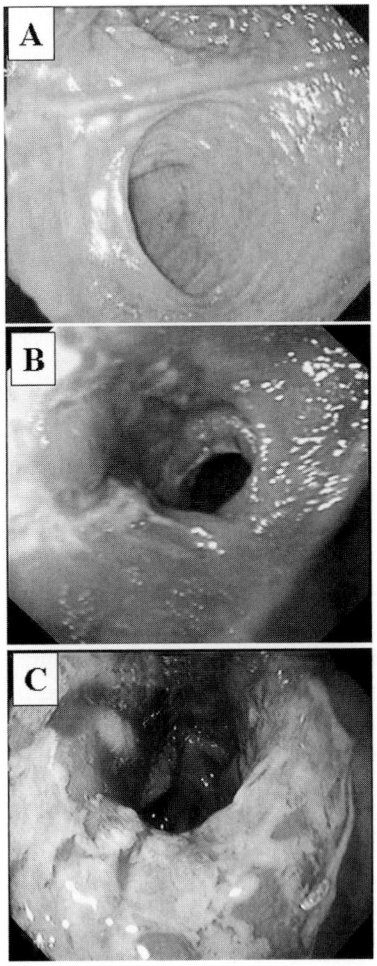

Figure 20–26. Endoscopic images of a pelvic ileal J-pouch. **A.** Appearance of a normal pouch 5 years after IPAA. The mucosal surface glistens and has a velvety appearance indicative of normal villi. **B.** Mild pouchitis. **C.** Severely inflamed pouch showing characteristic signs of pouchitis. The mucosal surface appears erythematous and edematous with numerous shallow ulcers and a mucous exudate. Presence of a stricture may be indicative of Crohn's disease. (Reproduced, with permission, from Becker JM, Stucchi AF. Management of acute and chronic pouchitis. In: Lichtenstein G [ed]. *Inflammatory Bowel Disease: The Complete Guide to Medical Management.* Thorofare, NJ: Slack Inc.; 2006:chapter 36.)

For ulcerative colitis patients having undergone IPAA, pouchitis is not an absolutely certain outcome. Based on the current reporting standards, approximately one out of two to five of these patients will suffer from at least one episode. A review of the literature through 2005 indicates that the incidence of pouchitis can vary from just 6%[128] to upwards of 58%[127] and 59%.[129] In our own series, the overall incidence of pouchitis is approximately 22%, although the majority of patients experience only acute episodes with few chronic or refractory cases (Table 20–9). As one would

TABLE 20–9. INCIDENCE OF POUCHITIS AND ILEAL POUCH DYSPLASIA AFTER ILEAL POUCH–ANAL ANASTOMOSIS[a]

Incidence of pouchitis (overall)	22.2%
Chronic ulcerative colitis: single or acute episode	12.1%
Chronic ulcerative colitis: multiple or chronic episodes	10.1%
Chronic ulcerative colitis: refractory	<1%
Familial adenomatous polyposis	0.2%
Incidence of ileal pouch dysplasia	0%

[a]Follow-up from 590 patients.

expect, the cumulative risk rises significantly as follow-up approaches 10 years.[56,77] However, patients with preoperative extraintestinal manifestations experience a significantly higher incidence, frequency, and severity of pouchitis,[130] especially those with primary sclerosing cholangitis.[131] In a series from the Mayo Clinic, the cumulative risk of pouchitis in 1,097 ulcerative colitis patients without preoperative primary sclerosing cholangitis following IPAA at 1, 2, 5, and 10 years postoperatively was 16%, 23%, 36%, and 45%, respectively. However, in patients with preoperative primary sclerosing cholangitis, the risk of pouchitis rose to 22%, 43%, 61%, and 79% at 1, 2, 5, and 10 years, respectively.[132] Although pouchitis can occur at any time, the greatest risk for experiencing an episode is during the initial 6-month period following closure of the temporary diverting loop ileostomy. After that, the risk continues to rise steadily for the next 18–36 months before leveling off at around 4 years.[133]

While the etiology of pouchitis is unknown, causes that have been investigated include undetected Crohn's disease, bacterial overgrowth or bacterial dysbiosis, either primary or secondary malabsorption, stasis, ischemia, and nutritional or immune deficiencies.[134] At present, pouchitis remains a clinically defined syndrome. Clinical, endoscopic, and histological criteria have all been applied without clear controls or norms. Although a pouchitis disease activity index encompassing these diagnostic parameters and providing a simple, objective, and quantitative criteria for pouch inflammation has been proposed,[135] it is not widely used diagnostically.

Historically, the medical management of pouchitis has been primarily empirical and predicated more on individual clinical experiences than evidence-based knowledge. Broad-spectrum antibiotics continue to be the mainstay of treatment, especially for patients with acute or episodic flare-ups. In our experience,[136] rapid relief is often achieved with a 10-day combination course of ciprofloxacin (250 mg twice a day) and metronidazole (250 mg four times a day). A significant portion of these patients experience an improvement in clinical symptoms within several days, especially in stool frequency. Those patients that either do not respond or show partial improvement to this initial trial will undergo at least one more 10-day course at the same dose before further diagnostic evaluation is undertaken. For the approximately 30% of patients that experience recurrence and the 10–15% that suffer from chronic episodes or unremitting pouchitis, current treatment strategies are inadequate. However, we have devised a treatment algorithm that has proven to be successful for even the most chronic cases.[136]

The management of chronic or relapsing pouchitis can be a challenging and frustrating task for the practitioner and patient as well. Antibiotics, especially in combination, are certainly still appropriate and effective in treating these patients, many of whom often require nearly continuous antibiotic treatment with either low maintenance doses or full-dose pulse therapy in order to remain in remission.[137] Some patients in our series with recurring episodes of pouchitis require a long-term, low-dose combination antibiotic regimen with ciprofloxacin (250 mg once daily) plus metronidazole (250 mg once daily) for up to 90 days to achieve a response. The dose will be increased to two times per day in nonresponsive patients, and in other cases the dosing interval is reduced to every other day.[136] For those patients that are either resistant to antibiotics or relapse shortly after antibiotic therapy is discontinued, therapy with oral or topical anti-inflammatory agents, corticosteroids, and immunomodulators are reasonable, and in some cases effective alternatives, especially given their efficacy for ulcerative colitis.[137]

Severe, unremitting, or refractory pouchitis is rare, occurring in our series in less than 1% of patients. After ruling out more atypical possibilities including several less common but documented viral pathogens such as primary cytomegalovirus,[138] the focus must turn to undiagnosed Crohn's disease. Although uncommon, a patient with refractory pouchitis can present with clinical, endoscopic, and pathological features resembling Crohn's disease that may include complex perianal or pouch fistulizing disease and ileitis proximal to the pouch. At this point, serologic testing for P-ANCA or ASCA titers may be beneficial. In our own cohort, serologic profiles showed some utility in differentiating between ulcerative colitis and Crohn's disease, and were useful in predicting the development of fistulas postoperatively.[139] In other cases, the original colectomy records must be carefully re-reviewed by an experienced gastrointestinal pathologist. As discussed earlier, the confirmation of Crohn's disease of the ileal pouch often results in severe morbidity and significant risk of pouch excision. Until recently, these patients could only be treated with standard Crohn's disease therapies. However, the advent of anti–tumor necrosis factor-α antibody therapy (infliximab), which has markedly improved the treatment of Crohn's disease, has also been shown to benefit patients who develop Crohn's disease of the ileal pouch. A recent study of 26 patients with Crohn's-related complications of the ileal pouch showed that infliximab was beneficial in both the short and long term.[126]

Several mechanical problems such as outlet obstructions and anastomotic strictures as well as Crohn's disease (discussed above) can also mimic the clinical symptoms of pouchitis. In addition, cuffitis resulting from retained rectal mucosa can also present with pouchitis-like symptoms. Therefore, patients that do not respond to antibiotic therapy require a further work-up including a flexible ileal pouchoscopy with biopsy.

Other Complications

Perhaps one of the more infrequent complications reported in patients with IPAA ulcerative colitis is dysplasia and carcinoma of the ileal pouch. We have reported that although the ileal pouch mucosa goes through morphologic changes called colonic metaplasia, these adaptative responses are in response to inflammation and do not precede dysplasia or adenocarcinoma.[140] In addition to our own series (see Table 20–9), others have also shown that dysplastic transformations within the ileal pouch mucosa are rare, even after a long follow-up.[141] Although these findings can be reassuring for both patients and surgeons, we still advocate routine surveillance with endoscopic biopsy every 5 years for dysplasia in the ileal pouch mucosa.

Recurrent disease and rectal cancer have been essentially nonexistent in our own series; however, we are encountering more patients with high-grade dysplasia and adenocarcinomas of the anal canal who had undergone a double-stapled IPAA. As mentioned earlier, some surgeons believe that preservation of the mucosa in the anal transition zone significantly improves function. Resting pressures do tend to be somewhat higher following stapled IPAA;[76] however, this does not necessarily translate into significantly better long-term function. Thus, to alleviate further and unwarranted risk, we advocate that mucosectomy should be recommended in all patients undergoing IPAA for ulcerative colitis.[142]

▪ CONCLUSION

The surgical management of ulcerative colitis requires a comprehensive understanding of all the surgical options. While ileorectal anastomosis and proctocolectomy with Brooke ileostomy or Kock pouch have a role in the surgical management of select patients with ulcerative colitis, IPAA has become the definitive procedure in most cases. IPAA has evolved through many phases prior to arriving at the highly successful procedure currently utilized in major centers. Continued technical advances and greater surgeon experience can only further improve function, outcome, and patient satisfaction. Despite some opposition,[143] under elective conditions, IPAA remains an excellent option for patients with ulcerative colitis once the decision for surgery has been mutually reached by the patient, gastroenterologist, and surgeon.[144] With experience, mucosal proctectomy and IPAA can now be performed with a low complication rate, good functional results, and good quality of life, and with excellent long-term outcome. Optimal results can be obtained by careful patient selection, appropriate preoperative management, meticulous standardized surgical technique, appropriate postoperative education, and rigorous follow-up.

REFERENCES

1. Joossens S, Reinisch W, Vermeire S et al. The value of serologic markers in indeterminate colitis: a prospective follow-up study. *Gastroenterology* 2002;122:1242–1247
2. Kirsner JB. Historical origins of current IBD concepts. *World J Gastroenterol* 2001;7:175–184
3. Binder V. Epidemiology of IBD during the twentieth century: an integrated view. *Best Pract Res Clin Gastroenterol* 2004;18:463–479
4. Andres PG, Friedman LS. Epidemiology and the natural course of inflammatory bowel disease. *Gastroenterol Clin North Am* 1999;28:225–281
5. Bonen DK, Cho JH. The genetics of inflammatory bowel disease. *Gastroenterology* 2003;124:521–536
6. Hugot JP. Genetic origin of IBD. *Inflamm Bowel Dis* 2004; 10(Suppl 1):S11–S15
7. Oostenbrug LE, van Dullemen HM, te Meerman GJ et al. IBD and genetics: new developments. *Scand J Gastroenterol Suppl* 2003;63–68
8. Orchard T. Extraintestinal complications of inflammatory bowel disease. *Curr Gastroenterol Rep* 2003;5:512–517
9. Danese S, Sans M, Fiocchi C. Inflammatory bowel disease: the role of environmental factors. *Autoimmun Rev* 2004;3:394–400
10. Sartor RB. Therapeutic manipulation of the enteric microflora in inflammatory bowel diseases: antibiotics, probiotics, and prebiotics. *Gastroenterology* 2004;126: 1620–1633
11. Cosnes J. Tobacco and IBD: relevance in the understanding of disease mechanisms and clinical practice. *Best Pract Res Clin Gastroenterol* 2004;18:481–496
12. McGrath J, McDonald J, Macdonald J. Transdermal nicotine for induction of remission in ulcerative colitis. *Cochrane Database Syst Rev* 2004:CD004722
13. Hallas J, Gaist D, Sorensen HT. Does appendectomy reduce the risk of ulcerative colitis? *Epidemiology* 2004;15: 173–178
14. Wen Z, Fiocchi C. Inflammatory bowel disease: autoimmune or immune-mediated pathogenesis? *Clin Dev Immunol* 2004;11:195–204

15. Yantiss RK, Sapp HL, Farraye FA et al. Histologic predictors of pouchitis in patients with chronic ulcerative colitis. *Am J Surg Pathol* 2004;28:999–1006
16. Loftus EV Jr. Management of extraintestinal manifestations and other complications of inflammatory bowel disease. *Curr Gastroenterol Rep* 2004;6:506–513
17. Fefferman DS, Farrell RJ. Endoscopy in inflammatory bowel disease: Indications, surveillance, and use in clinical practice. *Clin Gastroenterol Hepatol* 2005;3:11–24
18. Carter MJ, Lobo AJ, Travis SP. Guidelines for the management of inflammatory bowel disease in adults. *Gut* 2004;53(Suppl 5):V1–V16
19. Hanauer SB, Present DH. The state of the art in the management of inflammatory bowel disease. *Rev Gastroenterol Disord* 2003;3:81–92
20. McLeod R. Surgery for ulcerative colitis. *World Gastroenterology News* 2002;6:35–36
21. Larson DW, Pemberton JH. Current concepts and controversies in surgery for IBD. *Gastroenterology* 2004;126: 1611–1619
22. Becker JM. Surgical therapy for ulcerative colitis and Crohn's disease. *Gastroenterol Clin North Am* 1999;28: 371–390
23. Cheung O, Regueiro MD. Inflammatory bowel disease emergencies. *Gastroenterol Clin North Am* 2003;32:1269–1288
24. Cima RR, Pemberton JH. Surgical indications and procedures in ulcerative colitis. *Curr Treat Options Gastroenterol* 2004;7:181–190
25. Gan SI, Beck PL. A new look at toxic megacolon: an update and review of incidence, etiology, pathogenesis, and management. *Am J Gastroenterol* 2003;98:2363–2371
26. Turnbull RB Jr, Hawk WA, Weakley FL. Surgical treatment of toxic megacolon. Ileostomy and colostomy to prepare patients for colectomy. *Am J Surg* 1971;122:325–331
27. Remzi FH, Oncel M, Hull TL et al. Current indications for blow-hole colostomy:ileostomy procedure. A single center experience. *Int J Colorectal Dis* 2003;18: 361–364
28. Cima RR, Pemberton JH. Protagonist: Early surgical intervention in ulcerative colitis. *Gut* 2004;53:306–307
29. Munkholm P. Review article: the incidence and prevalence of colorectal cancer in inflammatory bowel disease. *Aliment Pharmacol Ther* 2003;18(Suppl 2):1–5
30. Sharan R, Schoen RE. Cancer in inflammatory bowel disease. An evidence-based analysis and guide for physicians and patients. *Gastroenterol Clin North Am* 2002;31: 237–254
31. Sjoqvist U. Dysplasia in ulcerative colitis-clinical consequences? *Langenbecks Arch Surg* 2004;389:354–360
32. Odze R. Diagnostic problems and advances in inflammatory bowel disease. *Mod Pathol* 2003;16:347–358
33. Gorfine SR, Bauer JJ, Harris MT et al. Dysplasia complicating chronic ulcerative colitis: is immediate colectomy warranted? *Dis Colon Rectum* 2000;43:1575–1581
34. Loftus EV Jr, Harewood GC, Loftus CG et al. PSC-IBD: a unique form of inflammatory bowel disease associated with primary sclerosing cholangitis. *Gut* 2005;54:91–96
35. Brooke BN. The management of an ileostomy, including its complications. *Lancet* 1952;2:102–104
36. Crile G Jr, Turnbull RB Jr. The mechanism and prevention of ileostomy dysfunction. *Ann Surg* 1954;140:459–466
37. Aylett SO. Ileorectal anastomosis: review 1952–1968. *Proc R Soc Med* 1971;64:967–971
38. Baker WN, Glass RE, Ritchie JK et al. Cancer of the rectum following colectomy and ileorectal anastomosis for ulcerative colitis. *Br J Surg* 1978;65:862–868
39. Kock NG. Intra-abdominal "reservoir" in patients with permanent ileostomy. Preliminary observations on a procedure resulting in fecal "continence" in five ileostomy patients. *Arch Surg* 1969;99:223–231
40. Meagher AP, Farouk R, Dozois RR et al. J ileal pouch-anal anastomosis for chronic ulcerative colitis: complications and long-term outcome in 1310 patients. *Br J Surg* 1998;85:800–803
41. Lepisto AH, Jarvinen HJ. Durability of Kock continent ileostomy. *Dis Colon Rectum* 2003;46:925–928
42. Borjesson L, Oresland T, Hulten L. The failed pelvic pouch: conversion to a continent ileostomy. *Tech Coloproctol* 2004;8:102–105
43. Berndtsson IE, Lindholm E, Oresland T et al. Health-related quality of life and pouch function in continent ileostomy patients: a 30-year perspective. *Dis Colon Rectum* 2004;47:2131–2137
44. Stryker SJ, Dozois RR. The ileoanal anastomosis: historical perspectives. In: Dozois RR (ed). *Alternatives of Conventional Ileostomy.* Chicago, IL: Yearbook Medical; 1985:255
45. Ravitch MM, Sabiston DL Jr. Anal ileostomy with preservation of the sphincter: a proposed operation in patients requiring total colectomy for benign lesions. *Surg Gynecol Obstet* 1947;84:1095–1099
46. Martin LW, LeCoultre C, Schubert WK. Total colectomy and mucosal proctectomy with preservation of continence in ulcerative colitis. *Ann Surg* 1977;186: 477–480
47. Beart RW Jr, Dozois RR, Kelly KA. Ileoanal anastomosis in the adult. *Surg Gynecol Obstet* 1982;154:826–828
48. Pemberton JH, Heppell J, Beart RW Jr et al. Endorectal ileoanal anastomosis. *Surg Gynecol Obstet* 1982;155:417–424
49. Heppell J, Kelly KA, Phillips SF et al. Physiologic aspects of continence after colectomy, mucosal proctectomy, and endorectal ileo-anal anastomosis. *Ann Surg* 1982; 195:435–443
50. Parks AG, Nicholls RJ. Proctocolectomy without ileostomy for ulcerative colitis. *BMJ* 1978;2:85–88
51. Utsunomiya J, Iwama T, Imajo M et al. Total colectomy, mucosal proctectomy, and ileoanal anastomosis. *Dis Colon Rectum* 1980;23:459–466
52. Taylor BM, Beart RW Jr, Dozois RR et al. Straight ileoanal anastomosis v ileal pouch–anal anastomosis after colectomy and mucosal proctectomy. *Arch Surg* 1983; 118:696–701
53. Taylor BM, Cranley B, Kelly KA et al. A clinico-physiological comparison of ileal pouch-anal and straight ileoanal anastomoses. *Ann Surg* 1983;198:462–468

54. Becker JM, Stucchi AF. Inherited colorectal polyposis syndromes. In: Cameron JL (ed). *Current Surgical Therapy*, 8th ed. Philadelphia, PA: Elsevier Mosby; 2004:200–211
55. Panis Y. Is there a place for ileal pouch-anal anastomosis in patients with Crohn's colitis? *Neth J Med* 1998;53:S47–S51
56. Farouk R, Pemberton JH, Wolff BG et al. Functional outcomes after ileal pouch-anal anastomosis for chronic ulcerative colitis. *Ann Surg* 2000;231:919–926
57. Tan HT, Connolly AB, Morton D et al. Results of restorative proctocolectomy in the elderly. *Int J Colorectal Dis* 1997;12:319–322
58. Gorgun E, Remzi FH, Goldberg JM et al. Fertility is reduced after restorative proctocolectomy with ileal pouch anal anastomosis: a study of 300 patients. *Surgery* 2004;136:795–803
59. Hahnloser D, Pemberton JH, Wolff BG et al. Pregnancy and delivery before and after ileal pouch-anal anastomosis for inflammatory bowel disease: immediate and long-term consequences and outcomes. *Dis Colon Rectum* 2004;47:1127–1135
60. Becker JM, Dayton MT, Fazio VW et al. Prevention of postoperative abdominal adhesions by a sodium hyaluronate-based bioresorbable membrane: a prospective, randomized, double-blind multicenter study [see comments]. *J Am Coll Surg* 1996;183:297–306
61. Parks AG, Nicholls RJ, Belliveau P. Proctocolectomy with ileal reservoir and anal anastomosis. *Br J Surg* 1980; 67:533–538
62. Nicholls RJ, Pezim ME. Restorative proctocolectomy with ileal reservoir for ulcerative colitis and familial adenomatous polyposis: a comparison of three reservoir designs. *Br J Surg* 1985;72:470–474
63. Fonkalsrud EW. Endorectal ileoanal anastomosis with isoperistaltic ileal reservoir after colectomy and mucosal proctectomy. *Ann Surg* 1984;199:151–157
64. Menzies D. Peritoneal adhesions. Incidence, cause, and prevention. *Surg Annu* 1992;24:27–45
65. Fevang BT, Fevang J, Lie SA et al. Long-term prognosis after operation for adhesive small bowel obstruction. *Ann Surg* 2004;240:193–201
66. Reed KL, Fruin AB, Bishop-Bartolomei KK et al. Neurokinin-1 receptor and substance P messenger RNA levels increase during intraabdominal adhesion formation. *J Surg Res* 2002;108:165–172
67. Becker JM, LaMorte W, St. Marie G et al. Extent of smooth muscle resection during mucosectomy and ileal pouch-anal anastomosis affects anorectal physiology and functional outcome. *Dis Colon Rectum* 1997;40:653–660
68. Knight CD, Griffen FD. An improved technique for low anterior resection of the rectum using the EEA stapler. *Surgery* 1980;88:710–714
69. Tekkis PP, Fazio VW, Lavery IC et al. Evaluation of the learning curve in ileal pouch-anal anastomosis surgery. *Ann Surg* 2005;241:262–268
70. Ziv Y, Fazio VW, Church JM et al. Stapled ileal pouch anal anastomoses are safer than handsewn anastomoses in patients with ulcerative colitis. *Am J Surg* 1996;171: 320–323
71. Deen KI, Williams JG, Grant EA et al. Randomized trial to determine the optimum level of pouch-anal anastomosis in stapled restorative proctocolectomy. *Dis Colon Rectum* 1995;38:133–138
72. Hallgren TA, Fasth SB, Oresland TO et al. Ileal pouch anal function after endoanal mucosectomy and handsewn ileoanal anastomosis compared with stapled anastomosis without mucosectomy. *Eur J Surg* 1995;161:915–921
73. McIntyre PB, Pemberton JH, Beart RW Jr et al. Double-stapled vs. handsewn ileal pouch-anal anastomosis in patients with chronic ulcerative colitis. *Dis Colon Rectum* 1994;37:430–433
74. Choen S, Tsunoda A, Nicholls RJ. Prospective randomized trial comparing anal function after hand sewn ileoanal anastomosis with mucosectomy versus stapled ileoanal anastomosis without mucosectomy in restorative proctocolectomy. *Br J Surg* 1991;78:430–434
75. Luukkonen P, Jarvinen H. Stapled vs hand-sutured ileoanal anastomosis in restorative proctocolectomy. A prospective, randomized study. *Arch Surg* 1993;128:437–440
76. Reilly WT, Pemberton JH, Wolff BG et al. Randomized prospective trial comparing ileal pouch-anal anastomosis performed by excising the anal mucosa to ileal pouch-anal anastomosis performed by preserving the anal mucosa. *Ann Surg* 1997;225:666–676
77. Fazio VW, Ziv Y, Church JM et al. Ileal pouch-anal anastomoses complications and function in 1005 patients. *Ann Surg* 1995;222:120–127
78. Shen B, Lashner BA, Bennett AE et al. Treatment of rectal cuff inflammation (cuffitis) in patients with ulcerative colitis following restorative proctocolectomy and ileal pouch-anal anastomosis. *Am J Gastroenterol* 2004;99: 1527–1531
79. Becker JM, Stucchi AF. Proctocolectomy with ileoanal anastomosis. *J Gastrointest Surg* 2004;8:376–386
80. Sugerman HJ, Sugerman EL, Meador JG et al. Ileal pouch anal anastomosis without ileal diversion. *Ann Surg* 2000;232:530–541
81. Heuschen UA, Hinz U, Allemeyer EH et al. One- or two-stage procedure for restorative proctocolectomy: rationale for a surgical strategy in ulcerative colitis. *Ann Surg* 2001;234:788–794
82. Hosie KB, Grobler SP, Keighley MR. Temporary loop ileostomy following restorative proctocolectomy. *Br J Surg* 1992;79:33–34
83. Jarvinen HJ, Luukkonen P. Comparison of restorative proctocolectomy with and without covering ileostomy in ulcerative colitis. *Br J Surg* 1991;78:199–201
84. Farouk R, Dozois RR, Pemberton JH et al. Incidence and subsequent impact of pelvic abscess after ileal pouch-anal anastomosis for chronic ulcerative colitis. *Dis Colon Rectum* 1998;41:1239–1243
85. Williamson ME, Lewis WG, Sagar PM et al. One-stage restorative proctocolectomy without temporary ileostomy for ulcerative colitis: a note of caution. *Dis Colon Rectum* 1997;40:1019–1022
86. Hay AR, Hay JW. Inflammatory bowel disease: medical cost algorithms. *J Clin Gastroenterol* 1992;14:318–327

87. Cohen RD. IBD indirect costs: the sleeping giant? *Gastroenterology* 2003;125:982–984
88. Longobardi T, Jacobs P, Bernstein CN. Work losses related to inflammatory bowel disease in the United States: results from the National Health Interview Survey. *Am J Gastroenterol* 2003;98:1064–1072
89. Sher ME, Weiss EG, Nogueras JJ et al. Morbidity of medical therapy for ulcerative colitis: what are we really saving? *Int J Colorectal Dis* 1996;11:287–293
90. McLeod RS. Surgery for inflammatory bowel diseases. *Dig Dis* 2003;21:168–179
91. Sagar PM, Lewis W, Holdsworth PJ et al. Quality of life after restorative proctocolectomy with a pelvic ileal reservoir compares favorably with that of patients with medically treated colitis. *Dis Colon Rectum* 1993;36:584–592
92. Kamm MA. Antagonist: Early surgical intervention in ulcerative colitis. *Gut* 2004;53:308–309
93. Kamm MA. Review article: maintenance of remission in ulcerative colitis. *Aliment Pharmacol Ther* 2002;16(Suppl 4):21–24
94. Odze RD. Pathology of indeterminate colitis. *J Clin Gastroenterol* 2004;38:S36–S40
95. Vernier G, Sendid B, Poulain D et al. Relevance of serologic studies in inflammatory bowel disease. *Curr Gastroenterol Rep* 2004;6:482–487
96. Dayton MT, Larsen KR, Christiansen DD. Similar functional results and complications after ileal pouch-anal anastomosis in patients with indeterminate vs ulcerative colitis. *Arch Surg* 2002;137:690–694; discussion 694–695
97. Delaney CP, Remzi FH, Gramlich T et al. Equivalent function, quality of life and pouch survival rates after ileal pouch-anal anastomosis for indeterminate and ulcerative colitis. *Ann Surg* 2002;236:43–48
98. Regimbeau JM, Panis Y, Pocard M et al. Long-term results of ileal pouch-anal anastomosis for colorectal Crohn's disease. *Dis Colon Rectum* 2001;44:769–778
99. Braveman JM, Schoetz DJ Jr, Marcello PW et al. The fate of the ileal pouch in patients developing Crohn's disease. *Dis Colon Rectum* 2004;47:1613–1619
100. de Oca J, Sanchez-Santos R, Rague JM et al. Long-term results of ileal pouch-anal anastomosis in Crohn's disease. *Inflamm Bowel Dis* 2003;9:171–175
101. Peters WR. Laparoscopic total proctocolectomy with creation of ileostomy for ulcerative colitis: report of two cases. *J Laparoendosc Surg* 1992;2:175–178
102. Dunker MS, Bemelman WA, Slors JF et al. Functional outcome, quality of life, body image, and cosmesis in patients after laparoscopic-assisted and conventional restorative proctocolectomy: a comparative study. *Dis Colon Rectum* 2001;44:1800–1807
103. Marcello PW, Milsom JW, Wong SK et al. Laparoscopic restorative proctocolectomy: case-matched comparative study with open restorative proctocolectomy. *Dis Colon Rectum* 2000;43:604–608
104. Kienle P, Z'Graggen K, Schmidt J et al. Laparoscopic restorative proctocolectomy. *Br J Surg* 2005;92:88–93
105. Ky AJ, Sonoda T, Milsom JW. One-stage laparoscopic restorative proctocolectomy: an alternative to the conventional approach? *Dis Colon Rectum* 2002;45:207–210
106. Kang JC, Chung MH, Chao PC et al. Hand-assisted laparoscopic colectomy vs open colectomy: a prospective randomized study. *Surg Endosc* 2004;18:577–581
107. Ballantyne GH, Leahy PF. Hand-assisted laparoscopic colectomy: evolution to a clinically useful technique. *Dis Colon Rectum* 2004;47:753–765
108. Targarona EM, Gracia E, Garriga J et al. Prospective randomized trial comparing conventional laparoscopic colectomy with hand-assisted laparoscopic colectomy: applicability, immediate clinical outcome, inflammatory response, and cost. *Surg Endosc* 2002;16:234–239
109. Targarona EM, Gracia E, Rodriguez M et al. Hand-assisted laparoscopic surgery. *Arch Surg* 2003;138:133–141
110. Nakajima K, Lee SW, Cocilovo C et al. Laparoscopic total colectomy: hand-assisted vs standard technique. *Surg Endosc* 2004;18:582–586
111. Rivadeneira DE, Marcello PW, Roberts PL et al. Benefits of hand-assisted laparoscopic restorative proctocolectomy: a comparative study. *Dis Colon Rectum* 2004;47: 1371–1376
112. Gill TS, Karantana A, Rees J et al. Laparoscopic proctocolectomy with restorative ileal-anal pouch. *Colorectal Dis* 2004;6:458–461
113. Maartense S, Dunker MS, Slors JF et al. Restorative proctectomy after emergency laparoscopic colectomy for ulcerative colitis: a case-matched study. *Colorectal Dis* 2004;6:254–257
114. Kienle P, Weitz J, Benner A et al. Laparoscopically assisted colectomy and ileoanal pouch procedure with and without protective ileostomy. *Surg Endosc* 2003;17: 716–720
115. Majewski WD. Long-term outcome, adhesions, and quality of life after laparoscopic and open surgical therapies for acute abdomen: follow-up of a prospective trial. *Surg Endosc* 2004;19:81–90
116. Delaney CP, Fazio VW, Remzi FH et al. Prospective, age-related analysis of surgical results, functional outcome, and quality of life after ileal pouch-anal anastomosis. *Ann Surg* 2003;238:221–228
117. Lehrmann J, Stucchi AF, LaMorte WW et al. Complications and outcomes after ileal pouch-anal anastomosis (IPAA): A meta-analysis of more than 8300 patients. *Gastroenterology* 2003;124:A814
118. Hahnloser D, Pemberton JH, Wolff BG et al. The effect of ageing on function and quality of life in ileal pouch patients: a single cohort experience of 409 patients with chronic ulcerative colitis. *Ann Surg* 2004;240:615–621; discussion 621–613
119. Muir AJ, Edwards LJ, Sanders LL et al. A prospective evaluation of health-related quality of life after ileal pouch anal anastomosis for ulcerative colitis. *Am J Gastroenterol* 2001;96:1480–1485
120. Michelassi F, Lee J, Rubin M et al. Long-term functional results after ileal pouch anal restorative proctocolectomy for ulcerative colitis: a prospective observational study. *Ann Surg* 2003;238:433–441
121. Fazio VW, Tekkis PP, Remzi F et al. Quantification of risk for pouch failure after ileal pouch anal anastomosis surgery. *Ann Surg* 2003;238:605–614; discussion 614–607

122. Saltzberg SS, DiEdwardo C, Scott TE et al. Ileal pouch salvage following failed ileal pouch-anal anastomosis. *J Gastrointest Surg* 1999;3:633–641
123. Wolf JM, Achkar JP, Lashner BA et al. Afferent limb ulcers predict Crohn's disease in patients with ileal pouch-anal anastomosis. *Gastroenterology* 2004;126:1686–1691
124. Sandborn WJ. How future tumor necrosis factor antagonists and other compounds will meet the remaining challenges in Crohn's disease. *Rev Gastroenterol Disord* 2004;4(Suppl 3):S25–S33
125. Ricart E, Panaccione R, Loftus EV et al. Successful management of Crohn's disease of the ileoanal pouch with infliximab. *Gastroenterology* 1999;117:429–432
126. Colombel JF, Ricart E, Loftus EV Jr et al. Management of Crohn's disease of the ileoanal pouch with infliximab. *Am J Gastroenterol* 2003;98:2239–2244
127. Kuisma J, Jarvinen H, Kahri A et al. Factors associated with disease activity of pouchitis after surgery for ulcerative colitis. *Scand J Gastroenterol* 2004;39:544–548
128. Reissman P, Piccirillo M, Ulrich A et al. Functional results of the double-stapled ileoanal reservoir. *J Am Coll Surg* 1995;181:444–450
129. Simchuk EJ, Thirlby RC. Risk factors and true incidence of pouchitis in patients after ileal pouch-anal anastomoses. *World J Surg* 2000;24:851–856
130. Hata K, Watanabe T, Shinozaki M et al. Patients with extraintestinal manifestations have a higher risk of developing pouchitis in ulcerative colitis: multivariate analysis. *Scand J Gastroenterol* 2003;38:1055–1058
131. Cheifetz A, Itzkowitz S. The diagnosis and treatment of pouchitis in inflammatory bowel disease. *J Clin Gastroenterol* 2004;38:S44–S50
132. Penna C, Dozois R, Tremaine W et al. Pouchitis after ileal pouch-anal anastomosis for ulcerative colitis occurs with increased frequency in patients with associated primary sclerosing cholangitis. *Gut* 1996;38:234–239
133. Stahlberg D, Gullberg K, Liljeqvist L et al. Pouchitis following pelvic pouch operation for ulcerative colitis. Incidence, cumulative risk, and risk factors. *Dis Colon Rectum* 1996;39:1012–1018
134. Stucchi AF, Becker JM. Pathogenesis of pouchitis. *Problems Gen Surg* 1999;16:139–150
135. Sandborn WJ. Pouchitis following ileal pouch-anal anastomosis: definition, pathogenesis, and treatment. *Gastroenterology* 1994;107:1856–1860
136. Becker JM, Stucchi AF, Bryant DE. How do you treat refractory pouchitis and when do you decide to remove the pouch? *Inflamm Bowel Dis* 1998;4:167–169; discussion 170–161
137. Shen B. Diagnosis and treatment of patients with pouchitis. *Drugs* 2003;63:453–461
138. Pfau PR, Lichtenstein GR. Cytomegalovirus infection as a cause of ileoanal pouchitis. *Dis Colon Rectum* 2000;43: 113–114
139. Dendrinos KA, Becker JM, Stucchi AF et al. Serologic markers (ANCA/ASCA) are associated with the development of postoperative fistulae in subjects with inflammatory bowel disease undergoing ileal pouch-anal anastomosis. *Gastroenterology* 2004;126:A212
140. Fruin AB, El-Zammer O, Stucchi AF et al. Colonic metaplasia in the ileal pouch is associated with inflammation and is not the result of long-term adaptation. *J Gastrointest Surg* 2003;7:246–254
141. Borjesson L, Willen R, Haboubi N et al. The risk of dysplasia and cancer in the ileal pouch mucosa after restorative proctocolectomy for ulcerative proctocolitis is low: a long-term term follow-up study. *Colorectal Dis* 2004;6: 494–498
142. Becker JM. What is the better surgical technique in ileal-pouch-anal anastomosis? Mucosectomy. *Inflamm Bowel Dis* 1996;2:151–154
143. Sandborn WJ. Does the surgical failure rate, increased incidence of pouchitis, and recent findings of dysplasia in pouches deter you from recommending an ileal pouch-anal anastomosis for ulcerative colitis. *Inflamm Bowel Dis* 1997;3:239–240
144. McLeod RS. The pelvic pouch procedure remains an excellent option for most patients with ulcerative colitis requiring surgery. *Inflamm Bowel Dis* 1997;3: 236–238

21

Appendix and Appendectomy

Douglas S. Smink ▪ *David I. Soybel*

▪ HISTORY

The first descriptions of the appendix date to the sixteenth century.[1–3] Although first sketched in the anatomic notebooks of Leonardo da Vinci around 1500, the appendix was not formally described until 1524 by da Capri[4] and 1543 by Vesalius.[5] Perhaps the first description of a case of appendicitis was by Fernel in 1554,[6] in which a 7-year-old girl with diarrhea was treated with a large quince. Soon thereafter she developed severe abdominal pain and died. Autopsy showed that the quince had obstructed the appendiceal lumen, resulting in appendiceal necrosis and perforation. For the next few centuries, such cases of appendicitis were typically diagnosed at autopsy.

Amyand is credited with the first appendectomy in 1736, when he operated on a boy with an enterocutaneous fistula within an inguinal hernia.[7] On exploration of the hernia sac, he discovered the appendix, which had been perforated by a pin resulting in a fecal fistula. As a result of his original description, an inguinal hernia containing the appendix carries Amyand's eponym to this day.[8] Nearly 150 years passed until Lawson Tait in London presented the first successful transabdominal appendectomy for gangrenous appendix in 1880.[9] Less than a decade later, in 1886, Reginald Fitz of Harvard Medical School first described the natural history of the inflamed appendix, coining the term "appendicitis."[10] In 1889, Charles McBurney of the Columbia College of Physicians and Surgeons in New York presented his series of cases of surgically-treated appendicitis and in so doing described the anatomic landmark that now bears his name. McBurney's point is the location of maximal tenderness "very exactly between an inch and a half and two inches from the anterior spinous process of the ileum on a straight line drawn from that process to the umbilicus."[11] In the 1890s, Sir Frederick Treves of London Hospital advocated conservative management of acute appendicitis followed by appendectomy after the infection had subsided;[12] unfortunately, his youngest daughter developed perforated appendicitis and died from such treatment.

Numerous advances in the diagnosis and treatment of appendicitis have emerged in the past 125 years. Nonetheless, acute appendicitis continues to challenge surgeons to this day.

▪ ANATOMY

Embryologically, the appendix and cecum develop as outpouchings of the caudal limb of the midgut loop in the sixth week of human development. By the fifth month, the appendix elongates into its vermiform shape. At birth, the appendix is located at the tip of the cecum, but due to unequal elongation of the lateral wall of the cecum, the adult appendix typically originates from the posteromedial wall of the cecum, caudal to the ileocecal valve. The appendix averages 9 cm in length,[3] with its outside diameter ranging from 3–8 mm and its lumen ranging from 1–3 mm. The base of the appendix is consistently found by following the teniae coli of the colon to their confluence at the base of the cecum. The appendiceal tip, however, can vary significantly in location (Fig 21–1). Although usually

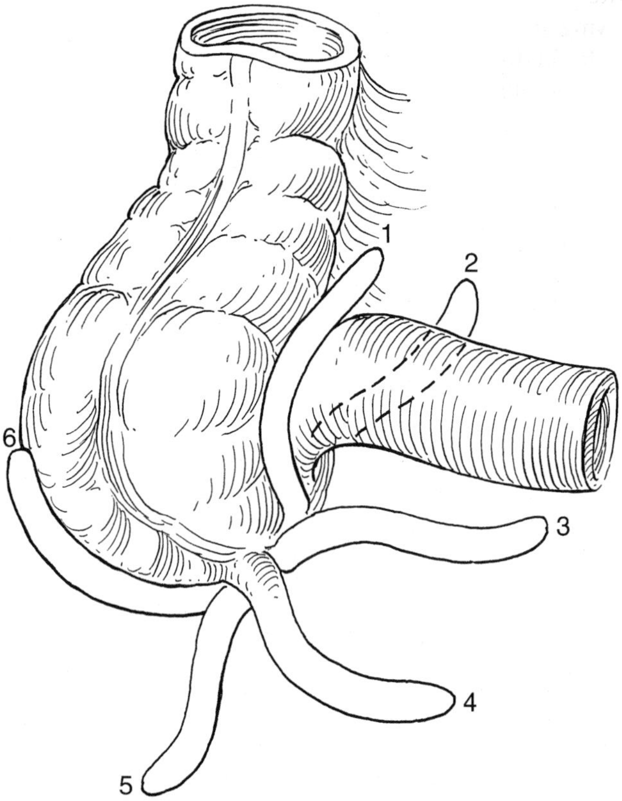

Figure 21–1. Anatomic variation in the position of the appendix. (1) Preilieal; (2) postilieal; (3) promontoric; (4) pelvic; (5) subcecal; (6) paracolic or prececal. (Redrawn from Wakeley CP. The position on the vermiform appendix as ascertained by analysis of 10,000 cases. *J Anat* 1933;67:277.) After Waldron.

located in the right lower quadrant or pelvis, the tip can occasionally reside in the left lower or right upper quadrants.

The arterial supply of the appendix comes from the appendicular branch of the ileocolic artery, which originates posterior to the terminal ileum and enters the mesoappendix near the base of the appendix (Fig 21–2). Lymphatic drainage flows to lymph nodes along the ileocolic artery.

▪ ACUTE APPENDICITIS

EPIDEMIOLOGY

Addiss and associates[13] estimated the incidence of acute appendicitis in the United States population to be 11 cases per 10,000 population annually. The disease is slightly more common in males, with a male:female ratio of 1.4:1. In a lifetime, 8.6% of males and 6.7% of females can be expected to develop acute appendicitis. Young age is a risk factor, as nearly 70% of patients with acute appendicitis are less than 30 years of age. The highest incidence of appendicitis in males is in the 10- to 14-year-old age group (27.6 cases per 10,000 population), while the highest female incidence is in the 15- to 19-year-old age group (20.5 cases per 10,000 population). Patients at extremes of age are more likely to develop perforated appendicitis. Overall, perforation was present in 19.2% of cases of acute appendicitis. This number was significantly higher, however, in patients under 5 and over 65 years of age. Although less common in people over 65 years old, acute appendicitis in the elderly progresses to perforation more than 50% of the time.[13]

ETIOLOGY AND PATHOPHYSIOLOGY

Appendicitis, diverticular disease, and colorectal carcinoma have been shown to be diseases of developed civilizations. Burkitt[14] found an increased incidence of appendicitis in Western countries compared to Africa, as well as in wealthy, urban communities compared to rural areas. He attributed this to the Western diet, which is low in dietary fiber and high in refined sugars and fat, and postulated that low-fiber diets lead to less bulky bowel contents, prolonged intestinal transit time, and increased intraluminal pressure. Burkitt theorized that

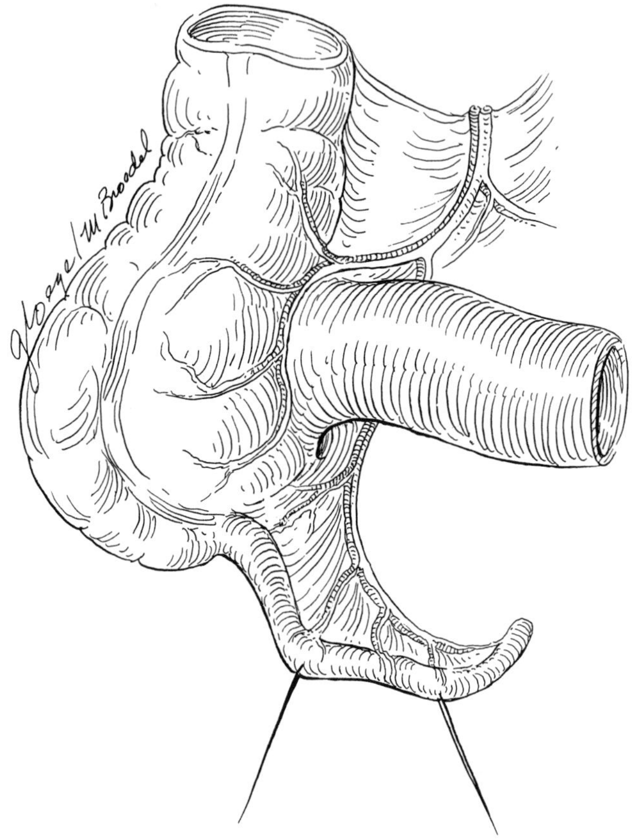

Figure 21–2. The appendix and its arterial supply.

the combination of firm stool leading to appendiceal obstruction and increased intraluminal pressure causing bacterial translocation across the bowel wall resulted in appendicitis. In examining appendixes removed for reasons other than appendicitis, he found fecaliths to be more prevalent in Canadian (32%) than in South African (4%) adults. In a group of patients with appendicitis, fecaliths were more common in Canadians (52%) than in South Africans (23%).[15] He felt this was confirmation that appendiceal obstruction resulted in appendicitis. Of note, however, the majority of patients with appendicitis in his study did not have evidence of a fecalith.

Wangensteen extensively studied the structure and function of the appendix and the role of obstruction in appendicitis.[16,17] Based on anatomic studies, he postulated that mucosal folds and a sphincterlike orientation of muscle fibers at the appendiceal orifice make the appendix susceptible to obstruction. He proposed the following sequence of events to explain appendicitis: (1) closed loop obstruction is caused by a fecalith and swelling of the mucosal and submucosal lymphoid tissue at the base of the appendix; (2) intraluminal pressure rises as the appendiceal mucosa secretes fluid against the fixed obstruction; (3) increased pressure in the appendiceal wall exceeds capillary pressure and causes mucosal ischemia; and (4) luminal bacterial overgrowth and translocation of bacteria across the appendiceal wall result in inflammation, edema, and ultimately necrosis. If the appendix is not removed, perforation can ensue.

Although appendiceal obstruction is widely accepted as the primary cause of appendicitis, evidence suggests that this may be only one of many possible etiologies. First, some patients with a fecalith have a histologically normal appendix.[15,18,19] Moreover, the majority of patients with appendicitis show no evidence for a fecalith.[15,18,19] Arnbjornsson and Bengmark[20] studied at laparotomy the appendixes of patients with suspected appendicitis. They found the intraluminal pressure of the appendix prior to removal to be elevated in only 8 of 27 patients with nonperforated appendicitis. They found no signs of obstruction in the remaining patients with nonperforated appendicitis, as well as all patients with a normal appendix. Taken together, these studies imply that obstruction is but one of the possible etiologies of acute appendicitis.

PRESENTATION

Perhaps the most common surgically correctable cause of abdominal pain, the diagnosis of acute appendicitis remains difficult in many instances. Some of the signs and symptoms can be subtle to both the clinician and the patient and may not be present in all instances. Arriving at the correct diagnosis is essential, however, as a delay in diagnosis may allow progression to perforation and significantly increased morbidity and mortality. Incorrectly diagnosing a patient with appendicitis, although not catastrophic, often subjects the patient to an unnecessary operation.

The classic presentation of acute appendicitis begins with crampy, intermittent abdominal pain, thought to be due to obstruction of the appendiceal lumen. The pain may be either periumbilical or diffuse and difficult to localize. This is typically followed shortly thereafter with nausea; vomiting may or may not be present. If nausea and vomiting precede the pain, patients are likely to have another cause for their abdominal pain, such as gastroenteritis. Classically, the pain migrates to the right lower quadrant as transmural inflammation of the appendix leads to inflammation of the peritoneal lining of the right lower abdomen. This usually occurs within 12–24 hours of the onset of symptoms. The character of the pain also changes from dull and colicky to sharp and constant. Movement or Valsalva maneuver often worsens this pain, so that the patient typically desires to lie still; some patients describe pain with every bump in the car or ambulance ride to the hospital. Patients may report low-grade fever up to 101°F (38.3°C). Higher temperatures and shaking chills should again alert the surgeon to other diagnoses, including appendiceal perforation or nonappendiceal sources. When questioned, patients who have appendicitis commonly report anorexia; appendicitis is unlikely in those with a normal appetite.

The surgeon is constantly reminded that in practice, the classic presentation of acute appendicitis is not present in all patients. Patients may have none or only a few of the symptoms just described. For instance, they may not notice or recall the initial colicky pain. When the pain becomes constant, it may localize to other quadrants of the abdomen due to an alteration in appendiceal anatomy as in late pregnancy or malrotation. In patients with a retrocecal appendix, the pain may never localize until generalized peritonitis from perforated appendicitis occurs. Urinary or bowel frequency may be present due to appendiceal inflammation irritating the adjacent bladder or rectum. Because appendicitis is so common, a high index of suspicion for appendicitis is warranted in all patients with abdominal pain.

PERFORATED APPENDICITIS

It is a commonly held belief that if left untreated, appendiceal inflammation will progress inevitably to necrosis, and ultimately to perforation. The time course of this progression varies among patients. In one study of the natural history of appendicitis, the authors questioned patients undergoing appendectomy for suspected appendicitis about their duration of symptoms.[21] Patients with nonperforated appendicitis reported an average of 22 hours of symptoms prior to presentation to the hospital, while patients with perforated appendicitis reported an average of 57 hours. However, 20% of cases of perforated appendicitis presented within 24 hours of the onset of symptoms; one of those patients had symptoms for only 11 hours. Although concern for perforation should be present when evaluating a patient with more than 24 hours of symptoms, the clinician must remember that perforation can develop more rapidly.

Some authors have questioned whether some perforations in acute appendicitis are attributable to delay in diagnosis after a patient seeks medical attention. Velanovich and Satava postulated a surgeon's misdiagnosis rate (the percentage of normal appendixes found at appendectomy) to be inversely related to the perforation rate (the percentage of perforated appendixes found at laparotomy).[22] They believed that surgeons are obliged to operate quickly when appendicitis is suspected, thus minimizing the likelihood of perforation in exchange for a higher rate of misdiagnosis. More recent studies suggest that this reasoning is flawed. Temple and colleagues showed that patients with perforated appendicitis were operated on more quickly than those with nonperforated appendicitis (6.5 hours versus 9 hours), but perforated patients had significantly longer prehospital symptoms (57 hours versus 22 hours).[21] These findings are confirmed by two other studies, both showing that longer duration of prehospital delay is the major contributor to perforation.[23,24] Perforation after presenting to surgical attention appears to be uncommon.

When acute appendicitis has progressed to appendiceal perforation, other symptoms may be present. Patients will often complain of two or more days of abdominal pain, but their duration of symptoms may be shorter, as previously discussed. The pain usually localizes to the right lower quadrant if the perforation has been walled off by surrounding intra-abdominal structures including the omentum, but it may be diffuse if generalized peritonitis ensues. The pain may be so severe that patients do not remember the antecedent colicky pain. Patients with perforation often have rigors and high fevers to 102°F (38.9°C) or above. A history of poor oral intake and dehydration may also be present.

Most patients with perforated appendicitis present with symptoms related to the inflamed appendix itself or to a localized intraperitoneal abscess from perforation. Other more rare presentations do occur, however. These are most likely to occur in the very young and very old, who cannot express their symptoms and often present late in the course of their disease. For instance, abscesses can also form in the retroperitoneum due to perforation of a retrocecal appendix, or in the liver from hematogenous spread of infection through the portal venous system. An intraperitoneal abscess could fistulize to the skin, resulting in an enterocutaneous fistula. Pylephlebitis (septic portal vein thrombosis) presents with high fevers and jaundice and can be confused with cholangitis; it is a dreaded complication of acute appendicitis and carries a high mortality.[25] Occasionally, patients will have bilious vomiting and obstipation due to a small bowel obstruction resulting from appendiceal perforation. Because appendicitis is so common, these rare presentations should alert the surgeon to the possibility of appendicitis.

DIAGNOSIS

History and Physical Examination

As always, the diagnosis begins with a thorough history and physical examination. The patient should be asked about the classic symptoms of appendicitis, but the surgeon should not be dissuaded by the absence of many of the symptoms. Many patients with acute appendicitis do not have a classic history. Because the differential diagnosis of appendicitis is extensive, patients should be queried about certain symptoms that may suggest an alternative diagnosis. Surgeons must also remember that a previous appendectomy does not definitively exclude the diagnosis of appendicitis, as "stump appendicitis" (appendicitis in the remaining appendiceal stump after appendectomy), although rare, has been described.[26]

On inspection, patients look mildly ill and may have slightly elevated temperature and pulse. They often lie still to avoid the peritoneal irritation caused by movement. The surgeon should systematically examine the entire abdomen, starting in the left upper quadrant away from the patient's described pain. Maximal tenderness is typically in the right lower quadrant, at or near McBurney's point, located one-third of the way from the anterior superior iliac spine to the umbilicus. This tenderness is often associated with localized muscle rigidity and signs of peritoneal inflammation, including rebound, shake, or tap tenderness. Right lower quadrant tenderness is the most consistent of all signs of acute appendicitis;[27,28] its presence should always raise the specter of appendicitis, even in the absence of other signs and symptoms. Because of the various anatomic locations of the appendix, however, it is possible for the tenderness to be in the right flank or right upper quadrant, the suprapubic region, or the left lower quadrant. Patients with a retrocecal or pelvic appendix may have no abdominal tenderness whatsoever. In such cases, rectal examination can be helpful to elicit right-sided pelvic tenderness.

Multiple signs can be detected on physical examination to contribute to the diagnosis of appendicitis. Rovsing's sign, pain in the right lower quadrant on palpation of the left lower quadrant, is further evidence of localized peritoneal inflammation in the right lower quadrant. Psoas sign, pain with flexion of the leg at the right hip, can be seen with a retrocecal appendix due to inflammation adjacent to the psoas muscle. The obdurator sign, pain with rotating the flexed right thigh internally, indicates inflammation adjacent to the obdurator muscle in the pelvis.

In cases of perforated appendicitis, patients can look gravely ill, appearing flushed with dry mucous membranes and considerable elevations in temperature or pulse. If sepsis has developed, blood pressure can be depressed. If the perforation has been walled off by surrounding structures to create an abscess or phlegmon, a mass may be palpable in the right lower quadrant. If free intraperitoneal rupture has occurred, the patient can have signs of generalized peritonitis with diffuse rebound tenderness.

Laboratory Studies

Laboratory studies can be helpful in the diagnosis of appendicitis, but no single test is definitive. A white blood cell count (WBC) is perhaps the most useful laboratory test. Typically, the WBC is slightly elevated in nonperforated appendicitis, but may be quite elevated in the presence of perforation. The clinician must remember, however, that the WBC can be normal in patients with acute appendicitis, particularly in early cases. Serial WBC measurements improve the diagnostic accuracy, with a rising value over time commonly seen in patients with appendicitis.[29] Urinalysis is performed to diagnose other potential causes for abdominal pain, specifically urinary tract infection and ureteral stone. Significant hematuria with colicky abdominal pain suggests ureterolithiasis, and testing directed at this diagnosis is indicated. A urinary tract infection, on the other hand, is not uncommon in patients with appendicitis. Its presence does not exclude the diagnosis of acute appendicitis, but it should be identified and treated. Although pyuria suggests urinary tract infection, it is not uncommon for the urinalysis in a patient with appendicitis to show a few white blood cells solely due to inflammation of the ureter by the adjacent appendix.

In certain patient populations, other laboratory tests are indicated. Measurement of serum liver enzymes and amylase can be helpful in diagnosing liver, gallbladder, or pancreatic disease in patients complaining of mid-abdominal or right upper quadrant pain. In women of childbearing age, the urine β-human chorionic gonadotropin should be checked to alert the clinician to the possibility of ectopic or concurrent pregnancy. Ectopic pregnancy is another cause of right lower quadrant pain that demands emergent diagnosis and treatment. Concurrent pregnancy should be known before a patient with suspected appendicitis is subjected to ionizing radiation from imaging studies or to general anesthesia.

Diagnostic Scores

Diagnostic scoring systems have been developed in an attempt to improve the diagnostic accuracy of acute appendicitis.[18,30] The most prominent of those scores, developed by Alvarado,[30] was based on a retrospective analysis of 305 patients with abdominal pain suspicious for appendicitis. This scoring system gives points for symptoms (migration of pain, anorexia, and nausea), physical signs (right lower quadrant tenderness, rebound tenderness, and pyrexia), and laboratory values (leukocytosis and a left shift). Although these scores can help guide clinical thinking, they do not markedly improve diagnostic accuracy.[31] With the recent improvement in imaging studies, these scores play a smaller role in diagnosis.

Imaging Studies

The potential imaging modalities for diagnosis of acute appendicitis include plain radiographs, ultrasound, and computed tomography. Prior to the widespread use of modern imaging techniques, plain abdominal films were often obtained in patients with abdominal pain, and a right lower quadrant fecalith (or appendicolith) was considered pathognomonic for acute appendicitis. A number of studies question this teaching, however. Teicher and colleagues[18] reviewed the abdominal radiographs of 200 appendectomy patients, 100 with pathologically proven appendicitis and 100 with a normal appendix. Of those with appendicitis, 10.5% had an appendicolith on x-ray, compared to 3.3% of those without appendicitis. An extensive review of appendectomy specimens at the Mayo Clinic[19] showed that fecaliths or appendiceal calculi were present in 9% of patients with nonperforated appendicitis and 21% of those with perforated appendicitis. Interestingly, fecaliths were also present in 7% of patients with suspected appendicitis who had a pathologically normal appendix, and 2% of patients who had an appendectomy for other reasons.

These studies show that fecaliths are not pathognomonic for appendicitis, as some patients with abdominal pain and a fecalith have a normal appendix. In addition, fecaliths are not common enough in patients with appendicitis to be used as a reliable sign. As a result, plain abdominal radiographs are neither helpful nor cost effective and are not recommended for the diagnosis of acute appendicitis. Plain radiographs are indicated in elderly patients with severe abdominal pain, in whom a perforated viscus is included in the differential diagnosis. In this patient population, an upright chest x-ray can assess for the presence of free air.

Abdominal ultrasonography is a popular imaging modality for acute appendicitis. Findings that suggest appendicitis include thickening of the appendiceal wall, loss of wall compressibility, increased echogenicity of the surrounding fat signifying inflammation, and loculated pericecal fluid (Fig 21–3). The advantages of ultrasound include its widespread availability, as well as the avoidance of ionizing radiation and the side effects of intravenous contrast such as renal toxicity and allergic reactions. In addition, ultrasound (both abdominal and transvaginal) is particularly useful in assessing obstetric and gynecological causes of abdominal pain in women of childbearing age. Ultrasound is highly operator-dependent, however, and it is frequently unable to visualize the normal appendix.[32] A recent meta-analysis of 14 prospective studies showed ultrasound to have a sensitivity of 0.86 and a specificity of 0.81.[33]

Computed tomography (CT) is yet another imaging modality for acute appendicitis. CT benefits from a high diagnostic accuracy for appendicitis[33] and visualization and diagnosis of many of the other causes of abdominal pain that can be confused with appendicitis. The radiographic findings of appendicitis on CT include a dilated (>6 mm), thick-walled appendix that does not fill with enteric contrast or air, as well as surrounding fat stranding to suggest inflammation (Fig 21–4).[34] In a meta-analysis of 12 prospective studies, CT demonstrated a sensitivity of 0.94 and a specificity of 0.95.[33] CT thus has a high negative predictive value, making it particularly useful in excluding appendicitis in patients for whom the diagnosis is in doubt. Appendicitis is highly unlikely if enteric contrast fills the lumen of the appendix and no surrounding inflammation is present. The clinician must remember, however, that a CT performed early in the course of appendicitis might not show the typical radiographic findings. In confusing cases, it is reasonable to repeat the CT after 24 hours of observation.

A number of recent prospective studies have compared the accuracy of CT and ultrasound in imaging the appendix (Table 21–1).[32,35,36] Balthazar and associates[35] performed CT and ultrasound on 100 consecutive pa-

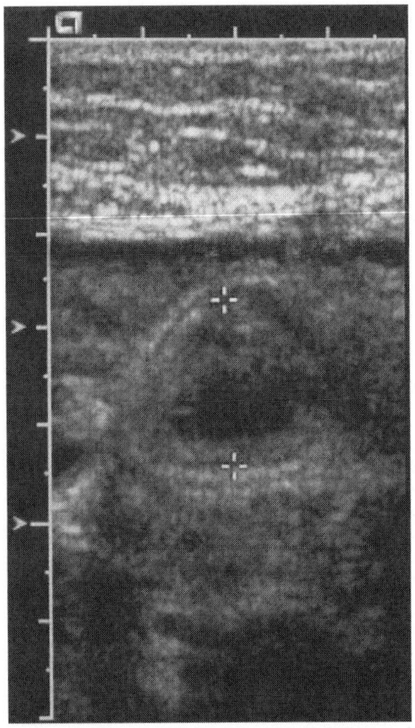

Figure 21–3. Appendiceal ultrasound showing distended, noncompressible appendix measuring 1.7 cm in transverse dimension (larger than 0.6 cm is abnormal). (Courtesy of M. Stephen Ledbetter, MD, Brigham and Women's Hospital, Boston, Mass.)

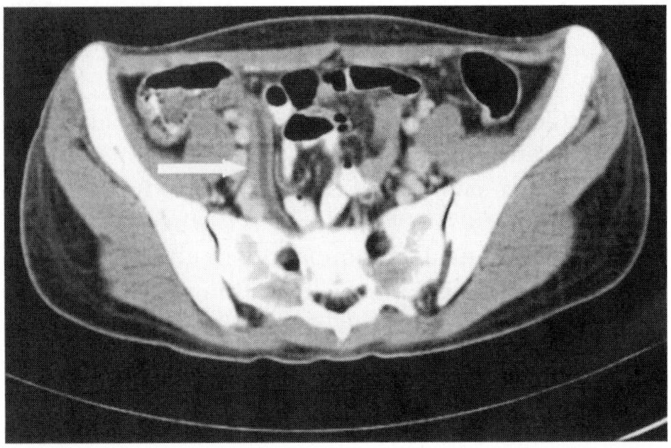

Figure 21–4. Computed tomography of acute appendicitis. The *arrow* points to an enlarged, fluid-filled appendix with wall hyperemia that does not fill with oral contrast. The paucity of intra-abdominal fat limits identification of fat stranding. (Courtesy of M. Stephen Ledbetter, MD, Brigham and Women's Hospital, Boston, Mass.)

TABLE 21–1. ACCURACY OF COMPUTED TOMOGRAPHY AND ULTRASOUND FOR THE DIAGNOSIS OF ACUTE APPENDICITIS

		Sensitivity (%)	Specificity (%)	Accuracy (%)
Balthazar et al[35]	CT	96	89	94
	US	76	91	83
Horton et al[36]	CT	97	100	98
	US	76	90	80
Wise et al[32]	CT	96	92	93
	US	62	71	69
Terasawa et al[33] (meta-analysis)	CT	94	95	N/A
	US	86	81	N/A

tients with suspected appendicitis. The sensitivity of CT was considerably higher (96% for CT, 76% for ultrasound), while the specificity was comparable (89% for CT, 91% for ultrasound), yielding a higher accuracy for CT (94% versus 83%). CT was also able to provide an alternative diagnosis in more patients and was better able to visualize abscesses or phlegmons (Fig 21–5). Horton and colleagues[36] randomized patients with suspected appendicitis to either CT or ultrasound. Their findings echo those of Balthazar, with both CT and ultrasound having high specificity (100% for CT, 90% for US) but CT having significantly higher sensitivity (97% versus 76%). Yet another prospective study showed similar results, with CT having higher sensitivity (96% versus 62%) and specificity (92% versus 71%) than ultrasound.[32] Again, CT was also better able to visualize other intra-abdominal pathology in the absence of appendicitis.

In a study of 100 patients evaluated by CT with rectal and intravenous contrast, Rao and coworkers[37] showed that CT can reduce the use of hospital resources and costs. CT changed the management of 59 patients, avoiding 13 unnecessary appendectomies and eliminating a total of 50 inpatient hospital days for observation of unexplained abdominal pain. Even factoring in the cost of the CT scans, the authors calculated a net savings of $447 (U.S. dollars) per patient.

Taken together, these studies suggest an algorithm for evaluation of patients with suspected acute appendicitis. Patients with a history, physical examination, and laboratory studies classic for appendicitis should undergo urgent appendectomy. In those with an evaluation suggestive but not convincing for appendicitis, further imaging is indicated. In women of childbearing age, this should begin with a pelvic ultrasound to evaluate for ovarian pathology. Following this, the study of choice is an abdominopelvic CT because of its accuracy in diagnosing both appendiceal and other intra-abdominal pathology. This can be supplemented with rectal contrast CT, if needed, to better visualize the appendix.[32,37] Patients with a CT showing appendicitis are taken for appendectomy. In many instances, patients with a normal CT do not require hospital admission. If symptoms persist, admission to the hospital for observation and perhaps a repeat CT scan is warranted.

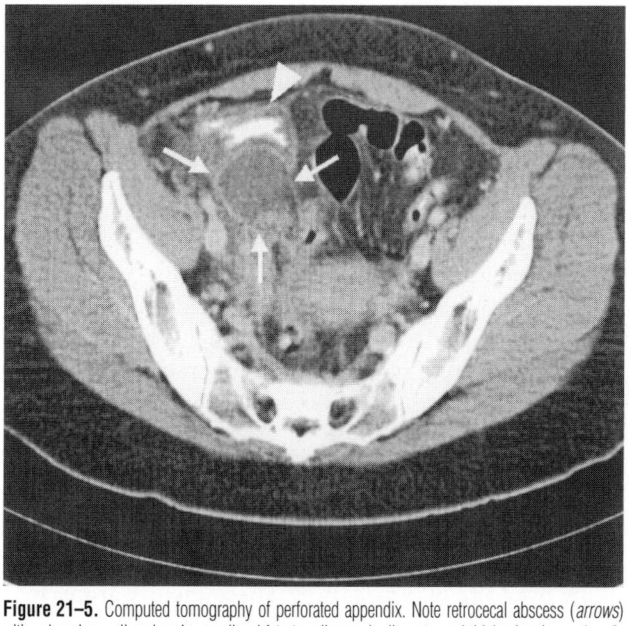

Figure 21–5. Computed tomography of perforated appendix. Note retrocecal abscess (*arrows*) with enhancing wall and periappendiceal fat stranding and adjacent cecal thickening (*arrowhead*). (Courtesy of M. Stephen Ledbetter, MD, Brigham and Women's Hospital, Boston, Mass.)

Differential Diagnosis

Because many of its signs and symptoms are nonspecific, the differential diagnosis of acute appendicitis is extensive and includes virtually all possible abdominal sources of pain, as well as some nonabdominal sources (Table 21–2). However, some diagnoses are more likely than others in certain patient groups. For instance, in young males with a suggestive history and physical examination, acute appendicitis is the most likely cause of right lower quadrant pain. Meckel's diverticulitis causes similar symptoms, but is relatively uncommon.[38] Gastroenteritis is considerably more common and should be expected when nausea and vomiting precede the abdominal pain, or when diarrhea is a prominent symptom. Crohn's disease affecting the terminal ileum may resemble appendicitis in its initial presentation, but on further questioning, the patient typically describes a subacute course including fever, weight loss, and pain.

In middle-aged and older adults, other inflammatory conditions should be considered, including peptic or duodenal ulcer (with fluid tracking into the right paracolic gutter), cholecystitis, and pancreatitis. In addition, cecal or sigmoid diverticulitis can be confused with acute appendicitis. Cecal diverticulitis is quite similar in pathogenesis and presentation to appendicitis, due to the fact that cecal diverticuli, like the appendix, are true diverticuli containing all layers of the intestinal wall. Because a redundant, floppy sigmoid colon can extend to the right side of the abdomen, patients with sigmoid diverticulitis can sometimes present with right lower quadrant pain. Those patients typically describe a quicker progression to localized tenderness, as well as a prodrome of an alteration in bowel habits. Malignancies can present with acute right lower quadrant pain due to perforation of a cecal carcinoma or appendicitis caused by a mass obstructing the appendiceal orifice.[39] These patients will also typically have guaiac-positive stools, anemia, and a history of weight loss.

In women of childbearing years, the diagnosis of right lower quadrant pain can be even more difficult.

TABLE 21–2. DIFFERENTIAL DIAGNOSIS OF ACUTE APPENDICITIS

Gastrointestinal Causes
Cecal diverticulitis
Sigmoid diverticulitis
Meckel's diverticulitis
Epiploica appendicitis
Mesenteric adenitis
Omental torsion
Crohn's disease
Cecal carcinoma
Appendiceal neoplasm
Lymphoma
Typhlitis
Small bowel obstruction
Perforated duodenal ulcer
Intussusception
Acute cholecystitis
Hepatitis
Pancreatitis
Infectious Causes
Infectious terminal ileitis (*Yersinia*, tuberculosis or cytomegalovirus)
Gastroenteritis
Cytomegalovirus colitis
Genitourinary Causes
Pyelonephritis or perinephric abscess
Nephrolithiasis
Hydronephrosis
Urinary tract infection
Nonabdominal Causes
Streptococcal pharyngitis
Lower lobe pneumonia
Rectus muscle hematoma
In Women
Ovarian cyst (ruptured or not ruptured)
Corpus luteal cyst (ruptured or not ruptured)
Ovarian torsion
Endometriosis
Pelvic inflammatory disease
Tubo-ovarian abscess
In Pregnancy
Ectopic pregnancy
Round ligament pain
Chorioamnionitis
Placental abruption
Preterm labor

In addition to the causes of right lower quadrant pain mentioned for young men, young women can also have pain from obstetric and gynecological causes such as ruptured ovarian cyst or follicle, ovarian torsion, ectopic pregnancy, acute salpingitis, and tubo-ovarian abscess. A complete history including recent menstrual history, as well as pelvic examination, can be helpful in differentiating these causes of pain from acute appendicitis. Nonetheless, appendicitis can be difficult to diagnose in this patient population, and higher rates of misdiagnosis have been described in women of childbearing age.[40]

Special Considerations

Children. Appendicitis most commonly affects children age 10–19, with an overall incidence of approximately 20 cases per 10,000 population annually.[13] Among those under age 20, infants age 0–4 have the lowest incidence of appendicitis (2 cases per 10,000 annually), but up to two-thirds will present with perforation.[41] Perforation is common because infants often present later in their disease course and because of the difficulty in obtaining an accurate history. The diagnosis is further complicated by diseases of childhood that can mimic appendicitis. For instance, mesenteric adenitis, an inflammation of the mesenteric lymph nodes secondary to upper respiratory tract infection, can present with fever and right lower quadrant pain. Streptococcal pharyngitis and bacterial meningitis can also present with fever, nausea, and abdominal pain. These diagnoses should be considered when evaluating children for suspected appendicitis.

In children with an equivocal history and physical examination, CT has been shown to be highly accurate in diagnosing appendicitis. Garcia Pena and associates compared ultrasonography and rectal contrast CT in 139 children with suspected appendicitis and found CT to be more sensitive (97% for CT, 44% for ultrasound), more specific (94% for CT, 93% for ultrasound), and more accurate (94% for CT, 76% for ultrasound).[42] CT correctly changed the management of 73% of patients, while ultrasound correctly changed 19%. The use of CT can be recommended for children with one caveat. The radiation from a CT in childhood theoretically causes a small increase in the lifetime risk of certain cancers.[43] Therefore, clinicians should consider the risks and benefits of CT, and efforts should be directed toward reducing radiation dose when imaging children.[44]

Elderly. Although appendicitis is more common in younger age groups, it is still an important cause of abdominal pain in the elderly. Perhaps due to a diminished inflammatory response, the elderly can present with less impressive symptoms and physical signs, longer duration of symptoms, and decreased leukocytosis compared to younger patients.[45] Perforation is thus more common, occurring in as many as 50% of patients over age 65.[13] These patients may have cardiac, pulmonary, and renal conditions resulting in considerable morbidity and mortality from perforation. In one series, the mortality from perforated appendicitis in patients over age 80 was 21%.[46] These factors argue that right lower quadrant pain in elderly patients must be aggressively investigated. Due to the multiple other possible causes of abdominal pain in this patient population (including malignancy, diverticulitis, and perforated peptic ulcer disease), prompt CT scan is advocated when the diagnosis is in question.

Pregnancy. The diagnosis of acute appendicitis in the pregnant patient can be particularly challenging, as nausea, anorexia, and abdominal pain may be symptoms of both appendicitis and normal pregnancy. In addition, the gravid uterus can displace the abdominal viscera, shifting the location of the appendix from the right lower quadrant. Appendicitis affects 1 in every 1,400 pregnancies, an incidence similar to that of the nonpregnant female population.[47] It can occur in any trimester, with perhaps a slight increase in frequency during the second trimester.[47,48] Perforation is more common in the third trimester, however, and results from a longer duration from the onset of symptoms to operation.[49] The differential diagnosis of appendicitis includes not only the conditions possible in nonpregnant women, but also certain conditions specific to pregnancy: ectopic pregnancy, chorioamnionitis, preterm labor, placental abruption, and round ligament pain.

In the first and early second trimesters, the presentation of appendicitis is similar to that seen in nonpregnant women. In the third trimester, women may not present with right lower quadrant pain due to displacement of the appendix by the gravid uterus. Baer and associates performed barium enemas on normal pregnant women and found the appendix to migrate superiorly towards the right upper quadrant in later stages of pregnancy.[50] His findings suggest that appendicitis should present with right upper quadrant or flank pain in late pregnancy. Two retrospective studies contradict this, however, showing that even in the third trimester, pain and tenderness are more common in the right lower than the right upper quadrant.[47,48] Nonetheless, right upper quadrant pain did predominate in some third-trimester patients with appendicitis in each study,[47,48] reminding the clinician that right upper quadrant and right flank symptoms could be due to appendicitis in an appendix displaced by the gravid uterus.

Ultrasound is accurate in pregnancy[51] and is a useful first radiological study because it has no known adverse fetal effects.[52] Rectal contrast CT has also been shown to be highly accurate in the pregnant population.[53] Although ionizing radiation has risks to the fetus, the radiation from a typical abdominopelvic CT is below the threshold of 5 rads at which teratogenic effects are seen.[54] When the diagnosis is in doubt, the risk of radiation should be weighed against the risk of spontaneous abortion from an unnecessary laparotomy or from undiagnosed appendicitis progressing to perforation. Hospital admission with close observation for progression of symptoms is a viable alternative if the risks of radiation from CT scan are deemed excessive.

The pregnant patient should proceed directly to appendectomy if appendicitis is suspected. A normal appendix is not an uncommon finding, as negative laparotomy has been reported in approximately one-third of cases due to the difficulty of diagnosis in this population.[47,48,55] Negative laparotomy should not be considered an error in diagnosis, because the risk to the fetus varies directly with the severity of appendicitis. In one series, fetal loss occurred in only 1 (3%) of 30 negative laparotomies.[47] Fetal mortality rises to 5% in cases of nonperforated appendicitis, and increases to 20% when the appendix perforates.[55] These data warrant an aggressive approach to appendectomy. Early negative exploration is justified to minimize the likelihood of progression to perforation.

Although laparoscopic appendectomy has become increasingly popular, its appropriateness during pregnancy remains in question. The gravid uterus can make laparoscopic visualization difficult, particularly if the appendix is located in the pelvis. In addition, carbon dioxide insufflation of the abdomen results in fetal hypercarbia and decreased placental blood flow, the effects of which have not been completely studied. Although case series of successful laparoscopy during pregnancy have been presented,[56] the overall safety of laparoscopic appendectomy in pregnancy is uncertain.[57] Until further research is available, the open approach is advised.

Immunocompromise. The immunocompromised state alters the normal response to acute infection and wound healing. Appendicitis affects all types of patients and must be considered in those who have undergone organ transplantation, are receiving chemotherapy, have hematological malignancy, or are infected with the human immunodeficiency virus. The differential diagnosis of abdominal pain in this population is broad and includes hepatitis, pancreatitis (from medications or cytomegalovirus infection), acalculous cholecystitis, intra-abdominal opportunistic infections (cytomegalovirus colitis or mycobacterial ileitis), secondary malignancies (lymphoma or Kaposi's sarcoma), graft-versus-host disease, and typhlitis. This broad differential diagnosis often results in delay in diagnosis and late presentation to surgical evaluation, at which time perforation may be more likely.[58,59]

Appendicitis in patients with human immunodeficiency virus (HIV) and acquired immunodeficiency syndrome (AIDS) presents unique challenges. Abdominal pain is not an uncommon symptom in these patients, making differentiation between surgical and nonsurgical causes difficult. Nonetheless, immunocompromised patients with appendicitis present with symptoms similar to those of the general population,[58] and appendicitis should be considered in patients with right lower quadrant pain, nausea, and anorexia. Fever and white blood cell count may not be helpful in this population, so imaging studies, particularly CT, have been supported by some authors.[59] There is no specific contraindication to operation in immunocompromised patients, so once diagnosed with appendicitis, appendectomy should be performed promptly.

■ TREATMENT

NONOPERATIVE MANAGEMENT

Appendectomy was one of the first intra-abdominal operations performed, and appendicitis has long been a surgically treated disease. Rare descriptions of nonsurgical management dot the surgical literature, however. Treves was an advocate of early nonoperative management of acute appendicitis, even prior to the advent of antibiotics.[12] In the post-antibiotic era, Coldrey presented his retrospective series of 471 patients with appendicitis treated with antibiotics.[60] This treatment failed in at least 57 patients, with 48 requiring appendectomy and 9 requiring drainage of an appendiceal abscess. Only one randomized controlled trial, performed by Eriksson and associates, addresses this issue.[61] Their results show a high rate of recurrence of appendicitis treated nonsurgically. The authors randomized 40 adults with presumed appendicitis to appendectomy or 10 days of intravenous and oral antibiotics. Eight (40%) of the 20 patients in the antibiotic group required appendectomy within 1 year: one patient for perforation within 12 hours of randomization, and another 7 for recurrent appendicitis (one of whom had perforation). Based on the high rate of failure with antibiotics alone, nonoperative management of acute appendicitis cannot be recommended. Antibiotic treatment may be a useful temporizing measure, however, in environments with no surgical capabilities such as in space flight and submarine travel.[62]

PREOPERATIVE PREPARATION

When the decision is made to perform an appendectomy for acute appendicitis, the patient should proceed to the operating room with little delay to minimize the chance of progression to perforation. Such occurrences are rare, however, as most cases of appendiceal perforation occur prior to surgical evaluation.[23,24] Patients with appendicitis may be dehydrated from fever and poor oral intake, so intravenous fluids should be begun, and pulse, blood pressure, and urine output should be closely monitored. Markedly dehydrated patients may require a Foley catheter to ensure adequate urine output. Severe electrolyte abnormalities are uncommon with nonperforated appendicitis, as vomiting and fever have typically been present for 24 hours or less, but may be significant in cases of perforation. Any electrolyte deficiencies should be corrected prior to the induction of general anesthesia.

Intravenous antibiotics have been shown to reduce significantly the incidence of postoperative wound infection and intra-abdominal abscess.[63] Antibiotics should be administered 30 minutes prior to incision to achieve adequate tissue levels. The typical flora of the appendix resembles that of the colon and includes gram-negative aerobes (primarily *Escherichia coli*) and anaerobes (*Bacteroides* spp.). No standardized antibiotic regimen exists. Acceptable options include a second-generation cephalosporin or a combination of antibiotics directed at gram-negatives and anaerobes. In nonperforated appendicitis, a single preoperative dose of cefoxitin suffices.[64] In cases of perforation, an extended course of at least 5 days of antibiotics is advocated.[65]

OPEN VERSUS LAPAROSCOPIC APPENDECTOMY

Once the diagnosis of appendicitis is made, the surgeon must decide whether to perform an open (OA) or laparoscopic (LA) appendectomy. Numerous randomized controlled trials have compared these two methods, sometimes with conflicting results.[66,67] Meta-analyses and systematic reviews have combined these studies to address the controversy (Table 21–3).[68–70] These meta-analyses have similar findings, which can be summarized as follows: (1) OA can be performed more quickly; (2) LA patients have less postoperative pain and reduced narcotic requirements; (3) there is a trend toward reduced length of stay with LA; (4) LA patients have fewer wound infections; (5) OA patients de-

TABLE 21–3. LAPAROSCOPIC VERSUS OPEN APPENDECTOMY

Favors Laparoscopy	Favors Open
Diagnosis of other conditions	
Decreased pain and lower narcotic requirement	Shorter operating room time
Reduced length of stay	Lower operating room costs
Fewer wound infections	Fewer intra-abdominal abscesses
Quicker return to usual activities	Lower hospital costs
Lower societal cost	

Adapted, with permission, from McCall JL, Sharples K, Jadallah F. Systemic review of randomized controlled trials comparing laparoscopic with open appendicectomy: a meta-analysis. *J Am Coll Surg* 1998; 186:545–553; and Sauerland S, Lefering R, Neugebaur EA. Laparoscopic versus open surgery for suspected appendicitis [see comment]. *Cochrane Database Syst Rev* 2004; 4.

velop fewer intra-abdominal abscesses; (6) LA patients return to work more quickly; (7) operating room and hospital costs are less with OA; and (8) societal costs may be less with LA.[68–70] Based on the data available, one cannot convincingly recommend either OA or LA over the other. Each method has its advantages and disadvantages that should be considered when deciding how to perform appendectomy.

One situation in which laparoscopic appendectomy may be advisable is when the diagnosis of appendicitis is in doubt. This can be particularly useful in women of childbearing age, in whom obstetric and gynecological pathology may also be likely. In this population, a normal appendix can be found in more than 40% of patients with suspected appendicitis.[71] Laparoscopy can thus be both diagnostic and therapeutic, and a laparotomy can be avoided if gynecologic pathology is found. The ovaries, fallopian tubes, and uterus can be examined for nonappendiceal causes of abdominal pain, including ovarian cyst or torsion, endometriosis, or pelvic inflammatory disease. Laparoscopy makes this evaluation considerably easier and less morbid for the patient. In one study, when a normal appendix was discovered, gynecological pathology was found in 73% of women explored laparoscopically, but only 17% of women who had an open appendectomy.[72] Although diagnostic accuracy will likely improve in young women with more widespread use of CT scans, this population will continue to provide diagnostic dilemmas that may be aided by laparoscopy.

Open Appendectomy

If open appendectomy is chosen, the surgeon must then decide on the location and type of incision. Prior to incision, a single dose of antibiotics should be administered, typically a second-generation cephalosporin.[64] The patient should be re-examined after the induction of general anesthesia, which enables deep palpation of the abdomen. If a mass representing the inflamed appendix can be palpated, the incision can be centered at that location. If no appendiceal mass is detected, the incision should be centered over McBurney's point, one-third of the distance from the anterior superior iliac spine to the umbilicus. A curvilinear incision, now known as a McBurney's incision, is made in a natural skin fold. It is important not to make the incision too medial or too lateral. An incision placed too medial opens onto the anterior rectus sheath, rather than the desired oblique muscles, while an incision placed too lateral may be lateral to the abdominal cavity.

The operation proceeds much as McBurney first described it in 1894.[73] The incision is carried down through the subcutaneous tissue, exposing the aponeurosis of the external oblique muscle, which is divided, either sharply or with electrocautery, in the direction of its fibers (Fig 21–6). A muscle-splitting technique is typically used, in which the external oblique, internal oblique, and transversus abdominis muscles are separated along the orientation of their muscle fibers. The peritoneum is thus exposed, grasped with forceps, and opened sharply along the orientation of the incision, taking care not to injure the underlying abdominal contents. Hemostats can be placed on the peritoneum to facilitate its identification at the time of wound closure. Cloudy fluid may be encountered on entering the peritoneum. Although some advocate bacterial culture of the peritoneal fluid, studies show that this neither helps direct the antibiotic regimen[74] nor reduces infectious complications.[75]

With a correctly placed incision, the cecum will be visible at the base of the wound. The incision should be explored with a finger in an attempt to locate the appendix. If the appendix is palpable and free from surrounding structures, it can be delivered into the incision. Frequently, the appendix is palpable but it adheres to surrounding structures. Filmy adhesions can be divided using blunt dissection, but thicker adhesions should be divided under direct vision. To facilitate this, the cecum can be partially delivered into the incision to provide better exposure of the appendix. If necessary to improve exposure, the incision can be extended medially by partially dividing the rectus muscle, or laterally by further dividing the oblique and transversus abdominis muscles. If the appendix cannot be visualized, it can be located by following the teniae coli of the cecum to the cecal base, from which the appendix invariably originates. Once located, the appendix is delivered through the incision. Grasping the mesentery with a Babcock clamp can sometimes facilitate this maneuver. Care should be taken to avoid perforation of the appendix, with spillage of pus or enteric contents into the abdomen.

The arterial supply to the appendix, which runs in the mesoappendix, is now divided between clamps and tied with 3-0 polyglactin suture. This is usually performed in an antegrade fashion, from the appendiceal tip toward the base. Division of the artery to the appendiceal base is necessary to ensure that the entire appendix can be removed without leaving an excessively long appendiceal stump.

In excising the appendix, the surgeon must decide whether or not to invert the appendiceal stump. Traditionally, the appendix was ligated and divided, and its stump was inverted with a purse-string suture for the theoretical purpose of avoiding bacterial contamination of the peritoneum and subsequent adhesion formation.[76,77] However, recent prospective studies show no advantages to appendiceal stump inversion.[78,79] In one such study, 735 appendectomy patients were randomly assigned to ligation plus inversion or simple ligation of the appendiceal stump. There was no difference between the two groups in the incidence of wound infection or adhesion formation, and operating time was shorter in the simple ligation group. Inversion may also have the deleterious effect of deforming the cecal wall, which could be misinterpreted as a cecal mass on future contrast radiographs.[79] Furthermore, the longstanding notion that stump inversion reduces postoperative adhesions was discredited by Street and colleagues.[80] In their analysis, postoperative adhesions requiring operation were significantly increased in the inversion group.

To divide the appendix, the surgeon can use either suture ligation or a gastrointestinal stapler. For ligation, two hemostat clamps are placed at the base of the appendix. The clamp closest to the cecum is removed, having crushed the appendix at that site. Two heavy, absorbable sutures such as 0 chromic gut is used to doubly ligate the appendix, and the appendix is subsequently divided proximal to the second clamp. The exposed mucosa of the appendiceal stump can be cauterized to minimize the theoretical risk of postoperative mucocele, although no data exist to support this. If appendiceal stump inversion is chosen, a seromuscular purse-string 3-0 silk suture is placed in the cecum around the appendiceal base after ligation but prior to division of the appendix. The purse-string suture should be placed approximately 1 cm from the base of the appendix, as placing it too close to the appendix makes stump inversion difficult. After the appendix is divided, the purse-string suture is tightened and tied while the assistant uses forceps to invaginate the appendiceal stump. Alternatively, the appendix can be divided at its base using a TA-30 stapler. Again, the stump

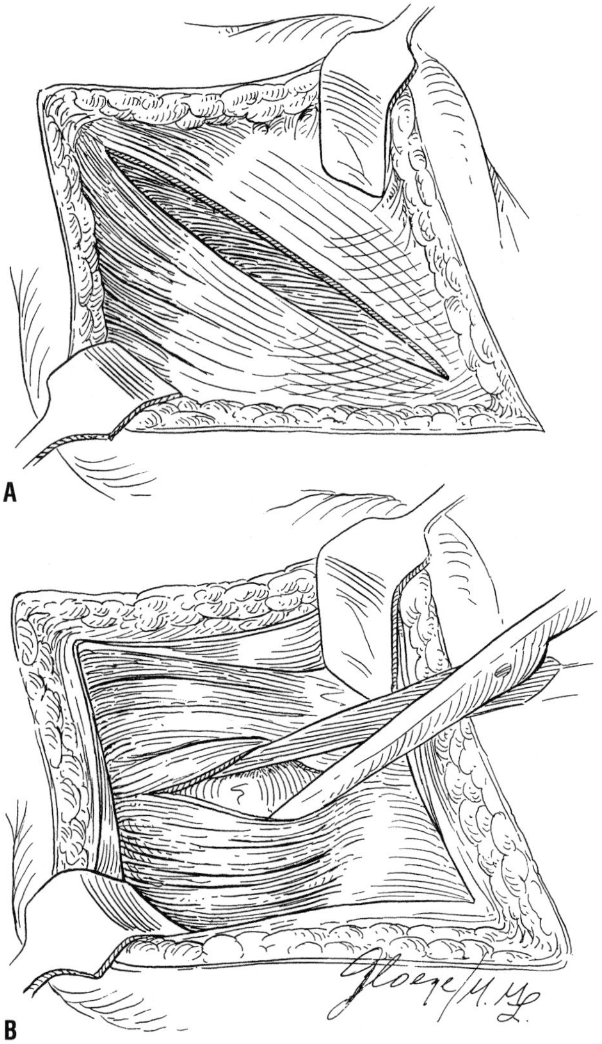

Figure 21–6. Open appendectomy technique. *Continued*

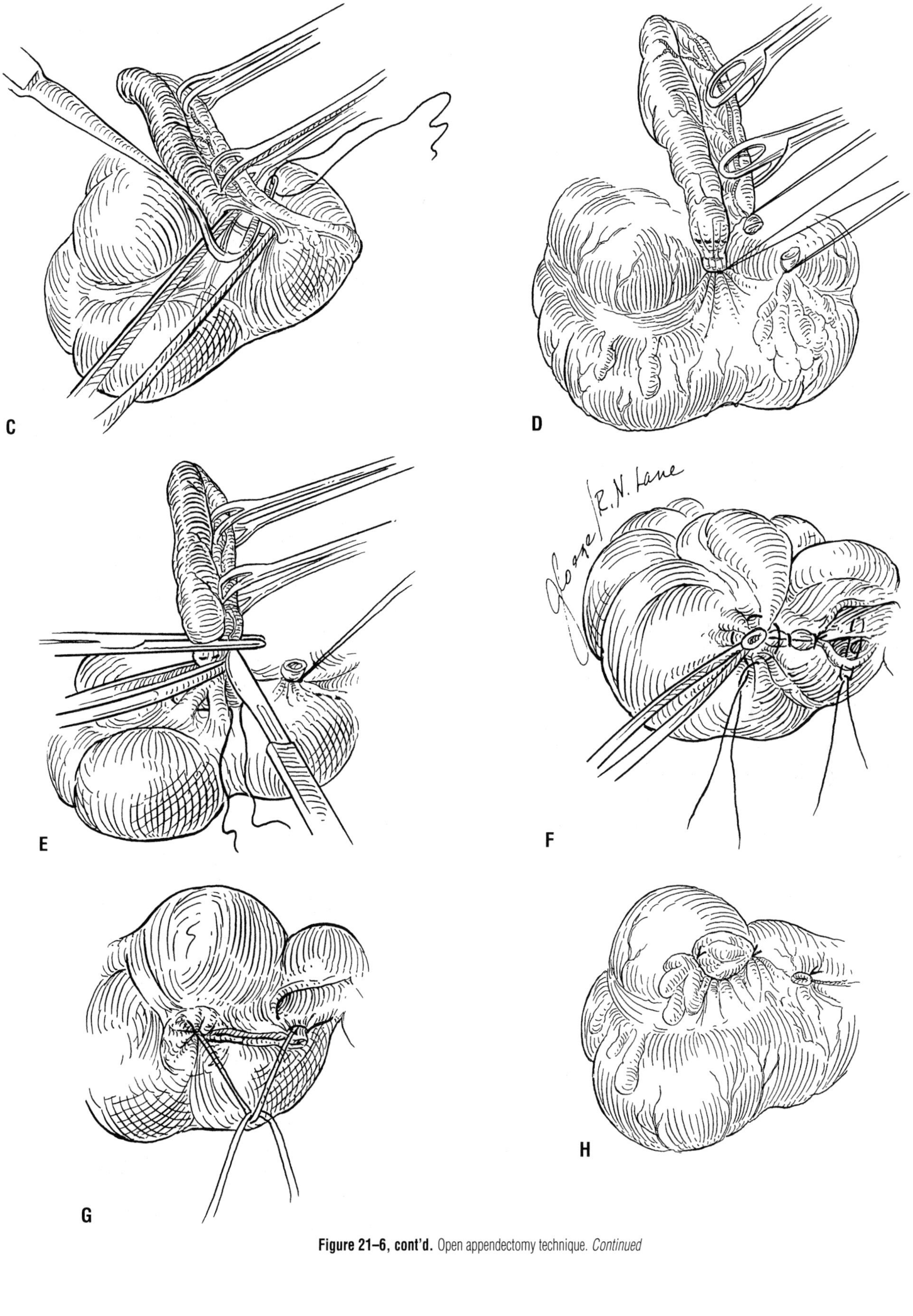

Figure 21–6, cont'd. Open appendectomy technique. *Continued*

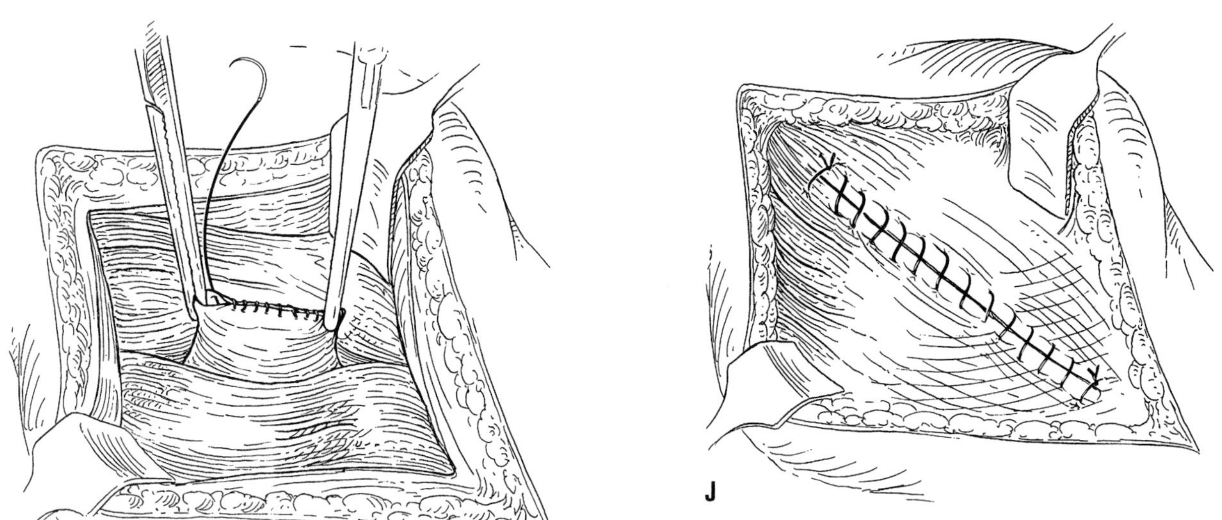

Figure 21–6, cont'd. Open appendectomy technique.

need not be inverted, but can be if desired, using interrupted Lembert sutures with 3-0 silk suture. No matter how the appendix is divided, the residual appendiceal stump should be no longer than 3 mm to minimize the possibility of stump appendicitis in the future.[26]

Occasionally, inflammation at the tip of the appendix makes antegrade removal of the appendix difficult. In such cases, the appendix can be removed in a retrograde fashion. In so doing, the appendix is divided at its base using one of the methods described previously. The mesoappendix is then divided between clamps, starting at the appendiceal base and progressing toward the tip (Fig 21–7).

In certain cases, the appendiceal inflammation extends to the base of the appendix or beyond to the cecum. Division of the appendix through inflamed, infected tissue leaves the potential for leakage of cecal contents with a resultant abscess or fistula. Ensuring that the resection margin is grossly free of active inflammation can minimize this risk. If the base of the cecum is also inflamed but there is sufficient uninflamed cecum between the appendix and the ileocecal valve, an appendectomy with partial cecectomy can be performed using a stapling device.[81] Care should be taken to avoid narrowing the cecum at the ileocecal valve. If the inflammation extends to the ileocecal junction, an ileocectomy with primary anastomosis may be necessary.

After the appendix is removed, hemostasis is achieved and the right lower quadrant and pelvis are irrigated with warm saline. The peritoneum is closed with a continuous 0 absorbable suture; this layer provides no strength but helps to contain the abdominal contents during abdominal wall closure. The internal and external oblique muscles are then closed in succession using continuous 0 absorbable suture. To decrease postoperative narcotic requirements, the external oblique fascia can be infused with local anesthetic. Interrupted absorbable sutures are typically placed in

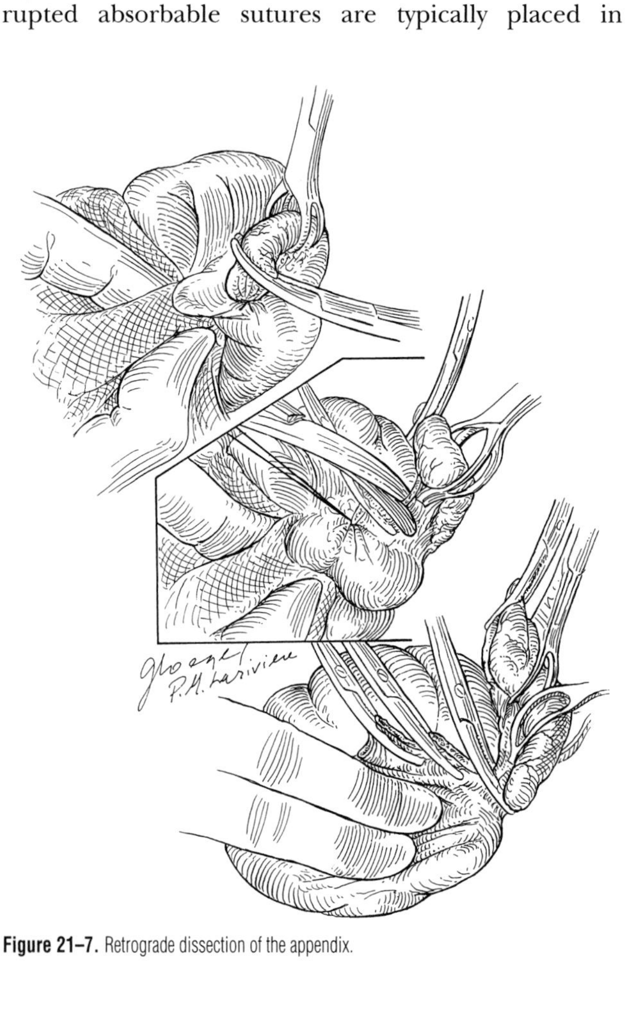

Figure 21–7. Retrograde dissection of the appendix.

Scarpa's fascia, and the skin can be closed with a subcuticular absorbable suture. With a preoperative dose of intravenous antibiotics and primary closure of the skin, fewer than 5% of patients with nonperforated appendicitis can be expected to develop a wound infection.[82]

Laparoscopic Appendectomy

We utilize a three-port technique, with one umbilical and one suprapubic port. Although the third port can be placed in either the left or right lower quadrant, we prefer the left lower quadrant. This follows the laparoscopic principle of triangulation, such that the port locations direct the camera and instruments toward the right lower quadrant for optimal visualization of the appendix.

The patient is positioned supine on the operating room table with the left arm tucked (Fig 21–8). The video monitor is placed at the patient's right side, because once pneumoperitoneum is performed, the surgeon and assistant both stand on the patient's left. A single dose of a second-generation cephalosporin is administered prophylactically. Prior to incision, a nasogastric tube and a Foley catheter are placed to decompress the stomach and urinary bladder. All midline incisions should be oriented vertically, in case conversion to an open midline incision is necessary. A 1- to 2-cm vertical incision is made just inferior to the umbilicus and carried down to the midline fascia. A 12-mm trocar is placed using either Hassan or Veress technique, depending on surgeon preference. After insufflation of the abdomen and inspection through the umbilical port, a 5-mm suprapubic port is placed in the midline, taking care to avoid injury to the bladder, and another 5-mm port is placed in the left lower quadrant. These port sites typically provide excellent cosmesis postoperatively due to their small size and peripheral location on the abdomen.

A 5-mm 30° laparoscope is inserted through the left lower quadrant trocar. Placing the laparoscope in the left lower quadrant allows triangulation of the appendix in the right lower quadrant by instruments placed through the two midline trocars. The surgeon operates the two dissecting instruments and the assistant operates the laparoscope. The appendix is identified at the base of the cecum, and any adhesions to surrounding structures can be lysed with a combination of blunt and sharp dissection supplemented with electrocautery. If a retrocecal appendix is encountered, division of the lateral peritoneal attachments of the cecum to the abdominal wall often improves visualization. Care must be taken to avoid underlying retroperitoneal structures, specifically the right ureter and iliac vessels. The appendix or mesoappendix can be gently grasped with a Babcock clamp placed through the suprapubic port and retracted anteriorly. A dissecting forceps placed through the umbilical port creates a window in the mesoappendix at the appendiceal base. Caution should be taken not to injure the appendiceal artery during this maneuver. As in the open procedure, the base of the appendix should be adequately dissected so that it can be divided without leaving a significant stump.[26] We try when possible to staple at the confluence of the appendix and cecum, or just onto the cecal wall, to avoid the possibility of stump appendicitis or mucocele (Fig 21–8).

The appendix can be removed in a retrograde fashion, first dividing the appendix, followed by division of the mesoappendix. A laparoscopic gastrointestinal anastomosis (GIA) stapler is placed through the umbilical port and fired across the appendiceal base. After reloading, the stapler is again inserted through the umbilical port and placed across the mesoappendix, which is divided with firing of the stapler. Alternatively, the appendix and mesoappendix can be secured using an endoloop.[83] If desired, the appendix can be removed antegrade, by first dividing the mesoappendix prior to directing attention to the base. The appendix should be placed in a retrieval bag and removed through the umbilical port site to minimize the risk of wound infection. The operative field is inspected for hemostasis and irrigated with saline. Finally, the fascial defect at the umbilicus is closed with interrupted 0 absorbable suture, and all skin incisions are closed with fine subcuticular absorbable suture.

Postoperative Care

Patients with nonperforated appendicitis typically require a 24- to 48-hour hospital stay. Postoperative care for both the laparoscopic and open approaches is similar. Patients can be started on a clear liquid diet immediately, and their diet can be advanced as tolerated. No postoperative doses of antibiotics are required. Patients can be discharged when they tolerate a regular diet and oral analgesics.

PERFORATED APPENDICITIS

When appendicitis progresses to perforation, management depends on the nature of the perforation. If the perforation is contained, a solid or semisolid periappendiceal mass of inflammatory tissue can form, referred to as a phlegmon. In other cases, contained perforation may result in a pus-filled abscess cavity. Finally, free perforation can occur, causing intraperitoneal dissemination of pus and fecal material. In the case of free perforation, the patient is typically quite ill and perhaps septic. Urgent laparotomy is necessary for appendectomy and irrigation and drainage of the peritoneal cavity. If the diagnosis of perforated appendicitis is

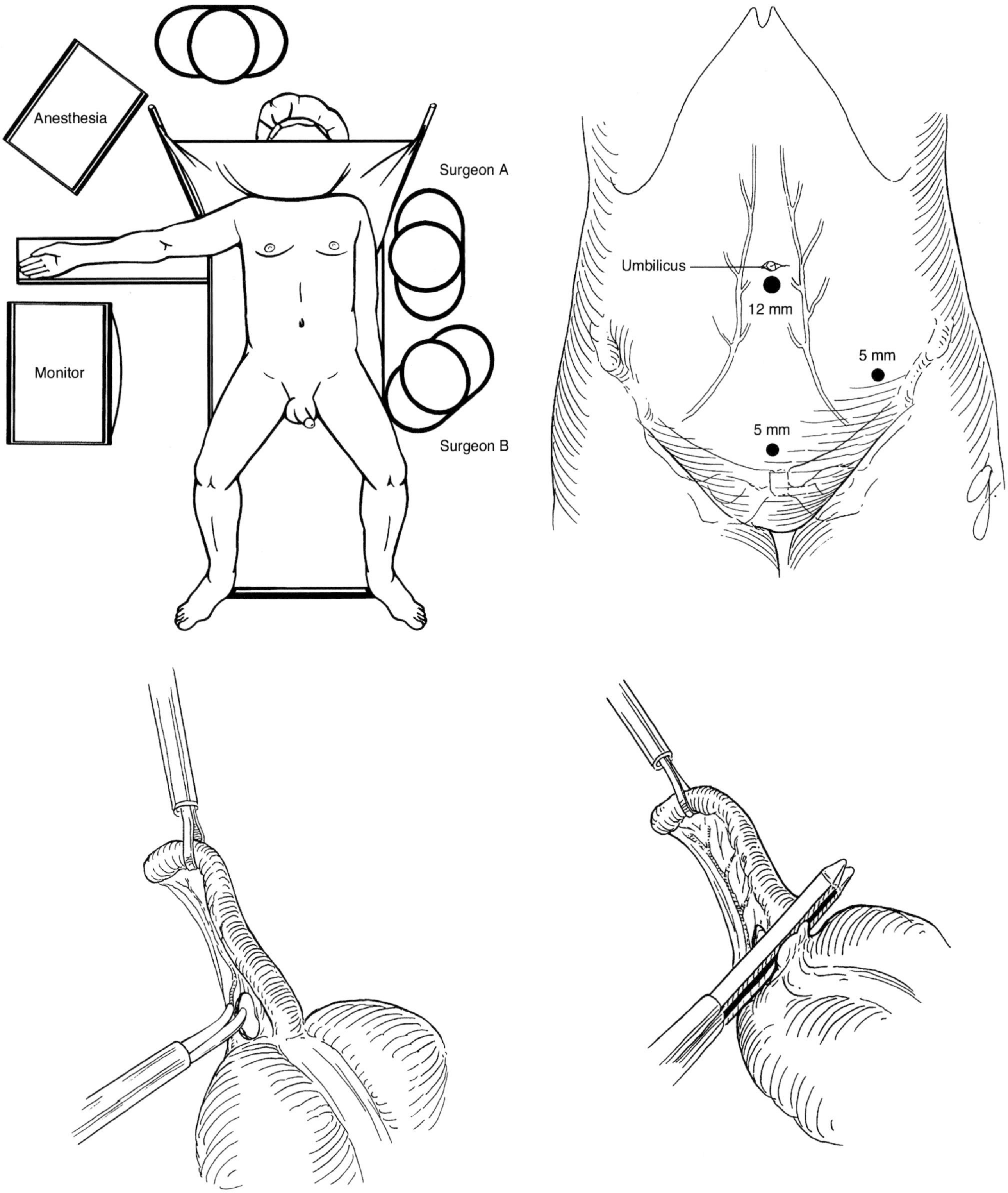

Figure 21–8. Laparoscopic appendectomy technique. *Continued*

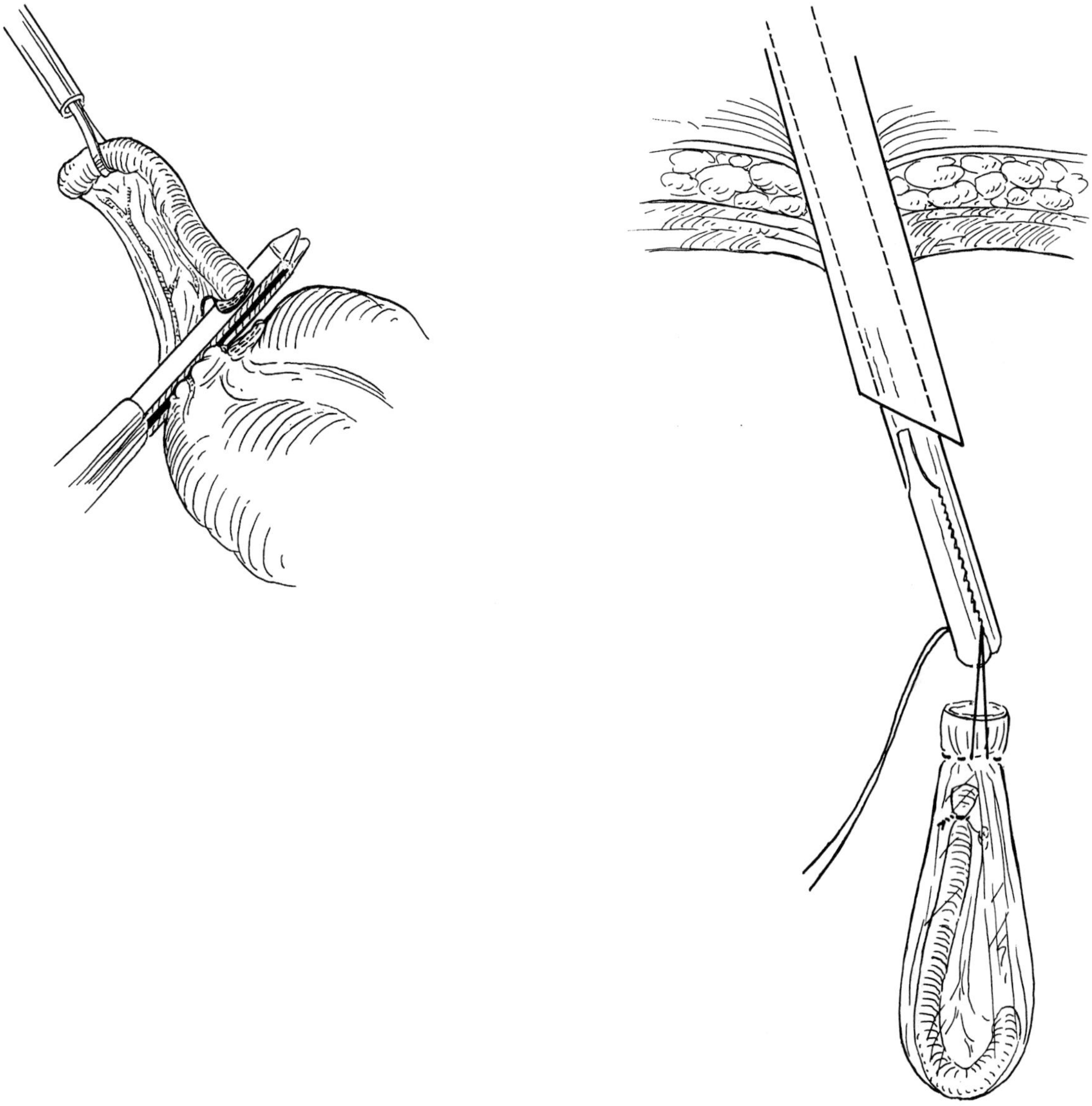

Figure 21–8, cont'd. Laparoscopic appendectomy technique.

known, the appendectomy can be performed through a right lower quadrant incision, and the technique follows that previously described for open appendectomy. Sometimes patients with free perforation present with an acute abdomen and generalized peritonitis, and the decision to perform a laparotomy is made without a definitive diagnosis. In such instances, a midline incision is prudent. Once perforated appendicitis is discovered, appendectomy again proceeds as described above. Peritoneal drains are not necessary, as they do not reduce the incidence of wound infection or abscess after appendectomy for perforated appendicitis.[84,85] The final operative decision is whether or not to close the incision. Because of wound infection rates ranging from 30–50% with primary closure of grossly contaminated wounds, many advocate delayed primary or secondary closure.[82,86] However, a cost-utility analysis of contaminated appendectomy wounds showed primary closure to be the most cost-effective method of wound management.[87] Our technique of skin closure is interrupted permanent sutures or staples every 2 cm with loose wound packing in between. Removal of the packing in 48 hours often leaves an excellent cosmetic result with an acceptable incidence of wound infection. Patients are often continued on broad-spectrum antibiotics for 5–7 days and should remain in the hospital until afebrile and tolerating a regular diet.

If the patient does not have signs of generalized peritonitis, but an abscess or phlegmon is suspected by history and physical exam, a CT scan can be particularly helpful to solidify the diagnosis. A solid, inflammatory mass in the right lower quadrant without evidence of a fluid-filled abscess cavity suggests a phlegmon. In such instances, appendectomy can be difficult due to dense adhesions and inflammation. Ileocecectomy may be necessary if the inflammation extends to the wall of the cecum. Complications such as inadvertent enterotomy, postoperative abscess, or enterocutaneous fistula may ensue. Because of these potential complications, many support an initially nonoperative approach.[88–90] Such an approach is only advisable if the patient is not ill-appearing. Nonoperative management includes intravenous antibiotics and fluids as well as bowel rest. Patients should be closely monitored in the hospital during this time. Treatment failure, as evidenced by bowel obstruction, sepsis, or persistent pain, fever, or leukocytosis, requires immediate appendectomy. If fever, tenderness, and leukocytosis improve, diet can be slowly advanced, usually within 3–5 days. Patients are discharged home when clinical parameters have normalized. Using this approach, more than 80% of patients can be spared an appendectomy at the time of initial presentation.[88,89]

If imaging studies demonstrate an abscess cavity, CT- or ultrasound-guided drainage can often be performed percutaneously or transrectally.[91,92] Studies suggest that this approach to appendiceal abscesses results in fewer complications and shorter overall length of stay.[90,93] Again, following drainage the patient is closely monitored in the hospital and is placed on bowel rest with intravenous antibiotics and fluids. Advancement of diet and hospital discharge progress as clinically indicated.

Interval Appendectomy

Treatment following initial nonoperative management of an appendiceal phlegmon or abscess is controversial. Some recommend interval appendectomy[93,94] (appendectomy performed approximately 6 weeks after inflammation has subsided), while others consider subsequent appendectomy unnecessary.[89,95] Authors who advise against interval appendectomy cite a relatively low incidence of future appendicitis (20% or less)[95] and complication rates from interval appendectomy as high as 16%.[90] Proponents of interval appendectomy point to the low morbidity relative to appendectomy for acute appendicitis, the likelihood of recurrence, and the possibility of ongoing appendiceal pathology,[94] including cancer. Because it can now be performed laparoscopically on an outpatient basis with low morbidity,[96] interval appendectomy should be considered for most patients who were initially treated with nonoperative management.

Normal Appendix

Because of the difficulty in diagnosing appendicitis, it is not uncommon for a normal appendix to be found at appendectomy. Sometimes referred to as misdiagnosis, this can occur more than 15% of the time, with considerably higher percentages in infants, the elderly, and young women.[40] Negative appendectomy is to be avoided when possible, due to the risk of surgical complications and the cost associated with unnecessary surgery.[97] Nonetheless, in certain instances, the diagnosis is in doubt, and a noninflamed appendix is found at laparotomy or laparoscopy. The surgeon must then decide whether or not to remove the appendix. For multiple reasons, it is advisable to remove the grossly normal appendix. First, if the pain recurs and the appendix has been removed, appendicitis will no longer be a possibility and can be removed from the differential diagnosis. If the patient suffers right lower quadrant pain in the future and the appendix has not been removed, but the patient has a classic right lower quadrant scar, a surgeon evaluating the patient may assume a history of appendectomy and erroneously remove appendicitis from consideration. As laparoscopic appendectomy becomes more popular, this may even be true for patients with port site scars suggestive of appendectomy. Finally, there is strong evidence that a surgeon's gross assessment of the appendix can be inaccurate. In one study, 11 (26%) out of 43 appendectomy specimens described as normal by the surgeon showed acute appendicitis on pathological examination.[98] As a result, removal of a grossly normal appendix at the time of appendectomy is recommended.

When a normal appendix is discovered at appendectomy, it is important to search for other possible causes of the patient's symptoms. The terminal ileum can be inspected for evidence of terminal ileitis, which could be from infectious causes (*Yersinia* or tuberculosis) or Crohn's disease. In the absence of perforation, resection should not be performed for Crohn's disease and appropriate medical therapy should be initiated postoperatively. The ileum should also be evaluated for an inflamed or perforated Meckel's diverticulum, which should be excised. In females, the ovaries, fallopian tubes, and uterus should be examined for pathology as well. Evaluation of the left adnexa can be difficult through a right lower quadrant incision, highlighting the utility of laparoscopy in female patients.

▪ CHRONIC APPENDICITIS

Although rare, chronic appendicitis can explain persistent abdominal pain in some patients. Patients do not present with the typical symptoms of acute appendicitis. Instead, they complain of weeks to years of right lower quadrant pain, and may have had multiple medical evaluations in the past. When queried, they may describe an initial episode with more classic symptoms of acute appendicitis, for which no treatment was delivered.[99] Diagnosis can be difficult, as laboratory and radiological studies are typically normal. Pathology evaluation revealing chronic inflammation confirms the diagnosis. Because the diagnosis is often uncertain preoperatively, laparoscopy can be a useful tool to allow exploration of the abdomen.[100]

▪ ASYMPTOMATIC APPENDICOLITH

As CT scans become more widely utilized, it is likely that an increasing number of asymptomatic appendicoliths will be discovered. As discussed above, appendicoliths are not pathognomonic for appendicitis but should only be considered in conjunction with the clinical presentation and other diagnostic studies. Lowe and associates[101] studied CT scans of children with suspected appendicitis and compared them to CT scans of children with abdominal trauma. Six (14%) of 44 patients with suspected appendicitis had an appendicolith but proved not to have appendicitis. In addition, 2 (3%) of the 74 trauma patients had an appendicolith on CT. These children were not followed to see if appendicitis developed later in life, but the considerable number of asymptomatic appendicoliths seen on adult abdominal radiographs suggest that many patients with an appendicolith will never develop appendicitis.[18,19] Based on this, appendectomy for asymptomatic appendicolith cannot be recommended.

▪ NEOPLASMS OF THE APPENDIX

Neoplasms of the appendix are rare, affecting less than 1% of appendectomies. Signs and symptoms of appendicitis prompt appendectomy in up to 50 percent of patients, and it is not uncommon for the patients with an appendiceal neoplasm to have acute appendicitis as well.[102] Patients may also present with a palpable mass, intussusception, urologic symptoms, or an incidentally discovered mass on abdominal imaging or at laparotomy for another purpose. Typically, the diagnosis is not known until laparotomy or pathologic evaluation of the appendectomy specimen, but preoperative diagnosis may become more common as imaging techniques become more widely used. Because of their common embryologic origin, the appendix and colon are susceptible to many of the same neoplastic growths. The most common appendiceal tumors include cystic neoplasms, carcinoid tumors, adenocarcinoma, and metastases. Other tumors have been reported but are extremely rare, such as lymphoma, stromal tumors (leiomyoma and leiomyosarcoma), and Kaposi's sarcoma.[103]

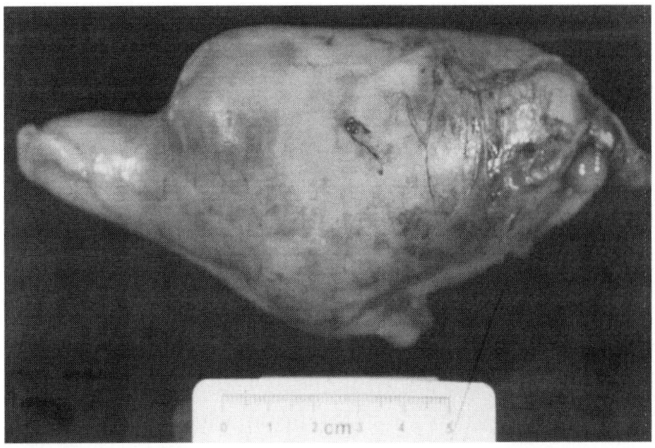

Figure 21–9. A 14-cm mucinous cystadenoma of the appendix. The appendiceal tip is to the left, the base to the right. (Courtesy Jacqueline M. Wilson, MD, PhD, Brigham and Women's Hospital, Boston, Mass.)

CYSTIC NEOPLASMS AND PSEUDOMYXOMA PERITONEI

Sometimes referred to as mucoceles, mucinous neoplasms of the appendix include a spectrum of diseases including simple cyst, mucinous cystadenoma, mucinous cystadenocarcinoma, and pseudomyxoma peritonei. Mucocele is not a true pathologic diagnosis and instead refers to the macroscopic appearance of an appendix distended with mucus. Any of the above conditions can form a mucocele, but the more specific diagnostic term is preferable.[104] A simple cyst results from non-neoplastic occlusion of the appendiceal lumen, is usually less than 2 cm in diameter, and is often an incidental finding at appendectomy. In contrast, mucinous cystadenomas, benign tumors that represent the majority of "mucoceles," can grow to 8 cm or larger (Fig 21–9).[105] They typically remain asymptomatic due to slow-growing distension of the appendix and instead present incidentally as a mass on physical exam or abdominal imaging (Fig 21–10). On plain radiograph or CT, wall calcification is characteristic.[104]

It is recommended that all mucinous appendiceal masses 2 cm or larger be surgically removed.[105] For mucinous cystadenoma, appendectomy is sufficient if the lesion does not involve the appendiceal base. Occasionally, the mass will rupture prior to or at the time of removal, but this rupture is typically contained to the right lower quadrant and is considered localized pseudomyxoma peritonei. If the mass is benign, appendectomy and removal of any residual mucin is curative.[106] Laparoscopic appendectomy is not currently recommended due to the possibility of malignancy and spillage of mucin-secreting cells throughout the abdomen.[107] Because of an association with colon and rectal carcinoma, a screening colonoscopy is recommended postoperatively.[105]

Mucinous cystadenocarcinoma represents the malignant form of cystic neoplasms of the appendix. In contrast to cystadenoma, patients are usually symptomatic with abdominal pain, weight loss, an abdominal mass, or signs of acute appendicitis. Increasing abdominal girth may also be present and suggests development of pseudomyxoma peritonei from perforation and peritoneal dissemination of mucin-secreting cells. Diffuse pseudomyxoma peritonei is highly predictive of malignancy; in one series, 95% of patients with pseudomyxoma had an associated mucinous cystadenocarcinoma.[105] The recommended treatment consists of right hemicolectomy with debulking of any gross spread of disease and removal of all mucin. It is not uncommon, however, for the diagnosis to be unknown until the time of pathologic evaluation of the appendectomy specimen. In such cases, reoperation with right hemicolectomy is recommended, as 5-year survival for mucinous cystadenocarcinoma is 75% after hemicolectomy and less than 50% after appendectomy alone.[108] Some referral centers advocate extensive initial resections including omentectomy, as well as repeated debulking procedures for recurrent disease.[109]

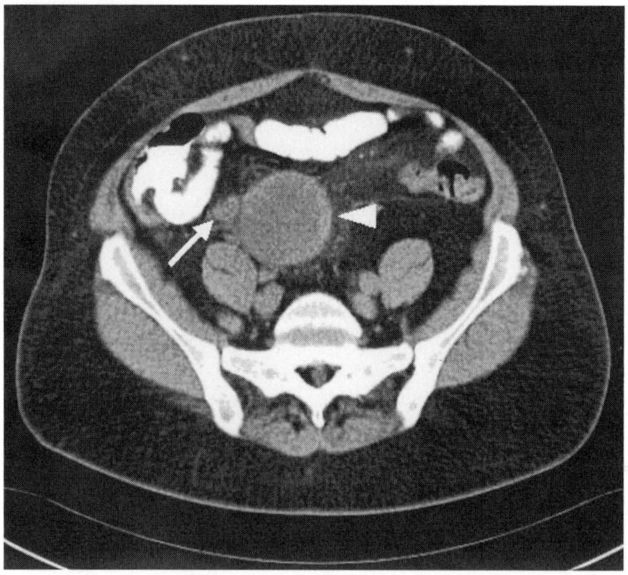

Figure 21–10. Computed tomography axial image at the level of the terminal ileum shows a fluid-filled mass (*arrowhead*) corresponding to the mucinous cystadenoma seen in Fig 21–8. The more proximal appendix (*arrow*) is seen between the mass and cecum. (Courtesy of M. Stephen Ledbetter, MD, Brigham and Women's Hospital, Boston, Mass.)

ADENOCARCINOMA

Primary adenocarcinoma of the appendix is classified into two types, mucinous (discussed above) and colonic. The colonic type is less common, less likely to secrete mucus, and more likely to present with acute appendicitis due to obstruction of the appendiceal lumen.[104] Because of similarities with colon carcinoma, appendiceal adenocarcinomas are classified as Dukes stage A, B, C, and D, with 5-year survival rates of 100%, 67%, 50%, and 6%, respectively. The colonic type has a less favorable prognosis, with only 41% 5-year survival after treatment, compared to 71% for the mucinous type. The optimal treatment is right hemicolectomy, and reoperation should be recommended if the diagnosis is made on pathologic evaluation of an appendectomy specimen.[108]

CARCINOID TUMORS

The most common neoplasm of the appendix, carcinoid tumors comprise more than 50% of all appendiceal tumors.[102] Among malignant tumors of the appendix, carcinoids are less aggressive and carry a much more favorable prognosis than adenocarcinomas, with 5-year survival approaching 90%.[110] Most appendiceal carcinoids are found incidentally at the time of appendectomy for appendicitis. However, because the majority of appendiceal carcinoids are located at the tip of the appendix, the carcinoid mass is the cause of appendicitis only 25% of the time.[103] Tumor size is the primary determinant of malignant potential. About 75% of carcinoids are less than 1 cm in size, and 5–10% are over 2 cm. Lymph node invasion and distant metastases are exceedingly rare except in tumors over 2 cm.[111] Histologically, carcinoids of the appendix are categorized as goblet cell and classical carcinoid. Mortality is higher for goblet cell, but is still lower than of adenocarcinoma.[110]

Treatment of appendiceal carcinoids is dictated primarily by tumor size. Simple appendectomy is sufficient for tumors less than 2 cm because of the low likelihood of lymph node involvement. For masses larger than 2 cm, right hemicolectomy is recommended. Because of a concern for increased metastatic potential, some authors also advocate right hemicolectomy in young patients and in carcinoids involving the appendiceal base.[111,112]

REFERENCES

1. Meade RH. *An Introduction to the History of General Surgery.* Philadelphia, PA: Saunders; 1968
2. Richardson RG. *The Surgeon's Tale.* New York, NY: Scribner's; 1958
3. Williams RA, Myers P. *Pathology of the Appendix.* London, England: Chapman & Hall; 1994
4. Da Capri JB. Commentaria cum Amplissimus Additionibus Super Anatomia Mundini Una cum Texta Ejusudem

in Pristinum et Verum Nitorem Redanto. 528 ff. Bolonial Imp. per H. Benedictus, 1521
5. Vesalius A. *De Humani Corporis Fabrica Liber V.* Basel, Switzerland: Johanes Oporinu; 1543
6. Thomas CG. *Classic Description of Disease.* Springfield; 1932
7. Amyand C. Of an inguinal rupture, with a pin in the appendix caeci, incrusted with stone, and some observations on wounds in the guts. *Philos Trans R Soc Lond* 1736;39:329–342
8. Tsoulfas G, Howe JR. Amyand's hernia: Appendicitis in an incarcerated hernia. *Surg Rounds* 2004;27:515–517
9. Tait L. Surgical treatment of typhlitis. *Birmingham Med Rev* 1890;27:26–34
10. Fitz RH. Perforating inflammation of the vermiform appendix; with special reference to its early diagnosis and treatment. *Am J Med Sci* 1886;92:321–346
11. McBurney CM. Experience with early operative interference in cases of disease of the vermiform appendix. *N Y Med J* 1889;50:676–684
12. Treves F. A series of cases of relapsing typhlitis treated by operation. *BMJ* 1893;i:835–837
13. Addiss DG, Shaffer N, Fowler BS, Tauxe RV. The epidemiology of appendicitis and appendectomy in the United States. *Am J Epidemiol* 1990;132:910–925
14. Burkitt DP. The aetiology of appendicitis. *Br J Surg* 1971; 58:695–699
15. Jones BA, Demetriades D, Segal I, Burkitt DP. The prevalence of appendiceal fecaliths in patients with and without appendicitis. A comparative study from Canada and South Africa. *Ann Surg* 1985;202:80–82
16. Wangensteen OH, Buirge RE, Dennis C, Ritchie WP. Studies in the etiology of acute appendicitis: The significance of the structure and function of the vermiform appendix in the genesis of appendicitis. *Ann Surg* 1937;106:910–942
17. Wangensteen OH, Dennis C. Experimental proof of the obstructive origin of appendicitis in man. *Ann Surg* 1939;110:629–647
18. Teicher I, Landa B, Cohen M et al. Scoring system to aid in diagnoses of appendicitis. *Ann Surg* 1983;198:753–759
19. Nitecki S, Karmeli R, Sarr MG. Appendiceal calculi and fecaliths as indications for appendectomy. *Surg Gynecol Obstet* 1990;171:185–188
20. Arnbjornsson E, Bengmark S. Obstruction of the appendix lumen in relation to pathogenesis of acute appendicitis. *Acta Chir Scand* 1983;149:789–791
21. Temple CL, Huchcroft SA, Temple WJ. The natural history of appendicitis in adults. A prospective study. *Ann Surg* 1995;221:278–281
22. Velanovich V, Satava R. Balancing the normal appendectomy rate with the perforated appendicitis rate: implications for quality assurance. *Am Surg* 1992;58:264–269
23. Hale DA, Jaques DP, Molloy M et al. Appendectomy. Improving care through quality improvement. *Arch Surg* 1997;132:153–157
24. Pittman-Waller VA, Myers JG, Stewart RM et al. Appendicitis: why so complicated? Analysis of 5755 consecutive appendectomies. *Am Surg* 2000;66:548–554
25. Baril N, Wren S, Radin R et al. The role of anticoagulation in pylephlebitis. *Am J Surg* 1996;172:449–452
26. Mangi AA, Berger DL. Stump appendicitis. *Am Surg* 2000;66:739–741
27. Wagner JM. Likelihood ratios to determine 'Does this patient have appendicitis?': Comment and clarification. *JAMA* 1997;278:819–820
28. Wagner JM, McKinney WP, Carpenter JL. Does this patient have appendicitis? *JAMA* 1996;276:1589–1594
29. Thompson MM, Underwood MJ, Dookeran KA et al. Role of sequential leucocyte counts and C-reactive protein measurements in acute appendicitis. *Br J Surg* 1992; 79:822–824
30. Alvarado A. A practical score for the early diagnosis of acute appendicitis. *Ann Emerg Med* 1986;15:557–564
31. Saidi RF, Ghasemi M. Role of Alvarado score in diagnosis and treatment of suspected acute appendicitis. *Am J Emerg Med* 2000;18:230–231
32. Wise SW, Labuski MR, Kasales CJ et al. Comparative assessment of CT and sonographic techniques for appendiceal imaging. *AJR Am J Roentgenol* 2001;176:933–941
33. Terasawa T, Blackmore CC, Bent S, Kohlwes RJ. Systematic review: computed tomography and ultrasonography to detect acute appendicitis in adults and adolescents. *Ann Intern Med* 2004;141:537–546
34. Rao PM, Rhea JT, Rattner DW et al. Introduction of appendiceal CT: impact on negative appendectomy and appendiceal perforation rates [see comment]. *Ann Surg* 1999;229:344–349
35. Balthazar EJ, Birnbaum BA, Yee J et al. Acute appendicitis: CT and US correlation in 100 patients. *Radiology* 1994;190:31–35
36. Horton MD, Counter SF, Florence MG, Hart MJ. A prospective trial of computed tomography and ultrasonography for diagnosing appendicitis in the atypical patient [see comment]. *Am J Surg* 2000;179:379–381
37. Rao PM, Rhea JT, Novelline RA et al. Effect of computed tomography of the appendix on treatment of patients and use of hospital resources. *N Engl J Med* 1998; 338:141–146
38. Cullen JJ, Kelly KA, Moir CR et al. Surgical management of Meckel's diverticulum. An epidemiologic, population-based study [see comment]. *Ann Surg* 1994;220: 564–568
39. Bizer LS. Acute appendicitis is rarely the initial presentation of cecal cancer in the elderly patient. *J Surg Oncol* 1993;54:45–46
40. Flum DR, Morris A, Koepsell T, Dellinger EP. Has misdiagnosis of appendicitis decreased over time? A population-based analysis. *JAMA* 2001;286:1748–1753
41. Bratton SL, Haberkern CM, Waldhausen JH. Acute appendicitis risks of complications: age and Medicaid insurance. *Pediatrics* 2000;106:75–78
42. Garcia Pena BM, Mandl KD, Kraus SJ et al. Ultrasonography and limited computed tomography in the diagnosis and management of appendicitis in children. *JAMA* 1999;282:1041–1046
43. Brenner D, Elliston C, Hall E, Berdon W. Estimated risks of radiation-induced fatal cancer from pediatric CT. *AJR Am J Roentgenol* 2001;176:289–296

44. Donnelly LF, Emery KH, Brody AS et al. Minimizing radiation dose for pediatric body applications of single-detector helical CT: strategies at a large Children's Hospital. *AJR Am J Roentgenol* 2001;176:303–306
45. Watters JM, Blakslee JM, March RJ, Redmond ML. The influence of age on the severity of peritonitis. *Can J Surg* 1996;39:142–146
46. Paajanen H, Kettunen J, Kostiainen S. Emergency appendectomies in patients over 80 years. *Am Surg* 1994; 60:950–953
47. Tamir IL, Bongard FS, Klein SR. Acute appendicitis in the pregnant patient. *Am J Surg* 1990;160:571–575
48. Mourad J, Elliott JP, Erickson L, Lisboa L. Appendicitis in pregnancy: new information that contradicts long-held clinical beliefs [see comment]. *Am J Obstet Gynecol* 2000;182:1027–1029
49. To WW, Ngai CS, Ma HK. Pregnancies complicated by acute appendicitis. *Aust N Z J Surg* 1995;65:799–803
50. Baer JL, Reis RA, Arens RA. Appendicitis in pregnancy with changes in position and axis of the normal appendix in pregnancy. *JAMA* 1932;98:1359–1364
51. Lim HK, Bae SH, Seo GS. Diagnosis of acute appendicitis in pregnant women: value of sonography. *AJR Am J Roentgenol* 1992;159:539–542
52. Anonymous. ACOG Committee Opinion: Guidelines for diagnostic imaging during pregnancy. *Obstet Gynecol* 2004;104:647–651
53. Ames Castro M, Shipp TD, Castro EE et al. The use of helical computed tomography in pregnancy for the diagnosis of acute appendicitis. *Am J Obstet Gynecol* 2001; 184:954–957
54. Brent RL. The effect of embryonic and fetal exposure to x-ray, microwaves, and ultrasound: counseling the pregnant and nonpregnant patient about these risks. *Semin Oncol* 1989;16:347–368
55. Mahmoodian S. Appendicitis complicating pregnancy. *South Med J* 1992;85:19–24
56. Curet MJMD, Allen D, Josloff RKMD et al. Laparoscopy during pregnancy. *Arch Surg* 1996;131:546–551
57. Fatum M, Rojansky N. Laparoscopic surgery during pregnancy. *Obstet Gynecol Surv* 2001;56:50–59
58. Whitney TM, Macho JR, Russell TR et al. Appendicitis in acquired immunodeficiency syndrome. *Am J Surg* 1992;164:467–470
59. Flum DR, Steinberg SD, Sarkis AY, Wallack MK. Appendicitis in patients with acquired immunodeficiency syndrome. *J Am Coll Surg* 1997;184:481–486
60. Coldrey E. Five years of conservative treatment of acute appendicitis. *J Int Coll Surg* 1959;32:255–261
61. Eriksson S, Tisell A, Granstrom L. Ultrasonographic findings after conservative treatment of acute appendicitis and open appendicectomy. *Acta Radiologica* 1995; 36:173–177
62. Campbell MR, Johnston SL 3rd, Marshburn T et al. Nonoperative treatment of suspected appendicitis in remote medical care environments: implications for future spaceflight medical care. *J Am Coll Surg* 2004;198:822–830
63. Andersen BR, Kallehave FL, Andersen HK. Antibiotics versus placebo for prevention of postoperative infection after appendicectomy. *Cochrane Database Syst Rev* 2004;4:4
64. Bauer T, Vennits B, Holm B et al. Antibiotic prophylaxis in acute nonperforated appendicitis. The Danish Multicenter Study Group III. *Ann Surg* 1989;209:307–311
65. Danish Multicenter Study Group. A Danish multicenter study: cefoxitin versus ampicillin + metronidazole in perforated appendicitis. *Br J Surg* 1984;71:144–146
66. Frazee RC, Roberts JW, Symmonds RE et al. A prospective randomized trial comparing open versus laparoscopic appendectomy. *Ann Surg* 1994;219:725–728
67. Martin LC, Puente I, Sosa JL et al. Open versus laparoscopic appendectomy. A prospective randomized comparison. *Ann Surg* 1995;222:256–261
68. McCall JL, Sharples K, Jadallah F. Systematic review of randomized controlled trials comparing laparoscopic with open appendicectomy. *Br J Surg* 1997;84:1045–1050
69. Golub R, Siddiqui F, Pohl D. Laparoscopic versus open appendectomy: a metaanalysis. *J Am Coll Surg* 1998;186: 545–553
70. Sauerland S, Lefering R, Neugebauer EA. Laparoscopic versus open surgery for suspected appendicitis [see comment]. *Cochrane Database Syst Rev* 2004;4
71. Cox MR, McCall JL, Padbury RT et al. Laparoscopic surgery in women with a clinical diagnosis of acute appendicitis [see comment]. *Med J Aust* 1995;162:130–132
72. Larsson PG, Henriksson G, Olsson M et al. Laparoscopy reduces unnecessary appendicectomies and improves diagnosis in fertile women. A randomized study. *Surg Endosc* 2001;15:200–202
73. McBurney CM. The incision made in the abdominal wall in cases of appendicitis, with a description of a new method of operating. *Ann Surg* 1894;20:38–43
74. Mosdell DM, Morris DM, Fry DE. Peritoneal cultures and antibiotic therapy in pediatric perforated appendicitis. *Am J Surg* 1994;167:313–316
75. Bilik R, Burnweit C, Shandling B. Is abdominal cavity culture of any value in appendicitis? *Am J Surg* 1998;175: 267–270
76. Kingsley DP. Some observations on appendicectomy with particular reference to technique. *Br J Surg* 1969; 56:491–496
77. Arnbjornsson E. Invagination of the appendiceal stump for the reduction of peritoneal bacterial contamination. *Curr Surg* 1985;42:184–187
78. Watters DA, Walker MA, Abernethy BC. The appendix stump: should it be invaginated? *Ann R Coll Surg Eng* 1984;66:92–93
79. Engstrom L, Fenyo G. Appendicectomy: assessment of stump invagination versus simple ligation: a prospective, randomized trial. *Br J Surg* 1985;72:971–972
80. Street D, Bodai BI, Owens LJ et al. Simple ligation vs stump inversion in appendectomy. *Arch Surg* 1988;123: 689–690
81. Poole GV. Management of the difficult appendiceal stump: how I do it. *Am Surg* 1993;59:624–625
82. Lemieur TP, Rodriguez JL, Jacobs DM et al. Wound management in perforated appendicitis. *Am Surg* 1999; 65:439–443

83. Motson RW, Kelly MD. Simplified technique for laparoscopic appendectomy [see comment]. *ANZ J Surg* 2002; 72:294–295
84. Greenall MJ, Evans M, Pollock AV. Should you drain a perforated appendix? *Br J Surg* 1978;65:880–882
85. Petrowsky H, Demartines N, Rousson V, Clavien P-A. Evidence-based value of prophylactic drainage in gastrointestinal surgery: a systematic review and meta-analysis. *Ann Surg* 2004;240:1074–1085
86. Cohn SM, Giannotti G, Ong AW et al. Prospective randomized trial of two wound management strategies for dirty abdominal wounds. *Ann Surg* 2001;233:409–413
87. Brasel KJ, Borgstrom DC, Weigelt JA. Cost-utility analysis of contaminated appendectomy wounds. *J Am Coll Surg* 1997;184:23–30
88. Skoubo-Kristensen E, Hvid I. The appendiceal mass: results of conservative management. *Ann Surg* 1982;196: 584–587
89. Nitecki S, Assalia A, Schein M. Contemporary management of the appendiceal mass. *Br J Surg* 1993;80:18–20
90. Oliak D, Yamini D, Udani VM et al. Initial nonoperative management for periappendiceal abscess. *Dis Colon Rectum* 2001;44:936–941
91. Bagi P, Dueholm S. Nonoperative management of the ultrasonically evaluated appendiceal mass. *Surgery* 1987; 101:602–605
92. Jeffrey RB Jr, Federle MP, Tolentino CS. Periappendiceal inflammatory masses: CT-directed management and clinical outcome in 70 patients [erratum appears in *Radiology* 1988;168:286]. *Radiology* 1988; 167:13–16
93. Brown CV, Abrishami M, Muller M, Velmahos GC. Appendiceal abscess: immediate operation or percutaneous drainage? *Am Surg* 2003;69:829–832
94. Mazziotti MV, Marley EF, Winthrop AL et al. Histopathologic analysis of interval appendectomy specimens: support for the role of interval appendectomy. *J Pediatr Surg* 1997;32:806–809
95. Hoffmann J, Lindhard A, Jensen HE. Appendix mass: conservative management without interval appendectomy. *Am J Surg* 1984;148:379–382
96. Nguyen DB, Silen W, Hodin RA. Interval appendectomy in the laparoscopic era. *J Gastrointest Surg* 1999;3:189–193
97. Flum DR, Koepsell T. The clinical and economic correlates of misdiagnosed appendicitis: nationwide analysis. *Arch Surg* 2002;137:799–804
98. Grunewald B, Keating J. Should the 'normal' appendix be removed at operation for appendicitis? *J R Coll Surg Edinb* 1993;38:158–160
99. Mattei P, Sola JE, Yeo CJ. Chronic and recurrent appendicitis are uncommon entities often misdiagnosed. *J Am Coll Surg* 1994;178:385–389
100. Klingensmith ME, Soybel DI, Brooks DC. Laparoscopy for chronic abdominal pain. *Surg Endosc* 1996;10:1085–1087
101. Lowe LH, Penney MW, Scheker LE et al. Appendicolith revealed on CT in children with suspected appendicitis: how specific is it in the diagnosis of appendicitis? *AJR Am J Roentgenol* 2000;175:981–984
102. Connor SJ, Hanna GB, Frizelle FA. Appendiceal tumors: retrospective clinicopathologic analysis of appendiceal tumors from 7,970 appendectomies. *Dis Colon Rectum* 1998;41:75–80
103. Deans GT, Spence RA. Neoplastic lesions of the appendix. *Br J Surg* 1995;82:299–306
104. Pickhardt PJ, Levy AD, Rohrmann CA Jr, Kende AI. Primary neoplasms of the appendix: radiologic spectrum of disease with pathologic correlation [erratum appears in *Radiographics* 2003;23:1340]. *Radiographics* 2003;23: 645–662
105. Stocchi L, Wolff BG, Larson DR, Harrington JR. Surgical treatment of appendiceal mucocele. Arch Surg 2003;138:585–589
106. Higa E, Rosai J, Pizzimbono CA, Wise L. Mucosal hyperplasia, mucinous cystadenoma, and mucinous cystadenocarcinoma of the appendix. A re-evaluation of appendiceal "mucocele." *Cancer* 1973;32: 1525–1541
107. Gonzalez Moreno S, Shmookler BM, Sugarbaker PH. Appendiceal mucocele. Contraindication to laparoscopic appendectomy. Surg Endosc 1998;12:1177–1179
108. Nitecki SS, Wolff BG, Schlinkert R, Sarr MG. The natural history of surgically treated primary adenocarcinoma of the appendix [see comment]. *Ann Surg* 1994;219:51–57
109. Smith JW, Kemeny N, Caldwell C et al. Pseudomyxoma peritonei of appendiceal origin. The Memorial Sloan-Kettering Cancer Center experience. *Cancer* 1992;70:396–401
110. McCusker ME, Cote TR, Clegg LX, Sobin LH. Primary malignant neoplasms of the appendix: a population-based study from the surveillance, epidemiology and end-results program, 1973–1998. *Cancer* 2002;94:3307–3312
111. Roggo A, Wood WC, Ottinger LW. Carcinoid tumors of the appendix. *Ann Surg* 1993;217:385–390
112. Gouzi JL, Laigneau P, Delalande JP et al. Indications for right hemicolectomy in carcinoid tumors of the appendix. The French Associations for Surgical Research. *Surg Gynecol Obstet* 1993;176:543–547

22

Tumors of the Small Intestine

Douglas Turner ■ *Barbara Lee Bass*

Tumors of the small intestine, both benign and malignant, are rare. With the potential to arise from virtually every cell type within the small intestine—the epithelium, neural tissues and lymphatic and mesenchymal cells—the small bowel may also be the site of metastases from other primary tumors. The variety and uncommon nature of these tumors makes generalizations regarding their management difficult. In this chapter we will review the epidemiology and clinical diagnostic and management strategies for benign and malignant neoplasms of the small bowel.

■ EPIDEMIOLOGY

While the small bowel accounts for 75% of the length and 90% of the mucosal surface area of the gastrointestinal tract, fewer than 3% of gastrointestinal malignancies arise in this organ. Most of these tumors are clinically silent. Autopsy series have identified incidental small bowel tumors in 0.2–0.3% of hospital deaths—a rate 15 times the operative incidence of small bowel resections for tumors.[1]

Given the rare nature of these tumors, most published reports are collections of relatively small series of tumors accrued over a period of many years. Hence, interestingly these reports differ in regard to the type of small bowel tumors, the distribution of tumors, and until the advent of molecular diagnostic criteria for GIST (gastrointestinal stromal tumors), in the classification of tumors of stromal origin. Nonetheless in most series adenocarcinoma, GIST, carcinoid tumor, and lymphoma comprise the most common malignant tumors and are approximately equally represented.[2,3] Small bowel tumors are more prevalent in older than in younger patients, and a recent analysis identified that over 65% of patients with small bowel adenocarcinoma were age 60 or older.[3] The proportion of small bowel tumors that are benign varies from 14–52% in different series, a disparity explained by the failure to detect the typically asymptomatic benign lesions.

There are no satisfactory explanations for the observed variation in prevalence of small bowel tumors around the world. Carcinoids are rare tumors in Asian series, while GIST comprise a higher proportion of reported series in the East.[4,5] Men are more likely to develop small bowel neoplasms than women, with a male preponderance of three to two reported for both benign and malignant tumors.

■ PATHOGENESIS

Given the length of the small bowel and its large mucosal surface, it is intriguing that it is such an uncommon site for malignancy. Unlike the adenoma-carcinoma sequence seen in the colon, a clear molecular progression sequence has not been defined in the small bowel. Only periampullary adenomas are known to be premalignant lesions with the potential to progress to adenocarcinomas. Adenomatous polyps arising elsewhere in the small bowel presumably have similar potential for malignant transformation, although the molecular traits of this transformation remain unknown. Such progression has not been definitively documented at other sites in the small bowel.

Based on theories of luminal injury defined in the colonic mucosa, several hypotheses are proposed regarding the pathogenesis of epithelial-derived small bowel tumors. Unlike the colon with its high bacterial luminal content, the lumen of the healthy small bowel is largely free of bacteria; bacterial metabolites implicated in the genetic alterations of colon carcinogenesis are absent. Transit through the small bowel is rapid—30 minutes to 2 hours—so exposure to potential toxins and metabolites is much more limited. The alkaline, mucus-rich succus entericus of the small bowel may have protective capacity and less noxious potential than the more solid contents of the colon. Enterocytes of the brush border epithelium express the enzyme benzopyrene hydroxylase, possibly protecting against mucosal damage by detoxifying the carcinogen benzopyrene. And lastly, high levels of luminal IgA and greater distribution of lymphoid tissue in the small intestinal epithelium and submucosa may provide an additional protective mechanism via an immune surveillance mechanism.

Bile acids and their metabolites have been implicated in the pathogenesis of small bowel adenocarcinoma. Postcholecystectomy patients may be at greater risk for the development of small bowel malignancy. In one study of patients with small-intestinal malignancy, 12% had a history of cholecystectomy, and of those with duodenal adenocarcinoma, 25% had prior cholecystectomy. However, a causative relationship between cholecystectomy and small intestinal adenocarcinoma remains unproven.

HIGH-RISK POPULATIONS

Several heritable and inflammatory gastrointestinal conditions are associated with an increased risk for development of small bowel tumors.

Familial Adenomatous Polyposis

Patients with familial adenomatous polyposis (FAP) carry a lifetime risk approaching 100% for the development of adenomatous polyps of the duodenum, and these lesions may progress to adenocarcinoma. FAP patients have a 331-fold increased risk for development of adenocarcinoma of the duodenum over the normal population,[3] and this is the leading cause of cancer death in patients with FAP previously treated by colectomy. These patients require regular screening esophagogastroduodenoscopy and endoscopic or surgical excision of enlarging adenomas.

Crohn's Disease

Patients with active jejunoileitis of Crohn's disease have a 100-fold increased incidence of adenocarcinoma. Active disease in the terminal ileum is the most frequent site of malignancy.[6] Abdominal complaints and symptoms consistent with their primary condition may delay evaluation and diagnosis, leading to detection of tumors at advanced stages. The prognosis for patients with adenocarcinoma arising in Crohn's disease is poor.[7] For patients undergoing bowel-preserving procedures such as stricturoplasty, a biopsy of the site of past or active disease is advocated to look for dysplasia or in situ carcinoma. Such findings, while rare, would warrant resection rather than bowel-preserving approaches.

Celiac Disease

Celiac disease is associated with increased risk of lymphoma and is seen in up to 14% of patients.[8] A gluten-free diet has been postulated to decrease this risk, although this has not been substantiated by a recent study.[16]

Miscellaneous Conditions Associated with Small Bowel Neoplasms

Patients with Peutz-Jeghers syndrome develop benign hamartomas throughout the intestinal tract. Surveillance is indicated, as these lesions are at risk of malignant transformation into adenocarcinoma.[9] Patients with von Recklinghausen's disease may develop neurofibromas in the gastrointestinal tract that can undergo malignant transformation. Patients on chronic immune suppression therapy are at particular risk for small bowel malignancies, especially lymphomas and sarcomas. Transplant recipients on immunosuppression have a 45- to 100-fold increase in non-Hodgkin's lymphoma (NHL), a condition termed posttransplant lymphoproliferative disorder (PTLD).[10] PTLD accounts for 30% of all malignancies in cyclosporine-treated patients, but accounts for only 12% of malignancies in patients without cyclosporine in their regimen. PTLD tends to develop rapidly, often within 12 months of transplantation. Greater degrees of immunosuppression carry greater risk for development of PTLD. HIV infection is also associated with the development of lymphoma in up to 30% of patients. Most are extranodal and the gastrointestinal tract is the involved site in 10–25% of cases. More than 90% of patients present with stage IV disease and the median survival is only 6 months.

▪ CLINICAL PRESENTATION

Patients with small bowel tumors present with nonspecific gastrointestinal and constitutional complaints. In hindsight, the gradual development of symptoms is usually evident. The most common symptoms include vague abdominal discomfort and cramps, gradual weight loss, anemia, nausea, and vomiting. These nonspecific complaints, and the fact that most patients are older and often on a variety of medications that may also elicit these complaints, result in a high rate of misdiagnosis and delay in diagnosis. In most series, the average duration of symptoms prior to diagnosis ranges from weeks to many months. Initial evaluation to exclude more common conditions, including evaluation of the gastroduodenum, colon, and biliary tract are completed, but when negative, further evaluation of the small bowel is delayed or deferred.

Benign lesions rarely cause abdominal pain or obstruction; rather, their presence is often heralded by acute gastrointestinal hemorrhage. Benign neoplasms may grow to a large size prior to detection and may simply be discovered incidentally on a radiological exam or at laparotomy.

■ DIAGNOSIS

Diagnosis of small bowel tumors is hampered by a number of factors. In addition to being rare tumors that elicit nonspecific and common gastrointestinal complaints, the ability to fully image and observe the small intestine is limited. Accurate preoperative diagnosis is in fact uncommon prior to surgery.[11,12]

History and physical exam are nonspecific. Abdominal mass, heme-positive stool, or signs of intestinal obstruction are usually absent. Laboratory data may demonstrate iron deficiency anemia in a minority of patients.

Plain abdominal films are an appropriate initial diagnostic test, although they are rarely helpful unless the patient presents with obstructive symptoms.

After ruling out more common conditions that could elicit similar gastrointestinal and abdominal complaints with endoscopic evaluation of the gastroduodenum and colon, computed tomography of the abdomen is the appropriate initial imaging test. CT may reveal bulky tumors (Fig 22–1) or more subtle findings suggestive of small bowel tumors, such as thickening of the small bowel wall. Thickening of the bowel wall to greater than 1.5 cm or the detection of discrete mesenteric lymph nodes or masses greater than 1.5 cm in diameter are highly suggestive of malignancy. If obstructing lesions are present, CT scan may reveal a transition zone demarcating dilated proximal bowel from decompressed distal bowel.

Tumors of the distal small bowel may cause jejunoileal or ileocolic intussusception. During intussusception, the small bowel tumor serves as the lead point to pull the small bowel into the distal small bowel or colonic lumen; the mass lesion precludes spontaneous reduction. CT findings of ileocolic or jejunoileal intussusception include the presence of concentric rings with a donut appearance involving the bowel. This sign is nearly pathognomonic for small bowel tumor. In adults, radiographic attempts to reduce an intussusception should not be done. Rather, prompt surgical exploration and resection of the non-reduced intussuscepted bowel segment with mesenteric resection should be completed.

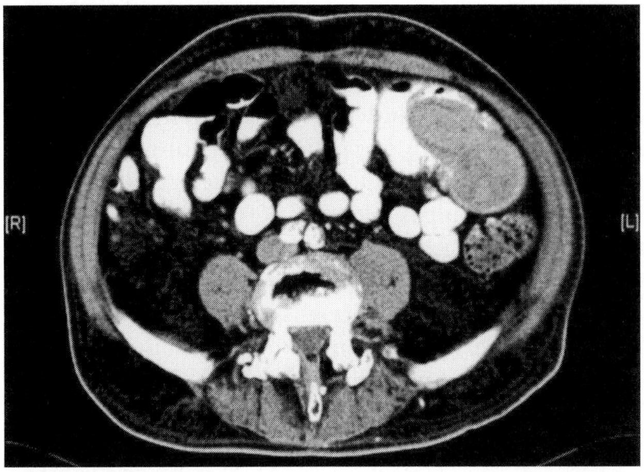

Figure 22–1. Adenocarcinoma in the ileum is obvious as a mass in the left mid-abdomen.

Luminal contrast radiographic studies may be used if abdominal CT imaging fails to reveal evidence of a small bowel tumor, usually an upper gastrointestinal contrast series with small bowel follow-through. A small bowel follow-through study will show an abnormality in 53–83% of cases, although direct evidence of a tumor is detected in only 30–44%.

While enteroclysis (a dynamic contrast technique using a slurry of barium and methylcellulose infused into the small bowel via a nasoduodenal tube to uniformly distend the small bowel lumen) was formerly utilized to study the mucosal surface of the small bowel lumen, this procedure has been largely replaced by video capsule endoscopy (VCE). Similarly, small bowel enteroscopy is far less commonly utilized with the advent of VCE.

For proximal jejunal lesions that cannot be visualized by routine esophagogastroduodenoscopy (EGD), "push" enteroscopy utilizes a pediatric colonoscope for direct examination of the lumen of the proximal 2–3 feet of small bowel.[13] Formerly utilized, Sonde "pull" small bowel enteroscopy, which relies on peristalsis to passively pull an enteroscope with a wide-angle lens into the distal ileum or colon, is now a procedure of only historical interest.

Intraoperative enteroscopy allows a much more complete evaluation of the small bowel. It is rarely required for the diagnosis of small bowel tumors, for most can usually be readily identified by careful palpation or visualization of the bowel once operation is pursued.

VCE with the Given wireless video capsule endoscope is now widely employed in the diagnosis of small bowel tumors in patients with otherwise negative diagnostic studies. The device is an ingestible 11 × 26 mm capsule swallowed by the patient, that contains a miniature video camera, light source, battery, and transmitter that sends images (up to 50,000 overall) to a recording device worn by the patient.[14] Currently the device does not have the capacity for biopsies or for precise localization of lesions, although such capability is in development. The device can be very useful in identifying lesions within the lumen of the small bowel (Fig 22–2). The major complication of VCE is capsule retention, which is reported in 5% of cases, although the rate of requirement of surgical retrieval is less than 1%.[15]

While diagnostic methods continue to improve, most patients with small bowel neoplasms still have initial presentation as a surgical emergency, and more than half of patients with malignant disease have metastatic spread at the time of operation.

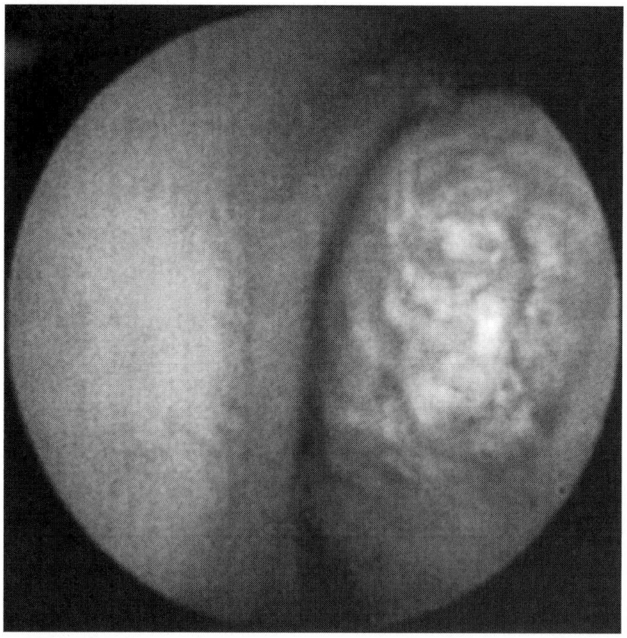

Figure 22–2. Video capsule endoscopy image of the adenocarcinoma.

▪ BENIGN TUMORS OF THE SMALL INTESTINE

Although accounting for 30–50% of primary neoplasms of the small bowel, benign tumors are poorly characterized. Half the patients with benign tumors are symptom free, and most will be diagnosed at the time of presentation with a surgical emergency such as obstruction, massive gastrointestinal hemorrhage, or perforation. Gastrointestinal bleeding is the most common presenting complication, presumably a consequence of spontaneous necrosis when the benign lesion outgrows the available blood supply.[5]

Once these lesions are diagnosed, surgical segmental intestinal resection is appropriate. While local excision via endoscopic mucosal resection or operative enterotomy with submucosal excision is feasible, it is generally not possible to grossly differentiate between benign and malignant lesions. Hence transmural resection is preferred for indeterminate lesions. Open and laparoscopic approaches have been described.

BRUNNER GLAND ADENOMAS

Brunner gland adenomas are rare tumors of the proximal duodenum.[17] Originating in the Brunner glands of the duodenal submucosa that secrete alkaline bicarbonate-rich fluid and mucus that function to neutralize gastric acid, the pathogenesis of glandular hyperplasia and subsequent adenoma formation from this cell population remains unknown. Although Brunner gland adenomas have not been described to transform into carcinomas, endoscopic mucosal resection is advised to prevent complications including acute and chronic bleeding.[17]

ADENOMAS

As in the colon, small bowel adenomas are histologically classified as tubular, tubulovillous, or villous. Most common in the periampullary region, they can develop throughout the small bowel mucosa. Increased size correlates with malignant potential and excision is advised when diagnosis is established, often as an incidental finding. Adenomas larger than 2 cm in diameter should be considered worrisome for malignancy.

Approximately one-third of adenomas in the duodenum present with obstructive jaundice. In these cases ultrasound will reveal evidence of biliary obstruction, prompting upper endoscopy for endoscopic retrograde biliary and pancreatic duct evaluation (endoscopic retrograde cholangiopancreatography), which will reveal the presence of the ampullary lesion. Without these physical signs to direct the workup, duodenal adenomas are detected during evaluation of gastrointestinal blood loss or other abdominal complaints, with either contrast upper gastrointestinal series or EGD, which are equally sensitive in most series. Adenomas usually appear as intraluminal filling defects and may be pedunculated (Fig 22–3). CT scan may differentiate adenoma from carcinoma, as carcinomas are often associated with bowel wall thickening.

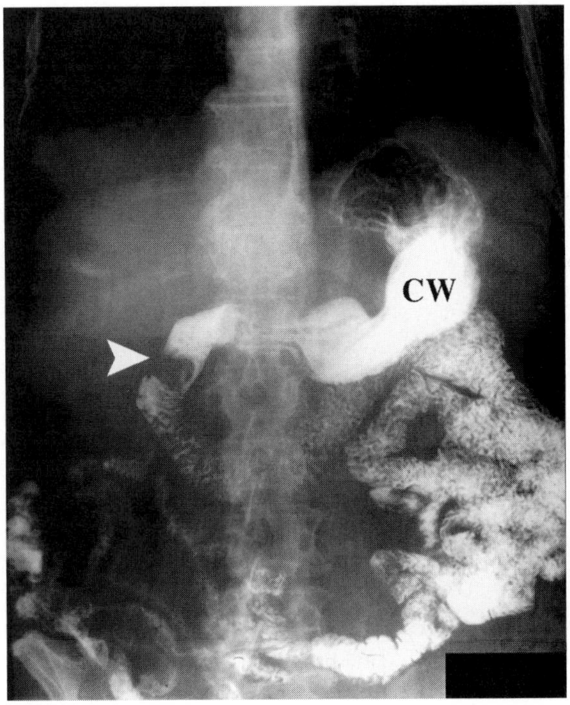

Figure 22–3. Filling defect in the duodenum caused by a large benign adenoma.

Endoscopic ultrasound is becoming essential in the evaluation of duodenal adenomas to evaluate depth, and to determine if mucosal excision or surgical resection is more appropriate. Transduodenal local excision for small lesions is appropriate, while lesions >3 cm in size have a high rate of associated malignancy and are most appropriately treated with either pancreas-sparing duodenectomy, or pancreaticoduodenectomy for larger lesions or periampullary tumors in suitable operative candidates.[18] Local recurrence is common for periampullary adenomas treated with excision only: 40% at 10 years, 25% of which were malignant, in a recent retrospective series from the Mayo clinic. For those treated with excision only, annual surveillance with endoscopy is appropriate.[19]

LIPOMAS

Lipomas of the gastrointestinal tract are typically identified as incidental findings on abdominal imaging. They rarely cause symptoms, although as polypoid, compressible intraluminal lesions, they may serve as lead points for intussusception. Lipomas are circumscribed lesions arising in the bowel wall appearing as fat density on CT imaging. Small tumors under 2 cm require no intervention, while larger lesions or growing lesions should be resected to rule out malignant liposarcoma.

HAMARTOMAS

The hamartoma is the characteristic lesion of Peutz-Jeghers syndrome, an autosomal dominant condition characterized by multiple gastrointestinal hamartomas and mucocutaneous pigmentation. The tumors are widely distributed throughout the bowel in affected individuals, and in rare cases are associated with intussusception, bleeding, or obstruction. While malignant transformation has been described, this is a rare event. Given the broad distribution of the tumors, prophylactic excision is not feasible and surgical intervention is appropriate only to treat complications caused by the tumors.[9]

HEMANGIOMAS

Hemangiomas are rare congenital lesions of the small bowel. They appear to grow slowly and may become symptomatic in midlife, when acute or chronic bleeding may develop. Arising from the submucosal vascular plexuses, hemangiomas are usually solitary and not at risk for malignant transformation. Hemangiomas associated with bleeding should be locally excised or resected with a limited small bowel resection. Endoscopic sclerotherapy or angiographic embolization has also been reported as a treatment option depending on the size and position of the tumor.

■ MALIGNANT NEOPLASMS

The small bowel can give rise to a number of different primary tumors and is also a site for metastasis from tumors of other origins. Primary malignancies include adenocarcinoma, GIST, carcinoid, lymphoma, and leiomyosarcoma, with rare reports of other lesions including liposarcoma, myxoliposarcoma, and lymphangiosarcoma. Metastatic tumors may come from any other cancer, but the most common metastatic lesions are from melanomas and lymphomas.

Malignant tumors are much more likely to elicit symptoms than benign tumors, including abdominal pain, weight loss, anorexia, and acute or chronic blood loss. As a group, patients with malignant small bowel tumors present at advanced stages and have a poor prognosis.

Up to 30% of patients with small bowel malignancy develop a second primary tumor in another organ. For patients with GI carcinoid tumors, the incidence of second primaries is 50%. The second primary cancer may arise in any organ, but the most frequent second primary sites are the colorectum and breast.[20,21]

ADENOCARCINOMA

Epidemiology

Adenocarcinoma accounts for about 35% of small bowel tumors, making it the most common primary malignancy.[7] The frequency of small bowel tumors decreases along the length of the small bowel, with 80% located in the duodenum and proximal jejunum. Men are slightly more likely to develop adenocarcinoma than women. Risk factors for development of adenocarcinoma include polyposis syndromes, Crohn's disease, and celiac disease.

Clinical Presentation

Clinical presentation is dictated by the size and position of the tumor. Large tumors form the classic circumferential annular "apple core" constriction leading to obstruction with symptoms of anorexia, vomiting, and crampy pain (Fig 22–4). Periampullary lesions may cause biliary obstruction with secondary jaundice. Absent advanced or strategically placed lesions with obstruction, the only complaint may be vague, persistent abdominal pain.

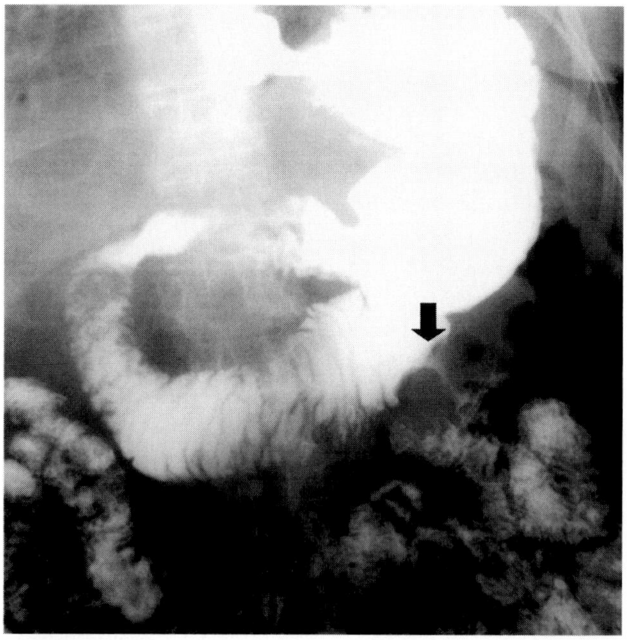

Figure 22–4. "Apple core" constricting adenocarcinoma of the proximal jejunum causing proximal partial bowel obstruction.

Diagnosis

For patients with advanced lesions, plain abdominal films may show gastric distention or proximal small bowel obstruction. For the jaundiced patient, ultrasound or abdominal CT or magnetic resonance retrograde cholangiopancreatography may demonstrate the duodenal mass and site of biliary obstruction. Upper gastrointestinal contrast studies or esophagogastroduodenoscopy have equal diagnostic rates of 85–90%, while EGD allows diagnostic tissue biopsy. CT reveals approximately 50% of small bowel adenocarcinomas and the appearance is that of a heterogeneous infiltrating mass. Despite diagnostic strategies, preoperative diagnosis of cancers beyond the duodenum is achieved in only 20–50% of cases.

Management

Surgical resection offers the only potential cure. Many patients have intra-abdominal metastases at initial surgery, with R0 resection (i.e., no gross or microscopic disease left) achieved in only 50–65% of cases. Pancreaticoduodenectomy is appropriate for proximal duodenal tumors. In the third and fourth portions of the duodenum and in the mesenteric small bowel, a segmental resection with lymphadenectomy should be performed. Palliative procedures to relieve obstruction or control hemorrhage should be completed at the time of exploration for patients with metastatic disease. Endoscopic expandable stents (Wall type) may be the best strategy to palliate proximal gastrointestinal obstruction from recurrent or metastatic disease. Gastrojejunal or gastrostomy tubes may be of palliative value for decompression or nutritional support in patients with carcinomatosis or unresectable disease.

Staging and Prognosis

The American Joint Committee on Cancer staging system applies to small bowel adenocarcinoma.[22] The tumor (T) classification describes depth of invasion with T1 and T2 within the bowel wall and T3 and T4 lesions penetrating the bowel wall. The node (N) classification is defined by the presence or absence of lymph node metastases, and distant metastases are classified by M. Most patients present with stage III (lymph node involvement) or stage IV disease (distant metastases), which carries a poor prognosis.

The most significant prognostic factor is lymph node metastases, with poor survival linked to node-positive disease. Likely due to limited reported experience with small series, the primary tumor features, including the degree of differentiation, do not appear to impact survival. For ampullary tumors, prognosis is improved if lymph nodes are negative and the tumor does not infiltrate the pancreas.[19] A recent retrospective analysis showed that positive margins, extramural venous spread, positive lymph nodes, and a history of Crohn's disease are associated with poor prognosis.[6]

Adjuvant therapies including chemotherapy and/or radiation therapy have not demonstrated efficacy, although clinical trials are ongoing.[20]

NON-HODGKIN'S LYMPHOMA

The gastrointestinal tract is the most common extranodal site for development of non-Hodgkin's lymphoma (NHL), comprising approximately 20% of all cases of NHL. Most GI lymphomas arise in the stomach (60%), followed by the small bowel (30%), and then the colon. Most small bowel lymphomas are distributed in the jejunum and ileum reflecting the distribution of lymphoid tissue in the bowel. Diagnostic criteria for primary GI NHL include the absence of superficial adenopathy on physical examination, absence of mediastinal adenopathy by chest imaging, normal peripheral blood cell counts, and absence of splenic or hepatic involvement. At surgery, disease must be restricted to the primary tumor with mesenteric lymph node involvement.[23]

The majority of cases of primary intestinal NHL are B-cell type with T-cell lymphoma comprising only 10–25%. Low-grade lymphomas derived from mucosal-associated lymphoid tissue typically arise in the stomach in association with *Helicobacter pylori* infection. These tumors may regress with treatment of this infection.[24] T-cell lymphomas tend to have a worse prognosis than B-cell tumors.

Clinical Presentation

The majority of patients present with nonspecific abdominal complaints. Malabsorption, obstruction, or palpable mass may be present. Although rare, small intestinal lymphomas may present with perforation.

Diagnosis

Lymphomas may grow to large size before clinical symptoms present. Most small bowel lymphomas will be demonstrable on CT scan as a mass, bowel wall thickening, displacement of adjacent organs, or luminal obstruction (Fig 22–5). Multiple lesions are present in 10–25% of patients. Tissue diagnosis requires biopsy of the submucosal lesion by endoscopy or CT guided biopsy.

Staging and Prognosis

Staging is based on site involvement as outlined in Table 22–1. Like tumors elsewhere in the small intestine, most patients present with stage III or IV disease. Fewer than 30% of patients have surgically resectable tumors and prognosis, although improving with new chemotherapy regimens, is poor.[22]

Treatment

With no randomized series and small numbers of cases at single institutions, the optimal treatment of GI NHL remains controversial. Most agree that surgical resection of isolated small bowel lymphoma for local control and prevention of perforation and bleeding are the cornerstones of treatment. For more extensive gastrointestinal lymphoma, there is no evidence-based consensus on optimal management, although a variety of chemotherapeutic regimens have been utilized.[23,24]

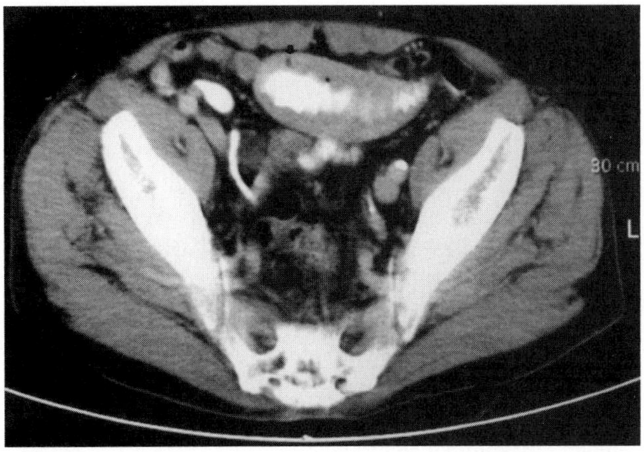

Figure 22–5. Thickening of the bowel wall on abdominal CT scan characteristic of lymphoma.

CARCINOID TUMORS

Carcinoid tumors arise from the enterochromaffin cells at the base of the crypts of Lieberkühn. Enterochromaffin cells are capable of amine precursor uptake and decarboxylation (APUD) and tumors derived from these can secrete vasoactive peptides responsible for the carcinoid syndrome. Eighty percent of carcinoids arise in the gastrointestinal tract, 10% in the bronchus

TABLE 22–1. STAGING FOR LYMPHOMA

Stage I	Involvement of a single lymph node region; or localized involvement of a single extralymphatic organ or site in the absence of any lymph node involvement
Stage II	Involvement of two or more lymph node regions on the same side of the diaphragm; or localized involvement of a single extralymphatic organ or site in association with regional lymph node involvement, with or without involvement of other lymph node regions on the same side of the diaphragm
Stage III	Involvement of lymph node regions on both sides of the diaphragm, which also may be accompanied by extralymphatic extension in association with adjacent lymph node involvement, or by involvement of the spleen, or both
Stage IV	Diffuse or disseminated involvement of one or more extralymphatic organs, with or without associated lymph node involvement; or isolated extralymphatic organ involvement in the absence of adjacent regional lymph node involvement, but in conjunction with disease in distant site(s); any involvement of the liver or bone marrow, or nodular involvement of the lungs

Reproduced, with permission, from American Joint Commission on Cancer. *Cancer Staging Handbook*, 6th ed. New York, NY: Springer; 2002.

or lung, and others in rare sites including the ovaries, testicles, pancreas, and kidneys. The appendix is the most common site in the GI tract for primary carcinoid tumors, followed by the small bowel. Thirty percent of GI carcinoids arise in the jejunum or ileum and have the most aggressive clinical features.

Carcinoids represent 5–35% of small bowel neoplasms; the mean age of presentation is 60 years with a slight male preponderance. Autopsy rates reveal an incidence of occult tumors approximately 2000 times that of the annual clinical incidence rate, indicating that the overwhelming majority never develop clinical findings.[24,25]

Clinical Presentation and Diagnosis

Most carcinoids grow slowly and have insidious clinical manifestations; in hindsight, symptoms may be present for 2–20 years prior to diagnosis. Carcinoid syndrome secondary to metastatic disease is the presenting sign in 40% of patients. Rarely, intestinal necrosis secondary to desmoplastic occlusion of the mesenteric vessels may develop, leading to initial presentation as a surgical emergency.

The most common presenting symptom for patients with small bowel carcinoid is abdominal pain. The polypoid lesions serve as a lead point for intussusception characterized by intermittent symptoms and signs of obstruction. Abdominal films often demonstrate a distal small bowel obstruction and the CT findings of intussusception are distinctive, demonstrating a multilayer ringed structure in the ileocolic region (Fig 22–6).

Appendiceal carcinoids are typically solitary lesions. However, for carcinoids arising in other areas of the gut, multiple tumors are observed in 30–40% of patients.[26] In addition, 30–50% of small bowel carcinoids are associated with second primary malignancies, most frequently of the breast and colon. Gastrointestinal carcinoids have the capacity to elicit a marked desmoplastic reaction in the mesentery of the small bowel. The fibrotic reaction can cause sclerosis of mesenteric vessels, leading to kinking of the bowel or intestinal ischemia and necrosis. The fibrosis affects not only peritumoral tissues, but distant tissues in the heart and lungs and is attributed to the humoral products of the tumors, although the specific factors are unknown.[27,28]

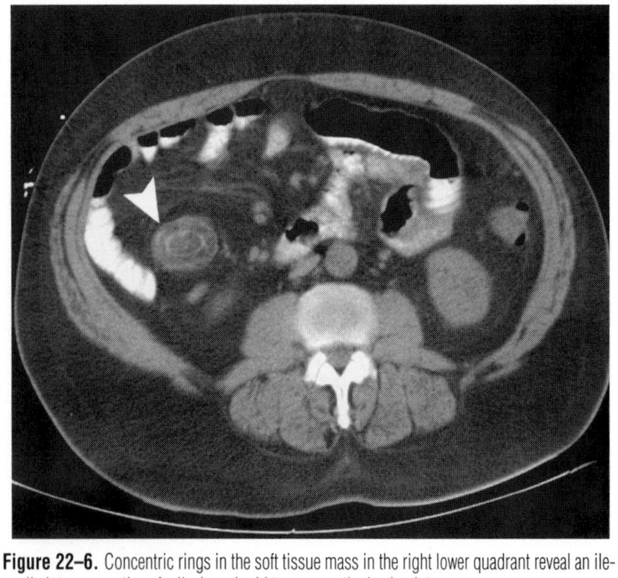

Figure 22–6. Concentric rings in the soft tissue mass in the right lower quadrant reveal an ileocolic intussusception. An ileal carcinoid tumor was the lead point.

Staging and Prognosis

Appendiceal carcinoids, even at a small size, may cause appendicitis due to luminal compression; hence early diagnosis of appendiceal carcinoid is common. In contrast, small bowel carcinoids exhibit a more aggressive phenotype and are frequently associated with lymph node spread and hepatic metastasis at initial presentation. Tumor size is proportional to the risk for metastatic spread. For jejunoileal carcinoids smaller than 1 cm, there is a 20–30% incidence of nodal and hepatic spread. Tumors 1–2 cm in size have nodal spread in 60–80% and hepatic disease in 20%. The rate of nodal and hepatic metastasis for tumors larger than 2 cm is >80% and 40–50%, respectively.[25] Only very small jejunoileal carcinoid tumors, those less than 1 cm, can be treated with local excision. All others should be treated with segmental bowel and mesenteric resection.[29]

Carcinoid Syndrome

Carcinoid syndrome refers to vasomotor, gastrointestinal, and cardiac manifestations induced by systemic circulation of peptides produced by carcinoid tumors. The APUD cells of carcinoid tumors can produce vasoactive products including serotonin, histamine, kallikrein, bradykinin, and prostaglandins, although the specific mediator or mediators of the syndrome remain unknown. Carcinoid syndrome is confirmed by finding elevated 24-hour 5-hydroxyindoleacetic acid (5-HIAA) urinary excretion, the primary stable metabolite of serotonin.

Attacks are characterized by intense flushing and tachycardia. Watery diarrhea, at times explosive and associated with cramping, may occur in some patients. Attacks may be spontaneous or precipitated by stress, alcohol, a large meal, or sexual intercourse. Flushing, a 5- to 10-minute sensation of heat associated with facial and truncal erythema, is the most common finding and affects approximately 80% of patients. Diarrhea occurs in most patients and is likely related to serotonin release, as serotonin antagonists can effectively treat this symptom. Abdominal cramps and malabsorption may occur. Cardiac manifestations are present in 60–70% of patients with advanced disease, due to tricuspid and pulmonary valve endocardial fibrosis, possibly secondary to high levels of 5-HIAA. As the disease progresses, the fibrotic plaque stiffens, leading eventually to right heart failure.

Carcinoid syndrome is due to metastatic disease in either the liver or retroperitoneum. Monoamine oxidase in the liver contains deactivated serotonin, one of the major effector hormones. Carcinoid syndrome occurs when metabolically active tumor is present in a site without portal drainage, such as a bronchial carcinoid or retroperitoneal tumor, or when hepatic metastatic tumor burden exceeds the capacity of hepatic monoamine oxidase to metabolize serotonin. Patients with gastrointestinal carcinoids that drain into the portal circulation must have metastatic disease prior to the development of the syndrome.

Management of patients with carcinoid syndrome is optimized by utilization of surgical, imaging-guided interventional procedures and medical therapies. Given the relatively slow growth of carcinoid tumors, including metastatic disease, surgical debulking of extensive hepatic disease or formal hepatic resection for resectable metastases can improve symptoms and prolong life. Five- and 10-year survival for patients with residual abdominal tumor and hepatic metastases approaches 60%, so while in general the initial surgery should involve attempts to debulk as much tumor as possible, it must also avoid catastrophic injuries such as those to the superior mesenteric vessels that may lead to short gut syndrome.[30] Hepatic artery embolization or radiofrequency ablation may be more appropriate for widespread hepatic metastases and can give marked symptomatic relief and durable tumor control.[31]

Medical therapy is based on somatostatin analogues (octreotide), including short- and long-acting peptides for relief of carcinoid syndrome symptoms. Carcinoid tumors express somatostatin receptors and the somatostatin analogues inhibit vasoactive peptide release from carcinoid tumors. Palliation of symptoms is effective in 90% of patients with octreotide. Some studies have demonstrated a tumorstatic or tumor reduction effect after the administration of somatostatin, although these latter findings have not been consistently reproduced. Efficacy of treatment can be documented by following excretion of the tumor marker 5-HIAA.

Chemotherapeutic agents for the treatment of metastatic carcinoid tumor include doxorubicin, 5-fluorouracil, dacarbazine, and interferon-α, with response rates of approximately 20%. Combination protocols most often utilize streptozotocin and 5-fluorouracil.

Preliminary reports on the use of targeted radiotherapeutics have been presented. Somatostatin analogues bind to somatostatin receptors on carcinoid tumors with high affinity. After binding, the ligand-receptor complex is internalized. This internalization has led to the development of "smart bombs"—radiolabeled somatostatin analogues that theoretically deliver radiation specifically to carcinoid cells. Indium-111-labeled-pentetreotide demonstrated an enhanced tumor regression response compared to unlabeled analogue in one study.[32]

GASTROINTESTINAL STROMAL TUMORS

Although gastrointestinal stromal tumors (GIST) are the most common non-epithelial tumors of the small bowel, they are in fact rare tumors of the GI tract representing only 0.2% of all GI tumors. Approximately 25% of GIST arise in the small bowel, with 50% gastric, 15% rectal, and 10% colonic in origin.[33] Men and women are equally at risk and peak incidence occurs in patients aged between 50 and 70 years. GIST arise from the interstitial cell of Cajal, the pacemaker cell of the GI tract intercalated between the intramural neurons and the smooth muscle cells. The molecular diagnostic feature of GIST is the presence of activating c-kit mutations, a transmembrane receptor tyrosine kinase involved in the regulation of cellular proliferation, apoptosis, and differentiation. Over 95% of GIST express kit (CD117) mutations, a molecular marker that distinguishes them from histologically similar mesenchymal tumors of the small bowel including leiomyomas, leiomyosarcoma, schwannomas, and others. Retrospective molecular analysis of mesenchymal tumors has led to reclassification of up to 70% small bowel tumors as GIST that had previously been classified as a variety of mesenchymal tumors.[35]

GIST are characterized by indolent clinical symptoms including vague abdominal pain, weight loss, and occult gastrointestinal bleeding. Of all small bowel tumors, GIST are typified by growing to massive size prior to surgical presentation. They tend to grow insidiously as extraluminal masses from their submucosal origin in a noninvasive manner, characteristically pushing adjacent organs away from the expanding mass. Gastrointestinal hemorrhage may develop in patients with necrotic GIST in communication with the bowel lumen.

Given the propensity of GIST to grow to a large size prior to diagnosis, CT scan is most likely to be the initial positive test. A characteristic finding is the presence of a large space-occupying mass, often with evidence of central necrosis and compression of adjacent organs and calcifications (Fig 22–7).

Regardless of size, all GIST tumors should be considered to be malignant.[33] Malignant potential is determined by two major criteria: tumor size and mitotic rate. Biologically aggressive tumors are large tumors with a high mitotic index, while tumors with benign features are small and exhibit a low mitotic index. Tumors are thus classified into very low- to high-risk for malignant potential, a classification that has prognostic significance.

Treatment

Surgery is the primary therapeutic option with the goal being complete resection. At operation, wide local excision of the primary tumor to achieve gross negative margins with incontinuity resection of adherent organs is appropriate to attain curative resection. Lymph node metastasis is rare, negating the need for wide mesenteric resection.

Molecular Therapeutics and Gastrointestinal Stromal Tumors

Given the central role of activating mutations in the tyrosine kinases KIT and more recently platelet-derived growth factor receptor alpha (PDGFRA) in the pathogenesis of GIST,[34] this tumor has served as a prototype for molecular therapeutic drug development. Activation of KIT leads to phosphorylation of a receptor substrate protein, initiating an intracellular phosphorylation cascade leading to nuclear activation of transcription events resulting in cell proliferation and survival. The discovery of a drug that inactivates KIT with a safe therapeutic margin has revolutionized the treatment of metastatic GIST. Imatinib mesylate is a small molecule that occupies the ATP binding pocket of the KIT kinase domain, blocking phosphorylation of the receptor and intracellular signaling. This binding arrests cellular proliferation and survival signaling.

Clinical use of imatinib is now routine in the management of GIST. This oral agent is well tolerated and highly effective for patients with metastatic GIST. While complete regression of tumor is rare, partial regression of disease and arrest of progression of disease can be achieved for durable intervals with continuous treatment in up to 80% of patients. Efficacy of treatment can be predicted and followed using fluorodeoxyglucose-positron emission tomography scanning; these highly biologically active tumors will become metabolically silent with imatinib therapy in those patients with responsive tumors. Emergence of resistant clones within tumors has been recognized with prolonged use of imatinib. Newer receptor tyrosine kinase inhibitors, including SU11248, which has activity against PDGFRA as well as KIT, are in clinical trials.[36]

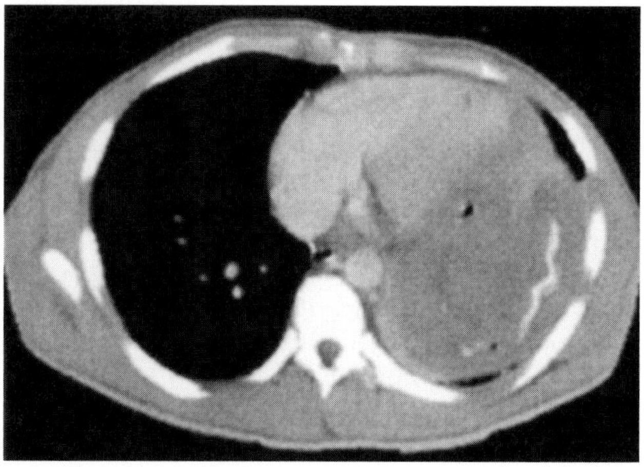

Figure 22–7. Large GIST arising from the stomach in the left upper quadrant. The diaphragm and the spleen were invaded by the tumor.

Neoadjuvant use of imatinib for unresectable or locally aggressive tumors is currently being evaluated in cooperative group clinical trials. The efficacy of imatinib in the adjuvant setting for high-risk or partially resected tumors is also being evaluated in ongoing trials. Given the favorable risk profile of the agent, such applications may prove useful in these settings as well, although definitive survival data are not yet available.

METASTATIC LESIONS TO THE SMALL BOWEL

While metastases to the small bowel are rare, as a group, they are in fact more common than primary small bowel neoplasms.

Metastatic spread can occur by direct invasion, hematogenous spread, or intraperitoneal seeding. Colon and pancreatic cancers are the most common primary sites for direct invasion. Hematogenous metastases spread most frequently from lung and breast carcinoma or melanoma. Peritoneal seeding may arise from any intra-abdominal malignancy including gastric, hepatic, ovarian, appendiceal, and colonic primary tumors.[37]

CT scan may identify metastatic lesions or reveal sites of partial or complete luminal obstruction. Metastases can be identified as bowel wall thickening or mesenteric masses. For small lesions, CT scan may be negative, while small bowel follow-through study may reveal an irregular luminal filling defect. Carcinomatosis is frequently not specifically identifiable on imaging studies.

Optimal palliative management is based on clinical criteria. Segmental intestinal resection or bypass to relieve hemorrhage, obstruction, or pain is indicated except in the most terminal stages of disease. While cases of prolonged survival after intestinal resection of solitary metastases have been reported, progression of metastatic disease is more common.

Management of patients with carcinomatosis, regardless of tumor origin, remains challenging. Endoscopic luminal stents for obstructing duodenal lesions may offer short-term palliation, while intestinal bypasses and decompressive gastrostomy tubes are indicated for patients with advanced or more distal disease to enhance palliative care.

REFERENCES

1. Ciresi DL, Scholten DJ. The continuing clinical dilemma of primary tumors of the small intestine. *Am Surg* 1995;61:698–703
2. Landis SH, Murray T, Bolden S, Wingo PA. Cancer Statistics, 1999. *CA Cancer J Clin* 1999;49:8–31
3. Howe JR, Karnell LH, Menck HR, Scott-Conner C. Adenocarcinoma of the small bowel: Review of the National Cancer Data Base, 1985–1995. *Cancer* 1999;86:2693–2706
4. Matsuo S, Eto T, Tsunoda T et al. Small bowel tumors: an analysis of tumor-like lesions, benign and malignant neoplasms. *Eur J Surg Oncol* 1994;20:47–51
5. Minardi AJ Jr, Zibari GB, Aultman DF et al. Small-bowel tumors. *J Am Coll Surg* 1998;186:664–668
6. Sigel JE, Petras RE, Lashner BA et al. Intestinal adenocarcinoma in Crohn's disease; a report of 30 cases with a focus on coexisting dysplasia. *Am J Surg Pathol* 1999;23: 651–655
7. Abrahams NA, Halverson A, Fazio VW et al. Adenocarcinoma of the small bowel: A study of 37 cases with emphasis on histologic prognostic factors. *Dis Colon Rectum* 2002;45:1496–1502
8. O'Boyle CJ, Kerin MJ, Feeley K, Given HF. Primary small intestinal tumors: increased incidence of lymphoma and improved survival. *Ann R Coll Surg Engl* 1998;80: 332–334
9. Dong K, Li B. Peutz-Jeghers syndrome: case reports and update on diagnosis and treatment. *Chin J Dig Dis* 2004; 5:160–164
10. Crump M, Gospodarowicz M, Shepherd FA. Lymphoma of the gastrointestinal tract. *Semin Oncol* 1999;26:324–337
11. Maglinte DDT, Reyes BL. Small bowel cancer: radiologic diagnosis. *Radiol Clin North Am* 1997;35:361–380
12. Buckley JA, Jones B, Fishman EK. Small bowel cancer; imaging features and staging. *Radiol Clin North Am* 1997; 35:381–402
13. Waye JD. Small-bowel endoscopy. *Endoscopy* 2003;35:15–21
14. Swain P. Wireless capsule endoscopy. *Gut* 2003;52(Suppl IV):iv48–iv50
15. Cave DR. Wireless video capsule endoscopy. *Clin Perspect Gastroenterol* 2002;5:203–207
16. Green PH, Fleischauer AT, Bhagat G et al. Risk of malignancy in patients with celiac disease. *Am J Med* 2003;115: 191–195
17. Adeonigbagbe O, Lee C, Karowe M et al. A Brunner's gland adenoma as a cause of anemia. *J Clin Gastroenterol* 1999;29:193–196
18. Beger HG, Treitschke F, Gansange F et al. Tumor of the ampulla of Vater. *Arch Surg* 1999;134:526–532
19. Sakorafas GH, Sarr MG, Tsiotos GG et al. Villous tumors of the duodenum; reappraisal of local versus extended resection. *Gastroenterology* 1999;116:S0069
20. Cunningham JD, Aleali R, Aleali M et al. Malignant small bowel neoplasms; histopathologic determinants of recurrence and survival. *Ann Surg* 1997;225:300–306
21. Marcilla JAG, Bueno FS, Aquilar J, Paricio PP. Primary small bowel malignant tumors. *Eur J Surg Oncol* 1994;20: 630–634
22. American Joint Committee on Cancer and TNM Committee of the International Union Against Cancer: Small intestine. In: Greene FL, Page DL, Fleming ID et al (eds). *Handbook for the Staging of Cancer.* Philadelphia, PA: JB Lippincott; 2002:119–125
23. Cooper DL, Daria R, Salloum E. Primary gastrointestinal lymphomas. *Gastroenterologist* 1996;4:54–64
24. Pandey M, Wadhwa MK, Patel HP et al. Malignant lymphoma of the gastrointestinal tract. *Eur J Surg Oncol* 1999;25:164–167
25. Memon MA, Nelson H. Gastrointestinal carcinoid tumors; current management strategies. *Dis Colon Rectum* 1997;40:1101–1118
26. Yantiss R, Odze R, Farraye F et al. Solitary versus multiple carcinoid tumors of the ileum: a clinical and pathological review of 68 cases. *Am J Surg Pathol* 2003;27:811–817
27. Modlin IM, Shapiro MD, Kidd M. Carcinoid tumors and fibrosis: An association with no explanation. *Am J Gastroenterol* 2004;99:2466–2478
28. Sheth S, Horton K, Garland M et al. Mesenteric neoplasms: CT appearance of primary and secondary tumors and differential diagnosis. *Radiographics* 2003;23:457–473
29. Rothmund M, Kisker O. Surgical treatment of carcinoid tumors of the small bowel, appendix, colon and rectum. *Digestion* 1994;55:86–91
30. Schell S, Camp E, Caridi J et al. Hepatic artery embolization for control of symptoms, octreotide requirements, and tumor progression in metastatic carcinoid tumors. *J Gastrointest Surg* 2002;6:664–670
31. Roche A, Girish B, de Baerre et al. Trans-catheter arterial chemoembolization as first-line treatment for hepatic metastases from endocrine tumors. *Eur Radiol* 2003;13:136–140
32. Anthony L et al. Indium-111-pentetreotide prolongs survival in gastroenteropancreatic malignancies. *Semin Nucl Med* 2002;32:123
33. Miettinen M, Lasota J. Gastrointestinal stromal tumors—definition, clinical, histological, immunohistochemical, and molecular genetic features and differential diagnosis. *Virchows Arch* 2001;438:1–12

34. Heinrich MC, Corless CL, Duensing A et al. PDGFRA activating mutations in gastrointestinal stromal tumors. *Science* 2003;299:708–710
35. Fletcher CD, Berman JJ, Corless C et al. Diagnosis of gastrointestinal stromal tumors: A consensus approach. *Hum Pathol* 2002;33:459–465
36. von Mehren M. New therapeutic strategies for soft tissue sarcomas. *Curr Treat Options Oncol* 2003;4:441–451
37. Ciplone G, Santarelli G, Quitadamo S et al. Small bowel metastases from lung cancer. *Chir Ital* 2004;56:639–648
38. American Joint Commission on Cancer. *Cancer Staging Handbook*, 6th ed. New York, NY: Springer; 2002

23

Tumors of the Colon

Andreas M. Kaiser ▪ *Joseph W. Nunoo-Mensah* ▪ *Robert W. Beart, Jr.*

Tumor is a descriptive term for an abnormal growth or mass of cells that are not linked to any physiologic function or demand. The two characteristic biologic growth patterns of tumors include the ability (1) to disrespect tissue boundaries and invade other structures (*invasiveness*) and (2) to gain access to blood and lymph vessels or other structures, spread tumor cells to distant locations, and allow these specially equipped cells not only to survive but also to seed and grow new remote tumors (*metastases*). If a tumor does not have either property, it is *benign;* if a tumor can invade locally but even at a large size does not have a tendency to metastasize, it is called *semimalignant;* and if a tumor has the ability to metastasize once a sufficient size is reached, it is a *malignant* tumor. Tumors of the colon are either benign—with or without a malignant potential—or they are malignant; the semimalignant variant with invasion only but no affinity to later form metastases is not common in the colon.

Colonic tumors are important for two reasons. First, they are frequent and account for both a significant mortality rate and high cumulative health care costs. Second, the sequence of events leading from a normal mucosa to a manifest cancer occurs largely through preventable precursor stages over the course of several years.

Colorectal lesions may be classified as either benign, potentially malignant, or malignant based on their pathologic features (Table 23–1). The overwhelming majority of colorectal tumors are of epithelial origin and arise from the mucosal surface, where they become visible descriptively as a polyp. Benign polyps include nonneoplastic polyps (e.g., hyperplastic, hamartomatous, or inflammatory polyps); the potentially malignant group consists of adenomatous polyps. Once dysplastic cells in a polyp cross the boundaries of the mucosa (basement membrane) and start to invade the submucosa, a true cancer (carcinoma) with the potential to metastasize is established. Tumors of nonepithelial or mesenchymal origin are comparably rare and include, among others, lymphoma, carcinoid, and sarcoma.

Since malignant tumors and lesions with a malignant potential (premalignant lesions) are of utmost clinical importance, this chapter focuses predominantly on the detection, management, and prevention of these conditions.

▪ EPIDEMIOLOGY

Colorectal cancer is the most common malignancy in the gastrointestinal tract. In the United States, colorectal cancer ranks third in terms of both gender-specific annual cancer incidence and cancer mortality (behind lung and prostate or breast, respectively).[1] With an estimated 147,000 newly diagnosed cases, this disease will be responsible for an estimated 57,000 deaths, or 10–15% of cancer-related deaths in the year 2004.[1] The lifetime risk of approximately 6% in our Western civilization means that 1 in 18 individuals of the general population will be affected by colorectal cancer, making it an important public health issue.[2] Worldwide, colorectal cancer shows large geographic differences, with a crude incidence of 6.5/7.7 cases per 100,000 females/males in less developed areas as opposed to 50.9/60.8 in more developed regions.[3]

TABLE 23–1. INTRODUCTION: CLASSIFICATION OF TUMORS OF THE COLON

A) Epithelial Tumors of the Colon

Type	Class	Subclassification
Benign lesions	Hyperplastic polyps	
	Noninherited gastrointestinal polyposis syndromes	Hyperplastic polyps
	Hamartomas	Juvenile polyps
		Cowden syndrome
		Bannayan-Riley-Ruvalcaba syndrome
		Cronkite-Canada syndrome
	Inflammatory polyps	
Potentially malignant lesions/syndromes	Inherited hamartomatous polyposis syndromes	Juvenile polyposis syndromes
		Peutz-Jeghers syndrome
	Hereditary polyposis syndromes	Familial adenomatous polyposis (FAP)
		Attenuated familial adenomatous polyposis (AFAP)
	Noninherited gastrointestinal polyposis syndromes	Cronkite-Canada syndrome
	Adenomatous polyps	Hereditary colon cancers
Malignant lesions	Epithelial tumors of the colon	Sporadic colon cancers
		Familial colorectal cancer
		Hereditary nonpolyposis colon cancers (HNPCC)
		Hereditary polyposis colon cancers

B) Nonepithelial Tumors of the Colon

Type	Class
Benign lesions	Lipomas and lipomatous polyposis
Potentially malignant lesions/syndromes	Carcinoid
	Gastrointestinal stromal tumors
	Nodular lymphoid hyperplasia of the colon
Malignant lesions	Lymphoma

C) Secondary Tumors to the Colon

Type	Class
Benign lesions	Endometriosis
Potentially malignant lesions/syndromes	Leukemia
	Carcinoma arising in endometriosis
Malignant lesions	Lymphoma
	Malignant melanoma
	Carcinomas from other primary sites

The colorectal cancer incidence has a negligible overall predominance of females, who represent in 51.6% of the cases.[4] Rectal cancer is somewhat more frequent in males, whereas colon cancer is slightly more frequent in women, resulting in almost identical overall mortality rates for both genders. Regardless of ethnicity, there is an age-dependent increase in incidence with each decade starting at age of 40 years, and the mean age at presentation is around 70–75 years.

In the period between 1977 and 2001, the Surveillance, Epidemiology and End Results (SEER) Registry of the National Cancer Institute (NCI) shows a gradual decline of all cases of colorectal cancer in the United States from 62.4 to 51.4 cases per 100,000.[5] However, although these numbers reflect the trend in Caucasians, the incidence of colorectal cancer in the United States for African Americans has remained at the same level of 62 cases per 100,000 individuals. African-American males therefore now represent the ethnic subgroup with the highest risk.[6,7]

■ RISK FACTORS, PREVENTION, AND SCREENING

The specific cause of colorectal cancer is not known. However, a number of genetic and environmental risk factors have been associated with the disease.[8] From a practical and screening standpoint, it has been helpful to group individuals into three risk categories (i.e., average risk, increased risk, high risk) based on their individual and family history.[9,10] The high-risk and increased-risk groups consist of patients with known hereditary syndromes or bowel diseases or patients with a personal/family history of polyps or cancer, all of which will be discussed in a later section of the chapter (Table 23–2).

The majority of cases, however, are sporadic colon cancers that typically arise within a polyp. Geographic and migrational studies have suggested that the Western lifestyle increases the risk for colon cancer, hence suggesting that nutritional and environmental factors may play a key role.[11] A large number of epidemiological studies have been undertaken to identify these individual, nutritional, lifestyle, genetic, and environmental factors that would either predispose to or prevent the development of colorectal polyps and cancer[12] (Table 23–3).

EXTRINSIC RISK FACTORS

Dietary Fiber, Meat, and Fat

One of the characteristics of a Western diet generally has been the lack of fiber as opposed to the increased amount of meat, total fat, and animal fats.[13,14] In view of the known geographic differences, with the highest colorectal cancer incidence in industrialized nations,[3] high-fat and low-fiber diet generally has been considered a risk factor for the development of colorectal

TABLE 23–2. COMPARISON OF MAJOR RISK CATEGORIES

	SCC	FAP	HNPCC	IBD
Variants		AFAP, Gardner, Turcot	Lynch I/II	Ulcerative colitis Crohn's disease
Genetics		+ Autosomal-dominant	+ Autosomal-dominant	?
Genes	Chromosomal deletions, K-*ras*, *DCC*, *p53*, *APC*	*APC*	*MSH2*, *MLH1*, *PMS1/2*, *MSH6*	?
Age of onset	>40 yrs Average 70–75	Polyps start after age 10–20, cancer in 100% at age 40	<50 yrs	Any, often young patients
Number of polyps	Variable, <10	>100	<10	Inflammatory pseudopolyps
Risk	5–6% of population	100%	>80%	Depending on age at onset, duration of disease, extent of active disease
Location	Left > right colon	Any location	Right > left colon	Active disease
Chemoprevention	NSAID? Vitamins? Calcium?	NSAID	?	IBD suppression?
Screening	> 50 yrs (45 yrs in African Americans)	>10–15 yrs Genetic counseling	>25 or 10–15 yrs before cancer onset in youngest family member Genetic counseling	7 yrs post onset, annually
Associated risks	?	Desmoids	Endometrium and other cancers	Extracolonic disease

SCC, sporadic colon cancer; FAP, familial polyposis syndromes; AFAP, attenuated FAP; HNPCC, hereditary nonpolyposis colon cancer; IBD, inflammatory bowel disease.

cancer. This concept gained support from epidemiological studies[15] and resulted in common recommendations of high-fiber supplements in order to increase the stool bulk, dilute toxins, and reduce the colonic transit time and thus the exposure time to fecal carcinogens.[16–19] More recent prospective trials, however, have questioned the benefit of dietary fiber supplementation in that they were at best inconclusive and did not reduce the incidence of colorectal cancer.[17,20,21] On the other hand, selected fats such as *n*-3 fatty acids found in fish oils may have a protective effect.[22] It therefore could be concluded that the total amount of fats or fibers is of lesser importance than their quality and origin.[13,23] The protective effect of vegetables and fruits[22,24] may come not only from their fiber content but also from the content of antioxidative and antiproliferative agents such as isothiocyanates in cruciferous vegetables (e.g., broccoli), which may enhance the expression of carcinogen-metabolizing enzymes and induce apoptosis in neoplastic cells.[25]

Calcium, Vitamins, and Micronutrients

Several prospective studies suggested that increased oral calcium intake may protect from colorectal polyps,[26–29] whereas other studies could not verify a significant benefit. The mechanism by which calcium supplements are thought to reduce the risk of colon cancer are twofold. First, calcium can bind bile and fatty acids in the stool to insoluble complexes that are less likely to attack the colonic mucosa, and second, it can interfere directly with the mucosal cells and decrease their proliferative potential on a cellular level.[15]

Several vitamins were found to have a cancer-protective effect. Vitamins A, C, and E have been shown to have antioxidant activity. Results from interventional studies, however, have remained somewhat disappointing or controversial.[30]

In a study on postmenopausal women, another correlation was found between dietary heme iron and an increased risk of proximal colon cancer, especially in conjunction with alcohol consumption, whereas intake of dietary zinc reduced the risk of both proximal and distal colon cancer.[31]

Aspirin and COX-2 Inhibitors

Aspirin and other nonsteroidal anti-inflammatory drugs (NSAIDs) may interfere with the development of

TABLE 23–3. RISK FACTORS ASSOCIATED WITH COLON CANCER

Risk Factor	Comment
Geographic variation	Highest risk in Western countries and lowest risk in developing countries
Age	Risk increase sharply after the fifth decade
Diet	Increased with total and animal fat diets
Physical inactivity	Increased with obesity and sedentary life style
Adenoma	Risk dependent on type and size
FAP penetrance in gene carriers	100%
HNPCC penetrance in gene carriers	80%
Hamartomatous syndromes	Risk increased with Peutz-Jeghers syndrome and juvenile polyposis but not isolated juvenile polyps
Previous history of colon cancer	Increased risk for recurrent cancer
Ulcerative colitis	10–20% after 20 years
Radiation	Associated with a mucinous histology and poor prognosis
Ureterosigmoidostomy	100–500 times increased risk at or adjacent to the uretero-colonic anastomosis

Reproduced, with permission, from Wu JS, Fazio VW, 2000.[220]

colorectal neoplasms by blocking the cyclooxygenase-dependent prostaglandin pathway. The targets are the constitutive COX-1, as well as the cytokine-inducible COX-2, which has been found at increased expression levels in both polyps and cancers.[32] Several trials therefore have studied these agents (e.g., aspirin and sulindac) for the chemoprevention of colorectal cancer both in sporadic polyps[33] and cancers and in familial adenomatous polyposis (FAP).[34–36] In both settings, controlled studies have provided contradictory results. Regular prophylactic medication with low-dose aspirin may reduce the risk of sporadic colorectal cancer if it is given for more than a decade.[33] Data from chemoprevention trials in FAP suggest that cyclooxygenase inhibition may delay the onset and number of adenomatous polyps, but it is not yet clear whether its is able to prevent the cancers overall or reduce their respective risk.[34–36] COX-2-independent mechanisms may play a role for the beneficial effect of some COX-2 inhibitors.[37] A major recent concern, however, has been the documented increased risk of serious cardiovascular events with the use of COX-2 inhibitors.[38,39]

Since data on the benefits remain conflicting, physicians must decide how to use these pharmacologic tools and calcium in the management of their patients. Based on the presumed small risks in general and the supporting data on a possible benefit, most physicians would be inclined to err on the side of a potential benefit in preventing colon polyp formation. However, recent concern about cardiovascular side effects and increased mortality has resulted in a withdrawal of COX-2 inhibitors until further redefinition of the indications and risk groups has been accomplished.[38,39]

Cholecystectomy and Bile Acids

Evidence that bile acids may act as cocarcinogens or tumor promotors comes from both experimental and epidemiological studies.[40,41] Bile acids can induce hyperproliferation of the intestinal mucosa via a number of intracellular mechanisms. Cholecystectomy, which alters the enterohepatic cycle of bile acids, has been associated with a moderately increased risk of proximal colon cancers.[42,43] It cannot be ruled out, however, that it is less the effect of the cholecystectomy than the impact of other, not yet identified factors in the lithogenic bile of such patients. A number of cofactors have been identified that may enhance or neutralize the carcinogenic effects of bile acids, e.g., the amount of dietary fat, fiber,[15] or calcium.[44] Calcium, in fact, binds bile acids and thus may reduce their negative impact. However, other more intrinsic mucosa-protective mechanisms of calcium supplements probably are more relevant for the demonstrated reduction of recurrent adenomatous colon polyps.

Smoking and Alcohol Consumption

The risk of colorectal cancer is increased, even though only modestly, among long-term smokers compared with nonsmokers.[19,45,46] The data suggested a dose-response relationship between pack-years of tobacco use and the development of adenomatous polyps.[47–49] Equally, excessive alcohol consumption has been associated with an increased risk for colon cancer.[19,45,46,49]

Other Factors

An ever-increasing number of other factors are accumulating that have been attributed to an increased risk of colon cancer, e.g., lack of physical activity, diabetes, serum insulin levels, elevated concentrations of insulin-like growth factor 1, and low concentrations of insulin-like growth factor binding protein 3 (IGFBP-3).[50] The complexity of interactions between these factors and the previously mentioned parameters, however, makes it difficult at the present time to draw conclusions that have an impact on the clinical practice.

INTRINSIC RISK FACTORS

Personal and Family History

There is generally little debate that the presence of an adenomatous or inflammatory colonic pathology in itself represents a risk factor for a subsequent colon cancer. In patients with a colon cancer, synchronous colorectal cancers are found in 5–10%, whereas about 10–20% of patients with a history of colorectal cancer will develop metachronous primary cancers in the large intestine. A personal history of adenomatous colonic polyps is an indicator for an increased colonic predisposition to develop subsequent adenomatous or cancerous changes.

Compared with the general population, relatives of patients with colon cancer have a two to four times increased risk of developing the disease themselves[19,51,52] (Table 23–4). A similar, even though proportionally lesser risk is observed for family members of individuals with colonic adenomatous polyps.[52]

TABLE 23–4. LIFETIME RISKS OF COLORECTAL CANCER IN FIRST-DEGREE RELATIVES OF PATIENTS WITH COLON CANCER

Population risk	1 in 50
One relative affected	1 in 17
One first-degree relative and one second-degree relative affected	1 in 12
One relative aged under 45 affected	1 in 10
Two first-degree relatives affected	1 in 6
Dominant pedigree	1 in 2

Reproduced, with permission, from Houlston RS et al, 1986.[77]

Inflammatory Bowel Disease

Inflammatory bowel disease is a strong risk factor for colorectal cancer. The risk correlates with the age of onset and extent and duration of active disease[53,54] (Table 23–5 and Fig 23–1). In contrast, however, the disease activity historically was not thought to be correlated with the risk, but recent studies have challenged this view.[55] In ulcerative colitis, the risk of colorectal cancer increases from approximately 3% in the first decade to 10–20% in the second decade.[54] In patients with Crohn's disease with colonic involvement, the disease-associated risk for colorectal cancer is also elevated, but generally to a lesser extent.[56–58]

Other Factors

Less frequent risk factors for colorectal cancers may include a history of a ureterocolostomy[59] or previous radiation treatment.[60] The former requires the combination of fecal bacteria and urine because the microbes degrade urinary metabolites into strong carcinogens.[61,62] When colonic mucosa is used for bladder augmentation, no increased cancer risk is observed owing to the absence of bacteria. Radiation-induced colorectal cancer is a little less clear, but it has been suggested that it may be associated with a mucinous histology and poor prognosis.[60]

PREVENTION AND SCREENING

Since symptoms are not reliable for early detection of colorectal cancer, risk-adjusted screening programs for asymptomatic individuals are important. Effective screening has to be based on an understanding of the adenoma-carcinoma sequence, which may take up to 5–10 years from the first molecular change to a clinically manifest cancer, and should reflect an individual's genetic and disease- or age-dependent risk for the development of colorectal cancer.[9,10,63] Any prevention program has to be sensitive but also practical and cost-effective in order to achieve a broad screening of the population at risk. The term *screening* is applicable only to asymptomatic people; if symptoms are present, it is not screening but diagnostic tests that are initiated. Common tools for screening include fecal occult blood tests, flexible sigmoidoscopies or colonoscopies, and contrast enemas. The American Cancer Society, endorsed by the major professional societies, recommends starting colorectal cancer screening in asymptomatic average-risk adults at age 50.[9,10,63] A slightly earlier screening start at age of 45 has been recommended recently for African-American patients based on their statistically increased risk.[7] A first baseline colonoscopy is to be performed and, if no pathology is found, repeated every 10 years. In addition, a fecal occult blood test (FOBT) should be done at an annual basis, and any positive result should precipitate a full colonic evaluation. Every 5 years, a limited endoscopy (flexible sigmoidoscopy) or barium enema is indicated. If precursor lesions are found, they should be removed and a colonoscopy be performed after 1–3 years to detect missed (20%) or recurrent polyps.[64]

In individuals at increased risk (e.g., personal/family history of polyps or cancer or African-Ameri-

TABLE 23–5. RELATIVE RISK OF COLORECTAL CANCER AMONG PATIENTS WITH ULCERATIVE COLITIS ACCORDING TO SEX, EXTENT OF DISEASE AT DIAGNOSIS, AND AGE AT DIAGNOSIS

Variable	Observed Cases	Person-Years of Follow-Up	SIR (95% CI)[a]
Sex			
Male	52	19,312	5.6 (4.2–7.4)
Female	39	16,268	5.9 (4.2–8.0)
Extent of disease			
Proctitis	9	11,170	1.7 (0.8–3.2)
Left-sided colitis	17	11,169	2.8 (1.6–4.4)
Pancolitis	65	13,241	14.8 (11.4–18.9)
Age at onset (yr)			
0–14	13	4,220	118.3 (63.0–202.3)
15–29	21	14,047	16.5 (10.2–25.2)
30–39	15	6,892	8.2 (4.6–13.6)
40–49	16	4,119	6.1 (3.5–9.8)
50–59	11	3,294	3.4 (1.7–6.1)
≥ 60	15	3,008	2.2 (1.2–3.6)

[a]SIR, standardized incidence ratio; CI, confidence interval. Reproduced, with permission, from Ekbom A et al, 1990.[53]

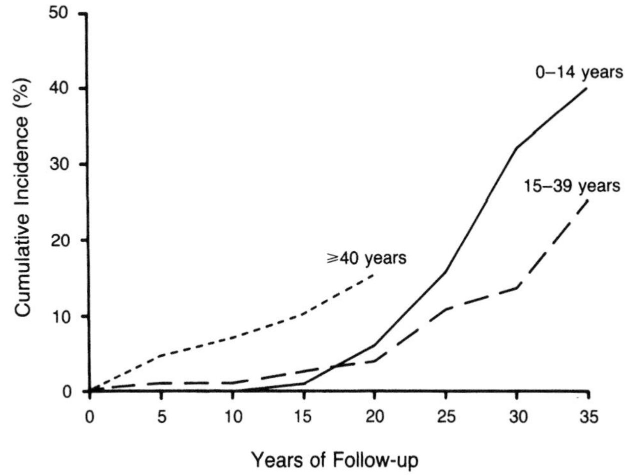

Figure 23–1. Impact of the age at diagnosis on the cumulative incidence of colorectal cancer in patients with pancolitis. Patients diagnosed with pancolitis when they were younger than 15 years of age are represented by solid line, when they were 15–39 years of age by dashed line, and when they were 40 years of age or older by the dotted line. (Reproduced, with permission, from Ekbom A, Helmick C, Zack M, Adami HO. Ulcerative colitis and colorectal cancer: A population-based study. *N Engl J Med* 1990;323:1228–1233.)

can ethnicity) or at high risk (e.g., cancer syndromes or inflammatory bowel disease), the screening has to start earlier (see Table 23–2) and has to be performed at a higher frequency.[7,65] Successful screening programs have been shown to reduce the colorectal cancer incidence by 76–90%.[66]

▪ PATHOGENESIS OF COLONIC CANCER

Carcinogenesis in the colon is a complex multistep process in which a multitude of alterations have to coincide in order to transform a normal cell into a malignant cell. Several categories of genes are involved that normally are regulated in a sophisticated network to keep a tight balance between cell growth and turnover, cell death, DNA replication, and mismatch repair. Disruption of the fine balance between oncogenes, which promote cell proliferation, and tumor suppressor genes, which inhibit excessive growth, results in a growth advantage and allows malignant cells to expand.

COLON CANCER: A GENETIC DISEASE

All cells of even such a complex organism as a human being have DNA that is virtually identical to the DNA found in the zygotes. DNA mutations can occur either as a germ-line mutation or as a somatic mutation. The former may be transmitted from one to the next generation as an inherited defect. More commonly, a spontaneous mutation occurs in a non-germ-line cell during the growth, development, and maintenance of a tissue or organ (somatic mutation). Even in the cycle of a normally functioning cell, there is a high chance of spontaneous gene mutations, most of which will not result in a growth advantage to the harboring cell. Genesis of a cancer therefore requires several independent accidents to occur in one cell. One can assume that a normal cell will be able to detect damage to its own DNA and maintain an effective repair mechanism. However, if the cell is too severely damaged, it might rather initiate the inherent suicide program called *apoptosis*. When a cell fails to recognize or correct a DNA damage and continues to replicate, accumulation of faulty gene products within the cell eventually may lead to a proliferative response. If that replication exceeds the growth potential of the neighboring normal cells, the mutation provides a growth advantage that will increase the state of "genetic instability" and hence lead toward a malignant cell.[67] Despite this potential, most mutations are silent or lethal to the cell rather than beneficial in terms of providing the cell a biologic advantage. The triggers and the step-by-step cumulative failures that lead to carcinogenesis still are relatively poorly understood.

Two types of genetic instability may occur: at the chromosome level or at the DNA level. A loss of chromosomal material, i.e., a chromosomal instability (CIN), results when the chromosomes are not divided symmetrically during mitosis such that one daughter cell receives both copies and the other cell receives none. On an electrophoretic gel, this can be visualized as a loss of one or more bands, which is described as *loss of heterozygosity* (LOH), and has been associated with a worse prognosis of colorectal cancer.[68] The second form of genetic instability, at the DNA level, occurs when replication errors in repetitive short polymorphisms lead to an additional band or bands.[69] This phenomenon is described as *microsatellite instability* (MSI), and it has been a characteristic feature of hereditary nonpolyposis colon cancers (HNPCCs).[70]

During the process of cell division, DNA is duplicated, with the original DNA serving as a template for the replicated copy. DNA polymerase serves as a "proofreader" that recognizes mismatched genes, halts the DNA synthesis, removes the defective sequence, and then resynthesizes the DNA. Failure of the DNA mismatch repair system predisposes to the development of mutations within daughter cells. Enzymes that monitor newly formed DNA and correct replication errors are called *DNA mismatch repair* (MMR) *systems*.

Specific gene functions are lost when both copies (alleles) of a gene are inactivated. Thus, when a germline mutation occurs in a suppressor gene, only the mutation of the remaining normal allele is required for the gene's loss of function. When both copies of the gene are normal, two mutational events are required for the gene's loss of function. This two-hit hypothesis may explain why inherited diseases usually manifest at an earlier age than sporadic disease.[2]

THE ADENOMA-CARCINOMA MODEL

After identifying several genetic alterations in colorectal specimens at various stages of their neoplastic transformation and progression, Vogelstein and colleagues in 1988 pioneered a genetic model for colorectal tumorigenesis that since has been known as the *adenoma-carcinoma sequence*[71] (Fig 23–2). This multistep model described the carcinogenesis as an accumulation of genetic events, uninhibited cell growth, and proliferation and clonal development. Gene mutations and chromosomal/gene losses that were observed in sporadic colon cancer include the *APC* gene (adenoma–polyposis coli), *MMC* gene (mutated in colon cancer), K-*ras*, *DCC* (deleted in colon cancer), and *p53*.[68,72,73] Mutations of the

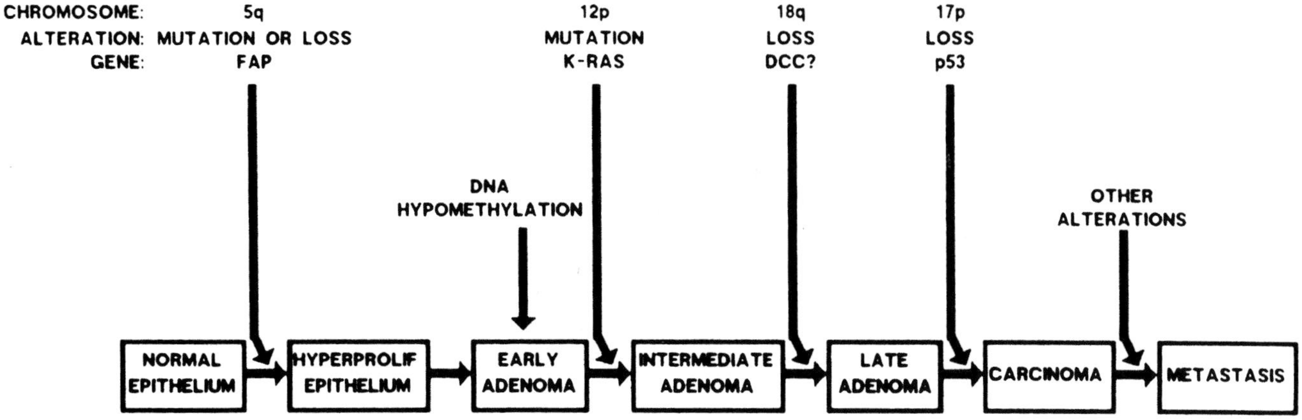

Figure 23–2. Genetic model for colorectal tumorigenesis (adenoma-carcinoma sequence). (Reproduced, with permission, from Fearon ER, Vogelstein B. A genetic model for colorectal tumorigenesis. *Cell* 1990;61:759–767.)

APC gene, which is involved in the control of cell-to-cell adhesions and intercellular communication, are found in 60% of even small adenomatous polyps, as well as in carcinomas,[74] and therefore are believed to occur as a very early event in carcinogenesis. Mutations of K-*ras*, which under normal function plays a role in intracellular signal transduction and stimulated cell division, occur in larger adenomas and carcinomas and are thought to stimulate cell growth. Deletion of the tumor suppressor gene *DCC* may be important in the progression from a benign polyp toward a malignant condition.[75] Mutations of the *p53* gene, which are among the most frequent gene mutations in human cancers, are also common in invasive colon cancers but rare in adenomas, suggesting that *p53* mutations occur as a late event in the development of the invasive phenotype.[76] The wide range of gene mutations, inactivations, and deletions in the progression to carcinoma seems to hold the secret code for the various tumor behaviors observed in the clinical setting. It is important to note, however, that an increasing number of other genetic events have been observed and reported and that no single event seems to be equally present in all colon cancers. One therefore should caution that the described sequence is only one possible model and that the scenario may not reflect all aspects of colonic carcinogenesis.

▪ HEREDITARY AND NONHEREDITARY COLON TUMORS

NONHEREDITARY COLON CANCER

Sporadic Colon Cancer

Sporadic colon cancer, i.e., colon cancer arising in individuals without a family history or an inherited predisposition, accounts for approximately 60% of all colorectal cancers and affects patients commonly above the age of 50. The risk factors associated with sporadic development of colon cancer have been discussed previously in the epidemiological section of this chapter (see Table 23–3).

Familial Colon Cancer

Familial colon cancer is the second most common (25–30%)[2] and at the same time least understood pattern of genetic colon cancer development. In affected families, colon cancer develops too frequently to be considered a sporadic colon cancer, but the pattern is not consistent with the known inherited syndromes.[77] An association of familial colon cancer has been found with polymorphisms, which reflect subtle genetic changes in the form of variations in the nucleotide base sequences but which do not affect protein structure.[2] Familial colon cancer in the Ashkenazi Jewish population probably is the result of an *APC* germ-line mutation on codon 1307 (I1307K). This mutation, which predisposes to sporadic mutations at distant sites of the gene and later results in structural protein abnormalities, is found in 6% of all Ashkenazi Jews and in 28% of Ashkenazi Jews with both a personal and a family history of colon cancer.[78]

HEREDITARY COLON CANCER

Familial Adenomatous Polyposis (FAP)

Familial adenomatous polyposis (FAP) is an autosomal dominant inherited syndrome with near-complete penetrance. The offspring of affected individuals thus have a 50% risk of inheriting FAP. However, up to 20% of patients with FAP are new mutations without a family history. This condition is attributed to a truncating mutation in the germ-line adenomatous polyposis coli (*APC*) gene on chromosome 5q21.[79] Variants of the polyposis syndrome are classified as Gardener's syndrome (i.e., osteomas, desmoid tumors, thyroid neoplasms, and congenital hypertrophy of the retinal pigment epithelium) and Turcot's syndrome (i.e., brain tumors).

The inherited syndrome of FAP and its variants accounts for less than 1% of all colon cancers. It is characterized by greater than 100 and often several thousands of adenomatous intestinal polyps that start to develop in the late teens and early twenties and turn into cancer by age 40–45. An attenuated variant of the disease is relatively rare and is characterized by a lower number and a later onset of both the polyps and the resulting cancer (see below). Nearly all FAP patients develop duodenal adenomas that are severe in 10% and account for the group's second-highest cancer risk, with adenocarcinoma developing in the periampullary region in 3–10% of patients.[80,81] Carcinoma arising in the antrum and duodenum after colectomy is the main cause of cancer-related deaths in FAP patients.[80,82,83] Nonadenomatous fundic gastric polyps develop in approximately 10–30% of patients with FAP[83] but usually do not have a malignant potential. Ten percent of FAP patients develop desmoid tumors either intra-abdominally or on the abdominal wall, extremities, and trunk.[84] Histologically, desmoids are fibromatous lesions consisting of large proliferation of myofibroblasts. Even though they do not necessarily carry features of a malignant lesion, the recent literature suggests a low-grade sarcoma-like behavior. Desmoids are lethal in 10% and are the third most frequent cause for mortality of FAP patients, mainly owing to the intra-abdominal variants, which cause small bowel and ureteral obstructions.[84,85]

Approximately 25% of FAP patients remain without an identified *APC* mutation (*APC*-negative),[86,87] and using a detailed analysis, they seem to differ in terms of lower polyp number, later age at diagnosis, and lower occurrence of extracolonic manifestations as compared with classic FAP patients.[83,88] This variant of FAP is known as *attenuated familial adenomatous polyposis* (AFAP).

Hereditary Nonpolyposis Colon Cancers (HNPCC)

Hereditary nonpolyposis colon cancer (HNPCC), also known as *Lynch I and II syndromes,* is an inherited autosomal dominant disease that accounts for 3–5% of all colorectal cancers.[89] It is characterized by an early onset of colorectal cancers predominantly but not exclusively on the right side of the colon with synchronous and metachronous cancers. Despite its name, these cancers typically arise from colonic polyps, but a diffuse polyposis is not present. The penetrance of the HNPCC predisposition is high and results in an 80–85% lifetime risk of colorectal cancer and a 40–50% risk of endometrial cancer.[90–92] Furthermore, HNPCC patients are at increased risk of developing extracolonic malignancies, such as cancer of the small bowel, stomach, hepatobiliary tract, urinary tract, ovary, and brain. The Lynch variants describe patients with predominantly colorectal cancer at a young age (Lynch I) and those with both colorectal and extracolonic cancers (Lynch II).[89]

An initial observation of expansions and contractions of microsatellite DNA in the genome of colorectal tumor specimens from HNPCC patients established a link between HNPCC and the DNA MMR system.[93–95] In contrast to the gatekeeper concept applicable to the *APC* gene in FAP, the DNA MMR genes belong to the so-called caretakers, which when inactivated do not promote tumorigenesis directly but rather lead to a genetic instability that then promotes tumor growth indirectly.[96]

In order to facilitate the clinical diagnosis off HNPCC, the International Collaborative Group on HNPCC (ICG-HNPCC) proposed the Amsterdam Criteria in 1990.[89] Linkage studies in HNPCC families fulfilling Amsterdam Criteria I (Table 23–6) led to the discovery of the first two human MMR genes—*hMSH2* and *hMLH1.* These genes accounted for 45–86% of all classic HNPCC families.[97] There also was a higher risk for *hMSH2* mutation carriers to develop extracolonic cancers, in particular endometrial cancer, as compared with *hMLH1* mutation carriers.[92,98] Several other MMR genes have been identified in conjunction with HNPCC and include *hPMS1, hPMS2,* and *hMSH6.* A recent study[99] reported that endometrial cancer represents the most common clinical manifestation of HNPCC among female *hMSH6* mutation carriers and that colorectal cancer cannot be considered an obligate requisite to define HNPCC. The ICG-HNPCC therefore revised the criteria (Amsterdam Criteria II), which now better weigh extracolonic manifestations (e.g., endometrial, breast, small bowel, and upper renal tract cancers) as part of the family history (see Table 23–6). In addition, the less restrictive revised Bethesda Criteria (Table 23–7) were adopted to better serve patients who carry *hMSH2* or *hMLH1* gene mutations but otherwise do not fulfill the Amsterdam Criteria. Testing for microsatellite instability (MSI) has become a valuable diagnostic tool to identify individuals with suspected HNPCC because 85–90% of HNPCC tumors have MSI as opposed to only 15-20% of sporadic colon cancers.[70]

Hamartomatous Polyposis Syndromes

Approximately 4% of colonic cancers are seen in the context of rare syndromes. Among these are inherited hamartomatous polyposis syndromes that are characterized by the presence of gastrointestinal hamartomatous polyps and an increased risk of gastrointestinal

TABLE 23–6. AMSTERDAM CRITERIA I AND II

Amsterdam Criteria I (1990)	Amsterdam Criteria II (1999)
At least three relatives with colorectal cancer, one of whom should be a first-degree relative of the other two.	There should be at least three relatives with HNPCC-associated cancer (colorectal cancer, cancer of the endometrium, small bowel, and ureter), of which one should be a first-degree relative of the other two.
At least two successive generations should be affected.	At least two successive generations should be affected.
At least one colorectal cancer should be diagnosed before the age 50 years.	At least one colorectal cancer should be diagnosed before the age 50 years.
FAP should be excluded.	FAP should be excluded.
Tumors should be verified by a pathologist.	Tumors should be verified by a pathologist.
	Benign tumors, by definition, do not invade adjacent tissue borders, nor do they metastasize to distal sites. By contrast, malignant tumors have the added property of invading contiguous tissues and metastasizing to distant size.
	A polyp is defined as a mass that protrudes into the lumen of the colon. They are subdivided according to the attachment to the bowel wall (e.g., sessile or pedunculated), their histologic appearance (e.g., hyperplastic or adenomas), and their neoplastic potential (i.e., benign or malignant).

Reproduced, with permission, from Vasen HFA, 2000.[221]

malignancy. Hamartomas result from a disordered differentiation during embryonic development and are characterized morphologically by disrupted representations of normal tissue components.

Peutz-Jeghers Syndrome. Peutz-Jeghers syndrome is the second most common hamartomatous syndrome, occurring as an autosomal dominant condition with variable penetrance. Genetic alterations in the *LKB1/STK* (19p13) gene are responsible for approximately 50% of the cases of Peutz-Jeghers syndrome.[100] The syndrome is associated with hamartomatous polyps of the gastrointestinal tract and cutaneous melanin deposition. The most common location of Peutz-Jeghers polyps is in the upper gastrointestinal tract, specifically the upper jejunum. One of the most characteristic features is the melanin depositions that is seen most frequently in the perioral region or buccal mucosa but which also can occur in the genital region and on the hands and the feet. While a majority of these patients remain relatively asymptomatic, some may present with abdominal pain secondary to obstruction or impending obstruction owing to an intussuscepted polyp and others with gastrointestinal bleeding. Patients with Peutz-Jeghers syndrome have a moderately increased risk in the range of 2–3% to develop gastrointestinal malignancies as well as extraintestinal malignancies.

Juvenile Polyposis Syndrome. Juvenile polyposis syndrome is the most common hamartomatous syndrome and is inherited as an autosomal dominant trait. The average age of onset is approximately 18 years, and there is an association with congenital birth defects in 15% of patients.[101] Although the diagnostic criteria for juvenile polyposis syndrome are somewhat controversial, the most commonly used criteria include three or more juvenile polyps of the colon, polyposis involving the entire gastrointestinal tract, or any number of polyps in a member of a family with a known history of juvenile polyps.[102]

In infancy, patients may present with acute or chronic gastrointestinal bleeding, intussusception, rectal prolapse, or a protein-losing enteropathy. In adulthood, patients commonly present with either acute or chronic gastrointestinal blood loss. Most of these patients will be found to have polyps, which are located most frequently in the rectosigmoid region.

A germ-line mutation in the *SMAD-4* gene (18q21) accounts for approximately 50% of the reported cases of the syndrome.[103] A significant risk of colorectal cancer is associated with juvenile polyposis syndrome, which should not be confused with isolated juvenile polyps because the latter have virtually no malignant potential.

TABLE 23–7. REVISED BETHESDA GUIDELINES (2002) FOR TESTING COLORECTAL TUMORS FOR MSI

Criterion	Comment
Colorectal cancer diagnosed in a patient less than 50 years of age	
Presence of synchronous, metachronous colorectal cancer, or other HNPCC-associated tumor, regardless of age	Stomach, ovarian, pancreas, ureter and renal pelvis, biliary tract, and brain, sebaceous gland adenomas and keratoacanthomas, and small bowel
Colorectal cancer with MSI-high histology diagnosed in a patient less than 60 years of age	Tumor infiltrating lymphocytes, Crohn's-like lymphocytic reaction, mucinous/signet-ring differentiation, or medullary growth pattern
Colorectal cancer diagnosed in at least on first-degree relative with an HNPCC-related tumor diagnosed under age 50	
Colorectal cancer diagnosed in two or more first or second-degree relatives with HNPCC-related tumors, regardless of age.	

Reproduced, with permission, from Omar A et al, 2004.[222]

Cowden Syndrome. Cowden's disease, first described in 1963, is known as multiple hamartoma-neoplasia syndrome. It is an autosomal dominant condition with nearly complete penetrance by age 20 that is caused by a germ-line mutations in the *PTEN* tumor suppressor gene located at 10q22.[104,105] Cowden's disease is unique among the hamartomatous syndromes because polyps arise more commonly from ectodermal rather than endodermal elements. Eighty percent of patients present with tricholemmoma, a benign tumor of the hair shaft. The central nervous system is the second most involved system, with approximately 40% of affected individual suffering from macrocephaly. Only 35% of patients who meet the diagnostic criteria for Cowden's disease have gastrointestinal polyposis, but no increased risk of invasive gastrointestinal malignancy has been reported to date. The majority of patients with Cowden's disease suffer from benign thyroid or breast disease, on top of which adds a projected lifetime risk of 10% for thyroid cancer and of 30–50% for breast cancer.

Bannayan-Riley-Ruvalcaba Syndrome. Formerly known as its subentity, the Ruvalcaba-Myhre-Smith syndrome, this rare autosomal dominant condition includes two other syndromes, both of which, like Cowden's disease, are associated with genetic alterations in the *PTEN* gene on chromosome 10q23 and may be considered a variant of juvenile polyposis coli.[106–108] It is characterized by hamartomatous polyps of the gastrointestinal tract, macrocephaly, mental retardation, delayed psychomotor development, lipid storage myopathy, Hashimoto's thyroiditis, and hyperpigmentation of the skin of the penis. No increased risk of colorectal carcinoma, other gastrointestinal malignancies, or extraintestinal malignancy has been documented in these patients.

Cronkite-Canada Syndrome. Cronkite-Canada syndrome is characterized by diffuse polyposis and ectodermal abnormalities such as alopecia, onychodystrophy, and skin hyperpigmentation. The syndrome can be distinguished by the diffuse distribution of polyps throughout the entire gastrointestinal tract with exception of the esophagus, which is spared.[109] Symptoms include diarrhea, weight loss, nausea, vomiting, and anorexia, as well as paresthesias, seizures, and tetany related to electrolyte abnormalities. Cancer occurs in the stomach, colon, and rectum, but it remains controversial whether polyps in Cronkite-Canada syndrome possess malignant potential. As many as 15% of patients with Cronkite-Canada syndrome have a malignant tumor at the time of diagnosis.

▪ PATHOLOGY AND STAGING

POLYPS

Polyp is a descriptive term for any mucosal elevation. Polyps are subdivided according to their attachment to the bowel wall (e.g., sessile or pedunculated), their nature (e.g., hyperplastic, hamartomas, or adenomas), their histologic appearance (e.g., tubulous, tubulovillous, or villous), and their neoplastic dignity (i.e., benign or malignant). A neoplastic lesion consists of cells that have the potential to acquire with time the ability to invade and to spread, i.e., metastasize, to another location in the body.

Hyperplastic Polyps and Hyperplastic Polyposis

A hyperplastic or metaplastic polyp is a small, sessile mucosal outgrowth of 3–6 mm diameter that displays an exaggerated crypt architecture. Only rarely (1–4%) are hyperplastic polyps larger than 1 cm; however, these larger polyps actually may be serrated adenomas rather than hyperplastic polyps.[110] Hyperplastic polyps are found commonly in the large bowel, predominantly in the rectum and sigmoid colon, and they have been reported in up to 75% of patients over age 60 at autopsy.[111] It is not unusual to find several of these polyps in a single individual.

Histologically, hyperplastic polyps display well-formed glands and crypts that are lined by nonneoplastic epithelial cells. These polyps may be confused with serrated adenomas because of their morphologic similarities. Because of their small size, hyperplastic polyps rarely cause symptoms. However, large or multiple hyperplastic polyps occasionally can be responsible for gastrointestinal symptoms. Although these asymptomatic polyps are not considered premalignant per se, they may—in a paradigm shift—be indicators for other premalignant conditions.[19]

Hyperplastic polyposis is a rare condition that was first described in 1980.[110] This condition is characterized by numerous hyperplastic polyps throughout the large bowel that give the mucosa a "studded" look. The endoscopic and radiologic appearance of the mucosal abnormalities closely resembles FAP, but hyperplastic polyposis is not heritable and does not have any extraintestinal manifestations. The World Health Organization (WHO) has defined this entity as follows: (1) at least five histologically diagnosed hyperplastic polyps of which two are greater than 20 mm or (2) any number of hyperplastic polyps occurring proximal to the sigmoid colon in someone who has a first-degree relative with hyperplastic polyposis, or (3) more than 30 hyperplastic polyps of any size that are distributed throughout the colon and rectum. Since patients with hyperplastic polyposis may have associated cancers and a family history of colorectal cancer, colonic surveillance should be recommended.

Adenomatous Polyps (Adenomas)

The most common epithelial neoplasm in the colon is the adenomatous polyp, which occurs as tubulous, tubulovillous, and villous variants. It may either be pedunculated (with a stalk) or sessile (broad-based).[112] By definition, the adenomatous polyps' neoplastic nature in itself is a manifestation of colonic dysplasia. However, different degrees of dysplasia are distinguished commonly that parallel the likelihood of cancerous transformation. The degree of dysplasia can be divided into three grades based on the histopathologic differentiation and the arrangement and architecture of the epithelial cells and the acinar complexes. Common terms for still benign polyps include *low-grade dysplasia, intermediate-grade dysplasia,* and *high-grade dysplasia* or *in situ adenocarcinoma.* Once there are clear microscopic features of tumor invasion through the basal membrane into the polyp stalk or base, an invasive cancer is present. The term *malignant polyp* is used often but in truth is a euphemism because tumor invading into the submucosa reflects a T1 cancer with a 7–10% risk of nodal metastasis.[113] The term *invasive adenocarcinoma* is appropriate for neoplastic lesions that have invaded through the basal membrane and the muscularis mucosae into the submucosa. The descriptive terms then switch to *well-differentiated* (grade I), *moderately differentiated* (grade II), or *poorly differentiated* (grade III) *adenocarcinoma* as additional criteria for staging (see later section in this chapter).

Flat and/or depressed adenomas are a subtype of colonic adenomata with a propensity for high-grade dysplasia (carcinoma in situ) in 10–41% of affected patients regardless of the small size of these lesions.[114] These lesions, which are flat or slightly raised to less than 2 mm and commonly less than 1 cm in size, may be overlooked easily on colonoscopy and turn into a cancer before having reached a size comparable with classic cancers.[114–116] The entity was first described in Japan, where they seem to occur at a regular frequency. However, more recent screening studies in other countries, which took advantage of chromoendoscopy techniques, have confirmed that flat adenomas represent up to 25–36% of all polyps found in a random cohort.[117] It is difficult to estimate the likelihood that a small adenoma will progress to a larger and more dysplastic adenoma and eventually into a cancer. A number of biologic and molecular markers have been analyzed at predictors of a malignant potential.[118] Longitudinal and comparative data suggest that polyps not only progress but also may regress.[119]

Invasive carcinoma is present in 5% of all adenomas, but the incidence correlates with the size and type of the adenoma[112,120] (Table 23–8). The Haggitt classification, which defines four levels within the polyp, has evolved as a useful tool to describe the degree of invasion into a pedunculated or sessile polyp adenoma.[121] This classification forms the basis of the management of malignant polyps (Fig 23–3). In Haggitt levels 1, 2, and 3, the risk of lymph node metastasis is less than 1%, whereas a level 4 invasion of the stalk behaves like a sessile lesion and carries a much higher risk of 12–25% of having lymph node metastases. A similar but less well-known classification was developed in 1993 by Kudo, who for prognostic purposes suggested to divide the submucosal invasion of sessile malignant lesions into three levels[122] (Fig 23–4). In other studies, multivariate analysis showed that the depth of invasion into the submucosa in the poorly differentiated carcinoma was correlated with the risk of lymph node metastases that posed the high risk.[113]

Management of Colonic Polyps. The majority of polyps can be removed colonoscopically, which will reduce the risk for an invasive neoplasm by 76–90%.[66] However, if there are too many polyps (e.g., polyposis or numerous sporadic polyps), or if a polyp is very large and sessile, endoscopic removal increasingly carries two associated risks—first that the polyp harbors a cancer despite negative biopsies (false-negative result owing to sampling error) and second that the broad and deep endoscopic removal causes a perforation that, in the case of a cancer, would be detrimental because a confined tumor would be allowed to spill into the intraperitoneal cavity.

When invasive cancer is found in a polyp, the management is based on the level of invasion and the completeness of polypectomy. Based on Haggitt's observations,[121] it has been suggested to treat pedunculated colonic cancers with Haggitt levels 1, 2, and 3 with complete endoscopic excision or snaring, whereas level 4 lesions should be treated as sessile T1 tumors. A sessile lesion, which can be snared adequately in one piece and on microscopic examination shows a clear margin of more than 2 mm, is con-

TABLE 23–8. ADENOMATOUS POLYPS AND VILLOUS ADENOMA: SIZE, HISTOLOGICAL TYPE, AND PERCENT OF CARCINOMA

Histologic Type	Size		
	<1 cm	1–2 cm	>2 cm
Tubular adenoma	1% (1382)	10.2% (392)	34.7% (101)
Intermediate type	3.9% (76)	7.4% (149)	45.8% (155)
Villous adenoma	9.5% (21)	10.3% (39)	52.9% (174)

Reproduced, with permission, from Muto T et al, 1975.[223]

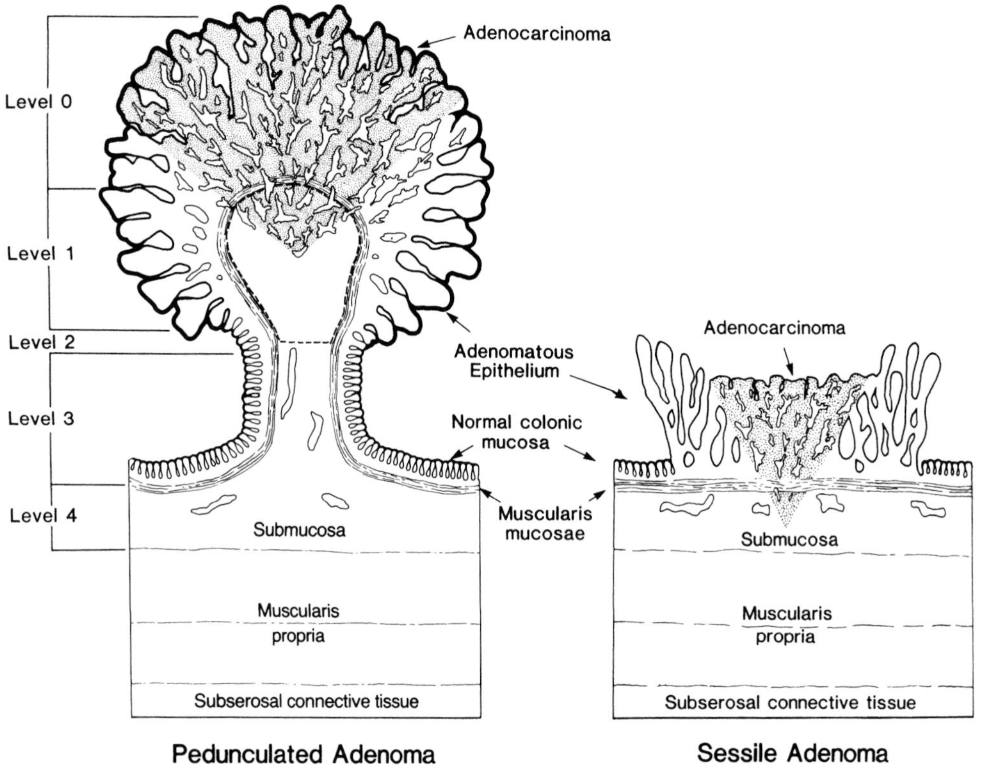

Figure 23–3. Haggitt's classification of tumor invasion in pedunculated or sessile polyp. Pedunculated polyps: level 0—not invasive carcinoma; level 1—invasion to the head of the pedunculated polyp; level 2—invasion to the neck of the pedunculated polyp; level 3—invasion to the stalk of the pedunculated polyp; level 4—invasion to the base of the pedunculated polyp. Sessile polyps: All lesions are level 4. (Reproduced, with permission, from Haggitt RC, Glotzbach RE, Soffer EE, Wruble LD. Prognostic factors in colorectal carcinomas arising in adenomas: Implications for lesions removed by endoscopic polypectomy. *Gastroenterology* 1985;89:328–336.)

sidered adequately managed. If a sessile lesion is removed in piecemeal technique and demonstrates lymphovascular invasion, deep invasion into level Sm3, or has a microscopically clear margin of less than 2 mm, the patient should undergo an oncologic colonic resection. It is advisable in any case to tattoo the area of a suspect polyp endoscopically with India ink for later identification.

CARCINOMA OF THE COLON

Carcinoma, i.e., a malignant epithelial tumor, is the most frequent malignancy of the gastrointestinal tract. Based on the endodermal glandular tissue origin, adenocarcinoma and its histologic variants are by far the predominant histopathology and account for 90–95% of all colorectal malignancies. Squamous and adenosquamous carcinoma are exceptionally rare and are located characteristically in the rectoanal junction. The histopathologic classification of colorectal cancer as defined by the WHO is illustrated in Table 23–9.

Macroscopically, most colorectal cancers have either a polypoid or an ulcerative-infiltrating appearance, but combinations are frequent. Very rarely, colorectal cancer may have a dissolute growth pattern and resemble linitis

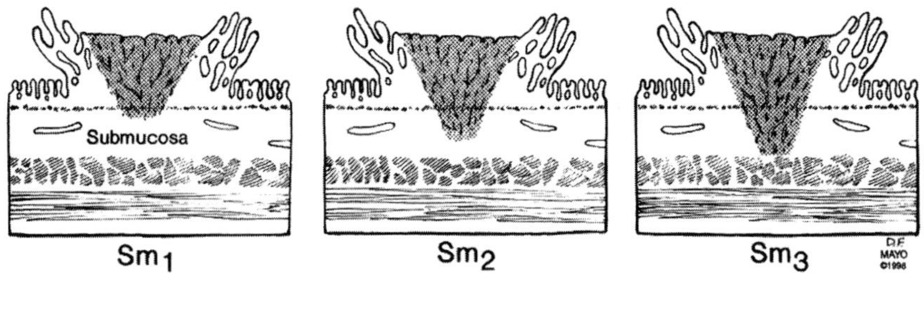

Figure 23–4. Depth of submucosal invasion in sessile malignant polyps. Sm1: invasion into upper third of submucosa; Sm2: invasion into middle third of submucosa; Sm3: invasion into lower third of submucosa. (Reproduced, with permission, from Nivatvongs S. Surgical management of early colorectal cancer. *World J Surg* 2000;24:1052–1055.)

TABLE 23–9. WHO HISTOPATHOLOGIC CLASSIFICATION OF COLORECTAL CANCERS AND THEIR SIGNIFICANCE

Histopathologic Types	Pathology	Prognosis
Adenocarcinoma	90–95% of the colorectal malignancies	
Mucinous adenocarcinoma	10% of all colorectal cancers; the extracellular type is more common than the intracellular type	Controversial whether mucinous histology itself is an independent negative prognostic factor
Signet ring cell carcinoma		
Small cell carcinoma (oat cell)	<1%; histologically identical to small cell carcinoma of the lung	Extremely poor prognosis and almost all cases have lymph node, liver and brain metastasis
Small cell adenosquamous carcinoma		
Squamous cell carcinoma		
Undifferentiated carcinoma (medullary)		

plastica of the stomach, in which case a metastatic lesion from another primary site (e.g., lobular breast cancer or stomach cancer) or a nonepithelial neoplasia (e.g., lymphoma or carcinoid) would have to be ruled out.

Adenocarcinoma

Adenocarcinoma, the exceedingly predominant histopathology of colon cancer, has a less frequent variant of mucinous adenocarcinoma that includes signet ring cell carcinoma and accounts for approximately 10% of all colorectal cancers. Compared with nonmucinous colon cancers, mucinous carcinomas usually present at a more advanced stage and thus have an overall poorer prognosis.[4,123,124]

A rare variant of colorectal cancer is small cell cancer, which accounts for less than 1% of all cases and, similar to small cell cancer of the lung, appears to be related to some degree to a neuroendocrine origin. These tumors have a high tendency to develop widespread metastasis early in the course and have an extremely poor prognosis.

The distribution of colorectal cancers among the various segments has seen a continued shift toward right-sided colon cancer.[125,126]. An estimated 45–55% of colorectal cancers are located in the rectum (10–15%) or sigmoid colon (40%) and 25–35% in the cecum or ascending colon, whereas the remaining are equally distributed through the rest of the colon. The local growth pattern for colorectal cancer involves circumferential and transmural invasion of the tumor through the intestinal wall into the peritoneal cavity or surrounding organ structures. Tumor dissemination occurs primarily through access to the lymphatic vessels into the locoregional lymph nodes or through access to the bloodstream as hematogenous metastasis to distant organs. The most common site of blood-borne spread is via the portal venous system to the liver; other secondary locations include the lung and, less frequently, kidneys, bone, etc. In addition, tumor dissemination can occur by transperitoneal seeding and result in peritoneal carcinomatosis.[127] Following gravity, peritoneal seeds may accumulate in the pelvic cul-de-sac or paracolic gutters, where they can grow to a considerable size (Blumer's shelf). Growth by perineural infiltration may be seen on microscopic examination and has a negative prognostic impact. About 20% of patients have evidence of distant metastases (stage IV disease) at the time of presentation.

Staging of Colon Cancer

Modern staging of colorectal cancer defines four clinical stages (I–IV) based on the TNM system[4,128] (Tables 23–10 and 23–11). Independent parameters are to the depth of tumor invasion into and through the layers of the intestinal wall (T), the number of regional lymph nodes involved (N), and the presence or absence of distant me-

TABLE 23–10. TNM STAGING OF COLON CANCER

Stage	Definition
Primary Tumor (T)	
TX	Primary tumor cannot be assessed
T0	No evidence of primary tumor
Tis	Carcinoma in situ: intraepithelial or invasion of lamina propria
T1	Tumor invades submucosa
T2	Tumor invades muscularis propria
T3	Tumore invades through muscularis propria into the subserosa or into nonperitonealized pericolic or perirectal tissues
T4	Tumor perforates visceral peritoneum or directly invades other organs or structures
Regional lymph nodes (N)	
NX	Regional lymph nodes could not be assesed
N0	No regional lymph node metastases
N1	Metastasis in one to three regional lymph nodes
N2	Metastasis in four or more regional lymph nodes
Distant metastasis (M)	
MX	Distant metastasis could not be assessed
M0	No distant metastasis
M1	Distant metstasis
Extent of resection	
RX	Presence of residual tumor cannot be assessed
R0	No residual tumor
R1	Microscopic residual tumor
R2	Macroscopic residual tumor

TABLE 23–11. STAGING SYSTEM BY AMERICAN JOINT COMMITTEE ON CANCER (AJCC, 6TH EDITION)

Stage	T	N	M
0	Tis	N0	M0
I	T1	N0	M0
	T2	N0	M0
IIA	T3	N0	M0
IIB	T4	N0	M0
IIIA	T1–T2	N1	M0
IIIB	T3–T4	N1	M0
IIIC	Any T	N2	M0
IV	Any T	Any N	M1

tastases (M). Additional modifiers are used to reflect the method of stage determination (p for pathology, c for clinical, u for ultrasound). Historical classifications such as Dukes and Astler-Coller still are in use sporadically but largely have been and should be abandoned.

Since the extent of tumor resection (complete versus incomplete) strongly correlates with prognosis, the American Joint Committee on Cancer (AJCC) released additional guidelines to reflect the extent of residual tumor after a surgical resection with the letter R[128] (see Table 23–10).

NONEPITHELIAL TUMORS OF THE COLON

Benign Nonepithelial Tumors

Lipomas and Lipomatous Polyposis. Lipomas are submucosal lesions that develop in the fifth or sixth decade of life and are more common in the large than in the small intestine. Whereas solitary lipomas tend to occur more frequently on the right side of the colon in the vicinity of the ileocecal valve or the ascending colon, lipomatous polyposis may involve the entire small and large intestines diffusely. Histologically, the polyps consist of a submucosal lump of adipose tissue that is covered with a normal colonic mucosa. Lipomas generally are asymptomatic but may be found incidentally on colonoscopy. Occasionally, when lipomas are big enough and tend to protrude into the lumen, they may cause symptoms such as gastrointestinal bleeding, diarrhea, intussusception, or bowel obstruction. Endoscopic removal of a lipoma with a snare often is possible but has a risk that the fat prevents the cautery from transmitting the energy well enough to the stalk vessel, resulting in postprocedure hemorrhage. Surgery may be required in such a complication or preemptively if the lesion is too large.

Potentially Malignant Nonepithelial Tumors of the Colon

Carcinoid or Neuroendocrine Tumors. Carcinoid tumors may occur anywhere in the entire body. A recent study on 11,427 patients found that the gastrointestinal tract is affected in 55%, with the most frequent locations being the small intestine (44.7%), the rectum (19.6%), the appendix (16.7%), and the colon (10.6%),[129] a finding that contrasts with traditional reports that the appendix is the most frequent site in the gastrointestinal tract. The annual incidences for the colon and rectum were reported to be 2.0 and 4.2 cases per 100,000 people per year, the risk of metastasis proportional to the size of the carcinoid.[129] Carcinoids less than 1 cm in size are considered benign, lesions greater than 2 cm are likely malignant, and the gray zone in between remains undetermined or potentially malignant.[130] Malignant carcinoids may spread locoregionally into the lymph nodes or directly to the liver. An oncologic resection should be performed in all carcinoids larger than 2 cm, whereas the management of tumors measuring 1–2 cm remains controversial.[130]

Patients with a gastrointestinal carcinoid tumor may be either completely asymptomatic or present with intestinal obstruction, bleeding, carcinoid syndrome, or carcinoid heart disease, i.e., acquired and commonly right-sided valvular heart disease.[131,132] Carcinoid syndrome is a bad prognostic sign because it is caused by metastatic lesions in the liver that release vasoactive substances (e.g., serotonin and 5-hydroxyindolacetic acid) directly into the systemic circulation. Diagnosis may be suspected clinically but is difficult to confirm histologically because the lesions are submucosal and not commonly reached with an endoscopic biopsy.

Gastrointestinal Stromal Tumors (GISTs). Gastrointestinal stromal tumors (GISTs) are the most common mesenchymal tumors of the gastrointestinal tract and originate from the intestinal pacemaker cells, the interstitial cells of Cajal.[133] Sixty percent of GISTs are found in the stomach; 29% in the small intestine; 2% in the colon, rectum, and rectovaginal septum; and 9% in the esophagus.[134] Symptoms are nonspecific and include pain, obstruction, bleeding, and a mass. Distinction from other mesenchymal tumors (e.g., leiomyosarcoma) is important from a prognostic point of view. Tumor size and light microscopic determination of the mitotic rate (mitotic figures per x number of high-power fields) are the most important conventional prognostic indicators.[133] The diagnosis of GISTs is based on morphologic features and immunohistochemical demonstration of *c-Kit* (CD117) expression. This marker is seen in almost all GISTs and is regarded as one of the key diagnostic elements, but a few otherwise characteristic tumors are found to be *c-Kit*-negative.[135] While the majority of GISTs have activating mutations of the KIT receptor tyrosine kinase, another subset of tumors show mutations in the KIT-related kinase gene PDGF receptor alpha (PDGFRA).[136] KIT and PDGFRA mutations appear to be alternative and mutually exclusive oncogenic mechanisms in GISTs.[137] Determination of CD117 expression is of practical importance because positivity correlates with a tumor response to treatment with imatinib (Gleevec), which inhibits KIT kinase activity. Surgical resection is the primary treatment for localized GISTs that are resectable without mutilation. Recurrent and locally advanced or metastatic tumors are treated increasingly with imatinib in a palliative, adjuvant, or neoadjuvant setting.

Nodular Lymphoid Hyperplasia. This condition is characterized by numerous lymphoid nodules that are protruding from the mucosa of the small and large intestine, rarely of the stomach. Associated diseases are immune deficiencies of various origins (e.g., tumors, hematoproliferative disorders, immunoglobulin A deficiency, and HIV infection), in which case recurrent infections (e.g., giardiasis) appear to promote the nodular lymphoid hyperplasia. Immunocompetent patients usually are asymptomatic, and the nodular lymphoid hyperplasia is an incidental finding. Nodular lymphoid hyperplasia has been associated with an increased subsequent incidence of small bowel lymphoma.[138]

Malignant Nonepithelial Tumors of the Colon

Lymphoma. Primary malignant lymphoma of the colon is uncommon and accounts for only 0.2–0.4% of all colonic malignancies and 10–15% of all primary lymphomas of the gastrointestinal tract, which themselves account for about 30% of extranodal lymphomas.[139] The most frequent colonic location is the cecum (70%), followed by the rectum and ascending colon. The gross appearance may be a circumferential or polypoid mass, an ulceration, or a diffuse infiltration with stricturing and bowel wall thickening.[140] Eighty-six percent of the lesions are solitary, but they can be multiple and diffuse in nature. The intestinal lymphomas may be subclassified into B-cell lymphomas (85%) and T-cell lymphomas (15%). Among the B-cell lymphomas, mantle cell lymphoma has a worse prognosis, whereas mucosa-associated lymphoid tissue (MALT) lymphomas have a better prognosis than other B-cell tumor types.[140] While surgical treatment may be indicated for some localized tumors, many authors consider medical management to be the primary treatment. It may include new approaches such as anti-infectious treatment for MALT lymphoma or reconstitution of the patient's immune status, e.g., by means of antiretroviral treatment in HIV-associated B-cell lymphoma.[141]

Multiple lymphomatous polyposis of the gastrointestinal tract is a distinct clinicopathologic entity. This rare form of primary gastrointestinal lymphoma occurs most often in elderly patients and accounts for 9% of all gastrointestinal lymphomas.[142] The polyps can be widespread throughout multiple segments of the gastrointestinal tract. Histopathologic and immunohistochemical techniques are required to differentiate lymphomatous polyposis from other forms of gastrointestinal polyposis.

Smooth Muscle Tumors. Smooth muscle tumors of the colon are rare and occur most commonly in the form of a pedunculated leiomyoma of the muscularis mucosa. Leiomyosarcomas, which consist histologically of spindle cells that resemble smooth muscle cells, are even less frequent but are characterized by an extremely aggressive and rapidly fatal growth pattern.

Secondary Tumors to the Colon

Endometriosis. Endometriosis may involve the colon or rectum in approximately 15–20% and may mimic colonic carcinoma. The lesions are rarely larger than 5 cm, involve the subserosa and muscle coats, and may project into the lumen of the bowel. When endometrial tissue extends through to the colonic mucosa, biopsy may be mistaken for adenocarcinoma.

Metastatic Cancer. Carcinomas from other primary sites may metastasize to the colon and occasionally mimic a primary colon cancer. Metastases originate most commonly from lobular breast cancer, stomach cancer, ovarian cancer, malignant melanoma, and leukemia, the latter of which can be diagnosed by the hematopoetic infiltrates.

▪ SURGICAL ANATOMY OF THE COLON

A fundamental knowledge of the surgical anatomy is of utmost importance for an adequate surgical technique that aims at the best oncologic outcome with minimized morbidity. The large intestine starts at the ileocecal junction and extends to the anus. It is about 5–6 ft (125–150 cm) long and can be divided into the cecum with the appendix, the ascending colon, the transverse colon, the descending colon, the sigmoid colon, and the rectum. Definitions of where the sigmoid colon ends and the rectum begins have not always been uniform and included (1) a distance of 12–15 cm above the anal verge, (2) the level of the peritoneal reflection, and (3) the level of the sacral promontory. The most useful landmark from a functional as well as surgical viewpoint is the confluence of the teniae coli at the rectosigmoid junction.[143] However, because this anatomic reference point cannot be visualized endoscopically, the National Cancer Institute recently has defined the rectum for the purpose of uniformity in clinical trials as the last 12 cm above the anal verge, as measured by rigid sigmoidoscopy.[144] This endoscopic definition is necessary because the increasing trend toward neoadjuvant chemoradiation for rectal but not sigmoid cancer demands a determination of whether a lesion is located in the rectum or in the sigmoid colon.[144]

The arterial and venous blood supply, as well as the lymphatics, of the colon are summarized in Figure 23–5. The arterial blood supply to the colon comes from the superior mesenteric artery (SMA) and the inferior mesenteric artery (IMA), which communicate in a watershed area in the splenic flexure (artery of Drummond). The rectum has additional branches from the internal iliac vessels. With a significant degree of anatomic variation, the major vascular stalks to the colonic segments consist of the ileocecal and right colic artery (last branch of the SMA), the middle colic artery (second branch of the SMA), the left colic artery (first branch of the IMA), and the superior hemorrhoidal artery (distal branch of the IMA, feeding the sigmoid colon and upper rectum). The venous blood supply peripherally follows the arterial branches but more centrally divides into the superior mesenteric vein and the inferior mesenteric vein, which connect at separate levels to the portal system. The lymphatic drainage starts with lymphatic follicles in the colonic submucosa, drains through the colonic muscle wall into the epicolic nodes, and continues to the paracolic lymph nodes that follow the blood vessels to the bowel, along the major arteries to the principal lymph nodes at the level of the arterial runoff from the aorta. These lymph node groups consist of the celiac, the superior mesenteric, and the inferior mesenteric groups of lymph nodes.

For a safe surgical technique, the relationship of the colon with adjacent structures, mostly in the retroperitoneum, has to be understood fully. The colon is only a partially intraperitoneal organ. Only the transverse colon and the sigmoid colon are fully peritonealized and have a free mesocolon; the ascending colon and the descending colon, including both flexures, are partially located in the retroperitoneum and therefore reside in proximity to essential anatomic structures. The structures most at risk during a right hemicolectomy include the right ureter and the duodenum; during a transverse colon resection, the SMA/SMV and the gastroepiploic vessels at the gastric curvature; during a takedown of the splenic flexure, the spleen and left kidney; and during a left colon or sigmoid resection, the left ureter, the gonadal vessels, and the hypogastric nerves.

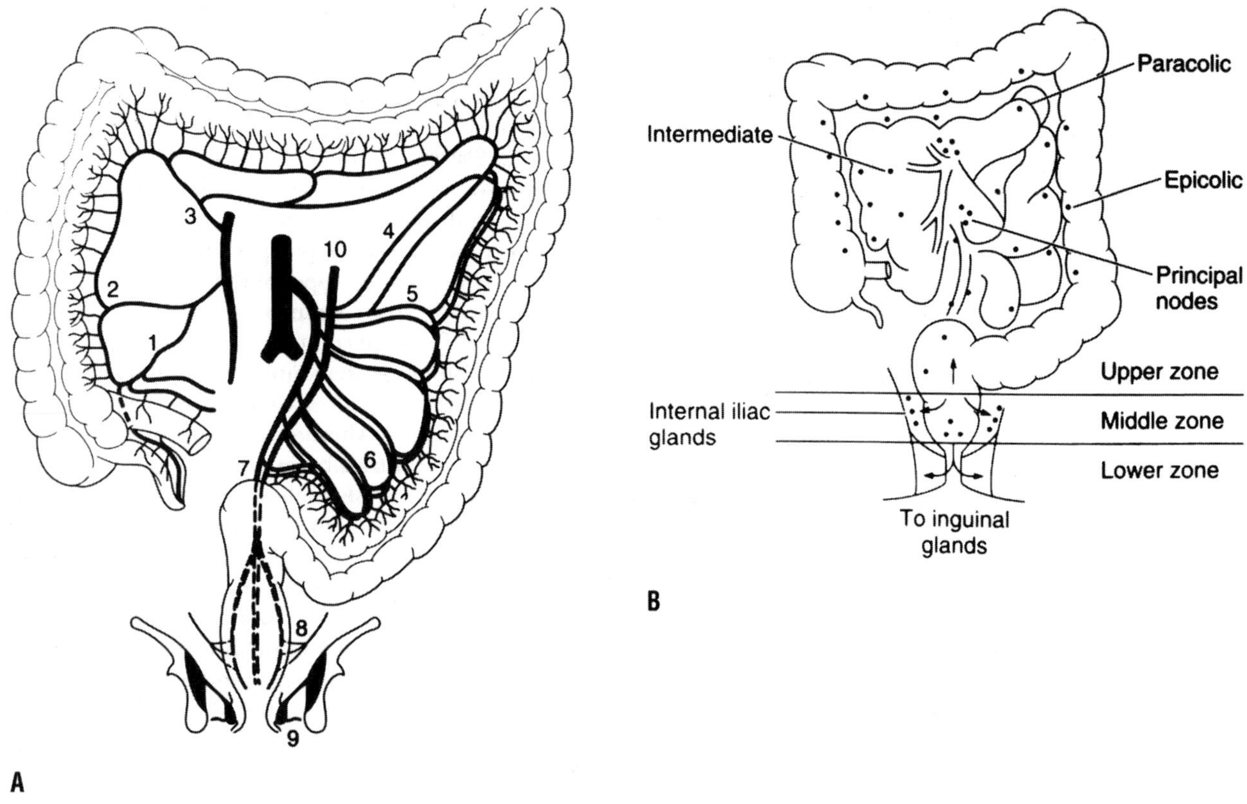

Figure 23–5. Anatomy of the colon. **A.** Arterial and venous supply of the colon. **B.** Lymphatic drainage of the colon.

▪ CLINICAL PRESENTATION OF COLORECTAL CANCER

SYMPTOMS

Colorectal cancer does not have any early signs. In fact, symptoms often are absent until a tumor has grown to a significant size. Unless a patient presents with a tumor complication (e.g., bowel obstruction, bleeding, perforation, or fistula formation), symptoms mostly are subtle or uncharacteristic and vague. They may consist of unexplained weight loss, anemia and weakness from chronic blood loss, flatulence, or episodes of colicky abdominal pain. If present, these symptoms therefore always should be suspicious for a locally relatively advanced tumor stage, which is also reflected by the fact that 20% of colorectal cancer patients at the time of first presentation have stage IV disease with distant metastasis (Table 23–12). Proximal colon tumors may grow relatively large before they interfere with the passage of the still liquid or semisolid stool. The more distal a lesion is localized (e.g., left colon or rectum), the more likely changes in bowel habits occur. These include bloody or mucous discharge in or with the stool, sudden onset of constipation, alternating periods of diarrhea and constipation, or a decreasing diameter of the stool. Pelvic or anal pain is an ominous sign because it may occur with increasing size or sphincter invasion of a rectal cancer.

Any large bowel obstruction, bleeding per rectum, gas or stool passage other than through the anus, or peritoneal signs should raise the index of suspicion for a colorectal malignancy until proven otherwise. Several other conditions and diseases have to be considered in the differential diagnosis. Obstructive symptoms may result from chronic diverticulitis, benign polyps, Crohn's disease, endometriosis, or a postischemic stricture. A fistula may suggest complicated diverticulitis, Crohn's disease, or tuberculosis. Bleeding per rectum also may be found in hemorrhoids, diverticular disease, endometriosis, and colitis. However, even if one of these benign diseases is found on clinical evaluation, the symptoms should not be attributed automatically to them before a malignant disease of the large intestine has been ruled out.

Since symptoms are not reliable for the prevention or early detection of colorectal cancer, risk-adjusted screening programs (as discussed in an earlier section of the chapter) are crucial to achieve a reduction in cancer mortality.

Management planning in a situation with acute cancer complications not only should include strategies to alleviate symptoms and minimize the morbidity from the complication but also should provide an oncologically adequate treatment for the tumor.

TABLE 23–12. DISTRIBUTION OF SINGLE COLON PRIMARY CANCER BY STAGE

Stage	Number	(%)
0,I	1845	(37.8)
II	1085	(22.2)
III	825	(16.9)
IV	955	(19.6)
Unspecified	168	(3.4)

Reproduced, with permission, from Passman MA et al, 1996.[219]

HISTORY AND PHYSICAL EXAMINATION

A careful history and physical examination remain the cornerstone in all patients presenting with gastrointestinal symptoms. Obtaining the history and review of systems should include questions about changes in bowel habits, time of last stool and gas passage, weight loss, and a personal or family history of cancer, particularly of colorectal cancer. Awareness of possible underlying diseases and genetics that predispose to colorectal cancer is of utmost importance not only for the management of the individual patient but also for adequate counseling of potentially affected family members.

A careful physical examination follows to identify any palpable tumor masses and/or signs of tumor complication or dissemination. Apart from vital signs and temperature, the patient's general appearance may reveal evidence of cachexia, dehydration, jaundice, and lymph node enlargements. For example, enlargement of the left supraclavicular nodes may be the first but late sign of a disseminated gastrointestinal malignancy (Troisier's sign). The abdomen is examined for a palpable primary tumor, hepatomegaly (liver metastasis?), distension, and tympanitic bowel sounds (partial/complete bowel obstruction?). Presence of peritoneal signs such as guarding with local direct and rebound tenderness or percussion tenderness may indicate a tumor perforation. A digital rectal examination and proctoscopy are mandatory to determine the exact distance of a palpable tumor from the anal verge, its axial and circumferential positions, and the mobility of the tumor against surrounding structures (e.g., sacrum, prostate/vagina, anal sphincter muscle). In addition, the checking finger may assess the rectal vault for the presence of stool, blood, or melena. A thorough general physical examination is necessary to evaluate the patient's general health status with regard to the ability to tolerate a major abdominal procedure under general anesthesia.

Particular attention has to be paid to patients who present with acute symptoms in an emergency setting. Prolonged fasting, nausea or vomiting, and translocation of fluids into the third space during a period of bowel obstruction or after a perforation will result rapidly in a state of malnutrition and dehydration. Developing sepsis or acute and recurrent blood loss potentially aggravates these symptoms and may result in a preshock. Alarming signs are a decrease in urine output, tachycardia, hypotension, elevated temperature, short-term weight loss, standing skin folds, dry oral mucosa, and acidosis. Immediate fluid and volume resuscitation has to parallel the further clinical work-up and monitoring. Falsely high hematocrit values that result from dehydration may mask a loss of blood.

INVESTIGATIONS

Patients with symptoms suggestive of colorectal cancer should undergo a series of timely investigations with three goals: (1) to assess the large bowel with regard to the primary lesion, concomitant lesions, and a potential underlying colonic disease, (2) to determine whether the tumor has metastasized, and (3) to assess the patient's operability (overall condition and comorbidities).

Complete Evaluation of the Large Intestine

Endoscopic and radiologic techniques are available for evaluation of the colon and rectum. Irrespective of the method, the primary goal is to document the presence of a malignant pathology and to rule out concomitant lesions in other segments of the large intestine.

Rigid Proctoscopy and Flexible Sigmoidoscopy. These are the first-line diagnostic tools in the outpatient clinic setting to assess rectosigmoidal lesions accurately. The two methods are rapid, widely available, and require only minimal bowel preparation (enema). However, they do not provide complete information about the rest of the colon, and therefore, a complementary study is indicated before surgery. Furthermore, the flexible sigmoidoscope is notorious for giving inaccurate measurements of the level of the tumor. Determination of the rectal versus colonic location of the tumor should be done with a rigid proctoscope.

Colonoscopy. Colonoscopy clearly has evolved as the method of choice because of its high sensitivity in detecting tumors and its ability to take biopsies. It provides accurate information about the entire colonic mucosa (i.e., polyps, synchronous cancer, colitis, melanosis, and diverticula), and it may be used to remove synchronous neoplastic polyps. Apart from determining the circumferential and longitudinal extent of a colonic lesion, colonoscopy addresses functional aspects such as active bleeding or an imminent obstruction by cauterization, laser ablation, or placement of a self-expanding wall stent and thus to turn an emergency situation into an elective one.

While the overall risk of colonoscopy is very low, with a much less than 1% incidence of a bowel perforation, there are some limitations to the technique. There is a 25% risk of smaller lesions escaping detection and an estimated 10% incidence that the cecum may not be reached for technical reasons. In addition, the precise position of a lesion seen on colonoscopy may not be determined adequately because the only reliable landmarks are the dentate line and the terminal ileum, and the length from the anal verge may vary considerably. In practical terms, however, this handicap may be overcome by India ink tattooing of the area of a lesion for better identification during surgery or repeat endoscopy.

Contrast Enema. Radiographic contrast enemas alternatively can be used for a colonic evaluation. They have the advantage of more accurately visualizing the anatomic position of a colonic lesion (road map). Most commonly, a barium-air double-contrast technique will be used; however, if there is suspicion of a colonic perforation, administration of barium is contraindicated (risk of barium peritonitis), and instead, a water-soluble contrast material (e.g., gastrografin) should be used. The typical aspect of a colon cancer is a fixed filling defect with destruction of the mucosal pattern in an annular configuration ("apple core"), as opposed to an intact mucosal pattern in a filling defect from an extramucosal compression or from chronic diverticulitis. Although preoperative histologic confirmation of a colon cancer is preferable, an unequivocal and characteristic morphology on a barium enema or endoscopy is sufficient evidence to proceed to surgery. Contrast studies have the advantages of a better passage through even severely obstructing lesions and that they commonly reach the cecum. In addition, they are superior in visualizing diverticula or a suspected fistula between the colorectum and other pelvic organs. The major disadvantage of contrast studies is the inability to take biopsies and to detect small lesions.[64]

Evolving Techniques. Virtual colonoscopy (or CT colonography)[145,146] and the microcapsule study have evolved in the last decade as high-tech alternatives to the two previously described methods. While there is certainly a lot of promise for both new approaches, which likely will continue to improve over time, some more recent studies suggest that CT colonography has a considerable rate of false-negative and false-positive results.[146,147] In addition, incidental extracolonic findings may precipitate a large number of unwarranted tests, which add tremendous cost to the health care system. The definite role of these techniques awaits further clarification.

Evaluation of the Local Tumor Extent and of Metastatic Dissemination

In contrast to rectal cancer, where endorectal ultrasound, computed tomographic (CT) scans, and magnetic resonance imaging (MRI) are used routinely in the preoperative work-up, a cancer of the colon does not necessarily require further imaging studies to determine the local extent of the tumor because in the majority of cases they do not change the local surgical approach. For a more general preoperative evaluation of the abdomen, however, abdominal sonography, CT scan, or MRI is indicated and equally accurate to check for the presence of liver metastases, hydronephrosis, or gross paraaortic lymph node involvement, as well as concomitant diseases such as gallstones, cysts, ascites, aortic aneurysm, etc. Preoperative involvement of other specialists (e.g., urologists) therefore may be initiated. CT scans are used most commonly in the United States and have a 90% and 95% sensitivity and specificity in detecting liver lesions greater than 1 cm.[148] However, in some patients with liver metastasis or undetermined liver lesions, intraoperative liver ultrasound may be an extremely helpful tool because several studies now have shown it to be superior to preoperative radiologic examination and intraoperative clinical assessment.[149]

In order to rule out extrahepatic metastases, a chest x-ray in two planes commonly is sufficient, although the yield of this test is relatively low. A CT scan of the chest may be necessary to substantiate a concern from conventional images. Only under special circumstances where the presence of previously unknown tumor manifestations (e.g., recurrence versus scar tissue, solitary versus multiple liver metastases, and presence of extrahepatic metastases) would have an impact on the treatment approach (e.g., operative versus non-operative) is a positron-emission tomographic (PET) scan indicated. Routine use of PET scanning in the primary management of colorectal cancer is not recommended.

Laboratory and Preoperative Tests

Preoperative laboratory tests are aimed at providing evidence for pathophysiologic effects of the tumor and ruling out general health problems that could have an effect on the patients' general operability. A comprehensive work-up includes a complete blood count, electrolytes, creatinine/blood urea nitrogen (BUN), glucose, liver function tests (alkaline phosphatase, AST, ALT, bilirubin, total protein, albumin), and coagulation parameters (PT, PTT, INR). Arterial blood gas analysis and additional tests will be ordered in an emergency setting or according to the individual patient's risk assessment (e.g., cardiac enzymes, etc).

Even though tumor markers such as carcinoembryonic antigen (CEA) are determined routinely, their role is limited because of the low sensitivity and specificity for colonic carcinoma and because the measured value virtually never changes the management. CEA can be elevated in proximal gastrointestinal cancers, benign inflammatory conditions of the bowel, lung and breast cancer, and smoking. Nonetheless, CEA level determination may prove helpful in some settings, e.g., when the return of an elevated preoperative CEA level to normal indicates a complete tumor resection or when a postoperatively elevated level may indicate residual or recurrent disease.[150]

Preoperative standard evaluation includes a chest x-ray in two planes for cardiopulmonary assessment and for detection of pulmonary metastases (see previous sections). Electrocardiogram (ECG) and pulmonary function tests (FVC, FEV_1, and RV diffusion capacity) are indicated in patients either older than 40 years of age or with a respective personal history. Specialized tests such as cardiac stress tests, echocardiogram, perfusion scintigraphy, or interventional cardiologic studies depend on the individual patient's history and risk assessment.

▪ TREATMENT

PRINCIPLES OF SURGICAL MANAGEMENT

As a basic principle, any colorectal cancer is an indication for surgery unless widespread tumor dissemination or general contraindications from the patient's overall health status are present. Furthermore, any precursor pathology with statistical or biopsy-proven risk for cancer (e.g., large sessile polyp in an otherwise healthy individual or dysplasia in a patient with ulcerative colitis) that cannot be managed nonoperatively is an indication for surgery.

The general goal for surgical management is either to achieve cure from the tumor and extension of survival or disease-free survival or, in the case of a precursor pathology with or without an underlying disease (e.g., ulcerative colitis or FAP), to prevent the cancer and to remove the risk-causing disease. In a palliative setting, the goal is to prolong the period of symptom-free survival.

Local tumor control generally is the primary treatment objective to prevent local tumor complications, i.e., obstruction, perforation, bleeding, and pain. Even in the presence of distant metastases in the liver or lung, resection of the primary tumor remains a reasonable priority. Since solitary or a limited number of metastases in the liver or lung often may be treated surgically by partial organ resection or metastasectomy with a cure rate of up to 35%, their presence should not necessarily alter the surgical approach at the primary site to do a curative resection. However, if there are extensive metastases or peritoneal carcinomatosis, surgical cure is not a reasonable goal, and alleviation of present or impending local complications by restoring the intestinal continuity is the best palliation.

The specific surgical and oncologic strategy planning is based on a number of factors. It has to take into account the exact localization of the tumor, the tumor stage, the presence of synchronous colonic lesions or an underlying colonic disease, the risk for metachronous lesions, the patient's age, the extent of the local procedure, and the timing. Only after the extent of the operation has been defined can the method and approach to be used be discussed as to whether the procedure is only suitable for an open laparotomy approach or laparoscopy may be reasonable and beneficial.

In contrast to rectal cancer, neoadjuvant treatment (i.e., preoperative chemoradiation) is not indicated in the overwhelming majority of colonic cases unless a locally very advanced lesion is treated with chemotherapy in anticipation of an otherwise unresectable mass. Adjuvant (i.e., postoperative) treatment will be discussed in a later section.

PREPARATION FOR SURGERY

When a patient is considered to be an operative candidate, several preparatory steps need to be addressed.

Transfusion. Even though many colonic operations can be performed without a blood transfusion, it is recommended to have the patient's blood typed and crossed-matched, with a minimum of 2 units of blood available at the beginning of the surgery. The indication for transfusion will depend on the starting hemoglobin, the patient's age and physiologic status, and the extent of intraoperative blood loss. There is some controversy as to the immunologic effect of blood transfusions on the overall prognosis of colorectal cancer. Since the initial report that transfusion may be associated with an increased likelihood of recurrence,[151] there have been many subsequent reports that have reached conflicting conclusions. Meta-analysis studies have strongly questioned whether there is a true causal effect present.[152] Other factors such as extent of resection required, location of tumor, and experience of the surgeon actually may be the cause for recurrence, but transfusion may be an indirect reflection of extensive disease and surgery. Furthermore, a randomized trial comparing the use of autologous versus allogenic blood in patients undergoing colorectal resections did not show any statistical difference in prognosis.[153]

Bowel Cleansing. Since the colon is a large reservoir for numerous anaerobic and aerobic bacteria, a reliable method of bacterial load reduction is required to reduce the incidence of infections such as wound infections and intra-abdominal abscesses. Mechanical bowel cleansing and antibiotic prophylaxis have been used as an integrative part of the preoperative management in colorectal surgery, even though there have been a few recent reports that question the benefit of bowel preparation.[154] There are a wide variety of laxatives, washouts, and enemas available on the market for mechanical cleansing, but the products used generally are based on either polyethylene glycol (e.g., GoLytely) or sodium phosphate (Fleet Phospho-soda), the latter of which is contraindicated in patients with renal failure. In the absence of a consensus regarding the best regimens (i.e., orthograde cleansing alone or combined with retrograde enemas), the choice often is a matter of personal preference. Recent prospective, randomized, controlled studies comparing mechanical preparation versus no preparation for elective colorectal surgery have failed to demonstrate any appreciable decrease in infection rates, anastomotic leaks, or mortality rates in patients undergoing mechanical bowel preparation.[155–158] Depending on an individual patient's constitution and the degree of obstruction, the bowel cleansing should be started 1 or even 2 days before surgery. The cathartic causes significant alterations in the patient's fluid and electrolyte balance, which may result in profound dehydration and electrolyte imbalances. Elderly patients, who are more prone to this adverse effect, therefore should be given intravenous fluids and electrolytes. Nasogastric whole-gut irrigation with an electrolyte solution obtains excellent results, but patients find this very unpleasant.

Antibiotic Prophylaxis. Reduction of colonic bacterial concentration can be achieved with antibiotics that target colonic aerobes including *Escherichia coli* and colonic anaerobes such as *Bacillus fragilis.* The combination of mechanical bowel preparation and oral antibiotics or parenteral antibiotics or a combination of both has yielded excellent results.[159] Oral antibiotics may include metronidazole combined with the nonabsorbable neomycin. Intravenous broad-spectrum antibiotics often contain a combination of intravenous second- or third-generation cephalosporin (cefoxitin or ceftriaxone) with metronidazole. Alternatively, a combination of ciprofloxacin and metronidazole may be used. The optimal timing for administration of antibiotics is to start their intravenous administration 1–2 hours before incision and continue for up to 36 hours. Special considerations according to national guidelines have to be followed for prophylaxis in patients at risk for endocarditis (e.g., patients with mechanical heart valve).

Thromboembolic Prophylaxis. Thromboembolic prophylaxis is recommended in all patients undergoing major surgical procedures to reduce the incidence of postoperative deep venous thrombosis and pulmonary embolism. Both pharmacologic and physical prophylaxies (e.g., pneumatic calf compression) have been proven to be effective,[160] but the use of pharmacologic prophylaxis has been endorsed recently by a task force recommendation.[161] Both low-dose unfractionated heparin and low-molecular-weight heparins (LMWHs) have been shown to be equally effective in reducing the incidence of postoperative thromboembolic events without resulting in significant complications.[162] A recent randomized study, however, showed that LMWHs have a slightly higher rate of minor bleeding events.[163] Based on economic analysis, the data favor the use of subcutaneous heparin as being more cost-effective than LMWHs.[164] It is recommended that these drugs be commenced at least 2 hours before surgery and continued postoperatively until the patient has obtained full ambulation. Intermittent pneumatic calf-compression boots are an alternative to heparin that has been demonstrated to be equally successful in preventing deep venous thrombosis and possessing the advantage of no risk of increased bleeding.[165] It remains to be determined whether a combination of chemical agents and pneumatic calf-compression boots for patients undergoing colonic resection will be an advantage.

Anticoagulated patients who need to take warfarin (e.g., owing to a mechanical heart valve) should be switched perioperatively to intravenous heparin to allow for stopping the warfarin medication and antagonizing its effect with vitamin K. Four hours before incision, the heparin may be discontinued and resumed within 24 hours postoperatively with a stepwise increase in the dose.

Urinary Catheters/Stents. After induction of general anesthesia, bladder catheterization should be performed in all cases to monitor the urine output adequately peri- and postoperatively. In selected patients with a previous history of colorectal or pelvic dissections, placement of ureteral stents allows better intraoperative identification and protection of these crucial structures.

Nasogastric Tube. Placement of a nasogastric tube is not necessary on a routine basis for patients undergoing resection of the colon or rectum unless they present with a complete or partial bowel obstruction.[166]

Preoperative Marking of Ostomy Site. In patients who may need permanent or temporary placement of an ostomy during the surgical procedure, preoperative marking of the ideal stoma site by a stoma nurse helps to facilitate postoperative ostomy handling by the patient.

Preemptive Pain Management. Effective pain management is an important factor to reduce the incidence of postoperative pulmonary complications. Preoperative placement of epidural analgesia is a very valuable strategy, which, in addition to its pain-relieving effect, promotes the earlier resumption of postoperative bowel function as a result of its suppression of sympathetic nerves. The relevant segments that need to be blocked for an abdominal incision are located at a thoracic level (T6–T12).

SURGERY

General Technical Principles

The objective of surgery for colonic cancer is to perform a curative resection by removing the cancerous segment of colon, the mesentery with the primary feeding vessel and the lymphatics, and any organ with direct tumor involvement. Since the lymphatics run with the arterial supply of the colon, the primary artery supplying the segment of the colon to be resected is divided at its origin. Ligation at the origin of the vessel ensures inclusion of apical nodes, which may convey prognostic significance for the patient.[167] The length of bowel and mesentery resected is dictated by tumor location and distribution of the primary artery (Table 23–13). Nevertheless, with radical excision of a colonic tumor, at least a 5-cm distal and proximal clearance is required. Extended resections have not been shown to confer additional survival benefit[168]; however, tumors located in "border zones" should be resected with both neighboring lymphatics to encompass possible bidirectional spread. When synchronous cancers are present in the colon, an extended resection or even total colectomy, with ideally only one anastomosis, should be performed. Occasionally, two separate resections (e.g., right hemicolectomy and low anterior resection) with two anastomoses are preferable to preserve colon length and to avoid postcolectomy diarrhea. Cancer on the basis of an underlying pancolonic disease (e.g., ulcerative colitis or FAP) requires a total proctocolectomy with either an ileoanal pull-through procedure or an ileostomy.[54]

A limited resection may be considered for an unfit patient or for palliative resection in those with widespread tumor. This will relieve the patient's symptoms and prevent future obstruction and bleeding from the primary tumor. If a tumor is adherent to or invading an adjacent organ such as the kidney or small bowel, an en-bloc resection should be performed where technically feasible.

TABLE 23–13. STANDARD RESECTIONS OF THE COLON

Tumor Location	Resection	Description of Extent	Major Blood Vessel	Safety Margin
Cecum	Right hemicolectomy	Terminal ileum to mid transverse colon, right flexure included	Ileocolic artery, Right colic artery, Right branch of mid colic artery	5 cm
Ascending colon	Right hemicolectomy	Terminal ileum to mid transverse colon, right flexure included	Ileocolic artery, Right colic artery, Right branch of mid colic artery	5 cm
Hepatic flexure	Extended right hemicolectomy	Terminal ileum to descending colon (distal to left flexure)	Ileocolic artery, Right colic artery, Mid colic artery	5 cm
Transverse colon	Extended right hemicolectomy	Terminal ileum to descending colon (distal to left flexure)	Ileocolic artery, Right colic artery, Mid colic artery	5 cm
	(Transverse colon resection)	Transverse colon (including both flexures)	Mid colic artery	
Splenic flexure	Extended left hemicolectomy	Right flexure to rectosigmoid colon (sigmoid, beginning of rectum)	Mid colic artery, Left colic artery, Inferior mesenteric artery	5 cm
Descending colon	Left hemicolectomy	Left flexure to sigmoid colon (beginning of rectum)	Inferior mesenteric artery, Left branch of mid colic artery	5 cm
Sigmoid colon	Rectosigmoid resection	Descending colon to rectum	Superior hemorrhoidal artery, Inferior mesenteric artery	5 cm

Since adhesions between the tumor and adjacent organ may not necessarily be inflammatory but due to carcinoma, mere division or "pinching" of a tumor from an adjacent organ is not an acceptable surgical technique because it may reduce the chance of cure. While careful dissection in the right place is the mainstay of a successful surgery, the historical Turnball no-touch technique with early vascular ligation and occlusion of the bowel with tapes to prevent embolization of tumor and improve survival has not shown any advantage.[169]

Intraoperative Surgical Technique

Positioning. For all left-sided colonic resections, it is advisable to place the patient in a modified lithotomy position, which gives access to the anus (e.g., for a stapled anastomosis) and allows an assistant or the surgeon to stand between the legs for retraction or an excellent view to mobilize the splenic flexure, respectively. The same positioning obviously also can be used for all other colon resections, but a supine position usually is sufficient and faster.

Incision. The peritoneal cavity is entered through a midline laparotomy incision. For a proctocolectomy, we usually recommend the use of an infraumbilical incision in order to provide good exposure for the pelvic dissection. For a more proximal segmental colon resection, however, an equally short but higher midline incision may be more convenient. In addition, a transverse incision or even a subcostal incision may give excellent exposure for a right hemicolectomy.

Exploration. After the peritoneal cavity is entered, the abdomen is explored systematically to determine the resectability of the tumor. Special attention is addressed to the presence of distant metastases in the liver, peritoneal carcinomatosis, or additional synchronous lesions throughout the large intestine. Other accessible organ systems are assessed equally, e.g., the gallbladder and the female reproductive organs.

Colon Resection. The surgical technique has been standardized for three segments: right colon, left colon, and rectosigmoid. Depending on the extent of the resection eventually needed in an individual patient, the technique for those segments may be combined (see Table 23–13). With a detailed description of the maximal resection, i.e., a total colectomy/proctocolectomy, all information therefore will be provided about the individual steps necessary to perform any colorectal resection of lesser extent.

On careful exploration of the abdomen, mobilization of the colon starts on the right side. Use of a mobile (e.g., Richardson retractor) instead of a fixed (e.g., Balfour or Bookwalter retractor) abdominal wall retractor in this first phase will allow a more flexible and unidirectional exposure according to rapidly changing needs. The small bowel is eviscerated from the abdomen and moved to the left. The abdominal wall is retracted to the right side while exerting countertraction on the cecum and ascending colon. A small incision is made at the exposed white line of Toldt to enter the retroperitoneum. Elevating the ascending colon from the retroperitoneal structures, the peritoneum is divided along the lateral gutter from the terminal ileum to the hepatic flexure. On the right side, the ureter is at fairly low risk and routinely falls away; however, special care is needed to avoid damage to the third part of the duodenum. The mobilization is facilitated by firm traction placed on the colon and the surgeon's left hand inserted into the retroperitoneum as a guide to divide along the peritoneal reflection. Because of the limited view around the hepatic flexure and the presence of small vessels at this level, transsection of the peritoneum with cautery often is advisable.

As the right edge of the gastrocolic ligament is reached, it may be easier to complete the dissection of the hepatic flexure in retrograde direction. The abdominal wall retractor is moved quickly into the upper end of the incision in order to pull in a cephalad direction. The lesser sac is entered far to the left in an avascular portion of the omentum, and the greater omentum is divided inferior to the gastroepiploic vessels between clamps and ligatures. While the omentum may be preserved in benign diseases, its resection with the respective colon segment is part of an oncologic resection. Dissection of the gastrocolic ligament is carried out from the left to the right. Connective tissue attachments between the antrum, duodenum, and transverse mesocolon and the hepatic flexure are divided stepwise by a combination of blunt digital tunneling and sharp dissection using both hands. Care should be taken at this point to avoid dissecting too deeply into the retroperitoneum, where large blood vessels can be encountered. Once the mobilization has been completed around the hepatic flexure, the right colon and transverse colon are attached only to their vascular supply and are ready for resection. This would be used for any standard right hemicolectomy or the first part of an extended transverse colectomy. For total colectomy, mobilization of the whole colon commonly is continued before dividing the major vessels.

At this point, the abdominal wall retractor is moved to the left side of the abdomen, and traction is placed to expose the left portion of the colon. The dissection is initiated at the level of the sigmoid, where the white line of Toldt again is incised and the retroperitoneum entered. Once the areolar tissues are identified, a small sponge is taken, and with firm pressure against the sigmoid mesentery, the retroperitoneal tissues are bluntly reflected, and the left ureter is exposed. Only after the ureter has been clearly identified and moved out of the way is incision of the peritoneum continued into the pelvis for a short distance and up to the splenic flexure along the left gutter. The colon is reflected bluntly from the retroperitoneal tissues, and with firm traction, the peritoneal incision is continued. Gentle traction on the transverse and descending colon will help to lower the splenic flexure until it can be visualized fully. A hand placed in the retroperitoneum will help to mobilize the splenic flexure, and under direct vision, the peritoneum over the splenic flexure can be incised. Care must be taken at this point to protect the spleen from direct or traction injury. The final attachments of the splenocolic ligament that hold the splenic flexure are clamped and divided in appropriate tissue portions. Clamping and ligating this tissue are recommended because even small vessels retracting into the left upper quadrant can be a nuisance.

After completion of the first two parts, the colon is mobilized completely from its retroperitoneal attachments from the terminal ileum to the upper rectum. Elevation of the colon allows identification of all primary feeding vessels. In order to ligate the inferior mesenteric vessels, the surgeon is on the patient's left, and the colon is reflected to the left. The attachments that run over the sacral promontory and up along the left gutter are incised, and a hand is used to dissect the tissues bluntly from behind the inferior mesenteric vessels. By identifying the inferior mesenteric vessels and making the window just under those, the hypogastric nerves going down into the pelvis are protected routinely. Sometimes, e.g., if there is concern about cancer in the rectum or if the patient is very obese, these structures need to be freed up more to elevate the nerves initially and later to dissect them out under direct vision. The avascular window around the origin of feeding vessels then is opened. In the case of the inferior mesenteric vessels, the left hand is placed behind the inferior mesenteric stalk, and the thumb and opposing index finger can clear a window of avascular tissue above it. Dissection of redundant adipose tissue around the vessels is carried out under direct vision, before the vessels are clamped. Before transsection and ligature of the vessels, the remote location of the ureter is confirmed once more. If the ureter is not identified properly before dividing the vascular pedicle, accidental dissection of the ureter can occur and requires a repair. If unrecognized intraoperatively, the ureter injury may result in a urinoma. In difficult cases (e.g., repeat operation or recurrence), it is therefore advisable to place preoperative ureteral stents to allow better identification. The whole vascular stalk may be ligated with a double ligature or a suture ligature. Individual ligature of the artery and vein is optional and has not been shown to provide an advantage. For the reason mentioned earlier, it is recommend to ligate the vessels as proximally as possible, but from an oncologic standpoint, a high ligation of the inferior mesenteric artery does not provide any advantage in comparison with a low ligature distal to the origin of the left colic artery.[170,171]

The vascular dissection then is continued around the colonic mesentery. The avascular tissue can be divided sharply while clamping is applied to vessels when they are encountered. The vascular anatomy of the colon is quite variable. However, if one is truly in the retroperitoneum and ligating named vessels at their origin, the colon can be taken out with as few as three to four clamps. In particular, the inferior mesenteric, middle colic, and ileocolic vessels need to be ligated. The presence of additional right and left colic vessels sometimes requires the use of five or six clamps. By taking the vessels closer to their origin, i.e., before they branch off into multiple subsegments, fewer clamps are necessary, and the dissection proceeds more rapidly.

Once the vessels have been ligated, the bowel may be divided by means of cutting linear stapling devices at the previously determined levels. In patients with an underlying disease (e.g., ulcerative colitis or FAP), the dissection at this point would be continued as a total mesorectal excision down into the pelvis to the pelvic floor (see respective chapters). It is strongly recommended to have the specimen assessed macroscopically to verify the pathology. Tumor in the resection margin means an inadequate cancer operation requiring a re-resection. Intraoperative frozen sections of the resection margins should be requested whenever there is any doubt about the completeness of the resection.

Reconstruction/Diversion. After the resection has been completed, either the bowel ends can be reanastomosed or the proximal end may be brought out as an ostomy. Prerequisite for a successful anastomosis are meticulous technique, well-vascularized tissue, apposition of bowel ends without any tension, and good nutritional status of the patient with an albumin level greater than 3.0 mg/dL. Constructing an anastomosis under tension and with poor blood supply may result in an anastomotic leak and cause an infection and sepsis. A protective diverting ostomy does not prevent the leak but should diminish the life-threatening complications of an anastomotic leak. While a stapled functional end-to-end anastomosis between the ileum and the colon (i.e., an enterocolonic anastomosis) is reasonable, this type of anastomosis usually is not recommended for an anastomosis between two colon segments (i.e., a colocolonic anastomosis) because it results in an iatrogenic giant diverticulum that may interfere with propulsion of the formed stool and with performance of a surveillance colonoscopy. Performing an end-to-end anastomosis, either hand-sewn or by means of a circular stapler, will avoid these problems. An ileocolonic anastomosis in most instances can be performed in unprepared bowel, whereas a colocolonic anastomosis on the left side generally require pre- or intraoperative reduction in the stool load unless a colostomy is performed.

Drains. Placement of drains is often more a matter of personal preference than of scientific objectiveness.[172–174] While most bowel anastomoses do not need to be drained, the use of drains generally is recommended by many surgeons when a pelvic dissection and anastomosis have been performed in order to avoid accumulation of fluid and blood in the dependent areas. Whether prospective but underpowered studies are sufficient evidence to effectuate a change in this practice needs to be determined.[175,176]

Technical Considerations

Laparotomy versus Laparoscopy. Laparoscopic surgery for colonic cancer has excited a great deal of interest in recent years.[177] Long before any larger studies came out, it was considered reasonable in a palliative setting to remove the primary tumor by a laparoscopic resection to allow a more rapid recovery of an individual with limited residual life span. With regard to curative resections, however, there were concerns as to whether the laparoscopic technique would affect the oncologic outcome and the incidence or patterns of cancer recurrence adversely. In contrast to one early report of a high incidence of port-site recurrences, it has become clear subsequently that with appropriate surgical technique, the incidence is in the range of 0.8–1.3% and, on a stage-by-stage comparison, not higher than wound implants after open surgery. Apart from accumulating data from nonrandomized studies, several randomized studies have been published since 1990 throughout the world,[178–183] the largest being a multicenter study by the National Cancer Institute.[179] This study, which enrolled 872 patients with stage I–III colon cancer, confirmed that there was a moderate quality-of-life benefit for the laparoscopic approach[184] but otherwise no difference in outcome and survival between the laparoscopic and open-resection groups.[179] This equality of the study results has offered the unique opportunity for both opponents and proponents of the laparoscopic approach to justify their personal preference for either the open or laparoscopic technique depending on their preference and skills. Two large-scale European studies (i.e., the COLOR trial and the CLASICC trial) have completed enrollment and have begun to publish their data recently.[182,183]

For the laparoscopic procedure, about 3–4 trocars are inserted. The colon should be mobilized to the same extent as during open surgery. The vascular pedicle is identified and transected. The technical equipment to perform an intracorporeal resection and anastomosis is available, but it is questionable whether there is any advantage to this because at some point an incision must be made anyway to retrieve the specimen. In the laparoscopically assisted technique, the segment, once it has been mobilized to the required extent, therefore is exteriorized through a small but sleeve-protected abdominal incision, and an extra-abdominal resection and anastomosis are performed. The bowels are returned into the abdomen, the fascia is closed, and the pneumoperitoneum may be reinstalled to inspect the peritoneal cavity again. To facilitate complex resections, some surgeons use hand-assisted laparoscopic surgery (HALS) to combine tactile sensation with a minimally invasive approach.

Sentinel Lymph Node Mapping. Although the interest in lymphatic mapping and sentinel lymph nodes has been derived from favorable experiences in breast cancer and melanoma,[185] most recent data do not support the value of this technique for colon cancer. In particular, analysis of the recent intergroup study 0114 demonstrated a lack of correlation in an alarming 54% of the patients.[186] Sentinel lymph node mapping not only may be misleading and therefore not useful in the management of colorectal cancer, but there also is simply no need for this technique in colon resections because the lymphadenectomy—in contrast to breast and melanoma surgery—is not associated with any morbidity.

Special Circumstances in Emergency Surgery

Approximately 20% of patients with colon cancer present as an emergency requiring an urgent operation for a tumor-related complication (e.g., bowel obstruction, perforation, or massive bleeding).[187] Morbidity and mortality are significantly higher than under elective conditions. Contributing factors are the lack of a mechanical bowel preparation and the patient's impaired overall status, which typically is characterized by dehydration, third spacing of fluids, anemia, a deranged metabolism with electrolyte imbalances, and possible sepsis. The risks for wound and intra-abdominal infections and anastomotic leakages are three to six times higher.[188]

Tumor Obstruction. Sixteen percent of patients with colon cancer present with a bowel obstruction and complain of colicky abdominal pain, abdominal distension, vomiting, constipation, and occasionally, paradoxical diarrhea. Imaging studies (abdominal x-ray or CT scan) characteristically demonstrate the features of a large or small bowel obstruction depending on how proximal in the colon the obstruction is located and whether the ileocecal valve is competent. Attention should be paid to the diameter of the cecum, which presents a risk of cecal perforation if the diameter reaches 12 cm or more. Urgent intervention is required in such circumstances to prevent cecal perforation. The most important differential diagnosis is pseudo-obstruction (Ogilvie's syndrome), which is seen as a result of various medical conditions and may mimic the features of bowel obstruction. Every patient therefore should have a rigid proctoscopy, followed by a water-soluble contrast enema, which should visualize only the colon up to the site of obstruction but not beyond the stenosis because the hyperosmolar nature of the contrast material can result in an increase in the intraluminal volume and trigger a perforation. If the level of obstruction in the colon is proximal enough, a resection with primary entero-colonic anastomosis, e.g., right hemicolectomy, extended right hemicolectomy, or subtotal colectomy, may be carried out. If the tumor is located on the left side of the colon, adjustments to the surgical approach are necessary because the stool load proximal to the obstruction is of concern for a colocolonic anastomosis and because that segment of the colon could not be cleared before the operation. Synchronous lesions, which in the setting of an obstructing lesion may occur in up to 15%, may be missed and necessitate further intervention in the future. Strategies then include either (1) a subtotal colectomy, (2) an on-table lavage with segmental colon resection, intraoperative colonoscopy, and primary anastomosis, or (3) performance of a two- or even three-stage procedure instead of the elective one-stage approach. Historically, obstructed left-sided tumors were treated with a three-stage approach starting with a defunctioning loop colostomy, followed by resection and anastomosis and last by closure of the defunctioning stoma. The Hartmann procedure, the classic example among several two-stage procedures, consists of a rectosigmoid resection with creation of a terminal colostomy and a blind rectal stump in the first stage, followed by a colostomy takedown and reanastomosis in a second operation.

More recently, there has been a trend toward attempting to relieve the acute obstruction at the tumor-bearing segment by colonoscopic insertion of a self-expanding metallic stent. Successful decompression of the prestenotic colon converts the emergency situation into an elective setting, allowing for stabilization of the patient and performance of bowel preparation. The risk of a colonic perforation during stent placement is relatively low but acceptable because an emergency operation would be necessary anyway if the stent could not be placed successfully. Several nonrandomized, noncontrolled case series have demonstrated that colonic stenting for acute obstruction is safe and highly successful.[189,190] A proximal diversion may be performed with this procedure.

Tumor-Related Perforation. Colonic perforation secondary to a tumor occurs in two different settings. Either a transmural tumor perforates itself, or the proximal colon becomes overdistended, particularly in the case of a competent ileocecal valve. Both conditions may result in diffuse fecal peritonitis with significant morbidity and mortality. In addition, the tumor perforation results in spillage of tumor cells and thus has to be considered a stage IV tumor. Surgical management is indicated in every case and requires not only addressing the site of colonic perforation but also removing the tumor in an oncologically correct fashion.[187] The same tactical principles described in the preceding section apply.

Massive Colonic Bleeding. Massive bleeding from a colonic tumor is a relatively rare complication. The general algorithms for the work-up and management of lower gastrointestinal bleedings apply, but most commonly, the bleeding site can be identified easily. If the bleeding is minor or self-limited, the standard work-up can be performed. If the patient is or remains unstable and requires repeated transfusions, surgical management is indicated.

Management of Advanced Disease

Locally Advanced Disease. It has been estimated that approximately 15% of colonic tumors will be adherent to adjacent organs.[191] With locally advanced colon tumors, it is still possible to achieve cure if the surgeon is prepared to resect involved adjacent organs. Unfortunately, it is often impossible to distinguish between malignant and inflammatory adhesions, but at least 40% of these adhesions harbor malignant cells. The surgeon therefore has to consider them malignant until proven otherwise and perform an en-bloc resection to achieve a tumor-free margin.[192]

Operable Metastases. Twenty percent of patients with colorectal cancer have stage IV disease at the time of presentation. Distant metastasis, particularly liver and lung, are a major cause of death in patients with colorectal carcinoma. However, patients with asymptomatic liver metastases may have a statistically natural life expectancy of several months up to almost 2 years without any treatment. Chemotherapy and surgical metastasectomy in selected patients may improve disease-free and overall survival substantially, resulting in a cure rate of 30%.[193] In the case of potentially resectable metastases, resection of the colonic primary tumor therefore should be performed in an oncologic fashion.

Inoperable Disseminated Disease. In patients with unresectable metastatic disease, the surgical treatment goal is to provide palliation and to prevent predictable complications. In contrast to the oncologically defined standard resections, a limited segmental wedge resection of the colon is acceptable in this setting. Particularly tumors located in the sigmoid colon or in the cecum and ascending colon are suitable for a laparoscopic or laparoscopically assisted resection because these segments can be mobilized easily to a sufficient extent to ensure a safe anastomosis. If a tumor in a patient with metastatic disease is too advanced locally to be resected safely (e.g., infiltration of other organs), palliation may be achieved by creating an internal bypass or a proximal diversion.

Postoperative Management

Postoperative management after a colorectal resection has become very straightforward and routine. The immediate postoperative monitoring of vital signs, fluids, and electrolytes, as well as adequate pain control, are not different from any other major surgery. However, there has been an increasing tendency among colorectal surgeons to encourage early mobilization and regular spirometry exercises, to avoid nasogastric tubes, and to resume oral intake on the first or second postoperative day with advancement to a regular diet as tolerated. Daily assessment of the abdomen and bowel activity is crucial, including careful auscultation and palpation of the abdomen to assess bowel sounds or peritoneal signs. Unless soaking, a wound dressing may be left in place until the second postoperative day or even for five days if a transparent dressing is used. The incision has to be checked daily for the presence of induration, hematoma, redness, dehiscence, or discharge of fluids (e.g., pus, hematoma, or serosanguineous fluid). Large amounts of serous fluids draining from the wound should not be mistaken for a seroma but indicates a fascial dehiscence until proven otherwise. The average length of stay after colorectal resections depends on the patient's constitution but generally is in the range between 5–7 days. Before discharge, further tumor treatment should have been addressed with the patient. Adjuvant chemotherapy or radiation therapy typically is not initiated before 3–4 weeks after surgery and may be delayed if infectious complications or anastomotic leaks occur.

COMPLICATIONS OF SURGERY

The overall perioperative mortality within 30 days of colorectal resections is between 3.5% and 6%,[194] with less than 2% after elective but up to 20% after emergency operations. Complications of surgery may be of a general or surgery-specific nature and can be classified with regard to the time of their occurrence as either early (within the first 30 days) or late (after 30 days). Intraoperative complications such as injury to relevant anatomic structures such as ureters, spleen, bowel, and duodenum are related to the surgical technique, to blurred anatomic landmarks and layers owing to the disease (e.g., peritonitis or massive adhesions), or to the patient's habitus (e.g., obesity). Early surgery-specific complications include bleeding, most frequently within the first few days of the resection, nonspecific infections, or infections related to an anastomotic dehiscence. Other more general complications in the early postoperative period (postoperative days 1–3) commonly are related to the cardiopulmonary system and include pulmonary problems (e.g., atelectasis, pneumonia, aspiration, and pulmonary embolism) and cardiac events (e.g., arrhythmia, myocardial ischemia, and dysfunction). Insufficient pain control has been recognized as an important factor promoting these conditions because it results in a poor respiratory effort by the patient and the inability to cough up sputum, leading to superficial respiration and suboptimal saturation. High fever in the 3 days therefore may be related to the development of an atelectasis rather than to an early infection.

Infectious complications usually occur after the third postoperative day and may be located either intra-abdominally, in the wound, in the urinary tract, or in the lungs. The primary work-up therefore includes bacteriologic cultures and stains, blood and urine analysis, and a chest x-ray.

Abdominal complications consist of delayed return of upper and lower gastrointestinal function (also referred to as *postoperative ileus*), fascial dehiscence, and anastomotic breakdown. Clinical leaks occur in 1–2% of all colonic resections, but subclinical leaks are more frequent and may be seen incidentally on contrast studies in otherwise asymptomatic patients. A leak may present with insidious symptoms such as fever, tachycardia, abdominal distension, ileus, feces draining through a drain or the wound, or local and generalized peritonitis. Occasionally, a leak may present with sudden deterioration, generalized peritonitis, and septic shock as the result of a significant and rapid contamination of the peritoneal cavity. Owing to the heterogeneous symptoms, a leak should be suspected in any patient who is not progressing to the expected degree. Blood parameters such as white blood cell counts and C-reactive protein may be elevated but are nonspecific and difficult to distinguish from a normal postoperative reaction. After an abdominal operation, normal free air should be resorbed within 7–10 days.[195] The presence of substantial free subdiaphragmatic air later in the course therefore should raise the index of suspicion for an anastomotic leak.

Imaging studies to define the presence of an anastomotic leak include a water-soluble contrast enema to visualize extravasation of the contrast material and/or a CT scan with oral, intravenous, and possibly rectal contrast material. Apart from antibiotic treatment, the management of an anastomotic leak depends on its presumed extent and the clinical presentation. A patient with generalized peritonitis requires a relaparotomy after appropriate resuscitation. Depending on its location, the anastomosis either should be taken down and the ends should be exteriorized or, in more favorable conditions, resected and a new anastomosis performed with healthy-looking bowel ends, either with or without proximal diversion. A local repair alone carries a high risk of failure but may succeed in combination with drain placement and a proximal diverting ostomy. By the time of the reexploration, the prolonged peritonitis in some cases already may have transformed the bowel loops into rigid pipes that would not allow any mobilization for an ostomy or for a new anastomosis. In such a case, creation of a confined leak by means of a catheter enterostomy may be a desperate attempt for local control. A fecal fistula can be managed in a conservative manner if there is no evidence of generalized peritonitis or uncontrolled sepsis. Under favorable conditions, including good nutritional support and absence of a distal obstruction or disease of the involved bowel segment, the fistula may close spontaneously. The surrounding skin will need special care, and a stoma therapist will be helpful in this regard.

ADJUVANT CHEMOTHERAPY AND RADIOTHERAPY

The rationale for adjuvant chemotherapy is based on the fact that we are clearly not as successful with surgical treatment as we would like. 5-Fluorouracil was the first and most extensively evaluated drug for the treatment of colorectal cancer. Multiple studies had been completed without proof of value until Krook's study.[196] Subsequently, a review of 29 randomized trails concluded that adjuvant chemotherapy for colon cancer resulted in a 5% improvement in survival.[197] When studies using 5-fluorouracil (5-FU)–based regimens are analyzed, there is a 2.3–5.7% absolute improvement in 5-year overall survival. However, when just those at high risk of recurrence are treated, the improvement in survival in this group is closer to 30%. Patients with stage III colon cancer are recognized to be at high risk for recurrence, and administration of 5-FU/leucovorin (LV) for 6 months after surgery has proven to decrease recurrence and improve long-term survival.[198] The combination treatment of 5-FU/LV for 6 months was proven to be equivalent in efficacy to 12 months, and the addition of levamisole to 5-FU/LV did not seem to add any benefit.[199] Low-dose LV also was demonstrated to be equally efficacious as high-dose LV when used in combination with 5-FU. Thus the first-line standard of treatment from 1998 to 2000 was a combination of 5-FU and low-dose LV (folinic acid) given for 6 months on either a weekly schedule or 5 consecutive days every 4 weeks. At present, there is not enough evidence to recommend the routine use of adjuvant chemotherapy in stage II disease. Lenz and colleagues have demonstrated that molecular or genetic markers may better identify subgroups of patients who are likely to benefit from adjuvant chemotherapy.[200,201]

Several new agents, e.g., irinotecan[202,203] (CPT-11) and oxaliplatin,[204–206] have demonstrated significantly superior activity in combination with 5-FU/LV in the metastatic setting. Irinotecan/5-FU/LV (IFL)[202] and oxaliplatin/5-FU/LV (FOLFOX) have been entered into randomized clinical trials against 5-FU/LV in resected stage III colon cancer.[207] Both these studies prove that the new agents in association with 5-FU/LV were superior to 5-FU/LV alone. Because of these successes, IFL was approved as first-line chemotherapy in 2000. In 2005, 5-FU/LV with oxaliplatin (FOLFOX) was approved for adjuvant therapy and has evolved in most centers as the treatment of choice. The FOLFOX regime has been compared in a large randomized, controlled trial with IFL and irinotecan/oxaliplatin (IROX) in patients with previously untreated metastatic colorectal cancer.[207] This study showed significantly superior results of the FOLFOX regime for all end points. The median time to progression observed for FOLFOX was 8.7 months, response rate was 45%, and the median survival time was 19.5 months. The FOLFOX regimen had significantly lower rates of severe nausea, vomiting, diarrhea, febrile neutropenia, and dehydration. Sensory neuropathy and neutropenia were common with the regimens containing oxaliplatin.

Capecitabine (Xeloda), an oral agent designed to generate 5-FU preferentially in tumor tissue, is an exciting new development with improved convenience. A randomized phase III study comparing oral capecitabine versus intravenous 5-FU/LV concluded that capecitabine demonstrated a statistically significantly greater response rate compared with 5-FU/LV (26% versus 17%; $p < 0.002$) and an equivalent time to progression and overall survival.[208] This study demonstrated that capecitabine is a suitable alternative to IV 5-FU and perhaps a replacement in the future. There are currently phase II trails being conducted on capecitabine/oxaliplatin (CAPEOX) and capecitabine/irinotecan (CAPEIRI).[209–213] Two of the most promising new targets in the treatment of colorectal cancer are the epithelial growth factor receptor (EGFR) and vascular endothelial growth factor (VEGF) blockers.[214,215] Agents that inhibit the EGFR or bind to VEGF have demonstrated clinical activity as single agents and in combination with chemotherapy in phase II and phase III clinical trials. The most promising of these agents are the monoclonal antibodies cetuximab, which blocks the binding of epithelial growth factor, and bevacizumab, which binds free VEGF.[214,215] We await future developments of these drugs and their impact in the fight against colorectal cancer. Both agents have proven benefit and seem to work best as first-line therapy.

Generally, radiotherapy does not play a primary role in the adjuvant treatment of colon cancer. However, it may be considered as a locoregional field radiation in selected locally advanced T4N0–N1 tumors.[216–218]

OUTCOME AND PROGNOSIS

Recent years have produced a trend toward better outcome and survival in patients diagnosed with colorectal cancer. This may be related to safer and more successful surgical treatment in combination with better nonoperative and adjuvant treatments. The perioperative mortality within 30 days of elective colorectal resections is less than 2% even though it still may be relatively high after an emergency operation, thus resulting in an overall mortality of 3.5–5.5%.[194] SEER data demonstrate an overall decline in colorectal cancer mortality. While the overall 5-year survival of patients with colon cancer was at 41% between 1950 and 1952, it has since increased steadily to 63.8% between 1995 and 2000. Analyzed for each stage as defined by the AJCC sixth edition system separately, 5-year survival was 93.2% for stage I, 84.7% for stage IIa, 72.2% for stage IIb, 83.4% for stage IIIa, 64.1% for stage IIIb, 44.3% for stage IIIc, and 8.1% for stage IV.[4] The prognosis of patients with synchronous primary colon tumors is not different from that of patients with solitary tumors if they are compared on the basis of the most advanced stage (Table 23–14).[219]

TABLE 23–14. FIVE-YEAR SURVIVAL FOR SINGLE AND SYNCHRONOUS COLON CANCER PRIMARIES

Stage	Single (n = 4817)	Synchronous by highest stage (n = 160)	*P* value[a]
	%	%	
0,I	83	87	NS[b]
II	71	67	NS
III	53	50	NS
IV	9	14	NS

[a]By long-rank test.
[b]Not significant.
Reproduced, with permission, from Passman MA et al, 1996.[219]

REFERENCES

1. Society AC. *Cancer Facts & Figures 2004,* www.cancerorg/docroot/stt/stt_0asp 2004; accessed on November 25, 2004
2. Calvert PM, Frucht H. The genetics of colorectal cancer. *Ann Intern Med* 2002;137:603–612
3. Ferlay J, Bray F, Pisani P, Parkin DM. GLOBOCAN 2002: Cancer incidence, mortality and prevalence. In *Worldwide IARC Cancer Base,* vol 5, version 2.0. Lyon: IARC Press, 2004
4. O'Connell JB, Maggard MA, Ko CY. Colon cancer survival rates with the new American Joint Committee on Cancer sixth edition staging. *J Natl Cancer Inst* 2004;96:1420–1425
5. Troisi RJ, Freedman AN, Devesa SS. Incidence of colorectal carcinoma in the US: An update of trends by gender, race, age, subsite, and stage, 1975–1994. *Cancer* 1999;85:1670–1676
6. Chen VW, Fenoglio-Preiser CM, Wu XC, et al. Aggressiveness of colon carcinoma in blacks and whites. National Cancer Institute Black/White Cancer Survival Study Group. *Cancer Epidemiol Biomark Prevent* 1997;6:1087–1093
7. Agrawal S, Bhupinderjit A, Bhutani MS, et al. Colorectal cancer in African Americans. *Am J Gastroenterol* 2005;100:515–523; discussion 514
8. Potter JD. Colorectal cancer: Molecules and populations. *J Natl Cancer Inst* 1999;91:916–932
9. Burt RW. Colon cancer screening. *Gastroenterology* 2000;119:837–853
10. Winawer S, Fletcher R, Rex D, et al. Colorectal cancer screening and surveillance: Clinical guidelines and rationale—Update based on new evidence. *Gastroenterology* 2003;124:544–560
11. Wynder EL, Reddy BS, Weisburger JH. Environmental dietary factors in colorectal cancer: Some unresolved issues. *Cancer* 1992;70:1222–1228
12. Schatzkin A, Kelloff G. Chemo- and dietary prevention of colorectal cancer. *Eur J Cancer* 1995;31A:1198–1204
13. Ghadirian P, Lacroix A, Maisonneuve P, et al. Nutritional factors and colon carcinoma: A case-control study involving French Canadians in Montreal, Quebec, Canada. *Cancer* 1997;80:858–864
14. Chao A, Thun MJ, Connell CJ, et al. Meat consumption and risk of colorectal cancer. *JAMA* 2005;293:172–182
15. Alberts DS, Ritenbaugh C, Story JA, et al. Randomized, double-blinded, placebo-controlled study of effect of wheat bran fiber and calcium on fecal bile acids in patients with resected adenomatous colon polyps. *J Natl Cancer Inst* 1996;88:81–92
16. McKeown-Eyssen GE, Bright-See E, Bruce WR, et al. A randomized trial of a low fat high fibre diet in the recurrence of colorectal polyps. Toronto Polyp Prevention Group. *J Clin Epidemiol* 1994;47:525–536 [erratum appears in *J Clin Epidemiol* 1995;48(2):i]
17. Kim YI. AGA technical review: Impact of dietary fiber on colon cancer occurrence. *Gastroenterology* 2000;118:1235–1257
18. Konings EJ, Goldbohm RA, Brants HA, et al. Intake of dietary folate vitamers and risk of colorectal carcinoma: Results from The Netherlands Cohort Study. *Cancer* 2002;95:1421–1333
19. Lieberman DA, Prindiville S, Weiss DG, et al. Risk factors for advanced colonic neoplasia and hyperplastic polyps in asymptomatic individuals. *JAMA* 2003;290:2959–2967
20. Fuchs CS, Giovannucci EL, Colditz GA, et al. Dietary fiber and the risk of colorectal cancer and adenoma in women. *N Engl J Med* 1999;340:169–176
21. Ferguson LR, Harris PJ. The dietary fibre debate: More food for thought. *Lancet* 2003;361:1487–1488
22. Modan B, Barell V, Lubin F, et al. Low-fiber intake as an etiologic factor in cancer of the colon. *J Natl Cancer Inst* 1975;55:15–18
23. Levi F, Pasche C, La Vecchia C, et al. Food groups and colorectal cancer risk. *Br J Cancer* 1999;79:1283–1287
24. Michels KB, Edward G, Joshipura KJ, et al. Prospective study of fruit and vegetable consumption and incidence of colon and rectal cancers. *J Natl Cancer Inst* 2000;92:1740–1752 [erratum appears in *J Natl Cancer Inst* 2001;93:879]
25. Trock B, Lanza E, Greenwald P. Dietary fiber, vegetables, and colon cancer: critical review and meta-analyses of the epidemiologic evidence. *J Natl Cancer Inst* 1990;82:650–661
26. Garland C, Shekelle RB, Barrett-Connor E, et al. Dietary vitamin D and calcium and risk of colorectal cancer: a 19-year prospective study in men. *Lancet* 1985;1:307–309
27. Wu K, Willett WC, Fuchs CS, et al. Calcium intake and risk of colon cancer in women and men. *J Natl Cancer Inst* 2002;94:437–446
28. Baron JA, Beach M, Mandel JS, et al. Calcium supplements for the prevention of colorectal adenomas. Calcium Polyp Prevention Study Group. *N Engl J Med* 1999;340:101–107
29. Grau MV, Baron JA, Sandler RS, et al. Vitamin D, calcium supplementation, and colorectal adenomas: Results of a randomized trial. *J Natl Cancer Inst* 2003;95:1765–1771
30. Greenberg ER, Baron JA, Tosteson TD, et al. A clinical trial of antioxidant vitamins to prevent colorectal adenoma. Polyp Prevention Study Group. *N Engl J Med* 1994;331:141–147
31. Lee DH, Anderson KE, Harnack LJ, et al. Heme iron, zinc, alcohol consumption, and colon cancer: Iowa Women's Health Study. *J Natl Cancer Inst* 2004;96:403–407
32. Sheehan KM, Sheahan K, O'Donoghue DP, et al. The relationship between cyclooxygenase-2 expression and colorectal cancer. *JAMA* 1999;282:1254-1257 [erratum appears in *JAMA* 2000;283:1427]
33. Baron JA, Cole BF, Sandler RS, et al. A randomized trial of aspirin to prevent colorectal adenomas. *N Engl J Med* 2003;348:891–899
34. teinbach G, Lynch PM, Phillips RK, et al. The effect of celecoxib, a cyclooxygenase-2 inhibitor, in familial adenomatous polyposis. *N Engl J Med* 2000;342:1946–1952

35. Cruz-Correa M, Hylind LM, Romans KE, et al. Long-term treatment with sulindac in familial adenomatous polyposis: A prospective cohort study. *Gastroenterology* 2002;122:641–645
36. Giardiello FM, Yang VW, Hylind LM, et al. Primary chemoprevention of familial adenomatous polyposis with sulindac. *N Engl J Med* 2002;346:1054–1059
37. Ferrandez A, Prescott S, Burt RW. COX-2 and colorectal cancer. *Curr Pharm Des* 2003;9:2229–2251
38. Solomon SD, McMurray JJ, Pfeffer MA, et al. Cardiovascular risk associated with celecoxib in a clinical trial for colorectal adenoma prevention. *N Engl J Med* 2005;352:1071–1080
39. Bresalier RS, Sandler RS, Quan H, et al. Cardiovascular events associated with rofecoxib in a colorectal adenoma chemoprevention trial. *N Engl J Med* 2005;352:1092–1102
40. Rainey JB, Davies PW, Bristol JB, Williamson RC. Adaptation and carcinogenesis in defunctioned rat colon: Divergent effects of faeces and bile acids. *Br J Cancer* 1983;48:477–484
41. Imray CH, Radley S, Davis A, et al. Faecal unconjugated bile acids in patients with colorectal cancer or polyps. *Gut* 1992;33:1239–1245
42. Linos D, Beard CM, O'Fallon WM, et al. Cholecystectomy and carcinoma of the colon. *Lancet* 1981;2:379–381
43. Lagergren J, Ye W, Ekbom A. Intestinal cancer after cholecystectomy: Is bile involved in carcinogenesis? *Gastroenterology* 2001;121:542–547
44. Reddy BS, Engle A, Simi B, Goldman M. Effect of dietary fiber on colonic bacterial enzymes and bile acids in relation to colon cancer. *Gastroenterology* 1992;102:1475–1482
45. Martinez ME, McPherson RS, Annegers JF, Levin B. Cigarette smoking and alcohol consumption as risk factors for colorectal adenomatous polyps. *J Natl Cancer Inst* 1995;87:274–279
46. Giovannucci E, Rimm EB, Ascherio A, et al. Alcohol, low-methionine–low-folate diets, and risk of colon cancer in men. *J Natl Cancer Inst* 1995;87:265–273
47. Kikendall JW, Bowen PE, Burgess MB, et al. Cigarettes and alcohol as independent risk factors for colonic adenomas. *Gastroenterology* 1989;97:660–664
48. Slattery ML, Curtin K, Anderson K, et al. Associations between cigarette smoking, lifestyle factors, and microsatellite instability in colon tumors. *J Natl Cancer Inst* 2000;92:1831–1836
49. Baron JA, Sandler RS, Haile RW, et al. Folate intake, alcohol consumption, cigarette smoking, and risk of colorectal adenomas. *J Natl Cancer Inst* 1998;90:57–62
50. Giovannucci E, Pollak MN, Platz EA, et al. A prospective study of plasma insulin-like growth factor-1 and binding protein-3 and risk of colorectal neoplasia in women. *Cancer Epidemiol Biomark Prevent* 2000;9:345–349
51. Cannon-Albright LA, Skolnick MH, Bishop DT, et al. Common inheritance of susceptibility to colonic adenomatous polyps and associated colorectal cancers. *N Engl J Med* 1988;319:533–537
52. Winawer SJ, Zauber AG, Gerdes H, et al. Risk of colorectal cancer in the families of patients with adenomatous polyps. National Polyp Study Workgroup. *N Engl J Med* 1996;334:82–87
53. Ekbom A, Helmick C, Zack M, Adami HO. Ulcerative colitis and colorectal cancer: A population-based study. *N Engl J Med* 1990;323:1228–1233
54. Kaiser AM, Beart RW Jr. Surgical management of ulcerative colitis. *Swiss Med Wkly* 2001;131:323–337
55. Rutter M, Saunders B, Wilkinson K, et al. Severity of inflammation is a risk factor for colorectal neoplasia in ulcerative colitis. *Gastroenterology* 2004;126:451–459
56. Weedon DD, Shorter RG, Ilstrup DM, et al. Crohn's disease and cancer. *N Engl J Med* 1973;289:1099–1103
57. Ekbom A, Helmick C, Zack M, Adami HO. Increased risk of large-bowel cancer in Crohn's disease with colonic involvement. *Lancet* 1990;336:357–359
58. Gillen CD, Walmsley RS, Prior P, et al. Ulcerative colitis and Crohn's disease: A comparison of the colorectal cancer risk in extensive colitis. *Gut* 1994;35:1590–1592
59. Azimuddin K, Khubchandani IT, Stasik JJ, et al. Neoplasia after ureterosigmoidostomy. *Dis Colon Rectum* 1999;42:1632–1638
60. Otchy DP, Nelson H. Radiation injuries of the colon and rectum. *Surg Clin North Am* 1993;73:1017–1035
61. Kalble T, Tricker AR, Mohring K, et al. The role of nitrate, nitrite and *N*-nitrosamines in carcinogenesis of colon tumours following ureterosigmoidostomy. *Urol Res* 1990;18:123–129
62. Husmann DA, Spence HM. Current status of tumor of the bowel following ureterosigmoidostomy: A review. *J Urol* 1990;144:607–610
63. Smith RA, von Eschenbach AC, Wender R, et al. American Cancer Society Guidelines for the Early Detection of Cancer: Update of Early Detection Guidelines for Prostate, Colorectal, and Endometrial Cancers; *also:* Update 2001—Testing for Early Lung Cancer Detection. *CA* 2001;51:38–75
64. Winawer SJ, Stewart ET, Zauber AG, et al. A comparison of colonoscopy and double-contrast barium enema for surveillance after polypectomy. National Polyp Study Work Group. *N Engl J Med* 2000;342:1766–1772
65. Hadley DW, Jenkins JF, Dimond E, et al. Colon cancer screening practices after genetic counseling and testing for hereditary nonpolyposis colorectal cancer. *J Clin Oncol* 2004;22:39–44
66. Winawer SJ, Zauber AG, Ho MN, et al. Prevention of colorectal cancer by colonoscopic polypectomy. The National Polyp Study Workgroup. *N Engl J Med* 1993;329:1977–1781
67. Gatenby RA, Vincent TL. An evolutionary model of carcinogenesis. *Cancer Res* 2003;63:6212–6220
68. Iino H, Fukayama M, Maeda Y, et al. Molecular genetics for clinical management of colorectal carcinoma: 17p, 18q, and 22q loss of heterozygosity and decreased *DCC* expression are correlated with the metastatic potential. *Cancer* 1994;73:1324–1331

69. Senba S, Konishi F, Okamoto T, et al. Clinicopathologic and genetic features of nonfamilial colorectal carcinomas with DNA replication errors. *Cancer* 1998;82:279–285
70. Boland CR, Thibodeau SN, Hamilton SR, et al. A National Cancer Institute Workshop on microsatellite instability for cancer detection and familial predisposition: Development of international criteria for the determination of microsatellite instability in colorectal cancer. *Cancer Res* 1998;58:5248–5257
71. Vogelstein B, Fearon ER, Hamilton SR, et al. Genetic alterations during colorectal-tumor development. *N Engl J Med* 1988;319:525–532
72. Kikuchi-Yanoshita R, Konishi M, Fukunari H, et al. Loss of expression of the *DCC* gene during progression of colorectal carcinomas in familial adenomatous polyposis and nonfamilial adenomatous polyposis patients. *Cancer Res* 1992;52:3801–3803
73. Takayama T, Ohi M, Hayashi T, et al. Analysis of K-*ras, APC,* and beta-catenin in aberrant crypt foci in sporadic adenoma, cancer, and familial adenomatous polyposis. *Gastroenterology* 2001;121:599–611
74. Powell SM, Zilz N, Beazer-Barclay Y, et al. *APC* mutations occur early during colorectal tumorigenesis. *Nature* 1992;359:235–237
75. Fearon ER, Vogelstein B. A genetic model for colorectal tumorigenesis. *Cell* 1990;61:759–767
76. Kikuchi-Yanoshita R, Konishi M, Ito S, et al. Genetic changes of both *p53* alleles associated with the conversion from colorectal adenoma to early carcinoma in familial adenomatous polyposis and nonfamilial adenomatous polyposis patients. *Cancer Res* 1992;52:3965–3971
77. Houlston RS, Murday V, Harocopos C, et al. Screening and genetic counselling for relatives of patients with colorectal cancer in a family cancer clinic. *BMJ* 1990; 301:366–368 [erratum appears in *BMJ* 1990;301:446]
78. Laken SJ, Petersen GM, Gruber SB, et al. Familial colorectal cancer in Ashkenazim due to a hypermutable tract in *APC. Nature Genet* 1997;17:79–83
79. Powell SM, Petersen GM, Krush AJ, et al. Molecular diagnosis of familial adenomatous polyposis. *N Engl J Med* 1993;329:1982–1987
80. Offerhaus GJ, Giardiello FM, Krush AJ, et al. The risk of upper gastrointestinal cancer in familial adenomatous polyposis. *Gastroenterology* 1992;102:1980–1982
81. Bjork J, Akerbrant H, Iselius L, et al. Periampullary adenomas and adenocarcinomas in familial adenomatous polyposis: Cumulative risks and *APC* gene mutations. *Gastroenterology* 2001;121:1127–1135
82. Jagelman DG, DeCosse JJ, Bussey HJ. Upper gastrointestinal cancer in familial adenomatous polyposis. *Lancet* 1988;1:1149–1151
83. Wallace MH, Phillips RK. Upper gastrointestinal disease in patients with familial adenomatous polyposis. *Br J Surg* 1998;85:742–750
84. Gurbuz AK, Giardiello FM, Petersen GM, et al. Desmoid tumours in familial adenomatous polyposis. *Gut* 1994; 35:377–381
85. Clark SK, Smith TG, Katz DE, et al. Identification and progression of a desmoid precursor lesion in patients with familial adenomatous polyposis. *Br J Surg* 1998;85: 970–973
86. Lynch HT, Smyrk T, McGinn T, et al. Attenuated familial adenomatous polyposis (AFAP): A phenotypically and genotypically distinctive variant of FAP. *Cancer* 1995; 76:2427–2433
87. Wang L, Baudhuin LM, Boardman LA, et al. *MYH* mutations in patients with attenuated and classic polyposis and with young-onset colorectal cancer without polyps. *Gastroenterology* 2004;127:9–16
88. Heinimann K, Mullhaupt B, Weber W, et al. Phenotypic differences in familial adenomatous polyposis based on *APC* gene mutation status. *Gut* 1998;43:675–679
89. Lynch HT, de la Chapelle A. Hereditary colorectal cancer. *N Engl J Med* 2003;348:919–932
90. Aarnio M, Mecklin JP, Aaltonen LA, et al. Life-time risk of different cancers in hereditary nonpolyposis colorectal cancer (HNPCC) syndrome. *Int J Cancer* 1995;64: 430–433
91. Aarnio M, Mustonen H, Mecklin JP, Jarvinen HJ. Prognosis of colorectal cancer varies in different high-risk conditions. *Ann Med* 1998;30:75–80
92. Vasen HF, Wijnen JT, Menko FH, et al. Cancer risk in families with hereditary nonpolyposis colorectal cancer diagnosed by mutation analysis. *Gastroenterology* 1996; 110:1020–1027 [erratum appears in *Gastroenterology* 1996;111:1402]
93. Thibodeau SN, Bren G, Schaid D. Microsatellite instability in cancer of the proximal colon. *Science* 1993;260: 816–819
94. Chung DC, Rustgi AK. DNA mismatch repair and cancer. *Gastroenterology* 1995;109:1685–1699
95. De Jong AE, Morreau H, Van Puijenbroek M, et al. The role of mismatch repair gene defects in the development of adenomas in patients with HNPCC. *Gastroenterology* 2004;126:42–48
96. Kinzler KW, Vogelstein B. Cancer-susceptibility genes: Gatekeepers and caretakers. *Nature* 1997;386:761
97. Lynch HT, de la Chapelle A. Genetic susceptibility to nonpolyposis colorectal cancer. *J Med Genet* 1999;36: 801–818
98. Lin KM, Shashidharan M, Thorson AG, et al. Cumulative incidence of colorectal and extracolonic cancers in *MLH1* and *MSH2* mutation carriers of hereditary nonpolyposis colorectal cancer. *J Gastrointest Surg* 1998;2:67–71
99. Wijnen J, de Leeuw W, Vasen H, et al. Familial endometrial cancer in female carriers of *MSH6* germline mutations. *Nature Genet* 1999;23:142–144
100. Hemminki A, Tomlinson I, Markie D, et al. Localization of a susceptibility locus for Peutz-Jeghers syndrome to 19p using comparative genomic hybridization and targeted linkage analysis. *Nature Genet* 1997;15:87–90
101. Haggitt RC, Reid BJ. Hereditary gastrointestinal polyposis syndromes. *Am J Surg Pathol* 1986;10:871–887
102. Giardiello FM, Hamilton SR, Kern SE, et al. Colorectal neoplasia in juvenile polyposis or juvenile polyps. *Arch Dis Child* 1991;66:971–975

103. Howe JR, Roth S, Ringold JC, et al. Mutations in the *SMAD4/DPC4* gene in juvenile polyposis. *Science* 1998; 280:1086–1088
104. Nelen MR, Padberg GW, Peeters EA, et al. Localization of the gene for Cowden disease to chromosome 10q22-23. *Nature Genet* 1996;13:114–116
105. Chi SG, Kim HJ, Park BJ, et al. Mutational abrogation of the *PTEN/MMAC1* gene in gastrointestinal polyps in patients with Cowden disease. *Gastroenterology* 1998;115: 1084–1089
106. Eng C. *PTEN:* One gene, many syndromes. *Hum Mutat* 2003;22:183–198
107. Zigman AF, Lavine JE, Jones MC, et al. Localization of the Bannayan-Riley-Ruvalcaba syndrome gene to chromosome 10q23. *Gastroenterology* 1997;113:1433–1437
108. Arch EM, Goodman BK, Van Wesep RA, et al. Deletion of *PTEN* in a patient with Bannayan-Riley-Ruvalcaba syndrome suggests allelism with Cowden disease. *Am J Med Genet* 1997;71:489–493
109. Johnson GK, Soergel KH, Hensley GT, et al. Cronkite-Canada syndrome: Gastrointestinal pathophysiology and morphology. *Gastroenterology* 1972;63:140–152
110. Williams GT, Arthur JF, Bussey HJ, Morson BC. Metaplastic polyps and polyposis of the colorectum. *Histopathology* 1980;4:155–170
111. Clark JC, Collan Y, Eide TJ, et al. Prevalence of polyps in an autopsy series from areas with varying incidence of large-bowel cancer. *Int J Cancer* 1985;36:179–186
112. O'Brien MJ, Winawer SJ, Zauber AG, et al. The National Polyp Study: Patient and polyp characteristics associated with high-grade dysplasia in colorectal adenomas. *Gastroenterology* 1990;98:371–379
113. Nascimbeni R, Burgart LJ, Nivatvongs S, Larson DR. Risk of lymph node metastasis in T1 carcinoma of the colon and rectum. *Dis Colon Rectum* 2002;45:200–206
114. Muto T, Kamiya J, Sawada T, et al. Small "flat adenoma" of the large bowel with special reference to its clinicopathologic features. *Dis Colon Rectum* 1985;28:847–851
115. Adachi M, Muto T, Okinaga K, Morioka Y. Clinicopathologic features of the flat adenoma. *Dis Colon Rectum* 1991;34:981–986
116. Jaramillo E, Watanabe M, Slezak P, Rubio C. Flat neoplastic lesions of the colon and rectum detected by high-resolution video endoscopy and chromoscopy. *Gastrointest Endosc* 1995;42:114–122
117. Rembacken BJ, Fujii T, Cairns A, et al. Flat and depressed colonic neoplasms: A prospective study of 1000 colonoscopies in the UK. *Lancet* 2000;355:1211–1214
118. Pilbrow SJ, Hertzog PJ, Linnane AW. The adenoma-carcinoma sequence in the colorectum: Early appearance of a hierarchy of small intestinal mucin antigen (SIMA) epitopes and correlation with malignant potential. *Br J Cancer* 1992;66:748–757
119. Loeve F, Boer R, Zauber AG, et al. National Polyp Study data: Evidence for regression of adenomas. *Int J Cancer* 2004;111:633–639
120. Nusko G, Mansmann U, Kirchner T, Hahn EG. Risk related surveillance following colorectal polypectomy. *Gut* 2002;51:424–428
121. Haggitt RC, Glotzbach RE, Soffer EE, Wruble LD. Prognostic factors in colorectal carcinomas arising in adenomas: Implications for lesions removed by endoscopic polypectomy. *Gastroenterology* 1985;89:328–336
122. Kudo S, Kashida H, Tamura T. Early colorectal cancer: Flat or depressed type. *J Gastroenterol Hepatol* 2000;15:66–70
123. Sasaki O, Atkin WS, Jass JR. Mucinous carcinoma of the rectum. *Histopathology* 1987;11:259–272
124. Kanemitsu Y, Kato T, Hirai T, et al. Survival after curative resection for mucinous adenocarcinoma of the colorectum. *Dis Colon Rectum* 2003;46:160–1607
125. Obrand DI, Gordon PH. Continued change in the distribution of colorectal carcinoma. *Br J Surg* 1998;85: 246–248
126. Cheng X, Chen VW, Steele B, et al. Subsite-specific incidence rate and stage of disease in colorectal cancer by race, gender, and age group in the United States, 1992–1997. *Cancer* 2001;92:2547–2554
127. Jayne DG, Fook S, Loi C, Seow-Choen F. Peritoneal carcinomatosis from colorectal cancer. *Br J Surg* 2002;89: 1545–1550
128. Compton CC, Greene FL. The staging of colorectal cancer: 2004 and beyond. *CA Cancer J Clin* 2004;54:295–308
129. Maggard MA, O'Connell JB, Ko CY. Updated population-based review of carcinoid tumors. *Ann Surg* 2004; 240:117–122
130. Kulke MH, Mayer RJ. Carcinoid tumors. *N Engl J Med* 1999;340:858–868
131. Pellikka P, Tajik A, Khandheria B, et al. Carcinoid heart disease: Clinical and echocardiographic spectrum in 74 patients. *Circulation* 1993;87:1188–1196
132. Fox DJ, Khattar RS. Carcinoid heart disease: Presentation, diagnosis, and management. *Heart* 2004;90:1224–1228
133. Koh JS, Trent J, Chen L, et al. Gastrointestinal stromal tumors: Overview of pathologic features, molecular biology, and therapy with imatinib mesylate. *Histol Histopathol* 2004;19:565–574
134. Ueyama T, Guo KJ, Hashimoto H, et al. A clinicopathologic and immunohistochemical study of gastrointestinal stromal tumors. *Cancer* 1992;69:947–955
135. Medeiros F, Corless CL, Duensing A, et al. KIT-negative gastrointestinal stromal tumors: Proof of concept and therapeutic implications. *Am J Surg Pathol* 2004;28:889–894
136. Corless CL, Fletcher JA, Heinrich MC. Biology of gastrointestinal stromal tumors. *J Clin Oncol* 2004;22:3813–3825
137. Heinrich MC, Corless CL, Duensing A, et al. PDGFRA activating mutations in gastrointestinal stromal tumors. *Science* 2003;299:708–710
138. Castellano G, Moreno D, Galvao O, et al. Malignant lymphoma of jejunum with common variable hypogammaglobulinemia and diffuse nodular hyperplasia of the small intestine: A case study and literature review. *J Clin Gastroenterol* 1992;15:128–135
139. Chim CS, Shek TW, Chung LP, Liang R. Unusual abdominal tumors: Case 3. Multiple lymphomatous polyposis in lymphoma of colon. *J Clin Oncol* 2003;21:953–955

140. Kohno S, Ohshima K, Yoneda S, et al. Clinicopathological analysis of 143 primary malignant lymphomas in the small and large intestines based on the new WHO classification. *Histopathology* 2003;43:135–143
141. Raderer M, Pfeffel F, Pohl G, et al. Regression of colonic low grade B cell lymphoma of the mucosa associated lymphoid tissue type after eradication of *Helicobacter pylori*. *Gut* 2000;46:133–135
142. Ruskone-Fourmestraux A, Delmer A, Lavergne A, et al. Multiple lymphomatous polyposis of the gastrointestinal tract: Prospective clinicopathologic study of 31 cases. Groupe D'etude des Lymphomes Digestifs. *Gastroenterology* 1997;112:7–16
143. Kaiser AM, Ortega AE. Anorectal anatomy. *Surg Clin North Am* 2002;82:1125–1138
144. Nelson H, Petrelli N, Carlin A, et al. Guidelines 2000 for colon and rectal cancer surgery. *J Natl Cancer Inst* 2001;93:583–596
145. Fenlon HM, Nunes DP, Schroy PC 3rd, et al. A comparison of virtual and conventional colonoscopy for the detection of colorectal polyps. *N Engl J Med* 1999;341:1496–1503 [erratum appears in *N Engl J Med* 2000;342:524]
146. Pickhardt PJ, Choi JR, Hwang I, et al. Computed tomographic virtual colonoscopy to screen for colorectal neoplasia in asymptomatic adults. *N Engl J Med* 2003;349:2191–2200
147. Spinzi G, Belloni G, Martegani A, et al. Computed tomographic colonography and conventional colonoscopy for colon diseases: A prospective, blinded study. *Am J Gastroenterol* 2001;96:394–400
148. Ward J, Naik KS, Guthrie JA, et al. Hepatic lesion detection: Comparison of MR imaging after the administration of superparamagnetic iron oxide with dual-phase CT by using alternative-free response receiver operating characteristic analysis. *Radiology* 1999;210:459–466
149. Stone MD, Kane R, Bothe A Jr, et al. Intraoperative ultrasound imaging of the liver at the time of colorectal cancer resection. *Arch Surg* 1994;129:431–435; discussion 435–436
150. Moertel CG, Fleming TR, Macdonald JS, et al. An evaluation of the carcinoembryonic antigen (CEA) test for monitoring patients with resected colon cancer. *JAMA* 1993;270:943–947
151. Burrows L, Tartter P. Effect of blood transfusions on colonic malignancy recurrent rate. *Lancet* 1982;2:18
152. Vamvakas EC. Perioperative blood transfusion and cancer recurrence: Meta-analysis for explanation. *Transfusion* 1995;35:760–768
153. Busch OR, Hop WC, Marquet RL, Jeekel J. Blood transfusions and local tumor recurrence in colorectal cancer: Evidence of a noncausal relationship. *Ann Surg* 1994;220:791–797
154. Bucher P, Gervaz P, Soravia C, et al. Randomized clinical trial of mechanical bowel preparation versus no preparation before elective left-sided colorectal surgery. *Br J Surg* 2005;92:409–414
155. Santos JC Jr, Batista J, Sirimarco MT, et al. Prospective randomized trial of mechanical bowel preparation in patients undergoing elective colorectal surgery. *Br J Surg* 1994;81:1673–1676
156. Burke P, Mealy K, Gillen P, et al. Requirement for bowel preparation in colorectal surgery. *Br J Surg* 1994;81:907–910
157. Miettinen RP, Laitinen ST, Makela JT, Paakkonen ME. Bowel preparation with oral polyethylene glycol electrolyte solution vs no preparation in elective open colorectal surgery: Prospective, randomized study. *Dis Colon Rectum* 2000;43:669–675; discussion 675–677
158. Zmora O, Mahajna A, Bar-Zakai B, et al. Colon and rectal surgery without mechanical bowel preparation: A randomized, prospective trial. *Ann Surg* 2003;237:363–367
159. Wolff BG, Beart RW Jr, Dozois RR, et al. A new bowel preparation for elective colon and rectal surgery: A prospective, randomized clinical trial. *Arch Surg* 1988;123:895–900
160. Ramirez JI, Vassiliu P, Gonzalez-Ruiz C, et al. Sequential compression devices as prophylaxis for venous thromboembolism in high-risk colorectal surgery patients: Reconsidering American Society of Colorectal Surgeons parameters. *Am Surg* 2003;69:941–945
161. Anonymous. Practice parameters for the prevention of venous thromboembolism. The Standards Task Force of the American Society of Colon and Rectal Surgeons. *Dis Colon Rectum* 2000;43:1037–1047
162. Collins R, Scrimgeour A, Yusuf S, Peto R. Reduction in fatal pulmonary embolism and venous thrombosis by perioperative administration of subcutaneous heparin: Overview of results of randomized trials in general, orthopedic, and urologic surgery. *N Engl J Med* 1988;318:1162–1173
163. McLeod RS, Geerts WH, Sniderman KW, et al. Subcutaneous heparin versus low-molecular-weight heparin as thromboprophylaxis in patients undergoing colorectal surgery. Results of the Canadian Colorectal DVT Prophylaxis Trial: A randomized, double-blind trial. *Ann Surg* 2001;233:438–444
164. Etchells E, McLeod RS, Geerts W, et al. Economic analysis of low-dose heparin vs the low-molecular-weight heparin enoxaparin for prevention of venous thromboembolism after colorectal surgery. *Arch Intern Med* 1999;159:1221–1228
165. Clagett GP, Reisch JS. Prevention of venous thromboembolism in general surgical patients: Results of meta-analysis. *Ann Surg* 1988;208:227–240
166. Wolff BG, Pembeton JH, van Heerden JA, et al. Elective colon and rectal surgery without nasogastric decompression: A prospective, randomized trial. *Ann Surg* 1989;209:670–673; discussion 673–675
167. Malassagne B, Valleur P, Serra J, et al. Relationship of apical lymph node involvement to survival in resected colon carcinoma. *Dis Colon Rectum* 1993;36:645–653
168. Rouffet F, Hay JM, Vacher B, et al. Curative resection for left colonic carcinoma: Hemicolectomy vs segmental colectomy. A prospective, controlled, multicenter trial. French Association for Surgical Research. *Dis Colon Rectum* 1994;37:651–659

169. Wiggers T, Jeekel J, Arends JW, et al. No-touch isolation technique in colon cancer: A controlled, prospective trial. *Br J Surg* 1988;75:409–415
170. Pezim ME, Nicholls RJ. Survival after high or low ligation of the inferior mesenteric artery during curative surgery for rectal cancer. *Ann Surg* 1984;200:729–733
171. Surtees P, Ritchie JK, Phillips RK. High versus low ligation of the inferior mesenteric artery in rectal cancer. *Br J Surg* 1990;77:618–621
172. Sagar PM, Couse N, Kerin M, et al. Randomized trial of drainage of colorectal anastomosis. *Br J Surg* 1993;80: 769–771
173. Urbach DR, Kennedy ED, Cohen MM. Colon and rectal anastomoses do not require routine drainage: A systematic review and meta-analysis. *Ann Surg* 1999;229:174–180
174. Fingerhut A, Msika S, Yahchouchi E, et al. Neither pelvic nor abdominal drainage is needed after anastomosis in elective, uncomplicated, colorectal surgery. *Ann Surg* 2000;231:613–614
175. Yeh CY, Changchien CR, Wang JY, et al. Pelvic drainage and other risk factors for leakage after elective anterior resection in rectal cancer patients: A prospective study of 978 patients. *Ann Surg* 2005;241:9–13
176. Galandiuk S. To drain or not to drain (comment). *Ann Surg* 2005;241:14–15
177. Kaiser AM, Corman ML. History of laparoscopy. *Surg Oncol Clin North Am* 2001;10:483–492
178. Lacy AM, Garcia-Valdecasas JC, Delgado S, et al. Laparoscopy-assisted colectomy versus open colectomy for treatment of nonmetastatic colon cancer: A randomised trial. *Lancet* 2002;359:2224–2229
179. Clinical Outcomes of Surgical Therapy Study G. A comparison of laparoscopically assisted and open colectomy for colon cancer. *N Engl J Med* 2004;350:2050–2059
180. Leung KL, Kwok SP, Lam SC, et al. Laparoscopic resection of rectosigmoid carcinoma: Prospective, randomised trial. *Lancet* 2004;363:1187–1192
181. Kaiser AM, Kang JC, Chan LS, et al. Laparoscopic-assisted vs open colectomy for colon cancer: A prospective, randomized trial. *J Laparoendosc Adv Surg Technol* 2004;14:329–334
182. Guillou PJ, Quirke P, Thorpe H, et al. Short-term endpoints of conventional versus laparoscopic-assisted surgery in patients with colorectal cancer (MRC CLASICC trial): Multicentre, randomised, controlled trial. *Lancet* 2005;365:1718–1726
183. Group TCcLoORS. Laparoscopic surgery versus open surgery for colon cancer: Short-term outcomes of a randomised trial. *Lancet Oncol* 2005;6:477–484
184. Weeks JC, Nelson H, Gelber S, et al, Clinical Outcomes of Surgical Therapy Study G. Short-term quality-of-life outcomes following laparoscopic-assisted colectomy vs open colectomy for colon cancer: A randomized trial. *JAMA* 2002;287:321–328
185. Patten LC, Berger DH, Rodriguez-Bigas M, et al. A prospective evaluation of radiocolloid and immunohistochemical staining in colon carcinoma lymphatic mapping. *Cancer* 2004;100:2104–2109
186. Bertagnolli M, Miedema B, Redston M, et al. Sentinel node staging of resectable colon cancer: Results of a multicenter study. *Ann Surg* 2004;240:624–628; discussion 628–630
187. Kaiser AM, Katkhouda N. Laparoscopic management of the perforated viscus. *Semin Laparosc Surg* 2002;9:46–53
188. Alves A, Panis Y, Mathieu P, et al. Postoperative mortality and morbidity in French patients undergoing colorectal surgery: Results of a prospective multicenter study. *Arch Surg* 2005;140:278–283
189. Binkert CA, Ledermann H, Jost R, et al. Acute colonic obstruction: Clinical aspects and cost-effectiveness of preoperative and palliative treatment with self-expanding metallic stents—a preliminary report. *Radiology* 1998;206:199–204
190. Dauphine CE, Tan P, Beart RW Jr, et al. Placement of self-expanding metal stents for acute malignant large-bowel obstruction: A collective review. *Ann Surg Oncol* 2002;9:574–579
191. Sugarbaker PH, Corlew S. Influence of surgical techniques on survival in patients with colorectal cancer. *Dis Colon Rectum* 1982;25:545–557
192. Lopez MJ, Monafo WW. Role of extended resection in the initial treatment of locally advanced colorectal carcinoma. *Surgery* 1993;113:365–372
193. Geoghegan JG, Scheele J. Treatment of colorectal liver metastases. *Br J Surg* 1999;86:158–169
194. Schrag D, Cramer LD, Bach PB, et al. Influence of hospital procedure volume on outcomes following surgery for colon cancer. *JAMA* 2000;284:3028–3035
195. Tang CL, Yeong KY, Nyam DC, et al. Postoperative intra-abdominal free gas after open colorectal resection. *Dis Colon Rectum* 2000;43:1116–1120
196. Krook JE, Moertel CG, Gunderson LL, et al. Effective surgical adjuvant therapy for high-risk rectal carcinoma. *N Engl J Med* 1991;324:709–715
197. Dube S, Heyen F, Jenicek M. Adjuvant chemotherapy in colorectal carcinoma: Results of a meta-analysis. *Dis Colon Rectum* 1997;40:35–41
198. O'Connell MJ, Laurie JA, Kahn M, et al. Prospectively randomized trial of postoperative adjuvant chemotherapy in patients with high-risk colon cancer. *J Clin Oncol* 1998;16:295–300
199. Anonymous. Comparison of flourouracil with additional levamisole, higher-dose folinic acid, or both, as adjuvant chemotherapy for colorectal cancer: A randomised trial. QUASAR Collaborative Group. *Lancet* 2000;355:1588–1596
200. Shirota Y, Stoehlmacher J, Brabender J, et al. ERCC1 and thymidylate synthase mRNA levels predict survival for colorectal cancer patients receiving combination oxaliplatin and fluorouracil chemotherapy. *J Clin Oncol* 2001;19:4298–4304
201. Stoehlmacher J, Park DJ, Zhang W, et al. A multivariate analysis of genomic polymorphisms: Prediction of clinical outcome to 5-FU/oxaliplatin combination chemotherapy in refractory colorectal cancer. *Br J Cancer* 2004; 91:344–354

202. Saltz LB, Cox JV, Blanke C, et al. Irinotecan plus fluorouracil and leucovorin for metastatic colorectal cancer. Irinotecan Study Group. *N Engl J Med* 2000;343:905–914
203. Douillard JY, Hoff PM, Skillings JR, et al. Multicenter phase III study of uracil/tegafur and oral leucovorin versus fluorouracil and leucovorin in patients with previously untreated metastatic colorectal cancer. *J Clin Oncol* 2002;20:3605–3616
204. de Gramont A, Figer A, Seymour M, et al. Leucovorin and fluorouracil with or without oxaliplatin as first-line treatment in advanced colorectal cancer. *J Clin Oncol* 2000;18:2938–2947
205. Becouarn Y, Gamelin E, Coudert B, et al. Randomized multicenter phase II study comparing a combination of fluorouracil and folinic acid and alternating irinotecan and oxaliplatin with oxaliplatin and irinotecan in fluorouracil-pretreated metastatic colorectal cancer patients. *J Clin Oncol* 2001;19:4195–4201
206. Grothey A, Sargent D, Goldberg RM, Schmoll HJ. Survival of patients with advanced colorectal cancer improves with the availability of fluorouracil-leucovorin, irinotecan, and oxaliplatin in the course of treatment. *J Clin Oncol* 2004;22:1209–1214
207. Goldberg RM, Sargent DJ, Morton RF, et al. A randomized, controlled trial of fluorouracil plus leucovorin, irinotecan, and oxaliplatin combinations in patients with previously untreated metastatic colorectal cancer. *J Clin Oncol* 2004;22:23–30
208. Van Cutsem E, Hoff PM, Harper P, et al. Oral capecitabine vs intravenous 5-fluorouracil and leucovorin: Integrated efficacy data and novel analyses from two large, randomised, phase III trials. *Br J Cancer* 2004;90:1190–1197
209. Borner MM, Dietrich D, Stupp R, et al. Phase II study of capecitabine and oxaliplatin in first- and second-line treatment of advanced or metastatic colorectal cancer. *J Clin Oncol* 2002;20:1759–1766
210. Scheithauer W, Kornek GV, Raderer M, et al. Randomized multicenter phase II trial of two different schedules of capecitabine plus oxaliplatin as first-line treatment in advanced colorectal cancer. *J Clin Oncol* 2003;21:1307–1312
211. Shields AF, Zalupski MM, Marshall JL, Meropol NJ. Treatment of advanced colorectal carcinoma with oxaliplatin and capecitabine: A phase II trial. *Cancer* 2004;100:531–537
212. Cassidy J, Tabernero J, Twelves C, et al. XELOX (capecitabine plus oxaliplatin): Active first-line therapy for patients with metastatic colorectal cancer. *J Clin Oncol* 2004;22:2084–2091
213. Bajetta E, Di Bartolomeo M, Mariani L, et al. Randomized multicenter phase II trial of two different schedules of irinotecan combined with capecitabine as first-line treatment in metastatic colorectal carcinoma. *Cancer* 2004;100:279–287
214. Cunningham D, Humblet Y, Siena S, et al. Cetuximab monotherapy and cetuximab plus irinotecan in irinotecan-refractory metastatic colorectal cancer. *N Engl J Med* 2004;351:337–345
215. Hurwitz H, Fehrenbacher L, Novotny W, et al. Bevacizumab plus irinotecan, fluorouracil, and leucovorin for metastatic colorectal cancer. *N Engl J Med* 2004;350:2335–2342
216. Amos EH, Mendenhall WM, McCarty PJ, et al. Postoperative radiotherapy for locally advanced colon cancer. *Ann Surg Oncol* 1996;3:431–436
217. Palermo JA, Richards F, Lohman KK, et al. Phase II trial of adjuvant radiation and intraperitoneal 5-fluorouracil for locally advanced colon cancer: Results with 10-year follow-up. *Int J Radiat Oncol Biol Phys* 2000;47:725–733
218. Taylor WE, Donohue JH, Gunderson LL, et al. The Mayo Clinic experience with multimodality treatment of locally advanced or recurrent colon cancer. *Ann Surg Oncol* 2002;9:177–185
219. Passman MA, Pommier RF, Vetto JT. Synchronous colon primaries have the same prognosis as solitary colon cancers. *Dis Colon Rectum* 1996;39:329–334
220. Wu JS, Fazio VW. Colon cancer. *Dis Colon Rectum* 2000;43:1473–1486
221. Vasen HF. Clinical diagnosis and management of hereditary colorectal cancer syndromes. *J Clin Oncol* 2000;18:81S–92S
222. Umar A, Boland CR, Terdiman JP, et al. Revised Bethesda Guidelines for hereditary nonpolyposis colorectal cancer (Lynch syndrome) and microsatellite instability. *J Natl Cancer Inst* 2004;96:261–268
223. Muto T, Bussey HJ, Morson BC. The evolution of cancer of the colon and rectum. *Cancer* 1975;36:2251–2270
224. Nivatvongs S. Surgical management of early colorectal cancer. *World J Surg* 2000;24:1052–1055

VI

RECTUM AND ANUS

24

Benign Disorders of the Anorectum (Pelvic Floor, Fissures, Hemorrhoids, and Fistulas)

Jennifer K. Lowney ▪ *James W. Fleshman Jr.*

Benign diseases of the anorectum range from relatively simple disorders such as hemorrhoids and fissures to extremely complex problems associated with pelvic floor abnormalities.

▪ ANATOMY

The beginning of any evaluation of anorectal problems is the examination; therefore, clinicians need to understand the anatomy. The normal anatomic relationships of the rectum and pelvis are important in understanding pelvic floor abnormalities and anorectal pathology. The rectum normally lies attached to its mesorectum within the curve of the sacrum with limited mobility. The junction of the rectosigmoid is most consistently found at the sacral promontory and descends only 2 or 3 cm during a Valsalva maneuver. The rectum exits the pelvis anteriorly surrounded by a sling of muscle from the pubis through a slit in the pelvic floor. The sling is created by the horseshoe-shaped puborectalis muscle that circles around behind the rectum and reinserts on the pubis anteriorly. Contraction of the muscle pulls the rectum forward, creating a more acute angle at the anal outlet. The anal canal itself measures 3–4 cm and is a funnel-shaped extension of the pelvic floor musculature. The pressure generated by this voluntary muscle prevents egress of rectal contents. The internal sphincter muscle is a continuation of the thickened circular muscle of the rectum. As such, it is an autonomic muscle and has no voluntary control.

The anorectum receives both sympathetic and parasympathetic nerves. The sympathetic nerves originate from thoracolumbar segments, and unite below the inferior mesenteric artery to form the inferior mesenteric plexus. These fibers then descend to the superior hypogastric plexus located just inferior to the aortic bifurcation. These purely sympathetic fibers bifurcate and descend as the hypogastric nerves. Parasympathetic fibers from S2, S3, and S4 (the nervi erigentes) join the hypogastric nerves anterolateral to the rectum to form the inferior hypogastric plexuses. Mixed fibers from the plexuses innervate the prostate, rectum, bladder, penis, and internal anal sphincter. These autonomic plexuses of the pelvic nerves run around the lateral aspect of the pelvic rim to enter the prostate and seminal vesicles anteriorly. The sympathetic innervation of the internal sphincter is motor, while the parasympathetic innervation is inhibitory. Injury to the pelvic autonomic nerves during pelvic surgery may result in bladder dysfunction, impotence, or both.

The innervation of the voluntary muscles of the pelvic floor is via direct fibers from S2, S3, and S4 in the pelvis from the sacrum (Fig 24–1). The nerves of the external sphincter are derived from S2, S3, and S4 nerve roots from the sacral plexus and arrive at the external sphincter via the pudendal nerve around the ischial spine at Alcock's canal. The uterus and vagina are closely approximated to the anterior surface of the rectum but not attached. There is no ligamentous suspension of the rectum or the uterus at the lower aspect of the pelvis. The slitlike defect in the pelvic floor through

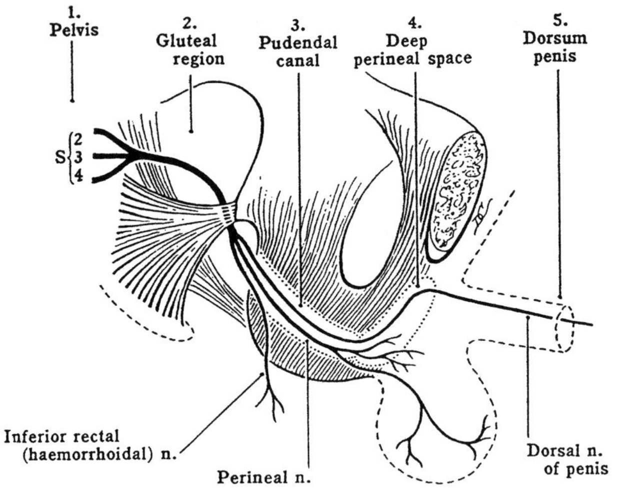

Figure 24–1. Diagram of the pudendal nerve. Note the five regions in which it runs, and the three divisions into which it divides. (Reproduced, with permission, from Anderson JE. *Grant's Atlas of Anatomy*, 8th ed. Baltimore, MD: Williams & Wilkins; 1983.)

which the rectum passes also provides an outlet for the vagina and the urinary bladder.

The alimentary tract terminates at the anus, which provides continence of flatus and feces. It is useful to consider the anus and surrounding structures as a single unit, the anorectum (Fig 24–2). The anorectum includes the perianal skin, the anal canal, the anal sphincters, and the distal rectum. The three main anatomic points of reference are the anal verge, the dentate line, and the anorectal ring. The distal external boundary of the anal canal is the anal verge, which is also the junction between the anal and perianal skin. Anal epithelium (anoderm) is devoid of the hair follicles, sebaceous glands, and apocrine glands that are present in the perianal skin, a fact worth remembering when attempting to distinguish between hidradenitis (inflammation of the apocrine glands in the perianal skin) and cryptoglandular anal disease.

The cephalad border of the anal canal is a true mucocutaneous junction, the dentate line. This union of the embryonic ectoderm with the endodermal gut resides approximately 1.0–1.5 cm above the anal verge. In a transitional zone of 6–12 mm in length, the columnar epithelium of the rectum changes to cuboidal epithelium which joins the squamous epithelium at the dentate line.

The upper border of the anal sphincteric complex is the anorectal ring. It may be palpated by digital examination about 1.0–1.5 cm above the dentate line.

Anatomists consider the anal canal to begin at the dentate line and end at the anal verge. However, most surgeons consider the anal canal to start at the anorectal ring and terminate at the anal verge. This latter conception of the anal canal will be used throughout this chapter.

Just above the dentate line, the rectal mucosa forms from 8–14 longitudinal folds known as the rectal columns. Between each two columns at the dentate line is a small pocket termed an anal crypt. Small, rudimentary anal glands open into some, but not all, of these anal crypts. The glands may extend through the internal sphincter as far as the intersphincteric plane, but they do not extend into the external sphincter.

Below the dentate line, cutaneous sensations of heat, cold, touch, and pain are conveyed by afferent fibers in the inferior rectal nerves. Cephalad to the dentate line, poorly defined dull sensations, elicited when the mucosa is pinched or internal hemorrhoids are ligated, are probably carried by parasympathetic fibers.

The superior rectal artery, the terminal branch of the inferior mesenteric artery, descends to the upper rectum where it divides into lateral branches. Subsequent smaller divisions penetrate the rectal wall. The middle rectal arteries arise from the internal iliac arteries and supply the distal rectum and upper anal canal. The inferior rectal arteries, branches from the internal pudendal arteries, cross the ischiorectal fossae to supply the anal sphincters (Fig 24–3).

There are two paths for venous blood return from the anorectum. Above the dentate line, venous blood flows into the portal system through the superior rectal vein and inferior mesenteric vein. Below the dentate line, the external hemorrhoidal plexus drains into the internal iliac vein via the middle rectal vein or via the pudendal vein, which receives blood from the inferior rectal vein.

▪ ANAL INCONTINENCE

PATHOPHYSIOLOGY

Mechanical disruption is usually due to obstetric injury, trauma, or fistula disease in which the external muscle is divided or damaged (Table 24–1). Neurogenic incontinence is due to stretching of the pudendal nerves during prolonged labor, descent of the perineum and nerve stretch during straining at stool or rectal prolapse, or systemic disease such as multiple sclerosis, scleroderma, or spinal cord injury. Idiopathic incontinence is due to medical disease such as diarrhea in a patient with limited rectal capacity, irritable bowel syndrome, or sedatives which cause poor sensation in the anal canal in patients with no evidence of heurogenic or mechanical incontinence.

The normal continence mechanism has several components. Rectal capacitance and compliance are essential. The rectum normally holds between 200 and 250 mL. It distends readily with filling and has limited mus-

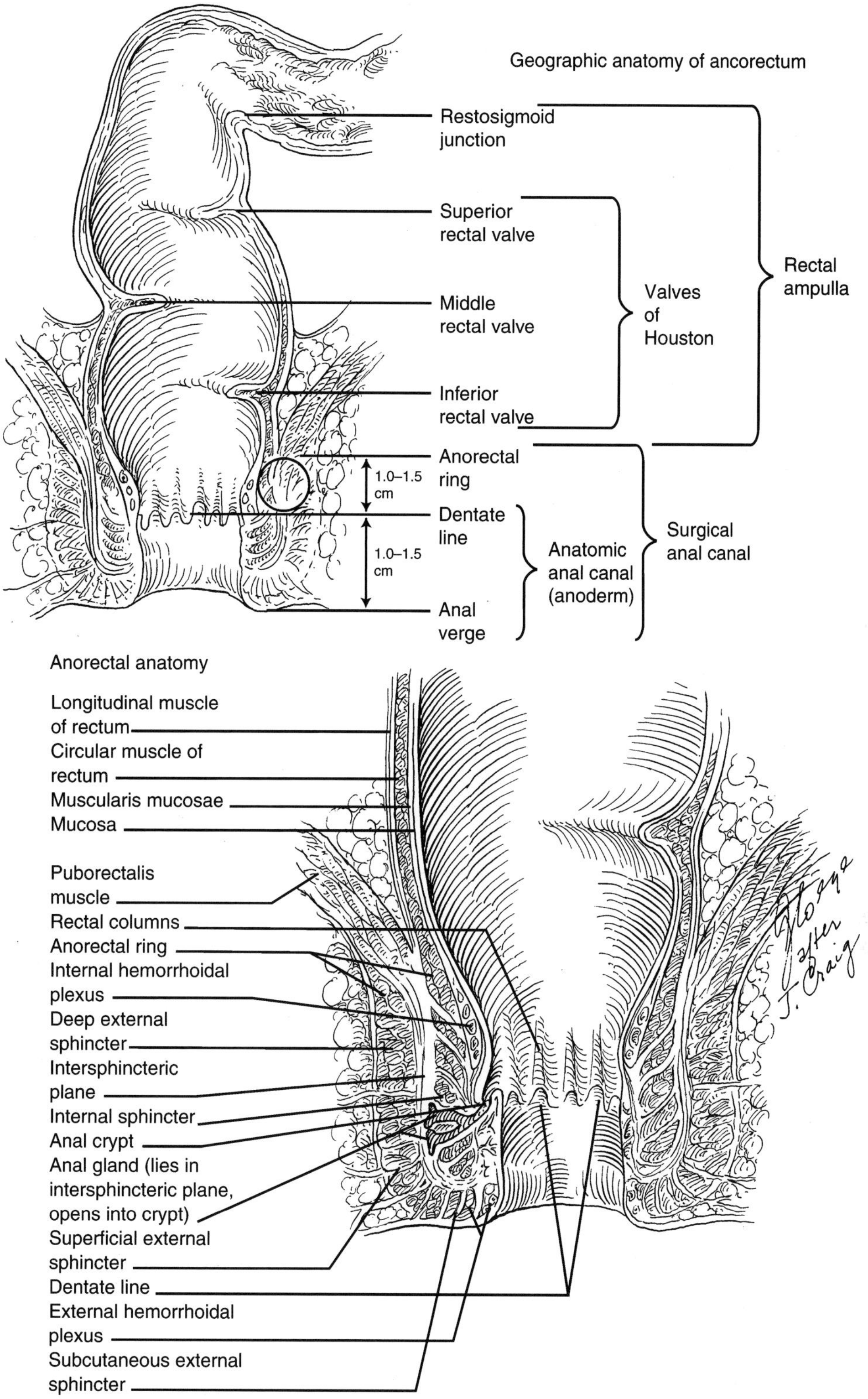

Figure 24–2. Anatomy of the anus and rectum: geographic anatomy of the anorectum and anorectal anatomy. (Redrawn, with permission, from Fry AD, Kodner IJ. Anorectal diseases. *Clin Symp* 1985; 37:3. Copyright 1985, CIBA-GEIGY. Originally illustrated by John Craig, MD.)

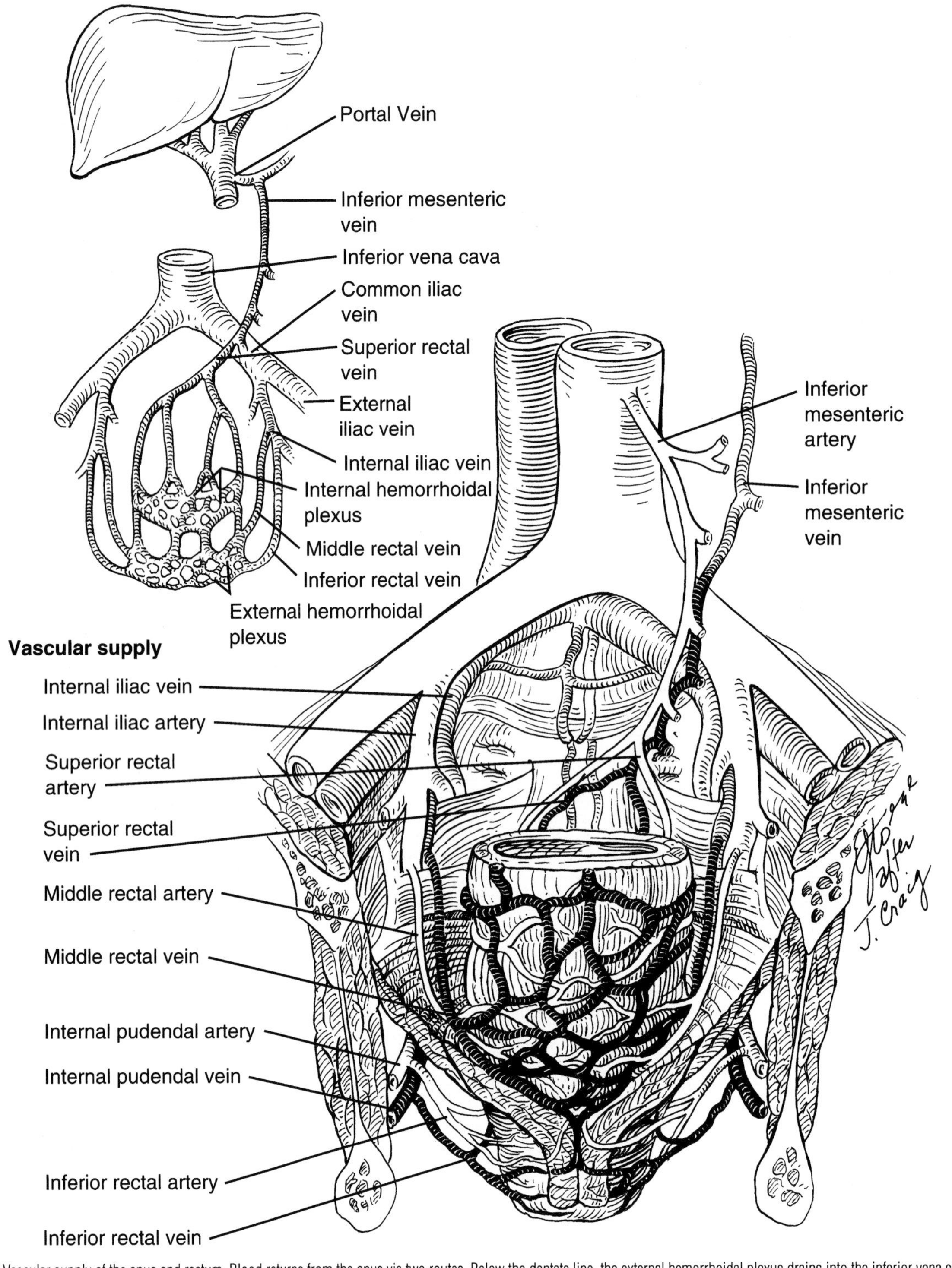

Figure 24–3. Vascular supply of the anus and rectum. Blood returns from the anus via two routes. Below the dentate line, the external hemorrhoidal plexus drains into the inferior vena cava via inferior pudendal veins. Above the dentate line, the internal hemorrhoidal plexus drains into the portal system via the superior rectal vein. (Redrawn, with permission, from Fry RD, Kodner IJ. Anorectal diseases. *Clin Symp* 1985;37:6. Copyright 1985, CIBA-GEIGY. Originally illustrated by John Craig, MD.)

cular activity intrinsically. The sampling reflex is a function of rectal distension allowing anal sphincter relaxation via an intramural reflex to the internal sphincter. The rectal contents can then be sensed in the sensory nerve–rich transitional zone and anoderm to discriminate the true nature of the rectal contents. This sampling reflex occurs frequently throughout the day to provide continence and also serves to initiate the defecation process. The voluntary external sphincter muscle contraction in response to this sampling reflex pro-

TABLE 24–1. ANAL INCONTINENCE ETIOLOGY

Mechanical	Neurogenic	Idiopathic
Obstetric injury	Pudendal nerve stretch	No clear etiology
Fistula disease	Strain	Medical illness
Trauma	Prolonged labor	Irradiation
Iatrogenic	Trauma	Irritable bowel syndrome
Systemic disease		Multiple sclerosis, diabetes mellitus, scleroderma
Diarrheal states		

vides the final active component of anal continence. The subconscious voluntary contraction of the external sphincter, puborectalis, and pelvic floor muscles provide complete control of rectal contents. The pelvic floor muscles maintain continual activity, even during sleep, to provide anal continence. This also seems to be a learned response since infants and children require 1–2 years to achieve control.

It is important to realize that the degree of incontinence affects the lifestyle of the patient. The frequency of incontinence may vary and the loss of control may involve solid stool, liquid stool, or gas only. Frequent episodes of incontinence of gas only may be as incapacitating as infrequent episodes of solid stool. It is essential to document the exact type of incontinence before planning treatment. It is especially important to clearly define the incontinence before attempting to report a series of patients who undergo a specific treatment. There is no universally accepted grading scale to assess severity and impact of fecal incontinence. Recently, the American Society of Colon and Rectal Surgeons validated a fecal incontinence severity index and a fecal incontinence quality of life index to help standardize the assessment of anal incontinence.[1,2]

DIAGNOSIS AND EVALUATION

Signs of anal incontinence in the office include a thin perineal body with scarring between the vagina and the anal canal and a poor squeeze on command. There is controversy regarding the adequacy of digital assessment of the anal sphincter mechanism. It is possible that an experienced examiner may be able to determine the adequacy of resting tone, but it is difficult to quantify and accurately evaluate the voluntary squeeze pressure generated by an anal sphincter mechanism. It is also essential to rule out the presence of a rectovaginal fistula in the setting of an anterior sphincter injury.

Anal manometry is useful to document reduced resting and squeeze pressures as well as sphincter length in individual sphincter quadrants. Three-dimensional vectorgrams may be more useful in research settings or for the very complicated patient who has confounded the examiner. Normal resting pressure is at least 40 mm Hg, normal squeeze pressure is 80 mm Hg, which is usually double the resting pressure, and sphincter length is greater than 3 cm. Normal sensation should allow detection of a balloon inflated with 10–20 mL of air. Maximal tolerable volume is usually over 100 mL of air-filled balloon distention.

Electromyography

Single fiber density determination is of historical interest and is also extremely painful for the patient. It is not routinely performed.

Pudendal nerve terminal motor latency determination measures the conduction velocity of the nerve action potential through the terminal 4 cm of the pudendal nerve between Alcock's canal and the external sphincter (Fig 24–4). A delay in conduction reflects injury to the fast-conducting fibers of the nerve. This injury usually is the result of stretch, direct trauma, or systemic disease. The normal terminal motor latency is 2.2 ± 0.2 ms. Any delay in conduction velocity greater than this indicates nerve injury.

Transrectal Ultrasound

The most sensitive method for documenting sphincter injury may be the anal ultrasound using a 360° rotating 10-MHz transducer covered with an anal cap and inserted into the anal canal. The focal length of the anal probe is approximately 1–2 cm and allows evaluation of the anal sphincter muscles in three dimensions as the probe is withdrawn from the rectum (Fig 24–5). Scarring at the site of an injury is usually easily seen by endoanal ultrasound. A rectovaginal fistula can also be detected. An algorithm for the evaluation and management of anal incontinence can be produced using these diagnostic techniques (Fig 24–6).

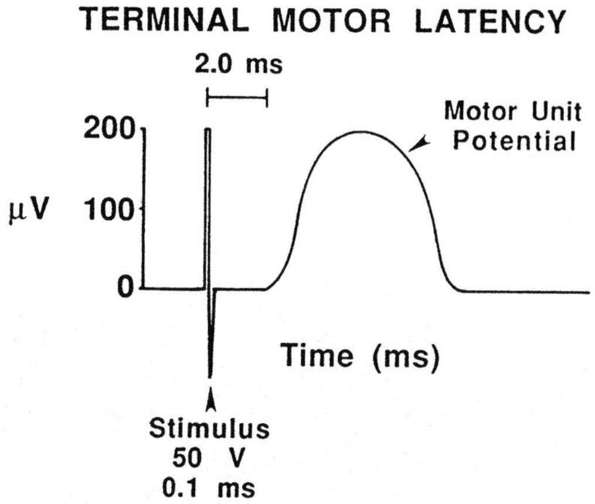

Figure 24–4. Normal tracing of pudendal nerve terminal motor latency. (Reproduced, with permission, from Fleshman JW, Kodner IJ, Fry RD. Anal incontinence. In: Zuidema GD (ed). *Shackelford's Surgery of the Alimentary Tract*, 3rd ed, Vol. 1. Philadelphia, PA: WB Saunders; 1991:349–361.)

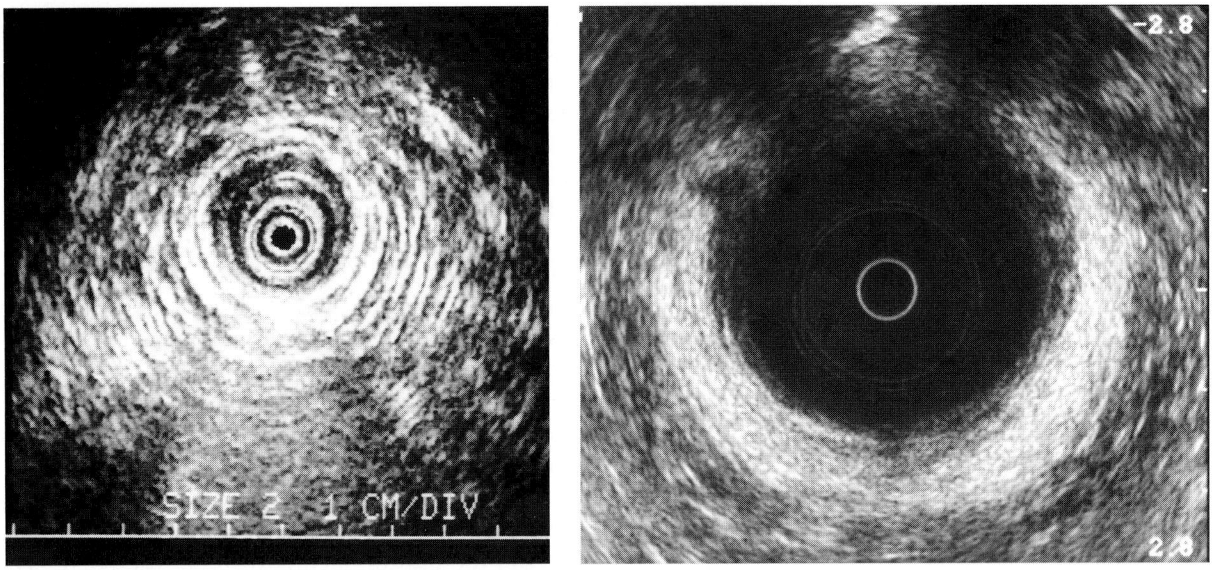

A B

Figure 24–5. A. Transrectal ultrasound of a normal male sphincter reveals internal and external sphincter muscles. An anal cap covers the 7.5- or 10-MHz rotating transducer of the Bruel and Kjaer ultrasound probe. The innermost dark layer is the mucosa of the anal canal. **B.** Image of anterior sphincter defect in a female patient with anal incontinence due to obstetric injury. (Part B reproduced, with permission, from Fleshman JW. Anorectal motor physiology and pathophysiology. *Surg Clin North Am* 1993;73:1256.)

High-resolution magnetic resonance imaging (MRI) with an endoanal coil is a newer diagnostic modality that can detect sphincter defects similarly to endoanal ultrasound. Endoanal coil MRI may also show sphincter atrophy or thinning not detectable by endoanal ultrasound that may have an impact on the success of surgical repair.[3]

TREATMENT

Anal Sphincter Reconstruction

Anal sphincter repair can be performed successfully in most patients who have an isolated mechanical sphincter defect. The patient requires a complete bowel preparation in order to avoid a colostomy at the time of the procedure. The ends of the injured sphincter are identified in the anterior perineum in patients with obstetric injury, and they are overlapped and secured or reefed in the midline to reconstruct the circular muscle (Fig 24–7). Control of solid and liquid stool will be adequate in 90% of patients after this type of repair. However, complete continence is usually only achieved in 75–90% of patients and the long-term results may even be less satisfactory.[4] Leakage of liquid, mucus, and gas may continue to affect patients after repair. Improvement in squeeze pressures has been shown to correlate best with functional outcome.[5] The presence of at least one normal pudendal nerve is necessary for an improvement after sphincter reconstruction. Complications of wound infection, fistula formation, and breakdown of the sphincter repair are reduced by leaving a drain in the perineal body after the repair. A repeat procedure is usually successful in those cases in whom the sphincter repair is disrupted.

Muscle Sensory Retraining or Biofeedback

Operant conditioning using manometric and balloon sensation techniques is possible in patients with a mechanical sphincter defect. Electromyographic anal plugs also provide biofeedback for conditioning. Much of the literature suggests a benefit to biofeedback, but it does not indicate which patients will benefit from which technique and which will not.[6] Pre- and postoperative biofeedback may aid in functional improvement. Obviously, patients with extremely poor pudendal nerve function or complete disruption of the anal sphincter will not benefit at all.

Other Treatments and New Modalities

New techniques have been developed, including implantation of an artificial sphincter of silicone or a neurostimulator that provides constant activity in a muscle transferred to the anal canal (i.e., dynamic graciloplasty).[7] "Pacemakers" implanted in the pelvis for sacral nerve stimulation of the anus have also been used, similar to a urologist's technique to cure urinary dysfunction.[8] These techniques are indicated for severe, idiopathic fecal incontinence when all else has failed. They are expensive procedures, and some have a high risk of complications, but patients with severe neuromuscular damage and even those who have had the

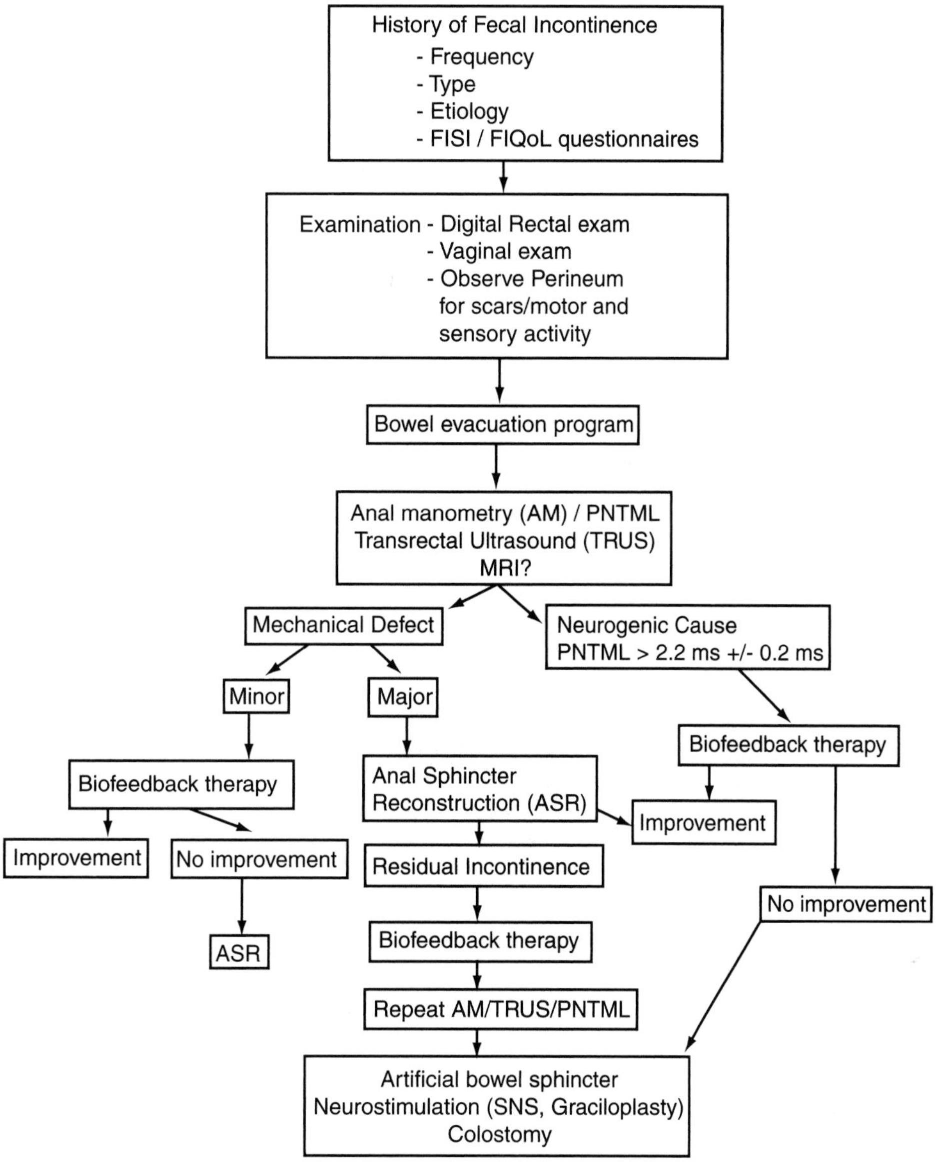

Figure 24–6. Algorithm for evaluation and management of anal incontinence. PNTML, pudendal nerve terminal motor latency; SNS, sacral nerve stimulation.

sphincter mechanism removed may benefit from reconstruction of the anal sphincter. The Parks posterior sphincter repair has been shown to yield poor results in patients with severe anal incontinence.

▪ RECTAL PROLAPSE AND INTERNAL INTUSSUSCEPTION

PATHOPHYSIOLOGY

Etiology and Physiology

The true etiology of rectal prolapse and intussusception is unknown. There are three components that require attention in both diagnosis and repair of rectal prolapse and internal intussusception. The rectum and rectosigmoid junction are unusually mobile from the sacrum. Descent of the rectosigmoid junction into the pelvis allows a funnel-shaped intussusception in the rectum as the rectum attempts to expel itself (Fig 24–8). Poor relaxation of the pelvic floor and external sphincter mechanism also occurs during straining. This outlet obstruction is eventually overcome by continued straining, resulting in descent of the perineum, expulsion of the rectum, and true rectal prolapse. There are no long-term data that document the progression of internal intussusception (funnel formation) to full rectal prolapse. However, there are anecdotal incidences in most practices that suggest that this occurs. The anal canal is injured by stretch of the internal sphincter during rectal

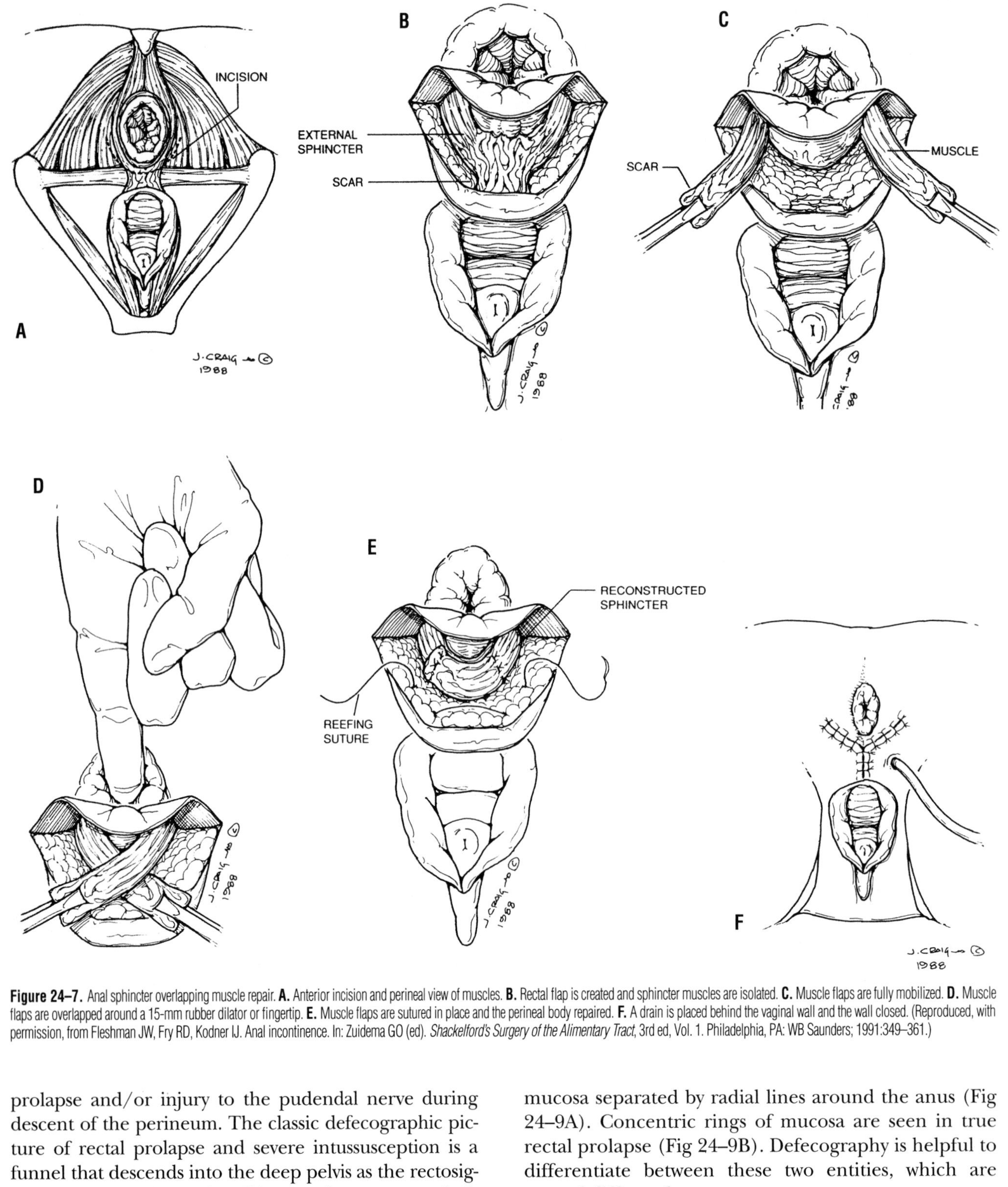

Figure 24–7. Anal sphincter overlapping muscle repair. **A.** Anterior incision and perineal view of muscles. **B.** Rectal flap is created and sphincter muscles are isolated. **C.** Muscle flaps are fully mobilized. **D.** Muscle flaps are overlapped around a 15-mm rubber dilator or fingertip. **E.** Muscle flaps are sutured in place and the perineal body repaired. **F.** A drain is placed behind the vaginal wall and the wall closed. (Reproduced, with permission, from Fleshman JW, Fry RD, Kodner IJ. Anal incontinence. In: Zuidema GO (ed). *Shackelford's Surgery of the Alimentary Tract*, 3rd ed, Vol. 1. Philadelphia, PA: WB Saunders; 1991:349–361.)

prolapse and/or injury to the pudendal nerve during descent of the perineum. The classic defecographic picture of rectal prolapse and severe intussusception is a funnel that descends into the deep pelvis as the rectosigmoid junction descends. This situation causes a ball-valve type obstruction at the level of the anal canal before being pushed through to the outside.

Distal mucosal prolapse is occasionally mistaken for full rectal prolapse. The typical appearance is that of mucosa separated by radial lines around the anus (Fig 24–9A). Concentric rings of mucosa are seen in true rectal prolapse (Fig 24–9B). Defecography is helpful to differentiate between these two entities, which are treated differently.

Diagnosis and Evaluation

Signs and symptoms of rectal prolapse include rectal pressure and pain, incomplete evacuation, outlet ob-

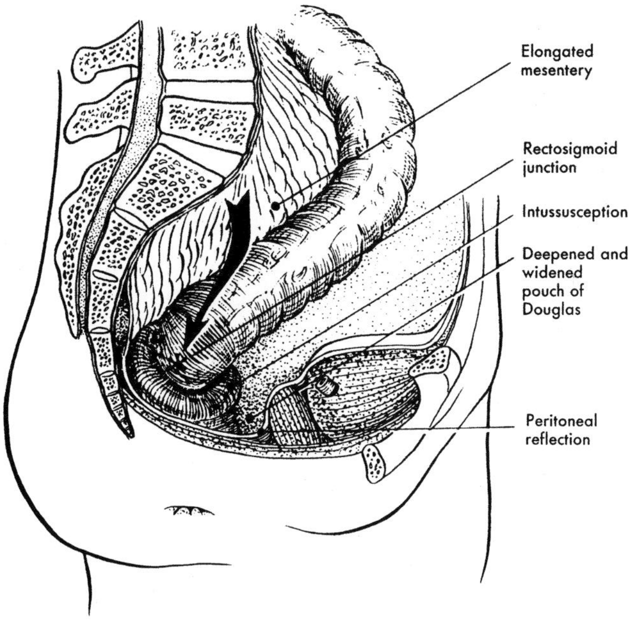

Figure 24–8. Rectum with internal intussusception. (Reproduced, with permission, from Hoffman MJ, Kodner IJ, Fry RD. Internal intussusception of the rectum: diagnosis and surgical management. *Dis Colon Rectum* 1984;27:435.)

struction, and constipation causing prolonged straining. Mucus discharge and bleeding from the fully prolapsed tissue may also be present. Examination most often reveals concentric rings of rectal tissue with a patulous anal canal, poor voluntary tone, and a very mobile rectum within the vault. Proctosigmoidoscopy reveals descent of tissue during straining and occasionally an ulcer on the anterior wall. Defecography reveals severe mobility of the rectum from its point of fixation to the sacrum, redundancy of the mesorectum, and funnel formation as the rectum prepares to descend through the anal canal opening at the pelvic floor. It is not essential to use defecography in obvious instances of rectal prolapse. It is most useful in cases that cannot be documented or visualized in an office setting. Thickened barium simulates stool and allows reconstruction of the defecating process during cinedefecography. It is helpful in cases in which mucosal prolapse is suspected and the intent is to rule out full rectal prolapse. Triple-contrast cinedefecography (rectum, vagina, and small bowel) also helps delineate complex pelvic floor abnormalities.

A grading system of intussusception has been developed to assist one in planning management

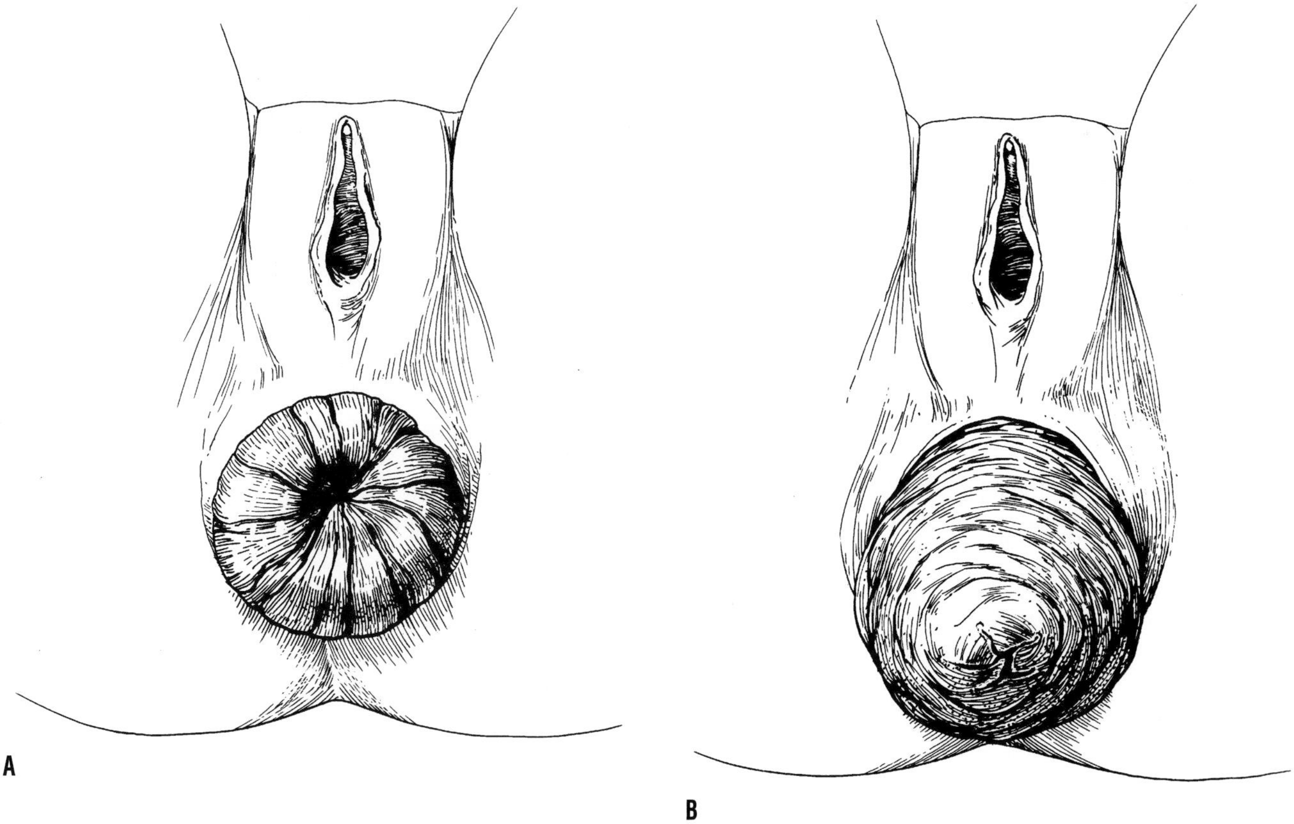

A

B

Figure 24–9. A. Radial folds of mucosal prolapse. **B.** Concentric rings of full-thickness rectal prolapse. (Reproduced, with permission, from Kodner IJ, Fry RD. Anorectal disorders. *CIBA Foundation Symposium* 1985;37. Copyright 1985, CIBA-GEIGY Corporation. Reprinted with permission from Clinical Symposia. Redrawn, with permission, from illustrations by John A. Craig, MD. All rights reserved.)

(Table 24–2). Mild to moderate intussusception with some mobility, some funnel formation, and descent of the rectum can usually be treated conservatively. However, grade 4 intussusception with severe outlet obstruction may require treatment using operative resection of the redundant rectum or rectopexy to fix the rectum to the sacrum.

Anal manometry is sometimes useful to document the preoperative function of the sphincter. The pudendal nerve latencies provide objective evidence of pudendal nerve injury and allow some prediction of outcome after repair.

Management

Rectal Prolapse. There are numerous techniques for management of rectal prolapse; over 100 procedures have been described. The procedures can be broken down into basic types which include rectopexy, low anterior resection, perineal proctectomy, and anal encirclement procedures.[11] The anal encirclement procedures using synthetic material such as nylon mesh should be limited to the extremely debilitated patient or the elderly patient who can not withstand perineal proctectomy. The other types of procedure rely on correction of the hypermobility of the rectosigmoid by refixation of the colon into the curve of the sacrum and removal of redundant sigmoid colon and rectum.

Rectopexy uses some means to fix the rectum to sacrum without removing a portion of the rectum. Foreign material or sutures attach the rectum to the sacrum. All of these procedures require complete mobilization of the rectum all the way to the pelvic floor, and stretching the rectum out of the pelvis to fit into the curve of the sacrum.

The low anterior resection technique uses the standard technique for removal of the middle and upper portions of the rectum and redundant sigmoid colon. The left colon is reattached to the middle to lower third of the rectum by using either a double-staple or hand-sewn technique (Fig 24–10). The rectum is mobilized to the level of the pelvic floor circumferentially, and the left colon and rectum (now in continuity) are returned to the curve of the sacrum. The incidence of anal incontinence may be higher after this procedure because the rectal capacitance is reduced. However, in patients who report constipation preoperatively this is an option, but it may lead to postoperative evacuation difficulties. Preoperative anal physiological testing may assist in the selection of patients who are candidates for the low anterior resection (i.e., no evidence of sphincter injury or dysfunction).

TABLE 24–2. DEFECOGRAPHY GRADING SYSTEM[a]

Grade	Description
N	Rectum remains fixed to sacrum, sphincter relaxes, and rectum empties
1	Nonrelaxation of puborectalis
2	Mild intussusception or mobility from sacrum
3	Moderate intussusception
4	Severe intussusception
5	Prolapse
R	Rectocele

[a]Lateral view on videofluoroscopy unit of patient in sitting position, passing thickened barium

(Reproduced, with permission, from Kodner IJ, Fry RD, Fleshman JW. Rectal prolapse and other pelvic floor abnormalities. *Ann Surg* 1992; 24:157–190)

The laparoscopic approach to rectal prolapse repair has gained wider acceptance in recent years. Laparoscopic rectopexy with or without sigmoid resection in patients with constipation-associated rectal prolapse have low recurrence rates in well-selected patients.

The use of a perineal proctectomy with anterior and posterior reefing of the sphincter muscle is becoming more popular for the treatment of rectal prolapse. This is a revival of the Altemeier perineal resection technique. The entire prolapsing rectum and redundant sigmoid are removed through a perineal approach beginning at the top of the transitional zone columns (Fig 24–11). The left colon or proximal sigmoid is sutured to the transitional zone 1–2 cm above the dentate line. The external anal sphincter and pelvic floor muscles can be reefed to the anterior and posterior midline to restore anal tone in patients with incontinence. The incidence of recurrence of prolapse is approximately 10% if the sphincter function has been adequate. Even though the operation has been recommended for elderly patients, it may be indicated for patients of all ages with severe compromise of sphincter tone and pronounced procidentia. This procedure is not technically possible in patients who do not evert the entire anal canal with the rectum.

Anal encirclement procedures have been mostly replaced by the perineal proctectomy. It is effective and safe to perform under local anesthesia in patients with prohibitive surgical risks and decreased life expectancy.

INTERNAL INTUSSUSCEPTION OF THE RECTUM

The treatment of internal intussusception of the rectum is initially a high-fiber diet and patient counseling. Once the patient is assured that there is no cancer, high doses of psyllium may prevent formation of the funnel and outlet obstruction. The bowel function is normalized and the need for operation is obviated. If the intussusception is severe or causes bleeding or incontinence, an operation may be the only satisfactory course of action. A low anterior resection or rectopexy is appropriate for these patients depending on whether they have constipation or incontinence, respectively. The use of perineal proctectomy is not recommended since the sphincter mechanism is intact and the resection of redundant rectum will be extremely difficult in patients with an incomplete prolapse. Prior to operation for internal intussusception, colonic transit times are essential to document normal colonic transit. Defecography shows the surgeon the level of the funnel formation within the rectum as he or she plans the operation. A balloon expulsion test is necessary to eliminate the possibility that the patient has pelvic floor outlet obstruction causing excessive straining and thereby exacerbating the rectal intussusception. This may also be the cause of postoperative constipation and persistent symptoms in a small number of patients.

■ PELVIC FLOOR OUTLET OBSTRUCTION AND SOLITARY RECTAL ULCER SYNDROME

PATHOPHYSIOLOGY

The presenting complaints of patients with pelvic floor outlet obstruction usually include some form of constipation and straining. Defecation is a learned process and pelvic floor outlet obstruction may be either a change in the defecating mechanism or a failure to learn the appropriate series of events to allow normal function. The muscle of the pelvic floor is completely normal but the function and control are abnormal. There may be a psychological influence in this syndrome since patients who have been sexually abused or who have been psychologically traumatized may develop this outlet obstruction. A need to dominate and control has also been documented in these

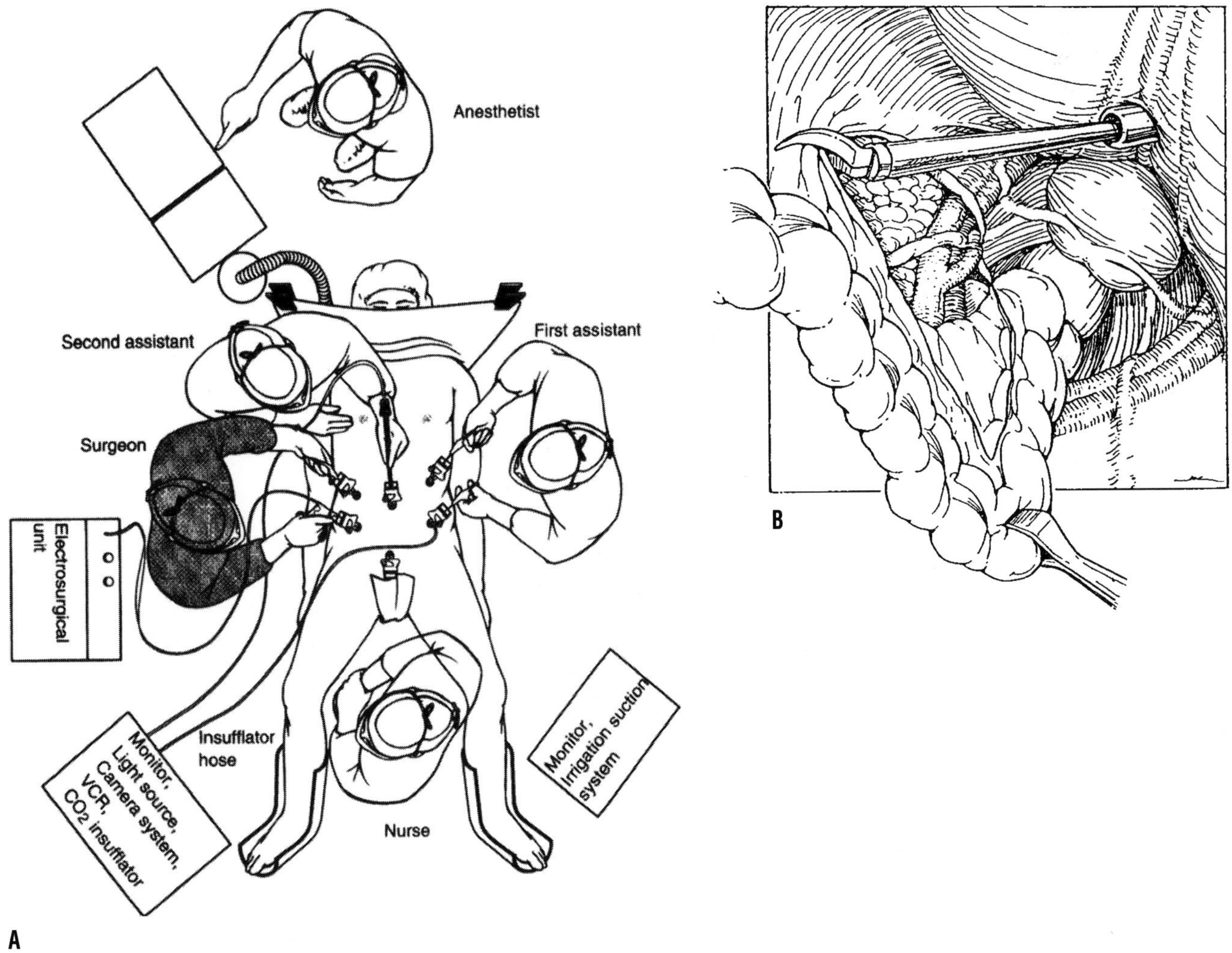

Figure 24–10. Laparoscopic low anterior resection with colorectal anastomosis—double-staple technique. **A.** Laparoscopic positioning of the patient and surgeon. The patient is secured to the table in modified lithotomy position. The operating surgeon stands to the right of the patient. Trocar placement is based on use of hand-assisting devices and surgeon preference. **B.** Lateral approach to mobilization of the sigmoid colon and identification of the left ureter. *Continued*

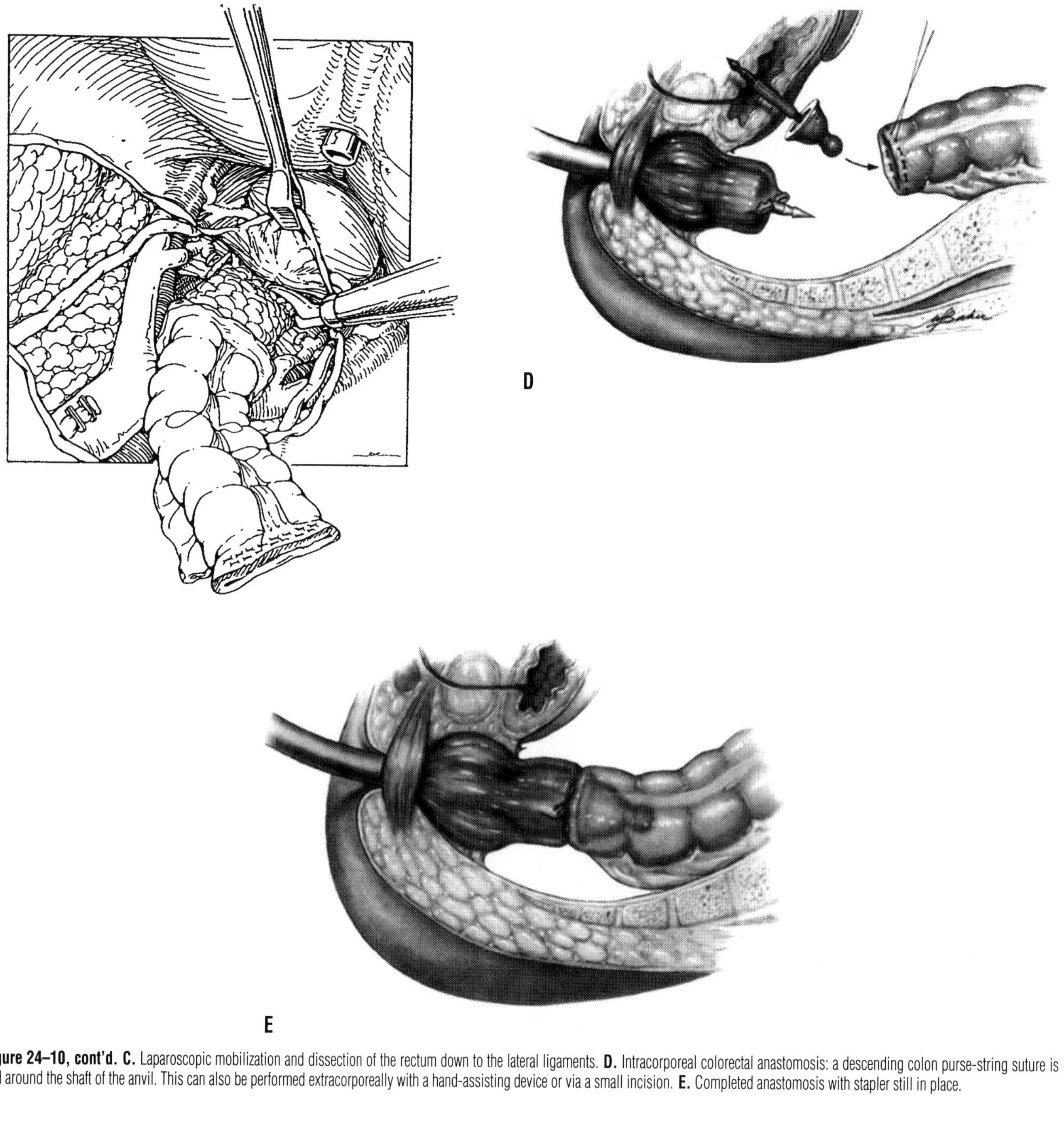

Figure 24–10, cont'd. C. Laparoscopic mobilization and dissection of the rectum down to the lateral ligaments. **D.** Intracorporeal colorectal anastomosis: a descending colon purse-string suture is tied around the shaft of the anvil. This can also be performed extracorporeally with a hand-assisting device or via a small incision. **E.** Completed anastomosis with stapler still in place.

patients. The syndrome results from an anterior displacement of the puborectalis muscle and contraction of the pelvic floor and external sphincter during straining to defecate that obstructs the anal canal. Attempts to defecate against a closed pelvic floor result in chronic funnel formation of the rectum and descent of the anterior rectal wall into the anal canal. This chronic trauma and ischemia may lead to the formation of an ulcer on the anterior wall of the rectum. The stimulus to defecate is often forgotten. The end result is an uncoordinated effort at defecation which causes the pelvic floor to obstruct the outlet, even when the rectum begins to distend and the autonomic muscles begin to relax.

It is possible that pelvic floor outlet obstruction is etiologically related to rectal prolapse and intussusception. However, no long-term studies have provided data as conclusive evidence. Patients may also present with megarectum from outlet obstruction, as well as anal incontinence due to nerve injury from chronic straining, or simply with severe mucosal prolapse or hemorrhoids.

The solitary rectal ulcer is assumed to be due to ischemia of an isolated portion of the anterior rectal wall, approximately 10 cm above the anal verge, which

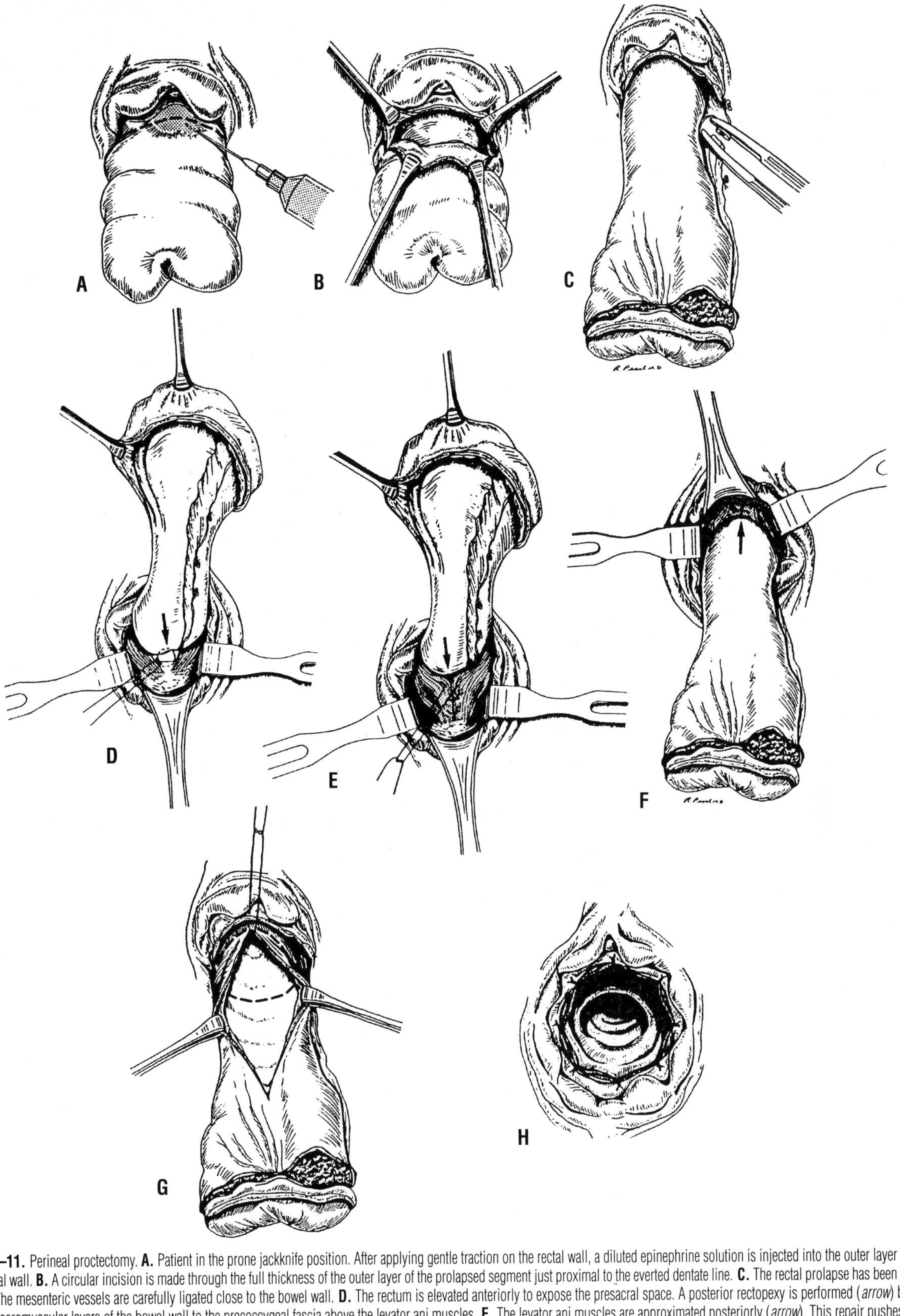

Figure 24–11. Perineal proctectomy. **A.** Patient in the prone jackknife position. After applying gentle traction on the rectal wall, a diluted epinephrine solution is injected into the outer layer of the prolapsed rectal wall. **B.** A circular incision is made through the full thickness of the outer layer of the prolapsed segment just proximal to the everted dentate line. **C.** The rectal prolapse has been completely unfolded. The mesenteric vessels are carefully ligated close to the bowel wall. **D.** The rectum is elevated anteriorly to expose the presacral space. A posterior rectopexy is performed (*arrow*) by approximating the seromuscular layers of the bowel wall to the precoccygeal fascia above the levator ani muscles. **E.** The levator ani muscles are approximated posteriorly (*arrow*). This repair pushes the bowel anteriorly to help recreate the anorectal angle. **F.** One or two sutures are used to approximate the levators anterior to the rectum to reinforce the pelvic floor. **G.** The prolapse is amputated and the colon is sutured to the dentate line in a circumferential fashion (*dotted line*). **H.** Completed anastomosis. (Reproduced, with permission, from Prasad ML, Pearl RK, Abcarian H, Orsay CP, Nelson RL. Perineal proctectomy, posterior rectopexy, and postanal levator repair for the treatment of rectal prolapse. *Dis Colon Rectum* 1986;29:547.)

prolapses partially into the anal canal and becomes ischemic during prolonged straining. The healing process may occasionally incorporate mucosal glands beneath the new mucosal surface and form a localized area of colitis cystica profunda. These entrapped glands continue to produce mucus and are occasionally mistaken for an early neoplasm of the rectum.

DIAGNOSIS AND EVALUATION

Patients with pelvic floor outlet obstruction complain of a number of problems which include constipation and straining at defecation, the need for digital maneuvers to evacuate the rectum, bleeding, mucosal prolapse, and hemorrhoids. They occasionally complain of chronic pain of the anal canal, and symptoms which have been designated in the past as amismus, proctalgia fugax, or levator ani syndrome. On examination, they have a normal exam but a paradoxical motion of the puborectalis muscle during attempts to expel the finger. Defecography generally shows a persistent puborectalis impression on the posterior rectum as the patient attempts to evacuate the rectal contents. Defecography tends to overdiagnose the problem of nonrelaxing puborectalis. This may be due to an unnatural setting in a cold radiology suite or possible embarrassment. The presence of nonrelaxing puborectalis muscle must therefore be confirmed using expulsion of a rectal balloon.[9] The method best suited to our practice has been to have the patient expel a 60-mL air-filled soft latex balloon while sitting in a private bathroom. This simple technique of expulsion of the balloon within the confines of a private bathroom seems to be adequate. Surface electromyography is also useful in the diagnosis and treatment of nonrelaxing puborectalis muscle, as it documents decreased electrical activity during proper straining techniques. A colonic transit time is essential to document outlet obstruction. The findings in this circumstance would be an accumulation of all of the administered radiopaque markers within the rectum after an elapsed period of time adequate for clearance (>7 days). An algorithm used to deal with pelvic floor disorders is shown in Figure 24–12.

TREATMENT AND MANAGEMENT

The initial steps in the treatment of outlet obstruction problems include high doses of fiber and establishment of a normal bowel routine with counseling. Outpatient biofeedback using surface electromyography, balloon expulsion, sensation techniques, and a simulated stool are also effective in severe cases of nonrelaxing puborectalis muscle.[10] Psychological counseling and relaxation techniques may be of help in patients who have a stressful or a psychological component to their problem.

RECTOCELE, ENTEROCELE, AND COMPLEX PELVIC FLOOR ABNORMALITIES

Outpouching or bulging of the rectum into the vagina (rectocele) can be seen on defecography in patients with symptoms of pelvic floor disorders. However, these findings can also be found in patients without any pelvic or bowel complaints. Surgical repair does not always lead to resolution of symptoms. There have been studies examining characteristics on defecography (depth of rectocele and problems emptying) and symptomatology to predict which patients will have successful outcomes of surgery; however, no predictors are universally accepted. Surgical technique is based on the surgeon's preference and can be performed via a transanal, vaginal, or perineal approach to bolster, pleat, and reconstruct the muscle in the rectovaginal septum. Thankfully, a majority of patients improve with medical management.[12,13]

Enteroceles or bulging of small bowel into the rectogenital area are also commonly detected on defecography. This is a common finding in post-hysterectomized patients, asymptomatic patients, and in patients with symptoms of obstructive defecation. These can be repaired transabdominally in the setting of surgical management of other pelvic abnormalities by reefing the pelvic peritoneum to obliterate the herniation of small bowel into the pelvic floor.

Pelvic floor disorders can also be seen in combination with bladder or gynecological complaints. A multidisciplinary surgical approach to complex pelvic floor abnormalities in combination with urology and gynecology, including vaginal and/or bladder suspensions, pelvic floor suspensions, and rectopexy/resection can be performed simultaneously as well. Dynamic MRI is a promising new modality for diagnosis of some of these challenging pelvic floor cases.[14]

▪ HEMORRHOIDS

Current theories about the development of hemorrhoids consider the nature of anal "cushions." Such cushions are aggregations of blood vessels (arterioles, venules, and arteriolar-venular communications), smooth muscle, and elastic connective tissue in the submucosa that normally reside in the left lateral, right posterolateral, and right anterolateral anal canal.[15] Smaller discrete secondary cushions may reside between the main cushions. Hemorrhoids

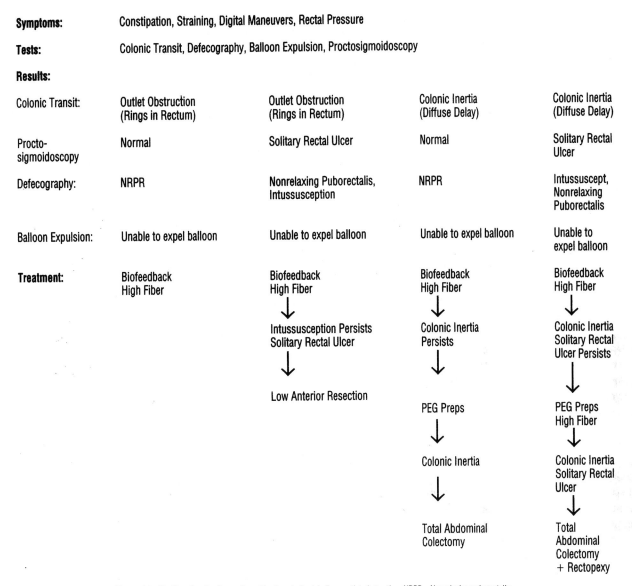

Symptoms: Constipation, Straining, Digital Maneuvers, Rectal Pressure

Tests: Colonic Transit, Defecography, Balloon Expulsion, Proctosigmoidoscopy

Results:

Colonic Transit:	Outlet Obstruction (Rings in Rectum)	Outlet Obstruction (Rings in Rectum)	Colonic Inertia (Diffuse Delay)	Colonic Inertia (Diffuse Delay)
Procto-sigmoidoscopy	Normal	Solitary Rectal Ulcer	Normal	Solitary Rectal Ulcer
Defecography:	NRPR	Nonrelaxing Puborectalis, Intussusception	NRPR	Intussuscept, Nonrelaxing Puborectalis
Balloon Expulsion:	Unable to expel balloon	Unable to expel balloon	Unable to expel balloon	Unable to expel balloon
Treatment:	Biofeedback High Fiber	Biofeedback High Fiber ↓ Intussusception Persists Solitary Rectal Ulcer ↓ Low Anterior Resection	Biofeedback High Fiber ↓ Colonic Inertia Persists ↓ PEG Preps ↓ Colonic Inertia ↓ Total Abdominal Colectomy	Biofeedback High Fiber ↓ Colonic Inertia Solitary Rectal Ulcer Persists ↓ PEG Preps High Fiber ↓ Colonic Inertia Solitary Rectal Ulcer ↓ Total Abdominal Colectomy + Rectopexy

Figure 24–12. Algorithm for diagnosis and treatment of pelvic floor outlet obstruction. NRPR = Nonrelaxing puborectalis.

are likely the result of a sliding downward of these anal cushions. Hemorrhoids provide tissue to close the anal canal during rest. It appears that the disintegration of the anchoring and supporting connective tissue and the terminal fibers of the longitudinal muscle above the hemorrhoids allows these structures to slide distally.

CLASSIFICATION

Anal skin tags are discrete folds of skin located at the anal verge. These may be the result of thrombosed external hemorrhoids, or more rarely may be associated with inflammatory bowel disease. Internal hemorrhoids reside above the dentate line and are covered by transitional and columnar epithelium (Fig 24–13). First-degree internal hemorrhoids cause painless bleeding with defecation. Second-degree hemorrhoids protrude through the anal canal at the time of defecation, but spontaneously reduce. Third-degree internal hemorrhoids protrude and bleed with defecation, but must be manually reduced. Fourth-degree internal hemorrhoids are permanently fixed below the dentate line and cannot be manually reduced.

External hemorrhoids consist of the dilated vascular plexus located below the dentate line and are covered by squamous epithelium. Mixed hemorrhoids are composed of elements of both internal and external hemorrhoids.

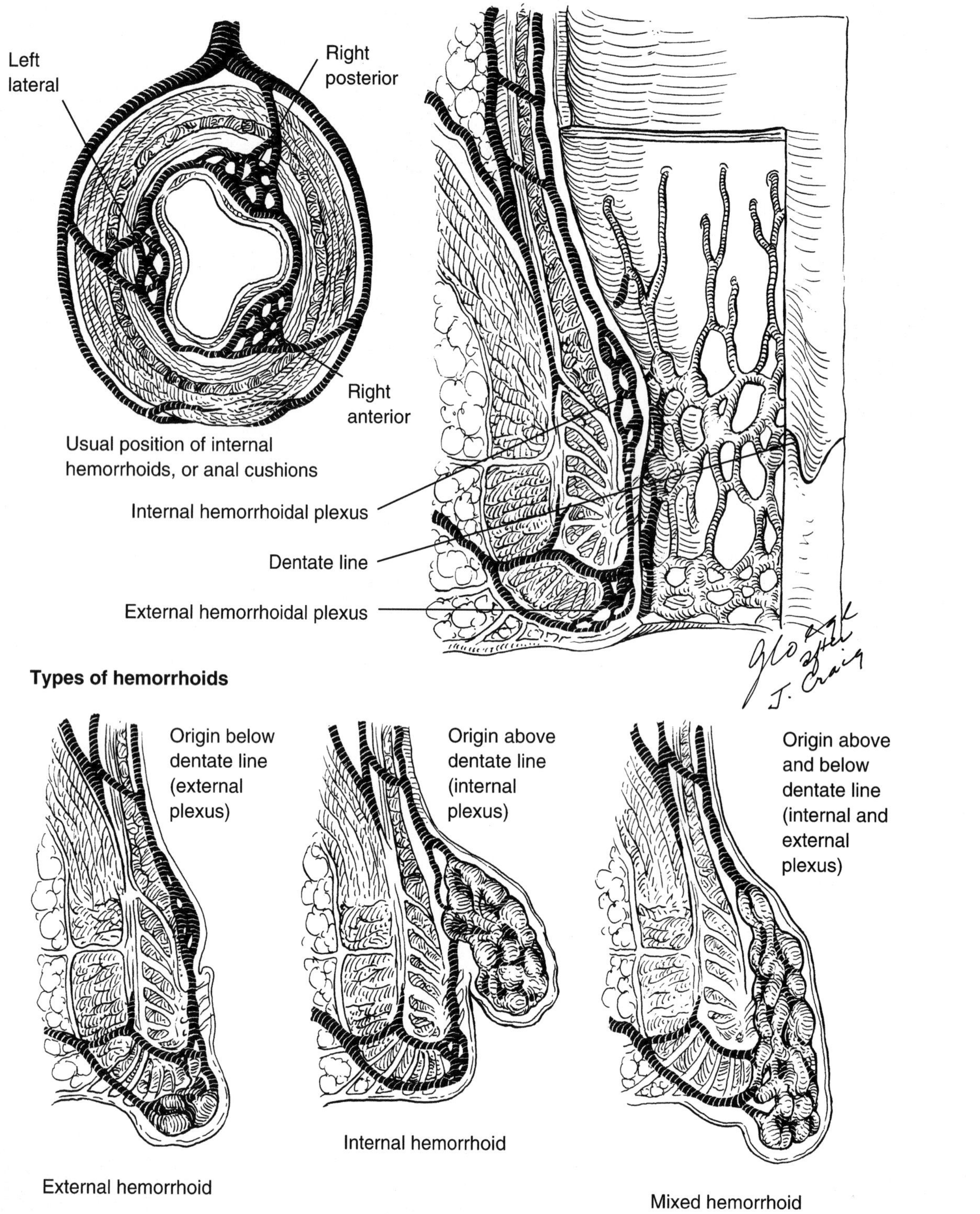

Figure 24–13. Location and types of hemorrhoids. (Redrawn, with permission, from Fry RD, Kodner IJ. Anorectal diseases. *Clin Symp* 1985;37:7. Copyright 1985, CIBA-GEIGY. Originally illustrated by John Craig, MD.)

Evaluation of Internal Hemorrhoids

Even though internal hemorrhoids are the most common source of rectal bleeding, it is imperative that other causes be excluded. Since internal hemorrhoids cannot be detected by digital examination, diagnosis can only be made by anoscopy. It is mandatory that colonoscopy be performed in high-risk patients to exclude other sources of bleeding, such as carcinoma or proctitis (e.g., for patients more than 40 years of age and those with a family history of colorectal neoplasia or a change in bowel habits).

TREATMENT

Regulation of diet and avoidance of prolonged straining at the time of defecation comprise the initial treatment of mild symptoms of bleeding and protrusion. Increasing the fiber content of the diet to at least 25–35 grams daily with raw vegetables, fruits, whole grain cereals, and hydrophilic bulk-forming agents can reduce and often alleviate all symptoms. If bleeding and protrusion persist, however, the hemorrhoids should be treated surgically.

Elastic ligation of the friable redundant hemorrhoidal tissue is quite satisfactory for first-, second- and third-degree hemorrhoids. The procedure is quite simple. The hemorrhoid is visualized with the aid of an anoscope and grasped with forceps. The redundant tissue is pulled into a double-sleeved cylinder on which there are two latex bands. The bands are discharged from the cylinder, and the hemorrhoidal bundle is ligated (Fig 24–14).

Certain precautions, however, must be taken with this form of treatment. The ligatures must be placed at least 1–2 cm above the dentate line to avoid extreme discomfort. Ideally, the ligatures should be placed at the top of the hemorrhoidal cushion. About 25% of patients experience mild, dull anorectal discomfort lasting for 2–3 days following the procedure. Mild analgesics and warm baths are usually sufficient to relieve the discomfort. In about 1% of patients, brisk bleeding that may require suture ligation occurs when the necrotic tissue sloughs off at 7–10 days. About 2% of patients treated with ligation of the internal hemorrhoid develop thrombosis of an external hemorrhoid, which may cause considerable discomfort.

Hemorrhoidal ligation is an office procedure, and no special preparation is required. Patients with a bleeding diathesis or with portal hypertension are not good candidates for ligation. Usually only one hemorrhoid is ligated on the first treatment visit. Ligations can be performed every 2–4 weeks until all symptoms of bleeding or prolapse are alleviated. The second ligation can be multiple if the first treatment is well tolerated.

Although diet, bowel regulation, or elastic ligation will alleviate most symptoms of internal hemorrhoids, occasionally further surgical treatment may be needed. Excisional hemorrhoidectomy is indicated for large, mixed (combined internal/external) hemorrhoids that are not amenable to ligation because the ligature would have to incorporate pain-sensitive tissue at or below the dentate line.

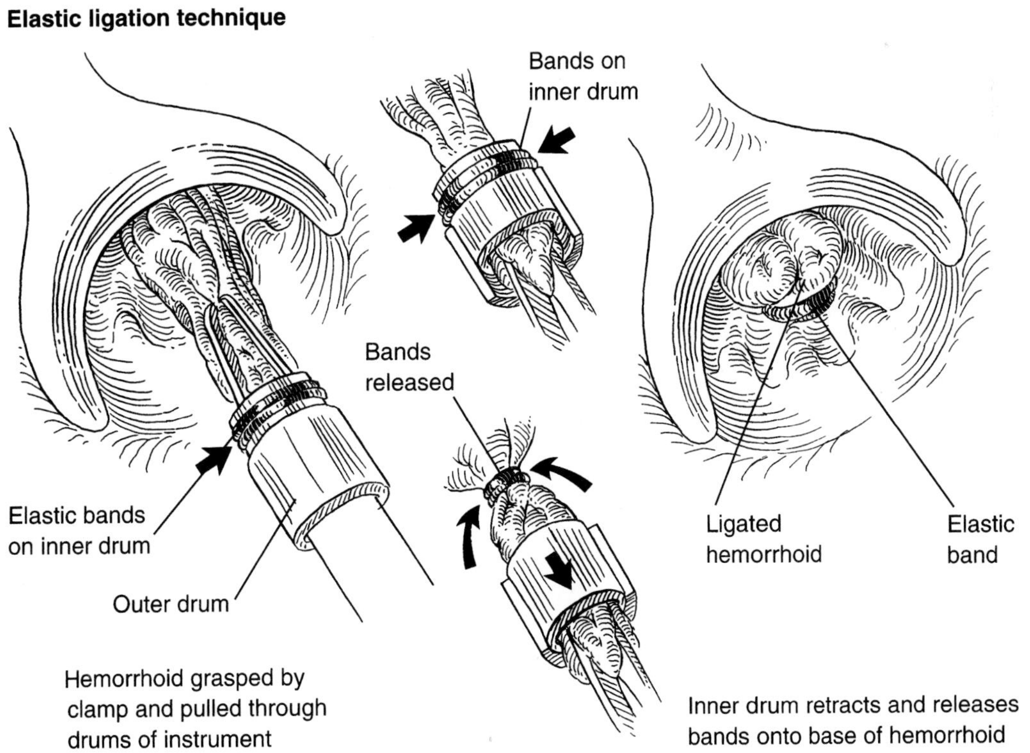

Figure 24–14. Elastic ligation technique. (Redrawn, with permission, from Fry RD, Kodner IJ. Anorectal diseases. *Clin Symp* 1995;37:9. Copyright 1985, CIBA-GEIGY. Originally illustrated by John Craig, MD.)

Circular stapled hemorrhoidectomy is a newer technique indicated for the elective treatment of circumferential third- and fourth-degree hemorrhoids that are not permanently prolapsed due to scar.[16] This entails a simple procedure of placing a purse-string suture incorporating only the mucosa above the anal canal in order to perform a stapled circumferential mucosectomy at a level 4–5 cm above the dentate line. This can be performed under regional anesthesia with minimal morbidity in experienced hands. Potential complications include bleeding if the staple line is incomplete, pain if the staple line is too close to the dentate line, rectovaginal fistula if the purse-string captures the rectovaginal septum, and return of symptoms if the purse-string is incomplete.

Occasionally the entire ring of internal hemorrhoidal tissue may be incarcerated outside the anal canal, resulting in spasm of the anal sphincter, massive local edema, and severe pain. In such circumstances, the edematous tissue may be injected with a local anesthetic containing epinephrine. Dissipation of the edema by manual compression then can be achieved, allowing reduction of the prolapsed tissue. Observation and stool softeners with tub soaks usually allow the acute episode to resolve without an operation. The thrombosed internal hemorrhoids will sclerose and may not require surgery. Only if symptoms persist will a three-quadrant hemorrhoidectomy then be necessary. If necrotic tissue is present at the time of acute thrombosis, an emergent excisional hemorrhoidectomy is necessary. Care should be taken to preserve the anoderm. The patient should be kept in the hospital after the procedure until the pain is minimal or until spontaneous voiding is possible.

Mixed Hemorrhoids

The mucosal component of mixed hemorrhoids occasionally can be treated by elastic ligation. Large symptomatic, nonreducing mixed hemorrhoids generally are treated by excisional hemorrhoidectomy. The patient is placed in the prone flexed position under local anesthesia using a perianal field block with 0.25% bupivacaine with or without epinephrine. The apex of the vascular pedicle is ligated first with a 3-0 chromic catgut suture. An elliptical excision incorporates the external and internal hemorrhoids from the perianal skin to the anorectal ring. The hemorrhoidal tissue is sharply dissected from the underlying internal sphincter (Fig 24–15). The entire wound is then closed by running the apex chromic catgut suture to the distal perianal skin edge. The largest hemorrhoid initially is excised, with care taken not to excise excessive tissue that may result in a stricture. If there is any question of leaving an adequate anal aperture covered by normal anoderm, it is best to modify a planned three-quadrant hemorrhoidectomy into a two-quadrant hemorrhoidectomy.

Thrombosed External Hemorrhoids

The external venous plexus is located at the anal verge and encircles the anal canal. A segmental thrombus is confined to the anoderm and perianal skin and does not extend above the dentate line. The problem presents as a painful perianal mass. The overlying skin may be stretched to 2 cm or more. Pain usually peaks within 48 hours, and generally becomes minimal after the fourth day. If untreated, the thrombus is absorbed within a few weeks. Occasionally, the pressure of the underlying clot will cause the adjacent skin to become necrotic, and the clot will be extruded through the area of necrosis. Generally, this is noted by the patient as rectal bleeding followed by relief of the anal pain. A partially extruded clot can be removed in the office to provide relief.

Treatment of thrombosed hemorrhoids is aimed at relief of the pain. If symptoms are minimal, mild analgesics, sitz baths, proper anal hygiene, and bulk-producing agents will suffice. However, if pain is severe, excision of the thrombosed hemorrhoid may be beneficial. Since numerous vessels usually are involved, it is necessary to excise the entire mass along with the overlying skin and subcutaneous tissue. The wound is left open, and packing is unnecessary. Postoperative care consists of mild analgesics and warm sitz baths or showers.

▪ ANAL FISSURE

An anal fissure is a split in the anoderm over the hypertrophied band of internal sphincter at the anal verge (Fig 24–16). The fissure is almost always located close to the midline of the anal canal; in men, 95% are close to the posterior midline and 5% near the anterior midline, whereas in women, about 80% will be located posteriorly and 20% anteriorly. The precise cause of an anal fissure has yet to be determined. However, fissures probably are related to tearing of the anoderm at the time of defecation. The increased anal canal pressure that accompanies an anal fissure is associated with ischemia in the area of the fissure and prevents healing, as spasm recurs with each bowel movement.[17] An anal ulcer is the chronic form of an anal fissure with heaped up edges, sentinel skin tag, and occasionally hypertrophied anal papilla.

CLINICAL FEATURES AND DIAGNOSIS

Most fissures are superficial and heal rapidly with no specific treatment. Occasionally, the fissure may extend

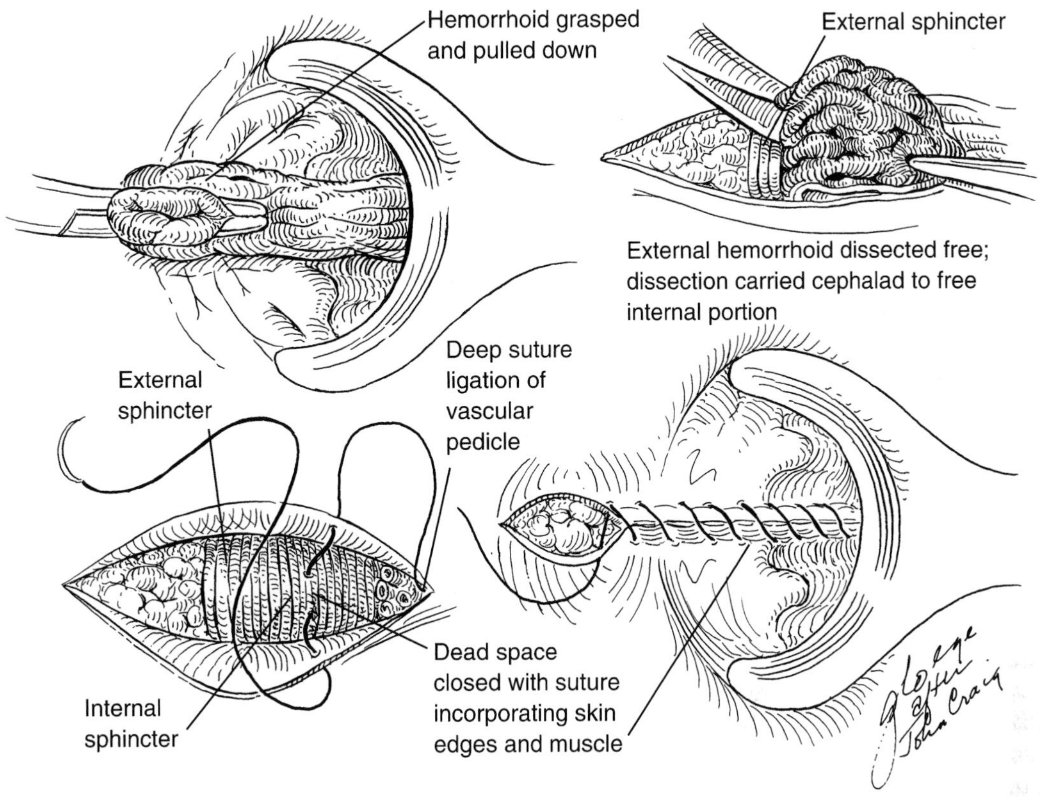

Figure 24–15. Excision technique for mixed hemorrhoids. (Redrawn, with permission, from Fry RD, Kodner IJ. Anorectal diseases. *Clin Symp* 1985;37:9. Copyright 1985, CIBA-GEIGY. Originally illustrated by John Craig, MD.)

deeply through the anoderm to expose the fibers of the internal sphincter. Surprisingly, secondary infection rarely occurs.

Fissures that are aberrantly located may be caused by previous anal operations that result in scarring, stenosis, and loss of anoderm. Individuals with chronic diarrhea may develop anal stenosis associated with a fissure. Crohn's disease often is complicated by anal fissures, which may be a primary manifestation of the disease. These fissures usually are associated with the shiny anal skin tags typical of anal Crohn's disease, and may lie laterally instead of close to the midline of the anus.

Patients with anal fissures usually complain of anal pain accompanying and following defecation. Bright red bleeding may accompany a bowel movement, although it is usually minimal. A slight discharge also may be present.

An anal fissure is detected by gently separating the buttocks to reveal the lower edge of the fissure at the anal verge, where a sentinel tag also may be seen. A soft touch of a cotton swab to this area will elicit the pain and help with the diagnosis. A deep gluteal cleft or tight spasm of the sphincter may sometimes obscure the fissure, and examination with a small anoscope may be required as the patient may tolerate.

Anal sphincter hypertonicity and an increase in ultraslow waves on anal manometry characterize typical anal fissures.

TREATMENT

Dietary recommendations and appropriate prescription of bulk agents to promote soft stools are beneficial, and warm tub soaks may provide comfort. The great majority of acute fissures will heal with this type of conservative management. The use of 2% nifedipine ointment applied to the anoderm outside the anal verge relaxes the sphincter and dilates local vessels to promote healing. Most of the remainder of acute fissures will heal with this added therapy.[18]

The injection of a total of 20–25 U of botulinum A toxin into both edges of an anal ulcer and directly into the internal sphincter muscle at the ulcer base is a simple procedure that has had some mixed success in healing anal fissures.[19] It can be done with local anesthesia as an outpatient procedure, with delay of symptomatic relief by approximately 1 week. Its paralysis of the internal sphincter completely reverses in several months, but the fissure may recur. Subsequent repeat treatments can be

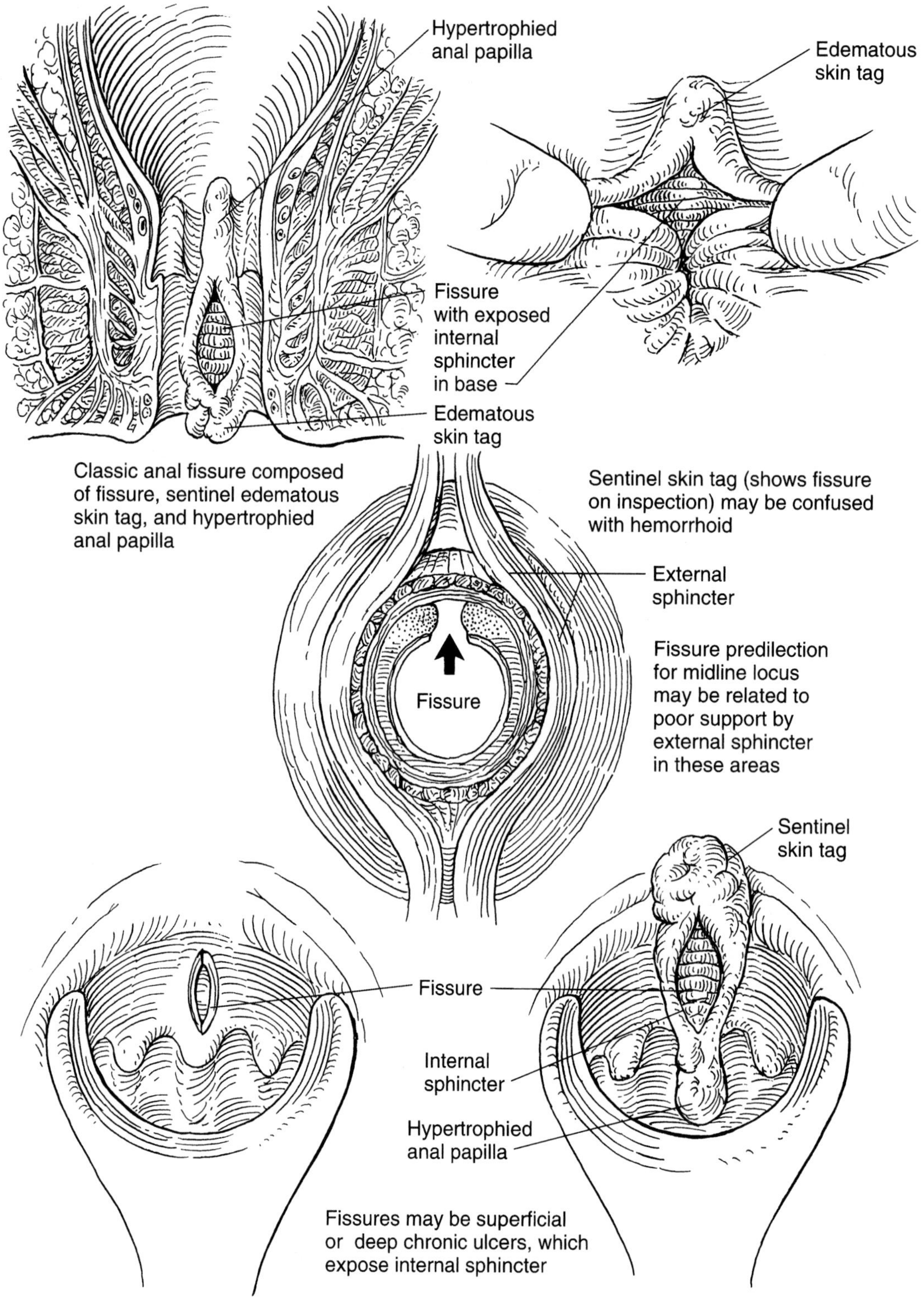
Hypertrophied anal papilla
Edematous skin tag
Fissure with exposed internal sphincter in base
Edematous skin tag
Classic anal fissure composed of fissure, sentinel edematous skin tag, and hypertrophied anal papilla
Sentinel skin tag (shows fissure on inspection) may be confused with hemorrhoid
External sphincter
Fissure
Fissure predilection for midline locus may be related to poor support by external sphincter in these areas
Sentinel skin tag
Fissure
Internal sphincter
Hypertrophied anal papilla
Fissures may be superficial or deep chronic ulcers, which expose internal sphincter

Figure 24–16. Anal fissure. (Redrawn, with permission, from Fry RD, Kodner IJ. Anorectal diseases. *Clin Symp* 1985;37:12. Copyright 1985, CIBA-GEIGY. Originally illustrated by John Craig, MD.)

performed if the initial response was adequate, but it is expensive with at best modest healing rates.

Surgical treatment may be required for deep, chronic fissures associated with a sentinel skin tag, hypertrophied anal papilla, and exposed internal sphincter. Excellent results can be achieved if the internal sphincter is divided laterally rather than in the midline. Furthermore, lateral sphincterotomy is not associated with keyhole deformity. Only the thickened band of the internal sphincter is divided (i.e., partial sphincterotomy), which

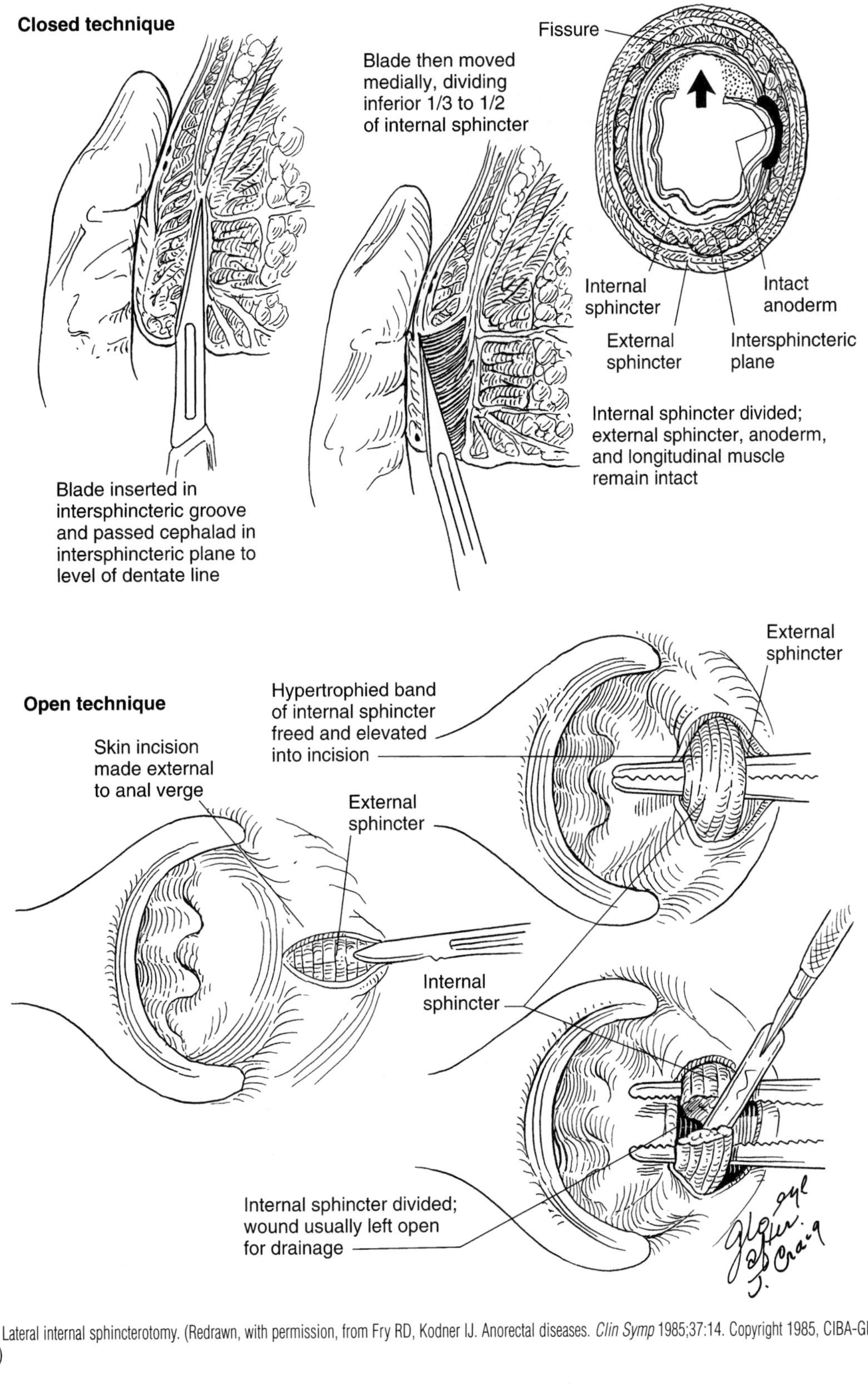

Figure 24–17. Lateral internal sphincterotomy. (Redrawn, with permission, from Fry RD, Kodner IJ. Anorectal diseases. *Clin Symp* 1985;37:14. Copyright 1985, CIBA-GEIGY. Originally illustrated by John Craig, MD.)

limits the amount of internal sphincter transection and reduces the potential for fecal incontinence.

Sphincterotomy can be performed under local anesthesia, using either an open or closed technique (Fig 24–17). The open technique consists of radial incision of the anoderm over the intersphincteric groove and division of the internal sphincter under direct vision. The closed method entails dividing the internal sphincter by a subcutaneous approach. Either technique may be used in the outpatient setting, and both operations afford rapid pain relief. Approximately 98% of fissures heal following sphincterotomy. However, there is a small incidence of minor anal incontinence following the procedure, so careful patient selection is mandatory. Elderly patients with decreased anorectal sensation are generally not ideal candidates for internal sphincterotomy because of this risk. Consideration should be given to a diamond skin advancement flap to cover the ulcer bed in women.

▪ ANORECTAL ABSCESS AND ANAL FISTULA

DIAGNOSIS AND CLASSIFICATION

More than 95% of all anorectal abscesses are caused by infections arising in the anal glands that communicate with the anal crypts (cryptoglandular disease). The acute phase of the infection causes an anorectal abscess, while the chronic stage is recognized as an anal fistula. The anal glands lie in the intersphincteric space between the internal and external anal sphincters. Inflammation of an anal gland leads to the formation of a local abscess in the intersphincteric plane. The clinical presentation, natural history, and proper treatment of anorectal abscess and fistula are understood easily if it is recognized that the disease originates as an intersphincteric abscess.

As the abscess enlarges, it escapes the confines of the intersphincteric plane and spreads in one of several possible directions (Fig 24–18). The most common of all anorectal abscesses is a perianal abscess, which presents as a tender, erythematous bulge at the anal verge. An ischiorectal abscess is formed when a growing intersphincteric abscess penetrates the skeletal muscle of the external sphincter below the level of the puborectalis and expands into the fat of the ischiorectal fossa. These abscesses can become quite large, because the levator ani (the upper border of the ischiorectal fossa) slopes upward. Thus an ischiorectal abscess may be palpated as a bulge above the puborectalis, although it actually lies below the levator ani musculature. In contrast to the perianal abscess, this abscess seldom presents as a visible bulge because of the large potential space in the ischiorectal fossa. Thus the abscess preferentially expands upward rather than protruding through the skin of the buttock. Rarely, an intersphincteric abscess may expand upward between the circular internal sphincter and the external sphincter, forming a supralevator abscess.

TREATMENT

Perirectal abscesses should be drained immediately, before fluctuance or erythema develops. Antibiotics are not indicated and should be used only in the presence of specific disorders: extensive cellulitis, valvular heart disease, diabetes, or states of compromised immunity. If the diagnosis is suspected but in doubt, examination under regional anesthesia should be performed.

With adequate anesthesia, the abscess can be detected and localized by digital examination. An intersphincteric abscess is treated definitively by excising the infected crypt and performing an internal sphincterotomy over the length of the abscess cavity, which serves to unroof and drain the abscess. However, if the infection has developed into a perianal or an ischiorectal abscess, adequate drainage of the abscess cavity first must be done by making a cruciate incision in the skin overlying the abscess as close to the anal canal as possible, or excising a small disc of overlying skin to permit complete evacuation of the contents of the abscess cavity. Incision and drainage alone will result in complete resolution of the infection in about half of patients. In the other half, an anal fistula occurs, which consists of a chronically infected tract with an internal opening located in a crypt at the level of the dentate line, and an external opening located at the drainage site of the earlier abscess.

The appropriate treatment for an anal fistula is dependent upon the anatomy and the location of the fistula tract. Goodsall's rule states that if the anus is bisected by a line in the frontal plane, an external opening anterior to the line will connect to an internal opening by a short, direct fistula tract (Fig 24–19). However, if the external opening is located posterior to this imaginary line, the fistula tract follows a curved course to the crypt in the posterior midline. This rule, while useful, is not infallible. Occasionally, an external opening located more than 2 cm from the anal verge anterior to the imaginary bisecting line connects to an internal opening in the posterior midline. Because of its shape this fistula is usually called a horseshoe fistula.

Horseshoe fistulas usually have an internal opening in the posterior midline of the anus and may extend anteriorly and laterally to both ischiorectal spaces by way of the deep space. The anterior extensions of the horseshoe tracts then can be drained by a secondary opening, avoiding a long skin incision that would unroof the entire tract (Fig 24–20).

If a perianal abscess develops into a fistula, the condition is appropriately treated by simple fistulotomy, which divides a portion of the internal sphincter and unroofs the tract entirely.

An anorectal fistula that persists after drainage of an ischiorectal fossa abscess usually is a transsphincteric fistula, since the tract crosses the lower portion of the external sphincter. The fistulotomy required to unroof this tract results in division of a portion of the internal sphincter as well as a portion of the lower external sphincter. If the tract lies below the posterior midline

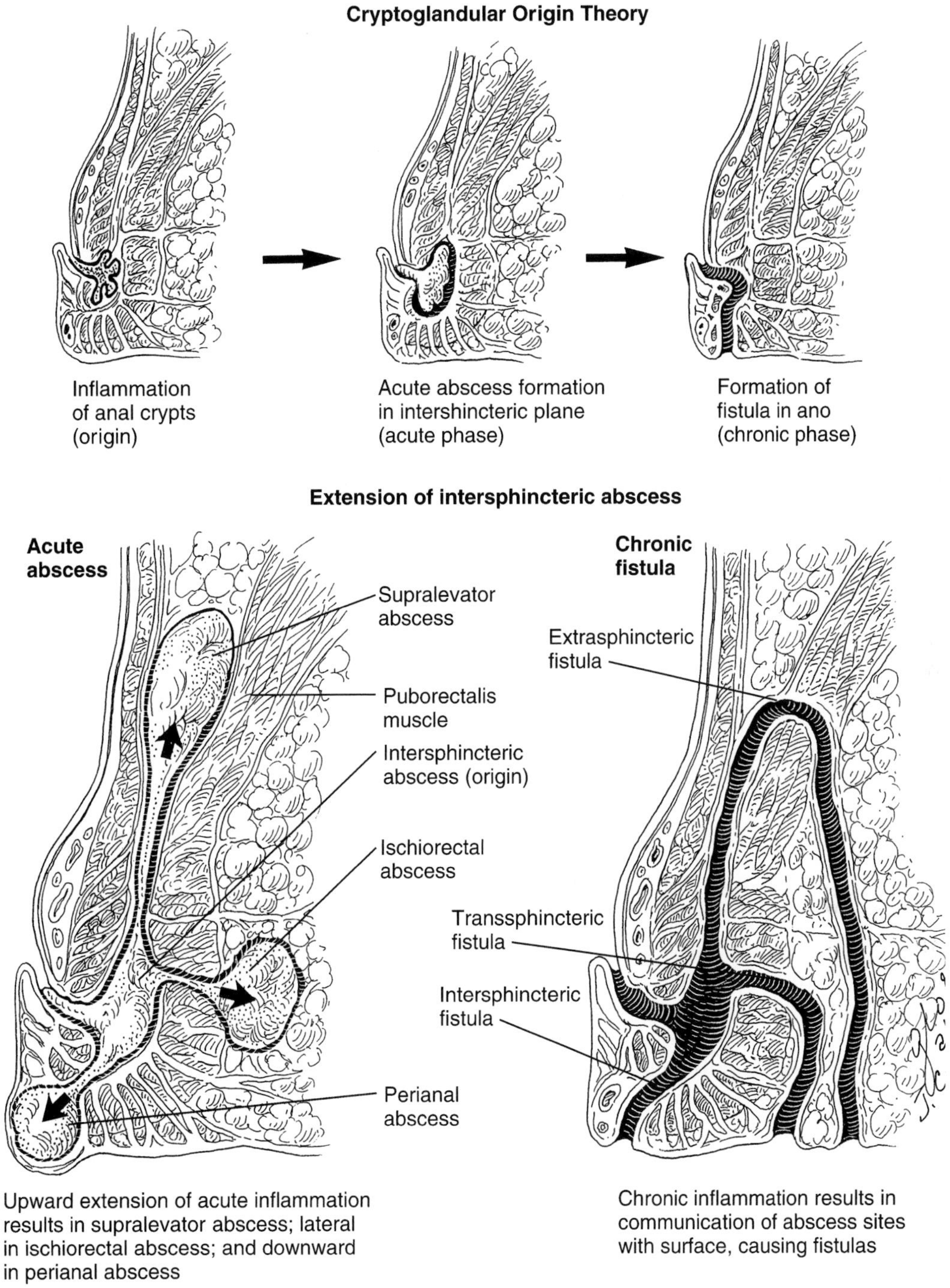

Figure 24–18. Anorectal abscess and fistula-in-ano cryptoglandular origin theory. (Redrawn, with permission, from Fry RD, Kodner IJ. Anorectal diseases. *Clin Symp* 1985;37:15. Copyright 1985, CIBA-GEIGY. Originally illustrated by John Craig, MD.)

puborectalis, the external sphincter usually can be divided at the site of the fistula tract without loss of continence. However, the puborectalis must not be divided, or incontinence will invariably ensue.

The external anal sphincter is much less prominent in the anterior midline. Thus fistulotomy as treatment for an anterior midline anal fistula is associated with an increased risk of anal incontinence, particularly in women. Consequently, treatment of such fistulas often involves eradicating the internal opening of the fistula at the level of the dentate line by advancing a flap of rectal mucosa. It is important to ensure adequate drainage of the fistula through the external opening until the suture line of the ad-

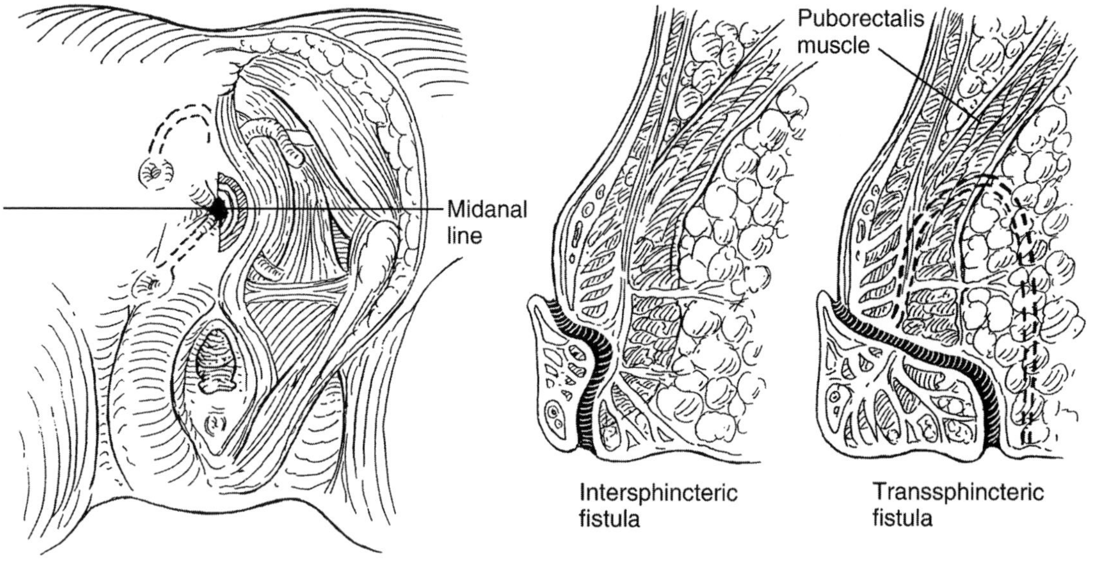

Goodsall's rule

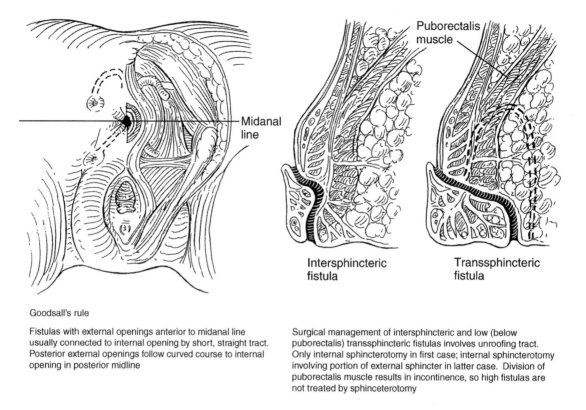

Fistulas with external openings anterior to midanal line usually connected to internal opening by short, straight tract. Posterior external openings follow curved course to internal opening in posterior midline

Surgical management of intersphincteric and low (below puborectalis) transsphincteric fistulas involves unroofing tract. Only internal sphincterotomy in first case; internal sphincterotomy involving portion of external sphincter in latter case. Division of puborectalis muscle results in incontinence, so high fistulas are not treated by sphinceterotomy

Figure 24–19. Surgical management of fistula-in-ano. (Redrawn, with permission, from Fry RD, Kodner IJ. Anorectal diseases. *Clin Symp* 1985;37:21. Copyright 1985, CIBA-GEIGY. Originally illustrated by John Craig, MD.)

vancement flap is well healed; otherwise an abscess can reform and disrupt the suture line, causing a recurrence of the fistula (Fig 24–21). The injection of Fibrin glue into the fistula tract is also an alternative with minimal morbidity and mixed success.[20,21]

The repair of rectovaginal fistulas after obstetric injury can also be performed in the same manner as the sliding advancement flap as diagrammed.[22,23] It is important to perform preoperative testing to rule out an associated external sphincter defect that can be repaired simultaneously with the advancement flap.

Although most anorectal abscesses originate in the anal crypts, other disease entities must be considered if the pathology appears atypical. Crohn's disease should be suspected if there are numerous complex fistula tracts associated with edematous skin tags, or if there is inflammation of the rectal mucosa. Tuberculosis is now a rare cause of anal abscesses and fistulas, but has recently been observed in immigrants to America. Hidradenitis suppurativa also may mimic cryptoglandular suppurative disease. However, close examination will reveal that the disease arises from the area of the perianal skin and not the anal crypts. Actinomycosis should be suspected if typical sulfur-like granules are seen in the abscess cavity or fistula tract. Pilonidal disease sometimes can be confused with a posterior perirectal abscess, but careful examination should reveal that there is no communication with the anus. Hair obtained from the abscess cavity when the pilonidal abscess is drained will indicate the true nature of the disease.

■ SEXUALLY TRANSMITTED ANAL DISEASE

During recent years there has been a profound change in the prevalence and types of sexually transmitted diseases. Genital-anal, oral-anal, and other anal-based erotic practices among homosexual or bisexual men and among women who engage in anal-receptive intercourse account for the transmission of most of these diseases. While the term "gay bowel syndrome" has been used to include all sexually transmitted diseases of the colon, rectum, and anus,[24,25] it should be recognized that these diseases also can occur in heterosexual women who practice anal intercourse.

The liberalization of sexual mores that occurred during the past two decades has now been tempered by the recognition of the acquired immunodeficiency syndrome (AIDS), which has led to public concern over the transmission of the causative agent, the human immunodeficiency virus (HIV). Surprisingly, the

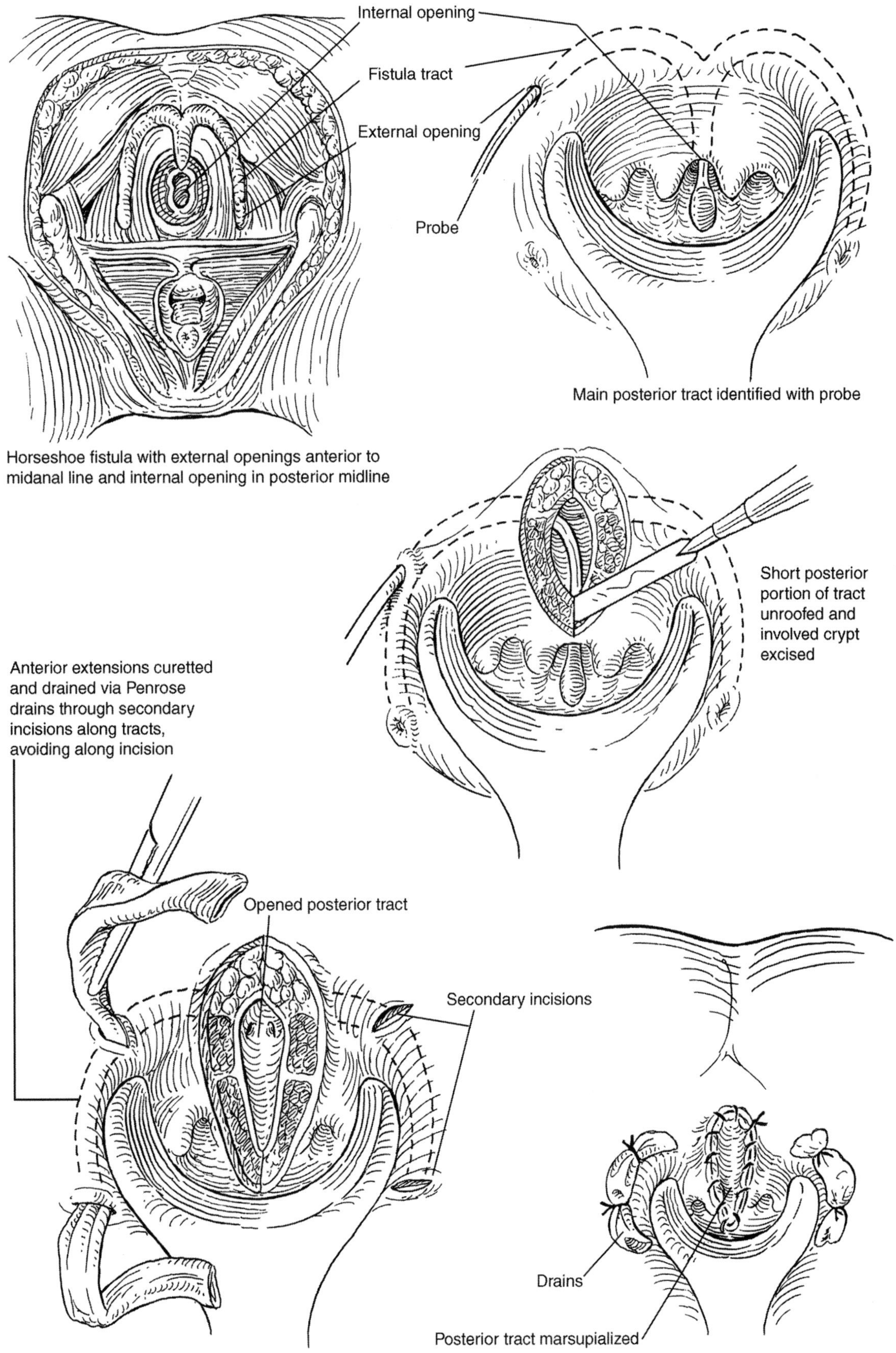
Internal opening
Fistula tract
External opening
Probe
Horseshoe fistula with external openings anterior to midanal line and internal opening in posterior midline
Main posterior tract identified with probe
Short posterior portion of tract unroofed and involved crypt excised
Anterior extensions curetted and drained via Penrose drains through secondary incisions along tracts, avoiding along incision
Opened posterior tract
Secondary incisions
Drains
Posterior tract marsupialized

Figure 24–20. Surgical management of horseshoe fistula. (Redrawn, with permission, from Fry RD, Kodner IJ. Anorectal diseases. *Clin Symp* 1985;37:18. Copyright 1985, CIBA-GEIGY. Originally illustrated by John Craig, MD.)

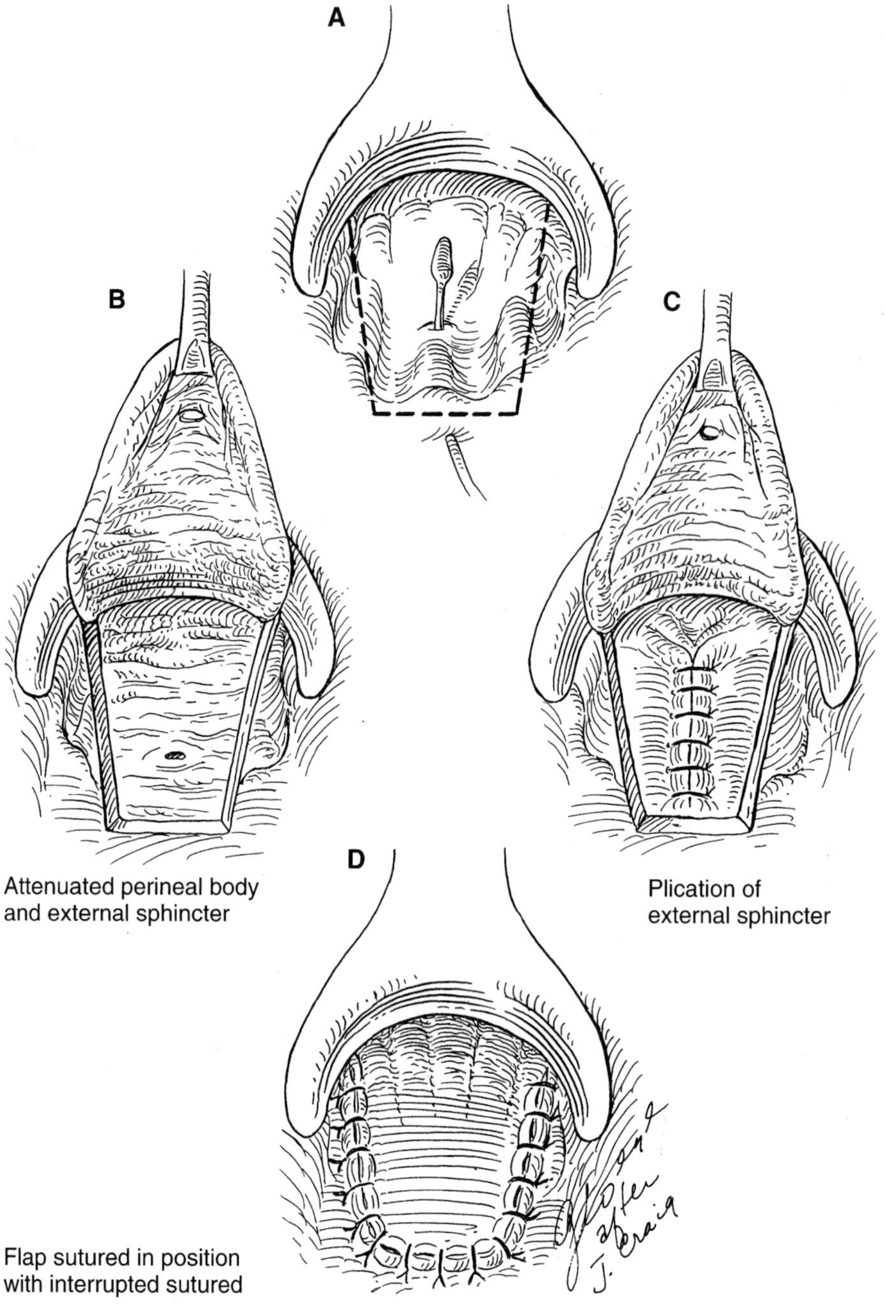

Figure 24–21. Endorectal advancement flap repair of complex anal-perineal or low rectal-perineal fistula. (Redrawn, with permission, from Kodner IJ, Mazor A, Shemesh EI et al. Endorectal advancement flap repair of rectovaginal and other complicated anorectal fistulas. *Surgery* 1993;114:682–690.)

incidence of other venereal diseases appears to be increasing. While a detailed discussion of these infections is beyond the scope of this textbook, the surgeon will often be consulted for evaluation of complications of these diseases.[30]

HUMAN PAPILLOMAVIRUS

Human papillomavirus (HPV) is the etiological agent causing venereal warts. These lesions are common in homosexual men, and can have a varied appearance, including (1) discrete warts: papillary or acuminate white lesions, usually occurring singly or in clusters at or below the dentate line; (2) circumferential wart ring lesions located at the dentate line and encompassing 60–100% of the anal canal; and (3) flat white epithelium: pale areas of smooth opaque epithelium that often extend cephalad to the dentate line. These latter lesions may be detected more easily by using a colposcope to magnify the anal canal. A high prevalence of histologically confirmed dysplasia in these internal lesions can be detected in asymptomatic homosexual men. Dysplasia was found in 70% of HIV-seronegative men and 85% and 90% of nonimmunosuppressed and immunosuppressed HIV-seropositive men, respectively. Biopsy of the lesions was necessary for detection, since it could not be predicted by the gross appearance of the warts.

The association of dysplasia with HPV is now well recognized. There are at least 60 different HPV types. Types 6 and 11 are associated with warts and low-grade dysplasia. Types 16 and 18 have been found in cervical cancer and high-grade cervical dysplasia, and type 16 has been found in high-grade anal dysplasia and invasive cancers. HPV types 31, 33, and 35 are thought to pose an intermediate cancer risk.

While it is clear that HPV is implicated in the pathogenesis of anal cancer in homosexual men, the rates of progression from dysplasia to cancer in the anal canal are unknown. It is likely that the progression is low, but further study is needed for documentation. At present the appropriate therapy seems to be ablation of the lesions, either by excision, cautery, or laser. It is still not known if such treatment will reduce the cancer risk.

CHLAMYDIAL INFECTIONS

Chlamydial infections are now the most common sexually transmitted disease in the United States, and they account for increasing numbers of cases of proctitis in patients who practice receptive anal intercourse. There are 15 recognized immunotypes of *Chlamydia trachomatis*, but for practical purposes it should be recognized that there are lymphogranulomatous (causing lymphogranuloma venereum; LGV) and nonlymphogranulomatous (non-LGV) and types. The non-LGV organisms are a common cause of urethritis, epididymitis, and pelvic inflammatory disease. At least half of the genital infections previously diagnosed as "nonspecific" or "nongonococcal" are caused by non-LGV *Chlamydia*. Chlamydial proctitis may coexist with other rectal infections, especially gonorrhea. Several serotypes are responsible for proctitis, and serotypes Ll, L2, and L3 are responsible for lymphogranuloma venereum. The pathogen is introduced by either genital-anal or oral-anal intercourse. The non-LGV organisms are obligate intracellular parasites that can penetrate only columnar or transitional epithelium. The LGV organisms also can penetrate mononuclear cells, which may account for the prominent lymphadenopathy in patients with lymphogranuloma venereum.

Infection may be asymptomatic, or may consist of nonspecific symptoms such as anal pain, pruritus, purulent discharge, and bleeding. More severe forms of infection, especially severe proctitis, usually indicate the presence of one of the LGV serotypes. Perianal fistulas and rectovaginal fistulas may develop, with untreated cases progressing to severe rectal stricture. Two weeks after the initial symptoms, inguinal lymphadenopathy becomes predominant and the inguinal nodes may fuse together in a large mass.

The organism is an obligate intracellular organism, and rectal cultures are usually inconclusive. A biopsy of the rectal mucosa is probably the most commonly used method to confirm the diagnosis. The diagnosis of chlamydial infections used to be difficult because satisfactory culture techniques were not widely available. Diagnosis usually required the detection of rising antibody titers. However, the organism now can be identified by using tissue culture techniques or DNA probes.

Chlamydial infections should be treated as soon as the diagnosis is suspected. The recommended treatment for non-LGV chlamydial infection is doxycycline, or alternatively, erythromycin for 7–14 days.[26] LGV chlamydial infection should be treated with tetracycline and sulfonamides for a minimum of 21 days.

As with all acute STDs, sexual abstinence until eradication is complete and education, testing, and treatment of sexual partners when appropriate is recommended.

HERPES SIMPLEX VIRUS

Anorectal herpes is usually caused by the type 2 herpes simplex virus (HSV-2), although the HSV-l virus is responsible for approximately 10% of anal infections. Patients who have been previously infected have virus-specific antibodies. The first symptoms of infection are perianal pruritus or paresthesia, followed by intense anal pain. Small vesicles surrounded by red areolas may appear. These vesicles subsequently rupture, leaving small ulcers which appear on the perianal skin, in the anal canal, or even on the rectal mucosa. Fever and malaise are frequently present. The ulcerated lesions may become secondarily infected, with increased pain and discharge.

The lesions usually heal in about 2 weeks. Unfortunately, a chronic relapsing course is common, although recurrent lesions are usually much less painful.

Scrapings from the base of a ruptured vesicle can be stained to show typical intranuclear inclusion bodies, but the diagnosis is most expeditiously made by viral HSV culture.

There is no known cure for herpes. Primary or initial infections are treated with oral acyclovir, famciclovir, or valacyclovir for 7–10 days.[29] Acyclovir should be taken at the onset of recurrent symptoms, which may reduce the formation of new vesicles. Chronic suppressive therapy or self-initiation of episodic treatment with these agents may be helpful in patients with more than 6 recurrences per year.

AIDS patients with perianal herpes resistant to acyclovir may benefit from two newer compounds, foscarnet or vidarabine.[27]

Patients are contagious while the lesions are present and should abstain from sexual activity until all lesions are completely healed. Even after the lesions have completely healed, a condom should be used during sexual intercourse.

GONORRHEA

Anorectal infections caused by the bacterium *Neisseria gonorrhoeae* are common in the male homosexual population and frequently accompany other venereal diseases. Over half of homosexual men seen in screening clinics have been found to be infected, with the rectum being the only site infected in about half of cases. The majority of these infections are asymptomatic.[28]

Symptoms vary from none to intense anorectal pain and tenesmus accompanied by a viscid, yellow anal discharge. Anoscopy may reveal anusitis or distal proctitis. Diagnosis is confirmed by obtaining cultures from the rectal discharge or mucosa, or more recently by DNA probes.

Treatment should be initiated if the disease is suspected. Untreated rectal gonorrhea can lead to septic arthritis, endocarditis, perihepatitis, and meningitis, as well as infection of sexual partners. Several drugs (penicillin, tetracycline, ampicillin, and spectinomycin) may be used for treatment, although increasing numbers of resistant strains are being recognized. Cultures should be repeated after treatment is completed, since antibiotic therapy may fail in as many as a third of the patients. All sexual contacts also must be treated. All patients with confirmed rectal gonorrhea should have a serologic test for syphilis 3 months after treatment is completed.

SYPHILIS

The classic lesion of primary syphilis is a chancre on the genitalia, but in homosexual males the chancre usually presents in the anal canal or at the anal verge.[31] These ulcerated lesions may mimic an anal fissure, but an aberrant location of the lesion (eg, lateral anus instead of midline) should arouse suspicion. Classic descriptions indicate that the syphilitic chancre is a painless lesion, but anal chancres may be extremely painful. The causative organism is the spirochete, *Treponema pallidum*, which may occasionally cause severe proctitis without an accompanying chancre. Inguinal adenopathy is common.

Early syphilis can be diagnosed by examining scrapings from the base of the chancre with dark-field microscopy; these lesions are teeming with spirochetes that can be seen as corkscrew-shaped motile fluorescent yellowish-green organisms. Serology is also very helpful in establishing the diagnosis. In untreated primary syphilis, the Venereal Disease Research Laboratory assay is reactive in about 75% of cases, in early latent syphilis about 95%, and in the secondary state it is 100% reactive. The fluorescent treponemal antibody absorption test usually becomes positive about 4–6 weeks after the initial infection. Rapid plasma reagin and darkfield microscopy are the appropriate tests for suspected early syphilis.

The second stage of anal syphilis appears 6–8 weeks after the chancre has healed in untreated patients. It may present as condyloma latum, a pale-brown or flesh-colored flat verrucous lesion, or as a mucocutaneous rash. All three serologic tests for syphilis will be positive at this stage. Skin lesions are highly contagious.

Benzathine penicillin G is the treatment of choice for syphilis. Alternate treatments include doxycycline, tetracycline, or erythromycin. Patients with syphilis must abstain from sexual contact until treatment is complete. All sexual contacts within the preceding 90 days should be prophylactically treated.

REFERENCES

1. Rockwood TH, Church JM, Fleshman JW et al. Patient and surgeon ranking of the severity of symptoms associated with fecal incontinence: the Fecal Incontinence Severity Index. *Dis Colon Rectum* 1999;42:1525
2. Rockwood TH, Church JM, Fleshman JW et al. Fecal Incontinence Quality of Life Scale: Quality of life instrument for patients with fecal incontinence. *Dis Colon Rectum* 2000;43:9
3. Rociu E, Stoker J, Eijkemans MJ et al. Fecal incontinence: endoanal US versus endoanal MR imaging. *Radiology* 1999;212:453
4. Halverson AL, Hull TL. Long-term outcome of overlapping anal sphincter repair. *Dis Colon Rectum* 2000;45:345
5. Ha HA, Fleshman JW, Smith M et al. Manometric squeeze pressure difference parallels functional outcome after overlapping sphincter reconstruction. *Dis Colon Rectum* 2001;44:655
6. Solomon MJ, Pager CK, Rex J, Roberts R, Manning J. Randomized, controlled trial of biofeedback with anal manometry, transanal ultrasound, or pelvic floor retraining with digital guidance alone in the treatment of mild to moderate fecal incontinence. *Dis Colon Rectum* 2003;46:703
7. Schoetz D Jr et al. Anal incontinence. *Semin Colon Rectal Surg* 2001;12:2
8. Matzel KE, Stadelmaier U, Hohenberger W. Innovations in fecal incontinence: Sacral nerve stimulation. *Dis Colon Rectum* 2004;47:1720

9. Fleshman JW, Drezmk Z, Cohen E et al. Balloon expulsion test facilitates diagnosis of pelvic floor outlet obstruction due to nonrelaxing puborectalis muscle. *Dis Colon Rectum* 1992;35:1019
10. Fleshman JW, Dreznik Z, Meyer K et al. Outpatient protocol for biofeedback therapy of pelvic floor outlet obstruction. *Dis Colon Rectum* 1992;35:1
11. Kim DS, Tsang CB, Wong WD et al. Complete rectal prolapse: evolution of management and results. *Dis Colon Rectum* 1999;42:460
12. Goei R. Anorectal function in patients with defecation disorders and asymptomatic subjects: evaluation with defecography. *Radiology* 1990;174:121
13. Selvaggi F, Pesce G, Scotto Di Carlo E et al. Evaluation of normal subjects by defecographic technique. *Dis Colon Rectum* 1990;33:698
14. Lienemann A, Fischer T. Functional imaging of the pelvic floor. *Eur J Radiol* 2003;47:117
15. Haas PA, Fox TA, Haas GP. The pathogenesis of hemorrhoids. *Dis Colon Rectum* 1984;27:442
16. Sutherland LM, Burchard AK, Matsuda K et al. A systematic review of stapled hemorrhoidectomy. *Arch Surg* 2002;137:1395
17. Schoeten WR, Briel JW, Auwerda JJ et al. Ischaemic nature of anal fissure. *Br J Surg* 1996;83:63
18. Orsay C, Rakinic J, Perry BW, et al. Practice parameters for management of anal fissures (revised). *Dis Colon Rectum* 2004;47:2003
19. Jost WH. One hundred cases of anal fissure treated with botulin toxin: early and long-term results. *Dis Colon Rectum* 1997;40:1029
20. Lindsey I, Smilgin-Humphreys MM, Cunningham C et al. A randomized, controlled trial of fibrin glue vs. conventional treatment for anal fistula. *Dis Colon Rectum* 2002;45:1608
21. Loungnarath R, Dietz DW, Mutch MG et al. Fibrin glue treatment of complex anal fistulas has low success rate. *Dis Colon Rectum* 2004;47:432
22. Kodner IJ, Mazor A, Shemesh EK et al. Endorectal advancement flap repair of rectovaginal and other complicated anorectal fistulas. *Surgery* 1993;114:682
23. Sonoda T, Hull T, Piedmonte MR, et al. Outcomes of primary repair of anorectal and rectovaginal fistulas using the endorectal advancement flap. *Dis Colon Rectum* 2002;45:1622
24. Weller IV. The gay bowel. *Gut* 1985;26:869
25. Wexner SD. Sexually transmitted diseases of the colon, rectum and anus: the challenge of the nineties. *Dis Colon Rectum* 1990;33:1048
26. Stoner BP. STD Clinical Practices Manual 2003–2004, fifth edition. St. Louis, MO: Washington University Infectious Disease Department; 2003
27. Apoola A, Radcliffe K. Antiviral treatment of genital herpes. *Int J STD AIDS* 2004;15:429
28. Janda WM, Bonhoff M, Morgello JA et al. Prevalence and site pathogen studies of *Neisseria meningitidis* and *Neisseria gonorrhoeae* in homosexual men. *JAMA* 1980; 244:2060
29. Corey L. The diagnosis and treatment of genital herpes. *JAMA* 1992;248:1041
30. Knapp JS, Zenilman JM, Thompson SE. Gonorrhea. In: Morse SA, Moreland AA, Thompson SE (eds). *Sexually Transmitted Diseases.* Philadelphia, PA: JB Lippincott; 1990:512–522
31. Golden MR, Marra CM, Holmes KK. Update on syphilis: Resurgence of an old problem. *JAMA* 2003;290:1510

25

Cancer of the Rectum

Kimberly Moore Dalal ■ *Ronald Bleday*

■ INCIDENCE

As we enter the twenty-first century, rectal cancer continues to be a significant medical and social problem. Currently, rectal cancer comprises nearly 30% of all colorectal cancers. Approximately 42,000 patients are diagnosed with adenocarcinoma of the rectum each year in the United States, and 8,500 people succumb to the disease within the same time period.[1]

■ HISTORY

The history of modern rectal cancer resection dates back to 1884, when Czérny described the first abdominoperineal resection (APR). In 1885, Kraske pioneered the transacral approach of rectal resection and anastomosis. In 1908, Miles improved on the APR by understanding that there was a "zone of upward spread."[2] He emphasized the importance of performing a wide perineal excision, including removal of the pelvic contents of the rectum, the abdominal attachments of the rectum with a high arterial ligation, and the iliac lymph nodes. Operative mortality in Miles' first series, however, exceeded 42%. During the last two decades, William Heald popularized the total mesorectal excision.[3] This surgical approach to rectal cancer appreciates the subtle fascial planes along with the lymphatic and neural anatomy of the pelvis. Heald describes a "zone of downward spread" within the mesorectum that requires proper excision in order to reduce local recurrence. Local excision of small rectal cancers, having been employed for a hundred years in selected patients, is being combined with other therapies to maximize local control with a minimally invasive approach.

■ ETIOLOGY AND RISK FACTORS

The average lifetime risk for an individual to develop colorectal cancer is approximately 6%. This risk increases two- to fourfold if the patient has a personal history of or a first-degree relative with colorectal cancer. Inflammatory bowel disease (IBD) is another risk factor. In the first 10 years after the initial diagnosis of ulcerative colitis (UC), the incidence of colorectal cancer ranges from 2–5%; however, this risk increases 1% for each year of disease thereafter. Pancolitis is associated with an earlier risk for colorectal cancer than left-sided colitis alone. For all patients with UC, the cumulative risk for colorectal cancer at 25 years is 25%. Screening the colon yearly starting at 10 years after the diagnosis with colonoscopy and multiple biopsies is used to predict when a patient is at risk for developing colorectal cancer. Ultimately, the most effective method for preventing colon cancer in patients with UC is to remove the colon once dysplasia has been identified. Crohn's colitis is associated with a similar risk for colorectal cancer. This is often not appreciated by clinicians because patients with severe Crohn's often undergo proctocolectomy before their long-term risk becomes an issue.

Genetic risk factors also have been implicated in the development of colorectal cancer. One is familial adenomatous polyposis (FAP), an autosomal dominant syndrome with 100% risk of developing colorectal cancer. The abnormality is caused by a defect in the *APC* gene located on chromosome 5q21. Patients with FAP develop hundreds or thousands of adenomas by their twenties, and colorectal cancer develops in all patients by age 50 if untreated. Extraintestinal manifestations of this genetic defect include desmoid tumors, periampullary masses, osteomas, and medulloblastomas. A second genetic abnormality associated with the development of colorectal cancer is related to defects in the mismatch repair genes *MSH2* and *MLH1*. Mismatch repair genes affect the repair of DNA replication errors and spontaneous base repair loss and contribute to hereditary nonpolyposis colorectal cancer (HNPCC). Despite the name, these cancers arise from adenomas and may account for 5% of all colorectal malignancies. In this autosomal dominant syndrome, cancers occur more often on the right side of the colon. Despite developing at a younger age, there is a better prognosis with these cancers than when compared with age-matched controls with non-HNPCC colorectal cancer. In theory, a patient with HNPCC living to age 80 would have an 80% risk for developing colorectal cancer; additionally, there is a risk of endometrial cancer (40%), gastric cancer (20%), biliary tract cancer (18%), urinary tract cancer (10%), and ovarian cancer (10%). Family members should be screened initially at age 20 with colonoscopy for the presence of polyps or colon cancer. After age 40, colonoscopies should be performed more frequently. If a polyp or cancer is detected, a subtotal colectomy with an ileorectal anastomosis is recommended.

Dietary fats, especially red-meat fats, have been implicated as risk factors for colon and rectal cancer.[4] Populations that consume less than 15% of their diet as fat have a lower incidence of colorectal cancer, whereas people who take in 20% of their diet as fat, either as unsaturated animal fat or as highly saturated vegetable oils, have an increased risk of cancer.

▪ POLYPS

The concept that colorectal cancers develop from polyps, or the "adenoma-to-carcinoma sequence," was first described by Dukes in 1926. The majority of patients with rectal cancer have no inherited component; instead, there is an initiating genetic mutation, such as of an oncogene like *ras*, that leads to abnormal cell growth. Subsequently, mutations resulting in inactivation of tumor suppressor genes, such as *p53*, allow for progression to cancer.

The time course for polyp development and transformation to cancer is thought to be 5–10 years. Most adenomas remain benign; however, histologic type, polyp size, and evidence of dysplasia are associated with transformation. Data from the National Polyp Study and St. Mark's Hospital show that approximately 75–85% of adenomas are tubular, 8–15% are tubulovillous, and 5–10% are villous. Tubular adenomas usually form a stalk, whereas villous adenomas have a broad base (Fig 25–1). Villous histology is associated with an increased risk of cancer development. Only 1% of polyps less than 1 cm in diameter show evidence of malignant transformation, whereas 50% of polyps greater than 2 cm in diameter harbor areas of carcinoma.

Clinically, it is important to diagnose the type, size, and number of polyps to risk-stratify patients for treatment and future surveillance. Endoscopic treatment likely reduces or eliminates the risk of colorectal cancer in patients. Rigid sigmoidoscopy and flexible sigmoidoscopy are all that are necessary to screen the rectum. Sigmoidoscopic screening should be followed by a complete colonoscopy if biopsy of a small rectal or sigmoid polyp shows adenomatous changes. Colonoscopic screening as the first study is indicated in high-risk populations. Autopsy studies have reported that adenomas are present in 20–60% of patients with a colorectal cancer, and synchronous cancers are found in 3–9% of patients. In patients who cannot undergo a preoperative colonoscopy, either a virtual colonoscopy or barium enema should be performed. If both procedures are contraindicated in these patients, colonoscopic evaluation should be performed 3 months after resection.

Treatment of the malignant rectal polyp is becoming more common with the increase in colonoscopic screening and the early diagnosis of small distal rectal cancers. Surgical treatment in part depends on the morphology of the polyp and the histologic evaluation of the resected lesion. Pedunculated malignant polyps are classified by Haggitt according to the depth of invasion of the cancer within the head of the polyp and stalk[5] (see Fig 25–1). Malignant polyps completely resected with greater than 2-mm margins and without stalk invasion are considered adequately treated with colonoscopic removal, provided there are no poor prognostic histologic features; tumors with poor differentiation or lymphatic or venous invasion are associated with an increased incidence of involved lymph nodes.[6]

▪ ANATOMY

ANATOMIC LANDMARKS

The type of therapy offered to a patient with rectal cancer depends not only on the stage of the tumor but also on its location within the pelvis and its rela-

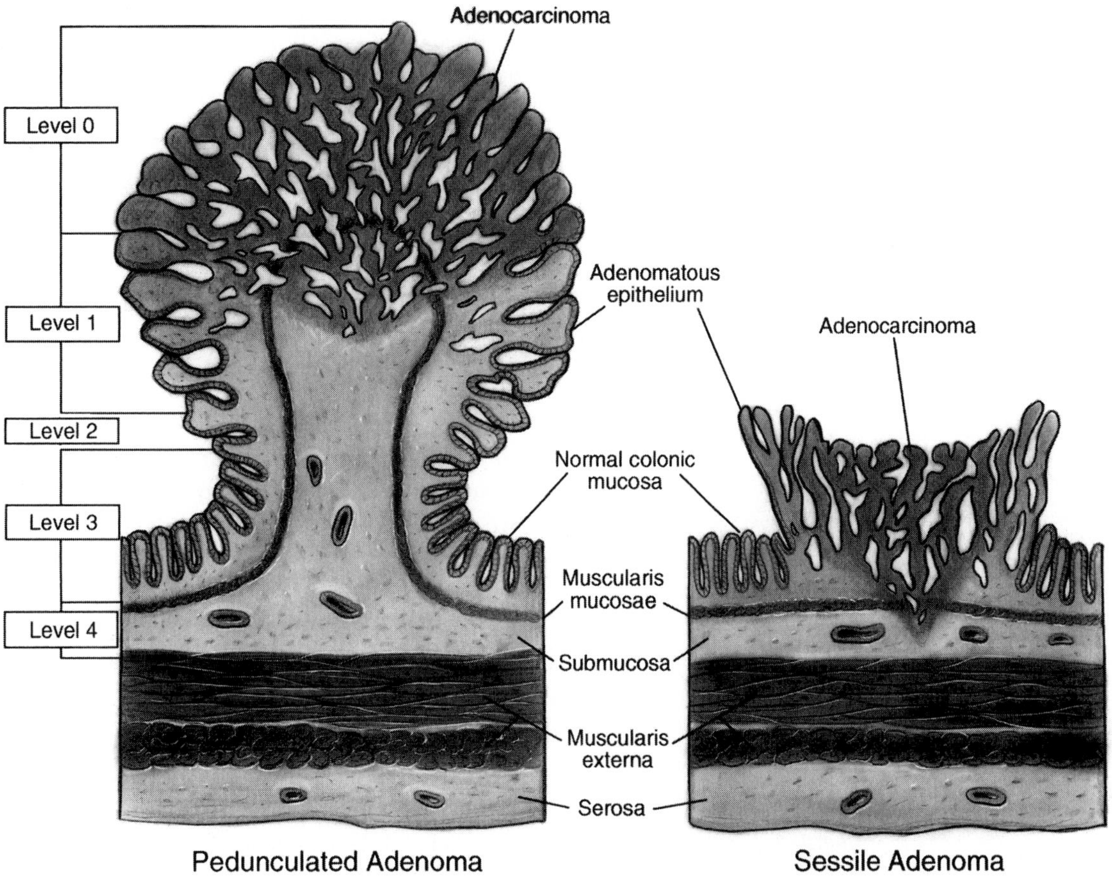

Figure 25–1. Haggitt classification of a pedunculated and sessile polyp, each of which contains an invasive cancer.

tion to the anal sphincters. Compared with colon cancer, knowledge and appreciation of anatomic landmarks are critical in determining resectability and sphincter preservation.

The rectum, usually 15 cm in length, extends from the rectosigmoid junction, marked by fusion of the taeniae coli into a completely circumferential muscular layer, to the anal canal. The rectum transitions from being intraperitoneal to being completely extraperitoneal 6–8 cm from the anus. The rectum is "fixed" posteriorly and laterally by Waldeyer's fascia and the lateral stalks, respectively. In the male patient, the anterior rectum is fixed to Denonvillier's fascia, a fold of two layers of peritoneum that separates the rectum from the posterior prostate and seminal vesicles. In the female patient, the peritoneal cavity descends to the pouch of Douglas, with its most dependent point being adjacent to the cervix anteriorly and midrectum posteriorly.[7] When seen endoscopically, the rectum has three valves of Houston, the middle of which corresponds to the anterior peritoneal reflection (Fig 25–2A).

While many surgical descriptions for rectal cancer refer to the distance of the lesion from the anal verge, a more reliable landmark is the *dentate line,* the distal end of the rectum. This line is clearly visible on anoscopy, but histologically, the junction between the columnar mucosa of the rectum and the transitional or squamous mucosa of the anal canal can be quite variegated. At the muscular level, the anal canal starts at the top of the "high-pressure zone" that is at the proximal aspect of the anorectal ring, a muscular structure consisting of the internal sphincter, external sphincter, and puborectalis (see Fig 25–2A, B). The high-pressure zone descends beyond the dentate line to the junction of the anal mucosa and the perianal skin; this junction is often referred to as the *anal verge.* In order to achieve an adequate distal margin ($\geq$ 2 cm) with sphincter preservation, the lower border of a tumor must be located high enough above the top of the anorectal ring. If curative resection compromises perfect function of the sphincter apparatus, or if an inadequate distal margin cannot be obtained while preserving the anorectal ring, an abdominoperineal resection (APR) with a permanent colostomy should be constructed. Although a patient may assume that a colostomy indicates a hopelessly incurable cancer, we must emphasize that the colostomy is necessary because of the anatomic location, not necessarily the severity of the rectal cancer.

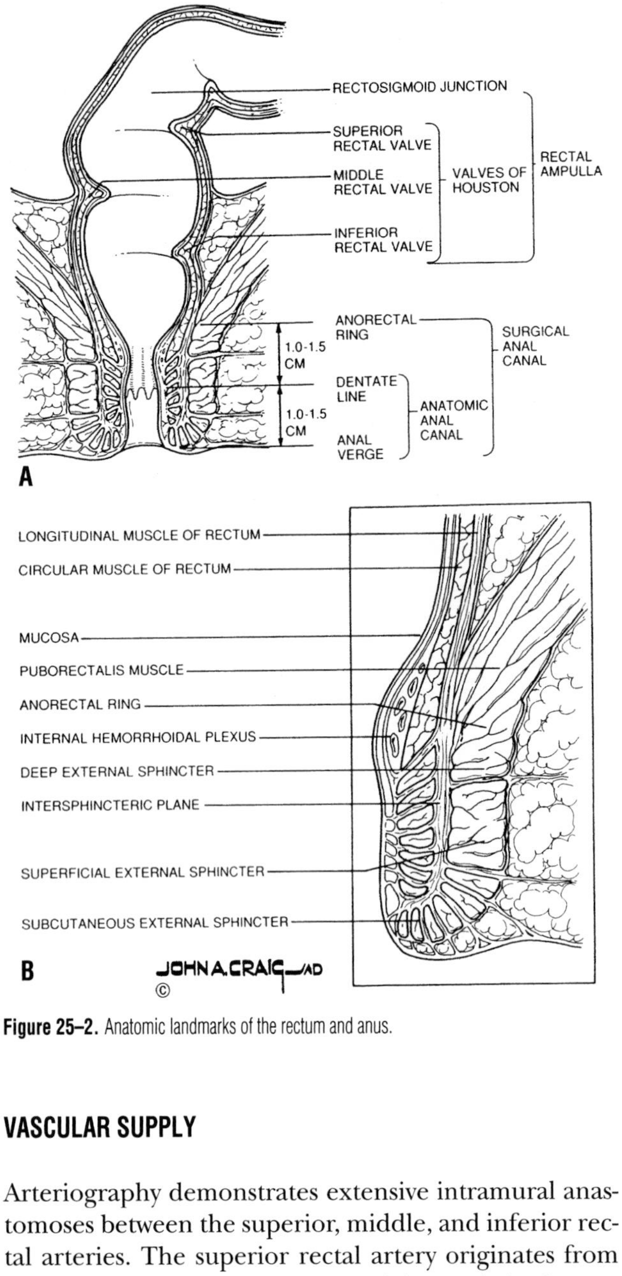

Figure 25–2. Anatomic landmarks of the rectum and anus.

VASCULAR SUPPLY

Arteriography demonstrates extensive intramural anastomoses between the superior, middle, and inferior rectal arteries. The superior rectal artery originates from the inferior mesenteric artery and descends in the mesorectum to supply the upper and middle rectum (Fig 25–3). The inferior rectal arteries, branches of the internal pudendal arteries, enter posterolaterally and provide blood supply to the anal sphincters and epithelium. The middle rectal artery, often depicted in anatomic drawings as a large and significant artery branching off the internal iliac artery on each side, is seldom greater than 1 mm in diameter.[8] In one study, the middle rectal artery was observed in only 22% of cadaver specimens.[7] When actually present, the middle rectal artery is located near the lateral rectal stalks. These stalks are primarily nerves but have been confused previously as arterial supply.

The superior rectal vein drains the upper and middle thirds of the rectum and empties into the portal system via the inferior mesenteric vein. The middle rectal veins drain the lower rectum and upper anal canal into the internal iliac veins. The inferior rectal veins drain the lower anal canal, emptying into the internal iliac veins via the pudendal veins. Since the venous systems communicate, low rectal cancers may spread via the portal and systemic circulations.

LYMPHATIC DRAINAGE

Local recurrence after resection is common and can occur with and without distant metastatic disease. Rectal cancer can spread locally via lymphatics that follow cranially along the superior hemorrhoidal vessels. This "zone of upward spread" was described initially by Miles in his landmark paper describing the APR. Heald has described a "zone of downward spread" within the mesorectum[3]; this zone can encompass as much as 4 cm beyond the distal mucosal edge of the tumor.[9,10] Although some surgeons and pathologists describe tumor within this zone of downward spread as tumor implants, others believe that these implants are replaced nodes. Appreciation of the zones of upward and downward spread has influenced the extent of dissection surgeons now perform for curative resection of rectal cancers.

Lymph from the upper and middle rectum drains into the inferior mesenteric nodes (Fig 25–4). Lymph from the lower rectum may drain into the inferior mesenteric system or into the network along the middle and inferior rectal arteries, posteriorly along the middle sacral artery, and anteriorly through the channels to the retrovesical or rectovaginal septum, to the iliac nodes, and ultimately, to the periaortic nodes. In a Japanese study, the obturator nodes, external to the hypogastric nerve plexus, were found to be involved with cancer in 8% of tumors located in the distal rectum, whereas these nodes were rarely, if ever, involved with proximal tumors.[11] Lymphatics from the anal canal above the dentate line usually drain via the superior rectal lymphatics to the inferior mesenteric lymph nodes and laterally to the obturator and internal iliac nodes. Below the dentate line, lymph drains primarily to the inguinal nodes but may empty into the inferior or superior rectal lymph nodes.

INNERVATION

The pelvic autonomic nerves consist of the paired hypogastric (sympathetic), sacral (parasympathetic), and inferior hypogastric nerves (Fig 25–5). Sympathetic nerves

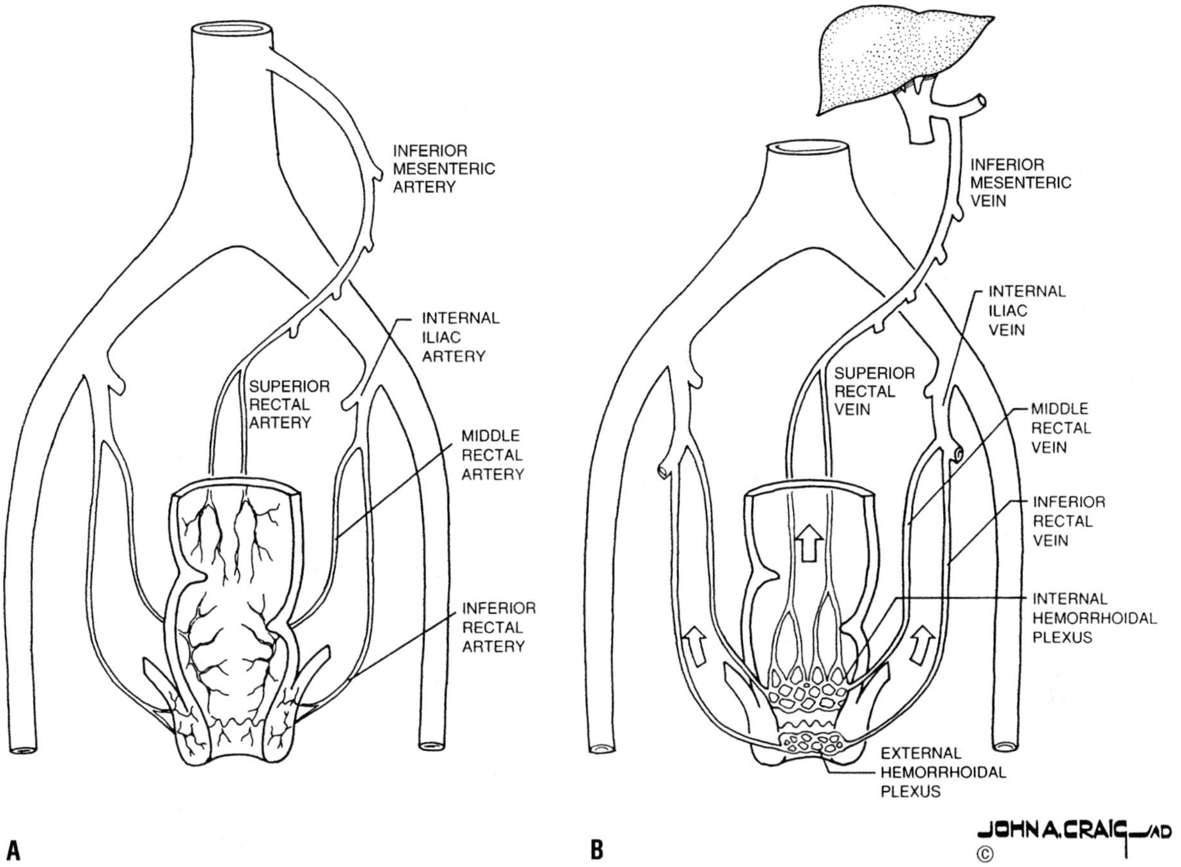

Figure 25–3. Vasculature of the rectum and anus. **A.** Arterial supply. **B.** Venous drainage.

originate from L1–L3, form the inferior mesenteric plexus, travel through the superior hypogastric plexus, and descend as the hypogastric nerves to the pelvic plexus. The parasympathetic nerves, or nervi erigentes, arise from S2–S4 and join the hypogastric nerves anterior and lateral to the rectum to form the pelvic plexus and ultimately the periprostatic plexus. The inferior hypogastric nerve plexus arises from interlacing sympathetic and parasympathetic nerve fibers and forms a fenestrated rhomboid plate on the lateral pelvic sidewall. Fibers from this plexus innervate the rectum as well as the bladder, ureter, prostate, seminal vesicles, membranous urethra, and corpora cavernosa. Therefore, injury to these autonomic nerves can lead to impotence, bladder dysfunction, and loss of normal defecatory mechanisms.

FASCIAL PLANES

The walls and floor of the pelvis are covered by the endopelvic, or parietal, fascia (Fig 25–6). The fascia propria, an extension of the endopelvic fascia, encloses the rectum and its mesorectal fat, lymphatics, and vascular supply as a single unit; forms the lateral stalks of the rectum; and connects to the parietal fascia on the pelvic sidewall. The presacral fascia is the parietal fascia that covers the sacrum and coccyx, presacral plexus, pelvic autonomic nerves, and the middle sacral artery. Posteriorly, a thickening of this fascia, called *Waldeyer's fascia,* is the anteroinferior fascial reflection from the presacral fascia at the level of S4. Anteriorly, *Denonvillier's fascia* separates the anterior rectal wall from the prostate and seminal vesicles in the male and is thought to be an entrapped extension of the peritoneum.[12]

▪ DIAGNOSIS AND EVALUATION

The preoperative evaluation is critically important to treat the cancer optimally and achieve sphincter preservation. With this information, surgeons must individualize the treatment and care of each patient.

HISTORY

The patient with rectal cancer usually presents to the surgeon after a definitive endoscopic diagnosis.

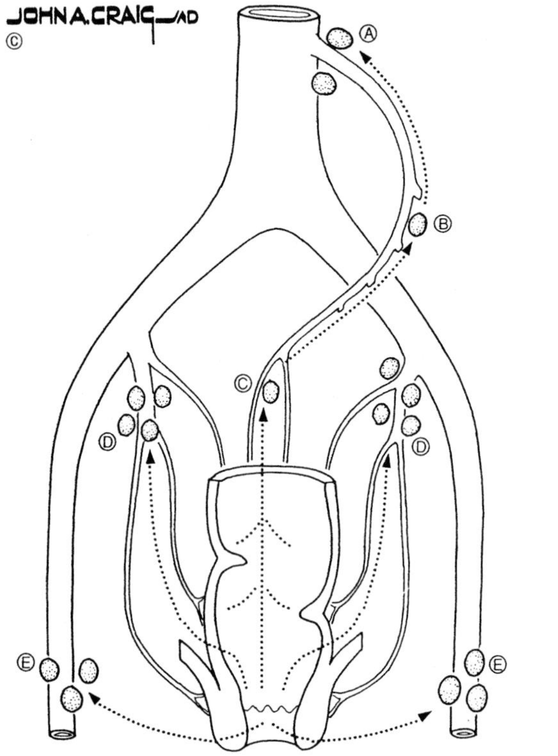

Figure 25–4. Lymphatic drainage of the rectum and anus. **A.** Nodes at the origin of the inferior mesenteric artery. **B.** Nodes at the origin of sigmoid branches. **C.** Sacral nodes. **D.** Internal iliac nodes. **E.** Inguinal nodes.

The patient's initial complaint may include rectal bleeding, a change in bowel habits or stool caliber, rectal pain, a sense of rectal "fullness," weight loss, nausea, vomiting, fatigue, or anorexia; however, many patients are completely asymptomatic. Specific symptoms may assist the surgeon in deciding on the optimal approach to therapy. Tenesmus, the constant sensation of needing to move one's bowels, usually is indicative of a large and possibly fixed stage II or III cancer. Pain with defecation suggests involvement of the anal sphincters; cancers growing directly into the anal sphincter usually are not amenable to sphincter-sparing procedures. Information pertaining to anal sphincter function is invaluable when one is contemplating a low anastomosis. If patients are incontinent, they are better served with an ostomy. Preoperative sexual function is important to know because one must discuss the risks of the procedure and possible diminution of sexual function postoperatively.

A comprehensive medical history should be aimed at identifying other medical conditions, such as cardiopulmonary, renal, and nutrition, that may require additional evaluation before surgical intervention and allow appropriate risk stratification. For patients with a cardiac history or symptoms, a stress test and cardiology evaluation are indicated.

Family history or factors predisposing the patient to rectal cancer, such as FAP, HNPCC, and IBD, are important to take into account as one plans the operative procedure.

PHYSICAL EXAMINATION

A careful and accurate digital rectal examination (DRE) is critical in determining the clinical stage and any plans for neoadjuvant therapy. DRE of a palpable lesion allows for the assessment of tumor size, mobility and fixation, anterior or posterior location, relationship to the sphincter mechanism and top of the anorectal ring, and distance from the anal verge.

Rigid proctoscopy is also essential to the evaluation of patients with rectal cancer because it demonstrates the proximal and distal levels of the mass from the dentate line, extent of circumferential involvement, orientation within the lumen, and relationship to the vagina, prostate, or peritoneal reflection. All this information aids in determining the feasibility of local excision. Rigid proctoscopy also allows one to obtain an adequate tissue biopsy. Flexible sigmoidoscopy is not used routinely because the flexibility of the instrument can give a false distance between the tumor and the dentate line.

A complete colonoscopy to the cecum is essential to rule out synchronous cancers, which occur 2–8% of the time. We prefer colonoscopy over virtual colonoscopy so that we may not only diagnose but also excise any amenable polyps.

Women should undergo a complete pelvic examination in order to determine vaginal invasion or spread to the ovaries. Men should be evaluated for extension into the prostate or bladder.

PREOPERATIVE STAGING

Following the initial history, DRE, and rigid proctoscopy, additional preoperative staging studies can help to determine the appropriate treatment for each patient, whether radical resection or local excision is warranted, and whether preoperative chemoradiation is recommended. Accurate preoperative staging is gaining increasing importance as combined-modality therapy and sphincter-preserving surgical approaches are considered.

Abdominal and pelvic computed tomographic (CT) scans can demonstrate regional tumor extension, lymphatic and distant metastases, and tumor-related complications such as perforation or fistula formation. Its accuracy in determining the depth of invasion, however, is less than that of endorectal ul-

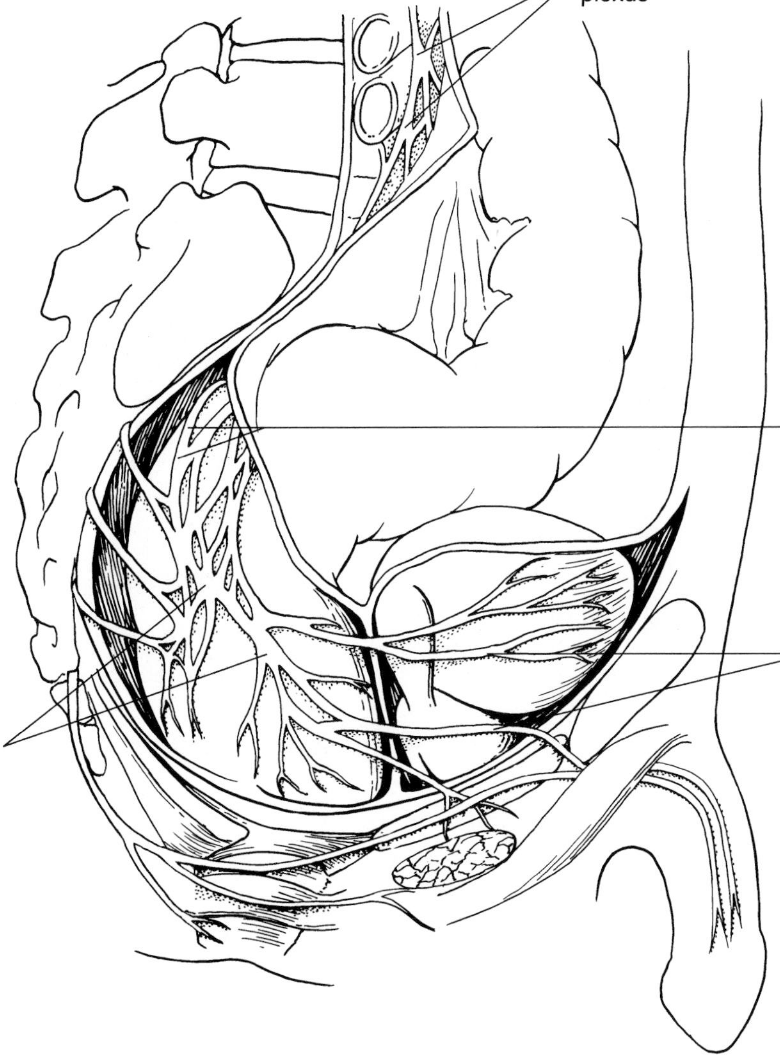

Figure 25–5. Nerve supply of pelvic organs.

trasound or endorectal magnetic resonance imaging (MRI). Pelvic CT scan therefore is not recommended as the only modality for evaluation of a patient's primary tumor. For example, the sensitivity of CT scan for detecting distant metastasis is higher (75–87%) than for detecting perirectal nodal involvement (45%) or the depth of transmural invasion (70%). If a node is seen on CT scan, it should be presumed to be malignant because benign adenopathy is not normally seen around the rectum.

Intravenous contrast material at the time of a CT scan is important to assess the liver for metastatic disease, as well as to evaluate the size and function of the kidneys. Ureteral involvement by the tumor can be assessed and allows for planning of ureteral stent placement preoperatively.

All patients should undergo a chest x-ray or chest CT scan to exclude pulmonary metastases. Although useful information for assessing long-term prognosis, the extra information obtained from a chest CT scan often does not influence the decisions that need to be made to treat the local/regional disease.

Laboratory Studies

Complete blood count and electrolytes often are obtained. Liver enzymes may be normal in the setting of small hepatic metastases and are not a reliable marker for liver involvement.

Guidelines published by the American Society for Clinical Oncology (ASCO) recommend that serum carcinoembryonic antigen (CEA) levels be obtained preoperatively in patients with rectal cancer to aid in staging, surgical treatment planning, and assessment of prognosis. Although neither sensitive nor specific enough to serve as a screening method for the detection of colorectal cancer, preoperative CEA levels

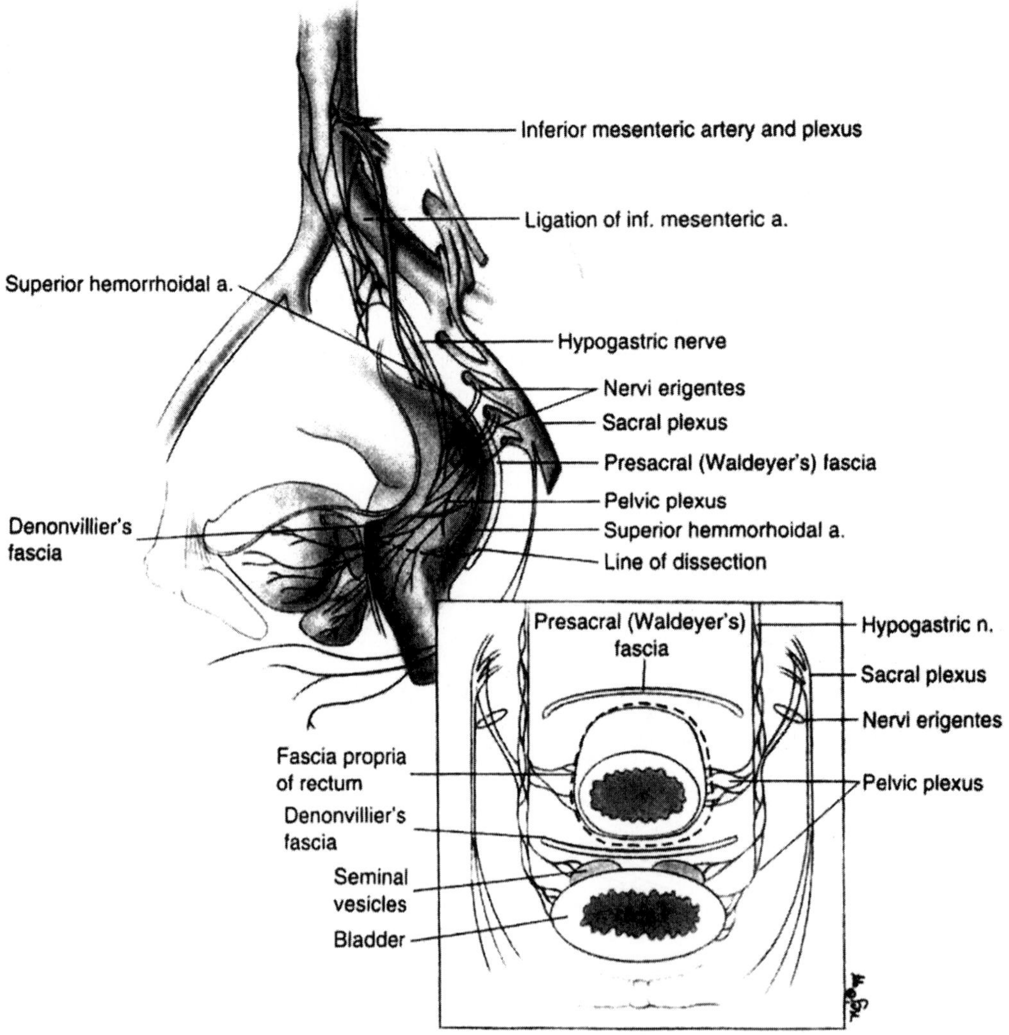

Figure 25–6. Fascial planes. (Used, with permission, from Michelassi F, Milsom JW (eds). *Operative Strategies in Inflammatory Bowel Disease.* New York: Springer-Verlag, 1999.)

greater than 5 ng/mL signify a worse prognosis, stage for stage, than those with lower levels. Additionally, elevated preoperative CEA levels that do not normalize following surgical resection imply the presence of persistent disease and the need for further evaluation. Furthermore, CEA is most helpful in identifying recurrent disease with an overall sensitivity rate of 70–80%.

Endoluminal Ultrasound

Compared with CT scanning, transrectal endoluminal or endoscopic ultrasound (TRUS) permits a more accurate characterization of the primary tumor and the status of the perirectal lymph nodes. Localized cancers involving only the mucosa and submucosa usually can be distinguished from tumors that penetrate the muscularis propria or extend through the rectal wall into the perirectal fat.

Endorectal ultrasound is an office-based procedure that is well tolerated and can be performed by the surgeon for preoperative planning. Figure 25–7 shows the schematic layers seen in TRUS.

T Stage. Several studies comparing the accuracy of TRUS with CT scan and MRI suggest that TRUS is superior for T staging of rectal cancer. The accuracy of TRUS ranges from 80–95% compared with 65–75% for CT scan, 75–85% for MRI, and 62% for DRE. In one review, the accuracy of TRUS was greatest (95%) in distinguishing whether a tumor was confined to the rectal wall (T1, T2) versus invading into the perirectal fat (T3 or greater) and less able to distinguish accurately T1 from T2 cancers.[13] Figure 25–8 demonstrates a uT2 lesion. Additionally, in patients who have received prior radiation, the accuracy decreases owing to edema and fibrosis.

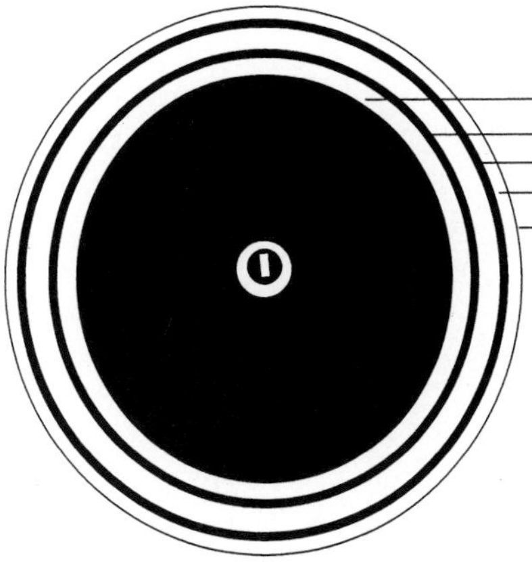

Figure 25–7. Schematic of transrectal endoluminal ultrasonography illustrates the five layers seen on ultrasound.

Despite these data, there is considerable interobserver variability and a significant learning curve associated with performing TRUS. For these reasons, TRUS understages more frequently than overstages the primary rectal tumor. However, TRUS understages the cancer less often than CT scan (15% versus 39%). A modified TNM classification for rectal cancer has been proposed based on TRUS-derived T stage (Table 25–1).

N Stage. TRUS is less useful in predicting the status of perirectal lymph nodes. In a number of comparative studies, the accuracy of TRUS (70–75%) was similar to that of CT scan (55–65%) and MRI (60–65%). The accuracy of nodal staging with TRUS requires the nodes to be larger than 5 mm. The contribution of TRUS-guided fine-needle aspiration (FNA) biopsy to N-staging accuracy for rectal cancer is controversial.

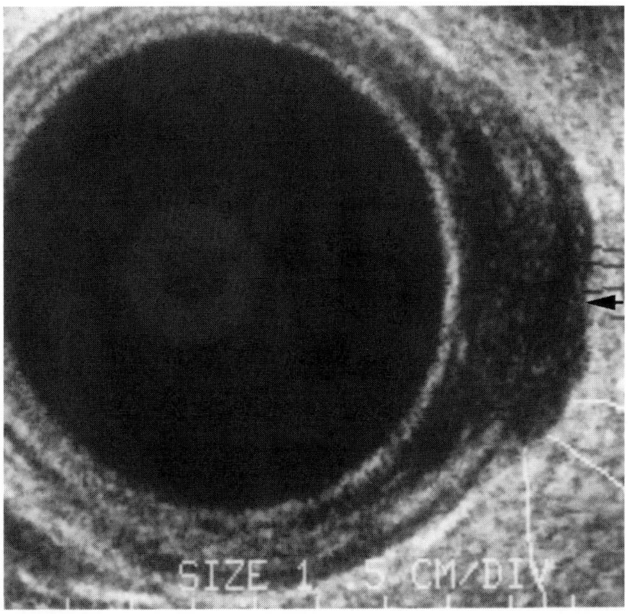

Figure 25–8. Transrectal endoluminal ultrasonography of a uT2 lesion. The *arrow* indicates the intact serosa.

Magnetic Resonance Imaging (MRI)

Both endorectal coil (ecMRI) and surface coil MRI are becoming more useful in the pretreatment evaluation of patients with rectal cancer. ecMRI offers some advantages compared with TRUS: It permits a larger field of view, it may be less operator- and technique-dependent, and it allows study of stenotic tumors that may not be even amenable to DRE.[14] Figure 25–9 illustrates a T_3 lesion. Like TRUS, ecMRI can discriminate small-volume nodal disease and subtle transmural invasion. EcMRI can identify involved perirectal nodes on the basis of characteristics other than size, with reported accuracy rates of 50–95%. Another advantage over TRUS is identification of foci not only within the mesorectum but also outside the mesorectal fascia, such as the pelvic sidewall. We prefer ecMRI and have demonstrated 88% accuracy in predicting the correct pathologic stage of disease.

TABLE 25–1. ENDOSCOPIC ULTRASOUND STAGING OF RECTAL TUMORS

uT1	Invasion confined to the mucosa and submucosa
uT2	Penetration of the muscularis propria but not through to the mesorectal fat
uT3	Invasion into the perirectal fat
uT4	Invasion into the adjacent organ
uN0	No enlargement of lymph nodes
uN1	Perirectal lymph nodes enlarged

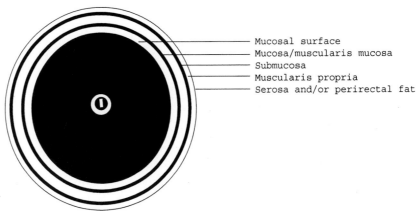

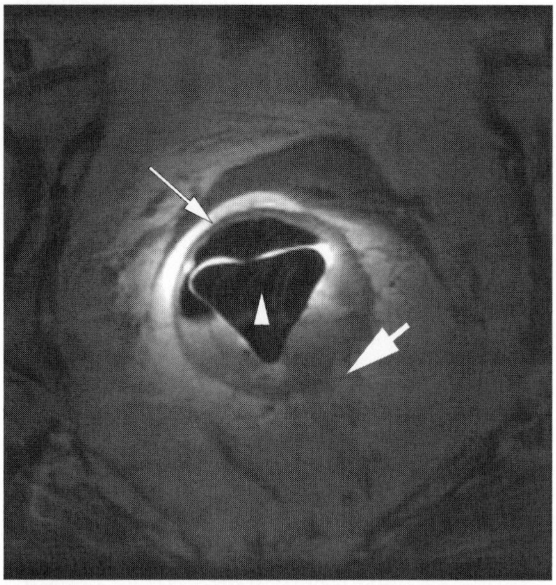

Figure 25–9. Endorectal MRI of a T3 lesion. *Arrowhead* indicates the site of the endorectal coil. *Large arrow* demonstrates finger-like projections of carcinoma invading into the mesorectal fat. *Small arrow* points to the radial margin of the mesorectum along the mesorectal fascia. (Courtesy of Koenraad J. Mortele, M.D., Department of Radiology, Brigham and Women's Hospital.)

Double-contrast MRI may permit more accurate T staging of rectal cancer by allowing better distinction between normal rectal wall, mucosa, muscularis, and perirectal tissues. In one report, the specificity and sensitivity of ecMRI with combined intravenous and endorectal contrast material to predict infiltration of the anal sphincter were 100% and 90%, respectively. However, N staging was not improved with this approach.

Phased-array surface coil MRI also may be beneficial in predicting the likelihood of a tumor-free resection margin by visualizing tumor involvement of the mesorectal fascia. If confirmed in other series, preoperative MRI may prove useful in selecting patients at high risk of local recurrence for therapy prior to resection.

Positron-Emission Tomography (PET)

Fluorine-18 fluorodeoxyglucose positron-emission tomography (FDG-PET) is effective in assessing the extent of pathologic response of primary rectal cancer to preoperative chemoradiation and may predict long-term outcome.[15] Additionally, it has an accuracy of 87% for detecting recurrence of rectal cancer after surgical resection and full-dose external-beam radiation therapy.[16] While PET scans are positive in 90% of primary and recurrent tumors and in distant metastatic disease, they are relatively inaccurate for nodal metastases. Rectal cancer rarely metastasizes to the bones or to the brain, and without symptoms, these two areas are not included routinely in surveillance imaging. They will, however, light up on PET scan.

▪ TNM STAGING

The purpose of staging any cancer is to describe the anatomic extent of the lesion. Staging by clinical examination, radiology, and pathology aids in planning treatment, evaluating response to treatment, comparing the results of various treatment regimens, and determining prognosis. Currently, the most widely accepted staging system for rectal cancer in the United States is the TNM classification system.

In 1987, the American Joint Committee on Cancer (AJCC) and the International Union against Cancer (IUC) introduced the TNM staging system for colorectal cancer; this system was updated in 2002 (Table 25–2). The TNM staging system is based on depth of tumor invasion as well as presence of lymph node or distant metastases. In stage I disease, the tumor may invade into the muscularis propria. In stage II disease, the tumor invades completely through this layer. Depth of invasion is an important prognostic variable. Even a small cancer extending into the muscularis mucosa (T1) will have a 10% incidence of metastasizing to perirectal lymph nodes.[17] Any lymph node metastasis represents stage III disease, and metastatic spread denotes stage IV disease.

The biologic behavior of rectal cancer cannot be predicted by it location or size. Poorly differentiated cancers have a worse long-term prognosis than well-differentiated or moderately differentiated tumors. Other factors that portend a poor prognosis include di-

TABLE 25–2. TNM CLASSIFICATION OF RECTAL CANCER

Primary Tumor (T)	
Tx	Primary tumor cannot be assessed
T0	No evidence of primary tumor
Tis	Carcinoma in situ
T1	Tumor invades submucosa
T2	Tumor invades muscularis propria
T3	Tumor invades through the muscularis propria into the subserosa or into nonperitonealized pericolic or perirectal tissues
T4	Tumor perforates the visceral peritoneum or directly invades other organs or structures
Regional Lymph Nodes (N)	
Nx	Regional lymph nodes cannot be assessed
N0	No regional lymph node metastasis
N1	Metastasis in 1–3 pericolic or perirectal lymph nodes
N2	Metastasis in 4 or more pericolic or perirectal lymph nodes
N3	Metastasis in 4 or more pericolic or perirectal lymph nodes
Distant Metastasis (M)	
Mx	Presence of distant metastasis cannot be assessed
M0	No distant metastasis
M1	Distant metastasis

rect tumor extension into adjacent structures (T4 lesions); lymphatic, vascular, or perineural invasion; and bowel obstruction.

■ PRINCIPLES OF TREATMENT

Surgical resection is the cornerstone of curative therapy. Following a potentially curative resection, the 5-year survival rate varies according to disease extent[18,19] (Table 25–3). However, these survival figures may improve with the increased use of adjuvant therapy.

Surgical and oncologic management varies greatly depending on the stage and location of the tumor within the rectum. Superficially invasive, small cancers may be managed effectively with local excision. However, most patients have more deeply invasive tumors that require major surgery, such as low anterior resection (LAR) or APR. Yet others present with locally advanced tumors adherent to adjoining structures such as the sacrum, pelvic sidewall, prostate, or bladder, requiring an even more extensive operation.

After establishing the diagnosis and completing the staging work-up, a decision is made whether to pursue immediate resection or administer preoperative chemoradiotherapy.

BOWEL PREPARATION

The high bacterial load in the intestinal tract requires preoperative bowel decontamination to reduce the incidence of infectious complications. Prior to the routine use of mechanical bowel preparation and preoperative antibiotics, the reported rate of infection following colorectal surgery was 60%.[20] A standard bowel prep includes a clear-liquid diet 1–3 days prior to surgery, laxatives and/or enemas, and gastrointestinal tract irrigation with a solution of polyethylene glycol electrolyte lavage (Go-lytely, Braintree Labs) or Fleet's Phospha-soda. In two separate surveys of North American colorectal surgeons, almost two-thirds preferred the polyethylene glycol electrolyte solutions because of the reliability of the cleansing results.[21,22] Certain preparations are contraindicated in patients with certain medical conditions. For example, patients with elevated creatinine or congestive heart failure should avoid the Phospha-soda preparations, whereas patients with gastroparesis should not take Go-lytely.

TABLE 25–3. SURVIVAL RATES

Stage I	80–90%
Stage II	62–76%
Stage III	30–40%
Stage IV	4–7%

Source: From Willett et al., 1992.

Oral antibiotics also are used to further decrease the incidence of postoperative infectious complications. Although mechanical cleansing decreases the total volume of stool in the colon, it does not affect the concentration of bacteria per milliliter of effluent. The most commonly used regimen is the Nichols/Condon prep: neomycin 1 g and erythromycin base 1 g by mouth at 1:00 PM, 2:00 PM, and 10:00 PM on the day prior to surgery. Many surgeons substitute metronidazole 500 mg for the erythromycin base because it is active against a greater percentage of gastrointestinal anaerobes.

Perioperative systemic antibiotics usually are combined with preoperative oral antibiotics for rectal procedures. A typical choice to cover both aerobic and anaerobic intestinal bacteria is cefazolin 1 g and metronidazole 500 mg administered intravenously just prior to the skin incision. A second dose of cefazolin is administered 4 hours into the case. Postoperative antibiotic prophylaxis usually is continued for 24 hours, although the perioperative dose is more critical.

Perioperative systemic antibiotic coverage is broadened in patients with high-risk cardiac lesions such as prosthetic heart valves, a previous history of endocarditis, or a surgically constructed systemic-pulmonary shunt and with intermediate-risk cardiac lesions such as mitral valve prolapse, valvular heart disease, or idiopathic hypertrophic subaortic stenosis. Intravenous ampicillin 2 g and gentamycin 1.5 mg/kg are administered 30–60 minutes before the procedure, and ampicillin is repeated once 6 hours postoperatively in place of cefazolin; metronidazole is administered as usual. Vancomycin is substituted for ampicillin if the patient is allergic to penicillin or cephalosporin.

GOALS OF SURGERY FOR RECTAL CANCER

The primary goal of surgical treatment for rectal cancer is complete eradication of the primary tumor along with the adjacent mesorectal tissue and the superior hemorrhoidal artery pedicle. Although reestablishment of bowel continuity at the time of surgery has become routine, cancer removal should not be compromised in an attempt to avoid a permanent colostomy.

For tumors located in the extraperitoneal rectum, resection margins are limited by the bony confines of the pelvis and the proximity of the bladder, prostate, and seminal vesicles in men and vagina in women. Although locoregional recurrence may be inevitable, local recurrence, cure, mortality, anastomotic leaks, and colostomy rates after rectal cancer surgery are related to surgical technique as well as to the experience and volume of the individual surgeon and institution.

RESECTION MARGINS

Distal Margins

The optimal distal resection margin for surgically treated rectal cancer remains controversial. Although the first line of rectal cancer spread is upward along the lymphatics, tumors below the peritoneal reflection can spread distally via intra- or extramural lymphatic and vascular routes.

The use of APR for low rectal cancers traditionally has been based on the need for a 5-cm distal margin of normal tissue. However, in retrospective studies, margins as short as 1 cm have not been associated with an increased risk of local recurrence.[23–25] Distal intramural spread usually is limited to within 2.0 cm of the tumor unless the lesion is poorly differentiated or widely metastatic. Data from a randomized, prospective trial conducted by the National Surgical Adjuvant Breast and Bowel Project demonstrated no significant differences in survival or local recurrence when comparing distal rectal margins of less than 2 cm, 2–2.9 cm, and greater than 3 cm.[23] Therefore, a 2-cm distal margin is acceptable for resection of rectal carcinoma, although a 5-cm proximal margin is still recommended.[26]

Radial Margins

The importance of obtaining an adequate circumferential or radial margin has been appreciated more in the last decade. In fact, the radial margin is more critical than the proximal or distal margin for local control. Tumor involvement of the circumferential margin has been shown to be an independent predictor of both local recurrence and survival. In one report of 90 patients undergoing resection for rectal cancer, when the radial margins were histologically positive, the hazard ratio (HR) for local recurrence was 12.2, and the HR for death was 3.2 when compared with those with clear circumferential margins. Furthermore, the length of mesorectum beyond the primary tumor that needs to be removed is thought to be between 3 and 5 cm because tumor implants usually are seen no further than 4 cm from the distal edge of the tumor within the mesorectum.[5,10] Therefore, in proximal rectal cancers, distal mesorectal excision 5 cm below the lower border of the tumor should be the goal.

■ LOCAL EXCISION

ONCOLOGIC RESULTS

A number of retrospective studies of local excision since the 1970s have demonstrated a local recurrence rate of 7–33% and survival rates from 57–87%. Many of these reviews are limited, small, single-institution studies, often combining patients with tumors of different depths, including T3 lesions, positive margins, or who underwent different forms of local therapy, such as fulguration and snare cautery. Despite these limitations, many of these studies have demonstrated that local excision for superficial tumors with negative margins may provide similar survival and local control but without the morbidity of the APR. Major risk factors for local recurrence include positive surgical margins, transmural extension, and poorly differentiated histology. These retrospective studies suggest that local excision of selected distal rectal adenocarcinomas may provide adequate oncologic control at considerably less morbidity than APR.

Several prospective studies have been published (Table 25–4). In a study from the M.D. Anderson Cancer Center, 46 patients underwent transanal excision of small distal rectal cancer followed by postoperative radiation treatment.[27] Patients with T3 lesions also were given chemotherapy. For patients with negative margins, there was only a 6.5% local recurrence rate (all were T3 tumors) with a 93% overall 3-year survival. Local treatments combined with radiation provided similar oncologic control for T1 or T2 small distal rectal adenocarcinomas as compared with APR.

From the New England Deaconess Hospital in Boston, patients with small distal cancers (<4 cm in diameter and <10 cm from the dentate line) with no evidence of metastatic disease were entered in a prospective study.[28] Patients with T_1 lesions were observed after local excision. Patients with T2 lesions treated with local excision were given postoperative chemoradiation. Sev-

TABLE 25–4. RECURRENCE RATES AFTER LOCAL EXCISION AND ADJUVANT THERAPY

	Patients (*n*)	Treatment	Follow-Up (months)	Local Recurrence	Survival
Ota[29]	46	LE & postop XRT and 5-FU for T2, T3	36 (median)	6.5% (3/46) All T3s	Overall 3-yr 93%
Bleday[28]	48	LE, Postop XRT and 5-FU for T2, T3	41 (mean)	8% (4/48)	Disease-specific 96%
Steele[31]	110	LE, Postop XRT and 5-FU for T2	48 (mean)	T—5.1% (3/59) T2—13.7% (7/51)	Overall 6-yr 85%; disease-specific 6-yr 78%

eral patients were found to have T3 lesions and all were recommended further radical surgery. Those who refused had adjuvant chemoradiation therapy and were followed. All patients were followed every 3 months for 2 years and then every 6 months for 5 years. The local recurrence rate in this study was 8%, and the cancer-specific mortality rate was 4%. Risk factors associated with recurrence were T3 cancers or lymphatic invasion. Surgery alone was adequate for T1 lesions, and surgery combined with chemoradiation was appropriate for T2 lesions excised with negative margins. Radical resection was and still is appropriate for tumors with positive margins after local excision or for T3 cancers. Patients with lymphovenous invasion deserve further therapy, although that therapy was not defined.

Steele and colleagues published the only large multicenter prospective trial of local excision.[29] Patients were eligible for the study if their cancer was within 10 cm of the dentate line and was less than 4 cm and involved less than 40% of the luminal circumference. All patients preoperatively were thought to have N0M0 disease, as determined clinically and by CT scan. All study patients had negative margins. T1 lesions had no further treatment, and T2 lesions were treated with chemoradiation. After 6 years of follow-up, the overall survival and disease-free survival were 85% and 78%, respectively. Disease-free survival was 84% and 71% for T1 and T2 lesions, respectively. Seven patients recurred with local disease only and underwent APR with a 70% salvage rate. This approach was no worse than that of radical resection.

PATIENT SELECTION AND CHOICE OF OPERATION

Preoperative staging, primarily with TRUS or MRI, is the most helpful in identifying appropriate patients for a local excision. Criteria for consideration for local excision are listed in Table 25–5. Patients with T3 or N1 disease are inappropriate for local excision. T1 lesions, given the low probability of microscopic nodal disease, are the best candidates for local excision. T3 and T4 lesions, having a high probability of nodal involvement, should be treated with radical resection. Controversy remains over the best therapy for T2 lesions. Some still would state that an APR remains the standard for T2 lesions. However, local excision combined with postoperative chemoradiation achieves similar rates of survival but not necessarily similar rates of disease-free survival; some patients require a salvage APR for ultimate cure.

Tumors less than 3 cm from the dentate line but not invading the sphincters usually can be resected via a transanal procedure. Tumors 5 cm from the dentate line may need a transcoccygeal approach or transanal endoscopic microsurgery (TEM). Tumors 7–10 cm from the dentate line require TEM or should be considered for a low anterior resection. Clearly, tumors tethered to the mesorectum or pelvic floor on physical examination, suggesting transmural involvement, are not amenable to local excision. Patients with such lesions should undergo preoperative radiation followed by a radical resection.

TABLE 25–5. CHARACTERISTICS OF TUMORS AMENABLE TO LOCAL EXCISION

T1N0 or T2N0 lesion
<4 cm in diameter
<40% circumference of the lumen
<10 cm from dentate line
Well to moderately differentiated histology
No evidence of lymphatic or vascular invasion on biopsy
Patients with extensive metastatic disease and poor prognosis who require local control
Adjuvant treatment for patients with lymphatic invasion, T1 with poor prognosis features, T2 lesions

Patients considered medically unfit for a major resection are good candidates for local treatment of most small, mobile tumors, including T2 and T3 lesions, accepting a higher rate of local recurrence. In these circumstances, adjuvant chemoradiation is advocated, and close follow-up is mandatory.

After local excision, if the pathology is unfavorable, the patient should be counseled to have further therapy, including chemoradiation therapy and either a low anterior resection or APR with total mesorectal excision. Local excision in these circumstances can be considered an open biopsy and not the definitive therapy.

TECHNIQUE

There are four approaches to local excision: transsphincteric, transanal, transcoccygeal, and TEM. The transsphincteric technique, however, leads to significant dysfunction of the anal sphincters with subsequent moderate to severe fecal incontinence. Therefore, the transanal, transcoccygeal, and TEM approaches are the preferred techniques.

TRANSANAL EXCISION

The majority of small distal rectal cancers can be excised locally via a transanal excision. Tumors amenable to this approach usually range from 3–5 cm above the dentate line.

Prior to the procedure, all patients should receive a full mechanical and antibiotic bowel preparation. Preoperative and perioperative medications are similar to those administered for radical resection. Most patients are placed in the prone jackknife position, and the buttocks are taped apart. For lesions that are directly posterior, the lithotomy position can be used. The surgeon wears a fiberoptic headlight. A pudendal nerve block using 0.5% marcaine with 1:100,000 units of epinephrine is administered to relax the sphincters and facilitate postoperative pain control. A lone-star retractor can be used to expose the dentate line. A Pratt bivalve retractor (Pilling-Weck Instruments, Ft. Washington, PA) or Parks retractor is inserted to dilate the anus and expose the lesion. Once the tumor is viewed adequately, traction sutures using 2-0 Vicryl (Ethicon, Somerville, NJ) are placed 2 cm proximal to the tumor. The circumferential dissection line is outlined on the mucosa using the cautery with a pinpoint Bovie tip approximately 1 cm from the border of the tumor; careful attention should be paid to maintaining a wide proximal margin. If an adequate view of the lesion cannot be obtained initially, serial traction sutures are used to prolapse the lesion into the field. Additional local anesthetic is injected submucosally circumferentially along the Bovie markings to provide hemostasis. Starting proximally and proceeding circumferentially, a full-thickness incision of bowel wall is made down to perirectal fat using the cautery along the previously marked mucosa (Fig 25–10). Once fat is reached, the dissection is made through the fat to undercut the specimen. Anteriorly in a female patient, one must not injure the posterior wall of the vagina. In a male patient, one must avoid the prostate. Once the specimen is free, carefully maintain and mark the orientation for the pathologist (e.g., proximal, anterior, left, right). Irrigate and check for hemostasis. After excision, the defect in the bowel wall is closed transversely with full-thickness bites using interrupted 3-0 Vicryl sutures. One stitch is placed in the center of the incision. One half is closed, followed by the other. A rigid sigmoidoscope is inserted to visualize the suture line and to ensure patency of the rectal lumen. The patient then is placed supine. A pad is applied to the rectal area and secured with mesh rectal shorts. A pack in the anal canal or rectum is not used. These procedures can be done either as an outpatient or with a short stay. Potential complications include urinary retention, urinary tract infections, fecal impaction, infections in the perirectal and ischiorectal spaces, and delayed hemorrhage. The incidence of these complications is quite low; mortality in most series is zero.

TRANSCOCCYGEAL EXCISION

Originally popularized by Kraske, the transcoccygeal excision is used for larger or more proximal lesions within the middle or distal third of the rectum. Bleday reported that the average distance of the distal margin of an appropriate tumor that was selected for the posterior or Kraske approach was approximately 4.8 cm from the dentate line.[28] This approach is useful for lesions on the posterior wall of the rectum but can be used for anterior lesions.

Patients undergo similar bowel preparation and thrombosis precautions as the transanal excision patients. The patient is placed in the prone jackknife position. The buttocks are taped apart for better exposure, but at closure the tape is released to facilitate approximation of the subcutaneous tissues and skin. After prep-

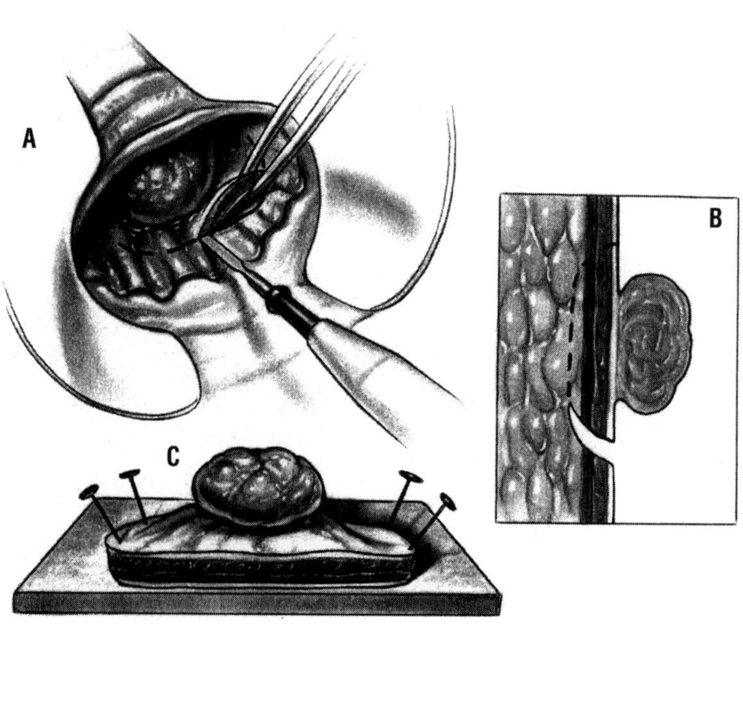

Figure 25–10. Approach to transanal excision of a rectal tumor. **A.** A 1- to 2-cm margin is marked circumferentially with Bovie electrocautery on the rectal mucosa. **B.** Full-thickness excision down to perirectal fat is performed. **C.** The specimen is oriented for the pathologist. (Reprinted, with permission, from Bleday R. Local excision of rectal cancer. *World J Surg* 1997;21:706–714.)

ping the skin, the rectum is irrigated with a Betadine solution. The incision is made in the intergluteal fold over the sacrum and coccyx down to the upper border of the posterior aspect of the external sphincter. After division of the skin and subcutaneous tissues, one encounters the coccyx and anal coccygeal ligament. In order to obtain optimal exposure, the coccyx is removed by cauterizing its attachments, including the anal coccygeal ligament, from each side and from its lower edge and then proceeding with the dissection on its undersurface. A cutting wire is used to transect the sacral coccygeal joint. With removal of the coccyx, bleeding from an extension of the middle sacral artery is controlled with electrocautery. The levator ani muscles are separated in the midline, exposing a membrane that is just outside the mesorectal fat. Once this membrane is divided, the rectum can be completely mobilized within the intraperitoneal pelvis. For anterior lesions, a posterior proctotomy is made; the anterior rectum is approached under direct vision, with removal of the tumor along with a 1-cm margin (Fig 25–11). For posterior-based lesions, after complete mobilization of the mesorectum, the distal margin of the tumor can be palpated via a rectal examination; the mesorectum and rectum are transected approximately 1 cm distal to the tumor (Fig 25–12). The tumor is excised with a 1-cm margin of normal tissue. The advantage of the posterior approach is that the immediate mesorectal tissue adjacent to the tumor is removed along with perirectal nodes. After removal, the specimen is oriented for the pathologist. The incision is closed in a transverse manner using an absorbable suture such as

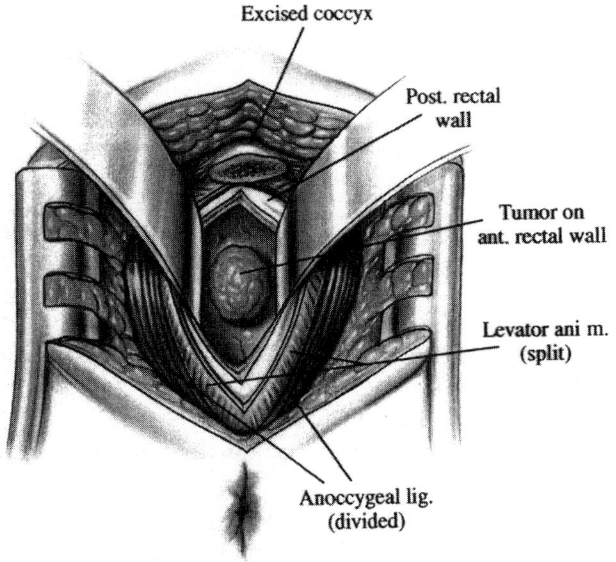

Figure 25–11. Kraske approach to an anterior lesion. The coccyx is excised, the levator is split in the midline, and the rectum is mobilized. The posterior rectal wall is opened to expose an anterior lesion. (Reprinted, with permission, from Bleday R. Local excision of rectal cancer. *World J Surg* 1997;21:706–714.)

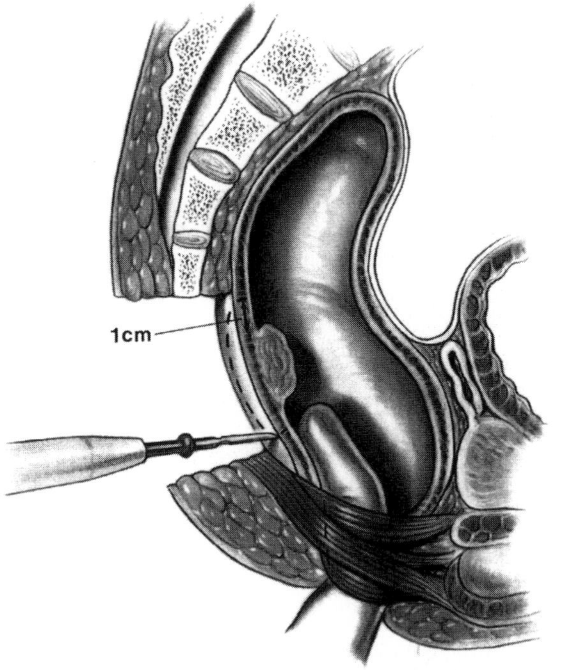

Figure 25–12. Kraske approach to a posterior lesion. After the rectum has been exposed, the surgeon may palpate the distal margin of the tumor. The tumor is excised with a 1-cm margin. (Reprinted, with permission, from Bleday R. Local excision of rectal cancer. *World J Surg* 1997;21:706–714.)

3-0 Vicryl or 3-0 PDS (Ethicon, Somerville, NJ). After closure of the rectum, an air test is performed by insufflating the rectum with air and filling the operative field with sterile saline. After all air leaks are controlled, the levator ani musculature is reapproximated, and the anal coccygeal ligament is reattached to the sacrum, followed by closure of the subcutaneous tissues and skin.

One of the most troubling complications of the transcoccygeal excision is a fecal fistula extending from the rectum to the posterior incision. The incidence of this complication ranges from 5–20%.[29] These fistulas usually heal after temporary fecal diversion.

TRANSANAL ENDOSCOPIC MICROSURGERY (TEM)

The TEM technique was first described by Buess in Germany. It is especially useful for small lesions in the rectum that are too high for a transanal excision. The instrumentation allows for performance of local excision in the middle and upper thirds of the rectum. A 4-cm Wolf operating proctoscope with binocular microscope and videoscope, a CO_2 insufflator, and long operating surgical instruments are needed. The surgeon must be trained in the technique, which follows the same principles as transanal excision described earlier using the pinpoint tip on the Bovie electrocautery. The patient is positioned using a beanbag and fixation to the table with tape, which allows the patient to be rotated laterally during the procedure. For an anterior lesion, the patient is placed in the prone jackknife position. For a posterior lesion, the patient is placed in a modified lithotomy position. For lateral lesions, the patient can be placed on the appropriate side so that the lesion is at the inferior quadrant of the visual field. Care must be taken to identify the peritoneal reflection, especially anteriorly. If dissection carries into the peritoneal cavity, the defect should be closed with interrupted 3-0 PDS sutures. In selected patients, temporary diversion is needed after entering the peritoneal cavity.

▪ LOW ANTERIOR RESECTION WITH TOTAL MESORECTAL EXCISION

ONCOLOGIC RESULTS

Local failures most often result from inadequate surgical clearance of the radial margin. The concept of total mesorectal excision (TME) proposed by Heald has been shown to improve both disease-free and overall survival.[3] TME in conjunction with an LAR or APR involves precise dissection and removal of the entire rectal mesentery, including that distal to the tumor, as an intact unit. Unlike conventional blunt dissection, which may leave residual mesorectum in the pelvis, TME involves sharp dissection under direct vision in the avascular, areolar plane between the fascia propria of the rectum, which encompasses the mesorectum, and the parietal fascia overlying the pelvic wall structures. This procedure emphasizes autonomic nerve preservation (ANP) and complete hemostasis and avoids violation of the mesorectal envelope. This results in a characteristic bilobed, smooth, glistening surface of the excised mesorectum.

Since rectal cancer spread appears to be limited to the mesorectal envelope, its total removal should encompass virtually every tumor satellite, thus improving the likelihood of local control. The excellent results with TME may be attributed to improved lateral clearance with removal of potential tumor deposits in the mesentery and decreased risk of tumor spillage from a disrupted mesentery.[30] The completeness of the mesorectal excision influences local control, even if the surgical margins are uninvolved. In one report, both local (11.4% versus 5.5%) and distant recurrence rates (19.2% versus 12.2%) were higher in patients with an incomplete as compared with a complete or nearly complete mesorectal resection. These favorable results have led some to question the need for routine postoperative radiation in patients undergoing complete resection of rectal cancer with TME. However, the Dutch neoadjuvant trial that randomly assigned 1861 patients with resectable rectal cancer to TME alone or a short course of preoperative radiation (5 Gy daily for 5 days, in the "Swedish style") followed by TME demonstrated a significantly decreased rate of local recurrence (2.4% versus 8.2%) at 2 years.[31]

Of greatest importance is that improved local control appears to result in better overall survival. In one of the earliest reports, Heald noted a local recurrence rate of 3.6% and a survival rate of 86% after 9 years of follow-up.[32] In 1994, the Norwegian Rectal Cancer Group was founded to improve the surgical standard by implementing TME on a national level and to evaluate the results; courses were arranged to teach surgeons the technique of TME. Optimized TME reduced the rate of local recurrence (6% TME versus 12% non-TME) and increased overall survival (73% TME versus 60% non-TME) within 2 years.[33] This led to a strategic change in both Norway and the United States to initiate quality assessment in the surgical treatment of rectal cancer.

Guillem recently demonstrated an improved overall and disease-free survival in patients with T3 or N1 tumors who underwent TME after preoperative combined-modality therapy.[34] With a median follow-up of 44 months, the estimated 10-year overall survival was 58% (Fig 25–13), and 10-year recurrence-free survival was 62% (Fig 25–14). On multivariate analysis, pathologic response greater than 95%, lack of lymphovascular invasion and/or perineural invasion (PNI), and lack of postoperative positive lymph nodes were significantly associated with improved overall and disease-free survival.

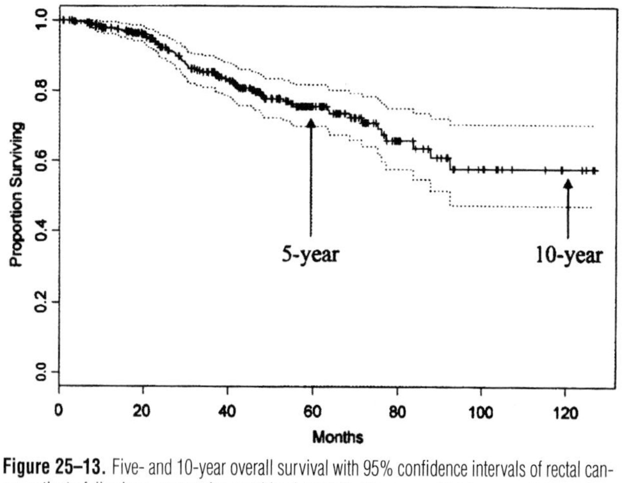

Figure 25–13. Five- and 10-year overall survival with 95% confidence intervals of rectal cancer patients following preoperative combined modality therapy and total mesorectal excision. (Used, with permission, from Guillem JG, Chessin DB, Cohen AM, et al. Long-term oncologic outcome following preoperative combined modality therapy and total mesorectal excision of locally advanced rectal cancer. *Ann Surg* 2005;241:829–838.)

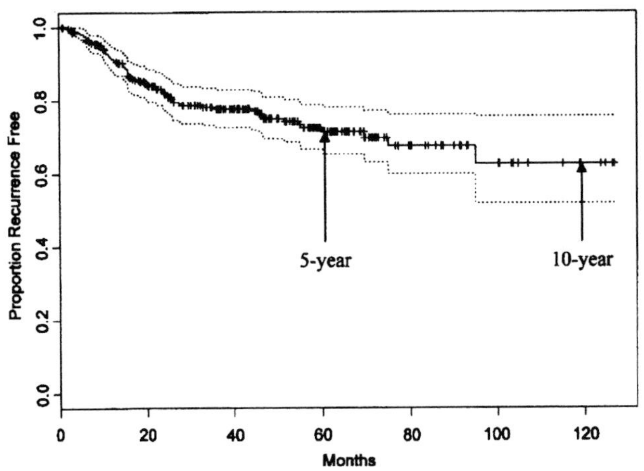

Figure 25–14. Five- and 10-year recurrence-free survival with 95% confidence intervals of rectal cancer patients following preoperative combined-modality therapy and total mesorectal excision. (Used, with permission, from Guillem JG, Chessin DB, Cohen AM, et al. Long-term oncologic outcome following preoperative combined modality therapy and total mesorectal excision of locally advanced rectal cancer. *Ann Surg* 2005;241:829–838.)

QUALITY OF LIFE

Quality of life has improved with TME and ANP. Conventional rectal surgery is associated with a significant incidence of impotence, retrograde ejaculation, and urinary incontinence, presumably owing to damage to the pelvic autonomic parasympathetic and sympathetic nerves by blunt dissection.[35] Postoperative impotence, retrograde ejaculation, or both are observed in 25–75% of conventionally treated patients compared with only 10–29% of patients after TME with its careful nerve-sparing dissection.[35]

Erectile capacity and normal ejaculation may be preserved in most male patients, especially those 60 years of age or younger. In one retrospective study of patients undergoing TME with ANP, 86% of male patients younger than 60 years of age and 67% of those 60 years of age or older were able both to engage in postoperative sexual intercourse and to achieve orgasm.[35] In female patients, sexual activity was maintained in 86%, sexual arousal with vaginal lubrication in 98%, and the ability to achieve orgasm in 91%. With the advent of pelvic dissections that preserve autonomic nerves, postoperative sexual dysfunction rates have been reduced from greater than 50% to 10–28%.[35]

Isolated urinary dysfunction is uncommon with preservation of the pelvic autonomic nerves. In a prospective study of rectal cancer patients undergoing TME with ANP, only 2 of 35 had difficulty with bladder emptying and possessed evidence of bladder denervation on postoperative studies.

Some studies, however, have demonstrated impaired quality of life owing to LAR with TME in part because of a temporary loop ileostomy or preoperative radiotherapy. Yet cost-utility analysis estimates that improved survival outweighs impaired quality of life.[36]

TECHNIQUE OF TOTAL MESORECTAL EXCISION

Prior to the procedure, all patients receive a full mechanical and antibiotic bowel preparation. The patient's abdomen is marked preoperatively by the enterostomal therapy nurse for potential stoma sites. An epidural catheter is placed by the anesthesia team for postoperative pain control. Sequential compression devices are applied to the lower extremities before general anesthesia is induced for deep vein thrombosis (DVT) prophylaxis. One dose of 5000 units of heparin is administered subcutaneously. Cefazolin 1 g and metronidazole 500 mg are infused. After anesthesia is induced, the patient is brought down on the table so that the buttocks are at the edge; a gel pad placed under the buttocks facilitates access to the anus. The patient is positioned in a modified lithotomy position using Allen or Yellow Fin stirrups (Fig 25–15). The hips are minimally flexed and abducted. The feet are positioned flat in the stirrups; an imaginary line is visualized keeping the ankle, knee, and contralateral shoulder in a straight line. Care is paid to having no pressure on the peroneal nerve or bony prominences; a hand should be able to be placed easily between the posterolateral aspect of each lower leg and its respective stirrup. If the patient has had previous pelvic surgery or evidence of hydronephrosis on CT scan, consider bilateral ureteral stent placement. A Foley catheter is placed, and it is draped over one leg. A nasogastric tube is inserted by the anesthesia team. A digital rectal examination is performed. If there is any question regarding the distal or proximal limits of the tumor, rigid proctoscopy may be performed at this time. Preoperatively, the lesion may have been marked by an injection of India ink. The surgeon should wear a headlight to help with visualization in the lower pelvis. Most surgeons stand on the patient's left, which allows them to operate more efficiently with their right hand in the lower pelvis. A low midline incision is made between the umbilicus and the pubis, keeping in mind potential stoma sites; cephalad extension may be necessary to mobilize the splenic flexure. The abdomen is explored to search for metastatic disease in the liver or peritoneal surfaces. The rectum is palpated to assess the primary mass. The colon is palpated for any synchronous lesions.

The abdominal self-retractor is set up. The patient is placed in slight Trendelenberg position. The sigmoid is mobilized laterally by scoring the white line of Toldt (Fig 25–16A). The left ureter is identified by several ways: visualizing it cross over the bifurcation of the

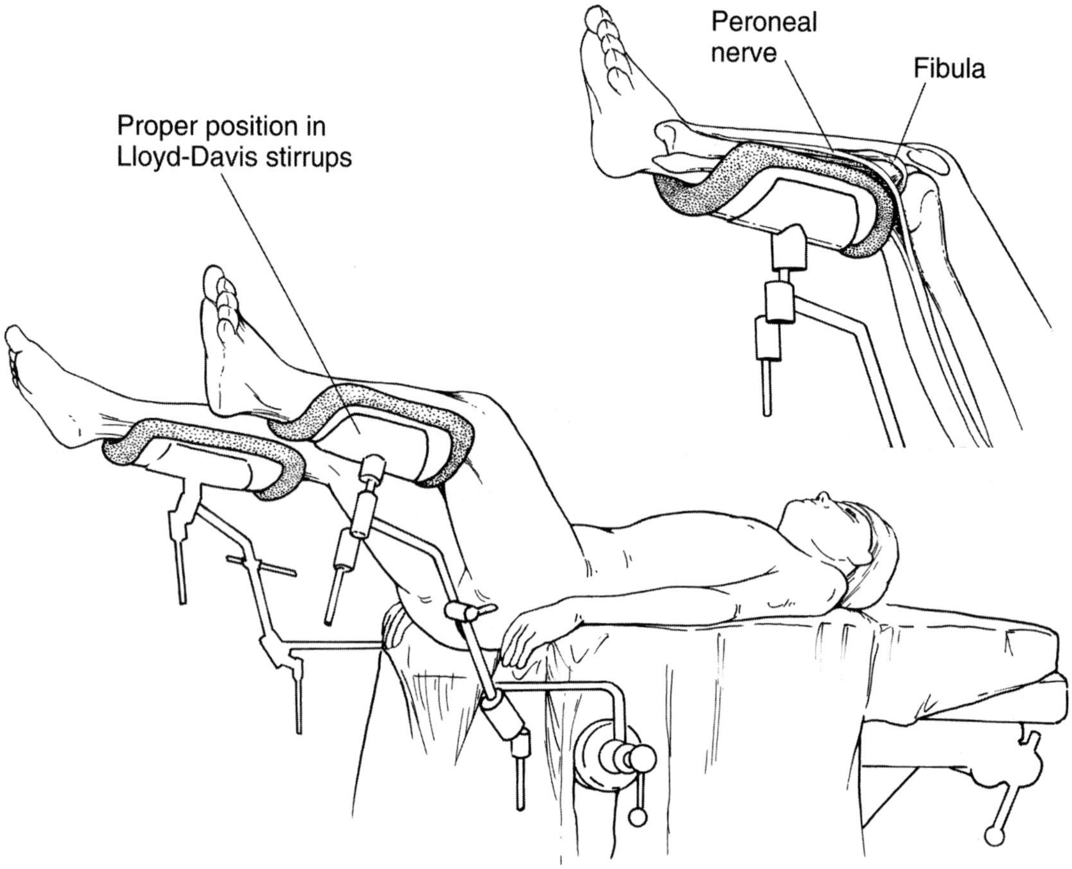

Figure 25–15. Position of patient for surgical treatment of rectal cancer allows access to both the abdomen and the perineum. (Redrawn, with permission, from Goldberg SM, Gordon PH, Nivatvongs S. *Essentials of Anorectal Surgery.* Philadelphia: Lippincott; 1980.)

common iliac artery, palpating the external iliac artery and pinching the tissue above it, locating it at the level where the sigmoid turns, or incising the peritoneum over the psoas muscle and finding the ureter on the medial aspect of the peritoneum (see Fig 25–16B). If it is clear that much length will be necessary for reconstruction, the splenic flexure is mobilized. Tension on the colon should be gentle but firm; too much traction on the colon or omentum can cause splenic injury. The transverse colon is freed from the omentum by sharp dissection along the avascular plane between the two structures. The bowel is packed into the upper abdomen. The sigmoid is held up in the air at the junction between the descending colon and sigmoid. Both sides of the mesentery are scored from this point down to the sacral promontory. The right ureter is identified. The colon usually is divided at the sigmoid–descending colon junction using a linear stapler (or may be divided between two bowel clamps, which would require a hand-sewn anastomosis). The sigmoidal vessels are isolated and divided using large Kelly clamps, two proximally and one distally. Metzenbaum scissors are used to divide the vessels. The vessels are doubly ligated. The colon is packed cephalad, out of the field. The superior hemorrhoidal artery then is divided at the junction with the left colic artery (see Fig 25–16C). A more proximal ligation of the inferior mesenteric vessel also can be performed if extra length on the colon is needed, but it is not necessary to ligate the IMA flush with the aorta for oncologic reasons. One usually suture ligates the superior hemorrhoidal vessels so as to ensure hemostasis.

After dividing the superior hemorrhoidal artery, it is important to find the proper plane of dissection at the sacral promontory. One first locates the sympathetic nerves along the pelvic brim. The rectum is retracted anteriorly. Electrocautery with a long Bovie tip is used to develop the loose areolar plane of avascular issue posteriorly (Fig 25–17B). The nerves are visualized and kept posterior to the plane of resection. The presacral fascia is incised down to Waldeyer's fascia, and the dissection is carried inferiorly to the coccyx. The St. Mark's abdominal retractor facilitates the deep pelvic dissection.

The anterior and lateral dissections then are started after the posterior dissection has been partially

MOBILIZATION OF THE LEFT COLON

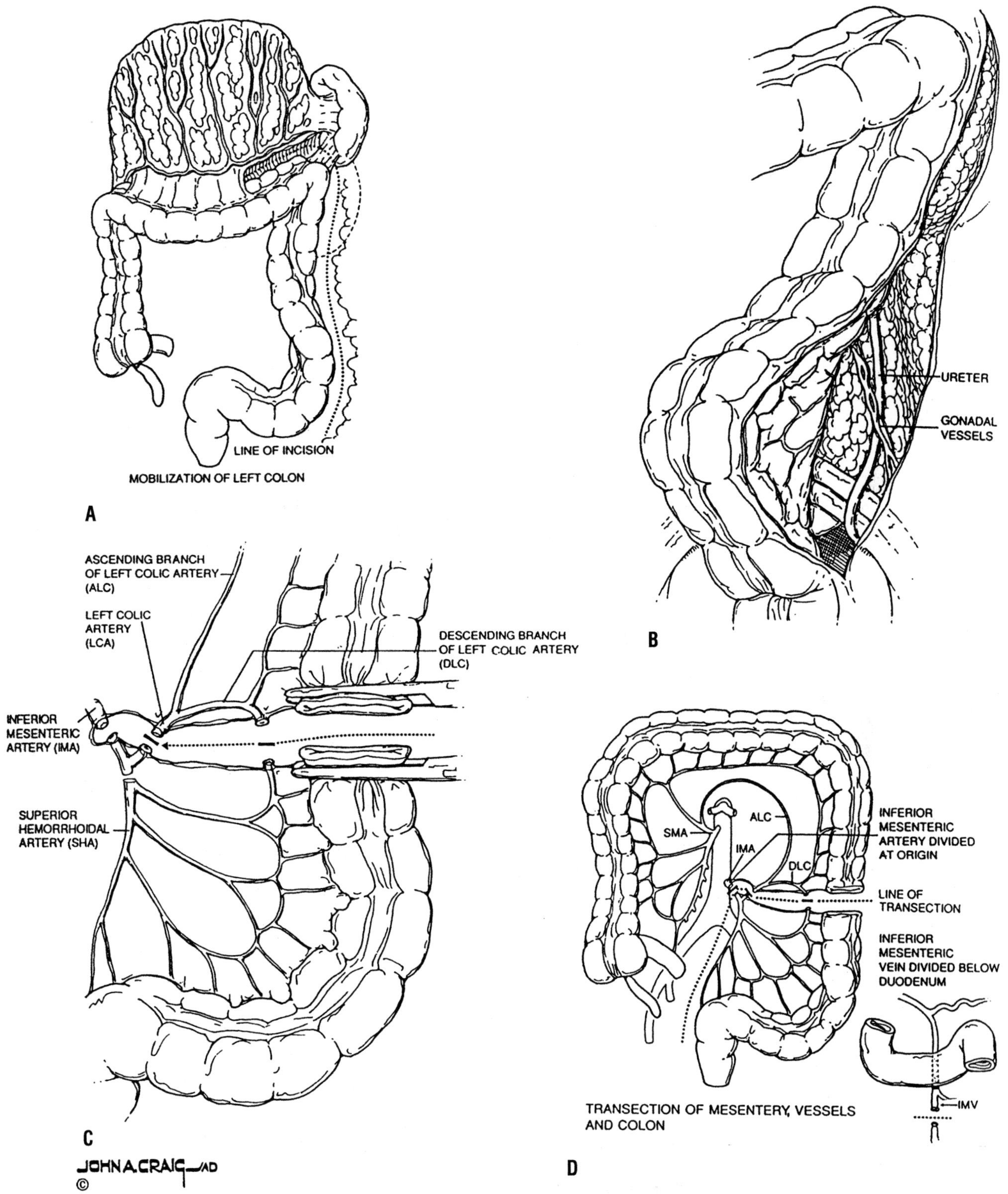

Figure 25–16. Mobilization of the left colon. **A.** Incision line around the left colon. **B.** Left colon reflected medially, exposing the ureter and gonadal vessels. **C.** Superior hemorrhoidal artery is divided close to the aorta to result in a high arterial ligation. The arcade of Riolan is preserved, and the left colon and mesentery are divided at the junction of the descending and sigmoid colon. **D.** Proximal ligation of the inferior mesenteric vein adds extra mobility.

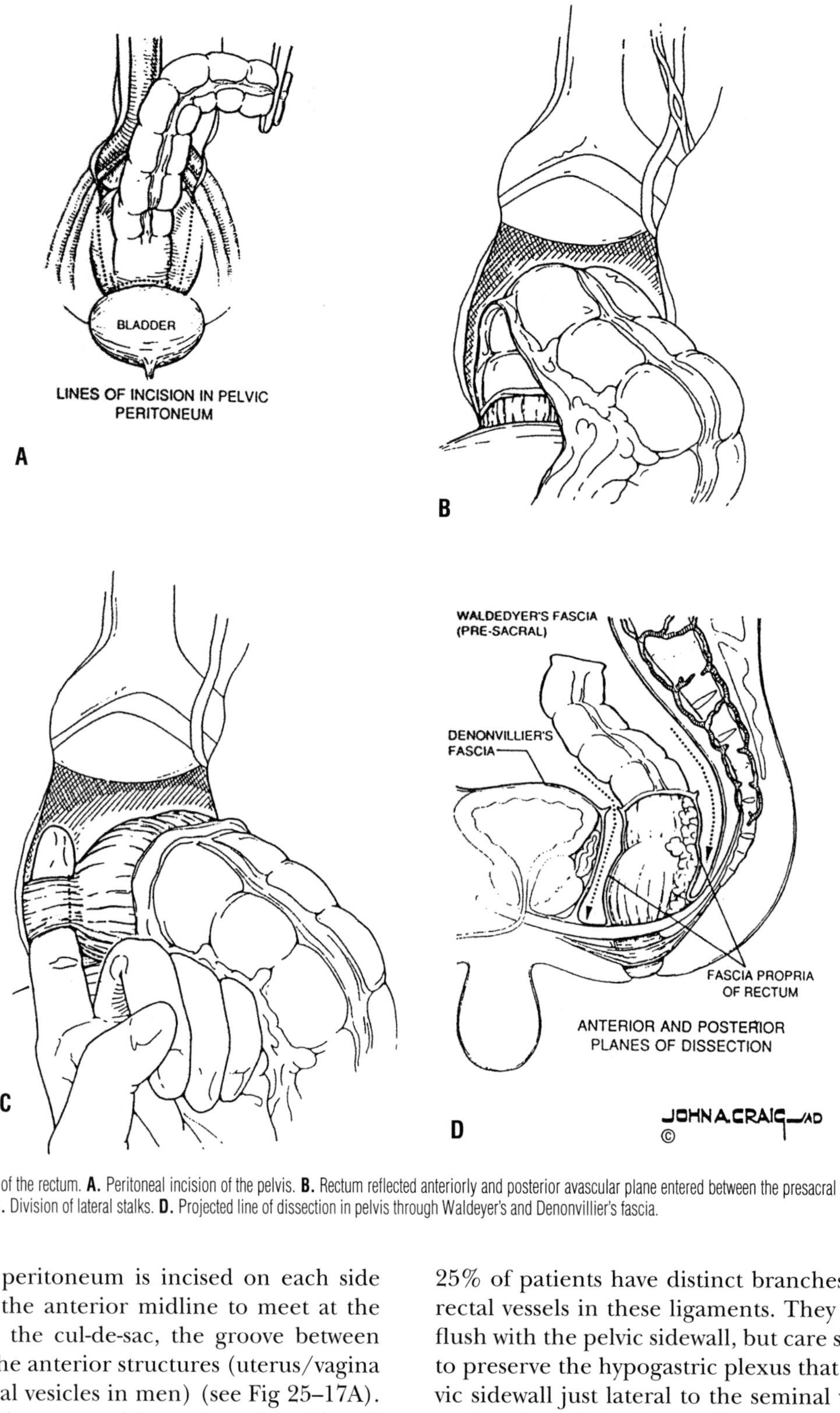

Figure 25–17. Mobilization of the rectum. **A.** Peritoneal incision of the pelvis. **B.** Rectum reflected anteriorly and posterior avascular plane entered between the presacral fascia of Waldeyer and the fascia propria of the rectum. **C.** Division of lateral stalks. **D.** Projected line of dissection in pelvis through Waldeyer's and Denonvillier's fascia.

completed. The peritoneum is incised on each side and then across the anterior midline to meet at the deepest point in the cul-de-sac, the groove between the rectum and the anterior structures (uterus/vagina in women, seminal vesicles in men) (see Fig 25–17A). The mesorectum is separated from the pelvic sidewall using the cautery to divide the thin areolar tissue that is found when one is dissecting in the proper plane. The dissection is carried down anterolaterally to the lateral ligaments or "stalks" (see Fig 25–17C). Only 25% of patients have distinct branches of the middle rectal vessels in these ligaments. They can be divided flush with the pelvic sidewall, but care should be taken to preserve the hypogastric plexus that lies on the pelvic sidewall just lateral to the seminal vesicles in men or just lateral to the cardinal ligaments in women. Preservation of the plexus helps with avoiding postoperative potency or urinary problems, and resection of the plexus is rarely helpful for oncologic reasons. Throughout the lateral dissection, one should be aware of the nerves and vessels along the pelvic sidewall. Too lateral a dissection causes bleeding from the pelvic sidewall.

Anteriorly, the planes are less distinct, and the fat of the mesorectum is thin. The vaginal wall or seminal vesicles are elevated anteriorly using the lipped St. Mark's retractor while the surgeon places posterior traction on the rectum. In the male patient, the dissection is continued through or anterior to Denonvillier's fascia (see Fig 25–17D). This fascia is often two layers of a thin membrane. When performing a cancer resection, one should take both layers of this membranous fascia off the seminal vesicles and upper prostate if possible.

Point of Transection

For middle to low rectal cancers, TME involves removing the entire mesorectum with its enveloping fascia as an intact unit. For tumors in the upper rectum (>10 cm from the anal verge), TME is extended to 5–6 cm below the level of the tumor, dividing the rectum and mesorectum at the same level. A number of pathologic studies demonstrate that tumor spread within the mesorectum rarely extends beyond 4 cm distal to the caudal edge of the tumor; usually most nodes or mesorectal implants are within 3 cm of the distal edge of the tumor.[5,10] However, multiple studies have shown that a 2-cm margin is adequate on the mucosa. Fewer than 2–4% of tumors will have mucosal or submucosal spread beyond 2 cm distally. Rigid sigmoidoscopy may be employed to identify the appropriate site for transection if the cancer is not palpable, especially after neoadjuvant therapy.

Once the rectum has been mobilized, a tumor measured at 5 cm by rigid proctoscopy often may be moved to 8 cm from the dentate line, a distance that permits an adequate resection margin and sphincter preservation (Fig 25–18).

When the distal extent of the tumor and the site of transection have been established, electrocautery is used to dissect the mesorectal fat away from the rectum. Vessels require ligation with 2-0 Vicryl ties. It is important to keep the dissection of the mesorectum perpendicular to the site of transection. "Coning in" as one divides the mesorectum prior to transection should be avoided.

Once the bowel has been cleared of mesorectal fat, a 30-, 45-, or 60-mm TA linear stapler is used to staple the rectum (Fig 25–19A). This is the first staple line in the "double-stapling technique." The bowel is clamped just proximal to this point. A #10 blade on a long handle is used to transect the bowel. The specimen is handed off the field.

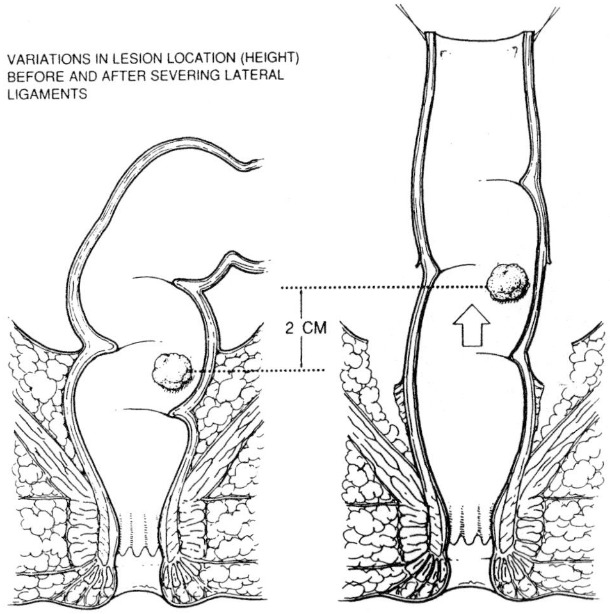

Figure 25–18. Tumor position relative to the dentate line after mobilization of the rectum. This may permit a sphincter-preserving resection.

Reconstruction: Double-Stapling Technique

The proximal colon is unpacked, and the length required for a tension-free anastomosis is determined. If more colon is needed, the splenic flexure is mobilized further. This may require an extension of the incision cephalad. Proximal ligation of the inferior mesenteric vein also adds extra mobility (see Fig 25–16D). The proximal bowel is cleaned by resecting residual fat and small vessels approximately 1 cm proximal to the staple line. The staple line is excised with Bovie electrocautery. Sizers may be inserted to select an end-to-end anastomosis (EEA) stapler diameter (25, 29, or 31 mm). A circular stapler then is chosen. The anvil is placed within the opened bowel. A 3-0 Prolene is used to take full-thickness 1–2-mm bites to fashion a purse-string stitch around the anvil. The purse-string suture is tied gently but firmly around the shaft so that the shaft is completely encircled by bowel (see Fig 25–19C). If there are any gaps, an additional 3-0 Prolene suture can be used to take another full-thickness bite, and this suture may be tied around the shaft as well. The serosa of the bowel is cleaned further of fat and small vessels within 1 cm of the shaft of the anvil to optimize bowel-to-bowel contact when the circular stapler is applied. One also can perform a similar placement of the anvil on the antimesenteric side of the colon for a side-to-end anastomosis. The optimal placement of the anvil in this case is such that only a small blind end of colon remains distal to the anastomosis (1–5 cm).

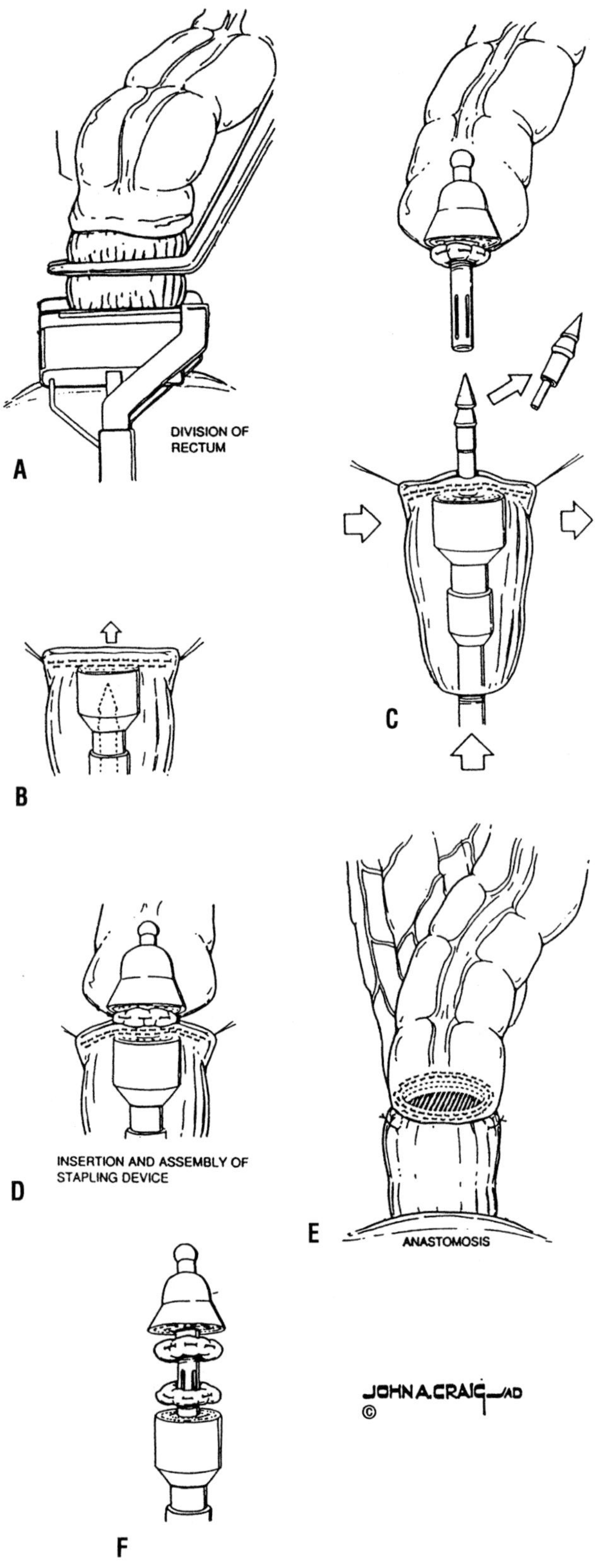

Figure 25–19. Colorectal anastomosis: double-staple technique. **A.** Transection of the distal rectum with a linear stapler. **B.** Stapling instrument introduced through rectum. **C.** Descending colon purse-string suture is tied around shaft of anvil. After the trocar of the circular stapler penetrates behind the staple line, the trocar is removed before reconnecting the anvil to the shaft. **D.** The circular stapler is reconnected, reapproximated, and fired. **E.** The anastomosis is complete. **F.** The proximal and distal staple lines are examined for intact inner "donuts."

Attention then is turned to the pelvis, which is irrigated and inspected for hemostasis. This is one's truly last opportunity to inspect this area because one's exposure will be compromised when the anastomosis is completed.

One member of the team then stands between the patient's legs. The circular stapler tip is coated with lubricant on the outside of the stapler; we do not place lubricant on the staples themselves. The tip is retracted fully. A rectal examination is performed, and the anus is dilated gently with two to three fingers in order to accommodate the stapler. The circular stapler is inserted gently following the curve of the rectum—initially straight in and then the stapler is tilted posteriorly. Using close communication with the surgeon overlooking the abdomen, the assistant positions the circular stapler tip so that the trocar will exit either 2–3 mm anterior or posterior (we elect to do this posteriorly in women in order to avoid the vaginal wall) to the staple line (see Fig 25–19B). The trocar then is advanced slowly; the bowel continues to be adjusted as necessary. When the trocar protrudes through the bowel wall, be sure that the trocar is fully advanced so that the its bottom is visualized (see Fig 25–19C). The trocar is removed. Ensuring that the proximal bowel is not twisted and that the remaining bowel, mesentery, and epiploicae are held away, the anvil is brought down gently to the stapler and connected. The colon is inspected again to verify that no adjacent tissue is entrapped. The stapler is closed slowly until both pieces of colon are fully approximated (see Fig 25–19D). The stapler is fired, opened slightly, and gently removed as directed according to the type of stapler. This is the second staple line in the double-stapling technique (see Fig 25–19E). The stapler is opened, and the tissues from the proximal and distal bowel are inspected to make sure that the two rings of tissue, or "donuts," are intact (see Fig 25–19F). If they are not intact, additional sutures are placed if a visible gap is apparent. All anastomoses are checked for integrity. The surgeon fills the pelvis with saline and clamps the bowel proximal to the anastomosis gently with his or her hands; the assistant introduces a rigid sigmoidoscope through the rectum and insufflates air. If bubbles cannot be detected, one can be confident that the anastomosis is intact. If bubbles are detected, additional sutures are placed in suspected areas, and a diverting loop ileostomy is constructed. If the anastomosis is disrupted completely, it must be refashioned.

Diverting Loop Ileostomy

A diverting loop ileostomy should be considered in any low anastomoses (<5 cm) from the dentate line, which are associated with anastomotic leak rates of up to 17%. Other risk factors for anastomotic breakdown include a history of radiation, perioperative steroid use, malnutrition, elderly females with a thin rectovaginal septum, or elderly patients undergoing preoperative combined-modality therapy with planned postoperative chemotherapy. Additionally, if there is any question regarding the integrity of the anastomosis, an ileostomy should be created.

Ileostomies can be closed within 8 weeks but often are left in place until the patient completes adjuvant chemotherapy. A Gastrografin enema is used to check the patency and integrity of the anastomosis prior to takedown of the anastomosis.

Drain Placement

Most surgeons continue to advocate routine use of drains after pelvic anastomoses. One prospective, randomized trial of 100 patients to receive either no drains or closed-suction drains demonstrated that the presence or absence of a drain did not influence the rate of morbidity and mortality. Although there is no evidence for the use of drains when an anastomosis has been made outside the pelvis, pelvic drainage may be important after anterior resection. We would strongly recommend placing a drain in extremely low resections, especially where the anastomosis was hand sewn or in patients who undergo an APR. For all other resections, placement of a drain may be determined on a case-by-case basis.

Closure

We prefer to close the abdominal fascia with a looped #0 PDS suture starting at the cephalad and caudad ends and to run the suture toward the middle. The deep dermal layer is closed with 3-0 Vicryl. The skin is closed with either staples or a 4-0 Vicryl subcuticular suture followed by benzoin and Steri-Strips. A 4 × 8 gauze dressing is applied and covered with Tegaderm.

POSTOPERATIVE CARE

The nasogastric tube is removed at the end of the procedure or on postoperative day 1, and the patient can drink sips of clear liquids. The diet is advanced to low residue after flatus is passed. Cefazolin and metronidazole are continued for 24 hours postoperatively. Heparin is administered subcutaneously at a dose of 5000 units bid or tid depending on the patient's weight. Low-molecular-weight heparin also can be used in appropriate doses. Sequential compression devices are worn by the patient unless the patient is ambulating well. Most patients ambulate on postoperative day 1. The Foley catheter is kept in place for 3–5 days. If an epidural has been used for postoperative pain control, it is usually left in place until the patient is started on oral pain medication when he or she is tolerating clear liquids well.

COLOANAL ANASTOMOSIS

Anastomoses at or just above the anorectal ring often result in increased frequency of stool, incontinence or soilage, and impaired quality of life owing to an insufficient reservoir. Diet restrictions and time after surgery usually will improve these symptoms, but two alternative techniques of reconstruction address these postoperative problems and often allow for improved function to be attained more quickly.

Colonic Pouch

A 6-cm limb of sigmoid or descending colon is folded, and the apex is brought down to reach the rectal stump without tension. The splenic flexure may require additional mobilization. A colotomy is made at the apex with Bovie electrocautery, and a #75 GIA linear cutter is used to staple the pouch on itself to create a common lumen. A second fire of the stapler may be necessary. This pouch now serves as the neorectum. A double-stapled anastomosis as described or a hand-sewn anastomosis then is performed. A diverting loop ileostomy is used routinely for these ultralow anastomoses.

Multiple prospective, randomized studies have demonstrated superior function of a coloanal J-pouch over a straight coloanal anastomosis, especially in the first 6 months after ileostomy takedown.

Transverse Coloplasty

When the pelvis is too narrow for a J-pouch or the length of the pouch is inadequate, a transverse coloplasty may be fashioned. This is performed by placing the anvil of a 29- or 33-mm circular stapler into the cut end of the sigmoid as described under "Low Anterior Resection." The colon should be mobilized to the level of the middle colic vessels. Beginning 2 cm proximal to the anvil, a 7–8-cm longitudinal colotomy is made. This colotomy then is closed transversely. The anastomosis is completed as described under "Low Anterior Resection." A diverting loop ileostomy is created.

▪ ABDOMINOPERINEAL RESECTION (APR)

Traditionally, distal rectal cancers have been treated with an APR, as first described by Miles, who noted high failure rates after local excision.[2] This procedure involves the en bloc resection of the tumor as well as the surrounding lymph nodes and the anal sphincters, resulting in a permanent colostomy.

The APR, although quite successful for early rectal cancers (stage I) in terms of survival, is associated with significant morbidity of 61% and mortality ranging from 0–6.3%.[37] Urinary complications can be as high as 50% and perineal wound infections 16%. In addition to these perioperative problems, significant long-term morbidity is associated with a permanent colostomy. In a patient survey, 66% of patients complained of significant leaks from their stoma appliance, 67% experienced sexual dysfunction, and only 40% of patients working preoperatively ultimately returned to work.[38] There is also a significant change in body image when compared with sphincter-saving procedures. The 5-year survival rates following an APR range from 78–100% for stage I, 45–73% for stage II, and 22–66% for stage III disease.[39] Despite radical resection, 20% recur locally. Variations in recurrence rates depend on location of the tumor within the rectum, changes in surgical technique, and the addition of adjuvant therapy.

For patients with cancers that involve the sphincter apparatus or for those who are incontinent of feces, an APR is performed to remove the rectal specimen.

TECHNIQUE

The patient is marked preoperatively by the enterostomal nurse for a permanent colostomy. Please see section "Low Anterior Resection with Total Mesorectal Excision" for details regarding additional preoperative care, positioning, incision, and rectal mobilization. The dissection proceeds down to the striated muscles of the levator ani; one can confirm muscle contraction by using electrocautery. Once this level is reached, the perineal excision field can begin either by the surgeon or by a second team. The two-team approach saves time.

PERINEAL DISSECTION

The anus is closed with a #0 silk suture in a purse-string fashion (Fig 25–20B). A marking pen is used to draw an ellipse 2 cm outside the superficial external sphincter and extending from the perineal body anteriorly, coccyx posteriorly, and ischial tuberosities laterally. The incision is made with a #10 blade and carried down through the dermis into ischiorectal fat (see Fig 25–20C). Two Gelpi retractors are placed at 45 degrees to the anus in order to facilitate deep dissection. The dissection is carried deep outside the external sphincter toward the tip of the coccyx, keeping in mind the planes of dissection (see Fig 25–20A, E). The anococcygeal ligament is palpated just anterior to the tip of the coccyx, and the palpating finger meets the fingers of a team member working from the abdominal field (see Fig 25–20D). A pair of large scissors is used to poke through the ligament; the scissors are fully spread and while wide open are pulled straight back. Hooking the index and middle fingers under the levator muscles and transecting with electrocautery frees the rectum laterally (see Fig 25–20F, G).

The anterior surface is dissected last (see Fig 25–20H, I). The rectum is delivered through the perineal opening. An assistant retracts the skin and subcutaneous tissue anteriorly with an army-navy retractor. Care is taken to keeping the posterior wall of the vagina or the prostate anterior to the plane of dissection. The surgeon cups his or her hand around the rectum with traction posteriorly and inferiorly and Bovies between the rectum and the anterior structures, often reassessing the plane of transection. Once freed circumferentially, the specimen is passed off the field.

The pelvic floor is irrigated and checked carefully for hemostasis. A tongue of omentum or omental pedicle flap may be used to cover the pelvis to prevent the small bowel from dropping deep into the pelvis if radiation is contemplated. Omentum also helps healing, especially in an irradiated perineum or when patients also have undergone prostate or vaginal resections. The descending colon is further mobilized in order to exit the skin without tension. The colostomy site is prepared similar to the diverting loop ileostomy as described under "Low Anterior Resection." The colon is drawn through the colostomy site using a Babcock clamp, but it is not matured until the midline incision is closed.

Two #10 Jackson-Pratt drains are placed in the pelvis and are brought anteriorly out through the abdominal wall and secured to the skin using 3-0 nylon suture (see Fig 25–20J). The abdomen is closed as described under "Low Anterior Resection." The colostomy is matured using interrupted 3-0 Vicryl suture.

If using a two-team approach, the perineal wound can be closed after the pelvis has been irrigated and hemostasis achieved. Two layers of interrupted 2-0 Vicryl suture are used to approximate the subcutaneous tissue. One layer of 3-0 Vicryl in a vertical mattress fashion is used to approximate the skin. Because this area is often radiated, multiple layers decrease the risk of the wound breakdown extending into the pelvis.

POSTOPERATIVE CARE

Postoperative care is similar to that described under "Low Anterior Resection." The patient is not allowed to

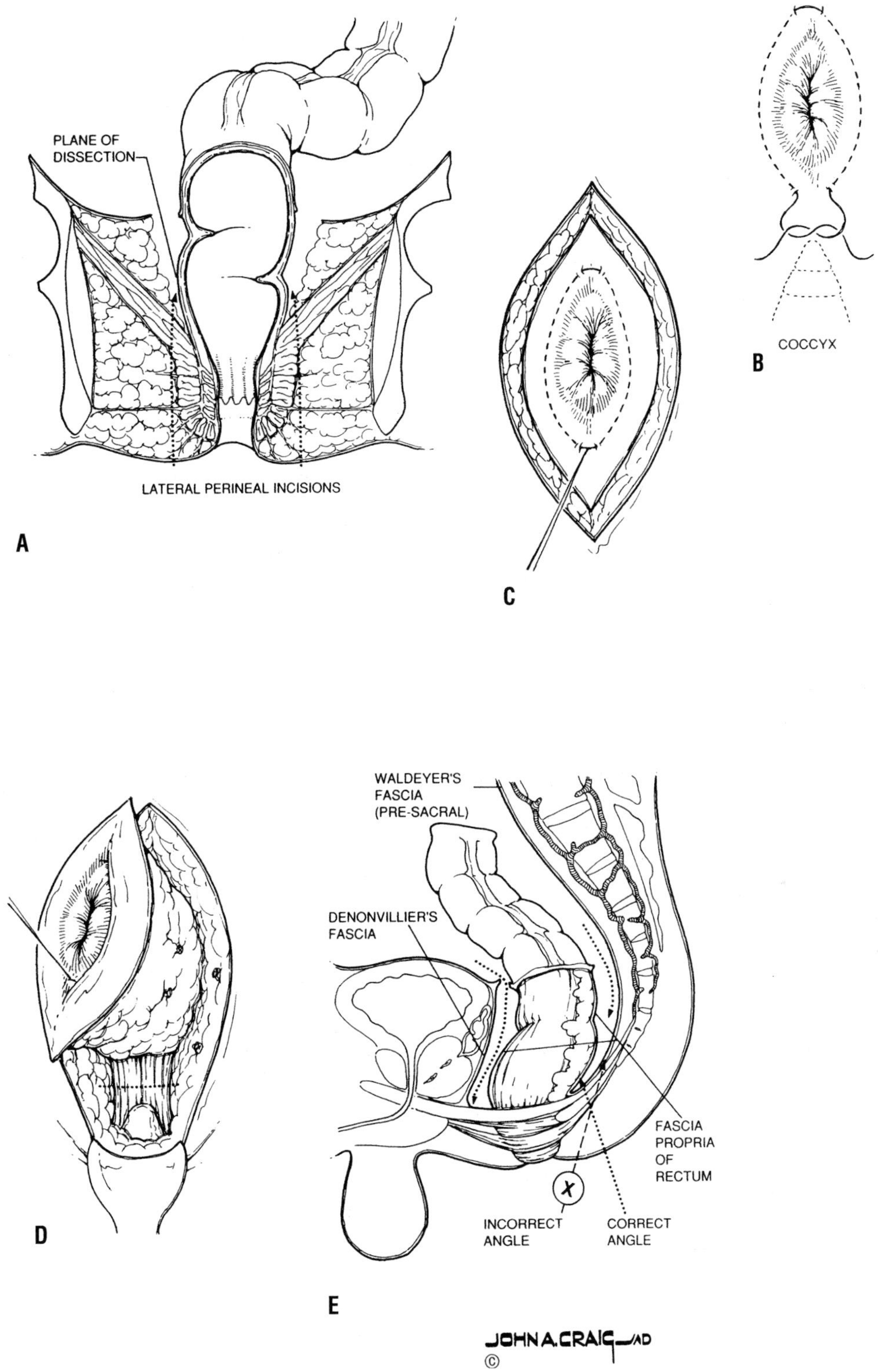

Figure 25–20. Perineal dissection: two team synchronous approach. **A.** Projected lines of pelvic floor resection in the vertical plane. **B.** Anal closure. **C.** Perineal incision. **D.** Incision line anterior to coccyx through anococcygeal ligament through which scissors are used to gain entrance to the pelvis. **E.** Planes of pelvic dissection and posterior plane of entry into pelvis through the pelvic floor. *Continued*

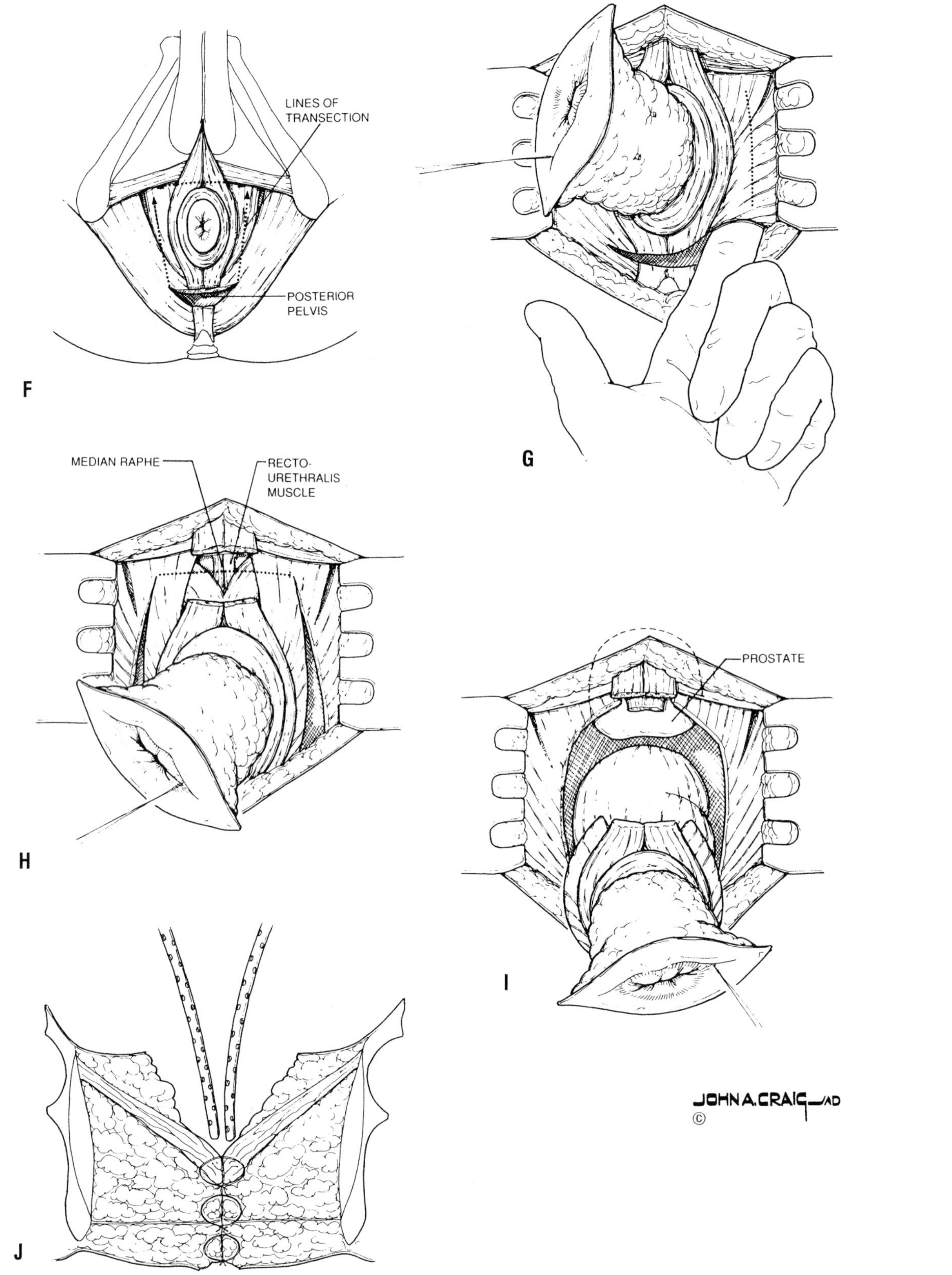

Figure 25–20 cont'd. **F.** Projected lines of pelvic floor transection. **G.** Lateral transection of levator ani muscle. **H.** Anterior transection of rectourethralis, puborectalis, and pubococcygeus. **I.** Completion of anterior dissection and removal of rectum through perineal wound. **J.** Pelvic floor closed with two drains in place.

sit for 5 days but may only recline and ambulate. Thereafter, the patient may sit on a soft pillow; we do not advocate using a "donut" because perineum is not supported. The perineum is cleaned daily with dilute hydrogen peroxide. The Foley catheter remains in place for 3–5 days.

COMPLICATIONS

Perineal wound complications are common following APR and occur in up to 25% of patients. While most of these wound complications are minor, some may require operative débridement. We demonstrated previously that preoperative radiation and primary closure were not associated with an increased incidence of wound complications compared with nonirradiated patients following APR for rectal cancer.[40]

Stoma complications include ischemia, retraction, hernia, stenosis, and prolapse. The construction of a good colostomy will provide a patient with a superb quality of life after APR. Early education in the immediate postoperative period allows the patient to adjust to life with a stoma. The stoma shrinks to its final size approximately 3 weeks postoperatively when the edema has subsided. An end colostomy may be irrigated to establish regularity of bowel movements and further improve the patient's quality of life. The operative mortality for APRs is less than 2%.

▪ EN BLOC EXCISION WITH RECTUM

POSTERIOR VAGINECTOMY

Partial vaginectomy is indicated for locally advanced low rectal cancers involving the vagina. One study demonstrated a 5-year survival of 46% and a median survival of 44 months, with most favorable results from negative surgical margins and node-negative disease.[41]

If the patient is undergoing an APR, the posterior wall of the vagina is removed as the anterior margin of the resection (Fig 25–21). After completing the posterior and lateral dissections, the rectum is delivered through the perineum. The anterior aspect of the perineal incision includes the posterior introitus and is extended around the posterior third to half of the vagina only to avoid denervation of the urethra. To achieve hemostasis during the procedure, one can place interrupted 2-0 absorbable full-thickness sutures through the vagina from either side, starting at the apex of the incision, and tie the sutures as the specimen is being excised.

If the patient is undergoing an LAR with a coloanal anastomosis, the partial vaginectomy may be performed through the abdominal approach. The involved area of the vagina is resected with a 1-cm margin and kept en bloc with the rectum. Subsequent closure of the vagina is completed by initially placing Allis clamps on the vaginal edges and then taking full-thickness bites with 2-0 Vicryl sutures in a figure-of-eight fashion.

Before abdominal closure, we recommend placing an omental flap around the vaginal cuff to prevent breakdown of the vaginal suture line. If a coloanal anastomosis is in place, we would position the omentum between the vaginal and the coloanal suture lines.

PROSTATECTOMY

In locally advanced rectal cancer in which there appears to be possible involvement of the prostate, urethra, bladder, or ureterovesicular junction on CT scan

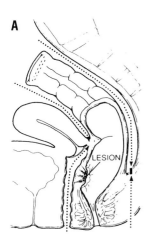

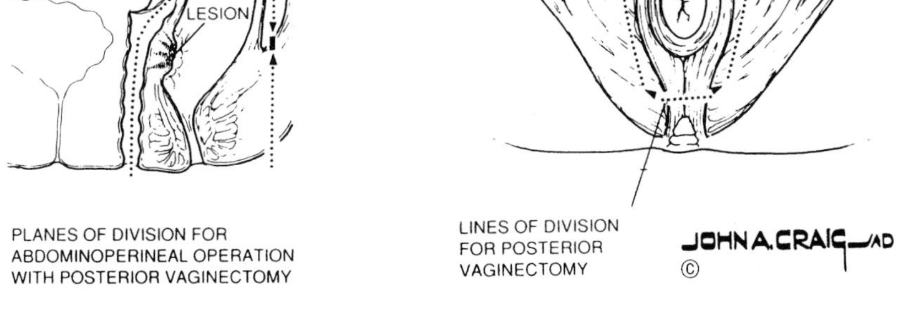

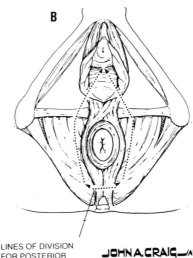

Figure 25–21. Posterior vaginectomy with APR. **A.** Line of dissection, including posterior wall of vagina for low anterior rectal cancer. **B.** Lines of transection, including posterior wall of vagina.

of the abdomen and pelvis, an MRI of the pelvis should be obtained. Urology consult should be made because one must be prepared for radical prostatectomy and/or cystectomy with ileal conduit diversion. A prostatectomy en bloc with rectal resection is an alternative to total pelvic exenteration in patients whose rectal cancer is fixed only to the prostate. The reasons for involving urology are in part due to the vascularity of the prostate. In addition, one should be concerned about constructing any genitourinary anastomosis (e.g., between bladder and urethra) in the presence of previous radiation and a rectal anastomosis. Attention should be paid to potential for autonomic nerve deficit if proximity and effacement of the neurovascular bundle are evident on MRI.

PELVIC EXENTERATION

Total pelvic exenteration is an alternative for patients with locally advanced rectal cancer in which the tumor is contiguous with adjacent organs, such as the prostate or bladder (Fig 25–22). Long-term survival rates range from 20–70% and are improved in younger patients with no lymph node metastases.[42] Local recurrence rates range from 3–8%. An argument against performing total pelvic exenteration is the considerable morbidity (20–40%) and 0–20% mortality associated with this procedure. The most common complications are infection, small bowel obstruction, and problems with urinary diversion.

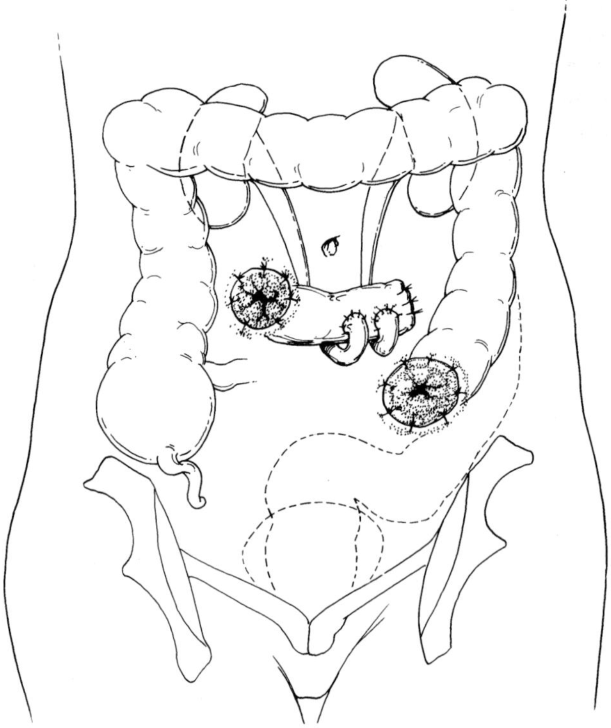

Figure 25–22. Pelvic exenteration. (Redrawn, with permission, from Craig JA, Kodner IJ, Fry RD, Fleshman JW, et al. Colon, rectum and anus. In: Schwartz DI (ed), *Principles of Surgery*, 6th ed. New York: McGraw-Hill, 1993, p 1296.)

PROPHYLACTIC BILATERAL OOPHORECTOMY

Carcinoma of the rectum metastasizes readily to the ovaries, and prophylactic oophorectomy during rectal resection may diminish the morbidity of carcinoma of the rectum in women. Additionally, the incidence of ovarian cancer in women with a history of colorectal cancer is roughly five times the incidence in women without such a history. Although prophylactic bilateral oophorectomy does not significantly affect survival, the prevention of primary ovarian cancer in postmenopausal women is considered to be the main benefit of this procedure. We discuss this with our postmenopausal patients and offer this to them at the time of operation.

▪ LAPAROSCOPIC SURGERY

Minimally invasive laparoscopically assisted surgery was first considered in 1990 for patients undergoing colectomy for cancer. The technical feasibility of performing laparoscopic TME was demonstrated in several prospective studies. Preservation of the autonomic nerves is also possible during laparoscopic TME. Early results confirmed complete resection of the mesorectum with intact visceral fascia in all patients.[43]

▪ OTHER TREATMENT OPTIONS

Besides surgical resection for rectal cancer, there are other options for patients who may not be candidates for surgery owing to their comorbidities, extent of disease, or preference. Endocavitary radiation may be delivered at doses of 50 cGy for palliation and for curative intent. Performed as an outpatient and well tolerated by patients, endocavitary radiation is delivered with sedation and local perineal block.

Electrocoagulation may be used via a transanal approach after administering general anesthesia and placing the patient in the lithotomy position. The rectal lesion and a 1-cm margin are fulgurated. Recurrence rates approach 50–80%; therefore, patients may require repeat treatments.

Cryotherapy, another alternative modality, results in a large amount of foul-smelling discharge. Photodynamic therapy has limited availability. Laser vaporization using neodymium:yttrium-aluminum-garnet laser provides palliation but is associated with a 14% recurrence rate and is costly.

▪ COMPLICATIONS

Complications of surgical management of rectal cancer may include those common to any major intra-abdominal operation, such as infection, bleeding, wound problems, deep venous thrombosis/pulmonary embolism, myocardial infarction, pneumonia, and renal failure. There are, however, several complications that are related to rectal cancer. There is a 50% incidence of impotence in men following resection for rectal cancer. Therefore, it is critical to discuss this situation with the patient before the resection and to record the preoperative status of his sexual function. If a man is impotent after surgery, it is advisable to wait 1 year before undergoing implantation of a penile prosthetic device. This delay is recommended not only to ensure that the malignancy has been cleared but also to allow the patient sufficient time to overcome psychological impediments such as a change in body image from pelvic surgery or from a colostomy. Women may also suffer from impaired sexual function, especially if the vagina is distorted during the rectal resection.

A possible permanent colostomy is often not preferred by patients. Its placement, however, must be explained in a way that the patient understands that he or she may be left with this if reconstruction is not technically possible.

Anastomotic leak, which occurs in up to 20% of patients, can be avoided by constructing the anastomosis with well-vascularized tissue without tension. Interestingly, young, muscular men have a higher incidence of anastomotic leaks, which may result from the technical challenge of operating in a narrow pelvis or from strong sphincters that may stress the anastomosis. The latter may be addressed by dilating the anal sphincter in the operating room at the end of the procedure. Anastomotic leaks usually present between 4 and 7 days postoperatively. Symptoms may include fever, tachycardia, arrhythmias, tachypnea, enterocutaneous fistula, or diffuse peritonitis. When a leak is suspected, the patient should be made NPO, and blood should be sent for a complete blood count, electrolytes, and type and cross-match. An upright chest x-ray will diagnose pneumoperitoneum. Abdominal series may demonstrate extraluminal air. CT scan of the abdomen and pelvis with water-soluble contrast material may demonstrate abscess formation, extraluminal air, and the actual leak. Barium should be avoided because leakage of barium creates a destructive peritonitis. A leak may be managed with intravenous antibiotics and bowel rest in a patient without peritonitis. An abscess may be drained percutaneously. An enterocutaneous fistula may be treated with total parenteral nutrition and local wound care. If a large leak is demonstrated or the patient experiences peritonitis, exploratory laparotomy with diverting ileostomy or colostomy should be performed. The anastomosis is rarely taken down and should not be reconstructed in the presence of sepsis.

Massive venous bleeding from the presacral space may result intraoperatively from lateral dissection onto the pelvic sidewall or sacrum. Ligation of the iliac vessels is discouraged and may be hazardous. If massive bleeding is encountered, a surgical metal "tack" may be driven into the sacrum to compress the venous space. Additionally, the pelvis may be packed for 24–48 hours, at which time the patient is returned to the operating room for pack removal and closure.

Urinary dysfunction may occur after rectal resection. Many men have coexisting prostatic hypertrophy. Because low rectal dissection approaches the membranous urethra, Foley catheters usually are kept in place for 5 days. Patients may be discharged with indwelling catheters, especially if they have undergone partial prostatectomies or seminal vesiculectomies. Women may experience urinary incontinence if the anterior aspect of the vagina, which contains the neurologic control of the urethra, is transected.

▪ OBSTRUCTING, METASTATIC, AND RECURRENT RECTAL CANCER

OBSTRUCTING CANCER OF THE RECTUM

For obstructing cancers of the rectum, a loop ileostomy, performed as an open or a laparoscopic procedure, is constructed for diversion. Usually, the tumor is staged as a T3 or N1 lesion; the patient is treated with neoadjuvant chemoradiation and considered for subsequent surgical resection.

METASTATIC RECTAL CANCER

The management of hepatic and pulmonary metastases will not be described in this chapter. Nonetheless, if a patient presents with incurable metastatic disease and life expectancy is greater than 6 months, it is reasonable to consider a palliative rectal resection. If the rectal lesion is staged as T3 or N1, we recommend neoadjuvant chemoradiation because this addresses both the primary lesion and the metastasis and may provide some palliation of obstruction, bleeding, or pain. Other options include rectal stents or laser destruction of the tumor to maintain an adequate lumen. It is important to understand the patient, his or her desires, and his or her general state of health when recommending treatment at this stage of cancer.

RECURRENT RECTAL CANCER

Local recurrence of rectal adenocarcinoma is seen in up to 30% of patients. Although recurrence may be seen at the distal margin of the anastomosis, most develop from residual cancer on the pelvic wall. The time course for recurrences to present through the anastomosis is approximately 18 months. By their nature, these tumors are fixed to the pelvic wall and surrounding viscera. They cause significant symptoms, such as intractable pelvic pain, bleeding, cramping or constipation, urinary tract dysfunction, and chronic pelvic sepsis.

When patients present with these symptoms or with a rising CEA level, a work-up including CT scan of the abdomen and pelvis, endorectal ultrasound, MRI of the pelvis, and PET scan may be helpful. A careful pelvic examination is mandatory. A biopsy, either via sigmoidoscopy or CT-guided, should be employed to confirm the diagnosis pathologically. If external radiation has not been used before, it should be considered. The surgeon should review the imaging studies and determine which organs are involved, such as the vagina, uterus, prostate, bladder, sacrum, and small intestine, which will require en bloc resection. Urology consult should be obtained if there is any question of prostate or bladder involvement; ureteral stents should be placed preoperatively. Removal of the rectum and urinary bladder with surrounding lymphatic tissue results in a permanent colostomy and ileal conduit.

Intraoperative Radiation Therapy

Intraoperative radiation therapy (IORT) may be considered in patients with pelvic sidewall recurrence. This is performed in an operating room–radiation therapy suite. Resection with negative microscopic margins and absence of vascular invasion independently predicts improved local control and survival after resection and IORT.[44] The major morbidities of IORT include peripheral neuropathy and ureteral stenosis.

Palliation

These tumors are difficult to palliate, let alone cure. Surgical resection combined with aggressive multimodality therapy is advocated to avert the morbidity of pelvic disease and to prolong survival in a subset of patients, with survival rates up to 30%.[45] Most patients, however, will not be offered curative surgery on the basis of comorbidities, poor performance status, distant metastases, or locally unresectable disease on preoperative imaging. These patients may be offered palliative intervention. Miner and colleagues demonstrated that in patients who underwent surgery with palliative intent, improvement was noted in 40% with bleeding, 70% with obstruction, and 20% with pain.[46] When considering the effective use of surgery for these patients, decision making is complex because one must balance palliation of symptoms, comorbidities, and patient desires and goals. Seeking the input of a multidisciplinary treatment group, including medical oncologists and radiation oncologists, is invaluable.

▪ CHEMORADIATION

Patients with rectal cancer who undergo surgery with intention to cure and without evidence of gross disease postoperatively still may develop local recurrence or distant metastases. Up to 10% of patients who undergo TME with tumor-free radial and distal margins may develop local failure. The goal of adjuvant therapy is to eliminate the micrometastatic disease present at the time of surgery.

ADJUVANT CHEMORADIATION

In 1990, the National Institutes of Health consensus statement concluded that "combined postoperative chemotherapy and radiotherapy improves local control and survival in stage II and III patients and is recommended." Most of the information regarding chemotherapy for colorectal cancer comes from trials of colon cancer rather than for rectal cancer. The NSABP C-04 trial studied stage II and III colon cancer patients and demonstrated that 5-fluorouracil (5-FU) and leucovorin treatment had a significantly better 5-year survival rate (74% versus 69%) compared with 5-FU and levamisole.[47]

Several trials have suggested a benefit for adjuvant chemoradiation for rectal cancer in patients with resected stage II or III cancers. The GITSG trial demonstrated that combined chemoradiation resulted in an improvement in overall survival as well as a decrease in local recurrence.[48] The NCCTG trial demonstrated that the addition of chemotherapy to radiation reduced both local recurrence (13% versus 25%) and distant metastases (28% versus 46%) and improved survival.[49]

Radiation therapy used alone as adjuvant therapy may improve local recurrence and survival rates. A theoretical reason to use postoperative radiation therapy is that more appropriate patient selection can be achieved because pathologic staging is performed prior to radiation. Disadvantages include radiating the neorectum and small bowel and a lower tendency of patients to complete their radiation. While none of the trials in the 1980s and 1990s demonstrated increased survival, one study did show a decrease in local recurrence.

NEOADJUVANT CHEMORADIATION

There are a number of potential advantages for using neoadjuvant chemoradiation. They include the ability to deliver higher doses of chemotherapy with radiation. Another advantage is not only to downstage the tumor, which has been noted in 60–80% of patients, but also to achieve a pathologic complete response, which occurs in 15–30% of patients. The ability to "shrink" the tumor facilitates surgical resection, thereby allowing one to achieve negative margins and perform a sphincter-preserving operation in patients who otherwise would require an APR. Additional advantages include radiating tissues with a greater oxygen supply, not radiating the anastomosis, and decreased likelihood of developing radiation enteritis because small bowel is less likely to enter the pelvis. Finally, patients are more likely to complete the course of radiation therapy because it precedes their surgical resection.

The Dutch Colorectal Cancer Group demonstrated a significantly decreased rate of local recurrence at 2 years in patients who received preoperative radiotherapy (20 Gy over 5 days) followed by TME compared with TME alone (2.4% versus 8%).[31] The Swedish trial was the first and only study to demonstrate a survival benefit (58%) for Dukes C patients receiving preoperative radiation (short course of 5 Gy over 5 days) followed by surgery compared with patients who underwent surgery alone (48%).[50] The Swedish trial also demonstrated a decreased rate of local recurrence in the radiation-treated group (11%) compared with 27% in the surgery-alone group. Furthermore, a meta-analysis concluded that preoperative radiation therapy plus surgery compared with surgery alone significantly reduced the 5-year overall mortality rate, cancer-related mortality rate, and local recurrence rate.[51]

Sauer randomly assigned patients with clinical stage II or III rectal cancer to preoperative or postoperative chemotherapy based on a concurrent long course of radiotherapy (5040 cGy delivered in fractions of 180 cGy per day, 5 days per week) and 5-FU (120-hour continuous intravenous infusion during the first and fifth weeks).[52] Six weeks later, TME was performed, followed by four cycles of 5-FU 1 month postoperatively. Despite the preponderance of distal tumors in the preoperative chemoradiation group, there was no difference in overall survival at 4 years. However, there was a significant decrease in the local recurrence rate (6% versus 13%), as well as toxicity, in the patients treated with the neoadjuvant protocol.

Our current practice is to recommend preoperative chemoradiation to our patients with T3 or N1 rectal carcinoma, as well as some patients with bulky T2 lesions near the sphincters (Table 25–6). Neoadjuvant therapy then is followed by TME with APR or TME with an end-to-side, colonic J-pouch, or coloplasty reconstruction.

▪ SURVEILLANCE

After curative resection, long-term follow-up includes routine screening for rectal recurrence and metachronous colorectal neoplasms. Between 60% and 84% of recurrences are seen in the first 24 months and 90% within 48 months. Median time to recurrence is 11–22 months. Local recurrence rates ranges between 4% and 50%. Survival rates vary according to stage (see Table 25–3). Median survival after recurrences are detected is 40 months.

Patients are seen postoperatively at 2 weeks and then every 3 months for 2 years. At each visit, the patient undergoes DRE and sigmoidoscopy, and a CEA level is obtained. At 1 year postresection, a colonoscopy and chest x-ray are performed. Patients continue to be followed every 6 months with CEA levels and physical examinations for a total of 5 years. Colonoscopy is continued yearly for 5 years. At 5 years, if the patient has had no recurrence, he or she may be followed yearly with

TABLE 25–6. CURRENT RECOMMENDATIONS FOR CHEMORADIATION IN RECTAL CANCER PATIENTS AFTER RADICAL RESECTION

Stage I	No adjuvant therapy
Stage II or III	Neoadjuvant chemoradiation for 5 weeks
Low/mid lesion	5-FU based chemotherapy with XRT (180 cGy 5 days/week × 5 weeks)
	Rest for 6 weeks
	Total mesorectal excision
	Rest for 4 weeks
	Continue 5-FU–based chemotherapy for 8 weeks
High lesion	Preop or postop chemotherapy
	Total mesorectal excision
Stage IV	LAR or APR for palliation/prevention of obstruction or bleeding
	Adjuvant chemotherapy
	5-FU + leucovorin ± irinotecan or oxaliplatin with individualized XRT

clinic visits and undergo colonoscopy every 3 to 5 years. Of course, closer observation is indicated for patients at high risk for subsequent cancer formation, such as patients with inflammatory bowel disease, polyposis syndromes, or a strong family history of colorectal cancer.

REFERENCES

1. Jemal A Murray T, Samuels A, et al. Cancer statistics, 2003. *CA Cancer J Clin* 2003;53:5
2. Miles WE: A method of performing abdominoperineal excision for carcinoma of the rectum and the terminal portion of the pelvic colon. *Cancer* 1908;2:1812
3. Heald RJ, Moran BJ, Ryall RD, et al. Rectal cancer: The Basingstoke experience of total mesorectal excision, 1978–1997. *Arch Surg* 1998;133:894–899
4. Wei EK, Giovannucci E, Wu K, et al. Comparison of risk factors for colon and rectal cancer. *Int J Cancer* 2004; 108:433–442
5. Haggitt RC, Glotzbach RE, Soffer EE, et al. Prognostic factors in colorectal carcinomas arising in adenomas: Implications for lesions removed by endoscopic polypectomy. *Gastroenterology* 1985;89:328–336
6. Masaki T, Muto T. Predictive value of histology at the invasive margin in the prognosis of early invasive colorectal carcinoma. *J Gastroenterol* 2000;35:195–200
7. Sato K, Sato T. The vascular and neuronal composition of the lateral ligament of the rectum and the rectosacral fascia. *Surg Radiol Anat* 1991;13:17–22
8. Jones OM, Smeulders N, Wiseman O, et al. Lateral ligaments of the rectum: an anatomical study. *Br J Surg* 1999;86:487–489
9. Scott N, Jackson P, al-Jaberi T, et al. Total mesorectal excision and local recurrence: A study of tumour spread in the mesorectum distal to rectal cancer. *Br J Surg* 1995; 82:1031–1033
10. Hida J, Yasutomi M, Maruyama T, et al. Lymph node metastases detected in the mesorectum distal to carcinoma of the rectum by the clearing method: Justification of total mesorectal excision. *J Am Coll Surg* 1997;184:584
11. Ueno H, Yamauchi C, Hase K, et al. Clinicopathological study of intrapelvic cancer spread to the iliac area in lower rectal adenocarcinoma by serial sectioning. *Br J Surg* 1999;86:1532–1537
12. Enker WE, Kafka NJ, Martz J. Planes of sharp pelvic dissection for primary, locally advanced, or recurrent rectal cancer. *Semin Surg Oncol* 2000;18:199–206
13. Garcia-Aguilar J, Pollack J, Lee SK et al. Accuracy of endorectal ultrasonography in preoperative staging of rectal tumors. *Dis Colon Rectum* 2002;45:10–15
14. Orrom WJ, Wong WD, Rothenberger DA, et al. Endorectal ultrasound in the preoperative staging of rectal tumors: A learning experience. *Dis Colon Rectum* 1990;33:654–659
15. Guillem JG, Moore HG, Akhurst T, et al. Sequential preoperative fluorodeoxyglucose–positron emission tomography assessment of response to preoperative chemoradiation: A means for determining long-term outcomes of rectal cancer. *J Am Coll Surg* 2004;199:1–7
16. Moore HG, Akhurst T, Larson SM, et al. A case-controlled study of 18-fluorodeoxyglucose positron emission tomography in the detection of pelvic recurrence in previously irradiated rectal cancer patients. *J Am Coll Surg* 2003;197:22–28
17. Morson BC, Whiteway JE, Jones EA, et al. Histopathology and prognosis of malignant colorectal polyps treated by endoscopic polypectomy. *Gut* 1984;25:437–444
18. Jessup JM, Stewart AK, Menck HR. The National Cancer Data Base report on patterns of care for adenocarcinoma of the rectum, 1985–1995. *Cancer* 1998;83: 2408
19. Willett CG, Lewandrowski K, Donnelly S, et al. Are there patients with stage I rectal carcinoma at risk for failure after abdominoperineal resection? *Cancer* 1992;69: 1651–1655
20. Clarke JS, Condon RE, Bartlett JG, et al. Preoperative oral antibiotics reduce septic complications of colon operations: Results of prospective, randomized, double-blind clinical study. *Ann Surg* 1977;186:251–259
21. Solla JA, Rothenberger DA: Preoperative bowel preparation: A survey of colon and rectal surgeons. *Dis Colon Rectum* 1990;33:154–159
22. Nichols RL, Smith JW, Garcia RY, et al. Current practices of preoperative bowel preparation among North American colorectal surgeons. *Clin Infect Dis* 1997;24: 609–619
23. Wolmark N, Fisher B. An analysis of survival and treatment failure following abdominoperineal and sphincter-saving resection in Dukes' B and C rectal carcinoma: A report of the NSABP clinical trials. National Surgical Adjuvant Breast and Bowel Project. *Ann Surg* 1986;204: 480–489
24. Vernava AM 3rd, Moran M, Rothenberger DA, et al. A prospective evaluation of distal margins in carcinoma of the rectum. *Surg Gynecol Obstet* 1992;175:333–336
25. Moore HG, Riedel E, Minsky BD, et al. Adequacy of 1-cm distal margin after restorative rectal cancer resection with sharp mesorectal excision and preoperative combined-modality therapy. *Ann Surg Oncol* 2003;10:80–85
26. Nelson H, Petrelli N, Carlin A, et al. Guidelines 2000 for colon and rectal cancer surgery. *J Natl Cancer Inst* 2001; 93:583–596
27. Ota DM, Skibber J, Rich TA. M.D. Anderson Cancer Center experience with local excision and multimodality therapy for rectal cancer. *Surg Oncol Clin North Am* 1992;1:147–152
28. Bleday R, Breen E, Jessup JM, et al. Prospective evaluation of local excision for small rectal cancers. *Dis Colon Rectum* 1997;40:388–392
29. Steele GD, Herndon JE, Bleday R, et al. Sphincter-sparing treatment of distal rectal adenocarcinoma. *Ann Surg Oncol* 1999;6:433–441
30. Guillem JG. Ultra-low anterior resection and coloanal pouch reconstruction for carcinoma of the distal rectum. *World J Surg* 1997;21:721–727
31. Kapiteijn E, Marijnen CA, Nagtegaal ID, et al. Preoperative radiotherapy combined with total mesorectal excision for resectable rectal cancer. *N Engl J Med* 2001;345: 638–646

32. Heald RJ, Husband EM, Ryall RD. The mesorectum in rectal cancer surgery: The clue to pelvic recurrence? *Br J Surg* 1982;69:613–616
33. Wibe A, Eriksen MT, Syse A, et al. Total mesorectal excision for rectal cancer: What can be achieved by a national audit? *Colorectal Dis* 2003;5:471–477
34. Guillem JG, Chessin DB, Cohen AM, et al. Long-term oncologic outcome following preoperative combined modality therapy and total mesorectal excision of locally advanced rectal cancer. *Ann Surg* 2005;241:829–838
35. Havenga K, Enker WE, McDermott K, et al. Male and female sexual and urinary function after total mesorectal excision with autonomic nerve preservation for carcinoma of the rectum. *J Am Coll Surg* 1996;182: 495–502
36. Van Den Brink M, Van Den Hout WB, Stiggelbout AM, et al. Cost-utility analysis of preoperative radiotherapy in patients with rectal cancer undergoing total mesorectal excision: A study of the Dutch Colorectal Cancer Group. *J Clin Oncol* 2004;22:244–253
37. Rothenberger DA, Wong WD. Abdominoperineal resection for adenocarcinoma of the low rectum. *World J Surg* 1992;16:478–485
38. Williams NS, Johnston D. The quality of life after rectal excision for low rectal cancer. *Br J Surg* 1983;70:460–462
39. Enker WE, Havenga K, Polyak T, et al. Abdominoperineal resection via total mesorectal excision and autonomic nerve preservation for low rectal cancer. *World J Surg* 1997;21:715–720
40. Christian CK, Kwaan MR, Betensky RA, et al. Risk factors for perineal wound complications following abdominoperineal resection. *Dis Colon Rectum* 2005;48:43–48
41. Ruo L, Paty PB, Minsky BD, et al. Results after rectal cancer resection with in-continuity partial vaginectomy and total mesorectal excision. *Ann Surg Oncol* 2003;10:664–668
42. Law WL, Chu KW, Choi HK. Total pelvic exenteration for locally advanced rectal cancer. *J Am Coll Surg* 2000; 190:78–83
43. Weiser MR, Milsom JW. Laparoscopic total mesorectal excision with autonomic nerve preservation. *Semin Surg Oncol* 2000;19:396–403
44. Shoup M, Guillem JG, Alektiar KM, et al. Predictors of survival in recurrent rectal cancer after resection and intraoperative radiotherapy. *Dis Colon Rectum* 2002;45:585–592
45. Salo JC, Paty PB, Guillem J, et al. Surgical salvage of recurrent rectal carcinoma after curative resection: A 10-year experience. *Ann Surg Oncol* 1999;6:171–177
46. Miner TJ, Jaques DP, Paty PB, et al. Symptom control in patients with locally recurrent rectal cancer. *Ann Surg Oncol* 2003;10:72–79
47. Wolmark N, Rockette H, Mamounas E, et al. Clinical trial to assess the relative efficacy of fluorouracil and leucovorin, fluorouracil, and levamisole, and fluorouracil, leucovorin, and levamisole in patients with Dukes' B and C carcinoma of the colon: Results from the National Surgical Adjuvant Breast and Bowel Project C-04. *J Clin Oncol* 1999;17:3553–3559
48. Gastrointestinal Tumor Study Group. Prolongation of the disease-free interval in surgically treated rectal carcinoma. *N Engl J Med* 1985;312:1465–1472
49. Krook JE, Moertel CG, Gunderson LL, et al. Effective surgical adjuvant therapy for high-risk rectal carcinoma. *N Engl J Med* 1991;324:709–715
50. Swedish Rectal Cancer Trial. Improved survival with preoperative radiotherapy in respectable rectal cancer. *N Engl J Med* 1997;336:980–987
51. Camma C, Guinta M, Fiorica F, et al. Preoperative radiotherapy for resectable rectal cancer: A meta-analysis. *JAMA* 2000;284;1008–1015
52. Sauer R, Becker H, Hohenberger W, et al. Preoperative versus postoperative chemoradiotherapy for rectal cancer. *N Engl J Med* 2004;351:1731–1740

26

Cancer of the Anus

Najjia N. Mahmoud ■ *Robert D. Fry*

Cancers of the anus are rare problems with diverse histology. While squamous cell carcinoma (SCC) of the anal canal remains by far the most common of these neoplasms and the main focus of this chapter, the anus may also harbor tumors such as adenocarcinoma, melanoma, and basal cell carcinoma. The treatment of anal cancer has undergone dramatic changes in the past 25 years. Multimodality treatment consisting of radiation and chemotherapy has replaced abdominoperineal resection or wide local excision as the mainstay of therapy. Five-year survival rates now exceed 80% and radical surgery is reserved for cancers of the anal canal that do not respond to chemoradiation or that subsequently recur locally. Our understanding of the etiology and epidemiology of anal SCC and its precursor lesions has also profoundly changed in the past few decades, yielding new initiatives in both therapy and prevention that may further alter the future treatment of this disease. The importance of the surgeon's role in the detection and diagnosis of anal cancer remains undiminished. The surgeon is the clinician most likely to diagnose the disease, delegate treatment, and provide follow-up care. Anal cancer is clearly a disease that benefits from multidisciplinary intervention. Because of this, the treatment of anal cancer serves as a paradigm for the multimodality treatment of cancer.

■ ANAL CANAL ANATOMY AND HISTOLOGY

Until recently, discrepancies in anatomic definitions and tumor locations in the anorectal region have made comparisons of therapeutic outcomes difficult. In addition, the evolution of anal canal cancer treatment has resulted in management differences between anal canal and margin tumors that make precise anatomic localization important. In 2000, the World Health Organization refined its definition of "anal canal" and "anal margin" in the context of histology, the American Joint Committee on Cancer (AJCC)/Union Internationale Contre le Cancer (UICC) staging system, and traditional anatomic landmarks. This standardized definition is currently used and endorsed by surgeons, pathologists, and radiologists.[1]

The anal canal extends from the top of the anorectal ring (a palpable convergence of the internal sphincter, deep external sphincter, and puborectalis muscle) to the anal verge (the junction of the anal canal and the hair-bearing keratinized skin of the perineum). The lining of the anal canal is comprised of transitional epithelium as well as non–hair bearing squamous epithelium. Tumors distal or beyond the verge are termed anal margin tumors (Fig 26–1).

The anal canal is divided by the anal transition zone (ATZ) into three histologically distinct areas. The ATZ is a circumferential band that extends above and below the dentate line in fingerlike projections that vary in length. Fenger defined the relationship of the ATZ to the dentate line by staining surgically excised specimens with alcian blue—a dye that renders mucin-rich columnar epithelium dark blue, mucin-poor transitional epithelium light blue, and squamous mucosa colorless.[2] He found that the dentate line ranges from 5–19 mm above the distal end of the anal

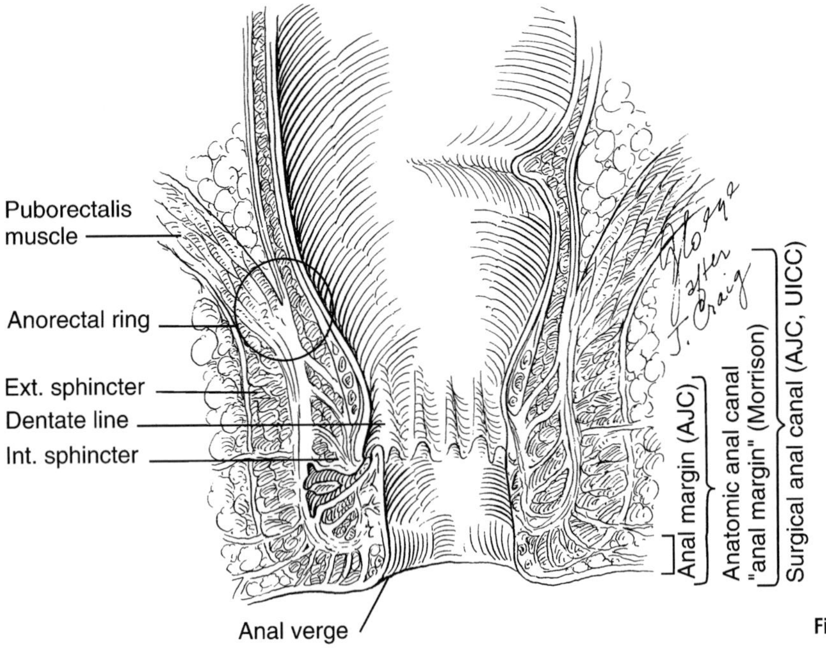

Figure 26–1. Anatomy of the anal canal and margin.

canal. The width of the ATZ is generally 1–2 cm, projecting 3–6 mm below the dentate line.[2] Columnar cells line the anal canal above the ATZ, and squamous epithelium resides below. The ATZ is an area of mixed histology where cuboidal cell types are prevalent. Tumors arising in the anal canal above and within the ATZ are typically nonkeratinizing squamous cell carcinomas. Those originating below this level are generally keratinizing.[2]

Because of the complex gross and histologic anatomy of this region, classification of anal neoplasms has been confusing and inconsistent. According to the World Health Organization classification, anal canal lesions consist of squamous cell (cloacogenic) variants, including keratinizing, nonkeratinizing, and basaloid tumors. Other anal canal neoplasms include adenocarcinoma, carcinoid, lymphoma, and melanoma.[3] Anal margin tumors include squamous cell carcinoma, giant condyloma (verrucous carcinoma), and basal cell carcinoma.[3]

The dentate line provides an anatomic reference point for lymphatic drainage of the anal canal and margin. Above the dentate line, drainage is primarily via the superior rectal lymphatics to the inferior mesenteric nodes and laterally along the middle and inferior rectal vessels to the internal iliac nodal basin. Lesions distal to the line drain to the inguinal and femoral lymphatics. Tumors in the ATZ may follow both lymphatic routes. Patients with unexplained inguinal lymphadenopathy should undergo a careful examination of the anal canal.

▪ ANAL SQUAMOUS CELL CARCINOMA

INCIDENCE AND EPIDEMIOLOGY

The incidence of anal cancer has nearly doubled in the past 20 years to 0.9 cases per 100,000.[4] Although this number represents only 1–2% of all large bowel cancers, the rise in incidence underscores a significant and serious change in the epidemiology of the problem.[5] Squamous cell cancers of the anus are thought to have a viral etiology that is similar to that of cervical cancer. There is much evidence to suggest that high-risk sexual activity in the era of the human immunodeficiency virus (HIV) is responsible for the potentiation of the viruses that cause anal SCC and that the rise in incidence is directly linked to this phenomenon. In the year 2000 approximately 3,400 new cases were reported in the United States, but this figure rose to 3,900 in 2002, reflecting a trend that mirrors increases in HIV infection.[4,5]

Until the past decade, the highest rates of anal SCC were described in women with numbers increasing after 30 years of age to plateau at an incidence of 5.0/100,000 after age 85.[6] The ratio of females to males affected was approximately 2:1.[7] However, in the past decade men under the age of 45 who have sex with men have constituted the group with both the greatest number of reported cases as well as the greatest increase in disease incidence. Currently in the United States, anal cancer occurs more frequently in males than in females.[7]

Considered as a group, men who practice anal-receptive intercourse have an incidence of anal SCC of 35/100,000—a rate identical to that of cervical cancer prior to routine cervical cytological screening.[7] Although not yet listed as an AIDS-defining illness like cervical cancer, the argument has been made that anal SCC should have similar emphasis. The United States AIDS-Cancer registry is a survey that linked AIDS-related cancer registries in 11 states or metropolitan areas for the period of time between 1995–1998 and included over 309,000 HIV-infected patients.[8] The relative risk of SCC-type anogenital cancers in this population was much higher than that of the general population. The relative risks for cervical, vulvar/vaginal, and penile cancers were 5.4, 5.8, and 3.7, respectively, while the risk for anal cancer in women was 6.8 and for men 37.9.[8] Subset analysis of affected individuals revealed that those less than 30 years of age had dramatically elevated relative risks of anal cancer of 134 for women and 162.7 for men. Analyzing the data by HIV exposure history showed that homosexual contact resulted in the highest relative risk of anal SCC, with other categories such as intravenous drug abuse, heterosexual contact among women, and blood transfusion somewhat less.[9]

ETIOLOGY, PATHOGENESIS, AND RISK FACTORS

Human Papillomavirus

Striking evidence, both circumstantial and direct, links human papillomavirus (HPV) infection with the development of both anal squamous cell carcinoma and cervical cancer, and it is accepted that these cancers have not only the same etiology and natural history, but a common mode of transmission.[10] Both anal SCC and cervical SCC arise in mucoepithelial histological transformation zones; both are associated with the same oncogenic HPV strains; and both have noninvasive precursor lesions. Sexual contact is the mode of transmission of HPV. Women with multiple sexual partners, other venereal diseases, or HIV have a significantly increased risk of developing cervical cancer.[11] Women with a prior history of cervical cancer have a relative risk of developing anal SCC of 4.6.[11]

HPV is a double-stranded DNA virus with a predilection for mucoepithelial tissues. More than 100 HPV strains have been identified, but only approximately 30 have been isolated in cancers of the anogenital region.[12] HPV infection results in either anogenital warts (condyloma acuminata) or squamous intraepithelial lesions (SILs).[12] Condylomata are generally associated with HPV 6 and 11 and their subtypes and consist of fleshy growths that harbor and generate infectious viruses and have virtually no malignant potential.[12] SILs are graded on the degree to which they exhibit cytologic atypia. In the U.S., the Bethesda criteria for anal intraepithelial lesions (AIN) lists two dominant categories—high-grade squamous epithelial lesions (HSIL) and low-grade squamous epithelial lesions (LSIL).[13] In the European literature, HSIL is known as AIN 3, whereas LSIL consists of AIN 1 and 2.[13]

The most commonly isolated oncogenic HPV viruses are HPV 16 and 18, which are strongly associated with invasive cancer and are commonly found in both anal and cervical cancer.[13] In a case-control study of 388 patients with anal cancer from Denmark and Sweden, 88% of anal cancers harbored HPV DNA.[14] HPV 16 was detected in 84% of these specimens, whereas no HPV DNA was found in the rectal cancer controls.[14] These investigations have been repeated in SIL with similar results.[15] Studies such as these provide good evidence to support a viral etiology for SIL and anal SCC. Further characterization of specific viral/cytologic changes have focused on defining the differences between LSIL (AIN 1 and 2) and HSIL (AIN 3). LSILs can be associated with both low- and high-risk HPV types, although there is a predominance of high-risk types.[13] It is likely that HSIL contains exclusively high-risk viruses.[13] It may be possible to base pharmacological prevention and intervention in SIL and cancer on the genetic differences between these viruses. Therapies may exploit the fact that on the cellular level, LSILs and condylomata support and tightly regulate the viral infectious cycle, resulting in completion of viral replication and production of intact virus.[13] In contrast, in HSIL certain genes essential to viral expression are lost, thereby facilitating integration into the host genome and producing incomplete viral replication and genetic instability leading to tumorigenesis.[13] It is unclear whether persistent viral infection produces increasing cellular atypia that supports this dysregulation, or whether there is something intrinsic and permissive about the anal epithelium itself that allows oncogenic viruses to exploit the cell cycle.

Human Immunodeficiency Virus Infection

There is an increased incidence of both anal squamous cell carcinoma as well as its precursor lesion HSIL in patients with HIV infection. Data collected in case-control studies among homosexual men and heterosexual women with high-risk behaviors show a direct correlation between HIV seropositivity, HPV prevalence, and anal cancer and its precursors. Epidemiological evidence among homosexual men in the San Francisco Bay area documents a dramatic rise in anal SCC between 1973 and 1999, when the relative risk increased from 3.7 to 20.6.[16] Similar studies conducted in New

York City between the years 1979 and 1985 show a 10-fold increase in anal SCC in men 20–49 years of age that coincided with the explosion of HIV in this population at this time.[11] However, HPV, HSIL, and anal cancer do not seem to be phenomena linked exclusively to homosexuality. Similar findings occur in HIV-infected male heterosexual IV drug users who deny anal-receptive sex. In this cohort, a high rate of HPV infection coincides with an elevated rate of HSIL as well as anal cancer.[17] Heterosexual women who are HIV-positive or have progressed to AIDS have high rates of HSIL as well.[8] When HIV-positive and HIV-negative cohorts (both male and female) with similar HPV risk factors are compared, the rates of both HSIL and anal cancer are dramatically increased in the HIV-positive groups.[8–11]

Although the resultant decline in cell-mediated immunity in HIV-infected patients seems to correlate with HPV infection, the exact mechanism of potentiation is unknown. In fact, there is evidence to support the hypothesis that HPV may represent an opportunistic infection assisted by retroviral preinfection.[8] It is uncertain whether the level of immunity and the severity of HIV infection as measured by CD4 counts directly correlate with HSIL or SCC rates in cervical or anal cancer. However, several studies done in the past 10 years have demonstrated an inverse relationship between CD4 counts and progression from LSIL to HSIL, supporting a causal relationship between cell-mediated immunosuppression and high-risk phenotypes.[12] Conversely, a recent subgroup analysis of a 202-member HIV-positive cohort receiving highly active antiretroviral therapy (HAART) for 6 months indicates that the rates of HPV infection, HPV levels, and progression of anal dysplasia remained unchanged in spite of significant improvement in CD4 counts.[8] Longer follow-up is certainly needed to determine whether advances in the treatment of HIV will correlate with lower rates of HPV positivity, anal dysplasia, and anal cancer.

Persistence of high-risk HPV types 16 and 18 in HIV-infected individuals is a well-documented problem. Lingering infection, immunosuppression, and the presence of the HIV virus may all be factors contributing to a lack of viral cell-cycle regulation, increased proliferation, diminished apoptosis, and faulty DNA repair. These individuals have a twofold increased risk over non-HIV infected patients of progression from LSIL to HSIL within 2 years of diagnosis, and have a relative risk of anal cancer of 63.4 over the general population.[13]

Smoking

Cigarette smoking is a well-known risk factor for anal squamous cell carcinoma that is independent of sexual practices. The risk increases two- to fivefold over that of the general population.[11,18] It is speculated based on data demonstrating an increased incidence in premenopausal women of 5.6 with a 6.7% linear increase per pack-year, that smoking may have some antiestrogenic effect permissive for the disease in the estrogen-sensitive tissues of the anal canal.[19] This hypothesis is supported by the finding that no risk increase was demonstrated by this study in either postmenopausal female or male smokers.

Chronic Inflammation

At one time, benign anorectal conditions such as hemorrhoids, fissures, and fistulas were thought to predispose to the development of squamous cell carcinoma (SCC). The etiology or common mechanism was presumed to be prolonged exposure of the anal canal epithelium and margin to chronic inflammatory conditions. Patients with inflammatory bowel disease were believed to be at increased risk, particularly when anal fistulas were present. In 1994, Frisch examined this issue in a large population and found no evidence to support a causal relationship between benign anorectal conditions and anal cancer up to 13 years after resolution of the benign condition.[20] In another large population study, Frisch and Johansen identified 9,602 Danish patients with a diagnosis of either Crohn's disease or ulcerative colitis with a mean follow-up of 10 years.[21] Only two patients developed anal squamous cell carcinoma during this time. Both patients had the disease longer than 15 years. Although long-term irritable bowel disease patients may be at slightly increased risk of anal SCC, short- and mid-term risk is not significantly different from that of the general population.[21]

ANAL INTRAEPITHELIAL NEOPLASIA

No discussion of anal squamous cell carcinoma would be complete without a consideration of its precursor lesion, anal intraepithelial neoplasia (AIN). The term high-grade squamous intraepithelial lesion (HSIL) is synonymous with AIN 3 (European designation), "carcinoma-in-situ," and "Bowen's disease." Bowen's disease is still a term frequently used to describe this entity and may refer to scaly, pruritic low-profile inflammatory perianal manifestations of AIN. Low-grade squamous intraepithelial lesions (LSILs) are called AIN 1 and 2 in Europe and describe a lesser degree of cellular atypia. Until recently, wide local excision had been the treatment of choice for HSIL (Bowen's disease). It was assumed, based on anecdotal evidence, that a percentage of patients with HSIL progress to invasive cancer. This led to attempts to surgically clear patients of the disease. Recent advances in the understanding of the natural history of LSIL, HSIL, and anal cancer have more clearly defined the risk of dysplasia, leading many to adopt a policy of either very specific ablative therapy or close and frequent observation.

The incidence of anal cancer among HIV-positive homosexual men is 75–80/100,000 (a rate of 0.8/100,000 in the general population), more than twice the incidence of cervical cancer in women (35/100,000) prior to the introduction of routine cervical Pap smear cytology evaluations.[8,16] Because of the dramatic reduction in cervical cancer (8/100,000 currently) attributed to the detection of dysplasia, it is widely believed that the same result could be seen in high-risk anal cancer populations if similar detection and ablation methods are used. A predicate to this hypothesis, however, is to better establish the role of equivalent potential precursor lesions in the development of invasive anal cancer.

There is a very high incidence of HSIL in the same population affected by high rates of anal cancer. In one study of 67 HIV-positive homosexual men (MSM) and 50 HIV-positive IV drug users who denied anal intercourse, HSIL was present in 85% of the MSM group and 46% of the IV drug users.[22] In a large group of HIV-positive women followed by the Women's Interagency HIV Study, 6% of HIV-positive and 2% of HIV-negative women had HSIL.[23] Seventy-nine percent of the HIV-positive women in this study were HPV-positive.[23] A similar result was documented in the University of California, San Francisco (UCSF) Anal Neoplasia Registry, where the vast majority of HIV-positive (93%) and HIV-negative (61%) homosexual men had HPV infection, whereas only 5% of the HIV-positive and only 1 HIV-negative man had HSIL.[24] Cytologic testing (anal Pap smears) in this group was abnormal in 60% of the HIV-positive and 21% of the HIV-negative men.[24] Clearly, abnormal anal cytology does not necessarily correlate with HSIL. Furthermore, it is clear that not all patients with HSIL progress to invasive cancer. Not enough longitudinal studies have been conducted, however, to specifically quantify the risk associated with either the presence of HPV or HSIL. The 4-year projected incidence of HSIL in HIV-positive men in the study mentioned is 49% and in HIV-negative homosexual men it is 17%.[24] Ongoing studies will help establish actual rates of conversion to invasion, associated risk factors, and high-risk populations.

Diagnosis and Treatment of High-Grade Squamous Intraepithelial Lesions

A growing awareness of the natural history of anal cancer has resulted in an increase in diagnosis of the problem in high-risk populations. Anal cytology (similar to cervical Pap smears) is currently being used by some physicians as a screening tool for the detection of anal dysplasia in high-risk populations. Prior to the present understanding of the pathogenesis of anal cancer, HSIL was most commonly (25–40% of cases) discovered as an incidental finding after hemorrhoidectomy.[25] Other patients came to attention with scaly, raised lesions at the anal margin. Because the majority of patients diagnosed are asymptomatic, the true incidence of HSIL is not presently known. Future studies following patients with abnormal anal cytology may clarify this number.

Anal screening (Pap smears) was first described in the 1990s as a direct corollary of cervical Pap smears and has since been promoted as a diagnostic and screening tool in high-risk populations.[26] However, evidence demonstrating a resulting decrease in the incidence of anal cancer similar to that of cervical cancer has not been forthcoming. Still, only a very short time has passed since the institution of the technique. The use of anal cytology as a screening technique has not gained the recognition afforded cervical Pap smears. Lack of recognition by clinicians of the increased incidence of anal cancer, limitation of the problem to high-risk populations, lack of knowledge of techniques, cost, and a dearth of supporting outcomes data may all conspire to limit the perceived usefulness of the technique. Ongoing outcome studies may clarify the role of anal Pap smear for high-risk patients.

A 1999 survey of the practice patterns of members of the American Society of Colon and Rectal Surgeons revealed that 86–95% of surgeons treated HSIL with wide local excision.[27] A distinction was made between "microscopic" disease and other manifestations. Most HSIL found incidentally in hemorrhoidectomy specimens were considered microscopic asymptomatic disease and simply followed without re-excision (74%).[27] This survey coincided with other investigations highlighting the multifocal nature of HSIL and the difficulty presented by wide local excision under these circumstances. In one review of 34 patients undergoing wide local excision for macroscopically evident HSIL, 19 had positive margins at the time of initial resection, and 12 of the 19 had recurrent HSIL within 1 year.[28] Even with a microscopically complete initial resection, 2 of 15 patients eventually developed HSIL. Although none of these individuals subsequently developed anal cancer, five developed significant surgical complications of resection including anal stenosis and incontinence.[28]

A growing recognition of the morbidity of surgery for HSIL, particularly asymptomatic microscopic disease, in light of the uncertain natural history of anal neoplasia and dysplasia has resulted in uncertainty concerning appropriate treatment. In the early 1990s high-resolution anoscopy (HRA) was developed at the UCSF. Like anal Pap cytologies, HRA is a direct application of the technology for cervical intraepithelial detection and ablation to anal dysplasia. The technique can be done in either the office, or for anal margin involvement or more extensive disease, in the operating room. After obtaining a Pap smear, a digital rectal exam is performed followed by placement of a cotton swab covered in gauze soaked in 3% acetic acid. The swab is held in place for 1 minute after which an anoscope is inserted, permitting examination of the anal canal by a colposcope providing 6- to 25-times magnification. Special attention is directed to the area surrounding the ATZ. Applying acetic acid causes these often inapparent lesions to become opaque or "acetowhite." Lugol's iodine solution is then placed in the anal canal to further highlight these areas. HSILs fail to take up Lugol's, rendering the area yellow to tan, whereas normal tissue or LSILs stain dark brown or black.[26] This approach, combined with the magnification, allows visualization of vascular changes such as punctate appearance, mosaicism, and atypical vessels characteristic of dysplastic change.[26] Suspicious lesions are then destroyed by electrocautery. Over 400 patients have been prospectively evaluated at UCSF with HRA. Patients with findings of HSIL have gone on to HRA with ablation. Over 75% of HIV-positive patients with "extensive" circumferential disease have had recurrent HSIL on follow-up (2.5 years). None of these patients have thus far developed anal cancer.[26]

There are no prospective studies or published reports documenting the rate of progression of HSIL to invasive cancer. While treatment strategies for anal HSIL vary widely, no approach has been conclusively shown to reduce anal cancer incidence. The rate of HSIL progression to anal cancer has, based on clinical models, been proposed as 1% per year.[12] Because the rate is so low and the natural history of HSIL as yet unknown, chemotherapy and radiation are unwarranted. Wide local excisional techniques that compromise form and function may also be too drastic given the apparent low malignant potential of HSIL. HRA with ablation may specifically eradicate early invasive lesions and aggressive precursors, but data supporting that position do not yet exist. Furthermore, HRA ablative therapy does not eliminate the need for follow-up.

While many clinicians advocate a program of close follow-up consisting of digital rectal exams and unmagnified anoscopy at regular intervals, this approach, too, is unvalidated. HRA may provide objective evidence of the presence of disease that office examination alone does not. Whether ablative therapies should follow documentation of HSIL by any method remains unknown and controversial.

Human Papillomavirus Vaccines

Both prophylactic and therapeutic vaccines to HPV are currently through Phase III trials targeting cervical cancer, testing both types of vaccine in high-risk populations.[13] Prophylactic or preventive vaccines are typically made from structural viral proteins, while therapeutic vaccines are made from the early viral replication proteins E6 and E7. In 2006, the FDA granted approval to the first vaccine designed to prevent cervical cancer. Gardisil (Merck & Co., Inc, Whitehouse Station, NJ) is a recombinant vaccine against HPV types 6, 11, 16, and 18. It is currently approved for use in females age 9–26 years of age and requires a series of three injections over a 6 month period. A total of 21,000 patients in four randomized trials demonstrated a dramatic, nearly 100% prevention rate in genital warts, and vulvar, vaginal, and cervical precancerous lesions caused by the serotypes against which the vaccine is directed. The vaccine is only effective, however, in patients not previously exposed to the viruses included in the vaccine, and it confers no protection against viruses not covered by the vaccine. Ongoing post-approval studies will focus on actual rates of cervical cancer prevention in this cohort, prevention of HPV infection in males, and other long-term safety and efficacy endpoints.

Other studies have combined aerosolized delivery mechanisms with intramuscular injections to maximize antibody titers against the virus. Although the practicality of prevention of dysplasia and cancer by vaccines is unclear at this time, results from these studies may clarify the situation in the near future.

Stressgen Biotechnologies, Inc. has developed a therapeutic vaccine for anal HSIL that has completed Phase II clinical trials in HIV negative patients.[13] The vaccine is a recombinant fusion protein called HspE7. The immune response generated by the vaccine seems to be CD8 dependent alone—CD4 cells do not seem to be involved. Of those patients receiving 500 mcg doses, 76% showed regression of their HSIL to LSIL, one of the primary endpoints of the study. Approximately 7 months elapsed before the first complete responses began to appear. Even so, results seem durable with 86% of this group remaining in remission at 15 months. Although the study samples are small and this approach has yet to be validated in HIV positive immunocompromised patients, early evidence supports an optimistic outlook for the field of HPV therapeutic vaccines.[13]

PATHOLOGY, DIAGNOSIS, AND STAGING OF ANAL SQUAMOUS CELL CANCER

Pathology

Nearly 80% of anal canal tumors are either squamous cell carcinomas or histologic variants of SCC. The great variation in terminology results from the histologically diverse microscopic anatomy and the fact that many tumors, especially in the anal transition zone, have a mixed histologic appearance, including squamous, basaloid, and rarely glandular elements. The World Health Organization designates all squamous carcinoma variants in this location as "cloacogenic."[3] Tumors of the distal anal canal, and particularly of the anal margin, are generally comprised predominantly of squamous cells, with fewer basaloid and no glandular characteristics.[29] The more distal in the anal canal the squamous tumor arises, generally the more likely it is to contain keratinizing cells. Tumors of the proximal anal canal and ATZ are usually composed of nonkeratinizing cells.[29] It is important to note that the difference in the cellular characteristics of these anal canal cancers does not result in a different mode of treatment. There are no data to suggest differences in outcome between squamous and basaloid histologic types in anal canal cancers. Anal margin tumors, however, are typically treated like skin cancers, by local excision.

The treatment of anal canal cancer has undergone major changes within the past 25 years. Currently chemotherapy and radiation is usually the sole treatment for patients with this disease. Prior to 1974, the standard of care was either wide local excision if the tumor was judged to be superficial, or abdominoperineal excision for (APR) tumors invading the sphincter. Outcomes were poor, with overall survival rates after APR ranging from 30–70%, depending on tumor grade, stage, and size.[30] The local recurrence rate after wide resection or APR was reported to be 25–35% with a 100% local recurrence rate for tumors invading through the submucosa in a series from Singh and associates at Roswell Park Memorial Institute.[31] Perineal or pelvic recurrence occurs in 50–70% of patients undergoing APR, with less than 10% dying of distant disseminated disease.[7] In 1974, Norman Nigro at Wayne State University used radiation and fluoropyrimidines in anal canal cancer as a way to reduce local recurrence following APR.[32] He observed that often there was no residual cancer in the resected specimen. Thus began an exciting and revolutionary time in the treatment of this disease that resulted in a radical shift in treatment.

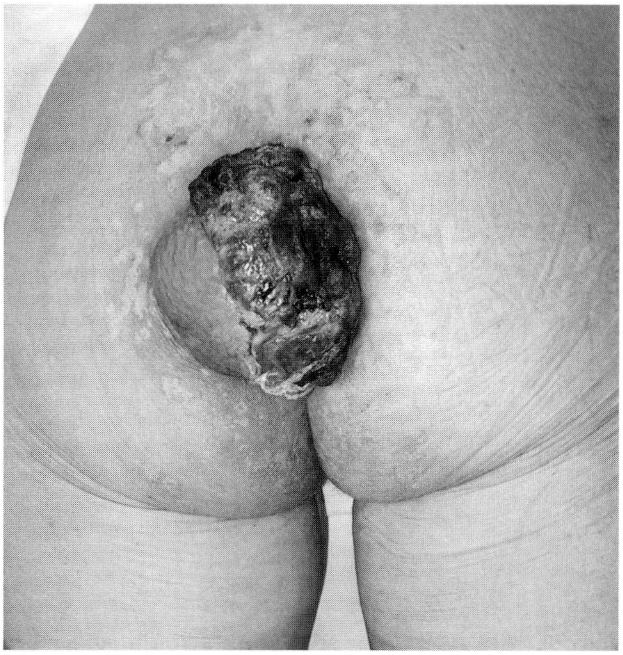

Figure 26–2. Large, fungating anal squamous cell carcinoma. (Courtesy Charles Friel, MD.)

Diagnosis and Staging

Over 50% of patients present with a complaint of rectal bleeding. Delays in diagnosis are common because the tumor is often mistaken by both patients and physicians for benign conditions such as hemorrhoids or fissures (Fig 26–2). Pain, tenesmus, and pruritus may be present. The initial physical examination should include a digital rectal exam, proctoscopy, and inspection of the inguinal lymph nodes. A biopsy of the anal mass is necessary to confirm the diagnosis. Inguinal masses should be aspirated with a fine needle for diagnosis and staging. Because the current nonoperative approach to anal cancer management is highly effective, excisional biopsy of suspected anal squamous cell cancers and inguinal node dissection for adenopathy should generally be avoided. The staging process is completed by computed tomography of the chest, abdomen, and pelvis, and a transanal ultrasound to assess depth of invasion and aid in establishing the size of the tumor (Figs 26–3A and B).

The IUCC staging system for anal cancer was updated in 1997 and adopted by the AJCC[7] (Table 26–1). In contrast to staging parameters for other gastrointestinal lesions, it is based upon size rather than depth of invasion. Anal margin tumors are staged and treated the same as skin cancers (Fig 26–4).

A number of reviews in the literature prior to and during the introduction of chemoradiotherapy for anal squamous cell carcinoma document the strong correlation between tumor size, lymphatic spread, and prognosis.[33] In a 1984 report from the M.D. Anderson Cancer Center, 132 patients treated by APR for anal squamous cell carcinoma were studied. For patients with tumors 1–2 cm in size, survival was 78%; 3- to 5-cm tumors had survival of 55%; and patients with tumors >6 cm experienced survival of only 40%.[33] Other reviews suggest that survival for large tumors is considerably worse, at less than 20%, and that generally overall survival is diminished when tumor size is greater than 5 cm, whether the tumor is treated by excision or chemoradiotherapy.[34–37]

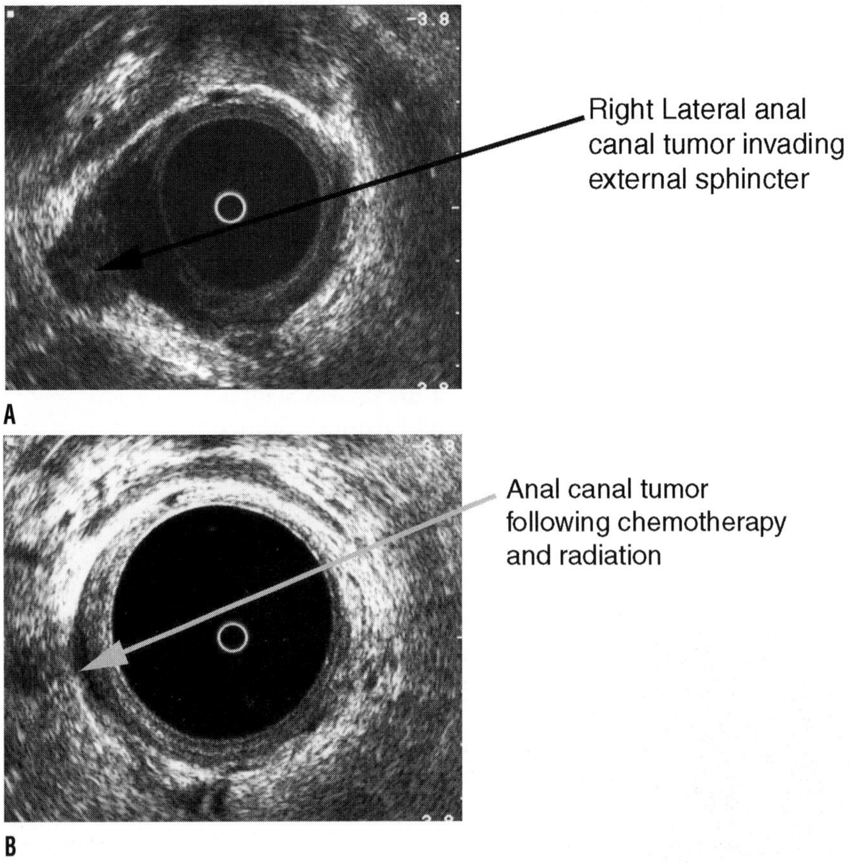

Figure 26–3. A. Endoanal ultrasound of a squamous cell carcinoma of the anal canal invading the anal sphincters prior to chemoradiation. **B.** The patient shown 4 months after 4,500 Gy radiation, cisplatin, and 5-fluorouracil. The patient has had a complete clinical response to therapy. (Courtesy Najjia N. Mahmoud, MD.)

The presence of regional nodal metastases is a poor prognostic indicator regardless of treatment modality. Although survival in the face of nodal metastases has improved significantly with the use of chemoradiation, patients who present with metastatic disease have a significant survival disadvantage.[33,34] Prior to the routine use of chemoradiotherapy, a report in which surgery was done with and without preoperative radiation demonstrated a 5-year survival rate of 44% for node-positive patients compared to 74% for node-negative patients.[33] Other studies confirm comparatively poor survival for patients with nodal metastases.[34]

SURGICAL MANAGEMENT

Operative therapy for anal canal squamous cell carcinoma has largely been supplanted by chemoradiation and is now the exception rather than the rule. Historically, the failure rate for APR has depended rather predictably on the size of the primary tumor. This procedure was often accompanied by prophylactic inguinal node dissection, but the morbidity and lack of efficacy caused inguinal lymphadenectomy to be abandoned. Failure rates for APR range from 40–70%, with local failure rates of 40% and median survival time after recurrence of only 1 year.[30]

Although chemotherapy and radiation have been shown to result in higher disease-free survival rates, there may still be a role for local excision in some cases of anal canal carcinoma. A retrospective analysis of local excision at the University of Minnesota revealed a direct correlation between survival and tumor size. For tumors greater than 2.5 cm, 5-year survival rates were 60%.[38] Although the sample size was small, the authors advocated local resection with curative intent for small (<1 cm) well-differentiated tumors confined to the submucosa.[38] Corman and Haggitt reported a similar experience, with all tumors confined to the submucosa being cured by local excision or APR, and those invading more deeply suffering eventual local recurrence.[39] Longo and colleagues recorded a 62% failure rate in stage I–III tumors undergoing solely local excision, in which all patients with stage II and III tumors recurred.[40] Tumor accessibility, full-thickness excision, depth of invasion, and negative margins seem imperative technical considerations when considering local resection. Even so, very few candidates are suitable for this approach.

TABLE 26–1. AJCC STAGING SYSTEM FOR ANAL CANAL CARCINOMA

PRIMARY TUMOR (T)
TX: Primary tumor cannot be assessed
T0: No evidence of primary tumor
Tis: Carcinoma in situ
T1: Tumor 2 cm or less in greatest dimension
T2: Tumor more than 2 cm but no more than 5 cm in greatest dimension
T3: Tumor more than 5 cm in greatest dimension
T4: Tumor of any size that invades adjacent organ(s) (e.g., vagina, urethra, or bladder[a])
REGIONAL LYMPH NODES (N)
NX: Regional lymph nodes cannot be assessed
N0: No regional lymph node metastasis
N1: Metastasis in perirectal lymph node(s)
N2: Metastasis in unilateral internal iliac and/or inguinal lymph node(s)
N3: Metastasis in perirectal and inguinal lymph nodes and/or bilateral internal iliac and/or inguinal lymph nodes
DISTANT METASTASIS (M)
MX: Distant metastasis cannot be assessed
M0: No distant metastasis
M1: Distant metastasis
STAGE GROUPINGS
Stage 0:
Tis, N0, M0
Stage I:
T1, N0, M0
Stage II:
T2, N0, M0
T3, N0, M0
Stage IIIA:
T1, N1, M0
T2, N1, M0
T3, N1, M0
T4, N0, M0
Stage IIIB:
T4, N1, M0
Any T, N2, M0
Any T, N3, M0
Stage IV:
Any T, any N, M1

[a]Direct invasion of the rectal wall, perirectal skin, subcutaneous tissue, or the sphincter muscle(s) is not classified as T4.
Adapted, with permission, from American Joint Committee on Cancer. *AJCC Cancer Staging Manual*, 6th ed. New York, NY: Springer; 2002:125-130.

CHEMORADIATION

The treatment of anal canal carcinoma has changed radically since the late 1970s, with the advent of chemoradiation protocols. In 1974 Norman Nigro defined a treatment protocol involving the administration of 5-fluorouracil (5-FU), mitomycin-C, and preoperative radiation to shrink anal canal tumors.[32] Fluoropyrimidines were known at the time to enhance the effect of radiation, and there was some evidence that mitomycin had an antineoplastic effect on squamous cell tumors. Nigro's protocol was neoadjuvant, and the radiation (30 Gy total) was given in 15 sessions over a 3-week period. The 5-FU was administered at a dose of 1,000 mg/m^2/day, for 4 days starting on the first day of radiation therapy, as a continuous infusion. It was then repeated on days 29 through 32. Mitomycin-C (15 mg/m^2) was administered as a single dose on treatment day one.[32] Of the three patients in the initial report, two underwent APR 6 weeks after treatment. The third refused surgery and remained disease-free. No evidence of tumor was found in the specimens of the two patients who underwent surgery.[32]

Following the dramatic results reported by Nigro's group, others followed suit, treating patients with both radiation alone and with multimodality therapy followed by surgical excision. In 1983, Michaelson and associates at Memorial Sloan-Kettering Cancer Center (MSKCC) reported that 52% of patients treated with both chemotherapy and radiation had a complete pathological response, and another 22% had only microscopic disease at operation.[41] All of these patients had undergone APR or wide local excision following treatment. After Nigro's 1974 publication, a number of other investigators examined the effects of multimodality therapy. Most used 5-FU and mitomycin-C as the chemotherapeutic regimen, although several made dose and infusion modifications, and nearly all increased the radiation dose. Maximal doses were in the range of 50 Gy. Because of such variability among therapies, meta-analysis is difficult. However, direct comparison between studies is useful.[30]

Preliminary studies done by Nigro and others set the stage for prospective Phase II studies. Among these, Martenson and colleagues reported on an Eastern Cooperative Oncology Group (ECOG) study of 50 patients receiving 40 Gy of radiation with a 10–13 Gy boost to the tumor.[42] Bolus 5-FU and mitomycin-C was given during radiation, and biopsy of the tumor or tumor site was performed 6–8 weeks later. APR was performed if the biopsy was positive. Of 46 patients completing treatment, 34 (74%) had a complete response and 11 had a partial response.[42] Eighty percent had no locoregional recurrence and 58% were disease-free at 7 years.[42]

The Radiation Treatment Oncology Group (RTOG) and ECOG reported on an intergroup trial of 79 patients treated with combined radiation and chemotherapy in 1989. The radiation dose was 40.8 Gy and only 8 patients had evidence of disease requiring APR at the completion of therapy. At 3 years, overall survival and local control rates were 73% and 71%, respectively.[43]

Further series from MSKCC supported the ECOG and intergroup study. Forty-two patients were treated with a total dose of 30 Gy and the 5-FU/mitomycin-C combination.[44] Eighteen patients had positive biopsy results after treatment but only half of these had local

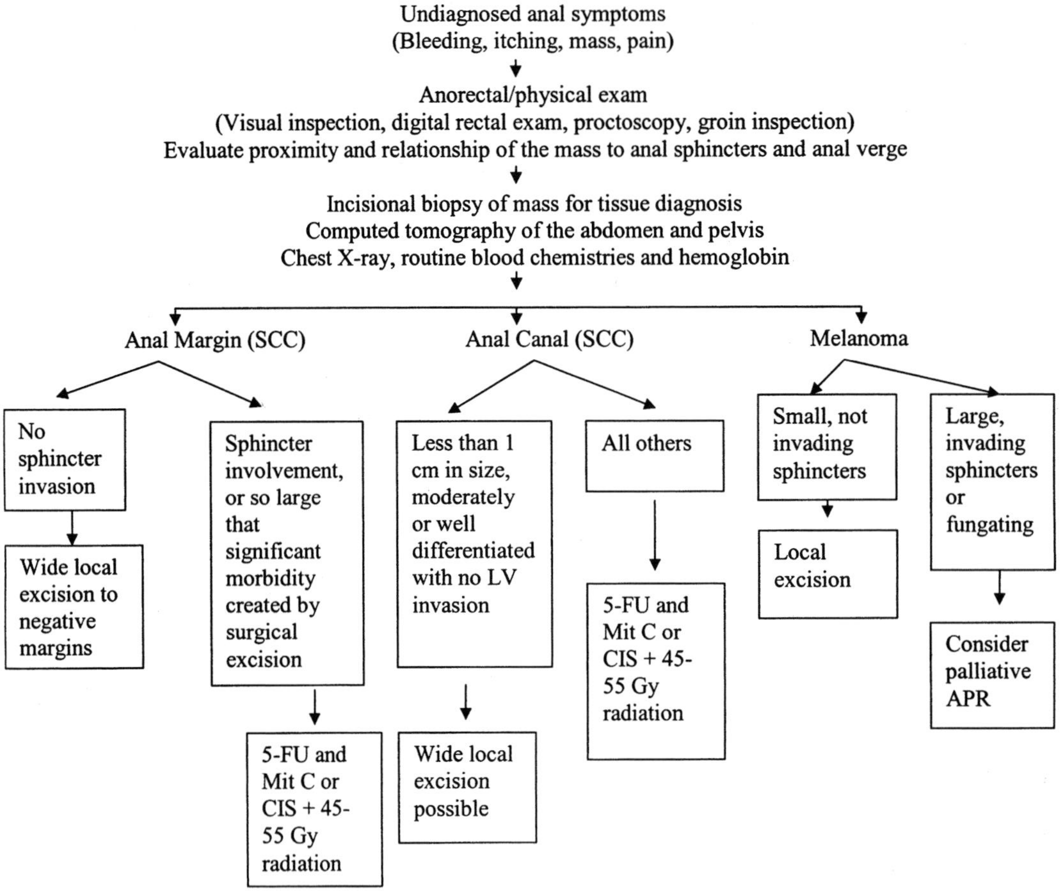

Figure 26–4. Basic treatment algorithm for most common anal neoplasms.

recurrence on follow-up. The 5 year disease-free survival rate was 82%.[44]

In all of these small Phase II trials, disease-free survival, colostomy-free survival, and local disease control compared very favorably to the standard surgical approach. However, the toxicities encountered were significant. In the ECOG study, 37% of patients suffered severe toxicities including severe neutropenia, moist desquamation of the perianal skin, and diarrhea.[42] Treatment toxicities like these gave rise to questions regarding the necessity of chemotherapy in anal cancer in spite of its early promise. Concurrent studies examined the role of radiation alone, often in doses substantially higher than those used with chemotherapy. At the Institute Curie, 183 patients receiving a dose between 60 and 65 Gy showed a 59% 5-year survival rate with a local control rate of 69%.[45] A similar 5-year survival rate of 61% was demonstrated in a review of 147 patients from the Hospital Tenon.[36] Local control in this study was 71%. Complications of higher-dose radiation included anal ulceration and stenosis requiring surgery in 5–15% of cases.

In the late 1990s three Phase III trials reported direct comparisons between radiation alone and radiation with concurrent chemotherapy (Table 26–2). In 1996, the United Kingdom Coordinating Committee on Cancer Research (UKCCCR) published the largest prospective randomized study of chemotherapy and radiation versus radiation alone.[46] The trial enrolled 585 patients, assigning them to either combined therapy or radiation, and then assessed them at 6 weeks. Poor responders were offered APR while those responding well received boost radiotherapy and reassessment. Those patients receiving only radiation had a local failure rate of 59%, whereas those with multimodality therapy recorded a 36% local failure rate with a mean follow-up time of 42 months. Although the early morbidity of combination therapy was higher than that with radiation alone (including two deaths from sepsis), the late morbidity rate was the same. Both the local failure rate as well as the number of patients requiring salvage surgery was halved compared to radiation alone. In all, 29/174 patients who had received combined therapy with a boost required salvage APR, compared to 72/188 who had received radiation alone. Although the local failure rate for radiation alone was higher, overall survival be-

TABLE 26–2. RANDOMIZED PHASE III TRIALS OF RADIATION AND CHEMOTHERAPY FOR ANAL CANAL CANCER

	Study Arms	Radiation Dose	Chemotherapy	Number of Eligible Patients	Stoma-Free Survival	Local Failure Rate	Overall Survival
EORTC[42]	Radiation alone	45 Gy + 15–20 Gy boost if CR/PR	None	103	22%	69%	56%
	Radiation + 5-FU/Mit-C	45 Gy + 15–20 Gy boost if CR/PR	5-FU, Mit-C	103	41% ($p = 0.002$)	42% ($p = 0.02$)	56% NSS
UKCCCR[41]	Radiation alone	45 Gy + 15–20 Gy boost if CR/PR	None	285	N/A	59%	58% (3-year)
		45 Gy + 15–20 Gy boost if CR/PR	5-FU, Mit-C	145	59%	36% ($p < 0.0001$)	65% (3-year) NSS
RTOG/ECOG[43]	Radiation + 5-FU	45 Gy	5-FU	145	59%	36%	67%
	Radiation + 5-FU/Mit-C	45 Gy	5-FU, Mit-C	146	71% ($p = 0.0019$)	18% ($p = 0.0001$)	76% ($p = 0.18$)

CR/PR, complete response/partial response; 5-FU, 5-fluorouracil; Mit-C, mitomycin-C; NSS, not statistically significant; N/A, not available.
Modified, with permission, from Chawla AK, Willett CG. Squamous cell carcinoma of the anal canal and anal margin. *Hematol Oncol Clin North Am* 2001; 15:321-344.

tween the groups was not statistically significant (58% radiation versus 65% chemoradiation at 3 years).[46]

The results of the European Organization for Research and Treatment of Cancer (EORTC) supported those of the UKCCCR trial.[47] Patients with locally advanced (T3–T4) cancers were randomized to radiation alone (45 Gy plus a boost of 15–20 Gy) versus combination therapy with 5-FU/mitomycin-C. With the addition of chemotherapy, the local failure rate dropped from 69% to 42% and colostomy-free survival increased from 22% to 41%. Early and late complication rates were similar except for anal ulcers, which were slightly increased in the combined group. As in the UKCCCR trial, although local control and colostomy-free survival rates were much improved over that of radiation alone, the rate of distant spread was unchanged. Overall survival between the two groups in this study was 56% at 5 years.[47]

In 1996, Flam and colleagues explored further the role of mitomycin-C as a radiation sensitizing agent in a phase III RTOG/ECOG trial.[48] Three hundred ten patients were enrolled and randomized to receive either radiation/5-FU or radiation/5-FU and mitomycin-C. They concluded that although the addition of mitomycin-C produced slightly greater toxicity, at 4 years the disease-free survival was higher (73% versus 51%; $p = 0.0003$) and the colostomy rate was lower (9% versus 22%; $p = 0.002$). While the 5-FU/mitomycin-C/radiation group had a good overall survival of 76%, this was not statistically different from that of the comparison group at 67% ($p = 0.18$). However, the role of mitomycin-C was validated.[48]

The RTOG/ECOG study also examined the ability to salvage patients with residual cancer in their post-treatment biopsy with additional chemotherapy and radiation. Of the 24 patients on the trial eligible to undergo salvage, 12 were rendered free of disease with a 9-Gy boost, 5-FU, and cisplatin (100 mg/m^2).[48] It has been suggested that the patients who underwent salvage chemoradiotherapy in this trial may have been free of disease secondary to radiation-induced apoptosis if the period prior to biopsy had been extended. It is unclear whether cisplatin was actually responsible for the results, but interest in the agent was sparked, given the treatment-limiting toxicities of mitomycin-C. Cisplatin is well-known as a radiation sensitizer and effective agent in the treatment of SCC in other areas such as cervix, head and neck, and esophagus. There have been two Phase II trials of high-dose radiation and 5-FU in combination with cisplatin for anal canal cancer. These studies showed complete response rates of 70–95% with reduced toxicity compared to mitomycin-C.[42,49] RTOG 98-11 is a Phase III study currently underway directly comparing mitomycin-C with cisplatin (Table 26–3).[50–53]

Based on these data, radiation (4500–5400 Gy), 5-FU, and either cisplatin or mitomycin-C constitutes primary treatment of most anal squamous cell carcinomas. At the University of Pennsylvania, cisplatin is the chemotherapeutic agent of choice. Small (<1 cm), well-differentiated cancers without evidence of lymphovascular invasion may be excised primarily if negative margins are achieved without sphincter compromise.

TREATMENT OF INGUINAL NODAL METASTASES

Palpable inguinal lymph nodes (LN) should be biopsied or evaluated by fine-needle aspiration at the onset of treatment for staging. Several reviews have confirmed the poor prognostic outlook conferred by in-

TABLE 26–3. RECENT TRIALS OF CHEMORADIATION FOR ANAL CANAL CANCER

Study	N	Stage	Follow-Up (Months)	Chemotherapy	Radiation	CR	Stoma-Free Survival	Local Control	Survival
Klass 1999[38]	122	T1–4	48	5-FU, Mit-C	35–45 Gy	N/A	N/A	N/A	57%[a]
Faynsod 2000[50]	30	Stage I–IV	40	5-FU, Mit-C	45–55 Gy	94%	N/A	64%	74%[a]
Mitchell 2001[51]	49	Stage I–IIIB	9.8 y	5-FU, Mit-C or CIS for tumors >3 cm (n = 26)	45–60 + 10–15 Gy boost	T1–2 74% T3–4 33%	81%	85%	Stage I[a] 62% Stage II 68% Stage IIIA 100% Stage IIIB 70%
Kapp 2001[52]	39	T1–4, N0–2, M0	31	5-FU, Mit-C for tumors >3 cm (n = 28)	Split-dose 50.4 with 6 Gy brachy-therapy	80%	73%	76%	76%[b]
Peiffert 2001[53]	80	>4 cm and/ or LN+	29	5-FU, CIS	45 Gy + 15–20 Gy boost	67%	73% (3 y)	84% (3 y)	86%[c]

[a]5-year overall survival.
[b]5-year disease-specific survival.
[c]3-year overall survival.
CR, complete response; 5-FU, 5-fluorouracil; Mit-C, mitomycin-C; CIS, cisplatin; LN, lymph node; N/A, not available.
Modified, with permission, from Chawla AK, Willett CG. Squamous cell carcinoma of the anal canal and anal margin. *Hematol Oncol Clin North Am* 2001; 15:321-344.

guinal LN metastases. In 1970, Stearns and Quan reviewed the MSKCC experience with anal canal cancer and noted that only 14% of patients with synchronous nodal metastases survived for 5 years.[54] Similarly, O'Brien and colleagues reported in 1982 that none of the 52% of patients presenting with synchronous LN involvement survived more than 3 years after diagnosis.[55] Both Stearns and O'Brien observed independently that patients presenting with metachronous LN metastases had better survival following therapeutic inguinal lymph node dissection. In the MSKCC review, 75% of patients survived longer than 5 years after groin dissection.

The use of radiation on the inguinal lymph nodes, both prophylactically and for treatment, was explored by Papillon.[56] In 1974, he reported on 19 patients with synchronous inguinal nodal involvement who underwent groin irradiation for disease control. Eleven of the 19 had no evidence of disease at 3 years. Cummings and associates treated nodal disease in a similar fashion and showed that 87% of patients had good disease control or cure without groin dissection.[57]

With the use of radiation fields expanded to include inguinal, internal, and external iliac nodes, the current treatment paradigm is to treat inguinal nodal metastases with chemotherapy and radiation concurrently with the primary tumor. Metachronous lymph node involvement is treated with salvage chemotherapy and radiation if dose limits have not been exceeded, as well as groin dissection if warranted.

MANAGEMENT OF HIV-POSITIVE PATIENTS

Treatment for anal cancer does not differ in the HIV-positive population. Combined chemotherapy and radiation is the best approach to this disease in the setting of HIV/AIDS. Studies have consistently documented responses to standard therapy that equal those in the HIV-negative population.[8,16] However, experience with treatment in this population is limited, confined mostly to retrospective reviews with historic comparisons. Therapy can be difficult under the best of circumstances. Although treatment duration is often only 6 weeks, it can be complicated by moist desquamation, diarrhea, perineal pain and tenderness, and severe anal pain. Late effects include anal stenosis, necrosis, chronic ulcer formation, and compromised continence. Severe toxicity may require diverting stomas in 6–12% of HIV-negative patients, with an even greater rate in the HIV-positive population.[8] Symptoms of acute toxicity are generally manageable with good skin care, antidiarrheals, and narcotic analgesics. Even so, there is widespread concern regarding the degree and management of these toxicities in the HIV-positive patient, and some evidence to suggest that they are significantly more severe, resulting in treatment delays or dose reductions. At UCSF toxicity requiring hospitalization, dose reduction, or treatment delays occurred in 82% of patients undergoing standard high-dose therapy.[8] For patients with a baseline CD4 count under 200, the rates of toxicity were especially severe—50% of these patients required fecal diversion.[8] A review of patients treated from 1985–1998 by Kim and associates compared treatment toxicity and tolerance of 13 HIV-positive with 60 HIV-negative patients.[58] Although demographics of the HIV-positive patients were different from those of the comparison group, there was no difference in treatment or stage at diagnosis. Acute toxicity occurred in 80% of the HIV-positive patients versus 30% of those who were HIV-negative. Late toxicity (40% versus 16%) and rates of local control (38.5% versus 15%) were also compromised in the HIV-positive cohort.[58]

The impact of HAART on the treatment of anal cancer in the HIV population is not well understood at this time. Several small series have published reports suggesting that HAART improves tolerance to anal cancer therapy. Stadler and colleagues at the University of Texas Southwestern Medical Center examined the effects of treatment in HIV-positive patients before and after the advent of HAART.[59] The group found the average CD4 count of the HAART patients was significantly higher, and that this seemed to correlate with better disease-free survival. All six pre-HAART patients died with active disease with a 2-year survival rate of 17%. Of those on HAART, the 2-year survival rate was 67% with 4/8 patients remaining free of disease.

A preliminary review of 11 HIV-positive patients at UCSF receiving both HAART and chemoradiation with baseline mean CD4 counts above 300 further delineates the difficulties in treating this population.[8] Although 10 patients completed therapy, 8 of 10 developed severe acute toxicity and 2 had chronic complications requiring colostomy. Three of the 11 have died of disease within 13 months of diagnosis and 2 have undergone APR for local recurrence.[8] It is clear that although HAART has extended and improved the lives of those infected with HIV, it has not necessarily provided protection against the toxicities of anal cancer treatment in those patients. A multinational, multi-institutional review of treatment response and effects is currently examining the issue of treatment of anal cancer in the HIV population with an aim toward the development of more specific recommendations. At this time, however, it seems prudent to deliver standard therapy (4500–5400 Gy and cisplatin, or mitomycin-C and 5-FU) to those HIV-positive patients in good health, and to monitor closely for side effects. HIV patients with very low CD4 counts (<200) and significant comorbidities may require individualized regimens, closer monitoring, or treatment breaks.

RECURRENT DISEASE AND SALVAGE THERAPY

The goal of early detection of local posttreatment recurrence is to prevent lymphatic spread of disease and maximize salvage. Most clinicians advocate a thorough physical exam including a digital rectal exam and anoscopy every 3–4 months for at least 2 years. An additional strategy involves the use of endoanal ultrasound (EAUS) inspection. At the Hospital of the University of Pennsylvania, the current protocol is EAUS inspection every 4 months for 3 years, followed by every 6 months for 2 years. Suspicious tissue or lymph nodes are biopsied with the aid of ultrasound guidance.

There is some evidence that local regression of disease following radiation therapy can occur up to 6–9 months following chemoradiation. Routine biopsy of the anal canal following treatment is no longer recommended within this time period. Rousseau and associates advise allowing the anal canal to heal completely, reserving biopsy for nonhealing ulcers and recurrent or enlarging anal canal masses after a period of at least 6 months following therapy.[60] After this point, any disease detected is residual and salvage therapy is warranted.

In spite of success with nonoperative anal canal cancer management, depending on the stage of disease, 10–30% of patients will recur, most locally. The treatment of recurrent or persistent disease is APR with negative margins. In a retrospective analysis of salvage therapy for recurrent disease following chemotherapy with radiation, Allal and colleagues found that APR results in a 53% actuarial 5-year survival rate versus 28% in those who did not receive additional treatment.[61] Pocard and colleagues' data from St. Antoine University Hospital examined salvage APR in 21 patients who had either residual disease after sphincter conservation or recurrence. The group found an actuarial 5-year survival benefit of 30%.[62] Factors resulting in failure were lymphadenopathy, positive margins, and distant disease. Longo and associates compared salvage with chemoradiation versus APR and found that only 27% of patients treated with additional combined therapy survived long-term, whereas 57% of those in the APR group did[63] (Table 26–4).[64–68]

Patients with recurrence die of locoregional complications including ureteral obstruction, perineal sepsis and necrosis, bowel obstruction, and venous thrombosis. Contraindications for salvage surgery include medical debilitation, known distant metastases, invasion of the pelvic sidewalls, and obvious inguinal lymphadenopathy. The preoperative assessment should include a chest x-ray and an MRI or CT scan of the abdomen and pelvis. A multidisciplinary approach is appropriate for local invasion of resectable structures such as the urinary bladder, cervix, vagina, or the sacrum. A team including a urologist, neurosurgeon, orthopedic surgeon, and plastic surgeon may be required. Recurrences close to the pelvic sidewall may be indistinguishable intraoperatively from fibrosis and scarring from prior ra-

TABLE 26–4. ABDOMINOPERINEAL RESECTION AFTER FAILURE OF RADIATION (WITH OR WITHOUT CHEMOTHERAPY) FOR ANAL CANCER

Review	Number of Patients	Median Follow-Up (Months)	Alive (%)	5-Year Survival Rate (%)
Zelnick 1992[37]	9	20	<10	—
Tanum 1993[65]	9	36	67	—
Lasser 1993[66]	14	36	50	—
Ellenhorn 1994[67]	38	47	—	44
Longo 1994[40]	11	25	18	—
Hill 1996[68]	11	25	18	—
Pocard 1989[62]	21	40	48	33

Modified, with permission, from Cummings BJ, Keane TJ, Hawkins NV et al. Treatment of perianal carcinoma by radiation (RT) or radiation plus chemotherapy (RTCT). *Int J Radiat Oncol Biol Phys* 1986; 12:170.

diation or surgery. An intraoperative frozen section may be useful if one is considering placing after-loading catheters or delivering intraoperative brachytherapy to these areas. The role and long-term outcomes of brachytherapy as a treatment adjunct for salvage surgery has not yet been validated.

The complications of salvage pelvic surgery may be severe and debilitating and include perineal wound dehiscence and necrosis. Tissue coverage in previously irradiated fields improves wound healing and many consider it essential for post-exenteration reconstruction. Pedicle and rotational flaps may be fashioned from the gluteus, gracilis, or rectus abdominis muscles.

Data documenting long-term follow-up in patients salvaged with radiation or chemoradiation following local excision are lacking. Patients who undergo primary excision for anal canal carcinoma do so for a number of reasons, including polypectomy, hemorrhoidectomy, or excisional biopsy, as well as local excision with intent to cure. Although it is unclear at this point whether further treatment for completely excised, early-stage lesions is appropriate, patients with positive margins, or those with tumors harboring vascular or lymphatic invasion with poorly differentiated characteristics are candidates for further therapy. A retrospective analysis from MSKCC in 1999 reviewed 14 patients who received postoperative chemoradiation (either 30 or 45–50 Gy) after local excision.[69] Actuarial 5-year local control rates were 93% with no differences between outcomes in the higher- and lower-dose groups. Longo and associates published the largest single retrospective analysis of outcomes in 1994, reviewing chemoradiation following local excision.[40] The overall local control rate at 5 years was 79% in 109 patients receiving a median dose of 42 Gy. Stratification of the data by stage revealed a 90% local control rate with stage I, 54% with stage II, and 100% with stage III (6/6 patients).[40] There have been no prospective studies comparing local excision alone versus chemoradiation for T1 favorable-histology tumors. However, current studies suggest that tumors that are incompletely excised, those with poor histologic characteristics, and those that are stage II and above are candidates for chemoradiation following excision.[60,63,69] As with primary therapy, giving chemotherapy (principally infusional 5-FU with mitomycin-C or cisplatin) seems to promote effective local control at lower radiation doses.

Anal canal carcinoma metastasizes in 10–20% of patients late in the course of disease and prognosis is exceedingly poor.[7] Liver and lung metastases predominate and cisplatin-based chemotherapy is the only strategy shown to be somewhat effective.[60]

▪ ANAL MARGIN CANCER

Squamous cell carcinoma of the anal margin is at least five times less common than anal canal carcinoma, and for the most part is treated by primary surgical excision similarly to skin cancers. These tumors arise on the perianal skin beyond the anal verge. They are usually well- or moderately-differentiated keratinized squamous cell carcinomas and generally have a favorable prognosis.[7] Metastases are late and rare, and recurrences are typically locoregional. Symptoms include pain, bleeding, itching, and palpable mass. In a study from Denmark, Jensen and associates noted a 6-month median duration of symptoms prior to diagnosis, with an erroneous initial diagnosis made in 29% of cases.[70] Because these tumors are fairly slow growing and uncommon, they are frequently mistaken for hemorrhoids or other benign conditions at initial presentation.

Diagnosis is often suspected by the experienced clinician on inspection, but biopsy prior to definitive treatment is imperative. If the lesion is small, excisional biopsy can be accomplished with adequate margins (1 cm). If the tumor is larger, a small incisional biopsy allows accurate classification of the tumor and appropriate preoperative counseling.

Metastases to the inguinal lymph nodes occurs in 15–25% of patients. The rate of nodal metastases is directly proportional to the size of the tumor. Papillon and Chassard reported that for tumors less than 2 cm in size, the rate of nodal metastasis was 0%, for those 2–5 cm 24%, and for those >5 cm 67%.[71] Cummings and colleagues found that those with tumors <5 cm in size had 0% nodal metastases, whereas metastases occurred in 25% of those with tumors 5 cm or larger.[72]

SURGERY

Although surgical excision (either local excision or APR, depending on location) is considered the standard of care for anal margin tumors, outcome data for this rare neoplasm are primarily retrospective. In most studies, overall and disease-specific survival are considered for all stages together and subgroup analysis for large numbers of patients is not available. Unfortunately, evaluation of local recurrence data is similarly limited by the small numbers of patients affected; however, in general a trend towards increased recurrence in larger tumors is apparent.[73]

Surgical treatment of the primary anal margin tumor is accomplished by wide local excision with 1-cm margins. At MSKCC, Greenall and associates reported a series of 51 patients with squamous cell carcinoma of the anal margin.[74] Five-year survival was 88%, although local recurrence was 46%. Local recurrences were amenable to re-excision. Inguinal nodal dissection was employed for metachronous inguinal nodal metastases. Thirteen patients in this series underwent APR as initial treatment. The local recurrence rates for these patients were identical to those of the local excision group. Tumor size was the most important factor for local control and survival (Fig 26–5). In 1979, Cleveland clinic reviewed their experience with surgery for anal margin tumors over a 20-year period.[75] Eight patients were identified for whom follow-up was available. A disease-specific survival rate of 70% was noted after 8 years, with a local recurrence rate of 30%. At the University of Chicago, a 19% local recurrence rate was noted in 16 patients undergoing surgical therapy alone.[76] Two of 11 patients recurred following local excision, and 1 of 3 recurred after APR. Of 27 patients with either stage I anal margin cancer or carcinoma-in-situ treated at the Mayo Clinic between 1950 and 1970, 5-year survival rates were 100%, although local recurrence rates were unavailable.[77]

After surgery alone (local excision or APR), the overall survival rate for all stages is 60–90% with a local recurrence rate of approximately 30%. Survival rates after surgery for recurrence are unknown.[7,73]

RADIOTHERAPY

The optimal treatment of anal margin tumors is dependent upon location. Significant challenges and functional problems may result when the anal sphincters are present within the boundaries of optimal surgery. If adequate excision compromises the sphincters, APR is an option. However, many surgeons and oncologists would advocate a more conservative approach and use

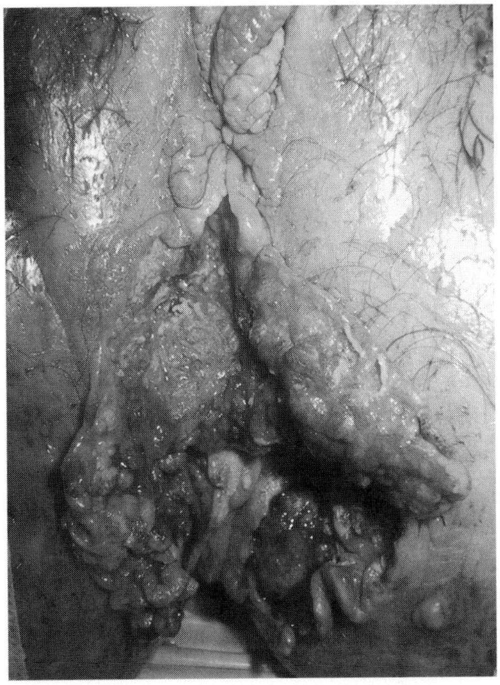

Figure 26–5. Deeply ulcerating anal margin tumor. (Courtesy Charles Friel.)

radiotherapy. Cummings and associates demonstrated local control rates of 100% for anal margin tumors less than 5 cm in size with a dose of 50 Gy over 4 weeks.[72] Local control rates were inversely proportional to the size of the tumor. For those tumors 5–10 cm, 70% local control was achieved, but for tumors >10 cm, only 40% sustained a durable response. Similar results were reported by Papillon and Chassard at Centre Leon Berard in France.[71] In this review, a 78% overall survival rate was achieved using external beam radiation (40 Gy cobalt 60 source) with a perineal field. Again, those with tumors greater than 5 cm in size fared considerably worse, with overall survival rates less than 50%.[71]

There have been numerous retrospective reviews of the response of anal margin tumors to radiation in the past 40 years documenting stage-specific local recurrence rates, disease-specific survival rates, and overall survival rates. Overall, local control rates of 52–87% are typical, with 5-year overall survival rates ranging from 52–90%.[73] T1 and T2 tumors have better local control rates with overall and disease-specific survival rates ranging from 82–100%.[73]

It is difficult to evaluate the sphincter preservation rate from these reviews. Small numbers and retrospective design limits direct comparison of this technique to surgery alone. There are no prospective studies comparing surgery alone to radiotherapy. Although the addition of chemotherapy (5-FU and mitomycin-C or cisplatin) seems logical, there are few data to support that approach. The rationale for these agents is extrapolated from the prospective trials of chemoradiation in the setting of anal canal carcinoma. Even so, it is reasonable to believe that primary radiotherapy with or without chemotherapy for anal margin tumors in close proximity to the anal sphincters, where adequate excision may compromise function, will result in both sphincter preservation and good local control. It is also reasonable to expect that surgical salvage for recurrence after primary radiotherapy is a possibility, with rates of local control of approximately 50%. Long-term disease-specific survival following this scenario is unknown.

■ ANAL MELANOMA

Melanoma of the anus and rectum is a rare malignancy accounting for less than 1% of all colorectal and anal neoplasms.[78] After the skin and eye the anorectum is the third most common site of melanoma. Although there is a female predominance with an almost 1:2 ratio, there is evidence that the median age of affected males is significantly less (57 versus 71 years of age).[79] Cagir and colleagues examined the epidemiology and demographics of anorectal melanoma using the Surveillance, Epidemiology and End Results (SEER) database. These investigators note a recent emergence of a bimodal age distribution of anorectal melanoma for all patients, with males occupying the younger aspect of the curve. Survival rates were slightly better in this group (63% versus 51% at 1 year and 41% versus 27% at 2 years; $p<0.01$).[79]

The most common symptoms include bleeding, itching, the presence of a mass, pain, tenesmus, or changes in bowel habits. Like anal squamous cell carcinoma, misidentification of the tumor as a hemorrhoid is a common mistake. Diagnosis is frequently made following hemorrhoidectomy or local excision of the perianal mass. The tumor can appear small and polypoid, or large and ulcerating. About 30% of these tumors are amelanotic and unpigmented making immediate recognition of the problem difficult.[78] On pathology, 70% of lesions show some evidence of melanin production either grossly or microscopically.[78] Commonly, anal melanoma arises at the mucocutaneous junction. Occasionally, the lesion arises more proximally, within the rectal mucosa. Although the origin of these tumors is speculative, they are believed to arise in areas of heterotopic anal canal epithelium in the rectum, or to start from proximal microscopic mucosal spread from a small lesion located more distally.[78]

STAGING AND PROGNOSIS

Like melanoma of the skin, anorectal melanoma is staged by depth or thickness of the lesion. Lymphatic metastases can occur in the inguinal, mesorectal, and internal iliac nodal distribution. Mesorectal lymph node metastases are found in 40–60% of patients at initial presentation and inguinal adenopathy is present in at least 20%.[80,81] Distant spread occurs to the bone, lung, and liver.

Regardless of stage, 5-year survival rates for patients diagnosed with anorectal melanoma are very poor, averaging about 6%. The median survival time following diagnosis is 12–18 months.[78]

SURGERY

In recent years, local excision has replaced APR for the treatment of anal melanoma. Outcomes data comparing local recurrence rates and survival do not demonstrate a survival difference between the two approaches; therefore the preservation of fecal continence is a priority when possible. A number of retrospective series published from 1990–2003 reviewing institutional experience with local excision and APR found that 5-year survival rates range from 0–29% for those undergoing wide local excision, and from 0–26% for those undergoing APR. Most authors now recommend wide local excision with negative margins for those patients without anal sphincter involvement.[78]

Even though survival differences are minimal between local and radical approaches, local recurrence rates may be higher after local excision. A study from the M.D. Anderson Cancer Center found that recurrence after local excision was significantly higher than recurrence after APR (58% versus 29%), and that median survival times were the same (approximately 19 months for both groups).[82] Patients with local recurrence in this study developed synchronous regional and distant disease. Roumen in the Netherlands also reported an increased rate of local recurrence with local excision, but no overall survival disadvantage.[83]

Inguinal lymph node dissection in anorectal melanoma is usually reserved for those with clinically positive nodes and is a palliative intervention. Prophylactic nodal dissection does not seem to provide a survival benefit and there currently is no clear indication for it. The role of sentinel lymph node mapping in this disease is not clear. The benefits of the technique are now well established in cutaneous melanoma, but it has not been investigated in anorectal melanoma and is not currently routinely performed.

ADJUVANT THERAPY

High-dose interferon-alfa is currently used in the treatment of cutaneous melanoma. It confers a survival benefit in this group, improving disease-free survival rates.[78] However, there are no data demonstrating its efficacy in anorectal melanoma, and current reports of adjuvant chemotherapy in this setting are anecdotal. External beam irradiation for symptomatic pelvic and local recurrences and metachronous inguinal nodal disease has been incorporated into the palliative treatment of anorectal melanoma, but again, no data are available to assess overall efficacy. It seems reasonable, however, to extrapolate treatment paradigms from cutaneous melanoma to anorectal melanoma in stage IV disease.

The surgical treatment of anorectal melanoma has changed over time, evolving from radical to local excision. No survival benefit is conferred by APR in most studies, and in most reviews survival is quite poor in spite of surgical excision, with median survival less than 20 months from the time of diagnosis. Although adjuvant chemotherapy is shown to be effective in cutaneous melanoma, lack of data hinders acceptance of this therapy in anorectal melanoma.

▪ ANAL ADENOCARCINOMA

Anal adenocarcinomas are uncommon, comprising 10% of all anal canal carcinomas.[78] Symptoms of bleeding, pain, and change in bowel habits are nonspecific and similar to other anal canal and distal rectal neoplasms. Anal adenocarcinomas may occasionally be found in chronic anal fistulas.

Although outcomes data are few, anal adenocarcinoma has a poor prognosis when compared to rectal cancers or anal squamous cell carcinoma. In small series, 5-year survival rates range from 64% to less than 5%.[84,85] These neoplasms have a high rate of both local and distant failure.[85]

Treatment is similar to therapy for adenocarcinoma of the rectum. Neoadjuvant chemoradiation followed by surgical excision is recommended. Postoperative adjuvant chemotherapy may be prudent, as it is in rectal adenocarcinoma, to reduce the risk of distant spread.

▪ PAGET'S DISEASE

Paget's disease was first described in 1874 by Sir James Paget, who reported 15 cases involving the nipple.[86] To date, less than 200 cases of perianal Paget's have been documented in the literature since Darier and Couillaud reported the first case in 1893.[86]

Paget's has a female predominance (1.5:1) with a median presentation age of 65 years.[87] The disease is usually present for an extended period of time prior to diagnosis because the symptoms are nonspecific and often mistaken for a benign dermatitis. Paget's occurs in apocrine, hair-bearing areas. Erythematous, pruritic, scaling plaques with well-defined serpiginous borders are a typical feature of the disease. These lesions may also appear ulcerated and crusty with a serous discharge. The disease can be found in both the anal canal and margin.[78,86] Histologically, Paget's disease is defined by the presence of large intraepidermal anaplastic tumor cells lying separately or in small clusters. Perianal Paget's cells are foamy and vacuolar in appearance and stain light blue with hematoxylin and eosin. They are positive for periodic acid-Schiff, mucicarmine, Alcian blue, and cytokeratin 7.[78]

The pathogenesis of Paget's disease is still somewhat unclear. Because it can be associated with the presence of rectal adenocarcinoma, it is speculated that Paget's represents a downward extension of the tumor or that a "neoplastic milieu" may create an environment hospitable to the presence of multiple gastrointestinal primary tumors. Another hypothesis holds that it is a primary tumor of the apocrine glandular elements of the distal anal canal and margin. Others have suggested that Paget's may arise from a neoplastic pluripotent epidermis basal cell.[78]

Perianal Paget's is associated with an underlying visceral malignancy in 20–86% of cases.[78,86,87] Colorectal adenocarcinoma is the most common synchronous tumor, but urogenital, breast, and bile duct carcinomas have also been reported. Screening for other malignancies is imperative. A colonoscopy and prostate exam are basic preventive and diagnostic tests that can be helpful. Some authors recommend computed tomography of the abdomen and pelvis as well.[86]

Complete excision is the treatment for Paget's disease. The extent of the disease is usually determined by taking circumferential biopsies of the anal canal and margin. After the disease is "mapped," wide local excision is performed. Often, the procedure creates large defects that may require skin grafts or flaps (rotational, island, or myocutaneous). Because excision to negative margins is critical to cure, techniques to ensure this may be required. Surgeons may obtain frozen sections of the margins of the specimen in the operating room prior to reconstruction. Others prefer to cover the wound with saline-soaked gauze, admit the patient to the hospital, and await permanent pathology results for up to 2–3 days prior to reconstruction. If a large flap reconstruction is placed in the anal canal, some recommend diversion with a colostomy or ileostomy at the time of the perineal excision.

Recurrence rates as high as 61% have been reported following excision of perianal Paget's disease.[88] Re-excision is the usual recommendation, although in cases in whom underlying rectal or anal adenocarcinoma exist, radiation followed by APR is advisable. Although recurrence rates are high, the prognosis of Paget's limited to the perianal area with no concomitant neoplasm is very good.[78] Because of the association with additional visceral neoplasms, continued surveillance is required for patients with perianal Paget's disease. Physical examination, including a prostate and pelvic examination, and periodic colonoscopy is probably prudent. Biopsies of new lesions at the edges of the flap or graft may reveal residual disease. Local excision of these recurrences and continued surveillance is required.

▪ BUSCHKE-LÖWENSTEIN TUMORS

Buschke-Löwenstein tumors are also referred to as giant condylomas and were first described in 1925 by Buschke and Löwenstein as "carcinoma-like condylomata acuminata."[89] They are rare entities belonging to a wider group of lesions called verrucous carcinomas, which includes oral and cutaneous fungating condylomata. The key feature of giant condyloma that differentiates it from benign anal condyloma is the presence of local invasion.

Although the natural history of these lesions is poorly understood, the etiology is assumed to be similar to that of condyloma.[89] Human papillomavirus has been isolated from the tumors. Histologically, the lesions are benign in appearance and do not invade the basement membrane as carcinomas do. Instead, they destroy surrounding tissue by expansion rather than direct invasion. The tumor does not metastasize. Deaths from untreated Buschke-Löwenstein tumors have occurred following deep invasion into unresectable pelvic structures followed by superinfection and recurrent sepsis. The overall mortality rate from this rare entity is 20%.[90]

Because there are so few cases reported, there are no consistent treatment guidelines. Primary treatment consists of surgical resection to clear margins.[90] However, adequate surgery may be impossible when the tumor deeply invades the pelvis. There have been several case reports demonstrating the efficacy of intralesional injection of interferon-alpha 2b.[89] At least three reported cases of deeply infiltrating giant condylomata have completely responded to long-term therapy, including one patient who would have required hemipelvectomy with limb amputation to achieve negative margins. Interferon-alpha 2b may be a good alternative or supplement to radical resection in select cases. Long-term outcomes are not available.

REFERENCES

1. American Joint Committee on Cancer. Anal cancer. In: *AJCC Cancer Staging Manual*, 6th ed. New York, NY: Springer-Verlag; 2002
2. Fenger C. The anal transitional zone. *Acta Pathol Microbiol Immunol Scand* 1979;87:379–386
3. World Health Organization. Anal cancer. In: *World Health Organization International Statistical Classification of Diseases and Related Health Problems*, 10th ed. 2003. http://www3.who.int/icd/vol1htm2003/fr-icd.htm
4. Greenlee RT, Murray T, Bolden S, Wing PA. Cancer statistics, 2000. *CA Cancer J Clin* 2000;50:7–33
5. Jemal A, Thomas A, Murray T et al. Cancer statistics, 2002. *CA Cancer J Clin* 2002;52:23–47.
6. Chawla AK, Willett CG. Squamous cell carcinoma of the anal canal and anal margin. *Hematol Oncol Clin North Am* 2001;15:321–344
7. Gervasoni JE, Wanebo HJ. Cancers of the anal canal and anal margin. *Cancer Invest* 2003;21:452–464
8. Klencke BJ, Palefsky JM. Anal cancer: an HIV-associated cancer. *Hematol Oncol Clin North Am* 2003;12:859–872
9. Goedert JJ, Cote TR, Virgo P et al. Spectrum of AIDS-associated malignant disorders. *Lancet* 1998;351:1933–1939
10. Goedert JJ. The epidemiology of acquired immunodeficiency syndrome malignancies. *Semin Oncol* 2000;4:390–401
11. Ryan DP, Compton CC, Mayer RJ. Carcinoma of the anal canal. *N Engl J Med* 2000;342:792–800
12. Palefsky JM. Anal squamous intraepithelial lesions in human immunodeficiency virus-positive men and women. *Semin Oncol* 2000;27:471–479
13. Stanley M. Genital human papillomavirus infections—current and prospective therapies. *J Natl Cancer Inst Monogr* 2003;31:117–124
14. Frish M, Glimelius B, vanden Brule AJC et al. Sexually transmitted infection as a cause of anal cancer. *N Engl J Med* 1997;337:1350–1358
15. Duggan MA, Boras VF, Inoue M et al. Human papillomavirus DNA determination of anal condylomata, dysplasias, and squamous carcinomas with *in situ* hybridization. *Am J Clin Pathol* 1989;92:16–21
16. Berry JM, Palefsky JM, Welton ML. Anal cancer and its precursors in HIV-positive patients: perspectives and management. *Surg Oncol Clin North Am* 2004;13:355–373
17. Frisch M, Biggar RJ, Engels EA et al. Association of cancer with AIDS-related immunosuppression in adults. *JAMA* 2001;13:1736–1745
18. Stephenson J. Health agencies update: anal cancer screening. *JAMA* 2000;283:3060
19. Frisch M, Glimelius B, Wohlfahrt J et al. Tobacco smoking as a risk factor in anal carcinoma: an antiestrogenic mechanism? *J Natl Cancer Inst* 1999;91:708–715
20. Frisch M, Olsen JH, Bautz A et al. Benign anal lesions and the risk of anal cancer. *N Engl J Med* 1994;331:300–307
21. Frisch M, Johansen C. Anal carcinoma in inflammatory bowel disease. *Br J Cancer* 2000;83:89–90
22. Piketty C, Darragh TM, Da Costa M et al. High prevalence of anal human papillomavirus infection and anal cancer precursors among HIV-infected persons in the absence of anal intercourse. *Ann Intern Med* 2003;138:453–459

23. Holly EA, Ralston ML, Darragh TM et al. Prevalence and risk factors for anal squamous intraepithelial lesions in women. *J Natl Cancer Inst* 2001;93:843–849
24. Palefsky JM, Holly EA, Ralson ML et al. Prevalence and risk factors for human papillomavirus infection of the anal canal in human immunodeficiency virus (HIV)-positive and HIV-negative homosexual men. *J Infect Dis* 1998;177:361–367
25. Scholefield JH. Anal intraepithelial neoplasia: clinical dilemma. *Br J Surg* 1999;86:1363–1364
26. Chang GJ, Berry JM, Jay N et al. Surgical treatment of high-grade anal squamous intraepithelial lesions, a prospective study. *Dis Colon Rectum* 2002;45:453–458
27. Cleary RK, Schaldenbrand JD, Fowler JJ. Treatment options for perianal Bowen's disease: Survey of American Society of Colon and Rectal Surgeons members. *Dis Colon Rectum* 2000;6:686–688
28. Brown SR, Skinner P, Tidy J et al. Outcome after surgical resection for high-grade anal intraepithelial neoplasia (Bowen's disease). *Br J Surg* 1999;86:1063–1066
29. Moore HG, Guillem JG. Anal neoplasms. *Surg Clin North Am* 2002;82:1233–1251
30. Chawla AK, Willett CG. Squamous cell carcinoma of the anal canal and anal margin. *Hematol Oncol Clin North Am* 2001;15:321–344
31. Singh R, Nime F, Mittleman A. Malignant epithelial tumors of the anal canal. *Cancer* 1981;48:411–415
32. Nigro ND, Vaitkevicius VK, Considine B. Combined therapy for cancer of the anal canal: A preliminary report. *Dis Colon Rectum* 1974;17:354–356
33. Frost DB, Richards PC, Montague ED et al. Epidermoid cancer of the anorectum. *Cancer* 1984;53:1285
34. Boman BM, Moertel CG, O'Connell MJ et al. Carcinoma of the anal canal: a clinical and pathologic study of 188 cases. *Cancer* 1984;54:114
35. Greenall MJ, Quan SHQ, Stearnes MW et al. Epidermoid cancer of the anal margin: Pathologic features, treatment, and clinical results. *Am J Surg* 1985;149:95
36. Toubouol E, Schlienger M, Buffat L et al. Conservative versus nonconservative treatment of epidermoid carcinoma of the anal canal for tumors longer than or equal to 5 centimeters: A retrospective comparison. *Cancer* 1995;75:786
37. Zelnick RS, Haas PA, Ajlouni M et al. Results of abdominoperineal resections for failures after combination chemotherapy and radiation therapy for anal canal cancers. *Dis Colon Rectum* 1992;35:574
38. Klas JV, Rothenberger DA, Wong WD et al. Malignant tumors of the anal canal: The spectrum of disease, treatment, and outcomes. *Cancer* 1999;85:1686–1693
39. Corman ML, Haggitt RC. Carcinoma of the anal canal. *Surg Gynecol Obstet* 1977;145:674
40. Longo WE, Vernava AM, Wad TP. Recurrent squamous cell carcinoma of the anal canal: Predicators of initial treatment failure and results of salvage therapy. *Ann Surg* 1994;220:40–49
41. Michaelson RA, Magill GB, Quan SHQ et al. Preoperative chemotherapy and radiation therapy in the management of anal epidermoid carcinoma. *Cancer* 1983;51:390
42. Martenson JA, Lipsitz SR, Wagner H Jr et al. Initial results of a phase II trial of high dose radiation therapy, 5-fluorouracil, and cisplatin for patients with anal cancer (E4292): An Eastern Cooperative Oncology Group study. *Int J Radiat Oncol Biol Phys* 1996;35:745
43. Sischy B, Doggett RLS, Krall JM et al. Definitive irradiation and chemotherapy for radiosensitization in management of anal carcinoma: Interim report on Radiation Therapy Oncology Group study no. 8314. *J Natl Cancer Inst* 1989;81:850
44. Miller EJ, Quan SH, Thaler T. Treatment of squamous cell carcinoma of the anal canal. *Cancer* 1991;67:2038
45. Salmon RJ, Fenton J, Asselain B et al. Treatment of epidermoid anal canal cancer. *Am J Surg* 1984;147:43
46. United Kingdom Coordinating Committee on Cancer Research Anal Cancer Trial Working Party. Epidermoid anal cancer: Results from the UKCCCR randomized trial of radiotherapy alone versus radiotherapy, 5-fluorouracil, and mitomycin. *Lancet* 1996;348:1049
47. Bartlink H, Roelofsen F, Eschwege F et al. Concomitant radiotherapy and chemotherapy is superior to radiotherapy alone in the treatment of locally advanced anal cancer: Results of a phase III randomized trial of the European Organization for Research and Treatment of Cancer Radiotherapy and Gastrointestinal Cooperative Groups. *J Clin Oncol* 1997;15:2040
48. Flam M, John M, Pajak TF et al. Role of mitomycin in combination with fluorouracil and radiotherapy, and of salvage chemoradiation in the definitive nonsurgical treatment of epidermoid carcinoma of the anal canal: Results of a phase III randomized intergroup study. *J Clin Oncol* 1996;14:2527
49. Doci R, Zucali R, La Moinic G et al. Primary chemoradiation therapy with fluorouracil and cisplatin for cancer of the anus: Results in 35 consecutive patients. *J Clin Oncol* 1996;14: 3121
50. Faynsod M, Vargas HI, Tolmos J et al. Patterns of recurrence in anal canal carcinoma. *Arch Surg* 2000;1:1090–1093
51. Mitchell SE, Mendenhall WM, Zlotecki RA et al. Squamous cell carcinoma of the anal canal. *Int J Radiat Oncol Biol Phys* 2001;49:1007–1013
52. Kapp KS, Geyer E, Gebhart FH et al. Experience with split-course external beam irradiation ± chemotherapy and integrated Ir-192 high-dose-rate brachytherapy in the treatment of primary carcinomas of the anal canal. *Int J Radiat Oncol Biol Phys* 2001;49:997–1005
53. Peiffert D, Giovannini M, Ducreux M et al. High-dose radiation therapy and neoadjuvant plus concomitant chemotherapy with 5-fluourouracil and cisplatin in patients with locally advanced squamous-cell anal canal cancer: final results of a phase II study. *Ann Oncol* 2001;12:397–404
54. Stearns MW, Quan SHQ. Epidermoid carcinoma of the anorectum. *Surg Gynecol Obstet* 1970;131:953
55. O'Brien PH, Jenrette JM, Wallace KM et al. Epidermoid carcinoma of the anus. *Surg Gynecol Obstet* 1982;155:745
56. Papillon J. Radiation therapy in the management of epidermoid carcinoma of the anal region. *Dis Colon Rectum* 1974;17:181

57. Cummings BJ, Thomas GM, Keane TJ et al. Primary radiation therapy in the treatment of anal canal carcinoma. *Dis Colon Rectum* 1982;25:778
58. Kim JH, Sarani B, Orkin BA et al. HIV-positive patients with anal carcinoma have poorer treatment tolerance and outcome than HIV-negative patients. *Dis Colon Rectum* 2001;44:1496–1502
59. Stadler RF, Gregorcyk SG, Euhus DM et al. Outcome of HIV-infected patients with invasive squamous-cell carcinoma of the anal canal in the era of highly active antiretroviral therapy. *Dis Colon Rectum* 2004;47:1305
60. Rousseau DL, Petrelli NJ, Kahlenberg MS. Overview of anal cancer for the surgeon. *Surg Oncol Clin North Am* 2004;13:249–262
61. Allal AS, Laurencet FM, Reymond MA et al. Effectiveness of surgical salvage therapy for patients with locally uncontrolled anal carcinoma after sphincter-conserving treatment. *Cancer* 1999;86:405
62. Pocard M, Tiret E, Nugent K et al. Results of salvage abdominoperineal resection for anal cancer after radiotherapy. *Dis Colon Rectum* 1989;41:1488
63. Longo WE, Vernava AM, Wade TP et al. Rare anal canal cancers in the US veteran: patterns of disease and results of treatment. *Am Surg* 1995;61:495–500
64. Zelnich RS, Haas PA, Ajlouni M et al. Results of abdominoperineal resections for failures after combination chemotherapy and radiation therapy for anal canal cancer. *Dis Colon Rectum* 1992;35:574–578
65. Tanum G. Treatment of relapsing anal carcinoma. *Acta Oncol* 1993;2:33–35
66. Lasser P. Chirurgie de rattrapage dans le traitement des epitheliomas du canal anal. *Bull Cancer Radiother* 1993; 80:361–363
67. Ellenhorn JD, Enker WE, Quan SH. Salvage abdominoperineal resection following combined chemotherapy and radiotherapy for epidermoid carcinoma of the anus. *Ann Surg Oncol* 1994;1:105–110
68. Hill J, Slade A, Schofield P et al. Salvage abdominoperineal resection for anal carcinoma. *Int J Colorect Dis* 1996;11:133
69. Hu K, Minsky BD, Cohen AM et al. 30 Gy may be an adequate dose in patients with anal cancer treated with excisional biopsy followed by combined modality therapy. *J Surg Oncol* 1999;70:71–77
70. Jensen SL, Hagen K, Harling H et al. Long-term prognosis after radical treatment of squamous-cell carcinoma of the anal canal and anal margin. *Dis Colon Rectum* 1988;31:273–278
71. Papillon J, Chassard JL. Respective roles of radiotherapy and surgery in the management of epidermoid carcinoma of the anal margin. Series of 57 patients. *Dis Colon Rectum* 1992;35:422–429
72. Cummings BJ, Keane TJ, Hawkins NV et al. Treatment of perianal carcinoma by radiation (RT) or radiation plus chemotherapy (RTCT). *Int J Radiat Oncol Biol Phys* 1986;12:170
73. Newlin HE, Zlotecki RA, Morris CG et al. Squamous cell carcinoma of the anal margin. *J Surg Oncol* 2004;86:55–62
74. Greenall MJ, Quan SH, Stearns MW et al. Epidermoid cancer of the anal margin. Pathologic features, treatment, and clinical results. *Am J Surg* 1985;149:95–101
75. Al-Jurf AS, Turnbull RP, Fazio VW. Local treatment of squamous cell carcinoma of the anus. *Surg Gynecol Obstet* 1979;148:576–578
76. Schraut WH, Wang CH, Dawson PJ et al. Depth of invasion, location and size of cancer of the anus dictate operative treatment. *Cancer* 1983;51:291–296
77. Beahrs OH, Wilson SM. Carcinoma of the anus. *Ann Surg* 1976;184:422–428
78. Billingsley KG, Stern LE, Lowy AM. Uncommon anal neoplasms. *Surg Oncol Clin North Am* 2004;13:375–388
79. Cagir B, Whiteford MH, Topham A. Changing epidemiology of anorectal melanoma. *Dis Colon Rectum* 1999;42: 1203–1208
80. Goldman S, Glimelius B, Pahlman L. Anorectal malignant melanoma in Sweden. Report of 49 patients. *Dis Colon Rectum* 1990;33: 874–877
81. Brady MS, Kavolius JP, Quan SH. Anorectal melanoma. A 64-year experience at Memorial Sloan-Kettering Cancer Center. *Dis Colon Rectum* 1995;38:146–151
82. Ross M, Pezzi C, Pezzi T et al. Patterns of failure in anorectal melanoma. A guide to surgical therapy. *Arch Surg* 1990;125:313–316
83. Roumen RM. Anorectal melanoma in the Netherlands: a report of 63 patients. *Eur J Surg Oncol* 1996;22:598–601
84. Jensen SL, Shokouh-Aminri MH, Hagen K et al. Adenocarcinoma of the anal ducts. A series of 21 cases. *Dis Colon Rectum* 31(4): 268–72, 1988.
85. Papagikos M, Crane CH, Skibber J et al. Chemoradiation for adenocarcinoma of the anus. *Int J Radiat Oncol Biol Phys* 2003;55:669–678
86. Delaunoit TH, Neczyporenko F, Duttmann R et al. Perianal Paget's disease: case report and review of the literature. *Acta Gastroenterol Belg* 2004;67:228–231
87. Amin R. Case report. Perianal Paget's disease. *Br J Radiol* 1999;72:610–612
88. Sarmiento JM, Wolff BG, Burgart LJ. Paget's disease of the perianal region—an aggressive disease? *Dis Colon Rectum* 1997;40:1187–1194
89. Geusau A, Gertraud H-P, Voc-Platzer B et al. Regression of deeply infiltrating giant condyloma following long-term intralesional interferon alfa therapy. *Arch Dermatol* 2000;136:707–710
90. Chu DC, Vezeridis MP, Libbey NP et al. Giant condyloma acuminatum of the anorectal and perianal regions: analysis of 42 cases. *Dis Colon Rectum* 1994;37:950–957

27

Complications following Anorectal Surgery

Mark Lane Welton ■ *Andrew A. Shelton*

Complications following anorectal surgery are often very distressing to the patient and surgeon alike. The problems that arise are frequently infectious in nature, or functional, occurring as a result of problems with the continence-maintaining function of the rectum and anal canal. With proper patient selection, a thorough understanding of the pathophysiology of the disease processes and of the anatomy and physiology of the anal canal, these complications can often be avoided.

■ COMPLICATIONS FOLLOWING HEMORRHOIDECTOMY

Hemorrhoidectomy is the most commonly performed anorectal procedure. Given the various approaches available to surgeons, gastroenterologists, and primary care physicians, the actual rates cannot be quantified. Nonsurgical therapies include injection, freezing, infrared coagulation, and banding, but these nonsurgical approaches have the same associated complications including pain, bleeding, urinary retention, constipation, abscess, fistula-in-ano, perineal sepsis (Fournier's gangrene), fissure, anal stenosis, incontinence, and recurrence.

Patient education regarding postoperative pain expectations, the use of stool bulk-forming agents, and mild laxatives are important components of optimizing the patient experience. Monitored anesthesia care (MAC) is safe in the prone jackknife position and may provide improved early postoperative pain control when compared to general anesthesia.[1] This benefit is particularly pronounced with the preemptive use of ropivacaine, dextromethorphan, or ketorolac.[2–7] Results for sphincter relaxants as an adjunct to improve postoperative pain control have been contradictory but largely disappointing.[8–12] Finally, postoperative pain control appears improved with a subcutaneous morphine pump, but urinary retention is increased at 50%.[13]

Postoperative bleeding may occur after hemorrhoidectomy as a normal course of the treatment, such as the small amount of bleeding seen 7–10 days after a banding procedure, when the tissue within the band sloughs. In contrast, it may represent poor control of the vascular pedicle post–excisional hemorrhoidectomy, where the bleeding is often pronounced and generally occurs within the first 24–48 hours. Patients with persistent bleeding or clots per anus may require examination under anesthesia and suture ligation of the offending vessel. Some surgeons prefer to limit anticoagulation from nonsteroidal anti-inflammatory drugs, warfarin, and low-molecular-weight heparins. We have not found this to be routinely necessary and would only routinely hold clopidogrel prior to hemorrhoidectomy. Should the patient develop delayed bleeding 1–2 weeks after the procedure, then these anticoagulant medications should be held and the rectum packed.[14]

Urinary retention was a common complication following hemorrhoidectomy with up to 50% of patients being affected. However by limiting intraoperative intravenous fluid volume, optimizing pain control, and avoiding spinal anesthetics, the incidence has been decreased 100-fold.[15,16]

Incontinence following hemorrhoidectomy may result from compromise of the internal or external sphincters during excisional hemorrhoidectomy. The risk of this complication can be minimized by identifying the white fibers of the internal sphincter as the hemorrhoidal cushions are elevated off the internal sphincter. The intersphincteric groove should be palpable and the external sphincter should not be violated if these landmarks are identified.

Care should be taken to avoid aggressive dilatation of the sphincters while attempting to optimize exposure. This may occur as the inexperienced assistant retracts vigorously or if the Pratt bi-valve retractor is forcefully opened.

Despite these maneuvers, patients may note compromised continence post-hemorrhoidectomy. Qualification and quantification of the nature and frequency of the postoperative incontinence is critical to planning appropriate intervention. Patients presenting with complaints of incontinence post-hemorrhoidectomy may note a range of symptoms from occasional spotting, to seepage, leakage, urgency, and incontinence to gas, liquid stool, or solid stool.

Early postoperative complaints of occasional mucus seepage, spotting, and urgency generally resolve without intervention. Mucus seepage may occur initially, as the inflexible fresh scar does not allow proper sealing of the anus. Spotting may be related to the fresh scar or edematous skin tags which complicate perianal hygiene. Urgency is secondary to the initial loss of rectal compliance due to the local inflammation in the healing wound.

Incontinence to gas, liquid stool, and solid stool represent potential injury to the internal and external sphincters. Postoperative complaints of incontinence should be compared to the preoperative condition. Suspected injury to the sphincters may be documented with careful digital rectal examination and endoanal ultrasound, but it should be remembered that sphincter injuries are much more common post–anorectal surgery than might be expected, and ultrasound documentation of presence or severity of injury do not correlate with fecal continence.[17]

Internal sphincter injuries are problematic because they have not been considered amenable to surgical repair despite small reports of direct repair or anoplasty.[18,19] Injections that provide bulk have been investigated while others have studied pharmacological agents to augment function.[20–22]

External sphincter injuries may be approached surgically with a standard overlapping sphincter repair. In contrast to the classic injury seen in the anterior midline after childbirth, the sphincter injury after hemorrhoidectomy may be particularly challenging in that injuries in right posterolateral and left lateral locations may overlie the innervation to the sphincter complex. Care must be exercised to avoid denervation of the sphincter during the repair. Given these concerns, the surgeon may choose to minimize the dissection of the sphincter muscle that would be necessary for an overlapping repair and chose rather to re-approximate the disrupted muscle. This is often feasible, as the injuries may be smaller and more focal when compared to an obstetric injury. In the rare situation in which injuries are found at all three hemorrhoidectomy sites, a staged repair may be necessary to avoid distracting forces on the repairs.

Stenosis after hemorrhoidectomy may occur when a circumferential hemorrhoidectomy is performed and is called a whitehead deformity if associated with an ectropion. Stenosis can be avoided if mucosal/skin bridges are preserved between the excised complexes, and the incidence of the whitehead deformity can be minimized with attention to surgical detail and anatomic landmarks.[23,24] This complication may also occur after hemorrhoidectomy performed with the Ligasure device, where the lateral burn may be underappreciated by the surgeon. This may be avoided by creating a skin incision first with cautery or knife allowing the hemorrhoidal cushion to retract from the surrounding skin and mucosa prior to sealing the tissues with Ligasure. Treatment of the stenosis is directed at advancing normal skin into the anal canal. The stenosis is released by incising the scar. The tissues are prevented from reapproximating by the island of skin that is brought in and sewn to the edges of the disrupted stenosis.[25] A Y-V advancement flap or house flap is effective and is discussed elsewhere.[26]

Despite counseling regarding the importance of fiber and water in the immediate postoperative period, fissures may occur as the relatively narrowed and edematous anal canal is presented with the firm bowel movement of the patient on postoperative analgesics. These are best treated with standard sitz baths (warm water in a bathtub, not a pan), fiber, water, and reassurance.

Simple infections occurring in the wounds after hemorrhoidectomy are quite rare, but perirectal abscesses, fistula-in-ano, and even Fournier's gangrene may occur after these procedures. The infrequent nature of the infectious complications attests to the importance of blood supply in prevention of wound complications. No wound is "dirtier," but the tissues are well perfused and infections are rare. The mechanism for a perirectal abscess and/or fistula post–closed excisional hemorrhoidectomy is easily understood, with a collection developing under the re-approximated wound edges. Some advocate minimizing the dead space under the edges by including the underlying muscle while closing the defect. Nonetheless, should the infection develop, prompt unroofing of the abscess should allow for resolution. If significant cellulitis exists, antibiotics should be considered. In the case of a fistula-in-ano, the tract should be superficial and easily unroofed without concern for injury to the sphincters.

Fournier's gangrene, perineal necrotizing fasciitis, may occur following excisional, banding, injection, and stapler hemorrhoidectomy.[27–30] Infection may occur under the re-approximated mucosal edges after excisional hemorrhoidectomy. The rectal wall may be inadvertently encompassed in the band during banding hemorrhoidectomy. This particular complication can be avoided by excluding rectal prolapse masquerading as hemorrhoids prior to performing the procedure. At the time of the procedure the surgeon should take care to grasp only the vascular complex of the hemorrhoidal cushion and avoid prolapsing the full thickness of the rectal wall into the band applicator. Patients are counseled to contact their physician immediately should they develop severe pain, high fever, and inability to void.[31] Injection sclerotherapy may also result in full-thickness injury if the sclerosant is injected into or through the rectal wall muscle.[32] Regardless of which procedure was performed, immediate reopening of the wound, débridement of all devitalized tissue, and broad-spectrum antibiotic coverage is mandatory. Imaging studies are unnecessary and may delay operative intervention. Frequently multiple trips to the operating room are required.

Recurrent disease should be treated initially with dietary and bowel habit counseling, as subsequent surgeries may be difficult and complication rates may be increased.

▪ COMPLICATIONS FOLLOWING INTERNAL SPHINCTEROTOMY

Lateral internal sphincterotomy is the surgical procedure of choice for the treatment of a chronic, nonhealing anal fissure. The internal anal sphincter is divided laterally up the to proximal extent of the fissure to prevent a keyhole deformity of the anus. Division of the sphincter results in decreased sphincter tone, increased blood flow to the anal mucosa, and healing of the fissure.

Persistent fissure disease following internal sphincterotomy should be approached with caution. Consideration should be given to malignancy, Crohn's disease, dermatological diseases, sexually transmitted diseases, and supratentorial processes prior to repeat sphincterotomy.

Exam under anesthesia and biopsy of the nonhealing ulcer for histopathology and culture should be routine. Malignancy, Crohn's disease, and dermatologic conditions may be excluded with the biopsy. Cultures may exclude infectious and sexually transmitted diseases. Colonoscopy and an upper gastrointestinal series may also be indicated to exclude infectious etiologies and inflammatory bowel disease.

If the above work-up is negative, anorectal manometry and endoanal ultrasound may document persistent hypertonicity and presence of significant internal sphincter, respectively. If these conditions do not exist, caution should be exercised when proposing surgical intervention. If the patient appears to have persistent fissure disease post–surgical intervention, strong consideration may be given to medical therapies such as botulinum toxin and isosorbide dinitrate.[33,34]

Although rare, abscess and fistula may complicate the lateral sphincterotomy. The subcutaneous sphincterotomy is performed through a small stab incision created with a no. 11 blade and may therefore be particularly susceptible to this complication. As in all other abscesses, adequate drainage is mandatory. If no cellulitis exists, antibiotics are not necessary. A fistula may complicate the abscess or actually occur when the no. 11 blade disrupts the rectal mucosa but not the anal mucosa, leaving a bridge between the two openings. In either case, simple unroofing of the tract is sufficient.

The rate of incontinence after lateral sphincterotomy is difficult to ascertain and is quite controversial. This is particularly true because the presence of a demonstrable injury does not correlate with symptoms.[35] Furthermore, the preoperative condition may be associated with incontinence, often not well documented, such that postoperative incontinence may be unrelated to surgical intervention.[36] Finally, an expertly performed sphincterotomy may uncover an occult injury.[37] Incontinence may occur in 5–10% of patients but the impact on quality of life seems minor.[38,39] The distal one-third of the internal sphincter should be divided so that the muscle underlying the fissure is disrupted, allowing the fissure to heal. If the muscle is divided up to the level of the dentate line, the rate of incontinence may be increased.[40] The chance of injury to the external sphincter is minimized by placing the no. 11 blade accurately in the intersphincteric plane and sweeping medially.

▪ COMPLICATIONS FOLLOWING FISTULOTOMY

Recurrent or persistent fistulous disease can be particularly challenging and requires the surgeon to explore other sources of the fistula-in-ano. Recurrent disease may be prevented with simple marsupialization of the fistulous tract at the first operation, which minimizes the effort the patient needs to expend "packing" the tract to promote healing from the bottom up. However, in other circumstances recurrent disease actually represents persistent unrecognized and untreated disease in the deep post-anal space. In particular, patients with a history of multiple drainage procedures often have overlooked deep post–anal space disease. The experienced surgeon assesses the deep post-anal space in every patient presenting with an abscess or fistula. This is done with careful bi-digital palpation of the anus, trapping the perianal tissues between the index finger in the rectum and thumb compressing the sphincter and associated soft tissues in the posterior midline. The deep post-anal space is palpated by compressing the tissues extending from the anus to the coccyx between the thumb and index finger. Indurated woody tissue is often palpated representing an uncontrolled deep post–anal space abscess, the source of the "recurrent" disease. A posterior midline internal opening is often identified. Unroofing the deep post-anal space is the critical intervention. This may involve division of a considerable amount of skeletal muscle tissue that has the appearance of sphincter muscle, but is actually the anococcygeal raphe and not the external sphincter muscle, which is found more centrally next to the rectum. Management of the external openings and the posterior midline internal opening is often staged and may be individualized to include placement of setons, Penrose drains, or extensive unroofing of the fistulous tracts.[41]

Incontinence following fistulotomy must be quantified and qualified as to frequency of episodes and nature of substance passed. Unroofing of a chronic deep post–anal space abscess may be prominent, as division of muscle into the deep post-anal space may result in a "keyhole" deformity caused by the anococcygeal raphe pulling the tissues posteriorly. Incontinence may be minimized with an understanding of where the fistulous tracts pass.[42] If it is necessary to divide significant sphincter muscle because a flap procedure cannot be performed or if the amount of muscle divided is underappreciated, then direct immediate or staged repair may be considered. Immediate reapproximation of healthy well-vascularized muscle after débridement of the tissue involved with the tract may have the best chance at healing.

▪ COMPLICATIONS FOLLOWING RECTOVAGINAL FISTULA REPAIR

Recurrence of a rectovaginal fistula occurs in roughly 15% of patients after the initial repair and essentially half of the patients who undergo a second repair.[43] Keys to minimizing this complication are control of the underlying disease process (i.e., Crohn's disease), a tension-free anastomosis, adequate blood supply, and avoidance of overlapping suture lines. Patients being considered for mucosal or skin advancement flaps should be evaluated in the operating room or office with particular attention paid to mobility of the tissues. If the inflammation following the first repair has not resolved significantly, then the tissues will not be adequately mobile to allow advancement of the rectal mucosa down to the dentate line or the anal mucosa up into the distal rectum. This may require waiting 6–12 months.[44] Fecal diversion is not mandatory during this time period but may help the patient manage symptoms from the fistula. Mobility of the tissues can be assessed by sliding an anoscope across the rectal mucosa. If the tissue folds up underneath the scope as the scope is moved distally in the rectum, then the tissue should be mobile enough for a mucosal advancement flap repair. Counter-drainage through a separate stab incision may minimize the chance of a hematoma collecting under the flap which may subsequently become infected. Bowel confinement is not routinely practiced following this procedure, but a low-fiber, low-residue diet may limit the trauma for the first 2 weeks. A broad-based, well-vascularized flap is an important part of all repairs. Overlapping suture lines can be avoided with the mucosal advancement flaps. In fact the vaginal mucosa does not need to be approximated and may be allowed to drain freely decompressing the undersurface of the flap if a drain is not used.

Recent reports suggest that Surgisis mesh may be useful in recurrent rectovaginal fistulas as material that separates the suture lines and provides a framework for collagen deposition between the two mucosal surfaces.[45] We have experience with Alloderm applied through a trans-perineal extrasphincteric approach separating the vagina from the rectum. The rectum and vagina are débrided and repaired and the Alloderm is sutured in place to the sphincter complex and deep and superficial perineal bodies. The subcutaneous tissues and skin are reapproximated. Our short-term results have been encouraging.

Fibrin glue repair has a low success rate but essentially no morbidity, making this a reasonable choice for the management of recurrent fistulous disease including the broad, short, well-epithelialized tracts that tend to exist between the anorectum and vagina.[46–48]

▪ COMPLICATIONS FOLLOWING SPHINCTERPLASTY

The most significant complication following sphincterplasty is breakdown of the repair and worsened fecal incontinence. In this circumstance the patient may require fecal diversion while the wounds heal. The tissues should be débrided and allowed to granulate. Once the wounds have healed, consideration may be given to alternative repairs such as graciloplasty or an artificial sphincter. Although initial series suggested high success rates with overlapping sphincterplasty, more long-term studies suggest that the repair may not be as durable.[49]

Stenosis may result from reapproximating the tissues too rigorously. This complication can be avoided by placing a finger in the anus to calibrate the closure during the repair. This may initially be somewhat snug, but as the edema resolves functionality improves and stenosis is avoided.

Patients may initially complain of a perineal mass that is painful while sitting. This may improve with time as the overlapped muscle become less edematous. However, in some this never resolves to the patient's satisfaction and this has led a few surgeons to advocate reapproximation rather than an overlapping repair to minimize the chance of a painful bulky mass being created in the perineum.

Graciloplasty may be considered after failed sphincterplasty but these are complicated multistage procedures that many patients are reluctant to undergo after other procedures have failed with their associated complications.[50,51]

Implantation of an artificial sphincter is less complicated but there is a high infection rate and explantation rates are 25% in most series.[52]

▪ COMPLICATIONS FOLLOWING SURGERY FOR ANAL STENOSIS

Persistent stenosis following surgical repair may represent a need for a contralateral repair. The success of the second repair is not compromised by an initial contralateral repair.[53] In fact, both repairs may be performed at the first operation if the need is appreciated.

Impaired continence may be experienced as the perianal skin, which lacks the exquisite sensitivity of the anal mucosa, is advanced into the anal canal. However, enough anal mucosa should persist such that this is not a significant issue.

Infection may develop under the flap and may result in a superficial fistula that can be unroofed. The flap itself may necrose. It should be débrided and the wound allowed to granulate.[54,55] A repeat flap on the contralateral side may be created should stenosis persist.

▪ COMPLICATIONS FOLLOWING PERINEAL PROCTECTOMY

Early complications following perineal proctectomy are uncommon, but include bleeding, pelvic hematoma, and pelvic abscess.[56,57] The mesentery of the colon may be difficult to control in the transperineal approach and a hematoma may accumulate. Postoperatively a pelvic abscess may also develop. Both of these complications may be minimized with adequate exposure and hemostasis. The Ligasure device has proven advantageous in this procedure because it allows the surgeon to seal and divide the vessels and decreases the risk of loss of control of the vessels in the proximal pelvis.

The most frequent complication of perineal proctectomy is recurrent rectal prolapse. The advantage of the approach is that it avoids an abdominal incision in these often-debilitated patients who may have multiple comorbidities. The disadvantage is a somewhat higher recurrence rate of 20–30% versus 10–20% for the abdominal approaches.[58] Another disadvantage is the loss of rectal reservoir function with the perineal proctectomy. The abdominal procedures mobilize but spare the rectum thereby preserving rectal function.

▪ COMPLICATIONS FOLLOWING TREATMENT OF CONDYLOMATA ACUMINATA

The most common complication is that of recurrence. Condylomata are caused by the human papillomavirus, and as with many viruses, the trigger for recurrence is unknown. The virus may recur at any time and recurrence rates are higher in the immunocompromised.[59]

Anal stenosis may become a significant concern with repeated treatments. Care should be exercised to minimize destruction of normal, healthy tissue preserving bridges of normal uninvolved skin and mucosa while destroying the condyloma. Additional measures such as the use of acetic acid and the operating microscope to highlight involved tissues may help spare normal tissue.[60]

Bleeding requiring reoperation may occur immediately postoperatively but is exceedingly rare with a rate of less than 0.2% in our experience. However, a small amount of bleeding should be expected over the first month or two postoperatively.

Infection and abscess fistulous disease have not been seen in our experience after surgery for condylomata, but may complicate interferon injection of the lesions and may be seen as a result of locally aggressive condylomatous disease known as Buschke-Löwenstein tumors.

REFERENCES

1. Li S et al. Comparison of the costs and recovery profiles of three anesthetic techniques for ambulatory anorectal surgery. *Anesthesiology* 2000;93:1225–1230
2. Vinson-Bonnet B et al. Local infiltration with ropivacaine improves immediate postoperative pain control after hemorrhoidal surgery. *Dis Colon Rectum* 2002;45: 104–108

3. Luck AJ, Hewett PJ. Ischiorectal fossa block decreases posthemorrhoidectomy pain: randomized, prospective, double-blind clinical trial. *Dis Colon Rectum* 2000;43: 142–145
4. Chang FL et al. Postoperative intramuscular dextromethorphan injection provides postoperative pain relief and decreases opioid requirement after hemorrhoidectomy. *Acta Anaesthesiol Sin* 1999;37:179–183
5. Liu ST et al. Premedication with dextromethorphan provides posthemorrhoidectomy pain relief. *Dis Colon Rectum* 2000;43:507–510
6. O'Donovan S et al. Intraoperative use of Toradol facilitates outpatient hemorrhoidectomy. *Dis Colon Rectum* 1994;37:793–799
7. Coloma M et al. The effect of ketorolac on recovery after anorectal surgery: intravenous versus local administration. *Anesth Analg* 2000;90:1107–1110
8. Davies J et al. Botulinum toxin (Botox) reduces pain after hemorrhoidectomy: results of a double-blind, randomized study. *Dis Colon Rectum* 2003;46:1097–1102
9. Ho YH et al. Randomized controlled trial of trimebutine (anal sphincter relaxant) for pain after haemorrhoidectomy. *Br J Surg* 1997;84:377–379
10. Wasvary HJ et al. Randomized, prospective, double-blind, placebo-controlled trial of effect of nitroglycerin ointment on pain after hemorrhoidectomy. *Dis Colon Rectum* 2001;44:1069–1073
11. Elton C, Sen P, Montgomery AC. Initial study to assess the effects of topical glyceryl trinitrate for pain after haemorrhoidectomy. *Int J Surg Invest* 2001;2:353–357
12. Coskun A et al. Nitroderm TTS band application for pain after hemorrhoidectomy. *Dis Colon Rectum* 2001;44: 680-685
13. Goldstein ET, Williamson PR, Larach SW. Subcutaneous morphine pump for postoperative hemorrhoidectomy pain management. *Dis Colon Rectum* 1993;36:439–446
14. Rosen L et al. Outcome of delayed hemorrhage following surgical hemorrhoidectomy. *Dis Colon Rectum* 1993; 36:743–746
15. Bleday R et al. Symptomatic hemorrhoids: current incidence and complications of operative therapy. *Dis Colon Rectum* 1992;35:477–481
16. Hoff SD et al. Ambulatory surgical hemorrhoidectomy—a solution to postoperative urinary retention? *Dis Colon Rectum* 1994;37:1242–1244
17. Felt-Bersma RJ et al. Unsuspected sphincter defects shown by anal endosonography after anorectal surgery. A prospective study. *Dis Colon Rectum* 1995;38:249–253
18. Morgan R et al. Surgical management of anorectal incontinence due to internal anal sphincter deficiency. *Br J Surg* 1997;84:226–230
19. Abou-Zeid AA. Preliminary experience in management of fecal incontinence caused by internal anal sphincter injury. *Dis Colon Rectum* 2000;43:198–202; discussion 202–204
20. Cook TA, Brading AF, Mortensen NJ. The pharmacology of the internal anal sphincter and new treatments of ano-rectal disorders. *Aliment Pharmacol Ther* 2001;15: 887–898
21. Tjandra JJ et al. Injectable silicone biomaterial for fecal incontinence caused by internal anal sphincter dysfunction is effective. *Dis Colon Rectum* 2004;47:2138–2146
22. Kumar D, Benson MJ, Bland JE. Glutaraldehyde cross-linked collagen in the treatment of faecal incontinence. *Br J Surg* 1998;85:978–979
23. Devien CV, Pujol JP. Total circular hemorrhoidectomy. *Int Surg* 1989;74:154–157
24. Wolff BG, Culp CE. The Whitehead hemorrhoidectomy. An unjustly maligned procedure. *Dis Colon Rectum* 1988; 31:587–590
25. Habr-Gama A et al. Surgical treatment of anal stenosis: assessment of 77 anoplasties. *Clinics* 2005;60:17–20
26. Angelchik PD, Harms BA, Starling JR. Repair of anal stricture and mucosal ectropion with Y-V or pedicle flap anoplasty. *Am J Surg* 1993;166:55–59
27. Atakan IH et al. A life-threatening infection: Fournier's gangrene. *Int Urol Nephrol* 2002;34:387–392
28. Lehnhardt M et al. Fournier's gangrene after Milligan-Morgan hemorrhoidectomy requiring subsequent abdominoperineal resection of the rectum: report of a case. *Dis Colon Rectum* 2004;47:1729–1733
29. Bonner C, Prohm P, Storkel S. [Fournier gangrene as a rare complication after stapler hemorrhoidectomy. Case report and review of the literature]. *Chirurg* 2001;72: 1464–1466
30. Guy RJ, Seow-Choen F. Septic complications after treatment of haemorrhoids. *Br J Surg* 2003;90:147–156
31. Quevedo-Bonilla G et al. Septic complications of hemorrhoidal banding. *Arch Surg* 1988;123:650–651
32. Kaman L et al. Necrotizing fasciitis after injection sclerotherapy for hemorrhoids: report of a case. *Dis Colon Rectum* 1999;42:419–420
33. Parellada C. Randomized, prospective trial comparing 0.2 percent isosorbide dinitrate ointment with sphincterotomy in treatment of chronic anal fissure: a two-year follow-up. *Dis Colon Rectum* 2004;47:437–443
34. Arroyo A. et al. Long-term results of botulinum toxin for the treatment of chronic anal fissure: prospective clinical and manometric study. *Int J Colorectal Dis* 2005; 20:267–271
35. Zbar AP et al. Fecal incontinence after minor anorectal surgery. *Dis Colon Rectum* 2001;44:1610–1619; discussion 1619–1623
36. Ammari FF, Bani-Hani KE. Faecal incontinence in patients with anal fissure: a consequence of internal sphincterotomy or a feature of the condition? *Surgeon* 2004;2:225–229
37. Tjandra JJ et al. Faecal incontinence after lateral internal sphincterotomy is often associated with coexisting occult sphincter defects: a study using endoanal ultrasonography. *Aust N Z J Surg* 2001;71:598–602
38. Hyman N. Incontinence after lateral internal sphincterotomy: a prospective study and quality of life assessment. *Dis Colon Rectum* 2004;47:35–38
39. Arroyo Sebastian A et al. Surgical (close lateral internal sphincterotomy) versus chemical (botulinum toxin) sphincterotomy as treatment of chronic anal fissure. *Med Clin (Barc)* 2005;124:573–575

40. Mentes BB et al. Extent of lateral internal sphincterotomy: up to the dentate line or up to the fissure apex? *Dis Colon Rectum* 2005;48:365–370
41. Inceoglu R, Gencosmanoglu R. Fistulotomy and drainage of deep postanal space abscess in the treatment of posterior horseshoe fistula. *BMC Surg* 2003;3:10
42. Westerterp M et al. Anal fistulotomy between Skylla and Charybdis. *Colorectal Dis* 2003;5:549–551
43. Kodner IJ et al. Endorectal advancement flap repair of rectovaginal and other complicated anorectal fistulas. *Surgery* 1993;114:682–689; discussion 689–690
44. Halverson AL et al. Repair of recurrent rectovaginal fistulas. *Surgery* 2001;130:753–757; discussion 757–758
45. Pye PK et al. Surgisis mesh: a novel approach to repair of a recurrent rectovaginal fistula. *Dis Colon Rectum* 2004;47:1554–1556
46. Venkatesh KS Ramanujam P. Fibrin glue application in the treatment of recurrent anorectal fistulas. *Dis Colon Rectum* 1999;42:1136–1139
47. Buchanan GN et al. Efficacy of fibrin sealant in the management of complex anal fistula: a prospective trial. *Dis Colon Rectum* 2003;46:1167–1174
48. Loungnarath R et al. Fibrin glue treatment of complex anal fistulas has low success rate. *Dis Colon Rectum* 2004;47:432–436
49. Barisic GI et al. Outcome of overlapping anal sphincter repair after 3 months and after a mean of 80 months. *Int J Colorectal Dis* 2006;21:52–56
50. Baeten CG et al. Anal dynamic graciloplasty in the treatment of intractable fecal incontinence. *N Engl J Med* 1995;332:1600–1605
51. Williams NS et al. Development of an electrically stimulated neoanal sphincter. *Lancet* 1991;338:1166–1169
52. Parker SC et al. Artificial bowel sphincter: long-term experience at a single institution. *Dis Colon Rectum* 2003;46:722–729
53. Liberman H Thorson AG. How I do it. Anal stenosis. *Am J Surg* 2000;179:325–329
54. Maria G, Brisinda G, Civello IM. Anoplasty for the treatment of anal stenosis. *Am J Surg* 1998;175:158–160
55. Aitola PT, Hiltunen KM, Matikainen MJ. Y-V anoplasty combined with internal sphincterotomy for stenosis of the anal canal. *Eur J Surg* 1997;163:839–842
56. Johansen OB et al. Perineal rectosigmoidectomy in the elderly. *Dis Colon Rectum* 1993;36:767–772
57. Williams JG et al. Treatment of rectal prolapse in the elderly by perineal rectosigmoidectomy. *Dis Colon Rectum* 1992;35:830–834
58. Madoff RD, Mellgren A. One hundred years of rectal prolapse surgery. *Dis Colon Rectum* 1999;42:441–450
59. de la Fuente SG, Ludwig KA, Mantyh CR. Preoperative immune status determines anal condyloma recurrence after surgical excision. *Dis Colon Rectum* 2003;46:367–373
60. Chang GJ et al. Surgical treatment of high-grade anal squamous intraepithelial lesions: a prospective study. *Dis Colon Rectum* 2002;45:453–458

Section VII

LIVER

28

Hepatic Abscess and Cystic Disease of the Liver

Kathleen K. Christians ▪ *Henry A. Pitt*

Hepatic abscesses and cystic disease of the liver are a spectrum of infectious, congenital, neoplastic, and traumatic hepatic lesions which differ in etiology, treatment options, and outcomes. Most of these lesions are uncommon although their relative incidence varies worldwide, and simple, small congenital cysts occur in 3–5% of the general population. Significant improvements have been made in the diagnosis, treatment, and outcome for many of these cystic hepatic lesions, but considerable controversy continues regarding the best treatment options. Several classification systems exist for these lesions, and the one used in this chapter is presented in Table 28–1.

▪ PYOGENIC LIVER ABSCESS

Hippocrates is credited with the first description of a hepatic abscess in the year 4000 BC. More recently, Ochsner's classic 1938 paper[1] described this disease as one that occurred in young males with underlying intra-abdominal infection. In the early 20th century, the inciting event was usually appendicitis, causing pylephlebitis and resultant hepatic abscess. Open surgical drainage was the recommended treatment for many years. In 1953, McFadzean and associates[2] in Hong Kong advocated closed aspiration and antibiotics for treatment of solitary pyogenic liver abscess; however, this treatment did not gain widespread acceptance until imaging advancements in the 1980s allowed for precise localization and a percutaneous approach to treatment. Modern times have seen a major shift in etiology, affected patient population, and treatment of pyogenic abscesses in the liver. Liver abscesses now rarely occur in young people secondary to appendicitis. They usually occur in older, more debilitated patients, often in the setting of malignancy. At present the most common source of a pyogenic liver abscess is biliary tract obstruction, and the current treatment includes antibiotics, usually with a percutaneous drainage procedure.[3–5]

ETIOLOGY

Kupffer cells act as a filter for the clearance of microorganisms in the liver. These organisms reach the liver via the bloodstream, the biliary tree, or by direct extension. Abscesses occur when normal hepatic clearance mechanisms fail or the system is overwhelmed. Parenchymal necrosis and hematoma secondary to trauma, obstructive biliary processes, ischemia, and malignancy also promote invasion of microorganisms.

In order to appropriately treat the abscess, source control must be achieved. Six distinct categories have been identified as potential sources: (1) bile ducts, causing ascending cholangitis; (2) portal vein, causing pylephlebitis from appendicitis or diverticulitis; (3) direct extension from a contiguous disease; (4) trauma due to blunt or penetrating injuries; (5) hepatic artery, due to septicemia; and (6) cryptogenic[3,4] (Fig 28–1).

Disease of the biliary system accounts for 35–40% of all pyogenic liver abscesses, and 40% of pyogenic liver abscesses of biliary origin are related to an un-

TABLE 28–1. CLASSIFICATION OF CYSTIC HEPATIC LESIONS

I. Infectious hepatic cysts
- A. Pyogenic liver abscess
- B. Amebic liver abscess
- C. Hydatid liver cysts

II. Congenital hepatic cysts
- A. Simple cysts
- B. Polycystic liver disease

III. Neoplastic hepatic cysts
- A. Cystadenoma
- B. Cystadenocarcinoma

IV. Traumatic hepatic cysts

derlying malignancy.[3] Obstruction of the biliary tree is the norm in these patients, with cholangitis present in up to one-half.[6] Intrahepatic stones and related biliary stricture are predominant in Eastern series whereas malignant biliary obstruction is more common in the West.[4] Any manipulation of the biliary tree—namely cholangiography, percutaneous transhepatic stents, endoscopic stent placement, and biliary-enteric anastomoses—also predispose patients to cholangitis and pyogenic hepatic abscess. Malignancy also contributes to poor nutrition and immunosuppression, potentiating the whole process.

Intestinal pathology is responsible for 20% of all pyogenic liver abscesses. Transient bacteremia due to bacterial translocation or frank gastrointestinal perforation cause overwhelming numbers of microorganisms to spread via the portal venous system to the liver. In the preantibiotic era, 43% of Ochsner's 622 patients seeded the liver via the portal vein, and appendicitis was the most common source (34%).[1] Today, appendicitis accounts for only 2% of all pyogenic liver abscesses. Diverticulitis, perforated colon cancers, and abscesses elsewhere in the abdomen and pelvis remain common causes of pyogenic liver abscesses. Primary and metastatic liver tumors may also become colonized with enteric flora.

Contiguous extension has also been reported as an abscess source in the setting of gangrenous cholecystitis, perforated ulcers, and subphrenic abscesses. Trauma to the liver causes parenchymal necrosis and clot, which creates an ideal milieu for the seeding and proliferation of microorganisms and subsequent abscess formation. Ablative procedures for tumors can create this same environment. Microorganisms can then seed these areas of necrosis through intraoperative contamination, biliary-enteric anastomoses, external drains involving the biliary tree, or percutaneous drains placed near the site of trauma or ablation.

Arterial embolization of bacteria via the hepatic artery causes approximately 12% of pyogenic liver abscesses. Intravenous drug abuse accounts for most of these cases, but hepatic artery chemoembolization and umbilical artery catheterization have also been cited. Arterial embolization can also occur from distant infection in the heart, lungs, kidneys, bones, ears, and teeth.[5]

Cryptogenic abscesses, those of unknown etiology, occur in 10–45% of patients, depending on the aggressiveness of investigation used to define the source.[5,7] Patients with cryptogenic abscesses usually have comorbidities such as diabetes, immunosuppression, or malignancy. Abscesses in these patients tend to be solitary, and usually contain a single anaerobe.

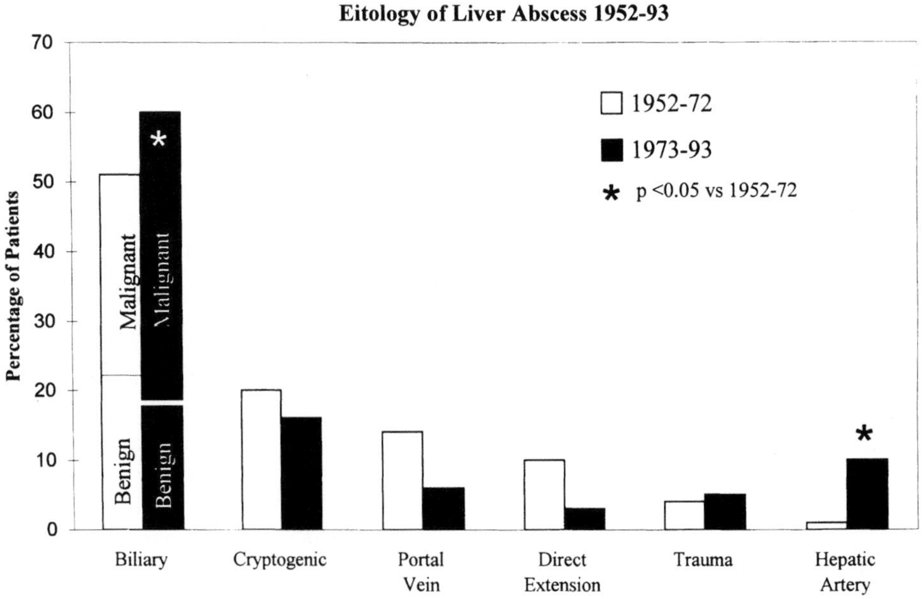

Figure 28–1. Comparison of etiology of pyogenic liver abscesses treated from 1952–1972 and 1973–1993 at the Johns Hopkins Hospital. (Reproduced, with permission, from Huang CJ, Pitt HA, Lipsett PA et al. Pyogenic hepatic abscess: Changing trends over 42 years. *Ann Surg* 1996;223:600–609.)

INCIDENCE

The incidence of pyogenic liver abscess is on the rise. Pyogenic liver abscess affected 5–13 patients per 100,000 admissions prior to 1970, and accounts for approximately 15 cases per 100,000 admissions today. Seeto and Rocky[9] reported an incidence nearly twofold that of earlier reports (22 per 100,000). This rising incidence is attributed to a more aggressive management approach to hepatobiliary and pancreatic cancers as well as major improvements in diagnostic imaging.[4,10]

PREDISPOSING FACTORS

Pyogenic liver abscesses occur more frequently in adults with comorbid conditions including diabetes mellitus, cirrhosis, pancreatitis, inflammatory bowel disease, pyelonephritis, and peptic ulcer disease. Solid organ cancers as well as lymphoma and leukemia are present in 17–36% of patients with liver abscesses.[5] Branum and associates from Duke[11] reported an increased incidence in patients with underlying malignancy and immunosuppression. Civardi and colleagues[12] as well as Lambiase and coworkers[13] have reported series of patients with liver abscesses and underlying acquired immune deficiency. The combination of chemotherapy and steroid use is thought to be responsible in these cases.

In children, pyogenic liver abscesses tend to occur in patients with host-defense abnormalities or immune disorders. Complement deficiencies, chronic granulomatous disease, and leukemia and other malignancies place these children at increased risk for liver abscess. Hepatic abscesses are also seen in sickle cell anemia, congenital hepatic fibrosis, polycystic liver disease, and after liver transplantation (Table 28–2).[5]

PATHOLOGY

The source of the liver abscess is predictive of the number, location, and size of the abscess affecting a given patient. In general, portal, traumatic, and cryptogenic hepatic abscesses are solitary and large, while biliary and arterial abscesses are multiple and small. Huang and associates[4] reported that 63% of patients had abscesses involving the right lobe, 14% had abscesses involving the left lobe, and 22% had bilobar disease. The number of bilateral and multiple abscesses have increased as more patients present with a biliary etiology. Bilateral disease may be seen in 90% of patients with an arterial or biliary source. In contrast, those with intra-abdominal infections frequently present with right lobe abscesses due to preferential flow from the superior mesenteric vein. Fungal abscesses are usually multiple, bilateral, and miliary.[5]

BACTERIOLOGY

Confirmation of pyogenic liver abscess involves aspiration of the abscess as well as positive blood cultures. Abscess cultures are positive for growth in the majority (80–97%), whereas blood cultures are positive in only 50–60% of cases.[9,14] *Escherichia coli*, *Klebsiella* species, enterococci, and *Pseudomonas* species are the most common aerobic organisms cultured in recent series, whereas *Bacteroides* species, anaerobic streptococci, and *Fusobacterium* species are the most common anaerobes.[10] Huang and colleagues[4] cited the increased use of indwelling biliary stents as the cause of an increasing incidence of *Klebsiella*, streptococcal, staphylococcal, and pseudomonal species in liver abscesses. They also noted the presence of fungi in 22% of cultures taken between 1973 and 1993 compared to only 1% between 1952 and 1972. Broad-spectrum antibiotic use in the treatment of cholangitis was thought to be the causative factor of this phenomenon. *Candida* fungal abscesses are also found in cancer patients that have undergone cytotoxic chemotherapy. *Mycobacterium tuberculosis* is a common infecting organism in the acquired immune deficiency syndrome[6] (Table 28–3).

The species of microorganism found in a hepatic abscess is related to the source of the abscess. The biliary tree gives rise to abscesses predominantly comprised of *E. coli* and *Klebsiella*. *E. coli*, enterococci, and anaerobes are the main organisms recovered from abscesses related to the intestinal tract. Anaerobes are the usual microorganisms found in cryptogenic liver abscesses. The reasons for negative cultures may relate to poor anaerobic culture technique or the use of broad-spectrum antibiotics prior to abscess drainage. If suspected bacte-

TABLE 28–2. PREDISPOSING FACTORS FOR PYOGENIC LIVER ABSCESSES

Children	Adults
Chronic granulomatous disease	Diabetes mellitus
Complement deficiencies	Cirrhosis
Leukemia	Chronic pancreatitis
Malignancy	Peptic ulcer disease
Sickle cell anemia	Inflammatory bowel disease
Polycystic liver disease	Jaundice
Congenital hepatic fibrosis	Pyelonephritis
Posttransplant liver failure	Malignancy
Necrotizing enterocolitis	Leukemia and lymphoma
Chemotherapy and steroid therapy	Chemotherapy and steroid therapy
Acquired immunodeficiency syndrome	Acquired immunodeficiency syndrome

TABLE 28–3. ORGANISMS ISOLATED FROM PYOGENIC LIVER ABSCESSES

Category of Organism	% of Patients
Gram-Negative Aerobes	50–70
Escherichia coli	35–45
Klebsiella	18
Proteus	10
Enterobacter	15
Serratia	Rare
Morganella	Rare
Acinetobacter	Rare
Gram-Positive Aerobes	55
Stretococcal species	20
Enteroccocus faecalis	10
β-Streptococci	5
α-Streptococci	5
Staphylococcal species	15
Anaerobes	40–50
Bacteroides species	24
Bacteroides fragilis	15
Fusobacterium	10
Peptostreptococcus	10
Clostridium	5
Actinomyces	Rare
Fungal	26
Sterile	7

rial cultures are repeatedly negative, amebic and parasitic organisms must be considered because they are difficult to identify by routine staining and culture techniques.[5]

DIAGNOSIS

The clinical presentation of pyogenic liver abscess is usually subacute and nonspecific, leading to delays in presentation, diagnosis, and treatment. In Seeto and Rocky's review[9] of 142 patients with pyogenic liver abscesses, the classic triad of fever, jaundice, and right upper quadrant tenderness was present in less than 10% of patients overall.

CLINICAL PRESENTATION

Most patients have fever (92%) and 50% have abdominal pain, but only half have pain in the right upper quadrant. Diarrhea occurs in less than 10% of patients. The liver may be tender (65%) and enlarged (48%), and the patient may appear jaundiced (54%). Other nonspecific complaints include malaise, anorexia, and nausea. If the diaphragm is involved, pleuritic chest pain, cough, or dyspnea may occur. If the abscess ruptures, peritonitis and sepsis may be presenting features [4,6,9] (Table 28–4).

LABORATORY EVALUATION

Leukocytosis is present in 70–90%, an elevated alkaline phosphatase in 80%, and an elevated bilirubin and transaminases in 50–67% of patients. Anemia, hypoalbuminemia, and prolonged prothrombin time are seen in 60–75% of patients.[4,6,8–10]

RADIOLOGY

Plain films such as chest radiographs are abnormal in 50% of patients. Findings may include an elevated right hemidiaphragm, a right pleural effusion, and/or right lower lobe atelectasis. Abdominal films may show hepatomegaly, air-fluid levels in the presence of gas-forming organisms, or portal venous gas if pylephlebitis is the source (Fig 28–2). Ultrasound will distinguish solid from cystic lesions and is cost effective and portable. Ultrasound (US) is 80–95% sensitive but has limited utility in the morbidly obese and in lesions that are located under the ribs or in an inhomogeneous liver.

Computed tomography (CT) is more sensitive (95–100%) than US in detecting hepatic abscesses. On CT examination, an abscess is of lower attenuation than the surrounding liver, and the wall of the

TABLE 28–4. SYMPTOMS, SIGNS, AND LABORATORY DATA OF PYOGENIC LIVER ABSCESSES

	% of Pyogenic Abscesses
SYMPTOM	
Fever	83
Weight loss	60
Pain	55
Nausea and vomiting	50
Malaise	50
Chills	37
Anorexia	34
Cough or pleurisy	30
Pruritus	17
Diarrhea	12
SIGN	
Right upper quadrant tenderness	52
Hepatomegaly	40
Jaundice	31
Right upper quadrant mass	25
Ascites	25
Pleural effusion or rub	20
LABORATORY DATA	
Increased alkaline phosphatase	87
WBC count >10,000/mm^3	71
Albumin <3 g/dL	55
Hematocrit <36%	53
Bilirubin >2 mg/dL	24

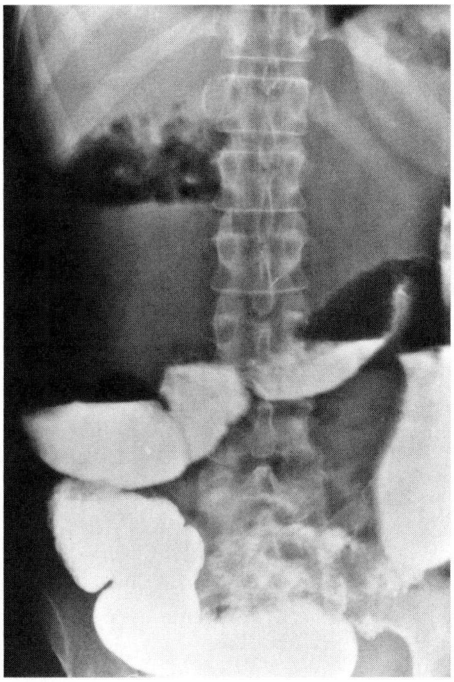

Figure 28–2. Plain film of a barium enema performed on a patient with a large gas-filled abscess located in the right hepatic lobe. (Reproduced, with permission, from Pitt HA. Liver abscess. In: Zuidema GD, Tureotte JG (eds). *Shackleford's Surgery of the Alimentary Tract*, 3rd ed. Philadelphia, PA: WB Saunders; 1991:444.)

abscess may enhance with intravenous contrast administration. Lesions are detectable to around 0.5 cm with CT and are not limited by shadowing from ribs or air. CT and US may also be used to evaluate and potentially treat the source of infection by percutaneous drainage (Fig 28–3). Radionuclide scanning with 99mTc is no longer used and has been completely replaced by CT and US. On the other hand, cholangiography, often via an indwelling biliary stent, may visualize the abscess (Fig 28–4).

TREATMENT

The appropriate treatment for pyogenic liver abscesses requires treatment of the abscess itself, and concomitant treatment of the source. Steps in management include antibiotic administration, radiologic confirmation by US or CT, and drainage. Exceptions to this strategy include multiple small abscesses and miliary fungal abscesses. These abscesses are treated with intravenous antibiotics and antifungals respectively, without a drainage procedure.

Antibiotics

After confirmatory imaging with US or CT, abscesses are aspirated, blood cultures are drawn, and broad-spectrum intravenous antibiotics are administered until sensitivities allow a more selective antibiotic choice. Serologic testing should also be performed if an amebic abscess is suspected.[6]

Classic antibiotic regimens include an aminoglycoside, clindamycin, and either ampicillin or vancomycin. Fluoroquinolones can replace aminoglycosides, and metronidazole can be used instead of clindamycin, especially if an amebic source is suspected. Single-agent therapy with ticarcillin-clavulanate, imipenem-cilastatin or piperacillin-tazobactam is also acceptable.[10] Treatment used to be given for 4–6 weeks; however, many

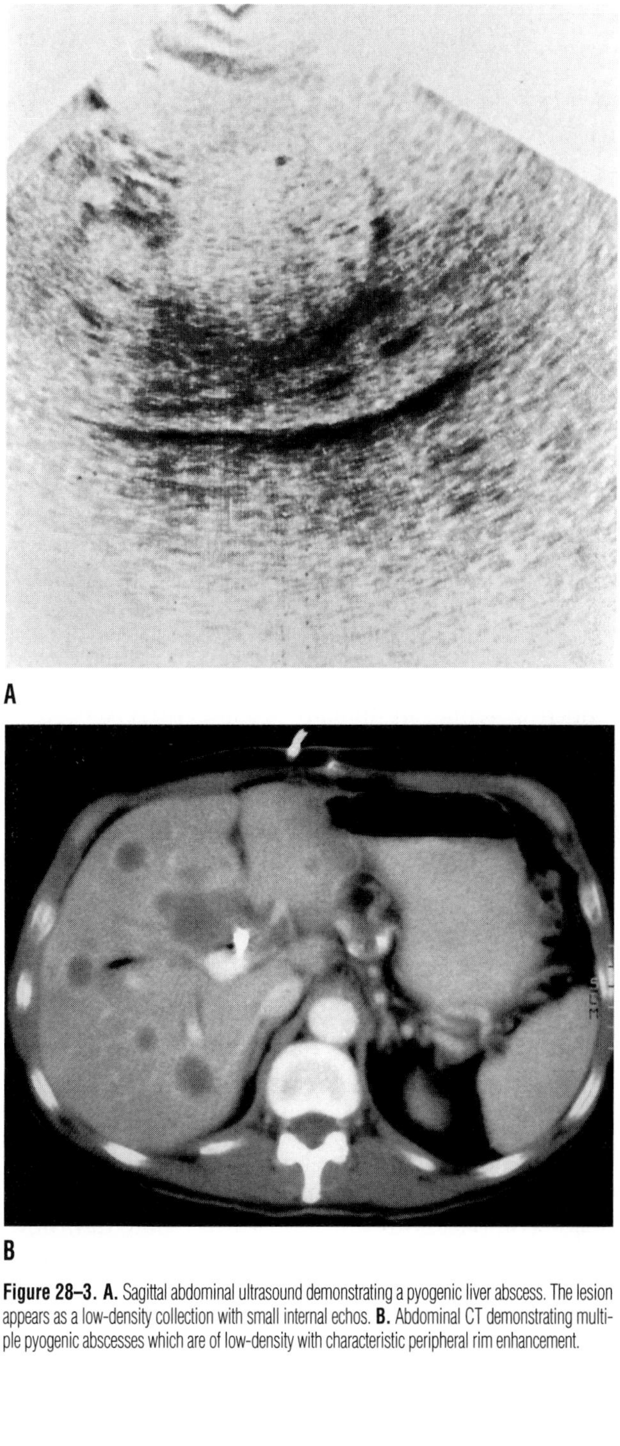

Figure 28–3. A. Sagittal abdominal ultrasound demonstrating a pyogenic liver abscess. The lesion appears as a low-density collection with small internal echos. **B.** Abdominal CT demonstrating multiple pyogenic abscesses which are of low-density with characteristic peripheral rim enhancement.

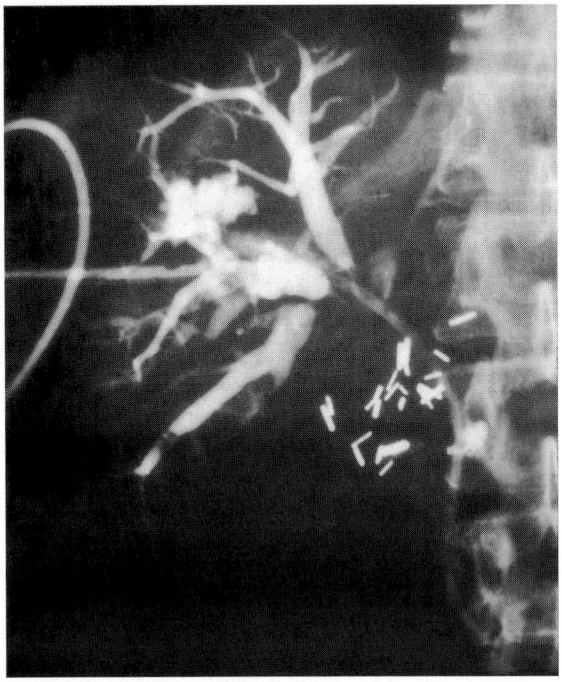

Figure 28–4. Cholangiogram via a transhepatic stent in a patient with biliary obstruction secondary to recurrent gastric cancer. It shows a communicating liver abscess.

studies now document success with only 2 weeks of antibiotic therapy.[5]

In the setting of multiple abscesses <1.5 cm in size and no concurrent surgical disease, patients may be treated with IV antibiotics alone. However, multiple small abscesses frequently imply biliary tract disease and may require biliary drainage for source control. Similarly, fungal abscesses are miliary in nature and not amenable to percutaneous or surgical drainage. Prolonged systemic antifungals are the preferred treatment for fungal abscesses.

Aspiration and Percutaneous Catheter Drainage

Needle aspiration and percutaneous catheter drainage of liver abscesses have similar mortality rates; however, recurrence rates and the requirement for surgical intervention may be greater in those who only undergo aspiration.[9] Needle aspiration is less invasive, less expensive, and avoids all of the complications associated with catheter care. Giorgio and colleagues[15] reported a series of 115 patients with a 98.3% success rate for needle aspiration, no mortality, and no procedure-related morbidity. A randomized controlled trial by Rajak et al[16] in 1998 compared percutaneous needle aspiration to catheter drainage and also found no major complications and no deaths. They did, however, report only 60% success with needle aspiration versus a 100% success rate with catheter drainage.[16] The highest rate of recurrence (15%) occurred in patients with biliary tract disease and obstructive lesions, whereas the recurrence rate with cryptogenic abscesses was less than 2%. This observation suggests that the underlying lesion should potentially influence the type of therapy chosen.[9]

Patients in whom percutaneous drainage is not appropriate include those patients with (1) multiple large abscesses; (2) a known intra-abdominal source that requires surgery; (3) an abscess of unknown etiology; (4) ascites; and (5) abscesses that would require transpleural drainage.[3] An example of a patient managed by percutaneous drainage is provided in Figure 28–5.

Surgical Drainage

Surgical drainage was the widely accepted treatment for liver abscesses for many years following Ochsner's 1938 report.[1] Abscesses were drained extraperitoneally via a 12th-rib resection to avoid contamination of the peritoneal cavity. With the advent of systemic antibiotics, transperitoneal surgical exploration also was considered a safe surgical approach. The transperitoneal approach has the advantages of the ability to: (1) treat the inciting pathology in the remainder of the abdomen/pelvis; (2) gain access and exposure of the entire liver for evaluation and treatment; and (3) access the biliary tree for cholangiography and bile duct exploration. Since the 1980s, treatment has shifted to a less invasive approach utilizing percutaneous needle aspiration or catheter drainage to treat pyogenic abscesses. Surgical drainage is currently reserved for patients that have failed nonoperative therapy, those who need surgical treatment of the underlying source, those with multiple macroscopic abscesses, those on steroids, or those patients with concomitant ascites.[4]

COMPLICATIONS

Up to 40% of patients develop complications from pyogenic liver abscesses, with the most common being generalized sepsis. In addition to sepsis, morbidity can include pleural effusions, empyema, and pneumonia. Abscesses may also rupture intraperitoneally, which is frequently fatal. Usually, however, the abscess does not rupture, but develops a controlled leak resulting in a perihepatic abscess. Pyogenic abscesses also can cause hemobilia and hepatic vein thrombosis.[5]

OUTCOME

From the 1950s to 1990, mortality rates varied from as low as 11% to as high as 88%.[3] The high mortality rates came from delay or failure to diagnose the abscess, failure to detect smaller intrahepatic abscesses, ineffective surgical

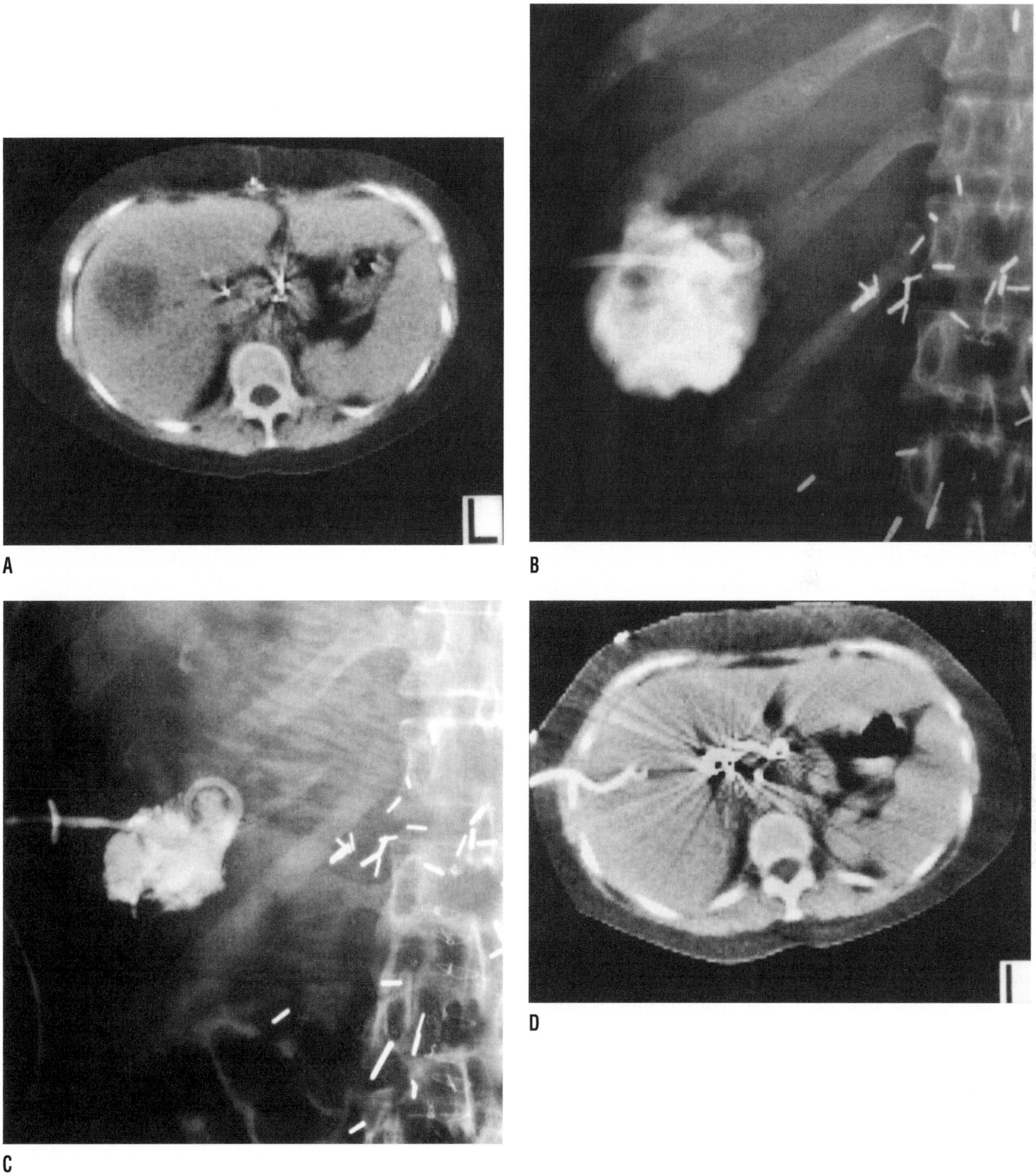

Figure 28–5. A. CT demonstrating a pyogenic abscess in the right hepatic lobe. **B.** Contrast injected into the abscess cavity through a percutaneously placed drainage catheter. **C.** Sinogram performed 2 weeks later revealing a decrease in the size of the abscess cavity. **D.** CT after 4 weeks demonstrating complete resolution of the abscess. (Reproduced, with permission, from Pitt HA. Liver abscess. In: Zuidema GD, Tureotte JG (eds). *Shackleford's Surgery of the Alimentary Tract*, 3rd ed. Philadelphia, PA: WB Saunders; 1991:444.)

drainage, lack of source control, associated malignancy, immune insufficiency, or other major comorbidities. Failure to (1) establish a diagnosis and (2) achieve adequate drainage were major factors that contributed to high mortality rates. No general consensus has been achieved regarding risk factors due to the variability of the patient population being studied and the presence of malignancy in the population (Table 28–5).

■ AMEBIC LIVER ABSCESS

Amebic liver abscess is caused by the parasitic protozoan *Entamoeba histolytica.* The disease was described in association with blood and mucus diarrheal stools in the 5th century BC by Hippocrates and other practitioners. In 1890, Sir William Osler described the first North American case when, after an attack of dysentery while in Panama, a physician's stool and abscess fluid were both found to contain amebae. Councilman and LaFleur of Johns Hopkins Hospital went on to detail the pathogenic role of amebae and coined the terms "amebic dysentery" and "amebic liver abscess" in 1891.[17] Today, invasive amebiasis is second only to malarial disease as a cause of protozoan-mediated death.[18]

ETIOLOGY

Two species of ameba infect humans. *E. dispar* is associated with an asymptomatic carrier state and not with disease. *E. histolytica* is responsible for all forms of invasive disease. The life cycle involves cysts, invasive trophozoites, and fecally contaminated food or water to initiate the infection.[18,19] Fecal-oral transmission occurs; the cyst passes through the stomach into the intestine unscathed, andthen pancreatic enzymes start to digest the outer cyst wall. The trophozoite is then released into the intestine and multiplies there. Normally, no invasion occurs, and the patient develops amebic dysentery alone or becomes an asymptomatic carrier. In a small number of cases, the trophozoite invades through the intestinal mucosa, travels through the mesenteric lymphatics and veins, and begins to accumulate in the hepatic parenchyma, forming an abscess cavity. Liquefied hepatic parenchyma with blood and debris gives a characteristic "anchovy paste" appearance to the abscess.[10]

TABLE 28–5. FACTORS ASSOCIATED WITH A POOR OUTCOME IN PATIENTS WITH PYOGENIC LIVER ABSCESSES

Age >70 years	WBC count >20.000/mm^3
Diabetes mellitus	Increasing bilirubin
Associated malignancy	Increasing SGOT
Biliary etiology	Albumin <2 g/dL
Multiple abscesses	Aerobic abscess
Septicemia	Significant complication
Polymicrobial bacteremia	

INCIDENCE

Worldwide, an estimated 500 million people are carriers of *E. histolytica* or *E. dispar*, 50 million people have active disease and 50,000–100,000 die annually. The vast majority of these infections are acquired in the developing world. Amebiasis is common in Africa, Indochina, and Central and South America. Up to 5% of diarrheal illness in Mexico is due to *Entamoeba* disease.[18] The overall prevalence in the United States is 4% per year. High-risk groups in the United States include sexually active homosexual men, immigrants, tourists who travel to endemic areas, institutionalized people, and those with HIV.[20] Children also have been known to infect entire families. Amebiasis follows a bimodal age distribution. One peak is at age 2–3 years, with a case fatality rate of 20%, and the second peak is at >40 years, with a case fatality rate of 70%.[18] Those living in developing countries have a greater risk and an earlier age of infection than do those in developed regions. Low socioeconomic status and unsanitary conditions are significant independent risk factors for infection.[20] Amebic liver abscess is ten times as common in men as in women and is a rare disease in children.[19]

PATHOLOGY

Roughly 90% of people that become infected with *E. histolytica* are asymptomatically colonized, and factors that control the invasiveness of this organism are not completely understood. *E. histolytica* cysts can last for days in a dried state at temperatures of 30°C. These cysts are resistant to the effects of gastric acid pH, but become stimulated to form trophozoites in the alkaline pH of the bowel. Trophozoites are found in the colon and in the feces of humans and mammals. Humans become reservoirs, and transmission occurs by ingesting food and water contaminated with amebic cysts, or occasionally through person-to-person contact. Incubation takes 1–4 weeks. Left untreated, asymptomatic individuals may shed cysts for many years.

Invasive amebiasis can include anything from amebic dysentery to metastatic abscesses. The most common form of the invasive disease is colitis. The majority (70–80%) of patients experience a gradual onset of symptoms with worsening diarrhea, abdominal pain, weight loss, and stools consisting of blood and mucus. Trophozoites invade and induce apoptosis in colonic mucosa resulting in "buttonhole" ulcers with undermined edges. Trophozoites are actually found in the edge of the ulcers.

The most common extraintestinal site of amebiasis is the liver, occurring in 1–7% of children and 50% of adults (usually males) with invasive disease.[18] Trophozoites reach the liver through the portal system, causing focal necrosis of hepatocytes and multiple microabscesses that coalesce into a single abscess. The central cavity of the lesion contains a homogenous thick liquid that is typically red/brown and yellow in color and similar to anchovy paste in consistency.[21]

DIAGNOSIS

The definitive diagnosis of amebic liver abscess is by *E. histolytica* trophozoites in the pus and by detection of serum antibodies to the ameba.[21] The differential diagnosis should include pyogenic liver abscess, necrotic adenoma, and echinococcal cyst.

Clinical Presentation

Ninety percent of amebic liver abscesses occur in young adult males. The presentation may be acute, with fever and right upper quadrant (RUQ) pain, or subacute, with weight loss and less frequent fever and abdominal pain. The usual case of amebic liver abscess does not present with concurrent colitis, but patients may have had dysentery within the last year. Alcohol abuse is common.[22] Eighty percent of patients with amebic liver abscess present with symptoms that develop within 2–4 weeks, including fever, cough, and a dull aching pain in the RUQ or epigastrium. Diaphragmatic involvement causes right-sided pleural pain or pain referred to the shoulder. Gastrointestinal symptoms of nausea, vomiting, abdominal cramping, abdominal distention, diarrhea, and constipation occur in 10–35%. Hepatomegaly with point tenderness over the liver or subcostal region is common[19] (Table 28–6). In contrast to pyogenic liver abscesses, amebic liver abscesses are more likely to occur in males under 50 years old who have immigrated or traveled to a country where the disease is endemic. The patient will also not be jaundiced or have biliary disease or diabetes mellitus[19] (Table 28–7).

Laboratory Evaluation

Patients may present with a mild to moderate elevation of the white blood cell count and anemia. Acutely, alkaline phosphatase will be normal and alanine aminotransferase levels will be elevated. The opposite is true of these values in patients with chronic disease.[19] Jaundice is rare. Because amebic abscesses involve destruction of liver parenchyma and are often larger than pyogenic liver abscesses on presentation, patients may have an elevated prothrombin time.[5] If colitis is present, wet mount preps of stool samples contain trophozoites 30% of the time in one sample and 70% if three samples are tested. Liver abscesses are associated with positive stool samples in 40–50% of cases.[18]

TABLE 28–6. SYMPTOMS, SIGNS, AND LABORATORY DATA OF AMEBIC LIVER ABSCESSES

	% of Amebic Abscesses
SYMPTOM	
Pain	90
Fever	87
Nausea and vomiting	85
Anorexia	50
Weight loss	45
Malaise	25
Diarrhea	25
Cough or pleurisy	25
Pruritus	<1
SIGN	
Hepatomegaly	85
Right upper quadrant tenderness	84
Pleural effusion or rub	40
Right upper quadrant mass	12
Ascites	10
Jaundice	5
LABORATORY DATA	
Increased alkaline phosphatase	80
WBC count >10,000/mm³	70
Hematocrit <36%	49
Albumin <3 g/dL	44
Bilirubin >2 mg/dL	10

Radiology

Chest radiographs are abnormal in two-thirds of patients with amebic liver abscess and frequently show pleural effusion, infiltrates, or an elevated hemidiaphragm.[5] Ultrasound, CT, and magnetic resonance imaging (MRI) are all excellent methods of detecting amebic liver abscesses but are nonspecific.[19]

In 75–80% of cases, only a single abscess is present and in the right lobe, 10% are in the left lobe, and the rest are multiple. Six percent may present as a caudate lobe abscess. Only 40% have typical sonographic features of amebic liver abscess, and serial scanning shows no change in the ultrasound features despite adequate treatment (Fig 28–6). The mean resolution time is 7 months, and 70% have findings that persist for more

TABLE 28–7. DISTINGUISHING CLINICAL CHARACTERISTICS OF PATIENTS WITH HEPATIC ABSCESSES

Amebic	Pyogenic
Age <50 years	Age >50 years
Male:female ratio 10:1	Male:female ratio 1:1
Hispanic descent	No ethnic predisposition
Recent travel to endemic area	Malignancy
Pulmonary dysfunction	High fevers
Abdominal pain	Pruritus
Diarrhea	Jaundice
Abdominal tenderness	Septic shock
Hepatomegaly	Palpable mass

than 6 months. Eventually, resolution may be complete or result in a small residual cystic cavity that resembles a simple cyst of the liver.[23]

Serology

Serum antibodies are positive in 85% of patients with invasive colitis, and 99% of patients with liver abscesses.[24] Countries with a high prevalence of amebiasis also have a high prevalence of positive serologies in asymptomatic individuals. Therefore serologies help exclude the diagnosis only in appropriately chosen populations. Patients with *E. dispar* infection will have negative serologies. Biopsies of the edge of an ulcer or the wall of an abscess reveal trophozoites with periodic acid-Schiff stain.[18]

Diagnostic Aspiration

Serologic data are usually available within 24–48 hours; therefore the need to aspirate a suspected amebic abscess is questionable. Diagnostic aspirations are usually done when amebic serologies are negative and a pyogenic cause needs to be ruled out. The fluid of an amebic abscess is odorless, and Gram's stain and cultures are negative. Amebae are recovered in 33–90% of aspirates, and wall scrapings increase the yield. Aspiration should not be done if an echinococcal cyst or a cancer is suspected. The former may result in anaphylactic shock, and the latter has the potential to seed the tract with malignant cells.[5]

The diagnosis of invasive amebiasis is most commonly attempted by a combination of stool testing for ova and parasites (O&P) and serologic testing, possibly coupled with colonoscopy and biopsy of intestinal lesions or drainage of liver abscesses. Numerous studies have demonstrated the inadequacies of microscopic examination for *E. histolytica* for the diagnosis of both amebic colitis and liver abscess. Antigen detection or polymerase chain reaction (PCR) to detect *E. histolytica* in the stool is a better approach than O&P, but requires fresh or frozen stool specimens (versus preserved), and PCR is impractical in the developing world. The detection of amebic markers in the sera of patients with amebic colitis and liver abscess remains only a research tool at the present time.[20]

TREATMENT

Since the introduction of metronidazole in the 1960s, surgical drainage of amebic liver abscesses has become virtually unnecessary. Drainage procedures, regardless of the approach, are reserved for those cases in whom the diagnosis is questionable or when complications occur.

Antibiotics

Noninvasive infections can be treated with paromomycin. Nitroimidazoles, especially metronidazole, are the mainstays of treatment for invasive amebiasis. Nitroimidazoles with longer half-lives (secnidazole, tinidazole, and ornidazole) are better tolerated and can be given for shorter periods of time, but are not available in the United States.[19] Metronidazole reaches high concentrations in the liver, stomach, intestine, and kidney. This antibiotic crosses the placenta and blood-brain barrier and is contraindicated in the first trimester of pregnancy. The drug is also excreted in milk; thus breastfeeding should be discontinued during use. Serious side effects are rare.

Positive responses to metronidazole should be seen by the third day of treatment. At 5 days, an 85% cure rate is achieved, and this response may be increased to 95% by 10 days. Five to fifteen percent of patients with amebic liver abscess may be resistant to

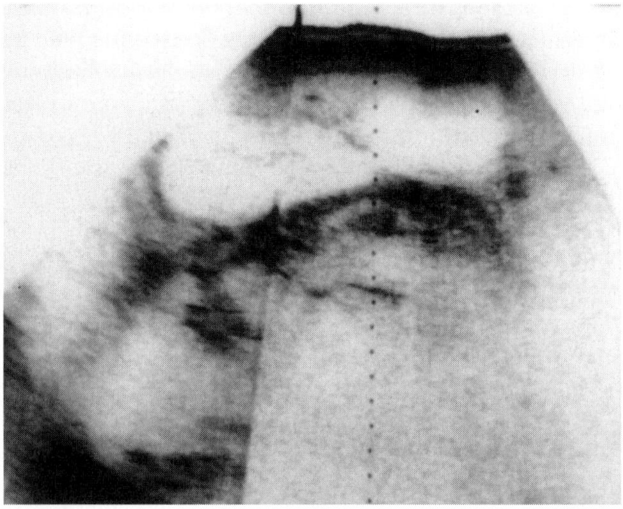

Figure 28–6. Abdominal ultrasound of two amebic abscesses located in the left hepatic lobe demonstrating a predominantly cystic fluid collection.

metronidazole.[23] Parasites persist in the intestine in up to 40–60% of patients who get a nitroimidazole; thus nitroimidazole treatment should be followed with paromomycin or diloxanide furoate to cure luminal infection or risk relapse from residual infection in the intestine.[19]

Therapeutic Aspiration

Blessmann and colleagues[25] reported a prospective, randomized trial of patients with amebic abscesses that were treated with metronidazole alone or with US-guided aspiration of the fluid plus medication. Fever, RUQ pain, liver tenderness, and laboratory studies such as erythrocyte sedimentation rate, white blood cell count, hemoglobin, C-reactive protein, and abscess size were obtained on admission and daily thereafter. Abscess aspiration resulted in improved liver tenderness within the first 3 days, but no other difference was demonstrable between the two groups. The authors concluded that this minor benefit was insufficient to justify routine needle aspiration. They advocated drug treatment alone for uncomplicated abscesses with a diameter up to 10 cm and located in the right lobe of the liver.

Therapeutic aspiration may occasionally be required as an adjunct to antiparasitic treatment. Drainage should be considered in patients that have no clinical response to drug therapy within 5–7 days or those with a high risk of abscess rupture defined as having a cavity >5 cm in diameter or by the presence of lesions in the left lobe.[26] Bacterial coinfection of amebic liver abscess has been observed; therefore addition of antibiotics, drainage, or a combination of both, to nitroimidazole therapy may be necessary.[19]

Drainage

Since the introduction of metronidazole in the 1960s, surgical drainage of most amebic abscesses has become unnecessary. Routine interventional drainage procedures do not have greater cure rates than amebicidal agents alone. Therefore aspiration or percutaneous or surgical drainage is usually reserved for cases in whom the diagnosis of amebic liver abscess is in question or when complications occur.

Percutaneous. Image-guided percutaneous treatment (aspiration or catheter drainage) has replaced surgical intervention as the procedure of choice for decreasing the size of an abscess. Percutaneous drainage remains most useful for treating pulmonary, peritoneal, and pericardial complications. The high viscosity of amebic abscess fluid, however, requires a large diameter catheter for adequate drainage, and this may cause more discomfort for the patient. Secondary infections related to the indwelling catheter are always a risk of this intervention.[5]

Surgical. Surgical drainage of amebic liver abscesses has largely been replaced by antibiotic therapy. The most common indication for surgical intervention is to manage abscesses that have failed to respond to more conservative therapy. Laparotomy is indicated for life-threatening hemorrhage that may or may not be related to abscess rupture, or when the amebic abscess erodes into a neighboring viscus and control of the involved viscus is necessary. Sepsis due to a secondarily infected amebic abscess also warrants operative intervention if percutaneous treatment fails.[5]

COMPLICATIONS

Complications from amebic abscesses occur secondary to rupture of the abscess into the peritoneum, pleural cavity, or pericardium (Fig 28–7). Extrahepatic sites also have been described in the lung, brain, skin, and genitourinary tract, presumably from hematogenous spread.[19] Ruptured amebic liver abscesses occur in 2–17% of patients and are associated with mortality rates between 12% and 50%.[23]

Peritonitis associated with amebiasis is due to rupture in the majority (78%), and secondary to necrotizing or perforated amebic colitis less frequently

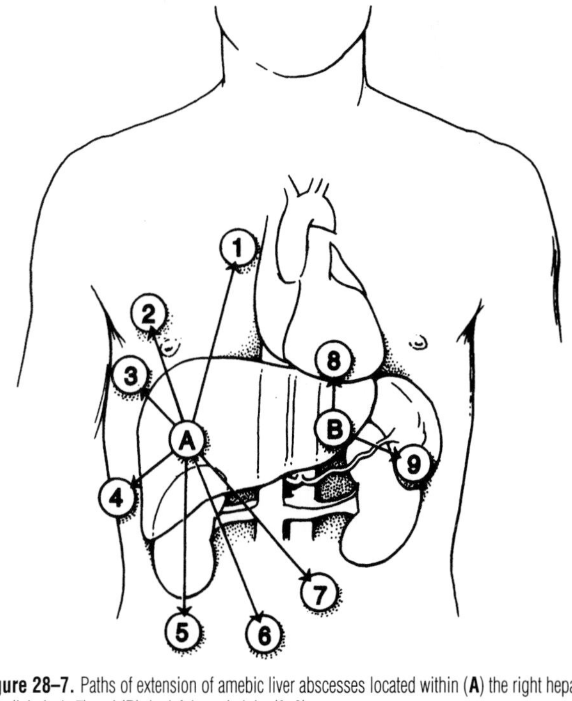

Figure 28–7. Paths of extension of amebic liver abscesses located within (**A**) the right hepatic lobe (labels 1–7) and (**B**) the left hepatic lobe (8, 9).

(22%). The liver abscess usually adheres to the diaphragm and the anterior abdominal wall, or the omentum and bowel tend to wall it off. Rupture into the colon or stomach also may occur. Free rupture into the peritoneal cavity is uncommon and occurs in patients with poor nutrition or those who are moribund.[23]

Thoracic amebiasis (empyema, bronchohepatic fistulas, and pleuropulmonary abscess) is the most common complication, followed by pericardial amebiasis (acute pericarditis with tamponade).[18] Transdiaphragmatic involvement manifests as dyspnea and dry cough. Right basilar crackles and a pleural rub may be heard on exam. Plain films show atelectasis and blunting of the costophrenic angle. If the abscess ruptures into the pleural cavity, it usually occurs suddenly, collapsing the lung, filling up the pleural space, and whiting out the lung on chest x-ray. Treatment requires drainage of the pleural cavity with tube thoracostomy. If the abscess ruptures into the bronchi, this complication causes sudden onset of coughing with expectoration of copious brown sputum. Surgical intervention is not required, as the abscess is usually walled off from the pleural and peritoneal cavities. Postural drainage, bronchodilators, and antiamebic drugs may suffice.

Left lobe abscesses are more likely to involve the pericardium. Complications range from asymptomatic effusions to cardiac tamponade to intrapericardial rupture. If pericardial thickening or effusion is noted on imaging, some experts believe that this complication is an indication for aspiration of a left lobe liver abscess. When tamponade develops, aspiration of the pericardium, drainage of the liver abscess, and antiamebic drugs are indicated.[23] Cerebral amebiasis is seen in up to 8% of autopsies. These patients are severely ill from sepsis, and may experience seizures.[18]

OUTCOME

The majority of patients with amebic liver abscess defervesce within 3–4 days of treatment;[22] however, left untreated amebic liver abscesses are often fatal. Mortality rates of 0–18% are reported, with higher rates occurring secondary to a delay in diagnosis, or when secondary bacterial infection or complications (abscess rupture) occur. Independent risk factors for mortality include serum bilirubin >3.5 mg/dL, encephalopathy, hypoalbuminemia defined as <2.0 g/dL, and multiple abscess cavities.[27] Abscess aspiration is a risk factor for secondary bacterial infection; however, secondary bacterial infection rates have decreased from 10–20% to 0–4% in the most recent reports (Table 28–8).

TABLE 28–8. FACTORS ASSOCIATED WITH A POOR OUTCOME IN PATIENTS WITH AMEBIC LIVER ABSCESSES

Increased age
Increased bilirubin level
Pulmonary involvement
Rupture or extension
Late presentation

■ HYDATID LIVER CYST

Echinococcosis (hydatid disease) is a zoonosis caused by the larval stage of *Echinococcus granulosus* (also known as *Taenia echinococcus*). Humans are accidental intermediate hosts, whereas animals can be both intermediate hosts and definitive hosts. The two main types of hydatid disease are caused by *E. granulosus* and *E. multilocularis.* The former is commonly seen in the Mediterranean, South America, the Middle East, Australia, and New Zealand, and is the most common type of hydatid disease in humans.[28] In humans, 50–75% of the cysts occur in the liver, 25% are located in the lungs, and 5–10% distribute along the arterial system. Infection with echinococcal organisms is the most common cause of liver cysts in the world.[29]

ETIOLOGY

The life cycle of *E. granulosus* has two hosts. The definitive host is usually a dog or some other carnivore. The adult worm of the parasite lives in the proximal small bowel of the definitive host attached by hooklets to the mucosa. Eggs are released into the host's intestine and excreted in the feces. Sheep are the most common intermediate host, and these animals ingest the ovum while grazing. The ovum loses the protective chitinous layer and is digested in the duodenum. The released hexacanth embryo (oncosphere) passes through the intestinal wall into the portal circulation and develops into cysts within the liver. The definitive host eats the viscera of the intermediate host and the cycle is completed (Fig 28–8).

Humans may become intermediate hosts through contact with the definitive host (usually a dog) or by ingestion of contaminated water or vegetables. Once in the liver, cysts grow to 1 cm in the first 6 months and 2–3 cm annually thereafter, depending on host tissue resistance. Once the parasite passes through the intestinal wall into the portal venous or lymphatic system, the

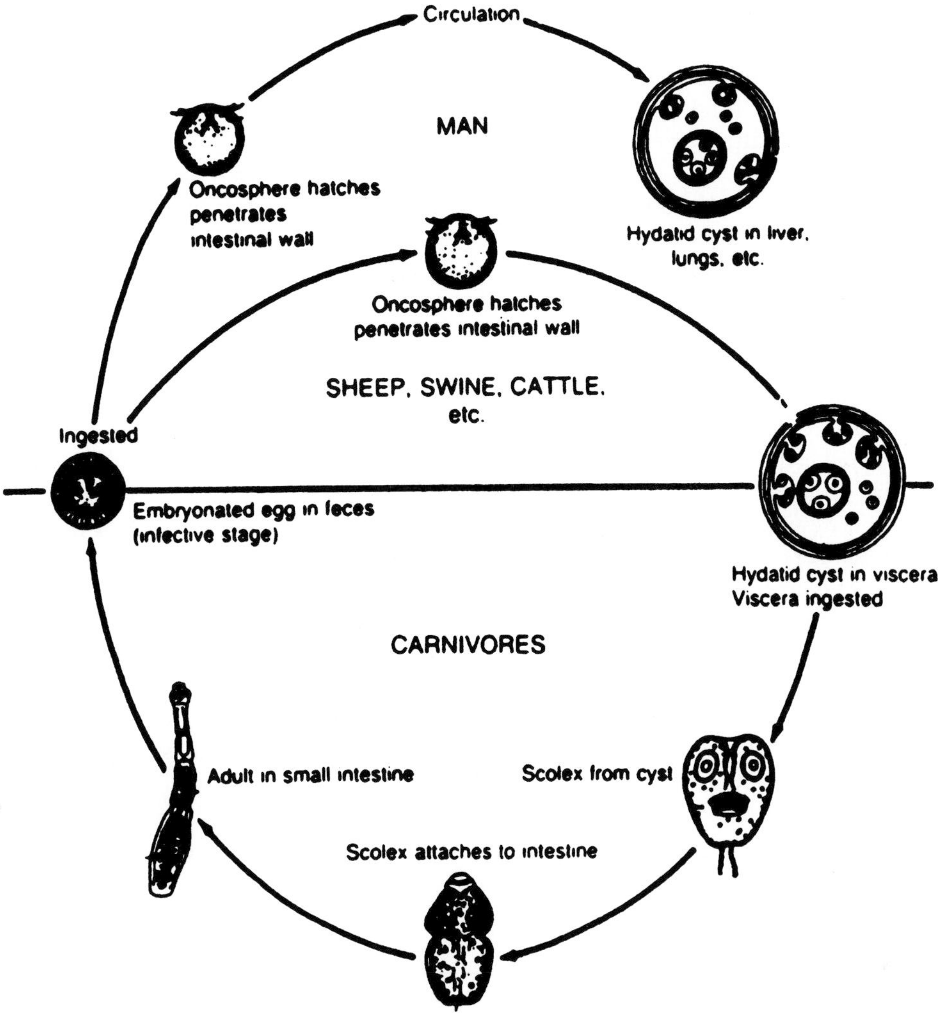

Figure 28–8. Life cycle of *Echinococcus granulosus.* (Reproduced, with permission, from McGreevy PB, Nelson GS. Larval cestode infections. In: Strickland GT (ed). *Hunter's Tropical Medicine.* Toronto, Canada: WB Saunders; 1984:771.)

liver acts as the first line of defense, and thus is the most frequently involved organ. The right lobe of the liver is the most commonly involved.[28]

INCIDENCE

The incidence of hydatid liver cysts in the United States is approximately 200 cases per year, with an increased frequency in immigrant populations. Hydatid liver disease affects all age groups, both sexes equally, and no predisposing pathologic conditions are associated with infection. Public education about the life cycle and transmission of the disease has helped decrease the incidence. Washing hands after contact with canines, eliminating the consumption of vegetables grown at ground level from the diet, and stopping the practice of feeding entrails of slaughtered animals to dogs have all aided in decreasing the incidence of the disease.[5]

PATHOLOGY

Hydatid liver cysts tend to expand slowly and without symptoms and are thus frequently very large on presentation. Single lesions are noted in 75% and are predominantly located within the right lobe (80%). Even though the lesion is single, half contain daughter cysts and are multilocular.

The typical hydatid cyst has a three-layer wall surrounding a fluid cavity. The outer layer is the pericyst, a thin, indistinct fibrous tissue layer representing an adventitial reaction to the parasitic infection. The pericyst acts as a mechanical support for the hydatid cyst and is the metabolic interface between the host and the parasite. As the cyst grows, bile ducts and blood vessels stretch and become incorporated within this structure, which explains the biliary and hemorrhagic complications of cyst growth and difficulties with resection. Over time, the pericyst calcifies.[5]

The outer layer of the cyst itself is the ectocyst or laminated membrane and is bluish-white, gelatinous, and about 0.5 cm thick. This membrane is a cuticular chitinous structure without nuclei and acts as a barrier for bacteria and an ultrafilter for protein molecules.

The inner layer or endocyst is the germinal membrane, responsible for the production of clear hydatid fluid, the ectocyst, brood capsules, scoleces, and daughter cysts. The endocyst is 10–25 μm thick and attached tenuously to the laminated membrane. The absorptive function of the inner layer is important for the nutrition of the cyst. The inner layer also has a proliferative function producing the ectocyst and scoleces.[30] This germinal layer forms small cellular masses that give rise to brood capsules, in which future worm heads develop. They enlarge and develop into invaginated protoscoleces with four suckers and a double row of hooks—a protoscolex. The protoscolex fully differentiates and matures attached by a pedicle to the capsule wall. Brood capsules and freed protoscoleces are released into the fluid of the original cyst and together with calcareous bodies, form hydatid sand.

Hydatid sand is made up of around 400,000 scoleces per milliliter of fluid. The protoscolex can differentiate in two directions. In the definitive host, the scolex becomes an adult tapeworm. In the intermediate host, including humans, each of the released protoscoleces is capable of differentiating into a new hydatid cyst. Development of brood capsules from the germinal layer indicates complete biologic development of the cyst, which occurs after 6 months of growth.

Daughter cyst formation is a defense reaction. Hydatid cysts in humans are long-standing, large, and liable to injury. Any injury may cause daughter cyst formation. Daughter cysts are replicas of the mother cyst, and their size and number are variable. In uncomplicated cysts, the cyst cavity is filled with sterile, colorless, antigenic fluid containing salt, enzymes, proteins, and toxic substances.[30] The formation of daughter cysts is called endogenic vesiculation.

Ectogenic vesiculation occurs when a small rupture or defect in the laminated membrane occurs and the germinal layer passes through and creates a satellite hydatid cyst. This process is uncommon in *E. granulosus*, but is characteristic for the larval stage of *E. multilocularis*. Because the liver parenchyma in humans cannot sequester *E. multilocularis* and the process of ectogenic vesiculation is fulminant, multiple vesicles are formed in all directions. The infected parenchyma has a multilocular appearance, and the center becomes necrotic, spongy, and filled with a gelatinous fluid similar to that of a mucoid liver carcinoma. Hepatic insufficiency is common and the disease is often lethal.[30]

DIAGNOSIS

The diagnosis of uncomplicated hydatid disease of the liver depends on the clinical suspicion. Uncomplicated hydatid cysts of the liver are usually asymptomatic. Symptoms may be secondary to a toxic reaction from the presence of the parasite, or the local mechanical effects, depending on the location and nature of the cysts.

Clinical Presentation

The clinical features of hydatid liver disease depend on the site, size, stage of development, whether the cyst is alive or dead, and whether the cyst is infected or not.[30] Pain in the RUQ or epigastrium is the most common symptom, whereas hepatomegaly and a palpable mass are the most common signs. Nonspecific fever, fatigue, nausea, and dyspepsia may also be present[31] (Table 28–9). Approximately one-third of patients will have eosinophilia, and only 20% will present with jaundice and hyperbilirubinemia.

Serology

No single biochemical test definitively establishes the diagnosis. The Casoni and Weinberg tests are no longer used due to their low sensitivities. Determination of specific antigens and immune complexes of the cyst with enzyme-linked immunosorbent assay (ELISA) give a positive result in more than 90% of patients. Specific IgE antibodies are demonstrated with ELISA and radioallergosorbent test (RAST) if active disease is present. The arc 5 antibody test involves precipitation during immunoelectrophoresis of the blood of patients with the antigen. Positivity for this test is 91%. Sbihi and colleagues[32] reported that purified fractions enriched in antigens 5 and B and glyco-

TABLE 28–9. SYMPTOMS, SIGNS, AND LABORATORY DATA OF HYDATID LIVER CYSTS

	% of Hydatid Cysts
SYMPTOMS	
Asymptomatic	75
Abdominal pain	20
Dyspepsia	13
Fever and chills	8
Jaundice	6
SIGNS	
Right upper quadrant mass	70
Right upper quadrant tenderness	20
LABORATORY DATA	
Eosinophilia	35
Bilirubin >2 mg/dL	20
WBC count <10,000/mm^3	10

proteins from hydatid fluid yielded a sensitivity of 95% with a specificity of 100%.

Radiology

Chest radiographs may show an elevated diaphragm and concentric calcifications in the cyst wall, but are of limited value. Ultrasound and CT are considered the first choice for imaging (Fig 28–9). Classic findings of hydatid cysts are calcified thick walls, often with daughter cysts.[33] Ultrasound defines the internal structure, number, and location of the cysts and the presence of complications. The specificity of ultrasound in hydatid disease is around 90%.[31] The classification proposed by Gharbi and associates[34] provides a morphologic description. Type I has a pure fluid collection. Type II has a fluid collection with a split wall (floating membrane). Type III reveals a fluid collection with septa (honeycomb image). Type IV has heterogenous echographic patterns and type V has reflecting thick walls. Differential imaging characteristics of hepatic cysts is presented in Table 28–10.

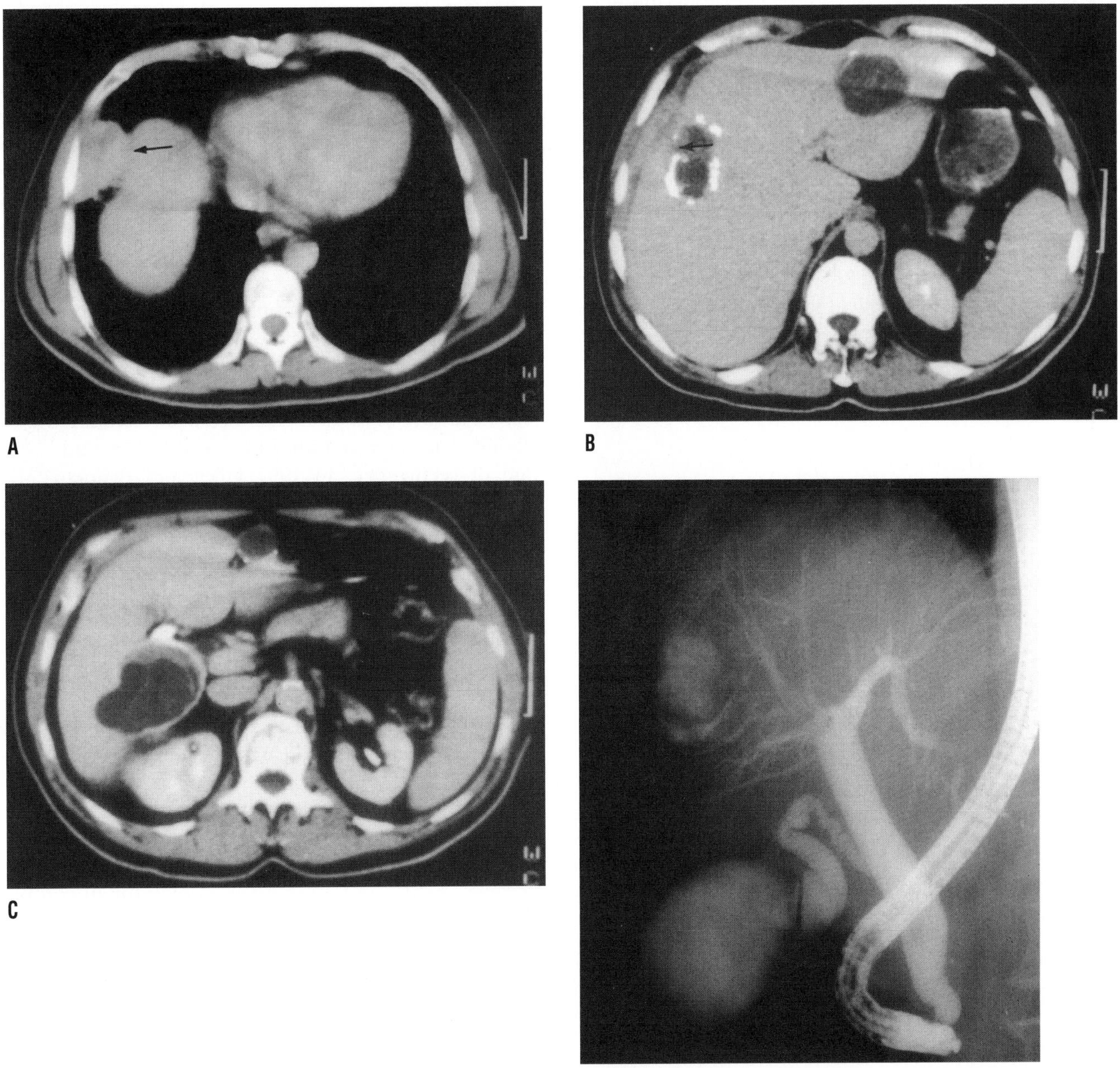

Figure 28–9. A. Computed tomography (CT) scan demonstrating rupture of hydatid cyst through the diaphragm (*arrow*) into the pleural space. **B.** CT scan in the same patient demonstrating a heavily calcified hydatid cyst (*arrow*) with diaphragmatic penetration and a lightly calcified cyst on the left. **C.** CT scan in the same patient showing a third calcified cyst near the gallbladder fossa and a small superficial fourth cyst on the left. **D.** Endoscopic retrograde cholangiopancreatography in the same patient demonstrating biliary communication in the cyst that also penetrates the diaphragm.

TABLE 28–10. DIFFERENTIAL IMAGING AND CHARACTER OF HEPATIC CYSTS

	Pyogenic	Amebic	Hydatid	Congenital	Cystadenoma
Number	Single or multiple	One or few	Usually single	Single or multiple	Single with loculations
Wall thickness	Thick	Thick	Thick	Thin	Variable
Wall character	Uniform or multiloculated	Usually uniform	Uniform, daughter cysts; 50% calcified	Uniform	Septations common may be irregular
Cyst contents	Usually pus with blood	Red-brown; like anchovy paste	Clear or bilious; gelatinous	Usually clear water density	Usually green-brown mucinous

Computed tomography gives similar information to ultrasound, but more specific information about the location and depth of the cyst within the liver. Daughter cysts and exogenous cysts are also clearly visualized, and the volume of the cyst can be estimated. CT is imperative for operative management, especially when a laparoscopic approach is utilized.[31] MRI provides structural details of the hydatid cyst, but adds little more than ultrasound or CT, and is more expensive. Endoscopic retrograde cholangiopancreatography (ERCP) may show communication between the cysts and bile ducts and can be used to drain the biliary tree before surgery. The routine use of ERCP is advocated by some to completely define the bile duct anatomy and to visualize any clinically silent connections between the bile ducts and cysts.[33]

TREATMENT

Most echinococcal cysts are asymptomatic on presentation, but complications such as pulmonary infection, cholangitis, rupture, and anaphylaxis give good reason to consider treatment for all. Medical, surgical, and percutaneous approaches may be part of the treatment armamentarium.[33] Small cysts (<4 cm) located deep in the parenchyma of the liver, if uncomplicated, can be managed conservatively.[31] Basic principles of treatment are: (1) eradication of the parasite within the cyst, (2) protection of the host against spillage of scoleces, and (3) management of complications.[33]

Anthelmintics

Medical therapy for echinococcosis is limited to the benzimidazoles (mebendazole and albendazole) and used alone is only 30% successful. Albendazole is readily absorbed from the intestine and metabolized by the liver to an active form. Mebendazole is poorly absorbed and is inactivated by the liver. Albendazole is thus the drug of choice for medical therapy. Greater success rates may be seen in extrahepatic manifestations of the disease and with the alveolar form caused by *E. multilocularis.* Given for at least 3 months preoperatively, albendazole reduces the recurrence rate when cyst spillage, partial cyst removal, or biliary rupture has occurred. Duration of therapy in these instances is at least 1 month.[33]

Percutaneous Aspiration and Drainage

Surgical dictum has stated that percutaneous puncture of a hydatid cyst is a dangerous and contraindicated activity. It was believed that the risk of anaphylaxis, communication with the biliary tree, and spillage outweighed any potential advantages with this nonoperative approach. In 1983, Fornage[35] challenged this axiom and reported an accidental puncture of a hydatid cyst by US that had no clinical consequences. Many successful reports followed thereafter.[30,36] The most frequently utilized protoscolecidal agents used for percutaneous treatment are 15–20% saline, 95% ethanol, a combination of 30% saline and 95% ethanol, and mebendazole solution. The PAIR technique (*p*ercutaneous *a*spiration, *i*njection and *r*e-aspiration) has also been combined with albendazole therapy with 70% success rates and a low rate of recurrence. In 1997 Filice and Brunetti[37] reported a series of 163 patients with 231 cysts treated percutaneously. No complications were reported and long-term results were good.

Despite these reports, percutaneous treatment is not benign. Spillage, anaphylaxis, and recurrence can be life-threatening. Complete aspiration of all cyst contents, especially multivesicular disease, is difficult, and complete sterilization with protoscolecidal agents is uncertain. If the protoscolecidal agent enters the biliary tree, serious damage also can occur within the liver. Exogenous vesiculation may also go undiscovered. Long-term results are unknown at this time.[30]

Surgery

Surgery is still the treatment of choice for uncomplicated hydatid disease of the liver. The objectives of surgical treatment are to: (1) inactivate the scoleces, (2) prevent spillage of cyst contents, (3) eliminate all viable elements of the cyst, and (4) manage the residual cavity of the cyst. The surgical procedure varies from a radical resective open approach (pericystectomy or hepatic resection) to a conservative approach (drainage or obliteration of the cavity or both) which can potentially even be done laparoscopically[31] (Fig 28–10).

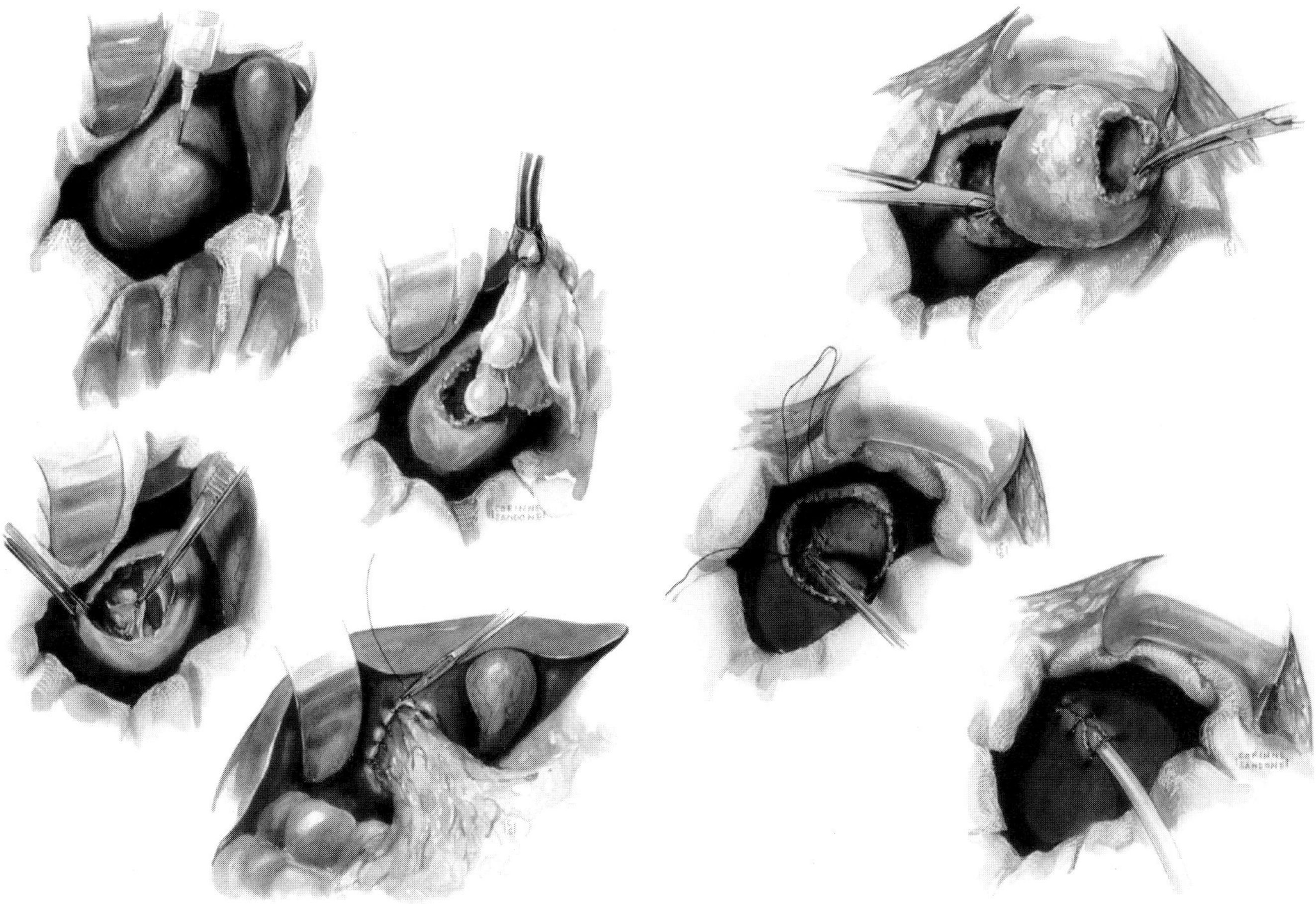

A B

Figure 28–10. A. Open cyst evacuation demonstrating cyst aspiration (*upper left*), removal of daughter cysts (*upper right*), resection of active cyst lining (*lower left*), and packing with omentum (*lower right*). **B.** Pericystectomy demonstrating removal of a calcified pericyst (*top right*), closure of a small bile duct (*middle left*), and closure of the cavity over a drain (*lower right*). (Reproduced, with permission, from Cameron JL, Sandove C. *Atlas of Surgery.* Philadelphia, PA: BC Decker; 1990:215–221.)

Scolecidal Agents. Early on, surgical management of hydatid cysts via cyst evacuation resulted in a high rate of peritoneal implantation. This problem prompted the use of scolecidal agents for injection into the cyst and for use in the surrounding peritoneum. Formalin, hypertonic saline, cetrimide, hydrogen peroxide, polyvinylpurrolidone-iodine, silver nitrate, and ethyl alcohol are among some of the many agents that have been used.[31,33] However, formalin caused sclerosing cholangitis when it entered the biliary tract. Hypertonic saline has to be used carefully to avoid biliary injection and hypernatremia. The safety of the other agents in the biliary tree has not been established. No agent should be injected pre-evacuation due to high intracyst pressure.

Open Cyst Evacuation. The safest surgical approach is open cyst evacuation. Peripherally located cysts are the most easily treated, and either abdominal or flank approaches may be utilized depending on cyst location. Prior to opening the cyst, the field is lined with hypertonic (20%) saline-soaked gauze to guard against spillage. The cyst is then opened, and the contents are aspirated with a suction device that is capable of generating high negative pressures. The cyst is then opened completely, and any remaining debris is meticulously cleared. The cavity may then be irrigated with a scolecidal agent.[33]

Laparoscopic Cyst Evacuation. Peripherally located echinococcal hepatic cysts may be safely managed by laparoscopic cyst evacuation.[38] The lesions best suited for this approach are situated anteriorly and do not have thick calcified walls. A right lateral approach also works for cysts in segments VI and VII. A trocar (11-mm) is inserted just above the cyst, and 10% povidone iodine–soaked sponges are placed as the scolecidal agent. The cyst is aspirated with a 14-gauge needle. The endocyst then shrinks back from the wall and rests at the bottom of the cyst. The 11-mm trocar is then exchanged for an 18-mm trocar, and the germinal membrane is aspirated. The laparoscopic camera is inserted directly into the cyst to explore for residual daughter cysts or biliary fistulae. The remaining cavity is irrigated with 20% saline solution, and the cyst wall is excised. The cavity may be plugged with omentum or closed over a closed suction drain.[38]

Pericystectomy. Pericystectomy involves complete resection of the cyst wall without entering the cyst cavity. This procedure is done through a plane outside of the pericyst or along the cyst wall itself. Preoperative localization of the bile ducts and vascular system is imperative. If a bile duct connection is suspected, preoperative ERCP should be obtained. Intraoperative ultrasound also should be utilized. Pericystectomy decreases the risk of spillage of cyst contents into the peritoneal cavity and also lowers the risk of recurrence. The disadvantage to this approach is the potential for bleeding or damage to bile ducts in proximity to the cyst wall.[33] Gunay and associates[29] reported 0% recurrence rates, a lower incidence of biliary fistulae, and shorter hospitalization compared with more conservative procedures. The procedure also precludes management of the cavity and facilitates detection of recurrence.

Liver Resection/Transplantation. Some experts have argued that formal resection for benign disease is excessive and unnecessary, whereas others have stressed that resection is very safe. Multiple cysts within proximity to a major blood supply or to each other, or a cyst in a relatively safe location (i.e., segments II/III) are candidates for resection provided a complete resection can be achieved. *E. multilocularis* infection may also lead to fulminant hepatic failure from sclerosing cholangitis, biliary sclerosis, or Budd-Chiari syndrome, and in these rare cases orthotopic liver transplantation may be necessary.[33] Among these various treatment options, criteria for uncomplicated and complicated patients are presented in Table 28–11.

COMPLICATIONS

Complications from hydatid cysts are seen in one-third of patients. Most commonly, the cyst ruptures internally or externally, followed by secondary infection, anaphylactic shock, and liver replacement, in order of decreasing frequency.[29] Viable hydatid cysts are space-occupying lesions with a tendency to grow. In confined areas such as the central nervous system, even small cysts can cause severe symptoms. In less confined areas, symptoms depend on the site and size of the cyst. Symptoms result from direct pressure or distortion of neighboring structures or viscera. Compressive atrophy of the surrounding hepatocytes and fibrosis occurs, and these cysts may grow to such an enormous size that they replace an entire lobe.

TABLE 28–11. TREATMENT OPTIONS FOR HYDATID LIVER CYSTS

Percutaneous or Laparoscopic Evacuation	Open Evacuation or Resection
UNCOMPLICATED PATIENTS	
Gharbi type I or II	Gharbi type IV or V
Anterior cysts	Posterior cysts
Peripheral cysts	Central cysts
One to three cysts	More than three cysts
Small cysts	Large cysts
No or minimal calcification	Heavy calcification
COMPLICATED PATIENTS	
Percutaneous or Laparoscopic Evacuation	**Open Evacuation or Resection**
Infected cysts meeting above criteria	Infected cysts meeting above criteria
Biliary communication—not indicated	Biliary communication—indicated
Pulmonary communication—not indicated	Pulmonary communication—indicated
Peritoneal rupture—not indicated	Peritoneal rupture—indicated

As the cysts enlarge, they may also rupture. If rupture of only the endocyst occurs, the content is retained within the pericyst. A communicating rupture is a rupture into the biliary or bronchial tree.[30] Frank intrabiliary rupture is the most common complication of hydatid cysts, and is reported in 5–25% of cases. T-tube drainage, cystojejunostomy, and choledochoduodenostomy are the main operations performed for this pathologic condition.[29] A free rupture occurs when hydatid contents rupture throughout the peritoneal, pleural, or pericardial cavity. Acute symptomatic rupture into the peritoneal cavity occurs in 1–4% of patients and may precipitate anaphylactic shock.[30]

OUTCOME

Uncomplicated cases undergoing elective procedures such as laparoscopic or percutaneous cyst aspiration should have morbidity rates between 15% and 30% and essentially no mortality. Outcomes should be similar for left lateral segment resections and wedge resections elsewhere within the liver. In patients with complicated disease that requires open evacuation, pericystectomy, or resection, morbidity is as high as 50%; however, mortality should still remain less than 5%. Septic shock, peritoneal rupture, and comorbid conditions (i.e., malnutrition) play a major role in increasing mortality rates.

Medical therapy used alone results in recurrence rates of 70–80% and is not recommended. Medical treatment is used in combination with a drainage procedure or in patients that are not surgical candidates. Uncomplicated cases that undergo open surgical, laparoscopic, and percutaneous drainage have recurrence rates around 10%. Since the disease is endemic to many locations, the potential for reinfestation remains, so long-term serologic and imaging studies are necessary. Rupture into the pleural or peritoneal cavity portends a recurrence rate of up to 25%.[33]

▪ CONGENITAL LIVER CYSTS

SIMPLE

The incidence of simple hepatic cysts in 1,695 patients referred for abdominal or pelvic ultrasound was 2.5% with a sharp increase noted at >60 years old.[39] In a separate European study[40] of more than 26,000 patients undergoing upper abdominal ultrasound, simple cysts were found in 2.8%, and most (more than 92 %) were over the age of 40. The female:male ratio was 1.5:1.

Solitary benign cysts are believed to be congenital and thought to arise from abnormal development of intrahepatic bile ducts in utero. The aberrant ducts enlarge slowly and result in symptoms later in life. In a study from the Mayo Clinic,[41] from 1907–1971 only 24% of simple cysts were symptomatic, and they usually became symptomatic in the fourth or fifth decade of life. Abdominal pain and mass were noted most frequently and were present in more than 50%. Less commonly, symptoms were related to mass effect resulting in nausea, vomiting, early satiety, and jaundice. Physical exam revealed hepatomegaly or a palpable abdominal mass. Laboratory values should be normal, but occasionally hyperbilirubinemia may be seen. Grossly, simple solitary cysts are bluish in color, and contain clear, straw-colored fluid. Echinococcal disease should be ruled out by serology.[42]

Ultrasound is the most accurate imaging modality, with a sensitivity and specificity for cysts of more than 90%. On ultrasound, the cysts appear as anechoic masses with smooth margins and thin, imperceptible walls. Ultrasound also differentiates between cystic and solid lesions and can assess for intra- and extrahepatic biliary dilatation in the jaundiced patient. CT imaging reveals nonenhancing, fluid (water) density lesions with a thin, uniform wall (Fig 28–11A). On MRI, simple cysts are well-circumscribed lesions that are hypointense on T1-weighted images and hyperintense on T2-weighted images.[40]

Most simple cysts are found incidentally and are asymptomatic, and 80–95% remain asymptomatic. In

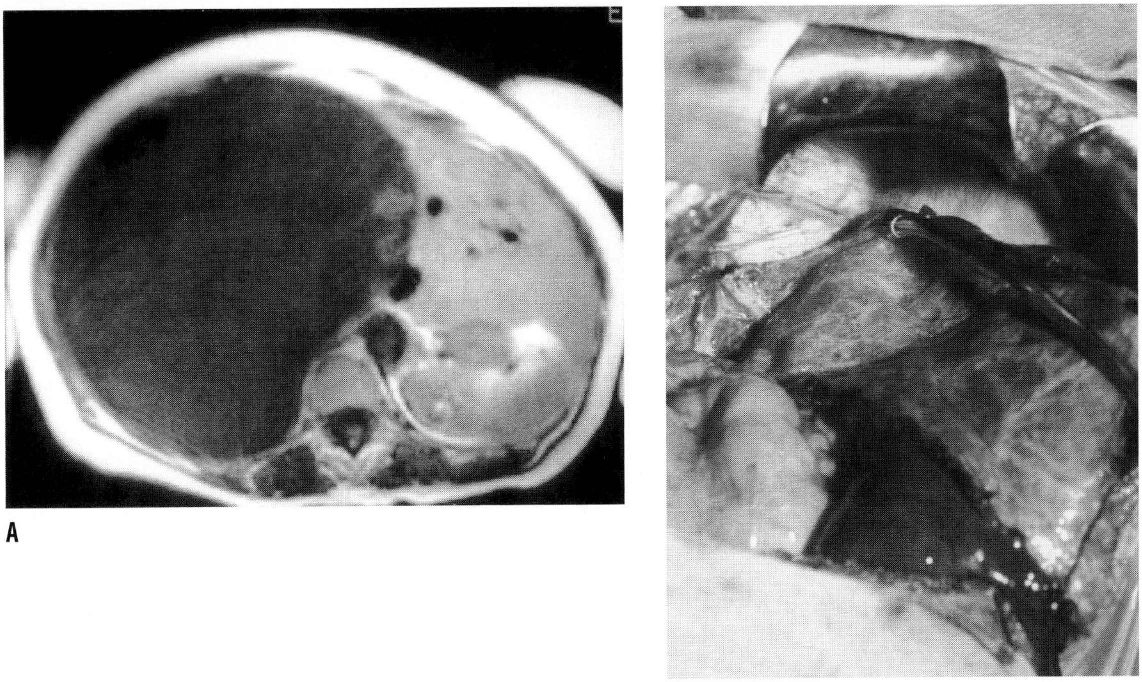

A

B

Figure 28–11. A. CT demonstrating a large simple cyst compressing the inferior vena cava. **B.** Operative picture demonstrating partial excision of the cyst.

the setting of symptoms, percutaneous aspiration can aid in diagnosis but is associated with 100% recurrence within a 2-year period. If sclerosants are added, a 17% recurrence rate can be achieved.[42]

Success of surgical treatment for cystic liver disease is judged by relief of symptoms rather than by complete disappearance of the cystic lesion on imaging studies. Once the benign nature of the cyst is established, a permanent internal cyst "drain" is the mainstay of surgical therapy, and complete cyst excision is not necessary.[43] If the cyst protrudes from the liver and no biliary connection is demonstrated, the accessible wall on the liver surface may be excised and the remaining cyst lining allowed to drain freely into the peritoneal cavity (Fig 28–11B). If the cyst has a biliary connection, suspicion should be high that the lesion is a biliary cystadenoma rather than a simple cyst. In general, cyst excision or unroofing and resection have a 0–20% recurrence rate and a mortality rate of 0–5%[42] (Table 28–12).

Unroofing the cyst by a laparoscopic approach also can be done with an overall success rate of more than 90% and a 10% rate of symptomatic cyst recurrence. Proponents of the laparoscopic approach report excellent exposure, less postoperative pain, and success rates similar to those of cases done open.[42] Tan and associates[44] reported a series of 11 patients treated by laparoscopic fenestration. Ten patients had solitary cysts, and one patient had polycystic liver disease (PCLD). The PCLD patient had two symptomatic recurrences, one of which was a cystadenoma. The others with solitary cysts had none, despite an overall radiographic recurrence rate of 28.5%. The authors concluded that long-term alleviation of symptoms can be achieved with a laparoscopic approach for solitary simple liver cysts, but not for PCLD or cystic tumors.

TABLE 28–12. TREATMENT OPTIONS FOR CONGENITAL LIVER CYSTS

I. Simple cysts
    A. Aspiration with sclerosis
    B. Open surgery
        1. Partial excision
        2. Complete excision
    C. Laparoscopic surgery
        1. Partial excision
        2. Complete excision
II. Polycystic liver disease
    A. Aspiration with sclerosis
    B. Open surgery
        1. Partial unroofing
        2. Unroofing with resection
        3. Liver transplantation

POLYCYSTIC

Polycystic liver disease (PCLD) is an autosomal dominant disorder often found in association with polycystic renal disease (40%).[45] PCLD commonly presents as the most frequent extrarenal manifestation of autosomal dominant polycystic kidney disease. PCLD also exists in an autosomal dominant pattern that is not associated with polycystic renal disease, but may have cysts that develop in other organs in addition to the kidneys.

Cysts in PCLD are epithelial-lined growths arising from biliary epithelium that usually do not communicate with the biliary tree. The majority of patients are asymptomatic and do not require treatment. Their prognosis is directly related to the severity of the accompanying renal disease.[46]

If PCLD becomes symptomatic, it is usually secondary to hepatomegaly. Symptoms may include abdominal fullness, distention and pain, or bowel and biliary obstruction. Complications such as bleeding, infection, rupture, portal hypertension, and Budd-Chiari syndrome have been reported, but are rare. Malignant transformation also has been reported but infrequently occurs. Function of the liver parenchyma is typically preserved, as is hepatic function, so progression to hepatic failure is uncommon.[46]

Routine imaging of cysts in PCLD is similar to that of simple cysts. Unenhanced CTs show multiple, homogenous, hypoattenuating lesions with a regular outline (Fig 28–12A). Contrast-enhanced CT images have no cyst wall or enhancement of cyst contents. MRI demonstrates very low signal intensity on T1-weighted images and does not enhance after administration of gadolinium. Since the cyst content is purely fluid and homogenous, high signal intensity is demonstrated on T2-weighted images.[45]

Development of symptoms in PCLD is most often due to hepatomegaly, and therefore treatment that addresses the cause needs to result in a reduction of liver size. Percutaneous aspiration with sclerotherapy may be used in those who are not surgical candidates or in lesions that are not surgically accessible, but long-term results of this approach are poor.

If a small number of large cysts exist, laparoscopic unroofing with the aid of intraoperative ultrasound may be successful (Fig 28–12B). Deeper cysts may be accessed and unroofed through the back wall of more superficially located cysts. Due to the rigid architecture found in PCLD, unroofing alone may not be enough to provide hepatic collapse and relief of symptoms. In addition, if too many cysts are unroofed, the peritoneum's absorptive capacity may be exceeded and cause ascites. Unroofing also has not

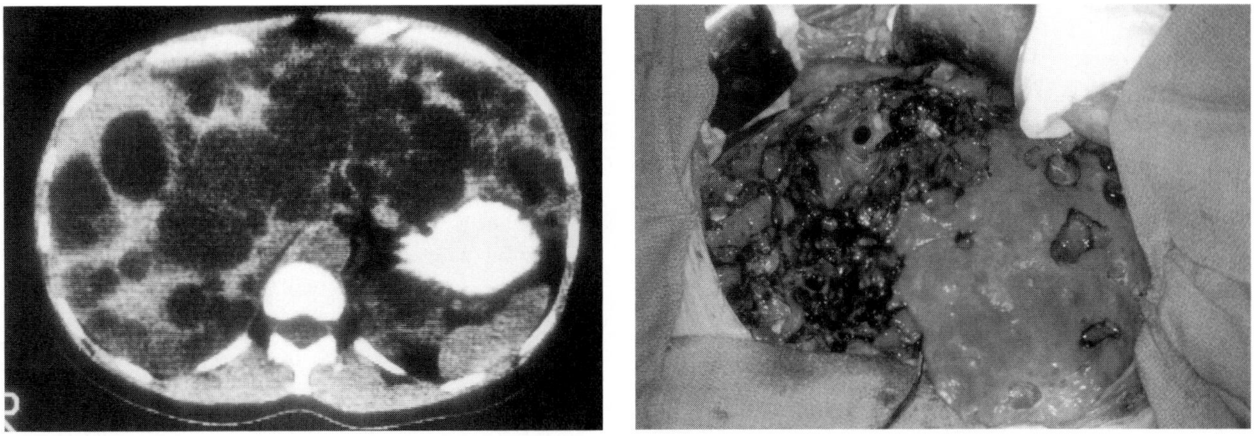

A B

Figure 28–12. A. CT demonstrating polycystic liver disease. **B.** Operative picture demonstrating unroofing of superficial cysts.

been shown to be useful in patients with a large number of smaller cysts because it cannot be adequately performed.

A combination of cyst unroofing and liver resection may achieve the best results in terms of reducing liver volume. Resection should include the most cysts with the least loss of hepatic function. Morbidity for this approach is greater, but long-term results are improved. Orthotopic liver transplant is occasionally indicated if symptoms are disabling or hepatic function is compromised. If patients have associated renal failure, the liver transplant may be combined with renal transplantation.[46]

▪ NEOPLASTIC CYSTS

Neoplastic cysts are acquired cysts that occur less commonly than simple cysts, usually in females, in the fifth decade of life. Their etiology is unknown. Cystic neoplasms are frequently large, resulting in abdominal discomfort and a palpable mass on examination. Cystic neoplasms appear as multiloculated lesions with papillary projections inside the cyst cavity. Invasion of the surrounding tissue suggests malignancy, as does the presence of a predominantly solid (versus cystic) component. Ten percent of neoplastic cysts are malignant. Definitive diagnosis requires intraoperative biopsy of the cyst wall. Incomplete resection will result in nearly 100% recurrence.[42]

Laboratory investigation is normal in most, although some patients present with elevated liver enzymes. Serum alpha-fetoprotein (AFP) and carcinoembryonic antigen (CEA) levels are usually normal. In some patients, CA 19-9 has been found to be elevated fivefold. In general, hemorrhagic cyst fluid suggests cystadenocarcinoma, whereas bilious or mucinous fluid suggests cystadenoma.[47]

CYSTADENOMA

Cystadenomas comprise less than 5% of all intrahepatic cysts of biliary origin. Fifty percent are located in the right lobe, 29% are found in the left lobe, and 16% are bilateral.[48] Hepatobiliary cystadenoma with mesenchymal stroma occurs exclusively in young and middle-aged women and has potential to transform into cystadenocarcinoma. In contrast, hepatobiliary cystadenoma without mesenchymal stroma occurs in both sexes equally, at a mean age of 50, and has no clear association with cystadenocarcinoma.[47] These tumors are lined with columnar epithelium and frequently have papillary infoldings[48] (Fig 28–13A).

Cystadenomas have a septated, multilocular appearance on US and CT (Figs 28–13B and C). The presence of the septae suggests a neoplastic cyst, whereas the presence of debris within the cyst cavity suggests malignancy.[42] MRI shows typical features for a fluid-containing loculated mass with homogeneous low signal intensity on T1-weighted images and homogeneous high signal intensity on T2-weighted images. Variable signal intensities depend on the presence of solid components, hemorrhage, and protein content.[45] ERCP will usually demonstrate communication with the biliary tree, often at the proximal left hepatic duct.

Neoplastic cysts with no signs of malignancy may be enucleated (Fig 28–13D). This technique requires removal of the entire cyst, the cyst's surrounding wall, and a small rim of liver parenchyma.[42] Formal hepatic resection also is an appropriate treatment.

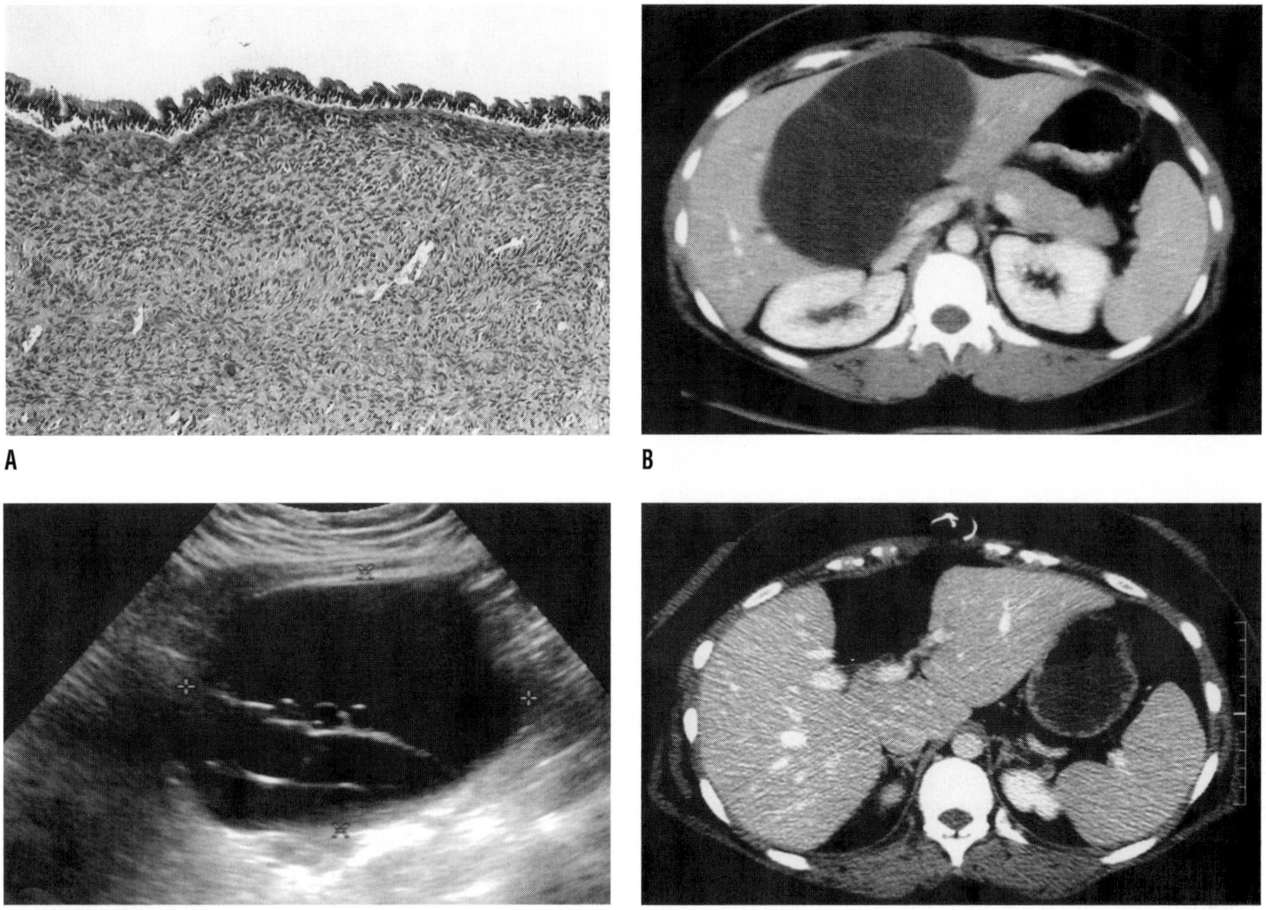
A B C D

Figure 28–13. A. Histologic section of biliary cystadenoma demonstrating columnar epithelium. B. CT scan in the same patient demonstrating a septated central hepatic cyst. C. Ultrasound in the same patient demonstrating septated central hepatic cyst. D. CT scan 6 months after enucleation of the biliary cystadenoma demonstrating no recurrence and the residual cavity.

Aspiration, sclerosis, marsupialization, and internal drainage must be avoided. Inadequate excision leads to recurrence in all cases[48] (Table 28–13).

CYSTADENOCARCINOMA

Devaney and colleagues[49] divided cystadenocarcinoma into three subtypes: (1) cystadenocarcinoma with mesenchymal stroma arising from cystadenoma with mesenchymal stroma, occurring exclusively in females and following a relatively indolent course; (2) cystadenocarcinoma without mesenchymal stroma not associated with cystadenoma, occurring in males and following an extremely aggressive course; and (3) cystadenocarcinoma without mesenchymal stroma, occurring in females and with a poorly understood clinical course.[50] Resection is the only appropriate treatment for malignant biliary cystadenocarcinoma.[42] After total resection, the clinical course for cystadenocarcinoma is better than that for hepatocellular carcinoma or cholangiocarcinoma.[50] In the rare patient with a symptomatic cystadenocarcinoma with peritoneal metastasis, palliative unroofing of the cyst may be indicated (Fig 28–14).

TABLE 28–13. TREATMENT OPTIONS FOR NEOPLASTIC LIVER CYSTS

I. Cystadenoma
- A. Enucleation
- B. Hepatic resection

II. Cystadenocarcinoma
- A. Hepatic resection
- B. Palliative unroofing

■ TRAUMATIC CYSTS

In recent years the management of hepatic trauma has undergone major changes. The frequent use of dual phase CT imaging to assess patients with ab-

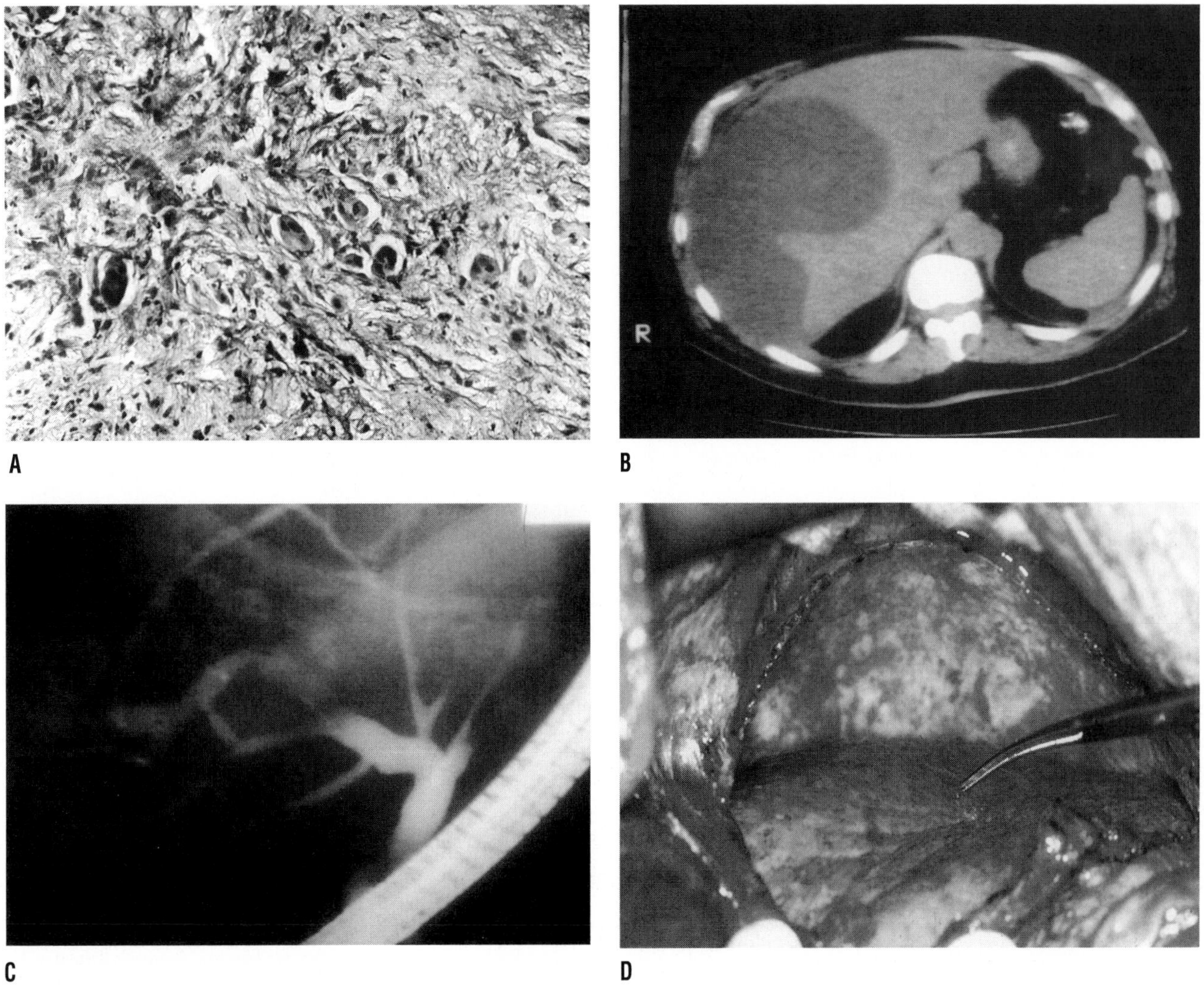

Figure 28–14. A. Histologic section of a biliary cystadenocarcinoma. **B.** CT scan in the same patient demonstrating a large hepatic cyst. **C.** ERCP in the same patient demonstrating biliary communication. **D.** Operative picture demonstrating palliative unroofing, as the patient had peritoneal metastases.

dominal trauma has resulted in the detection of even the most minor of liver injuries. In the hemodynamically unstable patient, damage control laparotomy—the control of bleeding and contamination with packing off of the abdomen to postpone definitive treatment—has gained popularity, while formal anatomic hepatic resection has fallen out of favor. More and more American Association for the Surgery of Trauma grade IV and V liver injuries are also being managed nonoperatively. Mortality rates have fallen to 7–12%,[51] but a different set of management problems is being created. One such problem is the traumatic cyst.

Traumatic cysts are acquired cysts that occur from continued bile leakage from an injured intrahepatic bile duct after abdominal trauma. When an injured biliary structure continues to leak into a hematoma cavity, a cyst containing bile and blood may form.[42] These cysts lack a true epithelial lining and are considered pseudocysts (Fig 28–15). Some traumatic cysts may resolve spontaneously,[46] while others may grow until compressive symptoms are caused. Presentation is typically delayed, and abdominal pain or fullness may occur months or sometimes years after the trauma.[42]

TREATMENT OPTIONS

Treatment is reserved for those who are symptomatic. Options include aspiration, unroofing, and excision. Bile leaks must be sought and controlled.[46] Small bilomas may be observed, whereas larger collections usually require percutaneous drainage at the time of diagnosis. Once the cavity is collapsed, spontaneous closure of the fistula is the rule.

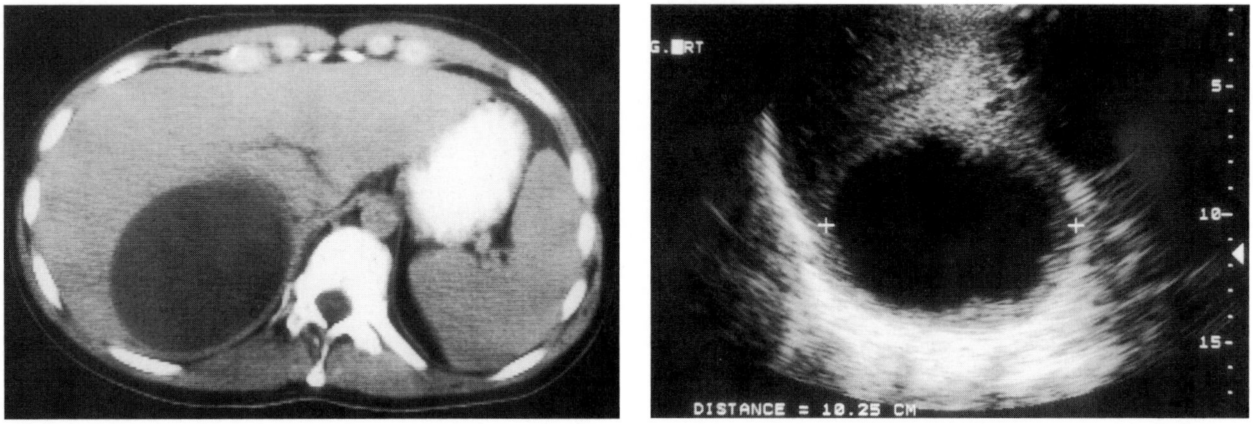

A B

Figure 28–15. A. CT scan demonstrating a traumatic hepatic cyst 4 months after blunt liver trauma. **B.** Ultrasound in the same patient demonstrating a thickened cyst wall.

REFERENCES

1. Ochsner A. Pyogenic abscess of the liver. *Am J Surg* 1938; 40:292
2. McFadzean AJS, Chang KPS, Wong CC. Solitary pyogenic abscess of the liver treated by closed aspiration and antibiotics: A report of 14 consecutive cases with recovery. *Br J Surg* 1953;41:141–152
3. Pitt HA. Surgical management of hepatic abscesses. *World J Surg* 1990;14:498–504
4. Huang CJ, Pitt HA, Lipsett PA et al. Pyogenic hepatic abscess: Changing trends over 42 years. *Ann Surg* 1996; 223:600–609
5. Barnes S, Lillemoe K. Liver abscess and hydatid cyst disease. In: Zinner M, Schwartz S, Ellis H, Ashley S, McFadden D (eds). *Maingot's Abdominal Operations,* 10th ed. Stamford, CT: Appleton & Lange; 1997:1513–1545
6. Pope IM, Poston GJ. Pyogenic liver abscess. In: Blumgart LH, Fong Y (eds). *Surgery of the Liver and Biliary Tract,* 3rd ed. London, England: WB Saunders; 2001: 1135–1145
7. Chu KM, Fan ST, Lai ECS et al. Pyogenic liver abscess: An audit of experience over the past decade. *Arch Surg* 1996;131:148–152
8. Wong E, Khardori N, Carrgsco CH et al. Infectious complications of hepatic artery catheterization procedures in patients with cancer. *Rev Infect Dis* 1991;13:583–589
9. Seeto RK, Rocky DC. Pyogenic liver abscess: Changes in etiology, management, and outcome. *Medicine* 1996;75: 99–113
10. Leslie DB, Dunn DL. Hepatic abscess. In: Cameron J (ed). *Current Surgical Therapy,* 8th ed. Philadelphia, PA: Elsevier Mosby; 2004:298–303
11. Branum GD, Tyson GS, Branum MA et al. Hepatic abscess: Changes in etiology, diagnosis and management. *Ann Surg* 1990;212:655–662
12. Civardi G, Filice C, Caremani M et al. Hepatic abscesses in immunocompromised patients: Ultrasonically guided percutaneous drainage. *Gastrointest Radiol* 1992;175:17–23
13. Lambiase RE, Deyoe L, Cronan JJ, Dorfman GS. Percutaneous drainage of 335 consecutive abscesses: Results of primary drainage with 1-year follow-up. *Radiology* 1992;184:167–179
14. Stain SC, Yellin AE, Donovan AJ, Brien HW. Pyogenic liver abscess: Modern treatment. *Arch Surg* 1991;126: 991–995
15. Giorgio A, Tarantino L, Mariniello N et al. Pyogenic liver abscess: 13 years of experience in percutaneous needle aspiration with U/S guidance. *Radiology* 1995; 195:122–124
16. Rajak CL, Gupta S, Jain S et al. Percutaneous treatment of liver abscesses: Needle aspiration versus catheter drainage. *Am J Roentgenol* 1998;170:1035–1039
17. Martinez Baez M. Historical introduction. In: Martinez-Palomo A (ed). *Amebiasis. Human Parasitic Diseases,* Vol. 2. Amsterdam, Holland: Elsevier; 1986:1–9
18. Yost J. Amebiasis. *Pediatr Rev* 2002;23:293–294
19. Haque R, Huston CD, Hughes M et al. Current concepts: Amebiasis. *N Engl J Med* 2003;348:1565–1573
20. Tanyuksel M, Petri WA. Laboratory diagnosis of amebiasis. *Clin Microbiol Rev* 2003;16:713–729
21. Salles JM, Moraes LM, Salles MC. Hepatic amebiasis. *Braz J Infect Dis* 2003;7:96–110
22. Petri WA Jr, Singh U. Diagnosis and management of amebiasis. *Clin Infect Dis* 1999;29:1117–1125
23. Thomas PG, Ravindra KV. Amebiasis and biliary infection. In: Blumgart LH, Fong Y (eds). *Surgery of the Liver and Biliary Tract,* 3rd ed. London, England: WB Saunders; 2001:1147–1165
24. Haque R, Mollah NU, Ali IKM et al. Diagnosis of amebic liver abscess and intestinal infection with the techLab *Entamoeba histolytica* II antigen detection and antibody tests. *J Clin Microbiol* 2000;38:3235–3239
25. Blessmann J, Binh HD, Hung DM et al. Treatment of amebic liver abscess with metronidazole alone or in combination with ultrasound-guided needle aspiration: A comparative, prospective and randomized study. *Trop Med Int Health* 2003;8:1030–1034

26. Weinke T, Grobusch MP, Buthoff W. Amebic liver abscess—rare need for percutaneous treatment modalities. *Eur J Med Res* 2002;7:25–29
27. Sharma MP, Dasarthy S, Verma N et al. Prognostic markers in amebic liver abscess: A prospective study. *Am J Gastroenterol* 1996;91:2584–2588
28. Pedrosa I, Saiz A, Arrazola J et al. Hydatid disease: Radiologic and pathologic features and complications. *Radiographics* 2000;20:795–817
29. Gunay, K, Taviloglu K, Berber E et al. Traumatic rupture of hydatid cysts: A 12-year experience from an endemic region. *J Trauma* 1999;46:164–167
30. Milicevic MN. Hydatid disease. In: Blumgart LH, Fong Y (eds). *Surgery of the Liver and Biliary Tract*, 3rd ed. London, England: WB Saunders; 2001:1167–1204
31. Sayek I, Onat D. Diagnosis and treatment of uncomplicated hydatid cyst of the liver. *World J Surg* 2001;25:21–27
32. Sbihi Y, Janssen D, Osuna A. Serologic recognition of hydatid cyst antigens using different purification methods. *Diagn Microbiol Infect Dis* 1996;24:205
33. Goldblatt M, Pitt H. Hepatic echinococcosis. In: Cameron J (ed). *Current Surgical Therapy*, 8th ed. Philadelphia, PA: Elsevier Mosby; 2004:306–311
34. Gharbi HA, Hassine W, Brauner MW et al. Ultrasound examination of hydatic liver. *Radiology* 1981;139:459
35. Fornage B. Fortuitous diagnosis by fine needle puncture under real-time ultrasound control of an atypical hydatid cyst of the liver. *J Radiologie* 1983;64:643–645
36. Khuroo MS, Wani NA, Javid G et al. Percutaneous drainage compared with surgery for hepatic hydatid cysts. *N Engl J Med* 1997;337:881–887
37. Filice C, Brunetti E. Use of PAIR in human cystic echinococcosis. *Acta Trop* 1997;64:95–107
38. Ertem M, Karahasanoglu T, Yavuz N et al. Laparoscopically treated liver hydatid cysts. *Arch Surg* 2002;137:1170
39. Gaines PA, Sampson MA. The prevalence and characterization of simple hepatic cysts by ultrasound examination. *Br J Radiol* 1989;62:335–337
40. Caremani M, Vincenti A, Benci A et al. Echographic epidemiology of non-parasitic hepatic cysts. *J Clin Ultrasound* 1993;21:115–118
41. Sanfelippo PM, Beahrs OH, Weiland LH. Cystic disease of the liver. *Ann Surg* 1974;179:922–925
42. Cowles RA, Mulholland MW. Solitary hepatic cysts. *J Am Coll Surg* 2000;191:311–321
43. Schacter P, Sorin V, Avni Y et al. The role of laparoscopic ultrasound in the minimally invasive management of symptomatic hepatic cysts. *Surg Endosc* 2001;15:364–367
44. Tan YM, Ooi LL, So KC, Mack POP. Does laparoscopic fenestration provide long-term alleviation for symptomatic cystic disease of the liver? *ANZ J Surg* 2002;71:743–745
45. Mortele KJ, Ros PR. Cystic focal liver lesions in the adult: Differential CT and MR imaging features. *Radiographics* 2001;21:895–910
46. Knauer E, Sweeney JF. Cystic disease of the liver. In: Cameron J (ed). *Current Surgical Therapy*, 8th ed. Philadelphia, PA: Elsevier Mosby; 2004:303–306
47. Maruyama S, Hirayama C, Yamamoto S et al. Hepatobiliary cystadenoma with mesenchymal stroma in a patient with chronic hepatitis C. *J Gastroenterol* 2003;38:593–597
48. Tsiftsis D, Christodoulakis M, DeBree E et al. Primary intrahepatic biliary cystadenomatous tumors. *J Surg Oncol* 1997;64:341–346
49. Devaney K, Goodman ZD, Ishak KG. Hepatobiliary cystadenoma and cystadenocarcinoma: A light microscopic and immunohistochemical study of 70 patients. *Am J Surg Pathol* 1994;18:1078–1091
50. Akiyoshi T, Yamaguchi K, Chijiiwa K, Tanaka M. Cystadenocarcinoma of the liver without mesenchymal stroma: Possible progression from a benign cystic lesion suspected by follow-up imagings. *J Gastroenterol* 2003;38:588–592
51. Pachter HL, Spencer FC, Hofstetter SR et al. Significant trends in the treatment of hepatic trauma: Experience in 411 injuries. *Ann Surg* 1992;215:492–502

29

Benign and Malignant Primary Liver Neoplasms

Peter J. Allen ▪ *Yuman Fong*

▪ INTRODUCTION

Benign tumors of the liver include hepatic hemangioma, liver cell adenoma, focal nodular hyperplasia (FNH), and less common lesions that arise from the hepatic epithelial or mesenchymal tissue (Table 29–1). The incidental diagnosis of benign liver tumors is rising because of the increased availability and use of abdominal CT imaging and MRI. Benign tumors of the liver are more than twice as common as malignant lesions, and may occur in up to 20% of the population.[1] Autopsy series have identified hepatic hemangiomas, the most common benign tumor of the liver, in as many as 7% of all patients.[2] Some of these lesions have a completely benign natural history and do not need to be resected, while others carry a risk of growth, hemorrhage, or malignant transformation and should be operatively removed. Obtaining a preoperative diagnosis is therefore critical, and this single factor remains the primary challenge in managing patients with benign tumors of the liver.

Diagnostic uncertainty is common, and has been reported to be the indication for operation in as many as 40% of resected patients.[3,4] Current clinical, laboratory, and radiographic studies are frequently unable to differentiate benign from malignant lesions of the liver. Symptoms, physical findings, and liver function tests are not specific. Tumor markers are normal in many patients with malignancy, and therefore should not be relied upon to identify a benign process. Ultrasound is commonly used, but also not specific. Currently, the most accurate radiographic tests are CT and MRI. These scans are complimentary tests that are often diagnostic for hemangioma, but are less helpful in differentiating focal nodular hyperplasia from hepatic adenoma.[4,5] In the setting of a hemangioma however, MRI is becoming the diagnostic test of choice with recent studies demonstrating an accuracy of 85–95%.[6] Table 29–2 presents the MRI and CT characteristics of the more common benign lesions.

A liver biopsy may be indicated when non-invasive tests are not diagnostic. The precise indications for preoperative liver biopsy remain controversial; in our practice, however, liver biopsy is generally reserved for cases in which there is diagnostic uncertainty after a thorough clinical and radiographic evaluation. Biopsy may be performed by percutaneous fine-needle aspiration (FNA), percutaneous core biopsy, or by laparoscopic techniques. The diagnostic accuracy of liver biopsy may be as low as 40%, and therefore the potential benefits of biopsy must be balanced with the risk of bleeding, and the potential for seeding the peritoneal cavity if the lesion is malignant.[7,8] In a recent study from our institution, 30 of 68 patients (44%) who underwent resection of a benign liver tumor had a preoperative percutaneous biopsy, and in only 11 of the 30 cases (37%) did the preoperative biopsy provide the correct diagnosis.[9]

The indications for resection of benign tumors include an uncertain diagnosis with a suspicion of malignancy, severe symptoms secondary to the size of the lesion, and in the case of hepatic adenoma, the risk of hemorrhage, rupture, or malignant degeneration. The decision to resect is usually based upon a combination of the patient's history, the radiographic appearance,

TABLE 29–1. BENIGN TUMORS OF THE LIVER

Epithelial tumors		
	Hepatocellular	
		Focal nodular hyperplasia
		Hepatocellular adenoma
		Nodular regenerative hyperplasia
	Bile duct	
		Bile duct adenoma
		Bile duct cystadenoma
Mesenchymal tumors		
	Blood vessel	
		Hemangioma
		Hemangioendothelioma
	Adipose	
		Lipoma
	Muscle	
		Leiomyoma
Others		
		Infectious lesions
		Focal fat

and the surgeon's clinical judgment. Because of the predominance of hemangioma within this group of patients, the majority of patients with benign liver tumors may be safely observed.[3,9] Asymptomatic patients with FNH or hemangioma do not require resection. In a large study by Weimann and colleagues, 388 patients who were diagnosed with either hemangioma or FNH by thorough radiographic evaluation were followed nonoperatively.[3] The median follow-up in this study was 32 months, and in 87% of patients the tumor remained stable in size and none of the 388 patients experienced tumor rupture. Figure 29–1 presents a flow diagram of our basic management approach for presumed benign tumors of the liver.

When surgical resection is indicated, a variety of approaches should be considered. These approaches include open resection, enucleation, and laparoscopic techniques. Whenever there is a concern for malignancy, resection should be performed with a margin of normal surrounding parenchyma. Resection is also necessary when the tumor lies deep within the liver, as enucleation is not feasible in this circumstance. Enucleation for benign tumors is often appropriate, and is our preferred approach for tumors known to be hemangiomas. Laparoscopic resection is another approach that is currently appropriate for selected patients with benign tumors. Data is now available from moderate-sized retrospective studies that suggest laparoscopic subsegmental, segmental, and lobar resections are safe and appropriate.[10,11]

■ HEMANGIOMA

EPIDEMIOLOGY AND ETIOLOGY

Hemangiomas are the most common benign tumors of the liver and may be present in up to 7% of the population.[2] The cause of hemangiomas is unknown. Hemangiomas of the liver may be associated with hemangiomas of other organs, and may be multiple within the liver.[12] There have been some reports of a higher incidence of hepatic hemangioma in women, but the data is conflicting. The most recent data would suggest that there is no difference in the incidence of liver hemangioma between men and women, and that sex hormones do not play a role in the growth of these lesions.[13,14] The most recent review from our institution of 153 patients with liver hemangioma found that 45% of the patients were male.[15] A recent case-control study from Israel found no association between liver hemangioma, and either the patient's reproductive history or use of oral contraceptives.[13]

PATHOLOGY

The typical cavernous hemangioma is a red-blue, soft, spongy mass approximately 1 to 2 cm in diameter. When

TABLE 29–2. RADIOGRAPHIC FEATURES OF BENIGN TUMORS OF THE LIVER

	Triphasic Contrast Enhanced CT			MRI	
	Pre-contrast	**Arterial phase**	**Delayed**	**T1**	**T2**
Hemangioma	Well-defined Hypodensity	Peripheral nodular enhancement		Hypointense	Hyperintense
FNH	Well-defined Hypo- or iso-dense	Homogenous enhancement	Increased scar uptake delayed images	Hypo- or iso-intense	Isointense with possible increased scar signal.
Hepatocellular adenoma	Iso-dense Fat, hemorrhage or necrosis may be evident	Homogenous enhancement	Possible prolonged hyperdense enhancement	Mixed, may be hyperintense	Mixed, may be hyperintense

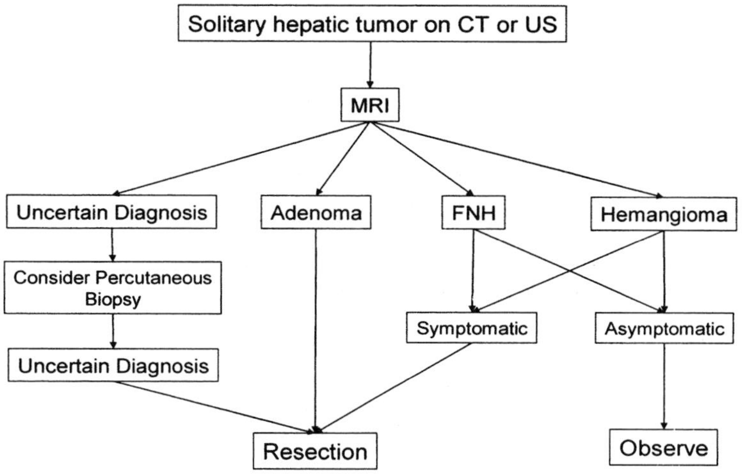

Figure 29–1. Treatment algorithm for patient presenting with presumed solitary benign tumor of the liver.

these lesions are greater than 4 cm in size, they are referred to as giant hemangiomas. Histologically these lesions are sharply defined, but not encapsulated, and are made up of large, cavernous vascular spaces, partly or completely filled with blood separated by minimal connective tissue stroma. The amount of stromal tissue is variable, however, and some lesions may exhibit extensive areas of necrosis and fibrosis. Thrombosis is common, and dystrophic calcification may also be present within the lesion.

The microscopic interface between hemangioma and the surrounding liver parenchyma is one that has been well-described, and may be a factor in the ease at which the hemangioma can be enucleated.[16,17] Zimmermann has described four different patterns of tumor-parenchymal interface. These patterns include: (1) fibrous interface characterized by a relatively avascular capsule-like fibrous lamella, (2) interdigitating interface characterized by a mixture of parenchymal and hemangioma components without a capsule-like interface, (3) compression interface characterized by direct apposition between hemangioma and parenchyma, and (4) irregular/spongy interface characterized by a highly irregular border with numerous parenchymal foci interspersed between dilated blood channels.[17] Zimmermann has reported that the fibrous interface is the most common interface in large hemangiomas. This capsule-like fibrous, and avascular, interface facilitates the enucleation these lesions.

DIAGNOSIS

Although cavernous hemangioma can be diagnosed on biopsy material, percutaneous biopsies should not be performed because of the risk of hemorrhage, and because of the low diagnostic accuracy of biopsy for hemangioma. In a recent study from our institution, 13 of 52 patients (25%) resected for hemangioma underwent preoperative percutaneous biopsy.[15] The diagnosis of hemangioma was established by biopsy in only three of the 13 patients (23%) with hemangioma who underwent resection.

The diagnosis of hemangioma is most often obtained through the use of high-quality CT and MRI. Non-contrast CT images will reveal a well-defined hypodense mass that may contain areas of calcification or central scarring. Contrast-enhanced images, both on arterial and portal venous phase series will usually demonstrate typical peripheral nodular enhancement.[18,19] In a study by Ashida and associates of 38 patients with 50 liver hemangiomas, there were five specific CT criteria found to be diagnostic of hemangioma. These criteria included: (1) a low density lesion on unenhanced scan, (2) early peripheral contrast enhancement, (3) progressive opacification from the periphery to the center, (4) a delay of at least three minutes before total opacification, and (5) eventual isodense appearance. In this study, 38 of the 50 lesions (76%) demonstrated all five of the criteria, and the presence of criteria 4 and 5 plus any other two of the criteria was considered diagnostic.

When hemangioma is suspected, and CT fails to confirm the diagnosis, an MRI should be performed. Hemangiomas typically have hypointense signal intensity compared to the surrounding liver tissue on T1-weighted imaging, and hyperintense signal intensity on T2-weighted imaging. The pattern of enhancement on gadolinium images is similar to that seen on contrast enhanced CT imaging. MRI may be more sensitive than CT in detecting subtle enhancement, and recent studies have demonstrated that MRI has a diagnostic accuracy as high as 96% for hepatic hemangioma [6,20]

Several other radiographic tests are available for the diagnosis of liver hemangioma, but are generally not indicated. Because of the high level of accuracy of CT and MRI, Tc-99m-labeled red blood cell scans are infrequently necessary. When CT and MRI are not diagnostic however, this test may be helpful, and is certainly superior to ultrasound or even biopsy.[21] Positron emission tomography (PET) has also been reported in the diagnosis of hepatic, as well as peripheral, hemangiomas.[15,22] Limited data so far have demonstrated that hemangiomas are not PET avid. Therefore, PET may be helpful in differentiating hemangioma from metabolically active malignancies.

TREATMENT

The majority of patients with hepatic hemangiomas should be managed nonoperatively. The natural history of these lesions is usually one of stability. Rarely do patients develop symptoms, and spontaneous rupture should be reported. Only 30 reports of spontaneous intra-abdominal rupture of hepatic hemangiomas have been reported in the literature.[23] Size alone should no longer be used as a criterion for resection as recent reports have demonstrated that even large lesions may be safely managed nonoperatively.[3,24] In a recent study from the Netherlands, 38 of 49 patients who were discovered to have hepatic hemangiomas were followed nonoperatively. In this study, the median diameter of the tumors managed nonoperatively was 6 cm. The median follow-up for these patients was 52 months, and during that time no patient experienced a complication from the lesion, or developed symptoms.

The three criteria we use as indications for resection include severe symptoms, inability to exclude malignancy, and the development of complications from the hemangioma. Controversy remains as to whether resection is advisable for symptom relief. Bismuth's group reported that seven of 14 patients (50%) who underwent treatment of hemangioma for symptom relief had persistent symptoms following treatment, and they therefore cautioned against resection.[25] It should be noted, however, that in this study, six of the 14 patients who were treated for symptomatic hemangioma underwent embolization or hepatic arterial ligation, rather than surgical excision; and of the seven total patients with persistence of symptoms, five of them were from the embolization/ligation group. Data from our institution, and others, suggests that between 75% and 90% of carefully selected patients who have undergone resection or enucleation for symptoms will have relief.[9,12,26,27] These patients however, must be carefully selected. Other pancreaticobiliary and upper gastrointestinal (GI) causes for the symptoms must be investigated, and the symptoms should be carefully matched to the size and nature of the hemangioma. The size of the lesion appears to be associated with the presence of symptoms. The median size for patients at our institution resected for symptoms was 14 cm.[15] In our experience, hemangiomas less than 4 cm in size are almost exclusively asymptomatic, and symptomatic lesions tend to be larger within the right liver than within the left.[15]

Another indication for surgical resection of hepatic hemangioma is the development of complications from the lesion. As noted above, intra-abdominal hemorrhage is extremely uncommon, but when it does occur, it should be considered as a life-threatening emergency and treated with a combination of angiography with embolization and surgery. Intratumoral bleeding has been reported more frequently as a complication of hemangioma, and is often thought to be associated with the development of symptoms. This complication is not life-threatening, but if symptoms develop it will often lead to the diagnosis of the lesion and eventual surgical evaluation. The Kasabach-Merritt syndrome is another complication of large hemangiomas that consists of thrombocytopenia and consumptive coagulopathy.[28] The pathophysiology is thought to be secondary to activation of the clotting cascade by trapped platelets within the hemangioma. Controversy exists as to the most appropriate treatment of this condition. Recommended treatments include immunosuppressive agents, radiation, surgical resection, and even transplantation.[28,29]

When surgical treatment is indicated, both resection and enucleation have been advocated. Multiple studies however, have documented that enucleation is performed in the majority of cases.[15,26,30] In a recent study from our institution, enucleation was performed for 31 of 52 patients (60%) undergoing operative treatment for hemangioma.[15] We feel that this technique decreases both operative time and operative blood loss. In a recent study by Lerner and colleagues of 52 patients undergoing surgical treatment for hemangioma, enucleation was associated with a lower postoperative complication rate, and similar rate of transfusion.[30] Hepatic hemangioma is suited for enucleation because of its benign nature, and the often associated fibrous cleavage plane that exists between the hemangioma and the surrounding hepatic parenchyma.

The technique for enucleation of hepatic hemangiomas has been described in detail previously.[15,31] In general, inflow control is initially achieved by use of the Pringle maneuver. The hepatic artery ipsilateral to the tumor is then identified and dissected proximally to the level of the proper hepatic artery. For large lesions of the right or left hepatic lobes, ligation of the ipsilateral artery will result in a gradual reduction in the size of the lesion. Smaller lesions do not require ligation of the lobar artery, and may be adequately devascularized with a more selective ligation of distal branch vessels. Once arterial inflow has been controlled, a small hepatotomy should be performed just a few millimeters from the edge of the hemangioma. Division of this parenchyma will allow entry into the compressed sheath of liver tissue that usually defines the border between hemangioma and normal parenchyma. Gentle dissection within this sheath is usually possible, and small blood vessels or bile ducts that are encountered may be easily controlled with clips or suture ligature.

▪ FOCAL NODULAR HYPERPLASIA

EPIDEMIOLOGY AND ETIOLOGY

FNH is defined as a nodule composed of benign-appearing hepatocytes within a liver that is otherwise histologically normal.[32] FNH is the second most common benign tumor of the liver, usually presents as a solitary lesion, and is often discovered incidentally. The lesion most commonly occurs in young women, and the male-to-female ratio is 1:8. The average age of patients at the time of diagnosis is 35 years of age.[33]

The pathogenesis of this lesion is not well understood, but in general it is thought to be a reactive process to either a vascular injury or malformation. The presence of large arteries within a central fibrous scar, and the absence of portal venous structures, is characteristic of FNH. Some have postulated that this abnormal vascular anatomy results in chronic malperfusion, and secondary hyperplasia of the surrounding hepatocytes.[34] Controversy exists as to whether this lesion, or its natural history, is associated with the use of oral contraceptives.[35,36] Current data suggests that neither the presence, the size, nor the number of lesions is influenced by the use of oral contraceptives.[37] In a study by Mathieu and associates of 216 women with FNH, the use of oral contraceptives, and even pregnancy, was not associated with lesion growth.[37] During follow-up, only four lesions (2%) were found to increase in size, and none of the 12 patients who became pregnant during follow-up experienced growth or other complications of the lesion.

PATHOLOGY

FNH grossly appears as a discrete pale mass, which is lobulated with abundant septae. A thin capsule will often be evident, and the tumor is usually without evidence of necrosis or hemorrhage. A central scar is characteristic. More than one central scar may be apparent, and within the scar dilated blood vessels are often evident. These vessels are representative of the dilated central artery that is typical of this lesion.

FNH is not a neoplastic process, but a hyperplasia. Currently, FNH is divided into two types: typical and atypical. Typical, or classic FNH, is characterized by a central stellate fibrous region, which contains abnormal arteries but not portal veins, and is multinodular with nearly normal appearing hepatocytes and mildly proliferative bile ducts.[36] These bile ducts are typically located at the junction of the abnormal hepatocytes and fibrous regions. Atypical lesions may be histologically classified as FNH, but lack one of the classic features such as a central scar, or have the presence of a portal vein within the central vascular region. These atypical lesions have been divided into three subtypes: (1) telangiectatic, (2) FNH with cytologic atypia, and (3) mixed hyperplastic/adenomatous FNH.[33,36]

DIAGNOSIS

FNH does not require surgical resection, and it is therefore critical to differentiate this lesion from other hypervascular lesions such as hepatocellular adenoma, hepatocellular carcinoma, and various metastatic lesions. Radiographic imaging is the current mainstay for diagnosis; however percutaneous biopsy may be warranted in situations where radiographic diagnosis is not definitive. Currently, the most sensitive test for the diagnosis of FNH is MRI with reported sensitivity and specificity rates of about 75% and 98% respectively.[36,38]

The increased availability of CT imaging, and the recent improvements in contrast administration and image detection, have resulted in an increased utilization and accuracy of this modality for FNH. The typical FNH will appear as a well demarcated hypo-intense lesion on noncontrast images. In the arterial phase the lesion will become uniformly hyperattenuating because of the homogenous enhancement of the entire lesion, except for the central scar. This pattern is similar to that of hemangioma, however within an FNH, the enhancement is uniform throughout the lesion rather than from the periphery. In the portal phase the lesion will become more iso-intense, and the central scar may show enhancement as a result of gradual diffusion of the contrast material into the fibrous scar.[39]

MRI should also be performed with gadolinium enhancement as this will enhance the sensitivity of the test.[38] Typically, FNH is hypointense on T1-weighted images, and slightly hyperintense on T2-weighted images. Similar to CT findings, FNH will show brisk and homogenous enhancement with gadolinium. During the later phases the central scar will enhance as well, and may even become hyperintense as contrast washes out of the lesion. Other tissue-specific contrast agents have been recently investigated.[36] These agents are specific for Kupffer cells and hepatocytes and may further increase the ability to differentiate FNH with MRI.

Data suggest that when imaging studies are equivocal, percutaneous biopsy will be able to diagnose FNH in the majority of cases.[36,40] In a study by Fabre and associates, the histologic diagnosis of FNH by percutaneous biopsy was made in 58% of lesions that had nondiagnostic radiographic imaging.[40] The typical FNH can be diagnosed with core biopsy when benign-appearing hepatocytes, a prominent arterial supply, the absence of a portal vein, and peripheral bile duct hyperplasia are observed.

TREATMENT

When the diagnosis of FNH is confirmed, the treatment should be nonoperative in the vast majority of patients. FNH is not a neoplastic process and therefore cannot be considered premalignant. As noted above, the growth of these lesions is uncommon, and does not appear to be related to the use of oral contraceptives or pregnancy.[37] Therefore, resection should not be recommended as a prophylactic measure against tumor enlargement and rupture. Occasionally, patients have been reported to present with symptoms secondary to FNH.[9,41] After careful diagnostic review, in this setting resection may be warranted. Subsegmental resections are often used for FNH, and minimally invasive approaches should be considered.

▪ HEPATOCELLULAR ADENOMA

EPIDEMIOLOGY AND ETIOLOGY

Hepatocellular adenoma also occurs predominantly in young women, however unlike FNH, hepatocellular adenoma is a neoplastic process that is clearly associated with the use of oral contraceptives (OCPs), and is also associated with type 1 glycogen storage disease and diabetes.[42] Hepatocellular adenoma was rarely reported before the development of oral contraceptives, and is believed to be four times more common in women who use OCPs than in those who do not.[42] The longer OCPs are used, the higher the risk of developing a hepatocellular adenoma. Patients who have used OCPs for longer than 9 years have an increased risk of 25 times that of the general population. Complications from hepatocellular adenoma have also been associated with the use of OCPs. A review of 237 patients by Klatskin in the 1970s found that patients taking OCPs presented with larger tumors (97% >5 cm vs. 75% >5 cm) and were more likely to present with tumor rupture and bleeding (65% vs. 25%) than patients not taking OCPs.[43]

The majority of these lesions will be symptomatic at presentation, and complications associated with hepatocellular adenomas include tumor growth, rupture with intraperitoneal hemorrhage, and malignant transformation. Hepatocellular adenoma should be considered a premalignant condition. Reports have been published of patients who have been followed with serial radiographic studies and developed hepatocellular carcinoma within a previous hepatocellular adenoma.[44–46] Within these studies, an increase in the serum alpha-feto protein (AFP) level was found to be an indicator of this malignant transformation.[7,44–46] Tumor growth and rupture is another complication of this lesion. The risk of rupture and intraperitoneal hemorrhage may be as high as 30–50%.[46,47] Foster published on 54 patients with hepatocellular adenoma in 1977.[48] In this review, 21 of the 54 patients (39%) were diagnosed after hemorrhage into the tumor or peritoneal cavity, and only four patients (7%) had the lesion discovered incidentally. When hemorrhage does occur, intra-abdominal bleeding may be observed in up to 60% of the patients.

PATHOLOGY

Hepatocellular adenomas will present as solitary lesions in approximately 75% of cases. Multiple adenomas are common in patients with glycogen storage disease or liver adenomatosis. Adenomas may vary from 1 cm to greater than 20 cm in size. Grossly the tumors are sharply demarcated from the normal parenchyma and are light in color. Unlike FNH, hemorrhage is common and may be evident on gross examination.

Microscopically adenomas consist of cords of cells that closely resemble normal hepatocytes, and histologic differentiation between adenoma and normal liver tissue may be difficult. Adenoma cells, however, are larger than normal hepatocytes and may contain large amounts of glycogen and lipid.[49] Adenomas are devoid of bile ducts, and this key histologic feature helps to distinguish hepatocellular adenoma from FNH on biopsy. The hepatocytes within an adenoma are separated by dilated sinusoids that represent the arterial blood supply of the lesion, which like FNH, typically lack a portal venous supply. The lesions characteristically have little fibrous connective tissue support and generally lack a tumor capsule.

DIAGNOSIS

The most important diagnosis to exclude in the evaluation of hepatocellular adenoma is FNH, as treatment for the majority of adenomas should be resection, and the treatment for the majority of FNH should be observation. Hepatocellular adenomas are often detected first by ultrasound during evaluation for right upper quadrant abdominal symptoms.[49] Often adenomas will be hyperechoic on ultrasound, which may be secondary to their high lipid content. Other findings may include significant heterogeneity secondary to intratumoral hemorrhage, or calcifications secondary to hemorrhage and necrosis. These findings may identify the lesion, but are not specific enough to diagnose an adenoma.

Multiphasic CT scan is more specific than ultrasound for adenoma.[50] Nonenhanced images may identify areas of fat or hemorrhage that is typical of adenoma. The majority of adenomas will appear sharply demarcated and be hypo- or iso-attenuating. The areas of old hemorrhage and necrosis will appear as discrete areas of hypoattenuation on nonenhanced images. Arterial phase contrast images may show some degree of peripheral enhancement secondary to the larger peripheral feeding vessels, however approximately 80% of cases will show homogenous rapid enhancement.[49] Unlike FNH, the enhancement in adenoma will often not persist secondary to a component of arteriovenous shunting.

Findings on MR imaging are reported to be more variable than those of CT.[49,51,52] Adenomas have been described as hyperintense, isointense, and hypointense on T1-weighted images.[51,52] Heterogeneity is common, with regions of increased signal intensity occurring secondary to fat, hemorrhage, and necrosis. Inconsistency is also reported for T2-weighted images but it appears that the majority of adenomas will be hyperintense relative to the liver on T2 imaging.[52] Dynamic gadolinium-enhanced MRI may also be used to demonstrate early arterial enhancement. Since adenomas have a sparse presence of Kupffer cells, Kupffer cell–specific agents will result in decreased signal intensity on T2-weighted imaging.

If diagnostic uncertainty remains after thorough imaging, then percutaneous biopsy should be considered. Biopsy should certainly be performed if FNH is within the differential. Percutaneous fine-needle aspiration, as well as core biopsy have been shown to be accurate in the diagnosis of hepatocellular adenoma.[42] As noted above, the absence of bile ducts within the lesion is one of the critical elements that histologically differentiates FNH from hepatocellular adenoma.

TREATMENT

Generally, patients with hepatocellular adenoma should undergo surgical resection in order to prevent the risk of tumor enlargement and rupture, and to prevent the risk of malignant degeneration. Some have recommended initial discontinuation of OCP use with follow-up imaging to look for evidence of regression.[9] This approach may be reasonable in selected patients, however it must be emphasized that regression is unpredictable, and reports exist of continued growth, rupture, and malignant transformation even after discontinuation of OCPs.[42–44]

MISCELLANEOUS BENIGN TUMORS

Nodular Regenerative Hyperplasia

Nodular regenerative hyperplasia is an uncommon lesion that is associated with chronic liver diseases. Cirrhosis and portal hypertension may be present in up to 50% of cases.[53] Radiographically these lesions appear similar to those of FNH, however portal venous phase images may show almost complete contrast washout and the lesion may be almost imperceptible on these images.[35] Given the rarity of this entity, the natural history of these lesions is poorly understood, however tumor growth and rupture are extremely rare. Adequate biopsy should be obtained to confirm diagnosis followed by nonoperative management.

Peliosis Hepatitis

Hepatic peliosis is an uncommon disorder characterized by multiple, small, blood-filled sinuses. Peliosis most commonly occurs in immunocompromised posttransplant patients, AIDS patients, and patients taking long-term steroids.[54,55] Radiographically these lesions present as diffuse hypodense areas spread throughout the liver. CT and MRI typically will show enhancement on early images, which may progress from central to peripheral on delayed imaging.[56] Rupture with intraperitoneal bleeding has been reported from this condition.[57,58] The reported treatment for bleeding from this lesion has been angiographic embolization. Given that this is a diffuse condition of the liver with known etiology, the treatment should be directed toward the specific etiology.

▪ MALIGNANT TUMORS

INTRODUCTION

Malignant tumors of the liver may arise from the hepatocyte, the bile duct epithelium, and the endothelial cells within the liver. The most common primary liver malignancy is hepatocellular carcinoma (HCC), and this tumor represents the most common of the solid organ cancers. As a group, these tumors present major diagnostic and therapeutic challenges. Though surgery can be potentially curative for these tumors, most patients with hepatobiliary cancer are discovered at a stage too advanced for complete excision. These tumors are also highly resistant to chemotherapy, limiting options for palliative treatment.

Over the last two decades however, great advances have been made in the diagnosis and treatment of these tumors. Advances in imaging have allowed for earlier detection, and more accurate staging of disease. The morbidity associated with surgical resection has improved, and more favorable short- and long-term results are now being achieved by extensive, but rational resections. These resections are being guided by both improved imaging techniques, and a better understanding of the biology of disease. Palliative treatments such as radiotherapy and other ablative techniques have extended the limits of tumor eradication and treatment.

TABLE 29–3. AGENTS KNOWN TO BE ASSOCIATED WITH THE DEVELOPMENT OF HCC

Infections	
	Hepatitis B virus
	Hepatitis C virus
Cirrhosis	
	Alcohol induced
	Autoimmune hepatitis
	Primary biliary cirrhosis
Environmental	
	Aflatoxins
	Pyrrolizidine alkaloids
	Thorotrast
	N-nitrosylated compounds
Metabolic diseases	
	Hemochromatosis
	Alpha$_1$-antitrypsin deficiency
	Wilson's disease
	Porphyria cutanea tarda
	Type 1 and 3 glycogen storage disease
	Galactosemia
	Citrullinemia
	Hereditary tyrosinemia
	Familial cholestatic cirrhosis

HEPATOCELLULAR CARCINOMA

Hepatocellular carcinoma is responsible for more than 1 million deaths annually worldwide. The difficulties in treatment of this cancer, and reason for the high mortality, result from three factors. Firstly, this cancer is usually associated with cirrhosis, which both limits the treatment options and increases the morbidity of any given therapy. Secondly, HCC is usually asymptomatic at early stages, and has a great propensity for intravascular or intrabiliary extension, even when the primary tumor is small. As a result, HCC is usually at an advanced stage when discovered. Thirdly, this tumor has been resistant to most conventional forms of cytotoxic chemotherapy.

EPIDEMIOLOGY AND ETIOLOGY

There are at least 1 million new cases of HCC yearly.[59] The incidence of HCC increases with age, and is four to eight times more common in males than in females. This cancer is strongly associated with chronic liver injury, and therefore the geographic distribution of HCC closely mirrors that of viral hepatitis (Table 29–3). The etiologic association between hepatitis B (HBV) infection and HCC is well established. In a landmark study examining HBV infection and HCC, Beasley followed 22,707 male subjects in Taiwan, 15.2% of whom were HBV chronic carriers as exhibited by detection of Hb_sAg in the serum.[60] Of the 116 cases of HCC that occurred during a mean follow-up period of 7 years, 113 occurred in patients positive for HB_sAg. This study demonstrated that HCC was related not simply to a history of HBV infection, but to the chronic carrier states, and that the relative risk of developing HCC was 200-fold greater in individuals with evidence of HBV infection than in noninfected individuals.[60]

The hepatitis C virus (HCV) has also been associated with HCC. Antibodies to HCV have been found in as many as 76% of patients with HCC in Japan, Italy, and Spain[61] and in 36% in the United States.[62] In contrast to HCV-associated HCC however, HCC rarely occurs in HBV carriers before the development of cirrhosis. Additionally, the incidence of HCC in chronic carriers of HCV is estimated to be as high as 5% per year, compared to 0.5% per year for HBV carriers.[63]

Chemical carcinogens have also been linked to primary liver cancers. Chemicals such as nitrites, hydrocarbons, solvents, organochlorine pesticides, primary metals, and polychlorinated biphenyls have been implicated in development of HCC.[64] Colloidal thorium dioxide (Thorotrast), which emits high level α, β, and γ radiation, and was used as an angiographicagent in the 1930s, has been linked to angiosarcoma, cholangiocarcinoma, and HCC.

Of all the chemicals linked to development of HCC, the most important is ethanol. Alcohol abuse has been liked not only to the development of HCC, but also carcinomas in the larynx, mouth, and esophagus. With regard to HCC, ethanol is thought to produce HCC through development of hepatic cirrhosis, or as a co-carcinogen with other agents such as HBV, HCV, hepatotoxins, and tobacco[65–70] rather than through direct effect on the hepatocytes.

Aflatoxins produced by the fungi *Aspergillus flavus* and *A. parasiticus* have also been linked to HCC. These are fungi that grow on grains, peanuts, and other food products, and are the most common cause of food spoilage in the tropics. These fungi produce aflatoxins designated B_1, B_2, G_1, and G_2. Aflatoxin B_1 is the most hepatotoxic, and chronic exposure to these mycotoxins leads to development of HCC.[71]

Congenital conditions may also lead to the development of HCC. Genetic diseases such as hemochromatosis, Wilson's disease, hereditary tyrosinemia, type 1 glycogen storage disease, hepatic porphyria of both intermittent and cutanea tarda types, familial polyposis coli, ataxia telangiectasia, familial cholestatic cirrhosis, biliary atresia, congenital hepatic fibrosis, neurofibromatosis, situs inversus, fetal alcohol syndrome, α-antitrypsin deficiency, and Budd-Chiari syndrome[72] have all been linked to a higher incidence of HCC. Ultimately though, the unifying etiology of HCC is the chronic injury and inflammation.

PATHOLOGIC FEATURES

HCC has been graded as well differentiated, moderately differentiated, and poorly differentiated. The well differentiated variety may be difficult to distinguish from a regenerating nodule on fine needle biopsy. No firm correlation of grade to prognosis has been established. HCC can be classified generally into three different growth patterns, which are associated with the ability to perform resection, and therefore have a significant influence on long-term outcome (Fig 29–2). The hanging type tumor, are tumors that are attached to the normal liver by a small vascular stalk, even when tumors are large. These are easily excised with little loss in functional parenchyma. The pushing type are generally well demarcated and often encapsulated by a fibrous capsule. These displace normal vasculature rather than infiltrate and invade the major vessels. These are often resectable even when there is substantial bulk. Finally, the infiltrative variety has a very indistinct tumor-live interface, and tends to have a much greater degree of vascular infiltration and invasion even when the tumor is small. Excising the infiltrative variety is often complicated by positive margins. The practical nature of this gross pathologic classification is reinforced by the distinctive radiologic appearance of these three different growth patterns on imaging.

The most important pathologic issue is the distinct appearance and clinical behavior of the fibrolamellar variant of HCC (Table 29–4). On gross and radiologic inspection, fibrolamellar HCC is generally well demarcated and often encapsulated and with a central fibrotic area. It is a variant that generally occurs in young patients without underlying cirrhosis. AFP, which is commonly elevated in the usual case of HCC is not elevated in fibrolamellar HCC. Other serum markers that are often elevated in fibrolamellar HCC include neurotensin, and vitamin B-12 binding protein.[73] The fibrolamellar variant of HCC has a prolonged survival compared with typical HCC likely because of the well demarcated nature of the tumor and the greater range in treatment for patients without underlying cirrhosis.[74]

CLINICAL PRESENTATION

Even though hepatocellular carcinoma is generally a slow growing tumor, the majority of patients present at an advanced stage and most are beyond curative treatments. Because the liver is relatively hidden behind the right costal cartilages, tumors have to reach substantial size before they are palpable. Furthermore, the large functional reserve of the liver masks any small impairment produced by local parenchymal disturbances. Small tumors are therefore most often asymptomatic, and are usually discovered during screening programs[75–77] or incidentally during imaging performed for other abdominal conditions.

The majority of cases therefore present when the tumor is large, at a stage when local symptoms are common. Patients usually complain of a dull, vague, right upper quadrant pain, sometimes referred to the shoulder. Hepatomegaly is a frequent accompanying finding. The liver edge is hard and irregular, because of both the tumor and the usual accompanying cirrhosis. A vascular bruit can be heard in about 25% of cases.[78] General symptoms of malignancy, including anorexia, nausea, lethargy and weight loss, are common. The most common clinical presentation is the triad of right upper quadrant pain, mass, and weight loss.[79–81] Central necrosis of large tumors can also lead to fever, and HCC can present as pyrexia of unknown origin. For the majority of patients, the presentation of HCC will also be the first presentation of the underlying cirrhosis. In one study, even though 90% of patients were eventually found to have cirrhosis, less than 10% were thought at first evaluation for HCC to have chronic liver disease on the basis of history and clinical examination.[80]

Hepatic decompensation is another common presentation for HCC, with patients seeking medical attention as a result of typical symptoms of liver failure

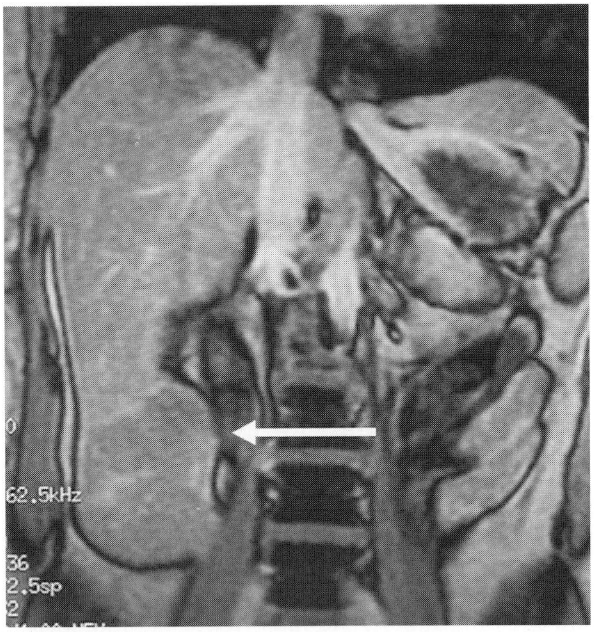

A

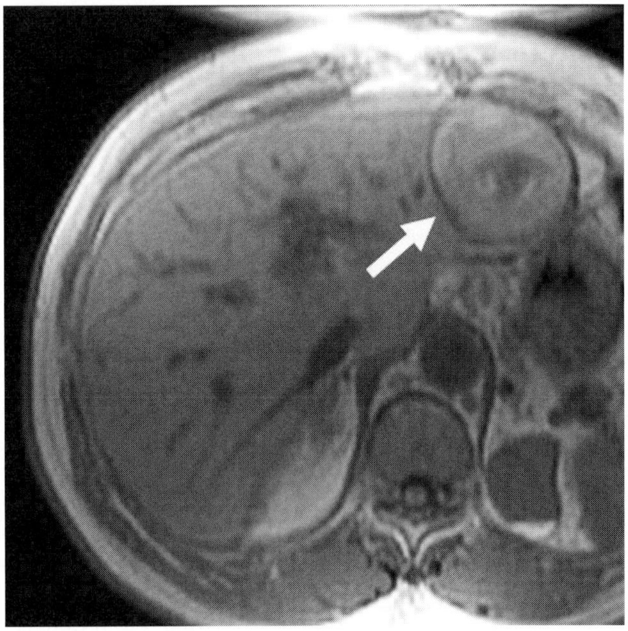

B

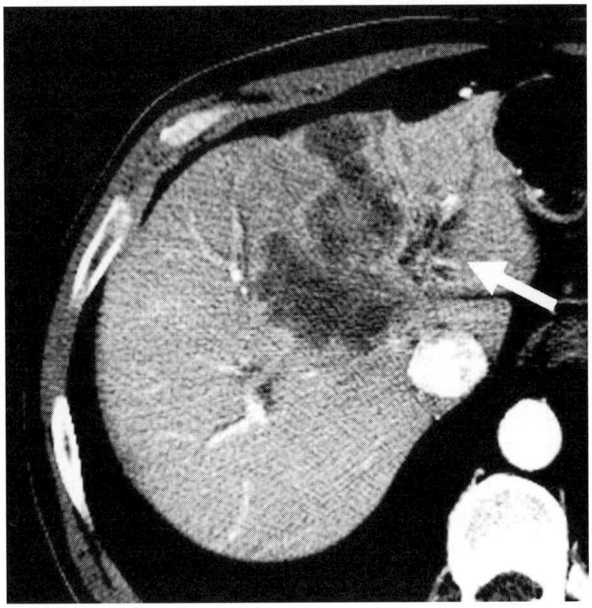

C

Figure 29–2. Growth patterns of HCC. **A.** "Hanging" type. MRI demonstrating a mass (*arrow*) that is attached by a stalk to the right lobe of the liver. **B.** "Pushing" type. These are generally encapsulated, well-circumscribed tumors (*arrow*). **C.** "Infiltrating/Invading" type. This lesion has diffusely infiltrated the entire left two thirds of the liver. Note the left biliary ductal dilation (*arrow*).

such as ascites, jaundice, or encephalopathy. This decompensation of liver function is most often because of tumor replacement of functional parenchyma in a patient with previously compensated cirrhosis. HCC also has a great propensity for vascular invasion and intravascular growth. Hepatic failure may therefore also be a result of portal vein occlusion secondary to intravascular tumor thrombus.[82–84] A much more rare cause of liver failure is a result of Budd-Chiari syndrome resulting from direct invasion and occlusion of the hepatic vein and inferior vena cava by tumor and tumor thrombus.

GI bleeding often complicates the clinical course of patients with HCC and in 10% of cases is the presenting finding.[84] In approximately half of these cases, bleeding is from esophageal varices,[84] which can result from portal hypertension because of cirrhosis alone or with an added contribution of intraportal thrombus.

TABLE 29–4. COMPARISON OF STANDARD HCC WITH FIBROLAMELLAR VARIANT

Characteristic	HCC	Fibrolamellar HCC
Male: Female	4:1–8:1	1:1
Median age	55	25
Tumor	Invasive	Well circumscribed
Resectability	<25%	50–75%
Cirrhosis	90%	5%
AFP +	80%	5%
HepB+	65%	5%

Patients with GI bleeding from esophageal varices have an extraordinarily poor prognosis, with a median survival measurable in weeks.[83] The particularly poor prognosis of variceal bleeding complicating HCC is a result of the common finding of intraportal thrombus, which further increases the portal pressure and makes bleeding varices more difficult to control. In one study, nearly a quarter of patients with HCC died from massive variceal hemorrhage.[82] GI bleeding can also occur from other causes, such as a benign peptic ulcer or direct invasion of the GI tract by tumor.[84] The most dramatic presentation of HCC is tumor rupture. This is the initial presentation in 2–5% of patients with HCC. Patients present with acute abdominal pain and swelling, and are found to have abdominal swelling, guarding, rebound tenderness, and ileus. The patient also commonly has signs of hemodynamic instability or overt hypovolemic shock. Diagnosis is confirmed either by findings of tumor mass and peritoneal blood through imaging, laparotomy, or paracentesis.[85–90]

Jaundice as a presenting symptom of HCC occurs in up to half the patients. The most common cause of the jaundice is, however, hepatic parenchymal insufficiency.[79,91–93] On rare occasions (<10% of jaundiced patients), jaundice associated with HCC results from biliary obstruction.[79,94–98] The biliary obstruction can occur from intraluminal tumor, from hemobilia, or because of extraluminal bile duct obstruction. In the clinical evaluation of jaundice for a patient with HCC, it is enormously important to distinguish hepatocellular failure from obstruction. The former usually indicates that the patient is beyond any therapy, while the latter can be treated often with good palliation and even potential cure.[94,97,99–103]

In rare cases (<5%), HCC can present with paraneoplastic syndromes because of hormonal or immune effects of the tumors.[104] The most important of these are hypoglycemia, erythrocytosis, hypercalcemia, and hypercholesterolemia. Porphyria cutanea tarda, virilization and feminization syndromes, carcinoid syndrome, hypertrophic osteoarthropathy, hyperthyroidism, and osteoporosis can also occur.[105–107]

DIAGNOSIS

For patients suspected of suffering from HCC, the aims of diagnostic investigations are (1) verification of diagnosis, (2) determine extent of disease, (3) determine functional liver reserve, and (4) assess biologic determinants that are predictors of long-term prognosis.

Diagnosis

Diagnosis of HCC can usually be positively established noninvasively by a combination of history, physical, imaging, and blood tests. There is little diagnostic doubt in a patient with a liver mass consistent with a HCC on CT or MRI and a serum AFP of >500 ng/dL. This combination is diagnostic and treatment can be instituted without tissue diagnosis. The presence of cirrhosis, or hepatitis infection as documented by presence of HB_sAg or HCV in the blood, is further confirmation.

In the patient with a space-occupying lesion on ultrasound or CT with a nondiagnostic AFP level, the role of a percutaneous needle biopsy is often debated. There is no doubt that needle biopsy is diagnostic for HCC. However, complications are also not infrequent. Hemorrhage or tumor rupture can occur. Furthermore, there is also a small but finite risk of tumor spillage and seeding of the needle biopsy tract.[108] In cases of potentially resectable HCC, where the diagnostic certainty is high, we would proceed to surgical exploration without tumor biopsy. Indeed, in this clinical scenario, the histologic appearance of the nonneoplastic liver may have a greater impact on surgical planning. If advanced cirrhosis will preclude safe resection, we often biopsy the portion of the liver not containing tumor for histologic evaluation.

In patients with nondiagnostic AFP who are not surgical candidates, and therefore not candidates for curative therapy, tumor biopsy is performed if they are candidates for palliative therapy. In that case, fine-needle aspirate for cytologic evaluation is usually performed in preference to core needle biopsy for histology, since comparative studies indicate that smear cytology yields a much higher percentage of correct diagnosis compared to microhistology (86 vs. 66%).[109] Patients who are not candidates for palliative therapy do not need a definitive diagnosis, and biopsy is discouraged.

Extent of Disease Evaluation

The two issues to be resolved by the extent of disease evaluation is (1) whether the disease is isolated to the liver, and (2) whether distribution of tumor in the liver is amenable to surgical excision. The most common sites of metastases of HCC include lung, peritoneum, adrenal, and bone. Chest radiograph is therefore mandatory. Cross-sectional imaging such as CT or MRI of the abdomen should be scrutinized for peritoneal and adrenal sites of disease. Many centers consider bone scans mandatory prior to liver resection. Certainly, in patients with pain attributable to bony metastases, a bone scan should be performed. Finding extrahepatic disease changes the prognosis of the patients greatly, since such findings preclude the possibility of hepatectomy as curative therapy.

The extent of liver involvement is usually determined by CT scanning. This diagnostic imaging modality is widely available and relatively inexpensive. In interpreting any cross-sectional imaging modality for the patient with HCC, the number and distribution of liver tumors must be determined, as well as the degree of vascular invasion. The triple phase (noncontrast enhanced, arterial phase, and portal phase) CT images should be obtained. HCC are generally highly vascular tumors, and tumors on images with contrast-enhancement may become isodense with the surrounding liver, and tumors are sometimes only visible during the noncontrast-enhanced phase. This tumor also has a great propensity for vascular invasion and extension. Tumor thrombus in the portal vein, hepatic vein, or vena cava is therefore not unusual. Scans should therefore be scrutinized for evidence of such invasion, since therapy and prognosis can significantly be altered by such findings. If such invasion is suspected but not proven by CT, doppler ultrasound or MRI is indicated.

At some centers hepatic angiography is standard.[110,111] Some have even advocated routine use of lipiodol injected angiographically to further delineate hepatic extent of disease.[112] This lipid is preferentially retained in HCC because of the particle size. There is no doubt that these angiographic methods are highly sensitive for the presence of tumor. With current helical CT or MRI however, there is only minor incremental yield. We only rely on angiography when we suspect small tumors not visible by conventional cross-sectional imaging, such as for a patient with small amounts of disease seen on CT who has a very high AFP.

Determination of Functional Liver Reserve

Various liver function tests, alone or in combination, have been touted as useful for predicting risks of liver resection and other treatments for HCC. Various single serum measures of liver function have been suggested to be useful predictors of perioperative outcome, including serum bilirubin,[113] and serum alanine aminotransferase (ALT).[114] A doubling of bilirubin has been suggested as a contraindication for liver resection.[113] Others have used a platelet count <50 K, or a prolonged prothrombin time >4 seconds over control to be relative contraindications for hepatic resection.[115] Most investigators, however, have not relied on a single parameter, but rather used a combination of clinical and biochemical parameters to gauge safety of hepatectomy and other treatments. The most clinically useful system is the Pugh-Child's classification, which is a point scoring system for evaluation of liver function based on the levels of serum bilirubin, coagulation profile, serum albumin, presence or absence of ascites and encephalopathy, and nutritional status (Table 29–5).[116,117] Functionally well compensated cirrhosis is classified as Pugh-Child's classification grade A; decompensating cirrhosis is grade B; and decompensated cirrhosis is grade C. Generally, partial hepatectomy is only offered to patients who are Pugh-Child's A and the most favorable class B patients.[118] In general, Child's class C patients are only offered supportive care, since even nonsurgical ablative methods such as embolization is associated with a procedure related mortality in one-third of patients.[119]

Many sophisticated dynamic measures of liver function have also been used in attempts to quantitate hepatic function. Investigators have attempted to use elimination of certain dyes that are exclusively cleared by the liver, such as bromosulphthalein or indocyanine green, as measures of hepatic function. Galactose clearance or [^{14}C] aminopyrine clearance, have also been used to evaluate specific metabolic capacity of the liver. Of these, the most commonly utilized evaluations in clinical practice are indocyanine green retention at 15 minutes[120] and the [^{14}C] aminopyrine breath test,[121] though controversy still exist concerning their usefulness.[122] We do not use these tests on a routine basis in our care of the patient with HCC. We have found clinical Child's classification sufficiently discriminatory for selecting patients for therapies.

Another relatively simple test that may be predictive of perioperative outcome is the hepatic venous wedge pressure. By passing a venous catheter through the vena cava into the hepatic vein, the hepatic venous pressure can be directly ascertained. By balloon occlusion of the hepatic vein, the hepatic venous wedge pres-

TABLE 29–5. PUGH'S MODIFICATION OF CHILD'S GRADING OF CIRRHOSIS

Measurements	1 point	2 points	3 points
Bilirubin (mg/dL)	1–1.9	2–2.9	>2.9
Prothrombin time prolongation (secs)	1–3	4–6	>6
Albumin (g/dL)	>3.5	2.8–3.4	<2.8
Ascites	none	mild	moderate to severe
Encephalopathy	none	grade 1 or 2	grade 3 or 4

Child's A: 5–6 points; B: 7–9 points; C: 10–15 points.

sure, which is a reflection of the portal pressure, can be determined. These measurements have been touted as useful in segregating Child's B patients who may have favorable results from resection versus those likely to have major complication.[123]

▪ POTENTIALLY CURATIVE TREATMENTS

Therapies for HCC can be separated into resectional, ablations, radiation therapy, systemic chemotherapy or immunotherapy, and supportive care. Resectional therapy represents the only potentially curative option. We will begin with a discussion of these, particularly emphasizing recent advances and comparison of partial hepatectomy with total hepatectomy/liver transplantation.

PARTIAL HEPATECTOMY

Partial hepatectomy represents the most common procedure for HCC performed with curative intent. The liver is normally a very resilient organ with remarkable regenerative capacity. In a noncirrhotic liver, routine recovery can be expected even after resection of over two thirds of functional parenchyma.[124] In the United States, near half the patients with HCC will have no associated cirrhosis.[125] Operative mortality at most major centers is generally less than 5%, and very extensive procedures are justified by the low risk and the potential for long-term survival and cure. Resection is associated with a 5-year survival in excess of 30% (Fig 29–3).[126–130] For a patient without cirrhosis, partial hepatectomy is a relatively safe procedure, and is the treatment of choice for eradication of HCC (Table 29–6).

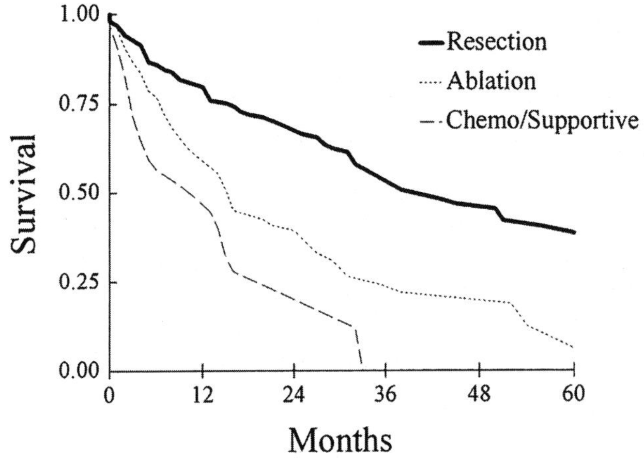

Figure 29–3. Survival curve for 154 patients undergoing hepatectomy for HCC at Memorial Sloan-Kettering Cancer Center. (With permission, from Fong Y, Sun RL, Jarnagin W, Blumgart LH. An analysis of 412 cases of hepatocellular carcinoma at a Western center. *Ann Surg* 1999;229(6):790–799.)

Worldwide, however, most cases of HCC are associated with cirrhosis. The associated cirrhosis greatly increases the risk for partial hepatectomy. This increase in risk is partly a result of intra-operative factors. These patients will usually have rigid and hard parenchyma and established varices that are difficult to manipulate and prone to bleeding. Additionally, these patients will have thrombocytopenia and coagulation defects that further exacerbate the risk of hemorrhage. Postoperatively, the liver may not regenerate and result in liver failure. Furthermore, postoperative exaggeration of portal hypertension may lead to ascites and variceal bleeds. It is understandable therefore, that resection is associated with increased morbidity and mortality in these patients. Even for a cirrhotic patient with well compensated liver function, we are reluctant to remove more than 20–25% functional parenchyma.[121,131–134] Until recently, even at centers with a low mortality for partial hepatectomy in the noncirrhotic population, partial hepatectomy for patients with cirrhosis was associated with a 10% mortality or more.[127,129,135–137] This explains the nihilistic view adopted by some for this disease, and explains the interest in treating this disease by total hepatectomy and liver transplantation. Nevertheless, even in this period of time, cirrhotic patients who survive the operation have a 5-year survival of approximately 30%.[126–130,135,136] Over the last decade, a number of series have demonstrated increasing safety of partial hepatectomy in cirrhotic patients. The mortality at most major centers treating HCC has been reduced to the 5% level.[125,135,138,139] This is because of improvements in patient selection, perioperative support, and surgical technique.

Patient selection for surgery depends first and foremost on hepatic function. As discussed above, the most commonly used clinical selection criteria for patient's fitness for surgery relies on the Pugh-Child's score. Few surgeons are willing to perform hepatic resection for patients with Child's C liver status. Most surgeons will only consider resection for patients with Child's A liver functional reserve, and the best Child's B patients.

The major changes in operative conduct that has improved perioperative outcome include willingness to use inflow occlusion during resection, as well as willingness to accept nonanatomic resection. Temporary occlusion of the hepatic artery and portal vein during liver resection by clamping the gastrohepatic ligament has been a useful technique for reducing blood loss during hepatectomy for patients with no cirrhosis.[140] In the past, surgeons have been reluctant to use such inflow occlusion, called the Pringle Maneuver, in cirrhotic patients because of fears that cirrhotic parenchyma will not tolerate the transient ischemia. Recent studies have indicated that the reluctance to use this

TABLE 29–6. SURVIVAL RATES AFTER LIVER RESECTION FOR HCC

Author / Year	*n*	Survival 1-yr (%)	Survival 2-yr (%)	Survival 5-yr (%)	Survival 10-yr (%)	Comments
Kanematsu, et al. 1984[135]	37	80	60	33	—	Limited resection
Okuda, et al. 1984[248]	98	62	43	—	—	—
Hsu, et al. 1985[249]	49	96	91	—	—	HCC <5 cm
Lee, et al. 1986[250]	109	84	72	—	—	—
Nagao, et al. 1987[137]	94	58	—	20	—	—
Kanematsu, et al. 1988[251]	107	83	—	26	—	—
Franco, et al. 1990[252]	72	68	55	—	—	100% cirrhosis
Yamanaka, et al. 1990[253]	295	76	—	31	—	—
The LCSG of Japan 1990[254]	2,174	67	—	29	—	—
Ringe, et al. 1991[255]	131	68	54	36	—	—
Sasaki, et al. 1992[256]	186	—	—	44	—	Cirrhosis
	57	—	—	68	—	Noncirrhotic
Nagasue, et al. 1993[133]	229	80	—	26	19	—
Ouchi, et al. 1993[257]	47	89	—	43	—	—
Takenaka, et al. 1994[258]	229	89	—	76	—	<70 yr old
	39	87	—	52	—	>70 yr old
Suenaga, et al. 1994[259]	134	100	—	68	—	—
Bismuth, et al. 1995[260]	68	74	—	40	26	Noncirrhotic
Lai, et al. 1995[261]	343	60	—	24	—	1987–1991
Vauthey, et al. 1995[126]	106	—	—	41	—	—
Takenaka, et al. 1996[262]	280	88	—	50	—	—
Nadig, et al. 1997[263]	71	—	—	20	—	—
Fong, et al. 1999[125]	154	80	—	39	—	67% cirrhosis

technique is largely unfounded, and that cirrhotic liver can tolerate a Pringle maneuver for well over 30 minutes.[141,142] The most important change in operative technique, however, is a willingness to use limited, nonanatomic resections. For patients without cirrhosis, most major centers adhere to the anatomic boundaries of the various segments during liver resection for cancer. Lobectomies, sectorectomies, and segmentectomies are preferred over wedge and other nonanatomic resection because limited resections are more likely to result in a positive microscopic margin.[143] In the cirrhotic liver, however, a smaller resection margin is acceptable if it will reduce the chance of postoperative liver failure. The smallest resection that will remove all gross tumors is generally used at most centers.

As safety of resections has improved, increasingly large experiences in treatment of HCC provide long-term results that allow for the analysis of prognostic factors. Many factors that in years past were thought to be contraindications to surgical resection have not been substantiated by data. It is now clear that multiple lesions do not preclude surgical resection,[130,144] with 5-year survival in patients resected of multiple tumors expected to be between 24%[126] and 28%.[130] Presentation with intraductal tumor and obstructive jaundice does not preclude long-term survival after surgical resection. Therefore, it is very important in a patient who presents with HCC and jaundice to distinguish biliary obstruction from hepatic insufficiency as the cause for the jaundice. Synchronous direct invasion of adjacent organs such as the diaphragm by HCC is also not an absolute contraindication to resectional surgery.[145,146]

One group that has particularly poor prognosis is the patient with major intravascular extension of tumor (Fig 29–4). Even though tumor thrombus can be treated with liver resection and thrombus extraction, the risks of disseminated disease is extremely high in these patients.[147] If the tumor thrombus involves the vena cava or main portal vein, liver resections accompanied by venous tumor thrombectomies are unlikely to yield long-term survival.

Neo-Adjuvant Treatment of Tumors

Many groups have attempted to treat HCC with local or systemic therapies prior to attempts at surgical resection. The rationale for such neo-adjuvant therapies is that (1) large primary tumors may be sufficiently reduced in bulk to make resection safer, and (2) local and systemic microscopic disease may be reduced or eradicated and improve long-term outcome. In this regard, methods that have been employed to achieve these goals include transarterial chemoemboliza-

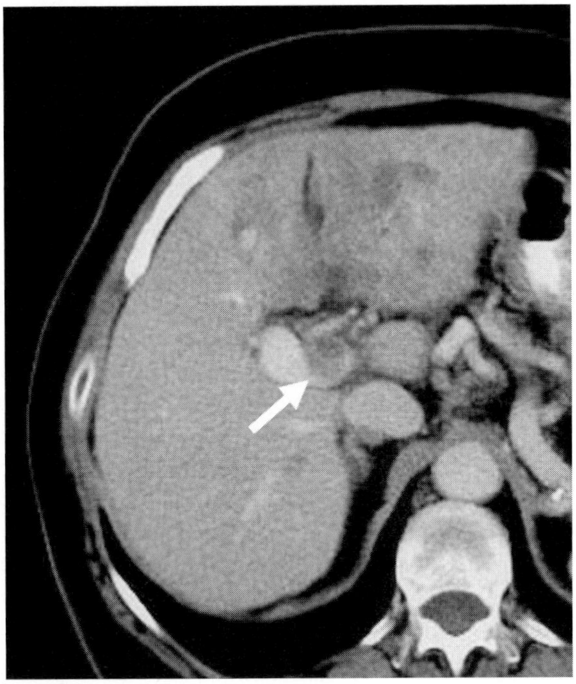

Figure 29–4. Vascular invasion of HCC. These tumors have propensity for intravascular extension. Note the tumor thrombus in the portal vein (*arrow*).

tion,[148,149] combined chemotherapy (doxorubicin and 5-fluorouracil) and radiation therapy (2,100 cGy), a combination of hepatic artery ligation, hepatic artery infusion of chemotherapeutic agents, radioimmunotherapy, and fractionated regional radiotherapy,[150] and transarterial yttrium 90 microspheres.[151]

In a French study, radiolabeled lipiodol with iodine 131 was given intra-arterially for two preoperative treatments. Fifty percent of patients developed stable disease. After surgery, pathology showed eight cases with complete tumor necrosis (23%). Survival at 1, 2, and 3 years was 82%, 70%, and 61%, and disease-free survival at 2 years was 62%. Another form of preoperative treatment is immuno-embolization. Neoadjuvant transarterial immmuno-embolization was also tested with OK-432, a Streptococcus preparation. In a comparison of 22 patients who underwent transarterial immmuno-embolization versus transarterial embolization alone, the 1- and 2-year disease-free survivals after resection were 85% and 85% for transarterial immmuno-embolization and 62% and 56% for transarterial embolization[152,153] randomized 91 patients with HCC to resection alone or with neo-adjuvant chemoembolization/immunotherapy. Two patients out of 20 had complete necrosis of tumor prior to surgery from preoperative therapy. The chemotherapy was mitomycin-C, carboplatin, farmorubicin, FU, and LV. Lipiodol was mixed with immukin and proleukin. Overall survival was 18 months for resection alone and 36 months for the group receiving chemoembolization.

There has also been promising data from neo-adjuvant use of a combination of systemic chemoimmunotherapy consisting of cisplatin, 5-fluorouracil, adriamycin, and interferon α.[154] In a regimen modified from that initially suggested by Patt, Lau and Leung[155] were able to produce objective response in tumors thought not to be resectable, and converted one quarter of these tumors to resectability.[154] Whether preoperative use of this regimen by Lau and Leung would help select the patients most favorably treated with resection, and continuing such chemotherapy as adjuvant therapy after resection will improve long-term outcome, awaits prospective studies. Overall, though, each of these studies consisted of only a few patients, and though such neo-adjuvant therapy seems promising, a definitive role for any of these treatments in the neo-adjuvant setting has not been demonstrated.

An alterative neo-adjuvant approach that attempts to improve outcome of resections involves embolization of the portal vein nourishing the side of liver to be removed. Compensatory pre-operative hypertrophy of the side of the liver not involved by the tumor will ensue, and potentially allows a safer hepatic resection.[156] Whether such theoretical advantage is sustained by clinical data awaits prospective randomized trials.

Adjuvant Therapy

Though up to one third of patients can expect to remain disease free long-term after hepatectomy for HCC, the majority will recur indicating the presence of microscopic residual disease at the time of liver resection.[157–159] This explains the keen interest in developing adjuvant therapy directed at microscopic residual disease.

In a study from China, 61 patients with resected HCC were randomized to no further therapy or postoperative hepatic infusion of lipiodol and cisplatin with systemic epirubicin. The treated group seemed to have a higher extrahepatic recurrence and a worse outcome.[160] Another study of 57 patients with resected HCC randomized to hepatic arterial infusional and systemic epirubicin versus no further treatment again demonstrated no difference in overall and disease-free survival.[161]

Though transarterial chemo-embolization is used extensively for the treatment of unresectable disease, randomized studies have not supported the use of this modality in the adjuvant setting. In fact, three different studies have demonstrated worse survival for those treated after resection with chemoembolization.[162–164] To date, no study has demonstrated any systemic chemotherapy or immunotherapy to improve survival after hepatectomy for HCC.

There have been two positive randomized trials of adjuvant therapy after resection for HCC. The first involves the use of the retinoid-derivative polyprenoic acid, which had been shown to inhibit hepatocarcinogenesis in rodents.[165] In a study randomizing patients after curative resection or percutaneous ethanol injection for HCC to polyprenoic acid or placebo, significantly higher numbers of patients receiving placebo developed additional HCC. Currently, this compound is not available in the United States, but these data encourage further study of this and other retinoid derivatives in adjuvant treatment for HCC and in chemoprevention of patients at high risk for development of HCC.

The other positive adjuvant study involved the use of radio-embolization employing transarterial delivery of ^{131}I-lipiodol. This compound has demonstrated significant activity against small HCC, but problems with dosimetry have limited its use for patients with bulky unresectable disease. In a prospective, randomized study, Lau and colleagues[166] compared 21 patients who received 50 mCi of transarterial ^{131}I-lipiodol within 6 weeks of liver resection with 22 patients receiving no adjuvant therapy. The 3-year survival rates for the treated group and the control group were 85% versus 46% respectively. These results await multicenter studies not only to confirm with bigger numbers the long-term survival results, but also the feasibility of using such radioembolization in diverse centers.

TOTAL HEPATECTOMY AND LIVER TRANSPLANTATION

From a theoretical standpoint, total hepatectomy and liver transplantation is the most attractive treatment for hepatocellular carcinoma. This treatment allows for removal of the liver cancer with the widest margin possible. It also allows for removal of diseased parenchyma that may contain microscopic metastatic disease as well as parenchyma that may be predisposed to formation of second primary tumors. A number of studies have in fact attempted to define the biologic parameters predicting good long-term outcome after liver transplantation. The best results are seen in patients with fibrolamellar histology, and in patients with small incidental tumors found unexpectedly within the explanted liver. Characteristics associated with poor long-term outcome include advanced stage, the presence of a margin involved by tumor, large tumors, multiple tumors, microscopic and/or macroscopic vascular invasion, and bilobar disease.[167,168] Patients with tumors smaller than 5 cm have a mean survival of 55 months while those with tumors larger than 5 cm have a mean survival of only 24 months.[169,170] Therefore, most transplant centers will not consider patients with tumors larger than 5 cm for transplantation. Currently, at most centers, only patients with tumors less than 5 cm, and fewer than three tumors, with no main portal vein or vena caval involvement are considered for liver transplantation.

It has been difficult to compare results of partial hepatectomy with liver transplantation for HCC. The major reason is that patients with very distinct clinical characteristics are usually selected for each treatment. Patients selected for partial hepatectomy generally have good liver function and may have tumors of enormous size. Patients selected for transplantation almost always have small tumors, but may have advanced liver failure. In the past, the reported 1-, 3- and 5-year survival rates of liver transplantation for HCC were 40–82%, 16–71% and 19.6–36% respectively (Table 29–7).

TABLE 29–7. RESULTS OF LIVER TRANSPLANTATION FOR HCC

Author / Year	*n*	Operative Mortality	Survival 1 yr (%)	Survival 3 yr (%)	Survival 5 yr (%)
O'Grady, et al. 1988[264]	50	23%	40	—	—
Ringe, et al. 1989[265]	52	15%	—	37	—
Yokoyama, et al. 1990[169]	80	13%	64	45	45
Iwatsuki, et al. 1991[266]	71	NR	—	43	—
Pichlmayr, et al. 1992[267]	87	24%	—	—	20
Haug, et al. 1992[170]	24	17%	71	42	—
Bismuth, et al. 1993[119]	60	5%	—	49	—
Romani, et al. 1994[268]	27	11%	82	71	—
Chung, et al. 1994[269]	29	14%	61	46	—
Dalgic, et al. 1994[270]	39	NR	56	32	26
Farmer, et al. 1994[271]	44	17%	71	42	—
Selby, et al. 1995[168]	105	NR	66	39	36
Pichlmayr, et al. 1995[272]	36	19%	57	31	27
Schwartz, et al. 1995[171]	57	0	72	57	—
Mazzaferro, et al. 1996[172]	48	6%	—	75% at 4 year	—

NR, not reported.

These results are very comparable to those achieved with partial hepatectomy, and indicate that long-term survival can be obtained by either treatment when patients are carefully selected.

Recently, two series of studies have encouraged a renewed comparison of these two treatment options. In a series of studies from the transplant literature, operative mortality appears to have been dramatically reduced such that it is well less than 5%.[167,171–173] With such low operative mortality, Mazzaferro and colleagues are reporting 3-year survival after transplantation of 85% for small HCC.[172] This has fueled enthusiasm for liver transplantation in this clinical setting. At the same time, a number of papers examining partial hepatectomy for HCC have been published with sufficient data in the subset of patients with small tumors to allow comparison.[125,174] It appears partial hepatectomy for patients with small tumors also results in very favorable outcomes. For a patient with a tumor that is less than 5 cm is size, the 5-year survival can be expected to be 45–57%.[125,174,175] In fact, disease-free survival can be expected in 44% of patients.[125] These results are comparable to the best results for liver transplantation. Therefore, given the organ shortage and costs of liver transplantation, partial hepatectomy should still be regarded as the curative treatment of choice. For patients without cirrhosis or with Child's A classification cirrhosis, partial hepatectomy should be considered first. Total hepatectomy with transplantation may be necessary in this group if removal of tumor requires extensive resection of nonneoplastic liver. For patients with severe liver dysfunction, total hepatectomy and transplantation is a better option and may indeed be the only viable option.

Because the incidence of recurrence of HCC after liver transplantation is high, many investigators have attempted to improve long-term results by use of adjuvant therapies. Cherqui and associates[176] used an adjuvant regimen combining neo-adjuvant chemoembolization and radiotherapy with posttransplant chemotherapy. Stone and associates[177] used a regimen of aggressive neo-adjuvant, intra-operative, and postoperative chemotherapy. Farmer and associates[178] used adjuvant chemotherapeutic regimen combining 5-fluorouracil, cisplatin, and doxorubicin. These are all small studies based upon sound understanding of HCC and represent promising approaches. All use neo-adjuvant therapy because patients often spend a considerable amount of time awaiting availability of a liver for transplantation. However, given the small number of transplants performed yearly for HCC, the role, timing, and regimens to be used is far from settled.

▪ PALLIATIVE TREATMENT MODALITIES

The majority of patients presenting with HCC will have disease not treatable by partial hepatectomy. Even if the disease is confined to the liver, the likelihood of treatment with total hepatectomy and transplantation is low because of the reasons outlined above. If the disease is nevertheless confined completely or largely to the liver, local tumor ablative therapies can be performed and result in good local control of disease. The ablative methods with the longest track record include ethanol injection, embolization, and cryotherapy. When a patient has widely disseminated disease, only systemic therapies make sense. However results of chemotherapeutic therapy or other systemic therapies for HCC have been dismal.

▪ CHOLANGIOCARCINOMA

EPIDEMIOLOGY AND ETIOLOGY

Cancers of the bile duct are uncommon tumors. Within the United States, approximately 4000 cases will be diagnosed annually.[179] Bile duct carcinoma may occur anywhere along the biliary tree and is commonly divided into distal, proximal, and intrahepatic varieties. It is a disease of the elderly, with the majority of patients diagnosed older than 65 years of age, and the peak incidence occurs in the eighth decade of life.[180] Untreated, bile duct cancers are rapidly fatal diseases, and the majority of patients will die within a year of diagnosis. Death usually results from liver failure or biliary sepsis.[179,181–183] Long-term survival is highly dependent on the effectiveness of surgical therapy. Indeed, it has been shown that location within the biliary tree has no impact on survival provided that complete resection is achieved.[184] However, it is more likely that a patient with distal bile duct cancer is resected with curative intent. This explains the relatively more favorable prognosis of distal tumors.

A number of conditions are associated with an increased incidence of cholangiocarcinomas:

Primary Sclerosing Cholangitis

In western nations, the disease most often associated with development of cholangiocarcinoma is primary sclerosing cholangitis (PSC). This is an auto-immune disease characterized by inflammation of the periductal tissues, and at advanced stages is characterized by multifocal strictures of the intrahepatic and extrahepatic bile ducts.[185–187] The majority (70–80%) of patients with PSC also have associated inflammatory bowel disease in the form of ulcerative colitis.[185] In a longitudinal study of patients with PSC, 8% of patients developed clinically apparent cholangiocarcinoma over a 5-year period.[185] This explains the high incidence (30–40%) of occult cholangiocarcinoma found in autopsy or explant specimens from patients with PSC.[185–187] Cholangiocarcinomas presenting in patients with PSC are often multifocal and not amenable to treatment by partial hepatectomy. Liver transplantation is often the only treatment possible for these patients, not only because of multifocal cancer, but also because of the baseline hepatic insufficiency from the underlying inflammatory disease.

Choledochal Cysts/Caroli's Disease

The increased risk of cholangiocarcinoma in patients with congenital cystic disease of the biliary tree is well recognized.[188,189] The reason for the malignant transformation is thought to be related to chronic inflammation and bacterial contamination within the cystic areas.[188,190–192] Early excision of the choledochal cyst significantly reduces the risk of cancer.[188,190] Fifteen percent to 20% of adult patients with unexcised choledochal cysts, or cysts previously treated with bypass, will be found to have a cholangiocarcinoma.[188,190]

Pyogenic Cholangiohepatitis and Other Hepatic Infections

In Asia, chronic infections of the liver can predispose to development of cholangiocarcinoma. Pyogenic cholangiohepatitis or oriental cholangiohepatitis results from chronic portal bacteremia and portal phlebitis, which gives rise to intrahepatic pigment stone formation. This hepatolithiasis leads to recurrent episodes of cholangitis and stricture formation.[193–196] Those that do not succumb to sepsis will have approximately a 10% chance of developing cholangiocarcinoma.[194–196] In southeast Asia, biliary parasites (*Clonorchis sinensis, Opisthorchis viverrini*) are also associated with an increased risk of cholangiocarcinoma.[187] In areas where these parasites are endemic, the incidence of cholangiocarcinoma is as high as 87 per 100,000.[197]

Environmental

Several radionuclides and chemical carcinogens, including thorium, radon, nitrosamines, dioxin and asbestos, have also been implicated in the development of cholangiocarcinomas.

PATHOLOGY AND CLASSIFICATION

Cholangiocarcinoma can arise anywhere within the biliary tree. Approximately 10% of cholangiocarcinoma cases arise within the intrahepatic bile ducts.[198–202] These usually present as hepatic masses that are first thought to be hepatocellular carcinomas, or metastatic tumor from unknown origin.

The extrahepatic variety is more common and can occur along the entire length of the bile duct from the confluence of the hepatic ducts to the ampulla. Some have classified these extrahepatic tumor into proximal (hilar), mid, and distal bile duct tumors. We agree with Nakeeb and colleagues who proposed dividing cholangiocarcinomas into intrahepatic, perihilar, and distal subgroups, thus eliminating the midduct group.[203] This segregation of extrahepatic cholangiocarcinomas into proximal and distal is much more practical. Those that are proximal to the cystic duct-common duct junction usually require a liver resection for extirpation. These represent approximately 40–60% of cases of cholangiocarcinoma and include the hilar cholangiocarcinomas or Klatskin tumors.[183,184,203–208] Those tumors distal to the cystic duct usually require pancreatectomy for treatment. Less than 10% of patients will present with multifocal or diffuse involvement of the biliary tree.[209]

Peripheral or intrahepatic cholangiocarcinoma is diagnosed in 1000 to 2000 patients in the United States annually.[210] Clinical presentation is similar to that for HCC, with the most common symptoms being right upper quadrant pain, epigastric pain, and weight loss.[198,210]

Jaundice occurs in only 24% of patients with peripheral cholangiocarcinoma compared with 71% of patients with hilar or Klatskin tumors.[210] Because the tumor is usually asymptomatic in early stages, most patients have advanced disease at presentation. On cross-sectional imaging by CT or MRI, peripheral cholangiocarcinoma is often confused with HCC or metastatic tumor from unknown primary. Unlike HCC, AFP levels will be normal. Search for alternative primary cancers that may have produced liver metastases will be unfruitful. A solitary lesion not associated with the gallbladder, in a patient with no cirrhosis and no other primary cancer, and with a normal serum AFP, should raise suspicion of a peripheral cholangiocarcinoma. Intrahepatic metastases and tumor growth along the biliary tract frequently occur, and can make it even more difficult to distinguish these tumors from metastatic disease originating from a distant site.

Lymph node involvement is also common with peripheral cholangiocarcinoma, and more so than in hilar bile duct tumors. In a series of 65 peripheral and 27 hilar cholangiocarcinomas, Nakajima and colleagues found lymph node involvement in 86% of peripheral compared with 33% of hilar tumors.[211] Intrahepatic and systemic metastases were found in 68% and 71%, respectively. The (primary) tumor, (regional lymph) node, (remote) metastases (TNM) staging of intrahepatic or peripheral cholangiocarcinoma is the same as that for HCC.

TREATMENT

Conventional surgical resection when possible is the treatment of choice. In a series of 42 patients with peripheral cholangiocarcinoma, Altaee and colleagues[212] reported that survival was indistinguishable from that of 70 patients with hilar cholangiocarcinomas. The median survival was 12 months, and no patient survived more than 42 months. Others have reported more favorable results. Chen and colleagues reported on 20 patients with peripheral cholangiocarcinoma undergoing surgery over a 10-year time period who had a median survival of 21 months.[210] Four patients lived more than 3 years, and a single patient was alive 5 years after resection. In our own report of 32 cases of resected peripheral cholangiocarcinoma, median survival was 59 months with an actuarial 5-year survival of 42%. Vascular invasion and intrahepatic satellite lesions were predictors of worse survival ($p < 0.05$).[198]

Transplantation has also been utilized for this disease, but the limited data available suggest that this approach does not offer improved survival. Penn and associates reported a 17% actuarial 5-year survival rate for 109 intrahepatic and extrahepatic cholangiocarcinoma patients transplanted at various centers throughout the world. In this series also, there was no significant difference between the recurrence rates of hilar and peripheral tumors.[213]

Data for chemotherapy or radiation in treatment of this disease is even less encouraging. Stillwagon and colleagues reported a 5% complete response and 46% partial response for the treatment of peripheral cholangiocarcinoma with a regimen of initial whole-liver irradiation to 2100 cGy in seven fractions, doxorubicin, cisplatin, and ^{131}I anti-CEA antibody.[70] Although the median survival was 14 months from diagnosis and 10 months from treatment, no patient survived more than 2 years from the onset of diagnosis.

▪ OTHER PRIMARY MALIGNANCIES OF THE LIVER

HEPATOBLASTOMA

Hepatoblastoma affects approximately 1 in 100,000 children and is the most common primary malignant liver tumor in children.[214,215] It is usually diagnosed before the age of 3 years, with a 2:1 male predominance. Patients usually present with abdominal swelling,[214,215] and are found to have an elevated serum AFP (>75% of patients). CT scans will reveal a vascular mass that is often (50%) speckled with calcifications.[216] Overall long-term survival varies between 15% and 37%.[216–219] Poor prognosis is associated with irresectable tumors, and tumors demonstrating aneuploidy and anaplastic characteristics.[217,220,221]

Complete resection is possible in 50% to 65% of children with hepatoblastoma and is associated with cure rates between 30% and 70%.[220,221] Unlike adult primary liver tumors, chemotherapy may produce response in a significant number of patients with hepatoblastomas. Preoperative chemotherapy has been used with some success in converting unresectable tumors to resectable lesions.[222,223] Adjuvant chemotherapy has also been used following resection of hepatoblastoma.[224] Evans and colleagues reported that 20% of 24 patients with hepatoblastoma were relapse-free 8 to 42 months after surgical resection coupled with adjuvant vincristine, doxorubicin, 5-FU, and cyclophosphamide.[224] Radiation therapy has been used in the treatment of unresectable hepatoblastomas, but its utility is far from proven.[222,225] Orthotopic liver transplantation should be considered in children with unresectable hepatoblastoma if the tumor does not become resectable after preoperative chemotherapy. Penn and associates reported on 18 patients undergoing liver transplantation for unresectable hepatoblastoma.[213] Though tumors recurred in six patients, five have survived disease-free for more than 2 years with actuarial survival rates of approximately 50%.

ANGIOSARCOMA

These malignant mesenchymal tumors of the liver are also referred to as hemangiosarcomas. Approximately 25 cases occur in the United States each year.[226] Peak incidence is in the sixth and seventh decades, with a predominance in males (85%).[227] Symptoms are as for any liver tumor, and are most commonly abdominal pain, abdominal swelling (usually because of liver enlargement), liver failure, nausea, anorexia, vomiting, and jaundice. These malignant tumors have been associated with exposure to thorotrast, arsenic, or vinyl chloride exposure.

Angiosarcomas are aggressive neoplasms. Partial hepatectomy can result in long-term survival, but most patients present with advanced tumors not treatable by excision. Distant metastases are found at initial presentation in half the patients. Most patients die within 6 months of diagnosis. Even with surgical excision, few patients survive more than 1 to 3 years after complete resection because of metastatic disease. Results of radiation therapy and chemotherapy or both have been disappointing.[227] The results of orthotopic liver transplantation for treatment of angiosarcoma has also been poor. Penn and his colleagues reported development of tumor recurrences in 9 of 14 transplant patients with tumors classified as either angiosarcomas or epithelioid tissue sarcomas. Two-year survival rate was

15%, with no patient surviving more than 28 months after surgery.[213]

The liver can occasionally be the primary site for rhabdomyosarcoma,[228] though this is more common in children than adults. Hepatic metastases from a GI or uterine primary need to be ruled out before the diagnosis of primary leiomyosarcoma of the liver can be made. Surgical resection is the treatment of choice for these primary hepatic sarcomas.[228] Unresectable disease can carry an unfavorable prognosis.

Undifferentiated sarcomas of the liver are very rare and usually occur in children between the ages of 6 and 15 years.[229,230] Most undifferentiated sarcomas of the liver are found at an advanced stage, when surgical resection is not possible. These patients rapidly succumb to the sarcoma, since these are usually not responsive to radiotherapy or chemotherapy.[230]

EPITHELIOID HEMANGIOENDOTHELIOMA

Epithelioid hemangioma is another malignant soft tissue tumor of endothelial cell origin.[226,228,231] Factor VII staining differentiates hemangioendothelioma from other nonvascular tumors. Unlike infantile hemangioendothelioma, which is benign, the adult variety is malignant and highly aggressive. Average age of presentation is 50 years of age. The patient usually presents with nonspecific complaints that include pain, and an abdominal mass. In contrast to angiosarcoma, there is a female predominance (63% of patients).[228] Epithelioid hemangioendothelioma has also been related to vinyl chloride exposure in some patients.[231]

Weiss and Ezinger recommended radical surgery if possible.[226] However, these tumors are almost always diffuse and multifocal, and therefore unlikely to be cured by partial hepatectomy. If this tumor is suspected, a percutaneous biopsy is performed for diagnosis. Frozen section analysis is not usually helpful at open surgery because special stains are required for diagnosis of this tumor. Patients with hemangioendotheliomas should be considered for total hepatectomy and liver transplantation. Penn reported a series of 21 patients who underwent orthotopic liver transplantation for treatment of epithelioid hemangioendotheliomas; 7 of 21 patients recurred with tumor.[213] The actuarial survival rate was 82% at 2 years and 43% at 5 years.

▪ TECHNICAL CONSIDERATIONS IN HEPATIC RESECTION

The past two decades have seen a dramatic improvement in perioperative outcome after hepatic resection. High-volume centers now routinely report operative mortality rates of less than 5%, and often as low as 2–3%.[1225,232–234] A recent review of over 1800 resections from our institution also documented a significant improvement in blood loss, transfusion requirements, and postoperative length of stay in patients undergoing hepatic resection over a 10-year time period.[234] There is no single factor responsible for this reduction in morbidity and mortality; however better patient selection, the evolution of hepatobiliary surgery as an area of specialization, improvement in anesthetic technique, and an improvement in operative technique have all contributed to these improved results.

Perhaps the single most important development in operative technique has been one that has resulted from a better appreciation of the segmental nature of hepatic anatomy. This improved understanding of anatomy has resulted in an increasing use of anatomically based resections and, more importantly, an increased use of parenchymal-sparing segmental resections. In a study from our institution, the number of hepatic segments resected was a strong predictor of outcome and, along with operative blood loss, was an independent predictor of both the morbidity and mortality of hepatic resection.[234] As the number of segments resected increased, there was an almost linear rise in the rate of complications and post-operative deaths (Fig 29–5). This study also documented a significant increase in the proportion of segmental resections performed over the last decade, resulting in a decline in the number of segments resected. Both of these factors correlated closely with the observed reduction in mortality and the overall improvement in perioperative outcome.

Data from this and other studies suggest that measures aimed at preserving hepatic parenchyma, without compromising the integrity of the resection, have a significant influence on operative morbidity and mortality. In selected patients, parenchymal sparing segmental resections offer the same benefit as more extensive lobar

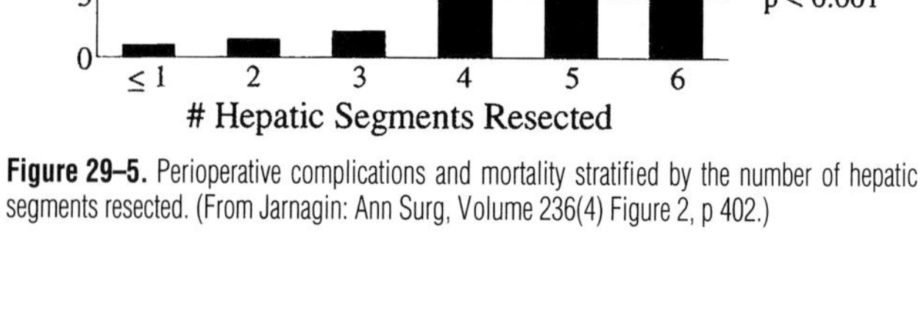

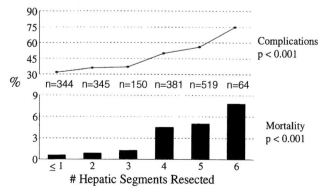

Figure 29–5. Perioperative complications and mortality stratified by the number of hepatic segments resected. (From Jarnagin: Ann Surg, Volume 236(4) Figure 2, p 402.)

resections with less risk. The use of segmental resections allows a complete but less extensive resection to be performed in patients with limited disease and allows for greater flexibility in those with more extensive disease or decreased hepatic functional reserve. Additionally, anatomically based segmental resections have been shown to be superior to nonanatomical wedge resections with respect to blood loss and tumor clearance.[235–237]

For major hepatic resections, we generally first achieve control of the vascular inflow. Several different techniques for vascular inflow control during hepatic lobectomy have been described.[238] In the 1950s, the technique of extrahepatic portal dissection and transection, prior to parenchymal division, became a common practice.[239] This technique consists of individual dissection and ligation of the ipsilateral hepatic artery and portal vein within the hilus of the liver. This extrahepatic technique is still commonly employed today, with division of the inflow being performed with the use of either stapling devices or suture ligation.[240,241] Some have noted, however, that this extrahepatic method for inflow control is time consuming, and in the setting of variant anatomy may result in inadvertent injury to aberrant vascular or biliary structures.[236]

The technique of intrahepatic vascular inflow control was first reported by Couinaud and Launois.[238,242,243] This technique is based on the anatomical finding that the structures of the portal triad enter the liver together as a pedicle, and carry Glisson's capsule with them into the hepatic parenchyma. Thus, within the liver all three structures of the porta are contained within a very strong and well-formed sheath (pedicle), which can be isolated and divided "en masse" within the liver. Outside of the liver no well-characterized sheath exists, and therefore the structures are isolated and divided individually. The technique of pedicle ligation is ideally suited for right-sided tumors that are situated away from the hilus and require a right hepatectomy. For tumors close to the hilus, pedicle ligation may compromise the resection margin and is therefore inappropriate. For major left hepatectomies, pedicle ligation may be used, but extrahepatic control is typically employed because the longer extrahepatic course of the portal triad allows for relatively easy extrahepatic dissection.

Two different methods have been reported for intrahepatic ligation of the portal pedicle during hepatic lobectomy.[242,243] These methods differ with respect to the direction from which the pedicle is approached, and the sequence for division of the parenchyma and the pedicle. In the posterior approach (or hepatotomy method), hepatotomies are created both anterior and posterior to the hilum on the side of resection (Fig 29–6). A clamp or other instrument is then used to isolate the pedicle sheath, and the pedicle is then transected with a vascular stapler prior to division of the hepatic parenchyma (Fig 29–7). In the anterior approach (or transection method), the hepatic parenchyma is initially divided along the line of the main hepatic fissure under Pringle control until the pedicle is identified. Once the pedicle has been identified, the pedicle is isolated from within the liver and divided. Regardless of approach, both techniques obviate the need for extrahepatic dissection within the hilus of the liver.

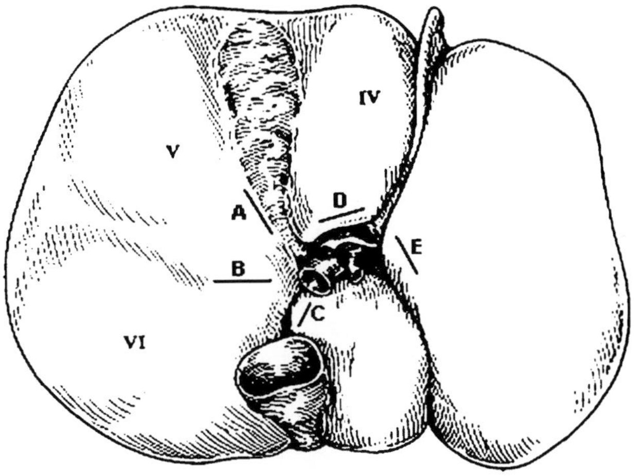

Figure 29–6. Hepatotomy placement for pedicle ligation. Right hepatectomy: A and C. Right anterior sectorectomy: A and B. Right posterior sectorectomy: B and C. Left hepatectomy: D and E.

With either approach, the technique of pedicle ligation for a right hepatectomy first involves mobilization of the right liver off the vena cava. Initial division of the lower most retrohepatic veins draining the caudate process is essential. Failure to do this can result in tearing of these veins during isolation of the pedicle.[244] Once the liver has been mobilized, the gallbladder is removed and the hilar plate lowered. A hepatotomy is then created anterior to the hilum, extending from the right side of the gallbladder fossa. A second parallel incision is made in the caudate process just posterior to the hilum. The hepatic parenchyma is then further dissected and a finger or clamp is passed to connect the two hepatotomies and encircle the portal pedicle with a tape or vessel loop. With traction, the right and left main pedicles can be exteriorized. After confirming adequate and appropriate isolation with clamping, the pedicle can then be divided with either an Endo GIA or TA-stapler.[236] This technique may also be used for sublobar segmental resections, since with further dissection of the hepatic parenchyma after initial isolation of the main pedicle, pedicle branches to individual segments can be isolated (Fig 29–7).

Once inflow control has been achieved, control of the hepatic venous outflow is then sought, which again can be achieved intrahepatically during parenchymal transec-

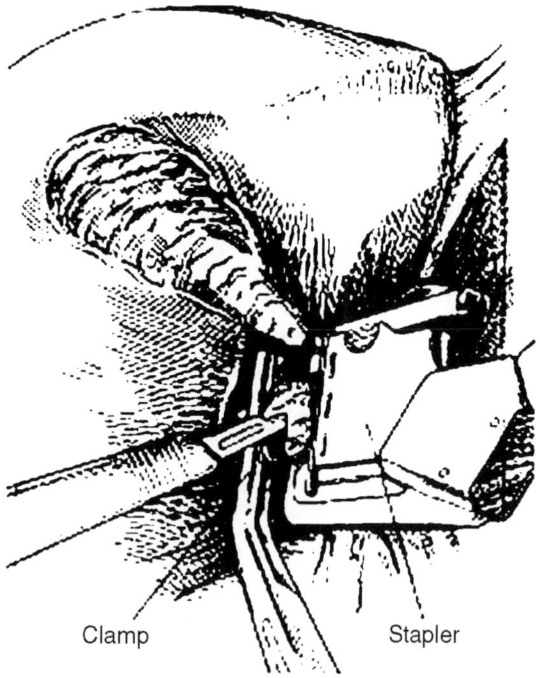

Figure 29–7. Placement of stapling device after isolation of the right portal pedicle.

tion, or outside of the liver. In general, we prefer to obtain extrahepatic control except for bulky tumors that involve the junction of the hepatic vein with the inferior vena cava, in which case hepatic vascular isolation may be appropriate. In almost all cases with good control of central venous pressure, as well as with careful dissection of the major veins, extrahepatic control can be achieved.

Once the vascular inflow and outflow have been controlled, the liver parenchyma may be transected with any variety of techniques or instruments. Our preferred approach is to crush the parenchyma with a clamp to expose the intrahepatic bile ducts and vessels, which are then ligated and divided. Over the past decade a number of devices have been described which can be used to transect the hepatic parenchyma. The ultrasonic dissector, water-jet dissector, harmonic scalpel, stapling devices, and most recently radiofrequency coagulators have all been used for parenchymal transection. The majority of reports regarding the use of these instruments are descriptive, and little data exist to suggest that one technique is better than another with respect to intraoperative blood loss.[31,236,245–247] In the setting of cirrhosis the crushing technique for parenchymal transection is probably not ideal, since the liver tissue tends to fracture and small vascular or biliary structures are more easily torn. In this situation, the use of noncrushing instruments such as the harmonic scalpel, which simultaneously coapt and coagulate may be beneficial.

REFERENCES

1. Karhunen PJ. Benign hepatic tumours and tumour like conditions in men. *J Clin Pathol* 1986;39(2):183–188
2. Ishak KG, Rabin L. Benign tumors of the liver. *Med Clin North Am* 1975;59(4):995–1013
3. Weimann A, Ringe B, Klempnauer J, et al. Benign liver tumors: differential diagnosis and indications for surgery. *World J Surg* 1997;21(9):983–890
4. Whitney WS, Herfkens RJ, Jeffrey RB, et al. Dynamic breath-hold multiplanar spoiled gradient-recalled MR imaging with gadolinium enhancement for differentiating hepatic hemangiomas from malignancies at 1.5 T. *Radiology* 1993;189(3):863–870
5. Soyer P, Gueye C, Somveille E, et al. MR diagnosis of hepatic metastases from neuroendocrine tumors versus hemangiomas: relative merits of dynamic gadolinium chelate-enhanced gradient-recalled echo and unenhanced spin-echo images. *AJR Am J Roentgenol* 1995; 165(6):1407–1413
6. Mitchell DG, Saini S, Weinreb J, et al. Hepatic metastases and cavernous hemangiomas: distinction with standard- and triple-dose gadoteridol-enhanced MR imaging. *Radiology* 1994;193(1):49–57
7. Abdelli N, Bouche O, Thiefin G, et al. Subcutaneous seeding on the tract of percutaneous cytologic puncture with a fine needle of a hepatic metastasis from colonic adenocarcinoma. *Gastroenterol Clin Biol* 1994;18(6–7):652–656
8. Vergara V, Garripoli A, Marucci MM, et al. Colon cancer seeding after percutaneous fine needle aspiration of liver metastasis. *J Hepatol* 1993;18(3):276–278
9. Charny CK, Jarnagin WR, Schwartz LH, et al. Management of 155 patients with benign liver tumours. *Br J Surg* 2001;88(6):808–813
10. Descottes B, Glineur D, Lachachi F, et al. Laparoscopic liver resection of benign liver tumors. *Surg Endosc* 2003; 17(1):23–30
11. Rogula T, Gagner M. Current status of the laparoscopic approach to liver resection. *J Long Term Eff Med Implants* 2004;14(1):23–31
12. Metry DW, Hawrot A, Altman C, et al. Association of solitary, segmental hemangiomas of the skin with visceral hemangiomatosis. *Arch Dermatol* 2004;140(5):591–596
13. Gemer O, Moscovici O, Ben Horin CL, et al. Oral contraceptives and liver hemangioma: a case-control study. *Acta Obstet Gynecol Scand* 2004;83(12):1199–1201
14. Reddy KR, Kligerman S, Levi J, et al. Benign and solid tumors of the liver: relationship to sex, age, size of tumors, and outcome. *Am Surg* 2001;67(2):173–178
15. Yoon SS, Charny CK, Fong Y, et al. Diagnosis, management, and outcomes of 115 patients with hepatic hemangioma. *J Am Coll Surg* 2003;197(3):392–402
16. Zimmermann A, Baer HU. Fibrous tumor-liver interface in large hepatic neoplasms: its significance for tumor resection and enucleation. *Liver Transpl Surg* 1996;2(3):192–199
17. Zimmermann A. Tumours of the liver: pathological aspects. In: Blumgart LH, (ed). *Surgery of the liver and biliary tract,* 2nd ed. Edinburgh: Churchill Livingstone; 1994:1277–1323

18. Quinn SF, Benjamin GG. Hepatic cavernous hemangiomas: simple diagnostic sign with dynamic bolus CT. *Radiology* 1992;182(2):545–548
19. Ashida C, Fishman EK, Zerhouni EA, et al. Computed tomography of hepatic cavernous hemangioma. *J Comput Assist Tomogr* 1987;11(3):455–460
20. Itai Y, Ohtomo K, Furui S, et al. Noninvasive diagnosis of small cavernous hemangioma of the liver: advantage of MRI. *AJR Am J Roentgenol* 1985;145(6):1195–1199
21. Tsai CC, Yen TC, Tzen KY. The value of Tc-99m red blood cell SPECT in differentiating giant cavernous hemangioma of the liver from other liver solid masses. *Clin Nucl Med* 2002;27(8):578–581
22. Hatayama K, Watanabe H, Ahmed AR, et al. Evaluation of hemangioma by positron emission tomography: role in a multimodality approach. *J Comput Assist Tomogr* 2003;27(1):70–77
23. Cappellani A, Zanghi A, Di Vita M, et al. Spontaneous rupture of a giant hemangioma of the liver. *Ann Ital Chir* 2000;71(3):379–383
24. Terkivatan T, Vrijland WW, Den Hoed PT, et al. Size of lesion is not a criterion for resection during management of giant liver haemangioma. *Br J Surg* 2002;89(10):1240–1244
25. Farges O, Daradkeh S, Bismuth H. Cavernous hemangiomas of the liver: are there any indications for resection? *World J Surg* 1995;19(1):19–24
26. Kammula US, Buell JF, Labow DM, et al. Surgical management of benign tumors of the liver. *Int J Gastrointest Cancer* 2001;30(3):141–146
27. Fioole B, Kokke M, Van Hillegersberg R, et al. Adequate symptom relief justifies hepatic resection for benign disease. *BMC Surg* 2005;5(1):7
28. Hall GW. Kasabach-Merritt syndrome: pathogenesis and management. *Br J Haematol* 2001;112(4):851–862
29. Hochwald SN, Blumgart LH. Giant hepatic hemangioma with Kasabach-Merritt syndrome: is the appropriate treatment enucleation or liver transplantation? *HPB Surg* 2000;11(6):413–419
30. Lerner SM, Hiatt JR, Salamandra J, et al. Giant cavernous liver hemangiomas: effect of operative approach on outcome. *Arch Surg* 2004;139(8):818–821
31. Baer HU, Dennison AR, Mouton W, et al. Enucleation of giant hemangiomas of the liver. Technical and pathologic aspects of a neglected procedure. *Ann Surg* 1992;216(6):673–676
32. Terminology of nodular hepatocellular lesions. International Working Party. *Hepatology* 1995;22(3):983–993
33. Nguyen BN, Flejou JF, Terris B, et al. Focal nodular hyperplasia of the liver: a comprehensive pathologic study of 305 lesions and recognition of new histologic forms. *Am J Surg Pathol* 1999;23(12):1441–1454
34. Bioulac-Sage P, Balabaud C, Wanless IR. Diagnosis of focal nodular hyperplasia: not so easy. *Am J Surg Pathol* 2001;25(10):1322–1325
35. Gibbs JF, Litwin AM, Kahlenberg MS. Contemporary management of benign liver tumors. *Surg Clin North Am* 2004;84(2):463–480
36. Hussain SM, Terkivatan T, Zondervan PE, et al. Focal nodular hyperplasia: findings at state-of-the-art MR imaging, US, CT, and pathologic analysis. *Radiographics* 2004;24(1):3–17
37. Mathieu D, Kobeiter H, Cherqui D, et al. Oral contraceptive intake in women with focal nodular hyperplasia of the liver. *Lancet* 1998;352(9141):1679–1680
38. Mortele KJ, Praet M, Van Vlierberghe H, et al. Focal nodular hyperplasia of the liver: detection and characterization with plain and dynamic-enhanced MRI. *Abdom Imaging* 2002;27(6):700–707
39. Mortele KJ, Praet M, Van Vlierberghe H, et al. CT and MR imaging findings in focal nodular hyperplasia of the liver: radiologic-pathologic correlation. *AJR Am J Roentgenol* 2000;175(3):687–692
40. Fabre A, Audet P, Vilgrain V, et al. Histologic scoring of liver biopsy in focal nodular hyperplasia with atypical presentation. *Hepatology* 2002;35(2):414–420
41. Herman P, Pugliese V, Machado MA, et al. Hepatic adenoma and focal nodular hyperplasia: differential diagnosis and treatment. *World J Surg* 2000;24(3):372–376
42. Shortell CK, Schwartz SI. Hepatic adenoma and focal nodular hyperplasia. *Surg Gynecol Obstet* 1991;173(5):426–431
43. Klatskin G. Hepatic tumors: possible relationship to use of oral contraceptives. *Gastroenterology* 1977;73(2):386–394
44. Gordon SC, Reddy KR, Livingstone AS, et al. Resolution of a contraceptive-steroid-induced hepatic adenoma with subsequent evolution into hepatocellular carcinoma. *Ann Intern Med* 1986;105(4):547–549
45. Gyorffy EJ, Bredfeldt JE, Black WC. Transformation of hepatic cell adenoma to hepatocellular carcinoma due to oral contraceptive use. *Ann Intern Med* 1989;110(6):489–490
46. Foster JH, Berman MM. The malignant transformation of liver cell adenomas. *Arch Surg* 1994;129(7):712–717
47. Foster JH, Berman MM. Solid liver tumors. *Major Probl Clin Surg* 1977;22:1–342
48. Foster JH. Primary benign solid tumors of the liver. *Am J Surg* 1977;133(4):536–541
49. Grazioli L, Federle MP, Brancatelli G, et al. Hepatic adenomas: imaging and pathologic findings. *Radiographics* 2001;21(4):877–892
50. Ichikawa T, Federle MP, Grazioli L, et al. Hepatocellular adenoma: multiphasic CT and histopathologic findings in 25 patients. *Radiology* 2000;214(3):861–868
51. Gabata T, Matsui O, Kadoya M, et al. MR imaging of hepatic adenoma. *AJR Am J Roentgenol* 1990;155(5):1009–1011
52. Arrive L, Flejou JF, Vilgrain V, et al. Hepatic adenoma: MR findings in 51 pathologically proved lesions. *Radiology* 1994;193(2):507–512
53. Trenschel GM, Schubert A, Dries V, et al. Nodular regenerative hyperplasia of the liver: case report of a 13-year-old girl and review of the literature. *Pediatr Radiol* 2000;30(1):64–68
54. Ishak KG. Hepatic lesions caused by anabolic and contraceptive steroids. *Semin Liver Dis* 1981;1(2):116–128
55. Relman DA, Falkow S, LeBoit PE, et al. The organism causing bacillary angiomatosis, peliosis hepatis, and fe-

ver and bacteremia in immunocompromised patients. *N Engl J Med* 1991;324(21):1514
56. Ferrozzi F, Tognini G, Zuccoli G, et al. Peliosis hepatis with pseudotumoral and hemorrhagic evolution: CT and MR findings. *Abdom Imaging* 2001;26(2):197–199
57. Wang SY, Ruggles S, Vade A, et al. Hepatic rupture caused by peliosis hepatis. *J Pediatr Surg* 2001;36(9): 1456–1459
58. Omori H, Asahi H, Irinoda T, et al. Peliosis hepatis during postpartum period: successful embolization of hepatic artery. *J Gastroenterol* 2004;39(2):168–171
59. Okuda K, Kojiro M. Neoplasms of the liver. In: Schiff L, Schiff ER (eds). *Diseases of the Liver,* 7th ed. Philadelphia: J.B. Lippincott Co.; 1993:1236–1296
60. Beasley RP, Hwang LY. Epidemiology of hepatocellular carcinoma. In: Vyas GH, Dienstag JL, Hoofnagle JH (eds). *Viral Hepatitis and Liver Disease.* New York: Grune & Stratton; 1984: 209–224
61. Simonetti RG. Prevalence of antibodies to hepatitis C virus in hepatocellular carcinoma. *Lancet* 1989;ii:1338–1340
62. Hasan F, Jeffers LJ, DeMedina M, et al. Hepatitis C-associated hepatocellular carcinoma. *Hepatology* 1990;12: 589–591
63. Di Bisceglie AM. Hepatitis C and hepatocellular carcinoma. *Semin Liver Dis* 1995;15:64–69
64. Forman D. Editorial Ames, the Ames test and the causes of cancer. *Br Med J* 1991;303:428–429
65. Austin H, Delzell E, Grufferman S, et al. A case-control study of hepatocellular carcinoma and the hepatitis B virus, cigarette smoking and alcohol consumption. *Cancer Research* 1986;46:962–966
66. Naccarato R, Farinati F. Hepatocellular carcinoma, alcohol and cirrhosis: facts and hypothesis. *Dig Dis Sci* 1991; 36:1137–1142
67. Nalpas B, Pol S, Theopot V, et al. Hepatocellular carcinoma in alcoholics. *Alcohol* 1995;12:117–120
68. Saunder J, Latt W. Epidemiology of alcoholic liver disease. *Bailleres Clin Gastroenterol* 1993;7:555–579
69. Schiff ER. Hepatitis C and alcohol. *Hepatology* 1997;26(3 Suppl 1):S39–S42
70. Trichopoulos D, Day NE, Kaklamani E, et al. Hepatitis B virus, tobacco smoking and ethanol consumption in the etiology of hepatocellular carcinoma. *Int J Cancer* 1987;39:45–49
71. Yu SZ. Primary prevention of hepatocellular carcinoma. *J Gastroenterol Hepatol* 1995;10:674–682
72. Leong ASY, Liew CT. Epidemiology, risk factors, etiology, premalignant lesions and carcinogenesis. In: Leong ASY, Liew CT, Lau JWY, Johnson PJ (eds). *Hepatocellular Carcinoma, Diagnosis, Investigation and Management.* London: Arnold; 1999:1–17
73. Collier NA, Bloom SR, Hodgson HJF, et al. Neurotensin secretion by fibrolamellar carcinoma of the liver. *Lancet* 1984;1:538–540
74. Craig JR. Fibrolamellar carcinoma: Clinical and pathological features. In: Okuda K, Tabor E (eds). *Liver Cancer.* New York: Churchill Livingstone; 1999:255–262.
75. Heyward W, Lanier A, McMahon B, et al. Early detection of primary hepatocellular carcinoma. *J Am Med Assoc* 1985;254:791–794
76. Johnson PJ, Leung N, Cheng P, et al. 'Hepatoma-specific' alphafetoprotein may permit preclinical diagnosis of malignant change in patients with chronic liver disease. *Br J Cancer* 1997;75:236–240
77. Lok ASF, Lai CL. Alpha-fetaprotein monitoring in Chines patients with chronic hepatitis B virus infection: role in early detection of hepatocellular carcinoma. *Hepatology* 1989;9:110–115
78. Sherman H, Hardison J. The importance of a coexistent hepatic rub and bruit. *JAMA* 1979;241:1495
79. Ihde DC, Sherlock P, Winawer SJ, et al. Clinical manifestations of hepatoma. A review of 6 years experience at a cancer hospital. *Am J Med* 1974;56:83–91
80. Lai CL, Wu PC, Chan GC, et al. Clinical features of hepatocellular carcinoma review of 211 patients in Hong Kong. *Cancer* 1988;47:2746–2755
81. Shiu W, Dewar G, Leung N, et al. Hepatocellular carcinoma in Hong Kong: clinical study on 340 cases. *Oncology* 1990;47:241–245
82. Ho J, Wu PC, Kung TM. An autopsy study of hepatocellular carcinoma in Hong Kong. *Pathology* 1981;13:409–415
83. Ng WD, Chan YT, Ho KK, Kong CK. Injection sclerotherapy for bleeding esophageal varices in cirrhotic patients with hepatocellular carcinoma. *Gastrointest Endosc* 1989;35:69–70
84. Yeo W, Sung JY, Ward SC, et al. A prospective study of upper gastrointestinal haemorrhage in patients with hepatocellular carcinoma. *Digestive Disease Sciences* 1995; 40:2516–2520
85. Dewar GA, Griffin SM, Ku KW, et al. Management of bleeding liver tumours in Hong Kong. *Br J Surg* 1991;78: 463–466
86. Chearanai O, Plengvanit U, Asavanichi C, et al. Spontaneous rupture of primary hepatoma: report of 63 cases with particular reference to the pathogenesis and rationale treatment by hepatic artery ligation. *Cancer* 1983; 51:1532–1536
87. Chen MF, Hwang TL, Jeng LB, et al. Surgical treatment for spontaneous rupture of hepatocellular carcinoma. *Surg Gynecol Obstet* 1988;167:99–102
88. Kew MC, Dos Santos HA, Sherlock S. Diagnosis of primary liver cancer of the liver. *Br Med J* 1971;4:408–411
89. Nagasue N, Inokuchi K. Spontaneous and traumatic rupture of hepatoma. *Br J Surg* 1979;66:248–250
90. Leading Article. Spontaneous rupture of the liver. *Br Med J* 1976;2:1278–1279
91. Edmondson HA, Steiner PE. Primary carcinoma of the liver: A study of 100 cases. *Cancer* 1954;7(462):503
92. Kappel DA, Miller DR. Primary hepatic carcinoma. A review of thirty seven patients. *Am J Surg* 1972;124:798–802
93. Kew MC, Geddes EW. Hepatocellular carcinoma in rural Southern African Blacks. *Medicine* 1982;61:98–108
94. Kojiro M, Kawabata K, Kawano Y, et al. Hepatocellular carcinoma presenting as intrabile duct tumor growth. A clinicopathologic study of 24 cases. *Cancer* 1982;49:2144–2147
95. Lai EC, Ng IO, Ng MM, et al. Long-term results of resection for large hepatocellular carcinoma: a multivariate analysis of clinicopathological features. *Hepatology* 1990; 11:815–858

96. Lau WY, Leung KL, Leung TW, et al. Obstructive jaundice secondary to hepatocellular carcinoma. *Surg Oncol* 1995;4:303–308
97. Lee NW, Wong KP, Siu KF, Wong J. Cholangiography in hepatocellular carcinoma with obstructive jaundice. *Clinical Radiology* 1984;35(119):123
98. Okuda K. Clinical aspects of hepatocellular carcinoma-analysis of 134 cases. In: Okuda K, Peters F (eds). *Hepatocellular Carcinoma.* New York: Wiley; 1976:387–436
99. Roslyn JJ, Kuchenbecker S, Longmire WP, et al. Floating tumor debris. A cause of intermittent biliary obstruction. *Arch Surg* 1984;119:1312–1315
100. Afroudakis A, Bhuta SM, Ranganath KA, et al. Obstructive jaundice caused by hepatocellular carcinoma. Report of three cases. *Digestive Diseases* 1978;23:609–617
101. Lau WY, Leow CK, Li AKC. A logical approach to hepatocellular carcinoma presenting with jaundice. *Ann Surg* 1997;225:281–285
102. Van Sonnenberg E, Ferucci J. Bile duct obstruction in hepatocellular carcinoma (hepatoma)-clinical and cholangiographical characteristics. Report of 6 cases and review of the literature. *Radiology* 1979;130:7–13
103. Wu CS, Wu SS, Chen PC, et al. Cholangiography of icteric type hepatoma. *Am J Gastroenterol* 1994;89:774–777
104. Kew MC, Dusheiko GM. Paraneoplastic manifestations of hepatocellular carcinoma. In: Berk PD, Chalmers TC (eds). *Frontiers Liver and Disease.* New York: Thieme-Stratton; 1981:305–319
105. Helzberg JH, McPhee MS, Zarling EJ, Lukert BP. Hepatocellular carcinoma : an unusual course with hyperthyroidism and inappropriate thyroid-stimulating hormone production. *Gastroenterology* 1985;88:181–184
106. McFrazean AJS, Yeung RRT. Further observations on hypoglycaemia in hepatocellular carcinoma. *Am J Med* 1969;47:220–235
107. Shapiro E, Bell GI, Polonsky K, et al. Tumor hypoglycemia: relationship to high molecular weight insulin-like growth factor II. *J Clin Invest* 1990;85:1672–1679
108. Lau JWY, Leow CK. Surgical management (including liver transplantation). In: Leong ASY, Leiw CT, Lau JWY, Johnson PJ (eds). *Hepatocellular Carcinoma. Diagnosis, Investigation and Management.* London: Arnold; 1999:147–172
109. Caturelli E, Bisceglia M, et al. Cytology versus microhistological diagnosis of hepatocellular carcinoma. Comparative accuracies in the same fine-needle biopsy specimen. *Dig Dis Sci* 1996;41:2326–2331
110. Voyles CR, Bowley NJ, Allison DJ, et al. Carcinoma of the proximal extrahepatic biliary tree radiologic assessment and therapeutic alternatives. *Ann Surg* 1983;197:188–194
111. Williamson BW, Blumgart LH, Mckellar NJ. Combined use of arteriography and venography in the assessment of resectability especially in hilar tumours. *Am J Surg* 1980;139:210–215
112. Lau WY, Arnold M, Leung NW, et al. Hepatic intraarterial lipiodol ultrasound guided biopsy in the management of hepatocellular carcinoma. *Surg Oncol* 1993;2: 119–124
113. Hasegawa H, Yamazaki S, Makuuchi M, et al. Hepatectomies pour hepatocarcinome sur goie cirrhotique: schemes desionnels et principes de reanimation peri-operatoir. Experience de 204 cas. *Journal de Chirurgie* 1987;124:425–431
114. Noun R, Jagot P, Farges O, et al. High preoperative serum alanine transferase levels: effect on the risk of liver resection in child grade A cirrhotic patients. *World J Surg* 1997;21:390–395
115. Lau WY, Leow CK, Li AKC. Hepatocellular carcinoma-current management and treatment. *GI Cancer* 1996;2: 35–42
116. Child CG, Turcotte JG. Surgery and portal hypertension. In: Child CG (ed). *The liver and portal hypertension.* Philadelphia: W.B. Saunders; 1964:50–62
117. Pugh RN, Murray-Lyon IM, Dawson JL, et al. Transection of the oesophagus for bleeding oesophageal varices. *Br J Surg* 1973;60:646–649
118. Franco D, Borgonovo G. Liver resection in cirrhosis of the liver. In: Blumgart LH (ed). *Surgery of the Liver and Biliary Tract,* 1st ed. Edinburgh: Churchill Livingstone; 1994:1539–1555
119. Bismuth H, Chiche L, Adam R, et al. Liver resection versus transplantation for hepatocellular carcinoma in cirrhotic patients. *Ann Surg* 1993;218(2):145–151
120. Hemming AW, Scudamore CH, Shackleton CR, et al. Indocyanine green clearance as a predictor of successful hepatic resection in cirrhotic patients. *Am J Surg* 1992; 163:515–518
121. Gill RA, Goodman MW, Golfus GR, et al. Aminopyrine breath test predicts surgical risk for patients with liver disease. *Ann Surg* 1983;198:701–704
122. Takenaka K, Kanematsu T, Fukuzawa K, et al. Can hepatic failure after surgery for hepatocellular carcinoma in cirrhotic patients be prevented? *World J Surg* 1990;14:123–127
123. Bruix J, Castells A, Bosch J, et al. Surgical resection of hepatocellular carcinoma in cirrhotic patients: prognostic value of preoperative portal pressure. *Gastroenterology* 1996;111(4):1018–1022
124. Bismuth H, Houssin D, Mazmanian G. Postoperative liver insufficiency: prevention and management. *World J Surg* 1983;7:505–510
125. Fong Y, Sun RL, Jarnagin W, Blumgart LH. An analysis of 412 cases of hepatocellular carcinoma at a Western center. *Ann Surg* 1999;229(6):790–799
126. Vauthey JN, Klimstra D, Franceschi D, et al. Hepatic resection for hepatocellular carcinoma. *Am J Surg* 1995; 169:28–35
127. Mnegchao W, Han C, Xiaohua Z, et al. Primary hepatic carcinoma resection over 18 years. *Chin Med J* 1980;93: 723–728
128. Chen MF, Hwang TL, Jeng LBB, et al. Hepatic resection in 120 patients with hepatocellular carcinoma. *Arch Surg* 1989;124:1025–1028
129. Tsuzuki T, Sugoika A, Ueda M, et al. Hepatic resection for hepatocellular carcinoma. *Surgery* 1990;107:511–520
130. Bagasue N, Kohno H, Chang YC, et al. Liver resection for hepatocellular carcinoma. *Ann Surg* 1993;217:375–384
131. Nagasue N, Yukaya H, Ogawa Y, et al. Human liver regeneration after major hepatic resection. A study of normal liver and livers with chronic hepatitis and cirrhosis. *Ann Surg* 1987;206:30–39

132. Vauthey JN, Klimstra D, Franceschi D, et al. Factors affecting long-term outcome after hepatic resection for hepatocellular carcinoma. *Am J Surg* 1995;169(January):28–35
133. Nagasue N, Kohno H, Chang YC, et al. Liver resection for hepatocellular carcinoma: results of 229 consecutive patients during 11 years. *Ann Surg* 1993;217(4):375–384
134. Tanabe G, Sakamoto M, Akazawa K, et al. Intraoperative risk factors associated with hepatic resection. *Br J Surg* 1995;82:1262–1265
135. Kanematsu T, Takenaka K, Matsumata T, et al. Limited hepatic resection effective for selected cirrhotic patients with primary liver cancer. *Ann Surg* 1984;199:51
136. Okuda K, The Liver Study Group of Japan. Primary liver cancer in Japan. *Cancer* 1980;71:19–25
137. Nagao T, Goto S, Kawano N, et al. Hepatic resection for hepatocellular carcinoma: clinical features and long-term prognosis. *Ann Surg* 1987;205:33–40
138. Capussotti L, Borgonovo G, Bouzari H,et al. Results of major hepatectomy for large primary liver cancer in patients with cirrhosis. *Br J Surg* 1994;81:427–431
139. Fuster J, Garcia-Valdecasas JC, Grande L, et al. Hepatocellular carcinoma and cirrhosis—results of surgical treatment in a European series. *Ann Surg* 1996;223(3):297–302
140. Melendez JA, Arslan V, Fischer ME, et al. Perioperative outcomes of major hepatic resections under low central venous pressure anesthesia: blood loss, blood transfusion, and the risk of postoperative renal dysfunction. *J Am Coll Surg* 1998;187(6):620–625
141. Kim YI, Nakashima K, Tada I, et al. Prolonged normothermic ischaemia of human cirrhotic liver during hepatectomy: a preliminary report. *Br J Surg* 1993;80:1566–1570
142. Man K, Fan ST, Ng IO, et al. Prospective evaluation of Pringle maneuver in hepatectomy for liver tumors by a randomized study. *Ann Surg* 1997;226(6):704–711
143. DeMatteo RP, Palese C, Jarnagin WJ, et al. Segmental resection is superior to wedge resection for colorectal liver metastases. *J Gastrointest Surg* 2000;4(2):178–184
144. Piehler JM, Crichlow RW. Primary carcinoma of the gallbladder. *Surg Gynecol Obstet* 1978;147:929–942
145. Lau WY, Leung KL, Leung TW, et al. Resection of hepatocellular carcinoma with diaphragmatic invasion. *Surg Oncol* 1995;82:264–266
146. Sitzmann JV, Abrams R. Improved survival for hepatocellular cancer with combination surgery and multimodality treatment. *Ann Surg* 1993;217:149–154
147. Yamanaka N, Okamoto E, Fujihara S, et al. Do the tumor cells of hepatocellular carcinomas dislodge into the portal venous system during hepatic resection? *Cancer* 1992;70:2263–2267
148. Fan J, Tang ZY, Yu YQ, et al. Improved survival with resection after transcatheter arterial chemoembolization (TACE) for unresectable hepatocellular carcinoma. *Dig Surg* 1998;15:674–678
149. Harada T, Matsuo K, Inoue T. Is preoperative hepatic arterial chemoembolization safe and effective for hepatocellular carcinoma? *Ann Surg* 1996;224:4–9
150. Tang ZY, Yu YQ, Zhou XD, et al. Cytoreduction and sequential resection for surgically verified unresectable hepatocellular carcinoma: evaluation with analysis of 72 patients. *World J Surg* 1995;19:784–789
151. Lau WY, Ho S, Leung TW, et al. Selective internal radiation therapy for nonresectable hepatocellular carcinoma with intraarterial infusion of 90 yttrium microspheres. *Int J Radiat Oncol Biol Phys* 1998;40:583–592
152. Lygidakis NJ, Tsiliakos S. Multidisciplinary management of hepatocellular carcinoma. *Hepatogastroenterology* 1996 Nov;43(12):1611–1619
153. Sakon M, Yoshida T, Kanai T, et al. Transcatheter Arterial Immunoembolization for Hepatocellular Carcinoma. *Proc Am Soc Clin Oncol* 1999;18:456A
154. Leung TW, Lau WY, Ho SK, et al. Final report on a phase II study of combination cisplatin, interferon alpha, doxorubicin and 5-fluorouracil for inoperable hepatocellular carcinoma. *Hepatology* 1998;28:227A
155. Patt YZ, Hoque A, Lozano R, et al. Systemic therapy with platinol, interferon a 2B, Doxorubicin and 5-fluorouracil (5-FU) (PIAF) for treatment of non-resectable hepatocellular carcinoma (HCC). *Proc Am Soc Clin Oncol* 1998;17[supp]:301A
156. Borzutzky CA, Turbiner EH. The predictive value of hepatic artery perfusion scintigraphy. *J Nucl Med* 1985;26: 1153–1156
157. Okuda K, Ohtsuki T, Obata H, et al. Natural history of hepatocellular carcinoma and prognosis in relation to treatment. *Cancer* 1985;56:918–928
158. Dewar GA, Griffin SM, Ku KW, et al. Hepatocellular carcinoma. *Ann Intern Med* 1991;108:390–401
159. Friedman M. Primary hepatocellular cancer: present results and future prospects. *Int J Radiat Oncol Biol Phys* 1983;9:1841–1850
160. Lai EC, Choi TK, Tong SW, et al. Treatment of unresectable hepatocellular carcinoma: results of a ranadomised controlled trial. *World J Surg* 1986;10:501–509
161. Carr BI, Zajko A, Bron K, et al. Phase II study of Spherex (degradable starch microspheres) injected into the hepatic artery in conjunction with doxorubicin and cisplatin in the treatment of advanced-stage hepatocellular carcinoma: interim analysis. *Semin Oncol* 1997; 24(2 Suppl 6):S6
162. Izumi R, Shimizu K, Iyobe T, et al. Postoperative adjuvant arterial infusion of lipiodol containing anticancer drugs in patients with hepatocellular carcinoma. *Hepatology* 1994;20:295–301
163. Lai EC, Lo CM, Fan ST, et al. Postoperative adjuvant chemotherapy after curative resection of hepatocellular carcinoma: A randomised controlled trial. *Arch Surg* 1998;133:183–188
164. Wu CC, Ho YZ, Ho WL, et al. Preoperative transcatheter arterial chemoembolization for resectable large hepatocellular carcinoma. A reappraisal. *Br J Surg* 1995;82:122–126
165. Muto Y, Moriwaki H, Ninomiya M, et al. Prevention of second primary tumors by an acyclic retinoid, polyprenoic acid, in patients with hepatocellular carcinoma. *N Engl J Med* 1996;334:1561–1567

166. Lau WY, Leung TW, Ho SK, et al. Adjuvant intra-arterial iodine-131-labelled lipiodol for resectable hepatocellular carcinoma: a prospective randomised trial. *Lancet* 1999;353(9155):797–801
167. Blumgart LH. Liver resection-liver and biliary tumours. In: Blumgart LH (ed). *Surgery of the Liver and Biliary Tract.* 1st ed. New York: Churchill Livingstone; 1988: 1251–1280
168. Selby R, Kadry Z, Carr B, et al. Liver transplantation for hepatocellular carcinoma. *World J Surg* 1995;19:53–58
169. Yokoyama I, Todo S, Iwatsuki S, Starzl TE. Liver transplantation in the treatment of primary liver cancer. *Hepatogastroenterology* 1990;37:188–193
170. Haug CE, Jenkins RL, Rohrer RJ, et al. Liver transplantation for primary hepatic cancer. *Transplantation* 1992; 53:376–382
171. Schwartz ME, Sung M, Mor E, et al. A multidisciplinary approach to hepatocellular carcinoma in patients with cirrhosis. *J Am Coll Surg* 1995;180:596–603
172. Mazzaferro V, Regalia E, Doci R, et al. Liver transplantation for the treatment of small hepatocellular carcinomas in patients with cirrhosis. *N Engl J Med* 1996; 334(11):693–699
173. Tan K, Rela M, Ryder S, et al. Experience of orthotopic liver transplantation and hepatic resection for hepatocellular carcinoma of less than 8 cm in patients with cirrhosis. *Br J Surg* 1995;82:253–256
174. Livraghi T, Bolondi L, Buscarini L, et al. No treatment, resection and ethanol injection in hepatocellular carcinoma: a retrospective analysis of survival in 391 patients with cirrhosis. Italian Cooperative HCC Study Group. *J Hepatol* 1995;22(5):522–526
175. Nonami T, Harada A, Kurokawa T, et al. Hepatic resection for hepatocellular carcinoma. *Am J Surg* 1997; 173(4):288–291
176. Cherqui D, Piedbois P, Pierga JY, et al. Multimodal adjuvant treatment and liver transplantation for advanced hepatocellular carcinoma. A pilot study. *Cancer* 1994;73: 2721–2726
177. Stone M, Klintmalm G, Polter D, et al. Neoadjuvant chemotherapy and liver transplantation for hepatocellular carcinoma: a pilot study in 20 patients. *Gastroenterology* 1993;104:196–202
178. Farmer DG, Rosove MH, Shaked A, et al. Current treatment modalities for hepatocellular carcinoma. *Ann Surg* 1994;219:236–247
179. Kuwayti K, Baggenstoss AH, Stauffer MH, Priestly JI. Carcinoma of the major intrahepatic and extrahepatic bile ducts exclusive of the papilla of Vater. *Surg Gynecol Obstet* 1957;104:357–366
180. Carriaga MT, Henson DE. Liver, gallbladder, extrahepatic bile ducts, and pancreas. *Cancer* 1995;75(1 Suppl): 171–190
181. Okuda K, Kubo Y, Okazaki N, et al. Clinical aspects of intrahepatic bile duct carcinoma including hilar carcinoma. A study of 57 autopsy proven cases. *Cancer* 1977; 39:232–246
182. Sako S, Seitzinger GL, Garside E. Carcinoma of the extrahepatic ducts. Review of the literature and report of six cases. *Surgery* 1957;41:416–417
183. Burke EC, Jarnagin WR, Hochwald SN, et al. Hilar Cholangiocarcinoma: patterns of spread, the importance of hepatic resection for curative operation, and a presurgical clinical staging system. *Ann Surg* 1998;228(3):385–394
184. Nagorney DM, Donohue JH, Farnell MB, et al. Outcomes after curative resections of cholangiocarcinoma. *Arch Surg* 1993;128:871–879
185. Broome U, Olsson R, Loof L, et al. Natural history and prognostic factors in 305 Swedish patients with primary sclerosing cholangitis. *Gut* 1996;38:610–615
186. Katoh H, Shinbo T, Otagiri H, et al. Character of a human cholangiocarcinoma CHGS, serially transplanted to nude mice. *Human Cell* 1988;1:101–105
187. Pitt HA, Nakeeb A, Abrams RA, et al. Perihilar cholangiocarcinoma. Postoperative radiotherapy does not improve survival. *Ann Surg* 1995;221:788–798
188. Vogt DP. Current management of cholangiocarcinoma. *Oncology* 1988;2:37–44, 54
189. Hewitt PM, Krige JE, Bornman PC, et al. Choledochal cyst in pregnancy; a therapeutic dilemma. *J Am Coll Surg* 1995;181:237–240
190. Becker CD, Glattli A, Maibach R, et al. Percutaneous palliation of malignant obstructive jaundice with the Wallstent endoprosthesis: follow-up and reintervention in patients with hilar and non-hilar obstruction. *J Vasc Inter Radiol* 1993;4:597–604
191. Jeng KS, Ohta I, Yang FS, et al. Coexisting sharp ductal angulation with intrahepatic biliary strictures in right hepatolithiasis. *Arch Surg* 1994;129:1097–1102
192. Tanaka K, Ikoma A, Hamada N, et al. Biliary tract cancer accompanied by anomalous junction of pancreaticobiliary ductal system in adults. *Am J Surg* 1998;175:218–220
193. Chu KM, Lo CM, Liu CL, Fan ST. Malignancy associated with hepatolithiasis. *Hepato-Gastroenterology* 1997;44:352–357
194. Kubo S, Kinoshita H, Hirohashi K, Hamba H. Hepatolithiasis associated with cholangiocarcinoma. *World J Surg* 1995;19:637–641
195. Meade CJ, Birke F, Metcalfe S, et al. Serum PAF-acetylhydrolase in severe renal or hepatic disease in man: relationship to circulating levels of PAF and effects of nephrectomy or transplantation. *J Lipid Mediators Cell Signaling* 1994;9:205–215
196. Winslet MC, Bramhall S, Neoptolemos JP, et al. Diffuse increase in renal uptake of technetium 99m methylene diphosphonate in association with disseminated cholangiocarcinoma. *Eur J Nucl Med* 1990;17:372–373
197. Wantanapa P. Cholangiocarcinoma in patients with opisthorchiasis. *Br J Surg* 1996;83:1062–1064
198. Harrison LE, Fong Y, Klimstra DS, et al. Surgical treatment of 32 patients with peripheral intrahepatic cholangiocarcinoma. *Br J Surg* 1998;85(8):1068–1070
199. Berdah SV, Delpero JR, Garcia S, et al. A western surgical experience of peripheral cholangiocarcinoma. *Br J Surg* 1996;83:1517–1521

200. Chu KM, Lai EC, al-Hadeedi SY, et al. Intrahepatic cholangiocarcinoma. *World J Surg* 1997;21:301–306
201. Severini A, Belloni M, Cozzi G, et al. Lymphomatous involvement of intrahepatic and extrahepatic biliary ducts. PTC and ERCP findings. *Acta Radiol Diagn* 1981; 22:159–163
202. Shimizu Y, Iwatsuki S, Herberman RB, Whiteside TL. Effects of cytokines in vitro growth of tumor-infiltrating lymphocytes obtained from human primary and metastatic liver tumors. *Cancer Immunol Immunother* 1991;32: 280–288
203. Nakeeb A, Pitt HA, Sohn TA, et al. Cholangiocarcinoma: A spectrum of intrahepatic perihilar, and distal tumors. *Ann Surg* 1996;224:463–475
204. Tompkins RK, Thomas D, Wile A, Longmire WP. Prognostic factors in bile duct carcinoma. Analysis of 96 cases. *Ann Surg* 1981;194:447–457
205. Fong Y, Blumgart LH, Lin E, et al. Outcome of treatment for distal bile duct cancer. *Br J Surg* 1996;83(12): 1712–1715
206. Haswell-Elkins MR, Sithithaworn P, Mairiang E, et al. Immune responsiveness and parasite-specific antibody levels in human hepatobiliary disease associated with Opisthorchis viverrini infection. *Clin Exp Immunol* 1991; 84:213–218
207. Kuo YC, Wu CS. Spontaneous cutaneous biliary fistula: a rare complication of cholangiocarcinoma. *J Clin Gast* 1990;12:451–453
208. Yeo CJ, Sohn TA, Lillemoe KD, et al. Six hundred fifty consecutive pancreaticoduodenectomies in the 1990s: pathology, complications and outcomes. *Ann Surg* 1997; 226:248–258
209. Saunders K, Longmire WP, Jr., Tompkins R, et al. Diffuse bile duct tumors: guidelines for management. *Am Surg* 1991;57:816–820
210. Chen MF, Jan YY, Wang CS, et al. Clinical experience in 20 hepatic resections for peripheral cholangiocarcinoma. *Cancer* 1989;64:2226–2232
211. Tong MJ, Hwang SJ. Hepatic B virus infection in Asian Countries. *Gastroenterol Clin North Am* 1994;23:523–536
212. Altaee MY, Johnson PJ, Farrant JM, Williams R. Etiologic and clinical characteristics of peripheral and hilar cholangiocarcinoma. *Cancer* 1991;68:2051–2055
213. Penn I. Hepatic transplantation for primary and metastatic cancers of the liver. *Surgery* 1991;110:726–735
214. Halpern E, Kun LE, Constine LS, et al. *Pediatric Radiation Oncology.* New York: Raven Press; 1989:280
215. Stocker JT, Ishak KG. Hepatoblastoma. In: Okuda K, Ihak KG (eds). *Neoplasms of the Liver.* New York: Springer-Verlag; 1987
216. Lack EE, Neave C, Vawter GF. Hepatoblastoma. A clinical and pathologic study of 54 cases. *Am J Surg Pathol* 1982;6(8):693–705
217. Mahour GH, Wogu GU, Siegel SE, Isaacs H. Improved survival in infants and children with primary malignant liver tumors. *Am J Surg* 1983;146(2):236–240
218. Weinberg AG, Finegold MJ. Primary hepatic tumors of childhood. *Hum Pathol* 1983;14(6):512–537
219. Schmidt D, Harms D, Lang W. Primary malignant tumors in childhood. *Virchows Archiv* 1985;407:387
220. Stevens WR, Johnson CD, Stephens DH, Nagorney DM. Fibrolamellar hepatocellular carcinoma: stage at presentation and results of aggressive surgical management. *AJR Am J Roentgenol* 1995;164:1153
221. Hata Y, Ishizu H, Ohmori K, et al. Flow cytometric analysis of the nuclear DNA content of hepatoblastoma. *Cancer* 1991;68(12):2566–2570
222. Filler RM, Ehrlich PF, Greenberg ML, Babyn PS. Preoperative chemotherapy in hepatoblastoma. *Surgery* 1991; 110(4):591–596
223. Ninane J, Perilongo G, Stalens JP, et al. Effectiveness and toxicity of cisplatin and doxorubicin (PLADO) in childhood hepatoblastoma and hepatocellular carcinoma: a SIOP pilot study. *J Med Ped Oncol* 1991;19:199
224. Evans AE, Land VJ, Newton WA, et al. Combination chemotherapy (vincristine, adriamycin, cyclophosphamide, and 5-fluorouracil) in the treatment of children with malignant hepatoma. *Cancer* 1982;50(5):821–826
225. Habrand JL, Pritchard J. Role of radiotherapy in hepatoblastoma and hepatocellular carcinoma in children and adolescents: results of a survey conducted by the SIOP Liver Tumour Study Group. *J Med Ped Oncol* 1991;19:208
226. Weiss SW, Enzinger FM. Epithelioid hemangioendothelioma: a vascular tumor often mistaken for a carcinoma. *Cancer* 1982;50(5):970–981
227. Makk L, Delmore F, Creech JL, et al. Clincial and morphological features of hepatic angiosarcoma in vinyl chloride workers. *Cancer* 1976;37:149
228. Ishak KG, Sesterhenn IA, Goodman ZD, et al. Epithelioid hemangioendothelioma of the liver: a clinicopathologic and follow-up study of 32 cases. *Hum Pathol* 1984;15(9):839–852
229. Leuschner I, Schmidt D, Harms D. Undifferentiated sarcoma of the liver in childhood: morphology, flow cytometry, and literature review. *Hum Pathol* 1990;21(1):68–76
230. Stocker JT, Ishak KG. Undifferentiated (embryonal) sarcoma of the liver. *Ann Surg* 1955;141:246
231. Shin MS, Carpenter JT, Jr., Ho KJ. Epithelioid hemangioendothelioma: CT manifestations and possible linkage to vinyl chloride exposure. *J Comput Assist Tomogr* 1991 May;15(3):505–507
232. Scheele J, Stang R, Altendorf-Hofmann A, Paul M. Resection of colorectal liver metastases. *World J Surg* 1995; 19:59–71
233. Gayowski TJ, Iwatsuki S., Madariaga JR, et al. Experience in hepatic resection for metastatic colorectal cancer: analysis of clinical and pathologic risk factors. *Surgery* 1994;116:703–711
234. Jarnagin WR, Gonen M, Fong Y, et al. Improvement in perioperative outcome after hepatic resection: analysis of 1,803 consecutive cases over the past decade. *Ann Surg* 2002;236(4):397–406
235. Billingsley KG, Jarnagin WR, Fong Y, Blumgart LH. Segment-oriented hepatic resection in the management of malignant neoplasms of the liver. *J Am Coll Surg* 1998; 187(5):471–481

236. DeMatteo RP, Fong Y, Jarnagin WR, Blumgart LH. Recent advances in hepatic resection. *Semin Surg Oncol* 2000;19(2):200–207
237. Fan ST, Lo CM, Liu CL, et al. Hepatectomy for hepatocellular carcinoma: toward zero hospital deaths. *Ann Surg* 1999;229(3):322–330
238. Couinaud CM. A simplified method for controlled left hepatectomy. *Surgery* 1985;97(3):358–361
239. Foster JH. History of liver surgery. *Arch Surg* 1991; 126(3):381–387
240. McEntee GP, Nagorney DM. Use of vascular staplers in major hepatic resections. *Br J Surg* 1991;78:40–41
241. Fong Y, Blumgart LH. Useful stapling techniques in liver surgery. *J Am Coll Surg* 1997;185(1):93–100
242. Launois B, Jamieson GG. The importance of Glisson's capsule and its sheath in the intrahepatic approach to resection of the liver. *Surg Gynecol Obstet* 1992;174(1):7–10
243. Launois B, Jamieson GG. The posterior intrahepatic approach for hepatectomy or removal of segments of the liver. *Surg Gynecol Obstet* 1992;174(2):155–158
244. Blumgart LH, Jarnagin W, Fong Y. Liver resection for benign disease and for liver and biliary tumors. In: Blumgart LH, Fong Y (eds). *Surgery of the Liver and Biliary Tract.* 3rd ed. London: WB Saunders; 2000:1639–1714
245. Yamamoto J, Kosuge T, Shimada K, et al. Repeat liver resection for recurrent colorectal liver metastases. *Am J Surg* 1999;178(4):275–281
246. Hodgson WJ, Morgan J, Byrne D, et al. Hepatic resections for primary and metastatic tumors using the ultrasonic surgical dissector. *Am J Surg* 1992;163(2):246–250
247. Rau HG, Buttler ER, Baretton G, et al. Jet-cutting supported by high frequency current: new technique for hepatic surgery. *World J Surg* 1997;21(3):254–259
248. Okuda K, Obata H, Nakajima Y, et al. Prognosis of primary hepatocellular carcinoma. *Hepatology* 1984;4:S3–S6
249. Hsu HC, Sheu JC, Lin YH, et al. Prognostic histologic features of resected small hepatocellular carcinoma (HCC) in Taiwan. A comparison with resected large HCC. *Cancer* 1985;56:672–680
250. Lee CS, Sung JL, Hwang LY, et al. Surgical treatment of 109 patients with symptomatic and asymptomatic hepatocellular carcinoma. *Surgery* 1986;99:481–490
251. Kanematsu T, Matsumata T, Takenaka K, et al. Clinical management of recurrent hepatocellular carcinoma after primary resection. *Br J Surg* 1988;75:203–206
252. Franco D, Capussotti L, Smadja C, et al. Resection of hepatocellular carcinomas: results in 72 European patients with cirrhosis. *Gastroenterology* 1990;98:733–738
253. Yamanaka N, Okamoto E, Toyosaka A, et al. Prognostic factors after hepatectomy for hepatocellular carcinoma. A univariate and multivariate analysis. *Cancer* 1990;65: 1104–1110
254. The Liver Cancer Study Group of Japan. Primary liver cancer in Japan. *Cancer* 1990;54:1747–1755
255. Ringe B, Pichlmayr R, Wittekind C, Tusch G. Surgical treatment of hepatocellular carcinoma: experience with liver resection and transplantation in 198 patients. *World J Surg* 1991;15:270–285
256. Sasaki Y, Imaoka S, Masutani S, et al. Influence of coexisting cirrhosis on long-term prognosis after surgery in patients with hepatocellular carcinoma. *Surgery* 1992; 112:515–521
257. Ouchi K, Matsubara S, Fukuhara K, et al. Recurrence of hepatocellular carcinoma in the liver remnant after hepatic resection. *Am J Surg* 1993;166:270–273
258. Takenaka K, Shimada M, Higahi H, et al. Liver resection for hepatocellular carcinoma in the elderly. *Arch Surg* 1994;129:846–850
259. Suenaga M, Sugiura H, Kokuba Y, et al. Repeated hepatic resection for recurrent hepatocellular carcinoma in eighteen cases. *Surgery* 1994;115:452–457
260. Bismuth H, Chiche L, Castaing D. Surgical treatment of hepatocellular carcinomas in noncirrhotic liver: experience with 68 liver resections. *World J Surg* 1995;19: 35–41
261. Lai EC, Fan ST, Lo CM, et al. Hepatic resection for hepatocellular carcinoma. An audit of 343 patients. *Ann Surg* 1995;221(3):291–298
262. Takenaka K, Kawahara N, Yamamoto K, et al. Results of 280 liver resections for hepatocellular carcinoma. *Arch Surg* 1996;131(1):71–76
263. Nadig DE, Wade TP, Fairchild RB, et al. Major hepatic resection. Indications and results in a national hospital system from 1988 to 1992. *Arch Surg* 1997; 132:115–119
264. O'Grady JG, Polson RJ, Rolles K, et al. Liver transplantation for malignant disease. *Ann Surg* 1988;207:373–379
265. Ringe B, Wittekind C, Bechstein WO, et al. The role of liver transplantation in hepatobiliary malignancy: a retrospective analysis of 95 patients with particular regard to tumor stage and recurrence. *Ann Surg* 1989; 209:88–98
266. Iwatsuki S, Starzl TE, Sheahan DG, et al. Hepatic resection versus transplantation for hepatocellular carcinoma. *Ann Surg* 1991;214:221–229
267. Pichlmayr R, Weimann A, Steinhoff G, Ringe B. Liver transplantation for hepatocellular carcinoma: clinical results and future aspects. *Cancer Chemother Pharmacol* 1992;21(Suppl 1):S157–S161
268. Romani F, Belli LS, Rondinara GF, et al. The role of transplantation in small hepatocellular carcinoma complicating cirrhosis of the liver. *J Am Coll Surg* 1994;178: 379–384
269. Chung SW, Toth JL, Rezieg M, et al. Liver transplantation for hepatocellular carcinoma. *Am J Surg* 1994;167: 317–321
270. Dalgic A, Mirza DF, Gunson BK, et al. Role of total hepatectomy and transplantation in hepatocellular carcinoma. *Transplant Proc* 1994;26:3564–3565
271. Farmer DG, Rosove MH, Shaked A, Busuttil RW. Treatment of hepatocellular carcinoma. *Ann Surg* 1994;219: 236–247
272. Pichlmayr R, Weimann A, Oldhafer KJ, et al. Role of liver transplantation in the treatment of unresectable liver cancer. *World J Surg* 1995;19:807–813

30

Colorectal Metastasis (Resection, Pumps, Radiofrequency Ablation, and Cryoablation)

Richard S. Swanson

Colorectal cancer (CRC) affects about 135,000 Americans per year and is the second-leading cancer killer. About half of those with CRC will develop metastases; only a percentage will have metastatic disease confined to the liver.[1] Of those with metastatic disease confined to the liver, the natural history of untreated disease demonstrates that median survival time depends on the amount of liver involved: 9–12 months for widespread liver disease, 15 months for multiple unilateral tumors, and 20 months for solitary nodules. Without treatment, only a rare patient will be alive at 5 years.[2,3] Resection allows the chance of long-term survival for a select subset. In the past, this group was limited to patients with four or fewer lesions, no extrahepatic disease, and a relatively long interval from diagnosis to the development of liver metastases. With resection, this group experienced about a 25% 5-year survival; without resection, only 2% in this group would live 5 years.[2] As will be discussed below, the indications for resection have expanded, and results have improved. Currently, about 10,000 patients per year with liver-only disease will be candidates for resection—the only treatment that offers a reasonable chance of long-term survival.[4,5] At the same time, other treatments for liver metastases have improved, such that survival times with these therapies have lengthened.

Systemic chemotherapy is the major alternative to resection for the treatment of CRC metastatic to the liver. It does not result in significant long-term (5-year) survival. In the past, systemic chemotherapy with 5-fluorouracil was associated with a 12-month median survival time—not substantially different from that achieved without treatment.[6] Recently, improvements in systemic chemotherapy have been associated with 20-month median survival times. These regimens include FOLFOX (5-fluorouracil, leucovorin, and oxaliplatin) and FOLFIRI (5-fluorouracil, leucovorin, and irinotecan).[7] Systemic chemotherapy is an option for patients with resectable CRC metastatic to the liver who decline surgery or who have significant comorbid disease that precludes resection. Systemic chemotherapy is suitable for patients with unresectable liver metastases or metastases involving the liver and other organs. An alternative or complement to systemic chemotherapy is chemotherapy given directly to the liver. This is known as *pump chemotherapy* or *hepatic arterial infusion* (HAI) *chemotherapy*. This treatment will be discussed below. CRC metastatic to the liver can be treated with hepatic arterial embolization to abolish the arterial inflow to the tumor. It results in shrinkage of the tumor, but this is usually short-lived. One study showed that chemotherapy added to the embolization resulted in the same 25% response rate as embolization alone. The survival time in this study was 9.3 months, similar to the 7- to 9-month survival times reported in other embolization studies.[8] Given the relatively short survival time associated with hepatic arterial embolization for CRC metastases to the liver, this treatment will not be discussed further. Discrete tumors in the liver can be killed with heat (radiofrequency ablation) or cold (cryoablation). These treatments will be discussed below.

▪ EVALUATION OF THE PATIENT WITH COLORECTAL CANCER METASTATIC TO THE LIVER

CRC metastatic to the liver can be detected at the time of diagnosis of the CRC or at a later date (synchronous versus metachronous detection). If it is detected intraoperatively at the time of surgery for the primary tumor, the abdomen should be evaluated thoroughly for other metastases. If no other disease is found, and if the liver lesion can be resected with negative margins and little morbidity, then a wedge resection is appropriate. If a major liver resection is required, and if this surgery had not been discussed preoperatively with the patient, then most surgeons would biopsy the liver lesion, complete the surgery for the primary tumor, and consider options for treatment of the liver disease postoperatively. In this case, a wait-and-watch approach for 3–6 months is reasonable to determine whether or not other sites of metastatic disease become obvious with this short "test of time." If after 3–6 months the patient has resectable disease in the liver, then a return to the operating room for a liver resection would be appropriate.

If CRC metastatic to the liver is detected before surgery for the primary tumor, then consideration should be given to a combined colorectal resection with liver resection. The assessment will be similar to that discussed below for patients with metachronous metastases. A partial hepatectomy can be performed safely at the time of colon resection. However, when synchronous liver metastases are discovered, many surgeons would resect the primary tumor and then wait 3–6 months as a short "test of time" to reevaluate the metastatic tumor burden prior to liver resection. One group found that those who had a delayed hepatic resection had a better outcome than those who had immediate combined resection of the liver metastases and the primary colorectal cancer. Specifically, they found that (1) no initially noted lesions became unresectable with the test of time, (2) 29% who had interval reevaluation were spared a laparotomy owing to growth of distant metastases or increased number of liver metastases, and (3) the 5-year survival rate of patients having a delayed hepatic resection was improved compared with all other patients with resectable metastases (45% versus 7%, respectively; $p = 0.02$).[9]

If metachronous liver metastases from CRC are detected, then examinations to assess extrahepatic disease and the extent of intrahepatic disease are appropriate. History, physical examination, a computed tomographic (CT) scan of the abdomen and pelvis, colonoscopy (to exclude an anastomotic recurrence or synchronous colorectal neoplasms), and a chest radiograph (CXR) are appropriate. Many would obtain a chest CT scan, although the yield is extremely small if the CXR is normal. [^{18}F]Fluoro-2-deoxy-D-glucose positron-emission tomography (FDG-PET) can detect additional tumors in 25% with CRC metastatic to the liver in patients who have standard imaging.[10] FDG-PET is being used increasingly for staging prior to planned hepatectomy. With identification of additional unresectable disease in 25% with FDG-PET, and with avoidance of hepatectomy in the 25%, one group found a presumed improved 5-year survival rate of 58% in patients who were staged with FDG-PET prior to planned hepatectomy.[11]

If the preceding examinations demonstrate potentially resectable disease in the liver, then evaluation of the liver to document the location and size of all metastases is appropriate. Usually, a high-quality CT scan will be the mainstay of the preoperative assessment of this issue. FDG-PET certainly can aid is this evaluation. If additional preoperative information about the liver is necessary, magnetic resonance imaging (MRI) can help; however, the best test to assess the extent of intrahepatic disease is intraoperative ultrasound (IUS). Several studies have examined the issue of the "best" test to detect liver metastases. A trial published in 1991 was unique in that it examined detection methods at the time of surgery and 6 months later. One-hundred and eighty-nine patients with CRC metastatic to the liver were studied. IUS was more sensitive in detecting liver tumors than surgical exploration and conventional CT scans (93% versus 66% versus 47%, respectively). Twenty-two of 104 liver metastases were detected solely by IUS in 10% of patients. During an 18-month follow-up period, liver metastases that were unrecognized at surgery were detected in 7% of patients. Accounting for the initially undiscovered metastases in the 7%, the sensitivity of IUS fell to 82%, which was significantly higher than the recalculated sensitivity for surgical exploration and CT scan (60% and 43%, respectively).[12]

Generally, up to 80% of the liver can be removed because the remaining 20% will grow. However, some data suggest that preresection chemotherapy or significant steatotosis can impair liver growth. Thus, if resection requires removal of 70% or more of the liver, it is possible that preoperative percutaneous transhepatic ipsilateral embolization of the portal vein will shrink the liver to be removed and stimulate growth in the segment that will remain (the future liver remnant). This procedure might reduce the risk of liver failure after resection. Whether this liver growth improves outcome is unclear. One randomized study examined this issue. Farges and associates randomized 55 patients who were candidates for right hepatectomy (removal of segments V, VI, VII, and VIII) to immediate surgery or preoperative right portal vein embolization (PVE) followed by resection. The mean increase in the future liver remnant 4–8 weeks after embolization was 44% for patients with normal liver function and 35% for those with chronic liver disease. After PVE, the future liver remnant grew in all the patients with normal liver function and 86% of those with chronic liver disease. The postoperative courses were similar for patients with normal liver function who did and did not have PVE; however, postoperative complications, intensive-care unit (ICU) stay, and total length of stay were decreased in patients with chronic liver disease who had PVE compared with those who did not. The investigators felt that if the liver did not grow with PVE, then major liver resection would not be safe.[13] It would be reasonable to consider PVE if 50% or more of the liver is being removed in a patient with chronic liver disease or if more than 70% of the liver is being removed in a patient with normal liver function.

If the preceding evaluation indicates that a patient has biologically and technically resectable metastases in the liver, then comorbid disease needs to be assessed carefully as it relates to the risk of surgery. Preoperative cardiopulmonary function should be evaluated thoroughly. Chronologic age is not as important as physiologic age in the prediction of risk.

▪ RESECTION

INDICATIONS

Resection of the liver for metastatic CRC is appropriate for patients with disease limited to the liver that can be resected safely with a negative margin. The number of tumor nodules that are appropriate for resection is controversial. Most surgeons feel that four or fewer nodules are reasonable for resection. Several reports suggest that there is no absolute number of lesions that contraindicate resection, but it is clear that prognosis after resection and the ability to resect safely and obtain a negative margin are inversely related to the number of nodules.[14,15] Most surgeons would not offer resection to a patient with over six nodules, but it is not uncommon to find more nodules in the specimen in the pathology laboratory than in the preoperative imaging study. One recent report focused on patients who had more than four nodules removed. In this study, patients with 9 to 20 metastases had a 14% 5-year survival rate with resection.[15] Since 5-year survival is close to zero without resection, and since the mortality rate for resection is less than 3%, many surgeons would consider liver resection if a 14% 5-year survival rate could be reached. The ideal patient has five preoperative characteristics: one nodule, size of the nodule less than 5 cm, a disease-free interval between detection of the primary and the liver disease of over 12 months, a lymph node–negative primary tumor, and a preoperative carcinoembryonic antibody (CEA) level of less than 200 ng/mL. If these five criteria are not met, prognosis will be inversely proportional to the number of criteria that are not met.[16]

ANATOMY

The division of the right and left liver is a plane through the liver from the gallbladder bed to the left side of the inferior vena cava. This plane is referred to as the *main portal fissure*, the *prinicipal plane*, or *Cantlie's line*. The middle hepatic vein is in this plane. The right hepatic artery and right portal vein supply the right liver; the corresponding vessels supply the left liver. The division of the portal vein occurs outside the liver, but the right portal vein quickly divides into anterior and posterior branches that can be injured easily during dissection. The left portal vein runs horizontally along the base of segment before it enters the umbilical fissure. There are branches from the left portal vein to the caudate lobe. The hepatic artery has variations in about 50% of patients. The most frequent variations are a replaced right hepatic artery from the superior mesenteric artery and a replaced left hepatic artery from the left gastric artery. Understanding the anatomy of these vessels is important for resection.

Couinaud has shown that there are eight segments of the liver, each with its own blood supply and bile duct drainage traveling as a triad in Glisson's sheath (Fig 30–1). Branching of the portal vein and the hepatic veins defines these segments. A right hepatectomy involves excision of Couinaud's segments V, VI, VII, and VIII. A left hepatectomy involves excision of segments II, III, and IV. Usually segment I will be removed with a left hepatectomy. A trisegmentectomy is based on the liver being divided into four segments (now referred to as *sectors*). With this terminology, the right liver is divided into an anterior segment (Couinaud's segments V and VIII) and a posterior segment (Couinaud's segments VI and VII). The left liver is divided into a lateral segment (Couinaud's segments II and III) and a medial segment (Couinaud's segment IV). The literature is somewhat confusing about the definition of a hepatectomy versus a lobectomy. For purposes of this chapter, a right and left hepatectomy will be a resection of the liver as defined by the main portal fissure. An extended right hepatectomy is a resection of Couinaud's segments IV, V, VI, VII, and VIII (also known as a *right trisegmentectomy*). An extended left hepatectomy is a resection of Couinaud's segments II,

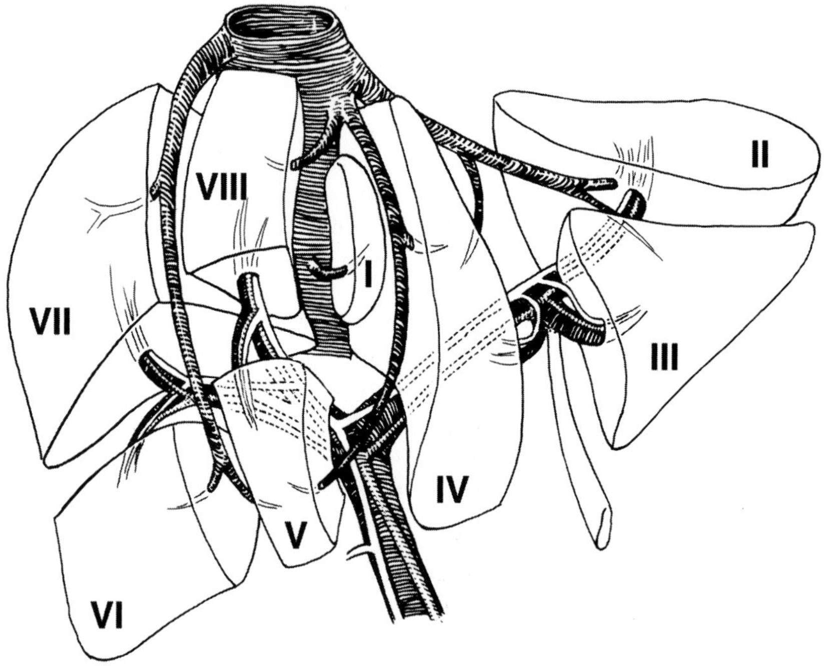

Figure 30–1. The functional division of the liver and the segments according to Couinaud's nomenclature. (Redrawn from Bismuth H: Surgical anatomy and anatomical surgery of the liver. *World J Surg* 1982;6:3.)

III, IV, V, and VIII (also called a *left trisegmentectomy*). These definitions follow the Brisbane 2000 terminology[17] and other reports in the literature[18–22]; they are summarized in Table 30–1.

The right liver is drained by a short right hepatic vein that usually can be secured outside the liver during right hepatectomy. The left hepatic vein usually joins the middle hepatic vein before entering the inferior vena cava. There commonly are about four pairs of small veins from the liver emptying directly into the inferior vena cava. There usually is a hepatocaval ligament just caudad to the right hepatic vein. This ligament frequently has small vessels in it.

Understanding the anatomy allows appropriate anatomic resection of the liver to minimize blood loss and maximize achievement of a negative margin.

TECHNIQUE

Most liver resections can be done with a right subcostal incision extended vertically in the midline to the xyphoid process. Occasionally, exposure can be improved with an extension to the left subcostal region. To improve exposure of the posterior liver at the diaphragm, an extension of the incision into the seventh intercostal space is appropriate but usually not necessary (Fig 30–2). Full exploration should exclude extrahepatic disease; suspicious lymph nodes should be biopsied. Next, the liver should be inspected and palpated. The ligamentum teres, the falciform ligament, the gastrohepatic ligament, the coronary ligament, and the triangular ligaments should be divided.

TABLE 30–1. DEFINITIONS OF LIVER RESECTION

Definition	Couinaud's Segments Removed
Right hepatectomy	V, VI, VII, VIII
Left hepatectomy	II, III, IV
Right trisegmentectomy (right lobectomy)	IV, V, VI, VII, VIII
Left trisegmentectomy	II, III, IV, V, VIII
Left lateral liver resection (left lobectomy)	II, III

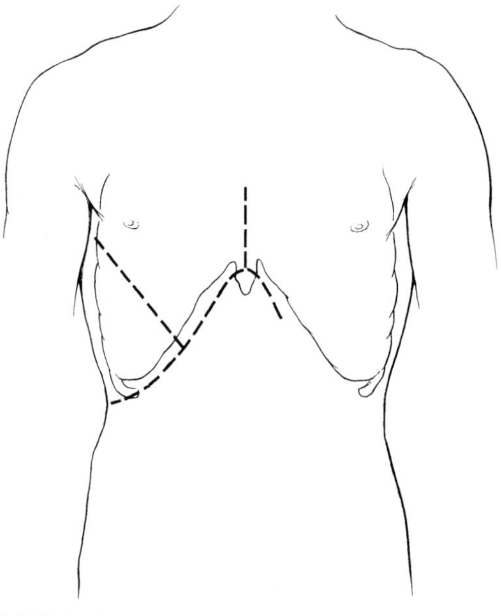

Figure 30–2. Choice of incisions for right hepatic lobectomy.

At this point, IUS should be performed to determine the size and location of all tumor nodules. IUS can help to plan the resection to maximize the chance of obtaining a negative margin. With no contraindication to resection, the appropriate resection can be performed.

Right Hepatectomy

The right side of the liver is mobilized by dividing the right triangular ligament and the anterior and posterior leaflets of the right coronary ligament. The inferior vena cava (IVC) is exposed, and small branches from the liver to the IVC are ligated and divided to facilitate exposure and avoid tearing. At this point, attention is focused on the porta hepatis for the hepatoduodenal dissection (Fig 30–3).

The gallbladder is removed, and the bile duct is traced to the liver. The hepatic artery is identified, and the right hepatic artery is isolated, usually anterior to the hepatic duct but occasionally posterior to the hepatic duct. The right hepatic artery is ligated and divided, carefully protecting the main and left hepatic arteries. The right hepatic duct is divided. At this point, the hepatic duct can be lifted anteriorly to the left to expose the portal vein. The junction of left and right portal veins is exposed cautiously, and a vessel loop is placed around the right portal vein. It is preferable to ligate and divide the right portal vein with sutures or a vascular stapler that ligates and cut, but if it bifurcates early, then simple ligation with a vascular stapler such as a TA-30 will achieve inflow control. When inflow control is achieved, the liver will quickly demarcate such that the right liver will discolor. At this point, it is reasonable to maximize outflow control.

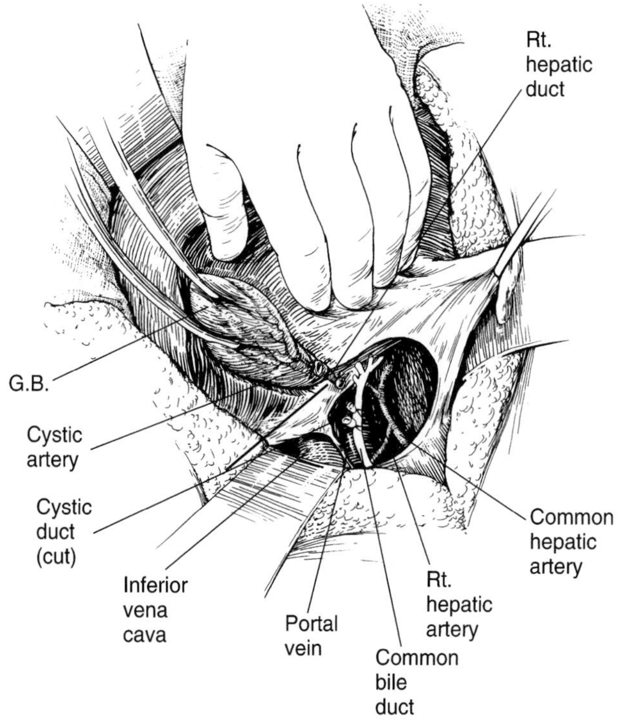

Figure 30–3. Hepatoduodenal dissection. (Redrawn from Schwartz SI. Liver resection. In: *Modern Technics in Surgery, Abdominal Surgery* 10:1. Mt. Kisco, NY: Futura; 1981.)

An alternative method to achieve inflow control is to isolate and ligate the right portal pedicle intrahepatically. This can be done by incising the capsule in segments IV and VI and placing a finger around the pedicle in the liver. IUS can monitor this technique. A vascular stapler can be applied to control the inflow.

The liver is rotated anteriorly and to the left. Small veins emptying directly from the liver into the IVC are ligated and divided (Fig 30–4A). This might require suture ligation of the veins at the IVC because these branches are quite short. The surgeon should work from caudad to cephalad to secure these branches; usually there are about four pairs. A broad fibrous band of tissue extends from the IVC to the liver just caudad to the right hepatic vein. This tissue has small veins in it or next to it. There can be a larger accessory right hepatic vein in or next to this tissue. This band needs to be divided to expose the right hepatic vein.

At this point, careful sharp and blunt dissection usually can isolate the right hepatic vein outside the liver such that it can be divided with clamps or a vascular stapler (see Fig 30–4B). If there is very little room to ligate and divide the vein, then it can be occluded by placing a vascular suture on a large needle (e.g., a 3-0 Prolene on an MH needle) around the vein. With the anterior, medial, and lateral aspects of the right hepatic vein exposed, the needle can be passed around the posterior aspect aiming to pass between the IVC and the right hepatic vein. If the needle inadvertently enters the vein, simply tying the suture should produce hemostasis.

With inflow and outflow control, the parenchyma is transected to obtain a 1-cm margin. If the central venous pressure (CVP) is kept low, then backbleeding will be minimized. To minimize the risk of air embolism when the central venous pressure is low during transection, the patient should be kept in a Trendelenberg position. There are several methods for parenchymal transection. The standard technique is "finger fracture" that requires fracturing the parenchyma with the index finger and thumb to define vessels and bile ducts. The vessels and ducts are ligated or clipped, and the liver is transected expeditiously (Fig 30–5). Variations of the finger-fracture technique use a Kelly clamp, closed scissors, or a metal suction device. The key is to use a method that works well for the surgical team such that one surgeon can do the "fracturing" while another surgeon secures the vessels. During this maneuver, bleeding can be minimized by occluding inflow at the porta hepatis as a Pringle maneuver with clamping for 10 minutes with 2 to 5 minutes of unclamping. This maneuver can be repeated until the liver has been divided. A nor-

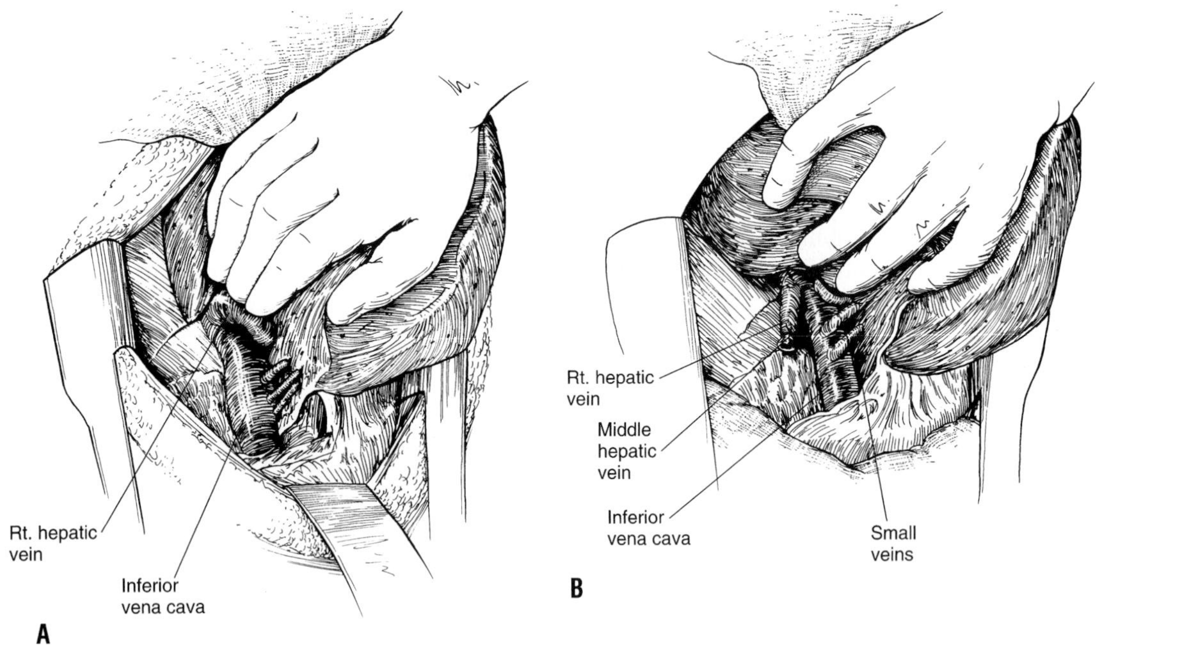

Figure 30–4. A and **B**. Retrohepatic dissection to achieve control of hepatic veins. (Redrawn from Schwartz SI. Liver resection. In: *Modern Technics in Surgery, Abdominal Surgery* 10:1. Mt. Kisco, NY: Futura; 1981.)

mal liver without steatohepatitis should tolerate 45 minutes of normothermic ischemia.

Other devices have been designed to divide the parenchyma. These include the ultrasonic dissector, the water-jet dissector, the saline-linked radiofrequency (RF) dissecting sealer, the bipolar vessel-sealing device, and the harmonic scalpel. Each device has its proponents. Some surgeons use these devices to meticulously and slowly divide the complete parenchyma of the liver. Others use these devices to divide a portion of the parenchyma; when they are deep in the parenchyma, and when the margin is not an issue, these surgeons switch to a finger fracture technique to finish the dissection. To expedite deep parenchymal division, many will use staplers—either vascular staplers or TA staplers.

The ultrasonic dissector or Cavitron ultrasonic surgical aspirator (CUSA) is the oldest of these devices. It has been used for over 25 years to fragment and aspirate hepatic parenchyma. It has no hemostatic properties, but it allows identification and control of vessels and ducts. It does not fragment fibrotic tissue or tumors. Whether it reduces blood loss depends on the skill and patience of the surgeon. One recent randomized trial using transesophageal echocardiography demonstrated that the CUSA resulted in a higher rate of venous air embolism than the finger fracture technique (100% versus 68%, respectively), although there were no differences in hemodynamics.[23] Another study showed a higher bile leak rate with no difference in blood loss for CUSA versus finger fracture.[24] A randomized, controlled trial involving 132 patients having liver resections found no difference between the ultrasonic dissector and finger fracture (or *clamp crush*) in median blood loss, transection time, and transection speed. Ultrasonic dissection was associated with an increased frequency of positive margins and postoperative morbidity.[25]

The harmonic scalpel divides the liver in a reasonably hemostatic manner such that it can be used to resect the liver laparoscopically. One retrospective review suggested that it was associated with decreased operative time and a trend toward decreased blood loss and transfusion requirements but an increase in bile leaks.[26]

The water-jet dissector was developed as another tool to clear the hepatic parenchyma and expose vessels and ducts for ligature. A prospective study involving 60 patients compared the harmonic scalpel with the water-jet dissector. The water-jet dissector was associated with a faster resection time and less blood loss than the harmonic scalpel.[27]

A bipolar vessel-sealing device has been developed for use in many areas of surgery, including liver surgery. A group in Italy used this device in 30 consecutive patients having liver surgery. A crush technique followed by application of this device was used to divide the parenchyma. The bipolar device was useful in 27 patients; 3 patients with cirrhosis did not achieve hemostasis with this device. Median blood loss was 250 mL. There was no evidence of postoperative hemorrhage, bile leak, or abscess.[28]

A saline-linked RF dissecting sealer was developed specifically for liver transection. It uses radiofrequency

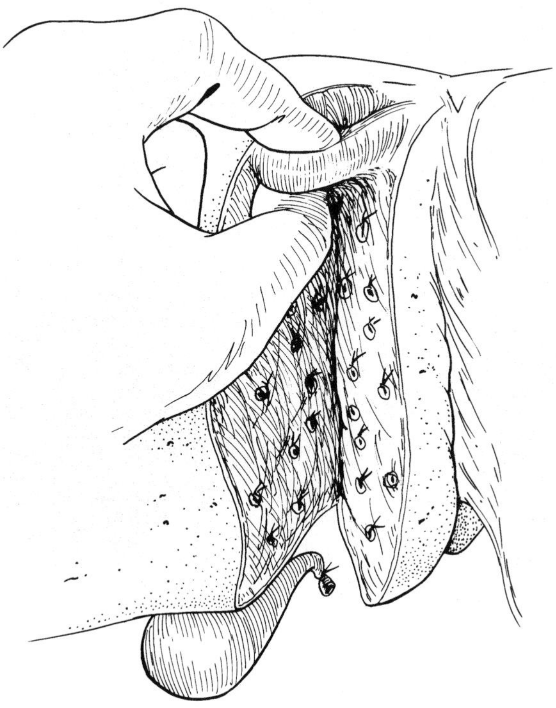

Figure 30–5. Finger fracture technique. Posterosuperior intraparenchymal dissection of the right hepatic vein.

energy to seal and divide the liver. Saline is dripped over the device to keep the tip cool and avoid coagulative necrosis. There is a considerable learning curve for this device that makes it difficult to use in a teaching hospital. The speed of transection, the rate of saline dripping, and the degree of aspiration of smoke need to be coordinated. A group in Hong Kong that normally uses a CUSA reported their results with the saline-linked RF dissecting sealer in 10 patients. Median transection time was 95 minutes; median blood loss was 100 mL (30–700 mL). Transection blood loss was 700 and 500 mL in cases of right and extended right hepatectomy, respectively. There were no blood transfusions.[29] This device and the others just described await further assessment before definitive statements about utility can be made.

Two new similar devices are under development and are being introduced for parenchymal transection using radiofrequency ablation (RFA) to ablate a plane of tissue. This ablated tissue should be hemostatic (vessels < 5 mm in diameter should be controlled with this technique), and if there are any microscopic tumor cells in this tissue, they should be killed with this device. After ablating the plane of tissue, it can be cut with a knife with little to no bleeding. These devices are particularly useful in a liver in which there are no large vessels. In areas where vessels are greater than 5 mm in diameter, the surgeon needs to use ultrasound to identify and avoid the larger vessels. A group in London used one of these RF resection devices in 15 patients to remove liver tumors. Blood loss was 30 ± 10 mL.[30] A group in Australia used a slightly different RF resection device that allows a 1-cm-thick plane of up to 6 × 6 cm of liver to be ablated per application. This in-line RF resection device was compared with the ultrasonic aspirator in eight patients. Blood loss was 6.5 mL/cm^2 with the RF resection device and 20.4 mL/cm^2 with the ultrasonic aspirator.[31] We have used the in-line RF resection device to perform two laparoscopic liver resections.[32]

After removing the right liver, the raw surface should be compressed temporarily to stop minor bleeding. The cautery, argon beam coagulator, or hemostatic agents such as fibrin glue and Surgicel can help at this point.

After resection, the surface should be examined to control bile leaks. The hepatic duct should be examined to ensure that it is intact; the stump of the right hepatic duct can be used to perform a cholangiogram or to perform cholangioscopy if there is any concern. The integrity of the left hepatic artery and the portal vein should be examined. Many surgeons close the falciform ligament to minimize the chance that the left liver will twist. Many surgeons also drain the right upper quadrant with closed suction drains, although randomized studies do not support this practice. Some surgeons drain, only if there is a concern about a bile leak from the surface of the liver.

Management after a right hepatectomy can be straightforward if blood loss is minimal, and in many cases, an ICU stay may not be necessary. Periodic hematocrit and international normalization ratio (INR) determinations should be done. Serum bilirubin might rise for a few days or 1 to 2 weeks, but with adequate hepatocellular function, it will return to normal. After removal of half the liver, drug metabolism is altered; thus the usual doses of narcotics and other drugs may result in abnormally high tissue concentrations. Glucose monitoring is important; occasionally, 10% dextrose is required for a short period because of loss of glycogen stores.

Left Hepatectomy

Left hepatectomy involves removal of segments II, III, and IV (Fig 30–6). Usually the caudate lobe is taken, depending on the location of the tumor in the left liver. The indications are for metastases in the left liver that can be removed as a left hepatectomy, achieving a negative margin. The incision, exploration, and IUS examination of the liver are similar to that in a right hepatectomy. The left triangular and coronary ligaments should be divided, and the left

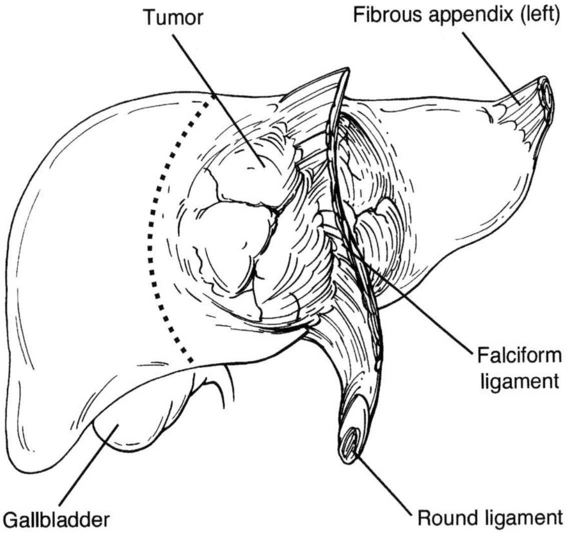

Figure 30–6. Left hepatectomy. Resection plane in left hepatectomy.

phrenic vein can be followed to the left hepatic vein. For large tumors, the right liver should be mobilized completely to expose the inferior vena cava and to take the small veins emptying directly into the IVC. This is especially important if the caudate lobe will be resected. This allows protection of the IVC during parenchymal transaction. The gastrohepatic ligament should be divided, and if present in the gastrohepatic ligament, a replaced or accessory left hepatic artery will be divided at this point.

Removal of the gallbladder facilitates dissection in the porta hepatis. The common hepatic artery is exposed. The cautery does not work well with this dissection; either ligation with fine ties or use of a device such as the harmonic scalpel is necessary. The artery is traced to expose the bifurcation of left and right hepatic arteries. This allows safe division of the left hepatic artery.

The left hepatic duct is exposed and divided at the base of segment IV, carefully protecting the right and common hepatic ducts. Vessel loops around the hepatic artery and hepatic duct allow exposure of the portal vein. The left portal vein is isolated and divided; the stump of the left portal vein is secured with vascular sutures such that it does not impinge on the right portal vein, causing stenosis (Fig 30–7).

At this point the liver will demarcate, and the parenchymal transection plane will be obvious, extending from the gallbladder fossa to the left of the IVC. If the tumor is close to the left hepatic vein, passing a vessel loop around the right hepatic vein for protection might be beneficial. The left hepatic vein can be secured outside the liver, although many surgeons do not bother with this step.

The parenchyma is divided using techniques described for right hepatectomy. The left hepatic vein is secured at the end of the parenchymal transaction with vascular clamps and sutures or the vascular stapler (Fig 30–8).

Trisegmentectomy

Trisegmentectomy can be performed by taking the right liver and the medial left liver (segments IV, V, VI, VII, and VIII) known as a *right trisegmentectomy* (or *extended right hepatectomy*) or by taking the left liver and the anterior (segments V and VIII) right liver known as a *left trisegmentectomy* (or *extended left hepatectomy*). A right trisegmentectomy, or extended right hepatectomy, removes the liver to the right of the falciform ligament or umbilical fissure. The initial exploration and dissection are similar to a right hepatectomy, taking the right hepatic artery and right portal vein and dividing the right hepatic duct. Mobilization of the liver off the IVC is similar to a right hepatectomy, and the right hepatic vein can be taken at this point. The positions of the left and middle hepatic veins should be noted to avoid injury during dissection. The left hepatic duct, the left hepatic artery, and the left portal vein are exposed and separated from segment four (Fig 30–9). The parenchymal bridge between segments III and IV is divided, usually with the cautery. Parenchymal transection should be at least 1 cm to the right of the umbilical fissure to avoid injury to the left portal vein in the base of the umbilical fissure. The portal vein branches to segment IV are multiple, coming back from the left portal vein in the umbilical fissure. The area of parenchyma to be divided will be significantly less than that of a right hepatectomy (Fig 30–10). Problems that should be avoided include (1) injury to the portal vein or hepatic arterial supply to segments II and III owing to dissection too close to the umbilical fissure, (2) injury to the left hepatic duct supplying segments II and III, and (3) injury to the left hepatic vein if the division of the middle hepatic vein is performed too close to the left hepatic vein (in most cases the middle hepatic vein empties into the left hepatic vein).

A right trisegmetaectomy removes 70–80% of the liver. Transient liver failure characterized by hyperbilirubinemia occurs often and usually improves after 1 week.

Left trisegmentectomy (or extended left hepatectomy) can be challenging because the plane of parenchymal transection is not as clear as it is for a right trisegmentectomy. This plane is at about 40 degrees when the right liver is mobilized completely (Fig 30–11). The right hepatic vein runs in this plane. IUS can help to determine the position of this plane between the anterior and posterior right liver. The initial phase of the operation is similar to a left hepatectomy in terms of exploration and division of vascular inflow to the left

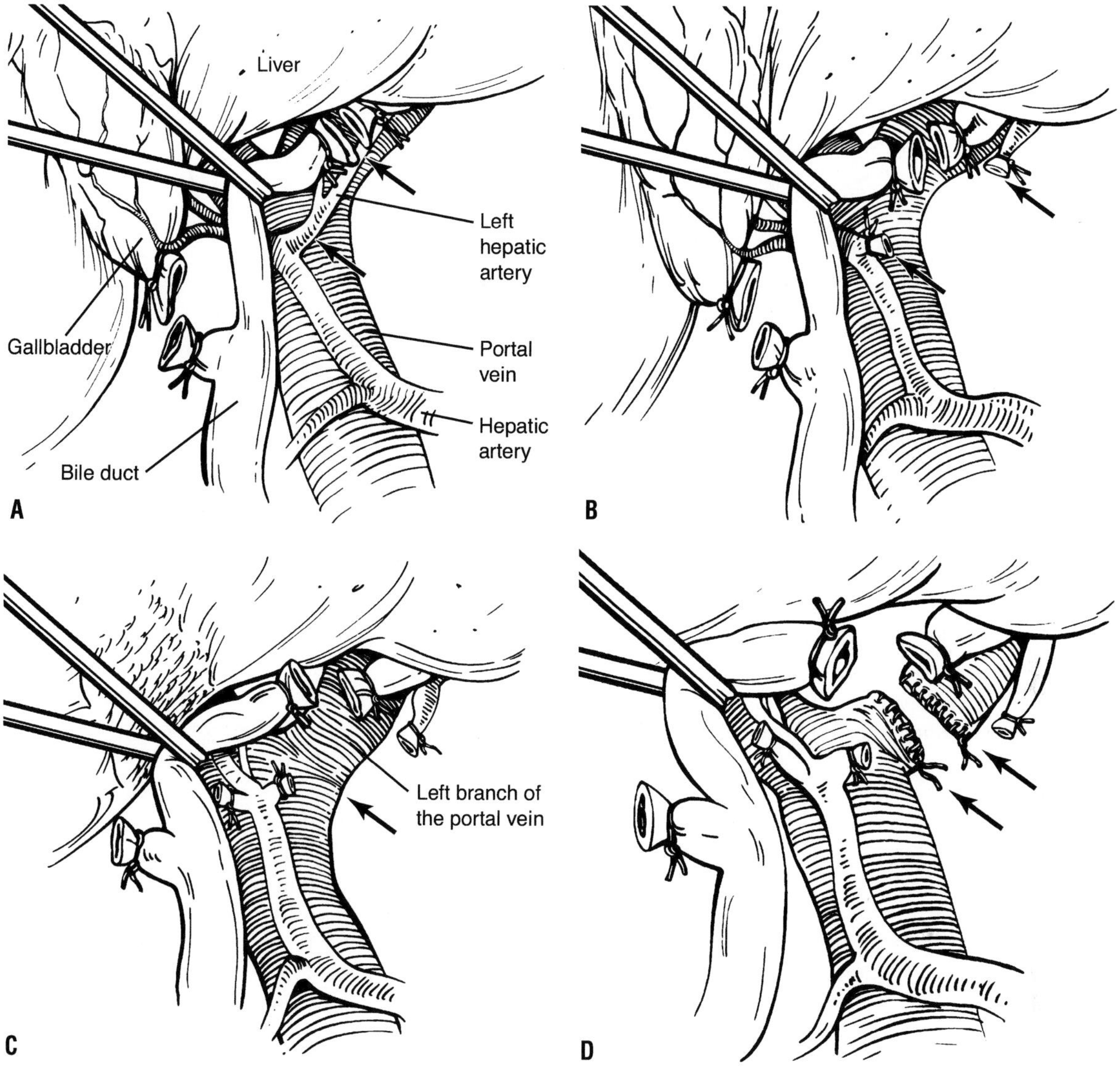

Figure 30–7. Hilar dissection in left hepatectomy.

liver. It is imperative that the liver be mobilized completely off the IVC to allow protection of the IVC during dissection. If possible, a vessel loop should be placed around the right hepatic vein. After dividing the left hepatic artery and portal vein, dissection proceeds to identify and ligate the anterior branch of the right hepatic artery. IUS can help at this point. The anterior branch of the right portal vein is identified and divided, if possible. If this branch can be identified but not divided safely, methylene blue can be injected into it to identify the portion of right liver that requires resection; IUS can help to identify this branch.

The liver parenchyma can be divided between the anterior (segments V and VIII) and the posterior (segments VI and VII) right liver. Protection of the inflow and outflow to the right posterior liver is mandatory. It will be critical to divide branches to the right hepatic vein, protecting the branches from the posterior right liver. Many surgeons will use the Pringle maneuver judiciously during parenchymal dissection to protect the vessels to and from the right posterior liver. If injury to the vessels of the right posterior liver occurs, total vascular inflow and outflow occlusion probably will be necessary to repair the injured vessel. If the hepatic duct to the right posterior liver is injured, a Roux-en-Y hepaticojejunostomy will be necessary. In most cases, the caudate lobe will be removed with the specimen.

Problems after left trisegmentectomy are similar to those after right trisegmentectomy and are related to the integrity of the inflow and outflow vessels, the integrity of the hepatic duct, bleeding from the raw surface, infection, and liver failure. Liver failure should be

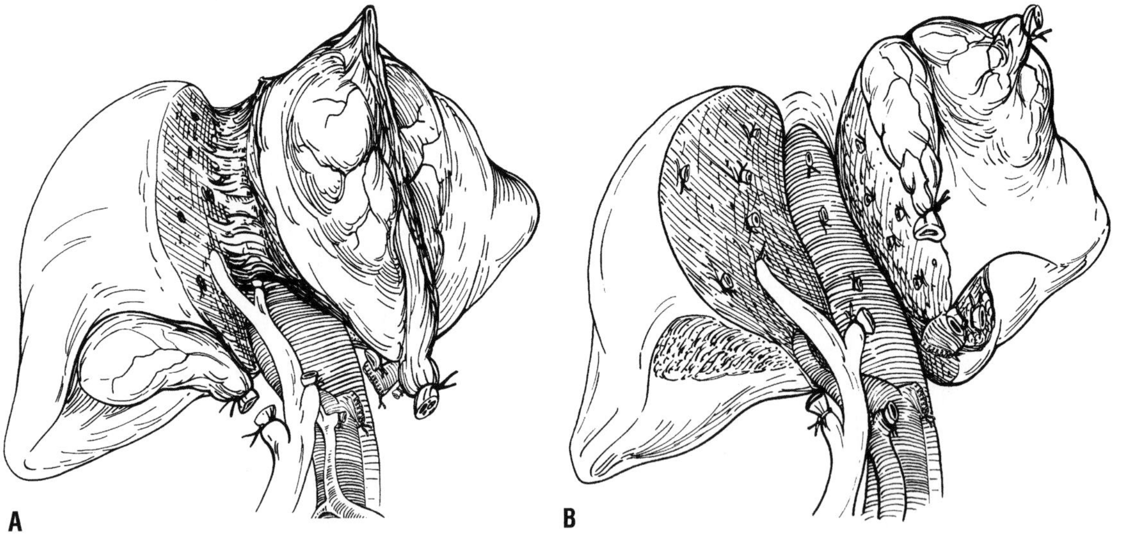

Figure 30–8. Completed transection of the parenchyma in left hepatectomy.

similar to that noted earlier for right trisegmentectomy. Of the small percentage of deaths after this procedure, liver failure is the predominant problem. It might be prevented by preoperative embolization of the portal vein of the half of the liver to be removed.

Segmentectomy

Given that each of the eight segments of the liver has its own portal triad with hepatic artery, portal vein, and bile duct and its own venous outflow, and given that no significant vessel runs through a segment, then theoretically each segment can be removed individually (Figs 30–12 and 30–13). Further, combinations of segments—such as segments IVB and V—also can be removed (Fig 30–14). As an example, if CRC metastasizes as two nodules, one in segment VI and one in segment IVB, then excising the two segments would be appropriate if a negative margin can be achieved. This approach allows the preservation of maximal liver mass that might be important in selected patients. IUS facilitates segmental resections; it can identify the pertinent blood supply to a segment, and it can determine whether or not a segmental resection will result in a negative margin. Performing a segmental resection requires mobilization and exposure of the segment in question. Using IUS, the portal vein branch in question can be identified and injected with methylene blue to outline the liver parenchyma that needs to be removed. The parenchyma of the segment can be divided using the techniques and tools noted earlier for hepatectomy. Many surgeons will use the Pringle maneuver during segment resection. Our practice is to use IUS, the harmonic scalpel, and—in selected patients—the RF resection devices discussed earlier to perform segmental resections. We use the Pringle maneuver sparingly.

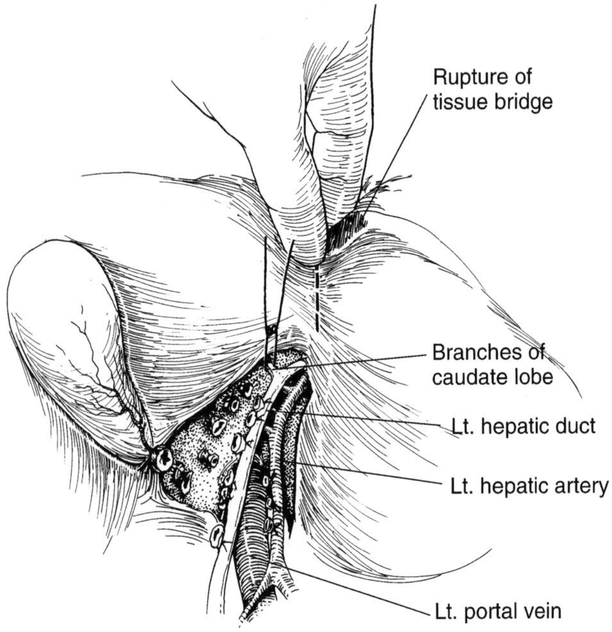

Figure 30–9. Nearly completed mobilization of the left branches of the portal triad. The tissue bridge is being broken down to permit access to the umbilical fissure. The final two branches before the main trunk reaches the umbilical fissure go to the left portion of the caudate lobe. These final branches, or at least the last one, should be preserved unless all of the caudate lobe is to be removed. Total caudate removal is not usually necessary. (Redrawn from Starzl T, Bell RH, et al. Hepatic trisegmentectomy and other liver resections. *Surg Gynecol Obstet* 1975; 141: 429. After J McC.)

RESULTS

The mortality rate of an elective liver resection for CRC metastatic to the liver should be less than 5%. Six published series with 208 to 1568 patients in each cohort demonstrate operative mortality rates of 1–4%, with slightly higher mortality rates for major versus minor liver resections.[33–38] A multi-institutional prospective

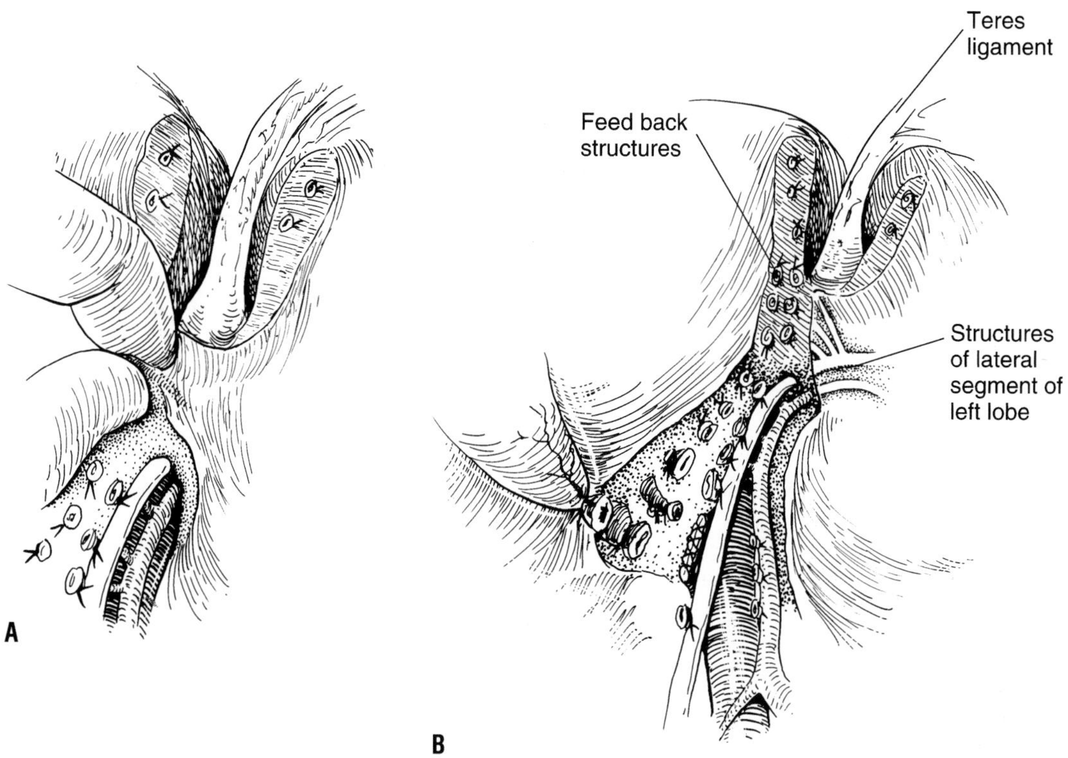

Figure 30–10. Structures feeding back from the umbilical fissure to the medial segment of the left lobe. **A.** These are encircled usually by blunt dissection within the liver substances just to the right of the falciform ligament and umbilical fissure without entering the fissure. Note that the hepatic tissue bridge concealing the umbilical fissure has been broken down. **B.** The three segments of the specimen now are devascularized. (Redrawn from Starzl T, Bell RH, et al. Hepatic trisegmentectomy and other liver resections. *Surg Gynecol Obstet* 1975; 141:429. After J McC.)

trial demonstrated a 2.7% mortality rate for attempted liver resection.[39] The morbidity for resection was addressed earlier for each technique. The rates of major morbidity range from 8–24% in the studies noted earlier.[33–39] The oncologic outcome depends on several factors. First, if the resection is associated with a positive margin, then survival will be no better than that associated with laparotomy without resection.[39] What constitutes a negative margin is open to debate. Most surgeons feel that resection to achieve a 1-cm negative margin is important.[37] Certainly, a negative margin greater than 1 mm is important.[33,37] Outcome with a margin between 1 and 10 mm is better than with a positive margin.[33,36,37] There is no obvious difference in outcome with 1- to 4-mm margins versus 5- to 9-mm margins.[33] Second, with a margin-negative resection, long-term survival will depend on a number of factors. Fong and colleagues analyzed 1001 patients who had a resection for CRC metastatic to the liver.[40] They found that five clinical criteria were important in predicting survival time: positive nodal status of the primary tumor, disease-free interval (DFI) from diagnosis of the primary tumor to detection of the metastases of less than 12 months, preoperative CEA level greater than 200 ng/mL, size of the largest lesion greater than 5 cm, and number of tumors more than 1. If each of these criteria were given one point for being present, then survival time was related to the number of points present, as noted in Table 30–2. From the data in the table, it is clear that when five risk factors are present, the 5-year survival rate is limited, but it gives one patient in seven a chance at long-term survival that would not be possible without resection.

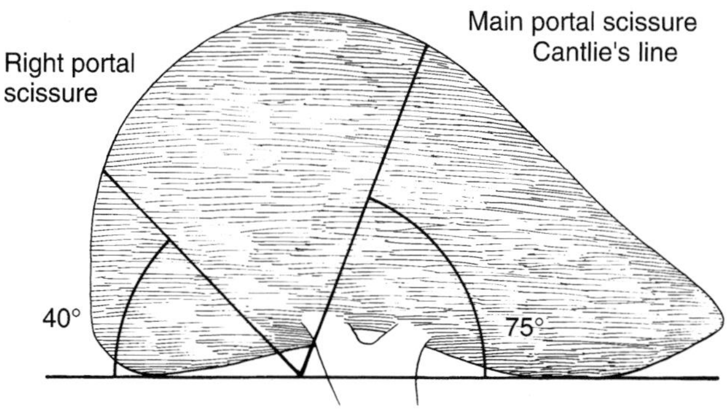

Figure 30–11. The obliquity of the middle and of the right portal scissurae. (Redrawn from Bismuth H. Surgical anatomy and anatomical surgery of the liver. *World J Surg* 1982;6:3.)

Liver resection traditionally has been done in an open fashion via relatively large incisions, as noted earlier. Advances in laparoscopic surgery have allowed major liver resections—including right hepatectomies and right trisegmentectomies—to be performed with a laparoscope using a handport in a manner similar to the

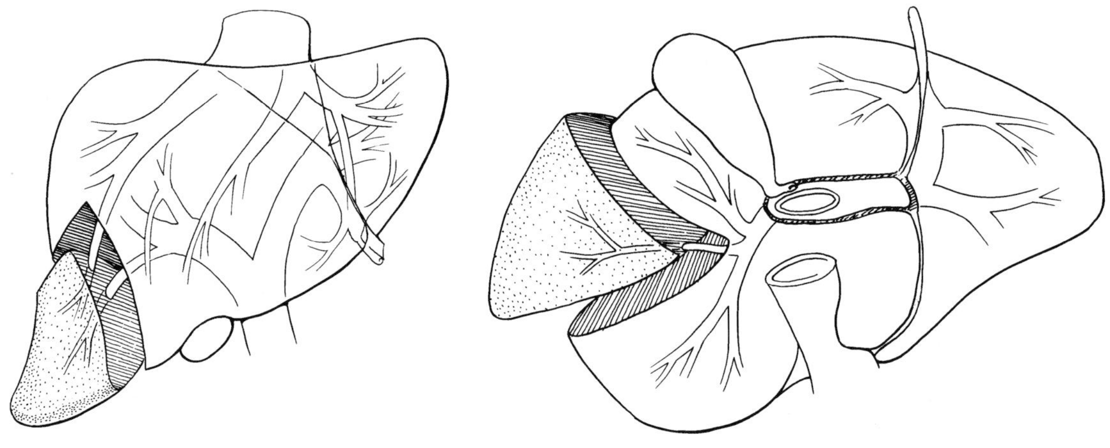

Figure 30–12. Segmentectomy VI. (Redrawn from Bismuth H, Houssin D, et al. Major and minor segmentectomies. "Reglees" in liver surgery. *World J Surg* 1982;6:10.)

open techniques noted earlier.[41,42] A report from Cincinnati stated that of 100 laparoscopic liver resections, 31 were formal right or left hepatectomies. Mean operative time was 2.2 hours. The mean length of stay was 3 days. Two patients required reoperation for bleeding, and one patient died.[42] These preliminary results certainly match the results of open liver resections.

▪ IMPLANTABLE PUMPS

Administering chemotherapy directly into the hepatic artery via a catheter introduced through the femoral artery has been practiced for over 30 years. Toward the end of the 1970s, a totally self-contained implantable pump was developed that allowed continuous arterial infusion of chemotherapy via a catheter placed in the gastroduodenal artery at the junction of the hepatic artery. The rationale for hepatic arterial infusion (HAI) chemotherapy takes advantage of the observation that CRC metastases in the liver derive the majority of their blood supply from the hepatic artery, not the portal vein.[43] Further, the drug used most commonly for HAI, fluorodeoxyxuridine (FUDR), has over 95% uptake in the liver on first pass as compared with 5-fluorouracil (5-FU), which has less than 50% uptake on first pass.[44] This major difference allows HAI with FUDR at 100–400 times the concentration of systemic 5-FU.

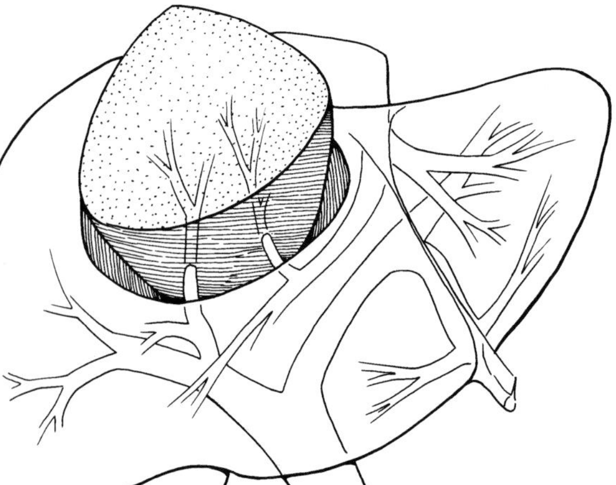

Figure 30–13. Segmentectomy VIII. (Redrawn from Bismuth H, Houssin D, et al. Major and minor segmentectomies. "Reglees" in liver surgery. *World J Surg* 1982;6:10.)

Randomized studies evaluating HAI with FUDR versus systemic 5-FU conducted in the 1980s showed response rates of 30–50% with HAI FUDR but did not demonstrate a survival benefit conclusively with this technique.[45–49] Thus the appropriate role for this treatment continues to be debated. The literature is clear that the frequency and severity of complications decrease with increasing experience of the surgeon. These complications include pump malfunction, pocket problems, catheter occlusion or dislodgment, and arterial complications (i.e., hemorrhage or thrombosis, or perfusion problems).[49] With no definitive randomized study showing a clear benefit to HAI chemotherapy, a multi-institutional trial of HAI with FUDR versus systemic 5-FU-based chemotherapy was conducted in the 1990s. The HAI chemotherapy group had about a 3-month median survival-time advantage over the systemic therapy group.[50] However, this trial was criticized by many medical oncologists because (1) the survival-time advantage was considered too short to argue for pump implantation and (2) newer systemic agents provide longer survival times than the systemic regimen used in this trial. A single-institution randomized trial from New York showed a survival advantage at 2 years with HAI chemotherapy after liver resection versus no HAI chemotherapy.[51] This trial was criticized be-

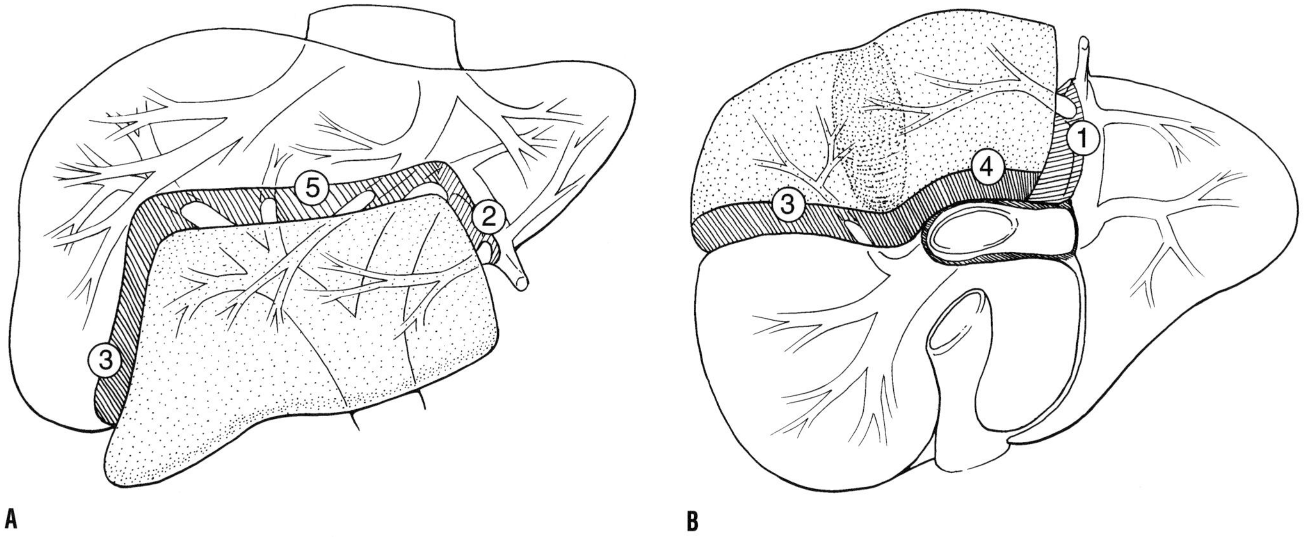

Figure 30–14. Bisegmentectomy IV and V. The different steps of the technique: 1. Opening of the umbilical fissure. 2. Splitting of the parenchyma to the right of the ligamentum teres. 3. Opening of the right portal scissura. 4. Ligation of the portal pedicles of the quadrate lobe and of the anterior portal pedicle of the right paramedian sector. (Redrawn from Bismuth H, Houssin D, et al. Major and minor segmentectomies. "Reglees" in liver surgery. *World J Surg* 1982;6:10.)

cause there was not a significant long-term survival advantage in the HAI group. At the moment, HAI chemotherapy is not used widely. Several protocols require this treatment. Outside protocol treatment, the main indication for this therapy is the treatment of liver-only disease in a patient who has progressed on the best systemic treatment available and who understands the risks and perhaps small benefit of HAI via an implantable pump.

TECHNIQUE OF PUMP IMPLANTATION

The technique of pump implantation begins before surgery with imaging studies to exclude extrahepatic disease. If no disease is found outside the liver, then either an angiogram or a CT-angiogram of the hepatic arteries is performed to ensure that any variation in anatomy is understood. Next, an exploratory laparotomy and search for disease outside the liver are performed. If extrahepatic metastases are found, then the pump is not placed. When disease outside the liver has been excluded, the gastroduodenal artery is isolated. The anterior leaf of the gastrohepatic and duodenohepatic ligament should be divided, and any arterial branches from the proper hepatic artery should be ligated to avoid infusion of chemotherapy to the stomach or duodenum. The gallbladder should be removed to avoid chemical cholecystitis. Next, a subcutaneous pocket is created for the pump, and the catheter from the pump is brought via a small stab incision into the abdomen. The pump is primed with heparinized saline, and the catheter is inserted into the gastroduodenal artery and secured such that the tip of the catheter is at the junction with—but not in—the hepatic artery. Then 5 mL of 10% fluorescein is injected through the sideport, and a Wood's lamp (ultraviolet light) is used to view the liver and right upper quadrant. Both lobes of the liver should show perfusion, and there should be no perfusion of the stomach or duodenum. If there is perfusion to the stomach or duodenum, the surgeon should search for and ligate an arterial branch to the stomach or duodenum from the hepatic artery distal to the gastroduodenal artery junction. The pump is secured in the pocket with heavy nonabsorbable sutures to the underlying fascia to minimize the chance that the pump will flip in the pocket. The abdomen and pump pocket incisions are closed in the usual manner. The procedure usually is performed via laparotomy, but it is possible to perform it laparoscopically. Postoperatively, the patient should have a nuclear medicine examination with technetium-99 macroaggregated albumin injected into the sideport of the pump that demonstrates flow to the liver with no extrahepatic flow. If this study shows perfusion of the stomach or duodenum, then an angiogram via

TABLE 30–2. CLINICAL RISK SCORE AND SURVIVAL RATES

Score	1 Year	5 Year	Median (mos.)
0	93%	60%	74
1	91%	44%	51
2	89%	40%	47
3	86%	20%	33
4	70%	25%	20
5	71%	14%	22

the femoral artery is performed, and any arterial branches from the hepatic artery to the duodenum or stomach are embolized.

With a normal postoperative nuclear medicine study of the pump, the pump can be filled with chemotherapy. Typical regimens of pump chemotherapy include cycles of FUDR infusion for 2 weeks followed by heparin infusions for 2 weeks. Generally, dexamethasone is added to reduce the risk of the complication of biliary sclerosis.[52] The dexamethasone also might enhance the activity of the chemotherapy regimen. Liver function studies are followed. Elevation in transaminases require a reduction in the dose of FUDR. Elevation of alkaline phosphatase or bilirubin should be evaluated with a magnetic resonance cholangiopancreatography (MRCP) or endoscopic retrograde cholangiopancreatography (ERCP). For bile duct stenoses, a stent should be placed.

Variations in the hepatic arterial anatomy can be challenging. A straightforward replaced right or left hepatic artery can be ligated; intrahepatic arterial collaterals will develop. When the pump no longer is useful, it can be removed under local anesthetic from the subcutaneous pocket; the catheter can be cut and ligated—it does not need to be removed.

COMPLICATIONS OF IMPLANTABLE PUMPS

Complications from the implantation of HAI pumps include infection (that might require removal of the pump), bleeding (especially from the arteriotomy in the gastroduodenal artery), and thrombosis of the hepatic artery if the tip of the catheter protrudes into this artery. These complications occur in over 20% of patients. Complications occurring fewer than 30 days from surgery usually can be corrected, but "late" complications usually preclude use of the pump.[51] Complications from HAI chemotherapy include chemical cholecystitis if the gallbladder is not removed, ulcers in the duodenum or stomach if an arterial branch was not ligated, and biliary sclerosis. Generally, HAI chemotherapy is well tolerated, and most patients return to work. Since the pump works by compression of gas in a closed space and expansion pushes the chemotherapy agent into the catheter, excessive heat and pressure changes can empty the pump too quickly; thus patients should talk with their medical oncologists before spending prolonged periods in a hot tub or an airplane.

■ RADIOFREQUENCY ABLATION

Radiofrequency (RF) ablation is a treatment that destroys tumors in situ by protein denaturation and thermal coagulation. It has been used to treat tumors since the early 1900s. Beer used RF coagulation through a cystoscope to treat bladder tumors in 1908. Cushing used RF ablation (RFA) to treat intracranial tumors in 1926. In 1990, two groups independently used ultrasound to guide RFA treatment of liver tumors. RFA uses alternating current with a frequency between 10 kHz and 900 MHz. Tissue adjacent to the electrode dies from the heat generated in the tissue by RF energy; the electrode itself does not become hot, but it delivers RF energy that causes mechanical friction in the tissue that leads to thermal ablation.[53] Several devices have been manufactured to perform RFA. One such device uses a multiprong electrode that allows treatment of tumors up to 5 cm in diameter. It uses thermocouples to monitor tissue heating. Typically, tissue needs to be heated to greater than 50°C to kill effectively.

Resection is the best treatment for CRC metastatic to the liver. RFA is used as an alternative to resection when (1) comorbid disease precludes resection or (2) anatomic considerations preclude resection. Examples of the latter indication principally are twofold. First, if a discrete number of metastases are located in different segments such that resection of the lesions would result in inadequate residual liver volume, then RFA would be reasonable. Second, if several lesions in one half of the liver can be removed with an ipsilateral hepatectomy but a lesion deep in the contralateral half of the liver cannot be removed, an ipsilateral hepatectomy with RFA of the lesion in the contralateral liver would be appropriate.

RFA can be performed percutaneously in an imaging suite with CT scan or ultrasound guidance or in the operating room either open or laparoscopically with ultrasound guidance. Using imaging guidance, RFA ablates the tumor with a 1-cm margin. Tumors close to the right and left hepatic ducts are difficult to treat because RFA can injure the ducts. If a tumor is close to the gallbladder or diaphragm, percutaneous ablation can injure those organs. If RFA is done in the operating room, the diaphragm can be protected, and the gallbladder can be removed, if necessary.

An advantage of RFA is hemostasis. After a lesion is ablated, the electrode is withdrawn while the tract is ablated. With this maneuver, bleeding rarely occurs.

If the procedure is performed in the radiology suite or laparoscopically, typically the patient will stay overnight in the hospital and will be discharged the morning after the procedure. Within 2 weeks of the procedure, a CT scan or MRI should be performed to evaluate the efficacy of the procedure. Three months after RFA, imaging is repeated and compared with the postprocedure CT scan or MRI. A homogeneous collection of necrotic tissue should be evident, and at 3 months the size of the collection should not be enlarging. If there is any concern about residual tumor, repeat RFA should be considered.

Complication rates associated with RFA in one large review and one single-institution study were 7% and 2.4%, respectively.[54,55] The reported procedure-related mortality rate is 0.5% (10 deaths in 1931 patients).[54] Complications are more frequent in those undergoing open RFA versus percutaneous RFA. Complications include abscess, biloma, bile duct injury, pleural effusion, and pain.

The results of RFA for CRC metastatic to the liver are difficult to discern because RFA results generally are reported for hepatomas together with metastases to the liver. The first question regarding RFA of CRC metastases is: Does RFA cause complete death of the treated tumor? One small study from Vancouver treated 12 metastatic tumors in 10 patients with percutaneous RFA. Resection was performed within 6 weeks. Nine of the 12 ablated tumors were removed. Microscopic examination showed successful ablation in 8 of 9.[56] Obviously, in this small group the local recurrence rate would be at least 11% if resection were not performed.

There are few reports in the literature that have adequate follow-up of adequate numbers of patients with CRC metastases to the liver treated with RFA. One study from M.D. Anderson Cancer Center examined 348 patients who were treated with resection and/or RFA for CRC metastatic to the liver. They were compared with 70 patients with CRC metastases who were found at surgery to be ineligible for resection or RFA. With a median follow-up time of 21 months, they noted a 9% recurrence rate at the RFA site in the liver as compared with a 2% recurrence rate for resection of CRC metastatic to the liver.[57] In this cohort, 110 tumors were treated with RFA in 57 patients. Survival at 4 years was 65% for resection, 36% for resection with RFA, and 22% for RFA alone ($p < 0.0001$). Survival for those having RFA ± resection was only slightly superior to nonsurgical treatment.

Some surgeons claim that RFA for solitary CRC metastases is associated with infrequent local recurrences. The M.D. Anderson group recently examined this issue. With a median follow-up time of 31 months, they found a 37% local recurrence rate for RFA treatment of solitary metastases as compared with a 5% local recurrence for resection ($p = 0.0001$).[58] The subset with smaller tumors—less than 3 cm in diameter—had a 31% local recurrence rate with RFA compared with 3% with resection. Clearly, RFA of CRC metastases to the liver is not equivalent to resection; RFA should be considered investigational or at best an inferior, second-choice treatment.

▪ CRYOABLATION

Cryoablation is similar to RF ablation with the important distinction that it uses freezing instead of heating to kill tumors in the liver. The technology has been known since the early 1960s, but it did not become practical until intraoperative ultrasound and adequately insulated cryoprobes became available.

The indications for cryoablation are similar to those for RFA. Typically, it is performed in the operating room either with open or laparoscopic technique; however, some centers such as our own have the ability to perform cryoablation in the radiology suite under magnetic resonance guidance.

The technique of intraoperative cryoablation begins with IUS evaluation of the liver to identify and measure all the metastases. If a lesion is close to a major bile duct, injury to the duct can occur. If a lesion is close to a major vascular structure, injury to the structure or inadequate freezing of the lesion owing to a "heat sink" effect can occur. A lesion that can be frozen safely with a 1-cm margin has a cryoprobe inserted under ultrasound guidance. The lesion typically is frozen with liquid nitrogen. It is then thawed, and the freeze-thaw cycle is repeated. The process can take over 30 minutes for one lesion; however, some units allow cryoablation of up to six lesions at the same time. Freezing can be monitored with IUS; a characteristic hypoechoic "iceball" is formed. During removal of the cryoprobe, the interface of the iceball and normal liver can "crack," resulting in significant bleeding. In the past, the cryoprobes were big and awkward to use, and bleeding was frequent; thus many surgeons switched to ablation with RFA. However, with smaller cryoprobes and more experience, significant bleeding with cryotherapy is an infrequent problem.

A postablation MRI or contrast-enhanced CT scan is done within days of the cryoablation. If the ablated volume is inadequate, repeat ablation should be considered.

Complications of cryoablation include (1) a right pleural effusion that usually does not need treatment, (2) an increase in transaminase that generally resolves within 7 days, (3) thrombocytopenia, (4) an elevated prothrombin time, (5) renal failure, (6) bleeding, (7) biliary leaks, and (8) multiple-organ failure.

Results of cryoablation for metastases to the liver from CRC are difficult to discern because few randomized studies exist, and most reports combine patients with different histologies [hepatocellular carcinoma (HCC)], CRC metastases, and other metastases) and different treatment combinations (cryoablation ± resection or ± chemotherapy). In 1997, Bismuth reported a local recurrence rate of 0% for HCC and 44% for CRC metastases with a 16-month mean follow-up time.[59] These results were not dissimilar to others in the literature at that time.[60,61] Bismuth obtained treated tumor for histopathologic analysis in nine cases; in seven of nine, there was viable tumor.[59] Clearly, these results are disappointing.

A report from Sydney was more encouraging.[62] In 1998, Morris reported results for cryotherapy in 116 patients with CRC metastases to the liver that were unresectable. All had partial double freeze-thaw cycles instead of complete freeze-thaw cycles to minimize the chance of cryoshock (a syndrome of multiple-organ failure and coagulopathy). The mean number of metastases was three (range one to nine), and the mean size was 3.5 cm (range 1 to 13 cm). Liver resection to remove additional lesions was done in 33 patients. Postoperative intra-arterial chemotherapy was given to 105 patients. Complications included acute renal failure, hemorrhage, liver failure, abscess, biloma or bile fistula, and pleural effusion. One patient (0.9%) died from a myocardial infarction. With a median follow-up time of 20.5 months, the median survival time was 26 months, and the 5-year survival rate was 13.4%. Multivariate analysis determined that several factors were associated with favorable prognosis, including complete cryotreatment and small size of the treated lesion. The authors felt that cryotherapy was a reasonable treatment for unresectable liver metastases but that it was not equivalent to resection. In 2006, the same group reported results for cryotherapy in a larger group of CRC patients (n = 224) with longer median follow-up time (26 months).[63] All were treated with postoperative intra-arterial chemotherapy. There was one death (0.4%), and the morbidity rate was 21%. Cryosite, remaining liver, and extrahepatic recurrence rates were 39%, 62%, and 67%, respectively. Median survival time was 31 months; 5-year survival rate was 23%. Ninety-one patients had more than four bilateral lesions. Median survival time was 31 months, and the 5-year survival rate was 26%. The authors concluded that cryotherapy and intra-arterial chemotherapy with or without resection can provide a long survival time in patients with unresectable CRC metastases to the liver. The 23% 5-year survival rate was impressive for a group expected to have a less than 2% 5-year survival rate, but the 39% cryosite recurrence rate was disappointing.

Many surgeons who ablate CRC metastases to the liver switched from cryotherapy to RFA because RFA is easier and quicker to perform; cryotherapy is associated with bleeding and multiorgan failure, whereas RFA stops (does not cause) bleeding and is not associated with multiorgan failure; and the local recurrence after cryotherapy was disappointing, whereas the early reports of local control with RFA were encouraging. With the recent M.D. Anderson report showing a 37% local recurrence rate of solitary CRC liver metastases and the Sydney report showing a 39% local recurrence with cryotherapy, it appears that cryotherapy and RFA are quite similar and substantially inferior to resection. Thus, until an appropriate randomized study is performed, the choice of cryotherapy versus RFA depends on the preference of the surgeon; neither treatment should be considered equivalent to resection.

SELECTIVE BIBLIOGRAPHY

Abdalla EK, Vauthey JN, Ellis LM, et al. Recurrence and outcomes following hepatic resection, radiofrequency ablation, and combined resection/ablation for colorectal liver metastases. *Ann Surg* 2004;239:818–825

Fong Y, Fortner J, Sun RL, et al. Clinical score for predicting recurrence after hepatic resection for metastatic colorectal cancer: Analysis of 1001 consecutive cases. *Ann Surg* 1999;230:309–321

Vauthey JN (ed). Primary and metastatic liver cancer. *Surg Oncol Clin North Am* 2003;12:135–220

REFERENCES

1. Jemal A, Tivari RC, Murray T, et al. Cancer statistics, 2004. *CA Cancer J Clin* 2004;54:8–29
2. Wagner JS, Adson MA, Heerden JA, et al. The natural history of hepatic metastses from colorectal cancer: A comparison with resective treatment. *Ann Surg* 1984; 199:502–508
3. Wanebo HJ, Semoglou C, Attiyeh F, Stearns MJ. Surgical management of patients with primary operable colorectal cancer and synchronous liver metastases. *Am J Surg* 1978;135:81–85
4. Foster JH, Lundy J. Liver metastases. *Curr Probl Surg* 1981;18:157–202
5. Altendorf-Hofmann A, Scheele J. A critical review of the major indicators of prognosis after resection of hepatic metastases from colorectal carcinoma. *Surg Oncol Clin North Am* 2003;12:165–192
6. Saltz LB, Cox JV, Blanke C, et al. Irinotecan plus fluorouracil and leucovorin for metastatic colorectal cancer. *New Engl J Med* 2000;343:905–914
7. Tournigand C, Andre T, Achille E, et al. FOLFIRI followed by FOLFOX6 or the reverse sequence in advanced colorectal cancer: A randomized GERCOR study. *J Clin Oncol* 2004;22:229–237
8. Martinelli DJ, Wadler S, Bakal CW, et al. Utility of embolization or chemoembolization as second-line treatment in patients with advanced or recurrent colorectal carcinoma. *Cancer* 1994;74:1706–1712
9. Lambert LA, Colacchio TA, Barth RJ. Interval hepatic resection of colorectal metastases improves patient selection. *Arch Surg* 2000;135:473–480
10. Abdel-Nabi H, Doerr RJ, Lamonica DM, et al. Staging of primary colorectal carcinomas with fluorine-18 fluorodeoxyglucose whole-body PET: Correlation with his-

topathologic and CT findings. *Radiology* 1998;206:755–760

11. Fernandez FG, Drebin JA, Linehan DC, et al. Five-year survival after resection of hepatic metastases from colorectal cancer in patients screened by positron emission tomography with F-18 fluorodeoxyglucose (FDG-PET). *Ann Surg* 2004;240:438–447
12. Machi J, Isomoto H, Kurohiji T, et al. Accuracy of intraoperative ultrasonography in diagnosing liver metastasis from colorectal cancer: Evaluation with postoperative follow-up results. *World J Surg* 1991;15:551–556
13. Farges O, Belghiti J, Kianmanesh R, et al. Portal vein embolization before right hepatectomy: Prospective clinical trial. *Ann Surg* 2003;237:208–217
14. Sasson A, Sigurdson ER. Surgical treatment of liver metastases. *Semin Oncol* 2002;29:107–118
15. Weber SM, Jarnagin WR, DeMatteo RP, et al. Survival after resection of multiple hepatic colorectal metastases. *Ann Surg Oncol* 2000;7:643–650
16. Fong Y, Fortner J, Sun RL, et al. Clinical score for predicting recurrence after hepatic resection for metastatic colorectal cancer. Analysis of 1001 consecutive cases. *Ann Surg* 1999;230:309–321
17. Terminology Committee of the International Hepato-Pancreato-Biliary Association. Brisbane 2000 terminology of liver anatomy and resections. *Hepatobil Pancreat Surg* 2000;2:333–339
18. Couinaud C. *Le foie: Etudes anatomiques et chirurgicales.* Paris: Masson, 1957
19. Goldsmith NA, Woodburne RT. Surgical anatomy pertaining to liver resection. *Surg Gynecol Obstet* 1957;195: 310–318
20. Starzl TE, Bell RH, Beart RW, Putman CW. Hepatic trisegmentectomy and other liver resections. *Surg Gynecol Obstet* 1975;141:429–437
21. Starzl TE, Koep LJ, Weill R III, et al. Right trisegmentectomy for hepatic neoplasms. *Surg Gynecol Obstet* 1980; 150:208–214
22. Starzl TE, Iwatsuki S, Shaw BW, et al. Left hepatic trisegmentectomy. *Surg Gynecol Obstet* 1982;155:21–27
23. Koo BN, Kil HK, Choi JS, et al. Hepatic resection by the Cavitron ultrasonic surgical aspirator increases the incidence and severity of venous air embolism. *Anesth Analg* 2005;101:966–970
24. Nakayama H, Masuda H, Shibata M. Incidence of bile leakage after three types of hepatic parenchymal transection. *Hepato-Gastroenterology* 2003;50:1517–1520
25. Takayama T, Masatoshi M, Kubota K, et al. Randomized comparison of ultrasonic vs clamp transection of the liver. *Arch Surg* 2001;136:922–928
26. Kim J, Ahmad SA, Lowy AM, et al. Increased biliary fistulas after liver resection with the harmonic scalpel. *Am Surg* 2003;69:815–819
27. Rau HG, Meyer G, Jauch KW, et al. Liver resection with the water jet: conventional and laparoscopic surgery. *Chirugie* 1996;67:546–551
28. Romano F, Franciosi C, Caprotti R, et al. Hepatic surgery using the Ligasure vessel-sealing system. *World J Surg* 2005;29:110–112
29. Poon RT, Sheung TF, Wong J. Liver resection using a saline-linked radiofrequency dissecting sealer for transection of the liver. *J Am Coll Surg* 2005;200:308–313
30. Weber JC, Navarra G, Jiao LR, et al. New technique for liver resection using heat coagulative necrosis. *Ann Surg* 2005;241:194–196
31. Haghighi KS, Wang F, King J, Daniel S, Morris DL. In-line radiofrequency ablation to minimize blood loss in hepatic parenchymal transection. *Am J Surg* 2005;190:43–47
32. Clancy TE, Swanson RS. Laparoscopic radiofrequency-assisted liver resection (LRR): A report of two cases. *Dig Dis Sci* 2005;50;2259–2262
33. Scheele J, Stang R, Altendorf-Hofmann A, Paul M. Resection of colorectal liver metastases. *World J Surg* 1995; 19:59–71
34. Doci R, Gennari L, Bignami P, et al. Morbidity and mortality after hepatic resection of metastases from colorectal cancer. *Br J Surg* 1995;82:377–381
35. Nordlinger B, Guiguet M, Vaillant JC, et al. Surgical resection of colorectal carcinoma metastases to the liver: A prognostic scoring system to improve case selection, based on 1568 patients. *Cancer* 1996;77:1254–1262
36. Fong Y, Cohen AM, Fortner JG, et al. Liver resection for colorectal metastases. *J Clin Oncol* 1997;15:938–946
37. Cady B, Jenkins RL, Steele GD, et al. Surgical margin in hepatic resection for colorectal metastasis: A critical and improvable determinant of outcome. *Ann Surg* 1998;227:566–571
38. Iwatsuki S, Dvorchik I, Madariaga JR, et al. Hepatic resection for metastatic colorectal adenocarcinoma: A proposal of a prognostic scoring system. *J Am Coll Surg* 1999;189:291–299
39. Steele G, Bleday R, Mayer RJ, et al. A prospective evaluation of hepatic resection for colorectal carcinoma metastases to the liver: Gastrointestinal Tumor Study Group Protocol 6584. *J Clin Oncol* 1991;9:1105–1112
40. Fong Y, Fortner J, Sun RL, et al. Clinical score for predicting recurrence after hepatic resection for metastatic colorectal caner: Analysis of 1001 consecutive cases. *Ann Surg* 1999;230:309–321
41. Gigot JF, Glineur D, Azagra JS, et al. Laparoscopic liver resection for malignant liver tumors: Preliminary results of a multicenter European study. *Ann Surg* 2002;236:90–97
42. Buell J, Koffron A, Thomas M, et al. Laparoscopic liver resection. *J Am Coll Surg* 2005;200:472–480
43. Ridge JA, Bading JR, Gelbard AS, et al. Perfusion of colorectal hepatic metastases: Relative distribution of flow from the hepatic artery and portal vein. *Cancer* 1987;59:1547
44. Ensminger WD, Rosowsky A, Raso V, et al. A clinical-pharmacological evaluation of hepatic arterial infusions of 5-fluoro-2′-deoxyuridine and 5-fluorouracil. *Cancer Res* 1978;38:3784–3789
45. Chang AE, Schneider PD, Sugarbaker PH, et al. A prospective, randomized trial of regional versus systemic continuous fluorodeoxyuridine chemotherapy in the treatment of colorectal liver metastases. *Ann Surg* 1987; 206:685–693

46. Hohn DC, Stagg RJ, Friedman MA, et al. A randomized trial of continuous intravenous versus hepatic intra-arterial floxuridine in patients with colorectal cancer metastatic to the liver: The northern California oncology group trial. *J Clin Oncol* 1989;7:1646–1654
47. Kemeny N, Daly J, Reichman B, et al. Intrahepatic or systemic infusion of fluorodeoxyuridine in patients with liver metastases from colorectal carcinoma. *Ann Intern Med* 1987;107:459–465
48. Martin JK, O'Connell MJ, Wieand HS, et al. Intra-arterial floxuridine vs systemic fluorouracil for hepatic metastases from colorectal cancer. *Arch Surg* 1990;125: 1022–1027
49. Allen PJ, Nissan A, Picon AI, et al. Technical complications and durability of hepatic artery infusion pumps for unresectable colorectal liver metastases: An institutional experience of 544 consecutive cases. *J Am Coll Surg* 2005;201:57–65
50. Kemeny N, Warren RS CALGB pump trial. Proc ASCO
51. Kemeny N, Huang Y, Cohen AM, et al. Hepatic arterial infusion of chemotherapy after resection of hepatic metastases from colorectal cancer. *N Engl J Med* 1999;228: 756–762
52. Kemeny N, Conti JA, Cohen AM, et al. Phase II study of hepatic arterial floxuridine, leucovorin, and dexamethasome for unresectable liver metastases from colorectal carcinoma *J Clin Oncol* 1994;12:2288–2292
53. Decadt B, Siriwardena AK. Radiofrequency ablation of liver tumors: Systematic review. *Lancet Oncol* 2004;5:550–560
54. Mulier S, Mulier P, Ni Y, et al. Complications of radiofrequency coagulation of liver tumours. *Br J Surg* 2002;89: 1206–1222
55. Curley SA, Francesco I, Delrio P, et al. Radiofrequency ablation of unresectable primary and metastatic hepatic malignancies. *Ann Surg* 1999;230:1–7
56. Scudamore CH, Shung IL, Patterson EJ, et al. Radiofrequency ablation followed by resection of malignant liver tumors. *Am J Surg* 1999;177:411–417
57. Abdalla EK, Vauthey JN, Ellis LM, et al. Recurrence and outcomes following hepatic resection, radiofrequency ablation, and combined resection/ablation for colorectal liver metastases. *Ann Surg* 2004;239:818–825
58. Aloia TA, Vauthey J-N, Loyer EM, et al. Solitary colorectal liver metastasis: Resection determines outcome. *Arch Surg* 2006;141:460–466
59. Adam R, Akpinar E, Johann M, et al. Place of cryosurgery in the treatment of malignant liver tumors. *Ann Surg* 1997;225:39–50
60. Onik G, Rubinsky B, Zemel R, et al. Ultrasound-guided hepatic cryosurgery in the treatment of colorectal metastatic colon carcinoma: Preliminary results. *Cancer* 1991; 67:901–907
61. Weaver ML, Atkinson D, Zemel R. Hepatic cryosurgery in treating colorectal metastases. *Cancer* 1995;76:210–214
62. Seifert JK, Morris DL. Prognostic factors after cryotherapy for hepatic metastases from colorectal cancer. *Ann Surg* 1998;228:201–208
63. Yan TD, Padang R, Morris DL. Long-term results and prognostic indicators after cryotherapy and hepatic arterial chemotherapy with or without resection for colorectal liver metastases in 224 patients: Long-term survival can be achieved in patients with multiple bilateral liver metastases. *J Am Coll Surg* 2006;202:100–111

31

Portal Hypertension

J. Michael Henderson

Portal hypertension is present when portal venous pressure exceeds 10 mm Hg. This chapter addresses the causes, evaluation, and treatment options for patients with portal hypertension. While the emphasis is on surgical aspects, this group of patients require a multidisciplinary approach and surgical therapy must inevitably be viewed in this context. The major clinical presentations that will be addressed are variceal bleeding, ascites, and end-stage liver disease. Whatever the presentation of portal hypertension, be it an incidental finding or one of the above clinical presentations, it demands full investigation. In the United States, the etiology is most commonly cirrhosis, but other etiologies such as prehepatic portal or splenic vein thrombosis or other intraparenchymal liver disease such as schistosomiasis or hepatic fibrosis should be considered. Definition of the cause is important as prognosis depends on the underlying liver disease, and a full evaluation to allow development of a treatment plan for variceal bleeding, ascites, or end-stage liver disease is paramount at initial presentation. The focus of this chapter is on emphasizing the role of a multidisciplinary team approach to managing patients with portal hypertension.

■ HISTORY[1,2]

Portal hypertension was recognized by the Greeks, was highlighted by Shakespeare in his character of Falstaff, and has played a role through much of history. The evolution of the treatment of portal hypertension was driven by surgeons until the 1980s. Nicolai Eck, a Russian Army surgeon, performed an end-to-side portocaval shunt in 1883 in an animal model. Pavlov, the great Russian physiologist, conducted animal studies that showed the detrimental effect of diverting portal flow, describing meat intoxication (encephalopathy) and liver failure. Vidal, a French surgeon is credited with performing the first portal systemic shunt in man in 1903. Morison and Talma operated on patients with portal hypertension with procedures such as omentopexy and splenic transposition, but their failure to recognize cirrhosis as the cause of portal hypertension led to poor results.

In the 1940s, Whipple and the Columbia Presbyterian group in New York initiated an era of success for portal decompression.[3] The next 40 years saw many refinements to decompressive shunts, Drapanas with mesocaval shunts,[4] Warren and Inochuchi with selective variceal decompression,[5,6] and Sarfeh with partial shunts.[7] This era saw many randomized trials documenting efficacy of shunts.

Endoscopic therapy was the next major advance in managing variceal bleeding, being first done by surgeons with rigid esophagoscopes.[8] In the 1980s, three surgeons Johnston, Terblanche,[9] and Paquet[10] bridged the gap from rigid to flexible variceal sclerotherapy. Another surgeon, Steigmann,[11] moved the field forward by introducing variceal band ligation.

Over the last three decades, the more recent advances have been made by nonsurgeons. A better understanding of the pathophysiology, the ability to better evaluate liver diseases, the introduction of pharmacologic therapy, development of the radiologic shunt, and coming of age of liver transplantation are the main contributors to this progress. Lebrec and his colleagues in the 1980s introduced beta-blockers to reduce portal hypertension,[12] and this has become the primary treatment for reducing the risk of an initial variceal bleed and first-line treatment for those who have bled. Transjugular intrahepatic portosystemic shunt (TIPS), pioneered by Rösch,[13] has led to shunts being more safely placed by the radiologist than the surgeon with lower early morbidity and mortality.

However, two surgeons, Starzl[14] and Calne,[15] revolutionized the whole field of hepatology with their persistence in developing liver transplantation through the 1960s to 1980s, and bringing it to a clinical reality. Transplant has not only offered a treatment for patients with end-stage liver disease and portal hypertension, but has also opened the doors to further investigation.

It is around this history of portal hypertension that many of the investigative and treatment options discussed in this chapter are built.

▪ PATHOPHYSIOLOGY[16,17]

The pathophysiology of portal hypertension has been clarified over the past two decades in animal models documenting the sequential changes in the splanchnic and systemic circulations. The sequence of events is:

- Block to portal flow leads to increased portal pressure.
- Splanchnic vascular bed response:
  - (a) initial increase vasoconstrictor and decrease vasodilator response increases intrahepatic resistance
  - (b) secondarily, the vasodilator response dominates, with increase in splanchnic inflow
- Collaterals develop between the portal circulation and the systemic circulation.
- Plasma volume expansion occurs, with the development of a systemic hyperdynamic circulation.

The splanchnic vascular response leads to increased flow in the gut and thus major clinical manifestations of collaterals in multiple locations: at the umbilicus, in the retroperitoneum, hemorrhoidal, and at the gastroesophageal junction.

The systemic hemodynamics changes result in cardiac outputs in the 10 to 15 L/minute range, systolic blood pressures in the 100 to 110 range, and a low calculated total systemic vascular resistance. These changes have significant management implications for fluid resuscitation and patient management. It is important for the managing physician to understand these pathophysiologic changes and their impact on patient care.

▪ COMPLICATIONS

The major complications of portal hypertension are:

- Variceal bleeding
- Ascites
- End-stage liver disease

This chapter will address the etiology, evaluation methods, specific therapies, and overall treatment strategies for each of these complications. An important distinction in patients with portal hypertension is between those with ascites and encephalopathy, which are markers of advanced liver disease, and patients with variceal bleeding, which may occur in patients with a normal liver (portal vein thrombosis) or early in the course of cirrhosis. The implication of this is that the range of treatment options is considerably broader for variceal bleeding than it is for patients with ascites and encephalopathy.

▪ ETIOLOGY[18]

Figure 31–1 illustrates the wide range of etiologies for portal hypertension. In the United States and Europe, approximately 90% of patients with portal hypertension have cirrhosis, with a small percentage having portal vein thrombosis or hepatic fibrosis. The latter are important to differentiate because they have normal liver function and a much better prognosis. Worldwide, schistosomiasis is an important etiology of portal hypertension, occurring mainly in the Middle and Far East and South America. It is characterized by fibrosis of the terminal portal venules, and in the absence of concurrent hepatitis, these patients have normal liver function.

Cirrhosis covers a broad spectrum of disease by etiology and severity. Alcoholic liver disease and hepatitis are the most common etiologies, with other causes, such as the cholestatic liver diseases of primary biliary cirrhosis (PBC) and primary sclerosing cholangitis (PSC), and the metabolic liver diseases such as hemochromatosis, Wilson's disease, and α1-antitrypsin deficiency, contributing a small percentage. Whatever the etiology of the cirrhosis, full evaluation of activity and stage of the disease is an important part of initial patient evaluation. Different etiologies may have different natural histories which is important in developing a treatment plan.

▪ EVALUATION

The evaluation of patients with portal hypertension has the following essential components, and should be done at initial presentation:

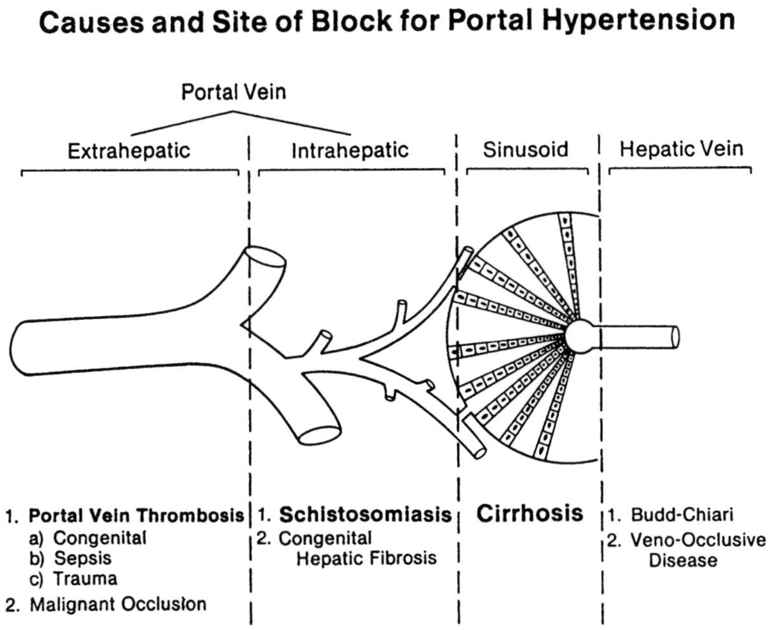

Figure 31–1. Sites for obstruction in portal hypertension. In the United States and Europe, most patients have a sinusoidal block secondary to cirrhosis. Other causes must be considered.

- Assessment of the liver disease
- Assessment of the portal circulation
- Upper gastrointestinal (GI) endoscopy

Liver evaluation[19,20] is based on clinical findings and laboratory studies. Jaundice, ascites, encephalopathy, and malnutrition define a patient with end-stage liver disease. Some patients with variceal bleeding do not show these clinical signs and have well-preserved liver function. Laboratory tests add objectivity, the most useful indicators being serum bilirubin, albumin, prothrombin time, and creatinine. The two main scoring systems for liver disease severity are the Child-Pugh score[19] (Table 31–1) and the Model for End-stage Liver Disease (MELD) Score[20] (Equation 31–1). Specific serologic markers may be useful in defining etiology for viral hepatitis, or for some of the metabolic diseases with antimitochondrial antibody, iron studies, 1-antitrypsin, or ceruloplasmin levels. In addition, alpha-fetoprotein (AFP) should be measured in all such patients as a screening test for hepatoma.

TABLE 31–1. CHILD-PUGH SCORE

Parameter	1 Point	2 Points	3 Points
Serum bilirubin (mg/dL)	<2	2–3	<3
Albumin (g/dL)	>3.5	2.8–3.5	<2.8
Prothrombin time (↑ S)	1–3	4–6	>6
Ascites	None	Slight	Moderate
Encephalopathy	None	1–2	3–4

Grades: A, 5 to 6 points
B, 7 to 9 points
C, 10 to 15 points

Equation 31–1.

MELD SCORE

$$\text{Score} = 0.957 \times \log_e \text{creatinine (mg/dL)} + 0.378 \times \log_e \text{bilirubin (mg/dL)} + 1.120 \log_e \text{INR}.$$

When a patient has portal hypertension, usually shown by varices, a cause must be found. If clinical and lab studies do not fit, imaging and a liver biopsy may be indicated. Quantitative liver testing with studies such as indocyanine green clearance, galactose elimination capacity, and MEG-X formation are advocated by some, but have not proved to be clinically useful.

Imaging is initially with ultrasound to show overall liver morphology and potentially to pick up focal lesions suggestive of hepatoma. Contrast-enhanced CT scan or MRI may be required for morphologic assessment. Liver biopsy may be required to confirm that some patients do have underlying cirrhosis, and in cases of focal lesions, to differentiate hepatocellular carcinoma from regenerative nodules. In the latter a biopsy of the uninvolved liver is performed as well as the focal lesion to assess for cirrhosis.

Vascular anatomy is evaluated with imaging modalities of escalating complexity depending on information required for management.[21–23] Doppler ultrasound can assess the hepatic artery, portal and hepatic veins and this may be all that is required. Documenting size, directional flow, velocities, and wave-form patterns of the portal and hepatic veins is a standard procedure. Tributaries to the portal vein—the superior mesenteric and splenic veins, and large collaterals such as the coronary and umbilical vein may also be readily defined. The most important information that the clinician needs to know is the patency (or thrombosis) of the portal vein. Hepatic artery patency, course, and resistive index can be assessed with Doppler ultrasound.

The next level of complexity for evaluating the liver circulation is with CT scan or MRI. These two modalities may be combined with CT or MR angiography (MRA). The speed of scanners, new contrast enhancing agents, and the increasingly advanced software for data reconstruction allows sophisticated imaging of the liver's arterial and venous anatomy. These methods have improved preoperative planning for living donor liver transplantation and liver resection.

Finally, angiography still plays a role for direct pressure measurement and clarification when the prior modalities are unclear. Portal pressure is measured indirectly from the hepatic veins by measuring wedged and free hepatic vein pressures, with the difference being the hepatic venous pressure gradient (HVPG).[24] This is done using a balloon occlusion technique akin to a Swan-Ganz catheter measurement in the pulmonary circulation. Normal HVPG is 6 to 8 mm Hg, and in cirrhosis will be >10 mm Hg. There has been resurgence of interest in HPVG to measure response to pharmacologic therapy. Direct portal pressure measurement also can be done by the transjugular, transhepatic route. This method, useful in the acute situation particularly when combined with TIPS, is not used for repeated measurements.

Upper GI endoscopy is used to assess varices. All patients with cirrhosis should have an upper endoscopy. This recommendation is based on epidemiologic studies that have shown:

- Thirty percent of patients with cirrhosis develop portal hypertension.
- Thirty percent of patients with portal hypertension will bleed from varices within 2 years.
- The rate of development of varices in patients with cirrhosis is approximately 8% per year.

Endoscopy should focus on the presence of varices; the size, extent, and tortuosity; and the presence or absence of red color signs. Large varices with red color signs are at greater risk of bleeding. In patients with cirrhosis and upper GI bleeding, endoscopy may be both diagnostic and therapeutic with banding. Following an acute variceal bleed, the extent of varices should be assessed after stabilization. Grading systems for varices have been developed and validated by the Japanese[25] and Italians.[26] Finally, the gastric mucosa should be evaluated for evidence of portal hypertensive gastropathy with congestion and cobble stoning.[27] Gastric varices may also be seen, with isolated gastric varices being more problematic than gastric varices in continuity with esophageal varicies.[28]

MANAGEMENT OF VARICEAL BLEEDING

Figure 31–2 illustrates a management algorithm for variceal bleeding that requires a multidisciplinary team, and may vary from center to center depending on available expertise. The team should have a predetermined, step-wise management plan for patients with variceal bleeding. This algorithm will form the basis for further discussion of patients.

The therapies available for treating variceal bleeding are:

- Pharmacotherapy
- Endoscopic therapy
- Decompressive shunts—radiologic or surgical
- Devascularization operations
- Liver transplantation

Pharmacologic therapy plays a role in preventing the initial bleed, managing the acute variceal bleed, and as first-line treatment in preventing rebleeding.

Non–cardioselective beta-blockers (Inderal [propranolol hydrochloride] or nadolol) were showed by Lebrec and his colleagues in the early 1980s to reduce portal hypertension.[12] This major contribution to the management of patients has stood the test of time and remains the mainstay of prophylactic therapy. Patients with moderate- to large-size varices should be placed on one of these drugs. Not all patients tolerate beta-blockers or are responsive to them, with a noncompliance or fallout rate of about 20%. It has been shown in the last decade that patients who have >20% reduction in their HVPG or who reduce their HVPG to <12 mm Hg will not bleed. These are the target treatment goals for beta-blockers in prophylaxis.[29]

Propranolol and Nadolol are used as initial therapy to prevent rebleeding, with the same caveats for tolerance, response rates, and targets for therapy. Many other pharmacologic agents have been evaluated over the last three decades such as long-acting nitrates, serotonin antagonists, 2-agonists, and calcium channel blockers. None of these have been shown to be as efficacious as the beta-blockers, and while combination therapy has been beneficial in some studies, it has been limited by side effects.[29,30] Continuing investigation of pharmacologic management of portal hypertension remains one of the important areas of clinical investigation.

Pharmacologic therapy for acute variceal bleeding has a longer history. Vasopressin was the first drug

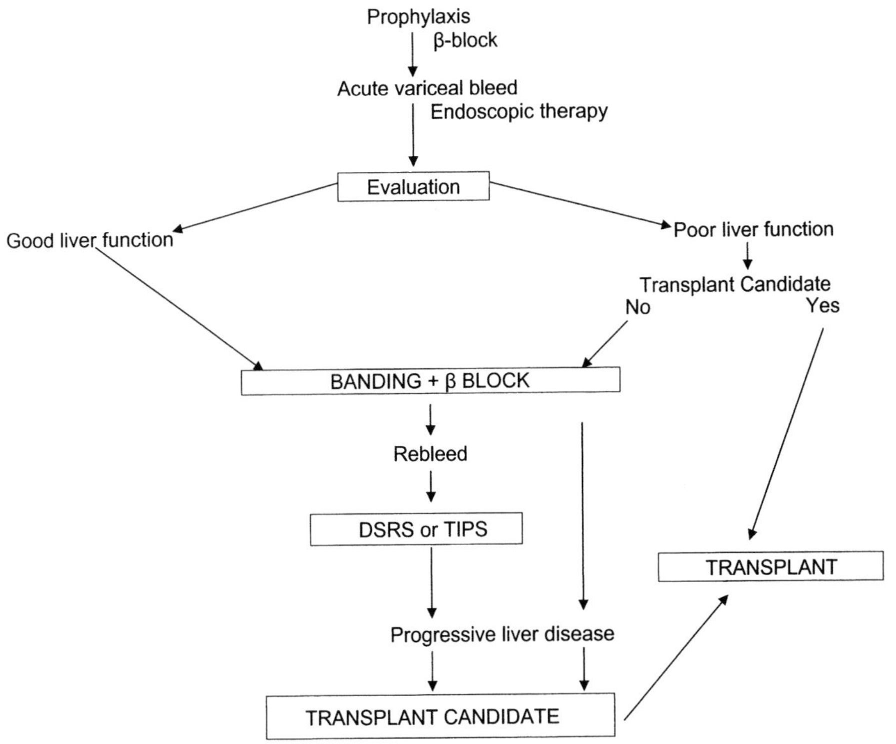

Figure 31–2. Algorithm for management of patients with variceal bleeding.

used and has been largely replaced by somatostatin or one of its analogs. Both of these drugs effectively reduce portal pressure in the patient with acute variceal bleeding. Vasopressin has significant side effects with systemic vasoconstriction, and although these can be minimized with a concomitant infusion of nitroglycerin, clinical practice has moved to the use of octreotide. Octreotide infused at 50 μg/hour is a safe and easy drug to use in this setting. In Europe, Terlipressin is available, has fewer side effects than vasopressin, and is widely used for acute variceal bleeding.

▪ ENDOSCOPIC THERAPY

The current standard for endoscopic therapy for esophageal varices is endoscopic banding.[11] This has largely replaced endoscopic sclerotherapy because it has fewer side effects, obliterates varices faster, and, with new technology, can be easily applied. Multiband ligators can be fitted on the end of the endoscope and allow the firing of six to eight bands in a spiral fashion on to columns of varices. The varix is sucked into the end of the applicator, and the band fired around its base. The bands will slough off in 5 to 7 days with less ulceration over the varices than induced by sclerotherapy, and hence a lower initial rebleeding rate. Endoscopic banding can be used in the patient with acute variceal bleeding providing the bleeding varix can be identified. A course of banding—usually 2 to 3 sessions—is then applied over the next month to 6 weeks in an attempt to obliterate the varices at the gastroesophageal junction. Occasionally, endoscopic sclerotherapy with injection of a sclerosing solution may be a useful adjunct to complete the obliteration of smaller varices that can not be banded.

Many prospective, randomized controlled trials have documented better control of bleeding with endoscopic banding than sclerotherapy, with lower morbidity. However, the mortality was not significantly different between banded or sclerosed patients in these trials.[31]

From a practical point of view, patients with an acute variceal bleed should have their bleeding controlled with an endoscopic session, have their varices obliterated with a course of banding, and be placed on a non–cardioselective beta-blocker for long-term management. This constitutes first-line treatment.

▪ DECOMPRESSIVE SHUNTS

This component of management of variceal bleeding has changed dramatically over the last two decades. Decompression is considered second line treatment and is reserved for patients who rebleed through endoscopic banding and beta-blockers or whose varices remain "high risk." Very few surgical shunts are performed at

rior wall and interrupted sutures to the anterior wall. The splenic vein stump is tied with a large clip placed behind it, which has been found to be the lowest risk for portal vein thrombosis. Portal vein thrombosis will occur in 4–5% of patients after DSRS and up to 20% may show some nonoccluding thrombus following this procedure. The operation is completed by interrupting the other collateral pathways between the portal vein and the shunt, most specifically the coronary vein needs to be ligated flush with the splenic or portal vein.

Postoperative management for all of these surgical procedures requires attention to detail. Patients should be managed in a monitored environment for 24 hours to make sure they are hemodynamically stable and there is no early postoperative bleeding. Under resuscitation is better than over resuscitation as one of the major risks in this group of patients, who still have a cirrhotic liver, is ascites. Attention to detail in fluid management, infection prophylaxis, nutrition, and careful monitoring of hepatic function are the key steps. It is this author's opinion that shunt patency should be documented prior to hospital discharge with further imaging studies of the portal circulation. Direct shunt catheterization is the most definitive way to document shunt patency and measure pressure gradients.

▪ TRANSJUGULAR INTRAHEPATIC PORTAL SYSTEMIC SHUNT

TIPS has gained increasing popularity over the last two decades, and is now the most widely used method for decompressing portal hypertension in patients with variceal bleeding or ascites.[42–44] It is an important part of the repertoire for the multidisciplinary team managing these patients. Figure 31–6 shows the principles of TIPS. The technical approach to TIPS is direct puncture of the internal jugular vein, passage of a catheter through the right atrium in to one of the major hepatic veins—usually the right vein—followed by a transparenchymal puncture of the liver to cannulate the portal vein. The catheter is passed in to the portal vein and pressure is measured. The portal vein puncture may be aided by ultrasound definition of its location. The intraparenchymal track is then dilated and the track stented with an expandable metal stent in the 10- to 12-mm-diameter range. Pressures are again measured and the goal is to decrease the gradient between the portal vein and the right atrium to <10 mm Hg. The technical success rate is high (>90%) with a low procedural morbidity and mortality (<10%). Patients are usually in the hospital for 1 to 2 days and the shunt patency should be documented the day after the procedure with a Doppler ultrasound.

The major issue with TIPS is its restenosis and thrombosis rates. This leads to the need for careful monitoring, and frequent repeat procedures with dilation and/or shunt extension. The risk of early thrombosis seems to be related to bile duct puncture as the parenchymal track is developed. Bile is extremely thrombogenic and occlusion of the TIPS occurring in the first 24 hours suggests this etiology. Covered TIPS stents reduce this risk. Late stenosis (over the next several months) occurs most commonly at the hepatic vein end of the stent, although it may be seen at the portal vein end or mid-shunt.

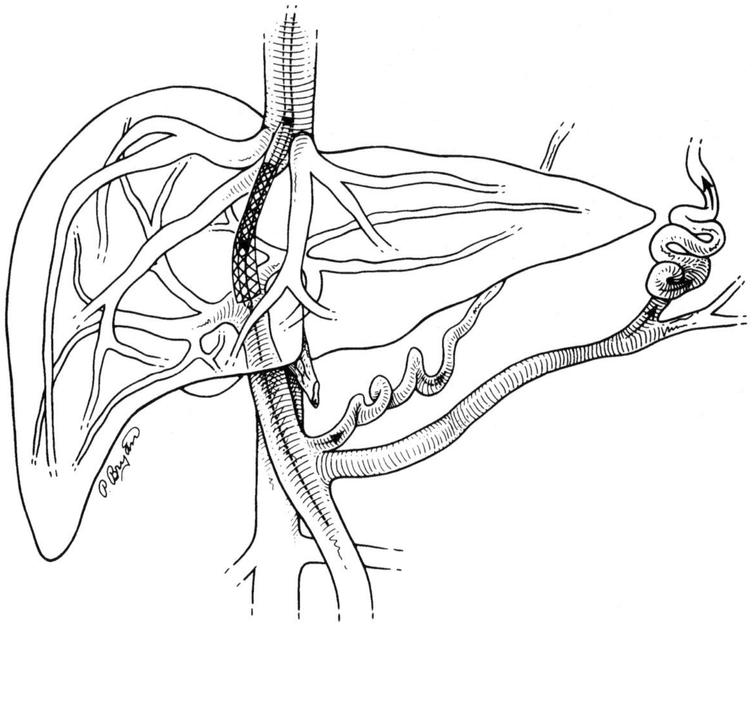

Figure 31–6. Transjugular intrahepatic portal systemic shunt (TIPS). This side-to-side shunt has variable hemodynamic effect depending on its diameter.

While a Doppler ultrasound will document patency, it has not proved to be a sensitive method for documenting stenoses. Changes in velocity may give some indication of hemodynamic changes within the stent, but direct measurement of the pressure gradient is required to document stenosis. Reintervention rates to maintain patency are high, ranging from 40–80%. The introduction of covered stents has reduced this stenosis rate with the rate of shunt dysfunction being significantly less in the covered stent group in a randomized, controlled study.[45] The overall published rebleeding rates for TIPS are around 20%, and this was reduced to 13% in the covered stent trial.[45]

Most centers have developed standard follow-up protocols to monitor TIPS, which call for repeated Doppler ultrasounds at 6 weeks, 3 months, and four times per year.[42] This should be supplemented by a protocol recatheterization of the shunt on an annual basis.

The initial reports of TIPS—which is a total portal systemic shunt—showed new encephalopathy rates around 30%. Most of this encephalopathy appears to be relatively easily controlled with lactulose and/or some minimal protein restriction.

▪ DEVASCULARIZATION PROCEDURES

These operations approach the problem of variceal bleeding by interrupting inflow to the varices. The components are splenectomy, gastric and esophageal devascularization, and possibly esophageal transaction (Fig 31–7).[46] The effectiveness of these procedures appears to depend on the aggressiveness of the operation. Popularized by Sugiura in Japan,[46] and Hassab in Egypt, good results have been obtained in these countries. The advantage of these procedures is that portal hypertension is maintained with portal flow to the cirrhotic liver. Control of variceal bleeding in the originators hands has been >90%,[47] but higher rebleeding rates (~30%) have been seen in Europe and the United States.[48] These results are probably related to applying this operation to poorer risk patients who are not candidates for other operations and inadequate operative devascularization. More recent application of devascularization procedures by Orozco and colleagues in Mexico has achieved good results with a 10% rebleeding rate.[49]

From a technical perspective, the original Sugiura operation combined an abdominal and a thoracic procedure either as a single or two-stage approach. More recently, most surgeons have approached devascularizations purely from an abdominal approach. Standard devascularization operations include splenectomy, but Orozco and colleagues have published data indicating this is not essential. The whole of the greater curve should be devascularized, at least 7 cm of the distal esophagus, and finally the upper two thirds of the lesser curve of the stomach. Attempts are made to keep the vagus nerve intact and the devascularization has the appearances of a proximal gastric vagotomy as the operation is completed. As many of these patients have received sclerotherapy or banding prior to operative intervention, most do not need an esophageal transection, which can be difficult with the thickened esophagus.

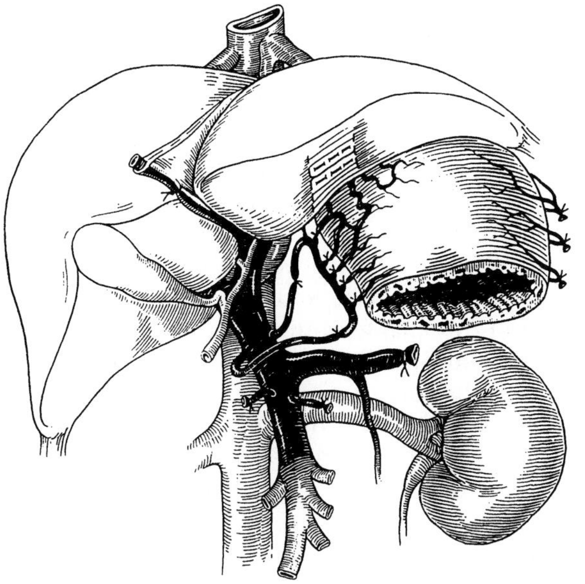

Figure 31–7. Gastroesophageal devascularization for variceal bleeding. Splenectomy, gastric and esophageal devascularization, and esophageal transection are the components of these operations.

Devascularization can be useful when patients have extensive portal and splenic venous thrombosis and there are no other operative or radiologic options. Extensive devascularization will reduce the risk of bleeding in such patients, and this remains the main indication for this operation.

Postoperative management requires attention to detail to minimize the risk of ascites as these patients still have portal hypertension. Follow-up endoscopy around 6 months is often helpful to document if there are any residual varices, treat them endoscopically at that time, or document the completeness of the devascularization procedure.

Overall, the bleeding rates can be reduced to <20% with this procedure and encephalopathy rates are low.

▪ LIVER TRANSPLANT

Liver transplant plays a key role in the management of patients with portal hypertension at the present time.[50–52]

This surgical treatment option has been THE major advance in the treatment of patients with advanced liver disease and sequelae of portal hypertension. The major issues are patient selection, timing of transplant, expanding the donor pool, and outcomes.

Patient selection for transplant is evolving. The indication for transplant is end-stage liver disease, but definition of this in the field of hepatology is a moving target. Variceal bleeding per se is not necessarily an indication of end-stage liver disease but, as indicated earlier in this chapter, other manifestations of portal hypertension such as ascites and encephalopathy are clinical indicators of end-stage liver disease. Patient selection also depends on other variables such as comorbid medical conditions and a psychosocial suitability for transplant particularly in the alcoholic and other chemical dependency patient populations. The increase in the incidence of hepatoma, particularly in the hepatitis C population, has also changed indications for patient selection for liver transplant. In many of these patients, there are other concomitant manifestations of portal hypertension such as variceal bleeding. Standards for patient listing have been set by United Network for Organ Sharing (UNOS), with evolving indications proposed by individual liver centers considered by regional review boards. This remains a field in evolution.

The timing of transplant is dictated by the severity of the underlying liver disease. Prioritization occurs on the basis of MELD scores, with sickest patients receiving cadaveric organs first. Variceal bleeding no longer gives a patient priority, nor does the clinical syndrome of ascites. Objective criteria, based on bilirubin, prothrombin time, and serum creatinine, have to show sufficient indications of end-stage disease for patients to receive a high enough priority score for transplant. Timing is therefore dictated by objective criteria rather than individual physician decisions in day-to-day patient management. The donor pool for liver transplant has changed over the last several years. The increasing public awareness of the need for organ donation, the use of "expanded donor" criteria with concomitant documentation that these organs do work, and the application of living donor transplant have gone some way to alleviate the donor shortage. The direct impact of these changes on the donor pool, the systems of organ allocation and prioritization, and individual center philosophies and priorities for their patients have changed and will continue to change the role of liver transplantation in portal hypertension.

The outcomes with liver transplant have continued to improve. The fear that pushing organs to the sickest patients would lead to poorer outcomes has not been fulfilled over the last 2 to 3 years. Hospital mortality remains at less than 10%, despite transplanting sicker and sicker patients and despite using more "marginal" organs. This is testimony to the advances in the fields of organ preservation and overall patient management during and following liver transplantation. The expectation therefore for outcomes is a less than 10% hospital mortality and an 80+% 1-year survival with a 60–65% 5-year survival for liver transplant.

Technical aspects of liver transplant are beyond the scope of this chapter other than a few brief pointers. Liver transplant has become the major role for the surgeon interested in managing patients with portal hypertension. Whole organ grafts, partial segmental grafts, living donor grafts, techniques of caval preservation, alternative methods of revascularization, and improved methods for biliary reconstruction have all contributed to technical advances in liver transplantation over the past decade. In addition to these technical advances in the transplant field itself, the increasing number of surgeons who have developed this expertise also represent the pool of surgeons with the ability to conduct some of the operative procedures described earlier in this chapter.

The management and longer-term follow-up of patients with portal hypertension coming to liver transplant is likewise an evolving field. Improvement in methods of immunosuppression, infection prophylaxis and treatment, patient monitoring to reduce the risk of transplant-related malignancy, and long-term health maintenance after transplant are ongoing fields of investigation and improvement. The net result of all of these advances is that patients with Child's Class C cirrhosis, variceal bleeding, and advanced liver disease can now look forward to a reasonable chance of long-term survival, whereas 15 to 20 years ago, they had a 15–20% chance of long-term survival.

■ MANAGEMENT STRATEGIES

VARICEAL BLEEDING

The treatment options just described need to be used appropriately in treatment strategies for:

- Prophylaxis
- Acute variceal bleeding
- Prevention of rebleeding

PROPHYLAXIS

Beta-blockers should be used for all patients with medium or large varices to reduce their risk of an initial bleed. Bleeding risk can be reduced from 30% to 18–20% with beta-blocker treatment. Multiple randomized controlled trials have documented this benefit. Patients with cirrhosis should have a screening endoscopy to assess for varices and initiate treatment if appropriate.[29,30]

Endoscopic therapy for prophylaxis does not have a proven role at this time.[53] Most data has been with trials using sclerotherapy, and the introduction of banding had raised questions of a role for prophylactic banding in patients with high-risk or large varices. This is acceptable management, but data are not yet clear as to proven advantages over beta-blocker alone. Surgical therapy or radiologic shunts are not indicated in prophylaxis prior to an initial variceal bleed.[30]

ACUTE VARICEAL BLEEDING

Acute variceal bleeding may require several treatment modalities and outcome has improved in the past decade.[54] Most important is the overall management of the patient rather than the specific therapies. Airway protection, appropriate fluid resuscitation, adequate monitoring, and antibiotic prophylaxis are all now standard of care for such patients. Transfusion of blood for bleeding, blood products for coagulopathy must be carefully monitored with a target of under rather than over resuscitation. Pharmacologic therapy with intravenous octreotide (50 μg/hour) will reduce portal pressure and should be initiated on suspicion of a variceal bleed. Early endoscopy, both for diagnosis and initial banding therapy, is the mainstay of treatment.[55] Endoscopic banding can be done provided the varix is visualized and can be sucked into the end of the scope. In the occasional patient in whom endoscopic therapy cannot be performed, balloon tamponade should be used to control bleeding. Inflation of the gastric balloon alone, pulled gently up into the gastric fundus, will usually suffice to control bleeding. If that fails to control the bleeding the esophageal balloon may need to be inflated to 40 mm Hg. Placement of a tamponade balloon mandates further reintervention within 24 hours, and this is usually an indication for an emergency TIPS procedure.

TIPS is required in less than 10% of patients with acute variceal bleeding.[42] Emergency TIPS placement needs to be treated in the same way as if the patient was going to the operating room. Airway protection, careful monitoring, and appropriate fluid management and resuscitation are required. While the radiologist is concentrating on the technical aspects of placing an accurate decompressing TIPS shunt, the patient overall management team needs to assure all other aspects of care are completed.

The patient with an acute variceal bleeding episode still carries a significant mortality risk, death most commonly resulting from decompensation of the underlying liver disease. A major bleed requires an ICU admission, but once the patient has been stabilized, they can be transferred to a regular hospital floor. Early evaluation and follow-up endoscopy to initiate an elective course of banding is the next step in overall patient management.

▪ PREVENTION OF REBLEEDING

The first-line treatment for prevention of rebleeding is a course of variceal banding and concomitant pharmacologic therapy with a beta-blocker no matter what the underlying cause.[29,30] The first elective banding episode should be performed within three or four days of the acute bleeding episode and as many bands placed as necessary to obliterate the columns of varices in the distal esophagus. Subsequently one or two banding sessions will probably be required to obliterate these varices. A beta-blocker is started with the target of reducing the pulse rate by 20% and with the plan to use this for long-term therapy.

Overall patient care also mandates a full evaluation of the patient at this timepoint.[56,57] An understanding of the etiology of the liver disease, its severity, its likely natural history, and looking for other complications of portal hypertension should be completed at this stage. Several possible case scenarios may emerge:

- Good risk patient—Child's A patient/MELD <10. If a patient still looks like a Child's A patient after a variceal bleed and has a MELD score less than 10, they probably have well-compensated liver disease. This patient should be treated with first-line treatment, but if they rebleed or have failure to obliterate their varices with banding, they may be a candidate for decompression with TIPS or distal splenorenal shunt.
- Indeterminate patient—Child's B/MELD 10 through 16. The majority of patients will fall into this category after their variceal bleed with some disturbance in their liver lab numbers, possibly developing ascites, and having an unpredictable course for their liver disease. From a management perspective, the question is whether the patient will improve to a Child's A patient, remain a Child's B patient, or move toward end-stage disease. Their initial treatment is with endoscopic banding and a beta-blocker. Subsequent treatment depends on their course.
- End-stage liver disease—Child's C/MELD >16. If initial evaluation shows the patient has Child's C

cirrhosis and clearly is not improving with routine clinical management, consideration needs to be given to full transplant evaluation. The severity of the bleeding episode may play some role in whether or not the patient's disease will return to a "compensated" level or whether they will continue to deteriorate secondary to the acute bleeding episode.

Failure of first-line treatment can occur in several scenarios. The main reasons are: (1) the patient may have a further acute variceal bleed, (2) the patient may have recurring small bleeding episodes that are not transfusion-requiring, or (3) the patient may fail to have their varices obliterated and continue to have large varices with risk factors. Patients with any of the above scenarios, who also have advanced liver disease, are candidates for liver transplantation, possibly using TIPS as a bridge. Any of the above occurring in patients with well-compensated liver disease (Child's class A) may lead to variceal decompression with DSRS or TIPS.

Decompression with TIPS versus a surgical shunt has recently been evaluated in two randomized controlled trials. Rosemurgy and associates[36] studied the relative benefits of TIPS versus the 8-mm portocaval H-graft shunt. In their "all comers" study of 132 patients, 50% of their population were Child's class C patients. They showed a significantly lower rebleeding rate, and significantly lower rate of need for transplant with the surgical shunt compared to the TIPS group, but no significant difference in survival.

A randomized trial compared DSRS to TIPS at five clinical centers in 140 Child's class A and B patients who failed first-line treatment.[58] Data showed no significant difference in rebleeding rates (5.5% DSRS group, 10.5% TIPS group), no significant difference in the times to first encephalopathy episode with 50% of patients in each group having at least one episode of encephalopathy by 5 years, and no significant difference in survival between the two groups. However, the reintervention rate in the TIPS group was significantly (p <.001) higher at 82% compared to a reintervention rate of 11% in the DSRS group. The rate of total thrombosis was significantly higher in the TIPS group compared to the DSRS group. This indicated the need for intensive surveillance in the TIPS group compared to the DSRS patients to achieve the low rebleeding rate seen in the TIPS group in this trial.

ASCITES

The management of ascites is primarily medical with dietary salt restriction and diuretics (spironolactone and furosemide).[59] When ascites becomes refractory to such a regimen, large volume paracentesis or TIPS may be considered, but these are a "bridge" to transplant. As indicated above, refractory ascites is one of the major clinical signs of end-stage liver disease. Four randomized trials have shown benefit and better control of ascites with TIPS compared to large volume paracentesis, but survival benefit was only shown in two of four studies.[60–63]

Surgical shunt is no longer indicated for management of ascites. The surgeon does, however, play a role in treating such patients as liver transplant is the best therapy for patients with intractable ascites. The issue is candidacy for and availability of transplant.

THE TEAM

As indicated at the beginning of this chapter, optimal management of portal hypertension, and particularly variceal bleeding, requires a multidisciplinary team approach. The members of the patient care team are:

- Nursing, nurse clinicians, and physician assistants who frequently coordinate all components, communicate with the patients and families, and help develop and implement diagnostic and management protocols
- Hepatologists who play a key role in diagnosis, prognosis, overall therapy strategies, and determining the timing for specific interventions
- Endoscopists who must be skilled and up to date in diagnostic severity grading, and therapeutic options for treating variceal bleeding
- Radiologists who have a diagnostic and therapeutic role in portal hypertension. As their diagnostic role becomes less invasive, their therapeutic role with TIPS has grown.
- Surgeons whose expertise in liver transplant is essential, with some residual role for surgical shunts in highly selected patients. Surgery must also bring overall patient management expertise to the team.
- Intensivists/Anesthesiologists who bring expertise in the differences these patients have in fluid/electrolyte/transfusion required in their ICU stays or for procedure management.

There is no question that the major advances in patient care in the past two decades in this field have been in bringing all these areas of expertise together. Variceal bleeding and portal hypertension remain difficult clinical problems. Advances discussed in this chapter are leading to improved care for all patients.

REFERENCES

1. Reuben A, Groszmann RJ. Portal Hypertension: A History. In: Sanyal AJ, Shah VH (eds). *Portal Hypertension: Pathobiology, evaluation, and treatment.* Totowa, NJ: Humana Press;2005:3–14
2. Donovan AJ, Covey PC. Early history of the portacaval shunt in humans. *Surg Gyn Obstet* 1978;147:423–430
3. Whipple AO. The problem of portal hypertension in relation to the hepatosplenopathies. *Ann Surg* 1945;122: 449–456
4. Drapanas T. Interposition mesocaval shunt for treatment of portal hypertension. *Ann Surg* 1972;176:435–448
5. Warren WD, Zeppa R, Fomon JJ. Selective trans-splenic decompression of gastroesophageal varices by distal splenorenal shunt. *Ann Surg* 1967;166:437–455
6. Inokuchi K. A selective portacaval shunt. *Lancet* 1968;ii: 51–52
7. Sarfeh IJ, Rypins EB, Mason GR. A systematic appraisal of portocaval H-graft diameters. Clinical and hemodynamic perspectives. *Ann Surg* 1986;204:356–363
8. Johnston GW, Rogers HW. A review of 15 years experience in the use of sclerotherapy in the control of acute hemorrhage from esophageal varices. *Br J Surg* 1973;60:797
9. Terblanche J, Northover JMA, Bornmann PC et al. A prospective controlled trial of sclerotherapy in the long term management of patients after esophageal variceal bleeding. *Surg Gynecol Obstet* 1979;148:323–333
10. Paquet KJ, Oberhammerk E. Sclerotherapy of bleeding esophageal varices by means of endoscopy. *Endoscopy* 1978;10:7–12
11. Steigmann GV, Goff JS, Sunn JH, et al. Endoscopic variceal ligation: an alternative to sclerotherapy. *Gastrointest Endoscopy* 1989;35:431–434
12. Lebrie D, Novel O, Corbic M, et al. Propanolol: a medical treatment for portal hypertension? *Lancet* 1980;2: 180–182
13. Rosch J, Hanafee W, Snow H, et al. Transjugular intrahepatic portacaval shunt. An Experimental work. *Am J Surg* 1971;121:588–592
14. Starzl TE, Groth CG, Brettschneider L, et al. Orthotopic homostransplantation of the human liver. *Ann Surg* 1968;168:392–415
15. Calne RY, Williams R. Liver transplantation in man. Observations on techniques and organization in 5 cases. *Br Med J* 1968;4:535–550
16. Bosch J, Pizcueta P, Fen F, et al. Pathophysiology of portal hypertension. *Gastroenterol Clin North Am* 1992;21:1–14
17. Groszmann RJ: Hyperdynamic circulation of liver disease forty years later: pathophysiology and clinical consequences. *Hepatology* 1994;20:1359–1363
18. Benhamou JP, Valla D: Intrahepatic portal hypertension. In Bircher J, Benhamou JP, McIntyre N, Rizzatto M, Rodes J (eds). *Clinical Hepatology.* Oxford: Oxford Univ Press; 1999:661–669
19. Pugh RN, Murray-Lyon IM, Dawson JL, et al. Transection of the esophagus for bleeding esophageal variceal. *Br J Surg* 1973;60:646–649
20. Kamath PS, Wiesner RH, Malinchoc M, et al: A model to predict survival in patients with end-stage liver disease. *Hepatology* 2001;33:464–470
21. Burns P, Taylor K, Biel AT. Doppler flowmetry and portal hypertension. *Gastroenterology* 1987;92:824–826
22. Oliver TW, Sones PH. Hepatic angiography: portal hypertension. In: Bernardino ME, Sones PH (eds). *Hepatic Radiology.* New York: Macmillan;1984:243–275
23. Bolondi L, Gatta A, Groszmann RJ, et al. Imaging techniques and hemodynamic measurements in portal hypertension. Baveno II consensus statement. In DeFrancis R (ed). *Baveno II Consensus Workshop.* Oxford: Blackwell Science;1996:67
24. Groszmann RJ, Wangcharatrawee S. The hepatic venous pressure gradient: anything worth doing should be done right. *Hepatology* 2004;39:280–282
25. Beppu K, Mokuchi K Kayanagi N, et al. Prediction of variceal hemorrhage by esophageal endoscopy. *Gastrointest Endoscopy* 1981;27:213–218
26. The North Italian Endoscopic Club for the Study and Treatment of Esophageal Varices. Prediction of the first variceal hemorrhage in patients with cirrhosis of the liver and esophageal varices. *N Engl J Med* 1988;319:983–989
27. Stewart C, Sanyal A. Grading portal gastropathy: a validation of a gastropathy scoring system. *Am J Gastroenterol* 2003;98:1758–1765
28. Hashizume M, Kitano S, Yamaga H, et al. Endoscopic classification and natural history of gastric varices: a long-term follow-up study in 568 portal hypertension patients. *Hepatology* 1992;16:1343–1349
29. D'Amico G, Pagliano L, Bosch J. Pharmacologic treatment of portal hypertension: an evidence based approached. *Semin Liver Dis* 1999;19:475–505
30. D'Amico G, Criscuoli V, Fili D, Pagliano L. Meta-analysis of trials for variceal bleeding. *Hepatology* 2002;36:1023–1024
31. Laine L, Cook D, Endoscopic ligation compared with sclerotherapy for treatment of esophageal variceal bleeding. *Ann Int Med* 1995;123:280–287
32. Orloff MJ, Orloff MS, Orloff SL, et al. Three decades of experience with emergency portacaval shunt for acutely bleeding esophageal varices in 400 unselected patients with cirrhosis of the liver. *J Am Coll Surg* 1995;180:257–272
33. Stipa S, Balducci G, Ziparo V, et al. Total shunting and elective management of variceal bleeding. *World J Surg* 1994;18:200–204
34. Henderson JM, Warren WD, Millikan WJ Jr, et al. Surgical options, hematologic evaluation, and pathologic changes in Budd-Chiari syndrome. *Am J Surg* 1990;159: 41–48; discussion 48–50
35. Collins CJ, Ong MJ, Rypins EB, et al. Partial portacaval shunt for variceal hemorrhage: longitudinal analysis of effectiveness. *Arch Surg* 1986;204:356–363
36. Rosemrugy AS, Serofini FM, Zweibal BR, et al: TIPS versus small diameter prosthetic H-graft protacaval shunt: extended follow-up of an expanded randomized prospective trial. *J Gastrointest Surg* 2000;4:589–597

37. Spina GP, Henderson JM, Rikkers LF, et al. Distal spleno-renal shunts versus endoscopic sclerotherapy in the prevention of variceal rebleeding. A meta-analysis of 4 randomized clinical trials. *J Hepatol* 1992;16:338–345
38. Henderson JM, Nagle A, Curtas S, et al. Surgical shunts and TIPS for variceal decompression in the 1990's. *Surgery* 2000;128:540–547
39. Jenkins RL, Gedaly R, Pomposelli JJ, et al. Distal splenorenal shunt: role, indications, and utility in the era of liver transplantation. *Arch Surg* 1999;134:416–420
40. Orozco H, Mercado MA, Garcia JG, et al. Selective shunts for portal hypertension current role of a 21 year experience. *Liver Transplant Surg* 1997;3:475–480
41. Rikkers LF, Jin G, Langnas AN, et al. Shunt surgery during the era of liver transplantation. *Ann Surg* 1997;226: 51–57
42. Boyer TD, Haskal ZJ. The role of transjugular intrahepatic portosystemic shunt in the management of portal hypertension. *Hepatology* 2005;41:386–400
43. Papatheodoridis GV, Goulis J, Leandro G, et al. Transjugular intrahepatic portosystemic shunt compared with endoscopic treatment for prevention of variceal rebleeding: a meta-analysis. *Hepatology* 1999;30:612–622
44. Burroughs AK, Vangoli M. Transjugular intrahepatic portosystemic shunt versus endoscopic therapy: randomized trials for secondary prophylaxis of variceal bleeding. An updated meta-analysis. *Scand J Gastroenterol* 2002;37:249–252
45. Bureau C, Garcia-Pagan JC, Otal P, et al. Improved clinical outcome using polytetrafluoroethylene-coated stents for TIPS: results of a randomized study. *Gastroenterology* 2004;126:469–475
46. Sugiura M, Futagawa S. Esophageal transaction with paraesophagogastric devascularizations (the Sugiura procedure) in the treatment of esophageal varices. *World J Surg* 1984;8:673–679
47 Idezuki Y, Kokudo N, Sanjo K, et al. Sugiura procedure for management of variceal bleeding in Japan. *World J Surg* 1994;18:216–221
48. Dagenais M, Langer B, Taylor BR, et al. Experience with radical esophagogastric devascularization procedures (Sugiura) for variceal bleeding outside Japan. *World J Surg* 1994;18:222–228
49. Orozco H, Mercado MA, Takahashi T, et al. Elective treatment of bleeding varices with the Sugiura operation over 10 years. *Am J Surg* 1992;13:585–589
50. Henderson JM. Liver transplantation for portal hypertension. *Gastroenterol Clin North Am* 1992; 21:197
51. Ringe B, Lang H, Tusch G, et al. role of liver transplantation in management of esophageal variceal hemorrhage. *World J Surg* 1994;18:233
52. Abu-Elmagd K, Iwatsuki S. Portal hypertension: role of liver transplantation. In: Cameron J (ed). *Current Surgical Therapy,* 7th ed. St. Louis, Mosby; 2001:406–413
53. Imperiale TF, Chalasani N. A meta-analysis of endoscopic variceal ligation for primary prophylaxis of esophageal variceal bleeding. *Hepatology* 2001;33:802–807
54. Chalasani N, Kahi C, Francois F, et al. Improved patient survival after acute variceal bleeding: a multi-center, cohort study. *Am J Gastroenterol* 2003;98:653–659
55. Banarus R, Albillos A, Rincon D, et al. Endoscopic treatment versus endoscopic plus pharmacologic treatment for acute variceal bleeding: a meta-analysis. *Hepatology* 2002;35:609–615
56. Zoli M, Merkel C, Magalotti D, et al. Natural history of cirrhotic patients with small esophageal varices: a prospective study. *Am J Gastroenterol* 2000;95:503–508
57. Defranchis R. Evaluation and follow-up of patients with cirrhosis and esophageal varices. *J Hepatology* 2003;38: 361–363
58. Henderson JM, Boyer TD, Kutner MH, et al. DSRS vs TIPS for refractory variceal bleeding: a prospective randomized controlled trial (abstract). *Hepatology* 40:725A
59. Moore KP, Wang F, Gines P, et al. The management of ascites: report on the consensus conference of the International Ascites Club. *Hepatology* 2003;38:258–266
60. Lebrie D, Giuily N, Hadenque A, et al. Transjugular intrahepatic portosystemic shunt: comparison with paracentesis in patients with cirrhosis and refractory ascites. A randomized trial. *J Hepatol* 1996;25:135–144
61. Rossle M, Oclis A, Gulberg V, et al: A comparison of paracentesis and transjugular intrahepatic portosystemic shunting in patients with ascites. *N Engl J Med* 2000;342:1701–1707
62. Sanyal A, Gennings G, Reddy KR, et al. A randomized controlled study of TIPS versus larger volume paracentesis in the treatment of refractory ascites. *Gastroenterol* 2003;124:634–643
63. Gines P, Uriz J, Calahorra B, et al. TIPS versus repeated paracentesis plus intravenous albumin for refractory ascites in cirrhosis: a randomized trial. *Gastroenerol* 2002; 123:1839–1847

VIII

GALLBLADDER AND BILE DUCTS

32

Cholecystectomy (Open and Laparoscopic)

Alexander P. Nagle ■ *Nathaniel J. Soper* ■ *James R. Hines*

Operations on the biliary tree are among the most common abdominal procedures performed in the United States, with more than 600,000 cholecystectomies performed annually. First described in 1882 by Langenbuch, open cholecystectomy (OC) has been the primary treatment of gallstone disease for most of the past century.[1] However, the prevailing public perception of this operation as one that resulted in pain, disability, and a disfiguring scar engendered many attempts over the past two decades at nonoperative treatment of gallstones.[2,3] Despite successful removal or dissolution of gallstones with some of these techniques, each is limited by the persistence of a diseased gallbladder. In 1985, the first endoscopic cholecystectomy was performed by Mühe of Böblingen, Germany. Although meeting early skepticism from the academic surgical community, laparoscopic cholecystectomy (LC) was adopted rapidly around the world, and has subsequently been recognized as the new "gold standard" for the treatment of gallstone disease.[4,5] In 1992, the National Institutes of Health (NIH) Consensus Development Conference stated that LC "provides a safe and effective treatment for most patients with symptomatic gallstones."[6] The advantages of LC over OC were immediately appreciated: earlier return of bowel function, less postoperative pain, improved cosmesis, shorter length of hospital stay, earlier return to full activity, and decreased overall cost.[7–11] There has been an increase in the rate of cholecystectomies subsequent to the introduction of LC accompanied by evidence of lower clinical thresholds for operative therapy of gallstones.[12–14] Currently it is estimated that 90% of cholecystectomies are performed by the laparoscopic approach. Indeed, LC as a now mature mode of therapy has introduced the general surgical world to the revolutionary advantages and unique perspectives and concerns of minimal access surgery.[14] However, the surgeon must also be facile with open biliary surgery for several reasons. First, the conversion rate to OC remains approximately 2–5% in most series. This is more common in the elderly and in the setting of acute cholecystitis. In these situations cholecystectomy will be more difficult and therefore experience and proper care are necessary to avoid technical errors that could lead to devastating complications. Secondly, there are specific instances when open surgery should be considered a wiser approach.

■ INDICATIONS FOR CHOLECYSTECTOMY

Experience with OC is vast and spans generations of surgeons. Traditionally, OC had been the standard treatment for all patients with symptomatic gallstone disease, regardless of whether the indication for intervention was recurring biliary colic, acute cholecystitis, or one of the complications of biliary stone disease. Although laparoscopic techniques have largely supplanted traditional methods of performing OC for most patients with chronic, uncomplicated cholecystitis and cholelithiasis, the open approach continues to be a safe and effective therapy for the treatment of complicated gallstone disease.

The indications for LC are, and should be, the same as those for OC (Table 32–1). Patients generally have documented cholelithiasis and symptoms attributable to a dis-

TABLE 32–1. INDICATIONS FOR LC

Symptomatic cholelithiasis
Biliary colic
Acute cholecystitis
Gallstone pancreatitis
Asymptomatic cholelithiasis
Sickle cell disease
Total parenteral nutrition
Chronic immunosuppression
No immediate access to health care facilities (e.g., missionaries, military personnel, peace corps workers, relief workers)
Incidental cholecystectomy for patients undergoing procedure for other indications
Acalculous cholecystitis (biliary dyskinesia)
Gallbladder polyps >1 cm in diameter
Porcelain gallbladder

eased gallbladder. Biliary colic is typically a severe and episodic right upper abdominal or epigastric pain that often radiates to the back. Attacks frequently occur postprandially or awaken the patient from sleep. Once a patient begins to experience symptoms, there is a greater than 80% chance that she will continue to have symptoms. There is also a finite risk of disease related complications such as acute cholecystitis, gallstone pancreatitis and choledocholithiasis. Therefore, elective cholecystectomy is indicated after the first episode of typical biliary symptoms.

On the other hand, patients with asymptomatic gallstones have less than a 20% chance of ever developing symptoms, and the risks associated with "prophylactic" operation outweigh the potential benefit of surgery in most patients.[15,16] Prophylactic cholecystectomy for asymptomatic cholelithiasis can be justified in certain circumstances, such as in patients with sickle cell disease, those undergoing open bariatric surgery, requiring long-term total parental nutrition, or patients who are therapeutically immunosuppressed after solid organ transplantation. Patients with sickle cell disease often have hepatic or vaso-occlusive crises that can be difficult to differentiate from acute cholecystitis.[17] In patients following bariatric surgery, the development of gallstones is markedly increased during the period of rapid weight loss to an incidence of about 30%.[18,19] A considerable percentage of these patients develop symptomatic cholelithiasis requiring cholecystectomy. Pharmacological prophylaxis with ursodeoxycholic acid during the period of rapid weight loss early after bariatric surgery is effective in decreasing the incidence of gallstone formation but is expensive (approximately $500 for 6-month therapy) and is associated with diarrhea (25%).[20] Removing the gallbladder at the time of bariatric surgery can abolish gallstone-related morbidity relatively easily. This approach has been adopted by many bariatric surgeons during open bariatric procedures, but not during laparoscopic bariatric surgery, because the potential morbidity of an added LC in the patient with morbid obesity appears greater than the potential later risk of cholelithiasis-related complications.[20–22] In transplant patients, there is concern that immunosuppression may mask the signs and symptoms of inflammation until overwhelming infection has occurred.[23] Recommendations in the literature range from mandatory screening and treatment of biliary disease before transplantation, to prophylactic cholecystectomy 6 months posttransplantation, to expectant management of all asymptomatic patients.[24–27] Other possible indications for prophylactic LC include individuals who may not have access to modern health care facilities for an extended time period, such as missionaries and military personnel, and patients who are already undergoing an abdominal operation for other reasons. Prophylactic cholecystectomy has been occasionally advocated in diabetics. There is no evidence to support this policy. There is good evidence to support a strategy of early cholecystectomy in the symptomatic patient. Diabetics tend to present with acute cholecystitis more frequently once they become symptomatic, and diabetics withstand complications less well. Individuals without gallstones but with typical biliary symptoms, i.e., acalculous cholecystitis or biliary dyskinesia, may also be considered for the procedure.[10] Other indications for cholecystectomy include gallstone pancreatitis and gallbladder polyps greater than 1 cm in size. In a patient with typical biliary colic, the only diagnostic study necessary prior to LC is an abdominal ultrasound revealing gallstones. Ultrasound demonstrates the size and number of stones, the thickness of the gallbladder wall, the presence or absence of pericholecystic fluid, and the diameter of the common bile duct (CBD) and other components of the biliary ductal system. Other nonbiliary disorders such as hepatic lesions or steatosis, masses in the pancreas, or renal tumors may also be diagnosed. When ultrasound is negative despite typical biliary symptoms, cholecystokinin-stimulated biliary scintigraphy demonstrating a low gallbladder ejection fraction with or without pain reproduction suggests acalculous cholecystitis.[28] If a patient with gallstones has atypical symptoms, however, a more extensive work-up including upper gastrointestinal contrast radiography or endoscopy, computerized tomography, or cardiac and pulmonary evaluation may be appropriate to rule out significant nonbiliary disease processes.

▪ CONTRAINDICATIONS TO LAPAROSCOPIC CHOLECYSTECTOMY

The number of absolute and relative contraindications to performing LC have decreased over the past 10 years as minimally invasive surgical equipment and skills have improved (Table 32–2). Absolute contraindications include the inability to tolerate general anesthesia or laparotomy, refractory coagulopathy, diffuse peritonitis with hemodynamic compromise, cholangitis, and potentially curable gallbladder cancer. Diffuse peritonitis with hemodynamic compromise represents a surgical urgency in which attempted LC is not prudent, because the etiology is less than clear or secure, and the pneumoperitoneum may lead to vascular collapse. Standard open laparotomy allows rapid determination of the etiology and more expeditious management of the disorder. Suspicion of gallbladder malignancy mandates that standard open resection be undertaken. This is because of persistent concerns with adequacy of resection and the possibility of gallbladder perforation with intraperitoneal dissemination of cancer.

Relative contraindications are dictated primarily by the surgeon's philosophy and experience. These include previous upper abdominal surgery with extensive adhesions, cirrhosis, portal hypertension, severe cardiopulmonary disease, morbid obesity, and pregnancy. In most patients, little is lost by initiating an LC with conversion to laparotomy if the laparoscopic approach is deemed to risky.

Pregnancy is a controversial relative contraindication to LC because of the unknown effects of prolonged CO_2 pneumoperitoneum on the fetus. LC can be performed safely during pregnancy but only with great care.[29] We limit this intervention to the second trimester of gestation after organogenesis is complete and prior to the uterine fundus reaching a size and height that encroaches on the operative field. Open insertion of the initial port or alternative location of the initial port in the right upper quadrant should be used to avoid injury to the gravid uterus and the insufflation pressure should be limited to less than 12 mm Hg to avoid respiratory embarrassment and decreased vena caval return. Also, maternal hyperventilation with close monitoring of end-tidal CO_2 should be undertaken to prevent fetal acidosis. When visualization of the biliary tree is required, laparoscopic ultrasound is used in place of cholangiography in order to limit fetal radiation exposure. And finally, perioperative consultation with an experienced obstetrician is advisable, as is perioperative monitoring of the fetal heart.

TABLE 32–2. CONTRAINDICATIONS TO LC

Absolute	
	Unable to tolerate general anesthesia
	Refractory coagulopathy
	Suspicion of gallbladder carcinoma
Relative	
	Previous upper abdominal surgery
	Cholangitis
	Diffuse peritonitis
	Cirrhosis and/or portal hypertension
	Chronic obstructive pulmonary disease
	Cholecystoenteric fistula
	Morbid obesity
	Pregnancy

Early experience suggested that acute cholecystitis was a relative contraindication to performing LC. A number of recent reports indicate that LC indeed can be done safely for patients with acute inflammation of the gallbladder, but should be performed in this setting only by experienced laparoscopic surgeons. There is clearly a higher rate of conversion in the setting of acute cholecystitis. In particular, after 72 hours the rate of conversion increases significantly. One should not hesitate to convert to an OC if significant adhesions or inflammation are identified during laparoscopy. The timing of cholecystectomy for acute cholecystitis has been a longstanding matter of debate. Based on several prospective studies, early surgical intervention has economic, social and medical benefits and therefore is the preferred approach for experienced laparoscopic surgeons in the management of acute cholecystitis. Our practice is to proceed with LC immediately after the diagnosis of acute cholecystitis has been made. In patients who present after 72 hours of symptoms, a LC is attempted only if the patient has no pre-existing medical conditions which preclude an OC. If the patient does have significant comorbid illnesses, we will continue with antibiotic therapy and possibly a percutaneous cholecystostomy tube and subsequent elective LC 6 to 8 weeks later. Surgeons must be comfortable in their ability to safely perform the procedure laparoscopically; significant concerns based on laparoscopic findings should prompt conversion to OC. Despite the advent of minimally invasive technology, OC continues to be a perfectly acceptable method for removal of the gallbladder under any circumstances and should certainly be considered if proper facilities for performance of laparoscopic surgery are not available or if the surgeon is not adequately trained in this technology.

▪ OPERATIVE TECHNIQUE

ANATOMY

The classic anatomy of the biliary tree is present in only 30% of individuals, so it may be said that anomalies are the rule, not the exception. As with any procedure, the knowledge of normal anatomy and common variants is critical to the success of surgical intervention. The cystic duct may join the common bile duct at an acute angle, travel parallel to the common duct for several centimeters prior to insertion, insert into the right hepatic duct, or be congenitally absent. The cystic artery usually arises from the right hepatic artery, but one must be absolutely sure that the cystic artery is visualized entering the gallbladder wall. Occasionally the right hepatic artery will loop up onto the surface of the gallbladder, and a very short cystic artery will arise. Furthermore, there can often be a posterior cystic artery, which can easily be injured if not recognized. The common bile duct begins at the junction of the cystic duct and the common hepatic duct and passes inferiorly to the ampulla of Vater. Its normal diameter is less than 6 mm, although it may be larger in elderly patients and those with biliary obstruction. It is important to clearly identify the structures forming the sides of Calot's triangle. The boundaries of Calot's triangle include the cystic duct, cystic artery, and the common hepatic duct. Distinction is here made with the hepatocystic triangle proper, which is the ventral aspect of the area bounded by the gallbladder wall and cystic duct, the liver edge, and the common hepatic duct; the cystic artery (and hence Calot's triangle) lies within this space. Aberrant anatomy is a well-recognized risk factor for biliary injury. The aberrant right hepatic duct anomaly is the most common problem. The most dangerous variant is when the cystic duct joins a low-lying aberrant right sectional duct. These injuries are underreported since occlusion of an aberrant duct may be asymptomatic and even unrecognized.

PATIENT PREPARATION

As with any abdominal operation, patients are fasted approximately 8 hours prior to the operation. Patients with no major comorbidity are admitted to the hospital on a same-day surgery basis. All patients are administered a single preoperative dose of intravenous broad-spectrum antibiotics. Sequential compression stockings are placed on both legs to avoid pooling of blood in the lower extremities by the reverse Trendelenburg position required for this operation. Following induction of general endotracheal anesthesia, an orogastric tube may be placed to decompress the stomach. The abdomen is shaved and prepared in standard sterile fashion with particular care taken to rid the umbilicus of all detritus.

OPEN CHOLECYSTECTOMY

The technical aspects of performing an OC have not changed significantly since Langenbuch's description of this procedure more than 100 years ago. Although this operation can be performed safely through a midline, paramedian, or right subcostal incision, most surgeons prefer the right subcostal (Kocher) incision. Adequate exposure of the gallbladder and the hepatoduodenal ligament is key to performing a safe cholecystectomy. Temporary sponges may be packed between the dome of the liver and the diaphragm and appropriate retractors should be inserted to optimize visualization of the hepatoduodenal ligament and its structures. The hepatic flexure of the colon is packed or retracted inferiorly and the medial segment of the left liver lobe is retracted superiorly. When a large distended gallbladder is encountered, removal can be facilitated by decompression of the gallbladder. Adhesions of omentum or viscera adjacent to the gallbladder are divided with sharp dissection or electrocautery. Meticulous dissection and positive identification of the cystic duct, its entry into the common bile duct, and the cystic artery are absolutely mandatory and significantly reduce the likelihood of bile duct injury. Most experienced surgeons prefer to identify these important structures before beginning dissection of the gallbladder from the hepatic bed. The fundus and infundibulum of the gallbladder are grasped with curved clamps. The fundus is retracted anteriorly and superiorly and the infundibulum inferiorly and laterally, exposing the structures of Calot's triangle. Caudal counter-retraction of the hepatoduodenal ligament stretches and exposes the porta hepatis, placing the peritoneum overlying the cystic duct and artery on tension. This maneuver may be accomplished with a retractor, although the left hand of the first assistant effectively retracts the duodenum, providing exposure of structure in Calot's triangle. The surgeon introduces the left index finger into the foramen of Winslow and thoroughly palpates for calculi in the common bile duct. Acute inflammation or chronic scarring may preclude approaching the infundibulum first; many surgeons prefer to dissect the fundus initially ("fundus first" technique), and the ductal and vascular structures subsequently, only after the organ has been separated from the liver. Careful ligation of the cystic duct is essential in preventing not only a biliary leak, but also in reducing the possibility of bile duct injury and stricture (Fig 32–1). Ligation of the cystic duct in close proximity to its junction with the common bile duct has long been considered an essential component of OC. However, experience with LC suggests that the length of the cystic duct stump is not a critical factor and probably does not significantly contribute to postcholecystectomy syndrome, a poorly defined clinical entity characterized by pain following gallbladder removal. The cystic artery should be dissected, secured, and divided near the surface of the gallbladder. This will reduce bleeding associated with division of the peritoneum investing the gallbladder and separation of areolar tissue between the gallbladder and the liver. Intraopera-

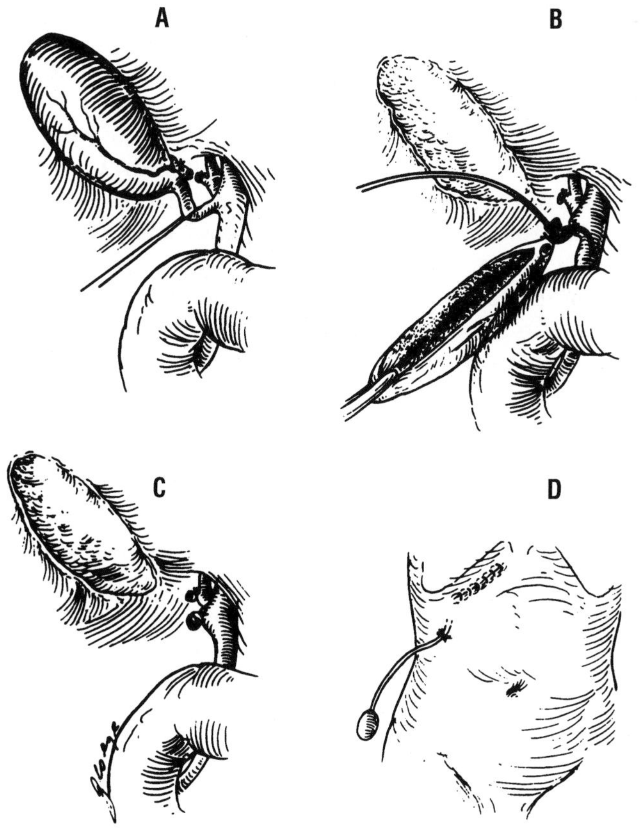

Figure 32–1. Technique of OC. **A.** Gallbladder in situ with the cystic duct isolated and the cystic artery ligated and divided. **B.** The gallbladder has been taken down from the liver bed and a catheter placed in the cystic duct for an intraoperative cholangiogram. **C.** Gallbladder completely removed with the cystic duct stump and proximal stump of the cystic artery remaining. **D.** The abdomen is closed with a closed-suction drain placed through a separate stab incision.

tive cholangiography can be performed at the discretion of the surgeon (Fig 32–1). Throughout the procedure, care should be exercised to minimize spillage of bile into the peritoneal cavity. Drains are not mandatory and are indicated only if the surgeon is concerned about identifying or controlling a possible bile leak. Common pitfalls are usually related to inadequate exposure, severe inflammation, bleeding and anatomic variants, which can lead to injury of portal structures, including the common bile duct and the hepatic artery or its branches. With a short cystic artery, the right hepatic artery must be carefully identified. Similarly with a short cystic duct, careful dissection and high ligation of the cystic duct near the gallbladder should be employed to avoid injury to the common bile duct. In fact, in the face of severe inflammation with obliteration of normal tissue planes it may be safest to perform a subtotal cholecystectomy, leaving a portion of the infundibulum in situ (after removing all stones) and suture ligating the mucosal side of the cystic duct origin. If there is unintentional gallbladder puncture, a second clamp or purse-string suture can be applied to prevent gallbladder bile and stone spillage. Before closure of the abdominal incision, bleeding and bilious drainage must be controlled. Structures in the porta hepatis are re-examined, with special attention to the cystic duct stump. The subhepatic space is irrigated with warm saline and all irrigation fluid is evacuated. The incision is usually closed in one or two layers. The skin can be closed with skin staples.

LAPAROSCOPIC CHOLECYSTECTOMY

Operating Room Set-Up

Most surgeons utilize two video monitors, one on each side of the operating table to facilitate visualization by both surgeon and assistant. Using the "American" technique, the surgeon stands to the left of the patient, the first assistant stands to the patient's right, and the laparoscopic video camera operator stands to the left of the surgeon (Fig 32–2). In the "French" technique, the patient's legs are abducted and the surgeon stands between the legs (Fig 32–3). The camera operator must always maintain the proper orientation of the camera and keep the operating instruments in the center of the video image.

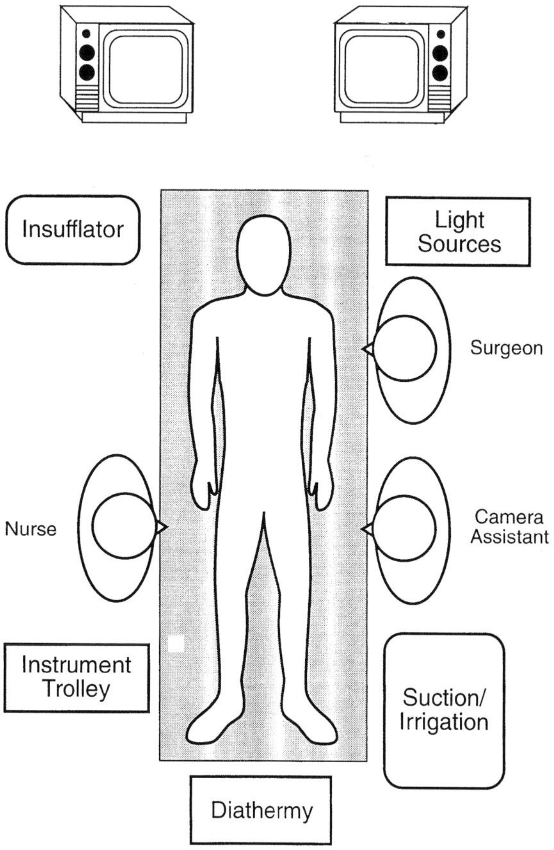

Figure 32–2. Diagrammatic representation of the position of the TV monitors, insufflator, and other equipment in relation to the surgeon. The English/American set-up.

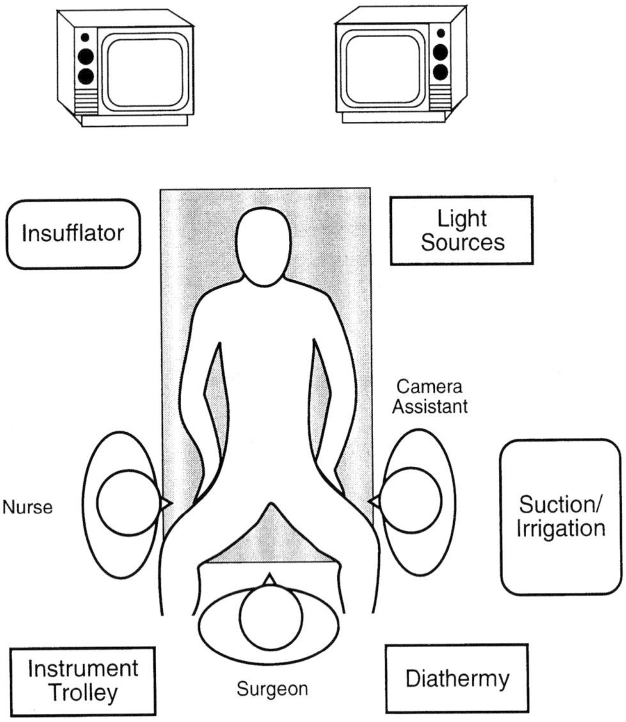

Figure 32–3. Diagrammatic representation of the position of the TV monitors, insufflator, and other equipment in relation to the surgeon. The French/European set-up.

Pneumoperitoneum

A working space, generally provided by a pneumoperitoneum, is essential for the surgeon to view and to operate within the abdominal cavity. $CO2$ has the advantage of being non-combustible and rapidly absorbed from the peritoneal cavity. It may, however, lead to hypercarbia in patients with significant cardiopulmonary disease.[30] Pneumoperitoneum can be established by either a closed or an open technique. In the closed technique, carbon dioxide is insufflated into the peritoneal cavity through a Veress needle, which is subsequently replaced with a laparoscopic port, placed blindly into the abdominal cavity. In the open technique, a laparoscopic port is inserted under direct vision into the peritoneal cavity via a small incision; only after ensuring definitive and safe peritoneal entry is the pneumoperitoneum established. There are advantages and disadvantages to both techniques. Surgeons performing LC should learn both and use them selectively.

Port Placement and Exposure

Depending on the surgeon's preference, a 5- or 10-mm laparoscope is inserted into the abdomen through the umbilical port. The patient is then placed in a reverse Trendelenburg position of 30 degrees while rotating the table to the left by 15 degrees. This maneuver allows the colon and duodenum to fall away from the liver edge. The falciform ligament and both lobes of the liver are examined closely for abnormalities. The gallbladder can usually be seen protruding beyond the edge of the liver.

Two small accessory subcostal ports are then placed under direct vision. The first 5-mm trocar is placed along the right anterior axillary line between the twelfth rib and the iliac crest. A second 5-mm port is inserted in the right subcostal area in the midclavicular line (Fig 32–4). Grasping forceps are placed through these two ports to secure the gallbladder. The assistant manipulates the lateral grasping forceps, which are used to elevate the liver and to expose the fundus of the gallbladder. The surgeon uses a dissecting forceps to raise a serosal "fold" of the most dependent portion of the fundus. The assistant's heavy grasping forceps are then locked onto this fold using either a spring or ratchet device. With these axillary grasping forceps, the fundus of the gallbladder is then pushed in a lateral and cephalad direction, rolling the entire right lobe of the liver cranially. This maneuver is complicated in patients with a fixed, cirrhotic liver or a heavy, friable liver because of fatty infiltration.

In patients with few adhesions to the gallbladder, pushing the fundus cephalad exposes the entire gallbladder, cystic duct, and porta hepatis. Most patients, however, have adhesions between the gallbladder and the omentum, hepatic flexure and/or duodenum. These adhesions are generally avascular and may be lysed bluntly by grasping them with dissecting forceps at their site of attachment to the gallbladder wall and gently "stripping" them down toward the infundibulum. After exposing the infundibulum, blunt grasping forceps placed through the midclavicular trocar are used to grasp and place traction on the neck of the gallbladder. The operative field is thereby established and the

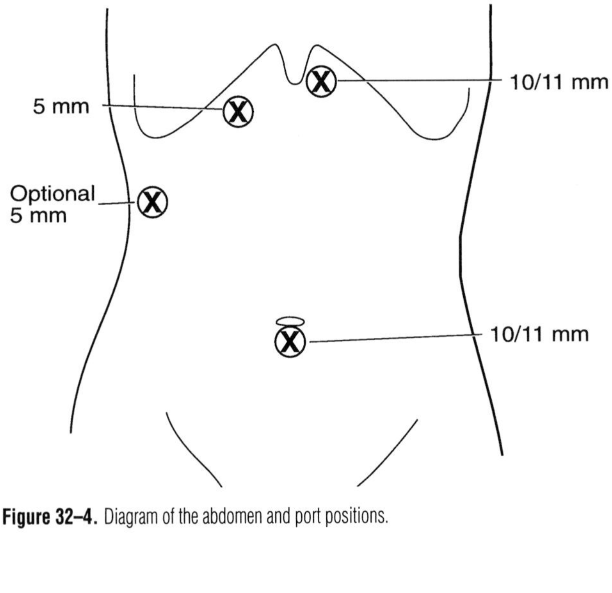

Figure 32–4. Diagram of the abdomen and port positions.

final working port is then inserted through an incision in the midline of the epigastrium. This trocar is usually inserted approximately 5 cm below the xiphoid process, but the precise position and angle depends on the location of the gallbladder as well as the size of the medial segment of the left lobe of the liver (Fig 32–4). Dissecting forceps are then inserted and directed toward the gallbladder neck. One should note that the orientation of the laparoscope is generally parallel to that of the cystic duct when the fundus is elevated, whereas the instruments placed through the other three ports enter the abdomen at right angles to this plane.

Dissection

The infundibulum is grasped, placing traction on the gallbladder in a lateral direction to disalign the cystic duct and common bile duct (CBD). Fine-tipped dissecting forceps are used to dissect away the overlying fibroareolar structures from the infundibulum of the gallbladder. The dissection should begin on a "known" structure, e.g., the gallbladder, rather than in an unknown area, to avoid damage to the underlying structures such as the bile duct or the hepatic artery.

It is important to clearly identify the structures forming the sides of Calot's triangle, which include the cystic duct, cystic artery, and common hepatic duct—the standard ventral aspect and its reverse (dorsal) aspect. Distinction is here made with the hepatocystic triangle which is the ventral aspect of the area bounded by the gallbladder wall and cystic duct, the liver edge, and the common hepatic duct; the cystic artery (and hence Calot's triangle) lies within this space. The hepatocystic triangle is maximally opened and converted into a trapezoid shape by retracting the infundibulum of the gallbladder inferiorly and laterally while maintaining the fundus under traction in a superior and medial direction (Fig 32–5). A lymph node usually lies adjacent to the cystic artery, and occasionally it is necessary to use a brief application of electrosurgical coagulation to obtain hemostasis as the lymph node is bluntly swept away. To expose the reverse of Calot's triangle, the infundibulum of the gallbladder is pulled in a superior and medial direction. After clearing the structures from the apex of the triangle, the junction between the infundibulum and the origin of the proximal cystic duct can be clearly identified. The strands of peritoneal, lymphatic and neurovascular tissue are stripped away from the cystic duct to clear a segment from the surrounding tissue. Curved dissecting forceps are helpful in creating a "window" around the posterior aspect of the cystic duct to skeletonize the duct itself. Alternatively, the tip of the hook cautery can be used to encircle and expose the duct. It is generally unnecessary and potentially harmful to dissect the cystic duct down to its junction with the CBD. The cystic artery is separated from the surrounding tissue by similar blunt dissection at this time. If the cystic artery crosses

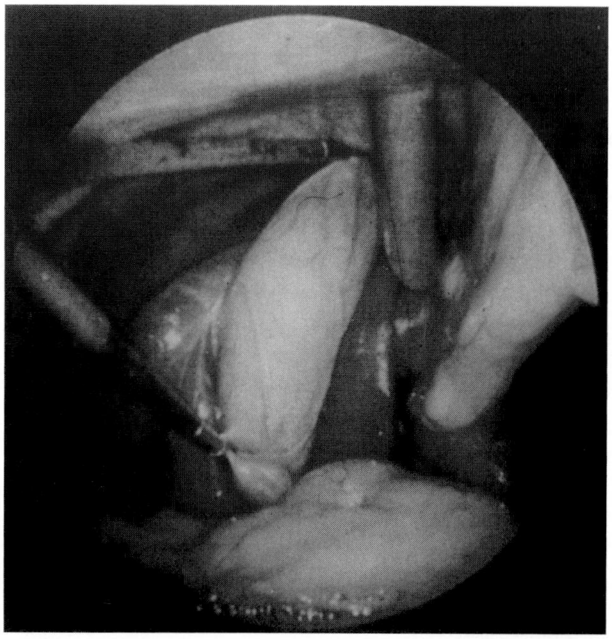

Figure 32–5. The gallbladder is elevated with the fundal grasper. Hartmann's pouch is held with a second grasping forceps.

anterior to the duct, the artery may require dissection and division prior to approaching the cystic duct. The neck of the gallbladder is thus dissected away from its liver bed, leaving only two structures entering the gallbladder—the cystic duct and artery. No structure should be divided until the cystic duct and cystic artery are unequivocally identified. This is the "critical view" of safety essential to prevent bile duct injury during LC (Fig 32–6).[30]

Intraoperative Evaluation for Choledocholithiasis

After initially dissecting the proximal cystic duct, the CBD should be imaged if there is any concern for choledocholithiasis or questions regarding the biliary anatomy. This can be achieved by radiographic intraoperative cholangiography (IOC) or intracorporeal laparoscopic ultrasonography (LUS). Prior to either procedure, a clip is applied high on the cystic duct at its junction with the gallbladder to prevent stones migrating down the duct. To perform IOC, the anterolateral wall of the cystic duct is incised and dissecting forceps are used to gently compress the cystic duct systematically back toward the gallbladder, thereby "milking" stones away from the CBD and out the ductotomy. A 4F or 5F catheter is inserted into the duct through a hollow, 5-mm metal tube that has an appropriate gasket to prevent carbon dioxide leakage around the catheter itself. The cholangiography catheter is inserted into the cystic duct and a clip is applied loosely to secure the catheter in place (Fig 32–7). If the introducer has grasping jaws, it can be used to secure the catheter into the duct (Fig 32–8). Alternatively, catheters equipped with balloons proximal to

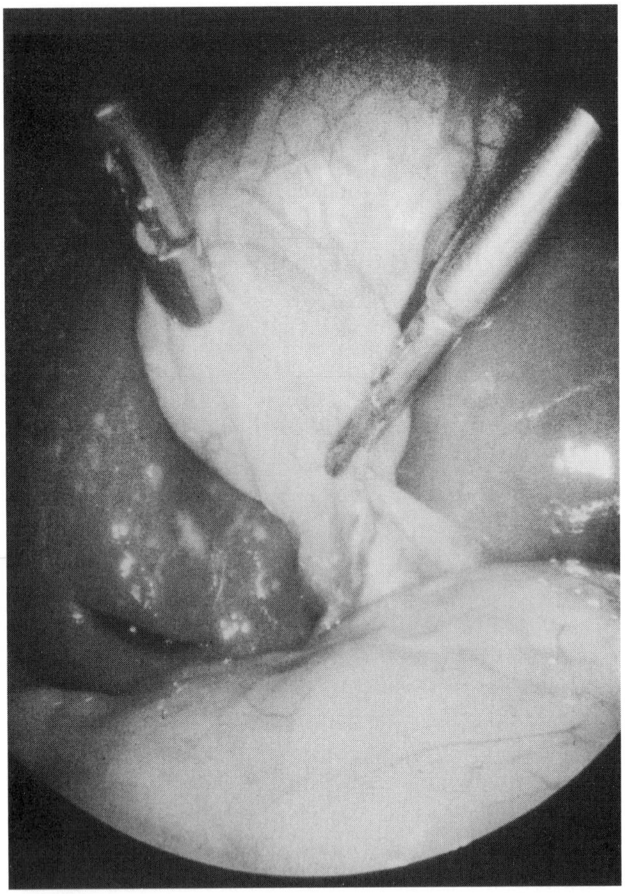

Figure 32–6. The cystic duct and artery are freed by blunt dissection.

the tip may be used for fixation. Cholangiography can be performed by either real-time fluoroscopy (dynamic IOC) or by obtaining two standard radiographs (static IOC) after injecting 5 and 10 mL of water-soluble contrast medium. The films should be inspected for the following: (1) the length of cystic duct and location of its junction with the CBD, (2) the size of the CBD, (3) the presence of intraluminal filling defects, (4) free flow of contrast into the duodenum, and (5) anatomy of the extrahepatic and intrahepatic biliary tree (Fig 32–9). After the cholangiocatheter is removed, the cystic duct is doubly clipped below the ductotomy with care to avoid the wall of the CBD, and then divided. The posterior jaw of the clip applier must be visualized prior to applying each clip in order to avoid injuring the surrounding structures. Great care should be taken so that the CBD is not "tented up" into the clip. If the cystic duct is particularly large or friable, it may be prefera-

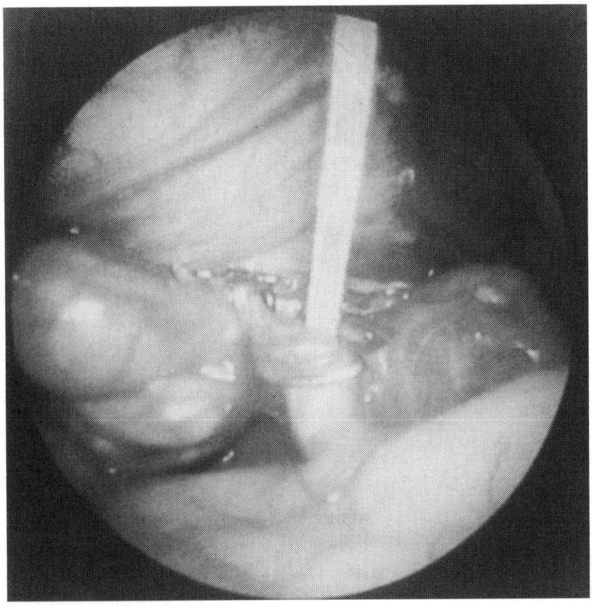

Figure 32–7. The Petelin method of performing operative cholangiography; the catheter is held in place using a snug clip across it and the cystic duct.

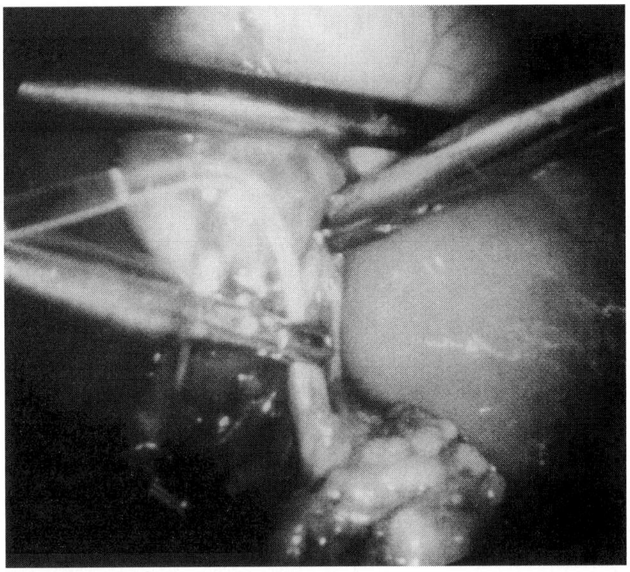

Figure 32–8. A clamp holds the cholangiogram catheter in the cystic duct.

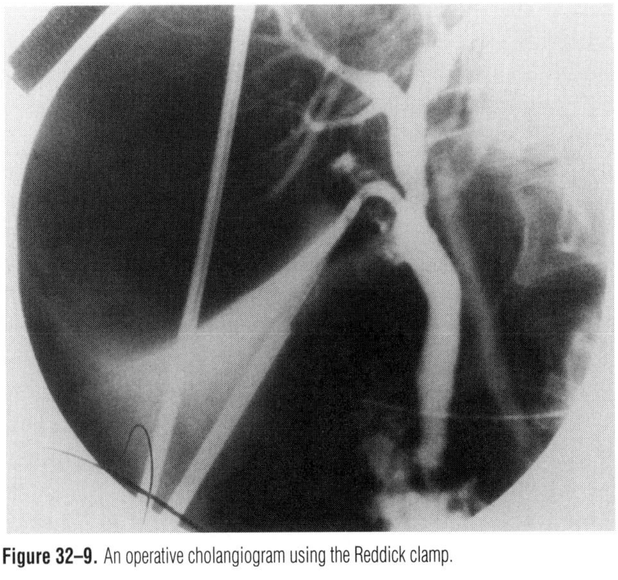

Figure 32–9. An operative cholangiogram using the Reddick clamp.

ble to replace one of the clips with a suture, either hand-tied or preformed.

Evaluation of the CBD by LUS is an alternative to cholangiography. Several studies performed at OC reported intracorporeal ultrasonography to be more accurate than operative cholangiography in assessing the CBD for stones (97–99% vs. 89–94%).[31–33] However, few surgeons adopted ultrasound for this purpose. Recently, LUS has been used in several centers during LC and is gaining popularity.[33–37] With LUS, the transducer has a higher frequency with improved resolution compared to that used with transabdominal ultrasonography. In experienced hands, LUS appears to be as accurate as cholangiography for demonstrating choledocholithiasis but can be performed more rapidly.[38] In a recent prospective multicenter trial with 209 LC patients, the time to perform LUS (7 ± 3 minutes) was significantly less than that of IOC (13 ± 6 minutes).[38] The study showed that LUS was more sensitive for detecting stones but that IOC was better in delineating intrahepatic anatomy and defining anatomical anomalies of the ductal system. The authors concluded that the two methods of duct imaging were complementary. Despite these promising data, more clinical experience will be necessary to establish the appropriate role of LUS for the detection of choledocholithiasis during LC.[39,40]

Completion of Cholecystectomy

Following clip ligation and division of the cystic duct, the cystic artery is dissected from the surrounding tissue for an adequate distance to permit placement of three clips. The surgeon must ascertain that the structure is indeed the cystic artery and not the right hepatic artery looping up onto the neck of the gallbladder or an accessory or replaced right hepatic artery. After an appropriate length of cystic artery has been dissected free, it is clipped proximally and distally prior to its transection. Electrocautery should not be used for this division, as the current may be transmitted to the proximal clips leading to subsequent necrosis and hemorrhage.

The ligated stumps of the cystic duct and the artery are then examined to ensure that there is no leakage of either bile or blood and that the clips are placed securely and compress the entire lumen of the structures without impinging on adjacent tissues. A suction-irrigation catheter is used to remove any debris or blood that has accumulated during the dissection. Separation of the gallbladder away from its hepatic bed is then initiated using an electrosurgical probe to coagulate small vessels and lymphatics. While maintaining cephalad traction on the fundus of the gallbladder with the axillary forceps, the midclavicular forceps pulls the neck of the gallbladder anterosuperiorly and then alternatively medially and laterally to expose and place the tissue connecting the gallbladder to the fossa under tension. An electrocautery spatula or hook is used in a gentle sweeping motion with low power (25 to 30 W) to coagulate and divide the tissue. Intermittent blunt dissection will facilitate exposure of the proper plane.

Dissection of the gallbladder fossa continues from the infundibulum to the fundus, progressively moving the midclavicular grasping forceps cephalad to allow maximal countertraction (Fig 32–10). The dissection proceeds until the gallbladder is attached by only a thin bridge of tissue. At this point, prior to completely detaching the gallbladder, the hepatic fossa and porta hepatis are once again inspected for hemostasis and bile leakage. Small bleeding points are coagulated and the right upper quadrant is liberally irrigated and then aspirated dry while checking for any residual bleeding or bile leakage. The final attachments of the gallbladder are divided, and the liver edge is again examined for hemostasis.

After the cholecystectomy has been performed, the gallbladder must be removed from the abdominal cavity (Fig 32–11). If the stone burden is small, the gallbladder can be extracted at the subxiphoid port site. Usually, the gallbladder is most easily removed at the umbilical port site where there are no muscle layers anterior to the fascial plane. Also, if the fascial opening needs to be enlarged because of large or numerous stones, extension of the umbilical incision causes less postoperative pain and has better cosmesis than does enlarging the subxiphoid incision. The laparoscope is removed from the umbilical port and placed through the epigastric port. Large "claw" grasping forceps are introduced through the umbilical port to grasp the infundibulum of the gallbladder. The forceps, trocar, and gallbladder neck are then retracted as a unit through the umbilical incision. The neck of the gallbladder is thus exteriorized through

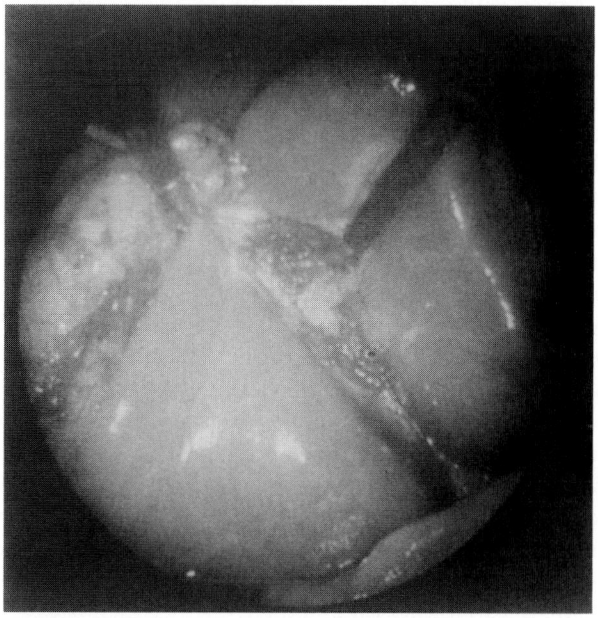

Figure 32–10. Dissection of the gallbladder from its liver bed.

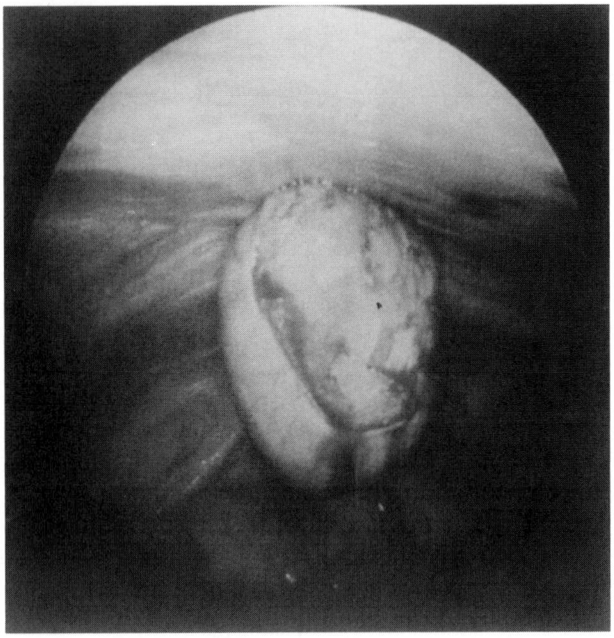

Figure 32–11. A tense gallbladder being taken through the anterior abdominal wall.

the anterior abdominal wall with the fundus remaining within the abdominal cavity (Fig 32–12). If the gallbladder is not distended with bile or stones, it can be simply withdrawn with gentle traction. In many cases, however, a suction catheter introduced through an incision in the gallbladder neck is used to aspirate bile and small stones. Stone forceps can also be placed into the gallbladder to extract or crush calculi if necessary. Occasionally, the fascial incision must be extended to extract larger stones or thick-walled gallbladders.

Each incision is infiltrated with bupivacaine for postoperative analgesia. The fascia of the umbilical incision is closed with one or two large absorbable sutures. Closure of the subxiphoid fascia is optional, as visceral herniation is unlikely to occur because of the oblique entry angle of the trocar into the abdominal cavity and its location anterior to the falciform ligament. The skin of the subxiphoid and umbilical incisions is closed with subcuticular absorbable sutures. The skin incisions at both 5-mm port sites can be closed with adhesive strips or skin closure adhesives. The orogastric tube is removed in the operating room, and the patient is transferred to the postanesthesia care unit. Patients are allowed out of bed as soon as they are fit enough to walk and >90% of patients are discharged from the hospital within 24 hours. Fit patients who have been preoperatively selected may be safely discharged within 6 hours following surgery.[41] Patients are evaluated 1 week following surgery and if sutures are present, they are removed (Fig 32–13). At this time, >95% of patients are back to a normal routine and most return to work immediately following their clinic visit.

■ ADVANTAGES AND DISADVANTAGES

The advantages of LC over other therapies for gallstone disease are multiple (Table 32–3). Unlike non-resective techniques for gallstone ablation, LC removes the diseased gallbladder along with its stones. Relative to traditional OC, postoperative pain and intestinal ileus are diminished with LC. The small size of the fascial incisions allows rapid return to heavy physical activities. The small incisions are also cosmetically more appealing than is the large incision used during traditional cholecystectomy. The patient can usually be discharged from the hospital either on the same day or the day following operation, and can return to full activity within a few days.[7,11] These factors lead to overall decreased cost of LC compared to its traditional open counterpart.[8]

There are, however, several potential disadvantages of LC (Table 32–3). As opposed to nonresective treatments for gallstones, patients must be acceptable candidates for general anesthesia and possible laparotomy. Three-dimensional depth perception is limited by the two-dimensional monocular image of the videoscope, and the operative field of view is usually directed by an individual other than the surgeon. It is more difficult to control significant hemorrhage using laparoscopic technology than in an open surgical field. There is also less tactile discrimination of structures using laparoscopic instruments as opposed to direct digital palpation during OC. CO_2 insufflation to create the pneumoperitoneum is associated with a number of potential risks, including reduction of vena caval flow and systemic hypercarbia with acidosis. Operative time is generally longer than for the traditional open operation, particularly during the early portion of the surgeon's experience. And finally, the videoscopic technology and minimal access instrumentation are costly, complex and continually evolving requiring the presence of appropriately trained support personnel.

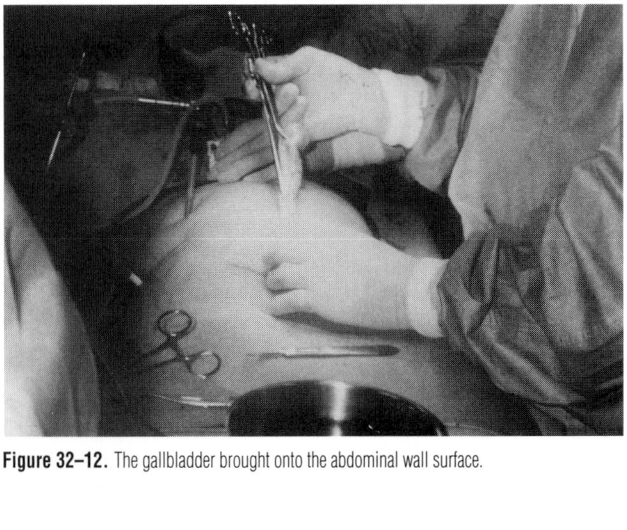

Figure 32–12. The gallbladder brought onto the abdominal wall surface.

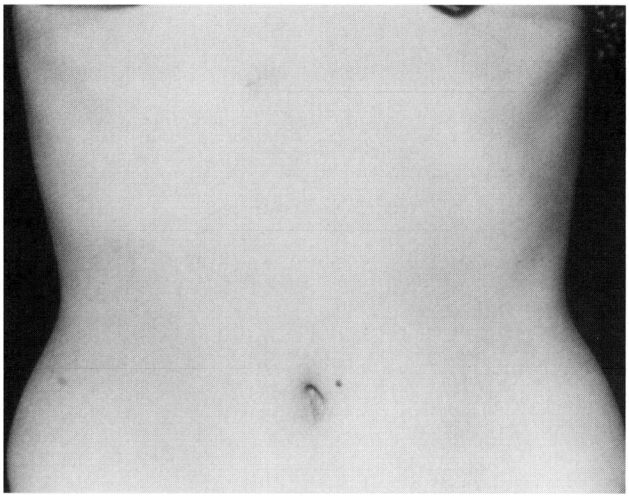

Figure 32–13. The abdominal incisions after removal of the sutures.

TABLE 32–3. ADVANTAGES AND DISADVANTAGES OF LC COMPARED TO OC

Advantages	Disadvantages
Less pain	Lack of depth perception
Smaller incisions	View controlled by camera operator
Better cosmesis	More difficult to control hemorrhage
Shorter hospitalization	Decreased tactile discrimination (haptics)
Earlier return to full activity	Potential CO_2 insufflation complications
Decreased total costs	Adhesions/inflammation limit use
	Slight increase in bile duct injuries

▪ SPECIAL CONSIDERATIONS

CONVERSION TO OPEN OPERATION

Surgeons performing LC should not think of conversion to open operation as a complication, but rather mature judgment, and hence not hesitate to convert to a traditional OC if the anatomy is unclear, if complications arise, or there is failure to make reasonable progress in a timely manner. It is "better to open one too many than to open one too few," even if it means a longer hospital stay for the patient. Some complications requiring laparotomy are obvious, such as massive hemorrhage or major injury to the bile duct. Open laparotomy allows the additional tool of manual palpation and tactile sensation and should be performed when the anatomy cannot be delineated because of inflammation, adhesions or anomalies. Fistulae between the biliary system and bowel are rare, but may require laparotomy for optimal management. The demonstration of potentially resectable gallbladder carcinoma also dictates an open exploration. Finally, CBD stones that cannot be removed laparoscopically and are unlikely to be extracted endoscopically (because of Billroth II anastomosis, previously failed endoscopic retrograde cholangiopancreatography [ERCP], or an inexperienced endoscopist) should be converted to open operation without hesitation.

ACUTE CHOLECYSTITIS

Acute cholecystitis may be treated successfully by LC. Intervention during the early phase reveals an inflamed, thick-walled, tensely distended organ. To gain adequate traction on the gallbladder with the grasping forceps, it may be necessary to decompress the gallbladder by aspirating its contents with a large-gauge needle. As long as the inflammation is limited to the gallbladder, LC is usually technically feasible. However, if inflammation extends to the porta hepatis, great care must be taken in proceeding with the operation. The normally thin, minimally adherent tissue that invests the cystic duct and artery is markedly thickened and edematous and may not readily separate from these structures with the usual blunt dissection techniques. The duct wall also may be edematous, thus making its external diameter similar to the gallbladder neck and CBD. If the anatomy is unclear, cholangiography must be performed before clipping or dividing tissue. When acute inflammation has been present for several days or weeks before operation, the pericholecystic tissue planes may be obliterated by thick, "woody" tissue that is difficult to dissect bluntly. The surgeon may therefore need to convert to OC if the minimal access approach is initially attempted during this subacute phase. There is no harm in inserting the laparoscope and assessing the right upper quadrant. The decision to convert to an open operation is a matter of judgment, based on the existing anatomy, local conditions, and the surgeon's experience and confidence in his or her ability to complete the procedure using minimal access techniques.

Several authors have reported performing LC in the face of acute inflammation with success but with a higher conversion rate than for elective LC.[42–46] Lo and associates reported in their prospective study (1996) that despite longer operative times and postoperative stays for early LC in patients with acute cholecystitis (treatment within 5 days) versus delayed LC (initial conservative treatment followed by LC 3 to 4 months later), the advantage of early LC was the reduction in the total hospital stay, from 15 to 7 days. In a second prospective study of 105 patients randomized to early LC (within 24 hours of diagnosis of acute cholecystitis) versus delayed LC (6 to 8 weeks later), there was no significant difference in conversion rate (early 21% vs. delayed 24%), postoperative analgesic requirement, or number of postoperative complications. The early group did have a longer operative time (123 min vs. 107 min; $p = 0.04$), but total hospitalization was shorter (8 days vs. 12 days; $p = 0.001$).[47] Rattner and associates retrospectively reviewed 20 patients who underwent attempted LC for acute cholecystitis and examined factors that were predictive of a successful procedure.[44] Seven of the 20 patients (35%) required conversion to OC. The interval from admission to cholecystectomy in the successful cases was 0.6 days versus 5 days in the cases requiring conversion to OC. Converted cases also had a significantly higher white blood cell count, alkaline phosphatase levels and Acute Physiology and Chronic Health Evaluation II (APACHE II) scores compared to those undergoing successful LC. Ultrasonographic findings such as gallbladder distention, wall thickness and pericholecystic fluid did not correlate with the success of LC. It can be concluded that LC should be performed immediately after the diagnosis of acute cholecystitis. Delaying surgery allows inflammation to become more intense and neovascularized, thus increasing the technical difficulty of LC.

INTRAOPERATIVE GALLBLADDER PERFORATION

Perforation of the gallbladder with bile or stone leakage can be a nuisance but should not ordinarily require conversion to OC. Perforation may occur secondary to traction applied by the grasping forceps or because of electrosurgical thermal injury during removal of the gallbladder from its bed. In our experience, almost one third of the patients have had intraoperative spillage of bile or stones.[48] Patients with a bile leak have not experienced an increased incidence of infection, prolongation of hospitalization or postoperative disability, nor adverse long-term complications (mean follow-up of 41 months in 250 consecutive LC patients). The only difference between those with and without bile leakage was that the operating time of patients with a gallbladder perforation was approximately 10 minutes longer, presumably because of the time spent cleaning up the operative field. When perforation does occur, the bile should be aspirated completely and irrigation used liberally. The hole in the gallbladder is best secured with a grasping instrument and then sutured or tied with an Endoloop. The stones should be retrieved and removed. Gallbladder spillage, when treated in this manner, results in no adverse short- or long-term complications. Escaped stones composed primarily of cholesterol pose little threat of infection. However, pigment stones frequently harbor viable bacteria and may potentially lead to subsequent infectious complications if allowed to remain in the peritoneal cavity.[49] The long-term complications of retained stones, either intra-abdominally with resultant abscess formation or intramurally with resultant port site abscess, have not been prospectively studied, but recent case reports and case series in the surgical literature document a clear potential for long-term infectious complications.[50–54] The relative infrequency of these complications probably does not justify conversion to open operation in the face of spilled stones, but vigilance in avoidance of perforation, a careful search for escaped stones, and liberal use of a plastic retrieval bag for large and friable gallbladders is recommended.[55]

▪ COMPLICATIONS

OPEN CHOLECYSTECTOMY

Experience with OC is vast, spanning generations of surgeons and having been practiced in virtually every country throughout the world. Over time, this operation has proved to be safe and effective. In a collected series of about 20,000 patients who underwent cholecystectomy between 1946 and 1973 at 10 different institutions, from the United States and throughout the world, the overall mortality rate was 1.6%. This figure is comparable to a 1.7% mortality rate reported for more than 12,000 patients operated on for calculous biliary tract disease between 1932 and 1979 at a single U.S. university center. In this latter group, the operative mortality rate for patients who underwent elective cholecystectomy was 0.1%. More recently, a U.S. population-based study examining the outcome of all open cholecystectomies performed in a 12-month period in two states reported an overall mortality rate of 0.17%. The morbidity rate was 14.7%, which includes all reported complications, including minor problems such as electrolyte imbalances, atelectasis, urinary retention, and other assorted difficulties that often occur following any surgical procedure. In this study, morbidity and mortality were dependent on age as well as disease status. Perhaps the most significant complication that can arise during open or LC is bile duct injury. Numerous reports in the literature, including this large population-based study indicate that the risk of bile duct injury during OC is between 0.1% and 0.2%. Similar morbidity and mortality data has been reported by other large series. These data confirm that OC continues to be a very safe operation that can be performed with a very low morbidity and mortality. In elective situations, OC is being performed in most hospitals throughout the world on patients who are admitted the day of surgery, with an overall stay of 2 to 4 days.

LAPAROSCOPIC CHOLECYSTECTOMY

Many complications related to laparoscopic removal of the gallbladder are similar to those occurring during traditional OC (Table 32–4). These complications include hemorrhage, bile duct injuries, bile leaks, retained stones, pancreatitis, wound infections, and incisional hernias. Other potential complications are pneumoperitoneum related (gas embolism, vagal reaction, ventricular arrhythmias, or hypercarbia with acidosis) and trocar related (injuries to the abdominal wall, intra-abdominal organ, or major blood vessels). The "protective" shield on disposable trocars is not an insurance against perforation of intestine or major vessels, especially after previous abdominal operations. Regardless of the make of trocar, during its insertion one should never aim toward the spine or the location of the great vessels, and a hand is used as a "brake" to prevent inadvertently introducing the trocar too far. Insertion of the initial trocar, especially when performed in a closed fashion, can cause iatrogenic injury to the bowel, bladder, aorta, iliac artery or vena cava.[56,57] When a trocar injury to a major blood vessel is suspected, the patient must be opened immediately without removing the trocar until the involved blood vessel is isolated. In contrast, if the small-bore Veress needle enters a viscus or blood vessel, the operation can generally be completed and the patient monitored closely for signs of complications in the postoperative period.

The laparoscopic trocars may also lacerate blood vessels in the abdominal wall. Prior to removal, each trocar should be visualized from the peritoneal aspect using the laparoscope. If significant hemorrhage is seen, it can generally be controlled with cautery, intraoperative tamponade with a Foley catheter, or a through-and-through suture on each side of the trocar insertion site.

TABLE 32–4. COMPLICATIONS OF LC

Hemorrhage
Bile duct injury
Bile leak
Retained stones
Pancreatitis
Wound infection
Incisional hernia
Pneumoperitoneum related:
CO_2 embolism
Vaso-vagal reflex
Cardiac arrhythmias
Hypercarbic acidosis
Trocar related:
Abdominal wall bleeding, hematoma
Visceral injury
Vascular injury

Most serious complications occur early in the surgeon's experience. For instance, in a multivariate regression analysis of 8839 LCs in which there were 15 bile duct injuries, the only significant factor associated with an adverse outcome was the surgeon's experience with the procedure.[58] The regression model predicted that a surgeon had a 1.7% chance of a bile duct injury occurring in the first case and 0.17% chance of a bile duct injury in the 50th case.

Of all the potential complications, biliary injuries have received the most attention and are discussed at length elsewhere in this text (Chapter 34). Most series quote a major bile duct injury rate of around 0.2% during OC, whereas the incidence of bile duct injuries during LC is 0.40% or higher.[30] These injuries can cause major morbidity, prolonged hospitalization, high cost and litigation.[59,60] In addition to the surgeon's experience and aberrant anatomy, a number of reports mention chronic inflammation with dense scarring, operative bleeding obscuring the field, or fat in the portal area contributing to the biliary injuries.[28,61–63] The classic biliary injury, however, occurs when the CBD or a right hepatic duct is mistaken for the cystic duct and is divided between clips. Many surgeons attribute this misidentification to the direction of traction of the gallbladder, i.e., pulling the CBD and the cystic duct into alignment, thus making them appear to be one. Other contributing factors to misidentification are a short cystic duct, a large stone in Hartmann's pouch (making retraction and display of the cystic duct difficult), or tethering of the infundibulum to the CBD by acute or chronic inflammation. Constant awareness of these potential misidentifications and technical causes of biliary injuries is the best method of prevention. If a bile duct injury occurs, an immediate repair should be performed. When a bile duct injury is discovered in the postoperative period, a coordinated effort by radiologists, endoscopists and surgeons is necessary to optimize management.[30] There should be no hesitation in asking for the help of a surgeon experienced in biliary repair.

▪ RESULTS OF CHOLECYSTECTOMY SERIES

There have been several prospective, randomized trials comparing OC with LC and results have been mixed in demonstrating advantages of LC over OC in treating elective symptomatic cholelithiasis (Table 32–5). The largest study prospectively randomized 310 patients to LC versus mini-laparotomy OC with 155 patients in each group. Conversion to large-incision cholecystectomy was significantly more common with LC (13% vs. 4%) and complications were significantly more frequent with LC (9% vs. 3%). When LC was successful, hospital

TABLE 32–5. PROSPECTIVE RANDOMIZED TRIALS OF OPEN VERSUS LC

Study	Number of Patients	Operating Room Time (min)	Complications (%)	Length of Stay (days)	Return to Work (days)
Barkun, et al. (1992)					
OC	25	73	8.0	4*	20*
LC	37	86	2.7	3	12
Trondsen, et al. (1993)					
OC	35	50*	20	4*	34*
LC	35	100	17	3	11
Berggren, et al. (1994)					
OC	12	69*	—	3*	24*
LC	15	87	—	2	12
McMahon, et al. (1994)					
OC	148	57*	20	4*	—
LC	151	71	17	2	—
Majeed, et al. (1996)					
OC	100	40*	—	3	35
LC	100	65	—	3	28
Kiviluoto, et al. (1998)					
OC	31	—	23*	6*	30
LC	32	—	3	4	14

* $p < 0.05$

stay was significantly shorter than for OC (2 vs. 3 days respectively), but overall the hospital stay was not significantly different. Postoperative analgesia requirements were reduced and return to normal activities and to work were faster after LC. There was no significant cost difference between the two procedures.[64] Similarly, another study prospectively randomized 200 patients in a single-blinded fashion (identical wound dressings were applied in both groups so that caregivers would be blinded to the type of operation) to LC versus minilaparotomy OC. Laparoscopic cholecystectomy took significantly longer than small-incision cholecystectomy (median 65 minutes vs. 40 minutes, $p < 0.001$). However, there was no significant difference in length of stay (median 3.0 for LC vs. 3.0 for small-incision OC, $p = 0.74$), return to work (median 5.0 weeks vs. 4.0 weeks; $p = 0.39$), and time to full activity (median 3.0 weeks vs. 3.0 weeks; $p = 0.15$).[65] A follow-up to this study prospectively randomized 200 additional patients to LC or minilaparotomy OC. Postoperative pain, analgesic and anti-emetic consumption, perceived health, and metabolic and respiratory responses were compared. Pain scores in both groups were low. Laparoscopic cholecystectomy, however, was associated with lower postoperative pain scores and analgesic requirements compared with small-incision OC, but the anti-emetic requirements were greater after LC. The duration of hospital stay and the perceived health after operation were the same, and both procedures were associated with a similar reduction of respiratory function. Twenty-four hours after operation the inflammatory (C-reactive protein, [CRP]) response to LC (22 ± 20 mg/L) was significantly lower than after small-incision OC (68 ± 30 mg/L), but the neuroendocrine (cortisol) response was similar (LC, 475 ± 335 nmol/L, compared with small-incision OC, 710 ± 410 nmol/L).[66] Numerous clinical series of LC, either accrued prospectively or retrospectively, have also been reported (Table 32–6).

Among the authors' personal series of >1500 LCs, there was a conversion rate of 2.1% and one perioperative death (<0.1%) because of myocardial infarction at 1 week postoperatively. Significant postoperative complications occurred in 2.7%, including three minor duct injuries (0.2%). The mean operative time decreased from more than 100 minutes in the first 100 patients to 85 minutes in the most recent 100 patients. The postoperative course in most patients was uneventful, with over 90% of patients discharged from the hospital within 24 hours of surgery, and only 10% required parental narcotics after leaving the recovery room. Similarly, the duration of disability was minimal, with the average postoperative interval to return to full activity being 10 days. These results compared favorably with those of traditional OC, in which the morbidity and mortality rates were similar but hospitalization for 3 to 5 days and return to work at 1 month after surgery were standard.[67] Our data mirror those from most series of LC reported to date. Morbidity rates range from 1.5–8.6%, and bile duct injuries range from 0.2–0.7%. Mortality is rare after this procedure, and is usually attributed to unrelated events. The conversion rates from laparoscopic to open operation in most series range

TABLE 32–6. RESULTS OF LARGE SERIES OF LC

Study	Number of Patients	Conversion (%)	Mortality (%)	Complications† (%)	Bile Duct Injuries (%)
Deziel, et al. (1993)	77,604	—	0.04	2.0	0.6
Scott, et al. (1992)	12,397	4.3	0.08	4.0	0.4
Deveney (1993)	9597	—	0.04	2.5	0.3
Croce, et al. (1994)	6865	3.1	0.06	2.5	0.3
Orlando, et al. (1993)	4640	6.9	0.13	8.6	0.3
Schlumpf, et al. (1994)	3722	7.0	0.08	4.8	0.6
Collett, et al. (1993)	2955	4.8	0.20	3.4	0.6
Airan, et al. (1992)	2671	4.6	0.15	—	0.2
Kane, et al. (1995)	2490	7.8	—	—	—
Litwin, et al. (1992)	2201	4.3	0.00	—	0.1
Kimura, et al.(1993)	1989	2.7	0.00	1.8	0.6
Larson, et al. (1992)	1983	4.5	0.10	2.1	0.3
Fullarton, et al. (1994)	1683	17.0	0.50	5.9	0.7
Newman, et al. (1995)	1525	2.2	0.26	4.1	0.0
Cuschieri, et al. (1991)	1236	3.6	0.00	1.6	0.3
Soper, et al. (1998)	1200	2.1	0.10	2.7	0.2
Brune, et al. (1994)	800	1.2	0.00	2.8	0.2
Perissat, et al. (1992)	777	5.5	0.10	3.3	0.4
Jatzko, et al. (1995)	740	5.4	0.14	1.9	—
Cappucino, et al. (1994)	563	4.8	0.00	6.9	0.3

†Includes intraoperative and postoperative complications.

from 1.8–7.8% and generally is greater early in the surgeon's experience with the procedure. Although a recent nationwide study reported that the conversion rate to an open procedure is as high as 5–10%.[68] Additionally, studies have shown that advanced age, longer duration of procedure, and acute cholecystitis significantly increase both postoperative morbidity and the length of stay.[69,70]

As would be predicted for this excisional procedure, LC effectively treats gallstone disease. However, postcholecystectomy problems occur in some patients. Kane and associates noted 89% of patients undergoing LC had preoperative biliary-type pain and only 10.6% of the patients had similar pain postoperatively.[71] Similarly, Ure and associates found that the percentage of patients with biliary colic was reduced from 83% before LC to 6.4% after LC.[72] Fenster and associates examined symptom relief in 225 patients undergoing LC followed postoperatively between 3 weeks and 3 months. They differentiated symptomatic gallstones from acalculous cholecystitis and discovered that 82% of patients with biliary colic and gallstones had complete relief of upper abdominal pain after the operation compared to only 52% of patients with acalculous cholecystitis.[73] These data are comparable to the data for OC in which biliary-type pain persisted at follow-up (<1 year) in 9–34% of patients with symptomatic gallstones.[74–76] In terms of cost-effectiveness, several studies have shown that LC is less expensive than the open procedure, while others have shown the contrary.[8,9,77]

▪ CONCLUSION

Cholecystectomy remains a common operation. Laparoscopic management of symptomatic gallstones has rapidly become the new standard for therapy throughout the world. Many patients can now undergo this operation in an ambulatory setting. There are numerous advantages of LC over OC. However, occasionally anatomical or physiological considerations will preclude the minimal access approach, and conversion to an open operation in such cases reflects sound judgment and should not be considered a complication.

REFERENCES

1. Beal JM. Historical perspective of gallstone disease. *Surg Gynecol Obstet* 1984;158:181–189
2. Schoenfield I, Lachin J, The Steering Committee TNCGSG. Chenodiol (chenodeoxycholic acid) for dissolution of gallstones: the national cooperative gallstone study. *Ann Intern Med* 1981;95:257–282
3. Schoenfield I, Berci G, Carnovale R, et al. The effect of ursodiol on the efficacy and safety of extracorporeal shockwave lithotripsy of gallstones. *N Engl J Med* 1990; 323:1239–1245
4. Soper NJ, Stockmann PT, Dunnegan DL, et al. Laparoscopic cholecystectomy: the new 'gold standard'? *Arch Surg* 1992;127S:917–921
5. Soper NJ, Brunt LM, Kerbl K. Laparoscopic general surgery. *N Engl J Med* 1994;330:409–419

6. Conference, NC. Gallstones and laparoscopic cholecystectomy. *JAMA* 1992;269:1018–1024
7. Barkun JS, Barkun AN, Sampalis JS, et al. Randomized controlled trial of laparoscopic versus mini-cholecystectomy. *Lancet* 1992;340:1116–1119
8. Bass EB, Pitt HA, Lillemoe KD. Cost-effectiveness of laparoscopic cholecystectomy versus open cholecystectomy. *Am J Surg* 1993;165:466–471
9. McMahon A, Russell I, Baxter J et al. Laparoscopic versus minilaparoscopic cholecystectomy: A randomized trial. *Lancet* 1994;343:135–138
10. Soper N. Laparoscopic cholecystectomy. *Curr Probl Surg* 1991;28:585–655
11. Soper N, Barteau J, Clayman R, et al. Laparoscopic versus standard open cholecystectomy: comparison of early results. *Surg Gynecol Obstet* 1992;174:114–118
12. Escarce J, Chen W, Schwartz J. Falling cholecystectomy thresholds since the introduction of laparoscopic cholecystectomy. *JAMA* 1995;273:1581–1585
13. Nenner R, Imperato P, Rosenberg C, et al. Increased cholecystectomy rates among medicare patients after the introduction of laparoscopic cholecystectomy. *J Community Health* 1994;19:409–415
14. Legorreta A, Silber J, Constantino G, et al. Increased cholecystectomy rate after introduction of laparoscopic cholecystectomy. *JAMA* 1993;270:1429–1432
15. Ransohoff D, Gracie W. Treatment of gallstones. *Ann Intern Med* 1993;119:606–619
16. Ransohoff D, Gracie W, Wolfenson L, et al. Prophylactic cholecystectomy or expectant management for silent gallstones: a decision analysis to assess survival. *Ann Intern Med* 1983;99:199–204
17. Tagge E, Othersen HJ, Jackson S, et al. Impact of laparoscopic cholecystectomy on the management of cholelithiasis in children with sickle cell disease. *J Pediatr Surg* 1994;29:209–212
18. Fobi M, Lee H, Igwe D, et al. Prophylactic Cholecystectomy with Gastric Bypass Operation: Incidence of Gallbladder Disease. *Obes Surg* 2002;12:350–353
19. Sugerman HJ, Brwer W, Shiffman M, et al. A Multicenter, Placebo-controlled, Randomized Double-Blind, Prospective Trail of Prophylactic Ursodiol for the Prevention of gallstone formation following Gastric-Bypass-Induced Rapid Weight Loss. *Am J Surg* 1995;169: 91–97
20. Hamad G, Ikramuddin S, Gourash W, et al. Elective cholecystectomy during laparoscopic Roux-En-Y gastric bypass: is it worth the wait? *Obes Surg* 2003;13:76–81
21. Villegas L, Schneider B, Provost D, et al. Is routine cholecystectomy required during laparoscopic gastric bypass? *Obes Surg* 2004;14:60–66
22. Liem R, Niloff P. Prophylactic cholecystectomy with open gastric bypass operation. *Obes Surg* 2004; 14:763–765
23. Hull D, Bartus S, Perdrizet G, et al. Management of cholelithiasis in heart and lung transplant patients: with review of laparoscopic cholecystectomy. *Conn Med* 1994; 58:643–647
24. Fendrick A, Gleeson S, Cabana M, et al. Asymptomatic gallstones revisited. Is there a role for laparoscopic cholecystectomy? *Arch Fam Med* 1993;2:959–968
25. Giradet R, Rosenbloom P, Deweese B, et al. Significance of asymptomatic biliary tract disease in heart transplantation recipients. *J Heart Transplant* 1989;8:391–399
26. Boline G, Clifford R, Yang H, et al. Cholecystectomy in the potential heart transplant patient. *J Heart Lung Transplant* 1991;10:269–274
27. Steck T, Castanfo-Nordin M, Keshavarzian A. Prevalence and management of cholelithiasis in heart transplant patients. *J Heart Lung Transplant* 1991;10:1024–1032
28. Soper NJ. Effect of nonbiliary problems on laparoscopic cholecystectomy. *Am J Surg* 1993;165:522–526
29. Soper N, Hunter J, Petrie R. Laparoscopic cholecystectomy during pregnancy. *Surg Endo* 1992;6:115–117
30. Strasberg S, Hertl N, Soper N. An analysis of the problem of biliary injury during laparoscopic cholecystectomy. *J Am Coll Surg* 1995;180:101–125
31. Machi J, Sigel B, Zaren A, et al. Operative ultrasonography during hepatobiliary and pancreatic surgery. *World J Surg* 1993;17:640–646
32. Machi J, Sigel B, Zaren A, et al. Technique of ultrasound examination during laparoscopic cholecystectomy. *Surg Endo* 1993;7:545–549
33. Orda R, Sayfan J, Levy Y. Routine laparoscopic ultrasonography in biliary surgery. *Surg Endo* 1994;8:1239–1242
34. Jakimowicz J. Review: Intraoperative ultrasonography during minimal access surgery. *J R Coll Surg Edinb* 1993; 38:231–238
35. John T, Banting S, Pye S, et al. Preliminary experience with intracorporeal laparoscopic ultrasonography using a sector scanning probe. A prospective comparison with intraoperative cholangiography in the detection of choledocholithiasis. *Surg Endo* 1994;8:1176–1180
36. McIntyre R, Stiegmann G, Peralman N. Update on laparoscopic ultrasonography. *Endosc Surg Allied Technol* 1994;2:149–152
37. Steigmann G, McIntyre R, Pearlman N. Laparoscopic intracorporeal ultrasound. An alternative to cholangiography? *Surg Endo* 1994;8:167–171
38. Steigmann G, Soper N, Filipi C, et al. Laparoscopic ultrasonography as compared with static or dynamic cholangiography at laparoscopic cholecystectomy. *Surg Endo* 1995;9:1269–1273
39. Soper NJ. The utility of ultrasonography for screening the common bile duct during laparoscopic cholecystectomy. *J Laparoendosc Adv Surg Tech* 1997;7:271–276
40. Wu J, Dunnegan D, Soper N. The utility of intracorporeal ultrasonography for screening of the bile duct during laparoscopic cholecystectomy. *J Gastrointest Surg* 1998;2:50–59
41. Curet MJ, Contreras M, Weber DM, et al. Laparoscopic cholecystectomy. *Surg Endo* 2002;16(3):453–457
42. Cooperman A. Laparoscopic cholecystectomy for severe acute, embedded, and gangrenous cholecystitis. *J Laparoendosc Surg* 1990;1:37–40
43. Hermann R. Surgery for acute and chronic cholecystitis. *Surg Clin North Am* 1990;70:1263–1275
44. Rattner D, Ferguson C, Warshaw A. Factors associated with successful laparoscopic cholecystectomy for acute cholecystitis. *Ann Surg* 1993;217:233–236

45. Reddick E, Olsen D, Spaw A, et al. Safe performance of difficult laparoscopic cholecystectomies. *Am J Surg* 1991; 161:377–381
46. Unger S, Edelman D, Scott J, et al. Laparoscopic treatment of acute cholecystitis. *Surg Laparosc Endo* 1991;1:14–16
47. Lai PBS, Kwong KH, Leung KL, et al. Randomized trial of early versus delayed laparoscopic cholecystectomy for acute cholecystitis. *Br J Surg* 1998;85:764–767
48. Jones D, Dunnegan D, Soper N. The influence of intraoperative gallbladder perforation on long-term outcome after laparoscopic cholecystectomy. *Surg Endo* 1995;9:977–980
49. Deziel D, Millikan K, Economou S, et al. Complications of laparoscopic cholecystectomy: A national survey of 4,292 hospitals and an analysis of 77,604 cases. *Am J Surg* 1993;165:9–14
50. Carlin CB, Kent RB, Laws HL. Spilled gallstones—complications of abdominal wall abscesses. *Surg Endo* 1995;9: 341–343
51. Horton M, Florence MG. Unusual abscess patterns following dropped gallstones during laparoscopic cholecystectomy. *Am J Surg* 1998;175:375–379
52. Parra-Davila E, Munshi IA, Armstrong JH, et al. Retroperitoneal abscess as a complication of retained gallstones following laparoscopic cholecystectomy. *J Laparoendosc Adv Surg Tech* 1998;8:89–93
53. Shocket E. Abdominal abscess from gallstones spilled at laparoscopic cholecystectomy. *Surg Endo* 1995;9:344–347
54. Zamir G, Lyass S, Pertsemlidis D, et al. The fate of the dropped gallstones during laparoscopic cholecystectomy. *Surg Endo* 1999;13:68–70
55. Berci G, Sackier JM. Laparoscopic cholecystectomy and laparoscopic choledocholithotomy. In Blumgart LH (ed). *Surgery of the Liver and Biliary Tract.* Edinburgh: Churchill Livingstone; 1994:633–662
56. Hanney RM, All KM, Cregan PC, et al. Major vascular injury and laparoscopy. *Aust N Z J Surg* 1995;65:533–535
57. Cogliandolo A, Monganaro T, Saitta FP, et al. Blind versus open approach to laparoscopic cholecystectomy: a randomized study. *Surg Laparosc Endo* 1998;8:353–355
58. Moore M, Bennett C. The learning curve for laparoscopic cholecystotomy. The Southern Surgeons Club. *Am J of Surg* 1995;170:55–59
59. Cates J, Tompkins R, Zinner M, et al. Biliary complications of laparoscopic cholecystectomy. *Am Surg* 1993;59: 243–247
60. Asbun HJ, Rossi RL, Lowell JA, et al. Bile duct injury during laparoscopic cholecystectomy: mechanism of injury, prevention, and management. *World J Surg* 1993;17: 547–552
61. Adams DB, Borowicz MR, Wootton FTI, et al. Bile duct complications after laparoscopic cholecystectomy. *Surg Endo* 1993;7:79–83
62. Davidoff A, Pappas T, Murray E, et al. Mechanisms of major biliary injury during laparoscopic cholecystectomy. *Ann Surg* 1992;215:196–202
63. Moosa A, Easter D, vanSonnenberg E, et al. Laparoscopic injuries to the bile duct. *Ann Surg* 1992;215:203–208
64. McGinn FP, Miles AJ, Uglow M, et al. Randomized trial of laparoscopic cholecystectomy and mini-cholecystectomy. *Br J Surg* 1995;82;1374–1377
65. Majeed AW, Troy G, Nicholl J P, et al. Randomised, prospective, single-blind comparison of laparoscopic versus small-incision cholecystectomy. *Lancet* 1996;347:989–994
66. Squirrell DM, Majeed AW, Troy G, et al. A randomized, prospective, blinded comparison of postoperative pain, metabolic response, and perceived health after laparoscopic and small incision cholecystectomy. *Surgery* 1998; 123:485–495
67. Wu JS, Dunnegan DL, Luttmann DR, et al. The evolution and maturation of laparoscopic cholecystectomy in an academic practice. *J Am Coll Surg* 1998;186:554–561
68. Livingston EH, Rege RV. A nationwide study of conversion from laparoscopic to open cholecystectomy. *Am J Surg* 2004;188(3):205–211
69. Lyass S, Perry Y, Venturero M, Muggia-Sullam M, et al. Laparoscopic cholecystectomy: what does affect the outcome? A retrospective multifactorial regression analysis. *Surg Endo* 2000;14(7):661–665
70. Pessaux P, Tuech JJ, Derouet N, et al. Laparoscopic cholecystectomy in the elderly: a prospective study. *Surg Endo* 2000;14(11):1067–1069
71. Kane R, Luie N, Borbas C, et al. The outcomes of elective laparoscopic and open cholecystectomy. *J Am Coll Surg* 1995;180:136–145
72. Ure B, Troidl H, Spangenberger W, et al. Long term results after laparoscopic cholecystectomy. *Br J Surg* 1995; 82:267–270
73. Fenster L, Lonborg R, Thirby R, et al. What symptoms does cholecystectomy cure? Insights from an outcome measurement project and review of literature. *Am J Surg* 1995;169:533–538
74. Bates T, Ebbs S R, Harrison M, et al. Influence of cholecystectomy on symptoms. *Br J Surg* 1991;78:964–967
75. Gilliland T, Traverso L. 1990 Modern standards for comparison of cholecystectomy with alternative treatments for symptomatic gallstones with emphasis on long term relief of symptoms. *Surg Gynecol Obstet* 1990;170:39–44
76. Scriven M, Burgess N, Edwards E, et al. Cholecystectomy: a study of patient satisfaction. *JR Coll Surg Edinb* 1993;38:79–81
77. Fullarton G, Darking K, Williams J, et al. Evaluation of the cost of laparoscopic and open cholecystectomy. *Br J Surg* 1994;81:124–126

33

Choledocholithiasis and Cholangitis

David W. McFadden ■ *Ankesh Nigam*

With advanced endoscopic and laparoscopic techniques being readily accessible to the treating surgeon, determining the wisest path to the successful treatment of choledocholithiasis and cholangitis has become more challenging and difficult. Nevertheless, a large number of options allows one to tailor specific therapy to each individual clinical situation so as to achieve the highest probability of success. In this chapter we hope to give the reader a better understanding of the methods available for the diagnosis and treatment of common bile duct stones and cholangitis so that he or she can develop treatment plans that are patient-specific and with the highest chance of success.

■ CHOLEDOCHOLITHIASIS

CLASSIFICATION AND EPIDEMIOLOGY

A common entity in Western societies, gallstones are found in approximately 15% of Americans and result in 700,000 cholecystectomies a year. The annual cost of medical care for gallstones is almost $6.5 billion (1.3% of U.S. health care costs) compared with chronic liver disease and cirrhosis ($1.6 billion), chronic hepatitis C ($0.8 billion), and diseases of the pancreas ($2.2 billion).[1] Common bile duct stones have been noted in 10–15% of patients with cholelithiasis, and this incidence increases with age to over 80% in those who are over 90 years old.[2] Choledocholithiasis in Western countries usually results from stones originating in the gallbladder and migrating through the cystic duct. These *secondary bile duct stones* are cholesterol stones in 75% and black pigment stones in 25% of patients. Cholesterol stones are formed in the presence of cholesterol saturation, biliary stasis, and nucleating factors. Behavioral factors associated with cholesterol gallstones include nutrition, obesity, weight loss, and physical activity. Biologic factors linked to gallstones include increasing age, female sex and parity, serum lipid levels, and the Native American, Chilean, and Hispanic race.[1] The formation of black pigment stones is associated with hemolytic disorders, cirrhosis, ileal resection, prolonged fasting, and total parenteral nutrition.[2] *Primary bile duct stones*, on the other hand, form within the bile ducts and usually are of the brown pigment variety. These tend to be lower in cholesterol content and higher in bilirubin content as compared with secondary stones. Unlike secondary stones, primary stones are associated with biliary stasis and bacteria.[3] In fact, in the pathogenesis of brown pigment stones, bile infection appears to be the initial event leading to stone formation.[4] Moreover, bacteria have been found in brown pigment stones by electron microscopy but not in black pigment stones. Primary bile duct stones are more common in Asian populations, and these often are associated with *primary intrahepatic stones* in this population.[1] These intrahepatic stones usually are calcium bilirubinate and mixed stones and contain more cholesterol and less bilirubin than the extrahepatic bile duct pigmented stones. The pathogenesis of these intrahepatic stones appears to involve bile infection; biliary stasis; low-protein, low-fat diets and malnutrition; and parasitic infections. However, the role of *Ascaris lumbricoides* and *Clonorchis sinesis* in the formation of intrahepatic stones is controversial. While these parasites are found in many geographic areas, primary intrahepatic stones are found mainly in Southeast Asia. Therefore, in addition to parasitic infections, other factors must play a role in the formation of these stones.[1]

CLINICAL PRESENTATION AND NATURAL HISTORY

Asymptomatic bile duct stones may be found incidentally during evaluation of patients with suspected gallstones. In fact, 5% of common duct stones found during surgery may be unsuspected by preoperative findings and discovered only during intraoperative evaluation of the biliary tree. In one autopsy study of 615 patients over age 60, 1% were found to have bile duct stones.[2] Patients with choledocholithiasis may present with biliary colic, bile duct obstruction, bilirubinuria (or tea-colored urine), pruritus, acholic stools, and jaundice. However, the biliary obstruction usually is incomplete. There may be nausea and vomiting with intermittent or constant epigastric or right upper quadrant pain.[5] The clinical course may be complicated by acute gallstone pancreatitis, cholangitis, or rarely, hepatic abscess. Infected patients may present with back pain, fever, hypotension, and mental status changes.

Common bile duct stones are covered by a bacterial biofilm of adherent quiescent bacteria residing in a hermetic environment. When stones cause obstruction of the ducts, cytokines released by epithelial cells activate these bacteria to the planktonic and virulent forms.[1] Therefore, bile duct obstruction secondary to stones often is accompanied by bacterial sepsis resulting from activation of the bacterial biofilm on these stones. Sepsis is much less likely to occur in the context of malignant obstruction without choledocholithiasis.

Although a majority of stones will pass spontaneously into the duodenum within hours, prolonged biliary obstruction can lead to biliary cirrhosis and portal hypertension. The average time for choledocholithiasis to lead to biliary cirrhosis is about 5 years, depending on the extent of obstruction.[1] Even with cirrhosis, however, the obstruction should be relieved because some reversal of portal hypertension and secondary biliary cirrhosis may be possible.

Physical examination of patients with choledocholithiasis may be normal or reveal jaundice, scleral icterus, and abdominal tenderness over the right upper quadrant without peritoneal signs. Early in the course, physical examination may not be very different from that of patients with cholecystitis. Severe tenderness may point to acute gallstone pancreatitis, whereas fever, hypotension, and confusion may suggest cholangitis.[6]

Blood tests may reveal elevation of serum alkaline phosphatase, gamma-glutamyl transpeptidase, and bilirubin. Mild elevations of aspartate aminotransferase and alanine aminotransferase can be seen, whereas these are particularly abnormal in the situation of cholangitis. Although bilirubin and aminotransferase levels are high in 70–90% of patients at the onset of symptoms, almost all patients have elevation of alkaline phosphatase and gamma-glutamyl transpeptidase.[6] Elevated amylase and lipase may suggest pancreatitis. White blood count elevation may be seen with cholangitis, pancreatitis, or associated acute cholecystitis. It is worth noting that laboratory evaluation of patients with bile duct stones can be normal repeatedly, and this should not dissuade further evaluation of patients suspected to harbor duct stones.[7]

EVALUATION AND MANAGEMENT

The evaluation and treatment of choledocholithiasis are best discussed by considering the three clinical circumstances in which patients who may have bile duct stones are seen: prior to cholecystectomy, during cholecystectomy, or some time after cholecystectomy.

Preoperative

The diagnosis of choledocholithiasis cannot be made on the basis of history, physical examination, and laboratory investigations alone. Moreover, the distinction between the symptoms of bile duct stones and gallbladder stones often is difficult. Increasing age, history of fever, cholangitis, and pancreatitis are risk factors for bile duct stones, whereas elevations of serum bilirubin, aspartate aminotransferase, or alkaline phosphatase are independent positive predictors.[1,8]

Transcutaneous ultrasound has been the traditional method of evaluating patients with biliary disease. It is highly accurate in identifying acute calculous cholecystitis and the presence of gallstones greater than 2 mm. Sensitivities and specificities of 48–100% and 64–100%, respectively, have been reported.[9] However, the ability of transcutaneous ultrasound to establish the diagnosis of choledocholithiasis is only about 50%, varying from 30–90%.[6,10] The role of ultrasound as a screening test for bile duct stones was evaluated prospectively by Gross and colleagues.[11] Patients who were about to undergo endoscopic retrograde cholangiopancreatography (ERCP) were examined by right upper quadrant sonography to assess the size of the intra- and extrahepatic ducts and for the presence or absence of bile duct stones. The findings were compared with ERCP, percutaneous transhepatic cholangiography, or surgical follow-up. Ultrasound was not found to be accurate in the diagnosis (sensitivity of 25%) or the exclusion (73% value of negative study) of choledocholithiasis.

Meanwhile, Costi and colleagues studied the usefulness of the number and size of gallbladder stones for predicting asymptomatic choledocholithiasis.[12] Ultrasound data of 300 consecutive patients undergoing laparoscopic cholecystectomy were analyzed. Patients were divided into two groups: those with multiple small (<5 mm) gallbladder stones or variable (≤5 mm and >5 mm) stones and those with large (>5 mm) stones only. The classification of stone size was confirmed by surgery in 95% of patients. Moreover, the presence of multiple small and variable gallbladder stones represented a risk factor for synchronous asymptomatic bile duct stones (9.5%) as compared with large stones only (2.5%). In another study, ultrasound was found to have a positive predictive value of 69% and a negative predictive value of 78% for choledocholithiasis in patients suspected to have bile duct stones.[13] This compared with liver function tests having predictive values of 68% and 93%, respectively. On the other hand, when compared with altered liver function tests and/or increased amylase levels, ultrasound evidence of common bile duct dilatation (>7 mm) has been described to be the best predictor of choledocholithiasis.[14] Nonetheless, it is worth noting that almost half the patients with common bile duct stones do not have dilated ducts by ultrasound, so no dilatation is not the same as no bile duct stones.[15]

In order to predict the presence of bile duct stones more accurately, the combination of clinical, laboratory, and ultrasound risk factors has been used by several investigators.[1,16,17] In one study, multivariate logistic regression analysis revealed that when a dilated common bile duct with stones was found by ultrasound in combination with cholangitis and elevated aspartate transaminase and bilirubin, the likelihood of having stones in the bile duct was 99%. If all these factors were absent, the chance of synchronous choledocholithiasis in patients with cholelithiasis was only 7%. Unfortunately, many patients present with only some of these findings, and the prediction of bile duct stone based on these criteria becomes difficult. Moreover, ultrasound sensitivity is in part operator-dependent and altered by bowel gas, making the findings inconsistent.[18]

In 1968, ERCP was introduced as a diagnostic tool to aid in the management of biliary and pancreatic diseases.[19] Five years later, with the development of endoscopic sphincterotomy, ERCP was transformed into a therapeutic modality.[20] More than 150,000 endoscopic biliary sphincterotomies are done annually today in the United States. Short of intraoperative examination, ERCP has long been considered the standard reference for the establishment of common bile duct stones.[18] The specificity and sensitivity of ERCP were reported in 1982 by Frey and colleagues.[21] ERCP was compared with findings on common duct exploration or cystic duct cholangiography in 72 patients and was found to have a sensitivity of 90% and specificity of 98%, with a 96% accuracy. Interestingly, the interval between performance of the procedure and operation was particularly important in patients with multiple small stones. Since small stones pass more readily from the gallbladder to the common duct and from the common duct to the duodenum, the longer the interval between ERCP and operation, the greater was the chance of discordant findings. With improvements in technique and better radiologic equipment, ERCP certainly has improved over time.

Along with the ability to diagnose bile duct stones, ERCP has the advantage of offering therapeutic intervention options in the same setting of diagnosis (Figs 33–1 and 33–2). That is, after stones in the bile duct are identified, endoscopic sphincterotomy and stone extraction can be performed at the same setting. If stones are not found, bile can be collected to test for microlithiasis if clinically appropriate.[18] *ERCP stone extraction* is successful 80–90% of the time using the techniques of sphincterotomy and balloon catheter or Dormia basket stone retrieval.[20,22] The addition of mechanical, electrohydraulic, laser, or extracorporeal shockwave lithotripsy for large stones increases the success rate to over 95%.

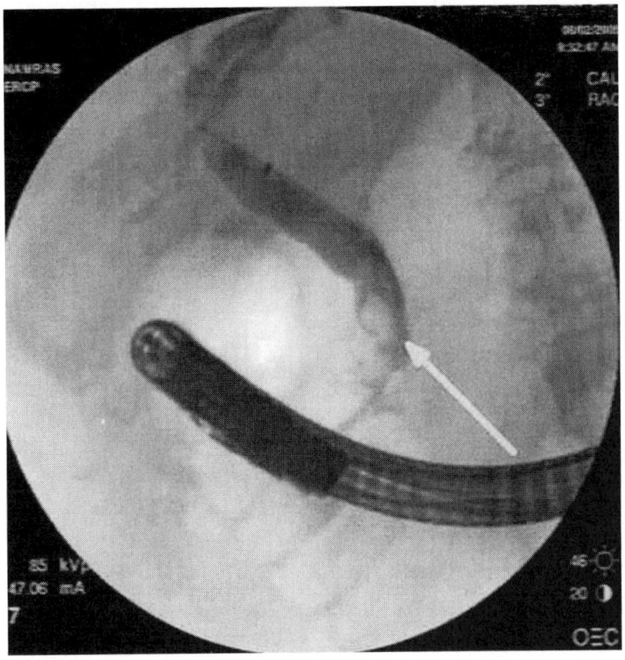

Figure 33–1. ERCP with distal common bile duct stone prior to cholecystectomy.

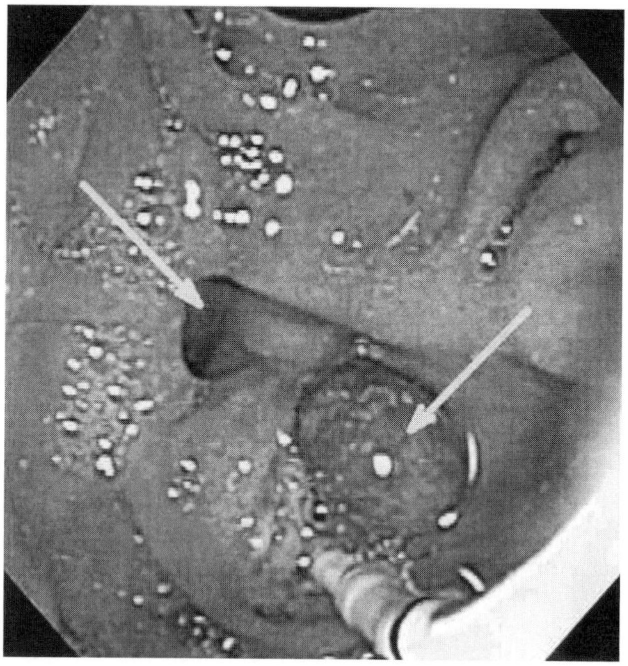

Figure 33–2. ERCP and common bile duct stone extraction.

Sphincterotomy entails division of the papilla and sphincter muscles to widen the distal end of the common bile duct with the use of a sphincterotome, a device consisting of a Teflon catheter with exposed cautery wire at the tip. The length of the intraduodenal part of the common bile duct limits the extent of the cut. *Balloon sphincteroplasty* is a sphincter-preserving alternative to sphincterotomy that uses a high-pressure hydrostatic balloon of either 6 or 8 mm diameter to dilate the papilla. One drawback of sphincteroplasty is the limited size of the papillary opening created as compared with sphincterotomy. Failure rates of 22% for stone extraction with balloon dilatation and the need for mechanical lithotripsy in 31% have been reported.[22] Furthermore, sphincteroplasty has been associated with a pancreatitis rate of 19 times greater than the rate associated with sphincterotomy.[23] A recent study evaluating the use of sphincteroplasty, on the other hand, found that severe pancreatitis only occurred in 1 patient out of 63, whereas the successful stone extraction rate was 84%.[24]

Once the sphincter has been divided, most stones can be removed using a Dormia basket or a balloon catheter. The Dormia basket has better traction than the balloon and consequently is recommended for larger stones (>1 cm). The balloon catheter occludes the bile duct lumen after inflation and therefore is useful for removal of small stones and gravel. The catheter also can be inserted over a guidewire, making it useful for intrahepatic duct stones. Three situations that may lead to a difficult extraction are stone size greater than 1.5 cm, stone location proximal to a stricture, and multiple stones that are impacted. Alternative approaches to these situations include mechanical lithotripsy, electrohydraulic or laser lithotripsy, and extracorporeal shock wave lithotripsy. Monooctain and methyl-tertiary butyl ether have been used in the past to dissolve bile duct stones through nasobiliary drainage catheters or T-tubes. The practice largely has been abandoned because of high complication rates, poor results, and the technical difficulty of performing the dissolution.[22]

Mechanical lithotripsy is the most commonly used and simplest means of fragmenting large bile duct stones or when a significant discrepancy between the stone size and the diameter of the exit passage exists.[25] A large, strong basket is used to trap the stone. The stone then is crushed against a metal sheath by applying tension to the wires by the use of a crank handle. Reimann and colleagues first described the technique in 1982, and since then, many variations in design have become available.[26,27] When stones are extremely large, repeat application of the technique may be needed to further break the stone fragments and thus allow removal. Success rates between 80% and 90% have been reported for clearing the bile duct using the procedure.[28–30] One retrospective study of 162 patients undergoing mechanical lithotripsy found that the probability of bile duct clearance was over 90% for stones less than 1 cm diameter versus 68% for stones greater than 2.8 cm.[31] Meanwhile, Garg and colleagues recently presented their data on 87 patients with stones greater than 1.5 cm that required mechanical lithotripsy.[32] They analyzed various predictive factors, including size and number of stones, stone impaction, serum bilirubin, presence of cholangitis, and bile duct diameter, in relation to the success or failure of lithotripsy. Impaction of the stones in the bile duct was found to be the only significant factor that predicted failure of mechanical lithotripsy and subsequent bile duct clearance. The composition of the stone also has been found to affect the success of stone removal. Soft stones, such as those found in Oriental cholangitis, are large but amenable to crushing, sometimes with even the Dormia basket.[25] One the other hand, stones that are calcified are hard and resist mechanical crushing.

When mechanical lithotripsy fails, *intraductal shock wave lithotripsy* can be performed using a cholangioscope that is inserted into the bile duct through the instrument channel of the duodenoscope. A flexible lithotripsy probe then is passed into the bile duct through the working channel of the cholangioscope. Shock waves are generated at the tip of the lithotripsy probe using electrical (*electrohydraulic lithotripsy*) or light energy (*laser lithotripsy*).[22] Impulses are fired on the surface of the stones under cholangioscopic guidance until the needed fragmentation is achieved. The main risk of intraductal shock wave therapy is bile duct injury resulting from a misguided shock wave. The avoidance of this complication makes cholangioscopic guidance necessary. Newer devices have a scattered light sensor located at the tip of the probe that allows automatic interruption of the laser pulse when tissue is detected. Nevertheless, the cost of intraductal shock wave lithotripsy and the requirement for two endoscopists experienced in the mother-baby scope system makes the availability of this technique limited to a few major referral centers.[22] Success rates of electrohydraulic and laser lithotripsy have been in the 80–95% range.[33] In a recent report by Arya and colleagues, the use of electrohydraulic lithotripsy was evaluated in 94 patients, with 81 having large stones and 13 having average-sized stones located above a narrow bile duct.[34] A total of 96% had successful fragmentation of their stones, with fragmentation failure secondary to hard stones in two patients and trouble with targeting in two patients. Seventy-six percent of the patients required one treatment session, 14% needed two sessions, and 10% underwent three or more treatments. Complications included cholangitis and/or jaundice in 13 patients, hemobilia in one, mild post-ERCP pancreatitis in one, biliary leak in one, and bradycardia in one patient. No deaths were reported, and the final stone clearance achieved was 90%.

Not approved for bile duct stones in the United States, *extracorporeal shock wave lithotripsy* has gained popularity in Europe and Japan for the treatment of bile duct stones in patients with major medical comorbidities and technical difficulties encountered using the standard methods of endoscopic stone extraction. A drawback with this technique is the need for multiple sessions to achieve complete stone fragmentation.[22] There have been several reports from various countries on extracorporeal shock wave lithotripsy to break down bile duct stones.[33,35–41] Shackman and colleagues, from Germany, reviewed their experience with 313 patients who had failed endoscopic stone extraction with mechanical lithotripsy and subsequently underwent high-energy extracorporeal shock wave lithotripsy.[35] Stone targeting was performed by either fluoroscopy (99%) or ultrasonography. Using the technique, complete clearance of the bile duct was achieved in 90% of the patients, with 80% requiring fragment extraction by endoscopy after the shock wave therapy. Spontaneous passage, however, was observed in 10% of the patients. No difference in outcome was noted with regard to size or number of stones, intrahepatic or extrahepatic stone location, or presence or absence of bile duct strictures. Four cases of cholangitis and one case of acute cholecystitis were the rare adverse effects noted. On the other hand, another study from Switzerland found that in their 54 patients treated with extracorporeal shock wave therapy for difficult bile duct stones, an intrahepatic location of stones was significantly associated with treatment failure.[37] Interestingly, the study found microhematuria in 95% of the patients treated. In a randomized, prospective study to evaluate extracorporeal shock wave lithotripsy versus laser-induced shock wave lithotripsy for retained bile duct stones, laser therapy achieved stone disintegration more rapidly and with significantly fewer treatment sessions, resulting in a lower cost for therapy.[39] Yasuda and colleagues, from Japan, presented the use of extracorporeal shock wave lithotripsy without preliminary endoscopic sphincterotomy for choledocholithiasis.[42] Fifty-two patients underwent endoscopic nasobiliary tube insertion followed by extracorporeal therapy. Fragmentation and complete clearance of stones were achieved in 67% without the need for additional treatment. In 25%, fragmentation was not achieved, and endoscopic extraction was required. A favorable response to extracorporeal shock wave therapy was noted in patients with smaller (<1.5 cm) "floating" stones.

In addition to lithotripsy, *large-balloon dilatation* of the distal bile duct has been reported as a means of removing difficult bile duct stones after standard extraction has been unsuccessful.[43] In a retrospective analysis, 58 patients who failed standard sphincterotomy and standard basket/balloon extraction underwent dilation with a 10–20-mm-diameter balloon (esophageal type) followed by standard basket/balloon extraction. The patients were divided into two groups: 18 patients with a tapered distal bile duct (group 1) and 40 patients with square, barrel-shaped, and/or large (>15 mm) stones (group 2). Stone clearance was successful in 89% of group 1 patients and 95% of group 2 patients. In the two patients in each group in whom extraction was not possible after dilatation alone, mechanical lithotripsy allowed for stone removal. Complication rates were 33% for group 1 and 7.5% for group 2. Complications included mild pancreatitis (two patients), mild cholangitis (two patients), and bleeding (five patients). Although bleeding was mild in two patients, moderate bleeding was noted in three patients in group 1 and was treated without surgery. Interestingly, hyperamylasemia was noted in all patients, and perforation was seen in none. Large-balloon dilatation offers an alternative in managing difficult bile duct stones, and further studies are needed to establish its role as compared with other lithotripsy options.

The management of complicated situations of choledocholithiasis may require several procedures or several sessions of the same procedure for successful clearance of the common bile duct. In such situations, partial stone impaction may lead to biliary stasis and cholangitis. Along with the administration of broad-spectrum antibiotics to cover gram-negative and gram-positive bacteria, it is important to decompress the biliary tree with either a nasobiliary catheter or a biliary stent as a temporizing measure pending more definitive treatment.[22,25] By doing this, serum bilirubin levels are allowed to decrease, and the rate of postprocedure cholangitis becomes similar to that after stone clearance. Interestingly, up to 30% of patients in whom a stent has been left in place for large stones have spontaneous disintegration of the stones, as noted on subsequent ERCP. [25] This may be secondary to the frictional movement of stone against the stent or as a result of improved bile flow with dissolution effects. Furthermore, by adding oral ursodeoxycholic acid to stent placement, 9 of 10 patients have been reported to become stone-free by this combination as compared with 0 of 40 with stent placement only.[44] Although long-term stent placement is an alternative management option for patients with large, inextricable stones who are at high risk for surgical intervention, this approach should be used with caution. In a long-term follow-up study of 58 elderly patients, 40% of patients treated with "permanent" stents for endoscopically irretrievable stones developed 34 complications in 23 patients, with cholangitis being the most frequent.[45] At median follow-up of 36 months, 44 patients had died, 9 as a result of biliary-related causes. Hui and colleagues prospectively evaluated 36 high-risk patients with difficult common bile duct stones.[46] Of these, 19 underwent stent placement, and 17 underwent complete stone clearance with electrohydraulic lithotripsy. The actuarial incidence of recurrent acute cholangitis was 8% in the lithotripsy group versus 63% in the stent group. The actuarial mortality also was higher in the stent group compared with the lithotripsy group: 74% and 41%, respectively.

Although ERCP has developed over the years as a relatively safe endoscopic diagnostic and therapeutic tool, there are well-defined, potentially severe life-threatening complications associated with it. The reported rates of complications vary widely in different studies, and this may be related in part to study design, with retrospective studies being prone to underreporting. Furthermore, the complication rates may diverge depending on the patient mix in the study and may be influenced in part by the definitions used for these complications.[19]

Mortality rate after diagnostic ERCP is about 0.2%, and this rate is nearly doubled by therapeutic interventions, to 0.5%.[18,19] Cardiopulmonary complications are the leading cause of death and include cardiac arrhythmia, hypoventilation, and aspiration. These may be the result of premorbid conditions or related to medications used during sedation and analgesia. Other significant complications include perforations (0.3–0.6%), bleeding related primarily to sphincterotomy (0.8–2%), cholecystitis (0.2–0.5%), and cholangitis (1%). Interestingly, in a recent meta-analysis, prophylactic antibiotics were not found to be beneficial in reducing infectious complications of ERCP. Moreover, another study failed to show a fall in the rate of cholangitis in patients with distal bile duct stones or biliary strictures receiving antibiotic prophylaxis.[19]

Pancreatitis is the most common complication seen after ERCP. The consensus definition for ERCP-induced pancreatitis is new or worsened abdominal pain, serum amylase that is three or more times the upper limits of normal 24 hours after the procedure, and a requirement of at least 2 days of hospitalization. Although the transient elevation of serum pancreatic enzyme levels is frequent, based on the consensus definition of ERCP pancreatitis, the expected rate of this complication is typically between 1% and 7%. Risk factors associated with ERCP-induced pancreatitis include a prior history of ERCP pancreatitis, nondilated biliary ducts, normal bilirubin, young age, female gender, and suspected sphincter of Oddi dysfunction. In fact, the risk of pancreatitis in women with normal bilirubin and suspected sphincter of Oddi dysfunction is 18% compared with 1.1% for the low-risk patient.[19,47] Moreover, one of five episodes of pancreatitis in this setting will be severe, requiring more than a 10-day hospital stay and resulting in necrosis or pseudocyst or abscess formation needing surgery or percutaneous drainage or resulting in death. Since the highest rate of complications appears to exist in the group of patients that is least likely to benefit from ERCP, the most effective method of reducing post-ERCP pancreatitis would be avoid unnecessary ERCP.

Pharmacologic methods of pancreatitis prophylaxis have been attempted to reduce this complication after ERCP.[19] Although meta-analyses have suggested that somatostatin and gabexate are useful in reducing pancreatitis rates, multicenter randomized, controlled trials have failed to show effect over that of placebo. Meanwhile, interleukin 10 (IL-10) with its anti-inflammatory activity has been found to have conflicting results in two controlled, prospective trials. The use of nonionic contrast agents has not reduced the rate of pancreatitis. On the other hand, glyceral trinitrate administered by both sublingual and transdermal routes has been shown to decrease post-ERCP pancreatitis in two placebo-controlled trials, supposedly by decreasing sphincter of Oddi pressure. Use of nitrates, however, is limited by their hypotensive effects.

The placement of pancreatic stents has been found to reduce the incidence of postbiliary sphincterotomy pancreatitis in patient suspected of sphincter of Oddi dysfunction. However, in a case-controlled evaluation of pancreatic stent placement after balloon dilatation of major papillae for bile duct stone removal, a decreased postprocedure hyperamylasemia did not result in a decreased pancreatitis rate.[19]

Based on clinical, laboratory, and ultrasound criteria for common bile duct stones, as many as 70% of patients may be found to not have duct stones at the time of preoperative ERCP.[17,48,49] Given this, a large number of patients may be subjected to an unnecessary ERCP and incur its risks and costs. In order to more firmly establish the presence of common bile duct stones prior to having patients under go ERCP or operative interventions for both therapeutic and diagnostic purposes, several methods have become available to diagnose the presence of bile duct stones accurately. The most important of these are magnetic resonance cholangiopancreatography (MRCP), endoscopic ultrasound (EUS), and computed tomography (CT).

Sensitivities of conventional *computed tomography* (CT) for choledocholithiasis in the setting of suspected bile duct stones is 76–90%, whereas unenhanced helical CT has been shown to have a sensitivity of 88%, a specificity of 97%, and an accuracy of 94%.[18] When compared with ERCP as the reference standard, CT without biliary contrast material showed poor concordance with ERCP (sensitivity 65% and specificity 84%) but compared better when oral biliary contrast material was given (sensitivity and specificity greater than 90%).[50] CT with intravenous biliary contrast material in other studies has been found to have a sensitivity of 71–85% and a specificity of 88–95%.[50] Patel and colleagues reported a comparison between non-contrast-enhanced helical CT and the reference standard of EUS and found that CT had both a sensitivity and a specificity of 83% for the detection of common bile duct dilatation in the setting of choledocholithiasis.[51] However, when CT was evaluated for identifying duct stones, it had a sensitivity only 22% and a specificity of 83%.

Since its introduction over a decade ago, *magnetic resonance cholangiopancreatography* (MRCP) has changed the way in which common bile duct stones are detected and excluded tremendously. With sensitivities and specificities that approach those of ERCP, MRCP has emerged as a diagnostic alternative to ERCP for the detection and exclusion of choledocholithiasis.[18] Performed with T_2-weighted sequences, the biliary tract is seen as a bright structure with high signal intensity without the use of contrast material, instrumentation, or ionizing radiation. Common duct stones are seen as low-signal-intensity filling defects surrounded by high-intensity bile. Improvements in hardware and software for MRCP over the last 10 years have resulted in the ability to image the entire biliary tract in a single breath-hold of 20 seconds with a resolution that allows visualization of fourth-order intrahepatic bile ducts and small stones. Stones as small as 2 mm can be detected even in the absence of biliary dilatation.[18] In one study of 97 patients, sensitivity of MRCP was 100% for stone diameters of 11–27 mm, 89% for stone diameters of 6–10 mm, and 71% for stone diameters of 3–5 mm.[47] In this study, MRCP had a 91% sensitivity compared with 100% for ERCP, whereas both tests had a specificity of 100%. Although earlier studies noted MRCP sensitivities ranging from 81–92% and specificities from 91–100% for choledocholithiasis, recent studies with state-of-the-art techniques have found sensitivities of 90–100% with specificities of 92–100%.[18] In a prospective analysis by Ke and colleagues, 267 patients felt to have common bile duct stones were evaluated by MRCP and ERCP.[52] MRCP was found to have a sensitivity of 100% and a specificity of 96% and a negative predictive value of 100%. Kejriwal and colleagues retrospectively examined patients with cholelithiasis who underwent MRCP for suspected choledocholithiasis.[53] Patients were considered not to have clinically relevant common duct stones if they had a negative MRCP and did not present for readmission for choledocholithiasis after treatment of their cholelithiasis. MRCP was negative for bile duct stones in 74% of patients (60 of 81) and missed clinically relevant stones in two patients, giving a positive predictive value of 95% and a negative predictive value of 97%. With its ability to exclude bile duct stones, MRCP may allow the avoidance of unnecessary diagnostic ERCP. Demertines and colleagues found that even in patients with high and moderate risk of common bile duct stones based on laboratory findings, the performance of MRCP could have resulted in the avoidance of ERCP in 52% and 80% of patients, respectively.[54] A three-dimensional (3D) virtual cholangioscopic software system to reconstruct a 3D image from MRCP data has been described recently, but experience is limited.[55]

One of the limitations of MRCP is that its resolution remains less than that of ERCP, and therefore, it cannot detect small stones and crystals consistently. Claustrophobia also may influence the use of MRCP, and patients may need sedation or even general anesthesia for its performance. Patient obesity may diminish the quality of images, whereas morbid obesity, pacemakers, and aneurysm clips precludes entry into the scanner.[18] On the other hand, ERCP may be limited by an inability to access and cannulate the papilla and opacify the ductal system. Failed ERCP rates vary greatly among endoscopists and vary from 5–20%.[18] Moreover, alterations in the gastrointestinal tract anatomy, such as a Billroth II gastrojejunostomy, may preclude access to the ampulla. MRCP offers a method of evaluating the biliary system for bile duct stones with sensitivities and specificities that approach those of ERCP in a manner that is noninvasive and avoids the risks and limitations of ERCP. Patients with a positive MRCP then may be considered for more invasive therapeutic procedures.

Another sensitive method of evaluating the biliary system for common bile duct stones is *endoscopic ultrasound* (EUS). EUS has been shown to have a diagnostic accuracy of 95% for bile duct stones.[56] With the high ultrasound frequencies used (7.5 and 12 MHz), EUS has a resolution of less than 1 mm, making it the best imaging technique available for extrahepatic biliary tract. Several studies have found EUS to be similar to ERCP in sensitivity and specificity for the evaluation of choledocholithiasis, with some showing ERCP to be better and others showing EUS to be better.[50] Compared with ERCP, EUS is semi-invasive with almost no procedure-related complications and negligible failure rate. In fact, several series consisting of over 1000 patients have reported no complications.[56] In a prospective study by Buscarini and colleagues, 485 patients suspected to have choledocholithiasis based on clinical, laboratory, and ultrasound, or CT findings underwent EUS.[56] Positive EUS findings were confirmed by surgery or ERCP with sphincterotomy; negative findings were confirmed by clinical follow-up of at least 6 months. EUS findings were verified in 463 patients as follows: 237 true positive, 216 true negative, 2 false positives, and 4 false negatives and in 4 patients EUS was incomplete (sensitivity 98%, specificity 99%, positive predictive value 99%, negative predictive value 98%, accuracy 97%). No complications were noted in the study. EUS offers higher resolution than MRCP and therefore is better able to detect small stones. It is able to identify bile duct stones as well as microlithiasis and is able to detect pathology that is not seen by ERCP. EUS prior to performing invasive diagnostic or therapeutic techniques would lower the rate of procedure-related complications in patients suspected of having bile duct stones. Cost analysis of EUS followed by ERCP versus ERCP alone is also in favor of EUS as a pretherapeutic procedure.[56]

In patients for whom ERCP is not available, not possible secondary to anatomic considerations, or not successful, an alternative method of cholangiography and nonsurgical therapy is *percutaneous transhepatic cholangiography* (PTC) followed by transhepatic methods of stone removal. A needle is introduced into the intrahepatic bile ducts through the skin, and a cholangiogram is performed, followed by wire insertion and then a catheter over the wire for external biliary drainage and access to the biliary system. The method was introduced in Denmark in the 1970s and has been refined over the years with the addition of several therapeutic options.[57] This technique is particularly useful for evaluating intrahepatic stones or other proximal bile duct disease. After diagnosis of bile duct stones, several therapeutic options are available through the percutaneous route. In 1981, the removal of an 8-mm common bile duct stone by percutaneous transhepatic technique was reported by Fernstrom and colleagues.[58] In 1990, Stokes and colleagues, from Boston, reported a series of 53 patients in whom surgery was contraindicated and ERCP unsuccessful.[59] By inserting a modified Dormia basket via a percutaneous transhepatic route, stones were advanced whole or after fragmentation into the duodenum. Monooctanoin or methyl tertiary butyl ether was used in 30 patients to reduce stone size or remove debris. Morbidity and mortality were 12% and 4%, with a success rate of 93%. Transhepatic cholangioscopy and lithotripsy can be performed after PTC and dilatation of the intrahepatic channel with success rates of 90–100% and 5–8% complications.[60] In a series of 12 patients with bile duct stones, percutaneous transhepatic cholangioscopy in combination with laser or electrohydraulic lithotripsy to deliver stone fragments into the duodenum was found to be successful in all the patients.[61] In another series of 13 patients, laser lithotripsy was used with percutaneous cholangioscopy performed either transhepatic (12 patients) or through T-tube track.[62] Stone fragmentation was successful in 92%, and stone clearance was possible in all patients. However, 11 patients required the addition of sphincterotomy (either by ERCP or by antegrade method with fluoroscopic monitoring) or stent insertion. Bleeding in two patients accounted for a 15% severe complication rate. Percutaneous transhepatic papillary balloon dilatation was reported recently by a Japanese group for the management of choledocholithiasis.[63] In the five patients in whom the method was used, bile duct stones were able to be pushed into the duodenum in all, with no complications or deaths. Ponchon and colleagues reported percutaneous choledochoscopy for stone extraction in 75 patients, with the transhepatic route used in 48 patients and T-tube tract used in 27 patients.[64] Complete clearance of bile duct stones was accomplished in 69 patients (92%).

After bile duct clearance is achieved by nonoperative methods, cholecystectomy generally is recommended in younger patients to decrease the risk of future cholecystitis and recurrent biliary colic. As many as 24% of patients have been found to require cholecystectomy at follow-up after endoscopic papillotomy at an average of 14 months.[65] Others have argued that sphincterotomy results in gallbladder stasis, bacterial overgrowth, and an increase in bile acids, and these may increase the risk of gallbladder cancer in 10–20 years.[2] On the other hand, Dhiman and colleagues studied the changes in gallbladder emptying and lithogenicity of bile following endoscopic sphincterotomy in patients with choledocholithiasis and gallbladder in situ.[66] Sphincterotomy was found to decrease stasis of gallbladder bile, improve gallbladder emptying, and decrease the lithogenicity of bile as measure by prolongation of nucleation time. Meanwhile, there is much evidence to support leaving the gallbladder in situ after bile duct clearance in high-risk or elderly patients.[67–76] In a study of 191 patients (median age 76 years) in whom the gallbladder was left in situ post-ERCP, 10 patients (5%) required subsequent uneventful cholecystectomy.[70] Twenty-six percent (49 patients) died during the review period from nonbiliary pathology. Kwon and colleagues followed 146 patients without elective cholecystectomy after endoscopic common bile duct stone removal for a period of 3 months or more to see if they could identify factors that predict subsequent gallbladder-related symptoms and need of cholecystectomy.[72] Fifty-nine patients had cholelithiasis, whereas 87 patients had no gallbladder stones. During a mean follow-up of 24 months, seven patients (5%) underwent cholecystectomy, on average, 18 months after ERCP as a result of acute cholecystitis (four patients), biliary pain (two patients), and acute pancreatitis (one patient). Nine patients (6%) died of causes unrelated to biliary disease. Interestingly, Cox regression analysis revealed that the need of subsequent cholecystectomy did not correlate with age, sex, presence of gallbladder stones, number of gallbladder stones, or underlying disease. On the other hand, Kullman and colleagues found that at a median observation time of 42 months, cholecystectomy was needed in 11% (13 patients) of 118 patients with an in situ gallbladders after ERCP bile duct clearance.[73] Forty-nine (42%) died 2–87 months after ERCP during the follow-up period. In another study of 33 elderly patients who were followed for an average of 42 months with gallbladders in situ after successful ERCP for choledocholithiasis, 3% (one patient) required cholecystectomy for acute cholecystitis, and 6% (two patients) had mild right upper quadrant pain, whereas 91% remained asymptomatic.[74] Over the time of the study, 30% of the patients died from nonbiliary causes. The impact of gallbladder status on patient outcome after extracorporeal shockwave lithotripsy for complicated common bile duct stones was studied by a German group.[71] One-hundred and twenty patients with an average age of 68 years (range 28–86 years) were followed for 3–9 years (mean 4 years). Thirty-seven had their gallbladder in situ, 27 had had a cholecystectomy after ESWL, and 56 had already undergone cholecystectomy prior to diagnosis of choledocholithiasis. During the follow-up period, 30% (36 patients) experienced biliary symptoms. However, there was no significant difference in the incidence of these symptoms between the three groups. Repeat ERCP revealed 28 cases of recurrent bile duct stones. Although not reaching statistical significance ($P = 0.077$), these, in fact, occurred more often in the cholecystectomy groups. Given the multiple studies supporting leaving the gallbladder in situ after common bile duct clearance, it seems reasonable to perform cholecystectomies on high-risk or elderly patients as needed rather than prophylactically following nonoperative treatment of bile duct stones.

Intraoperative

When patients present to the operating room for cholecystectomy, they either have common bile duct stones confirmed by preoperative studies (e.g., ERCP, MRCP, or EUS), or they are suspected to have common bile duct stones by clinical presentation, laboratory values, or transabdominal ultrasound, or they have no suspicion of bile duct stones. At the time of surgery, *intraoperative cholangiography* (IOC) is the method used most often to establish the presence of bile duct stones. IOC was first introduced to open biliary surgery by Mirizzi in the 1930s.[77] With the universal acceptance of laparoscopic cholecystectomy as the treatment of choice for symptomatic gallbladder stones, laparoscopic IOC has developed into a very useful method to evaluated the biliary tree. The technique may be performed by injecting contrast material through a catheter introduced into the cystic duct via a 14-gauge IV catheter placed through the abdominal wall 3 cm medial to the midclavicular port.[78] Cannulation rates with successful cholangiography are from 75–100%, and the use of fluoroscopy has become standard because it is faster, more detailed, and allows real-time surgeon interaction.[78,79] The reported sensitivity, specificity, positive and negative predictive values, and accuracy for laparoscopic cholangiography are 80–90%, 76–97%, 67–90%, 90–98%, and 95%, respectively, and these are comparable with the values for open IOC.[77] The rate of false-positive IOC results in a recent large review was found to be 0.8% (34 of 4209 patients).

Although approximately 10–15% of patients undergoing laparoscopic cholecystectomy harbor common bile duct stones, the need for routine IOC is a matter of much debate.[80] In a large Medline literature review, Metcalfe and colleagues found a 4% rate of common bile duct stones in 8 laparoscopic cholecystectomy trials in which routine IOC was performed on 4209 patients without suspected bile duct stones preoperatively.[79] This finding was felt to be consistent with previous reviews. On the other hand, in a total of 5179 patients without suspicion for bile duct stones who did not undergo IOC during laparoscopic cholecystectomy, 32 (0.6%) proceeded to develop symptoms from residual bile duct stones. Therefore, by extrapolating the data, it would seem that of the 4% of patients with silent common bile duct stones at laparoscopic cholecystectomy, only 15% go on to develop symptoms from retained stones. In other words, 167 IOCs would have to be done during laparoscopic cholecystectomy in order to detect one common bile duct stone that would go on to cause symptoms in patients without preoperative evidence of duct stones. This would result in eight unnecessary bile duct explorations or ERCPs.[79] It is possible that stones that are not manifested preoperatively are of the size that can pass spontaneously into the duodenum, never presenting with symptoms.

An important argument that is made for the use of routine IOC during laparoscopic cholecystectomy is for the prevention of bile duct injuries because variations in biliary anatomy occur in 10–20% of patients.[79] However, there is no association between the occurrence of bile duct injuries and anomalous anatomy. In the review by Metcalfe and colleagues, the incidence of complete common duct transection in 6024 patients undergoing routine IOC during laparoscopic cholecystectomy (0.02%) was not significantly different from that in the 3258 patients undergoing selective IOC (0.09%).[79] Moreover, the review found that 821 routine IOC would have to be done to detect one minor duct injury (defined by duct injury that is managed without choledochojejunostomy) at the time of surgery. Although IOC does not appear to prevent common bile duct injury, others argue that it allows for earlier detection of such injuries and thus more successful initial repair.[77]

Intraoperative ultrasound (IOUS) is a noninvasive way to evaluate the biliary system at the time of surgery. First introduced in the mid-1980s in the time of open cholecystectomy, laparoscopic IOUS came into use in the mid-1990s.[77] Recent experience with laparoscopic IOUS has suggested that it is a very sensitive test for common bile duct stones and roughly equivalent to IOC in evaluating the biliary ductal system. Moreover, it lacks the potential of common bile duct injury that exists with placement of the cholangiography catheter during IOC and will not cause a false-positive test owing to air introduced into the biliary tree.[79] The use of laparoscopic IOUS has been limited, however, possibly secondary to equipment availability and cost, as well as the expertise and experience required for its use. In fact, there appears to be a considerable learning curve associated with the use of laparoscopic IOUS.[81,82]

Once the presence of common bile duct stones has been established at the time of surgery, there are several treatment options. Depending on local availability and expertise, these may include open or laparoscopic duct exploration and postcholecystectomy nonoperative techniques such as ERCP or PTC. However, before embarking on a means of eradicating the biliary tree of stones, it is worth remembering that only 15% of patients with silent bile duct stones at the time of cholecystectomy present with symptoms of retained stones.[79] In fact, the natural history of choledocholithiasis was revisited in a recent prospective study by Collins and colleagues.[83] Operative cholangiography was attempted in 997 patients undergoing laparoscopic cholecystectomy and was successful in 962. Patients with cholangiogram-positive stones were restudied in 48 and 72 hours and 6 weeks after laparoscopic cholecystectomy through a cystic duct cholangiocatheter left in the cystic duct at the time of surgery. Of the 962 patients, 46 (4.6%) had at least one filling defect, but 12 had normal cholangiograms 48 hours later, giving a 26% possible false-positive cholangiogram rate. At 6 weeks, a further 12 had a normal cholangiogram, giving a 26% spontaneous passage rate of bile duct stones. This spontaneous passage was not predictable by either the number or size of stones or the diameter of the bile duct. Only 2.2% of the total population (22 patients) required postoperative endoscopic retrograde cholangiopancreatographic retrieval of persistent common duct calculi. Thus a treatment decision based on the findings of IOC alone would have resulted in 52% of patients with positive findings undergoing unnecessary intervention.

The first surgical exploration of the common bile duct was done in 1890 by Ludwig Courvoisier, a Swiss surgeon who made an incision in the common bile duct and removed a gallstone.[78,84] Prior to the development of laparoscopic cholecystectomy, patients found to have bile duct stones at surgery underwent *open common bile duct exploration* with greater than 90% duct clearance. ERCP was used for retained stones postoperatively or for patients who would not be able to tolerate extended general anesthesia. At the time of open cholecystectomy, the common duct is opened in the longitudinal direction so as to not compromise the blood supply to the duct. The bile duct is cleared of stones with the use of Fogarty balloons, saline irrigation, stone forceps, and scoops placed into the biliary tract through the opening. Choledochoscopy is particularly useful in evaluating the duct system during and after the clearance of residual stones and in making sure that there is no other ductal pathology. Moreover, a basket can be passed through the working channel of the scope and used under direct vision for stone removal. Although used commonly in the management of common bile duct stones in the era of open cholecystectomy, open bile duct exploration is used infrequently in the present age of minimally invasive surgery. In a recent series of 326 patients who underwent laparoscopic common bile duct exploration (LCBDE) for choledocholithiasis at the time of cholecystectomy, only five patients were converted to laparotomy and only two for open bile duct exploration and stone extraction.[78]

Over a hundred years after Langenbuch performed the first open cholecystectomy in 1882, laparoscopic cholecystectomy was introduced and soon became the standard treatment of cholecystitis and symptomatic gallstones.[78,84] In the early years after the development of laparoscopic cholecystectomy, *laparoscopic common bile duct exploration* (LCBDE) was used infrequently, and reliance on alternatives methods of duct clearance was widespread.[78] With increasing experience in laparoscopic techniques and the demand for single-procedure minimally invasive duct clearance, the use of LCBDE gained greater acceptance among experienced biliary surgeons. Since the development of the technique, thousands of successful LCBDEs have been reported in the literature, and success rates of duct clearance are between 80% and 90%, comparable with the open method of bile duct exploration.[77] The morbidities range from 8–10% and are typical of laparoscopic procedures, including nausea, diarrhea, ileus, atelectasis, phlebitis, urinary retention and infection, biliary leak, dislodgement of the T-tube, fluid collections, pulmonary embolus, and myocardial infarctions. Reported mortalities are from 0–2%.

The technique of LCBDE has been well described by Petelin.[77,78] Access to the biliary system, after obtaining a cholangiogram, can be either transcystic or transductal using a choledochotomy. Use of the transcystic approach varies from 5–98% depending on the series. With this method, the gallbladder is retracted toward the right hemidiaphragm, and if needed, the cystic duct is dilated with either over-the-wire mechanical or pneumatic dilators. Factors favoring the transductal approach include stones greater than 6 mm in diameter, intrahepatic stones, cystic duct diameter less than 4 mm, and cystic duct entrance either posterior or distal. When using the transductal method, a choledochotomy is made on the anterior surface of the common bile duct with a scissors or scalpel and is limited to 1 cm or the size of the largest stone.

Once the biliary tree has been accessed, choledocholithotomy is performed using several different techniques and is guided by either fluoroscopy or choledochoscopy. Although separate monitors may be used with a choledochoscope, the use of a video mixer to place the laparoscopic and choledochoscopic images on the same screen is helpful. Newer choledochoscopes with 3 mm diameters even can be passed through the cystic duct. Common bile duct clearance is started with irrigation, which allows the flushing of small, less than 3-mm stones and sludge. The administration of 1–2 mg intravenous glucagon allows relaxation of the sphincter of Oddi and facilitates the irrigation process. Fogarty-type balloons (4F) then can be inserted into the bile duct for retrograde extraction of stones with withdrawal of the inflated balloon. Stones also may be captured with a Dormia-type basket inserted directly through the cystic duct or choledochotomy or through the working port of the choledochoscope. Intraoperative electrohydraulic or laser lithotripsy is useful for large stones or stones that are impacted and not responsive to other methods. Care is needed, however, to avoid injury to the duct by inaccurate application of the lithotripsy device.

If a choledochotomy is used to perform the LCBDE, frequently a T-tube is left in place for later study of the biliary system, decompression if the biliary tree is not cleared, or access to the biliary system for recurrent stones. On the other hand, laparoscopic suturing with 4-0 or 5-0 Vicryl can be done instead to close the choledochotomy primarily. A recent study found that hospital stay was shorter in a group of patients who underwent primary closure versus placement of a T-tube (5 versus 9 days).[85] There does not appear to be an increase in the incidence of bile leak or peritonitis in patients undergoing primary closure.[78] This further abrogates the complications of T-tubes, including dislodgement, bacteremia, fracture of the tube, and the possibility of bile leak and peritonitis at the time of T-tube removal. An alternative to T-tube placement is a stent placed in an antegrade fashion into the duct similar to an ERCP-placed stent.[86] A recently described option to a T-tube is a modified ureteral catheter placed through the cystic duct and brought out through the abdomen after closure of the choledochotomy.[87] In a study of 30 patients undergoing placement of this modified catheter, no complications related to the catheter were found, and removal was possible at a median of 5 days as compared with 29 days when a T-tube was used.

If LCBDE is unsuccessful, a transcystic catheter may be inserted through the abdominal wall to decompress the biliary system and allow for postoperative cholangiography. If the catheter is further advanced into the duodenum, it can aid in bile duct cannulation at the time of postoperative ERCP.[77] In addition to treating bile duct stones postoperatively following an incomplete laparoscopic duct clearance, the option of converting to an open duct exploration is also available to the operating surgeon.

There are several alternatives to laparoscopic or open duct exploration for bile duct stones encountered at the time of surgery. At the time of cholecystectomy, a *tran-*

scystic stent may be placed over a wire antegrade through the sphincter of Oddi as initial treatment.[88] This allows for decompression of the biliary tree and can be followed postoperatively by ERCP and sphincterotomy with stent removal. Another option is the use of *intraoperative ERCP* (IO-ERCP), allowing for the same anesthetic to be used for the both the cholecystectomy and the ERCP.[89–91] In one Swedish study by Enochsson and colleagues, 592 patients underwent IOC during laparoscopic cholecystectomy.[91] thirty-four of these were subjected to IO-ERCP with a 100% common bile duct cannulation rate. This was assisted by the fact that the surgeon, while waiting for the endoscopist, introduced a thin guidewire into the IOC catheter and through the sphincter of Oddi into the duodenum. Bile duct clearance was possible in 94%, and a stent was left in place in the two patients with remaining stones. Operative time was prolonged by 1.5 hours as compared with laparoscopic cholecystectomy, but the length of hospitalization was not significantly longer for IO-ERCP patients. There were no cases of postoperative pancreatitis. In a French report by Meyer and colleagues, 60 patients were treated with laparoscopic cholecystectomy and IO-ERCP for confirmed or suspected CBD stones.[90] The mean operative time for laparoscopic cholecystectomy was 60 minutes (range 40–90 minutes), and general anesthesia was prolonged only 40 minutes (range 30–60 minutes) for performing the IO-ERCP, including the time needed for setting up the endoscopic equipment. The papilla could not be catheterized in two patients. In one, postoperative ERCP was possible, and in the second patient, a small stone passed spontaneously. In one patient, secondary to multiple calculi in common bile duct, open surgery was performed immediately after IO-ERCP. Final duct clearance was achieved in 100% of patients. The argument for using IO-ERCP versus postoperative ERCP is that the former allows the identification of anatomic problems (such as duodenal diverticulum) that could make later ERCP unsuccessful. Thus the surgeon has the option to convert to open bile duct exploration at the same anesthetic.[89] If one chooses to use IO-ERCP, performing the cholecystectomy prior to the ERCP is important because this avoids endoscopy-induced small bowel distension from interfering with gallbladder visualization. Moreover, transcystic IOC at the time of cholecystectomy may avoid unnecessary ERCP if no stones are visualized by the cholangiogram.

Postoperative

Patients presenting with common bile duct stones after cholecystectomy generally are treated with ERCP[77] (Fig 33–3) The noninvasive imaging techniques, such as ultrasound and MRI, are not different from those used preoperatively. If a T-tube (or other transabdominal drainage catheter) had been left in place at prior surgery, a cholangiogram can be obtained after surgery to establish the presence of bile duct stones. In situations in which ERCP is not possible or successful, other nonoperative methods can be used. For patients with T-tubes, percutaneous instrumentation under fluoroscopic guidance through the T-tube tract can be used to remove bile duct stones. In one report, 23 of 25 patients underwent successful duct clearance through the T-tube tract for retained stones.[92] A choledochoscope also may be inserted through the T-tube tract to allow for either laser or electrohydraulic lithotripsy and stone extractions.[64] Other percutaneous transhepatic options described in the preoperative section of this chapter also may be used. Combinations and repeated techniques may be needed to achieve duct clearance. In the rare incidences where the biliary system cannot be cleared of stones nonoperatively, surgical duct exploration is considered, and the need for surgical drainage procedures must be addressed.

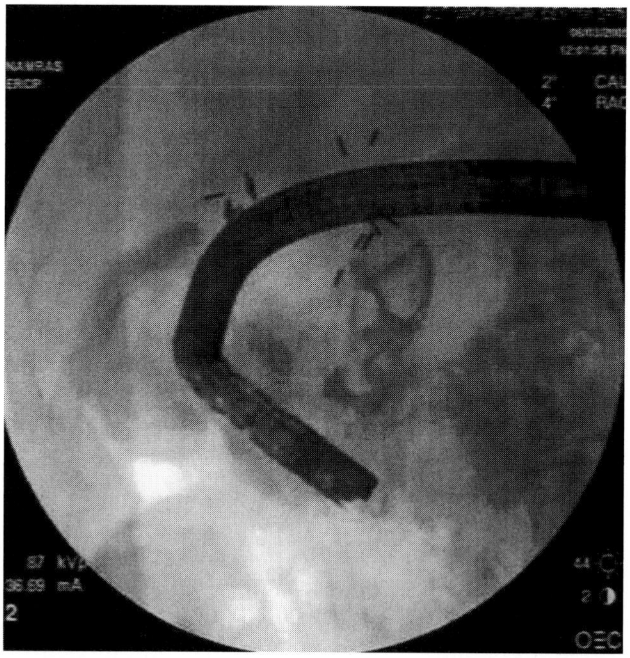

Figure 33–3. Multiple retained stones after cholecystectomy, seen on ERCP.

Surgical Biliary Drainage Procedures

Surgical biliary drainage procedures must be considered in situations of multiple stones; incomplete removal of all stones; impacted, irremovable distal bile duct stones; markedly dilated common bile duct; distal bile duct obstruction from tumor or stricture; and reoccurrence after previous bile duct exploration. The methods of surgical drainage include transduodenal sphincterotomy, choledochoduodenotomy, and choledochojejunostomy.

Transduodenal sphincterotomy (TDS) is useful in the management of choledocholithiasis when there is stone impaction in the ampulla of Vater, papillary stenosis, and multiple stones, particularly in the presence of a nondilated bile duct.[93–95] The duodenum is kocherized completely, and the ampulla is located by passing a biliary Fogarty catheter through the common bile duct into the duodenum. A longitudinal duodenotomy is made over the ampulla, and the entrance to the pancreatic duct is identified at the 4 o'clock position when possible. Intravenous secretin given at 0.2 g/kg over 1 minute sometimes is helpful in this identification. Absorbable sutures are placed on each side of the ampulla, and the sphincterotomy is started at 11 o'clock and extended with sequential placement of sutures along the incision. After the opening is wide enough to fit a biliary dilator the size of the common duct, the last ampullary suture is placed at the apex to prevent a duodenal leak. The duodenotomy then is closed in the transverse direction to prevent duodenal stenosis, and a drain is left in the event that the duodenotomy leaks.

In a French review by Suter and colleagues, of the 78 patients who underwent transduodenal sphincterotomy, 26 were operated on urgently.[95] Forty-seven (60%) were jaundiced, 15 (19%) had pancreatitis, and 12 (15%) had cholangitis before surgery. Three patients died, one from pulmonary embolism, one from pulmonary sepsis, and the other from multiorgan failure syndrome complicating preoperative necrotizing pancreatitis. Of the 30 patients (38%) with complications, 20 were directly related to the surgery and included 4 cases of hemorrhage not requiring transfusion, 17 instances of hyperamylasemia with 1 case of clinical pancreatitis, and 1 case of duodenal fistula that healed after conservative therapy. No deaths were noted that were directly attributable to the TDS. On the other hand, in a older review by Meyhoff, a 10% postoperative mortality was noted after TDS, with four patients developing fatal pancreatitis.[93]

Choledochoduodenostomy (CDD) was first performed by Riedel in 1888 in Europe.[96] Unfortunately, the patient died of anastomotic disruption secondary to a missed stone in the distal common bile duct. The first successful operation was done by Sprengel in 1891. Choledochoduodenostomy is indicated in patients with recurrent stones requiring repeated interventions, impacted or giant stones, biliary sludge, and ampullary stenosis. The funnel syndrome in which a distal bile duct stenosis exists in the presence of common bile duct stones is one of the most classic indications for CDD.[96] Most of the common bile duct stones in this situation are primary biliary stones forming as a result of biliary stasis. Any procedure done to remove only the stones has a temporary benefit if the stenosis is not addressed.

Choledochoduodenostomy can be performed either as an elective or an emergency operation, such as for cholangitis. The side-to-side anastomosis is the most commonly used technique, but an end-to-side is also an option. A common bile duct diameter of at least 1.2 cm is important in assessing the feasibility of CDD because this allows a wide enough stoma to ensure good biliary drainage and avert stenosis. The anastomosis is created in the most distal portion of the bile duct to decrease the chance of the well-described sump syndrome.[96] After opening the abdomen, the duodenum is kocherized widely to allow for a tension-free anastomosis, and the common bile duct is dissected completely along its distal anterior surface. A longitudinal duodenotomy is made close to the bile duct along the long axis of the duodenum, perpendicular to the choledochotomy. The common bile duct incision is made along the long axis of the bile duct as close to the duodenum as possible and of a 2-cm length to prevent stenosis. After performing a common bile duct exploration and clearing the duct of stones, a side-to-side single-layered anastomosis is made with absorbable suture, and a drain is placed for the possibility of an anastomotic leakage.

The morbidity and mortality rates associated with choledochoduodenostomy are 23% and 3%, respectively.[96] Mortality is most commonly from medical complications, such as pulmonary embolism, myocardial infarction, or heart failure. Among the specific operative morbidities, cholangitis and sump syndrome are described most commonly.

The incidence of cholangitis ranges from 0–6% in largest long-term follow-up series.[96] Although once thought to be caused by ascending reflux of duodenal contents into the biliary tree, cholangitis is now believed to be the result of stenosis of the anastomotic stoma. A wide anastomosis avoids stasis and stone retention by allowing entrance and egression of duodenal and biliary contents. Sump syndrome is caused by food and debris accumulating between the stoma and the papilla of Vater. This leads to contamination of the large and small bile ducts with resulting recurrent cholangitis and even secondary biliary cirrhosis.[96] Although the accumulation of debris in the blind segment of the bile duct may cause destruction of the stoma or cholangitis, some believe that the disease is caused by the stenosis of stoma. To avoid the problem, creating a stoma of at least 14 mm, along with placing the anastomosis near the duodenum, is important. Stomal patency is felt to be the most important factor for preventing both cholangitis and sump syndrome.[97] Other complications of CDD include wound infection, anastomotic leak, and intra-abdominal abscess. Long-term studies reveal that 70–80% of patients are asymptomatic 5 years after surgery.[96] In a review of 126 patients undergoing CDD after common bile duct exploration over a period of 19 years, Deutsch and colleagues reported a 4% mortality rate, with all deaths occurring in patients over 70 years old.[98] Morbidity included wound infections in 18 patients (14%) and bile leak through a drain for over 2 weeks in 4 patients (3%). Ninety-seven patients (94%) were symptom-free at a follow-up of 1–19 years.

Rameriz and colleagues reported their experience with choledochoduodenostomy and transduodenal sphincterotomy for the treatment of choledocholithiasis over a period of 10 years.[99] Of the 591 patients who underwent choledochotomy for bile duct stones, 240 (40.6%) were treated with primary closure over a T-tube, 126 (21.3%) received primary closure over a T-tube along with a transduodenal sphincterotomy, 216 (36.5%) had a supraduodenal choledochoduodenostomy, and 9 (1.5%) had both a choledochoduodenostomy and a transduodenal sphincterotomy. CDD was performed when the bile duct was more than 12 mm in diameter, and TDS was used if a stone was impacted in the papilla and/or papillary stenosis was noted. Complications included 6 abdominal abscesses and 3 external biliary fistulas in the patients undergoing CDD and 4 abscesses and 2 episodes of acute pancreatitis in the patients treated with TDS. There was no difference in mortality between the two groups, and after a mean follow-up of 5.6 years, 71.5% of the CDD group and 75.2% of the TDS group were asymptomatic. Symptoms noted in the remainder included dyspepsia, colicky pain, and episodes of cholangitis and resulted in reoperations for residual stones in 9 patients, 6 from the CDD group and 3 from the TDS group. The same authors had reported previously that of the patients who presented with symptoms after CDD and underwent endoscopy, no problems at the anastomosis were noted in those with dyspepsia, whereas 27% of those with colic had an anastomotic stenosis or sump syndrome, and all the patients with cholangitis had stenosis and residual stones.[100] On the other hand, in a comparison of 190 patients with CDD and 56 patients with TDS over a period of 10 years, Baker and colleagues found an overall mortality of about 5% in both groups.[94] The morbidity rates were 11.6% for CDD and 21.4% for TDS. With a mean follow-up of 4.5 years, 6 patients (3.3%) in the CDD group presented with sump syndrome or cholangitis or both, and 3 patients (5.7%) in the TDS group had cholangitis. In another report by the same authors, an elevated serum alkaline phosphatase level was noted in 22% of CDD patients and 3 % of the TDS patients, whereas radiologic studies showed that the CDD stoma admitted air and barium more often than the TDS stoma.[101] Interestingly, neither the biochemical nor the radiologic findings correlated with long-term symptomatic results after the two procedures.

An alternative to CDD is *choledochojejunostomy* (CDJ), which can be done with either a loop of jejunum or using a Roux-en-Y configuration. If a loop is used, a side-to-side jejunojejunostomy is used to divert the flow of intestinal contents from the biliary tree. The Roux-en-Y usually is brought retrocolic using a 60-cm afferent limb to protect against intestinal reflux and secondary cholangitis. In either case, an end-to-side choledochojejunostomy is created using interrupted absorbable suture. The anastomosis can be decompressed using a T-tube if the remaining bile duct is long enough to allow one, or a transhepatic stent can be used if the remaining bile duct is short. As in the other methods of surgical drainage, a drain is left in place to guard against possible anastomotic leakage.

Gouma and colleagues reported their experience with 43 patients undergoing Roux-en-Y choledochojejunostomy after complex clearance of the biliary tree for choledocholithiasis.[102] There were no mortalities and one major complication. Moreover, 98% of the patients had good long-term results with no signs or symptoms related to biliary obstruction or cholangitis. A comparison of CDD and CDJ for choledocholithiasis was evaluated by a French group.[103] One-hundred and thirty patients were included, of which 64 underwent CDD and 66 had a CDJ. No difference in morbidity or mortality was noted between the two groups. Of the 120 patients (58 CDD and 62 CDJ) available for a mean follow-up of 29 months, 107 were symptom-free. 13 patients (6 CDD and 7 CDJ) experienced biliary symptoms suggestive of cholangitis, and 8 presented in the first postoperative year, and 5 presented in the second postoperative year. In the CDD group, the cholangitis was secondary to sump syndrome (three patients), anastomotic stricture (one patient), or unknown causes (two patients). Anastomotic stricture (three patient), residual intrahepatic stones (one patient), or unknown causes (three patients) were felt to be the cause of cholangitis in the CDJ group. The authors concluded that CDD is preferable given the similar outcomes because it is easier and faster to perform than CCJ and allows for easy endoscopic interventions if needed in the future. However, often the choice between the two operations is dictated by the anatomy and feasibility of creating a tension-free anastomosis.[104]

One controversy in performing biliary anastomosis is the use of biliary stents. Earlier studies have argued that stents allow for decompression of the bile duct and decreased risk of bile leak, postoperative radiographic evaluation of the biliary tree, and reduced fibrotic narrowing of the anastomosis during early healing.[105] Pitt and colleagues noted a higher success rate with the anastomosis stented for more than 1 month compared with those stented for less than 1 month or not stented at all.[106] Others also have noted good results with the use of stents.[107,108] On the other hand, Bismuth and colleagues showed that excellent results could be obtained in 86% of 123 patients undergoing stentless hepaticojejunostomy for benign biliary disorders.[109] Pelligrini and colleagues found that stenting for more than 1 month postoperatively resulted in outcomes no different from anastomoses done without stents.[110] The argument has been raised that stents cause an inflammatory reaction that may predispose to stenosis. In a recent report, DiFronzo and colleagues found that of the 97 patients having either a choledochoduodenostomy (77%), choledochojejunostomy (8%), hepaticoduodenostomy (1%), or hepaticojejunostomy (13%) without the use of stents, only one patient developed an anastomotic leak that resolved spontaneously within 1 week.[105] In the mean follow-up period of 13 months, no postoperative strictures were noted. Meanwhile, Tocchi and colleagues presented their data on performing hepaticojejunostomy (48 patients), choledochojejunostomy (34 patients), and intrahepatic cholangiojejunostomy (8 patients) without stents in 84 patients over a period of 15 years for benign biliary strictures.[111] Excellent or good results were obtained in 83% of the patients. Anastomotic strictures occurred in 10 patients, 6 within 5 years and 4 at 62, 75, 85, and 96 months. By multivariate analysis, only postoperative complications and the degree of common bile duct dilatation proved to be significant independent predictors of outcome. A bile duct dilatation of less than 15 mm was noted in 60% of patients with poor outcome. Although not reaching statistical significance, higher complications and restrictures were noted in patients having a choledochojejunostomy versus hepaticojejunostomy, and the authors changed their practice to performing only higher anastomosis during the study period for even low strictures. Peptic ulcers were noted in only 2.3% of the patients in the entire series, which is not higher than the normal population and does not appear to be related to diverting the flow of bile from the duodenum, as others have suggest.

Laparoscopic approaches to both Roux-en-Y choledochojejunostomy and choledochoduodenostomy have been reported recently. Jeyapalam and colleagues reported 6 patients who underwent *laparoscopic choledochoduodenostomy* (LCDD).[112] While one patient died of comorbidities, the liver function tests returned to normal in all the remaining patients, and the average length of postoperative stay was 6 days. Meanwhile, Tang and colleagues selected 12 patients to undergo LCDD for recurrent pyogenic cholangitis.[113] A successful laparoscopic approach was used in all cases, with a mean operating time of 6 hours and a median postoperative length of stay of 7.5 days. One postoperative bile leak was noted and managed conservatively, whereas no patients developed cholangitis or sump syndrome at a mean follow-up of 38 months. Han and colleagues presented similar results in performing laparoscopic Roux-en-Y choledochojejunostomy for benign disease.[114] One episode of melena that resolved spontaneously was the only postoperative complication in six patients who underwent the surgery. All patients were symptom-free at a 27-month follow-up. With increasing experience in laparoscopy, the use of minimally invasive surgical drainage procedures is likely to become more widely used.

Summary

The evaluation and treatment of choledocholithiasis has changed many times over the last 100 years. As newer and less invasive techniques emerge, the surgeon finds that he or she has many options and many paths that can lead to the successful treatment of a patient with common bile duct stones. Evaluation and diagnosis may involve an examination and simple laboratory tests, or evaluation of the biliary tree accurately with MRCP or ERCP or an IOC. Treatment may be endoscopic, percutaneous, open, or laparoscopic. Given the multiple alternatives available, sometimes it is difficult to decide on the right one for a particular patient. Frequently, the best path is the one the surgeon is most adept at or the one that local expertise can accomplish most safely. Sometimes, however, the safest approach is a transfer to a center where multiple treatment options are available so that the treatment can be tailored to fit each individual situation.

▪ CHOLANGITIS

Cholangitis is the most rapidly fatal complication of gallstones and occurs as a result of biliary tract bacterial infection in the setting of biliary tree obstruction. Mortality approaches 100% in patients who after failing conservative therapy are not subjected to needed drainage interventions.[115] Early diagnosis and treatment are imperative for successful outcome.

PATHOPHYSIOLOGY

Although bile normally is sterile, when the biliary tree is compromised, such as by a stone, stricture or endoprosthesis, bacteria then often can be cultured from the bile.[116] Along with the sphincter of Oddi and the bacteriostatic properties of bile, bile flow is an important component of maintaining sterility. Bile duct obstruction results in decreased antibacterial defenses, allowing bacteria to gain access to the biliary tree. Although the route of infection is unclear, ascent from the duodenum or hematogenous seeding by way of the portal vein are felt to be possible sources.[115] Once colonization has occurred, stasis allows for exponential bacterial growth. As the biliary pressure rises with obstruction, bacteria and their products such as endotoxins leak into the systemic circulation and cause the septicemia of cholangitis.[116]

Patients with partial obstruction have a higher chance of developing cholangitis than those with complete obstruction, and bile duct stones are associated more often with cholangitis than neoplasms causing obstruction. In the United States, secondary choledocholithiasis is the most common cause of cholangitis. On the other hand, primary bile duct stones are common in areas where Oriental cholangiohepatitis is endemic, including Honk Kong and Southeast Asia.[115] Other causes of cholangitis include obstructing periampullary tumors, tumors metastatic to the porta hepatic or peripancreatic lymph nodes, benign strictures, and primary sclerosing cholangitis. Biliary tract interventions may lead to postprocedural cholangitis, and rare cases of cholangitis may be caused by hemobilia, parasites, and congenital abnormalities of the biliary tree.

Escherichia coli, Streptococcus spp., *Klebsiella* spp., and Enterobacteriaceae are the most common organisms cultured in cholangitis. *Pseudomonas* spp. and skin and oral flora are associated with biliary tract interventions, whereas anaerobes are noted most commonly in the elderly after biliary surgery.[115]

CLINICAL PRESENTATION AND DIAGNOSIS

Charcot's triad of fever, right upper quadrant pain, and jaundice is present in 50–70% of patients with cholangitis at presentation, with fever, abdominal pain, and jaundice occurring in 90%, 70%, and 60% of patients, respectively. Hypotension (20%) and altered mental status (30%) are seen in septic patients and are known as *Reynold's pentad* when presenting in the setting of Charcot's triad. Although peritonitis is uncommon, 65% of patients have right upper quadrant tenderness.[115] Laboratory and radiologic studies are important for distinguishing cholangitis from other conditions such as acute cholecystitis, liver abscesses, and pancreatitis. Elevations of serum alkaline phosphatase, gamma-glutamyl transpeptidase, and bilirubin are typical. Mild increases in transaminases may be seen, whereas hyperamylasemia is found in up to 30% of patients. A discussion of imaging studies for the evaluation of choledocholithiasis has been presented in the section on common bile duct stones. In a patient presenting with signs of cholangitis, the most widely used modalities are ultrasound and CT scan. Ultrasound is highly accurate in diagnosing acute cholecystitis and identifying gallstones. However, its ability to establish the diagnosis of choledocholithiasis is only 50%, varying from 30–90%.[6,10] Although the presence of bile duct stones can be inferred by associated bile duct dilatation, a normal ultrasound without duct dilatation does not exclude either choledocholithiasis or cholangitis.[15,115] On the other hand, a CT scan is better at determining the level of biliary tract obstruction and has a 94% accuracy in diagnosing choledocholithiasis in the setting of suspected bile duct calculi.[18] MRCP has sensitivities and specificities approaching ERCP in the diagnosis of bile duct stones and is useful in delineating biliary anatomy. However, its use in the setting of acute cholangitis is limited. ERCP is highly accurate in revealing the cause of biliary obstruction and at the same time allows for therapeutic intervention to occur at the same sitting.[115] Nonetheless, given the well-defined life-threatening complications associated with ERCP and the availability of other noninvasive imaging techniques, ERCP should not be used solely as a diagnostic tool in the setting of acute cholangitis.[115]

Treatment

Patients with cholangitis can become extremely ill in a short period of time, and rapid initiation of treatment can be lifesaving. Supportive measures are begun without delay and include fluid resuscitation, correction of electrolyte deficits and coagulopathy, and administration of analgesics.[117] Empirical broad-spectrum antibiotics are started while blood cultures, and when available, bile cultures are sent. Aminoglycosides and ampicillin are associated with gram-negative resistance and nephrotoxicity and are no longer felt to be the ideal regimen. Newer effective therapies include combinations of extended-spectrum cephalosporins, metronidazole, and ampicillin; fluoroquinolones as single-agent or in combination with metronidazole; and ureidopenicillins alone or with metronidazole.[115] Anaerobic coverage is felt to be more important in the elderly and those with biliary manipulations. Antibiotics usually are given for 7–10 days, even if biliary decompression has been accomplished during the interim. Whether continuation of antibiotics is needed after biliary drainage is achieved and signs of inflammation have subsided was evaluated in a retrospective study by van Lent and colleagues.[116] Eighty patients who were treated successfully for cholangitis with ERCP were included in the study and followed for 6 months. Forty-one patients received antibiotics for 3 days or less, 19 patients for 4–5 days, and 20 patients for more than 5 days. The three groups were well matched, and the rate of recurrent cholangitis (24%) was not different for the three groups. The authors felt that a 3-day duration of antibiotic therapy may be sufficient in treating cholangitis when adequate drainage has been achieved and fever is abating.

Drainage of the biliary tree is the mainstay of therapy for patients with acute cholangitis.[116] However, the timing and route of biliary decompression vary depending on the response of antibiotics, the cause of the obstruction, and the presence of morbidities.[117] Biliary sepsis will resolve in most patients with conservative therapy, allowing time for a detailed delineation of the biliary anatomy by noninvasive imaging (CT scan or MRI) in order to determine the cause and level of obstruction. On the other hand, urgent decompression is needed in the 10–15% of patients who fail to respond within 24 hours to supportive measures and antibiotic therapy.[116] When biliary decompression is not achieved, liver abscesses are an inevitable.[116] Mortality approaches 100% in patients who are not subjected to needed drainage interventions after failing conservative therapy.[118]

The methods of relieving biliary tract obstruction include endoscopic, percutaneous transhepatic, and surgical drainage techniques. With a success rate of 90–98%, ERCP with bile duct clearance is superior to the other methods and is the modality of choice for decompressing the biliary tree during acute cholangitis caused particularly by choledocholithiasis.[115,117] In a study of 83 patients with acute cholangitis randomized to undergo either endoscopic or surgical decompression, the mortality was 10% in the endoscopic arm versus 30% in the surgical group.[115] Meanwhile, in an evaluation of 65 patients undergoing endoscopic drainage verses 40 patients receiving traditional surgery for acute cholangitis, 5 operated patients and no individuals subjected to endoscopy died.[119] In comparison with percutaneous drainage, ERCP also has been shown to have lower morbidity, shorter hospitalization, and higher definitive success rates.[115] Sugiyama and colleagues found that in elderly patients (age 80 or older) with acute cholangitis, endoscopic drainage had lower morbidity (16.7%) and mortality (5.6%) than surgical (87.5% and 25%, respectively) or percutaneous drainage (36.4% and 9.1%, respectively).[120]

Various endoscopic treatment options are available from the placement of nasobiliary catheters or biliary stents to sphincterotomy and stone extraction. In patients who have responded to antibiotic therapy, sphincterotomy with bile duct clearance is preferred, whereas drainage catheters are used in those with ongoing sepsis and multiple large stones.[117] In critically ill patients or in those with coagulopathy, concerns about bleeding and increased procedure times are associated with endoscopic sphincterotomy.

On the other hand, in comparing nasobiliary catheters with biliary stents for the treatment of acute cholangitis, a randomized study found both to be equally effective, but stents were more comfortable and avoided the risk of accidental removal.[115]

Percutaneous transhepatic drainage is reserved for patients in whom the papilla is inaccessible or ERCP has failed and for those suspected of hilar cholangiocarcinoma, hepatolithiasis, and intrasegmental cholangitis.[115,117] Although successful in 90% of patients with biliary obstruction, percutaneous drainage has higher rates of morbidity (30–80%) and mortality (5–15%) than endoscopic techniques. As with ERCP, coagulopathy must be corrected prior to the procedure.

Used for almost 100 years, open surgery for acute cholangitis is associated with mortality rates of up to 40%.[115] Surgery maybe limited to choledochotomy, decompression, and T-tube insertion when performed for emergency situations. In patients who have undergone other methods of biliary drainage for the acute situations, surgery offers definitive treatment of the underlying disease and is associated with low mortality when performed electively after the initial treatment.

The need for cholecystectomy after common bile duct clearance in patients with cholelithiasis has been discussed in the section on choledocholithiasis. To prevent further biliary complications, some have advocated cholecystectomy for patients who are fit after the initial treatment of acute cholangitis. In nonrandomized and retrospective studies, the risk of developing subsequent biliary problems ranges from 4–12% in patients with common bile duct stones.[115] In a study by Boerma and colleagues, 47% of patients who were randomized to a wait-and-see approach after common duct clearance developed biliary symptoms compared with only 2% of patients who were allocated to cholecystectomy within 6 weeks of the endoscopic procedure.[121] Of the wait-and-see patients, 37% eventually needed cholecystectomy. Targarona and colleagues randomized 98 elderly (mean age 80) patients with biliary symptoms to either open cholecystectomy with operative cholangiography and (if necessary) bile duct exploration (48 patients) or to endoscopic sphincterotomy alone (50 patients).[122] There were no significant differences in immediate morbidity (23% and

16%) or mortality (4% and 6%) in the surgery versus endoscopic group. However, at a mean follow-up of 17 months, biliary symptoms recurred in 3 surgical patients, none of whom underwent repeat surgery, and in 10 endoscopic patients, 7 of whom had further biliary surgery. These studies suggest that patients with acute cholangitis should undergo elective cholecystectomy after bile duct clearance if they are able to tolerate an operation. On the other hand, in Asian patients in whom bile duct stones may originate from intrahepatic stones, cholecystectomy may not prevent future biliary complications.[115]

▪ HEPATOLITHIASIS

Hepatolithiasis is a primary disease of the biliary ducts and is more refractory to surgical treatment than most other benign diseases of the biliary system.[123,124] The relative incidence in Western countries is approximately 1%, whereas in Taiwan, South Korea, and China it has been reported to be 20%, 18%, and 40%, respectively.[125] Originally felt to be common only in Southeast Asia and referred to as *Oriental cholangiohepatitis,* the widespread immigration of Asians to the United States has resulted in an increasing number of patients with hepatolithiasis presenting to American general surgeon.[123,126] The pathogenesis of primary hepatic stones was discussed earlier in the section on choledocholithiasis and appears to involve bile infection; biliary stasis; low-protein, low-fat diets and malnutrition; and parasitic infections.[1] Hepatolithiasis presents with recurrent pyogenic cholangitis and sepsis, complicated by parenchymal infection and liver abscesses, obstructive cholangiopathy, and subsequent parenchymal destruction.[124,126,127] The natural course of the disease may lead to the development of biliary cirrhosis, portal hypertension, and liver failure and is complicated by cholangiocarcinoma in about 10% of patients.[123,124,128]

The diagnostic procedures used in establishing the diagnosis of hepatolithiasis include ultrasonography, CT scan, MRI, and direct (either endoscopic or percutaneous) cholangiography.[18,124,129,130] Characterizing features include varying combinations of ductal dilatation, intrahepatic and extrahepatic bile duct stones, segmental ductal strictures, and lobar or segmental atrophy. In acute exacerbation, parenchymal or ductal contrast enhancement, abscess formation, or biliary obstruction may be noted.[124]

The management of hepatolithiasis is difficult and far from satisfactory. More than two-thirds of patients undergo multiple surgical procedures, and 10% ultimately require liver transplantation for liver failure.[123] Initial biliary decompression usually can be achieved by endoscopic or percutaneous transhepatic drainage.[127] The goal of definitive treatment is complete removal of all bile duct stones and elimination of bile stasis at the sites of intra- or extrahepatic strictures.

If the stones and strictures are located in a single segment or lobe of the liver, hepatic resection generally is recommended.[123,127,131] Resection is particularly important for patients with parenchymal atrophy and stricture of the intrahepatic ducts who may have concomitant cholangiocarcinoma.[123] Even with resection, a significant number of patients will have recurrent disease. Kim and colleagues evaluated their experience with hepatectomy in 44 patients with hepatolithiasis by dividing them into two groups, those with intrahepatic biliary stricture and those without.[132] At a median follow-up of 65 months, the incidence of residual or recurrent stones was 36% for those with stricture and 11% for those without. The rate in late cholangitis was higher in the stricture group (54%) versus the no-stricture group (6%), as was the initial failure rate (50% versus 31%, respectively). Intrahepatic stricture recurred in 46% of the stricture group versus none in the no-stricture group, with stricture reoccurrence seen at the primary site in two-thirds. Therefore, the importance of including the strictured duct in the hepatic resection is emphasized by this study.

Nevertheless, the number of patients in whom resection is feasible is limited secondary to the diffuse and multifocal nature of the disease.[131] If stones are located predominantly in the extrahepatic ducts or at the primary convergence and there is minimal stenosis of the intrahepatic ducts, it may be possible to use endoscopic treatment. When stones or strictures are located at the secondary convergence or beyond, surgery and percutaneous transhepatic cholangioscopic lithotripsy have a complete stone clearance rate of 84–100% and 72–92%, respectively.[123] However, the stone recurrence rate is high, ranging from 33–40%. Hepaticojejunostomy has been used in the past to prevent biliary-enteric regurgitation and to decrease stagnation of debris and calculi in the intrahepatic ducts. The use of hepaticojejunostomy is controversial and refuted by others, who claim that increased biliary complications occur in patients with hepaticojejunostomies in the setting of hepatolithiasis.[123] However, adding cutaneous stoma to the roux limb of the hepaticojejunostomy creates an access point for entering the biliary system for treating future complications.[133]

With the advent of biliary endoscopy and radiologic intervention, percutaneous choledochoscopic removal of intrahepatic stones has been well established.[134] Stones can be removed through via cholangioscopic guidance with basket forceps or lithotripsy, and strictures can be dilated. In a study from Hong Kong, 79 patients with intrahepatic stones underwent percutaneous transhepatic choledochoscopy.[134] The success rate was 76.8%, with a complication rate of 21.5%. Cholangitis occurred within 3–5 years in a third of the patients after the procedure. Another study found that recurrent calculi are more common in the setting of bile duct strictures, and addressing the strictures is mandatory part of treatment.[135] Meanwhile, one study of percutaneous transhepatic cholangioscopic lithotripsy reported a biliary clearance rate of 100%, with a mean of two sessions required and a complication rate of 6.7%.[131] During the follow-up period of 1–127 months (mean 75 months), one recurrence was noted and treated by repeat choledochoscopy. Others have used percutaneous intracorporeal electrohydrolic lithotripsy for hepatolithiasis. Using this technique, in a series of 53 patients, complete clearance of stones was achieved in 92%, and during a mean follow-up of 5 years, 9% had recurrent symptoms of biliary obstruction.[136] On the other hand, in a recent publication, Han and colleagues described the use of laparoscopy in the treatment of intrahepatic stones.[128] A flexible choledochoscope, inserted through a choledochotomy, was used for stone removal in 12 patients, with a mean operating time of 288 minutes. Remnant stones were found in only one patient and removed by percutaneous choledochoscopy performed through the T-tube site. No cholangitis or recurrent stones were found at follow-up at 10–45 months. With the increasing demand for minimally invasive surgery, it is likely that laparoscopy will have a greater role in the difficult management of hepatolithiasis in the future.

REFERENCES

1. Ko, CW, Lee SP. Epidemiology and natural history of common bile duct stones and prediction of disease. *Gastrointest Endosc* 2002;56:S165–169
2. Tierney S, Pitt, HA. Choledocholithiasis and cholangitis. In: Bell RH, Rikkers LF, Mulholland MW (eds), *Digestive Tract Surgery: A Text and Atlas.* Philadelphia: Lippincott-Raven; 1996:407–431
3. Kaufman HS, Magnuson TH, Lillemoe KD, et al. The role of bacteria in gallbladder and common duct stone formation. *Ann Surg* 1989;209:584–592
4. Cetta F. Bile infection documented as initial event in the pathogenesis of brown pigment biliary stones. *Hepatology* 1986;6:482–489
5. Faust TW, Reddy KR. Postoperative jaundice. *Clin Liver Dis* 2004;8(1):151–166
6. Eisen GM, Dominitz JA, Faigel DO, et al. An annotated algorithm for the evaluation of choledocholithiasis. *Gastrointest Endosc* 2001;53:864–866
7. Goldman DE, Gholson CF. Choledocholithiasis in patients with normal serum liver enzymes. *Dig Dis Sci* 1995; 40:1065–1068
8. Abboud PA, Malet PF, Berlin JA, et al. Predictors of common bile duct stones prior to cholecystectomy: A meta-analysis. *Gastrointest Endosc* 1996;44:450–455
9. Yusoff IF, Barkun JS, Barkun AN. Diagnosis and management of cholecystitis and cholangitis. *Gastroenterol Clin North Am* 2003;32:1145–1168
10. Kohut M, Nowak A, Marek T, et al. [Evaluation of probability of bile duct stone presence by using of non-invasive procedures.] *Pol Arch Med Wewn* 2003;110:691–702
11. Gross BH, Harter LP, Gore RM, et al. Ultrasonic evaluation of common bile duct stones: Prospective comparison with endoscopic retrograde cholangiopancreatography. *Radiology* 1983;146:471–474
12. Costi R, Sarli L, Caruso G, et al. Preoperative ultrasonographic assessment of the number and size of gallbladder stones: Is it a useful predictor of asymptomatic choledochal lithiasis? *J Ultrasound Med* 2002;21:971–976
13. Tham TC, Collins JS, Watson RG, et al. Diagnosis of common bile duct stones by intravenous cholangiography: prediction by ultrasound and liver function tests compared with endoscopic retrograde cholangiography. *Gastrointest Endosc* 1996;44:158–163
14. Contractor QQ, Boujemla M, Contractor TQ, el-Essawy OM. Abnormal common bile duct sonography: The best predictor of choledocholithiasis before laparoscopic cholecystectomy. *J Clin Gastroenterol* 1997;25:429–432
15. Hunt DR. Common bile duct stones in non-dilated bile ducts? An ultrasound study. *Australas Radiol* 1996;40: 221–222.
16. Sarli L, Costi R, Gobbi S, et al. Scoring system to predict asymptomatic choledocholithiasis before laparoscopic cholecystectomy: A matched case-control study. *Surg Endosc* 2003;17:1396–1403
17. Alponat A, Kum CK, Rajnakova A, et al. Predictive factors for synchronous common bile duct stones in patients with cholelithiasis. *Surg Endosc* 1997;11:928–932
18. Fulcher AS. MRCP and ERCP in the diagnosis of common bile duct stones. *Gastrointest Endosc* 2002;56):S178–182
19. Mallery JS, Baron TH, Dominitz JA, et al, Standards of Practice Committee, American Society for Gastrointestinal Endoscopy. Complications of ERCP. *Gastrointest Endosc* 2003;57:633–638
20. Carr-Locke DL. Therapeutic role of ERCP in the management of suspected common bile duct stones. *Gastrointest Endosc* 2002;56:S170–174
21. Frey CF, Burbige EJ, Meinke WB, et al. Endoscopic retrograde cholangiopancreatography. *Am J Surg* 1982;144: 109–114
22. Binmoeller KF, Schafer TW. Endoscopic management of bile duct stones. *J Clin Gastroenterol* 2001;32:106–118
23. Disario JA, Freeman ML, Bjorkman DJ, et al. Endoscopic balloon dilation compared with sphincterotomy for extraction of bile duct stones. *Gastroenterology* 2004127:1291–1299

24. Watanabe H, Hiraishi H, Koitabashi A, et al. Endoscopic papillary balloon dilation for treatment of common bile duct stones. *Hepatogastroenterology* 2004;51:652–657
25. Leung JW, Tu R. Mechanical lithotripsy for large bile duct stones. *Gastrointest Endosc* 2004;59:688–690
26. Riemann JF, Seuberth K, Demling L. Mechanical lithotripsy of common bile duct stones. *Gastrointest Endosc* 1985;31:207–210
27. Riemann JF, Seuberth K, Demling L. Clinical application of a new mechanical lithotripter for smashing common bile duct stones. *Endoscopy* 1982;14:226–230
28. Hintze RE, Adler A, Veltzke W. Outcome of mechanical lithotripsy of bile duct stones in an unselected series of 704 patients. *Hepatogastroenterology* 1996;43:473–476
29. Leung JW, Neuhaus H, Chopita N. Mechanical lithotripsy in the common bile duct. *Endoscopy* 2001;33:800–804
30. Chung SC, Leung JW, Leong HT, Li AK. Mechanical lithotripsy of large common bile duct stones using a basket. *Br J Surg* 1991;78:1448–1450
31. Cipolletta L, Costamagna G, Bianco MA, et al. Endoscopic mechanical lithotripsy of difficult common bile duct stones. *Br J Surg* 1997;84:1407–1409
32. Garg PK, Tandon RK, Ahuja V, et al. Predictors of unsuccessful mechanical lithotripsy and endoscopic clearance of large bile duct stones. *Gastrointest Endosc* 2004;59:601–605
33. Hochberger J, Tex S, Maiss J, Hahn EG. Management of difficult common bile duct stones. *Gastrointest Endosc Clin North Am* 2003;13:623–634
34. Arya N, Nelles SE, Haber GB, et al. Electrohydraulic lithotripsy in 111 patients: A safe and effective therapy for difficult bile duct stones. *Am J Gastroenterol* 2004;99:2330–2334
35. Sackmann M, Holl J, Sauter GH, et al. Extracorporeal shock wave lithotripsy for clearance of bile duct stones resistant to endoscopic extraction. *Gastrointest Endosc* 2001;53:27–32
36. Neuhaus H, Zillinger C, Born P, et al. Randomized study of intracorporeal laser lithotripsy versus extracorporeal shock-wave lithotripsy for difficult bile duct stones. *Gastrointest Endosc* 1998;47:327–334
37. Meyenberger C, Meierhofer U, Michel-Harder C, et al. Long-term follow-up after treatment of common bile duct stones by extracorporeal shock-wave lithotripsy. *Endoscopy* 1996;28:411–417
38. Gilchrist AM, Ross B, Thomas WE. Extracorporeal shockwave lithotripsy for common bile duct stones. *Br J Surg* 1997;84:29–32
39. Jakobs R, Adamek HE, Maier M, et al. Fluoroscopically guided laser lithotripsy versus extracorporeal shock wave lithotripsy for retained bile duct stones: A prospective, randomised study. *Gut* 1997;40:678–682
40. Ragheb S, Choong CK, Gowland S, et al. Extracorporeal shock wave lithotripsy for difficult common bile duct stones: Initial New Zealand experience. *N Z Med J* 2000;113:377–378
41. Mora J, Aguilera V, Sala T, et al. [Endoscopic treatment combined with extracorporeal shock wave lithotripsy of difficult bile duct stones.] *Gastroenterol Hepatol* 2002;25:585–588
42. Yasuda I, Tomita E. Extracorporeal shockwave lithotripsy of common bile duct stones without preliminary endoscopic sphincterotomy. *Scand J Gastroenterol* 1996;31:934–939
43. Ersoz G, Tekesin O, Ozutemiz AO, Gunsar F. Biliary sphincterotomy plus dilation with a large balloon for bile duct stones that are difficult to extract. *Gastrointest Endosc* 2003;57:156–159
44. Johnson GK, Geenen JE, Venu RP, et al. Treatment of non-extractable common bile duct stones with combination of ursodeoxycholic acid plus endoprostheses. *Gastrointest Endosc* 1993;39:528–531
45. Bergman JJ, Rauws EA, Tijssen JG, et al. Biliary endoprostheses in elderly patients with endoscopically irretrievable common bile duct stones: report on 117 patients. *Gastrointest Endosc* 1995;42:195–201
46. Hui CK, Lai KC, Ng M, et al. Retained common bile duct stones: A comparison between biliary stenting and complete clearance of stones by electrohydraulic lithotripsy. *Aliment Pharmacol Ther* 2003;17:289–296
47. Cohen S, Bacon BR, Berlin JA, et al. National Institutes of Health State-of-the-Science Conference Statement: ERCP for diagnosis and therapy, January 14–16, 2002. *Gastrointest Endosc* 2002;56:803–809
48. Lakatos L, Mester G, Reti G, et al. Selection criteria for preoperative endoscopic retrograde cholangiopancreatography before laparoscopic cholecystectomy and endoscopic treatment of bile duct stones: Results of a retrospective, single center study between 1996–2002. *World J Gastroenterol* 2004;10:3495–3499
49. Tham TC, Lichtenstein DR, Vandervoort J, et al. Role of endoscopic retrograde cholangiopancreatography for suspected choledocholithiasis in patients undergoing laparoscopic cholecystectomy. *Gastrointest Endosc* 1998;47:50–56
50. Mark DH, Flamm CR, Aronson N. Evidence-based assessment of diagnostic modalities for common bile duct stones. *Gastrointest Endosc* 2002;56:S190–194
51. Patel P, Khodadadian E, Barawi M, et al. Noncontrast helical computed tomography versus endoscopic ultrasound for suspected choledocholithiasis and common bile duct dilation: A prospective blind comparison. *Gastrointest Endosc* 2002;56(4):101
52. Ke ZW, Zheng CZ, Li JH, et al. Prospective evaluation of magnetic resonance cholangiography in patients with suspected common bile duct stones before laparoscopic cholecystectomy. *Hepatobiliary Pancreat Dis Int* 2003;2:576–580
53. Kejriwal R, Liang J, Anderson G, Hill A. Magnetic resonance imaging of the common bile duct to exclude choledocholithiasis. *ANZ J Surg* 2004;74:619–621
54. Demartines N, Eisner L, Schnabel K, et al. Evaluation of magnetic resonance cholangiography in the management of bile duct stones. *Arch Surg* 2000;135:148–152
55. Simone M, Mutter D, Rubino F, et al. Three-dimensional virtual cholangioscopy: A reliable tool for the diagnosis of common bile duct stones. *Ann Surg* 2004;240:82–88

56. Buscarini E, Tansini P, Vallisa D, et al. EUS for suspected choledocholithiasis: Do benefits outweigh costs? A prospective, controlled study. *Gastrointest Endosc* 2003;57: 510–518
57. Buscharth F, Kruse A. Direct cholangiography and biliary drainage. *Scand J Gastroenterol* 1996;216:59–72
58. Fernstrom I, Delin NA, Sundblad R. Percutaneous transhepatic extraction of common bile duct stones. *Surg Gynecol Obstet* 1981;153:405–407
59. Stokes KR, Clouse ME. Biliary duct stones: Percutaneous transhepatic removal. *Cardiovasc Intervent Radiol* 1990;13:240–244
60. Petrtyl J, Bruha R. [Transhepatic cholangioscopy in the treatment of choledocholithiasis.] *Cas Lek Cesk* 2003; 142:603–605
61. Maier M, Kohler B, Riemann JF, et al. [Percutaneous transhepatic cholangioscopy (PTCS): An important supplement in diagnosis and therapy of biliary tract diseases (indications, technique and results).] *Zeitschrift Gastroenterol* 1995;33:435–439
62. Brambs HJ, Duda SH, Claussen CD, et al. Treatment of bile duct stones: Value of laser lithotripsy delivered via percutaneous endoscopy. *Eur Radiat* 1996;6:734–740
63. Nagashima I, Takada T,Okinaga K, et al. Percutaneous transhepatic papillary balloon dilatation as a therapeutic option for choledocholithiasis. *J Hepatobiliary Pancreat Surg* 2004;11:252–254
64. Ponchon T, Genin G, Valette P, et al. Methods, indications, and results of percutaneous choledochoscopy: A series of 161 procedures. *Ann Surg* 1996;223:26–36
65. Surick BG, Ghazi A. Endoscopic papillotomy while the gallbladder is in situ. *Am Surg* 1992;58:657–660
66. Dhiman RK, Phanish MK, Chawla YK, Dilawari JB. Gallbladder motility and lithogenicity of bile in patients with choledocholithiasis after endoscopic sphincterotomy. *J Hepatol* 1997;26:1300–1305
67. Reimann, JF, Gierth K, Lux G, Alterndorf A. [Retained cholelithiasis: A risk factor after endoscopic papillotomy?] *Zeitschrift Gastroenterol* 1984;22:188–193
68. Saraswat VA, Kapur BM, Vashisht S, Tandon RK. Duodenoscopic sphincterotomy for common bile duct stones in patients with gallbladder in situ. *Intern Surg* 1991;76: 142–145
69. Lamont DD, Passi RB. Fate of the gallbladder with cholelithiasis after endoscopic sphincterotomy for choledocholithiasis. *Can J Surg* 1989;32:15–18
70. Hill J, Martin DF, Tweedle DE. Risks of leaving the gallbladder in situ after endoscopic sphincterotomy for bile duct stones. *Br J Surg* 1991;78:554–557
71. Adamek HE, Kudis V, Riemann JF, et al. Impact of gallbladder status on the outcome in patients with retained bile duct stones treated with extracorporeal shockwave lithotripsy. *Endoscopy* 2002;34:624–627
72. Kwon SK, Lee BS, Park SM, et al. Is cholecystectomy necessary after ERCP for bile duct stones in patients with gallbladder in situ?. *Korean J Intern Med* 2001;16: 254–259
73. Kullman E, Borch K, Dahlin LG, Liedberg G. Long-term follow-up of patients with gallbladder in situ after endoscopic sphincterotomy for choledocholithiasis. *Eur J Surg* 1991;157:131–135
74. Moreira Vicente VF, Merono GE, Garcia PA, et al. [Choledocholithiasis in non-cholecystectomized patients: Endoscopic sphincterotomy and afterwards . . . cholecystectomy?] *Rev Espanola Enfermed Aparato Dig* 1989;76: 215–221
75. Boytchev I, Pelletier G, Buffet C, et al. [Late biliary complications after endoscopic sphincterotomy for common bile duct stones in patients older than 65 years of age with gallbladder in situ.] *Gastroenterol Clin Biologique* 2000;24:995–1000
76. Schreurs WH, Vles WJ, Stuifbergen WH, Oostvogel HJ. Endoscopic management of common bile duct stones leaving the gallbladder in situ: A cohort study with long-term follow-up. *Dig Surg* 2004;21:60–64; discussion 65
77. Petelin JB. Surgical management of common bile duct stones. *Gastrointest Endosc* 2002;56:S183–189
78. Petelin JB. Laparoscopic common bile duct exploration. *Surg Endosc* 2003;17:1705–1715
79. Metcalfe MS, Ong T, Bruening MH, et al. Is laparoscopic intraoperative cholangiogram a matter of routine? *Am J Surg* 2004;187:475–481
80. Ellison EC. What's new in general surgery: gastrointestinal conditions. *J Am Coll Surg* 2005;199:409–417
81. Catheline JM, Turner R, Rizk N, et al. Evaluation of the biliary tree during laparoscopic cholecystectomy: laparoscopic ultrasound versus intraoperative cholangiography: A prospective study of 150 cases. *Surg Laparosc Endosc* 1998;8:85–91
82. Falcone RA Jr, Fegelman EJ, Nussbaum MS, et al. A prospective comparison of laparoscopic ultrasound vs intraoperative cholangiogram during laparoscopic cholecystectomy. *Surg Endosc* 1999;13:784–788
83. Collins C, Maguire D, Ireland A, et al. A prospective study of common bile duct calculi in patients undergoing laparoscopic cholecystectomy: natural history of choledocholithiasis revisited. *Ann Surg* 2004;239:28–33
84. Tai CK, Tang CN, Ha JP, et al. Laparoscopic exploration of common bile duct in difficult choledocholithiasis. *Surg Endosc* 2004;18:910–914
85. Ha JP, Tang CN, Siu WT, et al. Primary closure versus T-tube drainage after laparoscopic choledochotomy for common bile duct stones. *Hepatogastroenterology* 2004;51: 1605–1608
86. Isla AM, Griniatsos J, Karvounis E, Arbuckle JD. Advantages of laparoscopic stented choledochorrhaphy over T-tube placement. *Br J Surg* 2004;91:862–866
87. Wei Q, Hu HJ, Cai XY, et al. Biliary drainage after laparoscopic choledochotomy. *World J Gastroenterol* 2004;10: 3175–3178
88. Martin CJ, Cox MR, Vaccaro L. Laparoscopic transcystic bile duct stenting in the management of common bile duct stones. *ANZ J Surg* 2002;72:258–264
89. Williams GL, Vellacott KD. Selective operative cholangiography and perioperative endoscopic retrograde cholangiopancreatography (ERCP) during laparoscopic cholecystectomy: A viable option for choledocholithiasis. *Surg Endosc* 2002;16:465–467

90. Meyer C, Le JV, Rohr S, et al. Management of common bile duct stones in a single operation combining laparoscopic cholecystectomy and peroperative endoscopic sphincterotomy. *J Hepatobil Pancreat Surg* 2002;9:196–200
91. Enochsson L, Lindberg B, Swahn F, Arnelo U. Intraoperative endoscopic retrograde cholangiopancreatography (ERCP) to remove common bile duct stones during routine laparoscopic cholecystectomy does not prolong hospitalization: A 2-year experience. *Surg Endosc* 2004;18:367–371
92. Becker C. [Percutaneous removal of residual calculi of the bile ducts by T-drainage tract.] *Bildgebung* 1992;59:179–182
93. Meyhoff HH. Sphincterotomy treatment for biliary tract stones: A retrospective review. *Acta Chir Scand* 1975;141:645–648
94. Baker AR, Neoptolemos JP, Leese T, Fossard DP. Choledochoduodenostomy, transduodenal sphincteroplasty and sphincterotomy for calculi of the common bile duct. *Surg Gynecol Obstet* 1987;164:245–251
95. Suter M, Jayet C, Richard A, Gillet M. [Current status of surgical transduodenal papillotomy.] *Helv Chir Acta* 1994;60:671–678
96. de Aretxabala X, Bahamondes JC. Choledochoduodenostomy for common bile duct stones. *World J Surg* 1998;22:1171–1174
97. de Aretxabala X, Bahamondes JC. Choledochoduodenostomy for common bile duct stones *World J Surg.* 1998;22(11):1171–1174
98. Deutsch AA, Nudelman I, Gutman H, Reiss R. Choledochoduodenostomy an important surgical tool in the management of common bile duct stones: A review of 126 cases. *Eur J Surg* 1991;157:531–533
99. Ramirez P, Parrilla P, Bueno FS, et al. Choledochoduodenostomy and sphincterotomy in the treatment of choledocholithiasis. *Br J Surg* 1994;81:121–123
100. Parrilla P, Ramirez P, Sanchez Bueno F, et al. Long-term results of choledochoduodenostomy in the treatment of choledocholithiasis: assessment of 225 cases. *Br J Surg* 1991;78(4):470–472
101. Baker AR, Neoptolemos JP, Leese T, et al. Long-term follow-up of patients with side-to-side choledochoduodenostomy and transduodenal sphincterosplasty. *Ann R Coll Surg Engl* 1987;69(6):253–257
102. Gouma DJ, Konsten J, Soeters PB, et al. Long-term follow-up after choledochojejunostomy for bile duct stones with complex clearance of the bile duct. *Br J Surg* 1989;76:451–453
103. Panis Y, Fagniez PL, Brisset D, et al. Long-term results of choledochoduodenostomy versus choledochojejunostomy for choledocholithiasis. The French Association for Surgical Research. *Surg Gynecol Obstet* 1993;177:33–37
104. Tocchi A, Costa G, Lepre L, et al. The long-term outcome of hepaticojejunostomy in the treatment of benign bile duct strictures. *Ann Surg* 1996;224:162–167
105. DiFronzo LA, Egrari S, O'Connell TX. Safety and durability of single-layer, stentless, biliary-enteric anastomosis. *Am Surg* 1998;64:917–920
106. Pitt HA, Miyamoto T, Parapatis SK, et al. Factors influencing outcome in patients with postoperative biliary strictures. *Am J Surg* 1982;144:14–21
107. Braasch JW, Bolton JS, Rossi RL. A technique of biliary tract reconstruction with complete follow-up in 44 consecutive cases. *Ann Surg* 1981;194:634–638
108. Cameron JL, Gayler BW, Zuidema GD. The use of silastic transhepatic stents in benign and malignant biliary strictures. *Ann Surg* 1978;188:552–561
109. Bismuth H, Franco D, Corlette MB, Hepp J. Long-term results of roux-en-Y hepaticojejunostomy. *Surg Gynecol Obstet* 1978;146:161–167
110. Pellegrini CA, Thomas MJ, Way LW. Recurrent biliary stricture: Patterns of recurrence and outcome of surgical therapy. *Am J Surg* 1984;147:175–179
111. Tocchi A, Costa G, Lepre L, et al. The long-term outcome of hepaticojejunostomy in the treatment of benign bile duct strictures. *Ann Surg* 1996;224:162–167
112. Jeyapalan M, Almeida JA, Michaelson RL, Franklin ME Jr. Laparoscopic choledochoduodenostomy: Review of a 4-year experience with an uncommon problem. *Surg Laparosc Endosc Percutan Tech* 2002;12:148–153
113. Tang CN, Siu WT, Ha JP, Li MK. Laparoscopic choledochoduodenostomy: An effective drainage procedure for recurrent pyogenic cholangitis. *Surg Endosc* 2003;17:1590–1594
114. Han HS, Yi NJ. Laparoscopic roux-en-Y choledochojejunostomy for benign biliary disease. *Surg Laparosc Endosc Percutan Tech* 2004;14:80–84
115. Yusoff IF, Barkun JS, Barkun AN. Diagnosis and management of cholecystitis and cholangitis. *Gastroenterol Clin North Am* 2003;32:1145–1168
116. van Lent AU, Bartelsman JF, Tytgat GN, et al. Duration of antibiotic therapy for cholangitis after successful endoscopic drainage of the biliary tract. *Gastrointest Endosc* 2002;55:518–522
117. Bornman PC, van Beljon JI, Krige JE. Management of cholangitis. *J Hepatobil Pancreat Surg* 2003;10:406–414
118. Yusoff IF, Barkun JS, Barkun AN. Diagnosis and management of cholecystitis and cholangitis. *Gastroenterol Clin North Am* 2003;32:1145–1168
119. Anselmi M, Salgado J, Arancibia A, Alliu C. [Acute cholangitis caused by choledocholithiasis: Traditional surgery or endoscopic biliary drainage.] *Rev Med Chili* 2001;129:757–762
120. Sugiyama M, Atomi Y. Treatment of acute cholangitis due to choledocholithiasis in elderly and younger patients. *Arch Surg* 1997;132:1129–1133
121. Boerma D, Rauws EA, Keulemans YC, et al. Wait-and-see policy or laparoscopic cholecystectomy after endoscopic sphincterotomy for bile-duct stones: A randomised trial. *Lancet* 2002;360:761–765
122. Targarona EM, Ayuso RM, Bordas JM, et al. Randomised trial of endoscopic sphincterotomy with gallbladder left in situ versus open surgery for common bileduct calculi in high-risk patients. *Lancet* 1996;347:926–929
123. Kusano T, Isa TT, Muto Y, et al. Long-term results of hepaticojejunostomy for hepatolithiasis. *Am Surg* 2001;67:442–446

34

Choledochal Cyst and Biliary Strictures

Genevieve B. Melton ■ Keith D. Lillemoe

Benign conditions of the extrahepatic bile duct can range from focal or diffuse dilatation (choledochal cyst) to obstructive strictures of the biliary tree. Choledochal cysts most commonly present in childhood but are increasingly being recognized in adults. In the United States, benign biliary strictures most commonly occur as a result of injury after cholecystectomy, but also occur in a number of diverse inflammatory conditions affecting the biliary tree. Both conditions represent significant clinical challenges where proper evaluation and management are paramount to prevent serious clinical sequelae.

■ CHOLEDOCHAL CYST

Choledochal cysts are focal or diffuse dilatations of the biliary tree that are believed to be congenital abnormalities. They may occur as single or multiple cysts within the extrahepatic or intrahepatic bile ducts. Diagnosis and treatment are essential because choledochal cysts may predispose patients to recurrent cholangitis, biliary stones, secondary biliary cirrhosis, or malignancy.

The incidence of choledochal cysts varies significantly throughout the world. The incidence in Asia may be as high as 1 in 1000, with reports from Japan comprising more than half the documented cases. In Western countries, choledochal cysts occur much less frequently, with reported rates that vary from 1 in 13,000 to 1 in 150,000.[1] There have been a few case reports of choledochal cysts occurring within families, but choledochal cysts generally do not have a hereditary pattern. The disorder occurs more commonly in females than males, with a ratio of approximately 3–4:1. Choledochal cysts classically present during childhood, but recent series report as many as 25% of cases presenting in adults.[1]

CLASSIFICATION

Proper management of choledochal cysts requires consideration of their classification. While the traditional classification system devised by Alonso-Lej and associates[2] exclusively involved the extrahepatic duct, the classification system was revised by Todani and colleagues[3] in 1977 to include intrahepatic cystic anomalies also known as Caroli's disease (Table 34–1 and Fig 34–1). A similar classification has been proposed based upon bile duct cholangiographic appearance.[4] More recently, Todani and colleagues have revised their classification further to reflect the presence or absence of pancreaticobiliary maljunction.[5] This further revision has yet to be broadly used.

While Todani's 1977 schema is the most widely accepted classification, it is not without controversy. Some have argued that the term "choledochal cyst" should refer to only type I and IV cysts (which comprise over 90% of biliary cysts).[6] This proposal is based upon current understanding of pathogenesis, treatment, malignancy risk, and natural history, which vary substantially with type I and IV cysts versus type II, III, or V cysts.

TABLE 34–1. TODANI CLASSIFICATION OF CHOLEDOCHAL CYSTS

Type I	Classic cyst type characterized by cystic dilatation of the common bile duct; most common, comprising 50–85% of all biliary cysts; subdivided into IA (cystic), IB (fusiform), and IC (saccular)
Type II	Simple diverticulum of the extrahepatic biliary tree, comprising less than 5% of all cysts; located proximal to the duodenum
Type III	Cystic dilatation of the intraduodenal portion of the extra hepatic common bile duct; also known as a choledochocele; comprise approximately 5%
Type IV	Involve multiple cysts of the intrahepatic and extrahepatic biliary tree; subdivided into type IVA (both intrahepatic and extrahepatic cysts) and IVB (multiple extrahepatic cysts without intrahepatic involvement); type IVA is the second most common type of biliary cyst (30–40%)
Type V	Isolated intrahepatic biliary cystic disease, also known as Caroli's disease; associated with periportal fibrosis or cirrhosis; can be multilobar or confined to a single lobe

PATHOGENESIS

The cause of choledochal cysts is not currently known. While there have been reports of acquired cysts in the literature, most are congenital in nature. It is unclear whether cases of choledochal cysts diagnosed in adults are acquired or late manifestations of congenital cysts.

There may be multiple mechanisms involved in the creation of biliary cysts, and several theories have been proposed. The high incidence of biliary cysts in Asia suggests a role for either genetic or environmental factors. Bile duct obstruction or distension in the prenatal or neonatal periods may contribute to biliary cyst formation. In animal models, bile duct ligation in neonates leads to cyst formation; in contrast, bile duct ligation in adult animals results in gallbladder distension.[7] Other proposed theories include congenital weakness in the bile duct wall and abnormal biliary epithelial proliferation during development.[8] Indirect evidence for a role of fetal viral infection includes the isolation of *Reovirus* RNA from biliary tissue in children with choledochal cysts.[9]

Pancreaticobiliary maljunction is defined as an extramural junction of the pancreatic and biliary ducts in the duodenum beyond the intramural sphincter function and is characterized by a long common channel (typically over 2 cm) (Fig 34–2). Pancreaticobiliary maljunction has been reported with high frequency associated with choledochal cysts, especially in the Japanese literature. Pancreaticobiliary maljunction is also thought to be a significant risk factor for the development of cholangiocarcinoma in the biliary cyst,[10] as well as the development of gallbladder cancer. Several investigators have speculated on the embryological etiology of pancreaticobiliary maljunction, hypothesizing that the development of pancreaticobiliary maljunction is a result of an arrest in the migration of the choledochopancreatic junction into the duodenal wall.[11,12]

Because of the long common channel, patients with pancreaticobiliary maljunction may have increased reflux of pancreatic juice into the biliary tree, since the ductal junction lies outside of the sphincter of Oddi.[13] Reflux of pancreatic juices may result in inflammation, activation of proteolytic enzymes, theoretical biliary epithelial damage, alterations in bile composition, and ductal distension. It is thought that a combination of these factors contributes to the development of malignancy within the choledochal cyst or gallbladder. Elevated sphincter of Oddi pressures have also been documented in patients with pancreaticobiliary maljunction, resulting in more reflux.[14,15]

On pathology, choledochal cysts have variable microscopic features, with appearance ranging from normal bile duct mucosa to carcinoma. In children, the classic histological appearance is a thick and dense fibrotic cyst wall with evidence of acute and chronic inflammation. In adults, common findings are inflammation, erosions, sparseness of mucin glands, and metaplasia.[1,16] Type III cysts are most often lined by duodenal mucosa, although they sometimes are lined by bile duct epithelium.[16] When malignancy is present, it is most commonly found along the posterior cyst wall.[17]

PRESENTATION

The classic triad of presentation for choledochal cysts is pain, jaundice, and abdominal mass. This triad is found in only a minority of children at the time of presentation. Infants commonly present with elevated conjugated bilirubin (80%), failure to thrive, or an abdominal mass (30%). In patients older than 2 years of age, abdominal pain is the most common presenting symptom. An abdominal mass becomes less common with increasing age and is rarely appreciated in adults. Intermittent jaundice and recurrent cholangitis are also common, as is pancreatitis, especially in patients with a type III cyst (choledochocele).[1,6,18] Rarely, choledochal cysts will present as intraperitoneal rupture or bleeding due to erosion into adjacent vessels.

DIAGNOSIS

The diagnosis of a choledochal cyst requires a high level of suspicion. Unless choledochal cyst is considered in the differential diagnosis in patients with ductal dilatation, type I cysts may go undiagnosed. Patients with biliary obstruction, either acutely or chronically, may also have biliary dilatation that can mimic a type I cyst. In contrast to a type I cyst, an obstructing lesion will often cause elevated alkaline phosphatase and bi-

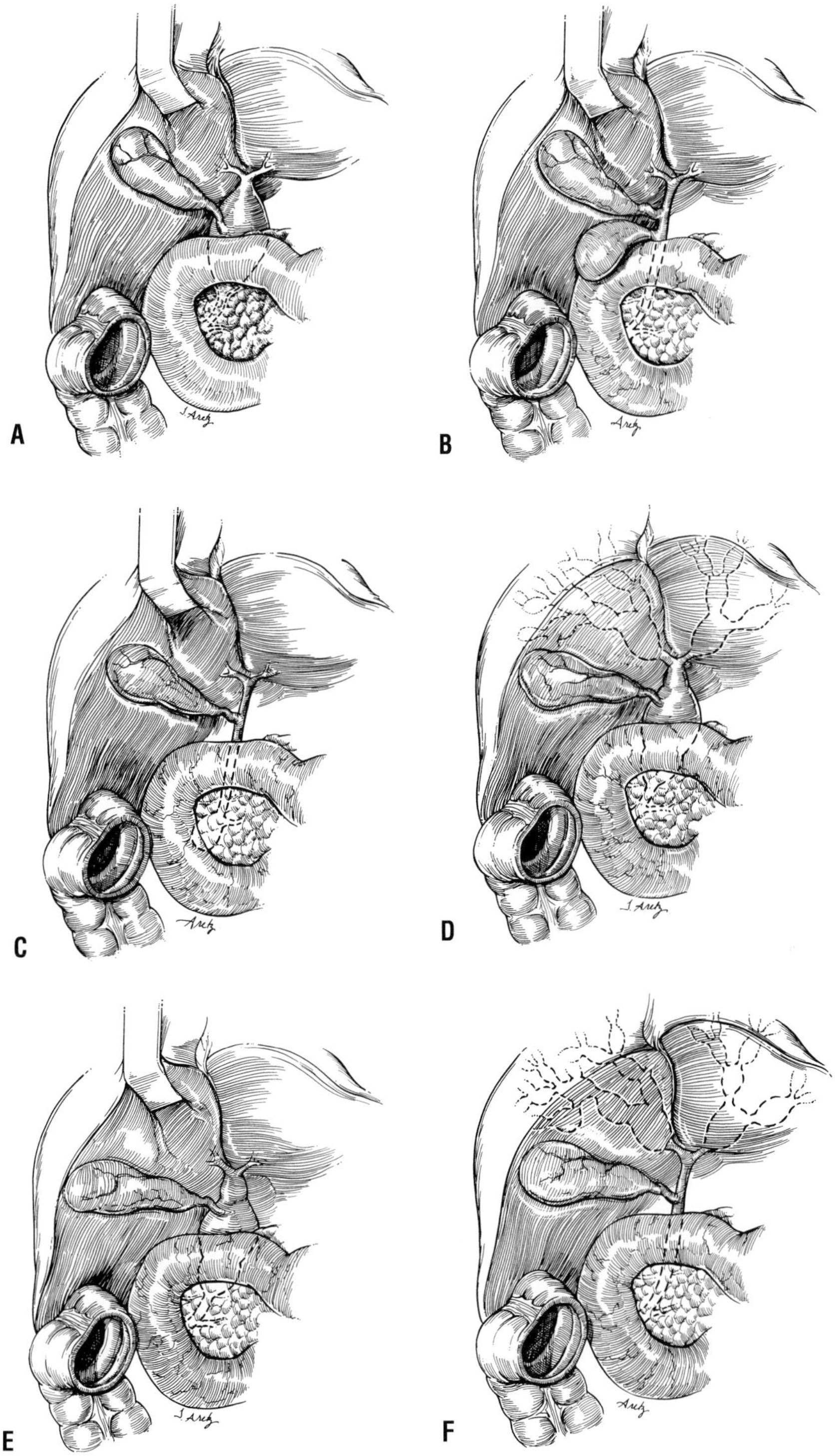

Figure 34–1. Illustrations of the Todani classification of choledochal cysts. **A.** Type IA. **B.** Type II. **C.** Type III. **D.** Type IVA. **E.** Type IVB. **F.** Type V.

lirubin, as well as improvement in biliary dilatation after appropriate treatment. The presence of pancreaticobiliary maljunction in uncertain cases can also be helpful in making the diagnosis of a type I cyst versus a biliary obstruction.

Ultrasound or CT scan imaging can be especially helpful in suggesting the presence of a choledochal cyst. While ultrasound is the standard for antenatal and childhood diagnosis, CT scan may be more appropriate in adult patients, in whom the differential diagnosis is

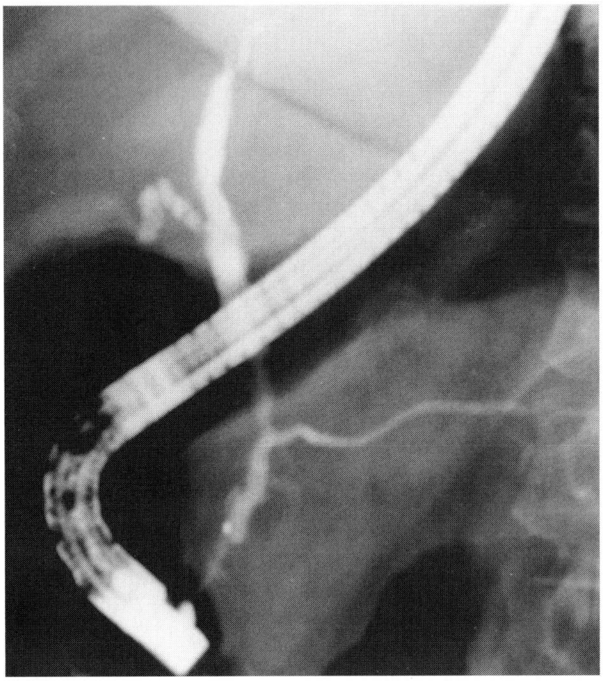

Figure 34–2. Pancreaticobiliary maljunction.

broader (Fig 34–3). Important considerations on CT scan include assessing the hepatobiliary and pancreatic anatomy, with evaluation for possible biliary malignancy, metastatic disease, and vascular encasement.

Magnetic resonance cholangiopancreatography (MRCP) may also be helpful in the diagnosis of choledochal cyst. While it appears to be superior to CT scan for defining pancreaticobiliary maljunction, MRCP is less sensitive than CT scan for examining intrahepatic biliary anatomy.

Cholangiography is considered the gold standard for diagnosis of choledochal cysts. Percutaneous transhepatic cholangiography (PTC) or endoscopic retrograde cholangiography (ERC) is typically performed on adults and larger children, while intraoperative cholangiography may be done on infants and small children. Cholangiography can demonstrate areas of cystic dilatation, the presence of stones, and excludes complete obstruction of the bile duct (Fig 34–4). It is also effective in demonstrating the presence of pancreaticobiliary maljunction.

In patients with type I or type IV cysts that extend to the hepatic bifurcation, PTC with placement of one or two transhepatic biliary catheters may be helpful to facilitate complete resection and biliary reconstruction (Fig 34–5). To decrease the high risk of pancreatitis in those patients with pancreaticobiliary maljunction and a long common channel, it is important to avoid placing the stent through the ampulla while performing PTC.

MANAGEMENT

Once the diagnosis of choledochal cyst is made and the patient's biliary anatomy is delineated through cholangiography and CT scan, several important clinical considerations must be taken into account. If a patient presents with pancreatitis or cholangitis, these problems must be treated supportively prior to considering definitive operative management of the biliary cyst. Because of the extensive sludge or stones that may be present within choledochal cysts and the high incidence of pancreaticobiliary maljunction, these patients are at espe-

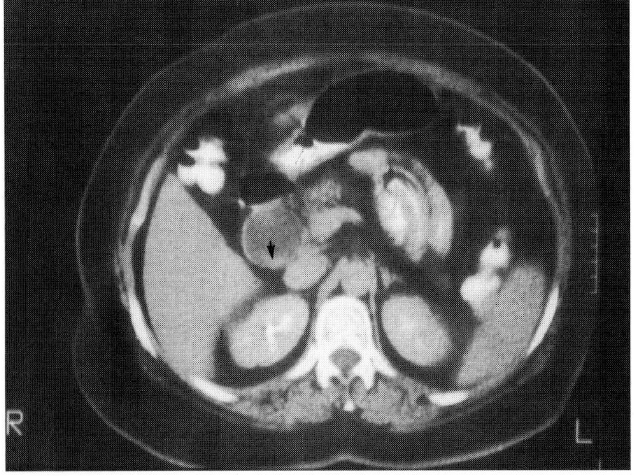

A

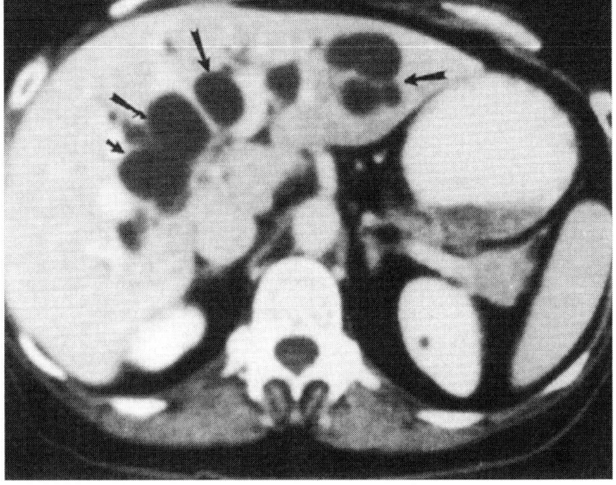

B

Figure 34–3. A. CT scan appearance of type IA choledochal cyst (*arrow* shows sludge within the cyst). **B.** CT scan appearance through the liver demonstrates multiple low-density structures (*arrows*) within the right and left lobe consistent with a type IVA choledochal cyst.

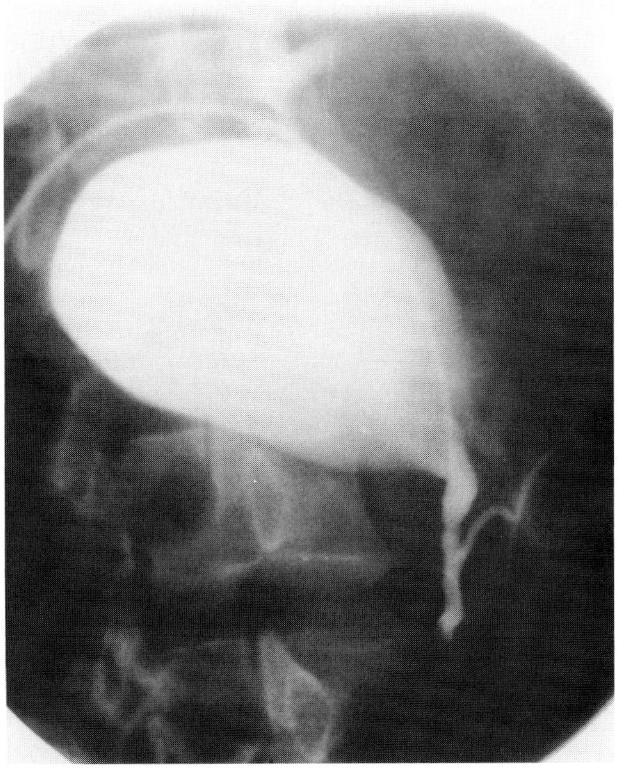

Figure 34–4. Percutaneous cholangiogram via the right hepatic duct. A large type I choledochal cyst is seen. Note the anomalous choledochopancreatic duct junction.

cially high risk for pancreatitis. Furthermore, there is a risk of pancreatitis during ERCP with ampullary stent placement.

Another important clinical consideration in patients with choledochal cyst is the presence of biliary or gallbladder malignancy. The incidence of malignancy with biliary cysts varies with patient age and cyst type. A 1983 review examining all published series of biliary cysts uncovered an incidence of cancer of 0.7% in patients under 10 years of age, 6.8% in patients aged 11–20 years, and 14.3% in patients over 20 years of age.[16] In older patients, the reported incidence is as high as 50%.[19] Type I and IV cysts have the highest risk of cancer, while cancer is rare in type II and III cysts. In type III cysts, cancer risk may be limited to those choledochoceles lined by biliary and not duodenal epithelium. Historically, choledochal cysts presenting in childhood were often treated with a cyst-enteric bypass leaving the cyst in situ. These patients remain at risk for the development of cancer within the retained cyst. Caroli's disease also carries a risk (about 7%) of cholangiocarcinoma. Most patients with Caroli's disease, however, will present first with compromised liver function or cholangitis before developing malignancy.

Speculated etiological factors in carcinogenesis associated with biliary cysts include bile stasis, reflux of pancreatic juice mixed with bile, superinfection, or inflammation.[19,20] Cholangiocarcinoma in choledochal cysts is strongly linked to patients with pancreaticobiliary maljunction.[10] Pancreaticobiliary maljunction on its own, even without associated choledochal cyst, is also associated with an increased risk of gallbladder cancer. Pancreaticobiliary reflux with the mixing of pancreatic and biliary secretions within the cyst has again been implicated in the pathogenesis. There is also strong pathological evidence of a hyperplasia-dysplasia-carcinoma sequence of carcinogenesis in patients with pancreaticobiliary maljunction. While the exact pathways have yet to be elucidated, cells with hyperplasia in patients with pancreaticobiliary maljunction have elevated expression of cellular proliferation markers, including cyclooxygenase-2 and vascular endothelial growth factor.[21] On a molecular level, hyperplastic cells also have a high incidence of K-*ras* mutations (13–63%),[22,23] while dysplastic cells frequently have microsatellite instability (60%)[24] and cancerous lesions often have overexpression of cyclin D1[25] and *p53* mutations.[26] Prophylactic cholecystectomy is also advised in all patients with either pancreaticobiliary maljunction or choledochal cyst.

Even after cyst resection, patients have a continued increased risk of carcinoma. Malignancy may develop with incompletely resected cysts, at the anastomotic site, or in residual cyst left within the pancreas. In addition to the continued increased risk of cancer after ex-

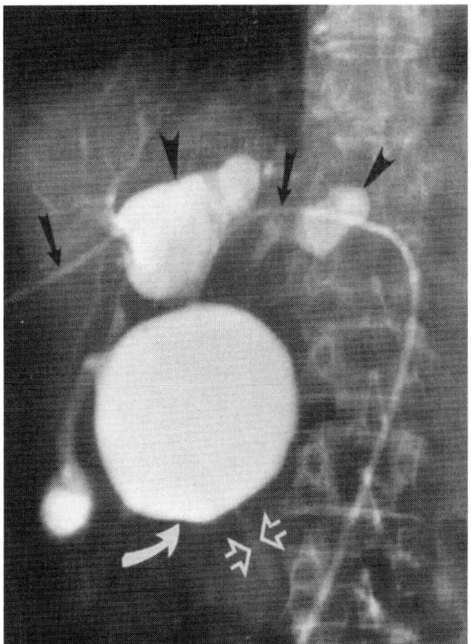

Figure 34–5. Type IVA choledochal cyst. Bilateral percutaneous biliary drainage catheters (*arrows*) were placed in this patient, who had extensive intrahepatic biliary duct dilatation (*arrowheads*) and a huge extrahepatic choledochal cyst (*curved arrow*). Note that the biliary catheters exit the cyst and enter the duodenum (*open arrows*).

cision, the most frequent long-term complication after biliary reconstruction is postoperative biliary stricture at the site of the anastomosis (approximately 25%).[27] Therefore, long-term follow-up should survey patients periodically for the development of an anastomotic stricture. Significant elevations in serum alkaline phosphatase levels merit further investigation and treatment to prevent long-term complications from postoperative biliary strictures.

Unfortunately, current methods for screening for malignancy within a choledochal cyst have not proved effective and therefore expectant management cannot be advised for most patients. Intraductal ultrasound and cytologic brushings of the cyst wall show promise for potentially detecting malignancy. Patients with choledochal cysts who are poor surgical candidates or who refuse biliary reconstructive surgery may be candidates for lesser interventions to treat symptoms caused by gallstones or sludge, such as cholecystectomy or endoscopic treatment.

Operative Management

Choledochal cysts were historically managed with biliary-enteric drainage via cyst-enterostomy. Recognition of an increased risk of bile duct and gallbladder cancer an average of 10 years after enteric drainage[19] has changed the recommended management to complete choledochal cyst excision. The main goal of management is therefore to prevent malignant degeneration of the cyst via surgical excision. In newly diagnosed adult patients with biliary cysts, the possibility of an existing cancer needs to be considered. Cyst excision can also reduce complications of choledochal cysts frequently seen with biliary-enteric drainage, including pancreatitis, choledocholithiasis, and cholangitis.[19]

The operative management of choledochal cysts should first consist of careful exploration of the patient. Upon entry to the abdomen via a midline incision, the initial step should be searching for possible metastatic disease.

Once metastatic disease has been excluded, management of the choledochal cyst consists of complete cyst excision and performance of cholecystectomy. If possible, excision should include all remnants of the cyst. Because of the extensive fibrosis that may be present, complete excision of the cyst can be technically challenging. Very rarely when there is severe pericystic inflammation, the back wall of the cyst may be left intact to prevent injury to the portal vein or hepatic artery.[28]

Following choledochal cyst excision and cholecystectomy, the bile duct is reconstructed. Standard methods to reconstruct the bile duct include hepaticojejunostomy or hepaticoduodenostomy, although Roux-en-Y hepaticojejunostomy is by far the most commonly used technique. Enteric interposition grafts have been proposed as an option due to the theoretical restoration of physiologic bile flow. Both jejunal interposition grafts and appendiceal interposition grafts between the duodenum and bile duct have been reported in the pediatric surgery literature. The value of these techniques, however, has been questioned because of graft dysfunction from stenosis and kinking.[29]

Successful resection and biliary reconstruction with type I and type II choledochal cysts has also been reported using laparoscopic techniques, particularly in children. While the choice of performing these procedures via an open or laparoscopic approach should be a matter of preference and technical ability for the surgeon, it is important that the procedure not be compromised by the use of laparoscopy.

Type I Cysts. Type I cysts can usually be identified without difficulty upon exploration and freed from attachments. A Kocher maneuver may be necessary to expose the distal portion of the cyst posterior to the duodenal wall (Fig 34–6A). After the cyst has been exposed, the gallbladder, which usually arises from the mid-portion of the choledochal cyst, should be dissected away from the hepatic bed (Fig 34–6B). The procedure then focuses on the distal portion of the choledochal cyst (Fig 34–6C). Type IB (fusiform) cysts are particularly prone to extend distally to the entrance of the common bile duct into the pancreas. The goal is then to excise the intrapancreatic portion of the cyst without injuring the pancreatic duct or the long common channel. The distal-most portion of the choledochal cyst is encircled and transected as it enters the pancreas. If the cyst extends distally into the pancreas, the mucosa of the intrapancreatic portion of the cyst should be stripped away prior to closure at the point of distal transection. Resection of the pancreatic head can usually be avoided unless there is documented malignancy.

Dissection is then carried proximally by elevating the cyst anteriorly (Fig 34–6D). This dissection may be facilitated by the presence of a preoperatively placed transhepatic stent. Since the cyst may need to be freed from both the portal vein and hepatic artery, the surgeon must be mindful of variant vascular anatomy that may be encountered and maintain careful hemostasis. Care must also be taken to recognize atypical biliary anatomy, which may be encountered at the most proximal portion of dissection near the hilum. The cyst is then transected at the bifurcation or more proximally if the cyst extends into the individual hepatic ducts (Fig 34–6E). The excised cyst should be examined grossly for malignancy, and then the specimen should be sent for frozen section. If malignancy is present, particularly at the surgical margin, the resection may need to be extended either proximally or distally, even including the performance of a pancreaticoduodenectomy to obtain a negative margin and adequate lymph node clearance.

Reconstruction of the biliary tree is typically performed with a Roux-en-Y hepaticojejunostomy at the bifurcation with a single anastomosis or multiple individual anastomoses with each of the hepatic ducts (Fig 34–6F). A suitable segment of intestine is mobilized with a Roux-en-Y jejunal limb, approximately 60 cm in length, and the anastomosis is created with a standard end-to-side Roux-en-Y hepaticojejunostomy, typically using a single layer of absorbable suture (Fig 34–6G and H).

Type II Cysts. Type II cysts are treated with simple cyst excision. After the cyst has been exposed, the common bile duct wall defect is closed transversely. A transverse closure helps to minimize potential narrowing or stricturing of the common bile duct. Patients with both a type II cyst and pancreaticobiliary malformation should

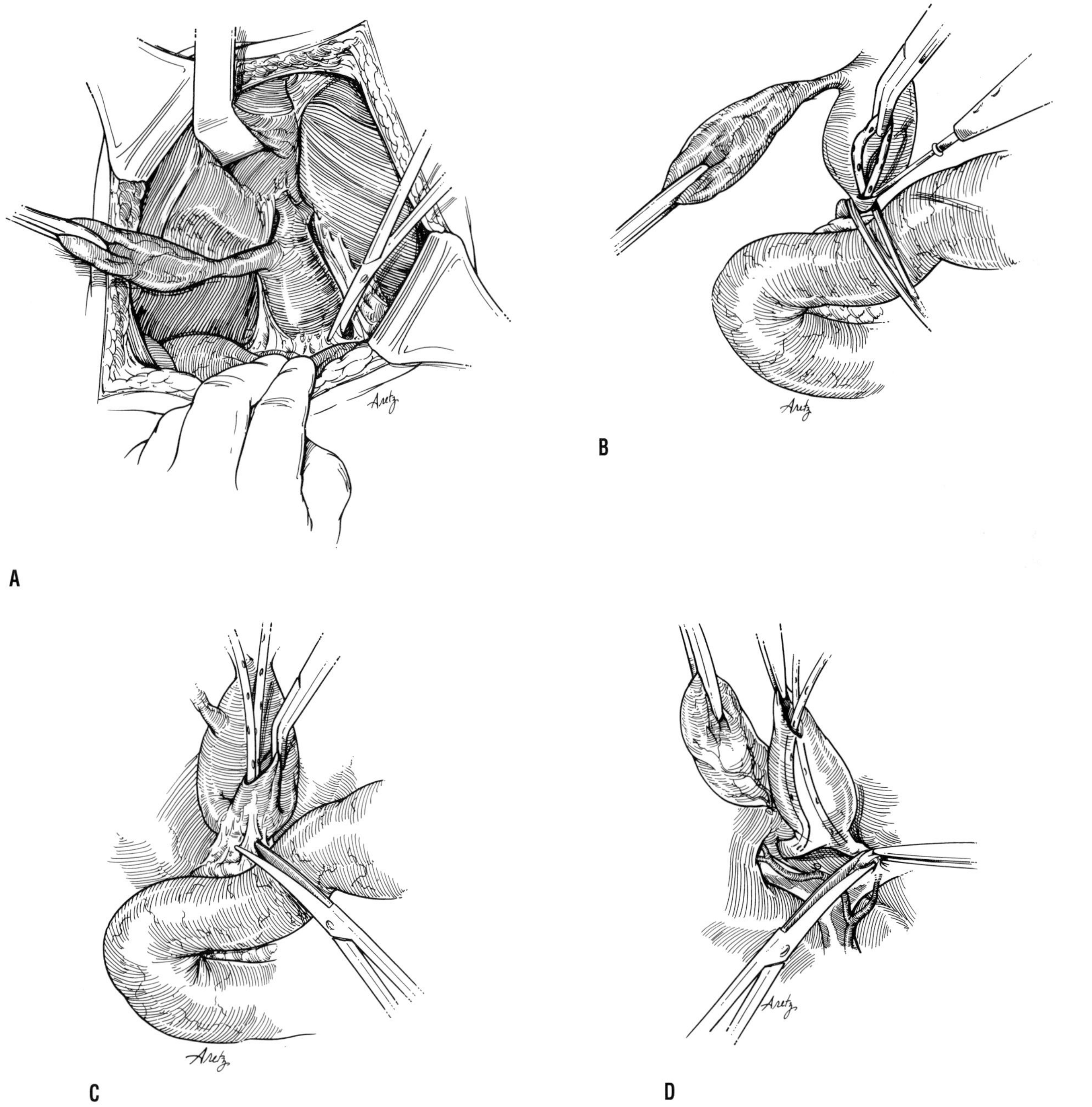

Figure 34–6. Type I choledochal cyst resection and biliary reconstruction with Roux-en-Y hepaticojejunostomy. **A.** Exposure of cyst and gallbladder. **B.** Cholecystectomy and anterior dissection of the distal choledochal cyst. **C.** Distal extent of the cyst identified, encircled, and opened. **D.** Posterior dissection proceeds caudad to cephalad. *Continued*

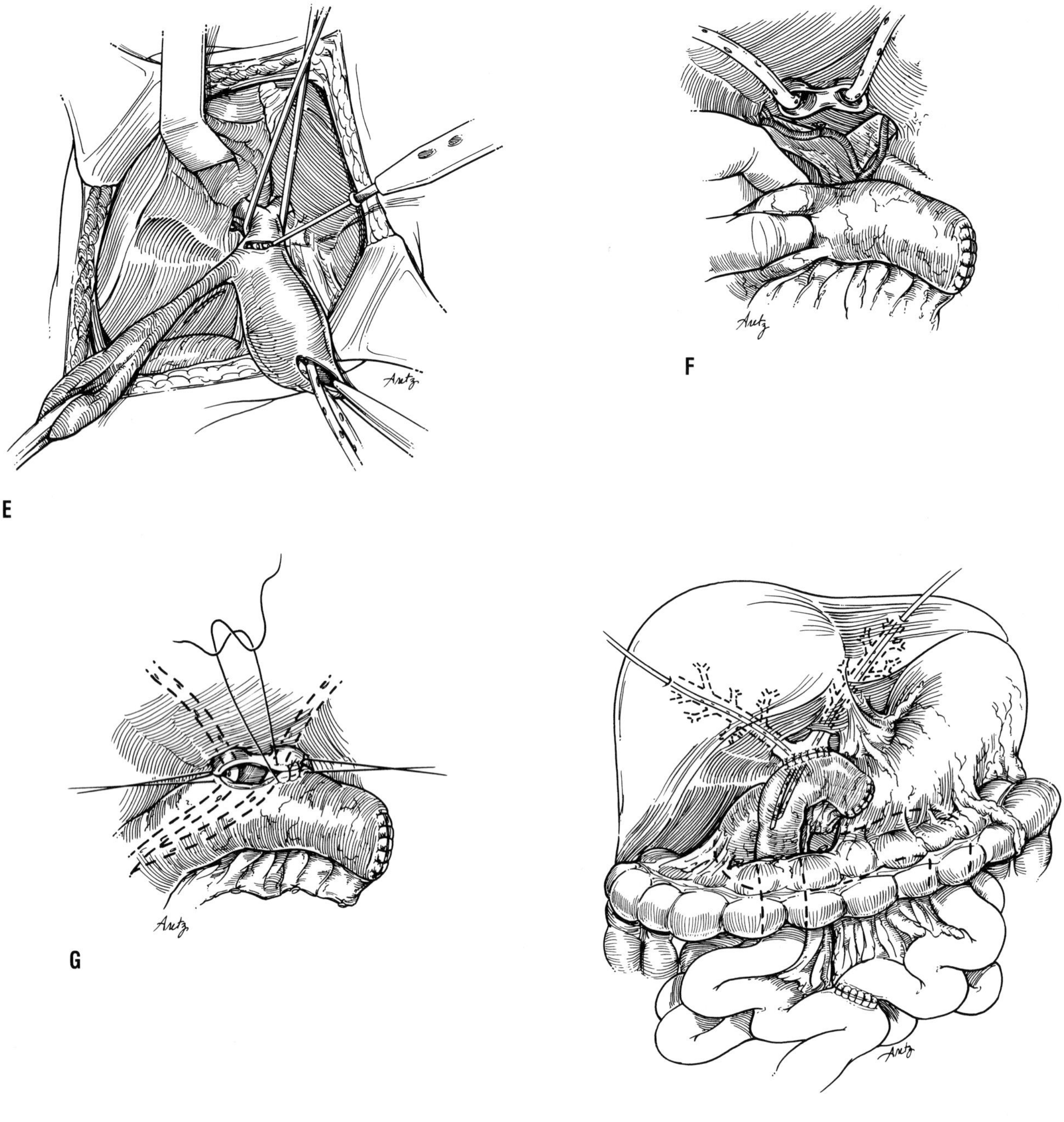

Figure 34–6, cont'd. E. Dissection proceeds until normal hepatic duct is identified. **F.** Cyst is transected and removed at normal duct. **G.** Excision is complete; reconstruction proceeds with a Roux-en-Y hepaticojejunostomy. If the bifurcation is involved, right and left hepaticojejunostomies can be performed. **H.** One-layer hepaticojejunostomy at the hepatic bifurcation.

also undergo cholecystectomy. Recently, resection of type II cysts has been completed successfully via a laparoscopic approach.

Type III Cysts. Because of their rarity and lower overall rate of malignant transformation, reports of choledochocele excision are uncommon. However, excision may be necessary in symptomatic patients, but many patients may benefit from endoscopic sphincterotomy. Surgical resection is typically approached via a transverse duodenotomy in the second or third portion of the duodenum. Prior to duodenotomy, cholecystectomy is performed and then the ampulla can be localized by passing a biliary Fogarty catheter into the duodenum via the transected cystic duct. The anatomy can also be better defined prior to duodenotomy by performing a Kocher maneuver and intraoperative ultrasound.

Duodenotomy allows both the biliary and pancreatic ducts to be identified individually. The pancreatic duct can be intubated using a small Silastic tube so that the intraduodenal biliary cyst can be excised. Both the bile duct mucosa and pancreatic duct mucosa are then sutured individually to the duodenal mucosa using interrupted absorbable sutures. A piece of 5F or 8F plastic tubing can be placed into the pancreatic duct and secured with a single absorbable suture as a temporary stent to prevent postoperative acute pancreatitis. Finally the duodenostomy is closed in a transverse fashion.

Type IV Cysts. Type IVA and type IVB cysts are managed similarly to type I cysts with regard to extrahepatic biliary resection, cholecystectomy, and biliary reconstruction. Because there may be proximally located cysts, reconstruction will be proximal to the bifurcation and involve anastomosing individual hepatic ducts. Preoperative transhepatic biliary stents may be especially helpful for managing patients with type IV cysts, particularly those with type IVA cysts that extend into the intrahepatic ducts. Specifically, the stents can facilitate proximal dissection intraoperatively and can help to manage postoperative anastomotic leaks and retained hepatic stones. Intraoperative choledochoscopy should be performed with stone extraction and biopsies of dominant strictures. Stone extraction can be tedious and involve extensive manipulation.

Intrahepatic disease in type IVA disease and Caroli's disease are prone to secondary biliary cirrhosis, hepatic atrophy, and portal hypertension. If the liver parenchyma is not cirrhotic and there is no evidence of intrahepatic duct malignancy, then hepatic parenchyma should be preserved, even in the setting of stones or strictures. If cirrhosis is unilateral or segmental, resection of the involved parenchyma is necessary.

Oncological principles should be followed in cases in whom malignancy is involved. If no metastatic disease is present and the vascular supply to the uninvolved hepatic parenchyma can be preserved, then resection of the involved bile ducts and adjacent parenchyma, along with regional lymph node dissection, is indicated. In rare cases, extensive resections involving combined hepatic and pancreatic resection may be necessary. In cases in whom metastatic disease is present, palliative stenting of the bile ducts is usually indicated.

Type V Cysts. While Caroli's disease may be diffuse and bilobar, it is often confined to a single lobe, more typically the left side. Similarly to type IVA cysts, Caroli's disease, if unilateral or segmental with cirrhosis, can be managed by resection of the involved parenchyma. Bilobar Caroli's disease represents an especially challenging problem. The use of ursodeoxycholic acid may improve bile flow, reducing the incidence of biliary sludge, stones, and cholangitis. In the absence of cirrhosis or malignancy, Roux-en-Y hepaticojejunostomy with bilateral transhepatic Silastic stents may be indicated to improve biliary drainage. Following operative management, the stents are left in place for 6–12 months, depending on the extent of intrahepatic stones and strictures. Patients that continue to have recurrent cholangitis or recurrent stones often require indefinite transhepatic stenting. Patients with Caroli's disease and liver failure may warrant liver transplantation.

Operative Results

Long-term results following resection of a benign choledochal cyst with biliary reconstruction are generally excellent, especially with type I cysts. The management of more proximal cysts can be more challenging, particularly in the presence of extensive intrahepatic stone disease and liver damage. A recent series by Tsuchida and associates[30] examined 103 patients with mean follow-up of 12.5 years. Patients with type IVA disease with dilated intrahepatic ducts developed strictures at a rate of 40%, with virtually all developing cholangitis. In contrast, management with large-bore Silastic transhepatic stenting results in 90% success without recurrent cholangitis.[31] Patients remain at long-term risk for recurrent cholangitis, postoperative biliary strictures, intrahepatic stones, pancreatitis, or malignancy.

SUMMARY

Choledochal cysts require proper diagnosis and treatment to address associated symptoms, risk of malignancy, and disease progression. The majority of cases of biliary cysts (type I and IVA) can be treated effectively with cyst resection, cholecystectomy, and biliary reconstruction. While operative therapy decreases the risk of subsequent cancer, patients continue to require long-term surveillance for recurrent cholangitis, intrahepatic stones, pancreatitis, postoperative biliary strictures, and malignancy.

▪ BENIGN BILIARY STRICTURES

Benign bile duct strictures include several diverse clinical entities that share the common characteristic of biliary obstruction. Although advances in medical technology have greatly improved their management, bile duct strictures continue to pose a significant clinical challenge. Complications of benign biliary strictures include cholangitis, portal hypertension, biliary cirrhosis, and end-stage liver disease. Proper diagnosis and treatment are essential in preventing these complications. In principle, the evaluation and treatment of all patients with bile duct strictures seeks to relieve bile duct obstruction. There are numerous etiologies of benign bile duct strictures (Table 34–2). The vast majority of strictures occur following injury to the bile duct during cholecystectomy. Inflammatory conditions such as pancreatitis, gallstone disease, and primary sclerosing cholangitis are also important causes of benign bile duct strictures.

POSTOPERATIVE BILIARY STRICTURE

The introduction and widespread use of laparoscopic cholecystectomy in the 1990s resulted in a significant increase in the frequency of biliary injuries and associated bile duct strictures. Postoperative bile duct injuries may present early in the postoperative period with biliary leak, or months to years later with jaundice or cholangitis from biliary stricture. Proper management begins with delineation of biliary anatomy followed by repair. Nonoperative balloon dilatation via percutaneous transhepatic or endoscopic routes is appropriate in select patients with intact biliary-enteric continuity. Operative repair, however, remains the mainstay of treatment in patients with benign strictures.

TABLE 34–2. ETIOLOGY OF BENIGN BILIARY STRICTURES

Postoperative Strictures
Laparoscopic cholecystectomy
Open cholecystectomy
Common bile duct exploration
Injury at other operative procedures
Gastrectomy
Hepatic resection
Portacaval shunt
Biliary-enteric anastomotic stricture
Blunt or penetrating trauma
Strictures Due to Inflammatory and Other Conditions
Primary sclerosing cholangitis
Chronic pancreatitis
Cholelithiasis and choledocholithiasis
Cholangiohepatitis and other parasitic disease
Sphincter of Oddi stenosis
Duodenal ulcer
Granulomatous lymphadenitis
Secondary sclerosing cholangitis
Toxic drugs
Infectious cholangiopathy from AIDS
Hepatic allograft rejection
Graft-versus-host disease in bone marrow transplantation
Histiocytosis X
Congenital biliary abnormality
Mast cell cholangiopathy

Classification

Strictures and injuries to the bile ducts vary widely in their complexity and nature. Injuries associated with laparoscopic cholecystectomy are often complex, located at or near the level of the hepatic duct bifurcation, and potentially include one or more hepatic duct branches. Minor injuries to the bile duct include lacerations of the bile duct, clip placement on an intact bile duct, injury via electrocautery, or avulsion of the cystic duct.

A number of classification systems for major bile duct strictures have been offered, with the traditional classification being that described by Bismuth, which classifies major injuries based on the level of obstruction of the biliary tree (Fig 34–7).[32] A drawback of the Bismuth classification is that patients with limited strictures, isolated right hepatic duct strictures, or cystic duct leaks cannot be classified. The Strasberg classification is able to classify all types of injury and is used extensively in describing bile duct injuries associated with laparoscopic cholecystectomy (Table 34–3).[33]

Pathogenesis

Most bile duct injuries and strictures occur in patients following abdominal surgery in the right upper quadrant. Cholecystectomy is performed on over 700,000 patients on an annual basis in the United States and accounts for over 90% of postoperative biliary strictures and injuries. Although the exact incidence of injuries is unknown because many cases go unreported, numerous studies have attempted to define the incidence and mechanisms of bile duct injuries associated with cholecystectomy. The incidence of injury following cholecystectomy can be estimated, however, using large databases comprising thousands of patients and hundreds of surgeons. An incidence of 1–3 major bile duct injuries per 1,000 cases was consistently reported during the era of open cholecystectomy. Roslyn and colleagues demonstrated a 0.2% incidence of major bile duct injuries from a series of over 42,000 open cholecystectomies.[34] A literature review by Strasberg and associates[33] of over 25,500 open cholecystectomies performed since 1980 revealed a 0.3% incidence of major bile duct injuries. The incidence of bile duct injury associated with laparoscopic cholecystectomy appears to be greater than that with open cholecystectomy. Multiple large surveys from numerous centers have estimated the rate of major bile duct injury with laparoscopic cholecystectomy to be 0.4–0.7%.[35–39]

In the early 1990s, many authors ascribed the increased incidence of bile duct injuries with laparo-

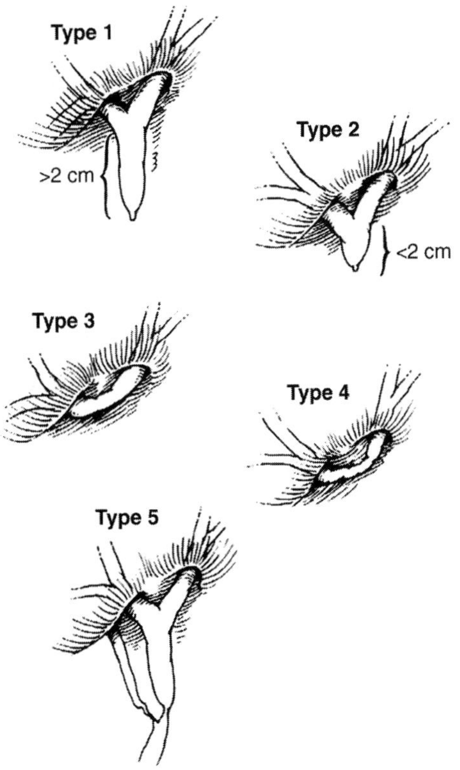

Figure 34–7. Bismuth classification system. Classification of bile duct strictures based upon the level of the stricture in relation to the confluence of the hepatic ducts. Types 3, 4, and 5 are usually considered complex injuries. (Reproduced, with permission, from Bismuth H. Postoperative strictures of the biliary tract. In: Blumgart LH (ed). *The Biliary Tract. Clinical Surgery International Series*, Vol. 5. Edinburgh, Scotland: Churchill Livingstone; 1983:209–218.)

scopic cholecystectomy as a "learning curve" associated with the new technique and projected that the rate of injury associated with laparoscopic cholecystectomy would decline with time. Unfortunately, these projections were not correct, and the rate of bile duct injuries appears now to have stabilized at a level still higher than that of the pre-laparoscopic era. A report of over 10,000 cases at United States military institutions[35] and nationwide reviews in New Zealand[36] and Denmark[37] have demonstrated no significant improvement in the incidence of injury as surgeons have passed through the learning curve. It is likely that the technology and technique associated with laparoscopic cholecystectomy will need fundamental enhancements for the current rate of injury to diminish.

Several technical factors associated with laparoscopic cholecystectomy make it prone to bile duct injury. First, the laparoscope gives a limited perspective from its end-viewing, two-dimensional picture of the operative field. The current operative technique also involves early identification and division of the cystic duct and cystic artery, creating the possibility of misidentification. The classic laparoscopic injury occurs when the cystic duct and the common bile duct are aligned in the same plane, leading to clipping and dividing the common bile duct (Fig 34–8). Retraction of the gallbladder infundibulum that is excessively cephalad may align the cystic and common bile duct, leading to misidentification and injury. As the operative dissection is carried cephalad, the common hepatic duct may also be transected, often without recognition, resulting in a postoperative bile leak. The right hepatic artery may also be injured, creating excessive bleeding. This classic injury is estimated to occur in over 75% of major bile duct injuries referred to major centers. The classic laparoscopic injury is usually also associated with excision of a segment of bile duct, making the proximal extent of the injury high, usually at or near the hepatic duct bifurcation.

A number of patient-related factors have been associated with bile duct injury. Patients with complicated gallstone disease have a higher risk of injury than patients with chronic cholecystitis, symptomatic cholelithiasis, or biliary colic. Acute cholecystitis is also associated with a higher rate of conversion to open cholecystectomy (29% versus 8%) and bile duct injury (1.3% versus 0.6%) than other indications for laparoscopic cholecystectomy.[37] Anatomic variations can also contribute to bile duct injury. A congenitally short cystic duct or a duct that appears shortened by an impacted stone may also lead to misidentification of the common bile duct, resulting in injury or transection. Other high-risk congenital anatomic anomalies include a long common wall between the cystic and common bile duct or a right hepatic duct inserting into the cystic duct. The risk of bile duct injury also appears to be increased in patients with obesity, chronic inflammation, excessive fat in the dissection area, inadequate exposure, poor or excessive clip placement, injudicious use of electrocautery, and bleeding into the operative field.

The role of intraoperative cholangiography in preventing bile duct injury remains controversial, with

TABLE 34–3. STRASBERG CLASSIFICATION OF BILIARY INJURY AND STRICTURE

Class A	Injury to small ducts in continuity with the biliary system, with cystic duct leak
Class B	Injury to sectoral duct with consequent obstruction
Class C	Injury to sectoral duct with consequent bile leak
Class D	Lateral injury to extrahepatic ducts
Class E_1	Stricture >2 cm distal to bifurcation
Class E_2	Stricture <2 cm distal to bifurcation
Class E_3	Stricture at bifurcation
Class E_4	Stricture involving right and left bile ducts; ducts are not in continuity
Class E_5	Complete occlusion of all bile ducts

Adapted, with permission, from Strasberg SM, Hertl M, Soper NJ. An analysis of the problem of biliary injury during laparoscopic cholecystectomy. *J Am Coll Surg* 1995;180: 101–125.

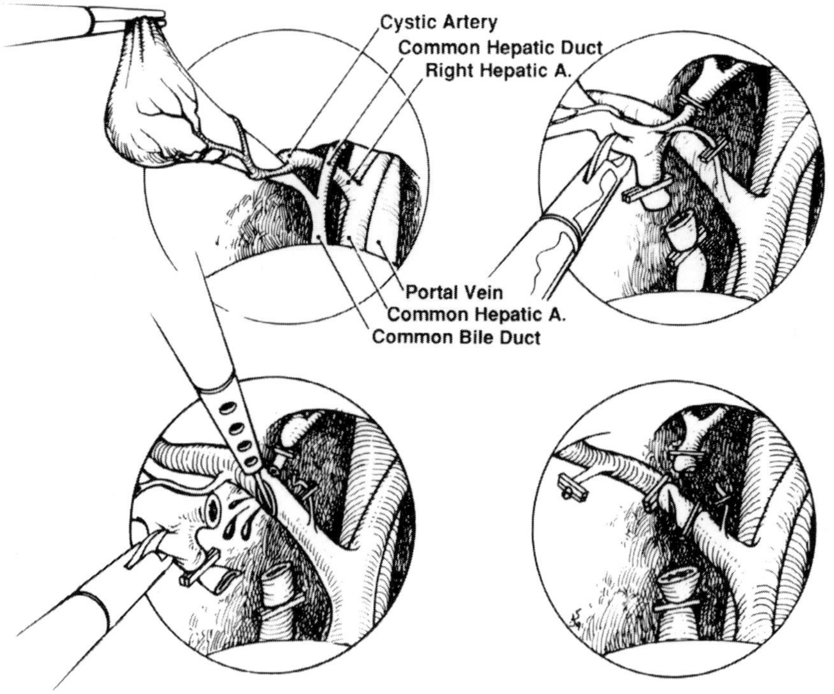

Figure 34–8. Classic laparoscopic bile duct injury. Confusion of the common bile duct with the cystic duct leads to clipping and division of the common bile duct. In many cases the common hepatic duct will not be clipped, but will instead be divided by scissors or cautery. (Reproduced, with permission, from Davidoff AM, Pappas TN, Murray EA et al. Mechanisms of major biliary injury during laparoscopic cholecystectomy. *Ann Surg* 1992;215:196.)

mixed results from reported series. A large series in Australia demonstrated a protective effect,[39] whereas a review from the Veteran's Administration Hospitals demonstrated that bile duct injury occurred more commonly in patients undergoing cholangiography (0.7% versus 0.2%).[35] Clinical information from patients in the Medicare claims database and surgeon data from the American Medical Association Physician Masterfile were recently used to examine the influence of intraoperative cholangiography on the rate of major bile duct injury, finding the rate of injury to be significantly higher when intraoperative cholangiography was not used.[40] In this study, surgeons who routinely performed intraoperative cholangiography had a lower rate of injuries than those who did not, and this lower rate disappeared when intraoperative cholangiography was not used by these surgeons. Whether or not intraoperative cholangiography actually prevents bile duct injury, the procedure can often lead to early recognition of the injury, and therefore potentially minimize the injury and its associated morbidity (Fig 34–9). The best technical approach in preventing and limiting bile duct injuries, regardless of the use of cholangiography, includes methodical dissection with careful exposure and identification of the structures of the triangle of Calot.[33]

There is also a growing understanding of surgeon cognitive factors associated with bile duct injury during laparoscopic cholecystectomy. A recent report examined 252 laparoscopic cholecystectomy bile duct injuries using human error factor and cognitive science techniques and found that 97% of injuries were due to a visual perceptual illusion or inadequate visualization.[41] In a subsequent study from the same group, one of the main explanations for the surgeon's frequent inability to recognize a bile duct injury associated with laparoscopic cholecystectomy appears to be confirmation bias, which is the propensity to seek cues to confirm a belief and to discount cues that might discount that belief.[42] While cognitive factors are important for understanding the psychological issues associated with bile duct injuries, surgeons must continue to have appropriate corrective mechanisms in place to minimize the chance of these injuries, including knowledge of anatomy, typical mechanisms of injury, appropriate level of suspicion, and logic.[43]

Several physiologic processes have been implicated in the formation of bile duct strictures. Ischemia of the bile duct may have an important role in the formation of postoperative anastomotic strictures. Anatomically, the major arteries of the common bile duct located at the 3- and 9-o'clock positions can be injured or divided by unnecessary dissection during cholecystectomy, or more commonly the bile duct can be excessively "skeletonized" while performing a bile duct anastomosis.

Fibrosis and scarring can be intense following a bile duct injury. In canine models, bile duct ligation results in an elevation of bile duct pressure that is immediate and sustained and is accompanied by an increased bile duct diameter.[44] A month following bile duct ligation, the bile duct wall is thickened, will have reduced mucosal folds, and has loss of surface microvilli with epithelial degeneration. On pathologic staining 2 weeks after

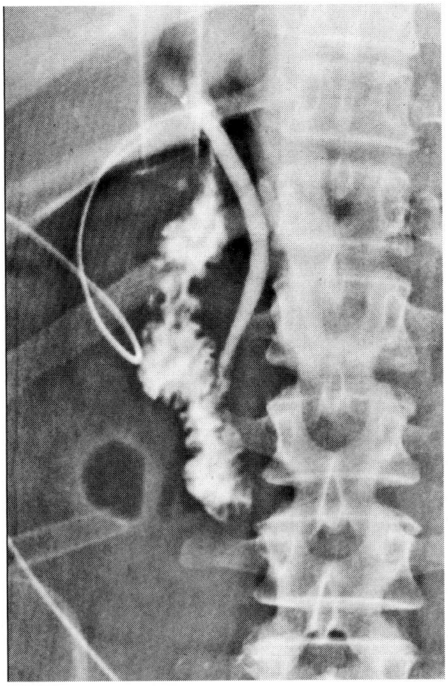

Figure 34–9. Intraoperative cholangiogram obtained during laparoscopic cholecystectomy. Cholangiogram demonstrates an injury to the common bile duct (which is clipped such that contrast does not fill the proximal biliary tree). Contrast fills the normal distal bile duct and duodenum.

ligation, there is evidence of increased synthesis of collagen and proline hydroxylase activation. Recently an animal model of bile duct injury demonstrated healing in traumatized bile duct tissue to occur in a mode of overhealing, implicating myofibroblasts as the main cause of contracture of scar and stricture of the bile duct.[45] Inflammation in the surrounding tissues compounds the problem by encouraging fibrosis, especially when associated with bile leakage.

Injuries and strictures of bile ducts occur less commonly in association with other operative procedures. After cholecystectomy, common bile duct exploration is the next most frequently associated procedure with stricture, typically occurring at the site of choledochotomy or an impacted stone. Gastrectomy and hepatic resection are the most common nonbiliary operations associated with postoperative strictures. Injuries associated with gastrectomy typically occur during pyloric and proximal duodenal dissection associated with closure of the duodenal stump or with creating a Billroth I gastroduodenostomy. Injuries during hepatic resection often take place during dissection of the hepatic hilum. Bile duct injury and stricture is also associated with hepatic transplantation, portacaval shunt, pancreatic procedures, and penetrating or blunt trauma. Finally, the recurrence of stricture after an initial attempt at repair is not uncommon and may occur over a decade following initial repair (Fig 34–10).[46]

Presentation

Most bile duct injuries unfortunately are not recognized at the time of laparoscopic cholecystectomy. Possible indications of intraoperative injury include a persistent and unexpected bile leak, atypical anatomy, or a second bile duct discovered during dissection. Injuries may also be discovered if the removed gallbladder specimen and cystic duct are carefully examined to ensure normal bile duct anatomy. Intraoperative cholangiography will also diagnose bile duct injuries at the time of cholecystectomy and may minimize injury, allowing early repair (see Fig 34–9).

In the early postoperative period, patients sustaining a bile duct injury following cholecystectomy present in one of two manners. The majority of patients present with symptoms associated with bile leak. Prompt investigation is required if patients have bilious drainage from incision sites or from intraoperatively placed drains. Bile leaks may also result in biliary ascites with associated chemical peritonitis if allowed to drain freely into the abdominal cavity. Alternatively, bile can become loculated resulting in biloma, or if infected, a subhepatic or subdiaphragmatic abscess. These patients may present in a subtle manner with persistent pain, abdominal distension, nausea and vomiting, or decreasing activity. It is especially important to appropriately evaluate these patients without delay for possible bile leak to prevent progression to frank sepsis. Failure to recognize a major bile leak or to institute appropriate treatment can result in life-threatening sepsis and the development of multisystem organ failure. In a recent series of 200 major bile duct injuries treated at The Johns Hopkins Hospital, three patients were transferred to this tertiary care center and died of complications of sepsis secondary to delayed or inadequate treatment.[47]

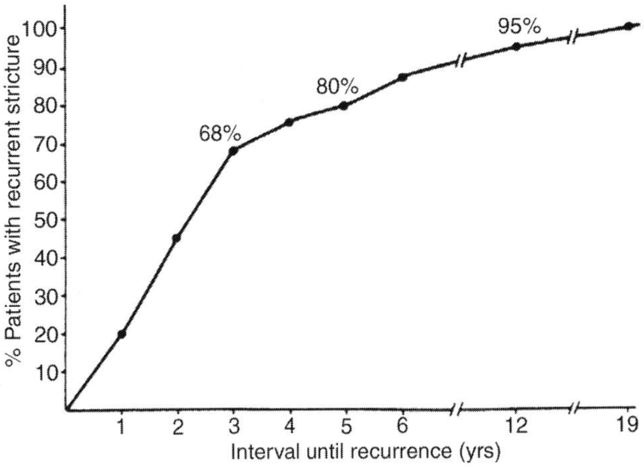

Figure 34–10. The cumulative percentage of recurrent strictures is shown with respect to the time interval from the initial repair to the next repair. (Adapted, with permission, from Pitt HA, Miyamoto T, Parapatis SK et al. Factors influencing outcome in patients with postoperative biliary strictures. *Am J Surg* 1982;144:14–21.)

Patients may also present in the early postoperative period with elevated liver function tests and jaundice if the divided bile duct is clipped completely at the time of injury. Patients typically do not present with cholangitis in the early postoperative period.

Bile duct strictures may also present months to years after the original operation. Most commonly, patients at this time present with symptoms of cholangitis, including abdominal pain, fever, and chills. These cholangitic episodes are typically mild and respond effectively to antibiotics. Less often, patients can present with painless jaundice, which can be confused with a malignant stricture.

Diagnosis

Patients with postoperative bile duct strictures typically reveal a stereotypical biochemical profile of cholestasis. In particular, liver function tests typically consist of an elevated alkaline phosphatase and normal or slightly elevated liver transaminases (alanine and aspartate aminotransferases). Serum bilirubin levels are usually elevated in the range of 2–6 mg/dL. Patients presenting with a biliary leak from injury usually present without evidence of biliary obstruction, and bilirubin levels are normal or slightly elevated due to absorption of bile from the peritoneal cavity. Patients with postoperative bile leak or cholangitis will also exhibit signs and symptoms of inflammation, including an elevated white blood cell count, pyrexia, or occasionally frank sepsis. In rare cases, patients with long-term obstruction will present late in the course of disease with cirrhosis, diminished serum albumin, and abnormal coagulation studies from altered hepatic synthetic function.

Definitive diagnosis for bile duct strictures and injuries requires radiographic imaging. Abdominal computed tomography and ultrasound are both helpful in patients who present in the early postoperative period for the detection of bilomas and biliary ascites (Fig 34–11), as well as bile duct dilatation from obstruction. Nuclear medicine imaging with technetium-HIDA scanning can demonstrate bile leakage noninvasively but typically does not have the sensitivity to define the specific anatomical site of injury. Magnetic resonance cholangiopancreatography (MRCP) has been demonstrated to be an effective noninvasive method for demonstrating biliary leakage or obstruction, as well as precisely defining biliary anatomy and the nature of the injury (Fig 34–12). Lastly, sinography, typically performed by injecting water-soluble contrast via operatively placed drains, can define the biliary anatomy and the source of bile leakage.

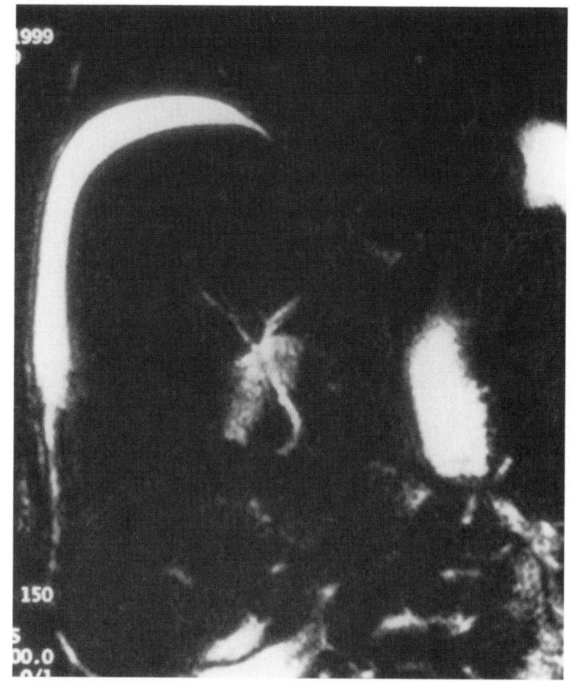

Figure 34–12. Diagnostic MRCP demonstrating biliary anatomy associated with a cystic duct leak after laparoscopic cholecystectomy. There is an intact biliary system with extravasation of contrast in the subhepatic space.

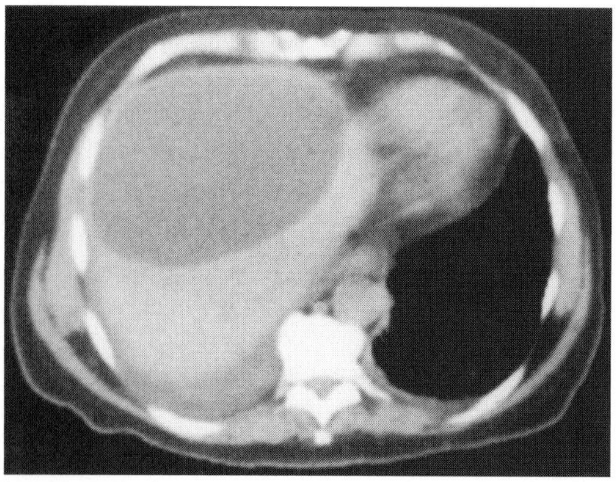

Figure 34–11. CT scan demonstrating biloma associated with biliary leak after bile duct injury. (Reprinted, with permission, from Lillemoe KD, Pitt HA, Cameron JL. Postoperative bile duct strictures. *Surg Clin North Am* 1990;70:1362.)

Cholangiography currently remains the gold standard for evaluating the biliary tree. Endoscopic retrograde cholangiography (ERC) is performed via a distal approach to the biliary tree and is useful in patients with partial injuries to the extrahepatic biliary tree or with cystic duct leaks (Fig 34–13A). In these cases, the biliary leak may be effectively controlled with the use of an endoprosthesis. Most cases of major bile duct injury, however, are associated with complete duct transection, and the cholangiogram via the retrograde endoscopic route will demonstrate a normal distal bile duct terminating in misapplied ligaclips (Fig 34–13B). Therefore, ERC will not define the site of bile leakage nor the proximal anatomy necessary for reconstruction. In such cases, percutaneous transhepatic cholangiography (PTC) is necessary to define the proximal biliary anatomy and the site of injury (Fig 34–14). In addition to delineating the anatomy, a percutaneous biliary drainage catheter may be placed

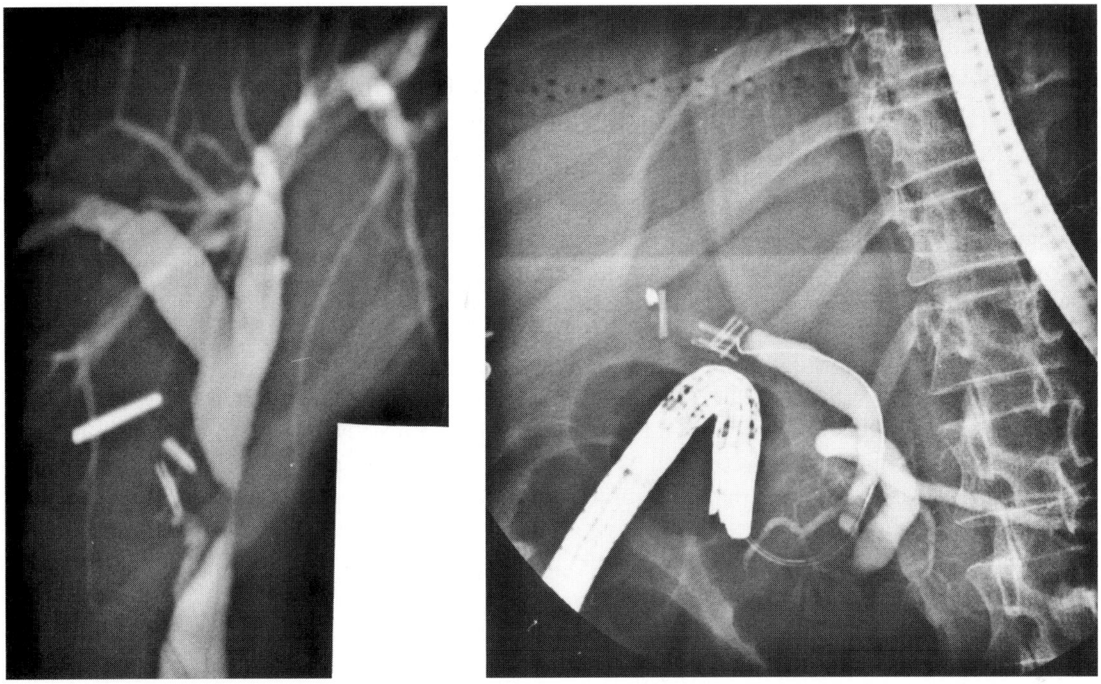

A B

Figure 34–13. A. Endoscopic retrograde cholangiopancreatogram demonstrating cystic duct leak. **B.** Endoscopic retrograde cholangiopancreatogram with multiple clips across the common bile duct without visualization of the proximal biliary tree in a patient with total transection of the common bile duct during laparoscopic cholecystectomy.

at the time of PTC to decompress the biliary tree, and treat cholangitis and control the biliary leak. Percutaneous biliary drainage catheters will also be useful at the time of operative repair as a guide for dissection and identification of the transected bile duct, which is often retracted high into the liver hilum. Finally, in those cases in which biliary-enteric continuity exists, percutaneous catheters allow access for balloon dilatation.

Preoperative Management

The timing of presentation is often a primary determinant of the preoperative management of a patient with a postoperative bile duct stricture or injury. In the early postoperative period, patients with a bile duct injury are often either septic due to intra-abdominal infections or otherwise manifesting a systematic inflammatory response from chemical peritonitis associated with the bile leak. Treatment and control of sepsis may require broad-spectrum parenteral antibiotics, percutaneous biliary drainage, and percutaneous or operative drainage of bilomas. Once sepsis is controlled, there is no hurry in proceeding with surgical reconstruction of the bile duct injury. Most biliary fistulae can be controlled with the combination of proximal biliary decompression and external drainage. After early control and clinical improvement the patient may be discharged home for several weeks to permit return of overall health and for the resolution of inflammation in the periportal region.

It should be stressed that despite the belief of many surgeons that a suspected bile leak warrants urgent reoperation, exploration with an attempt at repair should

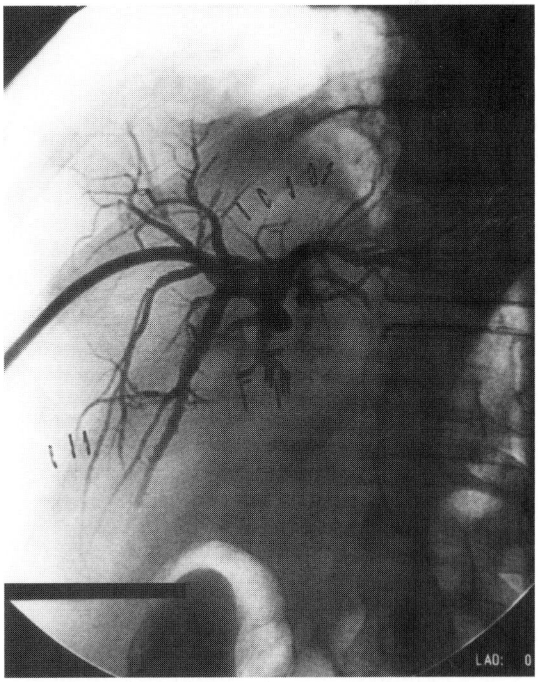

Figure 34–14. Percutaneous transhepatic cholangiogram in a patient with complete transection of the common hepatic bile duct. Note the surgical clips near the cutoff point.

be avoided early after presentation with a bile leak. In this situation exploration often reveals marked inflammation associated with bile spillage and small, decompressed bile ducts retracted high into the porta hepatis, making recognition of the injury and repair virtually impossible. Instead of proceeding to urgent exploration, a more prudent approach is to define biliary anatomy via preoperative cholangiography and to control the bile leak with percutaneous stents. Early operative intervention to deal with bile collections or ascites is not usually required because the intraperitoneal bile either can be drained percutaneously or is simply absorbed by the peritoneal cavity. Delayed reconstruction, with facilitation by percutaneous biliary catheters, allows for the most favorable operative results.

Patients who present with a biliary stricture remote from the initial operation usually experience symptoms of cholangitis that necessitate urgent cholangiography and biliary decompression. Transhepatic biliary drainage is the preferred approach for decompression, although endoscopic drainage with stent placement can sometimes be achieved if bile duct anatomy is intact. Both parenteral antibiotics and biliary drainage are central to controlling sepsis. Patients who present with jaundice without cholangitis should undergo either ERC or PTC to define the anatomy. As with patients presenting early in the postoperative period, ERC may not completely define the proximal biliary anatomy, making PTC the more favorable procedure. Preoperative biliary decompression in patients presenting with jaundice without cholangitis has not been demonstrated to improve outcome.

Operative Management

Operative repair for postoperative bile duct strictures is aimed at re-establishing a reliable, long-term conduit for bile flow from the biliary tree to the gastrointestinal tract. Complications of an unsuccessful operative procedure include sludge or stone formation, recurrent stricture, bile leak resulting in fluid collection or abscess, cholangitis, and biliary cirrhosis. To this end, the ideal technical procedure results in a tension-free, mucosa-to-mucosa repair to a segment of uninjured bile duct. Ideally, surgeons should also seek to maintain ductal length by not sacrificing tissue. Options for operative repair may include end-to-end repair, Roux-en-Y hepaticojejunostomy, choledochojejunostomy, choledochoduodenostomy, and mucosal grafting. The optimal operative procedure is contingent upon the timing of presentation, overall clinical status of the patient, level of injury, and type of injury.

Immediate Surgical Repair of Intraoperative Bile Duct Injury.

Immediate repair should generally be attempted if a bile duct injury is discovered at the time of initial operation. When the surgeon suspects an injury or variant anatomy, biliary anatomy must be clearly defined using intraoperative cholangiography and/or careful dissection, being cautious to avoid additional injury or devascularizing the bile duct. Conversion from laparoscopic to open cholecystectomy is often necessary to properly identify anatomy and the injury. Segmental or accessory duct injuries where the diameter of the bile duct is less than 3 mm and where the bile duct does not communicate with the major duct system or drain a large segment of hepatic parenchyma on cholangiography may be ligated. Bile ducts that are 4 mm or larger in diameter must be operatively repaired, as they likely drain multiple hepatic segments or an entire liver lobe.

Immediate intraoperative repair is indicated in most cases for a major injury of the common hepatic or common bile duct. Partial common duct transections, involving less than 180-degree circumference of the biliary tree, may be closed primarily over a T-tube using interrupted absorbable sutures (Fig 34–15). Transection of the common duct involving more than 180-degree circumference or complete transactions with an injury less than 1 cm in length can usually be repaired with an end-to-end anastomosis with a T-

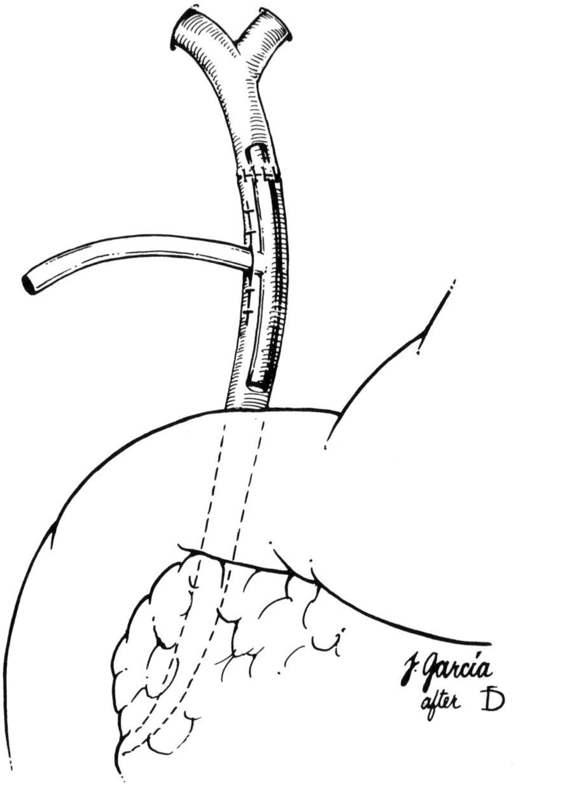

Figure 34–15. Primary end-to-end repair of the biliary tree over a T-tube. In general, this technique is used for partial transections of the bile duct, when there has been no associated loss of duct length. Note that the T-tube does not exit at the site of injury.

tube that exits either above or below the anastomosis via a separate choledochotomy. Primary reconstruction of the bile duct, however, should be used very selectively and should be avoided when the injury is near the bifurcation or when duct approximation cannot be accomplished without tension. In at least one series, a 100% re-stricture rate following primary end-to-end repair has been reported.[48] Transections of the bile duct high in the biliary tree or with significant loss of bile duct length cannot be repaired with a primary biliary anastomosis that remains tension-free. These injuries require reconstruction using a biliary-enteric anastomosis typically using Roux-en-Y hepaticojejunostomy to ensure a tension-free repair. This procedure involves oversewing the distal bile duct, débridement of injured tissue in the proximal tree, and then biliary-enteric end-to-side anastomosis to the Roux-en-Y jejunal limb. Transhepatic Silastic biliary stents should be placed to control potential anastomotic leaks and for postoperative cholangiography. A perianastomotic drain should also be placed in all cases.

Surgeons not experienced in complex biliary reconstruction should strongly consider not proceeding with immediate repair. Intraoperative, immediate biliary repair is often difficult with non-dilated bile ducts that may retract towards the liver or with injury involving multiple hepatic ducts. A failed attempt at repair may decrease the eventual chance of a successful outcome. If the surgeon does not feel that he or she can effectively repair the injury, intraoperative cholangiography should be performed to confirm the nature of the injury. A small, flexible catheter (such as a red rubber catheter) should be placed into the proximal hepatic duct, allowing for postoperative cholangiography and facilitating percutaneous access and drain placement. A closed suction drain should also be placed in the subhepatic space to control the bile leakage. The patient should then be referred to a tertiary care referral center experienced in hepatobiliary surgery for definitive repair. Similarly, in patients with an injury recognized in the postoperative period, surgeons with limited experience in complex biliary surgery should consider early transfer to a tertiary center with access to both surgeons and interventional radiologists experienced with these problems.

Elective Surgical Repair. Elective repair should generally occur only after preoperative clinical optimization of the patient. Cholangitic patients should be treated with broad-spectrum antibiotics followed by biliary drainage, typically with percutaneously placed drains. Those presenting with biliary leak should have the bile leak and sepsis controlled prior to having definitive repair. Biliary spillage and marked inflammation can make urgent laparotomy prior to biliary decompression problematic. Finally, the patient should be clinically stabilized prior to elective repair to correct fluid and electrolyte balances, anemia, and malnutrition.

The type of repair should be determined by several factors: previous history of attempted repair, location of stricture or injury, surgeon experience, and surgeon preference. Intraoperatively, biliary anatomy must be carefully defined followed by exposure of healthy proximal bile ducts. Care must be taken to avoid excessive dissection and devascularization of tissue. A biliary-enteric anastomosis is performed using a mucosa-to-mucosa technique in a tension-free manner.

The preferred technique, with few exceptions, is a hepatico- or choledochojejunostomy to a Roux-en-Y limb of jejunum. End-to-end anastomosis after excision of the stricture or area of injury is not prudent due to the loss of bile duct length and associated fibrosis. Significant loss of bile duct length is also a strict contraindication to performing choledochoduodenostomy, which is unlikely to be performed in a tension-free fashion and is also associated with duodenal fistula if leak occurs.

The use of percutaneous biliary stents with elective reconstruction of the biliary tree remains a topic of debate for hepatobiliary surgeons. Preoperatively placed stents act as intraoperative aids for defining anatomy, especially if the stricture is located proximally. Percutaneous biliary stents can also allow postoperative cholangiography and control early anastomotic leaks in the immediate postoperative period. Many surgeons also advocate extended postoperative transanastomotic stenting, with the purpose of minimizing fibrosis and risk of late anastomotic stricture. In this setting, follow-up cholangiography will reveal early evidence of anastomotic stricture and provide access for balloon dilatation if necessary.

Biliary reconstruction with the technique of hepaticojejunostomy with a Roux-en-Y limb and percutaneous transhepatic biliary stents is depicted in Figure 34–16. Dissection of the porta hepatis is performed to clear any adhesions between the duodenum or colonic hepatic flexure to the gallbladder fossa, subhepatic space, or Glisson's capsule. Preoperatively placed percutaneous stents are essential in assisting in dissection and bile duct identification in patients with a high bile duct transection. In patients with an intact but strictured bile duct, the duct is divided at the most distal portion of the stricture, and a segment of the strictured duct should be resected and sent to pathology for frozen section. The distal end of the stricture is then oversewn. The proximal extent of the duct should be débrided for a length not to exceed 5 mm to obtain healthy bile duct circumferentially for use in the anastomosis. Careful limited dissection is important to avoid vascular compromise to the bile duct. Preoperatively placed percutaneous transhepatic catheters, which now protrude from the proximal end, are usually ex-

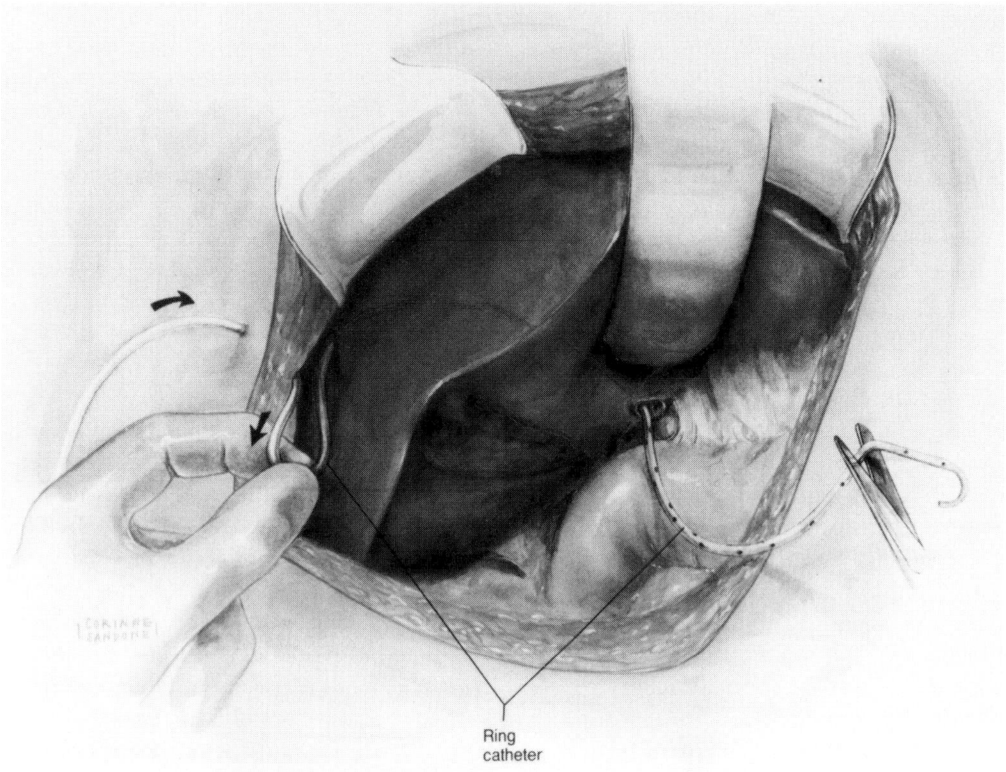

A

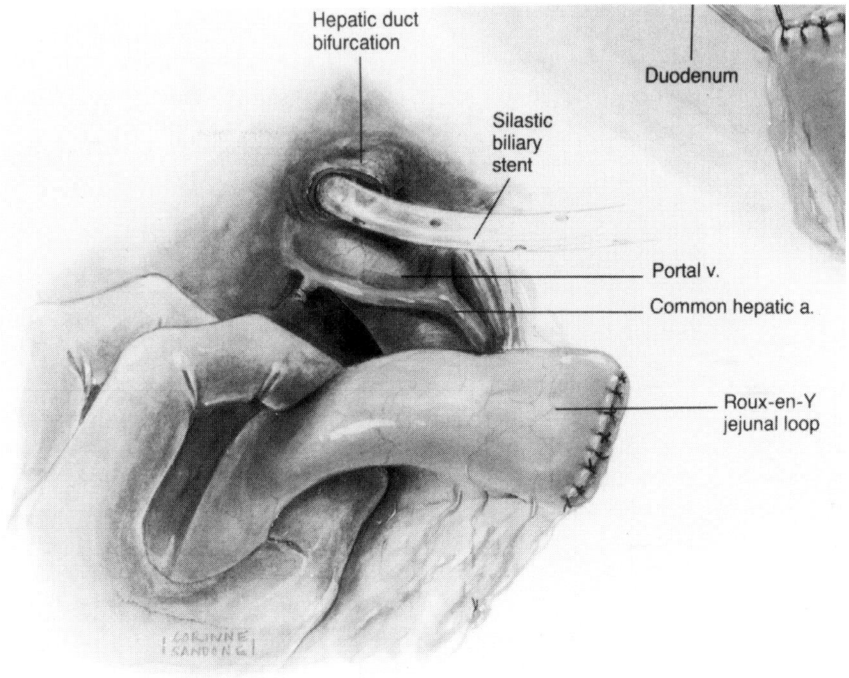

B

Figure 34–16. Roux-en-Y hepaticojejunostomy reconstruction of biliary tree. **A.** Repair of common hepatic duct stricture with transhepatic ring catheter exiting at the bifurcation. The stricture has been resected, and the distal biliary tree is oversewn. The hepaticojejunal anastomosis can then be performed over the ring catheter, or the ring catheter can be exchanged for a Silastic transhepatic stent. **B.** The Silastic transhepatic stent shown exiting the biliary tree, with the Roux-en-Y jejunal limb prepared for the hepaticojejunostomy. *Continued*

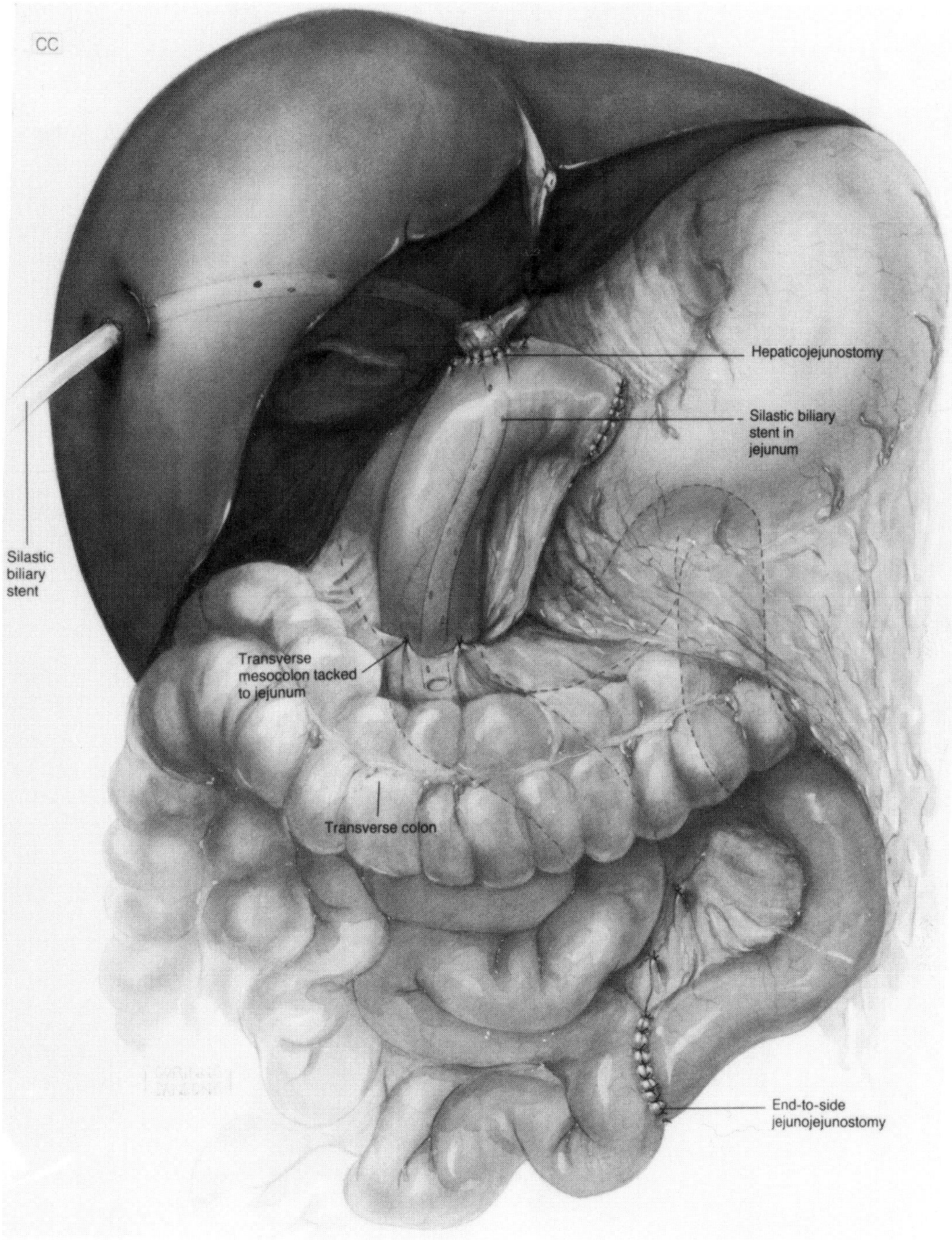

C

Figure 34–16, cont'd. C. Completed repair showing the Silastic biliary stent traversing the liver and the hepaticojejunostomy. The Roux-en-Y jejunal limb has been brought to the hepatic hilum in retrocolic position. (Reproduced, with permission, from Cameron JL (ed). *Atlas of Surgery*, Vol. I. Hamilton, Ontario, Canada: BC Decker; 1990:43, 53, 57.)

changed for soft Silastic stents. Silastic stents range from 12F–22F in size, with multiple side holes that are generally interspersed along 40% of the length of the catheter. A radiologic guidewire is placed through the percutaneous transhepatic catheter; using the Seldinger technique, a series of progressively larger coudé catheters are passed over the guidewire in order to dilate the system for Silastic stent placement. The Silastic stent is arranged with the side holes extending beyond the anastomosis distally and within the liver parenchyma proximally. The end of the Silastic stent without holes is brought through the hepatic parenchyma and out through the upper anterior abdominal wall. A Roux-en-Y jejunal limb is then created by mobilizing a suitable segment of intestine of approximately 60 cm in length. The anastomosis is then constructed with a standard end-to-side Roux-en-Y hepatico- or choledochojejunostomy, typically using a single layer of 4-0 or 5-0 absorbable sutures.

In the postoperative period, Silastic stents are left to external gravity drainage. Drip cholangiography is then performed on postoperative day four or five (Fig 34–17). If the biliary tree is adequately decompressed and no leakage is seen, the stents can be internalized, and the perianastomotic drain is removed.

The length of postoperative transanastomotic stenting is dependent on the individual patient, the clinical setting, and surgeon preference. Long-term stenting involves fluoroscopic exchange of stents at regular 2- to 3-month intervals. Timing of stent removal can be aided by biliary manometric flow studies that give objective data about the adequacy of the anastomosis, or by passing a clinical trial with the stent placed above the anastomosis.[49]

Nonoperative Therapy

Nonoperative interventional radiology and endoscopic techniques have also been developed for the management of select patients with bile duct strictures and injuries. The most common nonoperative technique in these patients is interventional radiology percutaneous stenting and balloon dilatation, which may be possible in patients with intact biliary-enteric continuity. With the administration of conscious sedation, the proximal biliary tree is accessed so that the stricture can be traversed using a guidewire under fluoroscopic guidance (Fig 34–18). Angioplasty-type balloon catheters are used to perform dilatation of the stricture to a goal diameter based upon the stricture location and the normal bile duct diameter. Following dilatation, a transhepatic biliary stent is left in place across the stricture. The stent allows for future cholangiography, repeat dilatation, and maintenance of the lumen while the bile duct heals. Complications of balloon dilatation include cholangitis, hemobilia, and bile leaks. Percutaneous management will usually require numerous dilatations.

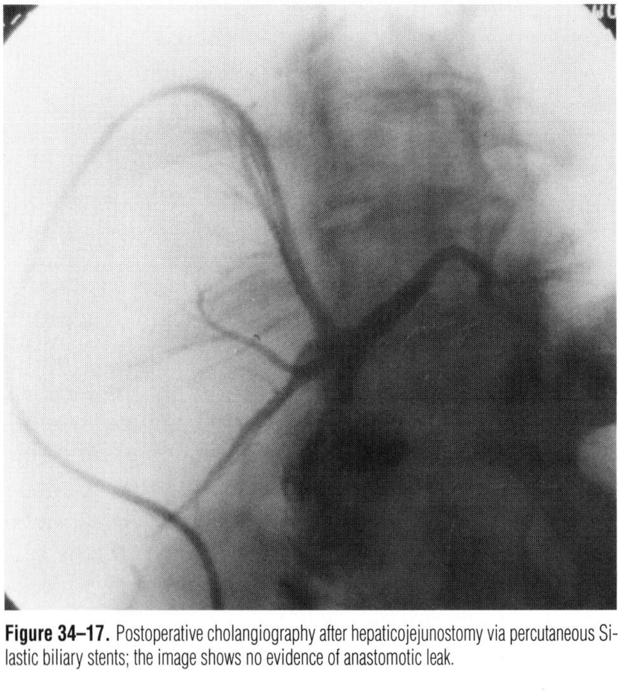

Figure 34–17. Postoperative cholangiography after hepaticojejunostomy via percutaneous Silastic biliary stents; the image shows no evidence of anastomotic leak.

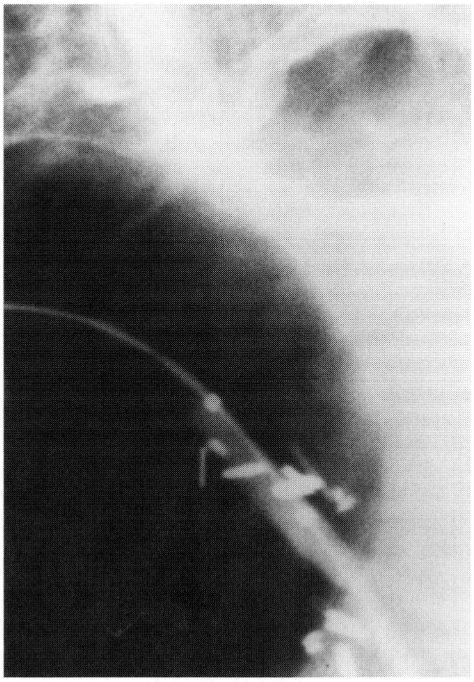

Figure 34–18. Percutaneous balloon dilatation of postoperative bile duct stricture using an angioplasty-type balloon catheter. Cholangiogram showing mid–bile duct stricture.

Results for the treatment of bile duct strictures using percutaneous balloon dilatation are limited. In a retrospective comparison, percutaneous balloon dilatation was compared to surgical repair in 43 patients with postoperative bile duct strictures treated at The Johns Hopkins Hospital between 1979 and 1987.[50] Twenty-five patients underwent surgical repair with postoperative stenting and 20 patients had percutaneous balloon dilatation with transhepatic stenting (mean: 4 dilatations). Three patients underwent both surgical management and balloon dilatation. Successful outcome was achieved in 89% and 52% of surgical and balloon dilatation patients, respectively. These results would appear comparable to other series in the pre-laparoscopic cholecystectomy era.[51–54]

Recently, a series of 51 patients undergoing percutaneous balloon dilatation therapy for bile duct strictures following laparoscopic cholecystectomy was reported by Misra and associates.[55] At a median 76-month follow-up, overall success with balloon dilatation, defined as stent-free without the need for further intervention, was 58%. With additional stenting and balloon dilatation for two patients and surgical reconstruction for the remaining patients, all but one patient (98%) had a successful long-term outcome. These results suggest that in highly selected patients, percutaneous balloon dilatation can provide long-term successful results.

Endoscopic balloon dilatation has a more limited application, since it is technically possible only in patients with primary bile duct stricture repair or with choledochoduodenal anastomosis. Endoscopic retrograde cholangiography is performed, followed by endoscopic sphincterotomy. Sequential balloon dilatation is performed after the stricture is traversed by a guidewire, often with an endoprosthesis left in place after dilatation. Complications associated with stent placement include cholangitis, pancreatitis, stent occlusion, migration, dislodgment, and ductal perforation, and have a reported incidence between 9% and 70%.[56–58]

Repeat cholangiography, often with repeat dilatations, may be performed at regular intervals of every 3–6 months. While most surgeons advocate regular follow-up and re-evaluation of the stricture, the risks of stent occlusion and replacement need to be weighed against the risks and costs of the repeat procedures, and there is still some debate about timing of stent change to avoid occlusion. Bergman and associates demonstrated a 70% re-obstruction rate with resultant jaundice or cholangitis when stents were not exchanged at 3-month intervals.[58] In contrast, De Masi and colleagues describe and advocate leaving the stents in place until patients were symptomatic.[59]

In addition, the rate of stent occlusion appears to vary with the type of stent used. While metallic stents provide a longer period of patency than plastic stents for patients with malignant obstruction, the indications for their use in patients with benign strictures are limited. Metallic stents cannot be routinely exchanged or removed, and several studies have demonstrated high re-occlusion rates at long-term follow-up.[60–62] In particular, one study demonstrated a 100% (6 out of 6) re-stricture rate at 50 months in patients with metallic stents compared to a 19% (7 out of 39) re-stricture rate at 44 months follow-up with plastic stents.[63] It would appear that metallic stents have no role in the management of benign bile duct stricture unless the patient is felt to have a very limited life expectancy from other causes.

While there have been no determinative studies for the length of time that stents should remain in place, most studies having excellent results have used larger bore stents (10F or greater) left in place 6–12 months.[57,58,64] Long-term studies reporting the endoscopic treatment of benign bile duct strictures are few. One of the few studies that directly compare endoscopic therapy to surgical reconstruction was done by Davids and colleagues from the Netherlands.[56] In 66 patients, endoscopic therapy consisted of dilatation and placement of an endoprosthesis, which was exchanged every 3 months. Surgical repair in 35 patients consisted of Roux-en-Y hepaticojejunostomy. Surgery was associated with excellent or good results in 29 patients (82%), with 6 patients (17%) developing a recurrent stricture at mean 40 months from initial surgery. In contrast, endoscopic stenting resulted in 81% with excellent or good outcome and 18% developing re-stricture at a mean of 3 months after stent removal. Recurrent strictures after stent removal in several other series have been reported to occur at a rate varying from 0–20% at median follow-up of 29–108 months.[57,58,64]

Results of Operative Repair

Biliary injury and stricture repair is associated with significant morbidity and mortality. With improved medical technology and experience, the incidence of operative mortality has decreased markedly. A recent series of 200 consecutive patients repaired at the Johns Hopkins Hospital reported a perioperative mortality of only 1.7%.[47] Advanced age, comorbid disease, and a history of major biliary tract infection are factors associated with operative mortality. Underlying liver disease is the most important correlated factor for operative mortality and morbidity, with advanced biliary cirrhosis and portal hypertension having mortality rates approaching 30%. Fortunately, in the modern era such advanced disease is uncommon.

A recent analysis of Medicare claims patient data examining mortality associated with major bile duct injuries over an 8-year period in 791 elderly patients demonstrated a mortality of 2.7% associated with repair.[65] In addition, survival decreased with increasing age, with decreasing surgical experience, and if the repairing surgeon was the same as the injuring surgeon. This study gives supportive evidence for improved survival in patients with major bile duct injuries treated by experienced hepatobiliary surgeons at tertiary referral centers.

In most series, postoperative morbidity rates are in the range of 20–40%. Morbidity nonspecific to biliary surgery includes hemorrhage, infection, and risks associated with general anesthesia. Complications specific to biliary repairs include anastomotic leak, cholangitis, and hepatic insufficiency associated with pre-existing liver disease. Anastomotic leaks can typically be managed via nonoperative means, especially when transanastomotic stenting has been utilized. Percutaneous transhepatic stenting may also have specific morbidity, including bile leaks from hepatotomy sites, hemobilia, and cholangitis from stent occlusion. Although one report found no difference,[66] several recent reports have found a significantly higher rate of postoperative complications associated with patients having combined bile duct and vascular injuries.[67,68]

The recent series reporting the outcomes in 200 patients undergoing surgical reconstruction at the Johns Hopkins Hospital demonstrated a 41% overall postoperative complication rate.[47] The most common complications were wound infection (8%), cholangitis (6%), minor stent-related complications (6%), and intra-abdominal abscess/biloma (3%). Postoperative cholangiography revealed an anastomotic leak in 5% of patients and extravasation at the liver dome–stent exit site in 10%. While interventional radiology drain placement, new biliary stent placement, or biliary stent exchanges were required in 7%, no patients required reoperation in the postoperative period. Despite the relatively high morbidity rate, median length of stay was similar to that in other reports (8 ± 4.6 days).

The ultimate goal of the repair of a bile duct stricture is a successful repair with no further symptoms, including jaundice, cholangitis, and preserved liver function. Excellent long-term results following operative repair of postoperative bile duct injuries have been reported with approximately 80–90% having a successful outcome (Table 34–4).[50,56,69–75] Early reports and observations from the laparoscopic era were less favorable than those previously reported with open cholecystectomy repairs. A seminal article published by Stewart and Way[48] reviewed 85 patients who had undergone 112 biliary repairs and defined four factors that influenced success or failure of operative repairs after laparoscopic cholecystectomy bile duct injury: (1) performance of preoperative cholangiography, (2) choice of surgical repair, (3) details of surgical repair, and (4) experience of the repairing surgeon. Procedures without preoperative cholangiography were unsuccessful 96% of the time, and those with incomplete cholangiography data had a success rate of only 31%. With complete cholangiography data, the success rate was 84%. All patients with complete transection of the bile duct who underwent primary end-to-end repair over a T-tube had a failed result. In contrast, 63% of Roux-en-Y hepaticojejunostomy repairs were successful. Initial repair by the original laparoscopic surgeon was successful in only 17% of cases. Repeat attempts at repair by the same surgeon were never successful. Finally, those patients whose first repair was by a tertiary care biliary surgeon achieved a 94% success rate.

The largest reported series providing long-term results after repair of bile duct injuries and strictures in the 1990s was reported by Lillemoe and associates.[75] A total of 156 consecutive patients underwent surgical reconstruction with a mean follow-up period of 57.5 months (range 11–119 months; median 54.7 months). The original operation consisted of laparoscopic cholecystectomy in 118 patients (76%), open cholecystectomy in 27 patients (17%), open cholecystectomy with bile duct exploration in 4 patients (3%), or other abdominal surgery or trauma in 7 patients (4%). Sixty patients (41%) had a previous attempt at repair prior to referral. Eight patients (5.5%) had more than one attempt at repair prior to referral. Of the 156 operatively repaired patients, 142 patients had completed treatment at the time of final evaluation with an overall success rate of 91%. Even though they were more likely to have had repair prior to referral and higher and more complex injuries, patients with repair of a stricture or injury associated with laparoscopic cholecystectomy had a better success rate than repair after other operations (94% versus 80%; $p<0.05$). There were 13 failures following surgical reconstruction. Ten had successful results following either surgical revision (1 patient) or percutaneous balloon dilatation (9 patients), resulting in an overall success rate of 98% including secondary intervention. Only three patients continued to require long-term biliary stents to prevent biliary obstruction symptoms and/or cholangitis. Outcomes after surgical repair for laparoscopic cholecystectomy injury from other series are outlined in Table 34–5.[75–79]

TABLE 34–4. RESULTS OF SURGICAL REPAIR OF POSTOPERATIVE BILE DUCT STRICTURES

Reference	Year	Number of Patients	Success Rate	Follow-Up (Months)
Lillemoe et al[75]	2000	156	91%	58
Tocchi et al[69]	1996	84	83%	108
McDonald et al[70]	1995	72	87%	<60
Chapman et al[71]	1995	104	76%	86
Davids et al[56]	1993	35	83%	50
Pitt et al[50]	1989	25	88%	57
Innes et al[72]	1988	22	95%	72
Genest et al[73]	1986	105	82%	60
Pellegrini et al[74]	1984	60	78%	102

Despite the overall high level of success in the surgical management of laparoscopic cholecystectomy bile duct injuries, there is an impression that patients may have an impaired quality of life even after a successful repair of their bile duct injury. Quality of life after laparoscopic cholecystectomy bile duct injury has been addressed in several recent reports, with differing results.[80–83] Two studies using the Short Form Health Survey quality of life instrument (SF-36) in patients with laparoscopic cholecystectomy injury found both the physical and mental quality of life aspects to be reduced compared to controls at approximately 5-year follow-up.[80,83] Decreased quality of life in one of these studies was not dependent on the type of treatment or the severity of injury.[80] A similar study with SF-36 found that patients with laparoscopic bile duct injury and subsequent biliary reconstruction had quality of life similar

TABLE 34–5. SURGICAL REPAIR OF LAPAROSCOPIC CHOLECYSTECTOMY BILE DUCT INJURIES

Reference	Number of Patients	Bismuth Level 3–5	Success Rate
Lillemoe et al[75]	118	63%	94%
Walsh et al[76]	34	80%	91%
Bauer et al[77]	32	24%	83%
Mirza et al[78]	52	53%	92%
Nealon et al[79]	23	26%	100%

to matched controls and national norms in all eight quality- of-life areas.[82] Melton and associates[81] assessed quality of life in 54 patients having undergone successful surgical repair of laparoscopic cholecystectomy bile duct injuries and compared these results to quality of life measures in patients after uncomplicated laparoscopic cholecystectomy and in healthy controls using a standard quality of life instrument, which was used to assess the physical, psychological, and social domains of health-related quality of life. Patients after surgical repair had overall quality-of-life scores comparable to those of controls. Only in the psychological dimension were patients post–bile duct injury repair found to have significantly worse scores compared to controls. Patients that reported pursuing a lawsuit following their injury (31%) had significantly worse quality-of-life scores in all domains when compared to those who did not entertain legal action ($p < 0.01$).

Summary

Postoperative bile duct strictures and major injuries remain a considerable surgical challenge. With proper diagnostic work-up, clinical optimization, and definitive treatment, the vast majority of patients can achieve satisfactory outcomes. With success rates of over 90% at long-term follow-up, the gold standard for managing patients with major bile duct injuries and strictures in the current era remains surgical reconstruction. In select patients with biliary-enteric continuity, percutaneous or endoscopic management with balloon dilatation may be an appropriate alternative, with success rates of approximately 50% at long-term follow-up.

■ INFLAMMATORY CAUSES OF BILIARY STRICTURE

Biliary strictures may occur in association with a wide range of processes causing fibrosis of the bile ducts. While inflammatory causes of bile duct strictures account only for a minority of biliary strictures in the United States, biliary strictures from these causes are important diagnostic and therapeutic challenges. Strictures from chronic pancreatitis, biliary calculous disease, sphincter of Oddi stenosis, and peptic ulcer disease can usually be managed with choledochoduodenostomy or Roux-en-Y hepaticojejunostomy without long-term stenting. The management of other infrequent causes of benign biliary strictures depends on the etiology, natural history, and severity of disease.

PANCREATITIS

Chronic pancreatitis is an infrequent cause of bile duct stenosis and stricture, accounting for less than 10% of benign biliary strictures. While acute pancreatitis is frequently associated with transient partial obstruction of the distal common bile duct from inflammation and edema, chronic pancreatitis can result in distal bile duct obstruction from inflammation and parenchymal fibrosis of the pancreatic gland. Strictures from chronic pancreatitis typically involve the entire intrapancreatic segment of the common bile duct, resulting in proximal dilatation of the biliary tree (Fig 34–19).

Chronic pancreatitis resulting in bile duct stricture is most commonly caused by alcoholism. Strictures more commonly present in patients that have advanced disease with pancreatic calcification, diabetes, or malabsorption at the time of presentation. The exact inci-

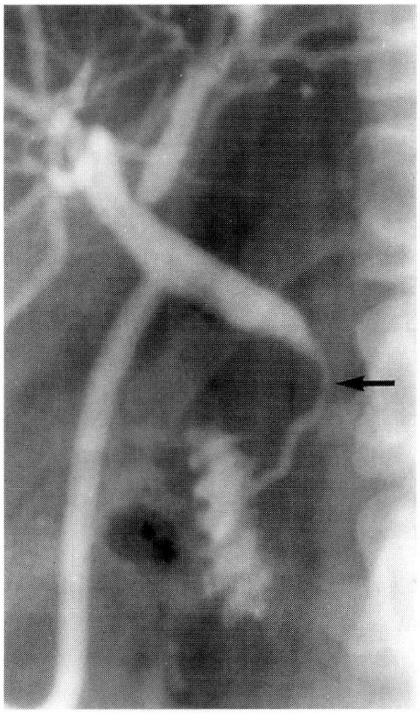

Figure 34–19. Stricture from chronic pancreatitis involving the entire intrapancreatic segment of the common bile duct, resulting in proximal dilatation of the biliary tree. (Reprinted, with permission, from Lillemoe KD. Biliary injuries and strictures and sclerosing cholangitis. In: Mulholland MW, Lillemoe KD, Doherty GM, Maier RV, Upchurch GR Jr (eds). *Greenfield's Surgery: Scientific Principles and Practice*, 4th edition. Philadelphia, PA: Lippincott Williams & Wilkins; 2006:1013.)

dence of common bile duct strictures is not known because cholangiography is not routinely performed in patients with chronic pancreatitis. With a review of several clinical series, common bile duct strictures associated with chronic pancreatitis occur in approximately 5% of patients with estimated ranges varying from 3–29% of patients.[84,85]

Common bile duct strictures due to chronic pancreatitis may have a wide range of clinical presentations. On one end of the spectrum, patients can be asymptomatic with only abnormal liver function tests. Serum alkaline phosphatase, the most sensitive liver function test, is elevated in over 80% of cases. Patients can also present with abdominal pain with or without jaundice. Importantly, abdominal pain from biliary strictures can be difficult to distinguish from pain caused by chronic pancreatitis. Patients with pain from biliary stricture that are not properly diagnosed and treated for their stricture may undergo inappropriate and unsuccessful operative procedures to address pain presumed to be from chronic pancreatitis. Finally, patients who develop jaundice in the setting of chronic pancreatitis may present a diagnostic dilemma, as an underlying periampullary malignancy must also be considered.[86]

Evaluation of bile duct strictures from chronic pancreatitis is most effectively accomplished with cholangiography. Both ERC and PTC are effective at delineating anatomy and allow decompression of the biliary tree in the setting of cholangitis or severe jaundice. ERCP has the advantage of demonstrating pancreatic ductal anatomy, including possible abnormalities, which is especially useful in surgical management, and is therefore the preferred diagnostic procedure. The most common cholangiographic image in chronic pancreatitis–associated bile duct strictures is a long (usually 2–4 cm), smooth, gradual tapering of the distal common bile duct (see Fig 34–19).

The most common accepted indications for operative management in common bile duct strictures from chronic pancreatitis are cholangitis, jaundice, or significant pain. It remains unclear, however, if biliary decompression in asymptomatic patients with elevated serum alkaline phosphatase is indicated. Many surgeons do advocate biliary bypass in this situation, as early biliary cirrhosis changes may be observed in liver biopsy specimens in patients with long-standing, significant biliary obstruction from chronic pancreatitis.[87,88]

Biliary bypass with choledochoduodenostomy or Roux-en-Y choledochojejunostomy represents the optimal form of management for bile duct strictures associated with chronic pancreatitis. Potential advantages of choledochoduodenostomy over Roux-en-Y choledochojejunostomy include maintenance of bile flow into the duodenum that may be more physiologic, increased technical ease, and no loss of small bowel length for formation of a Roux-en-Y limb. Operative management with pancreaticoduodenectomy is appropriate in those patients in whom periampullary malignancy cannot be ruled out by imaging studies or clinical course or in those patients with significant pain attributed to proximal pancreatic duct disease. Both long-term and short-term outcomes of surgically managed distal bile duct strictures from pancreatitis are usually excellent.[79,89]

The management of common bile duct strictures from chronic pancreatitis with either transduodenal sphincterotomy or endoscopic sphincterotomy is not recommended due to the stricture's long length. While long-term follow-up is lacking, several series have reported success in 60% of patients with follow-up at approximately 2 years after endoscopic balloon dilatation of distal bile strictures from chronic pancreatitis.[90,91] It would appear that in most cases when a benign process can be expected to require years of follow-up, that surgery would be the best form of management.

GALLSTONE DISEASE

Long-standing cholelithiasis with recurrent bouts of cholecystitis results in a progressively fibrosed, shrunken gallbladder. Eventually, the gallbladder lumen can lie alongside the common hepatic duct, resulting in inflammation and resultant bile duct stricture. Often referred to as Mirizzi's syndrome, this process is typically subdivided into two categories. Type I Mirizzi's syndrome occurs when the process results in either mechanical compression of the duct or an inflammatory stricture of the common hepatic duct. In contrast, type II consists of erosion of the stone in the duct, resulting in cholecystocholedochal fistula.

Mirizzi's syndrome usually presents as jaundice or recurrent cholangitis. In some long-standing cases, these findings exist in the face of chronic gallbladder symptoms. In cases of Mirizzi's syndrome associated with acute cholecystitis, care must be taken at the time of cholecystectomy to avoid bile duct injury during initial dissection. The presence of Mirizzi's syndrome obliterates the triangle of Calot and makes laparoscopic cholecystectomy particularly difficult and will often require conversion to an open procedure. If Mirizzi's syndrome is considered, intraoperative cholangiography should be performed.

If urgent cholecystectomy is not indicated, ERC or PTC can help to delineate the anatomy. Importantly, Mirizzi's syndrome can be difficult to distinguish from strictures that result from gallbladder cancer or cholangiocarcinoma.[92] ERC can also be helpful for obtaining brush biopsies in these patients.

Formal management of strictures from biliary stones varies according to the extent of disease. In cases in whom the bile duct is inflamed and no fistula is present (type I), patients can often be managed with cholecystectomy. The common hepatic duct almost always returns to normal after the offending stone has been removed by cholecystectomy and the inflammatory process has resolved. Care must be taken, however, during the dissection to avoid creating a defect in the common hepatic duct. Rarely, after the acute episode has resolved, a well-established stricture presents months to years after the acute episode. In such cases, management by Roux-en-Y hepaticojejunostomy is appropriate. If cholecystocholedochal fistula (type II) is present, partial cholecystectomy is recommended, and the cuff of remaining gallbladder is used to repair the bile duct over a T-tube.

In addition to Mirizzi's syndrome, calculous disease also rarely results in strictures due to choledocholithiasis. The pathogenesis of strictures from choledocholithiasis is thought to be from epithelial erosion of the distal bile duct from calculous disease, resulting in inflammation with subsequent fibrosis and stricture.

Nearly all stones remain entrapped in the intrapancreatic portion of the common bile duct because of the anatomic tapering of the common bile duct. These trapped stones are often difficult to remove via a supraduodenal approach during common bile duct exploration. In fact, common bile duct exploration to retrieve stones with forceps, scoops, and catheters can often result in additional trauma to the friable distal duct from excessive intraoperative manipulation. After stone removal, the distal bile duct should be gently sized with a soft rubber catheter to check for the presence of a stricture. Strictures often may not be recognized until the postoperative period when T-tube cholangiography is performed. When strictures are found postoperatively, stricture repair should be performed after inflammation has resolved, typically after 4–6 weeks. Stricture repair of the distal bile duct is indicated for persistent strictures using either Roux-en-Y choledochojejunostomy or choledochoduodenostomy biliary-enteric anastomosis. A choledochoduodenal anastomosis is preferable in patients with a large, dilated (>2 cm in diameter) proximal duct because of its technical ease and excellent results.

RECURRENT PYOGENIC CHOLANGITIS AND OTHER PARASITIC DISEASE

Recurrent pyogenic cholangitis, also known as Oriental cholangiohepatitis, is endemic is Southeast Asia. Recurrent pyogenic cholangitis occurs infrequently in Western countries but with immigration from Asia is now increasingly encountered. Most cases are due to parasitic infection (*Ascaris lumbricoides* or *Clonorchis sinensis*) of the biliary tree. The infection results in biliary stasis, bacterial overgrowth and inflammation, biliary sludge, and brown (calcium bilirubinate) stone formation. Patients will typically have multiple intrahepatic and extrahepatic stones and strictures, as well as recurrent cholangitis. Although strictures can occur throughout the biliary tree, they are most common in the main hepatic ducts, with disease in the left hepatic duct typically more frequent and more severe than the right. Classically, patients are young, thin, of Asian descent, of either gender, and present with recurrent bouts of cholangitis. Cholangitis can range in severity from subclinical chronic illness to life-threatening acute suppurative cholangitis.

Diagnostic imaging modalities for Oriental cholangiohepatitis include ultrasonography, CT scan, ERC, and PTC. While ultrasound is poor at showing biliary strictures reliably, ultrasound is effective at demonstrating biliary obstruction, biliary tract stones, pneumobilia from gas-forming organism infection, and liver abscesses. Intrahepatic stones on ultrasound have a characteristic posterior acoustic shadowing. CT scan is useful for delineating hepatic anatomy and parenchymal involvement in more advanced disease, which is helpful for guiding potential liver resection.

ERCP or PTC are the key diagnostic and therapeutic imaging modalities for Oriental cholangiohepatitis. Cholangiography performed via either method is the optimal method for evaluating biliary anatomy for the presence of strictures and stones (Fig 34–20). In addi-

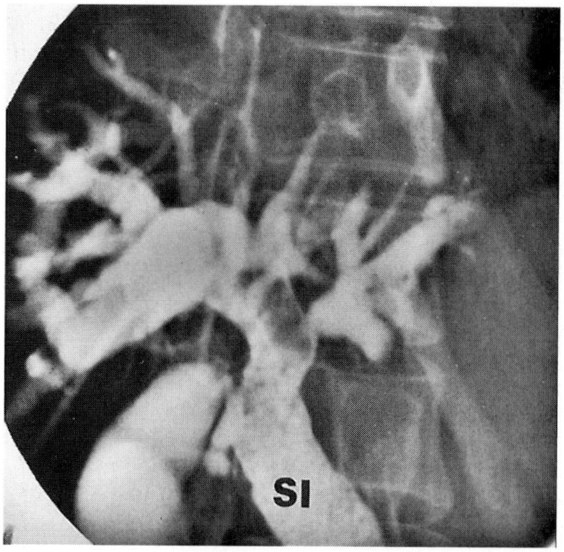

Figure 34–20. Cholangiogram in a patient with cholangiohepatitis with diffuse bile duct dilatation. The biliary tree is filled with sludge (*SI*) and stones. (Reprinted, with permission, from Lillemoe KD. Biliary injuries and strictures and sclerosing cholangitis. In: Mulholland MW, Lillemoe KD, Doherty GM, Maier RV, Upchurch GR Jr (eds). *Greenfield's Surgery: Scientific Principles and Practice*, 4th ed. Philadelphia, PA: Lippincott Williams & Wilkins; 2006:1014.)

tion, ERCP and PTC provide therapeutic biliary decompression in the setting of acute cholangitis.

Long-term management of recurrent pyogenic cholangitis is aimed at treating biliary strictures using improved biliary drainage via biliary reconstruction. Following temporary decompression of the biliary tree with ERCP or PTC for acute cholangitis, patients are allowed a period of several weeks for clinical optimization prior to further management. Attempts at percutaneous or endoscopic manipulations of the biliary tree for stone extraction and biliary stricture dilatation may be entertained. These interventions, however, have only temporary short-term benefit, and operative management will eventually need to be considered.

Standard operative management consists of Roux-en-Y hepaticojejunostomy, usually with a transhepatic stent. An attempt at complete clearance of stones from the intrahepatic ducts should be made, including the use of choledochoscopy. The stent is useful for follow-up cholangiography and further stone clearance after the initial procedure. One option for follow-up management is for the blind-end of the Roux-en-Y limb to be sutured to the peritoneal surface of the abdominal wall, along with a radiopaque marker. This creates an enteric portal for future access to the biliary tree and anastomosis. In cases in whom disease is confined to one portion of the liver with extensive fibrosis or hepatic abscess, hepatic resection may be considered.

Other causes of biliary strictures from parasites include various forms of echinococcal disease. Biliary strictures from echinococcal infection are primarily related to the compression of bile ducts by a thick-walled cyst. Because of its low rate of morbidity, long-term endoscopic stent therapy has become the initial therapy of choice in patients with biliary stricture from hydatid disease.[93,94] Operative therapy should be considered only in cases of failed previous repairs or failed endoscopic therapy. Surgical treatment of echinococcal liver and biliary disease is associated with a high rate of postoperative bile duct stricture, necessitating long-term clinical surveillance.

SPHINCTER OF ODDI STENOSIS

Also referred to as papillitis, stenosis of the sphincter of Oddi is a benign intrinsic obstruction of the common bile duct outlet. Papillitis is typically associated with inflammation, fibrosis, or muscular hypertrophy of the sphincter of Oddi. Patients with sphincter of Oddi stenosis are prone to (1) common bile duct obstruction from fibrosis and stenosis of the papilla, (2) recurrent pancreatitis, and (3) recurrent right upper quadrant abdominal pain in the absence of jaundice or pancreatitis. Initial presentation is most often jaundice or cholangitis. Patients can also sometimes present with an impacted stone at the ampulla.

The etiology of papillitis is unknown. Many cases are thought to be caused by trauma from the passage of multiple small stones or sludge from the common bile duct through the ampulla, resulting in inflammation, fibrosis, and stricture formation. There are other patients, however, that have papillary stenosis without gallstones. The cause in these cases is less clear; potential triggers include primary sphincter motility disorders and congenital anomalies.

Management consists of proper diagnostic imaging and therapeutic sphincterotomy. Cholangiography with either PTC or ERCP is the mainstay of diagnostic imaging. Therapeutic sphincterotomy can be performed either endoscopically or operatively in conjunction with cholecystectomy. The procedure of choice in patients with previous cholecystectomy is endoscopic sphincterotomy.

▪ PRIMARY SCLEROSING CHOLANGITIS

Primary sclerosing cholangitis (PSC) is an idiopathic condition characterized by a progressive, chronic cholestatic process resulting in diffuse inflammation, sclerosis, and obliteration of the intrahepatic and extrahepatic biliary duct systems. The diagnosis of PSC is confirmed by cholangiography, with findings of multiple areas of stricture and dilatation. The great majority of these patients have underlying ulcerative colitis or other autoimmune disease.

PSC has a variable course but can progress to biliary obstruction with secondary cirrhosis, portal hypertension with bleeding varices, or hepatic failure. Finally, PSC is a strong risk factor for the development of cholangiocarcinoma. Surgical management for symptomatic disease in patients with primarily extrahepatic and/or hilar disease and with no evidence of cirrhosis includes resection of the hepatic bifurcation with long-term transhepatic stenting. Although an uncommon disorder, PSC is a common indication for liver transplantation patients in several large series, with transplantation the treatment of choice in patients with primarily intrahepatic strictures or advanced cirrhosis.

PATHOGENESIS

The etiology of PSC remains unknown, and a variety of causal theories have been proposed. Inflammatory bowel disease, particularly ulcerative colitis, is present in 30–90% of patients with PSC in several large population-based studies.[95,96] This tight association with inflammatory bowel disease suggests an autoimmune process. Other mechanisms likely have a role in pathogenesis, however, since only a minority with ulcerative colitis have PSC.[95] Although both ulcerative colitis and PSC may occur in the same individual, the two disorders may occur at different times. PSC, for example, may occur years after colectomy for ulcerative colitis.

Due to the association between PSC and inflammatory bowel disease, several investigators have speculated that increased bacterial spread into the portal circulation from inflamed large or small intestine may lead to chronic or recurrent cholangitis. In support of this, an animal model of small intestinal bacterial overgrowth has biliary findings similar to PSC.[97] Although some studies have documented increased portal bacteremia in patients with PSC, other studies have not confirmed this finding.[98,99]

Correlating evidence for an immunological cause of PSC includes its association with hypergammaglobulinemia (30%) and an increase in IgM (50%). Patients with PSC can also have autoantibodies, with titers in the range associated with autoimmune hepatitis. In particular, anti–smooth muscle antibodies and antinuclear antibodies are present in approximately 75%.[100] Other autoantibodies commonly associated with the disease include cytoplasmic and nuclear antigens to neutrophils (p-ANCA); p-ANCA is often found in patients with PSC and no ulcerative colitis but is uncommon in patients with ulcerative colitis alone.[101]

Several genetic factors appear to give individuals a predisposition to PSC, including increased prevalence of HLA-B8, -DR3, and -Drw52a. The HLA-B8 and HLA-DR3 haplotypes are associated with other autoimmune diseases, including celiac disease, myasthenia gravis, and diabetes mellitus. A specific mutation of MICA (an MHC class I related molecule) is also strongly associated with PSC patients (58% compared to 22% in controls).[102]

In contrast to PSC, secondary sclerosing cholangitis has similar clinical characteristics but has identifiable causes. The inciting factors for secondary sclerosing cholangitis include infectious cholangiopathy associated with acquired immunodeficiency syndrome, congenital biliary abnormalities, ischemic cholangiopathy secondary to intrahepatic arterial infusion of 5-fluorouracil, hepatic allograft rejection, graft-versus-host disease in bone marrow transplantation, collagen vascular diseases, histiocytosis X, sarcoidosis, and mast cell cholangiopathy. Patients with diffuse stricturing from 5-fluorouracil are managed by simple discontinuation of infusion, and in some cases percutaneous transhepatic drainage. Surgery should be reserved for patients with persistent evidence of biliary obstruction. The pathogenesis of acquired immunodeficiency syndrome cholangiopathy is believed to be viral and related to cytomegalovirus infection. No experience in the surgical management of this condition has been reported.

PRESENTATION

PSC is predominantly a disease of young men. Approximately 70% of patients are male, and the average age at the time of diagnosis is 40 years. The typical presentation includes either an asymptomatic individual with abnormal liver function tests or an individual with intermittent jaundice. Other common symptoms may include right upper quadrant pain, weight loss, fever, pruritus, and fatigue. Despite its name, a minority have acute cholangitis and blood cultures are rarely positive. Asymptomatic patients, however, can have deceptively advanced disease. Approximately 10% are very symptomatic at the time of diagnosis. In addition to commonly occurring in patients with ulcerative colitis, PSC can occur with multifocal fibrosclerosis syndromes, including retroperitoneal, mediastinal, and/or periureteral fibrosis, Riedel's thyroiditis, or pseudotumor of the orbit.

DIAGNOSIS

Lab tests with PSC typically reveal a cholestatic picture. Patients will have an elevated alkaline phosphatase, and during exacerbations may have elevated bilirubin. Early in the disease course, patients will have a normal albumin.

The diagnosis is usually made through cholangiography. The typical study reveals multifocal strictures and dilatations, referred to as "beading," of the intrahepatic and extrahepatic ducts (Fig 34–21). The diagnostic modality of choice for cholangiography in suspected cases is endoscopic cholangiography. Percutaneous transhepatic cholangiography may be difficult since cannulation of nondilated and fibrotic ducts associated with PSC can be technically challenging via this approach. At the time of diagnostic cholangiography, brushings for cytology should be obtained to help distinguish between benign and malignant strictures.

MANAGEMENT

Management of PSC has several important treatment goals, including halting or reversing the disease process, managing disease progression, and symptom control. Unfortunately, there are no effective medical treat-

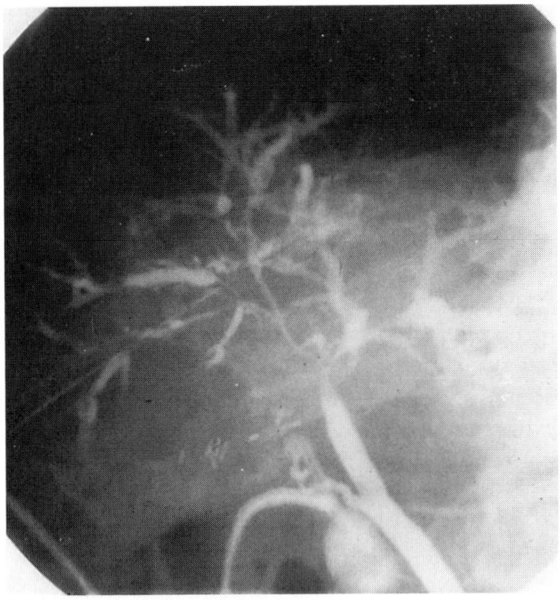

Figure 34–21. Cholangiographic appearance in primary sclerosing cholangitis. Multiple irregular strictures and dilatation (beading) of intrahepatic ducts. (Reprinted, with permission, from Lillemoe KD. Biliary injuries and strictures and sclerosing cholangitis. In: Mulholland MW, Lillemoe KD, Doherty GM, Maier RV, Upchurch GR Jr (eds). *Greenfield's Surgery: Scientific Principles and Practice*, 4th ed. Philadelphia, PA: Lippincott Williams & Wilkins; 2006:1011.)

ments that slow the progression of PSC. Patients should be monitored closely with cholangiography, liver biopsy and cytologic brushings, to detect disease progression and development of malignancy or biliary cirrhosis.

Most medical therapies are aimed at symptomatic relief or antibiotic treatment in the setting of cholangitis. Immunosuppression with glucocorticoids, methotrexate, azathioprine, 6-mercaptopurine, tacrolimus, or cyclosporine have not demonstrated efficacy for disease progression or survival. Recently, studies with ursodeoxycholic acid (UDCA) have demonstrated improvement of liver function tests and symptoms. Whether this translates into improvement in survival or end-organ failure is still unclear. A prospective, randomized, placebo-controlled trial of UDCA did not demonstrate long-term clinical benefit with UDCA.[103] High-dose UDCA in several small pilot studies has demonstrated decreased disease progression and improved survival;[104,105] larger-scale prospective trials with high-dose UDCA are underway.

A dominant extrahepatic biliary stricture (a high-grade, localized area of narrowing) occurs in approximately 20% of patients with PSC. These patients can be managed potentially with endoscopic therapy using dilatation with or without stenting. Cytologic brushings at the time of endoscopy should also be obtained to investigate for cholangiocarcinoma. Several retrospective reports have demonstrated benefit in relieving symptoms and improving liver function tests from endoscopic therapy,[106] and possible delay in disease progression.[107] The durability, however, of endoscopic therapy appears to be poor, with most patients requiring repeat dilatations at regular intervals. Whether patients should undergo stenting at the time of dilatation is not clear, with short-term results of stenting similar to those of dilatation treatment alone,[108] and with no long-term outcomes at present comparing the two techniques.

Operative biliary reconstruction with transhepatic stenting for primarily extrahepatic and/or hilar disease in noncirrhotic patients has been demonstrated to have excellent long-term outcomes.[109,110] Ahrendt and associates[110] reported 146 patients with PSC managed with either biliary reconstruction or nonoperative biliary dilatation. Survival was significantly longer in noncirrhotic patients with PSC managed surgically compared to patients managed nonoperatively, and time before requiring liver transplantation was significantly longer in the surgically-managed patients (Fig 34–22).

The natural history of PSC is typically progressive. Regardless of therapy, median survival is typically 12 years following diagnosis.[111,112] Survival is significantly worse in patients symptomatic at the time of diagnosis.[112] The incidence of cholangiocarcinoma of PSC patients at 5 years is 10–15% and at 10 years increases to 30%.

Hepatic transplantation provides excellent results in patients with PSC and end-stage liver disease, with 5-year actuarial survival and graft functioning of 85% and 72%, respectively.[113] Liver transplantation should be considered in patients with sclerosing cholangitis before the disease is too advanced. Primary indicators for referral for liver transplantation include persistently elevated bilirubin or decreased quality of life from disabling fatigue, severe pruritus, muscle wasting, or bacterial cholangitis. Biliary tract surgery prior to transplantation does not effect either short-term outcomes or survival following transplant.

Patients with preoperatively recognized cholangiocarcinoma have a poor prognosis. These patients are not

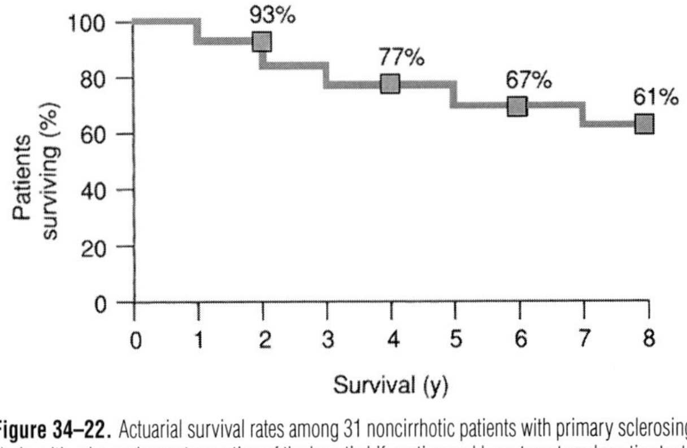

Figure 34–22. Actuarial survival rates among 31 noncirrhotic patients with primary sclerosing cholangitis who underwent resection of the hepatic bifurcation and long-term transhepatic stenting. (Reprinted, with permission, from Lillemoe KD, Pitt HA, Cameron JL. Primary sclerosing cholangitis. *Surg Clin North Am* 1990;70:1397.)

appropriate candidates for transplantation. On the other hand, the presence of a small (<1 cm) cholangiocarcinoma discovered incidentally on pathology at transplantation does not appear to portend a poor prognosis.

Patients transplanted for PSC are also at increased risk of postoperative biliary stricture compared to patients transplanted for other primary disease processes. Recurrent PSC occurs in approximately 10% of patients following transplantation, but with typically a less aggressive course.[113]

SUMMARY

PSC currently has no proven effective medical treatment. Resection of the hepatic duct bifurcation in conjunction with long-term transhepatic stenting in noncirrhotic patients with primarily extrahepatic and/or hilar disease can delay or even prevent the need for hepatic transplantation. This operation does not influence the outcomes associated with hepatic transplantation. Transplantation is recommended in patients with primarily intrahepatic strictures or advanced cirrhosis.

REFERENCES

1. Lipsett PA, Pitt HA, Colombani PM et al. Choledochal cyst disease. A changing pattern of presentation. *Ann Surg* 1994;220:644–652
2. Alonso-Lej F, Rever W, Pessagno DJ. Congenital choledochal cyst, with a report of 2, and an analysis of 94 cases. *Int Abstr Surg* 1959;108:1–30
3. Todani T, Watanabe Y, Narusue M et al. Congenital bile duct cysts: Classification, operative procedures, and review of thirty-seven cases including cancer arising from choledochal cyst. *Am J Surg* 1977;134:263–269
4. Savader SJ, Benenati JF, Venbrux AC et al. Choledochal cysts: classification and cholangiographic appearance. *Am J Roentgenol* 1991;156:327–331
5. Todani T, Watanabe Y, Toki A et al. Classification of congenital biliary cystic disease: special reference to type Ic and IVA cysts with primary ductal stricture. *J Hepatobiliary Pancreat Surg* 2003;10:340–344
6. Visser BC, Suh I, Way LW et al. Congenital choledochal cysts in adults. *Arch Surg* 2004;139:855–860
7. Spitz L. Experimental production of cystic dilatation of the common bile duct in neonatal lambs. *J Pediatr Surg* 1977;12:39–42
8. Hara H, Morita S, Ishibashi T et al. Surgical treatment for congenital biliary dilatation, with or without intrahepatic bile duct dilatation. *Hepatogastroenterology* 2001;48: 638–641
9. Tyler KL, Sokol RJ, Oberhaus SM et al. Detection of reovirus RNA in hepatobiliary tissues from patients with extrahepatic biliary atresia and choledochal cysts. *Hepatology* 1998;27:1475–1482
10. Song HK, Kim MH, Myung SJ et al. Choledochal cyst associated with the anomalous union of pancreaticobiliary duct (AUPBD) has a more grave clinical course than choledochal cyst alone. *Korean J Intern Med* 1999; 14:1–8
11. Wong KC, Lister J. Human fetal development of the hepato-pancreatic duct junction—a possible explanation of congenital dilatation of the biliary tract. *J Pediatr Surg* 1981;16:139–145
12. Ando H, Kaneko K, Ito F et al. Embryogenesis of pancreaticobiliary maljunction inferred from development of duodenal atresia. *J Hepatobiliary Pancreat Surg* 1999;6: 50–54
13. Kato T, Hebiguchi T, Matsuda K et al. Action of pancreatic juice on the bile duct: pathogenesis of congenital choledochal cyst. *J Pediatr Surg* 1981;16:146–151
14. Iwai N, Tokiwa K, Tsuto T et al. Biliary manometry in choledochal cyst with abnormal choledochopancreatico ductal junction. *J Pediatr Surg* 1986;21:873–876
15. Craig AG, Chen LD, Saccone GT et al. Sphincter of Oddi dysfunction associated with choledochal cyst. *J Gastroenterol Hepatol* 2001;16:230–234
16. Voyles CR, Smadja C, Shands WC et al. Carcinoma in choledochal cysts. Age-related incidence. *Arch Surg* 1983;118:986–988
17. Weyant MJ, Maluccio MA, Bertagnolli MM et al. Choledochal cysts in adults: a report of two cases and review of the literature. *Am J Gastroenterol* 1998;93:2580–2583
18. Swisher SG, Cates JA, Hunt KK et al. Pancreatitis associated with adult choledochal cysts. *Pancreas* 1994;9:633–637
19. Todani T, Watanabe Y, Toki A et al. Carcinoma related to choledochal cysts with internal drainage operations. *Surg Gynecol Obstet* 1987;164:61–64
20. Funabiki T, Sugiue K, Matsubara T et al. Bile acids and biliary carcinoma in pancreaticobiliary maljunction. *Keio J Med* 1991;40:118–122
21. Tsuchida A, Nagakawa Y, Kasuya K et al. Immunohistochemical analysis of cyclooxygenase-2 and vascular endothelial growth factor in pancreaticobiliary maljunction. *Oncol Rep* 2003;10:339–343
22. Iwase T, Nakazawa S, Yamao K et al. Ras gene point mutations in gallbladder lesions associated with anomalous connection of pancreatobiliary ducts. *Hepatogastroenterology* 1997;44:1457–1462
23. Tanno S, Obara T, Fujii T et al. Proliferative potential and K-ras mutation in epithelial hyperplasia of the gallbladder in patients with anomalous pancreaticobiliary ductal union. *Cancer* 1998;83:267–275
24. Nagai M, Kawarada Y, Watanabe M et al. Analysis of microsatellite instability, TGF-beta type II receptor gene mutations and hMSH2 and hMLH1 allele losses in pancreaticobiliary maljunction-associated biliary tract tumors. *Anticancer Res* 1999;19:1765–1768
25. Itoi T, Shinohara Y, Takeda K et al. Nuclear cyclin D1 overexpression is a critical event associated with cell proliferation and invasive growth in gallbladder carcinogenesis. *J Gastroenterol* 2000;35:142–149
26. Matsubara T, Sakurai Y, Zhi LZ et al. K-ras and p53 gene mutations in noncancerous biliary lesions of patients

with pancreaticobiliary maljunction. *J Hepatobiliary Pancreat Surg* 2002;9:312–321
27. Rothlin MA, Lopfe M, Schlumpf R et al. Long-term results of hepaticojejunostomy for benign lesions of the bile ducts. *Am J Surg* 1998;175:22–26
28. Lilly JR. The surgical treatment of choledochal cyst. *Surg Gynecol Obstet* 1979;149:36–42
29. Delarue A, Chappuis JP, Esposito C et al. Is the appendix graft suitable for routine biliary surgery in children? *J Pediatr Surg* 2000;35:1312–1316
30. Tsuchida Y, Takahashi A, Suzuki N et al. Development of intrahepatic biliary stones after excision of choledochal cysts. *J Pediatr Surg* 2002;37:165–167
31. Pitt HA, Venbrux AC, Coleman J et al. Intrahepatic stones. The transhepatic team approach. *Ann Surg* 1994;219:527–535
32. Bismuth H. Postoperative strictures of the biliary tract. In: Blumgart L (ed). *The Biliary Tract. Clinical Surgery International Series.* Edinburgh, Scotland: Churchill Livingstone; 1983:209–218
33. Strasberg SM, Hertl M, Soper NJ. An analysis of the problem of biliary injury during laparoscopic cholecystectomy. *J Am Coll Surg* 1995;180:101–125
34. Roslyn JJ, Binns GS, Hughes EF et al. Open cholecystectomy. A contemporary analysis of 42,474 patients. *Ann Surg* 1993;218:129–137
35. Wherry DC, Marohn MR, Malanoski MP et al. An external audit of laparoscopic cholecystectomy in the steady state performed in medical treatment facilities of the Department of Defense. *Ann Surg* 1996;224:145–154
36. Windsor JA, Pong J. Laparoscopic biliary injury: more than a learning curve problem. *Aust N Z J Surg* 1998;68:186–189
37. Adamsen S, Hansen OH, Funch-Jensen P et al. Bile duct injury during laparoscopic cholecystectomy: a prospective nationwide series. *J Am Coll Surg* 1997;184:571–578
38. Krahenbuhl L, Sclabas G, Wente MN et al. Incidence, risk factors, and prevention of biliary tract injuries during laparoscopic cholecystectomy in Switzerland. *World J Surg* 2001;25:1325–1330
39. Fletcher DR, Hobbs MS, Tan P et al. Complications of cholecystectomy: risks of the laparoscopic approach and protective effects of operative cholangiography: a population-based study. *Ann Surg* 1999;229:449–457
40. Flum DR, Dellinger EP, Cheadle A et al. Intraoperative cholangiography and risk of common bile duct injury during cholecystectomy. *JAMA* 2003;289:1639–1644
41. Way LW, Stewart L, Gantert W et al. Causes and prevention of laparoscopic bile duct injuries: analysis of 252 cases from a human factors and cognitive psychology perspective. *Ann Surg* 2003;237:460–469
42. Stewart L, Way LW. Cues associated with laparoscopic cholecystectomy bile duct injuries: confirmation bias may inhibit early diagnosis. *J Gastrointest Surg* (In press)
43. Lillemoe KD. To err is human, but should we expect more from a surgeon? *Ann Surg* 2003;237:470–471
44. Carlson E, Zukoski CF, Campbell J et al. Morphologic, biophysical, and biochemical consequences of ligation of the common biliary duct in the dog. *Am J Pathol* 1997; 86:301–320
45. Xu J, Geng ZM, Ma QY. Microstructural and ultrastructural changes in the healing process of bile duct trauma. *Hepatobiliary Pancreat Dis Int* 2003;2:295–299
46. Pitt HA, Miyamoto T, Parapatis SK et al. Factors influencing outcome in patients with postoperative biliary strictures. *Am J Surg* 1982;144:14–21
47. Sicklick JK, Camp MS, Lillemoe KD et al. Surgical management of bile duct injuries sustained during laparoscopic cholecystectomy: perioperative results in 200 patients. *Ann Surg* 2005;241:786–792; discussion 793–795
48. Stewart L, Way LW. Bile duct injuries during laparoscopic cholecystectomy. Factors that influence the results of treatment. *Arch Surg* 1995;130:1123–1128
49. Savader SJ, Cameron JL, Lillemoe KD et al. The biliary manometric perfusion test and clinical trial—long-term predictive value of success after treatment of bile duct strictures: ten-year experience. *J Vasc Intervent Radiol* 1998;9:976–985
50. Pitt HA, Kaufman SL, Coleman J et al. Benign postoperative biliary strictures. Operate or dilate? *Ann Surg* 1989; 210:417–425
51. Moore AV Jr, Illescas FF, Mills SR et al. Percutaneous dilation of benign biliary strictures. *Radiology* 1987;163: 625–628
52. Mueller PR, vanSonnenberg E, Ferrucci JT et al. Biliary stricture dilatation: multicenter review of clinical management in 73 patients. *Radiology* 1986;160:17–22
53. Vogel SB, Howard RJ, Caridi J et al. Evaluation of percutaneous transhepatic balloon dilatation of benign biliary strictures in high-risk patients. *Am J Surg* 1985;149:73–79
54. Williams HJ Jr, Bender CE, May GR. Benign postoperative biliary strictures: dilation with fluoroscopic guidance. *Radiology* 1987;163:629–634
55. Misra S, Melton GB, Geschwind JF et al. Percutaneous management of bile duct strictures and injuries associated with laparoscopic cholecystectomy: a decade of experience. *J Am Coll Surg* 2004;198:218–226
56. Davids PH, Tanka AK, Rauws EA et al. Benign biliary strictures. Surgery or endoscopy? *Ann Surg* 1993;217: 237–243
57. Smith MT, Sherman S, Lehman GA. Endoscopic management of benign strictures of the biliary tree. *Endoscopy* 1995;27:253–266
58. Bergman JJ, Burgemeister L, Bruno MJ et al. Long-term follow-up after biliary stent placement for postoperative bile duct stenosis. *Gastrointest Endosc* 2001;54:154–161
59. De Masi E, Fiori E, Lamazza A et al. Endoscopy in the treatment of benign biliary strictures. *Ital J Gastroenterol Hepatol* 1998;30:91–95
60. Bonnel DH, Liguory CL, Lefebvre JF et al. Placement of metallic stents for treatment of postoperative biliary strictures: long-term outcome in 25 patients. *Am J Roentgenol* 1997;169:1517–1522
61. Hausegger KA, Kugler C, Uggowitzer M et al. Benign biliary obstruction: is treatment with the Wallstent advisable? *Radiology* 1996;200:437–441
62. Maccioni F, Rossi M, Salvatori FM et al. Metallic stents in benign biliary strictures: three-year follow-up. *Cardiovasc Intervent Radiol* 1992;15:360–366

63. Dumonceau JM, Deviere J, Delhaye M et al. Plastic and metal stents for postoperative benign bile duct strictures: the best and the worst. *Gastrointest Endosc* 1998;47: 8–17
64. Costamagna G, Pandolfi M, Mutignani M et al. Long-term results of endoscopic management of postoperative bile duct strictures with increasing numbers of stents. *Gastrointest Endosc* 2001;54:162–168
65. Flum DR, Cheadle A, Prela C et al. Bile duct injury during cholecystectomy and survival in Medicare beneficiaries. *JAMA* 2003;290:2168–2173
66. Alves A, Farges O, Nicolet J et al. Incidence and consequence of an hepatic artery injury in patients with postcholecystectomy bile duct strictures. *Ann Surg* 2003;238: 93–96
67. Schmidt SC, Settmacher U, Langrehr JM et al. Management and outcome of patients with combined bile duct and hepatic arterial injuries after laparoscopic cholecystectomy. *Surgery* 2004;135:613–618
68. Stewart L, Robinson TN, Lee CM et al. Right hepatic artery injury associated with laparoscopic bile duct injury: incidence, mechanism, and consequences. *J Gastrointest Surg* 2004;8:523–530
69. Tocchi A, Costa G, Lepre L et al. The long-term outcome of hepaticojejunostomy in the treatment of benign bile duct strictures. *Ann Surg* 1996;224:162–167
70. McDonald ML, Farnell MB, Nagorney DM et al. Benign biliary strictures: repair and outcome with a contemporary approach. *Surgery* 1995;118:582–590
71. Chapman WC, Halevy A, Blumgart LH et al. Postcholecystectomy bile duct strictures. Management and outcome in 130 patients. *Arch Surg* 1995;130:597–602
72. Innes JT, Ferrara JJ, Carey LC. Biliary reconstruction without transanastomotic stent. *Am Surg* 1988;54:27–30
73. Genest JF, Nanos E, Grundfest-Broniatowski S et al. Benign biliary strictures: an analytic review (1970 to 1984). *Surgery* 1986;99:409–413
74. Pellegrini CA, Thomas MJ, Way LW. Recurrent biliary stricture. Patterns of recurrence and outcome of surgical therapy. *Am J Surg* 1984;147:175–180
75. Lillemoe KD, Melton GB, Cameron JL et al. Postoperative bile duct strictures: management and outcome in the 1990s. *Ann Surg* 2000;232:430–441
76. Walsh RM, Henderson JM, Vogt DP et al. Trends in bile duct injuries from laparoscopic cholecystectomy. *J Gastrointest Surg* 1998;2:458–462
77. Bauer TW, Morris JB, Lowenstein A et al. The consequences of a major bile duct injury during laparoscopic cholecystectomy. *J Gastrointest Surg* 1998;2:61–66
78. Mirza DF, Narsimhan KL, Ferraz Neto BH et al. Bile duct injury following laparoscopic cholecystectomy: referral pattern and management. *Br J Surg* 1997;84:786–790
79. Nealon WH, Urrutia F. Long-term follow-up after bilioenteric anastomosis for benign bile duct stricture. *Ann Surg* 1996;223:639–645
80. Boerma D, Rauws EA, Keulemans YC et al. Impaired quality of life 5 years after bile duct injury during laparoscopic cholecystectomy: a prospective analysis. *Ann Surg* 2001;234:750–757
81. Melton GB, Lillemoe KD, Cameron JL et al. Major bile duct injuries associated with laparoscopic cholecystectomy: effect of surgical repair on quality of life. *Ann Surg* 2002;235:888–895
82. Sarmiento JM, Farnell MB, Nagorney DM et al. Quality-of-life assessment of surgical reconstruction after laparoscopic cholecystectomy-induced bile duct injuries: what happens at 5 years and beyond? *Arch Surg* 2004; 139:483–488
83. Moore DE, Feurer ID, Holzman MD et al. Long-term detrimental effect of bile duct injury on health-related quality of life. *Arch Surg* 2004;139:476–481
84. Stahl TJ, Allen MO, Ansel HJ et al. Partial biliary obstruction caused by chronic pancreatitis. An appraisal of indications for surgical biliary drainage. *Ann Surg* 1988; 207:26–32
85. Vijungco JD, Prinz RA. Management of biliary and duodenal complications of chronic pancreatitis. *World J Surg* 2003;27:1258–1270
86. Nealon WH, Matin S. Analysis of surgical success in preventing recurrent acute exacerbations in chronic pancreatitis. *Ann Surg* 2001;233:793–800
87. Warshaw AL, Schapiro RH, Ferrucci JT Jr et al. Persistent obstructive jaundice, cholangitis, and biliary cirrhosis due to common bile duct stenosis in chronic pancreatitis. *Gastroenterology* 1976;70:562–567
88. Afroudakis A, Kaplowitz N. Liver histopathology in chronic common bile duct stenosis due to chronic alcoholic pancreatitis. *Hepatology* 1981;1:65–72
89. Escudero-Fabre A, Escallon A Jr, Sack J et al. Choledochoduodenostomy. Analysis of 71 cases followed for 5 to 15 years. *Ann Surg* 1991;213:635–642
90. Vitale GC, Reed DN Jr, Nguyen CT et al. Endoscopic treatment of distal bile duct stricture from chronic pancreatitis. *Surg Endosc* 2000;14:227–231
91. Pozsar J, Sahin P, Laszlo F et al. Medium-term results of endoscopic treatment of common bile duct strictures in chronic calcifying pancreatitis with increasing numbers of stents. *J Clin Gastroenterol* 2004;38:118–123
92. Principe A, Ercolani G, Bassi F et al. Diagnostic dilemmas in biliary strictures mimicking cholangiocarcinoma. *Hepatogastroenterology* 2003;50:1246–1249
93. Eickhoff A, Schilling D, Benz CA et al. Endoscopic stenting for postoperative biliary strictures due to hepatic hydatid disease: effectiveness and long-term outcome. *J Clin Gastroenterol* 2003;37:74–78
94. Saritas U, Parlak E, Akoglu M et al. Effectiveness of endoscopic treatment modalities in complicated hepatic hydatid disease after surgical intervention. *Endoscopy* 2001;33:858–863
95. Olsson R, Danielsson A, Jarnerot G et al. Prevalence of primary sclerosing cholangitis in patients with ulcerative colitis. *Gastroenterology* 1991;100:1319–1323
96. Bambha K, Kim WR, Talwalkar J et al. Incidence, clinical spectrum, and outcomes of primary sclerosing cholangitis in a United States community. *Gastroenterology* 2003;125:1364–1369
97. Lichtman SN, Keku J, Schwab JH et al. Hepatic injury associated with small bowel bacterial overgrowth in rats

is prevented by metronidazole and tetracycline. *Gastroenterology* 1991;100:513–519
98. Palmer KR, Duerden BI, Holdsworth CD. Bacteriological and endotoxin studies in cases of ulcerative colitis submitted to surgery. *Gut* 1980;21:851–854
99. Vinnik IE, Kern F Jr, Struthers JE Jr et al. Experimental chronic portal vein bacteremia. *Proc Soc Exp Biol Med* 1964;115:311–314
100. Angulo P, Peter JB, Gershwin ME et al. Serum autoantibodies in patients with primary sclerosing cholangitis. *J Hepatol* 2000;32:182–187
101. Lo SK, Chapman RW, Cheeseman P et al. Antineutrophil antibody: a test for autoimmune primary sclerosing cholangitis in childhood? *Gut* 1993;34:199–202
102. Norris S, Kondeatis E, Collins R et al. Mapping MHC-encoded susceptibility and resistance in primary sclerosing cholangitis: the role of MICA polymorphism. *Gastroenterology* 2001;120:1475–1482
103. Lindor KD. Ursodiol for primary sclerosing cholangitis. Mayo Primary Sclerosing Cholangitis-Ursodeoxycholic Acid Study Group. *N Engl J Med* 1997;336:691–695
104. Harnois DM, Angulo P, Jorgensen RA. High-dose ursodeoxycholic acid as a therapy for patients with primary sclerosing cholangitis. *Am J Gastroenterol* 2001;96: 1558–1562
105. Mitchell SA, Bansi DS, Hunt N et al. A preliminary trial of high-dose ursodeoxycholic acid in primary sclerosing cholangitis. *Gastroenterology* 2001;121:900–907
106. Baluyut AR, Sherman S, Lehman GA et al. Impact of endoscopic therapy on the survival of patients with primary sclerosing cholangitis. *Gastrointest Endosc* 2001;53: 308–312
107. Stiehl A, Rudolph G, Kloters-Plachky P et al. Development of dominant bile duct stenoses in patients with primary sclerosing cholangitis treated with ursodeoxycholic acid: outcome after endoscopic treatment. *J Hepatol* 2002;36:151–156
108. Kaya M, Petersen BT, Angulo P et al. Balloon dilation compared to stenting of dominant strictures in primary sclerosing cholangitis. *Am J Gastroenterol* 2001;96:1059–1066
109. Cameron JL, Pitt HA, Zinner MJ et al. Resection of hepatic duct bifurcation and transhepatic stenting for sclerosing cholangitis. *Ann Surg* 1998;207:614–622
110. Ahrendt SA, Pitt HA, Kalloo AN et al. Primary sclerosing cholangitis: resect, dilate, or transplant? *Ann Surg* 1998;227:412–423
111. Farrant JM, Hayllar KM, Wilkinson ML et al. Natural history and prognostic variables in primary sclerosing cholangitis. *Gastroenterology* 1991;100:1710–1717
112. Broome U, Olsson R, Loof L et al. Natural history and prognostic factors in 305 Swedish patients with primary sclerosing cholangitis. *Gut* 1996;38:610–615
113. Goss JA, Shackleton CR, Farmer DG et al. Orthotopic liver transplantation for primary sclerosing cholangitis. A 12-year single center experience. *Ann Surg* 1997;225:472–481

35

Cancer of the Gallbladder and Bile Ducts

Edward E. Whang ■ Michael J. Zinner

This chapter focuses on biliary tract cancers, including those of the gallbladder and intrahepatic and extrahepatic bile ducts. These cancers were once approached with great pessimism. During the past decade, however, there has been accumulating evidence that long-term survival can occur following complete (R_0) resection of these cancers, even in some patients with advanced lesions. As a result, there has been greater acceptance of extended radical resections designed to achieve this goal. Because the epidemiology, clinical presentation, and surgical approach associated with gallbladder cancer and bile duct cancer are distinct, these two cancers are discussed separately.

■ GALLBLADDER CANCER

EPIDEMIOLOGY

With an incidence of 5000 cases annually in the United States, gallbladder cancer is the fifth most common gastrointestinal tract malignancy. Incidence increases with age and is two to six times greater in women than in men. Worldwide, the highest incidence rates (up to 7.5 per 100,000 in men and 23 per 100,000 in women) occur among populations in the western part of South America (e.g., Chile and Peru) and in northern India and in North-American Indians and Mexican Americans.[1]

The best-characterized risk factor for the development of gallbladder cancer is the presence of gallstones (Table 35–1). Gallstones are present in 70–90% of patients diagnosed with gallbladder cancer, and the geographic pattern of gallbladder cancer incidence correlates with that of cholelithiasis. However, only 0.5–3% of patients with cholelithiasis will develop gallbladder cancer. There is some evidence that the risk of developing gallbladder cancer among patients with gallstones is correlated with increasing gallstone size and greater duration of cholelithiasis.[2]

Other factors implicated to increase the risk of gallbladder cancer include porcelain gallbladder (the incidence of gallbladder cancer is reported to range from 12.5–60% in patients with this condition[3]), adenomatous polyps of the gallbladder (cholesterol and inflammatory polyps and adenomyomas are not believed to be risk factors), chronic infection with *Salmonella typhi*, carcinogen exposure (e.g., increased risk has been reported for miners exposed to radon), and abnormal pancreaticobiliary duct junction (APBDJ). In this latter condition, a long common channel formed by an abnormally proximal junction between the pancreatic and common bile ducts and elevated sphincter of Oddi pressures predispose to reflux of pancreatic exocrine secretions into the bile ducts. APBDJ is most prevalent in Asian countries and appears to increase the risk for developing biliary cancers, especially gallbladder cancer.[4] Gallbladder cancers arising in patients with APBDJ tend to occur at a younger patient age, to have a lesser degree of female predominance, and to be associated less often with cholelithiasis than those arising in patients without APBDJ.

TABLE 35–1. RISK FACTORS FOR DEVELOPING GALLBLADDER CANCER

Cholelithiasis
Porcelain gallbladder
Adenomatous polyps of the gallbladder
Chronic *Salmonella typhi* infection
Carcinogens (e.g., radon)
Abnormal pancreaticobiliary duct junction (APBDJ)

PATHOGENESIS AND PATHOLOGY

Chronic irritation of the gallbladder mucosa related to gallstones is hypothesized to be the major factor leading to malignant transformation in most cases of gallbladder cancer. The progression from dysplasia to carcinoma in situ (CIS) and then to invasive cancer has been described for gallbladder cancer. The molecular changes associated with this progression are only beginning to be defined: K-*ras* mutations are relatively rare, whereas *p53* mutations are prevalent and tend to arise early during this progression.[1]

Gallbladder cancers arising in patients with APBDJ appear to be associated with a distinct pathogenetic mechanism. These cancers are associated with a high prevalence of K-*ras* mutations and a late onset of *p53* mutations.[1] In addition, there is a high prevalence of premalignant epithelial hyperplasia with a papillary or villous histology in the gallbladder mucosa of patients with APBDJ.

Eighty percent of primary gallbladder cancers are adenocarcinomas. Other histologic types include small cell cancer, squamous cell carcinoma, lymphoma, and sarcoma. Gallbladder cancers also are classified according to morphology as infiltrative, nodular, papillary, or a combination of these types. Papillary cancers tend to grow within the gallbladder lumen and are less likely to invade the liver or to metastasize to lymph nodes; these cancers are associated with the best prognosis. Infiltrative or nodular cancers have a more diffuse pattern of growth that is difficult to recognize on imaging studies. These lesions are more likely to have invaded the liver and to have metastasized to lymph nodes by the time of diagnosis.

Several staging systems for gallbladder cancer have been described. Although the Nevin staging system, originally put forth in 1976, is still referenced, the TNM system is preferred today (Table 35–2). The sixth edition of the American Joint Committee on Cancer (AJCC) staging system, published in 2003, contained important modifications to the staging of gallbladder cancer contained in the fifth edition.[5] T2N0 lesions (formerly stage II) have been reclassified as stage IB, T3N0 lesions (formerly stage III) have been reclassified as stage IIA, and T1–3N1 lesions (formerly stage III) have been reclassified as stage IIB. These changes reflect the increasing acceptance of the belief that locally advanced gallbladder cancers potentially are amenable to curative resection using aggressive surgical techniques.

CLINICAL PRESENTATION AND DIAGNOSIS

In the absence of advanced disease, patients with gallbladder cancer are asymptomatic or have symptoms, such as abdominal pain, anorexia, nausea, and vomiting, that may be indistinguishable from those of cholelithiasis or cholecystitis. With advanced disease, patients can present with weight loss, obstructive jaundice (owing to tumor invasion into the biliary tree or to liver metastases), and duodenal obstruction. Signs associated with advanced disease include palpable abdominal masses, hepatomegaly, and ascites.

Laboratory tests may suggest obstructive jaundice if this condition is present; otherwise, they are not helpful in the diagnosis of gallbladder cancer. Tumor markers carcinoembryonic antigen (CEA) and CA 19-9 may be elevated; however, they lack sufficient sensitivity or specificity to be useful in clinical decision making for individual patients.

Most patients with suspected gallstone- or gallbladder-related conditions undergo transabdominal ultrasonography (US). Findings suggestive of gallbladder cancer on US include mural thickening or calcification, a gallbladder mass greater than 1 cm in diameter, and loss of the normal gallbladder wall–liver interface (Fig 35–1). Relative to transabdominal US, endoscopic ultrasonography (EUS) offers greater accuracy in assessing depth of gallbladder wall penetration by masses and regional lymph node enlargement. Selective appli-

TABLE 35–2. TNM STAGING OF GALLBLADDER CANCER: AMERICAN JOINT COMMITTEE ON CANCER, 6TH EDITION

Stage 0	Tis	N0	M0
Stage IA	T1	N0	M0
Stage IB	T2	N0	M0
Stage IIA	T3	N0	M0
Stage IIB	T1–3	N1	M0
Stage III	T4	N0–1	M0
Stage IV	Any T	N0–1	M1

NOTE: Tis: carcinoma in situ; T1: cancer invades lamina propria and/or muscularis; T2: cancer invades perimuscular connective tissue but not beyond serosa or into liver; T3: cancer invades through gallbladder serosa and/or directly invades into the liver and/or one other adjacent organ or structure; T4: cancer invades main portal vein or hepatic artery or multiple extrahepatic organs or structures; N0: no regional lymph node metastasis; N1: regional lymph node metastasis present (regional lymph nodes defined as hilar, celiac, periduodenal, peripancreatic, superior mesenteric node groups); M0: no distant metastasis; M1: distant metastasis present.

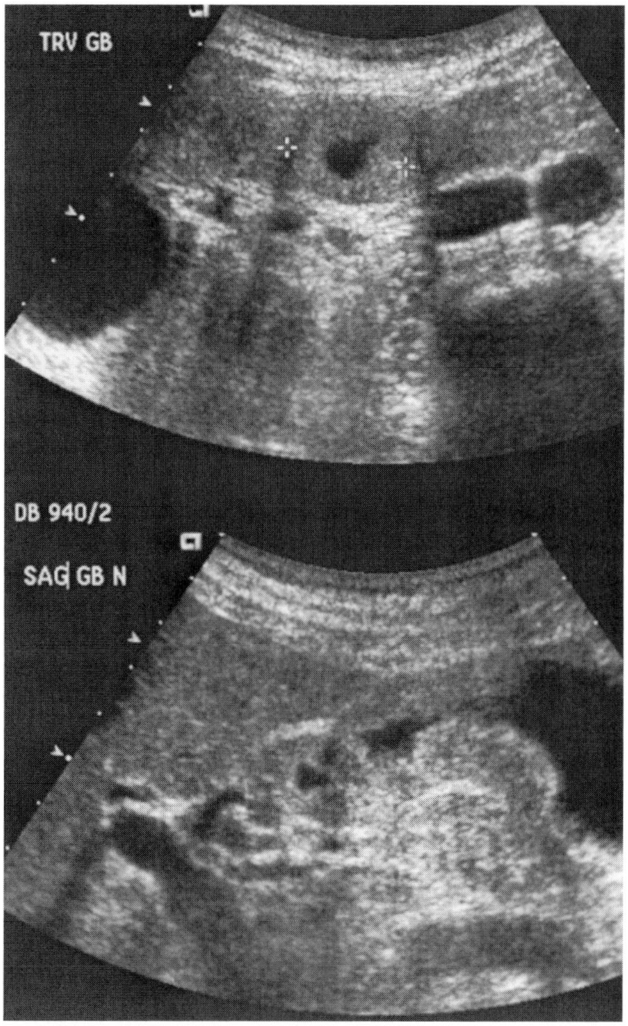

Figure 35–1. Ultrasound of gallbladder cancer. The images demonstrate asymmetric wall thickening of the body and neck of the gallbladder. (Courtesy of the Department of Radiology, Brigham & Women's Hospital, www.brighamrad.harvard.edu.)

cation of EUS in patients with a gallbladder mass can help in determining whether the mass is nonneoplastic (e.g., cholesterol pseudopolyp) or neoplastic. In addition, EUS-guided biopsy is an effective technique in cases in which a tissue diagnosis is required.

Computed tomographic (CT) scanning should be performed on all patients suspected of having gallbladder cancer. Findings of gallbladder cancer include a mass protruding into the gallbladder lumen or completely replacing the gallbladder and focal or diffuse thickening of the gallbladder wall (Fig 35–2). CT scanning also offers information on the presence or absence of distant metastases, regional lymph node involvement, and local invasion into the liver and porta hepatis.

Magnetic resonance imaging (MRI) and magnetic resonance cholangiopancreatography (MRCP) can offer additional information on local invasion, particularly into the porta hepatis. These tests are used selectively if CT findings are equivocal. Similarly, endoscopic or percutaneous cholangiography is not indicated routinely; these procedures are used primarily for palliation or preoperative management of obstructive jaundice.

SURGICAL THERAPY

Surgical resection is the only known curative form of therapy for gallbladder cancer. For patients in whom surgical exploration is contraindicated because of medical comorbidities or evidence of unresectable disease on imaging studies (e.g., metastatic disease), a percutaneous or endoscopic needle biopsy can be obtained to confirm the diagnosis. For patients in whom surgery is planned, a preoperative biopsy is contraindicated because gallbladder cancer has a propensity for dissemination along needle tracts.

Recommendations for extent of surgical resection according to disease stage are given in the following subsections. Specific technical issues are discussed subsequently.

Stages 0 and IA

For Tis (carcinoma in situ) and T1 (stage IA, cancer invasion that does not extend beyond the gallbladder muscularis) lesions, the available retrospective data suggest that simple cholecystectomy is sufficient in most cases. These lesions are detected most frequently on pathologic examination of gallbladders removed for presumed benign disease. Patients diagnosed with gall-

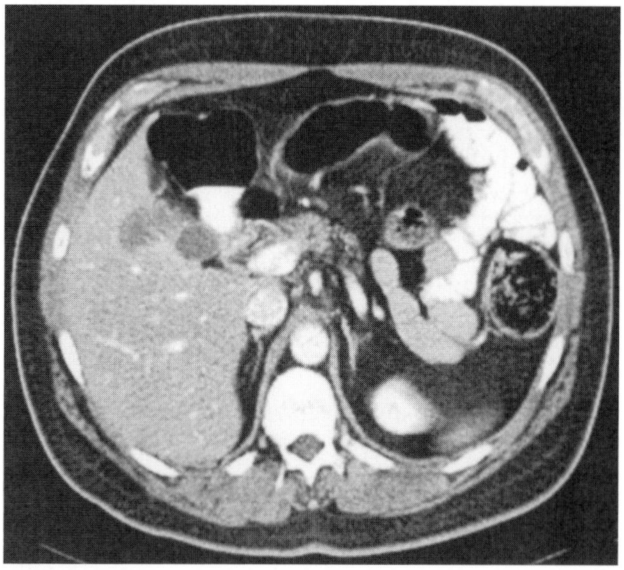

Figure 35–2. CT scan of gallbladder cancer. The image shows a 3.5 × 4 cm lesion arising from the gallbladder fundus and extending into segment 5 of the liver.

bladder cancer in this manner should undergo formal imaging-based staging, and the cholecystectomy specimen should be examined carefully to ensure that all margins are negative for cancer. Patients with imaging studies that reveal no evidence of residual or metastatic gallbladder cancer who are found to have a cystic duct margin that is positive for cancer should undergo reexploration with excision of the common bile duct, regional lymphadenectomy, and hepaticojejunostomy. In contrast, patients with negative margins and negative imaging studies who undergo no additional treatment for their gallbladder cancer have excellent outcomes that are unlikely to be improved by radical surgery.[6]

Stage IB

Patients found to have a T2 (cancer invasion into the perimuscular connective tissues of the gallbladder) lesion should undergo radical resection. Simple cholecystectomy usually is performed using a subserosal dissection plane and hence may leave positive margins in the gallbladder fossa. Indeed, reexploration reveals residual tumor in 40–76% of these patients.[7] In addition, the probability of regional lymph node metastasis in patients with T2 gallbladder cancer has been reported to range from 28–63%.[8] These findings provide a rationale for performing reexploration with liver resection and regional lymphadenectomy of the hepatoduodenal ligament. There is convincing, albeit retrospective, evidence that such radical surgery is associated with improved survival for patients with T2 gallbladder cancer.[8,9] Given the propensity of gallbladder cancer to seed wound sites, reexcision of all surgical wounds, including laparoscopic port sites, during reexploration traditionally has been recommended. However, reexcising port sites can be difficult (the trajectory through which ports had traversed the abdominal wall during the initial operation may be impossible to determine at the time of definitive surgery), and the value of this practice is unproven.

Patients suspected of having a T2 or more advanced gallbladder lesion preoperatively should undergo exploration with en bloc resection of the gallbladder and adjacent liver to a depth of at least 2 cm in addition to regional lymphadectomy of the hepatoduodenal ligament. Although a nonanatomic liver resection encompassing the gallbladder fossa can be applied at the time of reexploration or en bloc with the gallbladder during the initial procedure, anatomic resection of liver segments 4b and 5 may be associated with less intraoperative bleeding.

Stage II

A role for aggressive surgical resection of some stage II gallbladder cancers is being recognized increasingly. This stage includes T3 lesions (locally advanced cancers that perforate the gallbladder serosa or directly invade the liver and/or one adjacent organ) and T1–3 lesions associated with regional lymph node metastasis.

Surgery for patients with T3 lesions requires careful planning and must be tailored to individual patients. For some patients with liver invasion, hepatic resections encompassing segments 4b and 5 may be sufficient. However, because the gallbladder fossa bridges both the right and left hepatic lobes, trisegmentectomy often is required. Adjacent organs, such as the hepatic flexure of the colon, should be resected en bloc. Long-term survival rates ranging from 15–63% have been reported from some centers to be associated with these extended procedures for T3 lesions.[8] However, other centers have reported less favorable results.[8] Furthermore, the associated perioperative mortality rates have been reported to be as high as 18%.[8]

The value of radical surgery for patients with lymph node metastasis remains controversial. In some reports, 5-year survival rates among patients having undergone radical resection for lymph node–positive gallbladder cancer reach 60%.[10] However, other contemporary series report no long-term survivors among patients with lymph node metastases.[8]

Stages III and IV

Stage III (invasion of the main portal vein, common hepatic artery, or multiple extrahepatic organs) and stage IV (distant metastasis) disease meets criteria for unresectability. Anecdotal reports exist of super-radical procedures involving resection of the main portal vein and/or common hepatic artery exist, but these procedures are associated with substantial morbidity and mortality rates and are unlikely to confer any survival benefits.

If stage III disease is discovered at the time of exploration, radiopaque clips should be placed at the sites of gross tumor involvement to facilitate radiation treatment planning. There are no data to support the application of debulking cholecystectomy to prevent subsequent episodes of cholecystitis; we do not recommend it.

SURGICAL TECHNIQUE

For patients suspected of having resectable gallbladder cancer, we begin surgical exploration with laparoscopy. In the absence of disseminated disease, we proceed with open laparotomy. Because of the risk for gallbladder perforation and tumor spillage, we recommend against laparoscopic cholecystectomy in patients suspected of having gallbladder cancer. We also recommend early conversion to open laparotomy in patients undergoing laparoscopic cholecystectomy for presumed benign disease in whom the suspicion of gallbladder cancer arises intraoperatively.

We use a right subcostal incision because it can be extended easily to a chevron incision if necessary. We then conduct a thorough examination for metastases, especially in the liver and on the peritoneal surfaces. For patients in whom the suspicion of gallbladder cancer is low at this point, a simple cholecystectomy is done, and the gallbladder is examined using frozen-section analysis. Confirmation of T2 or T3 tumor should prompt radical resection, as described below. If the diagnosis based on frozen-section analysis is ambiguous (i.e., the presence of gallbladder cancer cannot be confirmed), radical surgery should be deferred. For patients in whom the suspicion of gallbladder cancer is high because of the presence of a firm mass, we obtain a small biopsy of the lesion. If the diagnosis of gallbladder cancer is confirmed on frozen-section analysis, the gallbladder is resected en bloc with the adjacent liver, as described below. Although determining depth of cancer invasion can be difficult on frozen sections, these grossly apparent cancers are likely to be T2 or more advanced lesions.

If radical resection is indicated, we then perform a Kocher maneuver to mobilize the duodenum and the head of the pancreas. Enlarged retropancreatic, celiac, superior mesenteric, or para-aortic lymph nodes are sampled and subjected to frozen-section analysis.

Presence of metastasis in lymph nodes beyond the regional ones (N1) is a contraindication to aggressive resection.

We then perform regional lymphadenectomy. We skeletonize the common bile duct (CBD) and common hepatic duct, hepatic artery, and portal vein from the superior border of the duodenum to the liver hilum. During this dissection, lymph node–bearing fibrofatty tissues are swept toward the gallbladder and removed as a specimen. Tumor invasion of the portal vasculature is assessed during this dissection. We do not perform major vascular resection for advanced gallbladder cancer at our institution.

In contrast, we do resect the CBD if the gallbladder cancer has invaded this structure. CBD resection also may facilitate resection of bulky nodal disease in the hepatoduodenal ligament. The CBD is transected at the superior border of the duodenum, and its distal stump is oversewn with a nonabsorbable monofilament suture. The proximal bile duct stump is also ligated at this point to prevent spillage of bile and cancer cells that may be present in the bile.

We then perform en bloc resection of the gallbladder and the adjacent liver (or the liver resection alone if the patient already has undergone cholecystectomy). If the CBD has not been transected, the cystic duct is divided near its junction with the CBD. Similarly, the cystic artery is ligated and divided near its origin. For T2 cancers, either a nonanatomic wedge resection of the liver that encompasses the gallbladder fossa to a depth of 2 cm or anatomic resection of liver segments 4b and 5 is acceptable (Fig 35–3). The capsule of the liver is scored with electrocautery to mark the resection plane. Overlapping chromic liver sutures then are placed around the periphery of the resection plane for hemostasis and retraction. The liver parenchyma then is transected using one of the standard methods (we usually use a combination of electrocautery and argon-beam laser coagulation). Care should be taken near the base of the liver resection margins to avoid injuring the right hepatic artery as it traverses inferiorly in the gallbladder fossa.

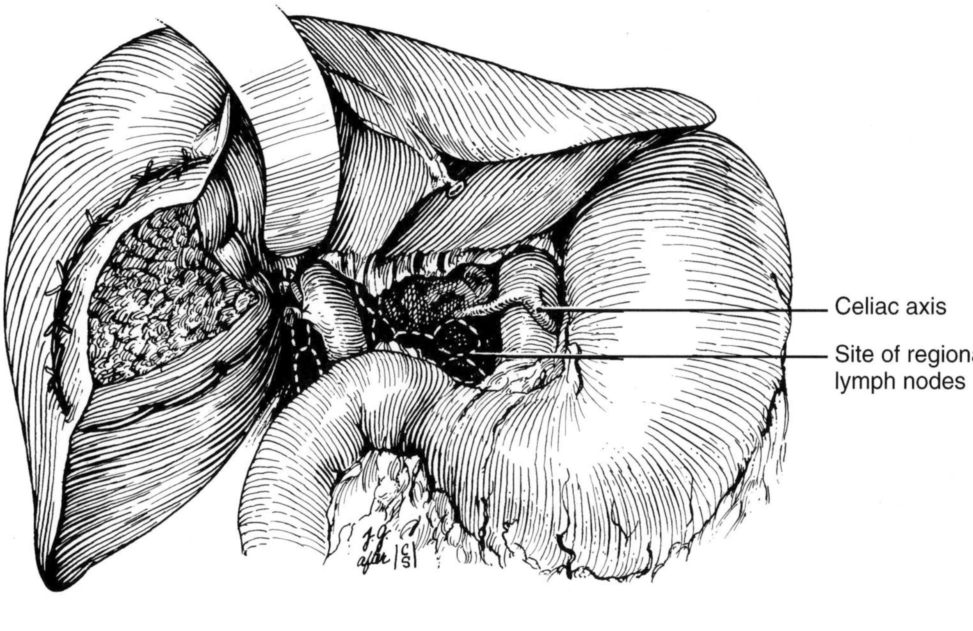

Figure 35–3. Radical resection of gallbladder cancer. This illustration depicts the operative field after radical cholecystectomy has been performed. The hatched line denotes the regions included in the lymphadenectomy.

If the CBD has been resected, a 60-cm Roux-en-Y limb of jejunum is used to create a hepaticojejunostomy. The anastomosis is constructed using a single layer of 5-0 absorbable sutures.

ADJUVANT THERAPIES

Adjuvant chemoradiotherapy is administered commonly after resection of gallbladder cancers. External-beam or intraoperative radiation therapy alone or in combination with 5-flourouracil (5-FU) is associated with diminished rates of local recurrence. The impact of these regimens on survival is unclear; no data derived from prospective, randomized clinical trials on the efficacy of these regimens exist.

PALLIATION

The goals of palliative therapy are relief of pain, of manifestations of biliary obstruction (e.g., pruritus and cholangitis), and of bowel obstruction. Given the limited expected survival duration of patients diagnosed with unresectable gallbladder cancer (weeks to months), endoscopic or percutaneous stenting rather than surgical bypass generally is recommended for relief of symptomatic biliary obstruction (Figs 35–4 and 35–5). Biliary stents are discussed in greater detail below in the section on palliation of bile duct cancers.

Palliative radiation therapy, regional intra-arterial chemotherapy, systemic chemotherapy, and chemoradiotherapy each have been applied in patients with advanced gallbladder cancer. The most commonly used chemotherapeutic agents in this setting are gemcitabine with either cisplatin or 5-FU/leucovorin. However, the value of any of these approaches in either locally advanced or metastatic gallbladder cancer has yet to be demonstrated in prospective, randomized clinical trials.

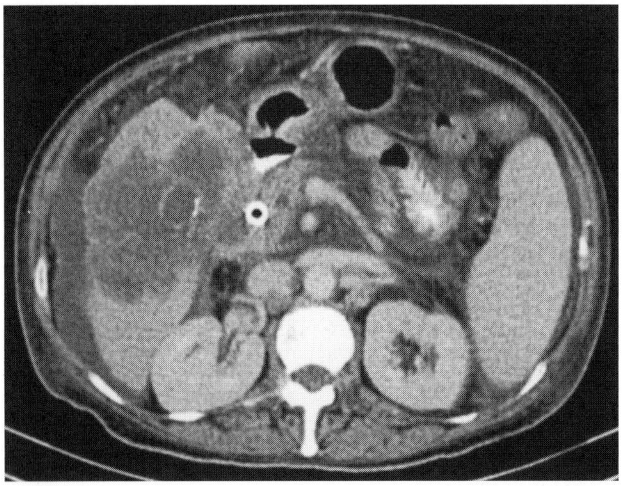

Figure 35–4. CT scan of advanced gallbladder cancer. The image demonstrates an advanced gallbladder cancer with extensive liver invasion. A stent has been placed for palliation of obstructive jaundice.

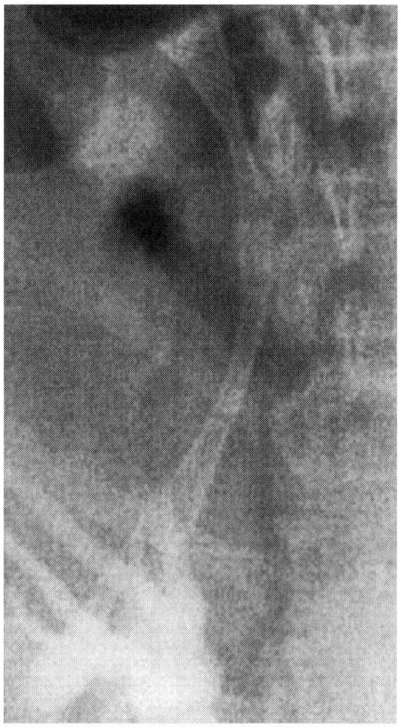

Figure 35–5. Palliation of gallbladder cancer. This radiograph depicts a Wallstent that has been placed for palliation of obstructive jaundice in a patient with advanced gallbladder cancer.

OUTCOMES

Data derived from the National Cancer Database support the nihilistic view traditionally associated with gallbladder cancer.[11] In these population-based data, 5-year survival rates for patients with T1N0, T2N0, and T3N0 (or node-positive) disease are 39%, 15%, and 5%, respectively.

However, contemporary surgical series suggest that substantially improved outcomes can be achieved by the application of surgical resection of gallbladder cancers.[12] In these reports, 5-year survival rates following resection of T1 lesions range from 85–100%. With radical resection of T2, T3, and T4 lesions, reported 5-year postoperative survival rates range from 80–90%, 15–63%, and 2–25%, respectively. Radical resection of node-positive disease has been reported to be associated with 5-year survival in as high as 60% of patients, although one recently reported series contained no patients who survived 2 or more years among those with lymph node metastasis.[8,10]

Reported morbidity and mortality rates associated with resection of gallbladder cancers range from 5–54%

and from 0–21%, respectively. In general, the highest morbidity and mortality rates are associated with series describing more extensive resections. The median survival associated with unresectable gallbladder cancer is less than 6 months.

■ BILE DUCT CANCER

EPIDEMIOLOGY

In this discussion, the term *cholangiocarcinoma* is used interchangeably with *bile duct cancer* and is used to denote cancers arising in the intrahepatic or extrahepatic biliary tree, exclusive of the ampulla of Vater and gallbladder. Approximately 5000 new cases of cholangiocarcinoma are diagnosed annually in the United States.[13] Most patients are diagnosed in the fifth through the seventh decades of life. Unlike gallbladder cancer, for which there is a clear female predominance, the incidence bile duct cancer is slightly greater in males than in females.

Although most patients diagnosed with cholangiocarcinoma have no identifiable predisposing factors, several conditions clearly increase the risk of developing this cancer (Table 35–3). In Western countries, primary sclerosing cholangitis (PSC) is the most important risk factor; indeed, approximately 30% of cases of cholangiocarcinoma in the West are diagnosed in patients with PSC. Among patients with PSC, the estimated lifetime incidence of cholangiocarcinoma ranges from 10–15%, with an annual incidence of 0.6–1.5%.[13] In addition, cholangiocarcinoma tends to be diagnosed at an earlier age (third through fifth decades of life) in patients with PSC than in the general population.

In Asian countries, infestation with the liver flukes *Opisthorchis viverrini* or *Clonorchis sinensis* and hepatolithiasis are important factors for cholangiocarcinoma. Other risk factors include choledochal cysts, Caroli's disease, and exposure to the radiologic contrast agent Thorotrast. Increased risk has been reported for workers in the auto, rubber, chemical, and wood-finishing industries and among patients with hepatitis C viral infection. Two genetic conditions (Lynch sydrome II and multiple biliary papillomatosis) have been identified as increasing the risk of bile duct cancer.

TABLE 35–3. RISK FACTORS FOR BILE DUCT CANCER

Primary sclerosing cholangitis
Liver flukes infestation (*Opisthorchis viverrini* and *Clonorchis sinensis*)
Choledochal cysts
Caroli's disease
Hepatolithiasis
Chemicals (e.g., Thorotrast and Dioxin)
Hepatitis C
Lynch syndrome II
Bile duct adenoma and multiple biliary papillomatosis

PATHOGENESIS AND PATHOLOGY

Malignant transformation in the bile duct epithelium, as in other regions of the gastrointestinal tract, is hypothesized to arise in association with a stepwise accumulation of genetic abnormalities. A range of mutations and other abnormalities involving oncogenes (e.g., K-*ras*, c-*myc*, c-*neu*, c-*erbB*-2, and c-*met*) and tumor suppressor genes (e.g., *p53*) have been reported to be prevalent in bile duct cancers; the biologic and clinical significance of these abnormalities remains to be characterized.[13]

Greater than 90% of bile duct cancers are adenocarcinomas. Other cancer types include squamous cell carcinoma, small cell carcinoma, and sarcoma. Adenocarcinomas of the bile duct are classified as sclerosing, nodular, or papillary (analogous to the classification scheme for gallbladder adenocarcinomas). Sclerosing (scirrous) tumors, which comprise over 80% of cholangiocarcinomas, are associated with an intense desmoplastic reaction, tend to be highly invasive, and are associated with low resectability rates. Nodular tumors have the appearance of constricting annular lesions and are also associated with low resectability rates. Papillary tumors are rare and present as bulky masses that project into the bile duct lumen. Because these lesions tend to cause symptomatic obstructive jaundice relatively early in their progression, they are associated with higher resectability rates than sclerosing or nodular tumors.

Cholangiocarcinomas are also classified into three groups according to their anatomic location: (1) intrahepatic or peripheral (10%), (2) perihilar (65%), and (3) distal (25%). The transition between perihilar and distal locations occurs where the common bile duct becomes a retroduodenal structure. Bile duct tumors involving the hepatic duct bifurcation are known as *Klatskin tumors*. An additional anatomic classification system for perihilar cholangiocarcinomas, originally proposed by Bismuth,[14] is useful in surgical planning (Table 35–4).

Cholangiocarcinomas arising in the intrahepatic bile ducts are staged in a manner similar to that of hepatocellular carcinoma[15] (Table 35–5). The TNM staging for extrahepatic cholangiocarcinomas is shown in Table 35–6.[16]

TABLE 35–4. CLASSIFICATION OF PERIHILAR BILE DUCT CANCERS ACCORDING TO ANATOMIC LOCATION

Type I: Tumors below the confluence of the left and right hepatic ducts
Type II: Tumors reaching the confluence
Type IIIa/IIIb: Tumors involving common hepatic duct and either the right or the left hepatic duct, respectively
Type IV: Tumors that are multicentric or involve the confluence and both the right and left hepatic ducts

CLINICAL PRESENTATION AND DIAGNOSIS

Intrahepatic cholangiocarcinomas typically present with nonspecific symptoms, such as abdominal pain, anorexia, weight loss, and malaise. Another mode of presentation for these cancers is the incidental detection of intrahepatic masses either on physical examination or on imaging studies. The most common presentation of extrahepatic cholangiocarcinomas is painless jaundice. Other manifestations of biliary obstruction, such as acholic stools, dark urine, and pruritus, also are prevalent. Abdominal pain, fatigue, malaise, and weight loss can occur with advanced disease. Signs of advanced bile duct cancer include right upper quadrant abdominal tenderness, hepatomegaly, and a palpable gallbladder. Cholangitis is unusual in the absence of prior biliary tract instrumentation.

The differential diagnosis for patients with these presentations includes primary and metastatic hepatobiliary and pancreatic neoplasms and benign biliary strictures due to conditions such as PSC, choledocholithiasis, Mirizzi's syndrome, and postoperative strictures.

In patients with intrahepatic cholangiocarcinoma, laboratory studies usually reveal an increased alkaline phosphatase level in the setting of normal bilirubin levels. In patients with extrahepatic cholangiocarcinoma, laboratory tests usually are consistent with the presence of obstructive jaundice. Tumor markers (e.g., CEA, CA 19-9, and CEA in combination with CA 19-9) may have utility in surveillance of patients with PSC; however, their sensitivities and specificities are too low for them to be applicable to screening or diagnosis in the general population.

Transabdominal ultrasonography is a useful initial test for patients with obstructive jaundice. Dilatation of the biliary tree in the absence of choledocholithiasis suggests a possible biliary or pancreatic malignancy and should prompt contrast-enhanced spiral CT scanning. CT scan findings of intrahepatic cholangiocarcinomas include a liver mass with or without peripherally dilated ducts (Fig 35–6). With perihilar cholangiocarcinomas, the primary tumor may not be visualized; their presence is suggested by the detection of dilated intrahepatic bile ducts (often bilateral), a normal or collapsed gallbladder (if the site of biliary obstruction is proximal to the cystic duct–bile duct confluence), a normal-caliber distal common bile duct, and a normal pancreas. Findings of distal cholangiocarcionomas include dilation of intra-

TABLE 35–5. TNM STAGING OF INTRAHEPATIC BILE DUCT CANCERS

Stage I	T1	N0	M0
Stage II	T2	N0	M0
Stage IIIA	T3	N0	M0
Stage IIIB	T4	N0	M0
Stage IIIC	Any T	N1	M0
Stage IV	Any T	N0–1	M1

NOTE: T1: solitary tumor without vascular invasion; T2: solitary tumor with vascular invasion or multiple tumors, each ≤ 5 cm in diameter; T3: multiple tumors >5 cm in diameter or tumor invasion of a major branch of the portal or hepatic vein(s); T4: direct tumor invasion of adjacent organs other than the gallbladder or with perforation of visceral peritoneum; N0: no regional lymph node metastasis; N1: regional lymph node metastasis present (hilar, hepatoduodenal ligament, and caval lymph node groups); M0: no distant metastasis; M1: distant metastasis present.

TABLE 35–6. TNM STAGING OF EXTRAHEPATIC BILE DUCT CANCERS

Stage 0	Tis	N0	M0
Stage IA	T1	N0	M0
Stage IB	T2	N0	M0
Stage IIA	T3	N0	M0
Stage IIB	T1–3	N1	M0
Stage III	T4	N0–1	M0
Stage IV	Any T	N0–1	M1

NOTE: Tis: carcinoma in situ; T1: cancer confined to bile duct wall; T2: cancer invades beyond wall of bile duct; T3: cancer invades liver, pancreas, and/or left or right branches of portal vein or hepatic artery; T4: cancer invades main portal vein or both its left and right branches, common hepatic artery, or other structures, such as colon, stomach, duodenum, or abdominal wall; N0: no regional lymph node metastasis; N1: regional lymph node metastasis present (regional lymph nodes consist of hilar, celiac, periduodenal, peripancreatic, and superior mesenteric groups); M0: no distant metastasis; M1: distant metastasis present.

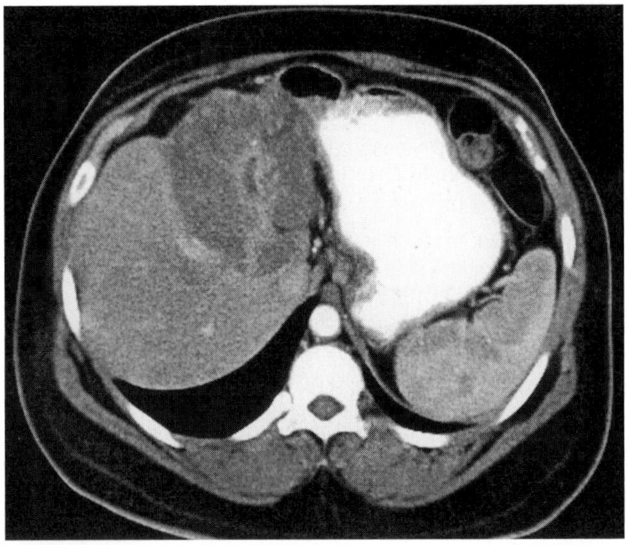

Figure 35–6. CT scan of intrahepatic cholangiocarcinoma. The image shows an intrahepatic cholangiocarcinoma primarily involving the left lobe of the liver.

and extrahepatic bile ducts and the gallbladder, with or without a mass in the head of the pancreas. In addition to offering information on the site of the primary lesion, the CT scan offers valuable information necessary for staging and planning of therapies, including the presence or absence of local vascular invasion, of regional lymphadenopathy, of distant metastasis, and of liver atrophy. Unilobar bile duct obstruction typically results in atrophy of the affected liver lobe together with hypertrophy of the unaffected lobe (atrophy-hypertrophy complex). Absence of the atrophy-hypertrophy complex can suggest vascular encasement by tumor.

For patients who are surgical candidates, an important goal of the preoperative evaluation is determining the proximal and distal tumor extent. If CT scanning fails to demonstrate the tumor itself (as is usually the case for resectable perihilar cholangiocarcinomas), additional imaging is helpful in surgical planning. In most centers, distal tumors are assessed by endoscopic retrograde cholangiopancreatography (ERCP) (Fig 35–7), whereas intrahepatic and perihilar tumors are best assessed by percutaneous transhepatic cholangiography (PTC). Recently, there has been increasing application of MRCP in this setting. Unlike conventional cholangiography, MRCP is noninvasive and does not require contrast material to be injected in the biliary ductal system. It also allows for visualization of the bile ducts both proximal and distal to a stricture. Some recent reports suggest that MRCP, when applied to patients with cholangiocarcinoma, offers information equivalent to that offered by CT scanning and traditional cholangiography combined.[17] For these reasons, MRCP has been supplanting traditional cholangiography in the evaluation of patients with suspected cholangiocarcinoma in some centers. Whether the initial experience with MRCP at these select centers is generalizable remains to be determined.

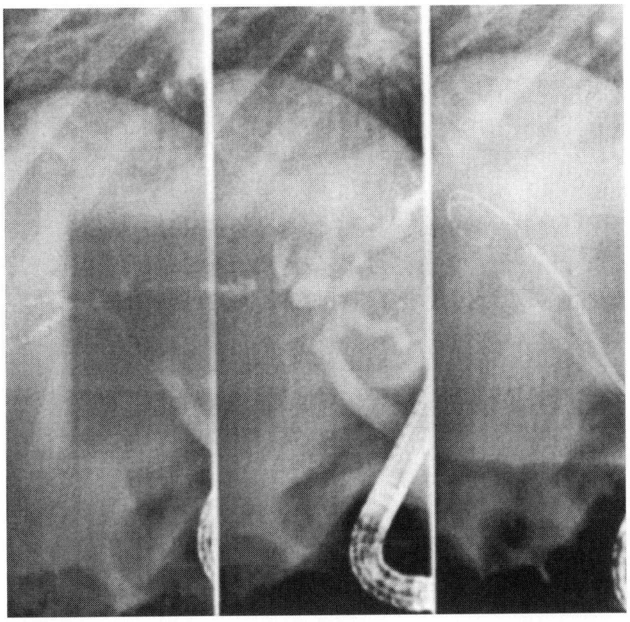

Figure 35–7. ERCP of hilar cholangiocarcinoma. The images depict a stricture at the confluence of the hepatic ducts in a patient with a Klatskin tumor.

Additional studies are not indicated routinely. Endoscopic ultrasonography (EUS) offers greater sensitivity than CT scanning in the detection of small periampullary tumors; there is little data with respect to the detection of perihilar and intrahepatic cholangiocarcinomas. The role of positron-emission tomographic (PET) scanning in the evaluation of patients with cholangiocarcinoma continues to be studied but is not yet established. If surgery is not planned, tissue diagnosis can be obtained through endoscopic or percutaneous biopsy. If surgical exploration is planned, a preoperative biopsy is not indicated.

SURGICAL THERAPY

As is the case for gallbladder cancer, complete surgical resection is the only potentially curative therapy for patients with cholangiocarcinoma. Therefore, all patients suspected of having cholangiocarcinoma should be offered exploration unless contraindications to surgical resection exist. These contraindications include (1) major comorbidities precluding safe surgery, including cirrhosis, (2) metastatic disease, (3) invasion of the main portal vein or hepatic artery proximal to their bifurcations, (4) bilateral invasion of portal vein and/or hepatic artery branches, (5) bilateral hepatic duct involvement (up to secondary radicles bilaterally), and (6) unilateral duct and/or vessel involvement with contralateral liver lobe atrophy.

The utility of preoperative biliary stenting in patients with cholangiocarcinoma is controversial. Available retrospective data suggest that among patients undergoing pancreaticoduodenectomy for periampullary cancers, routine preoperative biliary stenting is associated with increased perioperative morbidity rates, especially with respect to infectious complications. Therefore, we do not recommend routine preoperative stenting for patients with distal bile duct cancers. Instead, selective application of stenting in patients with obstructive jaundice who will experience significant delay until surgery is performed (e.g., those undergoing neoadjuvant therapy) is appropriate. However, this experience should not be extrapolated to patients with perihilar cholangiocarcinomas, for whom the relationship between preoperative stenting and operative outcomes is less clear. Some authors believe that stents placed preoperatively make intraoperative assessment of tumor extent more difficult.

In our experience, bilateral Ring catheters placed percutaneously into the left and right biliary systems shortly before the time of surgery greatly facilitate the resection of perihilar cholangiocarcinomas. Our approach is described in detail below.

SURGICAL TECHNIQUE

Resectable intrahepatic cholangiocarcinomas are treated using standard liver resections, and distal cholangiocarcinomas are treated by pancreaticoduodenectomy. These procedures are discussed elsewhere in this textbook. The following discussion focuses on our surgical approach to resectable perihilar cholangiocarcinomas.

We begin with exploratory laparoscopy to rule out the presence of disseminated disease that may have eluded detection on preoperative imaging. Recent reports suggest that 25–30% of patients undergoing laparoscopic exploration for cholangiocarcinoma are found to have unresectable disease during laparoscopy.[18] If laparoscopic examination fails to reveal metastasis, we proceed with laparotomy through either an upper midline or a right subcostal incision (that can be extended to the left as necessary). We then conduct a thorough examination for the presence of distant metastases. Enlarged regional lymph nodes are biopsied and subjected to frozen-section analysis. The presence of metastasis in lymph nodes beyond the regional ones (N1) is a contraindication to radical resection.

Next, we lower the hilar plate by incising the liver capsule at the base of the quadrate lobe (segment 4) between the gallbladder fossa and the umbilical fissure (Fig 35–8). This maneuver facilitates inspection of the porta hepatis. At this point we palpate the tumor in an attempt to assess its proximal and distal extent.

We then begin mobilization of the extrahepatic biliary tree from its surrounding structures. The gallbladder is mobilized, and the CBD is dissected circumferentially just proximal to where it assumes a retroduodenal location. We transect the CBD at this level and oversew the stump of the distal CBD with a nonabsorbable monofilament suture. We then dissect the extrahepatic biliary tree off the underlying vascular structures, starting distally and working proximally (Fig 35–9). During this step, cephalad and anterior traction is applied to the gallbladder, distal CBD, and distal ends of the preoperatively placed Ring catheters (which in combination form a convenient handle that can be grasped). The bile duct and surrounding lymph node–bearing soft tissues should be cleared en bloc from the portal vein and the hepatic artery. Only after this step is accomplished is the possibility of tumor vascular invasion definitely eliminated.

The most difficult step in this dissection is usually encountered at the hepatic duct bifurcation, the site of Klatskin's tumors. Dissection here is facilitated by plac-

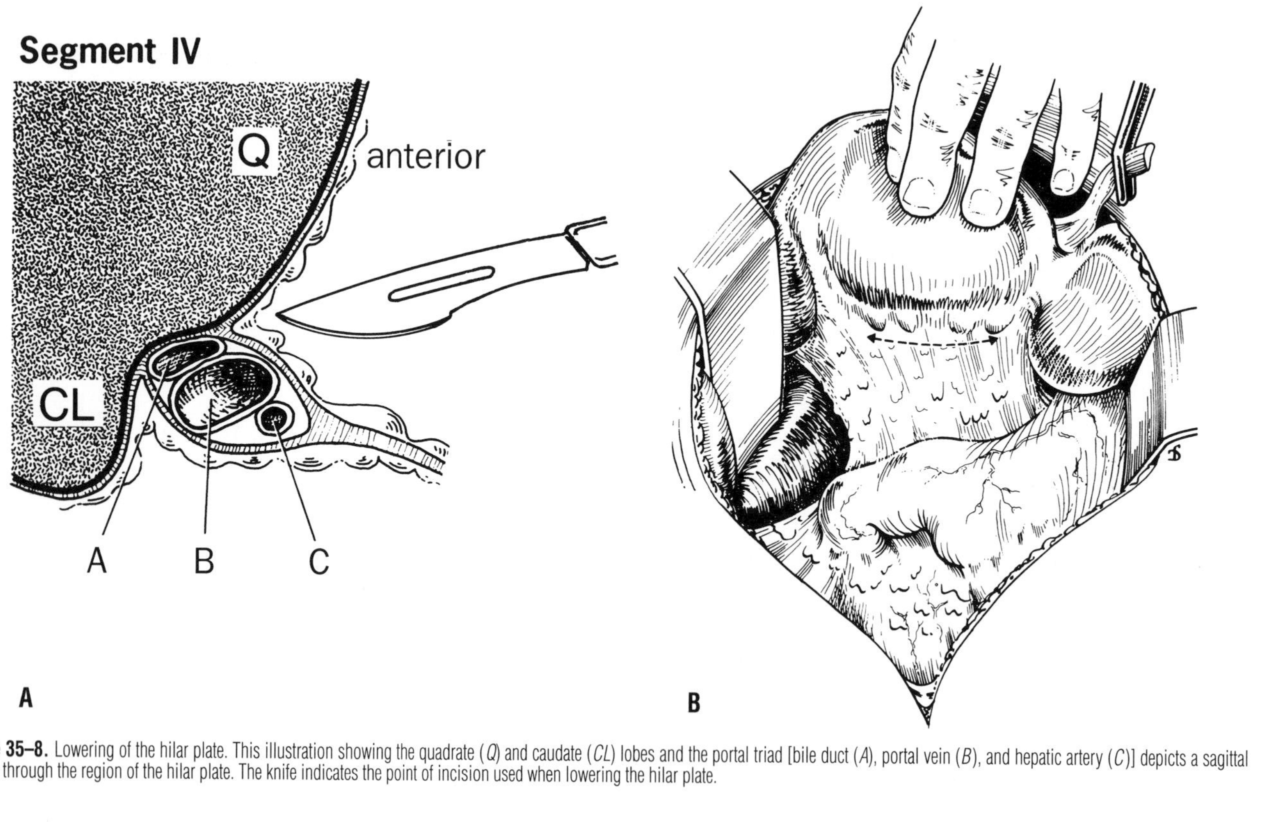

Figure 35–8. Lowering of the hilar plate. This illustration showing the quadrate (*Q*) and caudate (*CL*) lobes and the portal triad [bile duct (*A*), portal vein (*B*), and hepatic artery (*C*)] depicts a sagittal section through the region of the hilar plate. The knife indicates the point of incision used when lowering the hilar plate.

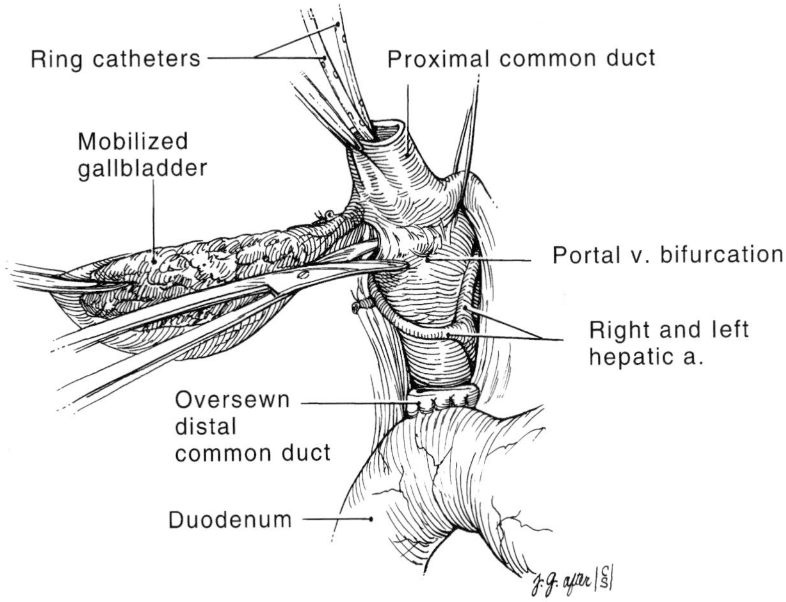

Figure 35–9. Resection of hilar cholangicarcinoma. This illustration shows the extrahepatic biliary tree being dissected off of the anterior surface of the portal vein. The dissection proceeds in a cephalad direction following transection of the distal bile duct.

ing vessel loops around the left and right hepatic ducts and placing them on traction as necessary. Because the left duct typically runs along the undersurface of the liver (segment 4) for a longer distance than the right duct, it is usually easier to dissect the left duct first and encircle it with a vessel loop prior to dissecting the right duct. We find that the Ring catheters are particularly helpful in the identification of the right and left hepatic ducts during this stage of the procedure. The resection is completed by transecting the biliary duct(s) proximal to the tumor (Fig 35–10). Frozen sections of the proximal and distal margins should be checked intraoperatively, with the goal of achieving negative microscopic margins (R_0 resection).

Reconstruction following resection of Klatskin's tumors consists of bilateral hepaticojejunostomies to a 60-cm retrocolic Roux-en-Y limb of jejunum. Small secondary or tertiary biliary branches should be incorporated into the anastamoses or ligated. Prior to performing the anastamoses, the Ring catheters are replaced with soft Silastic catheters (usually 14–18F) (Fig 35–11). Catheter exchange is performed as follows: The Silastic catheters are placed over the distal ends of the cut Ring catheters (the portions protruding from the transected bile ducts), and the Ring and Silastic catheters are sewn together with cross-sutures. The Ring catheters then are pulled proximally through the intrahepatic biliary tree and out the surface of the liver with the Silastic catheters attached. Finally, the Ring catheter is removed. If Ring catheters have not been placed preoperatively, the Silastic catheters can be placed as follows: Randall stone forceps are inserted into the intrahepatic biliary tree through the transected bile ducts and out the liver surface. The Silastic catheters then are sewn to the "eyelet" at the end of the forceps and pulled back down the duct. This maneuver is repeated so that a Silastic cather is present in each of the right and left biliary systems.

The hepaticojejunostomies are created using a single layer of interrupted 5-0 absorbable monofilament sutures (Fig 35–12). The posterior row of sutures is placed but not tied until the entire row can be "parachuted" closed. Using cautery, two small openings in

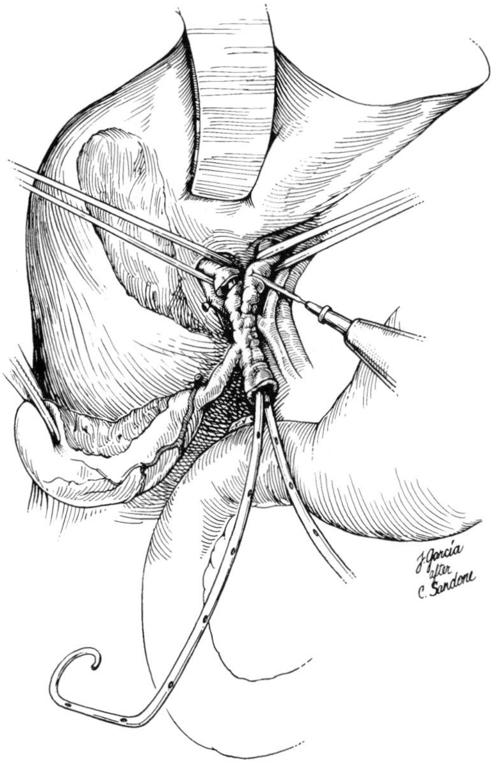

Figure 35–10. Transection of proximal bile ducts. This illustration depicts the transection of the left and right hepatic ducts proximal to the hilar cholangiocarcinoma. Note the vessel loops around each of the hepatic ducts and the Ring catheters.

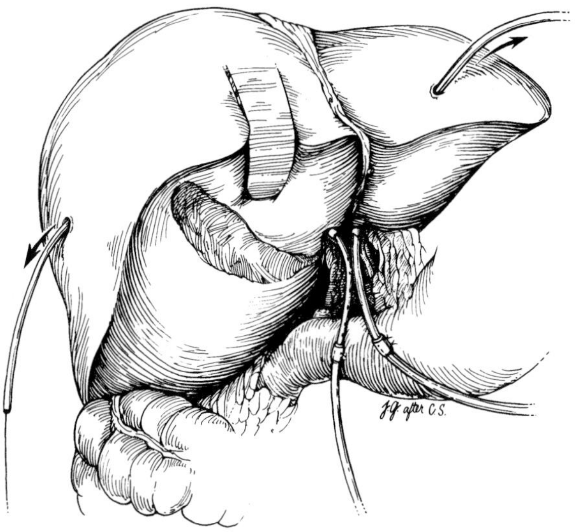

Figure 35–11. Replacement of biliary stents. Following completion of the resection, the Ring cathers are exchanged for Silastic catheters, as described in the text.

the distal portion of the Roux limb are made, through which the distal ends of the Silastic catheters are placed. The anterior row of sutures then is placed and tied to complete the anastomosis (Fig 35–13).

We then suture the roux limb to the undersurface of the liver and to the mesocolon. We suture two large radiopaque clips to the surface of the liver at the sites where each of the Silastic tubes exits. These clips serve as permament markers of the exit sites and allow for radiologic visualization of the relationship between the liver surface and the last radiopaque marker on the Silastic catheters.

Recently, more aggressive approaches that include routine application of liver resection and portal vein resection in select patients are being reported with increasing frequency. Addition of hepatic lobectomy can extend the possibility of R_0 resection to patients with Bismuth type III lesions (Fig 35–14). Because Bismuth type II and III tumors may involve the caudate lobe ducts, some authors recommend routine caudate lobectomy when resecting these lesions. Although the highest 5-year postoperative survival rates have been reported from centers using such aggressive surgical approaches, these extended procedures should be done only if they can be performed with low perioperative morbidity and mortality rates. In addition, some centers have reported the application of preoperative portal vein embolization to induce lobar hypertrophy and thereby extend the limits of liver resection in patients at risk of developing hepatic insufficiency postoperatively. To date, this approach has not been demonstrated conclusively to improve clinical outcomes and is not recommended for routine practice.

Finally, orthotopic liver transplantation has been applied to patients with intrahepatic and perihilar cholangiocarcinomas. However, cancer recurrence is seen in over 50% of patients, and 5-year survival rates average only 22%. Long-term survivors have been reported; most of these patients had small, peripheral cholangiocarcinomas discovered incidentally. For patients with known cholangiocarcinoma, liver transplantation should not be offered outside the context of a research protocol.

ADJUVANT THERAPIES

Adjuvant chemotherapy, radiotherapy, or chemoradiotherapy is offered commonly, based on results of retrospective series. However, clear efficacy data derived from prospective, randomized clinical trials are lacking. Similarly, neoadjuvant therapy, associated with anecdotal reports of tumor response sufficient to permit margin-negative resection in patients with advanced cholangiocarcinoma, needs to be studied further.

PALLIATION

The major goal of palliation is relief of symptoms of biliary obstruction. Endoscopic or percutaneous biliary stenting is associated with less morbidity than surgical biliary bypass and therefore is recommended except in patients who are found to have unresectable disease at the time of surgical exploration or those in whom nonsurgical stenting cannot be accomplished. Endoscopic stenting is the preferred approach for dis-

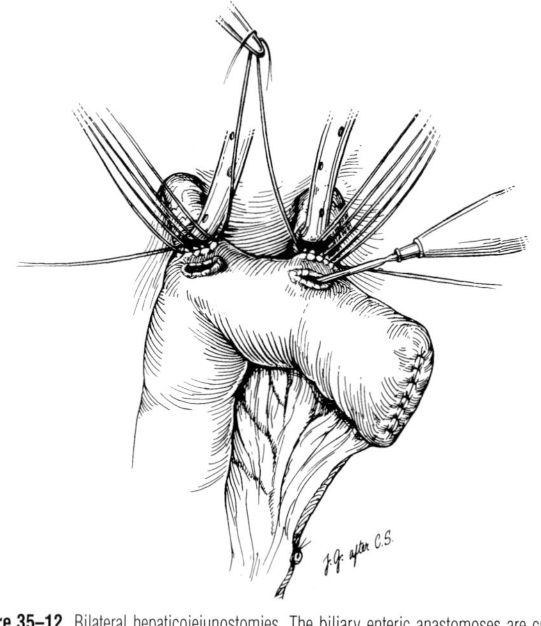

Figure 35–12. Bilateral hepaticojejunostomies. The biliary enteric anastomoses are created, starting with the posterior row of sutures.

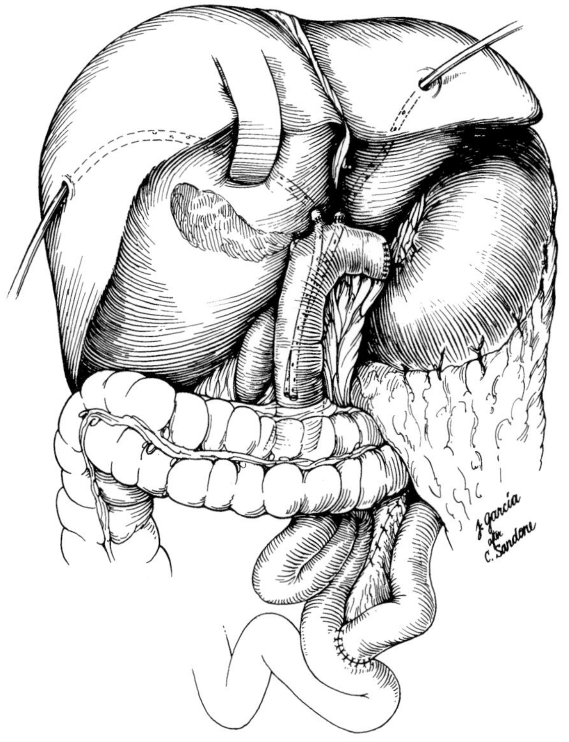

Figure 35–13. Completed reconstruction. This illustration depicts the operative field following completion of the bilateral hepaticojejunostomies.

tal bile duct cancers; proximal cancers are more difficult to stent endoscopically and usually require a percutaneous approach.

Patients with a Bismuth type I hilar cholangiocarcinoma usually are palliated effectively with a single biliary stent. Patients with Bismuth types II, III, and IV hilar cholangiocarcinomas may require two or more separate stents to decompress the entire biliary tree and prevent obstruction-related cholangitis. However, in a prospective, randomized, controlled trial of patients with hilar cholangiocarcinoma, unilateral biliary drainage was found to provide adequate palliation of obstructive jaundice; patients randomized to receive bilateral biliary stents had higher complication rates (cholangitis) but no detectable benefits.[18] The approach therefore needs to be individualized.

Metal stents tend to provide more durable palliation than plastic (polyethylene) stents (median stent patencies of 8–12 months versus 4.8 months) and generally are preferable in patients with malignant biliary obstruction. Plastic stents should be changed every 3–6 months to prevent episodes of cholangitis related to stent occlusion; these stents may be appropriate for patients with estimated survival durations of less than 3 months (e.g., patients with diffuse metastases).

For patients who are found to have carcinomatosis at the time of exploratory laparoscopy, laparoscopic cholecystectomy traditionally has been recommended to prevent subsequent development of acute cholecystitis related to biliary stent–induced cystic duct obstruction. The value of prophylactic cholecystectomy in this setting is unproven, and the procedure should be performed only if it can be done safely. Stenting should be performed using percutaneous or endoscopic techniques postoperatively.

For patients who are found to have unresectable disease at the time of open exploration, available retrospective evidence suggests that surgical biliary bypass offers more durable palliation than percutaneous or

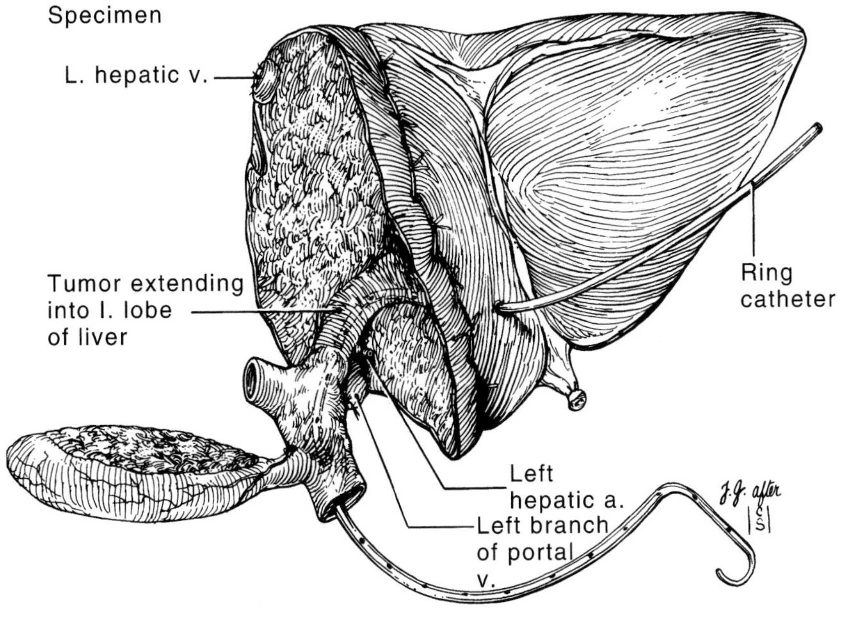

Figure 35–14. Extended resection of hilar cholangiocarcinoma. This illustration depicts of the resection specimen following removal of the extrahepatic bile duct en bloc with the left lobe of the liver.

endoscopic stenting. Patients with unresectable distal cholangiocarcinoma should undergo choledocho- or hepaticojejunostomy. The palliative options for patients with unresectable perihilar cholangiocarcinoma include (1) tumor debulking with Roux-en-Y hepaticojejunostomy and intraoperative placement of Silastic transhepatic catheters (as described earlier) and (2) Roux-en-Y hepaticojejunostomy using the segment 3 or 4 duct. Segment 3 or 5 bypass is used in patients with advanced perihilar cholangiocarcinoma with predominantly right- or left-sided disease, respectively. The segment 3 hepatic duct is approached by following the falciform ligament into the recess of the left lobe in the umbilical fissure (Fig 35–15). Localization of the segment 5 duct is difficult because no external anatomic landmarks exist, and considerable parenchymal dissection often is necessary. Intraoperative ultrasonography considerably facilitates this procedure. These unilateral bypasses should be avoided in the presence of ipsilateral liver lobe atrophy, a finding that indicates limited functional hepatic parenchyma.

External-beam radiation and transcatheter brachytherapy may contribute to pain relief and biliary decompression; however, the data on the effects of radiation on survival duration are conflicting. Palliative chemotherapy regimens include agents such as 5-FU/leucovorin alone or with gemcitabine, gemcitabine plus cisplatin, and gemcitabine alone. Clear efficacy in prolonging survival has not been demonstrated for any of these regimens.

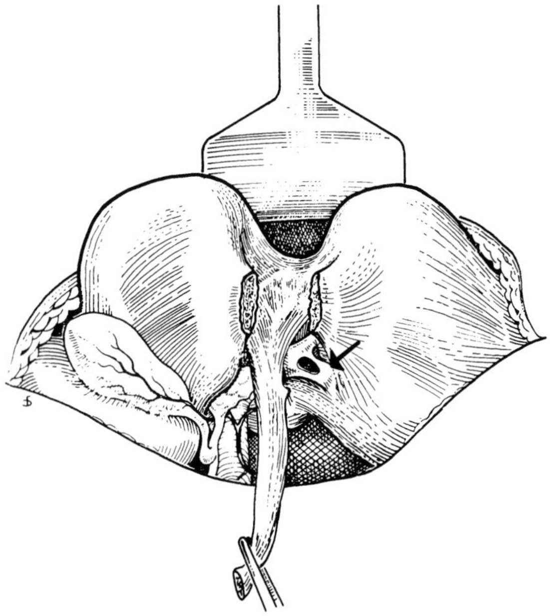

Figure 35–15. Segment 3 bypass. This illustration depicts the approach to the segment 3 duct (*arrow*) to which a Roux-en-Y limb of jejunum can be anastomosed for palliation of obstructive jaundice in patients with advanced perihilar cholangiocarcinoma primarily affecting the right biliary system.

Finally, photodynamic therapy (PDT), in which endoscopic application of light activates a photosensitizer, leading to local cell death, has been associated with promising results. One prospective, randomized trial in which 19 patients with advanced cholangiocarcinoma were randomized to stenting alone or stenting followed by PDT was terminated prematurely because patients randomized to the PDT arm were found to have a significantly longer survival (493 versus 98 days median survival) in addition to improved biliary drainage and quality of life.[20] Additional study of this modality is warranted.

OUTCOMES

Fewer than 50% of patients diagnosed with perihilar cholangiocarcinoma are able to undergo curative resection. Reported 5-year postoperative survival rates for patients with these cancers are highly variable; they range from 8% to greater than 50%.[17] In general, the highest survival rates are associated with series containing a high proportion of cases in which R_0 resection was achieved. Series containing the highest R_0 resection rates (>75% of cases in some published experiences) tend to be reported by institutions where liver resection is applied liberally to patients with cholangiocarcinoma.[17] A caveat that should be remembered is that these same series also tend to be associated with the highest perioperative mortality rates (up to 10% in some cases).

For patients with intrahepatic cholangiocarcinoma, reported 3-year survival rates following curative resection with negative margins range from 22–66%. For patients with distal cholangiocarcinoma, 5-year survival rates following pancreaticoduodenectomy range from 15–25% in most reported series. Among patients with node-negative disease, 5-year postoperative survival rates as high as 54% have been reported. Median survival durations associated with unresctable cholangiocarcinomas, regardless of anatomic location, range from 5–8 months.

REFERENCES

1. Wistuba II, Gazdar AF. Gallbladder cancer: lessons from a rare tumour. *Nature Rev Cancer* 2004;4:695
2. Misra S, Chaturvedi A, Misra NC, et al. Carcinoma of the gallbladder. *Lancet Oncol* 2003;4:167
3. Pandey M, Shukla VK. Lifestyle, parity, menstrual and reproductive factors and risk of gallbladder cancer. *Eur J Cancer Prevent* 2003;12:269
4. Elnemr A, Ohta T, Kayahara M, et al. Anomalous pancreaticobiliary ductal junction without bile duct dilatation in gallbladder cancer. *Hepatogastroenterology* 2001; 48:382

5. American Joint Committee on Cancer (AJCC), Greene FL, Page DL, Fleming ID, et al (eds), *Cancer Staging Manual,* 6th ed. New York: Springer-Verlag; 2002:139
6. Wakai T, Shirai Y, Yokoyama N, et al. Early gallbladder carcinoma does not warrant radical resection. *Br J Surg* 2001;88:675
7. Bartlett DL, Fong Y, Fortner JG, et al. Long-term results after resection for gallbladder cancer: Implications for staging and management. *Ann Surg* 1996;224:639
8. Ito H, Matros E, Brooks DC, et al. Treatment outcomes associated with surgery for gallbladder cancer: A 20-year experience. *J Gastrointest Surg* 2004;8:183
9. Fong Y, Jarnagin W, Blumgart LH. Gallbladder cancer: Comparison of patients presenting initially for definitive operation with those presenting after prior noncurative intervention. *Ann Surg* 2000;232:557
10. Chijiiwa K, Noshiro H, Nakano K, et al. Role of surgery for gallbladder carcinoma with special reference to lymph node metastasis and staging using Western and Japanese classification systems. *World J Surg* 2000;24:1271
11. Donohue JH, Stewart AK, Menck HR. The National Cancer Data Base report on carcinoma of the gallbladder, 1989–1995. *Cancer* 1998;83:2618
12. Dixon E, Vollmer C, Sahajpal A, et al. An aggressive surgical approach leads to improved survival in patients with gallbladder cancer. *Ann Surg* 2005;241:385
13. Lazaridis KN, Gores GJ: Cholangiocarcinoma. *Gastroenterology* 2005;128:1655
14. Bismuth H, Nakache R, Diamond T. Management strategies in resection for hilar cholangiocarcinoma. *Ann Surg* 1992;215:31
15. American Joint Committee on Cancer (AJCC), Greene FL, Page DL, Fleming ID, et al (eds), *Cancer Staging Manual,* 6th ed. New York: Springer-Verlag; 2002:131
16. American Joint Committee on Cancer (AJCC), Greene FL, Page DL, Fleming ID, et al (eds), *Cancer Staging Manual,* 6th ed. New York: Springer-Verlag; 2002:145
17. Clary B, Jarnigan W, Pitt H, et al. Hilar cholangiocarcinoma. *J Gastrointest Surg* 2004;8:298
18. Weber SM, DeMatteo RP, Fong Y, et al. Staging laparoscopy in patients with extrahepatic biliary carcinoma: Analysis of 100 patients. *Ann Surg* 2002;235:392
19. De Palma GD, Galloro G, Siciliano S, et al. Unilateral versus bilateral endoscopic hepatic duct drainage in patients with malignant hilar biliary obstruction: Results of a prospective, randomized, and controlled study. *Gastrointest Endosc* 2001;53:547
20. Ortner M, Caca K, Berr F, et al. Successful photodynamic therapy for nonresectable cholangiocarcinoma: A randomized, prospective study. *Gastroenterology* 2003; 125:1355

IX

PANCREAS

36

Management of Acute Pancreatitis

Thomas E. Clancy ▪ *Stanley W. Ashley*

Acute pancreatitis includes a wide spectrum of disease, from one with mild self-limiting symptoms, to fulminant processes with multiorgan failure and high mortality. Of the approximately 185,000 patients who develop acute pancreatitis each year in the United States, most experience relatively minor episodes of disease characterized by mild parenchymal edema without distant organ dysfunction and an uneventful recovery.[1] Severe episodes, however, may involve a progression to extensive pancreatic necrosis, development of the systemic inflammatory response syndrome (SIRS), multiorgan failure, rapid clinical deterioration, and even death.[2,3] Although the overall mortality rate for acute pancreatitis is 2–10%, this is related primarily to the 10–30% of patients with severe disease characterized by pancreatic and peripancreatic necrosis.

Given the wide spectrum of disease seen, the care of patients with pancreatitis must be highly individualized. Patients with mild acute pancreatitis generally can be managed with resuscitation and supportive care. Etiologic factors are sought and treated, if possible, but operative therapy essentially has no role in the care of these patients. Those with severe and necrotizing pancreatitis require intensive therapy, which may include wide operative débridement of the infected pancreas or surgical management of local complications of the disease. The precise indications for surgery in patients with pancreatitis have evolved in recent years. Whereas early aggressive débridement was used commonly for all patients with pancreatic necrosis in the past, now most pancreatic surgeons have adopted a more conservative algorithm of selective and delayed pancreatic débridement.[4,5] This chapter reviews current management strategies in acute pancreatitis, with particular attention to assessment of disease severity, timing and routes of supplemental nutrition, the role of prophylactic antibiotics, indications for and timing of surgery, methods of pancreatic débridement for necrotizing pancreatitis, and the role of endoscopic and minimally invasive techniques.

▪ ETIOLOGY

Acute pancreatitis has been attributed to a wide range of etiologic factors, some rare and rather obscure (Table 36–1). Intra-acinar activation of trypsinogen, with subsequent activation of other pancreatic enzymes, is thought to play a central role in the pathogenesis of the disease. Furthermore, ischemia-reperfusion injury is believed to be critical to disease progression. A local inflammatory response in the pancreas is associated with the liberation of oxygen-derived free radicals and cytokines including interleukin 1 (IL-1), IL-6, and IL-8; tumor necrosis factor a (TNF-α); and platelet-activating factor; these mediators play an important role in the transformation from a local inflammatory response to a systemic illness.

Approximately 80% of cases are associated with cholelithiasis or sustained alcohol abuse; the relative frequency of these two factors depends on the prevalence of alcoholism in the population studied. Of the mechanical causes of pancreatitis, choledocholithiasis is certainly the most common. The majority of nonalcoholic patients with acute pancreatitis will have gallstones on

TABLE 36–1. ETIOLOGIC FACTORS IN ACUTE PANCREATITIS

METABOLIC
Alcohol
Hyperlipoproteinemia
Hypercalcemia
Drugs
Genetic
Scorpion venom
MECHANICAL
Cholelithiasis
Postoperative
Pancreas divisum
Post-traumatic
Retrograde pancreatography
Pancreatic duct obstruction: pancreatic tumor, ascaris infestation
Pancreatic ductal bleeding
Duodenal obstruction
VASCULAR
Postoperative (cardiopulmonary bypass)
Periarteritis nodosa
Atheroembolism
INFECTION
Mumps
Coxsackie B
Cytomegalovirus
Cryptococcus

examination, and between 36% and 63% will develop recurrent acute pancreatitis if stones persist. Approximately 1% of patients undergoing endoscopic retrograde cholangiopancreatography (ERCP) develop clinically detectable pancreatitis. Several metabolic processes are associated with pancreatitis, particularly alcohol abuse. Symptoms and signs of pancreatitis are recognized in between 1% and 10% of alcoholic patients, usually after 10 years or more of heavy ingestion. The precise mechanism of this association is not well established but may be related to changes in pancreatic exocrine secretion and calculus formation in the pancreatic ducts. Several drugs are causally related to pancreatitis, particularly corticosteriods, thiazide diuretics, estrogens, azathioprine, and furosemide. Furthermore, in approximately 10% of cases, no underlying cause can be indentified. Some investigators have suggested that occult biliary microlithiasis may be the etiology in a majority of cases of idiopathic acute pancreatitis.[6]

■ DIAGNOSIS, STAGING, AND SEVERITY

The early diagnosis and precise staging of disease severity are important goals in the initial evaluation and management of pancreatitis. Pancreatitis not only must be differentiated from a myriad of other potential diagnoses, but patients also must be stratified to identify those with severe disease and to guide appropriate therapy. Unfortunately, despite our increased understanding of the pathophysiology of pancreatitis, diagnostic tools for pancreatitis have not changed much in recent years. Clinical signs and symptoms of pancreatitis, such as upper abdominal pain, back pain, vomiting, fever, tachycardia, and leukocytosis, are relatively nonspecific. Periumbilical and flank bruising may be seen with severe and hemorrhagic pancreatitis (Cullen and Grey-Turner signs), but these uncommon clinical signs are not pathognomonic of severe pancreatitis and are seen with any cause of retroperitoneal bleeding. Diagnosis therefore typically depends on a high level of clinical suspicion and the demonstration of elevated plasma concentrations of pancreatic enzymes. Levels of both amylase and lipase peak within the first 24 hours of symptoms, and amylase has a slightly shorter half-life in plasma. As a result, lipase levels may have a slightly greater sensitivity, particularly when measured late (>24 hours) after initial presentation.[7] Hyperamylasemia is neither specific for pancreatitis[8] nor perfectly sensitive because normal amylase levels have been described in some patients with acute pancreatitis.[9] Other pancreatic enzymes have not been shown to have any advantage over amylase and lipase for diagnostic purposes. Of note, plasma levels of pancreatic enzymes serve a purely diagnostic and not prognostic role; absolute levels have no direct correlation with disease severity. A common misconception is that amylase and lipase levels only slightly elevated above normal are associated with mild disease; in fact, such low levels also may be associated with severe disease.

Identification of patients with severe pancreatitis is crucial early in the course of the disease so that early goal-directed therapy may be instituted. However, an objective, reproducible, and universally accepted measure of disease severity is still lacking.[10] Early clinical evaluation is complicated by a relatively nonspecific presentation, and severe disease may present with a fulminant sepsis-like syndrome or in a manner that is deceptively innocuous. Initial signs and symptoms of necrotizing pancreatitis are only different in degree from edematous pancreatitis; likewise, both severe and mild forms of disease share the same etiologies.[11] Despite considerable experimental effort to identify differences in the pathogenesis of edematous and necrotizing pancreatitis,[12] no available clinical model is successful at predicting which patients will progress to severe disease.

Clinical scoring systems for pancreatitis, such as the Ranson[13] (Table 36–2) and Glasgow[14] scores, use multiple clinical variables to predict outcomes in groups of patients with acute pancreatitis. Patients are evaluated at admission and again during the subsequent 48 hours using de-

TABLE 36–2. THE RANSON SCORE: EARLY PROGNOSTIC SIGNS THAT CORRELATE WITH THE RISK OF MAJOR COMPLICATIONS OR DEATH IN ACUTE PANCREATITIS

At admission or diagnosis
1. Age over 55 years
2. White blood cell count over 16,000/mL
3. Blood glucose level over 200 mg/dL (100 mmol/L)
4. Serum lactic dehydrogenase concentration (LDH) > 350 IU/L
5. Serum glutamic oxaloacetic transaminase (SGOT) > 250 sigma-Frankel units/dL
During initial 48 hours
1. Hematocrit decrease > 10%
2. Blood urea nitrogen (BUN) increase > 5 mg/dL
3. Serum calcium level < 8 mg.dL (2 mmol/L)
4. Arterial PO_2 < 60 mmHg (8 kPa)
5. Base deficit > 4 mEq/L (4 mmol/L)
6. Estimated fluid sequestration > 6000 mL

mographic and laboratory parameters; the number of positive prognostic signs then is used to predict subsequent morbidity and mortality. In Ranson's report from the 1970s, for instance, the presence of five or six positive signs was associated with 40% mortality and prolonged intensive-care unit (ICU) stay in 50% of patients, whereas the presence of seven or eight signs was associated with virtually 100% mortality. Although these scoring systems are relatively successful in predicting disease severity, they require 48 hours from admission for full assessment. Furthermore, while higher scores suggest poorer outcomes, these scoring systems have not been reassessed adequately to reflect the substantial improvements in critical care since their introduction over two decades ago.[15]

The Acute Physiology and Chronic Health Evaluation II (APACHE II) score is another physiologic scoring system that attempts to estimate disease severity based on quantifying the degree of abnormality of multiple physiologic variables. Though not specific for pancreatitis and somewhat cumbersome to use, the APACHE II system is as accurate at 24 hours as other systems at 48 hours, and it is now therefore regarded as perhaps the optimal scoring system to assess disease severity in pancreatitis.[10] Twelve physiologic variables are measured and weighed based on their degree of abnormality: temperature, mean arterial pressure, heart rate, respiratory rate, arterial oxygen tension (PaO_2), arterial pH, serum sodium, serum potassium, serum creatinine, hematocrit, white blood cell count, and Glasgow coma scale. The score is determined from the most deranged physiologic value measured, and further points are added for increased age and chronic organ dysfunction. Unlike other systems, the APACHE II score may be recalculated continuously through the course of the disease. APACHE II scores also have been identified as prognostically important not only at admission but also after subsequent interventions such as pancreatic débridement.[16] The newer APACHE III system uses an additional five physiologic variables to improve accuracy, although the newer system may be less useful than the APACHE II score in distinguishing mild from severe pancreatitis.[17] A recent modification of the APACHE II system that includes a clinical assessment of obesity (APACHE-O score) has been suggested to further improve predictive accuracy, with a positive predictive value of 74%.[18] All versions of this scoring system are somewhat unwieldy for use with most patients and are more appropriately applied to critically ill patients.

Numerous individual markers have been investigated as possible indicators of prognosis in pancreatitis in both laboratory and clinical settings. With few exceptions, these have not gained widespread clinical application. Banks[19] and others[20] have shown that hemoconcentration predicts parenchymal necrosis, as well as the presence of organ failure, in acute pancreatitis. C-reactive protein (CRP) assays are readily available, and levels rise with disease severity. Based on the trajectory of CRP levels, however, this marker is useful to identify severe disease only 48 hours after the onset of symptoms.[21] Other inflammatory mediators such as IL-8 and IL-6 have shown promise as early indicators of severe disease but await general availability and further clinical validation.[22] Other inflammatory markers, including TNF soluble receptors, polymorphonuclear (PMN) elastase, serum procalcitonin, soluble IL-2 receptors, and soluble E-selectin, have shown potential in the investigative setting but await the availability of reproducible assays as well as clinical validation prior to their use as prognostic indicators.[23]

Trypsinogen-activating peptide (TAP) is an additional marker that may be useful in determining prognosis in acute pancreatitis. TAP is released, with activation of trypsinogen to trypsin, and plasma and urine levels are known to correlate with the severity of pancreatitis. However, the molecule is present in low concentrations in urine and is cleared rapidly from plasma. Recent data suggest that clinically useful TAP assays may be soon to come. Some authors have reported high sensitivity and specificity for elevated urinary TAP levels in severe pancreatitis.[24,25] Similarly, a recent report suggested that severe acute pancreatitis could be recognized with a sensitivity and specificity of 70% and 78%, respectively, using a plasma assay.[26]

Computed tomographic (CT) scans have proven invaluable in determining disease severity in acute pancreatitis. CT findings in pancreatitis include enlargement of the pancreas with loss of peripancreatic fat planes, areas of decreased density, and occasionally, the presence of fluid collections (Fig 36–1). The Balthazar scoring system and other similar grading systems have incorporated various CT findings such as pancreatic in-

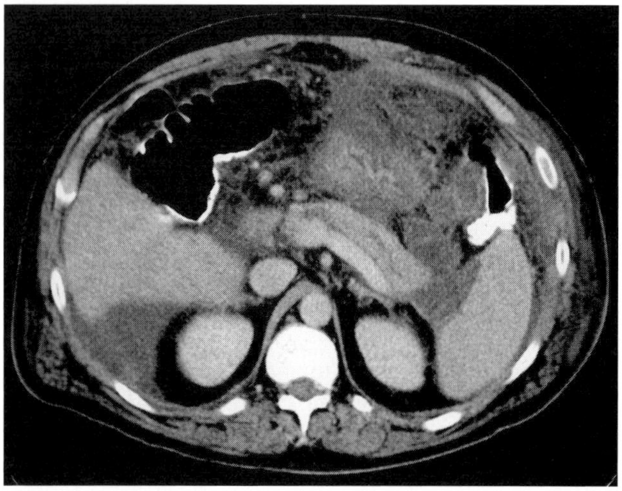

Figure 36–1. Contrast-enhanced abdominal CT scan in a 47-year-old man with acute pancreatitis. Relevant findings include significant fat stranding of the peripancreatic tissue, with a fluid collection at the tail of the pancreas measuring approximately 4 × 4 cm. Pancreatic parenchyma enhances with IV contrast, with no evidence of pancreatic necrosis. (Reprinted from Clancy TE, Benoit EP, Asley SW. Current management of acute pancreatitis. *J Gastrointest Surg* 9:440–452, copyright © 2005, with permission from Elsevier.)

flammation and peripancreatic fluid collections to correlate radiographic appearance with morbidity and mortality.[27,28] The contrast-enhanced CT scan is perhaps most useful in its ability to demonstrate pancreatic necrosis. From a baseline of 30–50 HU, viable pancreas typically will enhance by more than 50 HU with the administration of intravenous contrast material. Nonviable pancreas, however, will show no such enhancement with intravenous contrast administration (Fig 36–2). Various criteria used to diagnose necrosis include nonenhancement of more than 30% of the pancreatic parenchyma or an area of greater than 3 cm of the pancreas that does not enhance.[29] The sensitivity and specificity for diagnosing pancreatic necrosis increase with greater degrees of pancreatic nonenhancement, and complications also have been shown to correlate with the degree of nonenhancement.[28] In the patient with moderate renal impairment or allergy to intravenous contrast material, magnetic resonance imagining (MRI) may be used as an alternative. MRI has been shown to have comparable sensitivity and specificity to contrast-enhanced CT for detecting severe acute pancreatitis,[30] although MRI is currently less practical for the critically ill patient.

Clinical judgment rather than strict criteria often guides the timing of and indications for CT scans in acute pancreatitis, and precise recommendations are not universally accepted. Early CT scans often fail to identify developing necrosis until such areas are better demarcated, which may become evident only 2 to 3 days after the initial clinical onset of symptoms. The use of CT scans to diagnose necrosis or to predict severity within the first 24 hours of illness therefore is not recommended. Some authors have cautioned against the widespread use of CT scans in the setting of acute pancreatitis based on limited experimental evidence suggesting that intravenous contrast material may exacerbate early pancreatic necrosis.[31] However, clinical evidence to support this phenomenon in humans is lacking. The sensitivity for identifying pancreatic necrosis using contrast-enhanced CT scan approaches 100% 4 days from diagnosis.[10] It is therefore reasonable to recommend an abdominal CT scan with oral and intravenous contrast material in patients with clinical and biochemical features of acute pancreatitis who do not improve after several days of conservative management. Follow-up scans may be obtained with any signs of clinical deterioration.

CT scans also have been instrumental in facilitating the early diagnosis of infected pancreatic necrosis. Despite an increasing trend toward nonoperative management of sterile pancreatic necrosis, as reviewed below, infection remains an absolute indication for intervention.[1] Unfortunately, the precise diagnosis of infected pancreatic necrosis can be difficult to make. It is not possible to differentiate infected from sterile pancreatic necrosis based only on clinical and laboratory data because organ failure, significant leukocytosis, and fever are seen in both cases. Emphysematous pancreatitis, the demonstration of gas within the pancreatic parenchyma, is diagnostic of infection but is seen uncommonly (Fig 36–3). Using image-guided precise aspiration of the necrotic pancreas, however, infected pancreatic necrosis can be diagnosed with a high degree of accuracy (Fig 36–4). CT-guided pancreatic aspi-

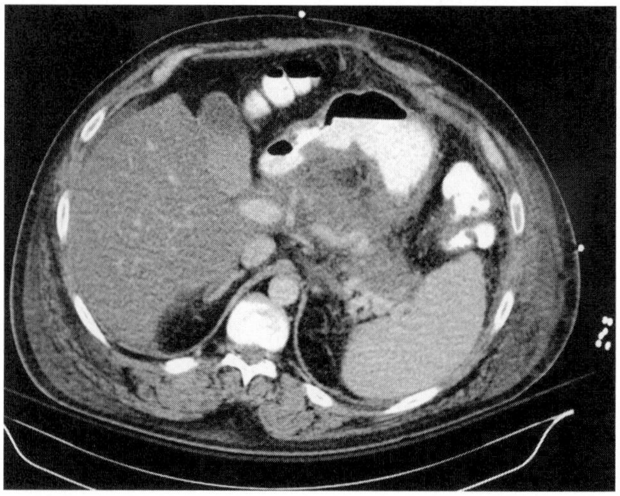

Figure 36–2. Contrast-enhanced abdominal CT scan in the same 47-year-old man with a second episode of acute pancreatitis. Scan shows stranding of peripancreatic fat consistent with acute pancreatitis. Most notable is the near-complete absence of pancreatic enhancement, diagnostic of pancreatic necrosis. (Reprinted from Clancy TE, Benoit EP, Asley SW. Current management of acute pancreatitis. *J Gastrointest Surg* 9:440–452, copyright © 2005, with permission from Elsevier.)

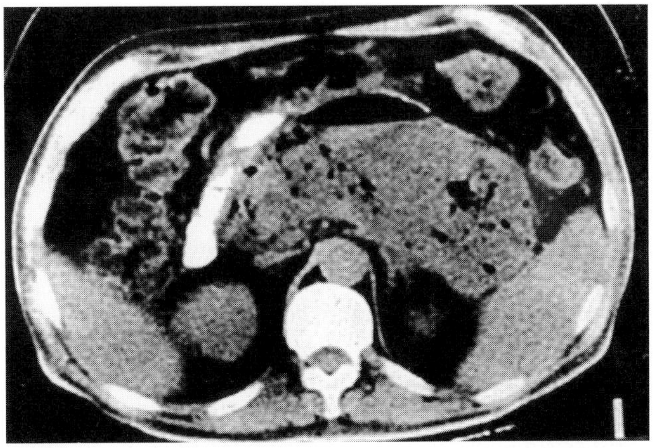

Figure 36–3. CT scan demonstrating emphysematous pancreatitis, pathognomonic for infected pancreatic necrosis. Operative débridement is indicated without additional confirmation of pancreatic infection.

ration usually is reserved for patients with documented pancreatic necrosis who are not improving clinically or who experience clinical decline. All patients should receive oral contrast material to opacify the gastrointestinal tract and avoid inoculating the pancreatic necrosum with gastrointestinal flora from an inadvertently perforated viscus.

The sensitivity and specificity for detection of infection using this method are reported as 96.2% and 99.4%, respectively, with a positive predictive value of 99.5% and a negative predictive value of 95.3%.[32] Areas of nonenhancing pancreas are aspirated under CT guidance, and samples are sent for aerobic, anaerobic, and fungal cultures. In most patients with infected necrosis, diagnosis may be made with a positive Gram's stain of the aspirate rather than waiting for confirmatory culture data. Gram's stains of the pancreatic aspirate are positive in most cases later documented to have infection, thus enabling rapid decision making.

Infection may occur at any point in the clinical course of a patient with pancreatic necrosis. The interval from presentation with necrosis to infection is variable, and the incidence of infection increases up to 3 weeks after presentation. In one study, infection was documented in 49% of patients in the first 14 days; less than 15% of patients had infection diagnosed after 35 days.[32] Infection may occur later in course of the disease, even after a prior negative aspiration. Repeat CT-guided aspirations therefore are necessary frequently in patients in whom a conservative strategy is adopted for sterile pancreatic necrosis until clinical improvement is documented. In a series at our institution with fine-needle aspirations (FNAs) demonstrating infection, the first aspirate was positive in 17 of 30 patients (57%); 7 patients (23%) required two procedures and 6 patients (20%) required three or more aspirations to demonstrate infection.[33]

▪ PRINCIPLES OF MANAGEMENT

RESUSCITATION AND MONITORING

Although patients with acute pancreatitis require management strategies specifically tailored to disease severity, the nonoperative management of acute pancreatitis has become increasingly standardized.[3,34–36] Aggressive fluid resuscitation is important to replenish extravascular, or "third space," fluid losses, which may be considerable. Intravenous fluids at rates of greater than 200 mL/h often are necessary to restore and maintain intravascular volume. This degree of fluid resuscitation is important to avoid systemic complications, particularly acute renal insufficiency, that may occur with hypovolemia. Furthermore, inadequate resuscitation has been shown recently to pose a significant risk for further pancreatic injury. Banks and colleagues have shown that while aggressive fluid resuscitation does not necessarily prevent the progression to pancreatic necrosis, patients with inadequate resuscitation have an increased risk of developing necrosis.[37] Close monitoring of respiratory, cardiovascular, and renal function is essential to detect and treat complications from hypovolemia. The degree and intensity of monitoring are tailored to disease severity. All patients require close assessment of fluid balance, including a Foley catheter. Monitoring for respiratory compromise and electrolyte imbalance is important in all, and any patient with severe disease should be admitted to an ICU with the capacity for continuous blood pressure and oxygen saturation monitoring. Intravenous narcotics often are essential for pain con-

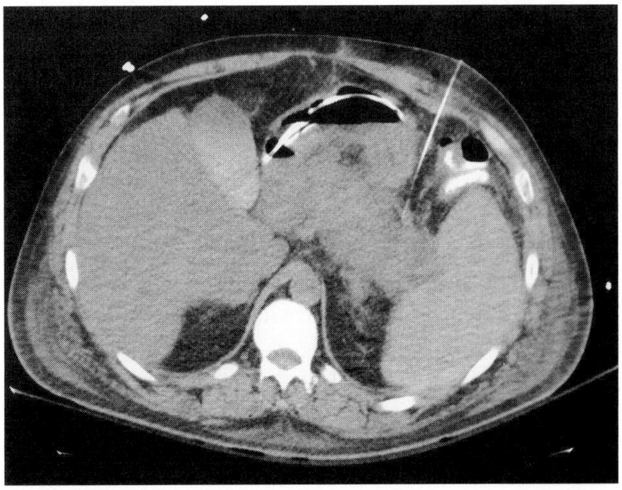

Figure 36–4. CT-guided percutaneous fine-needle aspiration of the pancreatic tail. The aspiration area had been identified previously as necrotic in the contrast-enhanced CT shown in Figure 36–2. Gram's stain and cultures were negative for organisms, consistent with sterile pancreatic necrosis. (Reprinted from Clancy TE, Benoit EP, Asley SW. Current management of acute pancreatitis. *J Gastrointest Surg* 9:440–452, copyright © 2005, with permission from Elsevier.)

trol in these patients. The use of nasogastric tubes to avoid pancreatic stimulation had been commonplace previously, although no clinical data support this practice, and the routine use of nasogastric suction probably should be abandoned. Paralytic ileus is not uncommon with acute pancreatitis, however, and nasogastric tubes should be used in this circumstance to prevent emesis and aspiration pneumonia.

NUTRITIONAL SUPPORT

Classic teaching in the management of pancreatitis has recommended the limitation of enteral feeding, theoretically to avoid stimulation of pancreatic exocrine function and thereby further pancreatic injury from release of proteolytic enzymes. Recent data, however, suggest that such strict limitations of enteral nutritrion may have been unnecessary. In mild cases of pancreatitis, brief periods without oral intake may be expected, and a full diet often is tolerated in several days with the resolution of pain. More severe cases of acute pancreatitis may have a prolonged disease course, hypercatabolic state, and ileus, which has led to a general use of parenteral nutrition in these patients.[38] Increasing evidence has accumulated to suggest that enteral nutrition may be feasible, safe, and even desirable in severe pancreatitis.[39] Enteral nutrition has the advantage of avoiding the high cost of total parenteral nutrition (TPN) as well as its associated catheter-related complications; furthermore, the use of enteral nutrition may support intestinal mucosal integrity and avoid the alterations to intestinal barrier function and intestinal permeability seen with TPN.[40] A small trial from 1997 randomized 38 patients with severe pancreatitis to TPN versus nasojejunal feeding.[41] In this cohort, enterally fed patients had significantly fewer septic and total complications. McClave and colleagues randomized 30 patients in a similar fashion and demonstrated only a trend toward fewer complications in the enterally fed group.[42] One significant advantage of enteral nutrition in this study was the lower cost; this was four times greater in the TPN group. Furthermore, Windsor and colleagues demonstrated that patients with pancreatitis randomized to enteral nutrition had significant improvement in CRP and APACHE II scores.[43] Recently, a larger study from China[44] randomized 96 patients with severe pancreatitis to TPN versus nasojejunal feeding. Measures of inflammation including CRP and IL-6 decreased earlier with enteral nutrition, as did APACHE II scores. Furthermore, mucosal permeability was improved, as inferred by urine endotoxin levels. Others have suggested that the addition of *Lactobacillus* preparations to enteral nutrition formulas may have a role in decreasing infectious complications in pancreatitis.[45] These studies all have involved nasojejunal feeding, although others have investigated the use of nasogastric feeding in pancreatitis. Investigators from Glasgow[46] have shown, in a nonrandomized cohort with severe pancreatitis, that nasogastric feeding is well tolerated in most patients. Whether this method is feasible and provides sufficient caloric support deserve further investigation.

A recent systematic review of the literature has concluded that there are insufficient data to definitively recommend preferential enteral nutrition in acute pancreatitis[47]; however, studies continue to accumulate demonstrating its safety and feasibility. The use of TPN will continue to have an important role in severe pancreatitis, particularly in patients with prolonged ileus. However, early enteral nutrition in the form of jejunal feeding should be considered for patients who will not resume oral intake early in the course of their disease.

THE ROLE OF ERCP

As noted earlier, the presence of gallstones leading to choledocholithiasis is recognized as a major cause of acute pancreatitis and the primary cause of acute pancreatitis in most populations. Endoscopic retrograde cholangiopancreatography (ERCP) therefore has been used as a diagnostic and potentially therapeutic modality in acute pancreatitis. The basis for selecting patients with pancreatitis who might benefit from ERCP lies predominantly in whether evidence exists for obstructive choledocholithiasis. The role of ERCP in cases of acute biliary pancreatitis with biliary obstruction or cholangitis is clear. Less obvious, however, is the role of early ERCP and papillotomy in acute biliary pancreatitis without evidence of obstruction. By randomizing patients with acute pancreatitis to early ERCP versus no ERCP, both Neoptolemos and colleagues[48] and Fan and colleagues[49] demonstrated a significant reduction in morbidity and nonsignificant trends to improved mortality with the routine use of ERCP. However, these studies were criticized for the inclusion of patients with known obstruction and cholangitis in the cohort, possibly accounting for the observed benefit from intervention. A more recent multicenter randomized study by Folsch and colleagues excluded patients with known biliary sepsis or obstruction and demonstrated increased complications and mortality in the ERCP group.[50] It therefore was suggested that early ERCP may be harmful in the absence of ongoing obstruction. Although diagnostic and management strategies continue to evolve, most surgeons and gastroenterologists would agree that it is generally not recommended to perform ERCP in acute pancreatitis in the absence of biliary obstruction or cholangitis.

Magnetic resonance cholangiopancreatography (MRCP) is an additional alternative to ERCP that avoids the risk of postprocedure pancreatitis. Although therapeutic maneuvers to clear identified stones cannot be performed with MRCP, its use as a diagnostic tool may allow ERCP to be used selectively for patients with known choledocholithiasis.[51] MRI poses unique challenges in the critically ill patient, including the need for prolonged scan times and compatible nonmetallic equipment for ventilators and intravenous fluid administration. Its use therefore is restricted currently primarily to patients outside the critical-care setting. As technology evolves, it is expected that MRI and MRCP will play an increased role in diagnosis of pancreatitis and ductal obstruction.

PROPHYLACTIC ANTIBIOTICS

Of patients with severe pancreatitis who succumb to the disease, most do so from local and systemic infectious complications. Local infection is increasingly common with larger amounts of pancreatic necrosis, and this increases in incidence as time progresses for at least the first 3 weeks in the course of the disease.[52] In one study, 24% of patients operated on for pancreatic necrosis had infection at 1 week, whereas 71% of patients were infected when exploration was performed at 3 weeks.[53] Aerobic and anaerobic gastrointestinal flora are the primary organisms involved, and infections may be monomicrobial or polymicrobial. In a collected series of over 1100 cases, the predominant microbes seen were *Eschericia coli* (35%), *Klebsiella pneumoniae* (24%), *Streptococcus* (24%), *Staphylococcus* (14%), and *Pseudomonas* (11%).[54] The association of pancreatic infection with mortality has been the rationale behind the widespread use of prophylactic systemic antibiotics in patients with pancreatic necrosis. The use of broad-spectrum antibiotics for this purpose is known to change the bacterial flora of pancreatic infections and has been demonstrated to encourage the development of antibiotic-resistant bacterial infections and fungal infections.[55,56] Antibiotic use to forestall pancreatic infection with pancreatic necrosis therefore has been the subject of considerable debate and clinical investigation.[57,58]

Several animal studies have shown a benefit from early antibiotic administration with pancreatitis,[57] although this benefit has not been demonstrated as consistently in humans. Early clinical studies suggested no benefit of prophylactic antibiotics for necrotizing pancreatitis, possibly owing to inclusion of patients at low risk for infection or to the use of antibiotics with poor pancreatic penetration. The precise relationship between antibiotic "penetration" into healthy pancreatic parenchyma and its efficacy in preventing or treating infection in necrotic pancreatic tissue is unclear. Still, considerable investigative effort has been made to characterize the penetration of various antibiotics into the pancreatic parenchyma,[59] and these studies have influenced the commonly used prophylactic antibiotic regimens.

There are conflicting recommendations from recent studies addressing the use of systemic antibiotic prophylaxis in severe pancreatitis. Pederzoli and colleagues randomized 74 patients with necrotizing pancreatitis to systemic imipenem or no antibiotics.[60] Pancreatic infection was decreased with imipenem (12% versus 30%), although there was no difference in the rate of multiorgan failure, need for surgery, or overall mortality. Antibiotic therapy was particularly useful with lesser degrees of necrosis; no patient with less than 50% necrosis developed septic complications with imipenem compared with 29% in the control group. Saino and colleagues, however, showed a decrease in complications and mortality with prophylactic antibiotics in the absence of any difference in local infection.[61] Patients with necrotizing alcoholic pancreatitis given cefuroxime in a randomized fashion showed a decrease in infectious complications, operations, and mortality. However, this apparent mortality benefit was not associated with any difference in local pancreatic infections between treated patients and controls. This study was subject to some criticism for the high incidence of antibiotic use in the control arm. Another small randomized study with 26 patients showed a nonsignificant trend toward improved mortality with intravenous ofloxacin and metronidazole for CT-confirmed pancreatic necrosis.[62] One further study that was not limited to patients with CT-confirmed pancreatic necrosis suggested no difference in mortality or the development of infected pancreatic necrosis with the use of ciprofloxacin and metronidazole.[63]

The inconsistencies among these small trials may result from the relatively small number of patients per study and a limited statistical power to detect such differences. Comparing results between studies is complicated by considerable heterogeneity between them. The studies do not share criteria for patient selection because some treat only those patients with CT evidence for pancreatitis and others have no such restriction. The studies use different antibiotic regimens for prophylaxis. The medical and surgical management of patients in these studies varies significantly with regard to fluid resuscitation, enteral nutrition, timing of surgery, and other factors. Despite their somewhat heterogeneous nature, several meta-analyses have been attempted to address the problem of insufficient statistical power. In one such meta-analysis,[64] early antibiotic use was associated with decreased mortality from pancreatitis for patients with severe disease receiving broad-spectrum antibiotics. A second study looked at randomized, controlled, nonblinded studies of prophylactic antibiotics in necrotizing pancreatitis. A nonsignificant trend toward decreased local infection was suggested with the use of imipenem, cefuroxime, or ofloxacin. Sepsis and overall mortality were significantly lower with antibiotic use, and the authors therefore supported prophylactic antibiotics for all patients with acute necrotizing pancreatitis.[65]

Despite variations in institutional practices, a consensus has emerged that broad-spectrum antibiotics should be used early in the course of necrotizing pancreatitis, particularly in patients with signs of organ failure or systemic sepsis.[66] The risks of superinfection with fungal or antibiotic-resistant organisms is well recognized[67] and is thought to be related to the length of treatment with prophylactic antibiotics.

The length of treatment therefore typically is limited. The optimal duration of antimicrobial therapy has not been defined, although the incidence of pancreatic infection increases for approximately the first 3 weeks after diagnosis.[52] A treatment course of 1–4 weeks therefore is recommended commonly, with many authors limiting treatment to 14 days.[5] Mortality is considerable when fungal infection complicates pancreatic necrosis. However, the precise role of prophylactic antifungal therapy is still undefined, with some authors recommending fluconazole for all patients receiving antibiotic therapy for necrotizing pancreatitis.[56] Prophylactic use of the antifungals garlicin or fluconazole has been shown to reduce fungal infection in a randomized study in severe acute pancreatitis.[68] Since the incidence of toxic side effects from fluconazole is relatively low, prophylactic antifungal treatment may be a useful addition to the prophylactic regimen in patients with necrotizing pancreatitis.

Since infection in necrotizing pancreatitis arises primarily from commensal organisms from the gastrointestinal tract, some investigators have suggested using gut decontamination to reduce intestinal bacterial load and thereby prevent pancreatic infection. Limited laboratory evidence does support the use of gut decontamination to decrease mortality in experimental pancreatitis,[69] although the use of selective gut decontamination has been reported in only one clinical study. Luiten and colleagues randomized patients with severe acute pancreatitis to oral and rectal administration of nonabsorbable antibiotics.[70] Mortality was decreased in the treatment group, predominantly via a reduction in late mortality and decrease in gram-negative pancreatic infection. However, patients also received a short course of intravenous antibiotics in the study, potentially confounding the results. Definitive recommendations regarding the use of gut decontamination await further studies.

SURGICAL MANAGEMENT: INDICATIONS AND TIMING

In the majority of patients with acute pancreatitis, the process is limited to parenchymal edema without necrosis. These patients require surgical therapy for very limited indications; specifically, intervention may be needed to address the etiology of pancreatitis or its complications. Interventions, either surgical or endoscopic, to prevent recurrent gallstone pancreatitis are recommended in any patient with suspected choledocholithiasis. Delayed surgery also is rarely needed for the delayed treatment of local complications such as pseudocysts. Patients with severe pancreatitis, however, may require surgical therapy as an integral part of their management. Between 10% and 30% of patients with pancreatitis develop severe illness, with pancreatic and peripancreatic necrosis and high associated morbidity and mortality.[2] The indications for surgical therapy with acute necrotizing pancreatitis have evolved in recent years. Prompt pancreatic débridement is the accepted standard of care for patients with infected pancreatic necrosis. As discussed below, an increasingly conservative surgical approach has been adopted in recent years toward the surgical management of patients with sterile pancreatic necrosis.

Occasionally, patients with severe disease may require urgent surgical intervention for reasons unrelated to their pancreatitis. For instance, at presentation, a surgical emergency such as a perforated viscus may be suspected. Diagnostic laparotomy may be appropriate in such circumstances. A patient managed conservatively also may require exploration for subsequent development of other intra-abdominal pathology. In other patients with severe pancreatitis or pancreatic necrosis, three indications for surgical intervention remain (Table 36–3). The first, documented pancreatic infection, is not disputed. Whether (and when) to operate for severe sterile necrosis is controversial. Finally, delayed intervention with symptomatic organized necrosis is recognized increasingly as a valid indication for drainage or débridement.

TABLE 36–3. INDICATIONS FOR SURGICAL INTERVENTION IN NECROTIZING PANCREATITIS

Diagnostic uncertainty
Intra-abdominal catastrophe unrelated to necrotizing pancreatitis such as perforated viscus
Infected necrosis documented by FNA or extraluminal gas on CT
Severe sterile necrosis
Symptomatic organized pancreatic necrosis

Abbreviations: FNA, fine-needle aspiration.

Infected Pancreatic Necrosis

The majority of deaths from acute pancreatitis occur in patients with infected pancreatic necrosis. The mortality rate is virtually 100% without intervention, although with appropriate surgical therapy it should approach the less than 15% mortality seen with sterile necrosis.[4,33,71] A minority of patients with infected pancreatic necrosis may demonstrate radiographic evidence of such, emphysematous pancreatitis, or intraparenchymal gas (Fig 36–3). In most patients, CT-guided percutaneous FNA is needed to diagnose infection. As noted previously, both severe sterile necrosis and infected pancreatic necrosis are associated with significant leukocytosis and fever, making clinical distinction impossible. Patients with severe pancreatitis or organ failure or those who fail to improve clinically in the first 2 weeks should be investigated for possible infected necrosis.

Severe Sterile Pancreatic Necrosis

The presence of pancreatic necrosis historically was considered sufficient justification for open surgical pancreatic débridement. This practice was called into question in 1991 when Bradley and Allen[53] published a small series of 11 patients with sterile pancreatic necrosis managed nonoperatively. This concept was introduced with some resistance because some authors have argued that all patients with pancreatic necrosis would benefit from débridement. Shortly after Bradley and Allen's study was published, Rattner and colleagues suggested that early pancreatic débridement was beneficial in pancreatic necrosis regardless of the status of infection.[72] With increased experience using nonoperative management and FNA of the pancreatic necrosum, clinicians have become increasingly comfortable with conservative therapy in stable patients. The indications for surgery in patients with sterile necrosis have continued to be refined since that time. Considerable effort has been made to identify criteria for débridement other than infection.[73,74] CT evidence of necrosis of more than 50% of the pancreas has been examined but is insufficiently specific for use in decision making.[74] Other indices are no more predictive.[75] Series using aggressive surgery regardless of pancreatic infection continue to be reported,[71,76] although most centers increasingly have managed sterile necrosis in a conservative manner.

Two large series have demonstrated the validity and analyzed the results of this approach. A group from Bern[4] prospectively studied 86 patients with necrotizing pancreatitis followed with a strict conservative protocol. In this cohort, the mortality rate was 10%, with only one patient undergoing operation in the absence of documented infection. A retrospective review from the Brigham and Women's Hospital analyzed 99 patients with CT-documented pancreatic necrosis (Fig 36–5). Six patients who had other reasons for surgery or who had their care withdrawn for severe underlying medical conditions were excluded from the analysis. Of the remaining 93 patients, 59 patients without infection were managed conservatively, with 7 deaths (11%). Thirty-four patients underwent open or percutaneous therapy for infected necrosis, with a mortality rate of 12%. Thirty-five patients did not have sufficient evidence of infection to warrant FNA. These 35 recovered relatively rapidly despite admission APACHE II scores similar to those of patients who required further intervention. Overall, these studies suggest that conservative strategies can be applied in most patients with necrotizing pancreatitis with reasonable outcomes. Furthermore, it is very difficult to identify prospectively which persons might benefit from more aggressive strategy. A randomized, controlled trial may be the only way to resolve this controversy definitively, although the small number of patients with this condition may preclude meaningful conclusions. Whether surgical management is ever indicated in this patient population and the precise timing of such intervention continue to be a matter of debate.

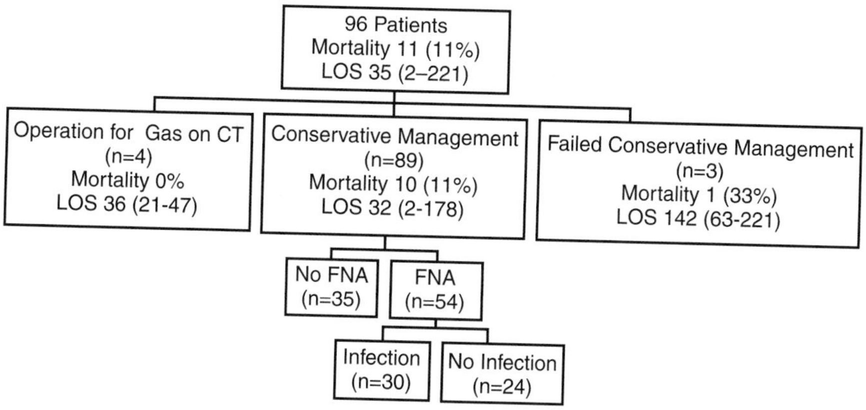

Figure 36–5. Management strategy in necrotizing pancreatitis used in Ashley et al.[33] (Reproduced, with permission, from *Ann Surg* 2001;234:529–575.)

Organized Pancreatic Necrosis

Despite increased acceptance among most authors of initial nonoperative management for sterile pancreatic necrosis, some have emphasized the eventual need to operate on patients who do not improve clinically. Among patients managed nonoperatively for pancreatic necrosis, some experience persistent pain, malaise, and inability to eat. Warshaw has described this phenomenon as "persistent unwellness."[77] The pathologic correlate of the pancreas later in the course of the disease is what Baron and colleagues describe as "organized pancreatic necrosis,"[78] a process of maturation of the inflammatory tissue with improved demarcation from healthy pancreatic and peripancreatic tissue. As is the case with sterile necrosis in the acute setting, the indications for and timing of surgery for this group of patients have not been defined precisely.

Several nonrandomized studies have demonstrated significantly better outcomes in patients undergoing late versus early débridement,[71,79] and surgical débridement is facilitated considerably by the demarcation that occurs later in the course of pancreatic necrosis. In the above-mentioned series of 99 patients with pancreatic necrosis at the Brigham and Women's Hospital, five patients underwent an operation for this indication at a mean of 29 days (23–34 days) after presentation. This group accounted for approximately one-fifth of the patients who had undergone a negative CT-guided FNA.[33] All patients were débrided, and two were found to have an inflammatory process sufficiently mature to add cystgastrostomy after the débridement. All patients recovered well and were discharged at a mean of 27 days (8–146 days) after surgery. The optimal timing for surgery in this group is unclear; Fernandez-del Castillo and colleagues suggest that there is no added benefit in delaying longer than 4 weeks from the onset of illness.[71] Such delayed procedures are an important part of a conservative management strategy that emphasizes nonoperative management for most cases of sterile necrosis and late operations if necessary.

An algorithm for management strategies in acute pancreatitis summarizing the principles just discussed is outlined in Figure 36–6. For patients requiring operative intervention, percutaneous drainage is employed increasingly as an adjunct to or in lieu of open surgical management.

SURGICAL MANAGEMENT: PROCEDURES

Surgical therapy for acute pancreatitis may address either the etiology of pancreatitis or its complications. Operations addressing etiology generally are limited to interventions to eliminate cholelithiasis and thus eliminate gallstone pancreatitis. For patients with known gallstone pancreatitis, cholecystectomy is recommended after resolution of the pancreatic inflammation. Preoperative endoscopic examination of the common bile duct is common in some institutions; if choledocholithiasis is detected on ERCP, endoscopic duct clearance often is attempted, with or without endoscopic papillotomy. In the absence of endoscopic interrogation and clearance of the biliary system, cholecystectomy should be combined with intraoperative cholangiogram, with or without common bile duct exploration.

The surgical management of the long-term complications of pancreatitis, such as pseudocysts and strictures, is addressed elsewhere. The primary surgical dilemma presenting in an acute or subacute fashion is surgical management of necrotizing pancreatitis. Surgical strategies for approaching the necrotic pancreas are addressed below, with particular attention to strategies for pancreatic débridement and postdébridement management and the use of minimally invasive techniques.

RESECTION

Pancreatic resection for acute pancreatitis is primarily of historical interest only and is not recommended currently. Several authors in the 1960s and 1970s recommended partial or total pancreatectomy for pancreatitis based on the possibility that the remaining pancreas could be a source of persistent inflammation.[80–82] Operative mortality was as high as 60% in one series.[82] Although others have reported more acceptable mortality, conventional imaging and staging systems were not applied universally. In addition to the hazards posed by the dissection of a highly vascularized organ amid an acute inflammatory process, resection risks overtreatment of many patients if performed for necrotizing pancreatitis. Viable tissue typically exists adjacent to necrotic tissue, and intraoperative differentiation between healthy pancreatic parenchyma and necrotic tissue can prove difficult. For instance, even with apparent total necrosis, the central pancreas surrounding the main pancreatic duct often is viable and is important for endocrine and exocrine function after resolution of the acute disease.[83] Resection therefore inevitably would risk the loss of viable, functioning parenchyma. Anatomic resection for pancreatitis, with or without associated pancreatic necrosis, therefore is thought to serve little utility and potentially may confer significant risk.

PANCREATIC DÉBRIDEMENT

All techniques of pancreatic débridement and postdébridement care are based on two principles: (1) wide removal of devitalized and necrotic tissue with thor-

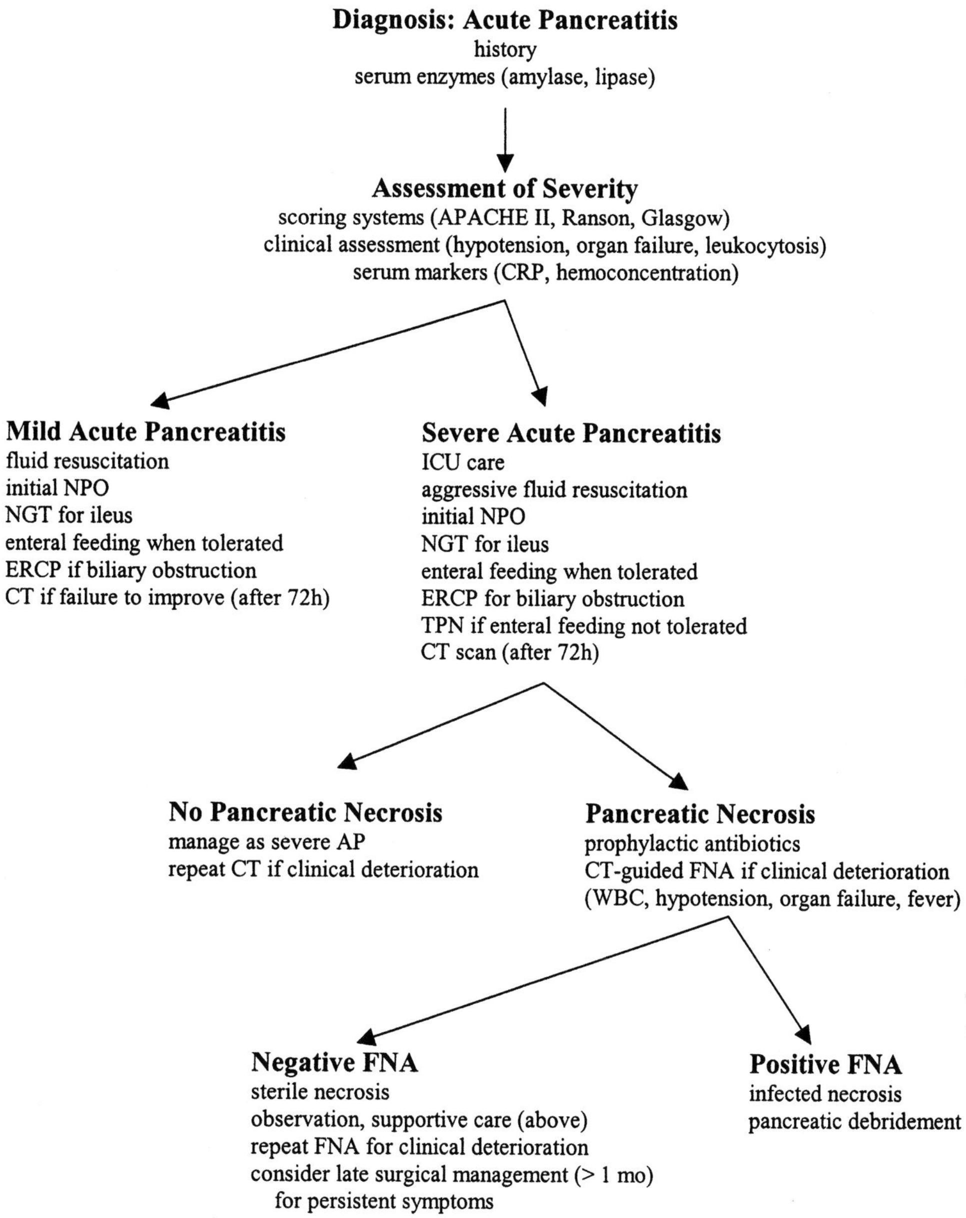

Figure 36–6. Management algorithm for acute pancreatitis. (Reprinted from Clancy TE, Benoit EP, Asley SW. Current management of acute pancreatitis. *J Gastrointest Surg* 9:440–452, copyright © 2005, with permission from Elsevier.)

ough exploration and unroofing of all collections of solid and liquid debris and (2) the assurance of postoperative removal of the products of ongoing local inflammation and infection that persist after débridement. Various techniques of open pancreatic débridement for necrotizing pancreatitis have been advocated in the literature.[71,76,84,85] While different approaches are fundamentally equal in terms of the method of débridement, postdébridement strategies differ considerably. Débridement with closure over drains, débridement with open packing, and débridement with closure over irrigation drains and postoperative lavage are the three methods commonly reported. Mortality and complication rates for several published series, representing each postoperative strategy, are shown in Table 36–4. Reported morbidity and mortality across these studies varies widely; however, comparisons between different studies are difficult given a lack of standardization in disease severity or criteria used for operative management.

Further complicating any comparison between studies is the lack of standard definitions in the earlier literature; many cases of pancreatic necrosis likely were incorrectly considered “pancreatic abscess.” Over the past decade

TABLE 36–4. PUBLISHED SERIES OF PANCREATIC DÉBRIDEMENT, POSTDÉBRIDEMENT MANAGEMENT WITH EITHER CLOSED DRAINAGE, OPEN PACKING OR CLOSED VOLUME AND LAVAGE. OPERATIVE MORTALITY IS LISTED AS WELL AS INCIDENCE OF REOPERATION, GI FISTULA, AND BLEEDING.

Author	*n*	Mortality	Reoperation	GI Fistula	Bleeding
Closed Drainage					
Fernandez[71] (1998)	64	6.2%	17%	16%	1%
Hwang[103] (1995)	31	48%	—	3%	19%
Teerenhovi[104] (1989)	12	17%	25%	—	—
Pemberton[90] (1985)	64	44%	n/a	14%	31%
Warshaw[86] (1985)	45	24%	16%	26%	
Aranha[87] (1982)	20	30%	40%	20%	—
Open Packing					
Hwang[103] (1995)	40	15%	100%	10%	5%
Fugger[105] (1995)	72	25%	100%	26%	18%
Bradley[89] (1993)	71	14%	100%	5%	5%
Orlando[106] (1993)	15	20%	100%	26%	26%
Sarr[85] (1991)	23	17%	100%	35%	26%
Garcia[107] (1987)	49	27%	100%	0%	—
Wertheimer[91] (1986)	10	20%	100%	40%	20%
Pemberton[90] (1985)	17	18%	100%	31%	29%
Closed Lavage					
Branum[76] (1998)	50	12%	48%	16%	—
Hwang[103] (1995)	15	33%	—	7%	13%
Pederzoli[108] (1990)	191	10.5%	18%	—	—
Beger[84] (1991)	95	8.4%	27%	12%	5%
Villazon[109] (1991)	18	22%	n/a (2.6 op. per pt. ave)	33%	6%
Nicholson[110] (1998)	11	27%	9%	9%	9%
Teerenhovi[104] (1989)	11	36%	64%	—	—
Larvin[111] (1989)	14	21%	—	43%	—

there has been increased precision in the definitions used to describe local complications of acute pancreatitis. The definitions proposed at the 1992 International Symposium on Acute Pancreatitis in Atlanta (Table 36–5) have proven useful for comparing data between studies and for standardizing treatment indications. However, these standards have been applied only recently. As a result of this lack of standardization and other difficulties listed earlier, recommendations for techniques of débridement and postdébridement management have not been uniform in the literature. No method is accepted universally, and the techniques have not been compared adequately in a randomized, prospective fashion. The method of postdébridement management used may be tailored to individual patients, and each method may have a role under specific circumstances.

TECHNIQUES OF DÉBRIDEMENT

Prior to surgical débridement, accurate preoperative imaging is essential. It is of paramount importance to identify all areas of necrosis or fluid collections to guide surgical exploration properly. To achieve this, a high-quality

TABLE 36–5. DEFINITIONS PROPOSED BY THE INTERNATIONAL SYMPOSIUM ON ACUTE PANCREATITIS (THE ATLANTA SYMPOSIUM), 1992[29]

Acute pancreatitis	Acute inflammatory process of the pancreas with variable involvement of other regional tissues or remote organ systems.
Severe AP	Association with organ failure and/or local complications, such as necrosis, abscess, or pseudocyst.
Acute fluid collection	Occurs early in the course of AP, located in or near the pancreas, always lacking a wall of granulation or fibrous tissue; bacteria variably present; occurs in 30–50% of severe AP; most acute fluid collections regress, but some progress to pseudocyst or abscess.
Pancreatic necrosis	Diffuse or focal area(s) of nonviable pancreatic parenchyma, typically associated with peripancreatic fat necrosis, diagnosed by CT scan with intravenous contrast enhancement.
Acute pseudocyst	Collection of pancreatic juice enclosed by a wall of fibrous or granulation tissue, which arises as a consequence of AP, pancreatic trauma, or chronic pancreatitis; formation requires 4 or more weeks form onset of AP.
Pancreatic abscess	Circumscribed intra-abdominal collection of pus usually in or near the pancreas, containing little or no pancreatic necrosis, arises as a consequence of AP or pancreatic trauma.

Note: The terms *phlegmon, infected pseudocyst, hemorrhagic pancreatitis,* and *persistent acute pancreatitis* are discouraged.

CT scan with intravenous contrast enhancement is essential to identify areas of pancreatic or peripancreatic tissue requiring drainage. Exploration of the pancreatic bed may be initiated via either a bilateral subcostal or midline incision (Fig 36–7). The pancreatic bed and lesser sac may be approached either through the gastrocolic ligament or through the transverse mesocolon. Some authors[71] have strongly advocated an approach to the lesser sac via the left side of the transverse mesocolon to avoid the dense inflammatory process that can obscure tissue planes between the stomach and transverse colon (Fig 36–8). If the anatomic plane between the stomach and colon is obliterated by inflammation, the transmesocolic approach avoids inadvertent injury to these structures. The middle colic vessels present a potential anatomic barrier to the transmesocolic approach, although these vessels often are thrombosed in the setting of necrotizing pancreatitis. If patent, these vessels often may be interrupted without consequence because the colon is supplied with collateral vasculature. An additional advantage of the transmesocolic approach is that drains may be placed in a dependent position after débridement. Other investigators have advocated an approach to the lesser sac via the gastrocolic ligament (Fig 36–9) for the primary reason that the inframesocolic space typically is uninvolved with peripancreatic inflammation and infection. Moreover, transmesocolic exposure opens the remainder of the abdomen to this inflammatory process.[76]

Pancreatic débridement is accomplished bluntly, primarily using finger dissection. The differentiation between necrotic tissue, which has a looser consistency, and viable tissue, which is firm, often is best made by palpation. Necrotic tissue should separate easily from the surrounding tissue without extensive dissection. While complete débridement is essential, efforts should be

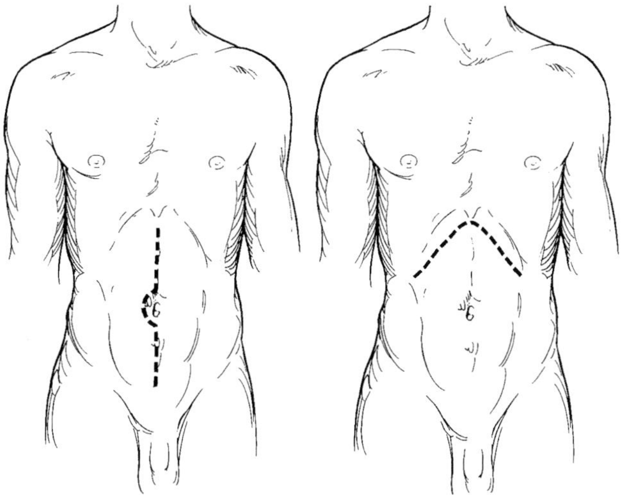

Figure 36–7. Operative approaches to open pancreatic débridement. Either a midline or bilateral subcostal approach is acceptable.

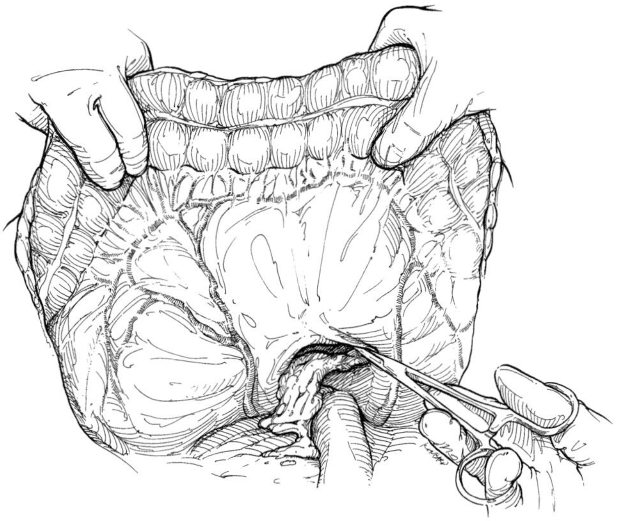

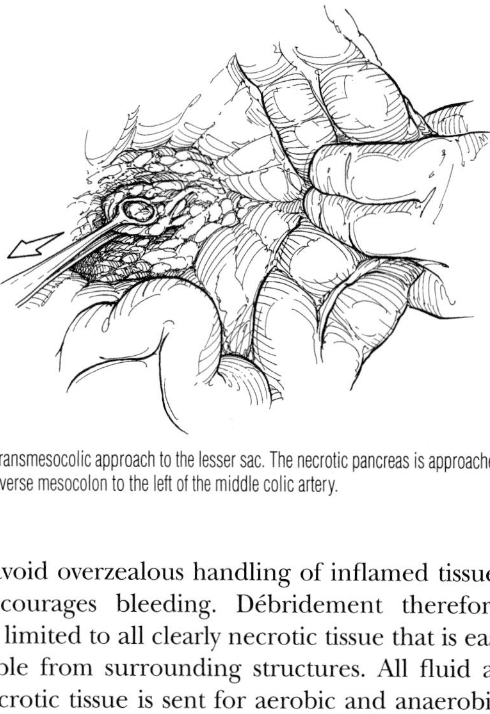

Figure 36–8. Transmesocolic approach to the lesser sac. The necrotic pancreas is approached through the transverse mesocolon to the left of the middle colic artery.

made to avoid overzealous handling of inflamed tissue, which encourages bleeding. Débridement therefore should be limited to all clearly necrotic tissue that is easily separable from surrounding structures. All fluid as well as necrotic tissue is sent for aerobic and anaerobic culture. Hemorrhage from diffuse oozing from inflamed retroperitoneal tissues is not uncommon; hemostasis may require packing of the cavity. Rapid hemorrhage from the intraoperative rupture of a major blood vessel, such as the splenic artery or vein, may require suture ligature. Precise vascular control in an inflamed tissue field can prove difficult if not impossible. If such is the case, hemostasis may require prolonged manual compression and possibly multiple sutures.

As the inflammatory mass is exposed during the course of the débridement, it may become necessary to extend the intra-abdominal dissection to fully expose all necrotic tissue. A complete search for and identification of all necrotic foci must take place. For necrosis of the head, improved exposure may be achieved either

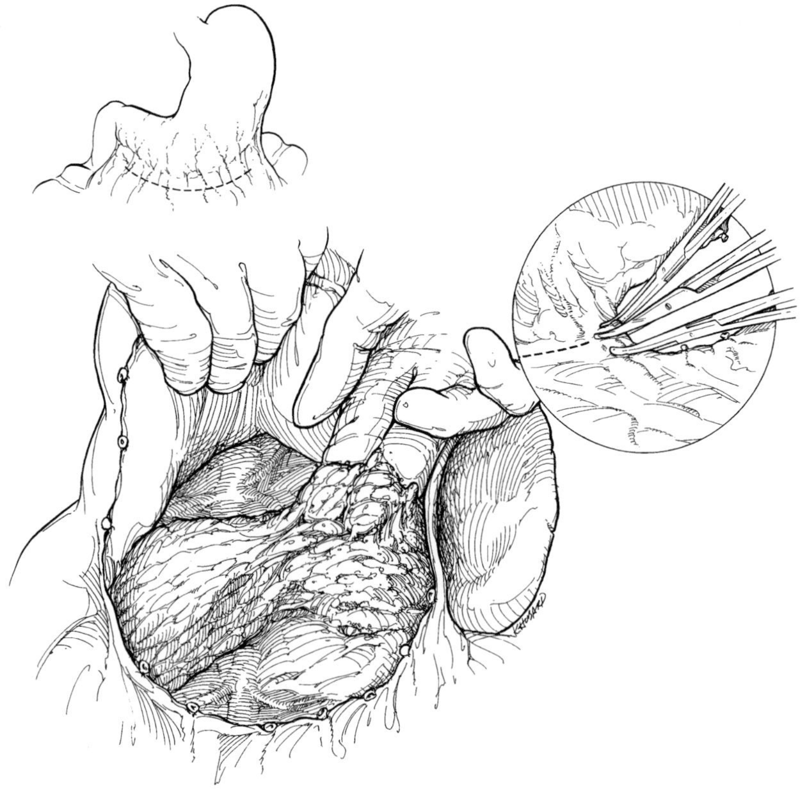

Figure 36–9. Approach to lesser sac via gastrocolic ligament.

through the right side of the mesocolon or via an approach posterior to the second and third portions of the duodenum. Additional exposure also may entail a release of the hepatic and splenic flexures of the colon. Thorough exposure of all necrotic tissue may involve opening both paracolic gutters, the pararenal spaces, the retroperitoneum into the pelvis, and the gastrohepatic omentum.

Débridement and Closed Drainage

Several authors have demonstrated very favorable results with débridement and closed drainage.[71,86] Proponents of this technique stress that the presence of residual necrotic pancreatic tissue is the most important factor dictating the need for subsequent reexplorations, each of which is associated with some morbidity and mortality. For this reason, the completeness of the initial débridement is the most crucial factor in avoiding subsequent reexplorations. In contrast to the open packing technique, a concerted effort is made to perform a complete débridement and drainage of fluid collections at the first surgical procedure. All necrotic tissue is débrided unless it is densely adherent to vital structures, and all spaces involved on preoperative imaging are opened and débrided.

Débridement is followed with gentle irrigation (Fig 36–10). The cavities left after débridement are drained with either closed-suction drains or Penrose drains stuffed with gauze. All drains are brought out through separate stab wounds in the abdomen. The placement of enteral feeding or drainage tubes (i.e., gastrostomy or jejunostomy) is optional. Drains are removed one at a time beginning 6 to 10 days after surgery in an effort to allow the cavity to collapse. If Penrose and closed-suction drains are used together, closed-suction drains are removed last and only when their output is minimal.

In some cases, complete débridement is not possible during the first exploration. If hemodynamic instability or coagulopathy prohibit further débridement, temporary closure is achieved after packing the necrotic cavity with Mikulicz pads and placing drains; repeat procedures may occur in 24 to 48 hours, along with additional procedures such as gastrostomy or jejunostomy.

Reported mortality for débridement and closure over drains has been as high as 40%. Recurrent pancreatic infection is an acknowledged complication of this technique, with early series reporting a recurrence rate of 30–40%.[87] However, a more recent series has reported significantly better results, with mortality of 6.2%.[71] In this series, an additional operation was required in 17% of patients, most of whom had persistent infected pancreatic necrosis. In addition, 20% required postoperative image-guided drainage of residual or re-

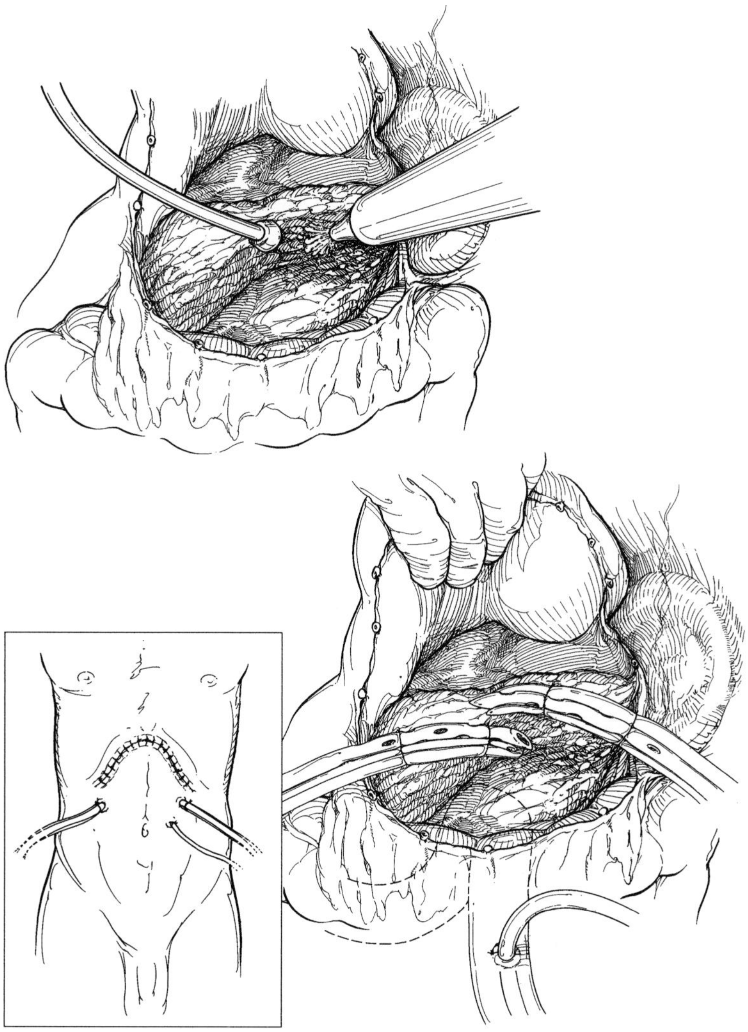

Figure 36–10. Irrigation and drainage of pancreatic bed. Drainage tubes are used for technique of closed drainage or postoperative saline lavage; for open packing technique, pancreatic bed is packed with sterile bandages.

current fluid collections. Overall, 69% required only one operation without further procedures.[71] The reported success of this procedure and rate of recurrence are attributed to thorough surgical débridement with maximal removal of necrotic tissue at the first operation.

Open Packing for Pancreatic Necrosis

As mentioned earlier, a recognized complication after an apparently adequate pancreatic débridement is recurrent pancreatic sepsis. While most necrotic debris is separated easily from surrounding structures, some borderline tissue may not be débrided so easily. Presumably, pancreatic necrosis is an ongoing process, and further demarcation of necrotic tissue after an initial débridement can result in a mass of particulate matter that is inadequately removed by sump drainage. Furthermore, the persistence of necrotic tissue is combined with the persistent postoperative leakage of activated pancreatic enzymes from the necrotic and inflamed tissue into the retroperitoneum. This combination of necrotic material and chemical inflammation may be responsible for the occasional failure of simple débridement and drainage. For this reason, some authors have advocated a process of open packing, or marsupialization, by which recurrent pancreatic débridement is facilitated.[88]

The surgical approach typically is a left subcostal incision, which is extended easily to a bilateral subcostal incision should additional exposure be necessary. This transverse incision optimally is situated above a transverse opening in the gastrocolic omentum to facilitate open packing. Advocates of open packing have preferred to access the lesser sac via the gastrocolic ligament, which may provide a more direct access to the entire pancreatic bed for future packing. Pancreatic débridement using blunt finger dissection is employed, with wide exposure of all areas of retroperitoneal necrosis. However, unlike procedures with planned closed packing, no effort should be made to remove every identifiable piece of necrotic tissue at the first procedure; rather, only tissues that are separated easily by blunt dissection should be dissected. Complete removal of all necrotic tissue is accomplished by multiple reexplorations and blunt débridements, limiting blood loss.

After débridement, the stomach and colon may be covered with a nonadherent gauze to prevent débridement of healthy tissue during dressing changes. This constructs a cone or cylinder with the pancreas at the base. Laparotomy pads or other gauze may be placed directly within this area, and some authors have recommended presoaking these packs in iodinated solutions. Some surgeons will suture the gastrocolic ligament to the skin, creating an inverted cone with the base consisting of the divided gastrocolic ligament at the skin level and the point at the pancreatic bed. However, in the setting of acute inflammation, this cavity may be ill defined, and suturing to the skin generally is not necessary. No attempts usually are made to close the fascia or skin, although occasionally a small number of extraperitoneal stay sutures of nylon may be tied loosely to discourage evisceration. This results in an open communicating defect for packing. Alternatively, some have used a separate retroperitoneal incision through which to bring packs, closing the abdominal incision. This method likely provides inferior access for future débridements.

Planned reexplorations are perfomed in the operating room at 2- to 3-day intervals for additional débridement. When retroperitoneal granulation tissue begins to form, daily dressing changes may be performed in the ICU using mild sedation and/or pain control. Although the majority of necrotic tissue is débrided with the first effort, significant amounts of tissue may be removed at the fourth or even fifth débridement procedure.[89]

After débridement has been achieved by open packing, the abdominal wound either may be left to heal entirely by secondary intention or may undergo delayed primary closure. In some cases, the open packing procedure may be combined with delayed closure over lavage catheters and continuous closed lavage of the lesser sac and abscess cavity. Catheters are withdrawn gradually over weeks after it is demonstrated that there is no pancreatic fistula.

DÉBRIDEMENT AND CONTINUOUS CLOSED POSTOPERATIVE LAVAGE OF THE LESSER SAC

After an initial pancreatic débridement, small amounts of residual necrotic tissue inevitably are present. Furthermore, the persistent soilage of the retroperitoneum with pancreatic enzymes and inflammatory mediators also may contribute to persistent systemic inflammation and sepsis. Removal of residual necrotic tissue, bacteria, and biologically active substances therefore is proposed to decrease persistent inflammation.

While some have advocated open packing and planned repeated operations to accomplish this goal, others report success with continuous postoperative high-volume lavage of the lesser sac.[83] Even an aggressive initial débridement therefore is not considered an end in itself but rather the first step of a thorough washout of the pancreatic bed.

Beger and colleagues have been written extensively on the procedure of débridement and continuous closed postoperative lavage.[84] With this technique, pancreatic débridement is performed in the standard fashion. Postoperative lavage is facilitated by the insertion of two to five large double-lumen tubes. After drain placement, the gastrocolic ligament may be sutured to form a closed compartment in the lesser sac. Continuous lavage is undertaken with hyperosmolar, potassium-free dialysate at approximately 2 L/h, although irrigation with normal saline is also employed.[83] Branum and colleagues describe the completion of one or more débridements, followed by the placement of multilumen sump drains for postoperative irrigation.[76] Irrigation continues until the effluent is free of particulate matter. These drains are downsized gradually and eventually withdrawn.

Beger and colleagues have published an overall operative mortality of 10.6% with this procedure and a mortality of 15% when the procedure is performed for infected pancreatic necrosis. These authors and others have argued that using postoperative continuous lavage results in decreased rates of postoperative pancreatic sepsis compared with closed drainage techniques, and the incidence of postoperative complications such as incisional hernia and gastrointestinal fistulas is said to be less than that with open packing and repeated débridements.

COMPARISON OF TECHNIQUES USED IN PANCREATIC DÉBRIDEMENT

As noted earlier, the benefits of various techniques of pancreatic débridement and postdébridement care have been debated in the literature. No strict criteria have been proposed to select patients adequately for different procedures, and the optimal method of débridement has not been examined in a prospective fashion. A number of case series have been reported in which patients with either pancreatic necrosis or severe acute pancreatitis have undergone pancreatic débridement followed by either closure over drains, open packing and redébridement, or closure over lavage catheters with postoperative continuous lavage (see Table 36–4). As seen in this table, reports of postoperative complications and mortality vary widely across different studies. Comparisons between these different studies can prove difficult for several reasons. Preoperative disease severity is difficult to standardize across different reports, as are the criteria for operative management employed. Earlier studies did not employ currently accepted criteria of disease severity, and the presence of pancreatic infection is not universally documented via preoperative studies. The various methods of pancreatic débridement have not been compared in a prospective, randomized fashion.

One small single-institution retrospective study compared surgical outcomes in 86 patients with acute pancreatitis after débridement and closed drainage, débridement with open packing, or débridement with continuous closed postoperative lavage. Patients were noted to have similar preoperative Ranson's scores. Mortality was significantly higher after closed drainage (48.4%) compared with 15% following open packing, and complications were not significantly different between the groups. However, pancreatic necrosis and the time to operation are not documented, so it is not clear that these results are applicable to current practice.

Several series in the literature have quoted a high rate of recurrent pancreatic sepsis and high rate of reoperation when the technique of débridement and closure over drains is used.[76] Bradley has quoted a rate of reexploration for recurrent sepsis of 30–40%,[87] and a review of large series suggests that the majority of postoperative deaths after closed drainage are due to persistent or recurrent infection.[54] These figures have been used to argue for either repeated pancreatic débridement via open packing or continuous postoperative pancreatic lavage. However, the Massachusetts General Hospital experience with the closed drainage technique reports a mortality of 6.2%, the lowest reported mortality rate in any series of pancreatic débridement for pancreatic necrosis.[71]

Bradley reported a favorable mortality rate of 14% mortality rate for the technique of open packing. Given a need for reoperation in up to 30–40% of patients after closed drainage or high-volume lavage, an argument then is made for controlled, planned reexploration to achieve thorough débridment. Others have suggested that the open packing technique might be particularly useful in patients with a larger mass of necrotic tissue.[90] However, postoperative morbidity can be considerable with the open packing technique. Bradley reported a rate of incisional hernia of 23% after open packing. Although this complication is not reported widely in other series, one other series has reported a hernia rate of 80%.[91] An increased rate of gastrointestinal fistulas has been reported in some series of open packing, although a brief review of published series shows that this complication is not universal. As with other complications, however, the precise definition of gastrointestinal fistula is not clarified in different series. Length of hospital stay, which is not reported commonly in different series, has been suggested to be prolonged after open packing.[92]

The recent trend toward delayed surgical therapy for pancreatic necrosis may facilitate atraumatic débridement because necrosis becomes increasingly organized and demarcated from viable tissue over time.[78] Some investigators have suggested that a policy of delayed exploration and débridement therefore may facilitate closed drainage without packing or postoperative lavage. In the previously mentioned 2001 series of 99 patients with pancreatic necrosis managed conservatively at the Brigham and Women's Hospital, operation was offered only for documented infection or for sterile pancreatic necrosis with persistent systemic illness. In this series, Ashley and colleagues demonstrated that most patients were managed with closed drainage.[33] The mean interval from presentation to surgery was 27 days. Of these patients, 31 (86%) were managed with débridement and closure over drains, 1 received postoperative irrigation, and 4 required open packing and planned reexploration. Nineteen patients (34%) developed complications, including 9% each with pancreatic or enteric fistulas and 15% with endocrine or exocrine insufficiency. Of patients managed with closure over drains, only 4 (13%) needed reexploration owing to inadequate persistent illness and presumed inadequate débridement. We continue to believe that each technique has its place. When early operation is mandated, open packing or lavage may be necessary to deal with the consequences of ongoing necrosis. If operation can be delayed, débridement with closed drainage and sometimes even internal drainage may be adequate.

MINIMALLY INVASIVE APPROACHES

Although mortality after open pancreatic débridement has decreased in recent years, many series still demonstrate a mortality rate of approximately 15%; in addition, the mortality in patients with established organ failure may exceed 75%.[93] Open approaches often are associated with initial postoperative deterioration requiring intensive physiologic support. Given the considerable morbidity, organ failure, and mortality associated with traditional open pancreatic débridement, some investigators have suggested that minimally invasive surgical procedures may be used successfully with pancreatic necrosis. Avoiding open débridement has the theoretical advantage of minimizing activation of systemic inflammatory processes and reducing respiratory and wound complications.

In recent years there has been a proliferation of reports describing minimally invasive approaches in necrotizing pancreatitis. Percutaneous, endoscopic, and laparoscopic techniques all have been described. Solid pancreatic debris traditionally has been thought to be too thick for adequate evacuation with percutaneous drains; still, small studies have demonstrated success with percutaneous catheter drainage as a primary treatment for infected pancreatic necrosis. Several series of successful percutaneous management in infected pancreatic necrosis have been reported in the literature.[94–96] For instance, Freeny and colleagues managed 16 of 34 such patients successfully with an aggressive protocol of percutaneous drainage.[94] This required a mean of four catheter insertions and lavage for a mean of 85 days. In 9 other patients, percutaneous intervention was not the sole means of therapy but allowed eventual open surgical intervention to be delayed. Thus, combined with the 52% of patients requiring elective or emergency surgery, approximately 75% of patients subsequently needed surgical intervention.[93] It is possible that percutaneous drainage in this case functioned just to delay an operation and prevent the need for laparotomy during the most acute phase of the illness. The concept that percutaneous drainage of infected necrosis may delay the need for early intervention, permitting surgery once the process has become more organized, is appealing but needs further validation.

An often-unstated principle of therapy for pancreatic necrosis in the past has been the need to externally drain the pancreatic bed. Necrotic tissue, pancreatic enzymes, bacteria, and inflammatory mediators in the infected milieu of the necrotic pancreas all were thought to be best drained outside the body. The concept of internal drainage, whereby inflammatory tissue and fluid are drained to the gastrointestinal tract directly, has been considered to be feasible only recently. In this regard, some investigators have suggested endoscopic therapy for pancreatic necrosis and have summarized these results recently.[97] Forty-four patients with pancreatic necrosis were treated for suspected or documented infection or for intractable symptoms from organized necrosis, including nausea, pain, or early satiety. Endoscopic transmural drainage was successful in 31 (72%) of patients with pancreatic necrosis, although 9 (29%) experienced recurrence, and 16 (37%) experienced complications. Transmural drainage was more successful with central rather than peripheral necrosis owing to the close proximity of the necrotic area to the gastric wall. Subsequent analysis has suggested that collections with solid debris of more than 1 cm are not suitable for endoscopic drainage.[98] In addition, up to 60% of patients drained successfully developed more collections over a 2-year period.

Seifert and colleagues have described a method of retroperitoneal endoscopy via transgastric fenestration.[99] Direct visual access to retroperitoneal collections thereby is obtained to allow optimal drainage. Few patients have been described using this method, and larger studies are necessary to validate this approach. These techniques also were not always performed for infected pancreatic necrosis. Of concern is the certainty that if sterile retroperitoneal collections are accessed via the gastrointestinal tract, these collections soon become contaminated with commensal gastrointestinal flora.[100] Inadequate drainage after endoscopic intervention clearly has the ability to complicate a troublesome but not life-threatening collection.

Various techniques of minimally invasive surgery have been adopted to treat pancreatic necrosis. Gambiez and colleagues have suggested using a retroperitoneal approach via dorsal lumbotomy and a 23-cm endoscope to explore and drain the peripancreatic area[101]; necrotic peripancreatic tissue could be removed by blunt dissection, and drains may be left for irrigation. These authors have employed this technique, repeating débridements at regular 5-day intervals until the resolution of necrotic debris, with a mean of five procedures. Purported advantages of this technique include an avoidance of peritoneal contamination. Furthermore, in the series reported by Gambiez and colleagues, subsequent laparotomy was required in just 2 patients for persistent collections.[101] Overall mortality in 20 patients with infected pancreatic necrosis was 10%, which compares favorably with historical controls.

Percutaneous necrosectomy and sinus tract endoscopy are techniques described by Carter and colleagues for minimally invasive débridement of the necrotic pancreas.[102] Briefly, methods borrowed from percutaneous nephroscopy are used to visualize the retroperitoneum directly. Under CT guidance, an 8F pigtail catheter is advanced into the pancreatic cavity either between the lower pole of the spleen and the splenic flexure or, for right-sided necrosis, through the gastrocolic omentum anterior to the duodenum. The cavity is accessed in the operating room under fluoroscopic guidance; the catheter tract is serially dilated first manually and then with a balloon dilator until a 34F sheath is accepted. An operating nephroscope then may be passed to the cavity, allowing irrigation, suction, and piecemeal removal of necrotic debris. Devitalized tissue is identified easily and may be removed by gentle traction in a piecemeal fashion. Large drains may be placed through the same access sites to allow postoperative drainage and/or lavage. Planned second-look procedures may be performed every 7–10 days until the cavity is clean. The technique of sinus tract endoscopy employs similar methods to inspect, débride, and drain residual collections after an initial open débridement. These techniques may achieve adequate débridement and adequate drainage and/or lavage of the pancreatic bed. Carter and colleagues, in an initial report with only 10 patients, reported mortality was 20%.[102] However, postoperative organ dysfunction was minimized, and the majority of patients were managed outside the ICU postoperatively.

The use of minimally invasive techniques undoubtedly can reduce the severity of systemic sepsis and organ dysfunction associated with open pancreatic débridement. The primary risk of these procedures is an inadequate débridement of solid necrosum and inadequate drainage of the pancreatic bed. No randomized studies exist to compare these techniques with traditional open débridement. Furthermore, studies are difficult to compare given small sample sizes, the retrospective nature of reports, and varying comorbidities and selection criteria. For the current time, open surgical débridement continues to be the "gold standard" treatment for surgical management of pancreatic necrosis. However, as management strategies become more nonoperative, it is likely that minimally invasive and percutaneous techniques will play an increasing role in the treatment of pancreatic necrosis in the future.

■ SUMMARY

While the treatment of mild pancreatitis has changed little in recent years, advances in the management of severe pancreatitis have been associated with significantly reduced morbidity and mortality. Improvements in the recognition of severe disease with scoring systems and serial CT scanning have allowed early goal-directed therapy in appropriate patients. Timely resuscitation and invasive monitoring are standard, and there is an increased recognition of the role of prophylactic antibiotics for pancreatic necrosis and image-guided FNA to diagnose infection. While the need for aggressive intervention in infected pancreatic necrosis remains unchanged, initial conservative management of most patients with sterile pancreatic necrosis has gained widespread acceptance. Some patients with sterile necrosis eventually may require delayed débridement either for persistent systemic illness or for failure to thrive, although accurate prospective identification on these patients has not been possible. For patients needing débridement, open surgical techniques remain the "gold standard" of management. Advances in minimally invasive technology hold promise as adjuncts to open procedures in the future, particularly as a means of delaying surgery to facilitate débridement when the necrotic pancreas becomes more organized.

REFERENCES

1. Banks PA. Acute pancreatitis: medical and surgical management. *Am J Gastroenterol* 1994;89:S78–85
2. Beger HG, Rau B, Mayer J, et al. Natural course of acute pancreatitis. *World J Surg* 1997;21:130–135
3. Yousaf M, McCallion K, Diamond T. Management of severe acute pancreatitis. *Br J Surg* 2003;90:407–420
4. Buchler MW, Gloor B, Muller CA, et al. Acute necrotizing pancreatitis: treatment strategy according to the status of infection. *Ann Surg* 2000;232:619–626
5. Clancy TE, Ashley SW. Current management of necrotizing pancreatitis. *Adv Surg* 2002;36:103–121
6. Sakorafas GH, Tsiotou AG. Etiology and pathogenesis of acute pancreatitis: current concepts. *J Clin Gastroenterol* 2000;30:343–356
7. Kazmierczak SC, Catrou PG, Van Lente F. Diagnostic accuracy of pancreatic enzymes evaluated by use of multivariate data analysis. *Clin Chem* 993;39:1960–1965
8. Sternby B, O'Brien JF, Zinsmeister AR, DiMagno EP. What is the best biochemical test to diagnose acute pancreatitis? A prospective clinical study. *Mayo Clin Proc* 1996;71:1138–1144
9. Clavien PA, Robert J, Meyer P, et al. Acute pancreatitis and normoamylasemia: Not an uncommon combination. *Ann Surg* 1989;210:614–620
10. Dervenis C, Johnson CD, Bassi C, et al. Diagnosis, objective assessment of severity, and management of acute pancreatitis: Santorini consensus conference. *Int J Pancreatol* 1999;25:195–210
11. Baron TH, Morgan DE. Acute necrotizing pancreatitis. *N Engl J Med* 1999;340:1412–1417
12. Lerch MM, Hernandez CA, Adler G. Acute pancreatitis. *N Engl J Med* 1994;331:948–949
13. Ranson JH, Rifkind KM, Roses DF, et al. Prognostic signs and the role of operative management in acute pancreatitis. *Surg Gynecol Obstet* 1974;139:69–81
14. Blamey SL, Imrie CW, O'Neill J, et al. Prognostic factors in acute pancreatitis. *Gut* 1984;25:1340–1346
15. Eachempati SR, Hydo LJ, Barie PS. Severity scoring for prognostication in patients with severe acute pancreatitis: Comparative analysis of the Ranson score and the APACHE III score. *Arch Surg* 2002;137:730–736
16. Connor S, Ghaneh P, Raraty M, et al. Increasing age and APACHE II scores are the main determinants of outcome from pancreatic necrosectomy. *Br J Surg* 2003;90:1542–1548
17. Williams M, Simms HH. Prognostic usefulness of scoring systems in critically ill patients with severe acute pancreatitis. *Crit Care Med* 1999;27:901–907
18. Triester SL, Kowdley KV. Prognostic factors in acute pancreatitis. *J Clin Gastroenterol* 2002;34:167–176
19. Brown A, Orav J, Banks PA. Hemoconcentration is an early marker for organ failure and necrotizing pancreatitis. *Pancreas* 2000;20:367–372

20. Lankisch PG, Mahlke R, Blum T, et al. Hemoconcentration: An early marker of severe and/or necrotizing pancreatitis? A critical appraisal. *Am J Gastroenterol* 2001;96: 2081–2085
21. de Beaux AC, Goldie AS, Ross JA, et al. Serum concentrations of inflammatory mediators related to organ failure in patients with acute pancreatitis. *Br J Surg* 1996;83: 349–353
22. Pezzilli R, Billi P, Miniero R, et al. Serum interleukin-6, interleukin-8, and b_2-microglobulin in early assessment of severity of acute pancreatitis: Comparison with serum C-reactive protein. *Dig Dis Sci* 1995;40:2341–2348
23. Kylanpaa-Back ML, Takala A, Kemppainen EA, et al. Procalcitonin, soluble interleukin-2 receptor, and soluble E-selectin in predicting the severity of acute pancreatitis. *Crit Care Med* 2001;29:63–69
24. Tenner S, Fernandez-del Castillo C, Warshaw A, et al. Urinary trypsinogen activation peptide (TAP) predicts severity in patients with acute pancreatitis. *Int J Pancreatol* 1997;21:105–110
25. Neoptolemos JP, Kemppainen EA, Mayer JM, et al. Early prediction of severity in acute pancreatitis by urinary trypsinogen activation peptide: A multicentre study. *Lancet* 2000;355:1955–1960
26. Kemppainen E, Mayer J, Puolakkainen P, et al. Plasma trypsinogen activation peptide in patients with acute pancreatitis. *Br J Surg* 2001;88:679–680
27. Balthazar EJ, Ranson JH, Naidich DP, et al. Acute pancreatitis: prognostic value of CT. *Radiology* 1985;156: 767–772
28. Balthazar EJ, Robinson DL, Megibow AJ, et al. Acute pancreatitis: value of CT in establishing prognosis. *Radiology* 1990;174:331–336
29. Bradley EL 3rd. A clinically based classification system for acute pancreatitis: Summary of the International Symposium on Acute Pancreatitis, Atlanta, GA, September 11 through 13, 1992. *Arch Surg* 1993;128:586–590
30. Arvanitakis M, Delhaye M, De Maertelaere V, et al. Computed tomography and magnetic resonance imaging in the assessment of acute pancreatitis. *Gastroenterology* 2004;126:715–723
31. Schmidt J, Hotz HG, Foitzik T, et al. Intravenous contrast medium aggravates the impairment of pancreatic microcirculation in necrotizing pancreatitis in the rat. *Ann Surg* 1995;221:257–264
32. Banks PA, Gerzof SG, Langevin RE, et al. CT-guided aspiration of suspected pancreatic infection: Bacteriology and clinical outcome. *Int J Pancreatol* 1995;18:265–270.
33. Ashley SW, Perez A, Pierce EA, et al. Necrotizing pancreatitis: Contemporary analysis of 99 consecutive cases. *Ann Surg* 2001;234:572–579; discussion 579–580
34. Toouli J, Brooke-Smith M, Bassi C, et al. Guidelines for the management of acute pancreatitis. *J Gastroenterol Hepatol* 2002;17:S15–39
35. Uhl W, Warshaw A, Imrie C, et al. IAP guidelines for the surgical management of acute pancreatitis. *Pancreatology* 2002;2:565–573
36. Tenner S, Banks PA. Acute pancreatitis: Nonsurgical management. *World J Surg* 1997;21:143–148
37. Brown A, Baillargeon JD, Hughes MD, et al. Can fluid resuscitation prevent pancreatic necrosis in severe acute pancreatitis? *Pancreatology* 2002;2:104–107
38. Goodgame JT, Fischer JE. Parenteral nutrition in the treatment of acute pancreatitis: Effect on complications and mortality. *Ann Surg* 1977;186:651–658
39. Lobo DN, Memon MA, Allison SP, et al. Evolution of nutritional support in acute pancreatitis. *Br J Surg* 2000;87: 695–707
40. uchman AL, Moukarzel AA, Bhuta S, et al. Parenteral nutrition is associated with intestinal morphologic and functional changes in humans. *JPEN J Parenter Enteral Nutr* 1995;19:453–460
41. Kalfarentzos F, Kehagias J, Mead N, et al. Enteral nutrition is superior to parenteral nutrition in severe acute pancreatitis: Results of a randomized prospective trial. *Br J Surg* 1997;84:1665–1669
42. McClave SA, Greene LM, Snider HL, et al. Comparison of the safety of early enteral vs parenteral nutrition in mild acute pancreatitis. *JPEN J Parenter Enteral Nutr* 1997; 21:14–20
43. Windsor AC, Kanwar S, Li AG, et al. Compared with parenteral nutrition, enteral feeding attenuates the acute phase response and improves disease severity in acute pancreatitis. *Gut* 1998;42:431–435
44. Zhao G, Wang CY, Wang F, et al. Clinical study on nutrition support in patients with severe acute pancreatitis. *World J Gastroenterol* 2003;9:2105–2108
45. Olah A, Belagyi T, Issekutz A, et al. Randomized clinical trial of specific *Lactobacillus* and fibre supplement to early enteral nutrition in patients with acute pancreatitis. *Br J Surg* 2002;89:1103–1107
46. Eatock FC, Brombacher GD, Steven A, et al. Nasogastric feeding in severe acute pancreatitis may be practical and safe. *Int J Pancreatol* 2000;28:23–29
47. Al-Omran M, Groof A, Wilke D. Enteral versus parenteral nutrition for acute pancreatitis. *Cochrane Database Syst Rev* 2003;1:CD002837
48. Neoptolemos JP, Carr-Locke DL, London NJ, et al. Controlled trial of urgent endoscopic retrograde cholangiopancreatography and endoscopic sphincterotomy versus conservative treatment for acute pancreatitis due to gallstones. *Lancet* 1988;2:979–983
49. Fan ST, Lai EC, Mok FP, et al. Early treatment of acute biliary pancreatitis by endoscopic papillotomy. *N Engl J Med* 1993;328:228–232
50. Folsch UR, Nitsche R, Ludtke R, et al. Early ERCP and papillotomy compared with conservative treatment for acute biliary pancreatitis: The German Study Group on Acute Biliary Pancreatitis. *N Engl J Med* 1997;336:237–242
51. Varghese JC, Farrell MA, Courtney G, et al. Role of MR cholangiopancreatography in patients with failed or inadequate ERCP. *AJR* 1999;173:1527–1533
52. Rau B, Uhl W, Buchler MW, et al. Surgical treatment of infected necrosis. *World J Surg* 1997;21:155–161
53. Bradley EL 3rd, Allen K. A prospective longitudinal study of observation versus surgical intervention in the management of necrotizing pancreatitis. *Am J Surg* 1991;161:19–24; discussion 24–15

54. Lumsden A, Bradley EL 3rd. Secondary pancreatic infections. *Surg Gynecol Obstet* 1990;170:459–467
55. Bassi C, Falconi M, Talamini G, et al. Controlled clinical trial of pefloxacin versus imipenem in severe acute pancreatitis. *Gastroenterology* 1998;115:1513–1517.
56. Grewe M, Tsiotos GG, Luque de-Leon E, et al. Fungal infection in acute necrotizing pancreatitis. *J Am Coll Surg* 1999;188:408–414
57. Ratschko M, Fenner T, Lankisch PG. The role of antibiotic prophylaxis in the treatment of acute pancreatitis. *Gastroenterol Clin North Am* 1999;28:641–659, ix–x
58. Bassi C, Larvin M, Villatoro E. Antibiotic therapy for prophylaxis against infection of pancreatic necrosis in acute pancreatitis. *Cochrane Database Syst Rev* 2003;4: CD002941
59. Buchler M, Malfertheiner P, Friess H, et al. Human pancreatic tissue concentration of bactericidal antibiotics. *Gastroenterology* 1992;103:1902–1908
60. Pederzoli P, Bassi C, Vesentini S, et al. A randomized, multicenter clinical trial of antibiotic prophylaxis of septic complications in acute necrotizing pancreatitis with imipenem. *Surg Gynecol Obstet* 1993;176:480–483
61. Sainio V, Kemppainen E, Puolakkainen P, et al. Early antibiotic treatment in acute necrotising pancreatitis. *Lancet* 1995;346(8976):663–667
62. Schwarz M, Isenmann R, Meyer H, et al. [Antibiotic use in necrotizing pancreatitis: Results of a controlled study.] *Dtsch Med Wochenschr* 1997;122:356–361.
63. Isenmann R, Runzi M, Kron M, et al. Prophylactic antibiotic treatment in patients with predicted severe acute pancreatitis: A placebo-controlled, double-blind trial. *Gastroenterology* 2004;126:997–1004
64. Golub R, Siddiqi F, Pohl D. Role of antibiotics in acute pancreatitis: A meta-analysis. *J Gastrointest Surg* 1998;2: 496–503
65. Sharma VK, Howden CW. Prophylactic antibiotic administration reduces sepsis and mortality in acute necrotizing pancreatitis: A meta-analysis. *Pancreas* 2001;22:28–31
66. Powell JJ, Campbell E, Johnson CD, et al. Survey of antibiotic prophylaxis in acute pancreatitis in the UK and Ireland. *Br J Surg* 1999;86:320–322
67. Gloor B, Muller CA, Worni M, et al. Pancreatic infection in severe pancreatitis: The role of fungus and multiresistant organisms. *Arch Surg* 2001;136:592–596
68. He YM, Lv XS, Ai ZL, et al. Prevention and therapy of fungal infection in severe acute pancreatitis: A prospective clinical study. *World J Gastroenterol* 2003;9:2619–2621
69. Lange JF, van Gool J, Tytgat GN. The protective effect of a reduction in intestinal flora on mortality of acute haemorrhagic pancreatitis in the rat. *Hepatogastroenterology* 1987;34:28–30
70. Luiten EJ, Hop WC, Lange JF, et al. Controlled clinical trial of selective decontamination for the treatment of severe acute pancreatitis. *Ann Surg* 1995;222:57–65
71. Fernandez-del Castillo C, Rattner DW, Makary MA, et al. Débridement and closed packing for the treatment of necrotizing pancreatitis. *Ann Surg.* 1998;228:676–684
72. Rattner DW, Legermate DA, Lee MJ, et al. Early surgical débridement of symptomatic pancreatic necrosis is beneficial irrespective of infection. *Am J Surg* 1992;163:105–109; discussion 109–110
73. McFadden DW, Reber HA. Indications for surgery in severe acute pancreatitis. *Int J Pancreatol* 1994;15:83–90
74. Rau B, Pralle U, Uhl W, et al. Management of sterile necrosis in instances of severe acute pancreatitis. *J Am Coll Surg* 1995;181:279–288.
75. Ashley SW. Sterile pancreatic necrosis: Is operation necessary? *J Am Coll Surg* 1995;181:363–364
76. Branum G, Galloway J, Hirchowitz W, et al. Pancreatic necrosis: Results of necrosectomy, packing, and ultimate closure over drains. *Ann Surg* 1998;227:870–877
77. Warshaw AL. Pancreatic necrosis: To débride or not to débride—that is the question. *Ann Surg* 2000;232:627–629
78. Baron TH, Morgan DE, Vickers SM, et al. Organized pancreatic necrosis: Endoscopic, radiologic, and pathologic features of a distinct clinical entity. *Pancreas* 1999; 19:105–108.
79. Mier J, Leon EL, Castillo A, et al. Early versus late necrosectomy in severe necrotizing pancreatitis. *Am J Surg* 1997;173(2):71–75
80. Watts GT. Total pancreatectomy for fulminant pancreatitis. *Lancet* 1963;13:384
81. Norton L, Eiseman B. Near total pancreatectomy for hemorrhagic pancreatitis. *Am J Surg* 1974;127:191–195
82. Alexandre JH, Guerrieri MT. Role of total pancreatectomy in the treatment of necrotizing pancreatitis. *World J Surg* 1981;5:369–377
83. Beger HG, Isenmann R. Surgical management of necrotizing pancreatitis. *Surg Clin North Am* 1999;79:783–800, ix.
84. Beger HG. Operative management of necrotizing pancreatitis: Necrosectomy and continuous closed postoperative lavage of the lesser sac. *Hepatogastroenterology* 1991;38:129–133
85. Sarr MG, Nagorney DM, Mucha P Jr, et al. Acute necrotizing pancreatitis: Management by planned, staged pancreatic necrosectomy/débridement and delayed primary wound closure over drains. *Br J Surg* 1991;78:576–581
86. Warshaw AL, Jin GL. Improved survival in 45 patients with pancreatic abscess. *Ann Surg* 1985;202:408–417
87. Aranha GV, Prinz RA, Greenlee HB. Pancreatic abscess: An unresolved surgical problem. *Am J Surg* 1982;144: 534–538
88. Davidson ED, Bradley EL 3rd. “Marsupialization” in the treatment of pancreatic abscess. *Surgery* 1981;89:252–256
89. Bradley EL 3rd. A fifteen year experience with open drainage for infected pancreatic necrosis. *Surg Gynecol Obstet* 1993;177:215–222
90. Pemberton JH, Nagorney DM, Becker JM, et al. Controlled open lesser sac drainage for pancreatic abscess. *Ann Surg* 1986;203:600–604
91. Wertheimer MD, Norris CS. Surgical management of necrotizing pancreatitis. *Arch Surg* 1986;121:484–487
92. Becker JM, Pemberton JH, DiMagno EP, et al. Prognostic factors in pancreatic abscess. *Surgery* 1984;96:455–461
93. Carter R. Management of infected necrosis secondary to acute pancreatitis: A balanced role for minimal access techniques. *Pancreatology* 2003;3:133–138

94. Freeny PC, Hauptmann E, Althaus SJ, et al. Percutaneous CT-guided catheter drainage of infected acute necrotizing pancreatitis: Techniques and results. *AJR* 1998; 170:969–975
95. Echenique AM, Sleeman D, Yrizarry J, et al. Percutaneous catheter-directed débridement of infected pancreatic necrosis: Results in 20 patients. *J Vasc Intervent Radiol* 1998;9:565–571
96. Endlicher E, Volk M, Feuerbach S, et al. Long-term follow-up of patients with necrotizing pancreatitis treated by percutaneous necrosectomy. *Hepatogastroenterology* 2003;50:2225–2228
97. Baron TH, Harewood GC, Morgan DE, et al. Outcome differences after endoscopic drainage of pancreatic necrosis, acute pancreatic pseudocysts, and chronic pancreatic pseudocysts. *Gastrointest Endosc* 2002;56:7–17
98. Morgan DE, Baron TH, Smith JK, et al. Pancreatic fluid collections prior to intervention: Evaluation with MR imaging compared with CT and US. *Radiology* 1997;203:773–778
99. Seifert H, Wehrmann T, Schmitt T, et al. Retroperitoneal endoscopic débridement for infected peripancreatic necrosis. *Lancet* 2000;356:653–655
100. Kozarek RA. Endotherapy for organized pancreatic necrosis: Perspective on skunk-poking. *Gastroenterology* 1996;111:820–823
101. Gambiez LP, Denimal FA, Porte HL, et al. Retroperitoneal approach and endoscopic management of peripancreatic necrosis collections. *Arch Surg* 1998;133:66–72
102. Carter CR, McKay CJ, Imrie CW. Percutaneous necrosectomy and sinus tract endoscopy in the management of infected pancreatic necrosis: An initial experience. *Ann Surg* 2000;232:175–180
103. Hwang TL, Chiu CT, Chen HM, et al. Surgical results for severe acute pancreatitis: Comparison of the different surgical procedures. *Hepatogastroenterology* 1995;42: 1026–1029
104. Teerenhovi O, Nordback I, Eskola J. High volume lesser sac lavage in acute necrotizing pancreatitis. *Br J Surg* 1989;76:370–373
105. Fugger R, Gotzinger P, Sautner T, et al. Necrosectomy and laparostomy: A combined therapeutic concept in acute necrotising pancreatitis. *Eur J Surg* 1995;161:103–107
106. Orlando R 3rd, Welch JP, Akbari CM, et al. Techniques and complications of open packing of infected pancreatic necrosis. *Surg Gynecol Obstet* 1993;177:65–71
107. Garcia-Sabrido JL, Tallado JM, Christou NV, et al. Treatment of severe intra-abdominal sepsis and/or necrotic foci by an "open-abdomen" approach: Zipper and zipper-mesh techniques. *Arch Surg* 1988;123:152–156
108. Pederzoli P, Bassi C, Vesentini S, et al. Retroperitoneal and peritoneal drainage and lavage in the treatment of severe necrotizing pancreatitis. *Surg Gynecol Obstet* 1990; 170:197–203
109. Villazon A, Villazon O, Terrazas F, et al. Retroperitoneal drainage in the management of the septic phase of severe acute pancreatitis. *World J Surg* 1991;15(1):103–107; discussion 107–108
110. Nicholson ML, Mortensen NJ, Espiner HJ. Pancreatic abscess: Results of prolonged irrigation of the pancreatic bed after surgery. *Br J Surg* 1988;75:89–91
111. Larvin M, Chalmers AG, Robinson PJ, McMahon MJ. Débridement and closed cavity irrigation for the treatment of pancreatic necrosis. *Br J Surg* 1989;76:465–471

37

Complications of Acute Pancreatitis (Including Pseudocysts)

John A. Windsor ▪ Patrick Schweder

Recovery from acute pancreatitis is now expected, which reflects the many improvements in supportive and intensive care. Complications still occur in a third of patients, and a quarter of these will die as a result. The protean nature of acute pancreatitis is illustrated in Figure 37–1,[1] where progression from mild edematous to severe necrotizing acute pancreatitis can be associated with a range of complications: local, regional, and systemic (Table 37–1). This chapter will focus on the diagnosis and management of the important complications of acute pancreatitis.

▪ FLUID COLLECTIONS

The accumulation of fluid in and around the pancreas is common with acute pancreatitis. This fluid can track widely and may take the form of peripancreatic fluid collections in the retroperitoneum and mediastinum, pancreatic ascites, and/or pleural effusions. Partly inflammatory exudates, the fluid collections also contain enzyme-rich pancreatic secretions as a consequence of parenchymal disruption. The most common routes of extension are into the lesser sac, behind the pancreatic head, behind the left and right colons on the psoas muscle, and into the small bowel mesentery and bulging through the transverse mesocolon. Fluid collections occur early (within 48 hours), resolve often, and are only important in and of themselves because they are the precursor of pancreatic pseudocysts. A fluid collection, when present for 4 weeks, is termed a *pseudocyst* (see below), as defined by the Atlanta conference.[2] The extent and number of fluid collections are included in the Balthazar grading of the severity of acute pancreatitis by computed tomographic (CT) scanning.[3] If spherical or ovoid with sharp margins, suggesting that they under some pressure from ongoing leakage, they are more likely to persist. It also has been noted that dark (or "prune juice") ascites is associated with more severe disease. Acute fluid collections are rarely symptomatic and do not require active treatment. Indeed, there is a risk of introducing infection if unnecessary percutaneous drainage is performed.

▪ PANCREATIC ASCITES AND PLEURAL EFFUSIONS

Pancreatic ascites and massive pancreatic pleural effusions are sometimes termed *internal pancreatic fistulas*. Significant pancreatic ascites is often due to the chronic leakage of a pseudocyst secondary to alcoholic pancreatitis in adults and traumatic pancreatitis in children. Weight loss may be a feature. Diagnostic aspiration will reveal a high amylase concentration. A trial of conservative treatment is indicated with nasojejunal tube feeding and treatment with a long-acting somatostatin analogue. Pancreatic ascites does not respond to diuretic therapy. Endoscopic retrograde pancreatography (ERCP) usually will identify the source of the fluid leak and enable a rational approach to treatment. Rarely, leakage from injury to the main pancreatic duct can be treated by a transsphincteric pancreatic duct stent. The operative approach is either a distal resection of the pancreas or

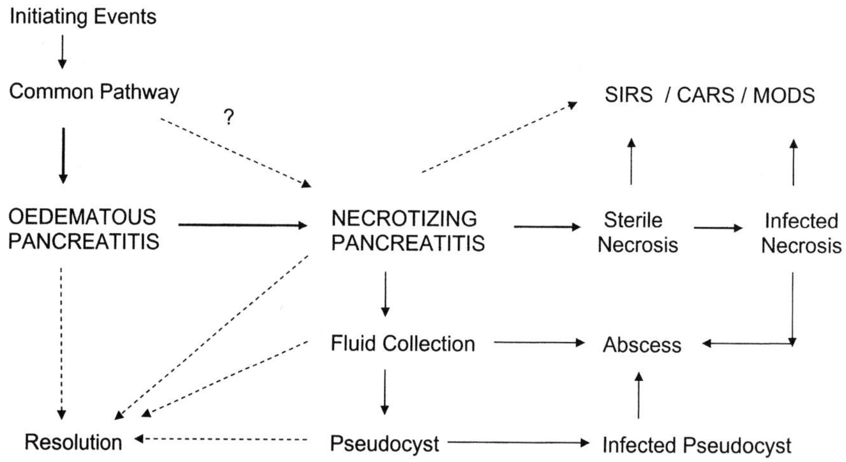

Figure 37–1. The protean nature of acute pancreatitis and related complications. SIRS = systemic inflammatory response syndrome; CARS = compensatory anti-inflammatory response syndrome; MODS = multiple-organ-dysfunction syndrome.

internal drainage into a Roux-en-Y limb of jejunum. There is some evidence that percutaneous peritoneal lavage of pancreatic ascites, in the context of acute pancreatitis, results in reduced abdominal pain, but this does not appear to alter the course of the disease and is not routine practice.

The drainage of pleural effusions in patients with acute pancreatitis should be considered if there is compromised respiratory function or inadequate oxygenation. Chronic pleural effusions owing to an internal pancreatic fistula often are treated with a chest tube, nasojejunal tube feeding, and somatostatin. Persistence or recurrence will require identification of a pancreatic leak and either drainage into a Roux-en-Y limb of jejunum or distal resection of the pancreas.

TABLE 37–1. THE COMPLICATIONS OF ACUTE PANCREATITIS

Local	Fluid collections Pancreatic ascites/pleural effusion Pancreatic pseudocyst Pancreatic necrosis Infected pancreatic abscess Hemorrhage/pseudoaneurysm
Regional	Venous thrombosis Paralytic ileus Intestinal obstruction Intestinal ischemia/necrosis Cholestasis
Systemic	Systemic inflammatory response syndrome Multiple-organ-dysfunction syndrome ARDS/pulmonary failure Renal failure Cardiovascular complications Hypocalcemia Hyperglycemia Disseminated intravascular coagulopathy Protein calorie malnutrition Encephalopathy

▪ PSEUDOCYST

A *pseudocyst* is defined as a peripancreatic fluid collection contained by a wall of fibrous granulation tissue that does not have an epithelial lining. This is in contrast to cystic neoplasms of the pancreas, which are characterised by an epithelial lining. It is salient to note that this is not an absolute distinction because there are reports of discontinuous epithelium in cystic neoplasms (probably owing to pressure atrophy) and of partial epithelialization of chronic pseudocysts (owing to communication with the main pancreatic duct). In fewer than 20% of cases, more than one pseudocyst is seen. With chronic pancreatitis, there is an increased tendency toward multiple, small, and intrapancreatic pseudocysts. Following acute pancreatitis, pseudocysts are located most often in close proximity to the pancreas, especially in the lesser sac (Fig 37–2) but also may be found in the pelvis, scrotum, mediastinum, and thorax.

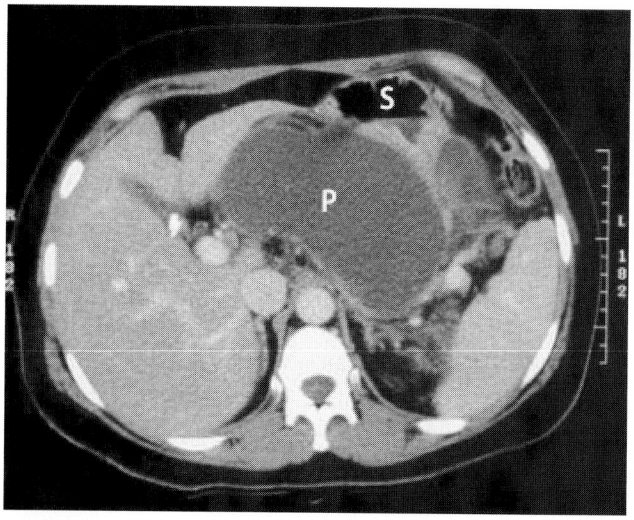

Figure 37–2. A CT scan of a pancreatic pseudocyst located in the lesser sac. (P = pseudocyst; S = stomach.)

The natural history of a pseudocyst is not easy to predict. Spontaneous resolution occurs frequently and usually within 6 weeks. When larger than 6 cm in diameter, and when it continues to enlarge during the first month, a pseudocyst is more likely to persist and develop complications. Size alone is a poor predictor because resolution can occur even with very large pseudocysts. Persistence is also more likely if there is a distal stricture of the main pancreatic duct and a proximal communication between the main pancreatic duct and the pseudocyst. Although not directly correlated, a large pseudocyst is more likely to cause discomfort and pain. Multiple pseudocysts and those associated with chronic pancreatitis are less likely to resolve.

PATHOGENESIS AND CLASSIFICATION

The development of a pseudocyst requires pancreatic duct disruption, and this occurs in the context of acute pancreatitis (2–10% of cases), trauma, or duct obstruction in chronic pancreatitis. The leakage of enzyme-rich secretion incites a marked inflammatory reaction of the peritoneum, retroperitoneal tissue, and serosa of adjacent viscera. As a result, the fluid is contained by a developing layer of fibrous granulation tissue that matures over time. If the communication between pancreatic duct and pseudocyst persists, the pseudocyst can continue to enlarge, sometimes reaching 20–30 cm in diameter. The contents of the pseudocyst usually consist of a relatively clear watery fluid. However, with hemorrhage, it may contain clot and become xanthochromic. In the presence of infection, a pseudocyst will contain pus. If the pseudocyst develops following pancreatic necrosis, it may contain a significant amount of solid tissue, both necrotic pancreas and peripancreatic fat necrosis. Pseudocyst rupture may result in free ascites, decompression into adjacent stomach or duodenum, or a pancreaticopleural/bronchial fistula.

Pseudocysts secondary to blunt trauma tend to develop anterior to the neck and body of the gland because the duct is injured where it crosses the vertebral column. In chronic pancreatitis, pseudocysts are considered to develop from a "blowout" of an obstructed pancreatic duct. The pseudocysts usually are located within the fibrotic gland and sometimes are difficult to distinguish from pancreatic retention cysts. The latter are formed by progressive dilatation of the pancreatic duct and tend to retain the epithelial lining of the duct.

The most useful classification of pseudocysts is that proposed by D'Egidio, and it incorporates the key features just discussed (Table 37–2). *Type I* are acute postnecrotic pseudocysts that occur after an episode of acute pancreatitis and are associated with normal duct anatomy and rarely communicate with the pancreatic duct. *Type II* are postnecrotic pseudocysts that occur after an episode of acute or chronic pancreatitis and have a diseased but not strictured pancreatic duct, and there is often a communication between the duct and the pseudocyst. *Type III* are also called *retention cysts,* occur in chronic pancreatitis, and are uniformly associated with a duct stricture and a communication between the duct and the pseudocyst.

COMPLICATIONS

The risk of pseudocyst complications is less than previously believed when pseudocysts were diagnosed on the basis of symptoms. With pervasive imaging, a higher proportion of asymptomatic pseudocsyts are diagnosed. Complications of pseudocysts include infection, leakage, and bleeding. By mass effect, a pseudocyst also can produce early satiety (stomach), stenosis (duodenum), cholestasis (bile duct), and thrombosis (portal, superior mesenteric and splenic veins) leading to portal or segmental hypertension and varices.

Infection of the pancreas can take several forms. Secondary infection of a simple pseudocyst is quite different from secondary infection of pancreatic necrosis, although the latter may develop into an abscess and be difficult to distinguish from the former on CT scan (see Fig 37–1). Sterile, organized pancreatic necrosis may appear as a mature pseudocyst on CT scan but be predominantly solid. These differences relate to the origin (isolated duct damage versus pancreatic necrosis) and to the amount of solid material contained within the collection. To fail to appreciate these differences may result in suboptimal treatment. In brief, the former requires drainage, whereas the latter, for resolution, requires drainage and débridement.

TABLE 37–2. THE D'EGIDIO CLASSIFICATION OF PANCREATIC PSEUDOCYSTS AND THE PRIMARY TREATMENT OPTIONS

	Context	Pancreatic duct	Duct-pseudocyst communication	Primary treatment
Type I	Acute postnecrotic pancreatitis	Normal	No	Percutaneous drainage
Type II	Acute-on-chronic pancreatitis	Abnormal (no stricture)	50:50	Internal drainage or resection
Type III	Chronic pancreatitis	Abnormal (stricture)	Yes	Internal drainage with duct decompression

The rupture of a pseudocyst can occur by erosion into the adjacent gastrointestinal tract, which may resolve the pseudocyst or leave a cystoenteric fistula. This term is not strictly accurate because the communication is not between two epithelial-lined structures. Rupture into the peritoneum leads to pancreatic ascites and can be a dramatic presentation with acute abdominal pain and rigidity from chemical peritonitis.

Bleeding associated with a pancreatic pseudocyst is a life-threatening complication. There are several causes of bleeding. Bleeding may occur secondary to erosion of the gut mucosa with the impending development of a cystoenteric fistula (as above). This may produce hematemesis and malena. More ominous is the direct erosion of a significant visceral vessel, including the splenic, gastroduodenal, and middle colic vessels. The action of pancreatic enzymes (especially elastase) on the vessel wall can lead to thinning of the vessel wall and aneurysm and pseudoaneursym formation (Fig 37–3). This situation carries a high mortality. The risk of bleeding is increased in the presence of local infection. If time and patient stability permit, emergency selective splanchnic angiography is performed to delineate the site of bleeding, and embolization is attempted (Fig 37–4A, B). Otherwise, emergency surgery is required, consisting of oversewing of the bleeding vessels and internal or external drainage of the pseudocyst. Sometimes it is possible to resect the pseudocyst, which is ideal because it prevents recurrent hemorrhage. Sometimes bleeding may be controlled only with packing at the first operation.

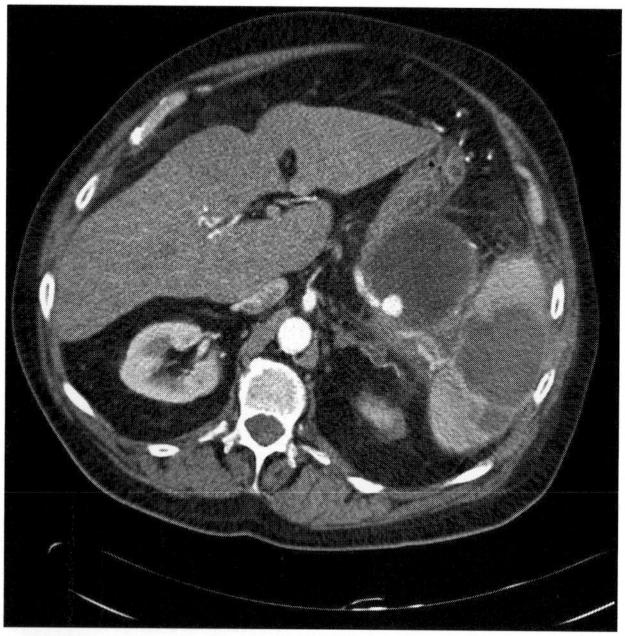

Figure 37–3. A contrast CT scan showing the pseudocysts, the medial one complicated by a pseudoaneurysm related to the splenic artery.

DIAGNOSIS AND INVESTIGATION

A pseudocyst should be suspected when a patient with acute pancreatitis fails to recover after a week of treatment or when, after improving for a time, symptoms return. Often the early stages of pseudocyst formation are observed radiologically before symptoms develop, and this provides some forewarning. Earlier imaging of a fluid collection, especially when associated with an area of pancreatic necrosis, increases the likelihood of the development of a pseudocyst. Most patients have epigastric discomfort or pain. There may be anorexia, early satiety, nausea, mild fever, back pain, and a palpable mass. Signs of sepsis usually are not overt. In about half the patients there is failure of the serum amylase level to return to normal or a mild (2–4 times normal) secondary rise.

The clinical diagnosis of a complication of a known pseudocyst is usually straightforward. The rupture of a pseudocyst into the peritoneal cavity is associated with the onset of acute abdominal pain and signs of peritonitis. This is in contrast to the spontaneous decompression of a pseudocyst into an adjacent organ, which usually results in the relief of symptoms. Infection of a pseudocyst is accompanied by signs of toxicity and leukocytosis. Infection can be confirmed with ultrasound-guided fine-needle aspiration for Gram's stain and bacterial culture. Bleeding usually results in an increase in abdominal pain and possible syncope, tachycardia, and hypotension. A drop in hemoglobin concentration is expected.

The clinical suspicion of a pseudocyst is best investigated by contrast-enhanced CT scan (Fig 37–5). While ultrasonography (US) is excellent for the detection of a pseudocyst, it is limited by operator skill, the patient's habitus, and overlying bowel gas. The advantage of US might be to better determine the extent of solid tissue within a pseudocyst, and it is used often to guide fine-needle aspiration. US (transabdominal or endoscopic) can be useful in distinguishing a pseudocyst from a cystic neoplasm because it often delineates internal septation better than CT scan.

Although cystic neoplasms are rare, they are mistaken commonly for pseudocysts. Absence of an antecedent history of acute pancreatitis, elevation of CEA or CA 19-9, and/or the presence of internal septation should suggest this diagnosis. If endoscopic US is available, it will enable the identification of septations (microscopic characteristics of serous lesions or macrocystic characteristic of mucinous lesions), mural nodules, echogenic debris, and calcification, and it also may allow aspiration of fluid content for analysis. Pseudocysts usually contain fluid with elevated amylase (>5000 units/mL) and an absence of tumour markers, but this should not be relied on for a definitive diagnosis.[4]

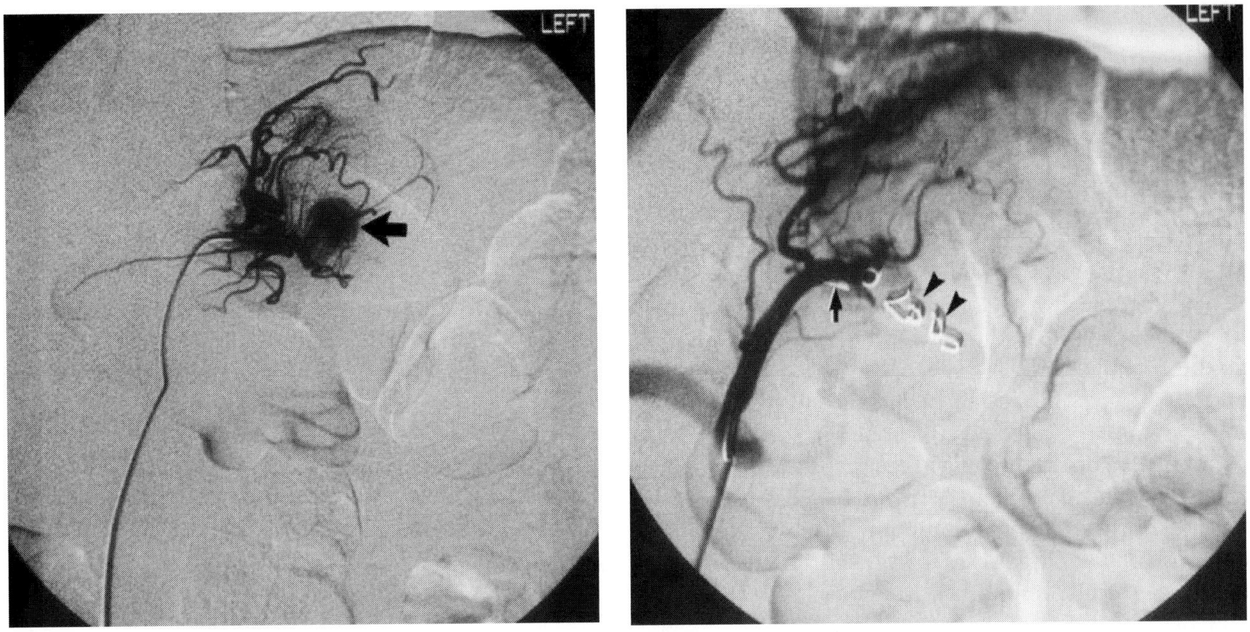

A B

Figure 37–4. Selective mesenteric angiogram showing a pseudoanuerysm related to the left gastric artery (**A**) and successful embolization (**B**).

Compared with US, CT scanning has an accuracy approaching 100% for the diagnosis of a pseudocyst, is not operator-dependent, and is more useful in planning therapy. It will demonstrate the key features of a pseudocyst (i.e., size, shape, wall thickness, and contents), the nature of the pancreas (i.e., presence and extent of necrosis, diameter of pancreatic duct, and features of chronic pancreatitis, including atrophy and calcification), and the relationship of these to the surrounding organs (see Fig 37–2), which can be critical in planning internal surgical drainage. Triphasic helical CT scanning will delineate the regional arteries (to look for pseudoanuerysm formation) and veins (to look for thrombosis, cavernous transformation, and formation of varices). MRI is not necessary for the diagnosis of pseudocysts, although, like US, it may be useful in determining the extent of solid content in the pseudocyst.

ERCP has both diagnostic and therapeutic roles. Because of the risks of exacerbating pancreatitis, perforation, bleeding, and introducing infection, it should not be a routine test and preferably is done within 48 hours of any planned drainage procedure. Over 90% of patients with a pseudocyst have some abnormality of the pancreatic duct, and most of these can be detected by MRCP. The unique diagnostic contribution of ERCP is to accurately delineate a communication between the main pancreatic duct and the pseudocyst, which occurs in over 60% of patients. A communication of this type is a relative contraindication to external drainage of a pseudocyst.[5] The classification of the main pancreatic duct by ERCP has been shown to assist in the selecting the type of treatment, where the presence or absence of a stricture, communication, and obstruction is an important feature to note.[6]

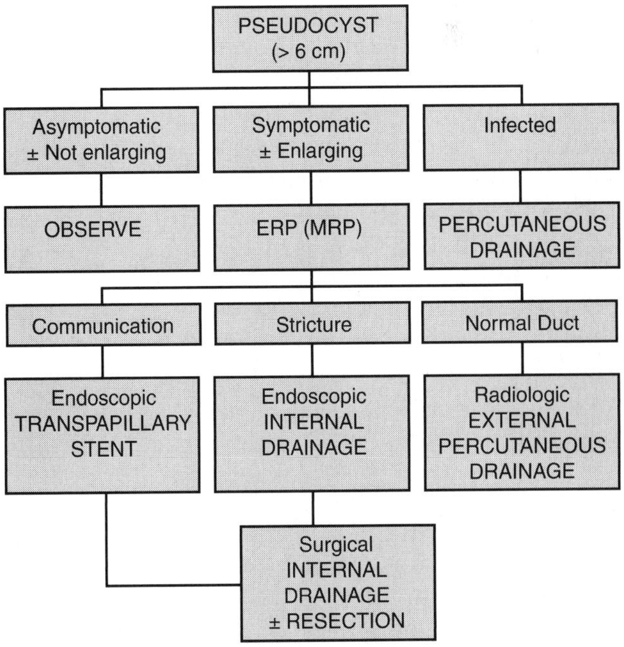

Figure 37–5. Algorithm for investigation and treatment of pancreatic pseudocysts. (ERP = endoscopic retrograde pancreatogram; MRP = magnetic resonance pancreatogram.)

TREATMENT

The principal indications for treating pancreatic pseudocysts are to relieve symptoms and to prevent complications. In the absence of symptoms or evidence of enlargement, expectant management usually is reasonable. The decision as to whether a pseudocyst in a particular patient requires active intervention can be difficult. The desire to allow time for spontaneous resolution to occur must be balanced against the risk of complications while waiting for cyst wall maturity. The traditional indications for treatment were the complications of a pseudocyst. Now the focus is on preventing complications. In many centers it has become less common to treat a pseudocyst solely on the grounds of a failure to resolve. An enlarging asymptomatic pseudocyst that has been present for 6 weeks usually is treated. This relatively conservative approach is based on the low risk of complications. A natural-history study from India indicates that asymptomatic pseudocysts less than 7.5 cm in diameter and without internal debris will resolve spontaneously at an average of 5 months.[7] At the same time as this trend toward conservatism, there has been an increase the number of treatment modalities, including endoscopic, percutaneous, and laparoscopic techniques.

There are two important rules in the treatment of pseudocysts. The first is that a cystic neoplasm must not be treated as a pseudocyst. The second is that elective external drainage of a pseudocyst must not be done if there is downstream and unrelieved pancreatic ductal obstruction because of the high risk of an external pancreatic fistula.

The approach to treatment (Table 37–3) depends on the nature of the pseudocyst, the pancreatic duct, and the fitness of the patient. Also important is the level of available expertise and experience with the various treatment modalities.

TABLE 37–3. THE TREATMENT APPROACHES FOR PANCREATIC PSEUDOCYST

Approaches	Examples
Open surgical	Cystogastrostomy Cystoduodenostomy Roux-en-Y cystojejunostomy Distal pancreatectomy ± splenectomy External drainage
Laparoscopic	Cystogastrostomy Cystoduodenostomy Roux-en-Y cystojejunostomy Distal pancreatectomy ± splenectomy External drainage
Radiologic	Percutaneous drainage Percutaneous transgastric drainage
Endoscopic	Transpapillary pancreatic duct stent Transgastric stent Transduodenal stent

The following features of a pseudocyst are important in considering the most appropriate treatment:

- *The thickness of the pseudocyst wall,* which is usually a function of the duration of the pseudocyst. This is important because the operative drainage of a pseudocyst requires that it safely accept sutures or staples. After 4–6 weeks, this will not be an issue.
- *The location of the pseudocyst.* If adherent to the stomach or duodenum, the options are different than if the pseudocyst is deep within the retroperitoneum and covered by bowel loops.
- *The contents of the pseudocyst.* Blood may require prior embolization of a pseudoanuerysm. Pus will require drainage, percutaneous or open. Infected necrosum will require débridement.
- The pancreas and the pancreatic duct need separate consideration in planning the treatment of a pseudocyst. The pancreas may warrant treatment in its own right, especially if there is a ductal stricture, a dilated duct, or regional disease warranting resection.

Open Surgical Treatment

There is no single surgical procedure that is appropriate for all pseudocysts. In principle, drainage procedures are preferred to resection because they preserve pancreatic function, are technically easier, and have a lower mortality rate. Despite the many alternatives and less invasive approaches, it is important to emphasize that the most effective and reliable means of treating a pseudocyst is internal drainage by an open surgical approach (see Table 37–3). The complication and mortality rates of internal drainage are half those of external drainage.

A D'Egidio type II pseudocyst is best treated by internal drainage or resection. When there is a mature wall, internal drainage is the best surgical option. Recurrence rates should be less than 5%, and mortality should be less than 2%. The pseudocyst can be drained into the stomach, the duodenum, or the jejunum. The choice of surgical procedure depends on the location of the pseudocyst and its relationship to these organs. A cystogastrostomy is ideal when the pseudocyst is adherent to the posterior stomach and indenting it (Fig 37–6). A longitudinal anterior gastrostomy is followed by the stepwise excision of a disk (>2 cm diameter) of stomach with subjacent pseudocyst wall. The tissue is sent for frozen section in all cases to exclude cystic neoplasia. Sutures are placed in stages to reduce the risk of edge bleeding as the disk is excised. Prior confirmation of the location of the pseudocyst may be required by needle aspiration, although it is usually obvious. The

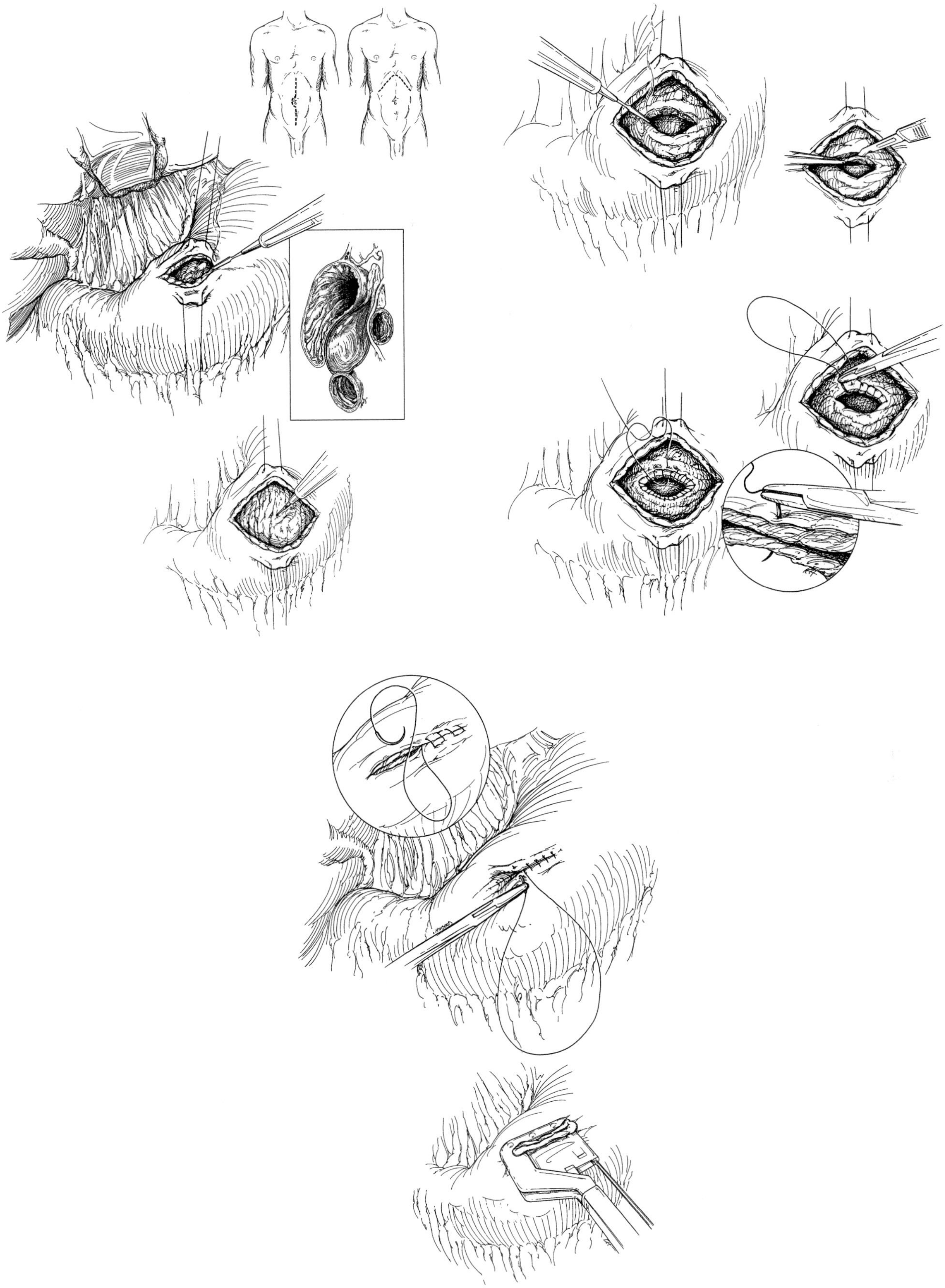

Figure 37–6. Internal drainage of a pseudocyst through the posterior wall of the stomach (cystogastrostomy).

stoma should be large enough to allow transgastric débridement of the pseudocyst cavity. A laparoscope can be used after open débridement to confirm that the cavity has been well débrided. A nasogastric tube can be left in the pseudocyst cavity for ongoing irrigation. The disadvantage of the cystogastrostomy is that it is not a dependent stoma, may act as a sump, and can become an abscess with very large pseudocysts. Where access permits, a roux en Y cystojejunostomy is ideal for internal drainage (Fig 37–7) and is particularly suited to drainage of pseudocysts arising from the body and tail of the pancreas, not adherent to the stomach and bulging through the left transverse mesocolon.

Combining internal drainage of a pseudocyst with a lateral pancreaticojejunostomy should be considered in patients with chronic pancreatitis and a dilated pancreatic duct because it will improve outcome without increasing the risk of the procedure. The blind end of the Roux limb should be placed toward the tail of the pancreas because this allows the head of the pancreas to be drained and the bile duct to be bypassed using the same limb should this be required.

Transduodenal drainage of a pseudocyst in the head of the pancreas is required occasionally, but only if it impinges the medial duodenal wall, because these pseudocysts may be difficult to drain by other techniques. Care must be taken to avoid the intrapancreatic portion of the common bile duct and the sphincter of Oddi.

Distal pancreatic resection has a role, particulary when the head of the pancreas is relatively preserved. An endoscopic retrograde pancreatogram will help to define the extent of resection. Provided that there is no pancreatic duct obstruction, the recurrence and fistula rates are very low. Specific ligation of the pancreatic duct will decrease the fistula rate.

External drainage of a pseudocyst has a limited role but is useful in the critically-ill patient and where a controlled external fistula is an acceptable goal. Other rare indications for external drainage at the time of laparotomy include the control of an immature ruptured pseudocyst and for some bleeding pseudocysts where there has been underrunning of the bleeding point. An external fistula may resolve more rapidly with placement of a transpapillary stent and with the use of a long-acting somatostatin analogue.

Radiologic Treatment

The first description of direct percutaneous aspiration and external drainage using ultrasound guidance was just 20 years ago. This technique has become widely practiced with a reported morbidity of between 10 and 30%. It can be used with an immature pseudocyst wall, although the risk of complications is higher in this setting. Percutaneous drainage is best suited to D'Egidio type I pseudocysts in which there is no significant underlying duct abnormality or communication between the duct and pseudocyst. In the setting of acute pancreatitis, catheter drainage is severely hampered by the inability to allow the ready egress of necrotic and viscous material. In the setting of chronic pancreatitis, the downstream obstruction of the duct gives rise to a high recurrence rate and/or a external fistula along the catheter tract. In simple, uncomplicated pseudocysts, percutaneous drainage usually is successful, although this is the group with the fewest symptoms, the lowest complication rate, and the best chance of spontaneous resolution.

The introduction of a transgastric approach to percutaneous drainage has almost abolished the problem of external pancreatic fistulas[8] (Fig 37–8A, B). This produces a percutaneous cystogastrostomy but requires an initial period of external transgastric drainage, clamping at 3 days, and then internalization at 2 weeks. Internalization can be helped with a concurrent endoscopic view, especially in the deployment of double pigtail catheters. The endoscopic approach is also used for the subsequent removal of the catheters. A well-matched population-based study comparing percutaneous (n = 8121) with open surgical drainage (n = 6409) in 14,914 patients with pancreatic pseudocysts revealed a longer length of hospital stay and twice the mortality (5.9 versus 2.8%) for the former.[9] A carefully considered selective approach to the use of percutanous drainage is required.

Endoscopic Treatment

There has been significant activity in the endoscopic treatment of pseudocysts over the last decade. Endoscopic transpapillary techniques include stenting the sphincter of Oddi to lower ductal pressures. The stent also can be advanced via the pancreatic duct into the pseudocyst when there is a demonstrable communication. Endoscopic transmural drainage is also possible and involves identifying the bulge into stomach or duodenum caused by the pseudocyst. The cyst generally is entered using a diathermy needle knife. Prior endoscopic ultrasonography allows greater accuracy and safety by confirming the anatomic route, and Doppler can be used to help avoid larger blood vessels. A number of pigtail stents can be inserted. The tract also can be dilated with a balloon catheter and the endoscope itself inserted into the cavity of the pseudocyst for direct visualization and retrieval of the cyst contents and wall biopsy (to rule out a cystic neoplasm).

These endoscopic methods are still evolving but have a reported success rate of up to 90% with experienced practitioners. But it must be remembered that the reports generally are in carefully selected patients. Caution needs to be exercised because of the risks of perforation, peritonitis, and infection through inadequate internal drainage. There is no reliable means of

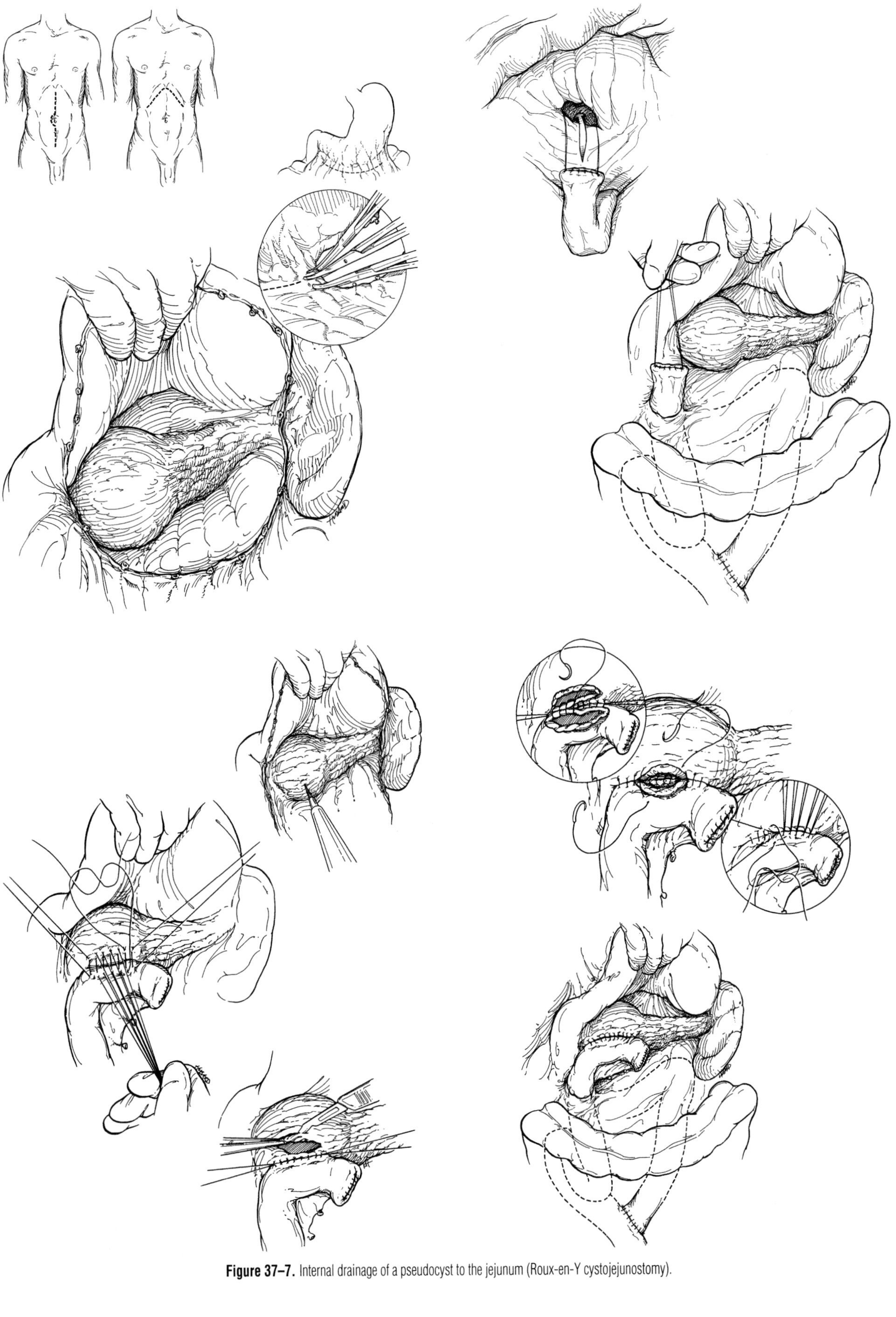

Figure 37–7. Internal drainage of a pseudocyst to the jejunum (Roux-en-Y cystojejunostomy).

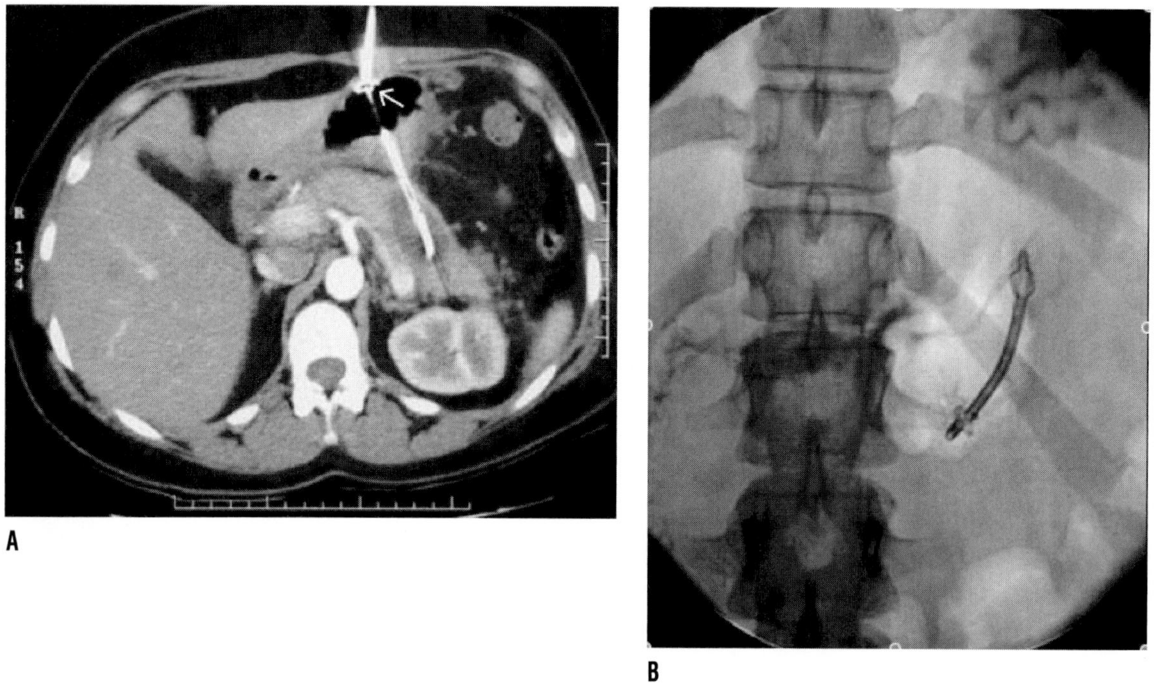

Figure 37-8. CT scans showing (**A**) percutaneous transgastric drainage of pseudocyst and (**B**) plain radiograph showing double Malecot-type stent cystogastrostomy. (Photographs courtesy of Dr. John Chen and Dr. Tom Wilson.)

obtaining a large tissue sample to exclude cystic neoplasia. There is also an increased risk of bleeding, reflecting the inability to place hemostatic sutures at the anastomotic edge. The real complication rate probably is higher than the reported 20%.

Minimally Invasive Surgery

All the open surgical techniques have been undertaken with a laparoscopic approach, and these will make a larger contribution with time.[10] Intraluminal laparoscopic surgery, where the trocars are placed through the abdominal and stomach walls, has been successful. The cystogastrostomy can be performed with a stapler or by suture. A more recent modification of this approach is the minilaparoscopic cystogastrostomy using a 2-mm intraluminal laparoscope. The view is augmented by the insertion of a flexible endoscope per os, which also can be used to explore the cyst cavity.

The balloon dilatation of a percutaneous catheter track using a similar approach to that used for percutaneous nephrolithotomy is feasible in many cases. It is worth considering this when the initial radiologic attempts have failed to bring resolution. The placement of a sheath then allows the insertion of an operating nephroscope to enable débridement of the pseudocyst and removal of organized pancreatic necrosis and infected necrosum. This procedure can be repeated and allows the placement of a soft large-bore external drain.

Summary of Treatment

The treatment of choice for pancreatic pseudocysts depends on a number of factors, including size, number, and location of pseudocysts; whether the main pancreatic duct is obstructed or communicates with the pseudocyst; and whether there are complications of the pseudocyst. The clinical context is important (see Table 37–2). With the range of approaches to treatment and the variation in the availability of equipment and expertise, it is necessary to develop a rational treatment algorthm that is appropriate for the clinical setting and the patient (see Fig 37–5). In practice, type I pseudocysts can be managed safely and effectively by percutaneous drainage. Type II pseudocysts are best managed by internal drainage, especially when there is communication between duct and pseudocyst. Endoscopic, laparoscopic, and radiologic approaches have an emerging role in expert hands.[11] With type III pseudocysts, consideration needs to be given to decompression of the pancreatic duct and relieving the stricture at the same time as drainage of the pseudocyst.

▪ PANCREATIC NECROSIS

From a clinical viewpoint, the development of necrosis is the most important event in the course of acute pancreatitis because subsequent complications, whether local or systemic, are associated with this. Pancreatic *ne-*

crosis is defined as a diffuse or focal area of nonviable pancreatic parenchyma that typically is associated with peripancreatic fat necrosis. Necrosis can be sterile or infected. Infected pancreatic necrosis is the leading cause of death associated with severe acute pancreatitis.

EPIDEMIOLOGY

The incidence of acute pancreatitis varies from 10–40 per 100,000 population. The proportion of patients that develop pancreatic necrosis is approximately 15–20%. Approximately 40% of these patients go on to develop infection of the necrosis. The overall mortality of edematous pancreatitis is 1% or less, that of sterile necrosis 5%, and that of infected necrosis 10–20% in centers of excellence.

The risk of infected necrosis increases with the duration of illness and the extent of necrosis. The risk of infection increases from 24% by the end of the first week of illness, to 36% at the end of the second week, and to 71% by the end of the third week.[12]

PATHOGENESIS

Pancreatic necrosis occurs within the first few days of the onset of acute pancreatitis. Of the patients who develop pancreatic necrosis, 70% have evidence of this by 48 hours of the onset of abdominal pain, and all of them by 96 hours. The premature activation of proteolytic enzymes within the acinar cells and interstitium of the lobule results in extensive necrosis of acinar cells and the substantial interstitial and intravascular accumulation and activation of leukocytes. There are a number of factors that contribute to the failure of the pancreatic microcirculation, which is evident histologically as stasis and/or thrombosis of intrapancreatic vessels. The failure of the pancreatic microcirculation leads to ischemia, which compounds the enzymatic and inflammatory injury and leads to the full syndrome of necrotizing pancreatitis. During this first week or two, in the so-called vasoactive phase, there is the release of proinflammatory mediators that contribute to the pathogenesis of pulmonary, cardiovascular, and renal insufficiency. This early systemic inflammatory response and multiorgan dysfunction are found frequently in the absence of pancreatic infection. In the later septic phase, which occurs in some patients after 3–4 weeks, these systemic events occur as a consequence of pancreatic infection.

There are five routes by which bacteria can infect pancreatic necrosis: (1) hematogenous through mesenteric vessels to the portal circulation, (2) transpapillary reflux of enteric content into the pancreatic duct, (3) translocation of intestinal bacteria and toxins via the mesenteric lymphatics to the thoracic duct and the systemic circulation, (4) reflux of bacteriobilia via a disrupted pancreatic duct into the necrotic parenchyma, and (5) transperitoneal spread.

Cultures of infected pancreatic necrosis yield monomicrobial flora in three-quarter of patients. Gram-negative aerobic bacteria usually are responsible (e.g., *Escherichia coli, Pseudomonas* spp., *Proteus,* and *Klebsiella* spp.), and this strongly suggests an intestinal origin, but gram-positive bacteria (e.g., *Staphylococcus aureus, Streptococcus faecalis,* and *Enterococcus*), anaerobes, and occasionally, fungi also have been documented.[13] The spectrum of bacteria cultured from infected necrosis has altered with the more widespread use of prophylactic antibiotics, with a shift toward gram-positive bacteria and fungal infections.[14]

The necrotizing process can extend widely to involve retroperitoneal fat, small and large bowel mesentery, and the retrocolic and perinephric compartments.

PREDICTION AND DIAGNOSIS

The clinical symptoms and signs of pancreatic necrosis are indistinguishable from those of other patients presenting with acute pancreatitis. Abdominal pain, distension, and guarding are associated with a low-grade fever and tachycardia. The severity of pain and the extent of hyperamylasemia do not correspond with the severity of acute pancreatitis. Patients presenting late with severe disease often will have established multiorgan dysfunction. The classic skin signs of retroperitoneal necrosis, including discoloration of the navel (Cullen's sign), the flanks (Grey-Turner's sign), and the inguinal region (Fox's sign), are rare and often not seen until the second or third week. The diagnosis of pancreatic necrosis requires more than clinical acumen.

The "gold standard" for the diagnosis of pancreatic necrosis is contrast-enhanced CT scanning demonstrating hypoperfusion in the arterial phase(see Fig 36–2). In the absence of a specific marker of pancreatic necrosis, many serum predictors have been proposed. An ideal predictor or prognostic indicator should be simple, cheap, reproducible, valid, available on admission, and specific for necrosis. While a full discussion of markers is beyond the scope of this chapter, there are several that fulfill most of these criteria, compare favorably with CT scanning, and have an established role in routine clinical practice.

C-reactive protein (CRP) is the most widely used predictor of pancreatic necrosis and is useful as a daily monitor of disease progress. The accuracy in detecting necrosis is about 85%, but it requires 3–4 days to reach this level. The threshold values depend on the assay and the study used. The most commonly used threshold is greater than 120mg/L.[15]

Other prognostic markers, none of which has been proven to outperform CRP, include interleukin-6 (threshold >14 pg/mL) which peaks a day earlier than CRP; polymorphonuclear elastase (threshold >120 μg/L), which peaks early and reflects neutrophil activation and degranulation; and phospholipase A_2 type II (threshold >15 units/L). Urinary trypsinogen-activating peptide may prove to be the most useful predictor as a quantitative dipstick.

In practice, the indications for a CT scan to diagnose and determine the extent of pancreatic necrosis are the prediction of severe pancreatitis (usually during the second week), when a patient fails to improve with initial resuscitation and/or when the CRP has crossed the diagnostic threshold (see above). The CT scan can be used to grade the severity of acute pancreatitis [CT Severity Index (CTSI)] based on the extent of extrapancreatic changes and pancreatic necrosis.[3]

The importance of the diagnosis of pancreatic necrosis is to initiate intensive-care management, which may necessitate transfer of the patient to a tertiary unit. The initiation of prophylactic antibiotics is the subject of considerable debate (see Chapter 36). The concerns with this approach relate to the increased risk of invasive fungemia,[16] which increases mortality,[17] and of the development of multiresistant organisms. The diagnosis of infected necrosis is imperative because it is an absolute indication for surgical intervention. Rarely, the early invasion of gas-forming organisms, such as *Clostridium perfringens,* makes the diagnosis of infection straightforward. It is more usual to suspect pancreatic infection with a secondary deterioration, often during the third and fourth weeks of admission. This is often heralded by a significant rise in CRP. A CT scan often will confirm the presence of a tense collection with rim enhancement arising from a region of pancreatic necrosis. The presence of gas within the tissues confirms infection, with an "air bubble" appearance (Fig 37–9), but this is present in the minority of cases. Infected necrosis usually is confirmed by fine-needle aspiration (FNA) for Gram's stain and bacterial culture. This can be guided by US or CT scan and is considered safe and reliable. Because of the risk of introducing infection, it is important not to perform the FNA unless it is going to make a difference in the way the patient will be managed. While there have been reports of conservative management (e.g., antibiotics + multiple and repeated percutaneous drainage) of infected necrosis, the confirmation of infection in a patient who had generated sufficient clinical concern to have warranted the test is an indication for surgical intervention. This removes the infected necrotic tissue that drives the systemic inflammatory response and multiorgan dysfunction.

STERILE NECROSIS

Over the last decade, there has been a trend toward the nonsurgical management of sterile necrosis, and this is now embedded within consensus guidelines.[2] The occa-

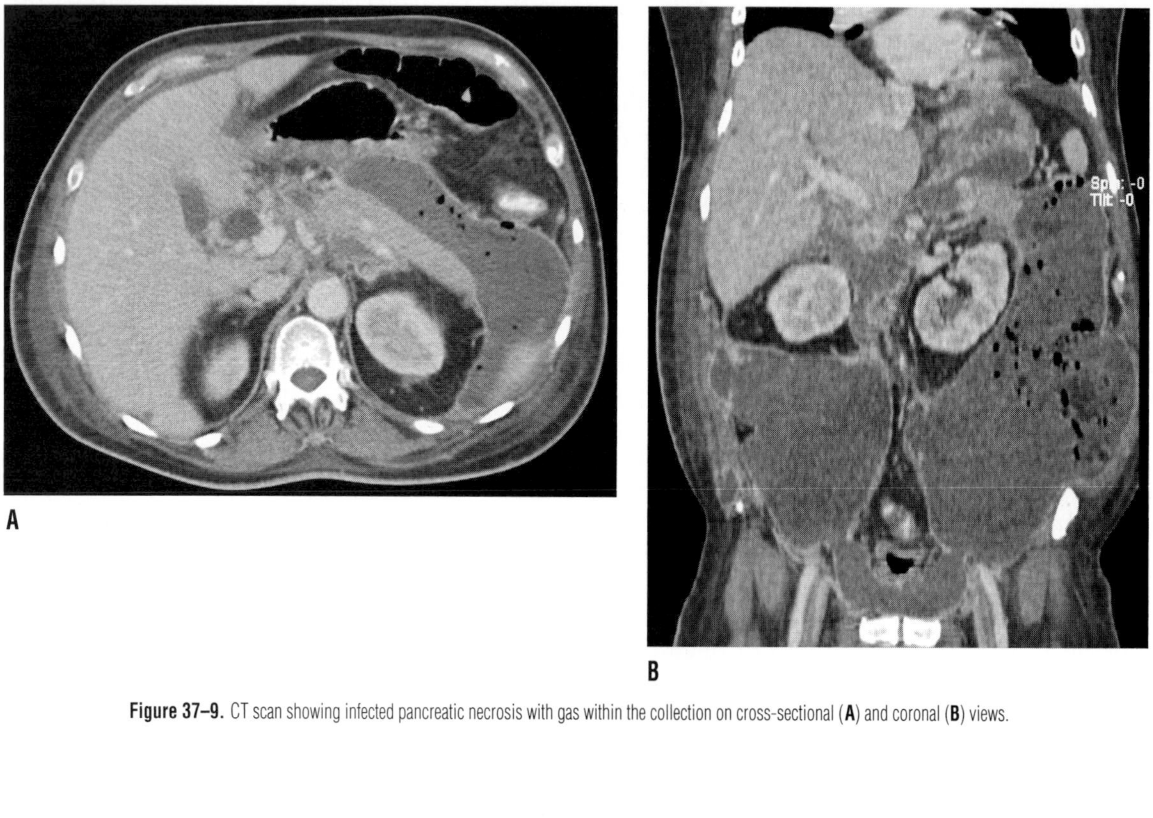

A

B

Figure 37–9. CT scan showing infected pancreatic necrosis with gas within the collection on cross-sectional (**A**) and coronal (**B**) views.

sional exception is when patients with negative aspiration cultures continue to deteriorate and develop multiorgan dysfunction, even with maximal intensive care. There are a few patients, usually with extensive sterile necrosis (grade D), who just fail to improve but who remain stable. These patients develop *organized pancreatic necrosis* or a *pancreatic sequestrum,* and a delayed necrosectomy is a straightforward procedure. The vast majority of patients with sterile necrosis can be managed without surgery.

TIMING OF SURGERY

There has been a change in the treatment standard for necrotizing pancreatitis from an aggressive policy favoring early surgical intervention to a more conservative strategy of delayed and less invasive intervention.[18] Early surgery was advocated in order to remove the focus of infection and terminate the inflammatory process. However, the inflammatory cascades are not easily switched off and are compounded by the surgery itself. Early surgery is more difficult because necrotic tissue is immature and not easily separated from viable tissue, resulting in a significant risk of bleeding. Additionally, early surgery may infect sterile necrosis. Delayed surgery may allow time for stabilization of the patient and the more easy removal of well-demarcated necrosum. There is a balance between operating too early and leaving it too late, and the decision needs to be individualized. The decision is aided by close surveillance of the patients' clinical trajectory with frequent clinical review and daily CRP measurements. From a review of published studies, the lowest mortality is associated with surgery after 3–4 weeks. However, the clinical picture (severity and evolution) should be the primary determinant of the timing of intervention.

PERCUTANEOUS DRAINAGE

Overreliance on percutaneous drains placed by the interventional radiologist in the treatment of infected necrosis is a mistake. The catheter size will not cope with the solid necrotic tissue. It achieves drainage and not necrosectomy. There are two settings in which percutaneous drainage is useful. The first is in an unstable septic patient with evidence of a tense rim-enhanced collection (pancreatic abscess) with a significant fluid component on CT scanning. Percutaneous drainage in this setting may take the "heat out of the fire," allow stabilization of the patient, and 'buy time' until necrosis is more amenable to surgical removal. The second setting in which percutaneous drainage is important is to establish the optimal route for dilatation and subsequent percutaneous necrosectomy, should this be appropriate. This will require careful discussion between the radiologist and surgeon. It usually involves a left-flank puncture and a route along the axis of the body/tail of the pancreas.

SURGERY FOR INFECTED NECROSIS

Figure 37–10 is an algorithm for the management of infected necrosis. The goals of surgical management are to remove necrotic and infected tissue, drain pus, lavage the

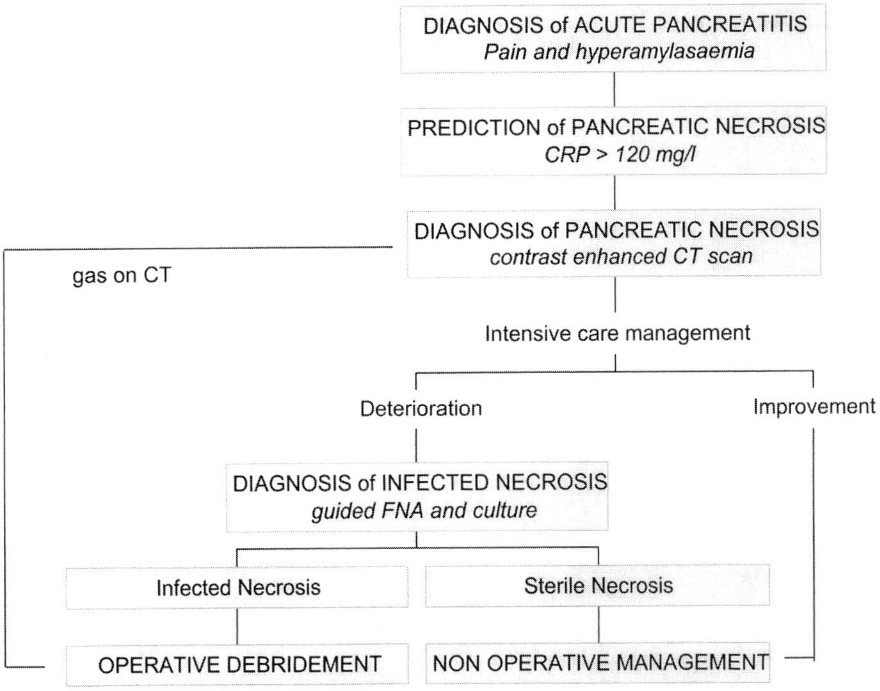

Figure 37–10. Algorithm for management of infected necrosis.

peritoneal cavity, and avoid blood loss and injury to other organs. Preservation of vital intact pancreatic tissue is important. The choice of operation is determined by the location, extent, and maturity the necrotic material; status of the infection; the patient's condition, the degree of organ dysfunction, and the preference and experience of the surgeon.[19] A number of different approaches have been described (Table 37–4; see also Table 36–4), some of which are only of historical interest. Necrosectomy is complex, fraught with potentially life-threatening complications, and should be left to the experienced surgeon. None of these surgical methods has been subjected to a randomized, controlled trial, and the minimally invasive approaches are still evolving.[10] The latter are best suited to treatment of well-demarcated and localized necrosis in the later stage of the disease. One possible benefit of this approach is a reduction in the number of patients who need intensive-care support.[20] The minimally invasive surgical approaches to pancreatic necrosectomy can be classified according to the type of optical system (flexible endoscope, laparoscope, or operating nephroscope) and the route used (via the stomach, peritoneum, or retroperitoneum) (Fig 37-11).

Pancreatic resection is a historical approach that has been associated with unacceptable complication and mortality rates. Pancreatic necrosectomy involves removing the devitalized pancreatic and peripancreatic tissue and drainage of associated pus. The usual approach to the pancreas is through the gastrocolic omentum into the lesser sac (Fig 37-12). Sometimes it is easiest to enter the region through the transverse mesocolon, from the greater sac, and to the left of the DJ flexure (Fig 37–13). At the same time, it is useful to take down both colonic flexures, providing better exposure and reducing the risk of subsequent injury to

TABLE 37–4. OPEN AND MINIMALLY INVASIVE APPROACHES TO THE TREATMENT OF PANCREATIC NECROSIS

Open surgery approaches
Pancreatic resection
Necrosectomy + wide tube drainage
Necrosectomy + relaparotomy (staged reexploration)
Necrosectomy + drainage + relaparotomy
Necrosectomy + laparostomy ± open packing
Necrosectomy + drainage + closed continuous lavage
Minimally invasive approaches
Laparoscopic necrosectomy
Laparoscopic intracavity necrosectomy
Laparoscopic assisted percutaneous drainage
Laparoscopic transgastric necrosectomy
Percutaneous necrosectomy and sinus tract endoscopy
MRI–radiologically assisted necrosectomy
Translumbar extraperitoneal retroperitoneoscopy
Video-assisted retroperitoneal débridement

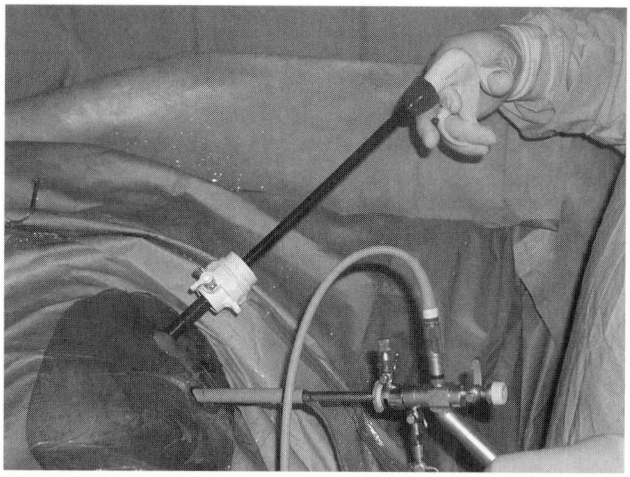

Figure 37–11. Large peripancreatic drains following necrosectomy and tube feeding jejunostomy.

the colon from tube drains. The head of the pancreas then can be approached anteriorly and posteriorly (after kocherization). If the abdomen is opened though a bilateral subcostal incision, in line with the opening to the lesser sac, subsequent laparotomies do not need to disturb the greater peritoneal sac or the upper abdomen. It is not necessarily a one-stage procedure, especially if an early necrosectomy is embarked on. Necrosectomy is a careful process, best accomplished by an educated finger. The extent of the cavity can be explored and the gentle separation of necrotic material accomplished. Necrotic extensions from the primary cavity need to be explored, often into the root of the small bowel mesentery and down the retrocolic gutters. Care must be taken to remove only what easily separates and to avoid injury to major vessels. The removal of necrotic material may be assisted by irrigation, pulsatile irrigation, gauze, and sponge forceps. When contained by a mature wall, it is advisable to avoid opening up the area too widely. The next step is placement of large-bore, soft, dependent drains to cover all the regions of what is often a complex area (Fig 37–14). Continuous lavage with peritoneal dialysis fluid, at flow rates of 300–1000 mL/h, may reduce the need to reoperate and often is continued for 2–3 weeks. The most common postoperative complications are hemorrhage and fistulization (pancreas, small and large intestine). The use of packing is lifesaving for major hemorrhage that occurs at the time of necrosectomy, but when used routinely, it is associated with a higher incidence of enteric fistulas.

PROGNOSIS

The prognosis of patients with necrotizing pancreatitis depends on the extent of necrosis and the onset of in-

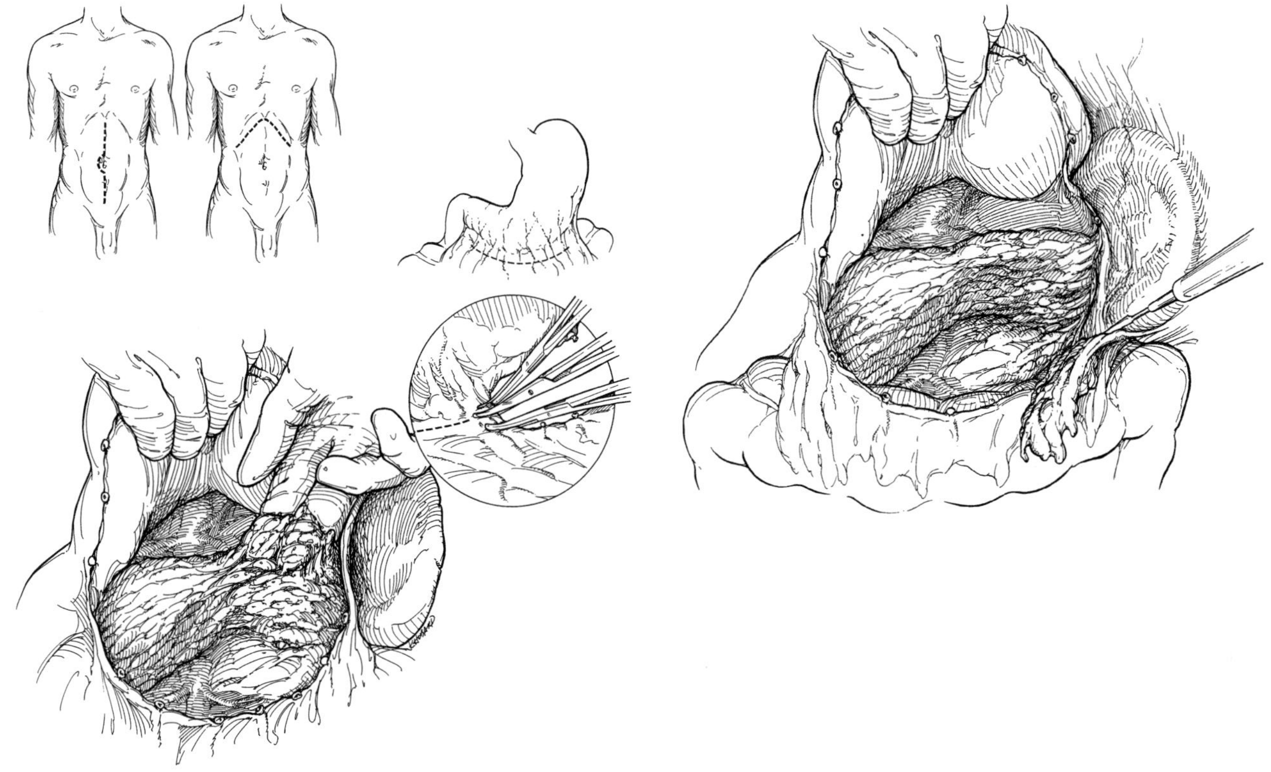

Figure 37–12. Necrosectomy via lesser sac.

fection. The overall mortality associated with pancreatic necrosis is 30–40%. This is an average of two major components—the mortality associated with sterile necrosis, which is 0–11%, and that for infected necrosis, which is usually 20–40% but may reach as high as 70%. Most deaths are in the context of multiorgan failure.

▪ PANCREATIC ABSCESS

The term *pancreatic abscess* has been used in different ways and can refer to an infected pancreatic pseudocyst or an abscess arising from infected necrosis (see Fig 37–1). The Atlanta definition[21] is a circumscribed intra-abdominal collection of purulent material containing little or no pancreatic necrosis. In contrast, infected necrosis is characterized by the extension of necrotic tissue in the pancreas and peripancreatic and/or retroperitoneal regions. The distinction between infected necrosis and pancreatic abscess is of importance because they are managed differently. The predominantly liquid contents of an abscess may be treated by percutaneous drainage (see above), whereas the solid contents of infected necrosis will require débridement (see above).

DIAGNOSIS

The clinical hallmarks of abscess are well recognized, with the development of fever, tachycardia, abdominal pain, and leukocytosis. Although these features may be present already, abscess formation often is accompanied by a secondary deterioration in the patient's clinical course. A secondary elevation in serum CRP level also may occur. Confirmation of a pancreatic abscess is best obtained by a contrast-enhanced CT scan. A rim-enhancing fluid collection arising from a region of previous pancreatic necrosis or pseudocyst is highly suggestive. The presence of bacterial (and fungal) infection can be confirmed by CT-guided FNA. The identification of the organism and its sensitivities allows rationalization of antibiotic therapy.

TREATMENT

The treatment of a pancreatic abscess involves the use of appropriate broad-spectrum antibiotics and drainage. The approach to drainage depends on whether the content of the abscess is predominantly liquid or solid and the available expertise. The percutaneous

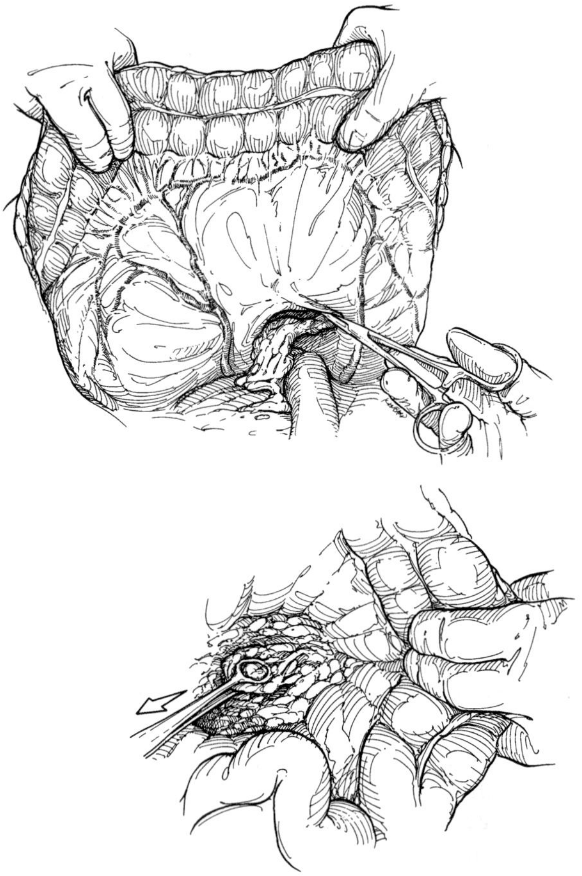

Figure 37–13. Necrosectomy via transverse mesocolon.

drainage of the abscess by an interventional radiologist is useful for infected pseudocysts with little solid content and in patients with an infected necrosis that has had time to undergo significant autolysis and liquefaction. The risk of pancreaticocutaneous fistula that arises owing to an underlying ductal disruption or stricture will be reduced if percutaneous drainage is performed through the stomach with subsequent internalization with a "double-mushroom" or "double-J" stent (see Fig 37–8). If the abscess can be identified readily with flexible gastroscopy as bulging into the lumen of the stomach or the duodenum, it may be feasible to consider endoscopic management. This is an evolving technique. Endoscopic US can confirm the safest route for confirmatory aspiration and drainage. When the abscess contains a significant proportion of necrosum, the radiologic and endoscopic drainage techniques usually are not definitive because the necrosum tends to block the 10–12F drains. Surgical drainage with débridement still may be required. The timing and techniques of necrosectomy were discussed earlier.

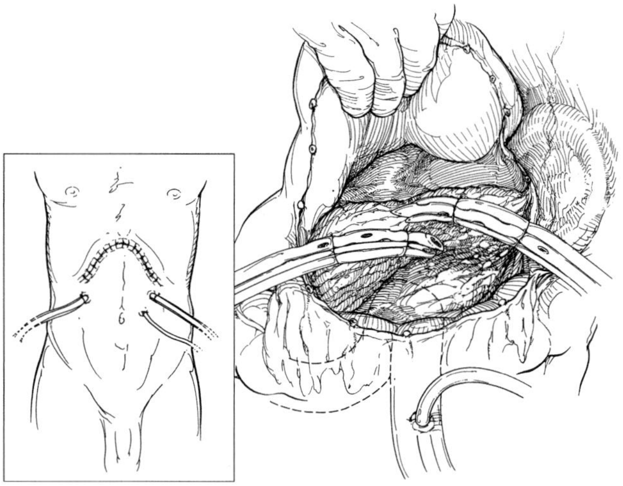

Figure 37–14. Percutaneous necrosectomy using operating nephroscope and supplemental laparoscopic port.

PROGNOSIS

The outcome of the treatment of pancreatic abscess depends on a number of factors. The premorbid fitness of the patient and the extent of comorbidities are important. Patients will do best if the abscess is mature with liquid content and treated late in the disease course. Early interventions in patients with significant comorbidity and an abscess associated with infected necrosis are less likely to do well.

▪ VENOUS THROMBOSIS

Venous thrombosis is a rare complication and one that usually develops a few weeks into a course of severe pancreatitis. The etiology is multifactorial, but extrinsic compression of the vein is important. Other factors include hypercoagulability and hemoconcentration. The consequences of splenic vein thrombosis are splenomegaly with discomfort and possible hypersplenism. Segmental venous hypertension may result in upper gastrointestinal bleeding from gastric varices. Because the risk of gastric variceal bleeding from pancreatitis-induced splenic vein thrombosis is low (5% for CT-identified varices and 18% for endoscopically identified varices), routine splenectomy is no longer recommended.[22] Portal vein thrombosis occurs insidiously and often is discovered after gastrointestinal hemorrhage has occurred. The consequences of superior mesenteric vein thrombosis are intestinal ischemia and venous infarction. CT scanning with contrast material is helpful in diagnosis and may show features of impaired mucosal enhancement, edematous swelling of the vessel wall, and filling defects within the vein. The goal of the initial treatment of venous thrombosis is to reduce extrinsic compression of the vein by drainage and/or débridement. The role of acute anticoagulation is controversial because of the risk of bleeding. If thrombosis occurs later in the disease course, it can be prescribed with less trepidation. Thrombolytic therapy and surgical thrombectomy have no established role in the context of acute pancreatitis. Acute venous thrombosis has a 30% mortality with a 25% recurrence rate without anticoagulant therapy. Anticoagulant therapy combined with surgery is associated with the lowest recurrence rate (3–5%).

▪ HEMORRHAGE/PSEUDOANEURYSM

Bleeding associated with severe acute pancreatitis is usually, but not always, due to a pseudoaneursym associated with a pancreatic pseudocyst. The splenic artery is the most commonly affected artery (30–50%) because of its proximity to the pancreas, followed by the gastroduodenal artery (10–15%), the inferior and superior pancreaticoduodenal arteries (10%), and all others to a lesser extent.

PATHOGENESIS

The disruption of the pancreas by necrosis and the damage to pancreatic ducts leads to the accumulation of activated proteolytic ezymes (e.g., elastase), weakening of the vessel wall, and aneurysmal dilatation. This process is accelerated in the presence of infection. The contained rupture of the aneurysm is a pseudoaneurysm, an extravascular hematoma communicating with the intravascular space.

DIAGNOSIS

Patients usually present with hypovolemic shock or with an unexplained drop in hemoglobin concentration. Bleeding may occur into a pseudocyst and tamponade, preventing any overt evidence of bleeding. Very rarely the diagnosis will be made in a patient with a known pseudocyst with the development of an abdominal bruit.

Selective mesenteric angiography is the best way to make the diagnosis of pseudoanuerysm (see Fig 37–4A), although it often can be detected on the arterial phase of CT scan. Angiography identifies the location of the pseudoaneurysm and its relationship to named vessels. The majority of patients will require surgical management, and the angiogram provides a useful guide.

TREATMENT

The approach to treatment depends on the hemodynamic stability of the patient. If the patient is anemic and stable, then angiography might enable embolization of the pseudoaneurysm (see Fig 37–4A, B). Transarterial catheter angioembolization will be considered. This procedure can be completed relatively quickly and is comfortable for the patient. If subsequent surgery is required, it can be performed under better conditions. Success is very operator-dependent but is over 90% in good centers. This approach is less likely to succeed with diffuse bleeding, bleeding from the pancreatic head, and bleeding after necrosectomy. Failure results from an inability to selectively cannulate the bleeding vessel or the poor placement of embolization material. Recurrent bleeding occurs in less than 40% of patients, and the overall mortality is under 20%.

If emergency laparotomy is required for bleeding, it may not be possible to arrange prior angioembolization. The lifesaving surgery may involve under-running the bleeding vessel (inside or outside the pseudocyst) and/or pancreatic resection. The mortality rate following surgical treatment of arterial hemorrhage during the acute phase of pancreatitis ranges from 28–56% and is higher from bleeding from the head of the pancreas. Hemostasis may require a Whipple procedure, which likely contributes to the higher mortality rate. The mortality rate with hemorrhage after operative débridement is usually over 50%.

Pancreatic or peripancreatic bleeding is one of the most formidable and life-threatening complications of pancreatitis. The standard of care in dealing with pseudoaneurysms has been surgical intervention; however, many interventional radiologists have reported excellent outcomes after angioembolization.

▪ CHOLESTASIS

Biochemical and clinical jaundice occur in approximately 20% of patient with acute pancreatitis, often during their hospital course. Mild cholestasis is more common and has been attributed to periductal edema and cholangitis. Long-term total parenteral nutrition will contribute to abnormal liver tests. Extrahepatic bile duct obstruction most often is due to choledocholithiasis or compression by a pseudocyst or pancreatic abscess.

▪ INTESTINAL COMPLICATIONS

PARALYTIC ILEUS

The proximity of the inflamed pancreas commonly results in regional self-limiting paralytic ileus affecting the duodenum, proximal jejunum, or transverse colon. This gives rise to the classic "sentinel loop" and "colon cutoff" signs on plain radiographs.

INTESTINAL OBSTRUCTION

Mechanical obstruction rarely complicates acute pancreatitis. The mechanism is usually inflammatory stenosis, and it is unusual to require surgery.

INTESTINAL ISCHEMIA AND NECROSIS

Subclinical mucosal ischemia is common in acute pancreatitis, particularly during the early phase, in response to the hypovolemia and reflex splanchnic vasoconstriction. This might be compounded by abdominal compartment syndrome, nonselective inotropes, and early and continuous enteral feeding. Full-thickness necrosis is rare and probably involves venous and/or arterial thrombosis at sites proximal to the inflammatory process. The middle mesocolic vessels and the transverse colon are most at risk.

▪ SYSTEMIC INFLAMMATORY RESPONSE SYNDROME

The systemic inflammatory response syndrome (SIRS) is common with acute pancreatitis and encompasses the hallmarks of a proinflammatory state (i.e., tachycardia, tachypnea or hyperpnea, hypotension, hypoperfusion, oliguria, leukocytosis or leukopenia, pyrexia or hypothermia, and the need for volume infusion) but without end-organ damage, identifiable bacteremia, or the need for pharmacologic support. SIRS is distinct from sepsis (where there is an identified pathogen) and septic shock (where there is associated hypotension). SIRS is best regarded as an exuberant host inflammatory response and the consequence of hypoperfusion.

There is no single trigger for SIRS. Instead, SIRS represents a whole-organism response to a variety of quite different challenges. Theories on the drivers for SIRS include the immunologic dissonance theory (where there is imbalance between the pro- and anti-inflammatory responses)[23] and the gut motor theory (where decreased intestinal perfusion and subsequent damage to the mucosal and immunologic barriers may allow the translocation of endogenous bacteria or their products into the systemic circulation).[24] More recently, the intestinal mucosa has been considered another source of inflammatory mediators activated by hypoperfused mucosa. Measurement of intramucosal pH (tonometry) can stratify mortality risk in acute pancreatitis.[25]

The mediation of SIRS is due to a number of well-described cytokines responsible for the proinflammatory state, a full description of which is beyond the scope of this chapter. In many patients with acute pancreatitis, SIRS progresses to multiple-organ-dysfunction syndrome (MODS) and possible end-organ damage. Occasionally, patients will be admitted with fulminant or early severe acute pancreatitis, often with respiratory and renal impairment from the outset, and these patients are responsible for early deaths. Organ failure on admission, which occurs in 30–40% of patients with necrotizing pancreatitis, is a very poor prognostic sign, doubling intensive-care stay and increasing mortality fourfold.[12] Early aggressive volume resuscitation has an important role in attenuating the systemic inflammatory response.[26]

▪ MULTIPLE-ORGAN-DYSFUNCTION SYNDROME (MODS)

The evolution of MODS is common in severe acute pancreatitis. MODS has been defined as the presence of altered organ function in a severely ill patient such that homeostasis cannot be maintained without intervention.[27] Many patients with early organ failure respond rapidly to supportive treatment and appear to have an otherwise uncomplicated outcome. Recently, it has been shown that organ failure in the first week of admission is a dynamic process and that the progression of early organ failure was attended by a mortality rate in excess of 50%. The response to the initial intensive care is an important determinant of outcome[28] (Fig 37–15).

The sequence of organ dysfunction is reasonably predictable. Initial pulmonary insufficiency and renal impairment are followed by circulatory failure and then metabolic dysfunction and liver failure.

Inflammation is the best explanation of MODS. Inflammation is the activation of circulating cells (leukocytes), the endothelium, the liver, and multiple mediator networks that normally are held in balance by corresponding anti-inflammatory mediators. Chemotactic agents attract, adhesion molecules focus, and cytotoxic agents assist these cells in driving the process. MODS occurs when either the host's inflammatory or anti-inflammatory response to injury (or both) is excessive; death may occur if the host response to injury is either excessive or insufficient.

A large body of work has demonstrated that the clinical manifestations of sepsis arise through the activation of a complex cascade of host-derived mediator molecules. Indiscriminate injury from these mediators may be the underlying mechanism to MODS. The possible

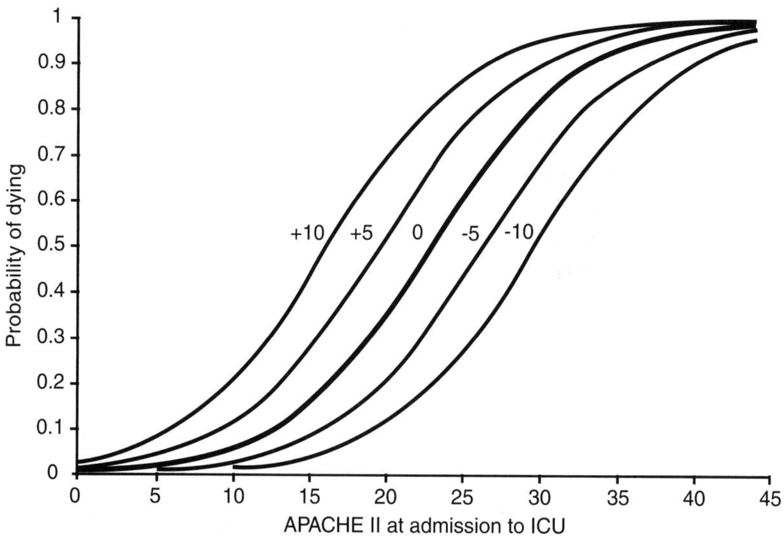

Figure 37–15. The relationship between the change in the severity of acute pancreatitis (APACHE II score) over the initial 48 hours of intensive-care management and the change in predicted mortality. (Reproduced from Flint R, Windsor JA. The physiological response to intensive care: A clinically relevant predictor in severe acute pancreatitis. *Arch Surg* 2004;139:438–443, copyright © 2004 American Medical Association. All rights reserved.)

mechanisms of injury are (1) excessive production of free radicals, (2) induction of elastase or endopeptidases, and (3) elevation of circulating soluble peptides that activate programmed cell death (apoptosis). However, opposing this etiologic concept is the finding that the serum concentration of these pleiotropic mediators does not always correlate directly with mortality.

Many potential predictors of organ failure early in the course of admission have been studied. MODS can be predicted with high accuracy at the time of hospital admission using a combination of the anti-inflammatory cytokine interleukin-10 (an early marker of systemic inflammation) and serum calcium (an early marker of organ dysfunction).[29]

MODS scoring systems can be classified using general physiologic critical-care scores, i.e., the Acute Physiologic and Chronic Health Evaluation (APACHE) score, the Simplified Acquired Physiological Score (SAPS), the Mortality Probability Model (MPM), a specific organ score to describe dysfunction [Multiple Organ Dysfunction Score (MODS)], developed by Bernard and colleagues as a descriptor of clinical outcome in MODS, the Sepsis-related Organ Failure Assessment (SOFA), and the Logistic Organ Dysfunction System (LODS). The specific organ dysfunction scores classify organs as failed (yes or no) or dysfunctional using an ordinal scale (graded score). The aggregate score quantitates severity in any one organ and the overall severity of organ dysfunction. The aggregate score then can be interpreted as the likelihood of predicted mortality based on the observed mortality in those study patients used to construct the original scoring system.

There exists no rationale to favor one scoring system over another. The scoring systems do not tell the clinician when specific organ dysfunction is reversible or irreversible. Practically, a simple count of organs affected and the duration of the dysfunction will stratify mortality within broad ranges between 60% and 98% depending on age, with dysfunction in three or more organs for at least a week.

Potentially, there is a therapeutic window between symptom onset and the development of distant organ damage in acute pancreatitis when anti-inflammatory therapy may be of use. Recent studies have established the critical role played by inflammatory mediators such as TNF-α, IL-1β, IL-6, IL-8, CINC/GRO-α, MCP-1, PAF, IL-10, CD40L, C5a, ICAM-1, and substance P in acute pancreatitis and the resulting MODS. Elucidation of the key mediators in acute pancreatitis, coupled with the discovery of specific inhibitors, may make it plausible to develop a clinically effective anti-inflammatory therapy. This will, of necessity, be a combination of modulators rather than a single "magic bullet."

RESPIRATORY COMPLICATIONS

Respiratory impairment can result from several causes, including atelectasis, pleural effusion, pneumonia, mediastinal pseudocyst/abscess, and/or adult respiratory distress syndrome (ARDS). Tachypnea, mild respiratory alkalosis, and mild hypoxemia are common within 2 days of the onset of acute pancreatitis. These clinical features usually can be corrected with analgesia, supplemental oxygen, and chest physiotherapy. A pleural effusion may require a chest drain. Impending respiratory failure is suggested when the arterial Po_2 remains less than 60 mmHg despite high-flow oxygen by mask. These patients should be considered for mechanical ventilation. Lung-protection ventilation strategies, with low tidal volumes for patients with ARDS, are recommended.[30] ARDS may occur within a few days of admission or after the development of infected necrosis and septicemia. ARDS results from the release of activated pancreatic enzymes vasoactive lysosomal enzymes and especially phospholipase A_2 (which destroys surfactant). Parenchymal injury appears to be due primarily to oxidative damage from the activated neutrophils in the lung.

RENAL COMPLICATIONS

Renal impairment usually is due to both hypovolemia (prerenal failure) and direct nephrotoxicity from the mediators of acute pancreatitis. Activation of the renin-angiotensin system may contribute to reduced perfusion. This manifests as oliguria (<30 mL/h) or anuria and as an increased serum concentration of creatinine and urea. The initial approach is aggressive intravenous crystalloid administration (of up to 10 L/24 hours). Then diuretics (furosemide 20–200 mg/24 h) and dopamine infusion (4 μg/kg per minute) should be considered. Further deterioration will necessitate continuous hemofiltration and/or hemodialysis.

CARDIOVASCULAR COMPLICATIONS

These include arrhythmias, pericardial effusion, impaired myocardial contractility, reduced peripheral vascular resistance, and increased permeability. Hypovolemia, from third-space fluid loss, is common during the first 12 hours and may be up to 30% in severe acute pancreatitis. This problem should be anticipated with aggressive intravenous fluid therapy in the first 24–48 hours. Circulatory failure (MAP <70 mmHg) requires prompt, aggressive fluid resuscitation plus or minus inotropic support. SIRS is characterized by decreased peripheral vascular resistance and is the reason for the preferred use of norepinephrine to increase vascular tone and blood pressure (dose 0.05–0.2 μg/kg per minute). Epinephrine (dose 0.05–0.2 μg/kg per minute) also may be used to support cardiac output. Unfortunately, these inotropes will compound splanchnic vasoconstriction.

If the patient with infected necrosis meets the criteria for severe sepsis, he or she should be managed by current sepsis guidelines.[31] Although not widely adopted, there is the evidence for the use of recombinant human activated protein C[32] and low-dose corticosteroids for vasopressor-dependent shock.[33] Recent evidence also has shown the importance of tight glycemic control in patients with severe sepsis.[34] These measures have yet to be widely adopted.

METABOLIC COMPLICATIONS

Hypocalcemia is the most frequent metabolic disturbance, and it usually occurs during the first week. Low serum albumin will make the hypocalcemia appear worse than it is, and therefore, replacement should be based on ionized calcium. There are several factors likely to be responsible for low calcium. Primarily, calcium is sequestered in areas of fat necrosis by the process of saponification. In addition, there is probably a contribution from altered calcium-regulating hormones (e.g., calcitonin, parathyroid hormone, and glucagon). Hypomagnesemia may inhibit parathyroid hormone and contribute to the hypocalcemia.

Hyperglycemia is a frequent finding but usually subsides rapidly without the need for treatment. It is an adverse prognostic sign. There are three contributing factors: a stress-induced increase in cortisol and catecholamines, hyperglucagonemia, and probably most important, an insulin deficiency that may reflect necrosis of the islet cells. Glucose intolerance, if not insulin-dependent diabetes, occurs in up to half of patients who have had severe necrotizing pancreatitis.

Disseminated intravascular coagulopathy is not common, but there is a tendency to hypercoagulability in acute pancreatitis. Other rare complications include subcutaneous fat necrosis and polyarthritis, which are also seen in patients with acinar cell carcinoma of the pancreas and thought to be due to increased serum lipase. There also have been reports of osteolysis and rhabdomyolysis in severe acute pancreatitis.

Protein-calorie malnutrition is a complication of acute pancreatitis, especially when severe and associated with infected necrosis. These patients have an elevated resting energy expenditure, and it has been shown that total parenteral nutrition is unable to reverse the catabolic insult on body protein[35] (Fig 37–16). The importance of and the approaches to nutritional support in patients with severe acute pancreatitis are discussed in the preceding chapter.

ENCEPHALOPATHY

Pancreatic encephalopathy is a rare complication of acute pancreatitis. Clinical features include focal neurologic signs and acute onset of dementia. This picture

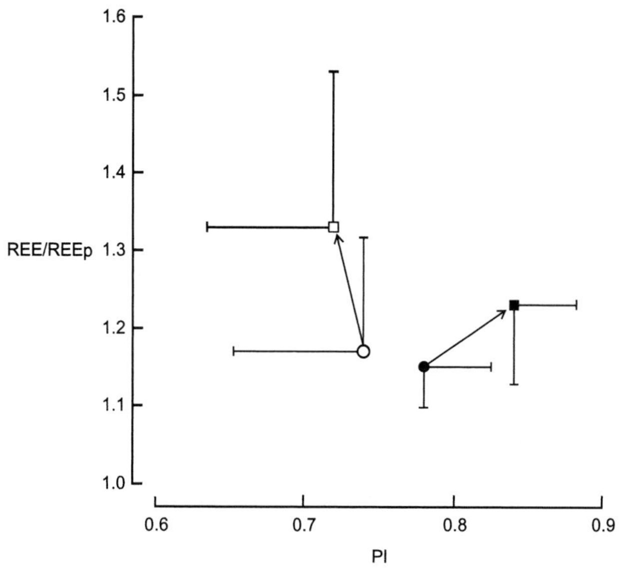

Figure 37–16. The changes in protein index (measured/predicted total-body protein, expressed as mean ± SEM) on day 0 (*circles*) and day 14 (*squares*) of total parenteral nutrition in acute pancreatitis patients with (*open symbols*) and without (*closed symbols*) sepsis and/or recent surgery. (Reproduced from Chandrasegaram MD, Plank LD, Windsor JA. The impact of total parenteral nutrition on the body composition of patients with acute pancreatitis. *JPEN J Parenter Enter Nutr* 2005;29:65–73, with permission from the American Society for Parenteral and Enteral Nutrition (ASPEN). ASPEN does not endorse the use of this material in any form other than its entirety.)

can fluctuate over time; cyclic progression with remission and relapses has been described. Although the exact mechanisms are unclear, postmortem examinations reveal amylase in the cerebrospinal fluid. MRI of the brain may be helpful. Patchy white matter signal abnormalities resembling the plaques seen in multiple sclerosis may reflect the lesions that are found in the cerebral white matter of postmortem confirmed cases. Treatment is supportive. Any patient with suspicious or unusual neurologic symptoms and signs associated with possible malnutrition, hyperemesis, or malabsorption should be given intravenous thiamine to avoid the potential morbidity and mortality associated with undiagnosed Wernicke's encephalopathy.

■ CONCLUSION

The many and varied complications of acute pancreatitis are responsible for the morbidity and mortality of this challenging disease. The prevention of pancreatic necrosis remains the fundamental goal of pancreatitis research because this complication is the basis for the others. Until such time as this is accomplished, it behoves the clinician to be on the alert for the development of the complications discussed in this chapter. By early detection and appropriate treatment, the clinical impact of these complications will be minimized.

REFERENCES

1. Windsor J, Hammodat H. The metabolic management of severe acute pancreatitis. *World J Surg* 2000; 24:664–672
2. Uhl W, Warshaw A, Imrie C, et al. IAP guidelines for the surgical management of acute pancreatitis. *Pancreatology* 2002;2:565–573
3. Balthazar E. Acute pancreatitis: Assessment of severity with clinical and CT evaluation. *Radiology* 2002;223:603–613
4. Brugge W, Lauwers G, Sahani D, et al. Cystic neoplasms of the pancreas. *N Engl J Med* 2004;351(12):1218–26.
5. Ahearne P, Baillie J, Cotton P, et al. An endoscopic retrograde cholangiopancreatography (ERCP)–based algorithm for the management of pancreatic pseudocysts. *Am J Surg* 1992;163:111–115
6. Nealon W, Walser E. Main pancreatic ductal anatomy can direct choice of modality for treating pancreatic pseudocysts (surgery versus percutaneous drainage). *Ann Surg* 2002;235:751–758
7. Mehta R, Suvarna D, Sadasivan S, et al. Natural course of asymptomatic pancreatic pseudocysts: A prospective study. *Ind J Gastroenterol* 2004;23:140–142
8. Davies R, Cox M, Wilson T, et al. Percutaneous cystogastrostomy with a new catheter for drainage of pancreatic pseudocysts and fluid collections. *Cardiovasc Intervent Radiol* 1996;19:128–131
9. Morton J, Brown A, Galanko J, et al. A national comparison of surgical versus percutaneous drainage of pancreatic pseudocysts: 1997–2001. *J Gastrointest Surg* 2005;9(1): 15–21
10. Kellogg T, Horvath K. Minimal access approaches to complications of acute pancreatitis and benign neoplasms of the pancreas. *Surg Endosc* 2003;17:1692–1704
11. Bhattacharya D, Ammori B. Minimally invasive approaches to the management of pancreatic pseudocysts. *Surg Laparosc Endosc Percutan Tech* 2003;13:141–148
12. Beger H, Rau B, Isenmann R. Natural history of necrotizing pancreatitis. *Pancreatology* 2003;3:93–101
13. Beger H, Bittner R, Block S, Buchler M. Bacterial contamination of pancreatic necrosis: A prospective clinical study. *Gastroenterology* 1986;91:433–438
14. Gloor B, Muller C, Worni M, et al. Pancreatic infection in severe pancreatitis: The role of fungus and multiresistant organisms. *Arch Surg* 2001;136:592–596.
15. Wilson C, Heads A, Shenkin A, et al. C-reactive protein, antiproteases and complement factors as objective markers of severity in acute pancreatitis. *Br J Surg* 1989;76:177–181
16. Isenmann R, Schwarz M, Rau B, et al. Characteristics of infection with *Candida* species in patients with necrotizing pancreatitis. *World J Surg* 2002;25:372–404
17. Connor S, Alexis N, Neal T, et al. Fungal infection but not type of bacterial infections is associated with a high mortality in primary and secondary infected pancreatic necrosis. *Dig Surg* 2004;21:297–304
18. Werner J, Feuerbach S, Uhl W, Buchler M. Management of acute pancreatitis: From surgery to interventional intensive care. *Gut* 2005;54:426–436

19. Buchler M, Gloor B, Muller C, et al. Acute necrotizing pancreatitis: Treatment strategy according to the status of the infection. *Ann Surg* 2000;232:619–626
20. Carter C, McKay C, Imrie C. Percutaneous necrosectomy and sinus tract endoscopy in the management of infected pancreatic necrosis: An initial experience. *Ann Surg* 2000;232:175–180
21. Bradley E. A clinically based classification system for acute pancreatitis: Summary of the International Symposium on Acute Pancreatitis, Atlanta, Ga, September 11 through 13, 1992. *Arch Surg* 1993;128:586–590.
22. Heider T, Azeem S, Galanko J, Behrns K. The natural history of pancreatitis-induced splenic vein thrombosis. *Ann Surg* 2004;239:876–882
23. Bone R. Immunological dissonance: A continuing evolution in our understanding of the systemic inflammatory response syndrome and the multiple organ dysfunction syndrome. *Ann Inter Med* 1996;125:680–687
24. Moore E, Moore F, Francoise R, et al. The postischemic gut serves as a priming bed for circulating neutrophils that provoke multiple-organ failure. *J Trauma* 1994;37:881–887
25. Bonham M, Abu-Zidan F, Simovic M, Windsor J. Gastric intramucosal pH as a predictor of mortaility in acute pancreatitis. *Br J Surg* 1997;84:1670–1674
26. Rivers E, Nguyen B, Havstad S, et al. Early goal directed therapy in the treatment of severe sepsis and septic shock. *N Engl J Med* 2001;345:1368–77
27. Bone R, Balk R, Cerra F, et al. Definitions of sepsis and organ failure and guidelines for the use of innovative therapies in sepsis. The ACCP/SCCM Consensus Conference Committee, American College of Chest Physicians/Society of Critical Care Medicine Consensus Conference, 1991, pp. 864–875
28. Flint R, Windsor J. The physiological response to intensive care: A clinically relevant predictor in severe acute pancreatitis. *Arch Surg* 2004;139:438–443
29. Mentula P, Kylanpaa M, Kemppainen E, et al. Early prediction of organ failure by combined markers in patients with acute pancreatitis. *Br J Surg* 2005;92:68–75
30. Brower R, Matthay M, Morris A, et al. Ventilation with lower tidal volumes as compared with traditional tidal volumes for acute lung injury and the acute respiratory distress syndrome. *N Engl J Med* 2000;342:1301–1308
31. Dellinger R, Carlet J, Masur H, et al. Surviving sepsis campaign guidelines for management of severe sepsis and septic shock. *Crit Care Med* 2004;32:858–873.
32. Bernard G, Vncent J, Laterre P, et al. Efficacy and safety of recombinant human activated protein C for severe sepsis. *N Engl J Med* 2001;344:699–709
33. Annane D, Bellissant E, Bollaert P, et al. Corticosteroids for severe sepsis and septic shock: A systematic review and meta-analysis. *Br Med J* 2004;329:1–9
34. van den Berghe G, Wouters P, Weekers F, et al. Intensive insulin therapy in critically ill patients. *N Engl J Med* 2001;345:1359–1367
35. Chandrasegaram M, Plank L, Windsor J. The impact of total parenteral nutrition on the body composition of patients with acute pancreatitis. *J Parenter Enter Nutr* 2005;29:65–73

38

Chronic Pancreatitis

Oscar Joe Hines ■ *Howard A. Reber*

Chronic pancreatitis is characterized by persistent and progressive fibrosis of the pancreas, resulting in the loss of both endocrine and exocrine tissue. Comfort gave the first modern description of this disease in 1946, when he recognized the relationship between alcohol intake and pancreatitis.[1] The incidence of this disease varies geographically. Data from Spain document an incidence of 14/100,000 during the 1980s.[2] In Japan the number of cases appears to be rising from 32,000 in 1994 to 42,000 in 1999 (5.7/100,000 incidence).[3] Recent basic laboratory investigations have begun to uncover information about the pathogenesis and genetic abnormalities associated with chronic pancreatitis and have identified factors that contribute to the development of this disease. This information is beginning to impact clinical decision making and the need for surgical intervention.

▪ ETIOLOGY

ALCOHOLIC PANCREATITIS

Excessive alcohol consumption appears to account for 70–80% of all cases of chronic pancreatitis worldwide. However, the mechanisms associated with alcohol-induced acute pancreatitis and the progression to chronic pancreatitis remain uncertain. This relationship is even more confounding considering the facts that less than 10% of alcoholics actually acquire chronic pancreatitis and that there does not appear to be any specific level of alcohol consumption below which pancreatitis does not occur. Epidemiologic studies confirm that there is a genetic basis for alcoholic pancreatitis. Therefore, genetic susceptibility, environmental exposures, and the interaction between these factors must all be critical to the development of alcohol-induced chronic pancreatitis.

Ethanol appears to have direct toxic effects on the pancreas. These include the reduction of pancreatic blood flow and microcirculation, generation of free oxygen radicals in the pancreas, direct effects on acinar cell viability, and, when combined with cigarette smoke, the creation of pancreatic ischemia.[4] Additionally, alcohol can directly activate pancreatic stellate cells—the main source of extracellular matrix in the pancreas.[5]

Recurrent subclinical episodes of pancreatitis induced by alcohol may ultimately lead to clinically evident inflammation and fibrosis. Since a small percentage of patients who drink ultimately present with chronic pancreatitis, a genetic susceptibility has been sought. To date, however, no candidate genes have been identified.

AUTOIMMUNE PANCREATITIS

Autoimmune pancreatitis is a unique form of chronic pancreatitis that must be distinguished from other forms of the disease since is treatable with steroids and may not require surgery.[6] This entity can be classified as either primary (no association with other autoimmune diseases) or secondary (associated with other autoimmune diseases, like Sjögren's syndrome, ulcerative colitis, Crohn's disease, or primary sclerosing cholangitis). In autoimmune pancreatitis, the gland does not contain calcifications. An abdominal CT scan often reveals what has been described as a "sausage"-shaped pancreas. Biopsy of the gland reveals infiltration with lymphocytes, plasma cells, and fibrosis. Often the serum level of immunoglobulin G4 (IgG4) is elevated. These patients usually respond quickly and completely to a course of corticosteroid therapy, and the pancreatic swelling and inflammation subside. The problem in many cases is that it may be impossible to determine whether pancreatic cancer is also present. Understandably, many patients are operated upon in an effort to avoid overlooking a malignant neoplasm. In this latter group, the diagnosis of autoimmune pancreatitis may only be made after the pathologist examines the pancreatic resection specimen.

PANCREAS DIVISUM

Pancreas divisum is an anatomic variation in which the dorsal and ventral pancreatic ducts fail to join, forcing the majority of the ductal drainage through the smaller duct of Santorini and the minor papilla. In some patients, this may result in increased ductal pressure and recurrent episodes of acute pancreatitis. It may be that recurrent episodes of inflammation over years eventually cause chronic pancreatitis in some. Nevertheless, large controlled studies failed to confirm pancreas divisum as a major risk for developing acute pancreatitis. The issue is still debated. From the surgeons' perspective, it is important to note that patients with established changes of chronic pancreatitis who have pancreas divisum and no other apparent etiology for the disease, will not respond to surgical sphincteroplasty. Surgical management of their chronic pancreatitis should be guided by the principles outlined later in this chapter.

GENETIC PREDISPOSITION

Recently, several genetic mutations have been identified as pathogenetic factors in chronic pancreatitis. Whitcomb and associates discovered the first of these, which was related to a mutation in the trypsinogen gene.[7] A number of these single point mutations have been identified and are clearly involved in many patients with hereditary pancreatitis, an autosomal dominant disorder. The mutations result in either an enzyme that is less susceptible to inactivation or more prone to activation. These patients typically present with episodes of recurrent acute pancreatitis early in life that lead to chronic fibrosis and pancreatic dysfunction. Over two thirds of patients with hereditary pancreatitis have one of these mutations.

A mutation in the serine protease inhibitor Kazal type 1 gene also known as the pancreatic secretory trypsin inhibitor, is associated with idiopathic chronic pancreatitis.[8] It is felt that this enzyme is responsible for the first line of defense against premature activation of trypsinogen in the gland. The incidence of mutations of the serine protease inhibitor Kazal type 1 gene in children with idiopathic pancreatitis is 15–25% and is only 5–10% in adult patients with the disease. Because of these low associations, it is felt that mutations in serine protease inhibitor Kazal type 1 serve as disease-modifying mutations worsening the severity of pancreatitis caused by other genetic or environmental factors.

The mutations in the cystic fibrosis transmembrane conductance regulator (CFTR) are also associated with idiopathic pancreatitis.[9] Patients with idiopathic chronic pancreatitis have a six times increased frequency of mutations of this gene without exhibiting other evidence of cystic fibrosis. This gene is involved in chloride and bicarbonate transport in pancreatic ductal epithelium. Loss of function of this gene leads to the accumulation of viscid mucus which becomes inspissated within the gland.

Other candidate mutations include those associated with hyperlipidemia syndromes, familial hyperparathyroidism, uniparental disomy (UPD) glucouronosyltransferases, glutathione S-transferase, and the HLA-DRB104 allele. Thus, it appears that genetic susceptibility is an important factor in the development of chronic pancreatitis, and that it will likely clarify our understanding of some fraction of the 20% of chronic pancreatitis currently deemed idiopathic.

▪ PATHOLOGY

This disease eventually impacts all elements of the pancreas, but initially the exocrine pancreas is affected. Acinar cells are lost and ductal cells eliminated. Ductal elements that remain are buried in a sea of connective tissue. Islets can be seen disconnected from acinar tissue and are also surrounded by fibrosis.

The fibrosis that is present includes collagen fibers, fibroblasts, and myofibroblasts. Recently, the identification and study of pancreatic stellate cells has contributed to our growing understanding of the biology of pancreatic fibrosis.[10] These cells in the normal pancreas reside at the base of acinar cells and harbor vitamin A-containing lipid droplets. They represent the main source of extracellular matrix and collagen in chronic pancreatitis. Ethanol can directly activate stellate cells and may also work through tumor growth factor (TGF)-beta and other proinflammatory cytokines. Transgenic mice overexpressing TGF-beta in islet cells develop severe fibrosis characterized by overabundant extracellular matrix and fibroblasts.[11]

Patients with long standing chronic pancreatitis demonstrate numerous nerves running throughout the fibrotic tissue (Fig 38–1). There is morphologic evidence that these nerves have lost their protective perineurium, which may make them more sensitive to various nociceptive substances. Often local inflammatory cells are seen near these nerves, which may be partially responsible for the significant pain these patients experience.

▪ DIAGNOSIS

The diagnosis of chronic pancreatitis is largely based on a history of abdominal pain and radiologic confirmation of fibrosis and calcification of the gland. The goals of imaging are to (1) gather anatomic evidence for the presence of chronic pancreatitis, (2) to assess the diameter of the duct, (3) to determine the presence of any associated disease (e.g., cysts, bile duct obstruction), and (4) to search for an unsuspected pancreatic malignancy. Patients can undergo a high resolution CT scan, endoscopic retrograde cholangiopancreatography (ERCP), MRI, magnetic resonance cholangiopancreatography (MRCP), and/or endoscopic ultrasound (EUS). We prefer high-resolution CT scan with fine cuts through the pancreas during the arterial phase of the study.

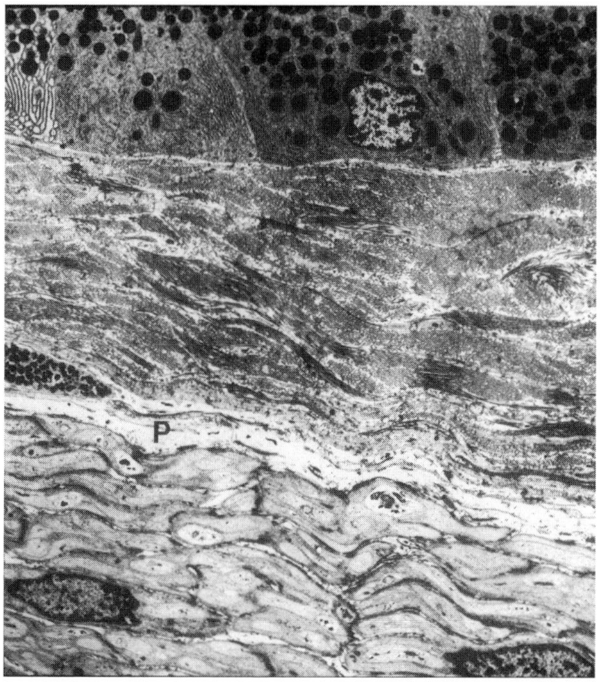

Figure 38–1. Histologic section of neural tissue in the midst of chronic pancreatitis. P = Perineurium.

ERCP has been considered the gold standard for the morphologic diagnosis of the chronic pancreatitis. Multifocal dilations, strictures, and irregular contours of the main duct along with calcifications and stones are hallmarks of the disease. More recently, MRCP images have been shown to provide similar information about duct anatomy, and MRCP has the advantage of being noninvasive.

The sensitivity of CT to make the diagnosis of chronic pancreatitis is as high as 95% in advanced disease, but the pancreas can appear normal in patients with early disease. CT scan is especially useful to reveal the complications of chronic pancreatitis (pseudocyst, the presence of bile duct and duodenal obstruction), and the presence of pancreatic ductal dilation. Three-dimensional reconstruction also can give additional information about the relationship of the gland to the surrounding vasculature. EUS with fine-needle aspiration (FNA) of any suspicious area may be indicated if the results of the CT scan raise a question about malignancy.[12]

Pancreatic function tests can be useful to delineate the severity of chronic pancreatitis and, occasionally, to make the diagnosis. The secretin-cholecystokinin test is the gold standard (Fig 38–2). The evaluation of pancreatic zinc output may also be useful.[13] The serum pancreolauryl test is the most sensitive noninvasive test for screening of patients for the presence of chronic pancreatitis (Fig 38–3). The problem with all of these tests is that they are least reliable in patients with mild disease, where there may be the greatest need for establishing the diagnosis. When the disease is advanced, and the tests are more likely to be positive, the diagnosis is usually evident on the basis of other less labor intensive studies.

▪ TREATMENT

The treatment of chronic pancreatitis requires an interdisciplinary approach involving the general practitioner, gastroenterologist, radiologist, and surgeon. The most common symptom in a patient with chronic pancreatitis is abdominal pain. The etiology of the pain is multifactorial and, in general, is not well understood. Factors include continued alcohol consumption that results in local release of oxygen-derived free radicals, elevated pancreatic ductal and parenchymal pressures that diminish pancreatic blood flow, perineural sheath destruction with exposure of the nerves to various nociceptive agents, and tissue acidosis.

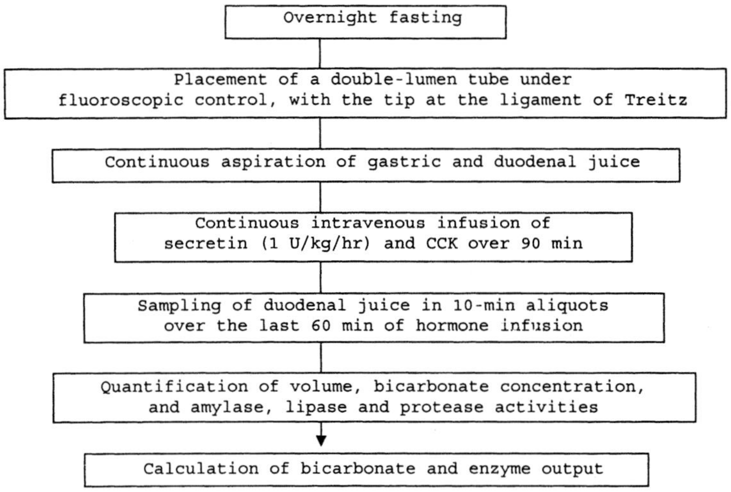

Figure 38–2. Secretin-cholecystokinin test. This test is used to quantify pancreatic function.

The initial treatment for pain in all of these patients should be nonoperative and includes recommendations for the cessation of alcohol intake, and the administration of oral analgesic agents. Analgesics are usually administered in a progressive fashion and begin with nonnarcotic medications including acetaminophen, ibuprofen, and cyclooxygenase-2 (COX-2) inhibitors. COX-2 is overexpressed in chronic pancreatitis and the degree of overexpression correlates with the stage of disease.[14] However, many of these patients soon need narcotics to control their pain. Tricyclic antidepressants at low doses may be adjuvants to these analgesics. Celiac plexus nerve block and transcutaneous electrical nerve stimulation generally are unsatisfactory.

Over the past decade, endoscopic treatment of pain in chronic pancreatitis has significantly advanced. There remains a bias in the surgical community against this approach, but some of the data are intriguing. Procedures available to the endoscopist for the treatment of pain include pancreatic sphincterotomy, pancreatic ductal stenting, extracorporeal shock wave lithotripsy (ESWL) of pancreatic stones, endoscopic drainage of pancreatic pseudocysts, and endoscopic celiac nerve block. Pancreatic sphincterotomy alone appears to be safe but the efficacy is unknown.[15] Pancreatic stenting and ESWL may eventually achieve complete or partial relief of pain in 80% of selected patients, but this approach requires multiple procedures and months of treatment (Table 38–1).

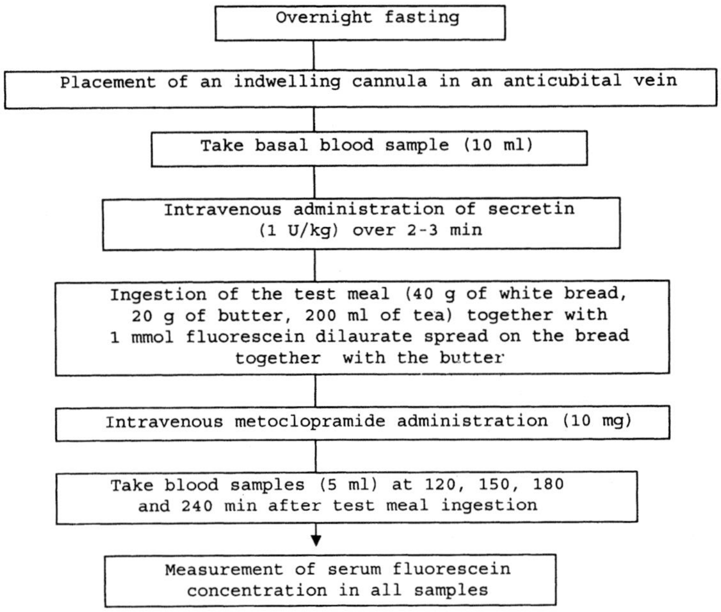

Figure 38–3. Serum pancreolauryl test. This test may be used to establish the diagnosis of chronic pancreatitis when this diagnosis is uncertain.

TABLE 38–1. RESULTS OF EXTRACORPOREAL SHOCK WAVE LITHOTRIPSY AND ENDOTHERAPY FOR CHRONIC PANCREATITIS

Study	Year	# Patients	Fragmentation (%)	Complete or Partial Pain Relief (%)	Need for Surgery (%)	Mean Follow-Up (mo)
Delhaye[17]	1992	123	99	85	8	14
Schneider[18]	1994	50	86	62	12	14
Johanns[19]	1996	35	100	83	14	23
Costamagna[20]	1997	35	100	72	3	27
Adamek[21]	1999	80	54	76	10	40
Brand[22]	2000	48	60	82	4	7
Farnbacher[23]	2002	125	85	48	13	29
Kozarek[24]	2002	40	100	80	20	30

A large multicenter study examining over a 1000 patients receiving endoscopic therapy for pain in the setting of chronic pancreatitis found that on an intention-to-treat basis, 65% of the patients can be expected to be completely or nearly free of pain after 5 years without needing surgery.[16] Nevertheless, there are problems with all of these studies that extol the virtues of endoscopic therapies. These include the lack of appropriate control groups (endoscopic treatment vs. surgical treatment vs. no treatment), the high frequency of spontaneous pain relief in this patient population, and the difficulty in precise quantification of pain severity.

In addition to pain, patients may present with exocrine or endocrine dysfunction which are managed medically. Diabetes usually requires insulin and dietary restrictions. Malabsorption is treated with pancreatic enzyme replacement in sufficient amount to provide at least 30,000 units of lipase with each meal. Antacid secretory medications also may be useful in patients with acid hypersecretion to avoid denaturation of the replacement enzymes. Rarely, fat intake must also be limited to decrease the bothersome diarrhea that accompanies excessive steatorrhea. Other reasons that a patient may present to a physician for care include various intra-abdominal complications of pancreatitis (e.g., bile duct, colonic or duodenal obstruction, pseudocyst), and the concern for pancreatic cancer.

▪ SURGICAL TREATMENT

Although chronic pancreatitis is not primarily a surgical disease, the surgeon is frequently asked to evaluate and treat patients with this problem. The most common indication for operation is pain, but there are several other indications for surgery in this group (Table 38–2).

Operation for persistent pain requires an assessment of the significance of the pain. Generally, operation may be indicated in patients whose pain interferes with the quality of their lives. For example, the attacks of pain may require frequent hospitalizations that interfere with school or employment. The patient may be unable to function productively because of the depression that often accompanies the chronic pain state. Nutrition may be impaired because the pain that eating produces, limits oral intake. The patient is often addicted to narcotics, but this may not be a contraindication to operation. For example, patients who undergo a pancreatic resection may develop exocrine insufficiency or diabetes if enough pancreas is removed. Although this may be an acceptable price to pay for pain relief in some patients, others might be unable to manage the dietary and insulin requirements that would ensue (e.g., patients who are addicted to narcotics and/or alcohol). However, even in patients with narcotic and/or alcohol addiction and a dilated duct, a duct decompression operation may be appropriate, because it almost never produces exocrine or endocrine insufficiency. Preoperative psychiatric evaluation may help the surgeon to decide about whether or not operation should be considered.

There are reports that duct decompression operations can postpone the progression of disease and prevent worsening diabetes or exocrine insufficiency. This remains unproven, and it should never be the reason that operation is considered.

The type of operation depends on the anatomy of the pancreatic ductal system, and whether or not the pancreas is diffusely involved with the disease or it in-

TABLE 38–2. INDICATIONS FOR SURGERY IN CHRONIC PANCREATITIS

Intractable pain
Pancreatic ductal stenosis
Biliary obstruction (Wadsworth syndrome)
Duodenal obstruction
Left sided portal hypertension from splenic vein thrombosis
Colonic obstruction
Pseudocyst
Pancreatic ascites
Pancreatic fistula
Pancreatic carcinoma

volves one part of the gland more than the others. Operations to relieve pain in these patients are designed to either (1) drain a dilated pancreatic ductal system, or (2) resect diseased pancreatic tissue if the duct is not enlarged. The main pancreatic duct normally measures 4 to 5 mm in the head, 3 to 4 mm in the body, and 2 to 3 mm in the tail of the pancreas. The duct is considered dilated when it is at least 7 mm in diameter in the body of the gland. Thus, patients with a dilated pancreatic duct (>7 mm in the body of the gland) are candidates for a drainage operation that decompresses the duct (longitudinal pancreaticojejunostomy, Puestow procedure). Those with a duct that is of normal caliber will probably require resection of a part of the pancreas, usually the head of the gland (pancreaticoduodenectomy, Frey or Beger procedure). Figure 38–4 depicts an algorithm.

LONGITUDINAL PANCREATICOJEJUNOSTOMY

In patients with a dilated pancreatic duct, a ductal drainage operation (longitudinal pancreaticojejunostomy, Puestow procedure) is likely to be effective. Table 38–3 summarizes the operative results for longitudinal pancreaticojejunostomy. The morbidity and mortality rates (<2%) are minimal and there is almost no risk of diabetes because little if any pancreatic tissue is resected. Pain is relieved in 85% of patients for the first several years. Most patients gain weight since they no longer experience pain with eating, although the degree of malabsorption does not change. The major drawback of this operation is that within 5 years, pain recurs in as many as 40–50% of patients. In a small number, this may be because of a stricture of the anastomosis, but in most, it is probably associated with disease progression or the development of a complication. Recurrence of pain may also herald the appearance of pancreatic cancer.

LONGITUDINAL PANCREATICOJEJUNOSTOMY—OPERATIVE TECHNIQUE

The pancreas is best exposed with a bilateral subcostal or chevron incision. The abdomen should be explored for any unforeseen pathology. An abdominal retractor is placed and dissection begun to expose the pancreas. This involves a complete Kocher maneuver and mobilization of the hepatic flexure of the colon. The lesser sac is opened through the gastrocolic ligament, and the posterior attachments of the stomach are dissected free to the point where the gastroduodenal artery (GDA) passes behind the duodenum and onto the head of the pancreas. The GDA and its branches on the surface of the head of the pancreas are suture ligated with vascular suture, which minimizes bleeding later when the pancreatic tissue in the head is cut in order to unroof the pancreatic duct. The superior mesenteric vein is identified where it passes under the neck of the pancreas but it is not necessary to separate it from the pan-

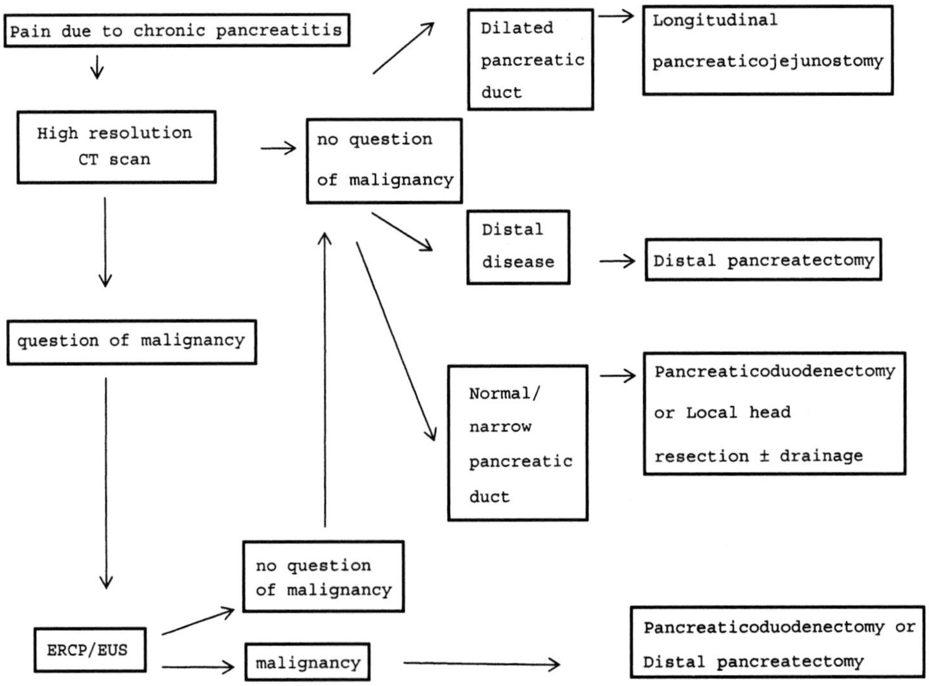

Figure 38–4. Surgery for Chronic Pancreatitis Algorithm.

TABLE 38–3. RESULTS OF LONGITUDINAL PANCREATICOJEJUNOSTOMY FOR CHRONIC PANCREATITIS

Author	Year	No. of Patients	Mortality (%)	Mean Follow-Up (Months)	Pain Relief (%)
Leger[25]	1973	45	4.5	—	63
Prinz[26]	1978	42	5	108	76
Prinz[27]	1981	43	4.5	95	65
Sarles[28]	1982	69	4.2	60	85
Warshaw[29]	1984	33	3	43	88
Bradley[30]	1986	48	0	69	66
Nealon[31]	1988	41	0	14.8	93

creas. The head of the pancreas should be completely exposed with the dissection.

Next, the pancreatic duct is identified by inserting a large bore needle through the parenchyma into the duct lumen. An incision is made with electrocautery following the needle shaft into the duct, and this incision is extended along the length of the duct into the head and back into the body and tail. Any stones are removed. When the head of the gland is large and the opened pancreatic duct dives deep into the parenchyma, we will remove some of the overhanging pancreatic tissue. We think this achieves a better decompression of the duct, and that the anastomosis is more likely to remain patent over time. This aspect of the operation is described more fully later (see Frey procedure).

A Roux limb of jejunum is then created and brought through the mesocolon in a retrocolic position. A side-to-side anastomosis is performed with an inner layer of continuous 3-0 (PDS) and an outer layer of interrupted 3-0 silk suture (Fig 38–5). A closed suction drain is placed near the anastomosis and the abdomen closed.

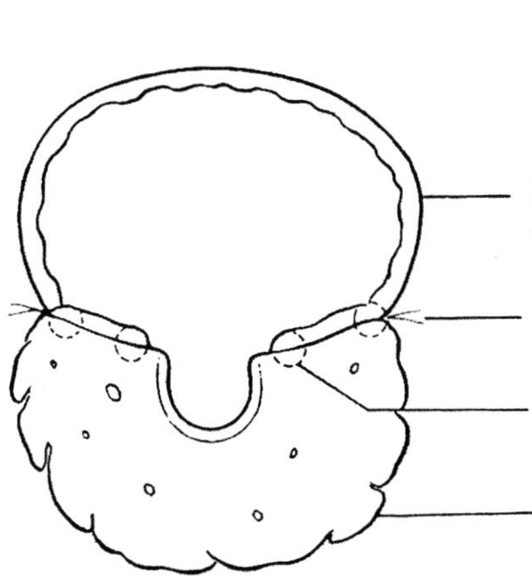

Figure 38–5. Cross-section of the anastomosis for a pancreaticojejunostomy. This also applies to the Frey procedure.

PANCREATICODUODENECTOMY

Patients with a normal diameter or narrowed duct may be candidates for pancreatic resection. This is especially true when the pancreatic head is enlarged and contains multiple cysts and calcifications. Pancreaticoduodenectomy (Whipple resection) or pylorus-preserving pancreaticoduodenectomy are performed most commonly. Pylorus preservation is felt by many to allow for better postoperative nutrition and weight gain, but little objective data support this. The operative mortality rate is <3% and permanent pain relief is to be expected in 85% to 90% (Table 38–4). These operations are more likely than pancreaticojejunostomy to produce endocrine (22%) and exocrine (55%) insufficiency, which is their major drawback. Of course, some patients develop these problems regardless as the disease progresses.

PANCREATICODUODENECTOMY—OPERATIVE TECHNIQUE

The operation is performed through a bilateral subcostal incision. After the abdomen has been entered, an initial assessment of its contents is performed. When exploring a patient for chronic pancreatitis, one should always remember that these patients may actually harbor an unsuspected pancreatic malignancy. Therefore, the liver, the peritoneum, and the root of the mesocolon must be carefully inspected, and a frozen section taken of suspicious lesions to rule out cancer.

The dissection is begun with an extensive Kocher maneuver. The hepatic flexure of the colon is mobilized and retracted inferiorly. The mobilization of the duodenum is carried past the aorta, opening through to the area of the proximal jejunum near the ligament of Treitz on the patient's left side. The head of the pancreas is palpated, the superior mesenteric vein is identified, and its tributaries from the head of the pancreas and stomach are divided. Then the gastrocolic omentum is opened to enter the lesser sac and the body of the pancreas is exposed. The duodenum is transected

TABLE 38–4. RESULTS OF RESECTION FOR CHRONIC PANCREATITIS

Study	Year		No. of Patients	Operative Mortality (%)	Pain Relief (%)	New Onset DM (%)	New Endo. Insuff. (%)
Heise[32]	2001	PPW	41	4.8	54	19	67
		Drainage	59	—	59	16	54
		DP	26	—	89	21	50
Jimenez[33]	2000	PPW	39	1.4	60	10	63
		SW	33	—	70	12	77
Martin[34]	1996	PPW	45	2.2	92	46	77
Beger[35]	1999	DPPHR	504	0.8	91	21	—
Frey[36]	1994	LRLPJ	50	0	87	11	11

PPW, pylorus-preserving Whipple; DP, distal pancreatectomy; SW, standard Whipple; DPPHR, duodenum-preserving pancreatic head resection; LRLPJ, local pancreatic head resection with longitudinal pancreaticojejunostomy; DM, diabetes mellitus; endo. insuff., endocrine insufficiency.

with an automatic stapling device about 2 cm distal to the pylorus. The stomach is retracted into the left upper abdomen.

A plane is developed between the anterior surface of the superior mesenteric vein and the undersurface of the neck of the pancreas, but the separation of the two is not pursued further at this time.

Attention is turned to the hepatoduodenal ligament where the distal common bile duct is freed circumferentially above the cystic-common duct junction and isolated with a vessel loop. The hepatic artery is isolated and the GDA and right gastric artery doubly ligated and divided. Inadequate control of these vessels can lead to serious postoperative bleeding. The portal vein is identified at the upper border of the pancreas. A plane is developed between the neck of the pancreas and the vein above and below the pancreas by a combination of finger dissection and the insertion of a blunt tipped instrument. When the opening is complete, a quarter inch Penrose drain is pulled through the hole where it remains in place until the neck of the pancreas is transected. Occasionally, especially with chronic pancreatitis, there may be some inflammatory adherence of the vein to the undersurface of the neck of the pancreas, which can make this maneuver problematic. If bleeding is encountered, it can almost always be controlled by compression of the superior mesenteric vein.

A cholecystectomy is performed, the common bile duct is divided, and a curved bulldog clip is placed temporarily to occlude the proximal hepatic duct. The distal duct is ligated.

The remainder of the fourth portion of the duodenum and proximal jejunum is mobilized by lifting the transverse colon and cutting the ligament of Treitz. The jejunum is transected with a stapler about 5 cm distal to the ligament, and the remaining mesenteric attachments to the proximal jejunum are divided close to the bowel wall with electrocautery. Then the entire duodenum and proximal jejunum is drawn through the peritoneal opening under the superior mesenteric vein and artery to the right side of the abdomen. This simplifies the final removal of the specimen, which is the next step of the operation.

We next place four 3-0 vascular sutures through the pancreatic tissue to occlude the transverse arteries before the pancreas is divided. Two are placed in the superior and two in the inferior border of the gland on either side of the proposed line of transection. During this maneuver, the neck of the gland is elevated by slight traction on the Penrose drain so that the underlying vessels are protected. One should avoid entering the pancreatic duct, which later can be incorporated into the pancreaticojejunal anastomosis. The duct normally is posterior and slightly superior in the neck of the pancreas, but often in patients with chronic pancreatitis, it is more anterior. The pancreas then is divided with electrocautery, and the Penrose drain, which is useful to protect the portal vein, is removed. Bleeders from the cut pancreatic surface are controlled and the pancreatic duct is identified.

Now the uncinate and duodenal mesentery is separated from the superior mesenteric vein and artery by successively ligating and dividing this tissue with 2-0 silk suture beginning superiorly. (Fig 38–6). If the tissue is particularly adherent to the portal or superior mesenteric veins, one can leave some of the soft tissue or even the uncinate process behind (this is not acceptable if the operation is being done for cancer). Any remaining attachments of the duodenum to the posterior abdominal wall are divided and the specimen is removed.

This final phase of the operation is often associated with some blood loss because of the vascularity of the tissues involved and the proximity to large vascular structures. This can be minimized by compression of the specimen, which is held in and retracted by the left hand of the surgeon as the dissection takes place, and by persistence and steady progression with removal of

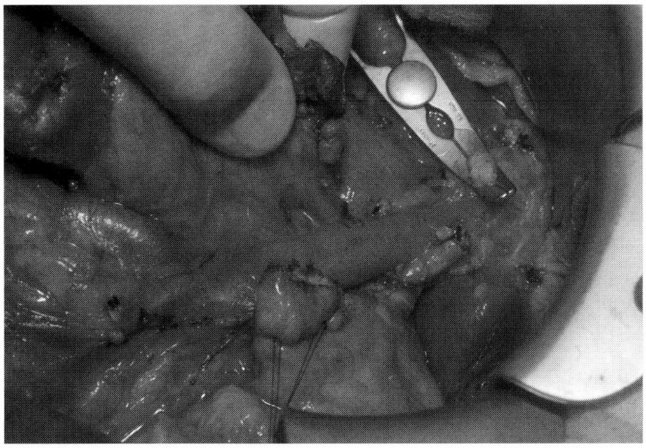

Figure 38–6. Intraoperative photo demonstrating the ligation of the duodenal mesentery during a pancreaticoduodenectomy.

the specimen in spite of the ooze of venous blood that often is present. This stops as the dissection progresses. Of course, if there is ever significant venous or arterial bleeding, this should be stopped immediately using vascular suture.

The operative field is copiously irrigated with saline and the specimen is sent for frozen section analysis to make certain that an unsuspected cancer is not present.

The pancreaticojejunal anastomosis is performed first. The jejunum is brought behind the superior mesenteric artery and vein. An end-to-side pancreaticojejunostomy is performed after the staple line of the jejunum is oversewn. We place a plastic stent into the duct so that it can be easily seen during the anastomosis, but the stent is removed after the anastomosis is completed. The anastomosis is performed in two layers—interrupted 3-0 silk for the outer and continuous 3-0 PDS for the inner. The pancreatic duct is incorporated into the running inner suture for a few of both the posterior and anterior row bites (Fig 38–7).

The choledochojejunal anastomosis is performed next at a sufficient distance from the pancreas to avoid tension on the suture line, but not too long to allow kinking of the bowel. A single layer anastomosis using interrupted sutures of 4-0 or 5-0 PDS is performed. Initially, the anterior sutures are placed through the duct wall from outside to inside the lumen, and the needles left attached. With the anterior duct wall retracted superiorly by those sutures, the posterior sutures are placed through both the duct and the jejunum, and tied after all of them have been inserted, with the knots inside the lumen. Then the anterior sutures are placed through the jejunum and they are tied after all have been placed, with the knots on the outside. If the duct is smaller than 1 cm in diameter, a small T tube inserted through the wall of the bile duct proximal to the anastomosis. The distal limb of the T-tube lies in the jejunal limb. The tube is removed 4 to 8 weeks later.

Finally, a retrocolic duodenojejunostomy is constructed approximately 30 cm distal to the choledochojejunostomy, in a standard two-layer fashion. This is performed through a separate defect created in the transverse mesocolon to the left of the middle colic vessels. Once the anastomosis is performed, the stomach is brought through the mesocolon and tacked to it with 3-0 silk suture.

Two closed suction drains are placed close to the pancreatic and hepatic duct anastomoses. These are brought through the abdomen separately on the right and left side. The T tube is also brought out of the abdomen on the right side and sutured to the skin with a nylon suture. After this, the abdomen is irrigated again, the adequacy of hemostasis reconfirmed, and the wound is closed in layers.

COMBINED RESECTION AND DRAINAGE PROCEDURES

In an effort to design an operation that would provide permanent pain relief and avoid the exocrine and endocrine insufficiency of a major resection, surgeons have designed several new procedures that combine limited resection of the head of the pancreas with a pancreaticojejunostomy. The so-called Beger (duodenal preserving resection of the head of the pancreas) or Frey (local resection of the head of the pancreas) operations remove most of the head of the pancreas except for a shell of pancreatic tissue posteriorly. The cavity thus created is drained into a Roux-en-Y limb of jejunum; gastroduodenal continuity is not disturbed. These operations can be performed whether or not the pancreatic duct is dilated. If it is, the pancreaticojejunostomy is extended over the

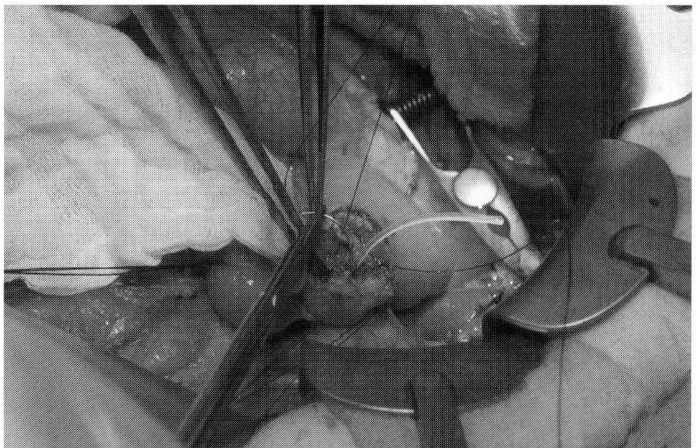

Figure 38–7. Intraoperative photo of the pancreaticojejunal anastomosis during a pancreaticoduodenectomy.

body of the pancreas to incorporate the dilated duct in that area. Early results suggest that pain relief is excellent in 85–90% of patients, that the relief persists beyond several years, and that exocrine or endocrine insufficiency are not precipitated by the surgery (Table 38–4). In those patients whose bile duct has also been obstructed by the fibrotic pancreas, this "coring" of pancreatic tissue from the head of the gland may decompress that duct as well. This operation is contraindicated if there is a concern about the presence of a malignant neoplasm in the head of the pancreas. Then, a pancreaticoduodenectomy should be performed.

LOCAL RESECTION OF THE HEAD OF THE PANCREAS (FREY PROCEDURE; CORING OF THE HEAD OF THE PANCREAS)—OPERATIVE TECHNIQUE

This operation may be indicated when the head of the pancreas is enlarged, e.g., 3 to 4 cm or more in anteroposterior diameter, and is an alternative to a Whipple type pancreatic resection. If the duct is dilated, the operation is performed in a fashion similar to that already described for a longitudinal pancreaticojejunostomy, including opening of the pancreatic duct in the head of the pancreas. That incision in the head of the pancreas is extended to within 1 cm of the duodenal border. Using electrocautery, we then begin removing pieces of pancreatic tissue starting from the opened main pancreatic duct. We extend the dissection out to within 1 cm of the duodenal border and posteriorly to within a few millimeters of the posterior capsule of the pancreatic head (Fig 38–8). A decision about when to stop the posterior dissection requires repeated assessment of the thickness of the remaining shell of tissue. This is accomplished by bimanual palpation of the cavity being created; the softness and pliability of the thin layer of remaining tissue stands in marked contrast to the firm parenchyma that existed at the start of the procedure. The superior mesenteric/portal vein often is not seen during this local resection, but the vein is protected from injury because its position is apparent. Thus, it always runs under the neck of the pancreas just medial to the point where the duct is seen to dive deeply posterior, and we do not excise tissue medial to that part of the duct.

During this local head resection, we occasionally may be concerned about the position of the intrapancreatic portion of the common bile duct. In order to identify it, a small Bakes dilator can be placed inside the duct. This can be removed after the dissection is complete, and a T tube placed at the site of the proximal choledochotomy. In some patients the intrapancreatic common duct may be obstructed by scar tissue. In about 70% of cases, local resection of the head of the pancreas also relieves the common duct obstruction. This should be confirmed by passage of a Bakes dilator, and if the obstruction cannot be relieved, a choledochojejunostomy can be performed in addition.

When the pancreatic parenchyma has been sufficiently resected, the ducts opened widely and the calculi removed, the Roux-en-Y limb of jejunum is prepared, and the pancreaticojejunostomy performed as already described (Fig 38–9).

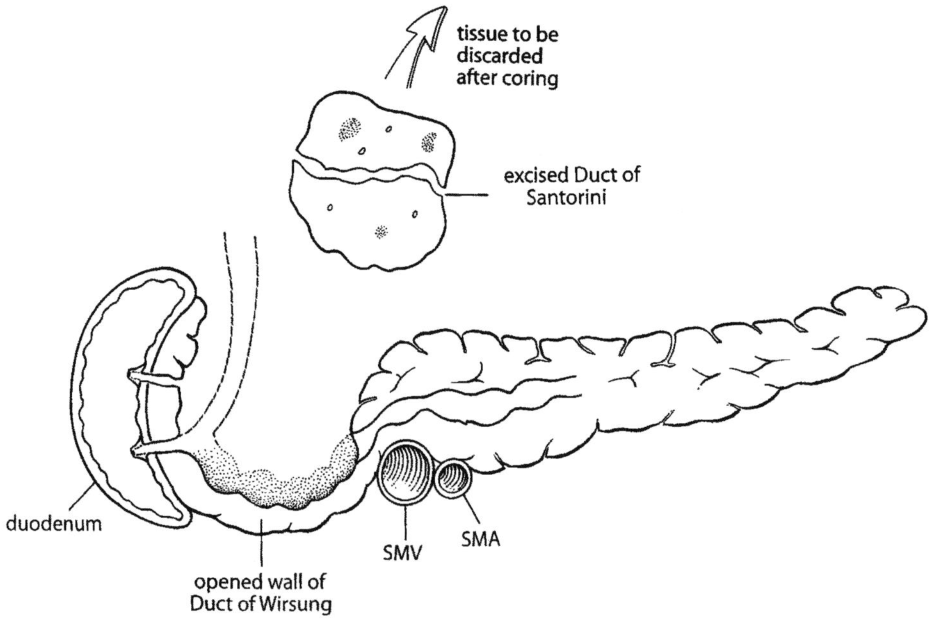

Figure 38–8. Cross-section drawing of the pancreas following the coring of the pancreatic head during a Frey procedure.

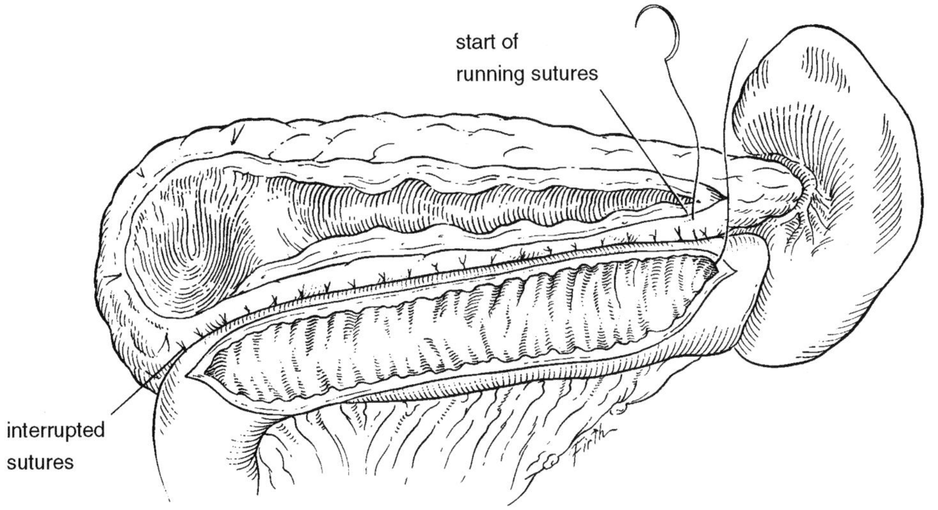

Figure 38–9. The pancreaticojejunostomy of the Frey procedure.

BEGER PROCEDURE (DUODENAL PRESERVING RESECTION OF THE HEAD OF THE PANCREAS)—OPERATIVE TECHNIQUE[37]

The operation is similar to the Frey operation, but the superior mesenteric/portal vein is exposed above and below the neck of the pancreas, freed from the posterior portion of the neck, and then the neck is divided, as done in a pancreaticoduodenectomy. The head of the pancreas is then resected in a fashion similar to that done in the Frey operation, preserving a shell of pancreas posteriorly. A bit more pancreas is usually removed with the Beger approach, since the neck of the gland is transected, and the portal vein is exposed (Fig 38–10). The operation may be challenging technically if there is inflammatory adherence of the pancreas to the vein. When the resection is complete, a pancreaticojejunostomy is done, incorporating both the transected end of the distal pancreatic segment and the cavity resulting from the head resection. If the pancreatic duct in the distal segment is dilated, the duct should be opened longitudinally and the pancreaticojejunostomy done as in a Puestow type anastomosis (Fig 38–11).

DISTAL PANCREATECTOMY

Uncommonly, chronic pancreatitis is localized predominantly in the body or tail of the pancreas. Then a distal pancreatectomy (with or without splenectomy) may be effective. The surgeon should investigate the possibility that an occult malignancy may have produced a more

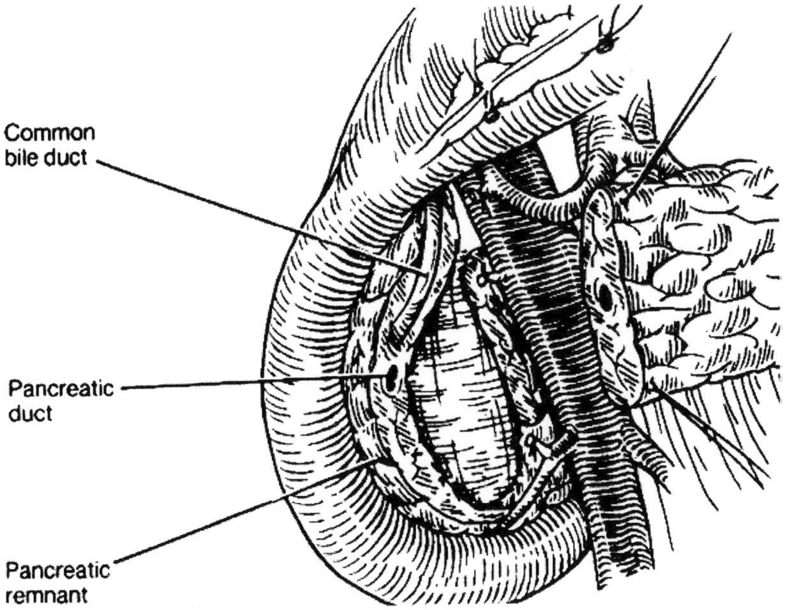

Figure 38–10. The anatomy following the transection of the neck of the pancreas and removal of the head during the Beger procedure.

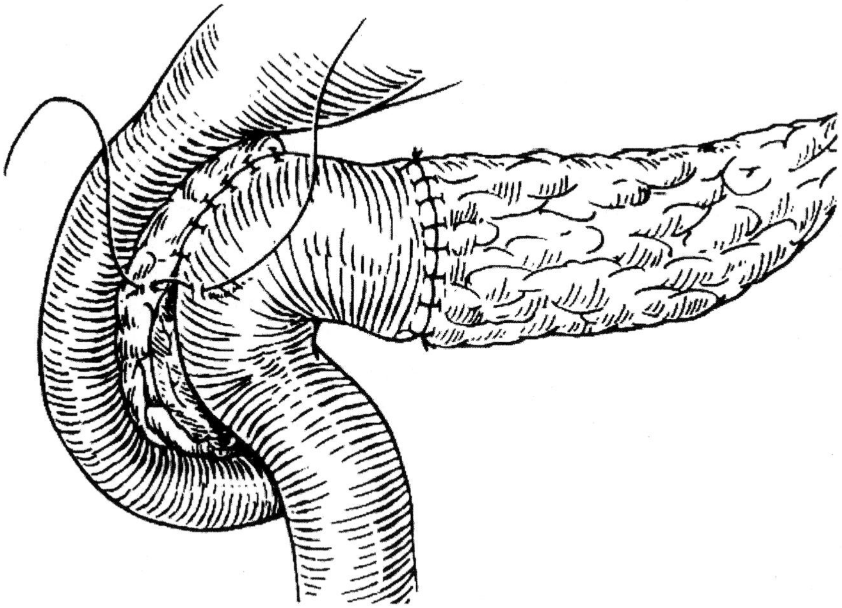

Figure 38–11. The final anatomy of the reconstruction following a Beger procedure.

proximal duct obstruction, and that a neoplastic duct stricture is the reason for such localized pancreatitis. Otherwise, in patients with predominantly distal disease, distal pancreatectomy is safe and pain relief can be expected in as many as 90% of patients after 4 years (Table 38–4). For the usual patient who has diffuse disease involving the entire pancreas, distal pancreatectomy is ineffective, however. Because it results in brittle diabetes that is often difficult to control, and because lesser procedures are likely to be effective, total pancreatectomy for chronic pancreatitis is almost never done today.

MINOR PAPILLA SPHINCTEROTOMY

In cases where pancreas divisum is thought to be the cause of recurrent episodes of pancreatitis, chronic pancreatitis, and pain, a minor papilla sphincterotomy is not appropriate. Once chronic pancreatitis has become established, the general principles of management outlined in the foregoing sections should be followed. Sphincteroplasty of the minor papilla may be effective in patients with pancreas divisum with recurrent episodes of acute pancreatitis early in the disease process before the changes of chronic pancreatitis have become established, however.

▪ COMPLICATIONS OF CHRONIC PANCREATITIS

PSEUDOCYST

A pancreatic pseudocyst is a collection of fluid, usually near the pancreas, which develops in association with a leak of pancreatic juice from the inflamed pancreatic parenchyma or from a disrupted duct. The wall of the pseudocyst is comprised of fibrous nonepithelialized tissue. Occasionally a pseudocyst may present at great distance from the pancreas (e.g., thorax, groin), when the fluid dissects through tissue planes. The majority of acute pseudocysts that appear during an episode of acute pancreatic inflammation resolve without intervention. However, most pseudocysts that develop on a background of chronic pancreatitis are unlikely to resolve spontaneously, and they may need treatment. Asymptomatic pseudocysts up to 5 to 6 cm in diameter may be safely observed, and are usually followed with either serial ultrasound or CT examinations. Larger cysts or pseudocysts of any size that are symptomatic require intervention. Symptoms are most often from gastrointestinal (GI) obstruction when the cyst distorts or compresses the stomach, duodenum, or bile duct, or produces abdominal pain. Serious complications also can occur, although they are uncommon (<5% of cases). These include hemorrhage into the cyst, perforation of the cyst, or cyst infection. Hemorrhage is usually caused by erosion of the splenic or gastroduodenal artery or other major vessel within the wall of the cyst, and the bleeding is often confined to the cyst lumen. The diagnosis should be suspected if there are clinical signs of hypovolemia, and a falling hematocrit. There may be abdominal pain, and a mass may be palpable. An abdominal CT scan shows the cyst with the contained blood clot. Angiography confirms the diagnosis, and the radiologist should attempt to embolize the bleeding vessel. If not, emergency surgery with ligation of the vessel or excision of the cyst is required. Perforation of a pseudocyst is a surgical emergency that is characterized by the sudden onset of intense abdominal pain with peritonitis. Patients require urgent surgery with irrigation of the peritoneal cavity and usually external cyst drainage. Infection of a pseudocyst should be suspected if signs of sepsis develop. Diagnosis by CT scan and treatment by percutaneous cyst aspiration and drainage are usually effective.

In the absence of a life-threatening complication, elective surgery of pseudocysts is usually delayed until the cyst has developed a mature wall that will hold sutures at the time of repair. For those cysts that develop following an episode of acute pancreatitis, this requires 4 to 6 weeks. In most cases the patient can eat and be discharged from the hospital during the interval. Pseudocysts that resolve spontaneously usually will do so during this time. If no episode of clinically significant acute pancreatitis preceded the development of the cyst, as is often the case in patients with chronic pancreatitis, usually no waiting period is necessary.

Pseudocysts may be treated surgically, or by endoscopic or radiologic drainage. Endoscopic methods require the placement of a plastic stent through the stomach or duodenal wall into the adjacent cyst. The stent is eventually removed, and in about 80% of cases, the cyst is permanently eradicated. Radiologic approaches usually consist of percutaneous external drainage of the cyst with eventual removal of the drainage catheter many weeks later. Many of these pseudocysts recur. Surgical treatment usually consists of drainage of the cyst internally to either the stomach (cystgastrostomy) or to a Roux-en-Y limb of jejunum (cystojejunostomy). Both are safe and effective, with recurrence rates <10%. If the pseudocyst is in the tail of the pancreas, a distal pancreatectomy with excision of the cyst may be best.

PANCREATIC FISTULA

In the setting of chronic pancreatitis, a pancreatic fistula is usually the result of a ductal disruption from an episode of acute pancreatitis. An internal pancreatic fistula causes pancreatic ascites, in which the leaking pancreatic fluid accumulates within the peritoneal cavity. Most fistulas are external, however, and are diagnosed when pancreatic fluid leaks from a healing incision or drain tract following the operative management of an episode of complicated pancreatitis. The diagnosis is made by finding a high amylase level (usually many thousands of U/L) in the fistula effluent. Some fistulas will close spontaneously, provided that ductal continuity can be re-established as healing occurs, infection is eradicated, and nutrition is adequate. However, the frequent presence of duct obstruction in chronic pancreatitis may make it less likely that the fistula will close. Parenteral nutrition is usually not required and most patients are able to eat a regular diet. There is no evidence that oral intake delays resolution of a fistula. The use of somatostatin does not appear to hasten fistula closure, although if it is a high output fistula (greater than 200 mL/day), the secretory inhibitor may simplify management of the patient. Almost all internal fistulas that cause pancreatic ascites, external fistulas that persist for as long as 1 year, or those whose anatomic characteristics preclude spontaneous closure (e.g., duct obstruction between fistula and duodenal lumen, duct discontinuity), will require operative repair. This is best done by creating an anastomosis between the pancreatic duct at the point of the leak and a Roux-en-Y limb of jejunum. The success rate of operative repair is >90%.

BILIARY STRICTURE OR OBSTRUCTION

Jaundice may occur in up to one third of patients with chronic calcific pancreatitis at some point during the disease, usually when there is pancreatic swelling at the time of an episode of acute pancreatitis. This often resolves as the acute inflammation subsides, but as many as 10% of patients are left with obstruction of the common duct. This is because of fibrosis of the head of the pancreas resulting in constriction of the duct as it passes through this portion of the gland. The stricture usually appears as a long, symmetrical narrowing when it is visualized by MRCP or ERCP. The proximal duct and gallbladder may be distended, but obstruction of the duct is almost never complete, which differentiates it from a malignant obstruction. A simple biliary bypass utilizing a Roux-en-Y choledochojejunostomy effectively treats such a biliary stricture.

INTESTINAL COMPRESSION OR OBSTRUCTION

A minority of patients will present with obstruction of the second or third portion of the duodenum. Upper endoscopy and CT scan should be performed to rule out the presence of a neoplastic process. Then a loop gastrojejunostomy can be done to bypass the obstruction.

Obstruction of the colon (usually the transverse or splenic flexure) can also occur from chronic pancreatitis. If this is a result of an episode of acute inflammation, the obstruction will likely resolve. If it persists, then a colonoscopy should be performed to rule out malignancy. Persistence of the obstruction requires a resection of the involved segment of colon and an end-to-end anastomosis.

▪ PANCREATIC CANCER

Patients with long-standing chronic pancreatitis are at a 10% lifetime risk for the development of pancreatic adenocarcinoma. During evaluation for surgery in a patient with chronic pancreatitis, imaging studies may show focal changes in the pancreas that suggest malignancy. Alternatively, other aspects of the clinical presentation (e.g., rising or markedly elevated CA 19-9, change in character of pain, accelerated weight loss) may have raised the clinician's index of suspicion about the possibility that cancer is present.

If there is concern about malignancy, we recommend EUS examination, which is currently the most sensitive diagnostic study to identify small cancers, and also can be used to obtain tissue from the lesion that could confirm the diagnosis. However, whether or not the diagnosis is confirmed preoperatively, patients in whom the surgeon suspects the coexistence of pancreatic cancer with underlying chronic pancreatitis require pancreatic resection. This means a pancreaticoduodenectomy for head and uncinate lesions and a distal pancreatectomy for body and tail lesions. Even if cancer is not found when the resected specimen is examined by the pathologist, this approach represents the current standard of care in such circumstances. This is because resection operations are safe, they are one of the standard operations normally done for chronic pancreatitis without coexisting cancer, and pancreatic cancer is uniformly fatal when it is not surgically resected.

▪ CONCLUSION

The surgical considerations for patients with chronic pancreatitis include procedures to address chronic pain, various complications of the disease, and pancreatic cancer. The decision to operate in any single patient with pain from the disease is complex, and should be based on a variety of factors that include the psychosocial makeup of the patient as well as pancreatic anatomy. If surgery is indicated, the type of operation hinges on the appearance of the pancreatic ducts. In patients with a dilated duct, a drainage procedure is often the best option since this offers good pain relief and the least long-term morbidity. If the ducts are not enlarged, prior ductal drainage has failed, or there is concern about the presence of cancer, resection should be performed. Newer operations that resect most of the head of the pancreas but still preserve GI continuity (Beger, Frey) may provide the best long-term pain relief with the least long-term morbidity. Patients with chronic pancreatitis can develop pseudocysts, pancreatic fistulas, and biliary or intestinal obstruction. The pancreatic surgeon must be prepared to deal with all of these issues.

REFERENCES

1. Comfort M, Gambill E, Baggenstoss A. Chronic relapsing pancreatitis. *Gastroenterology* 1946;6:653–658
2. De las Heras G, Pons F. Epidemiologia y aspectos etiopatogenicos de la pancreatitis alcoholica cronica. *Rev Esp Enferm Dig* 1993;84:253–258
3. Otsuki M. Chronic pancreatitis in Japan: epidemiology, prognosis, diagnostic criteria, and future problems. *J Gastroenterol* 2003;38:315–326
4. Gukovskaya AS, Mouria M, Gukovsky I et al. Ethanol metabolism and transcription factor activation in pancreatic acinar cells in rats. *Gastroenterology* 2003;122:106–118
5. Bachem MG, Schneider E, Gross H et al. Identification, culture and characterization of pancreatic stellate cells in rats and humans. *Gastroenterology* 1998;115:421–432
6. Gelrud A, Freedman SD. Autoimmue pancreatitis. *J Gastrointest Surg* 2005;9:2–5
7. Whitcomb DC, Gorry MC, Preston RA, et al. Mutations in the gene encoding the serine protease inhibitor. *Nat Genet* 100;25:213–216
8. Witt H, Luck W, Hennies HC, et al. Mutations in the gene encoding the serine protease inhibitor, Kazal type 1 are associated with chronic pancreatitis. *Nat Genet* 2000;25:213–216
9. Durie PR. Pancreatitis and mutations of the cystic fibrosis gene. *N Engl J Med* 1998;339:687–688
10. Apte, MV, Park S, Phillips PA, et al. Desmoplastic reaction in pancreatic cancer: role of pancreatic stellate cells. *Pancreas* 2004;29:179–187
11. Vogelmann R, Ruf D, Wagner M, et al. Development of pancreatic fibrosis in a TGFB1 transgenic mouse. *Gastroenterology* 1999;116:A1174
12. Kahl S, Glasbrenner B, Leodolter A, et al. EUS in the diagnosis of early chronic pancreatitis: a prospective follow-up study. *Gastrointest Endosc* 2002;55:507–511
13. Dominguez-Munoz JE, Martinez S, Leodolter A, et al. Quantification of pancreatic zinc output as pancreatic function test: making the secretin-caerulein test applicable to clinical practice. *Pancreatology* 2004;4:57–62
14. Koliopanos A, Friess H, Roggo A, et al. Cyclooxygenase-2 expression in chronic pancreatitis: correlation with stage of disease and diabetes mellitus. *Digestion* 2001;64: 240–247
15. Jakobs R, Benz C, Leonhardt A. Pancreatic endoscopic sphincterotomy in patients with chronic pancreatitis. *Endoscopy* 2002;34:551–554
16. Rosch T, Daniel S, Scholz M. Endoscopic treatment of chronic pancreatitis: a multicenter study of 1000 patients with long term follow-up. *Endoscopy* 2002;34:765–771
17. Delhaye M, Vandermeeran A, Baize M, et al. Extracorporeal shock wave lithotripsy of pancreatic calculi. *Gastroenterology* 1992;102:610–620

18. Schneider HT, May A, Benninger J, et al. Piezoelectric shock wave lithotripsy of pancreatic duct stones. *Am J Gastroenterol* 1994;89:2042–2048
19. Johanns W, Jakobeit C, Greiner L, et al. Ultrasound-guided extracorporeal chock wave lithotripsy of pancreatic ductal stones: a six years experience. *Can J Gastroenterol* 1996;10:471–475
20. Costamagna G, Gabbrielli A, Mutignani M, et al. Extracorporeal shock wave lithotripsy of pancreatic stones in chronic pancreatitis: immediate and medium-term results. *Gastrointest Endosc* 1997;46:231–236
21. Adamek HE, Jakobs R, Buttmann A, et al. Long term followup of patients with chronic pancreatitis and pancreatic stones treated with extracorporeal shock wave lithotripsy. *Gut* 1999;45:402–405
22. Brand B, Kahl M, Sidhu S, et al. Prospective evaluation of morphology, function, and quality of life after extracorporeal shock wave lithotripsy and endoscopic treatment of chronic calcific pancreatitis. *Am J Gastroenterol* 2000;95:3428–3438
23. Farnbacher MJ, Shoen C, Rabenstein T, et al. Pancreatic duct stones in chronic pancreatitis: criteria for treatment intensity and success. *Gastrointest Endosc* 2002;56: 501–506
24. Kozarek RE, Brandabur JJ, Ball JT, et al. Clinical outcomes in patients who undergo extracorporeal shock wave lithotripsy for chronic calcific pancreatitis. *Gastrointest Endosc* 2002;56:496–500
25. Leger L, Lenriot JP, Lemaigre G. Five to twenty year follow up after surgery for chronic pancreatitis in 148 patients. *Ann Surg* 1974;180:185–191
26. Prinz RA, Kaufman BH, Folk FA, Greenlee HB. Pancreaticojejunostomy for chronic pancreatitis: two- to 21-year follow-up. *Arch Surg* 1978;113:520–525
27. Prinz RA, Greenlee HB. Pancreatic duct drainage in 100 patients with chronic pancreatitis. *Ann Surg* 1981;194: 313–320
28. Sarles J-C, Nacchiero M, Garani F, Salasc B. Surgical treatment of chronic pancreatitis: report of 134 cases treated by resection or drainage. *Am J Surg* 1982;144: 317–321
29. Warshaw AL. Conservation of pancreatic tissue by combined gastric, biliary, and pancreatic duct drainage for pain from chronic pancreatitis. *Am J Surg* 1985;149:563–569
30. Bradley EL. Long-term results of pancreatojejunostomy in patients with chronic pancreatitis. *Am J Surg* 1987; 153:207–213
31. Nealon WH, Townsend CM Jr, Thompson JC. Operative drainage of the pancreatic duct delays functional impairment in patients with chronic pancreatitis: a prospective analysis. *Ann Surg* 1988;208:321–329
32. Heise JW, Katoh M, Luthen R, Roher H-D. Long-term results following different extent of resection in chronic pancreatitis. *Hepatogastroenterology* 2001;48:864–868
33. Jimenez RE, Fernandez-del Castillo C, Rattner DW, Chang Y, Warshaw AL. Outcome of pancreaticoduodenectomy with pylorus preservation or with antrectomy in the treatment of chronic pancreatitis. *Ann Surg* 2000;231:293–300
34. Martin RF, Rossi RL, Leslie KA. Long-term results of pylorus-preserving pancreatoduodenectomy for chronic pancreatitis. *Arch Surg* 1996;131:247–252
35. Beger HG, Schlosser W, Friess HM, Buchler MW. Duodenum-preserving head resection in chronic pancreatitis changes the natural course of the disease: a single-center 26-year experience. *Ann Surg* 1999;230:512–523
36. Frey CF, Amikura K. Local resection of the head of the pancreas combined with longitudinal pancreaticojejunostomy in the management of patients with chronic pancreatitis. *Ann Surg* 1994;220:492–507
37. Beger HG, Kunz R, Poch B. The Beger procedure—duodenum-preserving pancreatic head resection. *J Gastrointest Surg* 2004;8:1090–1097

39

Disorders of the Duodenal Ampullae

Michael Rosen ■ *Andrew L. Warshaw*

Clinical entities discussed in this chapter involve the orifice of the termini of the bile duct and the pancreatic ducts, either in producing a disease or in preventing its spontaneous resolution. Included are benign ampullary tumors, stenosis and dyskinesia of the sphincter of Oddi, stenosis of the orifice of the duct of Wirsung, and stenosis of the accessory papilla associated with pancreas divisum. Patients with these disorders have pain, pancreatitis, jaundice, or cholangitis, and malignancy must be excluded. Treatment of these conditions, in each instance, must consider elimination or bypass of the terminal sphincter mechanism.

■ ANATOMY

The duodenal papilla has both a major and minor component. The major papilla comprises the ampulla of Vater, the sphincter of Oddi, and the major duodenal papilla. The interchangeable use of eponyms to describe these anatomically unique structures leads to confusion and should be abandoned. The ampulla of Vater refers to the common channel of the bile duct and main pancreatic duct, which is sometimes slightly dilated to form a small chamber or ampulla. The sphincter of Oddi encompasses the smooth muscle fibers surrounding the termination of the bile duct and pancreatic duct, forming a true sphincter. This sphincter regulates pancreatic and biliary flow into the duodenum. The major duodenal papilla is the terminal protuberance of these elements, together with their associated glands and other structures, terminating in the ampullary orifice.

The minor duodenal papilla typically is located anterior and proximal to the major papilla. It represents the termination of the accessory pancreatic duct commonly referred to as the duct of Santorini. In up to 20% of patients this duct does not penetrate the duodenal wall. Smooth muscle fibers envelop the termination of this duct and are occasionally referred to as the sphincter of Helly. Occasionally in relapsing pancreatitis the accessory pancreatic duct can appear to have cystic dilatation and has been referred to as a Santorinicele.

■ TOOLS FOR DIAGNOSIS

BLOOD TESTS

The most sensitive blood test indicating biliary obstruction is determination of the serum alkaline phosphatase level. It is often elevated, whereas the bilirubin remains at normal levels. The levels of serum transaminase (alanine and aspartate aminotransferases; SGPT, SGOT) commonly rise modestly (up to 200 U, although they can reach levels of 1000 to 2000 U), which can cause diagnostic confusion by suggesting hepatitis. The serum amylase level remains the simplest and most useful index of acute pancreatitis. It is elevated in 70–95% of cases, the usual exceptions being those that come to medical attention late after the amylase level has already returned to normal, and flares of acute inflammation in chronic pancreatitis, in which the gland is thought to have insufficient remaining secretory capacity. There are many causes of hyperamylasemia, other than pancreatitis, that must by kept in mind for differential diagnosis (Table 39–1). Measurement of other pancreatic enzymes in the serum, including lipase, and determination of the amylase-creatinine clearance ratio have not contributed to diagnosis.

PANCREATIC FUNCTION TESTS

Ampullary stenosis, with the exception of iatrogenic injuries, is virtually never complete enough to cause clinical malabsorption. Pancreatic function (fecal fat measurement, pancrealauryl test) is usually normal.

RADIOGRAPHIC TESTS

Dilation of the biliary and pancreatic ducts can be demonstrated by ultrasonography and CT, but stones can be detected in the common duct in only 10–20% of cases, when present. Changes in diameter of a few millimeters of the bile duct, and as little as 1 mm of the pancreatic duct, are detectable. Real definition of the ducts, as well as the precise location and configuration of a blockage, requires opacification with contrast material (e.g., as used in transhepatic cholangiography [THC] and endoscopic retrograde cholangiopancreatography [ERCP]). ERCP (Fig 39–1) has the advantage of showing both systems, allowing visualization and biopsy of the ampulla, and providing at least an estimate of the ampullary orifice size. In competent hands, the papilla can be cannulated in >90% of cases. This success rate has led some to state that inability to cannulate the papilla is an indicator of stenosis. However, this statement generally has not correlated with surgical findings and can be attributed frequently to technical features of the procedure or the unique anatomy of the patient. When a retrograde cholangiogram is obtained, the presence of a dilated common bile duct (>12 mm) in the absence of structural causes for common duct dilation is a reliable indicator of ampullary disease. Delayed emptying of contrast material from the common bile duct (>45 minutes) also may indicate an element of ampullary obstruction (Fig 39–2). The absence of these findings does not exclude ampullary disease. In patients with suspected ampullary stenosis without evidence of biliary disease, information derived from pancreatograms may be useful in predicting the response to sphincteroplasty. Incomplete filling of the pancreatic duct, cyst formation, or changes compatible with chronic pancreatitis often predict sphincteroplasty failure. Biliary excretion scans also have been used to detect delayed emptying and may be abnormal in extreme cases. Shaffer used diisopropyl iminodiacetic acid (DISIDA) to measure tracer uptake and clearance by liver and biliary excretion. Patients with manometrically documented sphincter of Oddi dysfunction had prolonged times to peak excretion of the tracer. Endoscopic sphincterotomy shortened the time to peak excretion, although it did not return to normal values. This test is based on the premise that sphincter of Oddi dysfunction is defined best in terms of bile flow. With cholescintigraphy, delayed emptying can be detected and, therefore, this test may be a suitable screen for assessing persistent pain after cholecystectomy and the results of ampullary surgery.

TABLE 39–1. NONPANCREATIC CAUSES OF HYPERAMYLASEMIA

Renal disease	Acute and chronic renal failure
Salivary gland disease	Mumps, parotitis, sialadenitis, maxillofacial surgery, and other trauma
Liver disease	Cirrhosis, fulminant hepatitis, trauma
GI tract disorders	Common bile duct stones, acute cholecystitis, penetrating peptic ulcer, intestinal obstruction, afferent loop syndrome, acute appendicitis, Crohn's disease, ruptured aortic aneurysm, aortic dissection, mesenteric infarction, postoperative metabolic dysfunction
Diabetic ketoacidosis	
Pulmonary disorders	Pneumonia, pulmonary infarction
Neoplastic disease	Lung (primary and metastatic), prostate, parotid, colon, ovary, and breast carcinoma
Gynecologic disorders	Ruptured ectopic pregnancy, ruptured graafian follicle, ovarian cysts, salpingitis, endometritis
Intracranial trauma	Cerebral trauma
Macroamylasemia	
"Normal" hyperamylasemia	

EVOCATIVE TESTS

Evocative tests are intended to bring out a subtle abnormality that is not apparent on routine testing. In the morphine-prostigmin test championed by Nardi, prostigmin (1 mg intramurally) is given to increase pancreatic secretion, while morphine (10 mg intramurally) is given to induce sphincter spasm. A positive test result is defined as the reproduction of the patient's pain concomitant with a threefold rise of the serum amylase or lipase level. Several prospective studies have shown this test to have a low sensitivity and specificity in predicting the presence of sphincter of Oddi dysfunction coupled with a poor correlation with postsphincterotomy outcomes. These factors have limited the use of this provocative test, and it has been largely replaced with other more accurate tests.

Ultrasound can be used to assess the ductal diameter of the extrahepatic bile duct and/or the main pancreatic duct after secretory stimulation. In the ultrasound-

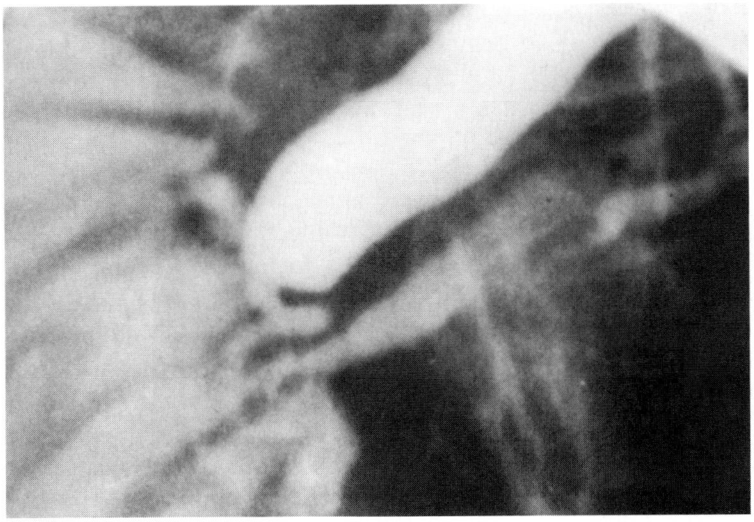

Figure 39–1. Detail of ERCP showing the bile duct and pancreatic duct entering the duodenum.

secretin test, secretin (1 U/kg) is given intravenously to induce pancreatic hypersecretion while the size of the pancreatic duct is monitored with ultrasonography. The normal response is a transient (up to 3 minutes) dilation followed by a return to baseline values. In the presence of outflow tract stenosis or dysfunction, the pancreatic duct has been observed to remain dilated for up to 30 minutes or longer (Fig 39–3), unless the gland is fibrotic and unable to respond. The sensitivity of the test has been estimated at 70% (Fig 39–4). Alternatively, after a lipid rich meal or cholecystokinin (CCK) administration, the gallbladder contracts, bile flow from the hepatocytes increases, and the sphincter of Oddi relaxes, resulting in bile entry into the duodenum. Again if there is either anatomic or functional obstruction the bile duct will tend to dilate. Provocation of typical pain symptoms should be noted during this test as well. Recently others have proposed the use of endoscopic ultrasonography in provocative testing with secretin stimulation. In one small series, this test proved useful with a positive predictive value of 93% and a negative predictive value of 62%.

Several groups have investigated the use of scintigraphy using various tracers including 99mTc-DISIDA with and without morphine provocation to determine the transit time from the hepatic hilum to the duodenum to detect biliary dysfunction. Results have been mixed and several prospective studies have reported sensitivities below 50%, positive predictive values of 40–60%, and negative predictive values of 75% when compared with standard manometry. Overall, noninvasive provocative testing for sphincter of Oddi dysfunction carries a relatively low yield and is not recommended for general clinical use except in situations where more definitive testing (e.g., manometry) is unavailable or unsuccessful.

The use of magnetic resonance cholangiopancreatography (MRCP) has greatly improved the noninvasive evaluation of the pancreaticobiliary tract. Likewise, the administration of secretin followed by magnetic resonance evaluation of the pancreatic duct has enabled a

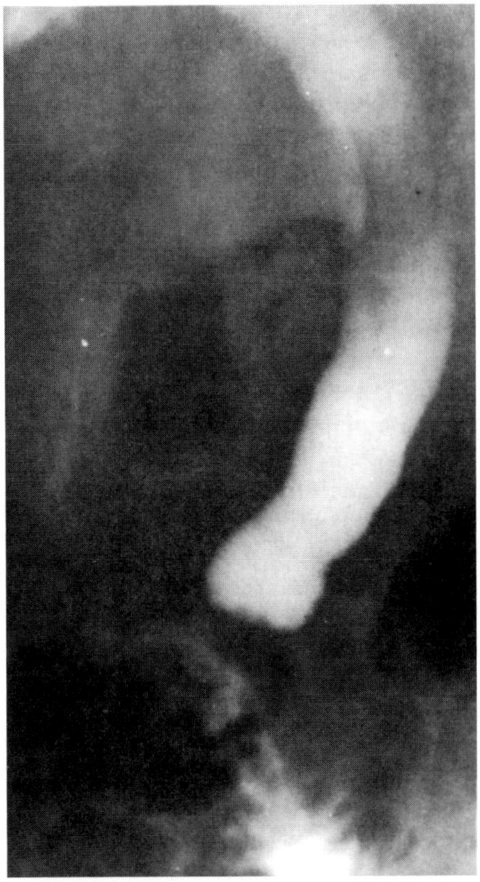

Figure 39–2. Endoscopic retrograde cholangiogram showing retention of contrast in the bile duct, which has not emptied 15 minutes after filling with contrast and removal of the catheter.

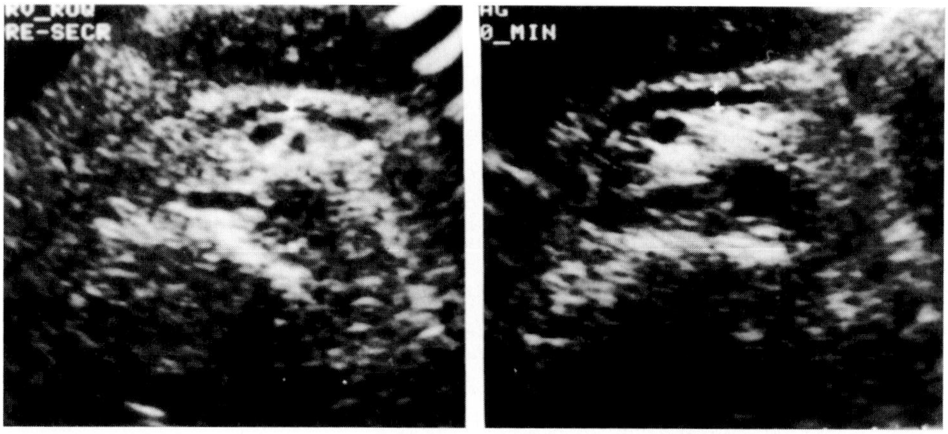

Figure 39–3. Ultrasound examination of the pancreas. The pancreatic duct in the body is indicated with markers before and 30 minutes after secretion. The prolonged 30-minute dilation is distinctly abnormal and probably indicates ampullary obstruction.

functional assessment of the pancreatic outflow. In several prospective trials evaluating secretin MRCP and standard sphincter manometry, magnetic resonance findings of pancreatic duct dysfunction correlated with manometry with a positive predictive value of 82% and a negative predictive value of 98–100%.

MANOMETRY

It has been widely accepted by biliary surgeons, but never verified, that the inability to pass a 3-mm Bakes dilator or 10F (French) rubber catheter through the ampulla during common duct exploration is indicative of ampullary stenosis. Whether one ought to proceed with sphincteroplasty solely on the basis of this finding is controversial. Intraoperative flow manometry can be used to measure the perfusion pressure in the common bile duct, the flow rate into the duodenum, and the opening pressure of the sphincter. These techniques depend on the assumption that obstruction at the ampullary level will cause an elevation of intrabiliary pressure or a reduction of flow through the sphincter. White found that the combination of abnormal resting pressure, decreased flow rate, and a dilated common duct was 99.1% accurate in detecting ampullary obstruction and that manometry detected abnormalities not appreciated on operative cholangiograms. Others have cast doubt on the utility of this technique, and few surgeons seem to use it. With the advent of preoperative endoscopic manometry, we see little use for intraoperative flow manometry.

ENDOSCOPIC TRANSAMPULLARY MANOMETRY

Sphincter of Oddi manometry is performed during ERCP. It is the only available method to measure sphincter of Oddi motor activity directly. While transampullary manometry is accepted by many as the gold standard for the diagnosis of sphincter of Oddi dysfunction, it is difficult to perform, invasive, not widely available, and associated with a relatively high complication rate. These factors have limited its widespread application in the work-up of presumed ampullary disorders.

The systems used for transampullary manometry consist of triple lumen catheters with continuous fluid

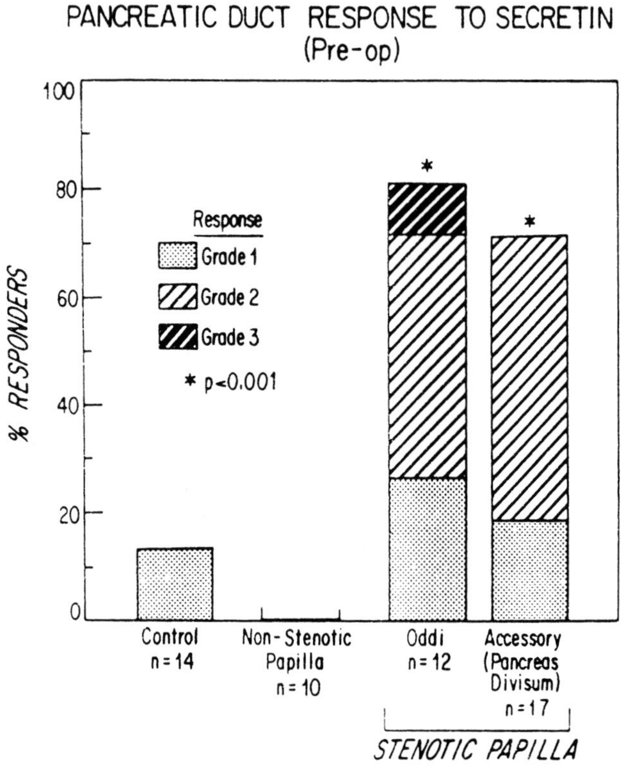

Figure 39–4. Pancreatic duct response to preoperative secretin ultrasound testing in 24 patients without ampullary stenosis and 2 patients with major and minor papilla stenosis.

perfusion (open system), or a pressure-sensitive microtransducer catheter (closed system). The closed systems measure pressure in the common bile duct or pancreatic duct, whereas the open triple-lumen system also records intrasphincteric pressure. It is important to remember that most reports of common duct manometry are based on patients who have had a prior cholecystectomy. If the gallbladder is present it acts as a low-pressure reservoir for the biliary system and may decrease elevations in common duct pressure induced by morphine.

Measurement of the sphincter pressures and contraction rhythms can be accomplished by introduction of transducers via an endoscope. The normal pressure within the sphincter of Oddi may reach 30 mm Hg with regular anterograde contraction waves. Abnormally high pressures and a variety of arrhythmias (e.g., "tachyoddia" or retrograde contractions) have been described. Elevated basal pressure, owing either to spasm or fibrosis, is the only manometric abnormality that has been associated with symptomatic relief following sphincterotomy. In a study of patients with suspected sphincter of Oddi dysfunction, Toouli and associates defined four types of manometric sphincter abnormalities. Most patients in this series were females between 30 and 60 years of age. If a patient had abnormal liver function tests and/or a dilated common bile duct, manometric abnormalities of the sphincter of Oddi invariably were found. The most common abnormality was excessively frequent retrograde propagation of phasic contractions. This abnormality is felt to prevent emptying from the ampulla of Vater and has been noted by other authors to be associated with common duct stones. Nearly as common was a high frequency of sphincter of Oddi phasic contractions, so called tachyoddia. The symptoms of these patients often correlated with bursts of phasic contractions. These contractions also have been shown to obstruct flow into the ampulla by shortening the diastolic interval, whereby filling of the intra-ampullary segment of the common bile duct ceases. Nearly one third of the study group demonstrated a paradoxical response to intravenous CCK, manifested by increased frequency of phasic contractions, by absence of change in the frequency of phasic contractions, or by an increase in basal pressure. These manometric changes occurred while the patients experienced pain. It is possible that these abnormalities represent a disordered control mechanism of the sphincter of Oddi such that bile flow is retarded after eating, with consequent common bile duct dilation and pain. Finally, as in most other series, there was a subgroup of patients with an abnormally elevated basal sphincter of Oddi pressure owing either to fibrosis or spasm. Unresponsiveness of the basal sphincter of Oddi pressure to CCK suggests the presence of a fixed structural stenosis. The implications for therapy of tachyoddia and retrograde contractions have not been established.

Hogan and Geenen developed a classification system based on clinical history, laboratory results, and ERCP findings to determine the appropriate use of sphincter of Oddi manometry prior to sphincterotomy. These authors found that patients with biliary type pain, abnormal SGOT or alkaline phosphatase >2 times normal documented on two or more occasions, delayed drainage of ERCP contrast >45 minutes, and dilated common bile duct (CBD) >12 mm diameter had a 95% chance of having pain relief after a biliary sphincterotomy regardless of the results of manometry. Therefore they deem manometry unnecessary in these patients. In patients with biliary type pain but only one or two of the above findings approximately 60% will have abnormal sphincter of Oddi manometry. Eighty-five percent of those patients with abnormal manometry will have pain relief if the preoperative manometry was abnormal versus only 35% of those with normal manometry. Thus, in patients with this constellation of findings manometry is recommended. Alternatively, patients with biliary type pain and no other abnormalities, only 25–55% will have an abnormal sphincter manometry, and only 60% will have a symptomatic improvement with biliary sphincterotomy. In this group these authors conclude manometry is mandatory prior to sphincterotomy.

In order to define the symptomatic success rate of sphincterotomy based on preoperative biliary manometry, Toouli performed a prospective randomized trial following biliary manometry. Patients were randomized to sphincterotomy or sham endoscopy based on having an abnormally elevated sphincter of Oddi basal pressure (>40 mm Hg). Patients were evaluated by blinded observers. After 2 years of follow-up this trial concluded that biliary sphincterotomy appears effective in those patients with an elevated sphincter of Oddi basal pressure (>40 mm Hg), but is no better than placebo in those patients with a normal basal pressure.

Finally, transampullary manometry has been associated with a high incidence of post-procedure pancreatitis in up to 31% of patients, particularly in patients being evaluated for causes of recurrent acute pancreatitis. In our practice, therefore, we have not found the benefits of manometry worth its risks of serious complications.

▪ AMPULLARY OBSTRUCTION, STENOSIS, AND DYSFUNCTION

The term ampullary stenosis is used in this discussion to include both fixed ampullary stenosis and motility disorders. Fixed ampullary stenosis most commonly is the result of inflammation and fibrosis. This situation usually develops in association with cholelithiasis and is postulated to be caused by chronic inflammation from repeated passage of small stones or sludge. Iatrogenic injury to the ampulla during common bile duct exploration also can produce fibrosis. Small ampullary tumors can create ampullary obstruction, either in a continuous fashion or by a "ball-valve" mechanism, with resultant right upper quadrant pain, jaundice, or recurrent pancreatitis. Such tumors include adenomas, villous adenomas, small adenocarcinomas, and a spectrum of neuroendocrine tumors. Infrequently, in patients with acquired immunodeficiency syndrome, infections with cytomegalovirus, cryptosporidium, or strongyloides species may produce sphincter of Oddi dysfunction. Motility disorders include muscular hyperplasia, dysfunction, or dyskinesia without a fixed fibrotic stricture. Patients without a demonstrable fixed obstruction or proximal dilation of the ducts are the most troublesome to treat. In the absence of any objective lesion, it is easier, and possibly safer, to be skeptical than overtreating a pain syndrome that is erroneously attributed to ampullary stenosis.

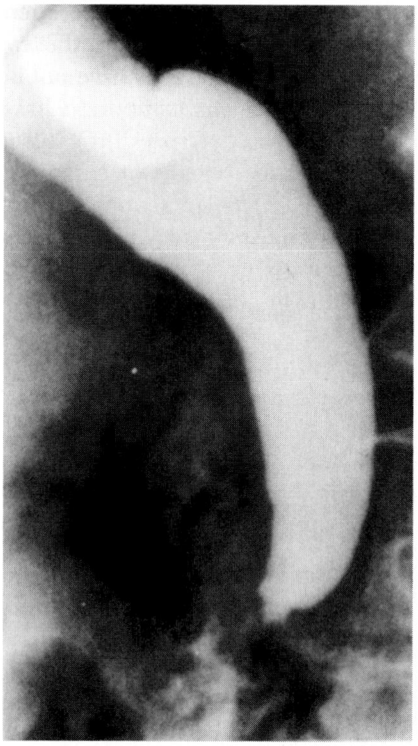

Figure 39–5. Biliary obstruction owing to fibrotic ampullary stenosis in a patient who presented with acute cholangitis.

MANIFESTATIONS

The presenting symptoms and signs of ampullary stenosis may be those of obstructive jaundice, cholangitis, pancreatitis, or pain. Pain is most often in the right upper quadrant of the abdomen, but also may be in the epigastrium and may radiate around the right side or straight through to the back. It is usually intermittent, but can be food-induced or constant.

Jaundice or cholangitis rarely occurs as a primary presentation (Fig 39–5). A dilated bile duct with or without an increased serum alkaline phosphatase level is more common. Ampullary stenosis, in combination with stasis, also may lead to formation of primary common duct stones.

Pancreatitis that is ascribed to ampullary stenosis is usually mild and recurrent. The symptom or recurrent pain, without accompanying signs or pancreatic inflammation or hyperamylasemia, is considered part of this syndrome (Nardi, Moody, Warshaw). Progression to chronic pancreatitis rarely occurs. The obstruction may involve the dorsal segment (duct of Santorini, accessory or minor papilla), the ventral segment (duct of Wirsung, major papilla, or papilla of Vater) or both, depending on ductal anatomy (Fig 39–6).

VENTRAL/MAJOR AMPULLARY STENOSIS

Ventral/major ampullary stenosis (Fig 39–7) has had its proponents and detractors for many years. The number of patients with unequivocal fibrosis of the duct orifice is small. It is unknown whether the fibrosis is congenital or acquired; the lesion responding to sphincterotomy has been described in children, but most cases are seen in adults. Some cases are attributed to the traumatic passage of gallstones. For the last 40 years, surgeons have treated ventral ampullary stenosis by transduodenal sphincterotomy/sphincteroplasty with varying success. Symptomatic improvement has been reported in no more than 70% of patients. Failures are due in part to the inclusion of patients in whom the diagnosis was either unproven or incorrect. Some writers have contended that the sphincterotomy is too short for ablation of the entire sphincter mechanism to include the duodenal wall component (sphincter of Boyden) (Figs 39–8 and 39–9). Others have emphasized the pathogenic role of the septum between the end of the duct of Wirsung and the terminal segment of the bile duct, and advocated the routine addition of septotomy-sphincterotomy of the pancreatic duct orifice in addition to the choledochal sphincter (Fig 39–10). Recently, the claim has been made that a misplaced pancreatic duct orifice, opening among the muscular fibers of the sphincter of Oddi, is an important cause of recurrent obstructive pancreatitis. Surgical transduodenal sphincteroplasty has largely been replaced with endoscopic sphincterotomy for the initial treatment of sphincter of Oddi dysfunction. However, certain circumstances including inability to cannulate the duct, failure of endoscopic papillotomy, and inability to perform an ERCP mandate open sphincteroplasty. In addition, a para-ampullary duodenal diverticulum may make endoscopic sphincterotomy more difficult or hazardous.

Electrosurgical papillotomy has been used widely. The relative safety of the procedure has been established. In addition to the difficulty of accurately identifying candidates for treatment when the objective indices are sparse or lacking, endoscopic papillotomy has two disadvantages: (1) it may be impossible to cannulate the papilla when it is genuinely stenotic, and (2) the usual papillotomy divides only the choledochal portion of the sphincter. Extending the procedure by cutting the septal segment of the duct of Wirsung greatly increases the risk of pancreatitis, which is sometimes severe. Conversely, if the pancreatic duct orifice is not opened the significant point of stenosis may elude treatment. At the Massachusetts General Hospital, we have seen several patients who continue to have recurrent pancreatitis after endoscopic papillotomy but who seem to have benefited from subsequent surgical septotomy.

The difficulties concerned with making an accurate diagnosis of sphincter of Oddi dysfunction limit the ability of comparing various trials evaluating either endoscopic or surgical series. Currently no prospective randomized trials comparing endoscopic sphincterotomy with transduodenal sphincteroplasty exist. However Tzovaras and Rowlands reviewed various trials evaluating outcomes in patients with sphincter of Oddi dysfunction. These authors found that open transduodenal sphincteroplasty series reported poor results in 7–35%, while endoscopic series documented poor results in between 20–39% of cases. While a statistical analysis was not provided, these authors concluded relatively little difference between the surgical and endoscopic treatment options. Toouli and associates performed a randomized controlled trial evaluating endoscopic sphincterotomy versus a sham endoscopy for manometrically documented sphincter of Oddi dysfunction. These authors noted a statistically significant symptomatic improvement in those patients with documented stenosis while there was no improvement in those patients with dyskinesia as compared to the sham group. However, repeated endoscopic interventions

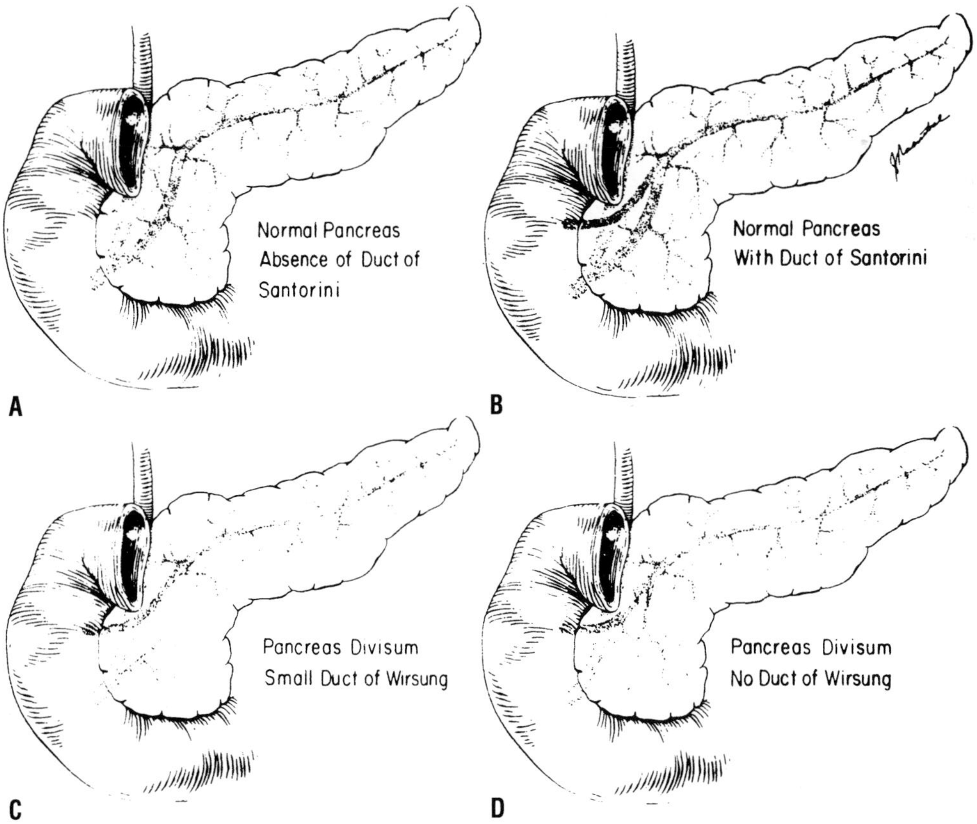

Figure 39–6. Variations of ventral (Wirsung) and dorsal (Santorini) duct anatomy. Small, functionally inadequate intercommunication is also common (10–20%). We use the term dominant dorsal duct for the latter, as well as **C** and **D**.

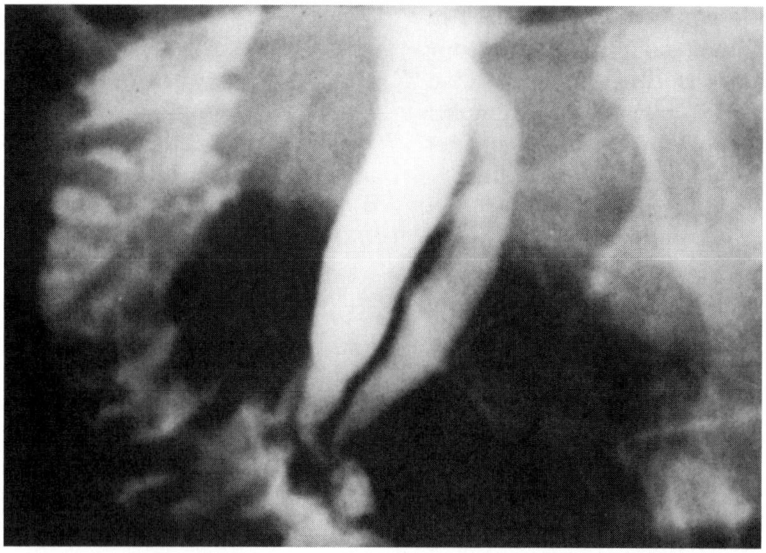

A

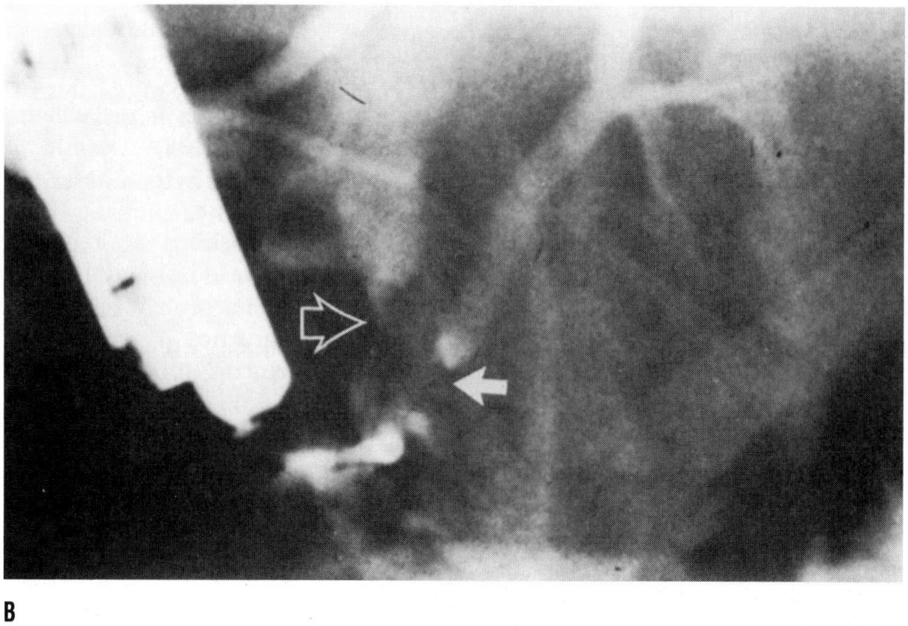

B

Figure 39–7. Two examples of ampullary stenosis. **A.** Dilated bile and pancreatic ducts in a man with recurrent discrete attacks of acute pancreatitis. **B.** Narrowed ampullary segments of the bile duct (open arrow) and pancreatic duct (closed arrow) in a woman with persistent pain, normal serum amylase, and a positive secretin-ultrasound test. Both were cured by transduodenal sphincteroplasty and transampullary septectomy.

were necessary in 23% of patients within 3 months as a result of incomplete sphincter division.

Safe attempts at relief of obstruction of the orifice of the pancreatic duct have been made with balloon dilation of the sphincter and placement of endoprosthetic stents. The benefits accruing from balloon dilation are short-lived and the incidence of postdilation pancreatitis is high. Therefore, this approach has been abandoned by most centers. However, enthusiasm persists for stenting the pancreatic duct orifice, championed by Geenen. In our view, a brief trial of stenting of the pancreatic duct may provide useful diagnostic information. Patients who are free of pain or who have relief of recurrent pancreatitis are likely to derive long-term benefit form surgical sphincteroplasty. If the stent remains in place for more than 2 months, granulation tissue forms in the pancreatic duct caused by the mechanical irritation of the stent, leading to fibrosis. When this occurs, the strictures are too proximal in the pancreatic duct to be opened via transampullary sphincteroplasty. Thus, we can endorse stenting as a diagnostic maneuver in patients without clear-cut objec-

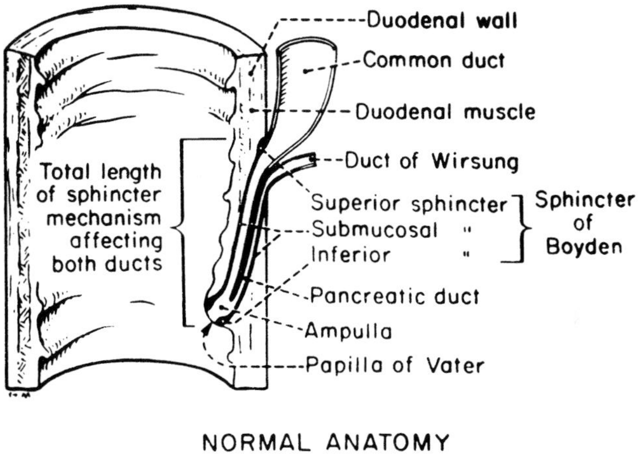

Figure 39–8. The duodenal wall and submucosal sphincter of Boyden together make up the constrictor mechanism of the major ampulla.

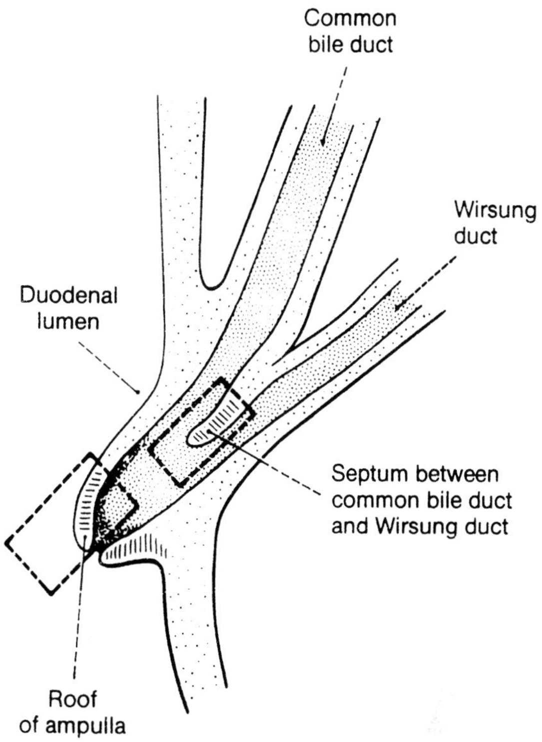

Figure 39–10. Abnormality of the septum between the common bile duct and the pancreatic duct may contribute to pancreatic duct obstruction in some patients. Sphincterotomy or sphincteroplasty of the choledochal (roof) portion of the ampulla may be inadequate.

tive parameters of ampullary stenosis, but condemn its use for long-term therapy. From what we have seen thus far, we are skeptical that stenting will be either as safe or as effective as surgical sphincteroplasty or endoscopic sphincterotomy.

Botulinum toxin is a potent inhibitor of acetylcholine release from nerve endings and has been applied in the treatment of various smooth muscle disorders of the gastrointestinal tract. Clinical evidence after injection of botulinum toxin into the sphincter of Oddi documents a 50% reduction in the basal biliary sphincter pressure and improved bile flow. In one small series, there was excellent correlation between symptomatic improvement after botulinum toxin injection into the major papilla in patients with sphincter of Oddi dysfunction and subsequent symptom resolution after biliary sphincterotomy.

DORSAL DUCT OBSTRUCTION

Dorsal duct obstruction may occur in patients with pancreas divisum (Fig 39–11). The later term originally described a failure of fusion of the duct system of the primitive embryologic dorsal and ventral pancreatic anlage (Fig 39–6). In this entity, the dorsal duct cannot

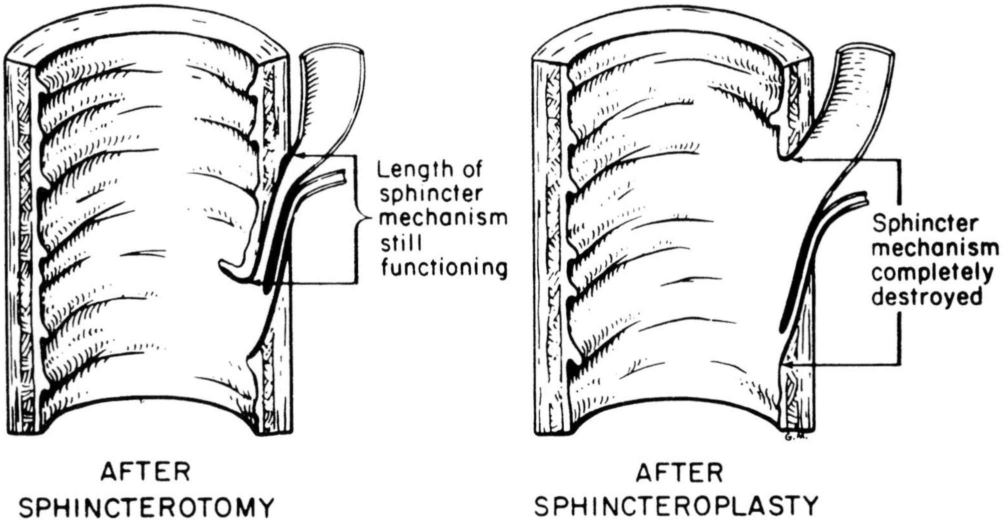

Figure 39–9. The difference between sphincterotomy and sphincteroplasty, according to Jones. The portion of the sphincter remaining after sphincterotomy is made incompetent by sphincteroplasty.

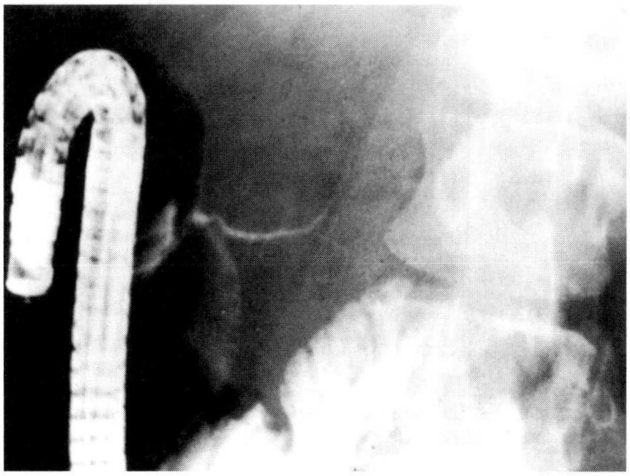

Figure 39–11. Pancreatogram via the major ampulla and duct of Wirsung, showing typical pancreas divisum. The duct is short (2–3 cm) and ends in a fine tapered arborization.

empty through the ampulla of Vater but must drain through the accessory or minor papilla. The concept since has been expanded to include other variants of dorsal duct dominance requiring the major fraction of pancreatic secretions to egress from the accessory papilla (Fig 39–12). A dominant dorsal pancreatic duct occurs in at least 9% of the population, as shown by both autopsy analyses and endoscopic pancreatography. The association of pancreas divisum and recurrent pancreatitis or pancreatic pain has been both upheld and disputed. Because the pancreas rarely is resected in this condition, histologic evidence is scarce. However, two reports have documented convincing chronic obstructive changes confined to the dorsal duct distribution in a few selected patients.

Cotton, summarizing the consensus of an international workshop held in London in 1984, indicated that pancreas divisum is probably a genuine factor in a syndrome of obstructed pancreatitis in some patients. Stenosis of the accessory papilla superimposed on pancreas divisum, rather than pancreas divisum alone, appears to be the critical combination. In addition, the term "pancreas divisum" is misleading because it does not include the other variants of dominant dorsal duct. Distinguishing patients with genuine accessory papillary stenosis from those with clinically insignificant pancreas divisum is difficult, and is the greatest cause of differing conclusions concerning the association of the dominant dorsal duct with pancreatitis and the efficacy of accessory papilla sphincteroplasty. MRCP has proven useful in defining the anatomy of the pancreatic ductal system as well as identifying the level of obstruction. However, the clinical significance of the obstruction cannot be determined. ERCP can readily establish the presence of a dominant dorsal duct, but endoscopic calibration of the papillary orifice size has not been successful. Recently, endoscopic measurements of dorsal duct pressure and sphincter function have suggested that hypertension of the sphincter and dorsal duct pressures may be a genuine phenomenon. Prolonged dorsal duct dilation after secretin administration has in our experience, correlated with accessory papillary stenosis and with subsequent response to sphincteroplasty. There is no medical treatment of accessory papillary stenosis. We have found oral pancreatic enzymes and spasmolytic drugs to be ineffective.

Small numbers of patients have been treated with a variety of endoscopic techniques, including balloon dilation, papillotomy, and stenting, but the overall experience has been disappointing. Analysis of collected anecdotes suggests that the attempted cannulation often is not possible, that pancreatitis follows the manipulations fairly frequently, that relief of symptoms is reported in only 27–59% of patients, and that restenosis is the rule. Some authors report up to 75% rates of pain relief in those patients with acute recurrent pancreatitis undergoing endoscopic minor papilla sphincterotomy. Signs of chronic pancreatitis and fibrosis reduce the success rate to less than one fourth of those treated with endoscopic minor papilla sphincterotomy. Furthermore, we have treated cases of stenosis of the minor papilla in which the stent has created a stricture of the dorsal duct 2 to 3 cm from its orifice, thereby creating an obstructive pancreatitis that cannot be treated by sphincteroplasty and may require pancreaticoduodenectomy. Despite these unsatisfactory results many patients undergo attempted sphincterotomy of the minor papilla prior to surgical referral for sphincteroplasty.

Surgical sphincteroplasty of the accessory papilla also has been advocated. Although results vary and

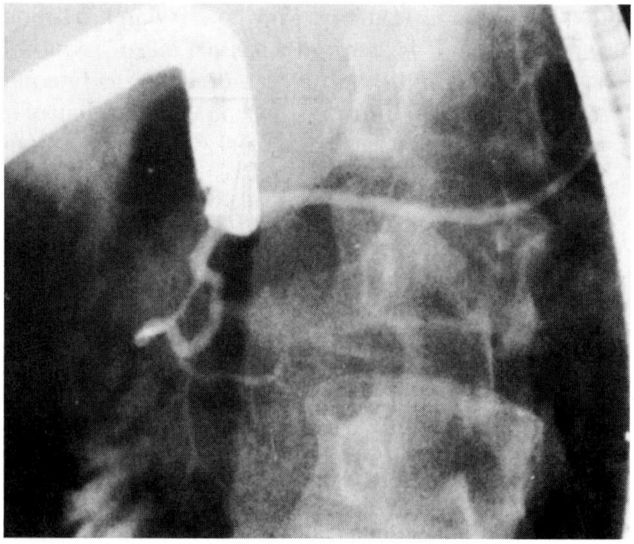

Figure 39–12. Pancreatogram showing a dominant dorsal duct. The dorsal duct in this case drains the entire pancreas, including the head. There is no duct of Wirsung.

some observations are negative, it is difficult to discount the good results. We have performed the operation on 130 patients, not including those with changes suggestive of chronic pancreatitis. Of those patients who have been followed for >2 years, 80% were judged at operation to have stenotic accessory papilla, and 85% of these have had a favorable response to the papillotomy. Only 15% who were judged to have a stenotic papilla have not had lasting benefit form the operation. Other series have confirmed these encouraging results in appropriately selected patients. Approximately 75% of patients with recurrent acute pancreatitis and pancreas divisum obtain symptomatic relief after sphincteroplasty. In patients with chronic abdominal pain suggesting pancreatitis, but lacking objective parameters, results of sphincteroplasty have been disappointing with only 20–50% symptomatic improvements reported. These results underscore the importance of proper patient selection prior to surgical intervention.

Most reported cases of pancreas divisum and pancreatitis have had acute recurrent disease without fibrosis or duct dilation. Changes of chronic pancreatitis may be seen in patients with pancreas divisum, but a causal relationship with accessory papilla stenosis has not been established. Confinement of the chronic fibrotic changes to the dorsal segment of the gland has been shown convincingly in a few exceptional instances. In any event, when there is established chronic pancreatitis, sphincteroplasty is inadequate and will fail. Resection of the pancreatic head or distal drainage by pancreaticojejunostomy has been advocated, and the decision depends on the degree of duct dilation.

TECHNIQUE OF TRANSDUODENAL SPHINCTEROPLASTY

In order to avoid confusion, what follows is a brief anatomic definition of the various surgical options. Sphincterotomy consists of simply cutting the sphincter without suturing of the bile duct mucosa to the duodenum. Sphincteroplasty implies incising the common portion of the sphincter of Oddi with subsequent suturing of the biliary mucosa to the duodenal mucosa. Occasionally in patients with recurrent pancreatitis a septectomy and septoplasty of the septum between the common bile duct and the pancreatic duct is necessary.

The operation may be performed through a right subcostal or midline incision. The duodenum is mobilized from the bile duct to the superior mesenteric vessels by an extensive Kocher maneuver.

If a cholecystectomy or common duct exploration is being performed, a small catheter may be passed down the cystic or common duct through the major papilla to identify its location along the length of the duodenum. The papilla of Vater is usually easy to palpate between the fingers, in the groove between the second portion of the duodenum and the pancreas. The duodenum is opened transversely opposite the papilla. Silk sutures are preplaced at either end of the incision, to elevate the duodenum and to limit the duodenotomy, and to keep it from extending too close to the pancreas for safe closure.

The orifice of the major papilla is cannulated with lacrimal duct probes and, if possible, a 5F pediatric feeding catheter. The secretions that fill the tube identify whether it is in the bile duct or pancreatic duct. If the bile duct cannot be entered, it may be safer to pass a catheter or instrument from above for identification of the orifice, rather than persist blindly form below. If ampullary obstruction is caused by an impacted stone, it is easy to cut down on it through the anterosuperior aspect of the papilla, opposite the pancreatic duct orifice and therefore, not endangering that structure. This procedure will release the stone.

Jones has advocated that the sphincteroplasty should be carried upward until the diameter of the stoma is equal to that of the largest diameter of the common duct. The entire sphincter mechanism, including the components derived from the intrinsic musculature of the duodenal wall, is thereby incapacitated (Fig 39–8). The sphincteroplasty may be up to 30 mm long and may reach the pancreatic substance outside the duodenal wall. Jones' argument is that such a complete elimination of the sphincter will maximize the freedom of bile drainage and minimize the chances for retention of missed stones, perhaps in the hepatic ducts, or formation of new primary common duct stones because of bile stasis (Fig 39–9).

The sphincteroplasty is carried out with sequential clamping and division and suture approximation of the duodenal mucosa and the bile duct mucosa (Fig 39–13). We prefer 4–0 synthetic absorbable sutures and carry the sphincteroplasty superiorly 2 to 3 cm to the end of the intramural segment. The pancreatic duct characteristically opens onto the anteromedial aspect of the ampulla (commonly described as the 5 o'clock position on the back wall) within a few millimeters of the lip, but it may be at, or even outside, the lip of the ampulla. Secretin (1 U/kg) given intravenously may be helpful in identifying the orifice. A probe is passed into the pancreatic duct, the septum between the bile duct space and pancreatic duct is incised, and the edges aresutured with interrupted fine synthetic absorbable sutures. The incision is carried far enough to produce a free flow of pancreatic secretions, generally 5 to 8 mm.

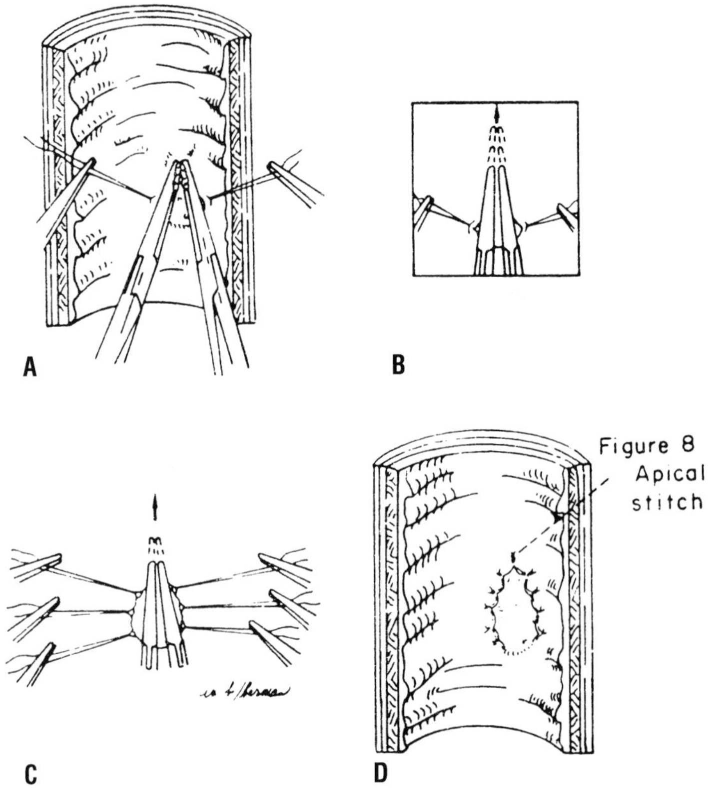

Figure 39–13. Technique of transduodenal sphincteroplasty; the roof of the ampulla is opened by serial clamping, division, and suture approximation of the common duct and duodenal walls until the opening created equals the maximum diameter of the intrapancreatic common bile duct.

We prefer to leave a 5F pediatric feeding catheter in the duct to ensure against impedance of flow by postoperative edema. The catheter exits through the wall of the duodenum and the abdomen and is removed after 10 days.

Accessory papillary sphincteroplasty follows most of the same principles (Fig 39–14). The accessory papilla lies 2 to 3 cm proximal and 1 cm anterior to the major papilla. It often is best identified by palpation against the duodenal mucosa and by administration of secretin. It courses perpendicularly through the duodenal wall, in contrast to the oblique path of the duct of Wirsung. The papilla is short and opens into the vestibule of the duct within a few millimeters. The papillotomy needs to be no longer than 7 to 9 mm.

RESULTS OF SPHINCTEROPLASTY

Adverse consequences of the operation should be minimal. Postoperative hyperamylasemia is common, but clinical pancreatitis has occurred in only 1% of patients. Mortality should be <1%. We have had one death in over 300 cases. Late restenosis is rare after sphincteroplasty of the major papilla, although it has occurred in approximately 6% of our patients after accessory papillotomy. Cure of clinical symptoms by the operation will depend largely on the accuracy with which patients are selected for surgery. Our current cure rate is approximately 80%.

■ LOCAL EXCISION OF AMPULLARY TUMORS

Local excision is suitable treatment for certain small tumors (<2 cm) arising from the ampulla of Vater or in the pancreatic or biliary duct within 2 cm of the ampulla. Some small adenomas (<1 cm) may even be removed endoscopically with stenting of the biliary and pancreatic duct orifice to allow healing without stenosis. These tumors include carcinoid tumors, islet cell tumors, tubulovillous adenomas, and small villous adenomas. Endoscopic options for resecting these lesions include snare papillectomy or ampullectomy and thermal ablation by laser, argon plasma coagulation, and monopolar or bipolar electrosurgery. According to Binmoeller, four criteria are necessary for eligibility for endoscopic snare papillectomy. The lesion must be less than 4 cm, and there must be no appearance of malignancy based on endoscopic appearance including a regular margin, no ulceration, and soft consistency. A minimum of six forceps biopsies must have benign histology, and there must be an absence of intraductal involvement confirmed by ERCP and/or endoscopic ultrasound.

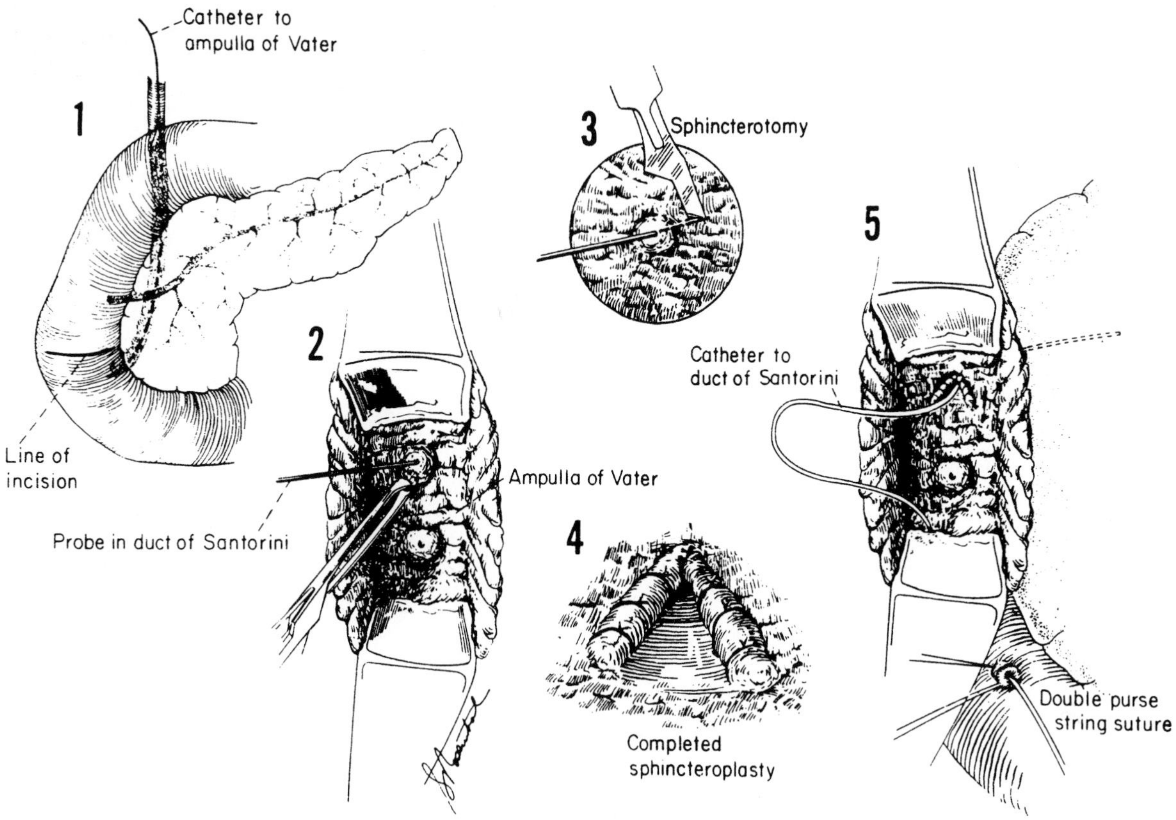

Figure 39–14. Technique of accessory papilla sphincteroplasty. Note the 5F catheter left in the pancreatic duct for postoperative drainage.

Current reported series are small with limited follow up. However, recurrence rates of up to 30% have been documented and multiple attempts are often necessary before complete eradication of the tumor. Additionally, major morbidity including pancreatitis and duodenal perforation has been reported in up to 20% of the cases. Recently endoscopic ultrasound has proven valuable in the work-up of ampullary tumors. The sensitivity and specificity of endoscopic ultrasonography for differentiating local from advanced ampullary tumors via depth of invasion were both over 80%. In fact, the use of EUS in the preoperative evaluation of patients with local ampullary tumors can result in significant cost savings and avoid the morbidity of a pancreaticoduodenectomy for localized disease.

Surgical options for ampullary tumors include transduodenal local excision or pancreaticoduodenectomy. In cases where there is a reasonable likelihood of malignancy, such as with villous adenomas, the risk of recurrent tumor and missed opportunity for cure must be balanced against the complications of a pancreaticoduodenectomy. It has been our preference to opt for a pancreaticoduodenectomy whenever there is suspicion of malignancy. Since recurrence rates are close to 100% when local resections are performed for malignancy, patients must be taken to the operating room with preparation for a pancreaticoduodenectomy if frozen section evaluation of the resected ampullary lesion demonstrates malignancy. While some authors have reported excellent concordance with frozen section and permanent analysis, the surgeon must recognize that the absence of malignancy on frozen section may not withstand a more rigorous evaluation on permanent section analysis. This situation is particularly true with respect to villous adenomas in which malignancy is found in >50% of cases even when biopsies have shown only a benign component. Notwithstanding these cautions, local resection may be an excellent treatment for benign lesions of the ampulla.

The Mayo Clinic recently reviewed their experience with local resection of villous adenomas of the duodenal ampulla. These authors performed 53 transduodenal local excisions over a 17-year period. Among these 53 patients, 32% recurred at 5 years and 43% recurred at 10 years. Interestingly, four of these recurrences (24%) were adenocarcinoma. In this series the recurrence rates were influenced by the presence of a polyposis syndrome and not on the size of the adenoma. While local resection of villous adenomas is appropriate in certain circumstances, these data reiterate the importance of diligent endoscopic follow-up. As minimally invasive surgery continues to improve, reports of laparoscopic transduodenal ampullectomy have shown this procedure to be technically feasible. However, further study with longer-term follow-up is necessary before this procedure can be endorsed.

A transverse or vertical duodenotomy can be used to expose the ampulla. A generous Kocher maneuver is essential to allow the second portion of the duodenum to be elevated into the wound. Normal duodenal mucosa 5 to 10 mm from the visible border of the tumor is tattooed with cautery to map out the margins of resections. A suture then is placed through the ampulla to provide traction. As the excision progresses, this suture can be replaced with an Allis clamp (Fig 39–15). The cautery is used to incise the mucosa circumferentially. One then works centripetally in a submucosal plane until the pancreatic and bile ducts are encountered and transected. As this occurs, it can be helpful to place traction sutures in the duct margins to prevent retraction (Fig 39–16). Placing catheters in the ducts also can aid in their dissection. The tumor then is lifted off the muscular layers of the medial wall of the duodenum. Maintenance of hemostasis during resection is critical to ensure good visualization and accurate dissection.

With the specimen resected, one must reconstruct the defect. The superior wall of the pancreatic duct is sutured to the inferior wall of the bile duct with fine interrupted synthetic absorbable sutures, thereby forming a common channel. The duodenum and cloacal neoampulla then are joined with interrupted full thickness 4–0 synthetic absorbable sutures to create a mucosa to mucosa anastomosis of the ducts to the duodenal wall (Fig 39–17). If the ducts are not dilated, the orifices of each duct can be enlarged by incising along one wall proximally, as in a sphincteroplasty. Stents may be placed and brought out through the common duct, the third portion of the duodenum, or both. These stents remain in place at least 10 days. The duodenotomy is closed transversely.

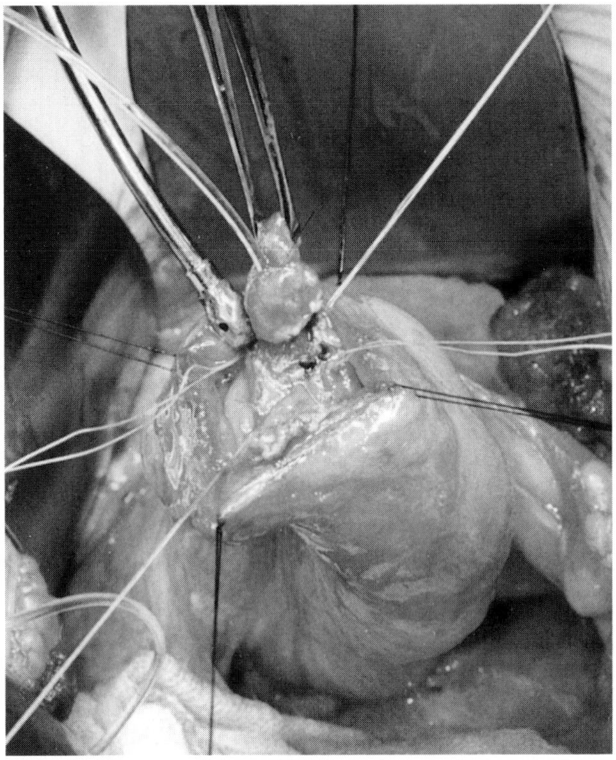

Figure 39–16. The ampullary tumor is dissected free centripetally in a submucosal plane.

After local resection of ampullary tumors, follow up endoscopy is performed 6 to 12 months postoperatively

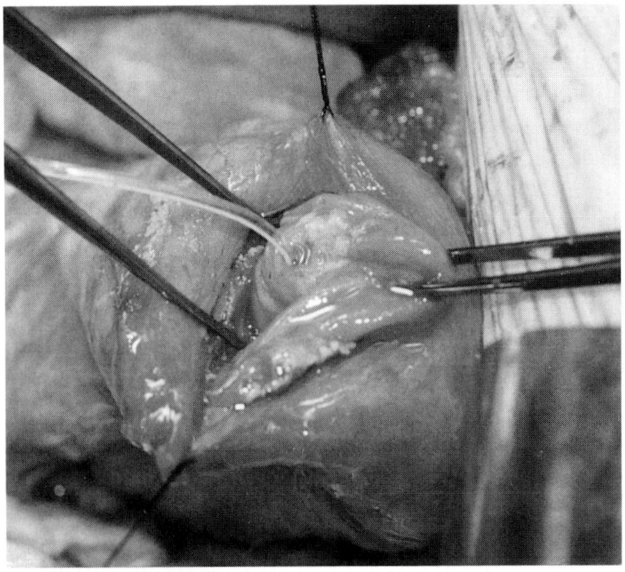

Figure 39–15. Early stage of the local resection of an ampullary carcinoid tumor. Stent is in the pancreatic duct and traction on the tumor is provided by an Allis clamp.

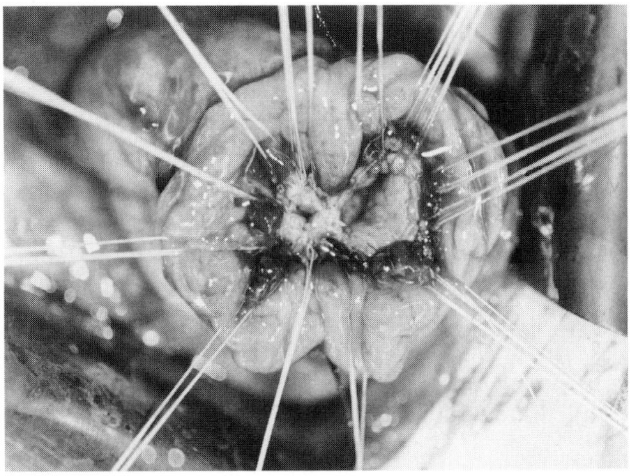

Figure 39–17. Anastomosis of the bile duct and pancreatic duct to the duodenal wall following local resection of an ampullary tumor.

to assess local recurrence. Patients who develop pancreatitis or jaundice months to years following local resection of ampullary tumors must be suspected of having local recurrence and should undergo repeat endoscopy with ERCP.

SUGGESTED READINGS

1. Boyden EA. The anatomy of choledochoduodenal junction in man. *Surg Gynecol Obstet* 1957;104:641–652
2. Bradley EL, Stephan RN. Accessory duct sphincteroplasty is preferred for long-term prevention of recurrent acute pancreatitis in patients with pancreas divisum. *J Am Coll Surg* 1996;183:65–70
3. Binmoeller KF, Boaventura S, Ramsperger K, Soehendra N. Endoscopic snare excision of benign adenomas of the papilla of Vater. *Gastrointest Endosc* 1993;39:127–131
4. Catalano MF, Lahoti S, Alcocer E, Geenen JE, Hogan WJ. Dynamic imaging of the pancreas using real-time endoscopic ultrasonography with secretin stimulation. *Gastrointest Endosc* 1998;48:580–587
5. Clary BM, Tyler DS, Dematos P, et al. Local ampullary resection with careful intraoperative frozen section evaluation for presumed benign ampullary neoplasms. *Surgery* 2000;127:628–633
6. Cotton PB. Congenital anomaly of pancreas divisum as a cause of obstructive pain and pancreatitis. *Gut* 1980; 21:105–114
7. Craig AG, Peter D, Saccone GT, et al. Scintigraphy versus manometry in patients with suspected biliary sphincter of Oddi dysfunction. *Gut* 2003;52:352–357
8. Delhaye M, Engelholm L, Cremer M. Pancreas divisum: congenital anatomic variant or anomaly? *Gastroenterology* 1985;89:951
9. Eisen G, Schultz S, Metzler D, et al. Santorinicele: new evidence for obstruction in pancreas divisum. *Gastrointest Endosc* 1994;40:73–76
10. Farnell MB, Sakorafas GH, Sarr MG, et al. Villous tumors of the duodenum: reappraisal of local vs. extended resection. *J Gastrointest Surg* 2000;4:13–21
11. Geenen JE, Hogan WJ, Dodds WJ, et al. Intraluminal pressure recording form the human sphincter of Oddi. *Gastroenterology* 1980;76:317–324
12. Geenen JE, Hogan WJ, Dodds WJ, et al. The efficacy of endoscopic sphincterotomy after cholecystectomy in patients with sphincter of Oddi dysfunction. *N Engl J Med* 1989;320:82–87
13. Glaser J, Stienecker K. Ultrasound secretin test in patients with pancreas divisum—an aid in the diagnosis of papillary or dorsal duct stenosis? *Z Gastroenterol* 1999;37:585–588
14. Griffin CA. Diagnosis of papillary stenosis by calibration. Follow-up 15 to 25 years after sphincteroplasty. *Am J Surg* 1982;143:717–720
15. Guelrud M, Siefel JH. Hypertensive pancreatic duct sphincter as a cause of pancreatitis: successful treatment with hydrostatic balloon dilation. *Dig Dis Sci* 1984;29:225
16. Hellerhoff KJ, Helmberger H, Rosch T, Settles MR, Link TM, Rummeny EJ. Dynamic MR pancreatography after secretin administration: image quality and diagnostic accuracy. *Am J Roentgenol* 2002;179:121–129
17. Heyries L, Barthet M, Delvasto C, et al. Long-term results of endoscopic management of pancreas divisum with recurrent acute pancreatitis. *Gastrointest Endosc* 2002 55:376–381
18. Hogan W, Sherman S, Pasricha P, Carr-Locke DL. Position paper on sphincter of Oddi manometry. *Gastrointest Endosc* 1997;45:342
19. Jones SA, Steedman RA, et al. Transduodenal sphincteroplasty (not sphincterotomy) for biliary and pancreatic disease: indications, contraindications and results. *Am J Surg* 1969;118:292
20. Khandekar S, Disario JA. Endoscopic therapy for stenosis of the biliary and pancreatic duct orifices. *Gastrointest Endosc* 2000; 52:500–505
21. Lans JI, Geenen JE, Johanson JF, Hogan WJ. Endoscopic therapy in patients with pancreas divisum and acute pancreatitis: a prospective, randomized, controlled clinical trial. *Gastrointest Endosc* 1992; 38:430–434
22. Lehman GA, Sherman S, Nisi R, Hawes RH. Pancreas divisum: results of minor papilla sphincterotomy. *Gastrointest Endosc* 1993; 39:1–8
23. Mariani A, Curioni S, Zanello A, Passaretti S, Masci E, Rossi M, Del Maschio A, Testoni PA. Secretin MRCP and endoscopic pancreatic manometry in the evaluation of sphincter of Oddi function: a comparative pilot study in patients with idiopathic recurrent pancreatitis. *Gastrointest Endosc* 2003;58:847–852
24. Marshall JB, Eckhauser ML. Pancreas divisum: a cause of chronic relapsing pancreatitis. *Dig Dis Sci* 1985;30: 582
25. Matos C, Metens T, Deviere J, et al. Pancreas divisum: evaluation with secretin-enhanced magnetic resonance cholangiopancreatography. *Gastrointest Endosc* 2001;53:728–733
26 Nardi GL, Acosta JM. Papillitis as a cause of pancreatitis and abdominal pain. *Ann Surg* 1966;164:611–618
27 Nussbaum MS, Warner BW, Sax HC, et al. Transduodenal sphincteroplasty and transampullary septotomy for primary sphincter of Oddi dysfunction. *Am J Surg* 1989; 157:38–42
28 Pasricha PJ, Miskovsky EP, Kalloo AN. Intrasphincter injection of botulinum toxin for suspected sphincter of Oddi dysfunction. *Gut* 1994;35:1319
29. Ponchon T, Berger F, Chavaillon A, et al. Contribution of endoscopy to diagnosis and treatment of tumors of the ampulla of Vater. *Cancer* 1989;64:161–167
30. Quirk DM, Rattner DW, Fernandez-del Castillo C, Warshaw AL, Brugge WR. *Gastrointest Endosc* 1997;46:334–337
31. Rattner DW, Fernandez-del Castillo C, Brugge WR, Warshaw AL. Defining the criteria for local resection of ampullary neoplasms. *Arch Surg* 1996; 131:366–371
32. Ricci JL. Carcinoid of the ampulla of Vater: local resection or pancreaticoduodenectomy. *Cancer* 1993;71:686–690
33. Rosen M, Zuccaro G, Brody F. Laparoscopic resection of a periampullary villous adenoma. *Surg Endosc* 2003;17: 1322–1323
34. Ryan DP, Shapiro RH, Warshaw AL. Villous tumors of the duodenum. *Ann Surg* 1986;203:301–306

35. Sarles H, Sarles JC, et al. Observations of 205 cases of acute pancreatitis, recurring pancreatitis, and chronic pancreatitis. *Gut* 1965;6:545
36. Shemesh E, Nass S, Czerniak A. Endoscopic sphincterotomy and endoscopic fulguration in the management of adenoma of the papilla of Vater. *Surg Gynecol Obstet* 1989;169:445–448
37. Sherman S, Ruffolo TA, Hawes RH, et al. Complications of endoscopic sphincterotomy. *Gastroenterology* 1991;101: 1068–1075
38. Staritz M, Meyer zum Buschenfelde KH. Elevated pressure in the dorsal part of pancreas divisum: the cause of chronic pancreatitis? *Pancreas* 1988;3:108
39. Stern CD. A historical perspective on the discovery of the accessory duct of the pancreas, the ampulla of "Vater", and pancreas divisum. *Gut* 1986;27:203–212
40. Tanaka M, Ikeda S, et al. Manometric diagnosis of sphincter of Oddi spasm as a cause of postcholecystectomy pain and the treatment of endoscopic sphincterotomy. *Ann Surg* 1985;202:712
41. Thomas PD, Turner JG, Dobbs BR, Burt MJ, Chapman BA. Use of (99m) Tc-DISIDA biliary scanning with morphine provocation for the detection of elevated sphincter of Oddi basal pressure. *Gut* 2000;46: 838–841
42. Toouli J, Roberts-Thomson IC, Kellow J, Dowsett J, Saccone GTP, Evans P. Manometry based randomized trial of endoscopic sphincterotomy for sphincter of Oddi dysfunction. *Gut* 2000;46:98–102
43. Tzovaras G, Rowlands BJ. Diagnosis and treatment of sphincter of Oddi dysfunction. *Br J Surg* 1998; 85:588–595
44. Tzovaras G, Rowlands BJ. Santoriniplasty in the management of symptomatic pancreas divisum. *Eur J Surg* 2000;166:400–404
45. Varshney S, Johnson CD. Surgery for pancreas divisum. *Ann R Col Surg Engl* 2002;84:166–169
46. Warshaw AL, Richter JM, Shapiro RH. The cause and treatment of pancreatitis associated with pancreas divisum. *Ann Surg* 1983; 198: 443–451
47. Warshaw AL, Simeone JF, Schapiro RH, et al. Evaluation and treatment of the dominant dorsal duct syndrome (Pancreas divisum redefined). *Am J Surg* 1990;159:59–66
48. Warshaw AL, Simeone J, Schapiro RH, et al. Objective evaluation of ampullary stenosis with ultrasonography and pancreatic stimulation. *Am J Surg* 1985;149:65–71
49. Warshaw AL. Dominant dorsal duct syndrome pancreas divisum redefined. *J Ped Gastroenterol Nutr* 1990;10:281–283
50. Wehrmann T, Schmitt T, Schonfeld A, Caspary WF, Seifert H. Endoscopic sphincter of Oddi manometry with a portable electronic microtransducer system: comparison with a perfusion manometry method and routine clinical application. *Endosocpy* 2000;32:444
51. Yamaguchi K, Enjoji M, Kitamura K. Endoscopic biopsy has limited accuracy in diagnosis of ampullary tumors. *Gastrointest Endosc* 1990;36:588–592
52. Zadorova Z, Dvofak M, Hajer J. Endoscopic therapy of benign tumors of the papilla of Vater. *Endoscopy* 2001;33: 345–347

40

Cystic Neoplasms of the Pancreas

Christopher J. Sonnenday ■ *Michael R. Marohn* ■ *Ralph H. Hruban*
Charles J. Yeo

Cystic lesions of the pancreas have long posed diagnostic and treatment dilemmas to surgeons and patients. While many identified lesions may prove to be inflammatory pseudocysts or other benign conditions, the possibility of malignancy within a cystic lesion necessitates a thorough diagnostic work-up. Advances in the medical disciplines of radiology, pathology, gastroenterology, and surgery have led to a recent reconsideration of the classification of cystic neoplasms of the pancreas, reflecting an improved understanding of diagnosis, prognosis, and treatment of these often challenging lesions.

Recent literature suggests either an increasing incidence of cystic pancreatic neoplasms, or more likely, improved detection and recognition of these lesions. Historically, autopsy studies have documented a significant prevalence of cystic lesions of the pancreas. Kimura and associates found cystic lesions in 24% of 300 consecutive autopsy specimens among an elderly Japanese population.[1] Approximately 52% of the cystic lesions identified were found to be either hyperplastic or carcinoma-in-situ, though there were no cases of invasive carcinoma.

While a large number of pancreatic cystic neoplasms may have previously gone undetected, the increased use of high resolution cross-sectional imaging, particularly computed tomography (CT) and high quality magnetic resonance imaging (MRI), has led to an increased discovery of cystic lesions of the pancreas as a clinical entity. Many of these lesions remain asymptomatic, and are thus detected incidentally.[2] Increasing use of "full body scans" and "screening" CT or MRI will only increase the number of patients with these lesions that are referred to surgeons for management decisions. Thus careful consideration must be given to the diagnosis and prognostic implications of these lesions.

The most significant recent change in the diagnosis and treatment of pancreatic cystic neoplasms is the recognition and description of the intraductal papillary mucinous neoplasm (IPMN) as a distinct pathologic entity.[3–6] In 1996, IPMNs were classified by the World Health Organization (WHO) as distinct from other mucin-producing cystic neoplasms of the pancreas.[7] In the span of one decade, IPMNs have become the second leading indication for pancreaticoduodenectomy at many large centers.[8] The prevalence of this disease, and the difficulty in preoperatively distinguishing this lesion from other cystic neoplasms, makes investigation of IPMN and similar tumors an important endeavor.

Surgical resection remains the only definitive treatment for cystic neoplasms of the pancreas. Unlike invasive ductal adenocarcinoma of the pancreas, many of the cystic neoplasms of the pancreas have quite favorable prognoses following surgical resection, even when invasive cancer is encountered. Thus there is an increasing population of patients who are survivors of pancreatic resection for cystic neoplasia. Furthermore, pancreatic resection is associated with improved outcomes when performed at high-volume referral centers,[9,10] thus making the proper diagnosis and referral of patients with resectable cystic lesions even more critical.

▪ CLINICAL PRESENTATION

The clinical manifestations of cystic neoplasms of the pancreas vary. A significant number of patients may have no symptoms at all, with the lesion being detected on imaging studies performed for another indication. When symptomatic, the location of the lesion in the head, body, or tail of the pancreas often dictates the signs and symptoms, and determines the degree of indolence of the clinical presentation. Published reviews of patients with cystic pancreatic neoplasms reveal that patients report abdominal pain as the most common presenting symptom, occurring in 60–70% of symptomatic patients.[2,11,12] A palpable abdominal mass and development of acute pancreatitis are other possible presentations. As cystic neoplasms of the pancreas may produce pancreatitis, the old surgical teaching that a cystic lesion of the pancreas in a patient with a history of pancreatitis represents a pseudocyst is no longer true. Jaundice and weight loss also may occur, though at a far lower frequency than is commonly seen in patients with ductal adenocarcinoma.

Increasingly, cystic lesions of the pancreas are detected incidentally, with no specific signs or symptoms. While the malignant potential of most pancreatic lesions is widely acknowledged, there is no current consensus on the appropriate evaluation and treatment of "incidentalomas" of the pancreas. Recent evidence suggests that pancreatic cystic lesions are common, occurring on 1.2% of 24,039 CT or MRI studies reviewed at the Medical College of Wisconsin.[13] Even exempting patients with a history of pancreatitis, the incidence of asymptomatic pancreatic cystic lesions approaches 1% in a population of patients undergoing imaging. While patient history, lesion size, and radiological characteristics may lend clues to the classification of these incidental lesions, over 60% of these lesions may be discovered to be either malignant or premalignant when resected.[2] Data from our unit at Johns Hopkins have identified approximately 100 recent patients with incidentally discovered pancreatic masses undergoing resection. Of these patients, 11% were determined to harbor invasive carcinoma and over 50% had premalignant lesions such as noninvasive IPMNs or mucinous cystic neoplasia (MCN) (Winter J, personal communication). Therefore a thorough diagnostic evaluation and treatment plan is necessary in all patients discovered to have pancreatic cystic lesions.

▪ DIAGNOSIS

The comprehensive evaluation of cystic lesions of the pancreas requires an understanding of the suitable role of individual imaging techniques, the proper interpretation of measured serum biochemical markers, and the judicious use of endoscopic ultrasonography with aspiration or biopsy in appropriate patients. Each of these modalities has unique advantages and limitations, and the application of any of these modalities in the diagnostic work-up of identified lesions should be selective.

Among imaging techniques, CT has become by far the most commonly utilized modality (Figs 40–1 and 40–2). High-resolution three-dimensional multidetector scanners have markedly improved the diagnostic sensitivity and specificity of CT in the detection of pancreatic lesions. CT characteristics of cystic lesions that may lend clues to a histopathologic diagnosis include the presence of septations, macrocystic or microcystic appearance, calcification, size, or presence of a central scar.[14,15] Studies performed at high-volume centers have demonstrated that experienced radiologists can somewhat accurately distinguish serous versus mucinous cystic neoplasms, particularly when the consensus of multiple radiologists is utilized.[14,15] Nevertheless, the radiographic diagnosis of specific histologic subtypes is difficult even in experienced hands, with an overall accuracy of 23–41% in a study of Johns Hopkins radiologists attempting to identify serous cystic neoplasms.[15]

The use of other diagnostic modalities as applicable to individual lesions is discussed below.

▪ PATHOLOGIC CLASSIFICATION

The accurate pathological description of pancreatic cystic neoplasms has evolved significantly in the past

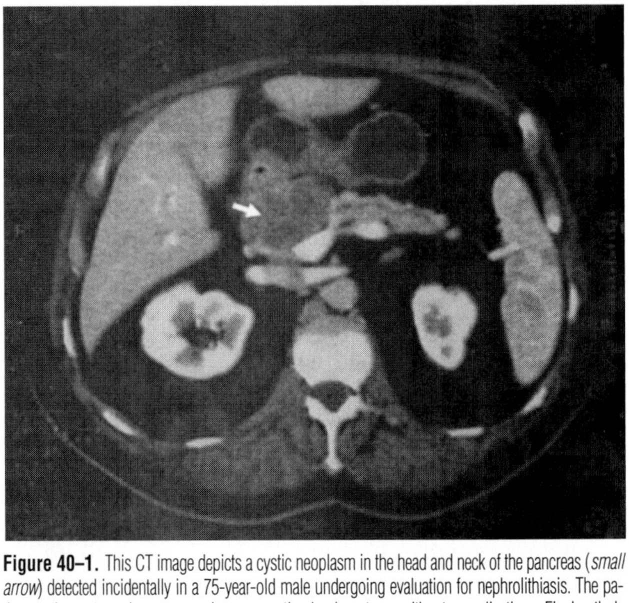

Figure 40–1. This CT image depicts a cystic neoplasm in the head and neck of the pancreas (*small arrow*) detected incidentally in a 75-year-old male undergoing evaluation for nephrolithiasis. The patient underwent a pylorus-preserving pancreaticoduodenectomy without complications. Final pathology revealed a 6-cm serous cystic neoplasm without evidence of malignancy.

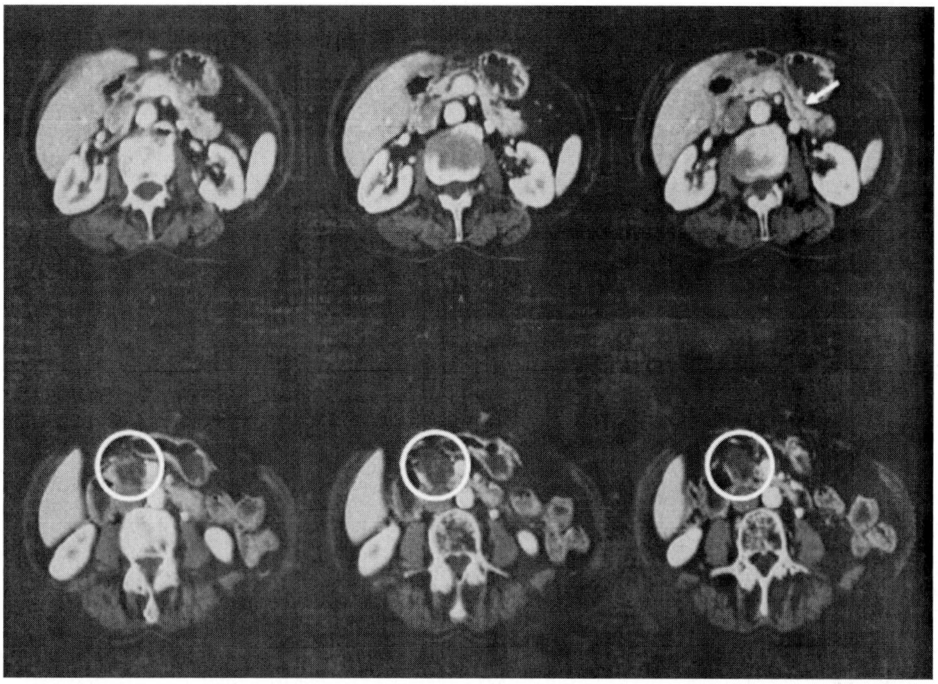

Figure 40–2. Abdominal CT of an 80-year-old female who presented with abdominal pain. The patient underwent a pylorus-preserving pancreaticoduodenectomy; final pathology revealed a 3.5-cm IPMN with a small focus of carcinoma-in-situ located in the head of the pancreas. Notable findings on this series of images that are characteristic of IPMN include the multiloculated cystic mass (*circle*) associated with mild to moderate pancreatic ductal dilatation (*arrow*).

two decades, influenced largely by an improved understanding of the malignant potential of mucinous cystic neoplasms (MCN), in comparison to the largely benign serous lesions, and the emergence of an understanding of the pathogenesis and behavior of IPMNs. Current classification of these tumors follows the WHO International Classification of Tumors as published in 2000 (Table 40–1).[16] While the diagnostic criteria and organizational schema for these tumors is likely to be adapted further in future editions, the current classification system provides a means to stratify these tumors in terms of prognosis and management. In this review, particular attention will be paid to the three most common lesions: serous cystic neoplasms, mucinous cystic neoplasms, and IPMNs.

■ SEROUS CYSTIC NEOPLASMS

Serous cystic neoplasms (SCNs), previously referred to as serous cystadenomas, glycogen-rich adenomas, and microcystic adenomas, are almost always benign. Unfortunately, failure to definitively identify SCNs preoperatively, and their inherent confusion with other more dangerous lesions, necessitates that the majority of these lesions be resected in appropriate operative candidates. Careful delineation of the radiological and pathological features that distinguish these lesions may facilitate nonoperative management (i.e., observation) of these lesions in selected patients who are compliant with follow-up imaging.

CLINICAL PRESENTATION

SCNs are notable for their significant tendency to occur in women in the sixth decade of life. In their comprehensive review of 398 cystic pancreatic neoplasms

TABLE 40–1. PATHOLOGIC CLASSIFICATION OF CYSTIC NEOPLASMS OF THE PANCREAS: THE WHO INTERNATIONAL CLASSIFICATION OF TUMORS, 2000

Serous cystic neoplasm (SCN)
Microcystic adenoma
Oligocystic adenoma
Mucinous cystic neoplasm (MCN)
Mucinous cystadenoma
Mucinous cystic tumor–borderline
Mucinous cystadenocarcinoma
Noninvasive (carcinoma-in-situ)
Invasive
Intraductal papillary mucinous neoplasm (IPMN)
Adenoma
Borderline
Carcinoma-in-situ
Invasive carcinoma

gathered from the French Surgical Association survey (1984–1996), Le Borgne and colleagues described 170 patients with SCN (45%) of which 86% were female, and the mean age at presentation was 56.6 years.[11] In other series of patients with cystic lesions of the pancreas, 12.5–20% of lesions eventually proved to be serous cystic neoplasms.[2,13] Nearly a third of patients (32%) were asymptomatic, while abdominal pain and the presence of a palpable mass were the most common complaints among symptomatic patients. Symptoms frequently associated with other more aggressive lesions, such as jaundice, weight loss, and acute pancreatitis, are unusual among patients with SCN (each less than 10%).[11]

Traditionally, SCNs have been described as having a predilection for the pancreatic body and tail, though Le Borgne an coworkers described a relatively even distribution throughout the gland (38% head, 41% body, 20% tail).[11] These lesions may be quite large in extreme cases,[17] though the mean size at presentation has been 4–5 cm.[11,18] Large SCNs located in the head are unlikely to cause biliary or duodenal obstruction, reflecting their slow pattern of growth and lack of invasive behavior. Rarely, extremely large tumors have been seen in elderly patients, with considerable symptoms of abdominal fullness, and occasionally gastroduodenal obstruction or jaundice.

One clinical condition that has been clearly associated with SCNs of the pancreas is the von Hippel-Lindau (vHL) syndrome. Simple pancreatic cysts or SCNs occur in 17–56% of patients with this heritable multisystem neoplastic syndrome.[19] In patients with vHL, these lesions typically present at a young age (mean of 37 years) as compared to sporadic SCNs.[19] Genetic analysis of DNA extracted from SCNs has revealed significant deletions and mutations of the *vHL* gene, located on the short arm of chromosome 3, perhaps suggesting a clue to the pathogenesis of these cystic lesions.[20]

DIAGNOSIS

As mentioned above, SCNs often have a characteristic imaging phenotype. Most are well demarcated multicystic masses composed of innumerable small cysts (Fig 40–3). Up to one-third have a central, calcified starburst scar (see Fig 40–1).[11,12] While these imaging characteristics can be suggestive, they are only present in 30–70% of cases, leaving the distinction from other cystic neoplasms with more malignant potential frequently in doubt (Fig 40–4). In order to gather more information on these neoplasms, further diagnostic evaluation with endoscopic ultrasound (EUS) and cyst aspiration (either under guidance of CT or EUS) has been proposed. In 2003, Fernandez-del Castillo and associates reported the retrospective experience of the Massachusetts General Hospital using such a diagnostic algorithm.[2] Of 212 patients with pancreatic cystic lesions evaluated over a 5-year period, 78 were incidental findings without symptoms. A total of 99 patients were evaluated with EUS, biopsy, and/or cyst aspiration. These methods had a sensitivity of 69% and specificity of 90% for the identification of malignant lesions. When lesions with malignant potential (i.e., IPMN and MCN) were included, the sensitivity of these methods rose to 81%. Based on these data, the authors proposed observation of asymptomatic lesions that were consistent with SCN, specifically those with microcystic architecture, no mucin, and low cyst fluid carcinoembryonic antigen (CEA) level (<20 mg/mL). Only one patient in the series with a confirmed pathologic diagnosis of SCN had a high cyst CEA level, the significance of which is not known. Of note, 19 of 23 patients with SCN in the series underwent resection, including all of the incidentally discovered lesions. This practice reflects the tendency to be aggressive in the resection of pancreatic cystic lesions because of the concern for missing malignant and premalignant lesions. To date, most diagnostic methods fail to identify SCNs with sufficient accuracy to satisfy patients and surgeons. Nevertheless, use of a diagnostic algorithm to identify low-risk lesions (i.e., SCNs or other benign pathology) may assist with patient counseling and allow nonoperative management of selected patients.

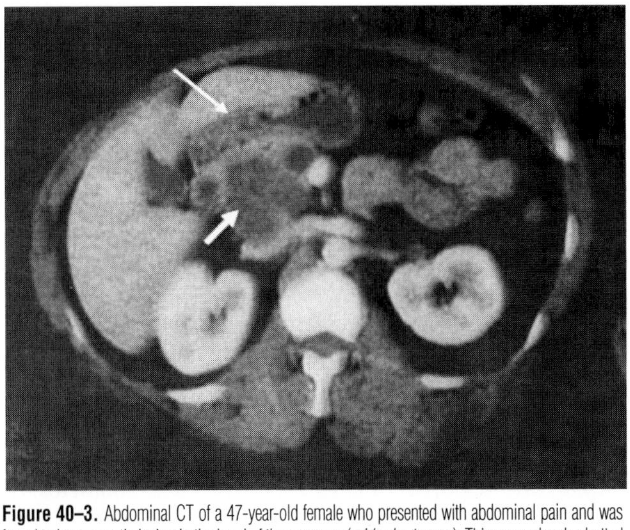

Figure 40–3. Abdominal CT of a 47-year-old female who presented with abdominal pain and was found to have a cystic lesion in the head of the pancreas (*wide short arrow*). This mass closely abutted the proximal duodenum and pylorus (*narrow long arrow*), necessitating a classic pancreaticoduodenectomy for complete resection. Final pathology revealed a benign serous cystic neoplasm.

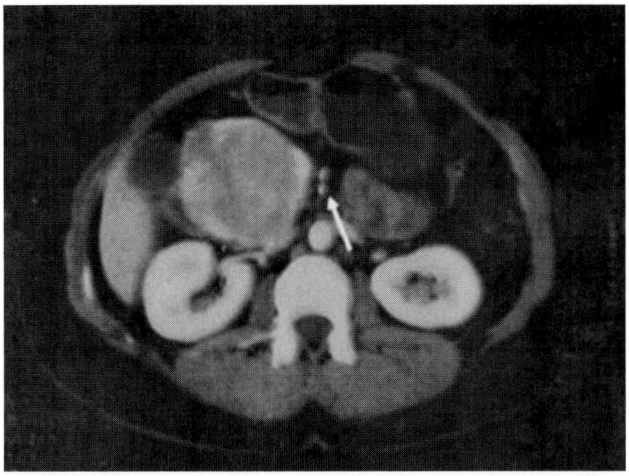

Figure 40–4. Abdominal CT of a large cystic mass with solid components arising from the head of the pancreas and extending into the root of the mesentery along the mesenteric vessels (*arrow*). The partially solid nature of the tumor raised concern of a malignant pancreatic tumor; however, at exploration the mass was found to be well-localized and easily separable from surrounding structures. A pylorus-preserving pancreaticoduodenectomy was performed; final pathology showed a 7-cm serous cystic neoplasm.

PATHOLOGIC FEATURES

The majority of SCNs (70–90%) are microcystic adenomas, characterized by a well-circumscribed, soft mass of numerous small cysts filled with clear serous fluid. Larger cysts may line the periphery of the lesion. The multiple small cystic loculations are well defined, often enhancing with intravenous contrast injection, and often focus on a central stellate scar with or without calcifications, features that may be highly suggestive of a SCN when seen on CT or MRI. A small number of SCNs ≤ 10%) are oligocystic adenomas, which present with one or more dominant cysts, rather than the multiple conjoined microcysts. These lesions may be more difficult to distinguish radiographically from MCNs, IPMNs, pseudocysts, and other cystic lesions.

Beyond these gross distinctions, both microcystic and oligocystic adenomas are composed of a single layer of simple cuboidal epithelium with rounded nuclei and clear cytoplasm (Fig 40–5). The cystic fluid is serous and glycogen-rich. The cyst fluid typically has no mucin content and has a low CEA level (<20 ng/mL), factors that may provide diagnostic information upon cyst aspiration. Unfortunately, aspiration or biopsy often fails to achieve a definitive pathological diagnosis because of sampling error or extensive denudation of the epithelial lining of these cysts.

The malignant potential of SCNs is so low that most experienced centers recommend management of these lesions as benign pathology. Certainly the argument can be made that clearly documented SCNs need not be resected, unless they are symptomatic or enlarging. The incidence of serous cystadenocarcinoma is extremely low, as fewer than 10 cases have been definitively documented in the literature.

TREATMENT

The principles of surgical therapy for SCNs are influenced by the inability to secure a confirmed pathological diagnosis prior to surgery. In cases in which the diagnosis of SCN is not certain, pancreatic resection should be performed according to oncological principles, as if the lesion were a possible malignancy. This practice avoids performance of an inadequate cancer operation in cases in which a malignancy is found on final pathological analysis. However, in cases in which the diagnosis of SCN is confirmed either preoperatively or with intraoperative biopsy, a less radical approach may be considered. Enucleation of SCNs has been shown to be technically feasible, though it may be associated with a significant risk of pancreatic fistula.[22] A central pancreatectomy, with reconstruction via pancreaticogastrostomy or Roux-en-Y pancreaticojejunostomy may be considered in select patients with lesions of the pancreatic neck. Distal pancreatectomy with splenic preservation may also be considered, particularly for small lesions in the tail, where the splenic hilum is more easily dissected. Lesions in the head of the pancreas that are not amenable to enucleation are best treated with pancreaticoduodenectomy, with particular caution paid to the pancreaticojejunostomy in these patients with an otherwise normal pancreas and thus a

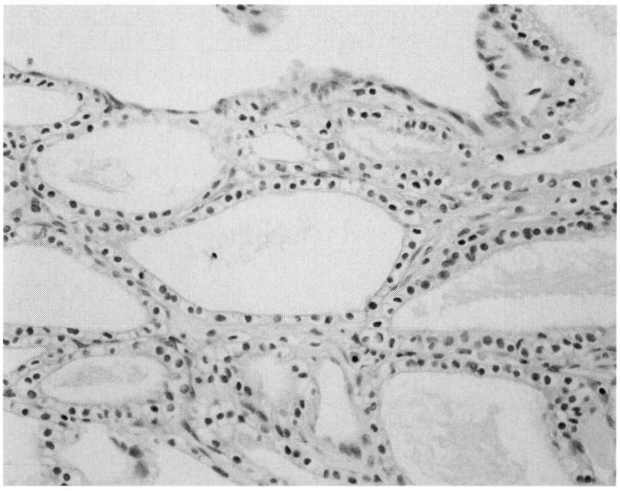

Figure 40–5. Photomicrograph of a typical SCN of the pancreas. Characteristic features include the single layer of cuboidal epithelial cells lining the microcysts within the lesion, uniform round nuclear architecture, and clear cytoplasm. The cyst cavities contain serous fluid and little cellular debris.

significant risk for pancreatic fistula. Patients with pathologically-proven, completely resected SCN do not require extensive serial imaging in follow-up.

Observation of patients with SCN may be appropriate in asymptomatic patients with small lesions (<2–3 cm) who are amenable to serial imaging. Significant documented growth of these lesions should be considered an indication for surgery, both for the concern of missing a malignant lesion and because of the potential of SCNs to grow extremely large in some cases.[17] Resection of a small SCN, particularly in young patients, may avoid a more technically difficult operation if the lesion grows substantially over time. Recommendations for appropriate monitoring of unresected SCNs vary, but serial imaging with either CT or MRI every 6 months for 2 years, and then annually seems reasonable.[23]

▪ MUCINOUS CYSTIC NEOPLASMS

The evolution of the diagnosis and management of pancreatic cystic neoplasms has been aided in large part by the recognition of distinct pathological features that distinguish mucinous cystic neoplasms (MCNs) from other cystic lesions. The distinction between MCN and SCN is critical, as the premalignant and malignant behavior of MCNs stands in stark contrast to the nearly universally benign SCN. Furthermore, the identification and characterization of MCNs with an associated invasive component is important, as patients with this disease have better survival than patients with invasive ductal adenocarcinoma not associated with a cystic neoplasm. Many of the same diagnostic challenges that exist for SCN are true for MCN, but the management decisions may be quite different, due to the differing clinical phenotype of these lesions.

MCNs account for approximately 20–30% of cystic neoplasms of the pancreas, at least as recorded in recent series in which the distinction of these lesions from IPMN has been clarified.[2,13,23] Clinical series published prior to the establishment of diagnostic criteria for IPMN in 1996 likely overestimated the relative prevalence of MCNs in comparison to other cystic lesions, since they included what are now categorized as IPMNs as "mucinous tumors."

CLINICAL PRESENTATION

MCNs are significantly more common in females than males, with over 90% of patients being female.[11,24] MCNs tend to present approximately a decade earlier than SCNs, with the mean age at presentation being 48–52 years.[11,24] Patients with MCNs with an associated invasive carcinoma present at a mean age of 64 years,[24] representing perhaps the longer time required to progress to overt malignancy within these neoplasms. Like other pancreatic cystic neoplasms, many patients with an MCN may be diagnosed incidentally, as 25–50% of patients will have no attributable symptoms (Fig 40–6).[2,11] Among symptomatic patients, abdominal pain is the most common patient complaint, with other symptoms such as jaundice and weight loss being unusual in patients with MCNs.[11,24] A history of acute pancreatitis may also be elicited in 4–17% of patients, though this is less common than in patients with IPMN.[11,24,25]

MCNs most commonly occur in the body or tail of the pancreas, as 72–83% of MCNs in recent studies were located to the left of the pancreatic neck.[11,24] MCNs present at a mean size of 5–6 cm, which is approximately 1 cm larger than SCNs and IPMNs.[5,11,24,25] MCNs with an associated invasive cancer tend to have a larger mean size, approaching 7 cm.[11]

DIAGNOSIS

Macroscopically, MCNs have some characteristic features that may become evident during imaging or operative evaluation. Classically, MCNs contain large septated cysts with thick irregular walls that may be well-detailed on CT, MRI, or ultrasound evaluation. Papillary projections from the epithelium often extend into the cystic cavities and may be visible, particularly on endoscopic ultrasound imaging. In a minority of cases, the wall of the MCN may contain calcifications, a characteristic that

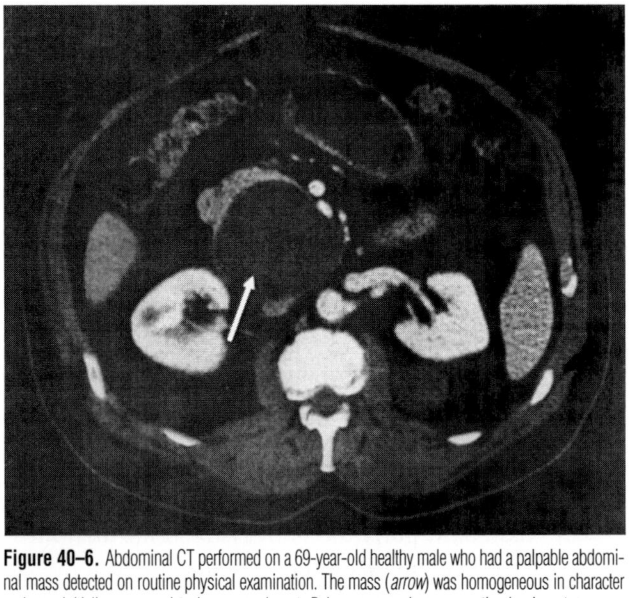

Figure 40–6. Abdominal CT performed on a 69-year-old healthy male who had a palpable abdominal mass detected on routine physical examination. The mass (*arrow*) was homogeneous in character and was initially presumed to be a pseudocyst. Pylorus-preserving pancreaticoduodenectomy was performed, revealing an 8.5-cm mucinous cystic neoplasm without malignancy.

may be associated with a higher likelihood of malignancy. MCNs may also present as large unilocular cysts that may appear similar on cross-sectional imaging to a pseudocyst. One distinguishing characteristic in this scenario is the lack of surrounding inflammatory changes beyond the wall of the neoplasm in MCN, a feature that is common in evolving pseudocysts related to pancreatitis.

Beyond these imaging features, the diagnosis of MCN is approached cautiously, as many of the available modalities suffer from a lack of sensitivity and specificity. Aspiration and biopsy, guided by CT or better EUS, may be considered when imaging studies are not adequately informative and/or the decision to operate is objectionable due to high surgical or medical risk. Serial imaging at 3- to 6-month intervals is an alternative strategy for lesions that cannot be distinguished radiographically from pseudocysts or other non-neoplastic conditions, but growth of a lesion that has not been definitively identified as a SCN should be an indication for surgical resection. Symptomatic patients should undergo resection without a preoperative biopsy, as all symptomatic cystic lesions should be resected in patients of appropriate operative risk. Measurement of biochemical markers in cyst aspirate may be suggestive of a diagnosis, as MCNs have been shown to be rich in CEA and low in amylase. Other tumor markers such as CA 72-4, CA 19-9, CA 125, and CA 15-3 have been investigated as adjuncts to diagnosis, but none has been prospectively validated.

PATHOLOGIC FEATURES

MCNs are cystic tumors of the pancreas characterized by a mucus-secreting columnar epithelium that is associated with a dense ovarianlike stroma. (Fig 40–7). This ovarianlike stroma serves as the pathognomonic feature of MCN. In addition to this unique stromal architecture, MCNs are also distinguished from IPMN by the nearly universal lack of a true communication with the pancreatic ductal system. MCNs are stratified histopathologically based on the degree of epithelial dysplasia, and the presence or absence of invasion. Over 40% of resected lesions are classified as mucinous cystadenoma without dysplastic features. Recurrence of disease or development of invasive carcinoma in patients with cystadenoma that is completely resected is extremely rare, with 5-year overall survival of 89% and disease-free survival approaching 100%.[24] Less than 10% of MCNs may be categorized as mucinous cystic tumor with moderate dysplasia (borderline features). These lesions also have an excellent long-term prognosis, with few documented recurrences after complete resection.

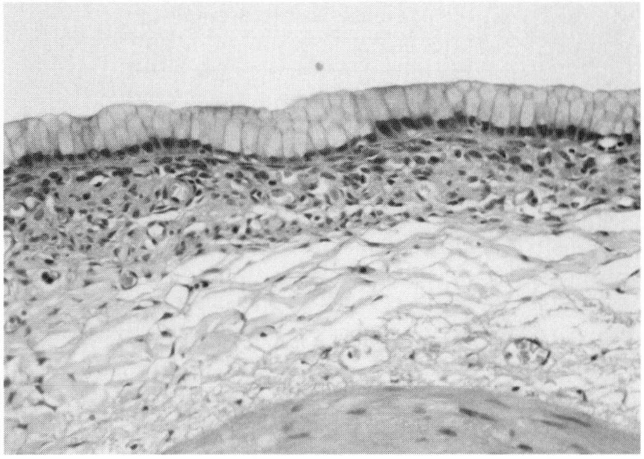

Figure 40–7. MCNs of the pancreas are distinguished by a uniform columnar epithelium associated with a dense underlying ovarianlike stroma.

Mucinous cystadenocarcinoma may be characterized as either noninvasive (carcinoma-in-situ) or invasive. As these two groups have often been considered together in published series, the relative prevalence of either is not clearly understood. However, approximately 25–33% of MCNs are associated with an invasive cancer.[11,13,23,24,26,27] When considered separately, MCNs with carcinoma-in-situ are associated with few recurrences and are appropriate for a lesser degree of serial imaging after complete resection.[27] Of note, MCNs with an associated invasive cancer are associated with a resectability rate of 65% and a significant rate of local recurrence.[11] Five-year survival for resected patients with invasive disease has been reported as high as 72%, though recent series report more modest 5-year survival data of 16–50%.[13,24,26] Our data at Johns Hopkins reveal a 50% 5-year survival postresection (Fig 40–8). The perioperative morbidity in patients with MCNs with an associated cancer is also increased relative to noninvasive MCNs, reflective of the increased aggressive behavior and the propensity of invasive tumors to be located in the pancreatic head and thus require pancreaticoduodenectomy for complete resection (approximately 50% of MCNs with an invasive cancer are located in the pancreatic head).[11,24]

Zamboni and colleagues have reported specifically on the clinicopathological features of 56 patients with MCNs in comparison to pancreatic ductal adenocarcinoma and mucinous tumors of other organs.[27] Specifically, pancreatic MCNs had increased malignant behavior when they were multilocular, when they had papillary projections or mural nodules, and when they labeled for *p53* by immunohistochemistry. Interestingly, these features correspond to a malignant phenotype also seen in mucinous tumors of the ovary, retroperitoneum, and the hepatobiliary tree, and are

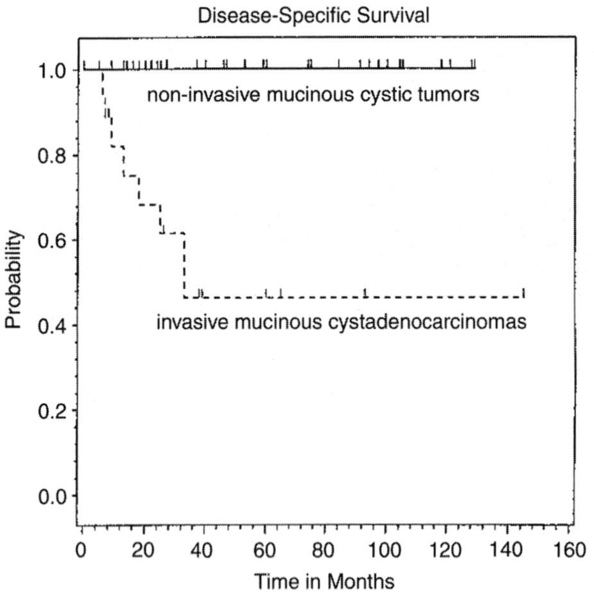

Figure 40–8. Kaplan-Meier disease-specific actuarial survival curves for invasive MCN and noninvasive MCN among 61 patients treated at the Johns Hopkins Hospital. The difference in survival between the two curves was statistically significant (p <0.005, log-rank test). Five-year survival for patients with invasive MCN is approximately 50%. (Reproduced, with permission, from Wilentz RE et al. Pathologic examination accurately predicts prognosis in mucinous cystic neoplasms of the pancreas. *Am J Surg Pathol* 1999;23:1320–1327.)

distinct from features of ductal adenocarcinoma of the pancreas. The authors of this study argue that MCNs may share a common origin with these mucinous tumors of other sites, which is distinct from the pathogenesis of ductal adenocarcinoma.[27]

TREATMENT

Due to the significant rate of malignancy and the risk of progression to malignancy associated with MCNs, all MCNs should undergo formal resection. As with SCNs, enucleation has been documented to be an effective strategy for resection in selected MCN cases.[22,26] However, the risk of performing an inadequate oncological resection for an occult MCN with an invasive cancer is significant, while it is virtually nonexistent for SCN. Therefore enucleation should only be applied to highly selected cases of small, peripherally located MCNs, with confirmation by extensive frozen section analysis. Likewise, segmental pancreatic resections for lesions in the pancreatic neck and body (central pancreatectomy) or tail (spleen-preserving distal pancreatectomy) should be performed cautiously in selected patients without any indication of invasive disease. Larger tumors in older patients (i.e., patients fitting the characteristics of MCNs with an associated invasive cancer) should be treated with formal pancreatic resection. Lesions in the pancreatic head are best treated with pancreaticoduodenectomy, while left-sided lesions are treated via distal pancreatectomy with en bloc splenectomy. Extended lymphadenectomy, which has not been shown to definitively improve locoregional control or survival in patients with ductal adenocarcinoma, has no role in the treatment of patients with cystic neoplasms.[28,29]

Failure to completely resect a noninvasive MCN may result in a later recurrence (persistence), and a missed opportunity for cure.

Adjuvant therapy for MCNs with an associated cancer has been poorly investigated and has no proven benefit. A single case report describes the use of neoadjuvant chemoradiation and treatment monitoring by serum CEA level, but no prospective clinical trials have been performed.[30] However, most experienced centers would likely offer adjuvant chemotherapy to patients with invasive cystadenocarcinoma, extrapolating from the experience with ductal adenocarcinoma.[31] There are no data to support adjuvant radiotherapy. Follow-up with serial imaging every 6 months for 2 years and annually thereafter appears reasonable for patients with resected MCNs with associated invasive cancer.[23]

▪ INTRADUCTAL PAPILLARY MUCINOUS NEOPLASMS

The past decade has seen a notable evolution in the understanding and recognition of the neoplasm now labeled intraductal papillary mucinous neoplasm (IPMN). Multiple centers around the world have described series of mucin-secreting cystic lesions of the pancreas, which are distinguished by their significant malignant potential. These lesions were variably referred to as mucinous ductal ectasia, intraductal papillomatosis, intraductal adenoma or adenomatosis, intraductal mucin-secreting tumor, and intraductal papillary mucinous tumor. However, the earliest report of this "new" lesion is attributed to Ohashi and Maruyama and was published in the Japanese literature in 1982.[32] This report described four malignant lesions associated with the main pancreatic duct and characterized by the now well-described copious amounts of mucus that distend and emanate from the ductal system. The authors noted the comparatively better survival of these patients compared to those with classic invasive adenocarcinoma of the pancreas. While many subsequent authors have helped to further characterize the subtleties of IPMNs, these initial observations accurately depict typical cases.

In 1996, the WHO first formally recognized IPMN as a distinct entity, establishing criteria for pathologic diagnosis of these lesions.[7] Characteristic features include a tall, columnar epithelium with marked mucin production, and cystic transformation of either the main pancreatic duct or one of its side branches. More recent versions of these diagnostic criteria have allowed the stratification of noninvasive IPMNs based on their degree of dysplastic change and the clear separation of noninvasive IPMNs from IPMNs with an associated invasive carcinoma.

CLINICAL PRESENTATION

IPMNs account for 7–35% of cystic neoplasms of the pancreas in published surgical series.[2,13,23] In comparison to patients with SCN or MCN, patients with an IPMN tend to be older, with a mean age of approximately 65 years. Patients with an IPMN with an associated invasive cancer are on average 4–6 years older than patients with noninvasive disease.[3,25,33] IPMNs are also believed to occur more frequently in males, though many recent series have a nearly even gender distribution.[3,5,25,33,34]

The presentation of IPMNs can be remarkably indolent in some cases. Approximately 25% of patients will be asymptomatic, with lesions detected incidentally on imaging studies performed for other reasons. A higher proportion of branch duct variant IPMN patients may be asymptomatic, as discussed below.[25] Among symptomatic patients, a history of vague abdominal pain is the most common presenting complaint. In the recent Johns Hopkins experience reported by Sohn and associates, 52% of 136 patients with IPMN presented with abdominal pain.[25] Acute pancreatitis was documented in 13% of patients, a characteristic presentation among patients with IPMN that is attributed to functional pancreatic ductal obstruction, secondary to excessive production of thick tenacious mucin. In a combined experience of the Massachusetts General Hospital and the University of Verona reported by Salvia and colleagues, acute pancreatitis occurred in 23% of 140 patients with main-duct variant IPMN.[33] These series and others have also documented pancreatic endocrine and exocrine insufficiency in a small number of IPMN patients (5–10%).

Approximately 25–40% of patients with IPMN will present with an invasive component.[24,25,35] Main-duct IPMNs more commonly harbor malignancy than do branch duct lesions, with 59% of the tumors in the MGH/Verona experience containing either carcinoma-in-situ or invasive carcinoma.[33] Of note, malignant IPMNs are more likely to present with symptoms typically attributed to ductal adenocarcinoma, such as obstructive jaundice and weight loss.[25,36]

DIAGNOSIS

Definitive diagnosis of IPMN presents challenges similar to those of all other cystic neoplasms of the pancreas, as no one modality or test often offers definitive information. Characteristic findings on CT include the presence of a focal, low-attenuation mass associated with dilatation of the pancreatic duct.[21] Lesions can in some cases appear lobulated with a "grapelike" appearance.[21] Larger lesions have been shown to be more likely invasive.[37] MRI, and specifically magnetic resonance cholangiopancreatography (MRCP), have been investigated in the diagnosis of IPMN. Specific findings that may be documented on MRCP that may be diagnostic include dilatation of the pancreatic duct, the presence of filling defects or mural nodules along the duct, and the presence of a communication between the duct and a cystic lesion.[38]

Endoscopy may be particularly helpful in the diagnosis of IPMN, with the ability to utilize direct visualization of the ampulla, use of EUS, and pancreatography via ERCP. A variable but pathognomonic feature of main-duct IPMNs is the obvious emission of mucin from a patulous ampulla of Vater. Other diagnostic features evident on contrast injection of the pancreatic duct include ductal dilatation, the presence of filling defects, and communication with the main duct or ectatic side branches. Documentation of a direct communication with the pancreatic duct definitively distinguishes IPMN from either MCN or SCN.[20,35] Pancreatoscopy has been utilized by some centers and may be helpful in distinguishing noninvasive from invasive disease.[39] EUS also may offer information suggesting invasive behavior and provides the opportunity for aspiration or biopsy. Cyst fluid from IPMN may be characterized by elevated CEA and amylase levels, as well as the presence of mucin.[20]

PATHOLOGIC FEATURES

By definition, IPMNs are mucin-producing neoplasms arising from the main pancreatic duct or one of its major branches (Fig 40–9). The prognosis of IPMN is tightly linked to the presence or absence of an associated invasive carcinoma. Recent efforts have focused on establishing an acceptable grading system for the degree of dysplastic change among these lesions.[40] Noninvasive IPMNs may be categorized histopathologically into one of three groups: IPMN adenoma, IPMN borderline (moderate dysplasia), or IPMN with carcinoma-in-situ. Differentiation between the three subtypes is based on the architectural and cytologic features of the papillary epithelium.[40,41] Tall mucin-producing columnar epithelial cells that remain well differentiated characterize IPMN adenoma. Little or

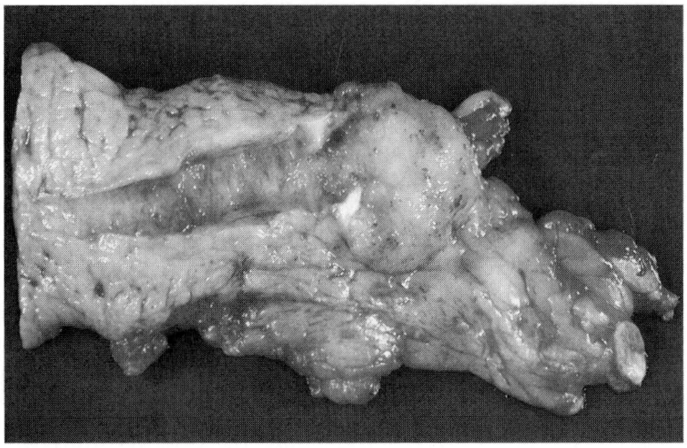

Figure 40–9. Gross photograph of a distal pancreatectomy specimen from a patient with an IPMN with carcinoma-in-situ. Characteristic features include the mass in direct communication with a markedly dilated main pancreatic duct.

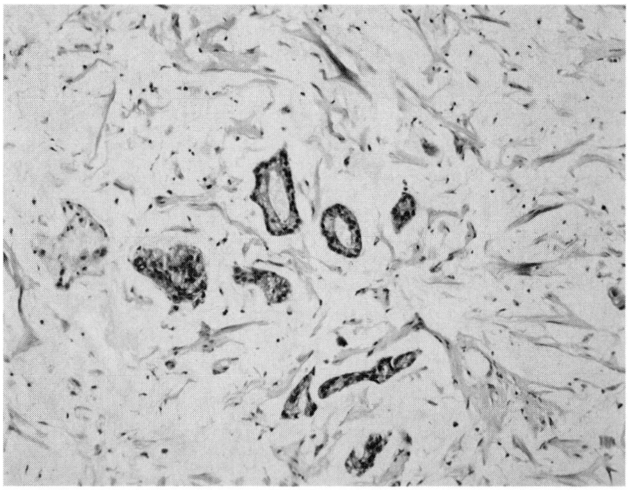

Figure 40–11. Photomicrograph of a colloid carcinoma within an IPMN. Note the largely acellular nature of these cancers and their abundant mucus production.

no dysplasia is present in these lesions. IPMN borderline lesions are described as lesions with moderate epithelial dysplasia, characterized by moderate loss of polarity, changes in nuclear morphology, and pseudopapillary formation (Fig 40–10). IPMNs with carcinoma-in-situ have severe dysplastic changes. These lesions may be papillary or micropapillary, and severely dysplastic lesions may lose the ability to secrete mucin. The invasive carcinomas associated with IPMNs are usually either colloid or tubular adenocarcinomas. Colloid carcinomas are associated with abundant extracellular mucin production (Fig 40–11), and tubular carcinomas are morphologically similar to invasive ductal adenocarcinomas.

Chari and associates reported on 113 patients from the Mayo Clinic with resected IPMN stratified according to the WHO criteria.[3] A total of 40 patients in the series (35%) had evidence of invasion on pathological analysis and were considered as a separate group. These patients had a significantly decreased survival compared to patients with noninvasive tumors (5-year survival 36% versus 88%, $p < 0.0001$), with 65% of patients developing recurrent disease at a median follow-up of 42 months. These data are corroborated by the experience at the Johns Hopkins Hospital and of the MGH/Verona groups, where 5-year survival rates of patients with IPMN and invasive carcinoma were 43% and 60%, respectively (Fig 40–12).[25,33] In the Hopkins experience, lymph node status was predictive of survival among patients with invasive carcinoma, as there were

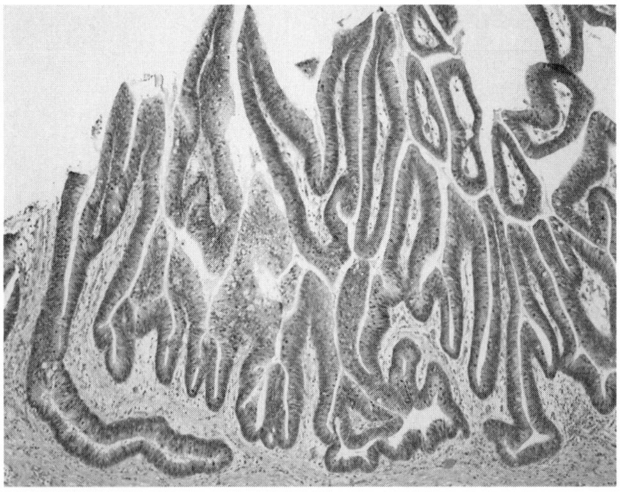

Figure 40–10. Photomicrograph of an IPMN with borderline features. Characteristic features include the tall columnar cells lining the papillary projections of the tumor, moderate dysplastic changes of the epithelium, and varied nuclear morphology.

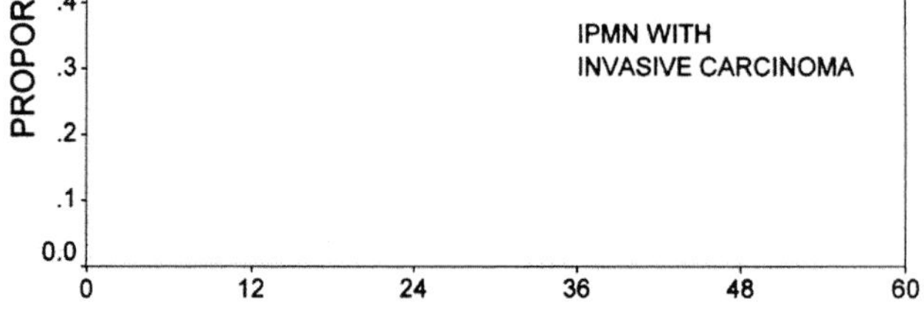

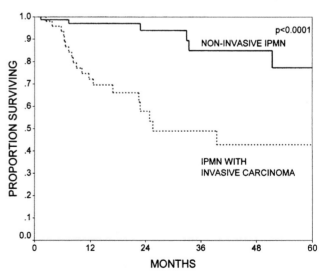

Figure 40–12. Kaplan-Meier actuarial survival curves comparing 84 patients with noninvasive IPMN to 52 patients with invasive IPMN following pancreatic resection at the Johns Hopkins Hospital (1987–2003). Patients with noninvasive IPMN have a significantly greater survival than those with invasive disease (p<0.0001).[25]

no long-term survivors among lymph node–positive patients and 85% 5-year survival among lymph node–negative patients. Histologic subtype of the invasive cancer also appears to be an important factor, as patients with colloid carcinomas had better survival than patients with tubular carcinomas (83% versus 24% 5-year survival, $p = 0.01$).

Among patients with noninvasive IPMN, the spectrum of adenoma, borderline, and carcinoma-in-situ has less dramatic influence on patient survival in current studies. The most troubling shortcoming of the current grading scheme for noninvasive IPMNs is the inability to accurately predict patient outcomes, and may be due to the presence of multifocal disease. Sohn and colleagues described four deaths from invasive adenocarcinoma during follow-up among 84 patients with noninvasive IPMN, and one additional patient treated with completion pancreatectomy for an invasive cancer diagnosed 5 years after his initial resection.[25] Two additional patients developed recurrent noninvasive disease in the pancreatic remnant. Both of these patients were treated with completion pancreatectomy and are free of disease. Importantly, invasive components appear to be distributed somewhat randomly within a given IPMN, creating a situation in which sampling error within the tumor may falsely underestimate the tumor grade. Interestingly, even when invasive cancers occur within an IPMN, the clinical behavior may be improved relative to ductal adenocarcinoma, arguing that the biology of these tumors may be distinct from other pancreatic cancers.

Establishment of a histopathologic diagnosis of IPMN must include consideration of two pathological conditions that may be confused for these lesions, MCN and pancreatic intraepithelial neoplasia (PanIN).[36,40,41] As discussed above, MCNs usually can be distinguished by the lack of pancreatic ductal involvement and their characteristic ovarianlike stroma.[27] Distinction of IPMNs from PanINs may be more challenging, and was the subject of an international consensus conference in August 2003.[41] PanINs tend to be smaller than IPMNs, and have shorter papillae. Like IPMNs, PanINs are graded according to the degree of dysplastic change and cellular architecture.[42] Low grade PanIN-1 lesions are common incidental findings in pathological analysis of pancreatic specimens resected for other conditions. Higher grade, PanIN-3 lesions are highly associated with ductal adenocarcinoma.[41] IPMNs, like PanINs, are intraductal lesions that may demonstrate a range of cellular atypia and malignant transformation. However, IPMNs may be distinguished based on their gross visibility and involvement of large ducts. PanINs should be considered a microscopic finding involving ducts less than 5 mm in diameter, while IPMNs are macroscopic findings.[41] In addition, IPMNs often express the mucin MUC-2, while PanINs usually express MUC-1.

IPMNs appear also to have distinct molecular events contributing to the clinical and pathological behavior that further distinguishes them from lesions in the PanIN–ductal adenocarcinoma sequence. Iacobuzio-Donahue and associates described the intact (normal) expression of the tumor suppressor gene *Dpc4* in the intraductal components of 79 IPMNs. *Dpc4* inactivation has been shown to be relatively specific for pancreatic adenocarcinoma,[43] and its persistence in both noninvasive and invasive IPMNs argues that these lesions may arise through a pathway that is distinct from PanIN–ductal adenocarcinoma. IPMNs also appear to have a significantly lower rate of *k-ras* and *p53* mutations, lesions that are common in ductal adenocarcinoma.[36,44] A recent study drawing on specimens from multiple institutions further argues that the epithelial lesions within IPMNs may represent a form of intestinal metaplasia associated with MUC2 and CDX2 expression.[45] These data and others suggest that IPMNs are unique pancreatic neoplasms, with a pathogenesis that is distinct from that of the PanIN–ductal adenocarcinoma.

As mentioned above, the malignant potential of IPMNs involving the main pancreatic ductal system appears to be greater than that of lesions involving only secondary ducts. In 1998, Traverso and associates reported on 33 patients with IPMN, 19 of which were identified as having branch-duct variants of IPMN without direct involvement of the main pancreatic duct.[6] Thirteen of these 19 patients had noninvasive disease, while only 4 of 13 main-duct IPMNs were found to be noninvasive. Even among patients with malignant disease, patients with branch-duct lesions were 25% less likely to die of recurrent disease following resection, as compared to patients with malignant main-duct IPMN. Terris and colleagues demonstrated similar findings in a pathological study of pancreatic specimens from 43 patients with resected IPMN. Patients with branch-duct IPMNs tended to be younger than those with main-duct lesions, and the neoplasms were located primarily in the head and neck of the pancreas (16 of 17 patients).[46] Interestingly, no cases of invasive IPMN were found among the branch duct variants. These reports are contrasted at least in part by the experience among resected patients at the Johns Hopkins Hospital, where the 5-year actuarial survival of patients with branch-duct variant IPMNs (N = 60) was identical to patients with main-duct or combined variants (N = 69), at 56% and 65%, respectively (Fig 40–13) ($p > 0.05$).[25] Further study of the clinicopathological differences between these two variants is necessary before prognostic and treatment decisions can be fully substantiated.

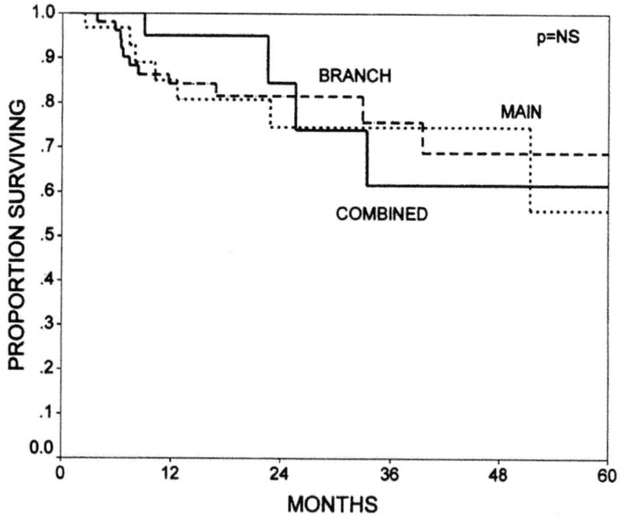

Figure 40–13. Kaplan-Meier actuarial survival curves comparing patients with main-duct (N = 36), side-branch (N = 60), and combined variants (N = 33) of IPMN resected at the Johns Hopkins Hospital (1987–2003). When analyzed by tumor location relative to the main pancreatic duct, there were no significant survival differences between groups (p>0.05).[25]

TREATMENT

Because of the significant risk of malignancy associated with IPMN, resection is the recommended treatment in virtually all patients without significant medical contraindications to surgery. A controversy clearly exists regarding the need for resection in patients with side-branch IPMN variants, particularly in the elderly and the very elderly patient populations. As at least 50% of IPMNs occur in the pancreatic head or uncinate process, pancreaticoduodenectomy has been the most common pancreatic resection performed for IPMN in published series.[3,5,25,33,34] In fact, IPMN has become the second leading indication for pancreaticoduodenectomy after invasive ductal adenocarcinoma, accounting for 20% of pancreaticoduodenectomies at some centers in recent years. Among 136 IPMNs resected at the Johns Hopkins Hospital between 1987 and 2003, 71% of patients were treated with pancreaticoduodenectomy, while only 12% underwent distal pancreatectomy.[25] In 21 patients (15%), total pancreatectomy was performed for diffuse IPMNs that involved the entire pancreas. Total pancreatectomy was associated with longer operative time (8.0 versus 6.6 hours), increased blood loss (1350 versus 700 mL), and increased transfusion requirement (1.5 versus 0 units of packed red blood cells) when compared to pancreaticoduodenectomy. However, patients treated with total pancreatectomy had equivalent length of stay and complication rates when compared to patients undergoing segmental pancreatic resections.[25]

While the role of resection has become well established in patients with large main-branch IPMN, the extent of resection may be controversial in the setting of extensive side-branch neoplasia that involves the majority of the pancreatic ductal system. Skip lesions clearly occur, such that a normal resection margin may not be indicative of a lack of neoplasia in the pancreatic remnant. Therefore the role of total pancreatectomy to achieve clearance of all dysplastic epithelium, even prophylactic total pancreatectomy, is controversial. In the Johns Hopkins experience, the presence of noninvasive IPMN at the resection margin of a patient with an invasive IPMN was not associated with decreased survival or increased risk of recurrence. Several patients with negative margins developed recurrent disease, regardless of what appeared to be a complete resection, again arguing that IPMNs are associated with diffuse neoplastic changes. Notably, of the 84 patients with noninvasive IPMN described by Sohn and colleagues,[25] 7 patients developed recurrent disease in the pancreatic remnant. Four of these patients eventually died secondary to invasive adenocarcinoma, but three underwent completion pancreatectomy and remain free of disease. Chari and coworkers report somewhat opposing results from the Mayo clinic.[3] Among 27 patients with invasive IPMN treated with partial pancreatectomy, six out of seven patients with dysplastic changes at the resection margin developed recurrent disease. Furthermore, none of the 13 patients treated with total pancreatectomy for noninvasive IPMN developed recurrent disease, while 4 patients treated via partial pancreatectomy and with negative margins developed local recurrence. Based on these results and the significant metabolic and physiological burden of total pancreatectomy, most experienced centers currently take a cautious approach towards total pancreatectomy. Segmental pancreatectomy resection is preferable in most cases, with a goal of achieving a negative margin of resection. Total pancreatectomy is indicated in patients in whom significant dysplasia remains on serial intraoperative frozen sections of the cut margin, or when tumor clearly involves the majority of the main pancreatic duct, as seen by preoperative EUS or intraoperative pancreatic ductoscopy. Prophylactic total pancreatectomy, without an attempt to achieve a negative margin with segmental resection, is not recommended. A final pathological report of noninvasive IPMN at a surgical margin is not a clear indication for re-exploration and completion pancreatectomy. Not all of these patients will develop invasive disease, and recurrent gross disease may be amenable to staged completion pancreatectomy if discovered on follow-up imaging. We typically recommend annual CT scan, or perhaps better annual MRCP, as a reasonable means to keep the pancreatic remnant under surveillance.

Based on the lower malignant potential of branch-duct IPMN, some centers have adopted a policy of observation with serial imaging for these lesions, rather than recommending surgical resection. Matsumoto and associates recently reported the serial observation of 11 patients with branch-duct IPMN with a mean follow-up time of 33 months.[47] No cases of progression or development of malignant disease have occurred to date in this small series. As the majority of branch-duct IPMNs occur in the head of the pancreas,[6,25,46–48] serial observation serves as an attractive option, as a means of avoiding pancreaticoduodenectomy. Of course, the contrast between recommending observation versus Whipple resection can be seen as problematic and troublesome for patient understanding. However, conflicting data about the rate of malignancy among patients with branch-duct IPMN and limited long-term survival information make a strategy of observation potentially of some risk to patients.[25,48] Therefore surgical resection is currently recommended for nearly all IPMNs, including obvious branch-duct variants, in appropriate operative candidates.

▪ UNUSUAL PANCREATIC CYSTIC NEOPLASMS

SOLID PSEUDOPAPILLARY TUMOR

These rare tumors are notable for several characteristic clinical and pathological features. They typically occur in women in the second or third decade of life and often present either with abdominal pain or a palpable abdominal mass. The lesions may be large, presenting in one series at a mean size of 13 cm.[49] On CT, these tumors often appear well-circumscribed with hypodense areas representing hemorrhage or necrosis. Lesions may be evenly distributed throughout the pancreas. Most of these lesions harbor β-catenin mutations. Though considered low-grade malignancies, local invasion into contiguous structures may occur, as may metastases. An aggressive surgical approach is warranted, as long-term survival in resected patients approaches 100%.[49]

CYSTIC NEUROENDOCRINE TUMOR

These lesions behave as other neuroendocrine lesions, but can present diagnostic difficulties when nonfunctional because their cystic appearance may lead to confusion with pseudocysts or other cystic neoplasms.[50] However, these lesions have a favorable prognosis if completely resected and should be treated aggressively in appropriate surgical candidates. Segmental pancreatic resection or enucleation are both appropriate therapies in selected patients. Ahrendt and associates published a series of four patients with this condition, all completely resected and free of disease.[50]

CYSTIC ACINAR CELL TUMOR

This describes a rare clinical entity for which descriptions and diagnostic criteria are evolving. Once thought to be degenerative cystic change within pancreatic acini, this tumor is now recognized by some as a true neoplasm.[51] Zamboni and colleagues recently described 10 patients treated for this lesion, described grossly as well-demarcated multilocular cystic lesions lined with columnar cells of acinar differentiation.[52] Patients in this series ranged in age from 16–66 years and were 70% female. All patients in the series were alive, regardless of whether the lesion was completely resected or biopsied. This lesion appears to be a benign cystic lesion without invasive behavior, which is notable because of its similar presentation and appearance to other cystic neoplasms. It is unclear if these lesions represent acinar metaplasia or if they are true neoplasms.

CYSTIC DEGENERATION OF DUCTAL ADENOCARCINOMA

While not truly a distinct lesion, it is important to realize that pancreatic ductal adenocarcinoma may present with cystic features. Thus all cystic lesions should at least be considered as potential pancreatic cancers until an alternative diagnosis is established. In a comparative review of symptomatic and incidental pancreatic cysts by Fernandez-del Castillo and colleagues, 9% of symptomatic lesions and 2% of incidental cysts proved to be ductal adenocarcinoma.[2] Adenocarcinomas that obstruct the pancreatic duct may be associated with retention cysts in up to 8% of patients.[53]

▪ SUMMARY

Cystic lesions of the pancreas should be considered as possibly malignant until proven otherwise. Improved diagnostic modalities and advances in histopathological analysis, molecular biology, and surgery have led to a significant evolution in our understanding of cystic neoplasms of the pancreas. Classification according to pathological criteria allows differentiation of the three major cystic neoplasms: SCN, MCN, and IPMN, thus providing important prognostic and therapeutic information. Further improvement in preoperative methods of diagnosis may in the future allow selective surgical management for high-risk lesions. At present, surgical resection remains the only curative modality for these lesions.

REFERENCES

1. Kimura W et al. Analysis of small cystic lesions of the pancreas. *Int J Pancreatol* 1995;18:197–206
2. Fernandez-del Castillo C et al. Incidental pancreatic cysts: clinicopathologic characteristics and comparison with symptomatic patients. *Arch Surg* 2003;138:427–430; discussion 433–434
3. Chari ST et al. Study of recurrence after surgical resection of intraductal papillary mucinous neoplasm of the pancreas. *Gastroenterology* 2002;123:1500–1507
4. Doi R et al. Surgical management of intraductal papillary mucinous tumor of the pancreas. *Surgery* 2002;132: 80–85
5. Sohn TA et al. Intraductal papillary mucinous neoplasms of the pancreas: an increasingly recognized clinicopathologic entity. *Ann Surg* 2001;234:313–321; discussion 321–322
6. Traverso LW et al. Intraductal neoplasms of the pancreas. *Am J Surg* 1998;175:426–432
7. Kloppel G. Histological typing of tumours of the exocrine pancreas. In: *World Health Organization International Classification of Tumors.* Berlin, Germany: Springer; 1996:11–20
8. Sarr MG et al. Primary cystic neoplasms of the pancreas. Neoplastic disorders of emerging importance—current state-of-the-art and unanswered questions. *J Gastrointest Surg* 2003;7:417–428
9. Sosa JA et al. Importance of hospital volume in the overall management of pancreatic cancer. *Ann Surg* 1998; 228:429–438
10. Birkmeyer JD et al. Hospital volume and surgical mortality in the United States. *N Engl J Med* 2002;346:1128–1137
11. Le Borgne J, de Calan L, Partensky C. Cystadenomas and cystadenocarcinomas of the pancreas: a multiinstitutional retrospective study of 398 cases. French Surgical Association. *Ann Surg* 1999;230:152–161
12. Brugge WR et al. Diagnosis of pancreatic cystic neoplasms: a report of the cooperative pancreatic cyst study. *Gastroenterology* 2004;126:1330–1336
13. Spinelli KS et al. Cystic pancreatic neoplasms: observe or operate. *Ann Surg* 2004;239:651–657; discussion 657–659
14. Curry CA et al. CT of primary cystic pancreatic neoplasms: can CT be used for patient triage and treatment? *AJR Am J Roentgenol* 2000;175:99–103
15. Johnson CD et al. Cystic pancreatic tumors: CT and sonographic assessment. *AJR Am J Roentgenol* 1988;151: 1133–1138
16. Aaltonen LA et al. Pathology and genetics of tumours of the digestive system. World Health Organization classification of tumours. Lyon Oxford, England: IARC Press, Oxford University Press (distributor); 2000:314
17. Moesinger RC et al. Large cystic pancreatic neoplasms: pathology, resectability, and outcome. *Ann Surg Oncol* 1999;6:682–690
18. Pyke CM et al. The spectrum of serous cystadenoma of the pancreas. Clinical, pathologic, and surgical aspects. *Ann Surg* 1992;215:132–139
19. Lonser RR et al. von Hippel-Lindau disease. *Lancet* 2003;361:2059–2067
20. Brugge WR et al. Cystic neoplasms of the pancreas. *N Engl J Med* 2004;351:1218–1226
21. Megibow AJ et al. Cystic pancreatic masses: cross-sectional imaging observations and serial follow-up. *Abdom Imaging* 2001;26:640–647
22. Talamini MA et al. Cystadenomas of the pancreas: is enucleation an adequate operation? *Ann Surg* 1998;227: 896–903
23. Allen PJ et al. Cystic lesions of the pancreas: selection criteria for operative and nonoperative management in 209 patients. *J Gastrointest Surg* 2003;7:970–977
24. Sarr MG et al. Clinical and pathologic correlation of 84 mucinous cystic neoplasms of the pancreas: can one reliably differentiate benign from malignant (or premalignant) neoplasms? *Ann Surg* 2000;231:205–212
25. Sohn TA et al. Intraductal papillary mucinous neoplasms of the pancreas: an updated experience. *Ann Surg* 2004;239:788–797; discussion 797–799
26. Kiely JM et al. Cystic pancreatic neoplasms: enucleate or resect? *J Gastrointest Surg* 2003;7:890–897
27. Zamboni G et al. Mucinous cystic tumors of the pancreas: clinicopathological features, prognosis, and relationship to other mucinous cystic tumors. *Am J Surg Pathol* 1999;23:410–422
28. Yeo CJ et al. Pancreaticoduodenectomy with or without distal gastrectomy and extended retroperitoneal lymphadenectomy for periampullary adenocarcinoma, part 2: randomized controlled trial evaluating survival, morbidity, and mortality. *Ann Surg* 2002;236:355–366; discussion 366–368
29. Yeo CJ et al. Pancreaticoduodenectomy with or without extended retroperitoneal lymphadenectomy for periampullary adenocarcinoma: comparison of morbidity and mortality and short-term outcome. *Ann Surg* 1999; 229:613–622; discussion 622–624
30. Wood D et al. Cystadenocarcinoma of the pancreas: neo-adjuvant therapy and CEA monitoring. *J Surg Oncol* 1990;43:56–60
31. Neoptolemos JP et al. A randomized trial of chemoradiotherapy and chemotherapy after resection of pancreatic cancer. *N Engl J Med* 2004;350:1200–1210
32. Ohashi K et al. Four cases of mucin-producing cancer of the pancreas on specific findings of the papilla of Vater. *Prog Dig Endoscopy* 1982;20:348–351
33. Salvia R et al. Main-duct intraductal papillary mucinous neoplasms of the pancreas: clinical predictors of malignancy and long-term survival following resection. *Ann Surg* 2004;239:678–685; discussion 685–687
34. Adsay NV et al. Intraductal papillary-mucinous neoplasms of the pancreas: an analysis of in situ and invasive carcinomas in 28 patients. *Cancer* 2002;94:62–77

35. Kozarek RA. Intraductal papillary mucinous tumors (IPMT) of the pancreas: the gastroenterologist's view (abstract). in Digestive Disease Week 2005, Combined Clinical Symposium; 2005: Chicago, IL
36. Adsay NV. Intraductal papillary mucinous neoplasms of the pancreas: pathology and molecular genetics. *J Gastrointest Surg* 2002;6:656–659
37. Nagai E et al. Intraductal papillary mucinous neoplasms of the pancreas associated with so-called "mucinous ductal ectasia". Histochemical and immunohistochemical analysis of 29 cases. *Am J Surg Pathol* 1995; 19:576–589
38. Irie H et al. MR cholangiopancreatographic differentiation of benign and malignant intraductal mucin-producing tumors of the pancreas. *AJR Am J Roentgenol* 2000;174:1403–1408
39. Yamaguchi T et al. Peroral pancreatoscopy in the diagnosis of mucin-producing tumors of the pancreas. *Gastrointest Endosc* 2000;52:67–73
40. Longnecker DS, Adler G, Hruban RH. Intraductal papillary mucinous neoplasms of the pancreas. In: *WHO Classification of Tumors of the Digestive System.* Geneva, Switzerland: WHO; 2000:237–240
41. Hruban RH et al. An illustrated consensus on the classification of pancreatic intraepithelial neoplasia and intraductal papillary mucinous neoplasms. *Am J Surg Pathol* 2004;28:977–987
42. Hruban RH et al. Pancreatic intraepithelial neoplasia: a new nomenclature and classification system for pancreatic duct lesions. *Am J Surg Pathol* 2001;25:579–586
43. Hahn SA et al. DPC4, a candidate tumor suppressor gene at human chromosome 18q21.1. *Science* 1996;271: 350–335
44. Hruban RH et al. Genetics of pancreatic cancer. From genes to families. *Surg Oncol Clin North Am* 1998;7:1–23
45. Adsay NV et al. Pathologically and biologically distinct types of epithelium in intraductal papillary mucinous neoplasms: delineation of an "intestinal" pathway of carcinogenesis in the pancreas. *Am J Surg Pathol* 2004;28: 839–848
46. Terris B et al. Intraductal papillary mucinous tumors of the pancreas confined to secondary ducts show less aggressive pathologic features as compared with those involving the main pancreatic duct. *Am J Surg Pathol* 2000; 24:1372–1377
47. Matsumoto T et al. Optimal management of the branch duct type intraductal papillary mucinous neoplasms of the pancreas. *J Clin Gastroenterol* 2003;36:261–265
48. Kobari M et al. Intraductal papillary mucinous tumors of the pancreas comprise 2 clinical subtypes: differences in clinical characteristics and surgical management. *Arch Surg* 1999;134:1131–1136
49. Zinner MJ, Shurbaji MS, Cameron JL. Solid and papillary epithelial neoplasms of the pancreas. *Surgery* 1990; 108:475–480
50. Ahrendt SA et al. Cystic pancreatic neuroendocrine tumors: is preoperative diagnosis possible? *J Gastrointest Surg*,2002;6:66–74
51. Adsay NV, Klimstra DS, Compton CC. Cystic lesions of the pancreas. Introduction. *Semin Diagn Pathol* 2000;17:1–6
52. Zamboni G et al. Acinar cell cystadenoma of the pancreas: a new entity? *Am J Surg Pathol* 2002;26:698–704
53. Itai Y, Moss AA, Goldberg HI. Pancreatic cysts caused by carcinoma of the pancreas: a pitfall in the diagnosis of pancreatic carcinoma. *J Comput Assist Tomogr* 1982;6: 772–726

41

Cancer of the Pancreas and Other Periampullary Cancers

Richard D. Schulick ▪ *John L. Cameron*

Periampullary cancers include a group of malignant neoplasms arising in the pancreas or in or near the ampulla of Vater. They are usually discovered because of obstructive jaundice or pain. The first successful resection of a periampullary tumor was performed by Halsted in 1898. He described a local ampullary resection with reanastomosis of the pancreatic and bile ducts into the duodenum of a woman who presented with obstructive jaundice.[1] Codivilla is often credited with performing the first en bloc resection of the head of the pancreas and duodenum for periampullary carcinoma but, unfortunately, the patient did not survive the postoperative period.[2] The first successful two stage pancreaticoduodenectomy was performed by Kausch in 1909.[3] In 1914, Hirschel reported the first successful one-stage pancreaticoduodenectomy.[4] In the first third of the 20th century, most periampullary cancers were managed by a transduodenal approach similar to that first reported by Halsted.

Pancreaticoduodenectomy was not popularized until 1935 with the report of Whipple and colleagues of three successful, two stage, en bloc resections of the head of the pancreas and the duodenum.[5] Over the next decade, a number of modifications and technical refinements were made in the procedure, including the first one-stage pancreaticoduodenectomy, reported in the United States by Trimble in 1941. The procedure was rarely performed despite technical advances, until the 1980s because of the formidable operative morbidity, mortality, and the poor prognosis associated with periampullary cancers. During the last two decades, significant advances have been made in understanding of the pathogenesis of periampullary carcinoma. There have been improvements in the ability to diagnose and stage these diseases, and the surgical and nonsurgical approaches to treating these patients have progressed.

▪ INCIDENCE

Periampullary carcinomas are major public health concerns throughout the world. Pancreatic cancer is the fourth leading cause of cancer death in the United States. In 2005, there were an estimated 31,800 deaths in the United States compared to 163,510 deaths for lung cancer, 56,290 for colorectal cancer, and 40,870 for breast cancer.[6] The incidence of pancreatic carcinoma rose dramatically from the 1930s until the mid-1970s, nearly doubling during this time period. Since 1973, the incidence in the United States has remained stable at about 8 to 9 per 100,000 of population. Unfortunately, the number of cases of pancreatic cancer, which is estimated be 32,180 in 2005, approximates the number of mortalities in the United States. The incidence in Western Europe is similar to that in the United States and has also remained stable during the past three decades. In Europe, pancreatic cancer is the sixth leading cause of cancer death. In Japan, however, a dramatic increase has been observed during the last three decades, although the overall incidence is still less than that observed in the West. The lowest incidence worldwide is seen in parts of the Middle East and in India. Worldwide over 200,000 people die annually of cancer of the pancreas.[7]

The incidence of periampullary carcinoma increases with age, and the majority of patients present in or beyond their sixth decade of life. There is a slight male preponderance, and African American males have the highest overall incidence in the United States.

▪ PATHOLOGY

Given the close proximity of the head of the pancreas, the distal bile duct, the ampulla of Vater, and the periampullary duodenum, the site of origin of a periampullary malignancy can be difficult to determine. At many large volume centers that perform significant numbers of pancreaticoduodenectomies, approximately 10–20% of the specimens contain only benign disease; therefore, the great majority of clinically significant periampullary tumors are cancers.[8,9] Local ampullary resections for presumed benign periampullary disease make up even a much smaller percentage of cases.

Pathologic examination of resected pancreaticoduodenectomy specimens reveal that 40–60% are adenocarcinomas of the head of the pancreas, 10–20% are adenocarcinomas of the ampulla of Vater, 10% are distal bile duct adenocarcinomas, and 5–10% are duodenal adenocarcinomas. Since these data represent resected specimens, and since the resectability rate of the nonpancreatic periampullary cancers is much higher, it is likely that pancreas cancer is the site of origin in up to 90% of cases.

Pancreatic ductal adenocarcinoma is by far the most common malignant histologic type of pancreatic carcinoma with more than two thirds of these tumors arising in the pancreatic head, neck, or uncinate process. Other rare histologies include acinar, squamous, islet cell tumors, or tumors of nonepithelial origin. Islet cell tumors, or neuroendocrine tumors, may be either benign or malignant and may be functional with hormone production resulting in clinical manifestations. Nonfunctional islet cell tumors either do not produce any hormone, or do so at a subclinical level and are usually detected because of their space-occupying characteristics. Obstructive jaundice is uncommon with benign islet cell tumors in head of the pancreas, but can occur with malignant lesions. Cystic neoplasms of the pancreas can also arise from the exocrine pancreas and are classified as either benign serous cystadenomas, potentially malignant mucinous cystadenomas, and an increasingly more commonly recognized entity, intraductal papillary mucinous neoplasms (IPMNs). Various sarcomas including gastrointestinal (GI) stromal tumors, fibrosarcomas, leiomyosarcomas, hemangiopericytomas, and histiocytomas may also arise in the periampullary region. Similarly, lymphomas can occur in these regions and present with less well-defined margins than the typical adenocarcinomas. Finally, the periampullary region can be the site of metastases from other primaries, including kidney, breast, lung, melanoma, stomach, colon, and germ cell primaries.

▪ ETIOLOGY

There are few established risk factors for cancer of the pancreas. They include tobacco smoking and inherited susceptibility (which account for only 5–10% of cases). Chronic pancreatitis, type II diabetes mellitus, and obesity have been consistently associated with pancreatic cancer, and are weak risk factors. Other possible risk factors include physical inactivity, certain pesticides, and high carbohydrate/sugar intake. Cholecystectomy, cholelithiasis, coffee consumption, and alcohol have been sporadically associated with the development of pancreatic cancer, but they are unlikely true risk factors.

MAJOR ENVIRONMENTAL FACTORS FOR CANCER OF THE PANCREAS

There is a significant amount of evidence that links cigarette smoking to pancreas cancer. Multiple animal studies have demonstrated the carcinogenic effects of tobacco smoke and nitrosamines on the pancreas. Human autopsy studies have revealed increases in hyperplastic changes with atypical nuclear patterns in pancreatic ductal cells of cigarette smokers. Several prospective studies have demonstrated an increased risk ratio of death from pancreatic cancer in smokers ranging from two- to 16-fold.[10] Many of the studies have demonstrated a dose-response relationship with either the number of cigarettes smoked or the duration of smoking.

There are often conflicting data in reviews examining the relationship of dietary factors and cancer of the pancreas.[10–12] Pancreas cancer seems to be associated with increased total calorie intake, as well as increased intake of carbohydrate, cholesterol, meat, salt, dehydrated food, fried food, refined sugar, and nitrosamines. Fat, beta carotene, and coffee are of unproven risk. Consumption of dietary fiber, vitamin C, fruits, vegetables, and unprepared food may have a protective effect, as may pressure and microwave cooking.

Alcohol, coffee, and radiation do not appear to be significant risk factors for development of pancreas cancer. When age, gender, smoking, amount of alcohol consumed, and socioeconomic class were controlled, three case-control studies from Europe did not demonstrate an increased risk of pancreatic cancer with coffee.[10] This is in disagreement with earlier reports of the association between pancreas cancer and coffee consumption.[13,14] Ionizing radiation does not seem to have a propensity to cause pancreas cancer when compared to other tissues. The survivors of the bombings of Hiroshima and Nagasaki have not shown an increased risk.[15,16]

MAJOR HOST FACTORS FOR PANCREAS CANCER

The most striking examples of host factors affecting the development of pancreatic cancer are the genetic syndromes with increased risk. Hereditary nonpolyposis colorectal cancer (HNPCC), familial breast cancer associated with the BRCA2 mutation, Peutz-Jeghers syndrome, ataxia-telangiectasia syndrome, familial atypical multiple mole-melanoma syndrome (FAMMM), and hereditary pancreatitis are the six genetic syndromes in which the afflicted family members have an increased risk of pancreas cancer. Members of families with two or more first-degree relatives affected by pancreatic cancer in the National Familial Pancreas Tumor Registry (NFPTR) have a 16-fold increased risk of developing pancreas cancer. This increased risk could be attributable to either a genetic basis or environmental exposure, but there is strong evidence that the familial aggregation has some genetic basis.[17]

Chronic pancreatitis has been associated with cancer of the pancreas.[10,18–20] It is hard, however, to separate out whether there is a common risk factor for the two diseases, or whether chronic pancreatitis may represent an indolent presentation of pancreatic cancer. The association of diabetes type II and pancreatic cancer is similarly implicated in multiple studies.[21,22] Again, it is difficult to distinguish whether diabetes is an early symptom of pancreas cancer or whether it is truly a causative factor.

RISK FACTORS FOR NONPANCREATIC PERIAMPULLARY CANCERS

Distal common bile duct, ampullary, and duodenal cancers are less common than pancreatic cancer and are less well characterized in terms of their risk factors. All are more common in the elderly with peak incidences in the 60- to 80-year range. Distal common bile duct cancers are associated with several known host factors in addition to advanced age, including inflammatory bowel disease, sclerosing cholangitis, choledochal cysts, and intrahepatic or common bile duct stones. Duodenal and ampullary cancers occur with increased frequency in patients with hereditary polyposis syndromes, including HNPCC, Peutz-Jeghers syndrome, familial adenomatous polyposis, and Gardner's syndrome.

GENETIC ALTERATIONS IN PANCREAS CANCER

Most malignancies are diseases of acquired and inherited mutations in protooncogenes, tumor suppressor genes, and or DNA mismatch repair genes. Mutations in these genes accumulate to yield invasive pancreas cancers. Rozenblum and associates analyzed pancreas cancers from 42 patients and found that all of them (100%) had mutations in the protooncogene K-ras, and 82%, 76%, 53%, and 10% had mutations in the tumor suppressor genes p16, p53, DPC4, and BRCA2, respectively.[23] Oncogenes are derived from normal cellular genes called protooncogenes that, when activated by a mutation or amplification, possess transforming properties. Tumor suppressor genes normally function to restrain cell proliferation. Loss of function of these genes by mutation, deletion, chromosome rearrangement, or mitotic recombination results in abnormally increased cell proliferation. Mutations in DNA mismatch repair genes are implicated in about 4% of pancreas cancers.[24] DNA mismatch repair genes encode for proteins that correct errors that occur during DNA replication. When these mismatch repair genes are mutated, errors in DNA replication are not efficiently repaired, causing simple repeated sequences located throughout the genome, known as cancer repeat and "microsatellite instability" and may lead to pancreas cancer.

■ DIAGNOSIS AND PREOPERATIVE EVALUATION

The diagnosis of periampullary cancer is made on the basis of clinical presentation, laboratory data, and radiologic work-up. Although in some situations a preoperative tissue diagnosis is available, treatment should not be delayed by attempts to obtain histologic confirmation of malignancy.

CLINICAL PRESENTATION

Patients with periampullary cancer often have vague symptoms early in the course of their disease. The symptoms at presentation are related to the location of the tumor. Lesions occurring near the bile duct are much more likely to present with obstructive jaundice, whereas those presenting in the body or tail are more likely to present with pain. Two thirds to three fourths of patients with pancreas cancer present with the classic constellation of symptoms indicative of obstructive jaundice: jaundice, pruritus, acholic stools, and tea-colored urine. Contrary to popular teaching, patients with pancreas cancer often experience pain as a part of their symptoms. Albeit early in the course of the disease, the pain is often vague and involving the upper abdomen, epigastrium, or back. Later in the course of the disease, this pain can progress to severe pain often radiating to the back. Patients may also present with other general symptoms including anorexia, fatigue, malaise, and weight loss. Nausea and vomiting may herald gastric outlet obstruction from duodenal involvement and is an ominous sign of locally advanced disease.

Patients may also present with very subtle signs such as having elevated liver function tests performed on routine laboratory screening, having new onset diabetes mellitus, or anemia from gastrointestinal blood loss, usually from tumor erosion into the duodenum. Patients may also present with acute pancreatitis from obstruction of the pancreatic duct. Therefore, elderly patients who present with acute pancreatitis but without a history of alcohol use or gallbladder stones should be screened for a pancreatic or periampullary cancer.

Patients with a distal common bile duct cancer are even more likely to present with obstructive jaundice than patients with pancreas cancer because the tumor does not have be very large to obstruct the duct. Patients with pancreas cancers involving the body or tail of the gland are more likely to have weight loss and abdominal pain rather than jaundice as their presenting complaints. Because tumors can grow to a larger size before producing noticeable symptoms, pancreas cancers in the body and tail are often diagnosed at a later stage and have a poorer prognosis.

Physical findings on examination include scleral icterus, jaundice, hepatomegaly, a palpable gallbladder (Courvoisier's sign), and skin excoriation from pruritus and scratching. Signs of advanced disease include cachexia, palpable nodules in the liver, palpable metastatic disease in the left supraclavicular fossa (Virchow's node), palpable metastatic disease in the periumbilical area (Sister Mary Joseph's node), and pelvic metastatic disease palpable anteriorly on rectal examination (Blumer's shelf).

Patients who present with obstructive jaundice have elevated serum levels of bilirubin and alkaline phosphatase, usually associated with only mild to moderate elevations in liver transaminases. Long term obstruction of the biliary tree may also lead to coagulopathy and prolongation of protime because of decreased absorption of vitamin K and the effect on the clotting factors of the intrinsic pathway. There are no great serum markers for pancreas cancer to facilitate early diagnosis. A marker commonly used is carbohydrate antigen 19–9 (CA 19–9) which is elevated in 75% of patients with pancreas cancer. Unfortunately, CA 19–9 levels are also elevated in benign conditions of the pancreas, liver, and bile ducts. CA 19–9 is neither sensitive nor specific enough to be used in population screening. It is sometimes of use in trying to measure response to therapy or for screening for recurrence in a patient who originally had an elevation of the marker.

Since approximately 90% of pancreatic cancers contain mutations in the K-ras protooncogene, several groups have tried to detect these mutations from duodenal aspirates, pancreatic duct aspirates, and stool.[25–27] These tests have not become commercially available, but this type of strategy will be necessary to detect disease at an earlier stage.

IMAGING STUDIES

The main imaging modalities used for patients with suspected periampullary neoplasms include right upper quadrant ultrasonography, CT, MRI with or without magnetic resonance cholangiopancreatography (MRCP), endoscopic retrograde cholangiopancreatography (ERCP), and percutaneous transhepatic cholangiography (PTC). The role of positron emission tomography (PET) has not been clearly established for pancreatic and the other periampullary cancers. Over the last 10 years, there has been a trend away from the invasive imaging studies (ERCP and PTC), toward the noninvasive imaging studies. This is especially true as surgeons have become more willing to operate on jaundiced patients based on clinical presentation and imaging studies.

Right upper quadrant ultrasonography is a commonly used initial test and is very sensitive for the detection of gallstones, the presence of a dilated biliary tree, and whether acute cholecystitis is causing a patient's right upper quadrant (RUQ) pain. This study is commonly available around the clock and heavily used in emergency departments. In addition to gallstones, dilatation of the biliary tree, and pericholecystic fluid, this imaging modality can also pick up hepatic metastases, pancreatic masses, peripancreatic and hilar lymphadenopathy, and ascites. The sensitivity for demonstrating pancreatic masses is not high and the absence of a pancreatic mass by RUQ ultrasonography does not rule out the presence of one in the patient.

The "workhorse" in the work-up of patients suspected of a pancreatic cancer or a periampullary neoplasm is a multidetector spiral CT and is probably the single most useful diagnostic and staging modality (Fig 41–1).[28] If a pancreatic mass is identified, spiral CT is often indicated, because CT provides more complete and accurate imaging of the pancreatic head and surrounding structures. It has largely supplanted ultrasound as the initial diagnostic procedure of choice. Pancreatic cancer is much more likely to be visible on a spiral CT than a distal common

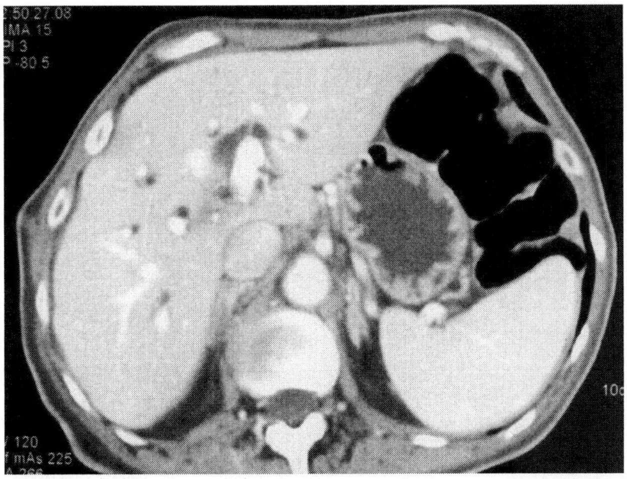

A

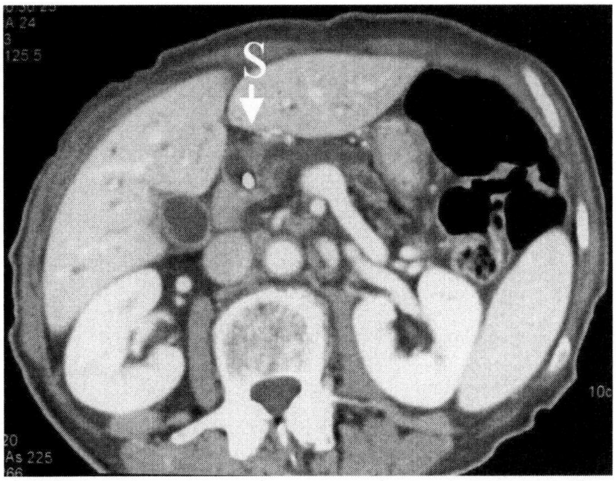

B

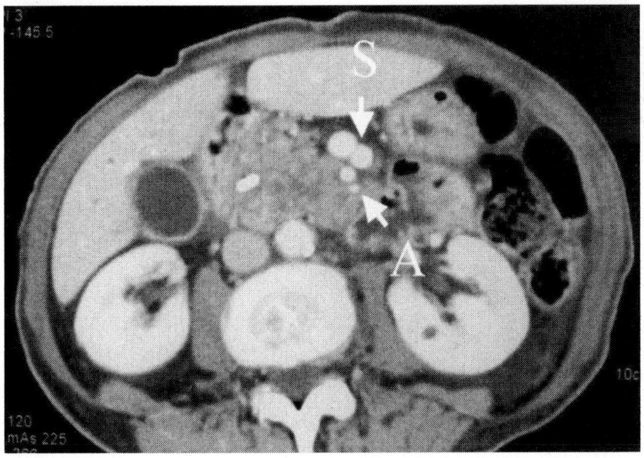

C

Figure 41–1. CT scan of a patient with obstructive jaundice from pancreas cancer. **A.** Dilated intrahepatic ducts. **B.** "Double duct sign" with dilated common bile duct and pancreatic ducts. There is a stent in the common bile duct (S). **C.** Pancreas cancer mass with stent through it (*arrow*). SMA (A) is adjacent to tumor.

bile duct, ampullary, or duodenal cancer. It gives very important information about the immediately adjacent vascular structures such as the portal, superior mesenteric, and splenic veins, as well as the superior mesenteric artery and celiac axis. Three-dimensional reconstruction of these vessels from thin cut multidetector spiral CT scans performed in both arterial and venous phase may also help in visualizing the anatomic relationships between the vessels and the mass (Fig 41–2). The involvement of periampullary lymph nodes and retroperitoneal structures may be demonstrated. Additionally, information about distant metastatic disease can be gleaned if metastatic deposits are seen in the liver or in the peritoneal cavity. The presence of ascites is usually an ominous sign.

When both intra- and extrahepatic ductal dilation are found on imaging studies, but no discrete mass lesion is seen on CT, cholangiography may be useful. Advances in MRI technology allow this modality to play an increasing role in hepatobiliary imaging (Fig 41–3). Ultrafast spin-echo MRI can also be quite sensitive, but it can be limited by motion artifact, lack of bowel opacification, compromised resolution, and patient discomfort from the longer scanning times.[28] MRCP is now being utilized to image the biliary tree and the pancreatic duct. It has the advantage of being completely noninvasive (Fig 41–4). This is also its main disadvantage secondary to the lack of immediate access to perform a therapeutic intervention such as removal of a stone, stenting of a lesion causing proximal biliary or distal pancreatic stasis and infection. The vascular structures can also be visualized with the use of the contrast agent gadolinium and the performance of a magnetic resonance angiogram (MRA). Thus a single (long) session in a scanner can provide information about tumor size and extent (MRI), the intraductal anatomy of the biliary and pancreatic system (MRCP), and the status of the nearby vasculature (MRA). The resulting scan has the potential to provide information about tumor size and extent, biliary and pancreatic ductal anatomy, and vascular involvement through a single, noninvasive procedure.

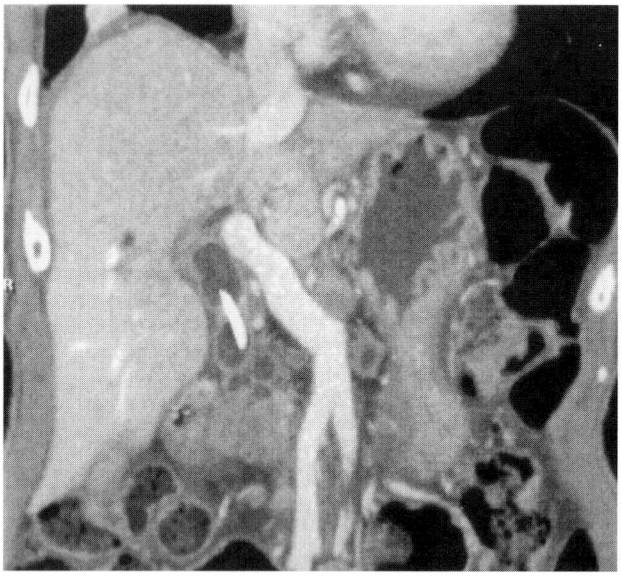

A

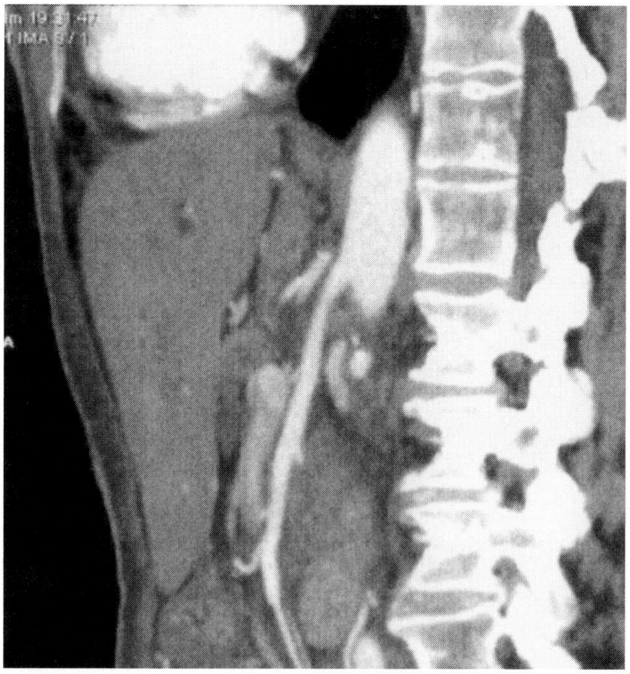

B

Figure 41–2. 3-D CT vascular reconstructions of same patient as in Figure 41–1. **A.** Portal and superior mesenteric veins do not appear involved. **B.** Superior mesenteric artery does not appear involved.

ERCP sometimes is required to solidify the diagnosis of pancreatic cancer. The classic findings of a long, irregular stricture in a pancreatic duct with distal dilation or a "double duct sign" in which there is cutoff of both the pancreatic duct and distal bile duct at the level of the genu of the pancreatic duct are pathognomonic (Fig 41–5). With the current imaging capabilities of CT and MRI, diagnostic ERCP is rarely necessary to guide treatment. However, many patients still show up in surgery clinic already having had an ERCP performed. ERCP may be of benefit in patients with biliary obstruction and cholangitis whereupon an en-

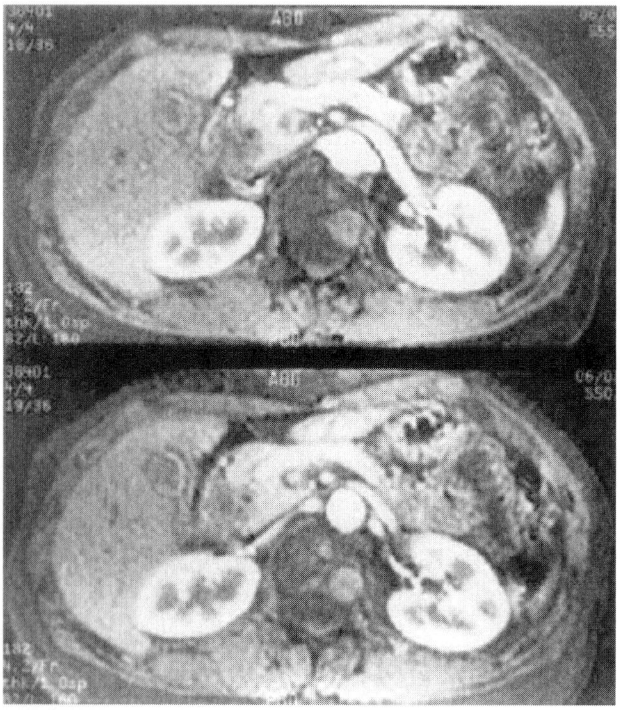

Figure 41–3. T1-weighted MR images with gadolinium contrast. A mass in the head of the pancreas appears hypodense. (From Yeo, et al. *Prob Surg* 199;36:57–152, Fig 17.)

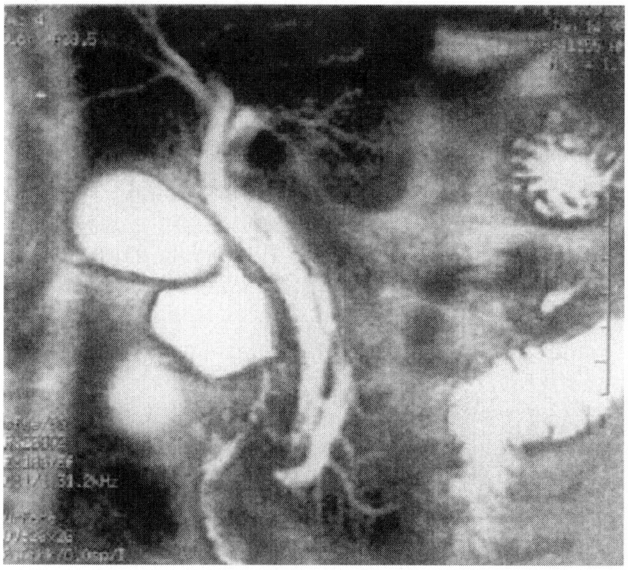

Figure 41–4. Single-shot spin-echo MR cholangiopancreatogram of patient with obstructive jaundice. Both the common bile duct and the pancreatic duct are dilated. The hypointense tumor is apparent in the periampullary region. (From Yeo et al. *Prob Surg* 199;36:57–152, Fig 18.)

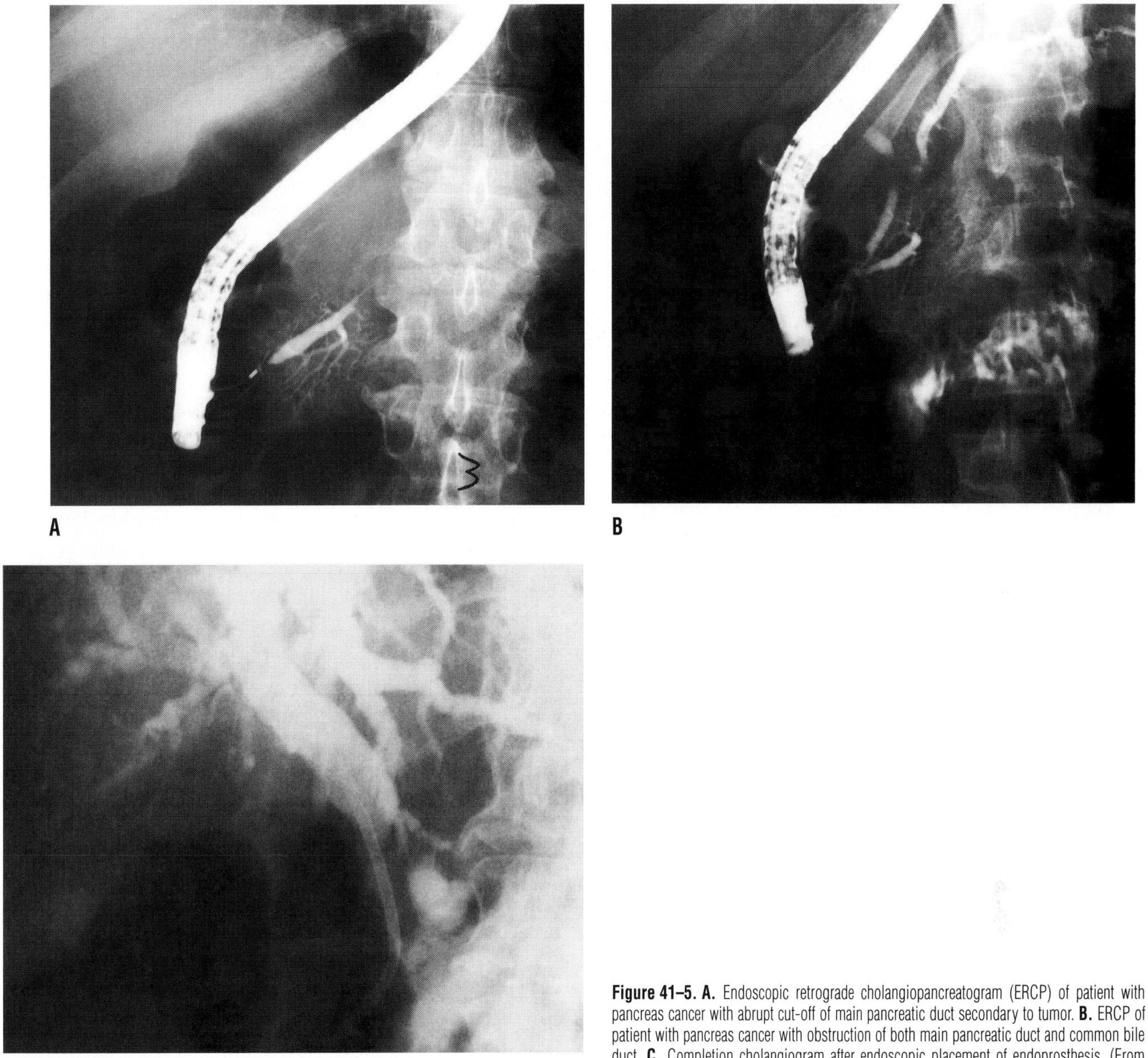

C

Figure 41–5. A. Endoscopic retrograde cholangiopancreatogram (ERCP) of patient with pancreas cancer with abrupt cut-off of main pancreatic duct secondary to tumor. **B.** ERCP of patient with pancreas cancer with obstruction of both main pancreatic duct and common bile duct. **C.** Completion cholangiogram after endoscopic placement of endoprosthesis. (From Lillemoe KD. *Ann Surg* 1995;221:133.)

doscopic stent can be placed for decompression. ERCP is most useful when there is pancreatic duct obstruction, but no mass is evident on either CT or MRI. In this situation, it is necessary to try to distinguish chronic pancreatitis from pancreatic cancer. A history of choledocholithiasis or heavy alcohol consumption in the setting of abdominal pain and multiple focal stenoses of the main pancreatic duct as well as radicals is more compatible with pancreatitis, whereas an abrupt cutoff of the pancreatic duct at a single location in an elderly patient without significant pain is more compatible with pancreas cancer.

PTC is another invasive means of defining the biliary anatomy and better defines the proximal biliary anatomy above the level of obstruction (Fig 41–6). During this procedure a percutaneous biliary drain (PBD) can also be left in place for the relief of cholangitis. The disadvantages of PTC are a result of the more invasive nature of this technique and include bleeding, hemobilia, and patient discomfort, as well as the inability to visualize the pancreatic duct. For periampullary cancer, ERCP is more commonly used than PTC or PBD.

At present the role of PET scanning is not well defined for pancreatic or other periampullary cancers. However, more recent reports support the conclusion that FDG-PET imaging may represent a useful adjunctive study in the evaluation of patients with suspected pancreatic cancer. A comprehensive review of the PET

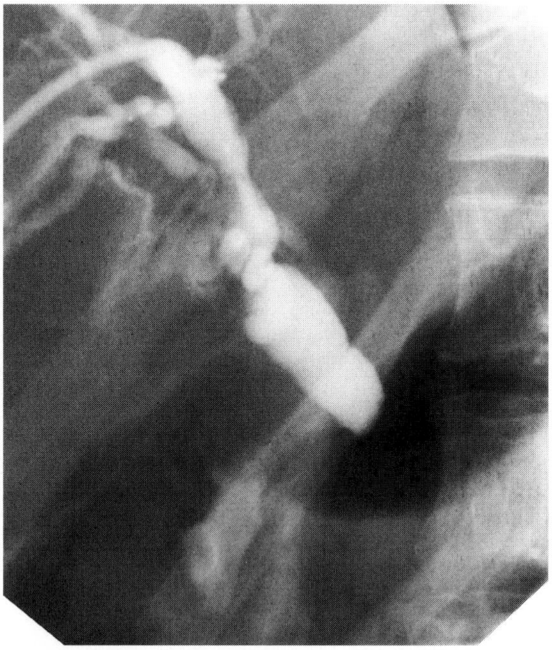

Figure 41–6. Percutaneous transhepatic cholangiogram of patient demonstrating a dilated intrahepatic biliary tree with complete obstruction at the genu of the common bile duct. (From Lillemoe KD. *Ann Surg* 1995;221:133.)

literature (387 patient's studies) has reported weighted averages for FDG-PET sensitivity and specificity of 94% and 90%, respectively, compared with 82% and 75% for CT.[29,30] PET scanning is not currently routinely used in patients suspected of pancreatic or periampullary cancers.

Upper endoscopy is useful in the diagnosis of ampullary and duodenal cancers as these lesions can be directly viewed through the endoscope. If visualized, it is relatively straight-forward to obtain a biopsy and tissue diagnosis. Additionally, endoscopic ultrasound may be performed during upper endoscopy. The duodenum, ampulla, head of the pancreas, and uncinate process of the pancreas are accessible with an ultrasound probe positioned in the duodenum. The body and tail of the pancreas are accessible with an ultrasound probe positioned in the stomach. Fine-needle aspiration (FNA) of any suspected lesions can be performed at the same time as endoscopic ultrasound if tissue diagnosis is of benefit.

TISSUE DIAGNOSIS

The use of percutaneous pancreatic biopsy in the evaluation of a patient with a pancreatic mass who appears resectable and is a good operative candidate remains somewhat controversial. Percutaneous pancreatic mass biopsies can easily be performed, but malignancy cannot be ruled out with certainty when no malignant cells are found in the FNA aspirate. They can be performed safely with rare complications including, fistula, pancreatitis, hemorrhage, abscess, tumor seeding, and death. A negative biopsy in a patient suspected of having pancreas cancer with a low operative risk and apparently resectable disease will not alter the decision to explore the patient. Percutaneous biopsies should only be performed in patients thought to have prohibitively high operative risks or who appear unresectable and are being considered for either neoadjuvant or palliative therapy. In special circumstances as a result of a patient presenting imaging characteristics where lymphoma or metastatic disease from another primary are suspected, percutaneous biopsy has value. These diseases are often best managed without resection. As discussed in the previous section, FNA may be performed at the same time as endoscopic ultrasound (EUS) and may be a more attractive means of obtaining a tissue diagnosis.

Tissue diagnoses of ampullary and duodenal cancers are relatively straightforward and can easily be performed through the endoscope. Due to their locations, the ability to obtain large and deep biopsies allows better sampling. However, the histologic finding of a benign villous adenoma with or without dysplasia cannot reliably rule out malignancy. Distal common bile duct lesions are sometimes scraped with brushes or biopsied via ERCP or PTC in order to obtain a tissue diagnosis. It is often difficult to preoperatively establish the histologic diagnosis of a distal bile duct cancer with false-negative rates nearing 50%.

PREOPERATIVE STAGING

The goal of preoperative staging of pancreas and other periampullary cancers is to determine the optimal treatment for each individual patient. Substantial overlap exists between diagnosis and staging. Multidetector thin slice spiral CT with intravenous contrast is useful in both diagnosis and staging. It can detect liver metastases with high sensitivity if they are over 1 cm, but it often misses those that are less than 1 cm in size. CT scans are not highly accurate in assessing retroperitoneal lymphadenopathy or carcinomatosis in the absence of ascites or large pockets of metastases.[28] Generally, a CT scan of the chest (with or without intravenous contrast) is often performed during the preoperative staging CT. The cost effectiveness of this approach is often questioned and some surgeons prefer a simple chest radiograph. However, when the patient is referred postoperatively for adjuvant or palliative therapy, a staging CT including the chest is usually required. It is rare for pancreas or the other periampullary cancers to metastasize exclusively to the lungs without any signs of dissemination in the abdominal cavity.

Three-dimensional reconstruction of CT scans has also increased the ability to predict resectable disease because of the capability to focus on the vasculature at risk. In a study of 140 patients who were thought to have resectable periampullary tumors after preoperative 3D-CT, 115 (82%) were subsequently determined to have periampullary cancer.[31] The remaining 25 patients had benign disease. Among the patients with periampullary cancer, the extent of local tumor burden involving the pancreas and peripancreatic tissues was accurately depicted by 3D-CT in 93% of the patients. 3D-CT was 95% accurate in determining cancer invasion of the superior mesenteric vessels. Preoperative 3D-CT accurately predicted periampullary cancer resectability and a margin-negative resection in 98% and 86% of patients, respectively. For patients with pancreatic adenocarcinoma (n = 85), preoperative 3D-CT resulted in a resectability rate and a margin-negative resection rate of 79% and 73%, respectively. The ability of 3D-CT to predict a margin-negative resection for periampullary cancer, including pancreatic adenocarcinoma, relies on its enhanced assessment of the extent of local tumor burden and involvement of the mesenteric vascular anatomy. Encasement of the portal or superior mesenteric vein over a distance not amenable to vascular reconstruction after resection, and/or encasement of the superior mesenteric, celiac, or hepatic arteries with or without occlusion are ominous signs and portend unresectability.

EUS is sometimes used to stage patients with periampullary lesions, especially if an FNA diagnosis is important in the decision to operate (Fig 41–7). It is highly accurate in assessing the size of the primary lesion. More information is needed to adequately assess its accuracy in predicting vascular involvement. It is very operator dependent and in borderline cases may lead to the overcall of vessel involvement. EUS is poor at predicting lymph node involvement or liver metastases unless they are quite sizable.

Depending on the medical institution, experienced surgeons will always use, never use, or selectively use staging laparoscopy in the management of periampullary cancers. Proponents of routine use of laparoscopy feel that its use will save significant numbers of patients from the morbidity and mortality of exploratory laparotomy only to find metastatic and/or locally unresectable disease. They feel that if a patient cannot be resected for potential cure, they are best palliated by nonoperative means.[32] The general arguments made against routine laparoscopy are that current cross-sectional imaging studies are good enough where it does not make sense to subject all patients to laparoscopy to pick up the few who have metastatic and/or locally unresectable disease. They further argue that as many as 20% of the unresectable patients will go on to develop gastric outlet obstruction requiring surgical intervention. They feel that the ability to perform a hepatojejunostomy will more durably relieve obstructive jaundice.[33] Additionally they feel that operative chemical splanchnicectomy will be of benefit. Yet others will selectively use staging laparoscopy.[34] The likelihood of finding disease that is unresectable is highest in those with pancreas cancers involving the body or tail or uncinate process. These lesions usually are larger and more advanced at the time of diagnosis because they do not tend to cause obstructive jaundice. The likelihood of finding disease that is unresectable is lower for duodenal, ampullary, and distal common bile duct cancer compared to pancreas cancer.

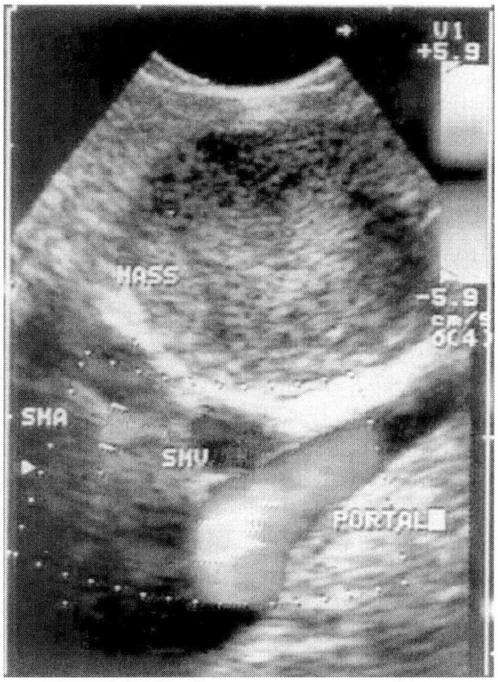

Figure 41–7. EUS image with linear array echoendoscope demonstrating a mass in the head of the pancreas with no vascular invasion of the superior mesenteric artery (SMA), superior mesenteric vein (SMV), or portal vein (PORTAL). (From Lillemoe KD. *Ann Surg* 1995;221:133.)

■ CLINICOPATHOLOGIC STAGING

Patients with exocrine pancreatic, distal bile duct, ampullary, and duodenal carcinomas are staged according to the American Joint Committee on Cancer (AJCC) staging system. These staging criteria are based on the size and extent of the primary tumor (T stage), lymph node involvement (N stage), and the presence of distant metastases (M stage). Based on these criteria, patients are stratified to the different stage groupings that guide prognosis and treatment. Pancreatic adenocarcinomas are staged using the AJCC exocrine pancreas guidelines. Distal common bile duct cancers are staged using the AJCC extrahepatic bile duct guidelines. Ampullary cancers are staged using the AJCC ampulla of Vater guidelines. Duodenal cancers are staged using the AJCC small intestine guidelines.

▪ RESECTION OF PERIAMPULLARY CANCERS

OPERATIVE TECHNIQUE OF PANCREATICODUODENECTOMY (WHIPPLE PROCEDURE)

Exposure for a pancreaticoduodenectomy can be performed through a vertical midline incision from the xiphoid process to several centimeters below the umbilicus. Alternatively, a bilateral subcostal incision can be used. Exposure is greatly enhanced with the use of a mechanical retracting device.

The first portion of a pancreaticoduodenectomy is devoted to assessing the extent of disease and resectability. The benefits and disadvantages of staging laparoscopy were discussed in the previous section. At open exploration, the entire liver is assessed for the presence of metastases not seen by preoperative imaging studies. The celiac axis is inspected for lymph node involvement. Tumor-bearing nodes within the resection zone do not contraindicate resection because long-term survival is sometimes achieved with peripancreatic nodal involvement. The parietal and visceral peritoneal surfaces, the omentum, the ligament of Treitz, and the entire small and intra-abdominal large intestine are carefully examined for the presence of metastatic disease. An extensive Kocher maneuver is performed by elevating the duodenum and head of the pancreas out of the retroperitoneum and into the midline, allowing the visualization of the superior mesenteric artery at its origin at the aorta (Fig 41–8). The porta hepatis is assessed by mobilizing the gallbladder and dissecting the cystic duct down to the junction of the common hepatic and common bile duct. The common hepatic artery and proper hepatic artery should also be assessed to determine that they are free of tumor involvement.

If the intraoperative assessment reveals localized disease without tumor encroachment upon resection margins, the resection is performed in relatively standard fashion. If assessment reveals evidence of local tumor extension giving the early impression of possible unresectability, the normal sequence for performing the pancreaticoduodenectomy should be modified. The easiest and safest portions of the resection should be performed first, and the more difficult portions later. Tumors that initially appear unresectable can be successfully resected by patiently working where it is easiest first and finishing the harder portions later.

The distal common hepatic duct is divided close to the level of the cystic duct entry site early during the operation. For distal common bile duct cancers or pancreatic cancers near this area, more margin on the bile duct into the hilus of the liver may be required. The bile duct is retracted caudally and a dissection plane is opened on the anterior surface of the portal vein. During these maneuvers, the portal structures should be assessed for a replaced right hepatic artery originating from the superior mesenteric artery. If found, this vessel should be dissected and protected from injury. If the patient appears to have an accessory right hepatic artery and a significant native right hepatic artery, the accessory vessel can often be taken without consequence. The gastroduodenal artery is next identified and clamped atraumatically. This maneuver confirms that the hepatic artery is not being supplied solely retrograde through the superior mesenteric artery collaterals (in the setting of celiac axis stenosis or occlusion).

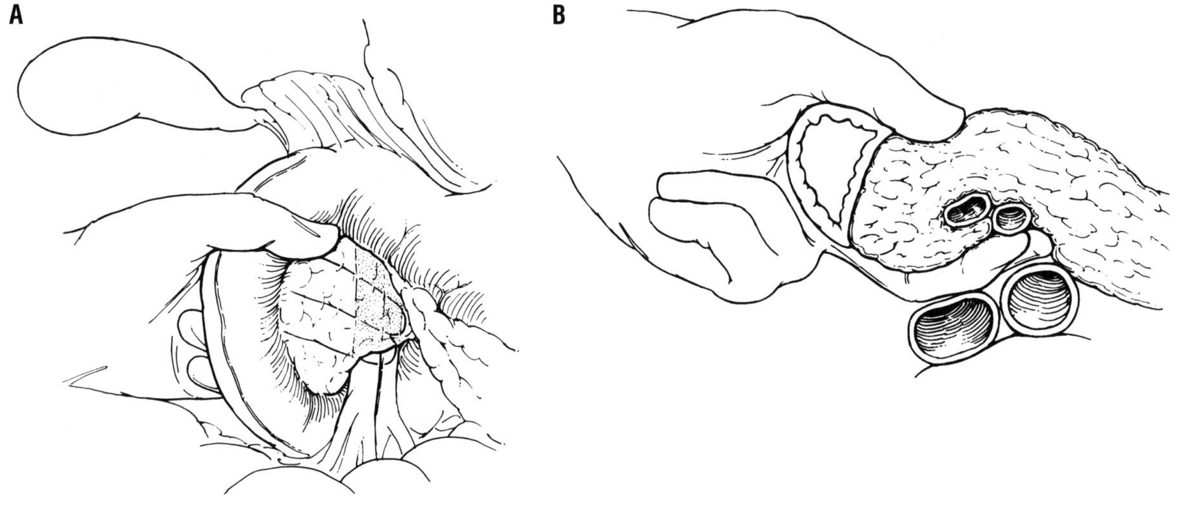

Figure 41–8. The uncinate process, head of the pancreas, and superior mesenteric artery are palpated between the thumb and index finger. This maneuver enables the surgeon to determine whether the tumor has extended into the uncinate process to involve the superior mesenteric artery. (From Crist DW, Cameron JL. The current status of the Whipple operation for periampullary carcinoma. *Adv Surg* 1992;25:21.)

For a classic Whipple procedure, a 30–40% distal gastrectomy is performed by dividing the right gastric and right gastroepiploic arteries. The antrectomy is then completed using a linear stapling device. For a pylorus-preserving pancreaticoduodenectomy, the proximal GI tract is divided 2 to 3 cm distal to the pylorus with a linear stapling device. The right gastric artery can often be spared, but may be taken if it allows better mobilization of the duodenum for reconstruction. The gastrointestinal tract is divided distally at a point of mobile jejunum, typically 20 cm distal to the ligament of Treitz. The mesenteric vessels to this initial portion of the jejunum are carefully divided over clamps and tied to avoid bleeding. Once the proximal jejunum is separated from its mesentery, it can be delivered dorsal to the superior mesenteric vessels from the left to the right side.

The superior mesenteric vein caudal to the neck of the pancreas can be identified by performing an extensive Kocher maneuver. The superior mesenteric vein is identified running anterior to the third portion of the duodenum and is frequently surrounded by adipose tissue as it receives tributaries from the uncinate process and neck of the pancreas, the greater curve of the stomach, and from the transverse mesocolon. In this location, the superior mesenteric vein is identified by dissecting the fatty tissue of the transverse mesocolon away from the uncinate process of the pancreas. Division of the branches emptying into the anterior surface of the superior mesenteric vein allows continued cephalad dissection. Often a vein retractor lifting the inferior edge of the neck of the pancreas is useful for visualization (Fig 41–9). The plane anterior to the superior mesenteric vein is developed under direct vision, avoiding branches and tumor involvement (Fig 41–10). Care should be taken to avoid inadvertent damage to the splenic vein as it joins the superior mesenteric vein posterior to the neck of the pancreas. After the plane anterior to the portal vein and superior mesenteric vein is complete, a Penrose drain is looped under the neck of the pancreas.

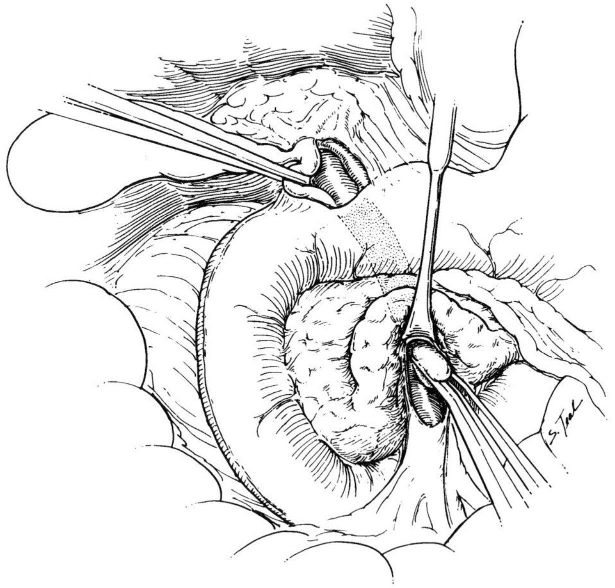

Figure 41–10. The SMV and portal veins are separated from the neck of the pancreas by dissection above and below the pancreas. The dissection should be limited to the anterior surface of these vessels, since there are usually no venous branches in this plane. (From Crist DW, Cameron JL. The current status of the Whipple operation for periampullary carcinoma. *Adv Surg* 1992;25:21.)

Stay sutures are placed superiorly and inferiorly on the pancreatic remnant to reduce bleeding from the segmental pancreatic arteries running in those locations. The pancreatic neck is then divided after confirming a free plane anterior to the portal and superior mesenteric veins. The Penrose drain previously placed behind the neck of the pancreas is used to elevate the pancreatic tissue to be divided and protect the underly-

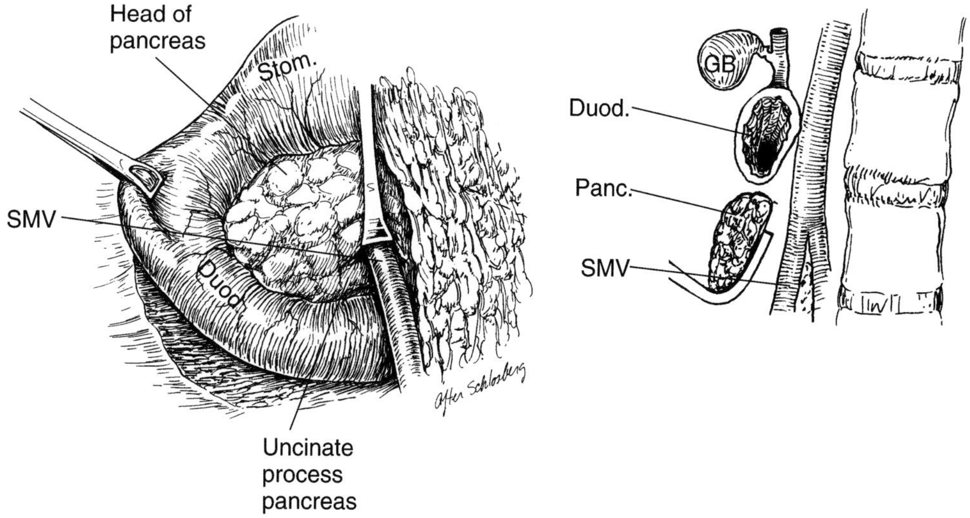

Figure 41–9. If one extends the Kocher maneuver of the duodenum along the third portion, the first structure one encounters anterior to the duodenum is the SMV. It can be cleaned quickly and visualized under direct vision from the posterior aspect of the pancreas (insert), and the dissection can be connected to that of the portal vein from above. Stom., stomach; Duod., duodenum; GB, gallbladder.

ing major veins. Some attention has been paid to identifying the blood supply of the resection margin of the pancreatic remnant and to not using electrocautery to divide the pancreas.[35] The site of the main pancreatic duct should be noted so it can be incorporated into the subsequent reconstruction.

The specimen now remains connected by the uncinate process of the pancreas. This structure is separated from the portal vein, superior mesenteric vein, and superior mesenteric artery. This is performed by serially clamping, dividing and tying the smaller branches off the portal and superior mesenteric vessels (Fig 41–11). Dissection should be performed flush with these structures to remove all pancreatic and nodal tissue in these areas. Great care is taken not to injure the superior mesenteric artery and vein at this level, but to remove completely the pancreatic tissue and lymph nodes near the vascular structures. With these areas dissected, the specimen is removed and the pancreatic neck margin, uncinate margin, and common hepatic duct margins are marked for the pathologists. To speed up analysis of these frozen section margins, the common hepatic duct margin and the pancreatic neck margin may be sampled earlier and sent to pathology while the main specimen is still being removed.

There are multiple options for reconstruction after pancreaticoduodenectomy. Most commonly the reconstruction first involves the pancreas, followed by the bile duct, and then the duodenum. The issues and controversies surrounding the pancreatic and biliary reconstructions are outlined by multiple papers specifically addressing these issues.

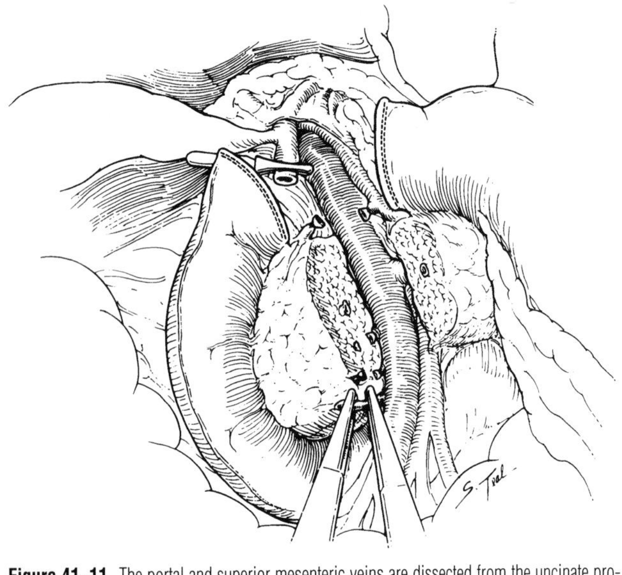

Figure 41–11. The portal and superior mesenteric veins are dissected from the uncinate process of the pancreas and the small venous branches between the veins and the uncinate process are ligated and divided carefully. (From Crist DW, Cameron JL. The current status of the Whipple operation for periampullary carcinoma. *Adv Surg* 1992;25:21.)

The most common reconstruction involves the end of the divided jejunum placed in retrocolic fashion with creation of a pancreaticojejunostomy, followed by hepaticojejunostomy, and then a duodenojejunostomy (Figs 41–12B and 41–12C). The pancreatic reconnection is the most problematic anastomosis out of the three and responsible for much of the morbidity and mortality associated with the procedure.

If the jejunum is used for reconstruction, some groups favor a separate Roux-en-Y reconstruction for the pancreas. Controversy continues regarding the best type of pancreaticojejunostomy, the importance of duct-to-mucosa sutures, and the use of pancreatic duct stents. The pancreatic reconstruction is typically performed with either a duct-to-mucosal anastomosis or with an invagination technique. With either technique the proximal jejunal stump is brought through a defect in the mesocolon to the right of the middle colic artery. The duct to mucosal anastomosis is constructed in an end-to-side fashion in which the outer back row consists of interrupted 3-0 silk sutures incorporating the capsule of the transected pancreas and seromuscular bites of the jejunum. A small defect is then made in the jejunum to which a duct-to-mucosa anastomosis is performed incorporating the pancreatic duct and the full thickness of the jejunum using interrupted 5-0 or 4-0 Maxon. Some surgeons prefer to stent this anastomosis with a 6-cm stent cut from a 5F or 8F (French) pediatric feeding tube. Three cm of the stent are placed into the pancreatic duct and the other half is placed into the jejunum. The stent is held in place with an absorbable stitch such as 4-0 Vicryl. This stent typically passes through the rest of the intestinal tract within a couple of weeks.

The invagination technique is typically performed with an end-to-end or end-to-side pancreaticojejunostomy. The pancreatic remnant should be circumferentially cleared and mobilized for 2 to 3 cm, to allow for an optimal anastomosis. The pancreaticojejunostomy is typically performed in two layers. The outer layer consists of interrupted silk sutures that incorporate the capsule of the pancreas and the seromuscular layers of the jejunum. The inner layer consists of a running 3-0 absorbable suture (or interrupted absorbable sutures) that incorporates the capsule and a portion of the cut edge of the pancreas and the full thickness of the jejunum. If possible, the inner layer should incorporate the pancreatic duct for several bites, to splay it open. When completed, this anastomosis nicely invaginates the cut surface of the pancreatic neck into the jejunal lumen.

If the stomach is used to reconnect the pancreas, it is invaginated into the back wall of the stomach as described previously for the jejunum (Fig 41–12A). In a

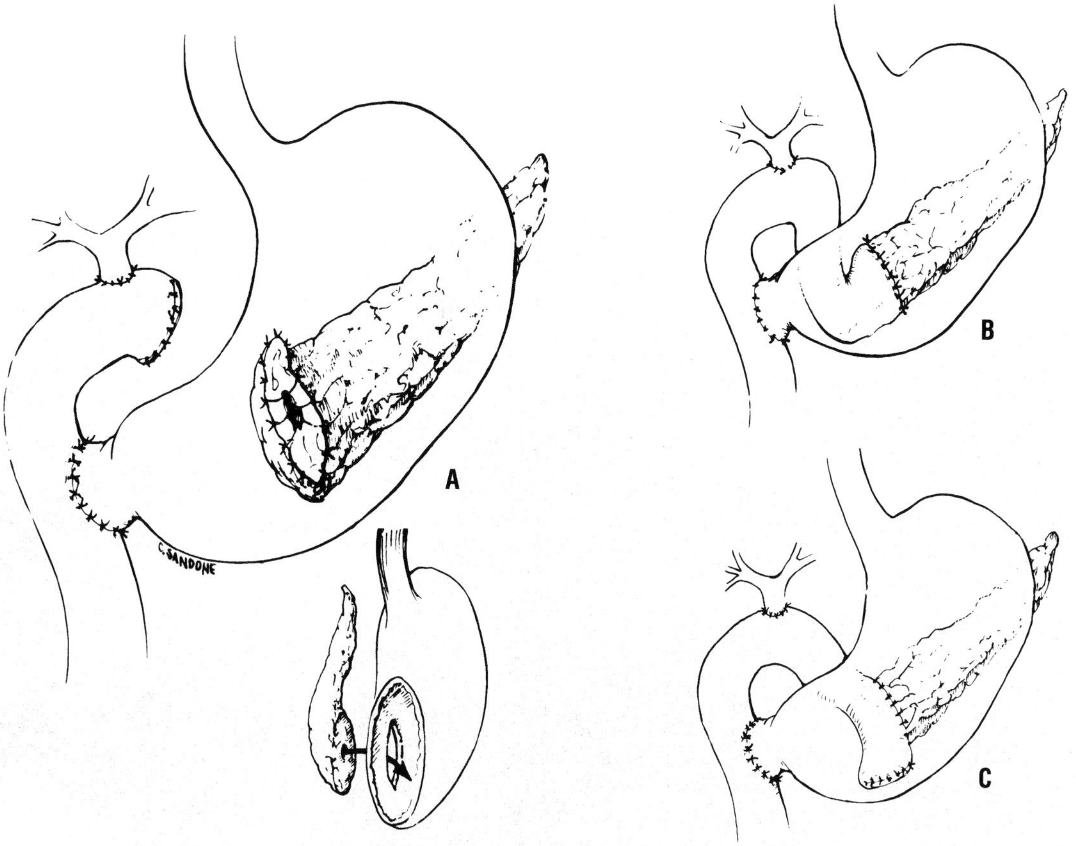

Figure 41–12. Schematic illustration of: **A.** pancreaticogastrostomy; **B.** end-to-end pancreaticojejunostomy; and **C.** end-to-side pancreaticojejunostomy. Insert: detailed pancreaticogastrostomy, indicating the location of the posterior gastrostomy. (From Yeo CJ, Cameron JL, Maher MM, et al. A prospective randomized trial of pancreaticogastrostomy versus pancreaticojejunostomy after pancreaticoduodenectomy. *Ann Surg* 1995;222:580.)

prospective randomized trial comparing pancreaticogastrostomy to pancreaticojejunostomy, there was no difference in the leak or fistula rate between the two types of anastomoses.[36]

The biliary anastomosis is typically performed with an end-to-side hepaticojejunostomy approximately 10 to 15 cm down the jejunal limb from the pancreaticojejunostomy. This anastomosis is typically performed with a single layer of interrupted absorbable sutures. If the patient has a percutaneous biliary stent, this is left in place, traversing the anastomosis. Preoperative biliary stenting remains controversial. Current data indicate that routine preoperative biliary stenting is of no benefit and carries potential risk, including an increased risk of wound or infectious complications, as well as an increased risk of pancreatic fistula formation.[37–39] Stenting should be used selectively in patients with obstructive jaundice who will have a substantial delay between initial presentation and definitive surgery, in patients who have undergone previous biliary-bypass surgery, and in rare patients with primary suppurative cholangitis. The method of stenting, endoscopic versus percutaneous, should be chosen based on local expertise.

The third anastomosis performed is the duodenojejunostomy in cases of pylorus preservation, or the gastrojejunostomy in patients who have undergone classic pancreaticoduodenectomy with distal gastrectomy. This anastomosis is typically performed 10 to 15 cm downstream from the hepaticojejunostomy, proximal to the jejunum traversing the defect in the mesocolon.

After the reconstruction is completed, closed suction drains are left in place to drain the biliary and pancreatic anastomoses. Some groups prefer not to place closed suction drains, accepting that, if a fluid collection becomes clinically evident postoperatively, percutaneous drainage by interventional radiology may be required.

The postoperative management following pancreaticoduodenectomy consists of keeping the patient with nothing by mouth for 1 or 2 days and advancing the diet with liquids and then solids as tolerated. The stomach is decompressed overnight after the day of surgery with a nasogastric tube which is usually removed the next morning unless there is an extraordinarily high output. The drains around the pancreatic anastomosis are typically removed once the patient has been on a regular diet. Drain amylase is typically checked prior to pulling the drains to check for leak or fistula.

▪ DISTAL PANCREATECTOMY FOR PANCREAS CANCER IN THE BODY OR TAIL

Staging with laparoscopy is often of benefit in patients with distal pancreatic cancers. If metastatic disease is found, distal pancreatectomy is unlikely to help in the palliation of the patient. The advantages of performing splenectomy with distal pancreatectomy include the ability to gain wider margins, removal of lymph nodes and lymphatic tissues at the tip of the pancreas and the hilum of the spleen, and avoidance of the tedious dissection of the splenic artery and vein away from the pancreatic parenchyma. The main disadvantage is the perceived increased incidence of postsplenectomy sepsis. For this reason, vaccines are given either preoperatively or after recovery postoperatively for pneumococcus, *Haemophilus meningitides*, and *H. influenza*.

Exposure for a distal pancreatectomy and splenectomy can be obtained through a vertical midline incision from the xiphoid process to several cm below the umbilicus. Alternatively, a bilateral subcostal incision can be used. Exposure is greatly enhanced with the use of a mechanical retracting device. Folded sheets placed behind the patient underlying the spleen can also enhance exposure, especially in patients with a deep body habitus.

The lesser sac should be entered by elevating the greater omentum off of the transverse colon. The splenic flexure of the colon should also be mobilized caudally and away from the spleen by dividing the ileocolic ligament. The spleen can technically be preserved for benign disease; however, for cancer most groups prefer to remove the spleen en bloc to gain a wider margin and incorporate the lymph nodes in the splenic hilum. The spleen is mobilized towards the midline by dividing the lienorenal ligament with the electrocautery device. The short gastric vessels in the lienogastric ligament should be also be isolated and ligated. A plane is then developed behind the pancreatic tail and body, also mobilizing the splenic artery and vein. This dissection is continued several centimeters beyond the tumor. The splenic artery and vein are isolated at this level and are suture ligated. A row of overlapping "U" stitches of absorbable suture should then be placed. The electrocautery device is then used to transect the pancreatic parenchyma distal to this suture line. A frozen section should be performed on the pancreatic margin to confirm clearance of the lesion.

▪ OPERATIVE PALLIATION

With accurate preoperative staging, the resectability rate for periampullary cancers is approximately 80%.[31,40–43] When a patient undergoes exploratory laparotomy (and sometimes exploratory laparoscopy) and is found to be unresectable, a decision must be made as to whether to operatively palliate the patient. Operative palliation is indicated in a patient without widespread metastatic disease and with a relatively long life expectancy. The added potential morbidity and mortality of operative palliation must be weighed against the more durable palliation achieved with hepaticojejunostomy and/or gastrojejunostomy (Fig 41–13). Additionally, chemical splanchnicectomy can be performed at the same time for relief of pain (Fig 41–14).

OPERATIVE PALLIATION OF OBSTRUCTIVE JAUNDICE

The most commonly performed operative procedure for the relief of obstructive jaundice is hepaticojejunostomy, and cholecystojejunostomy should no longer be performed. Simple drainage through a T tube inserted above the biliary obstruction should be avoided as this causes a high output biliary fistula and results in major electrolyte abnormalities. Hepaticojejunostomy provides more durable relief of obstructive jaundice than does cholecystojejunostomy because of the proximity of the cystic duct to most periampullary cancers.[44,45] The hepaticojejunostomy is performed after cholecystectomy in an end-to-side fashion to either a Roux limb or a loop of jejunum with a Braun jejunojejunostomy between the afferent and efferent limbs. Only 4% of patients with unresectable periampullary cancers palliated with hepaticojejunostomies develop recurrent jaundice prior to their deaths.[41] As operative palliation is attempted more with minimally invasive techniques, perhaps laparoscopic cholecystojejunostomies will be performed more often secondary to the relative ease with which they can be done and to avoid a major incision.

OPERATIVE PALLIATION OF DUODENAL OBSTRUCTION

Periampullary cancers may cause gastric outlet obstruction by compromising the duodenal lumen. Most patients with gastric outlet obstruction from a periampullary cancer that is not widely disseminated benefit from palliation, whether operative or with endoscopic stenting techniques. There remains controversy, however regarding the role of prophylactic gastrojejunostomy in a patient who is being explored but without symptoms of gastric outlet obstruction. Much of this controversy rests on the exact proportion of patients who actually develop gastric outlet obstruction requiring surgical intervention in the course of their disease.

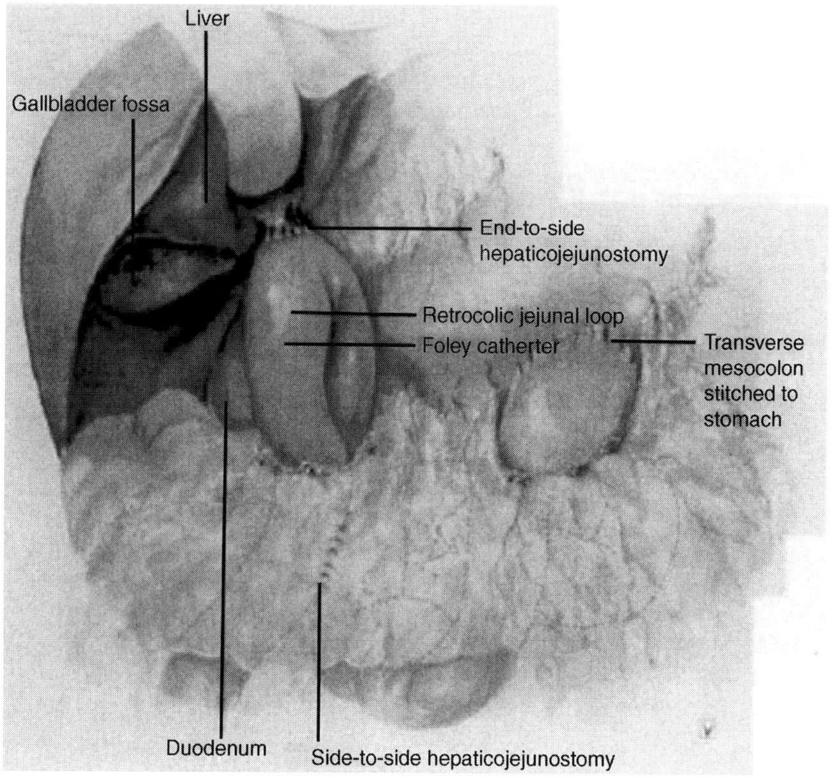

Figure 41–13. Anatomy after one method of palliative intervention. The biliary-enteric anastomosis is shown as a retrocolic end-to-side hepaticojejunostomy with a jejunal loop. A jejunojejunostomy is performed below the transverse mesocolon, to divert the enteric stream away from the biliary tree. Also shown is a retrocolic gastrojejunostomy. (From Cameron JL. *Atlas of Surgery,* Volume 1. Toronto: B.C. Decker; 1990:427, Image V.)

This number is surprisingly low in some series (3%),[46] and approaches 20% in other series.[47] In a prospective, randomized trial from the Johns Hopkins Hospital, 87 patients with unresectable periampullary cancers without signs of gastric outlet obstruction were randomized to either a retrocolic gastrojejunostomy or no gastric bypass.[49] None of the patients who underwent prophylactic gastrojejunostomy subsequently developed gastric outlet obstruction, whereas, 19% of the patients who did not have a gastric bypass subsequently developed gastric outlet obstruction requiring intervention. In this study, performance of the gastrojejunostomy did increase operative time, but it did not increase morbidity, mortality, or length of stay. The gastrojejunostomies were performed typically in a retrocolic (to the left of the middle colic vessels) and isoperistaltic fashion, using a loop of jejunum 20 to 30 cm beyond the ligament of Treitz. The gastrotomy is placed on the back wall of the stomach in the most dependent portion. Vagotomy is not routinely performed because of its contribution to delayed gastric emptying, the limited life expectancy of the patients, and the ability to control acid secretion medically.

OPERATIVE CHEMICAL SPLANCHNICECTOMY FOR PAIN

Operative chemical splanchnicectomy was first introduced in the 1960s to alleviate some of the pain associated with unresectable pancreas cancer.[48] A prospective, randomized trial compared intraoperative chemical splanchnicectomy to placebo in 137 patients with unresectable pancreatic cancer.[49] The procedure was performed by injecting 20 mL of 50% ethanol or saline through a spinal needle on either side of the aorta at the level of the celiac plexus. There were no differences in hospital morbidity, mortality, or length of stay. The group receiving the alcohol had significantly lower pain scores at 2, 4, and 6 months postoperatively. Even those patients who did not report pain preoperatively derived benefit from the splanchnicectomy as they appeared to have a delay in the onset of their pain and had lower pain scores as their disease progressed when compared to control patients.

▪ NONOPERATIVE PALLIATION

Only 15–20% of patients with pancreas cancer are found to be resectable for cure at the time of presentation because of disseminated disease or locally advanced disease. Patients with distal common bile duct, ampullary, and duodenal cancers are more likely to be resectable. For the majority of patients, palliation of symptoms is the primary goal of any invasive intervention. As discussed in the previous section, the three main problems that need to be palliated are obstructive jaundice, gastric outlet obstruction, and pain.

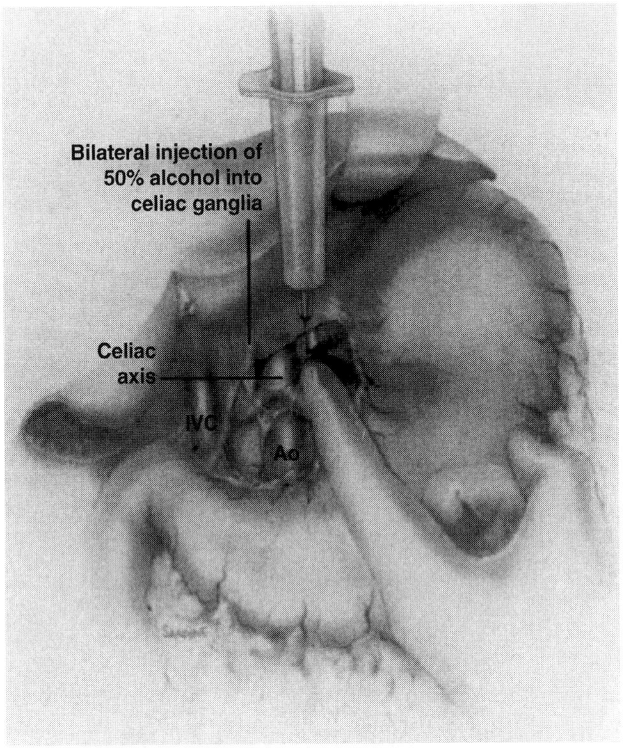

Figure 41–14. Technique of alcohol celiac nerve block. Twenty milliliters of 50% alcohol are injected on each side of the aorta (Ao) at the level of the celiac axis. IVC, inferior vena cava. (From Lillemoe KD, et al. *Ann Surg* 1993;217:447–57.)

NONOPERATIVE PALLIATION OF OBSTRUCTIVE JAUNDICE

Nonoperative biliary drainage can be achieved either through a percutaneous or an endoscopic approach (Fig 41–15). Percutaneous transhepatic approaches are aided by the fact that the intrahepatic ducts are usually dilated in patients presenting with obstructive jaundice. Endoscopic drainage has the advantage of not having any external catheters. In a randomized trial comparing endoscopic versus percutaneous stent placement in 70 patients, the success rate, overall complication rate, and procedure related mortality rate was significantly lower in the endoscopic group.[50] Endoscopic biliary stents may be either plastic or metal. Plastic stents are generally temporary and are available in different diameters and lengths. Because of the limitations in the diameter of the accessory channel of endoscopes, usually the largest plastic stent that can be placed is 12F. This relatively small diameter results in frequent occlusion and the necessity of periodically changing these stents. In an effort to improve on the rate of stent occlusion, self-expanding metallic stents have been developed and when deployed can reach a diameter of 30F. Randomized controlled clinical trials comparing 10F or 11.5F plastic stents to 30F metallic stents have shown metallic stents to have a longer patency rate (6.2 to 9.1 months compared to 4.2 to 4.6 months) and to be associated with lower rates of cholangitis, stent replacement/revision, and hospital days.[51,52] Metallic stents eventually fail because of tumor ingrowth at the ends and through the interstices. Polyurethane-covered stents are currently being developed and used and probably have better patency and results. The disadvantage of metallic stents is that they cost more and should be used in patients who are expected to live longer than 6 months.

NONOPERATIVE PALLIATION OF DUODENAL OBSTRUCTION

Until recently, duodenal obstruction in patients found to be unfit for surgical bypass was treated with placement of gastrostomy tubes. The development of expandable metallic bowel stents have provided an additional way of controlling gastric outlet obstruction in this group of patients. Gastroduodenal stenting is successful in 80–90% of patients and provides adequate relief of obstruction in most patients.[53,54]

NONOPERATIVE PALLIATION OF PAIN

In addition to opioids and nonsteroidal anti-inflammatory agents, several nonoperative palliative treatment modalities for pain with periampullary cancers have been developed including ultrasound or CT-guided celiac plexus nerve blocks and even external beam radiotherapy. Several randomized controlled clinical trials comparing percutaneous celiac plexus nerve blocks to standard oral analgesics have demonstrated significant diminution in pain and narcotic use in the majority of the patients.[55,56]

▪ COMPLICATIONS FOLLOWING PANCREATICODUODENECTOMY

The mortality rate after pancreaticoduodenectomy at centers specializing in pancreatic surgery is in the range of 2–3%. Despite low mortality rates, the incidence of postoperative complication remains high. In a series of 650 consecutive pancreaticoduodenectomies, the mortality rate was 1.4% with a complication rate of 41% (Table 41–1).[57] The three most common complications were delayed gastric emptying in 19%, pancreatic fistula in 14%, and wound infection in 10%. Delayed gastric emptying is not life-threatening and is usually self-limited. The condition, however, can significantly increase lengths of stay for the patient, as well as hospital costs. Patients are usually treated with parenteral nutritional support and nasogastric decompression until the condition resolves. Erythromycin, a motilin agonist, has been shown to improve gastric emptying after pancreaticoduodenectomy and is some-

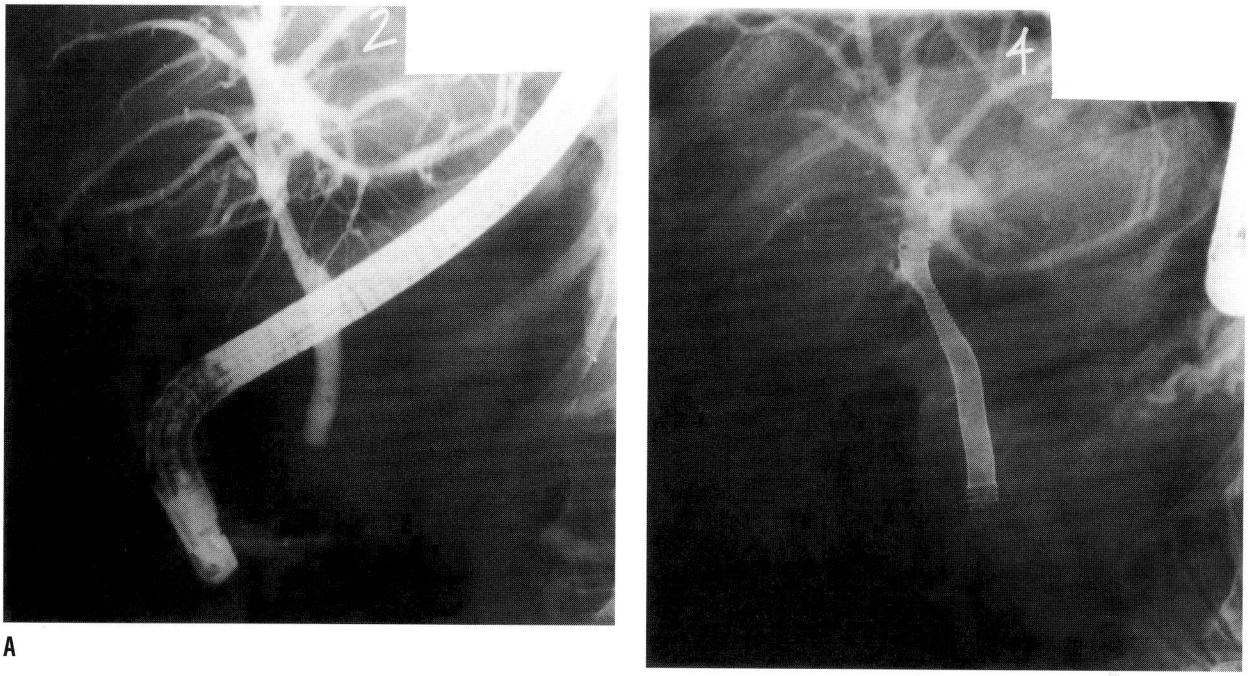

A

B

Figure 41–15. A. Endoscopic retrograde cholangiopancreatogram (ERCP) showing distal bile duct obstruction owing to pancreatic cancer. **B**. ERCP showing a metallic expandable stent in place.

times used.[58] Pancreatic fistulae are not uncommon after pancreaticoduodenectomy. The reported rates of pancreatic fistula vary and to some degree depend on how they are defined. In general, a pancreatic fistula exists if at 7 days postoperatively, there is amylase-rich fluid in excess of 50 mL per day. In the great majority of patients, the pancreatic leak will seal with conservative management. Most centers place intraoperative closed-suction drains near the pancreatic anastomosis to control potential leaks. Some centers do not place drains intraoperatively and prefer to have them placed postoperatively and by interventional radiological techniques should the patient become symptomatic with a pancreatic leak.[59] If the patient is relatively asymptomatic and the output is less than 200 mL per day while on a diet, consideration toward sending the patient home with outpatient drain management should be given. In most cases, the fistula will improve and cease within a couple of weeks. If the patient is symptomatic or the fistula is high output (>200 mL per day), consideration to making the patient NPO and using parenteral nutrition should be given.

TABLE 41–1. POSTOPERATIVE RESULTS OF 650 CONSECUTIVE PANCREATICODUODENECTOMIES AT JOHN HOPKINS HOSPITAL

	Number	%
Mortality		
Yes	9	1.4
No	641	98.6
Reoperation		
Yes	26	4
No	624	96
Complications		
No	384	59
Yes	266	41
Delayed gastric emptying	124	19
Pancreatic fistula	92	14
Wound infection	66	10
Intra-abdominal abscess	33	5
Cholangitis	31	5
Pneumonia	20	3
Bile leak	17	3
Pancreatitis	12	2
Marginal ulcer	6	1
Postoperative length of stay (days)		
Mean	16.5 ± 10.4	
Median	13	
Range	6–88	

(From Yeo et al. *Ann Surg.* 1997 Sep; 226(3):248-57.)

▪ LONG-TERM SURVIVAL AFTER RESECTION OF PERIAMPULLARY CANCERS

The percentage of patients with pancreas and other periampullary cancers that survive 5 years or longer after resection is dependent on multiple factors including site of primary and the stage of disease. A series of 616 patients who underwent resection of pancreatic cancers was recently reported.[60] In this series, 526 (85%) underwent pancreaticoduodenectomy for adenocarcinoma of the head, neck, or uncinate process of the pancreas, 52 (9%) underwent distal pancreatectomy for adenocarcinoma of the body or tail, and 38 (6%) underwent total pancreatectomy for adenocarcinoma extensively involving the gland. The overall survival of the entire cohort was 63% at 1 year and 17% at 5 years, with a median survival of 17 months. For right-sided lesions the 1- and 5-year survival rates were 64% and 17%, respectively compared to 50% and 15% for left-sided lesions (Fig 41–16). The factors that had favorable prognostic significance by univariate analysis were negative resection margins, tumor diameter less than 3 cm, negative lymph nodes, estimated blood loss less than 750 mL, lack of transfusion, well/moderate tumor differentiation, and postoperative chemoradiation (Table 41–2, Figs 41–17 and 41–18).

In an analysis of actual 5-year survivors from 242 consecutive patients with resected periampullary adenocarcinoma, of which 149 (62%) were pancreatic primaries, 46 (19%) arose in the ampulla, 30 (12%) were distal bile duct cancers, and 17 (7%) were duodenal cancers.[61] There were 58 actual 5-year survivors and the tumor specific actual 5-year survival rates were pancreatic 15%, ampullary 39%, distal bile duct 27%, and duodenal 59%. When compared with patients who did not survive 5 years, the 5-year survivors had a significantly higher percentage of well-differentiated tumors, negative resection margins, and negative lymph nodes. There is accumulating evidence suggesting that mutations in tumor suppressor genes, oncogenes, and DNA mismatch repair genes also influence prognosis in pancreas cancer. Patients who have pancreas cancers with p53 mutations have been shown to have a worse prognosis.[62] Additionally, the number of tumor suppressor gene mutations found in a pancreatic cancer correlates with the risk of death in patients.[23] In contrast to this and in line with improved prognosis in patients with hereditary nonpolyposis colorectal cancer (HNPCC), patients with pancreas cancers with DNA mismatch repair mutations seem to have a better prognosis.[24]

Technical factors related to the actual operative technique have been studied for their relationship to overall survival. Some groups have advocated that patients with node-positive pancreas cancers fared better after extended lymphadenectomies.[63] In contrast, a study recently performed involved 299 patients with periampullary adenocarcinoma enrolled in a prospective, randomized single-institution trial. After intraoperative verification (by frozen section) of margin-negative resected periampullary adenocarcinomas, patients were randomized to either a standard pancreaticoduodenectomy (removing only the peripancreatic lymph nodes en bloc with the specimen) or a radical (extended) pancreaticoduodenectomy (standard resection plus distal gastrectomy and retroperitoneal lymphadenectomy). The

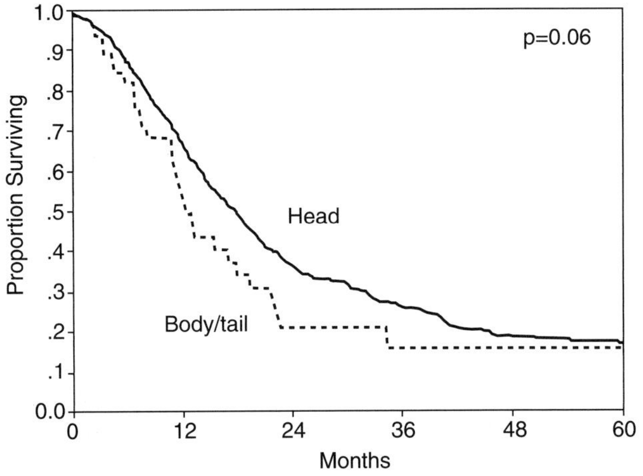

Figure 41–16. Survival curves of 616 patients who underwent resection of pancreatic cancers at Johns Hopkins Hospital. (From Sohn TA, et al. *J Gastrointest Surg* 2000;4:567–579.)

overall complication rates were 29% for the standard group versus 43% for the radical group ($p = .01$), with patients in the radical group having significantly higher rates of early delayed gastric emptying and pancreatic fistula and a significantly longer mean postoperative stay. With a mean patient follow-up of 24 months, there were no significant differences in 1-, 3-, or 5-year and median survival when comparing the standard and radical groups. Pylorus preserving versus standard pancreaticoduodenectomy have been compared and have not been shown to be a factor in long-term survival.[64]

There is also evidence that hospital volume is related to perioperative mortality, length of hospital stay, hospital cost, and long-term outcome in patients undergoing pancreatic resection.[65–68] These studies seem to suggest that regionalization of care of patients requiring pancreaticoduodenectomy and complex pancreatic procedures will affect both the cost and outcome.

▪ ADJUVANT THERAPY

In 1985, the Gastrointestinal Tumor Study Group (GITSG) trial was published.[69] This was a prospective randomized trial comparing observation (control) to split-course radiotherapy (4000 cGy, 20 fractions, over 6 weeks) with bolus 5-flourouracil (5-FU) 500 mg/m^2 intravenous daily on each of the first three days of radiotherapy of each 200-cGy sequence in patients with pancreas cancer. Additionally, patient receiving adjuvant therapy received bolus 5-FU every week for 2 years. The patients on this trial who received adjuvant therapy had better median and overall survival rates.

It has also been demonstrated that multiagent 5-FU chemotherapy regimens can be combined with radiotherapy. The group at the Virginia Mason Clinic have combined 5-FU, cisplatinum, gamma-interferon, and

TABLE 41–2. PROGNOSTIC FACTORS BY UNIVARIATE ANALYSIS IN 616 PATIENTS WHO UNDERWENT RESECTION OF PANCREATIC CANCERS AT JOHNS HOPKINS HOSPITAL

Factor	No. of Patients	1-Year (%)	5-Year (%)	Median (mo)	*P* Value
Overall	612	63	17	17	–
All patients					
Head, neck or uncinate	563	64	17	18	0.06
Body or tail	49	50	15	12	
Estimated blood loss <750 ml	294	71	20	20	0.003
Estimated blood loss ≥750 ml	095	55	14	14	
No transfusions	372	69	18	19	0.04
Transfusions	217	54	16	14	
Negative margins	423	69	21	19	<0.0001
Positive margins	184	49	6	12	
Negative nodes	166	68	22	20	0.006
Positive nodes	441	61	14	16	
Diameter <3 cm	268	72	22	21	<0.0001
Diameter ≥3 cm	325	56	12	14	
Well/moderate differentiation	380	67	18	19	0.0003
Poor differentiation	216	56	13	14	
Adjuvant therapy	333	71	20	19	<0.0001
No adjuvant therapy	119	48	9	11	
Head, neck, or uncinate lesions only					
Plyorus-preserving	395	64	16	17	NS
Classic	168	66	20	19	
Partial pancreatectomy	526	65	18	18	0.05
Total pancreatectomy	37	50	4	11	

(From Sohn et al. *J Gastrointest Surg.* 2000;4:567-579.)

radiotherapy and have shown significant activity in the adjuvant setting.[70] The effectiveness of delivering 5-FU as a continuous infusion, a manner of delivery associated with improved efficacy in rectal and colon cancer, is also being explored.[71] Gemcitabine has been compared to 5-FU for the nonradiotherapeutic components by the Radiation Therapy Oncology Group (RTOG) 97–04 (now closed with completion of accrual). This comparison was based on the observation that, in patients with metastatic pancreatic cancer, gemcitabine produced statistically superior survival results to 5-FU. We are likely to see more trials in the future combining gemcitabine with radiotherapy.

A randomized controlled trial was performed by the European Study Group for Pancreatic Cancer (ESPAC-1) in which 541 eligible patients with pancreas cancer were randomized to adjuvant chemoradiotherapy (20 Gy in 10 daily fractions over 2 weeks with IV 5-FU on days 1 through 3 and 15 through 17), chemotherapy (IV 5-FU and folinic acid for 5 days every month for 6 months), both, or observation. The study demonstrated no survival benefit for adjuvant chemoradiotherapy, but revealed a potential benefit for adjuvant chemotherapy over observation (median survival of 19.7 months vs. 14.0 months).[72]

The role of adjuvant chemoradiation in the treatment of distal bile duct, ampullary, and duodenal cancers is even less well understood than for pancreas cancer. This is because of the relative rarity of these diseases, especially in relation to pancreas cancer.

▪ NEOADJUVANT THERAPY

Neoadjuvant therapy has several theoretical advantages. It allows more timely administration of chemo- or chemoradiotherapy to patients who are at a high risk of failure following surgical resection. It has the potential to shrink the tumor and theoretically can decrease the extent of local disease. Patients who develop disseminated disease during neoadjuvant treatment are unlikely to have benefited from initial resection and are spared the time commitment, morbidity, and potential mortality of resection. It may allow better selection of patients who are most likely to benefit from surgical resection.

A recent series was reported from Duke University of 193 patients with biopsy-proven pancreatic adenocarcinoma who completed neoadjuvant chemoradiotherapy and 70 patients who underwent resection.[73] Exact treatment regimens varied, but 183 patients

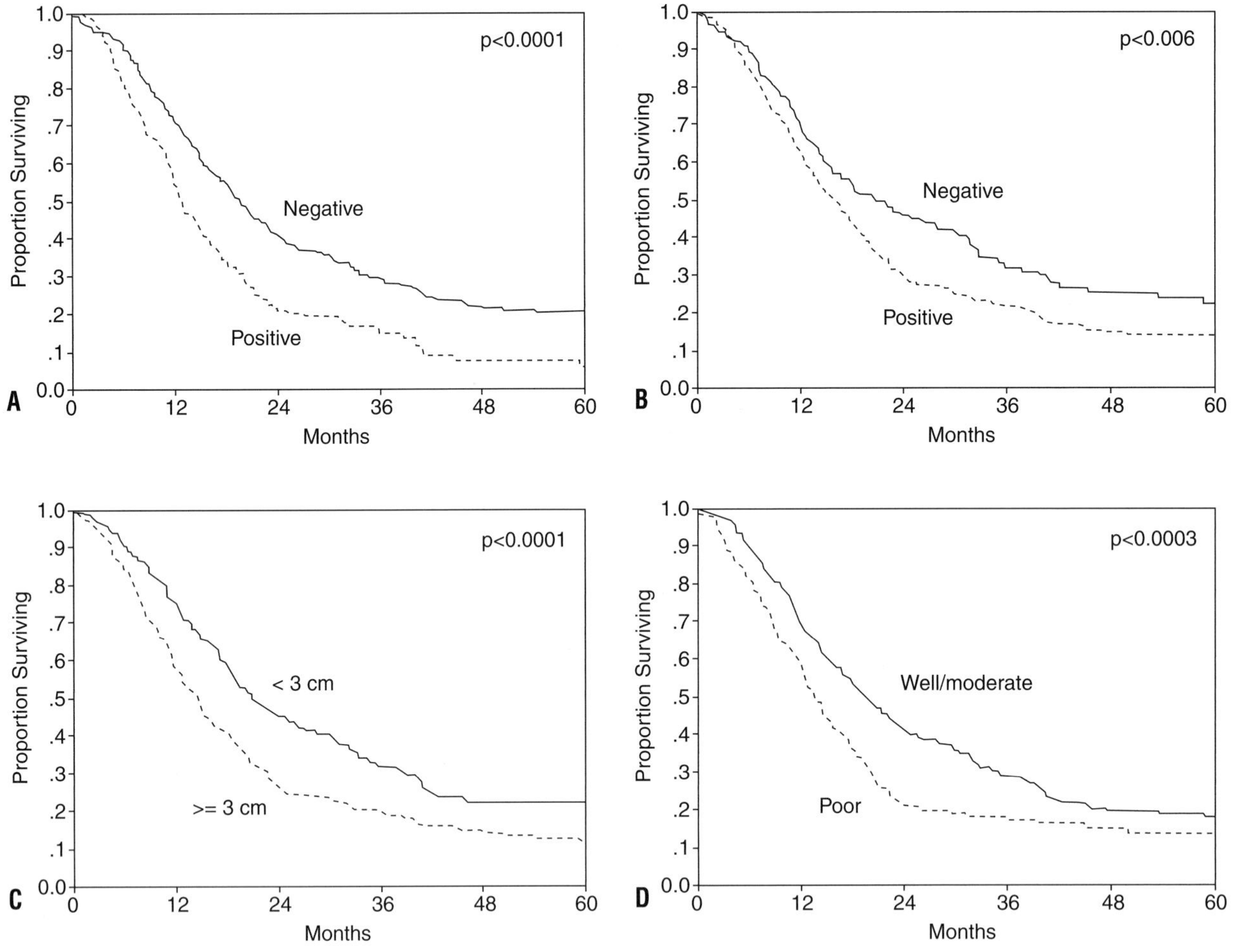

Figure 41–17. Survival curves comparing patients with: **A.** negative resection margins ($n = 442$) to those with positive resection margins ($n = 184$); **B.** negative lymph nodes ($n = 166$) to those with positive lymph nodes ($n = 441$); **C.** tumor diameter <3 cm ($n = 268$) to those with tumor diameter >3 cm ($n = 325$); and **D.** well/moderate tumor differentiation ($n = 380$) to those with poor tumor differentiation ($n = 216$). (From Sohn TA, et al. *J Gastrointest Surg* 2000;4:567–579.)

(95%) received 5-FU–based chemotherapy delivered concurrently with daily external beam radiotherapy for a planned total dose of 4500 cGy at 180 cGy per fraction over 5 weeks plus a 540-cGy boost to the tumor. Ten patients (5%) received gemcitabine chemotherapy with twice-daily external beam radiotherapy with a planned total dose of 3000 cGy at 150 cGy per fraction over 3 weeks. Complete histological responses occurred in 6% of patients. Patients who underwent resection with minimal residual disease, and those whose tumor specimens had significant tumor necrosis, enjoyed significantly better survival.

The MD Anderson Cancer Center experience with neo-adjuvant chemoradiation for resectable pancreatic cancer was recently summarized.[74] Since 1988 four prospective neoadjuvant trials have been completed at that institution with identical eligibility criteria using a CT-based definition of resectable disease, a uniform surgical technique for the performance of pancreaticoduodenectomy, and a standardized system for pathologic evaluation of the surgical specimens. All eligible patients were required to have biopsy proven adenocarcinoma of the pancreatic head. The trials have evolved with the first two using 5-FU as the chemotherapy component, the third using paclitaxel, and the fourth using gemcitabine. All four trials combined chemotherapy with radiotherapy in the neoadjuvant setting (Table 41–3).

■ PALLIATIVE CHEMOTHERAPY

Prior to the Food and Drug Administration (FDA) approval of gemcitabine, the antimetabolite 5-FU was considered standard therapy for advanced pancreatic cancer. Although response rates greater than 20% were reported for treatment with 5-FU, most of these reports predated the era of CT-imaging and were based primarily on clinical tumor evaluation. More modern phase II trials have reported response rates less than 10% for 5-FU alone or with leucovorin.[75,76]

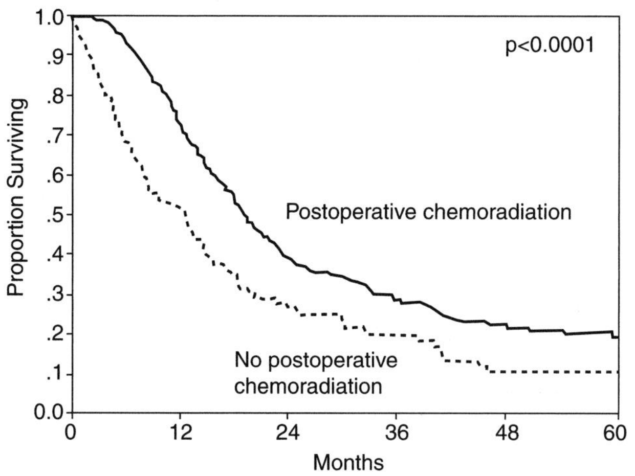

Figure 41–18. Survival curves comparing patients receiving postoperative chemoradiation ($n = 333$) to those not receiving postoperative chemoradiation ($n = 119$). (From Sohn TA, et al. *J Gastrointest Surg* 2000;4:567–579.)

Gemcitabine is a nucleoside analogue that is sequentially phosphorylated and incorporated into replicating DNA, resulting in premature chain termination and apoptosis. Through use of this agent, significant tumor shrinkage of greater than 50% was achieved in only about 5% of patients, but a substantial subset of patients had significant and sustained alleviation of tumor-related symptoms. As a result of these observations, a pivotal phase III trial was completed to quantify this effect in patients with metastatic, symptomatic pancreatic cancer.[77] One hundred twenty-six patients who had not received prior chemotherapy for metastatic disease were randomized to weekly gemcitabine ($n = 63$) or weekly bolus 5-FU ($n = 63$). Overall survival in patients treated with gemcitabine was significantly improved compared with patients treated with 5-FU (median survival, 5.7 vs. 4.4 months respectively; $p < .0025$). The 1-year survival rates were 18% for patients treated with gemcitabine versus 2% in patients treated with 5-FU.

Trials are currently ongoing combining gemcitabine with other chemotherapeutic agents such as topoisomerase I inhibitors, platinums, and taxanes. Additionally, gemcitabine is being combined with molecularly targeted agents such as antiangiogenic and epidermal growth factor receptor agents.[78]

▪ IMMUNOTHERAPY

Immune-based therapies can exploit both the cellular and humoral components of the immune system. Strategies aimed at the cellular components recruit and activate T cells that recognize tumor-specific antigens. Strategies using monoclonal antibodies are being designed to target tumor-specific antigens that can kill tumor cells by direct lysis or through delivery of a conjugated cytotoxic agent. Both approaches are attractive for several reasons. First, immune-based therapies act through a mechanism different from chemotherapy or radiation therapy, and would not be prone to cross-resistance in previously treated patients. Second, through the genetic recombination of their respective receptors, the B cells and T cells of the immune system are capable of recognizing a diverse array of potential tumor antigens. New knowledge into the mechanisms by which T cells are successfully activated and by which tumors evade immune recognition are driving the development of new combinatorial approaches. Also, recent advances in gene-expression analysis have allowed for the identification of new pancreatic targets, including candidate tumor antigens that might serve as T-cell and antibody targets. These advances now make it possible to exploit the immune system to recognize and destroy pancreas cancer.

TABLE 41–3. SUMMARY OF RECENT TRIALS OF PREOPERATIVE CHEMORADIATION FOR RESECTABLE PANCREATIC CANCER AT THE UNIVERSITY OF TEXAS M.D. ANDERSON CANCER CENTER

Author (Year)	n	Regimen	Hospitalization Rate	Resection Rate	Partial Response Rate	Median Survival (Months)
Evans (1992)[76]	28	5-FU 50.4 Gy	32%	61%	41%	18
Pisters (1998)[77]	35	5-FU 30 Gy	9%	57%	20%	25
Pisters (2002)[78]	35	Paclitaxel 30 Gy	11%	57%	21%	19
Wolff (2002)[79]	86	Gemcitabine 30 Gy	43%	74%	58%	36

(From Raut et al. *Surg Oncol Clin N Am* 2004;13:639-661.)

In a phase I trial of patients with surgically resected adenocarcinoma of the pancreas, 14 patients were treated with an allogeneic tumor cell vaccines transduced to secrete granulocyte-macrophage colony stimulating factor. No dose-limiting toxicities were encountered.[79] This vaccine approach induced dose-dependent systemic antitumor immunity as measured by increased postvaccination delayed-type hypersensitivity responses against autologous tumors. Moreover, the three long-term survivors had the strongest postvaccination responses. This strategy is currently being evaluated in a phase II trial at Johns Hopkins.

■ CONCLUSION

Pancreas and other periampullary cancers represent significant clinical problems. Although traditionally patients with these diseases had a dismal prognosis, proper staging and patient selection have led to improved results. When possible, surgical resection for cure should be attempted as this gives the only chance of long-term survival. Surgical resection should be performed by surgeons experienced in the management of these diseases and at centers that can aptly care for these patients to minimize morbidity and mortality. There are many developments on the horizon that have the potential to improve the survival and well-being of patients with these diseases.

REFERENCES

1. Halsted WS. Contributions to the surgery of the bile passages, especially of the common bile duct. *Boston Med Surg J* 1899;141:645–654
2. Sauve L. Des pancreatectomies et specialement de la pancreatectomie cephalique. *Rev Chir* 1908;37:335–385
3. Kausch W. Das carcinoma der papilla duodeni und seine radikale entfeinung. *Beitr Z Clinc Chir* 1912;78:439–486
4. Hirschel G. Die resection des duodenums mit der papille wegen karzinoims. *Munchen Med Wochenschr* 1914;61:1728–1730
5. Whipple AO, Parsons WB, Mullins CR. Treatment of carcinoma of the ampulla of Vater. *Ann Surg* 1935;102:763–779
6. American Cancer Society. *Cancer Facts and Figures 2005.* Atlanta: American Cancer Society; 2005
7. Michaud DS. Epidemiology of pancreas cancer. *Minerva Chir* 2004;59:99–111
8. Yeo CJ. The Whipple procedure in the 1990s. *Adv Surg* 1999;32:271–303
9. Bettschart V, Rahman MQ, Engelken FJ, et al. Presentation, treatment and outcome in patients with ampullary tumours. *Br J Surg* 2004;91(12):1600–1607
10. Gold EB, Goldin SB. Epidemiology of and risk factors for pancreatic cancer. *Surg Oncol Clin North Am* 1998;7:67
11. Gold EB. Epidemiology of and risk factors for pancreatic cancer. *Surg Clin North Am* 1995;75:819
12. Howe GR, Burch JD. Nutrition and pancreatic cancer. *Cancer Causes Control* 1996;7:69
13. MacMahon B, Yen S, Trichopoulos D, et al. Coffee and cancer of the pancreas. *N Engl J Med* 1981;304:630
14. Hseih C-C, MacMahon B, Yen S, et al. Coffee and pancreatic cancer (chapter 2). *N Engl J Med* 1986;315:587
15. Angevine DM, Jablon S. Late radiation effects of neoplasia and other diseases in Japan. *Ann N Y Acad Sci* 1964;114:823
16. Thompson DE, Mabuchi K, Ron E, et al. Cancer incidence in atomic bomb survivors. Part II: Solid tumors, 1958–1987. *Radiat Res* 1994;137:S17
17. Hruban RH, Peterson GM, Ha PK, Kern SE. Genetics of pancreatic cancer: From genes to families. *Surg Oncol Clin North Am* 1998;7:1
18. Lowenfels AB, Maisonneuve P, Cavallini G, et al. Pancreatitis and the risk of pancreatic cancer: International Pancreatitis Study Group. *N Engl J Med* 1993;328:1433
19. Bansal P, Sonnenberg A. Pancreatitis is a risk factor for pancreatic cancer. *Gastroenterology* 1995;109:247
20. Fernandez E, LaVecchia C, Porta M, et al. Pancreatitis and the risk of pancreatic cancer. *Pancreas* 1995;11:185
21. Chow H-W, Gridley G, Nyren O, et al. Risk of pancreatic cancer following diabetes mellitus: A nationwide cohort study in Sweden. *J Natl Cancer Inst* 1995;87:930
22. LaVecchia C, Negri E, D'Avanzo B, et al. Medical history, diet and pancreatic cancer. *Oncology* 1990;47:463
23. Rozenblum E, Schutte M, Goggins M, et al. Tumor-suppressive pathways in pancreatic carcinoma. *Cancer Res* 1997;57:1731
24. Goggins M, Offerhaus GJA, Hilgers W, et al. Pancreatic adenocarcinomas with DNA replication errors (RER+) are associated with wild-type k-ras and characteristic histopathology: Poor differentiation, a syncytial growth pattern, and pushing borders suggest RER+. *Am J Pathol* 1998;152:1501
25. Wilentz RE, Chung CH, Sturm PDJ, et al. K-ras mutations in duodenal fluid of patients with pancreas carcinoma. *Cancer* 1998;82:96
26. Berthelemy P, Bouisson, M, Escourrou J, et al. Identification of k-ras mutations in pancreatic juice early in the diagnosis of pancreatic cancer. *Ann Intern Med* 1995;123:188
27. Caldas C, Hahn SA, Hruban RH, et al. Detection of k-ras mutations in the stool of patients with pancreatic adenocarcinoma and pancreatic ductal mucinous cell hyperplasia. *Cancer Res* 1994;54:3568
28. Bluemke DA, Fishman EK. CT and MR evaluation of pancreatic cancer. *Surg Oncol Clin North Am* 1998;7:103
29. Gambhir SS, Czernin J, Schimmer J, et al. A tabulated review of the literature. *J Nucl Med* 2001;42(Suppl):9S–12S
30. Delbeke D, Pinson CW. Pancreatic tumors: role of imaging in the diagnosis, staging, and treatment. *J Hepatobiliary Pancreat Surg* 2004;11(1):4–10

31. House MG, Yeo CJ, Cameron JL, et al. Predicting resectability of periampullary cancer with three-dimensional computed tomography. *J Gastrointest Surg* 2004;8(3):280–288
32. Conlon KC, Dougherty E, Klimstra DS, et al: The value of minimal access surgery in the staging of patients with potentially resectable peripancreatic malignancy. *Ann Surg* 1996;223:134
33. Lillemoe KD: Palliative therapy for pancreatic cancer. *Surg Oncol Clin North Am* 1998;7:199
34. Vollmer CM, Drebin JA, Middleton WD, et al. Utility of staging laparoscopy in subsets of peripancreatic and biliary malignancies. *Ann Surg* 2002;235(1):1–7
35. Strasberg SM, Drebin JA, Mokadam NA, et al. Prospective trial of a blood supply-based technique of pancreaticojejunostomy: effect on anastomotic failure in the Whipple procedure. *J Am Coll Surg 2002*;194(6):746–758
36. Yeo CJ, Cameron JL, Maher MM, et al. A prospective randomized trial of pancreaticogastrostomy versus pancreaticojejunostomy after pancreaticoduodenectomy. *Ann Surg* 1995;222(4):580–588
37. Heslin MJ, Brooks AD, Hochwald SN, et al. A preoperative biliary stent is associated with increased complications after pancreaticoduodenectomy. *Arch Surg* 1998;133:149
38. Povoski SP, Karpeh MS, Conlon KC, et al. Association of preoperative biliary drainage with postoperative outcome following pancreaticoduodenectomy. *Ann Surg* 1999;230:131
39. Sohn TA, Yeo CJ, Cameron JL, et al. Preoperative biliary stents in patients undergoing pancreaticoduodenectomy: Increased risk of postoperative complications? *J Gastrointest Surg* 2000;4:258
40. Warshaw AL, Gu Z-Y, Wittenberg J, et al. Preoperative staging and assessment of resectability of pancreatic cancer. *Arch Surg* 1990;125:230
41. Sohn TA, Lillemoe KD, Cameron JL, et al. Surgical palliation of unresectable periampullary adenocarcinoma in the 1990s. *J Am Coll Surg* 1999;188:658
42. Sohn TA, Lillemoe KD, Cameron JL, et al. Reexploration for periampullary carcinoma: Resectability, perioperative results, pathology and long-term outcome. *Ann Surg* 1999;229:393
43. Awad SS, Colletti L, Mullholland M, et al. Multimodality staging optimizes resectability in patients with pancreatic and ampullary cancer. *Am Surg* 1997;63:534
44. Sarr MG, Cameron JL. Surgical management of unresectable carcinoma of the pancreas. *Surgery* 1982;91:123
45. Watanapa P, Williamson RCN. Surgical palliation for pancreatic cancer. Developments during the past two decades. *Br J Surg* 1992;79:8
46. Espat NJ, Brennan MF, Conlon KC. Patients with laparoscopically staged unresectable pancreatic adenocarcinoma do not require subsequent surgical biliary or gastric bypass. *J Am Coll Surg* 1999;188(6):649–655
47. Lillemoe KD, Cameron JL, Hardacre JM, et al. Is prophylactic gastrojejunostomy indicated for unresectable periampullary cancer? A prospective randomized trial. *Ann Surg* 1999;230(3):322–328
48. Lillemoe KD, Sauter PK, Pitt HA, et al. Current status of surgical palliation of periampullary carcinoma. *Surg Gynecol Obstet* 1993;176:1
49. Lillemoe KD, Cameron JL, Kaufman HS, et al. Chemical splanchnicectomy in patients with unresectable pancreatic cancer. A prospective randomized trial. *Ann Surg* 1993;217(5):447–455
50. Speer AG, Cotton PB, Russell RC, et al. Randomized trial of endoscopic versus percutaneous stent insertion in malignant obstructive jaundice. *Lancet* 1987;2:57–62
51. Knyrim K, Wagner HJ, Bethge N, et al. A controlled trial of an expansile metal stent for palliation of esophageal obstruction due to inoperable cancer. *N Engl J Med* 1993;329(18):1302–1307
52. Davids PH, Groen AK, Rauws EA, et al. Randomised trial of self-expanding metal stents versus polyethylene stents for distal malignant biliary obstruction. *Lancet* 1992;340(8834–8835):1488–1492
53. Kaw M, Singh S, Gagneja H. Clinical outcome of simultaneous self-expandable metal stents for palliation of malignant biliary and duodenal obstruction. *Surg Endosc* 2003;17(3):457–461
54. Maetani I, Tada T, Ukita T, et al. Comparison of duodenal stent placement with surgical gastrojejunostomy for palliation in patients with duodenal obstructions caused by pancreaticobiliary malignancies. *Endoscopy* 2004; 36(1):73–78
55. Polati E, Finco G, Gottin L, et al. Prospective randomized double-blind trial of neurolytic coeliac plexus block in patients with pancreatic cancer. *Br J Surg* 1998; 85(2):199–201
56. Bakkevold KE, Kambestad B. Palliation of pancreatic cancer. A prospective multicentre study. *Eur J Surg Oncol* 1995;21(2):176–182
57. Yeo C, Cameron JL, Sohn TA, et al. Six hundred fifty consecutive pancreaticoduodenectomies in the 1990s: pathology, complications, outcomes. *Ann Surg* 1997:248–260
58. Yeo CJ, Barry MK, Sauter PK, et al. Erythromycin accelerates gastric emptying following pancreaticoduodenectomy: A prospective, randomized placebo controlled trial. *Ann Surg* 1993;218:229
59. Conlon KC, Labow D, Leung D, et al. Prospective randomized clinical trial of the value of intraperitoneal drainage after pancreatic resection. *Ann Surg* 2001; 234(4):487–493; discussion 493–494
60. Sohn TA, Yeo CJ, Cameron JL, et al. Resected adenocarcinoma of the pancreas-616 patients: results, outcomes, and prognostic indicators. *J Gastrointest Surg* 2000;4(6): 567–579
61. Yeo CJ, Sohn TA, Cameron JL, et al. Periampullary adenocarcinoma: analysis of 5-year survivors. *Ann Surg* 1998;227:821–831
62. DiGuiseppe JA, Yeo CJ and Hruban RH. Molecular biology and the diagnosis and treatment of adenocarcinoma of the pancreas. *Adv Anat Pathol* 1996;3:139
63. Pedrazzoli S, DiCarlo V, Dionigi R, et al. Standard versus extended lymphadenectomy associated with pancreaticoduodenectomy in the surgical treatment of adenocarcinoma of the head of the pancreas: A multicenter, prospective, randomized study. *Ann Surg* 1998;228:508
64. Yeo CJ, Cameron JL, Lillemoe KD, et al. Pancreaticoduodenectomy for cancer of the head of the pancreas: 201 patients. *Ann Surg* 1995;221:721

65. Gordon TA, Burleyson GP, Tielsch JM, et al. The effects of regionalization on cost and outcome for one general high-risk surgical procedure. *Ann Surg* 1995;221:43
66. Sosa JA, Bowman HM, Bass EB, et al. Importance of hospital volume in the overall management of pancreatic cancer. *Ann Surg* 1998;228:429
67. Lieberman MD, Kilburn H, Lindsey M, Brennan MF. Relation of perioperative deaths to hospital volume among patients undergoing pancreatic resection for malignancy. *Ann Surg* 1995;222:638
68. Birkmeyer JD, Warshaw AL, Finlayson SRG, et al. Relationship between hospital volume and late survival after pancreaticoduodenectomy. *Surgery* 1999;126:178
69. Kalser MH, Ellenberg SS. Pancreatic cancer-adjuvant combined radiation and chemotherapy following curative resection. *Arch Surg* 1985;120:899–903
70. Picozzi VJ, Kozarek RA, Traverso LW. Interferon-based adjuvant chemoradiation therapy after pancreaticoduodenectomy for pancreatic adenocarcinoma. *Am J Surg* 2003;185(5):476–480
71. Abrams RA, Sohn TA, Zahurak ML, et al. A multivariate model for identifying risk of early death after pancreaticoduodenectomy and adjuvant therapy for periampullary adenocarcinoma: Importance for understanding post treatment outcomes. *Int J Radiat Oncol Biol Phys* 2002;54(2S):100–101
72. Neoptolemos JP, Dunn JA, Stocken DD, et al. European Study Group for Pancreatic Cancer. Adjuvant chemoradiotherapy and chemotherapy in resectable pancreatic cancer: a randomised controlled trial. *Lancet* 2001; 358(9293):1576–1585
73. White RR, Xie HB, Gottfried MR, et al. Significance of histological response to preoperative chemoradiotherapy for pancreatic cancer. *Ann Surg Oncol* 2005;12(3):214–221
74. Raut CP, Evans DB, Crane CH, et al. Neoadjuvant therapy for resectable pancreatic cancer. *Surg Oncol Clin N Am* 2004;13:639–661
75. Crown J, Casper ES, Botet J, et al. Lack of efficacy of high-dose leucovorin and fluorouracil in patients with advanced pancreatic adenocarcinoma. *J Clin Oncol* 1991;9:1682–1686
76. DeCaprio JA, Mayer RJ, Gonin R, Arbuck SG. Fluorouracil and high-dose leucovorin in previously untreated patients with advanced adenocarcinoma of the pancreas: results of a phase II trial. *J Clin Oncol* 1991;9:2128–2133
77. Carmichael J, Fink U, Russell RC, et al. Phase II study of gemcitabine in patients with advanced pancreatic cancer. *Br J Cancer* 1996;73:101–105
78. Lockhart AC, Rothenberg ML, Berlin JD. Treatment for pancreatic cancer: current therapy and continued progress. *Gastroenterology* 2005;128(6):1642–1654
79. Jaffee EM, Hruban RH, Biedrzycki B, et al. Novel allogeneic granulocyte-macrophage colony-stimulating factor-secreting tumor vaccine for pancreatic cancer: a phase I trial of safety and immune activation. *J Clin Oncol* 2001; 19(1):145–156

42

Endocrine Tumors of the Pancreas

Buckminster J. Farrow ▪ *James C. Thompson* ▪ *Courtney M. Townsend, Jr.*
B. Mark Evers

Pancreatic endocrine tumors are rare; however, unlike pancreatic adenocarcinomas, surgical excision for endocrine tumors offers an excellent chance for cure. Endocrine tumors elaborate active gastrointestinal (GI) hormones that produce clinical syndromes, which are defined by their cell of origin. The morbidity from pancreatic endocrine tumors results predominately from the severe derangements in GI physiology caused by the overproduction of these hormones. These tumors usually occur sporadically but may be associated with multiple endocrine neoplasia (MEN) syndromes. Compared with sporadic tumors, patients with MEN tend to have more aggressive and/or multifocal disease. Biochemical assays which demonstrate an abnormally high hormone level will establish the diagnosis; however, management of pancreatic endocrine tumors can be challenging since they can be difficult to localize prior to surgery. Surgical resection is the only treatment option that can provide a cure. Even when complete resection is not possible, removal of macroscopically evident disease often controls the debilitating sequelae of hormone overproduction. This chapter will review the pattern of symptoms and testing utilized to identify the clinical syndromes associated with pancreatic endocrine tumors, describe methods for tumor localization, and present the management options including surgical resection and adjuvant therapy.

▪ COMMON FEATURES

Pancreatic endocrine tumors occur with an incidence of approximately 5 per 1,000,000 per year. Autopsy series demonstrate an incidence of nearly 1%, suggesting that many nonfunctional, benign tumors remain asymptomatic. Additionally, 20% of pancreatic endocrine tumors that are diagnosed clinically are nonfunctional (i.e., do not secrete biologically active hormones). Functional tumors may be malignant or benign and the likelihood of malignancy varies with the cell type involved (e.g., insulinomas are usually benign while glucagonomas are almost always malignant). Any given tumor may produce multiple hormones, creating a mixed clinical picture which further complicates establishing a diagnosis. In these situations, syndromes are defined by the predominant hormone produced. For all types of pancreatic endocrine tumors, malignancy is defined by the presence of metastases to regional lymph nodes, the liver or elsewhere. In this regard, most malignant tumors are larger than their benign counterparts.

▪ ISLET CELL ANATOMY/PHYSIOLOGY

Endocrine tumors of the pancreas are thought to originate from hormone-producing islet cells, which arise from either neural crest cells or embryonic foregut endoderm. These islet cells normally constitute less than 2% of the adult pancreatic mass. There are four major cell types found within islets: alpha, beta, delta, and pancreatic polypeptide (PP) cells, each of which can produce more than one hormone (Table 42–1). Each cell type occupies a specific region of the islet; beta cells are found in the islet's center while alpha, delta, and PP cells line theperiphery (Fig 42–1). Islets are well vascularized,

TABLE 42–1. PANCREATIC ENDOCRINE TUMORS: HORMONES PRODUCED, CLINICAL SYNDROMES AND THE CELLS OF THE ORIGIN

Cell Type	Hormone Produced	Endocrine Tumor/Syndrome
Alpha	Insulin	Insulinoma
Beta	Glucagon	Glucagonoma
Delta	Somatostatin	Somatostatinoma
G	Gastrin	Gastrinoma/ZES
D_2	VIP	VIPoma/WDHA

containing a rich capillary bed, which drains into several collecting venules that carry secreted hormones into the portal and systemic circulations. These pathways are most important in regulating carbohydrate metabolism; beta cells release insulin to facilitate glucose uptake which is counterbalanced by glucagon released by alpha cells to maintain adequate glucose homeostasis.

HISTORY

The first description of an islet cell neoplasm was by Nichols in 1908 who reported finding a pancreatic adenoma composed of islet tissue. Several years later, Mayo was the first to establish the relationship between hyperinsulinemia and pancreatic islet cell carcinoma. In 1935, Whipple and Frantz described the diagnostic triad associated with insulin-secreting tumors: (1) symptoms of hypoglycemia, (2) low blood glucose, and (3) relief of symptoms by administration of glucose (Whipple's triad). In 1942, Becker described a patient with severe dermatitis, anemia, and diabetes who also had a pancreatic islet cell tumor. More than 20 years later, McGavran identified glucagon from an alpha cell tumor of the pancreas, which produced the same clinical presentation. In 1955, Zollinger and Ellison described a syndrome of severe peptic ulcer disease, massive acid hypersecretion and a non-beta islet cell tumor of the pancreas. It was later determined that production of a gastrin tumor was the cause of the syndrome; the clinical manifestations of gastrinomas are known as the Zollinger-Ellison syndrome (ZES). In 1958, Verner and Morrison described two patients with pancreatic islet cell tumors who died from watery diarrhea and hypokalemia. Later, patients with this same syndrome were found to have high circulating levels of VIP and Verner-Morrison syndrome (or VIPoma) was clearly defined. Also of historical note is the development of radioimmunoassay techniques by Yalow and Berson, which in 1956 greatly facilitated the understanding of pancreatic hormones and the diseases they cause by allowing the detection of minute concentrations of circulating peptides.

▪ ASSOCIATED SYNDROMES

MEN type 1 (MEN-1), also known as Werner syndrome, is the most common endocrinopathy associated with pancreatic endocrine tumors. MEN-1 is characterized by parathyroid hyperplasia, pituitary tumors, and pancreatic endocrine tumors that occur in 30–80% of patients with this syndrome. MEN-1 is inherited in an autosomal dominant fashion and occurs with equal incidence in both men and women. A mutation and allelic deletion in the tumor gene MENIN on chromosome 11q13 is believed to cause MEN-1; the deleted gene causes loss of tumor suppressor function predisposing afflicted patients to neoplastic growth in various tissues. In general, patients with MEN-1 develop pancreatic endocrine tumors earlier than those with sporadic tumors and are younger at the time of diagnosis (usually 30 to 40 years old). Pancreatic endocrine tu-

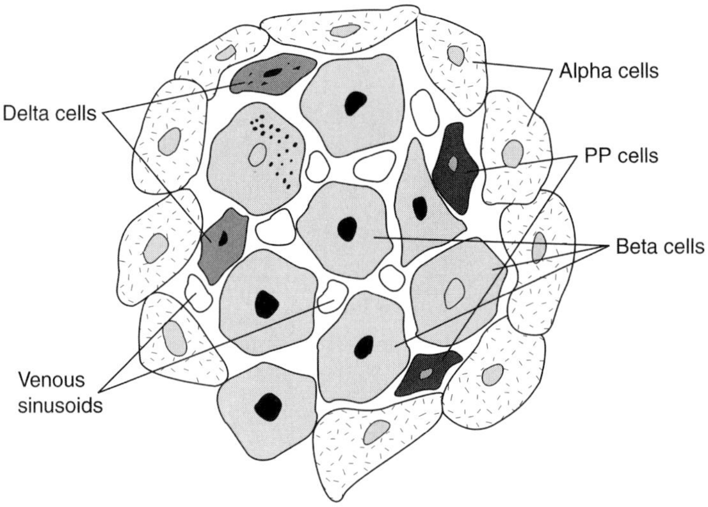

Figure 42–1. This diagram depicts the cells which compose a pancreatic islet and their typical location within the islet (i.e., alpha cells on the periphery and beta cells localized to the central region). The dots within the beta-cell cytoplasm depict the strong staining often seen from insulin-containing granules. Delta and PP cells constitute only a minority of the pancreatic islet endocrine cells. The rich blood supply is demonstrated by the abundance of venous sinusoids within the islet.

mors in MEN-1 are the most likely cause of death in gene carriers. Tumors associated with MEN-1 are also more likely to be malignant or multicentric and approximately 50% of patients with MEN-1 will have metastases at the time of diagnosis. PPomas are the most common nonfunctional pancreatic endocrine tumors in patients with MEN-1 occurring in >80% of cases. Gastrinomas are the most common functional pancreatic endocrine tumor noted in patients with MEN-1 (54% of patients), and, conversely, 20% of patients with ZES meet the diagnostic criteria for MEN-1. Insulinomas are the next most common functioning pancreatic endocrine tumor (21%), followed by glucagonomas (3%) and VIPomas (1%).

Management of patients with MEN-1 and pancreatic endocrine tumors requires recognition of associated tumors and staged treatment of each. Patients suspected of having MEN-1 should undergo biochemical screening for gastrin, insulin/proinsulin, pancreatic polypeptide, glucagon, and chromogranin A (a tumor marker elaborated by many pancreatic endocrine tumors). If hyperparathyroidism is present it should be treated first, as correction of hypercalcemia will improve the outcome of treatment for gastrinomas, the most common functional pancreatic endocrine tumor in MEN-1. ZES is more difficult to cure in patients with MEN-1 as it may involve multicentric, diffuse hyperplasia of islets in addition to discrete tumors, which are usually malignant. Gastrinomas in MEN-1 are more likely to be located within the duodenum than their sporadic counterparts. Treatment of insulinomas and VIPomas in patients with MEN-1 does not differ significantly compared to sporadic disease. Other endocrinopathies are also found in association with pancreatic endocrine tumors, including Von Hippel-Lindau syndrome and neurofibromatosis type 1, which is associated with duodenal somatostatinomas.

▪ INSULINOMA

Insulinomas account for 60% of all pancreatic islet cell tumors (Fig 42–2) and occur at an incidence of 1 per 1,000,000 patients per year. The average age of patients at the time of diagnosis is 45 years old; men and women are equally affected. Nearly all insulinomas are located in the pancreas with equal distribution in the head, body, and tail. Rarely (2–3%), these tumors are located in the duodenum, splenic hilum, or gastrocolic ligament. Ninety percent of insulinomas are less than 2 cm in size (average 1.0 to 1.5 cm) and weigh a few grams, but large tumors (>1 kg) have been reported. They are encapsulated, firm, yellow-brown nodules that are typically hypervascular, which can aid in their diagnosis by CT, MRI, or magnetic resonance angiography (MRA). Microscopically, insulinomas appear as clustered nests of normal appearing beta cells that stain positive for insulin. Malignancy, defined by the presence of local invasion or metastasis to distant sites, occurs in 10% of cases, but benign and malignant insulinomas appear similar histologically. Most occur as solitary lesions; however, multicentricity does occur in 10% of cases, and should raise suspicion of the possibility of MEN-1, which occurs in 4–7% of all patients with insulinoma.

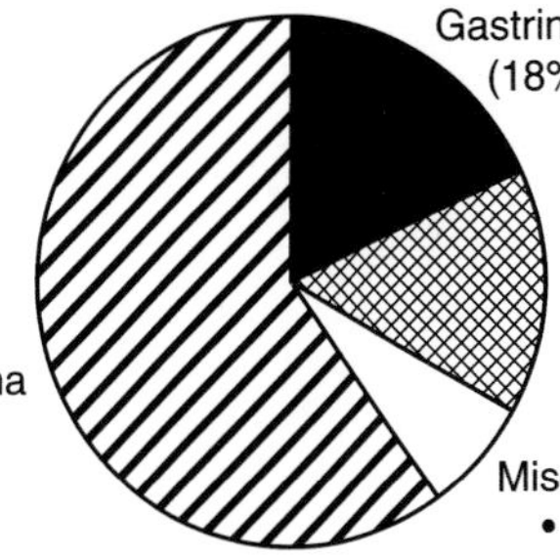

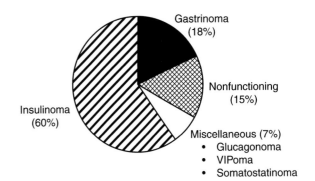

Figure 42–2. Relative incidence of pancreatic endocrine tumors.

Similar to their normal beta-cell counterparts, insulinoma cells release proinsulin composed of C-peptide and insulin. Normal regulatory pathways do not inhibit tumor overproduction of proinsulin and the high levels of circulating insulin cause hypoglycemia leading to the signs and symptoms associated with insulinomas. Neuroglycopenic symptoms are a result of the sympathetic nervous system response to profound hypoglycemia, resulting in catecholamine and glucagon release. Patients will commonly complain of headache, lethargy, dizziness, diplopia, or amnesia. Symptoms tend to occur in the early morning (before food ingestion) and after exercise. Release of catecholamines causes trembling, sweating, palpitations, nervousness, and hunger. These symptoms may partially resolve if glycogenolysis is also stimulated, thus increasing glucose levels and reducing the catecholamine surge by feedback inhibition. Patients will typically attempt to control their symptoms by eating frequent meals, leading to weight gain. Chronic hypoglycemia may have profound, even permanent neurologic consequences including apathy, clouded sensorium, behavioral changes, seizures, and coma.

Laboratory studies will usually confirm the diagnosis of insulinoma. Classically, patients will present with a low glucose level (<50 mg/dL) while having symptoms of hypoglycemia, which resolve with administration of glucose (Whipple's triad) (Table 42–2). Hy-

TABLE 42–2. DIAGNOSIS OF INSULINOMA

Whipple's triad:
Symptoms of hypoglycemia
Low (<45 mg%) blood sugar
Relief of symptoms with glucose

Triad precipitated by 12-hour fast in 37% of patients and by 24-hour fast in 73%.

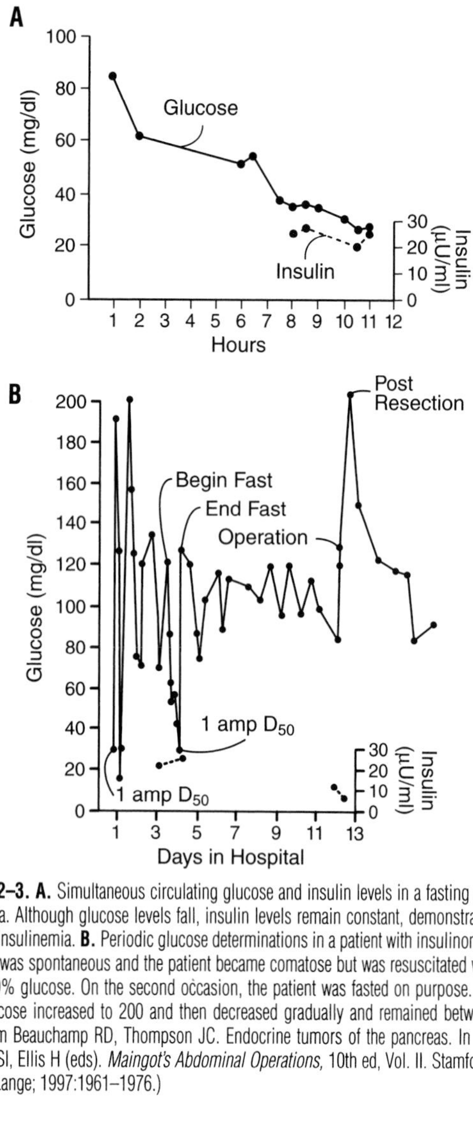

Figure 42–3. A. Simultaneous circulating glucose and insulin levels in a fasting patient with insulinoma. Although glucose levels fall, insulin levels remain constant, demonstrating a relative hyperinsulinemia. **B.** Periodic glucose determinations in a patient with insulinoma. The first major fall was spontaneous and the patient became comatose but was resuscitated with an ampule of 50% glucose. On the second occasion, the patient was fasted on purpose. Postoperatively, glucose increased to 200 and then decreased gradually and remained between 90 and 120. (From Beauchamp RD, Thompson JC. Endocrine tumors of the pancreas. In Zinner MJ, Schwartz SI, Ellis H (eds). *Maingot's Abdominal Operations,* 10th ed, Vol. II. Stamford, CT: Appleton & Lange; 1997:1961–1976.)

poglycemia (<50 mg/dL in men or <40 mg/dL in women) after a 72-hour fast occurs in 95% of patients; 75% of patients will achieve this degree of hypoglycemia within the first 24 hours (Fig 42–3). Insulin levels >7 μU/mL are highly suggestive of an insulinoma; however, these levels can also be found in patients with hyperinsulinemia from other causes. An insulin/glucose ratio greater than 0.3 occurs with insulinoma or less commonly with obesity, but obese patients should not be hypoglycemic. Levels of circulating proinsulin can be measured and compared to the total insulin present; a proinsulin level greater than 24% of total insulin is commonly found with insulinoma. Proinsulin may account for 40% of total insulin if the tumors are malignant. C-peptide levels should be measured to confirm an endogenous source of insulin if there is any suspicion of factitious hypoglycemia from insulin injections; levels >1.2 μg/mL with a glucose level <40 mg/dL are also highly suggestive of an insulinoma. Two other rare clinical syndromes may be difficult to distinguish from insulinoma, nesidioblastosis, and noninsulinoma pancreatogenous hypoglycemia. Nesidioblastosis will produce neuroglycopenic symptoms because of hyperplasia of pancreatic islets, but no pancreatic tumor is noted. Patients with noninsulinoma pancreatogenous hypoglycemia have high insulin levels and hypoglycemia; however, symptoms are rare even after a 72-hour fast. Islet cell hypertrophy may be seen with noninsulinoma pancreatogenous hypoglycemia, but no focal tumor is involved. Rarely, provocative testing is required to confirm the diagnosis of insulinoma. Since cerebrocytes use glucose as their sole source of energy, this must be done with extreme caution; profound hypoglycemia and subsequent permanent neurologic injury can occur. Insulin release can be stimulated with either calcium gluconate (given intravenously) or tolbutamide while insulin and glucose levels are measured. These techniques will produce hyperinsulinemia and hypoglycemia in >90% of patients with insulinoma.

Localization of insulinomas is successful pre-operatively in more than 90% of cases (Fig 42–4). The sensitivity of CT or MRI in localizing insulinomas ranges from 10–80% and is entirely dependent on the size of the tumor. Because of their hypervascularity, insulinomas will have a zone of peripheral enhancement noted with IV contrast on CT scan. This enhancement can also be seen by MRI studies performed with gadolinium (Fig 42–5). Initial non-invasive methods may fail to localize the tumor because 90% of insulinomas are <2 cm. The utilization of endoscopic ultrasound (EUS) has significantly improved the ability to localize even small insulinomas pre-operatively, detecting 77–93% of tumors within the pancreas (Fig 42–6). Detection using EUS is more successful for tumors in the pancreatic head compared to

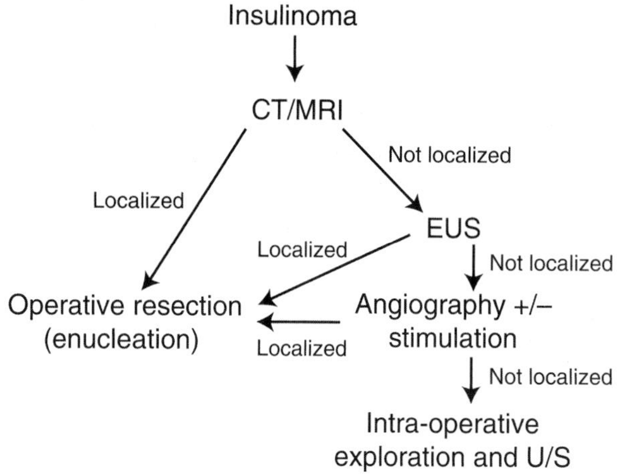

Figure 42–4. Localization of insulinomas. EUS = endoscopic ultrasound.

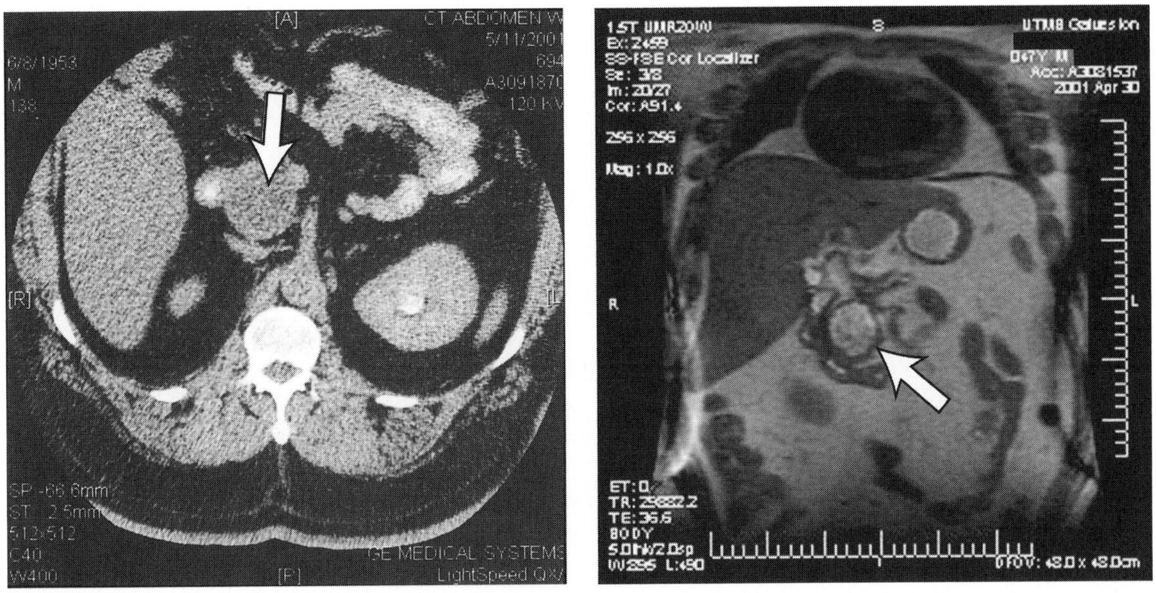

Figure 42–5. CT scan and MRI demonstrating an insulinoma in the uncinate process of the pancreas. The tumor shows increased contrast in both CT and MRI at the periphery a result of the hypervascularity of the insulinoma. (Courtesy of Aytekin Oto, M.D., The University of Texas Medical Branch.)

the body or tail. Angiography will detect approximately 70% of small insulinomas (>5 mm) (Fig 42–7), showing a characteristic "blush," which corresponds to the highly vascular nature of insulinomas. If standard radiographic techniques are unsuccessful, selective portal venous sampling for insulin levels may allow localization to a region of the pancreas (head, body, or tail) to aid in operative planning (Fig 42–8). Provocative testing, known as arterial stimulation venous sampling (ASVS), can further increase the likelihood of localization by injecting calcium into the celiac and superior mesenteric arteries with simultaneous portal venous sampling for insulin levels. ASVS has a sensitivity of over 90%. Somatostatin receptor scintigraphy using radiolabeled octreotide is not very useful in localizing insulinomas since fewer than 60% of tumors express somatostatin receptors. Somatostatin receptor expression may be higher in cases of malignant insulinoma. In the unlikely event that pre-operative studies cannot localize the tumor, intraoperative ultrasound combined with careful palpation and exploration of the entire pancreas accurately identifies nearly 100% of all tumors (Fig 42–9). Intraoperative portal venous sampling with rapid immunoassay for insulin may also be used if localization is still unsuccessful.

Surgical resection of insulinoma is usually curative as most tumors tend to be small, benign, and solitary. Preoperatively, it is important to prevent severe hypoglycemic attacks by administration of diazoxide which decreases beta-cell release of insulin (usually 3 mg/kg per day divided in two or three doses daily). Rarely, other

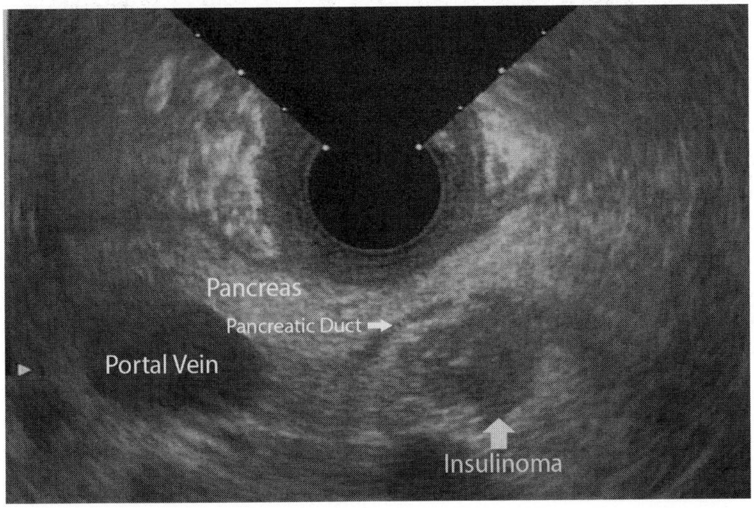

Figure 42–6. The EUS image shows a 1.1-cm insulinoma in the pancreas that was not seen by CT scan. The lesion was removed by enucleation. (Courtesy of John Deutsch, M.D., Saint Mary's/Duluth Clinic Health System, Duluth, MN.)

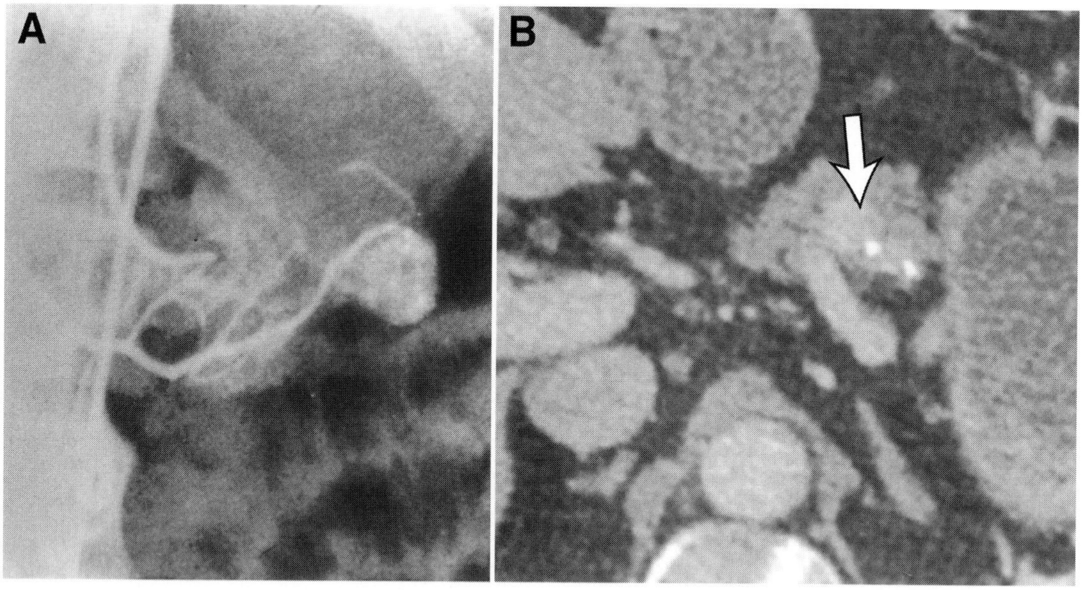

Figure 42–7. Localization studies demonstrating an insulinoma. **A.** Arteriographic demonstration of an insulinoma. Selective injection into the specific dorsal pancreatic artery demonstrates the tumor precisely. **B.** Insulinoma with triphasic enhancement on CT. The mass in pancreatic body (*arrow*) demonstrates early and prolonged enhancement with wash-out during the portal venous phase; note the maximal difference in enhancement between tumor and normal pancreas occurs during pancreatic phase (shown). (From Edis AJ, McIlrath DC, Van Heerden JA, et al. Insulinoma–Current diagnosis and surgical management. *Curr Probl Surg* 1976;13:1–45, and Ros PR, Mortele KJ. Imaging features of pancreatic neoplasms. *JBR-BTR* 2001;84:239–249, with permission.)

agents such as verapamil, glucocorticoids, and growth hormone may be required to maintain normoglycemia. Glucose infusions must be used in the peri-operative period especially when patients are nil per os. Surgical technique includes careful inspection of the liver and regional lymph nodes for evidence of metastatic disease. The pancreas is exposed and manual examina-

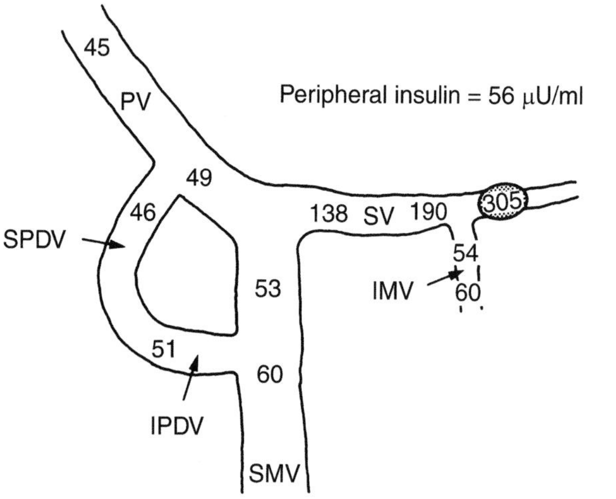

Figure 42–8. Schematic of transhepatic selective venous sampling of the portal vein and its tributaries for insulin. Venous insulin levels are greatly elevated in the distal splenic vein (shaded circle). Intraoperative ultrasound and palpation of the pancreas failed to reveal an insulinoma. A distal pancreatectomy was performed on the basis of the portovenous sampling gradient shown here, and the pathologists confirmed the presence of a 1-cm insulinoma. IMV, inferior mesenteric vein; IPDV, inferior pancreatic duodenal vein; PV, portal vein; SMV, superior mesenteric vein; SPDV, superior pancreatic duodenal vein; SV, splenic vein. Insulin concentrations are given in microunits per milliliter. (From Norton JA, Shawker TH, Doppman JL, et al. Localization and surgical treatment of occult insulinomas. *Ann Surg* 1990;212(5):615–620, with permission.)

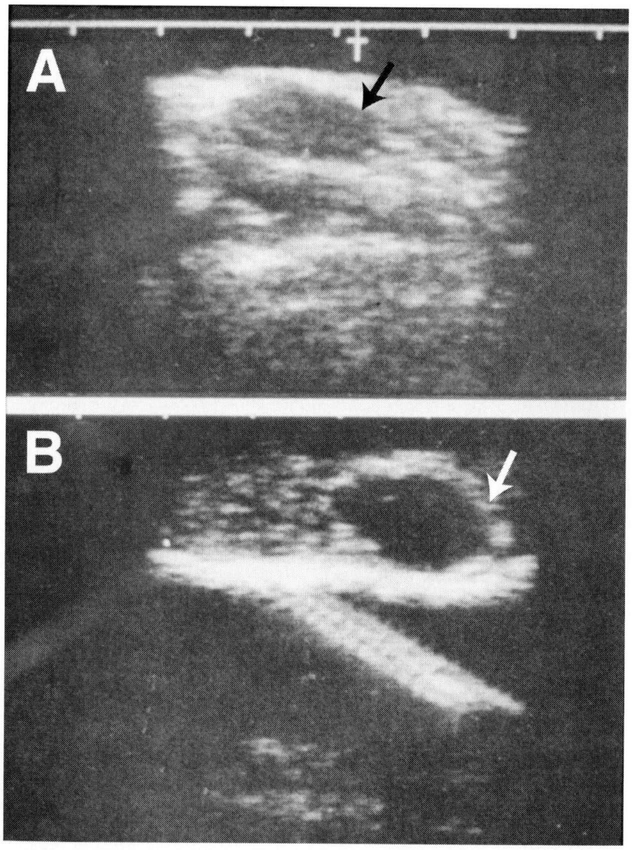

Figure 42–9. A and **B.** Intraoperative ultrasonographic demonstration of insulinoma using 7.5-MHz probe. Tumor of the midbody of the pancreas (*arrows*) is clearly shown in both panels; the horizontal (white) line beneath the tumor is the surgeon's glove. (From Thompson JC. Endocrine pancreas. In Townsend CM Jr, Beauchamp RD, Evers BM, Mattox KL (eds). *Sabiston Textbook of Surgery: The Biological Basis of Modern Surgical Practice,* 17th ed, Philadelphia: Elsevier Saunders; 2004:1001–1022, with permission.)

tion used to confirm the tumor location and determine whether any synchronous lesions are present. A generous Kocher maneuver and mobilization of the pancreatic tail are usually required to adequately inspect the entire pancreas (Fig 42–10). Enucleation is usually sufficient to remove the entire tumor as these are typically benign lesions (Fig 42–11). Careful dissection is necessary to avoid entry into the main pancreatic duct. Many surgeons advocate placement of a silastic drain adjacent to the enucleation site to control any leak of pancreatic secretions postoperatively. In the rare instance that the tumor cannot be localized with pre- or intraoperative techniques, blind resection of the pancreatic body or tail is not recommended, nor is blind pancreaticoduodenectomy. When no tumor can be identified, biopsies should be taken from the pancreatic tail to evaluate for nesidioblastosis.

Normal life expectancy is achieved by complete excision of a benign insulinoma. More extensive resec-

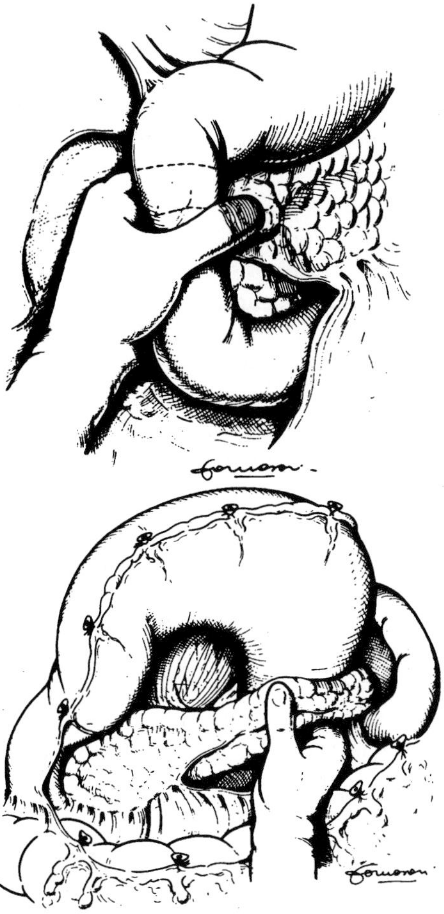

A

B

Figure 42–10. A. After a generous Kocher maneuver of the duodenum, the pancreatic head should be palpated between the thumb and fingers. **B.** The gastrocolic omentum is divided and the stomach is elevated. The body and tail of the pancreas are gently mobilized. The areas can now be visualized palpated carefully. (From Findley A, Arenas RB, Kaplan EL. Insulinoma. In Percopo V, Kaplan EL (eds). *GEP and multiple endocrine tumors.* Padova, Italy: Piccin Nuova Libreroa SpA; 1996:314, with permission.)

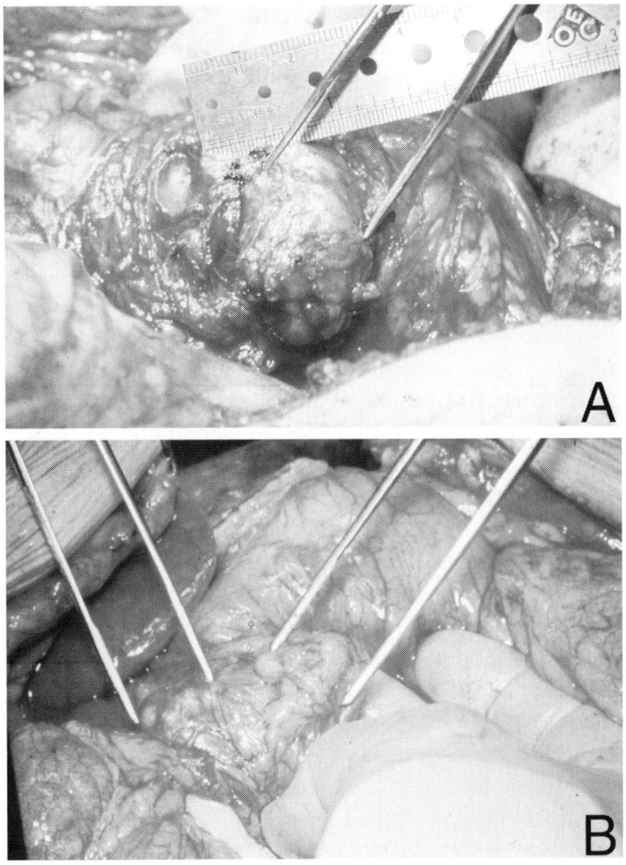

Figure 42–11. Intraoperative photographs demonstrating the enucleation of an insulinoma from within the body of the pancreas.

tions are required for complete excision of malignant insulinomas, which are typically much larger (approximately 6 cm), and in patients with MEN-1 or multifocal disease. These patients may require subtotal pancreatectomy, with enucleation of lesions in the head of the pancreas or pancreaticoduodenectomy with local resections of tumors in the body or tail. Tumor debulking may be useful even if all disease is not removed since some residual disease may not be functional. Median survival is 5 years after resection of malignant insulinoma; approximately 29% of patients are still alive 10 years after resection. For patients with metastatic insulinoma, resection of gross disease, along with octreotide for symptom control and systemic chemotherapy, is the appropriate treatment. Streptozotocin (with or without 5-fluorouracil) is associated with a response rate of 63%; however the survival benefit is not well established.

▪ GASTRINOMA

Gastrinomas are the second most common functional pancreatic endocrine tumor with an incidence of 1 per

2.5 million. The mean age of patients at diagnosis is 50 years and there is a slight male predominance (60%). Gastrinomas produce the ZES by overproduction of gastrin which is normally synthesized by G cells located in the antral mucosa of the stomach. Gastrin release by normal G cells is stimulated by amino acids and peptides in the stomach or gastric distension, whereas release is inhibited by low luminal pH and secretin that is released from endocrine cells in the duodenum. Gastrinomas produce gastrin without influence from normal stimulatory or inhibitory pathways. Specifically, these tumors are not suppressed by high luminal pH and can be stimulated (instead of inhibited) by secretin. The clinical manifestations of ZES are secondary to hypergastrinemia and high gastric acid secretion.

Over 60% of gastrinomas are malignant. Malignancy cannot be predicted by size or histology. Similar to other pancreatic endocrine tumors, malignancy is defined by the presence of lymph node or distant metastases. The liver is the most common site of spread but peri-pancreatic lymph nodes are also commonly involved. Between 70–80% of patients with malignant gastrinoma have metastases to the liver or lymph nodes at the time of diagnosis. Metastases may also involve the lungs or bone. Ninety percent of gastrinomas are located within the gastrinoma triangle, described originally by Stabile and Passaro (Fig 42–12). The triangle is formed by connecting lines between the cystic duct, the junction between the second and third portions of the duodenum, and the junction between the neck and body of the pancreas. Patients with MEN-1 are more likely to have lesions in the duodenum instead of the pancreas which is an important distinction to make since 20% of patients with ZES have MEN-1. These patients are also more likely to have multifocal disease, present at a younger age, and commonly have hyperparathyroidism, which can complicate the management of a gastrinoma.

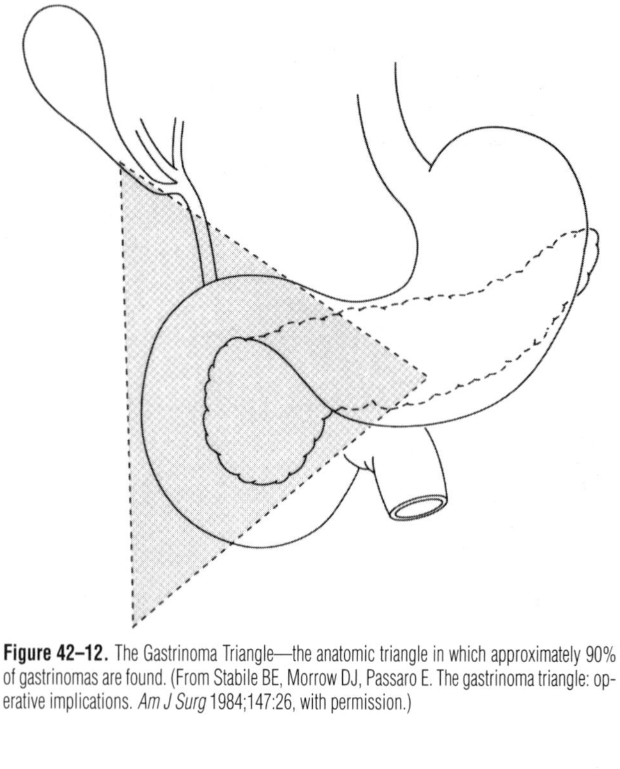

Figure 42–12. The Gastrinoma Triangle—the anatomic triangle in which approximately 90% of gastrinomas are found. (From Stabile BE, Morrow DJ, Passaro E. The gastrinoma triangle: operative implications. *Am J Surg* 1984;147:26, with permission.)

TABLE 42–3. CLINICAL MANIFESTATIONS OF ZOLLINGER-ELLISON SYNDROME

Virulent ulcer disease
Refractory to medical therapy
In atypical locations (e.g., jejunum)
Recurrent following vagotomy/antrectomy
Diarrhea
GI bleeding

The diagnosis of ZES (Table 42–3) is classically made after patients present with severe forms of peptic ulcer disease that are either refractory to standard treatment or are atypical in location. Ninety percent of patients with ZES have peptic ulcers, most in the duodenal bulb, with synchronous ulcers found in more distant portions of the duodenum or proximal jejunum. Jejunal ulcer perforations occur in 7% of patients. Patients may complain of upper abdominal pain and/or GI bleeding (melena or hematochezia), weight loss, or nausea and vomiting. Symptoms of gastroesophageal reflux are also common. High acid production can lower the normal pH of the duodenum and inactivate pancreatic enzymes, leading to diarrhea, which is relieved by nasogastric suction. Endoscopy performed in patients with ZES may show multiple ulcers, large gastric rugal folds, edema of the mucosa lining the duodenum or proximal jejunum, or jejunal hypermotility. ZES should be suspected in patients with ulcer disease and diarrhea, a strong family history of peptic ulcer disease, atypical or multiple ulcers, or recurrence of ulcers after acid-reducing operations or H_2 blocker therapy.

Laboratory testing for gastrin levels will usually confirm the diagnosis of ZES. A fasting serum gastrin level is typically 200 to 1000 pg/mL in patients with a gastrinoma, compared to 100 to 150 pg/mL in normal patients. Three normal fasting serum gastrin determinations should be done to exclude ZES. Acid-reducing medications can increase gastrin levels so H_2 blockers should be stopped for at least 1 week prior to testing and proton-pump inhibitors should be held for 3 weeks to ensure accurate results. Other conditions can also cause hypergastrinemia (Table 42–4) and should be excluded prior to making the diagnosis of ZES. A gastrin level of greater than 1000 pg/mL in a patient without gastric outlet obstruction or suppression of acid production is virtually diagnostic of ZES. Gastric acid production can also be measured, especially if achlorhydria is suspected

TABLE 42–4. CAUSES OF HYPERGASTRINEMIA

High gastric acid output	
	Gastric outlet obstruction
	G-cell hyperplasia
	Incomplete antrectomy
	Gastrinoma
Low gastric acid output	
H_2 receptor antagonists	
	Proton pump inhibitors
	Prior acid-reducing procedure
	Atrophic gastritis
	Achlorhydria
	Pernicious anemia
	Renal failure

to be causing hypergastrinemia, thus confounding the diagnosis. Basal acid output in patients with ZES is usually >15 mEq/hour which is not seen with achlorhydria. A gastric pH >3 without acid suppressing medications or prior acid reducing operations virtually excludes ZES as the potential cause of hypergastrinemia. A secretin stimulation test can also be used to confirm the diagnosis: 2 IU/kg of secretin is given intravenously and serum obtained for gastrin levels before injection and every 3 to 5 minutes thereafter for 30 minutes. ZES is present in approximately 85% of patients when gastrin levels rise above 200 pg/mL or >50% above baseline levels following administration of secretin.

Localization of gastrinomas can be challenging because of their small size and variable location (Fig 42–13). Most gastrinomas express somatostatin receptors, thus somatostatin receptor scintigraphy (SRS) with radiolabeled octreotide is often employed initially to localize the tumor. The radioisotope scan has an

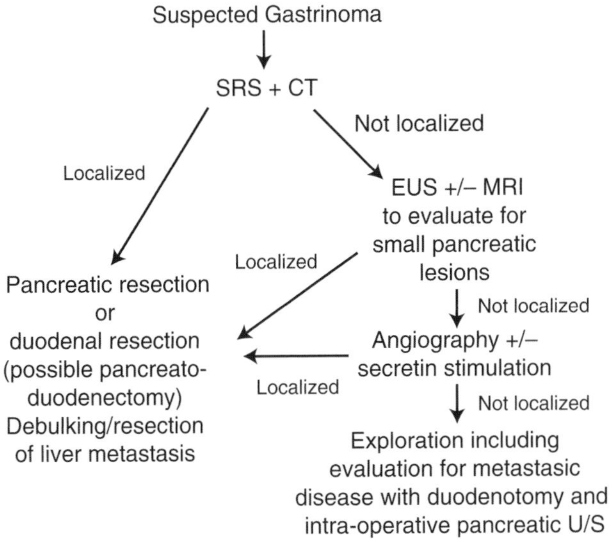

Figure 42–13. Localization of gastrinomas.

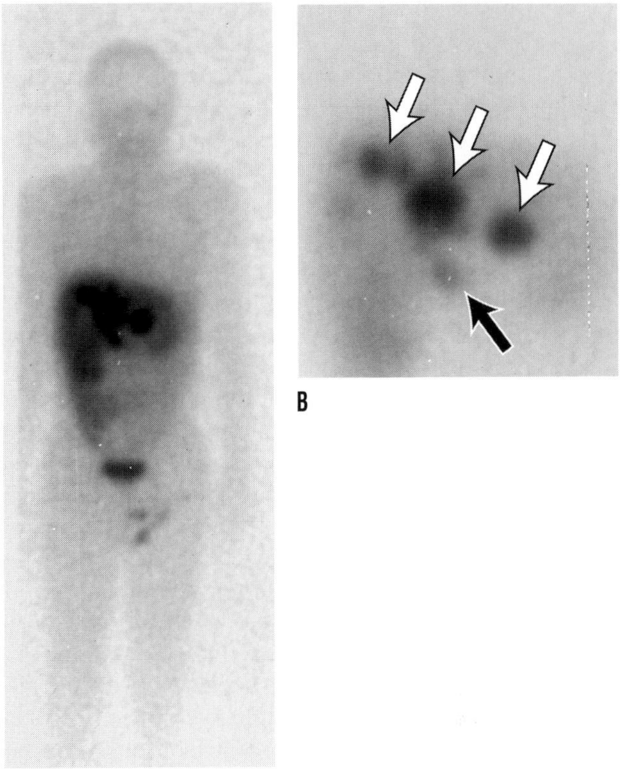

A B

Figure 42–14. Somatostatin receptor scintigram of a patient with metastatic gastrinoma. **A.** Whole body scan at 24 hours after injection of ^{111}In octreotide shows metastatic tumor in the liver with primary tumor in the head of the pancreas. **B.** Detail of hepatic metastases with pancreatic primary. White arrows denote hepatic metastases. The black arrow indicates the primary tumor in the pancreas. (From Thompson JC. Endocrine pancreas. In Townsend CM Jr, Beauchamp RD, Evers BM, Mattox KL (eds). *Sabiston Textbook of Surgery: The Biological Basis of Modern Surgical Practice,* 17th ed, Philadelphia: Elsevier Saunders; 2004:1001–1022, with permission.)

overall sensitivity of 80–100% and specificity of >90% for gastrinomas. SRS will also typically detect liver metastases when present (Fig 42–14). Gastrinomas not seen on the octreotide scan are typically small (<1 cm) and within the duodenal wall. Although sensitive, octreotide scanning may not show the exact location of a tumor, only its general vicinity within a few centimeters. More precise localization may be obtained by CT scanning, MRI, or other techniques. CT scanning has a 75–80% sensitivity overall but rarely detects tumors <1 cm and only 30% of tumors 1 to 3 cm. Gastrinomas within the pancreas are more readily detected by CT than in other locations, and liver metastases are usually detected if present. MRI is more sensitive than CT in detecting liver metastases. Less than 30% of sporadic gastrinomas are found within the duodenal wall; however, most are very small and are missed by CT scan. EUS may be useful to localize pancreatic gastrinomas not seen with other modalities (sensitivity approaches 90%), but detection of duodenal tumors with EUS is still poor (<50%). Some duodenal lesions may be seen on routine endoscopy, although its sensitivity is probably low. Angiography or ASVS with selective intra-arterial secretin injection has been used in select cases and may be useful in identifying which pancreatic lesions are functional when multifocal disease is present.

Duodenal gastrinomas are usually difficult to localize pre-operatively by any technique because of their small size. If not found by other techniques, it may be reasonable to proceed with operative exploration to definitively localize and treat the tumor at the same operation. Endoscopic transillumination of the duodenum will aid in the localization of small gastrinomas within the duodenal wall. Routine duodenotomy should also be utilized especially if the location of the tumor is at all in doubt or if multifocal disease is suspected as is common in MEN-1. Duodenotomy will detect 25–30% of tumors not seen on pre-operative imaging; therefore endoscopic transillumination of the duodenum and duodenotomy should be routinely performed.

Operative treatment of gastrinomas is indicated when curative resection appears possible based on pre-operative imaging or for palliative cytoreduction for symptom control. The surgical approach begins with careful inspection of the gastrinoma triangle to confirm the location of the tumor. Intraoperative ultrasound should be routinely applied to identify small pancreatic lesions or liver metastases. An extended Kocher maneuver and mobilization of the pancreatic body and tail allow for complete inspection of the pancreas. The duodenal wall can be gently palpated between the surgeon's fingers through a 3-cm duodenotomy on the anterior/lateral surface of the second portion of the duodenum allowing the detection of gastrinomas <1 cm in size. Small tumors within the duodenal wall should be excised by full thickness resection of the intestinal wall. Solitary gastrinomas of the liver should be resected, and enucleation of small pancreatic lesions is often curative even when malignant (Fig 42–15). Distal pancreatectomy should only be performed if the tumor is localized to the pancreatic tail; tumors in the pancreatic head should be enucleated. Pancreaticoduodenectomy is indicated only when necessary to completely excise gastrinomas in the head of the pancreas or adjacent duodenal wall. Pancreatic head resection in the presence of known metastatic disease is controversial, as the risk of surgical intervention may outweigh the morbidity associated with untreated disease. Pancreaticoduodenectomy may increase disease free survival in patients with MEN-1 because, following local excision, recurrent tumors are most commonly found within the duodenum. Blind resections of the pancreas are not indicated for gastrinomas, particularly since tumors not seen within the pancreas are likely to reside in another location within the gastrinoma triangle, which would not be removed with a pancreatic resection. Detailed inspection of peripancreatic, periduodenal, and portohepatic lymph nodes should be performed as resection of grossly positive lymphatic spread may increase disease free survival.

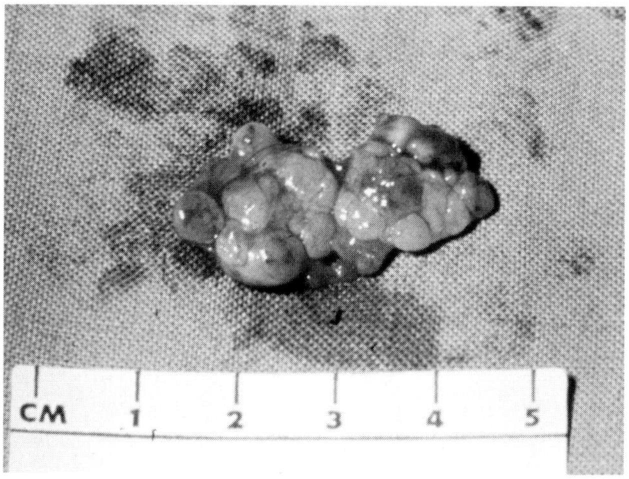

Figure 42–15. Gastrinoma excised from the gastrohepatic omentum. The tumor was excised from a patient with an elevated gastrin level after no lesions were found within the duodenum or pancreas. The patient's gastrin level fell from 800 to 72 pg/mL and has remained within normal limits on follow-up examinations.

Unfortunately, more than half of patients with gastrinomas have metastatic disease at the time of diagnosis. For these patients, treatment should focus on symptom control (i.e., reduction of acid production). The development of proton-pump inhibitors (PPIs) has reduced the need for surgical intervention for control of acid-related symptoms in patients with ZES. PPIs are so effective at reducing acid secretion that surgical procedures which had previously been superior to medications, are now rarely performed. Symptoms are controlled in >90% of patients starting with doses of 40 to 80 mg daily, although higher doses may be required. Efficacy can be demonstrated by measuring basal acid output (BAO); PPI dosage should be titrated to keep BAO <10 mEq/hour (or <5 mEq/hour if the patient had a prior acid reducing procedure). Octreotide can be used to decrease gastrin release and control acid secretion but is rarely effective without concurrent PPI use.

One of the few remaining indications for total gastrectomy in patients with ZES is the presence of gastric carcinoid tumors which may arise from prolonged hypergastrinemia. Gastric carcinoids probably occur in <10% of patients with MEN-1 and ZES; thus gastrectomy is rarely required. Gastrectomy may also be indicated for patients who are unable to tolerate PPIs and cannot achieve acid secretion control through other means. Total gastrectomy cures all symptoms produced by excessive acid.

The best predictor of survival for patients with gastrinoma is the presence of liver (not lymph node) metastases. Patients with bulky metastatic disease have a 5-

year survival <50%, while 90% of patients without metastases are alive after 5 years. Norton and colleagues showed that 58% of patients with gastrinomas had normalized gastrin levels following resection; however, approximately 50% of the patients in their series had recurred within 5 years yet 10-year survival was still >60% (Fig 42–16). Resection of all gross disease and metastases may provide palliation of symptoms and may prolong survival. Patients have been known to live more than 20 years with residual disease. Chemoembolization or radiofrequency ablation of hepatic metastases may be effective in reducing tumor burden within the liver. Cytotoxic chemotherapy has been used in patients with metastatic disease but does not provide a demonstrated survival benefit.

■ VIPOMA

Vasoactive intestinal peptide (VIP) is a small peptide normally found in the brain, G cells of the antrum, adrenal medulla, gut mucosa, pancreatic neurons, and the D_2 cells of the pancreas. VIPomas in the pancreas are believed to originate from neoplastic D_2 cells, which release high levels of VIP producing the Verner-Morrison syndrome. This syndrome is also known as WDHA syndrome, an acronym for its most prominent symptoms (Watery Diarrhea, Hypokalemia, and Achlorhydria). Overall, these tumors are exceedingly rare with an incidence of less than 1 per 2,000,000. There is a bimodal age distribution with most patients diagnosed at middle age but a small percentage (approximately 10%) diagnosed before the age of 10 years. Elevated VIP levels in these young patients are most commonly from ganglioneuromas, ganglioblastomas, or neuroblastomas, instead of pancreatic tumors. In the more common pancreatic form of VIPoma, lesions are usually solitary and 75% are found in the pancreatic body or tail (Fig 42–17). Two thirds of VIPomas are malignant and 50–60% of patients have liver or lymph node metastases at the time of diagnosis. Approximately 10% of patients with VIPomas have MEN-1.

Superphysiologic levels of VIP cause the symptoms associated with Verner-Morrison syndrome. VIP acts on intestinal epithelial cells to activate adenylate cyclase, thus increasing cyclic adenosine monophosphate (cAMP) levels within colonocytes, which stimulates hypersecretion of fluid into the lumen resulting in watery diarrhea. The diarrhea is further exacerbated as cAMP inhibits sodium reabsorption and stimulates chloride secretion causing increased fluid and electrolyte shifts into the intestinal lumen. Profuse, watery, iso-osmotic secretory diarrhea is the most common presenting symptom and may exceed a volume of 3 L/day. Stool volume less than 700 g/day is unlikely to be a result of VIPoma. This secretory diarrhea is independent of food intake and does not resolve with nasogastric suction, distinguishing it from the diarrhea associated with ZES. The liquid stool has the appearance of "weak tea" and is devoid of blood, fat, or inflammatory cells, which further distinguishes VIP-associated diarrhea from infectious, inflammatory, and malabsorptive conditions. Weight loss, crampy abdominal pain, dehydration, electrolyte abnormalities,

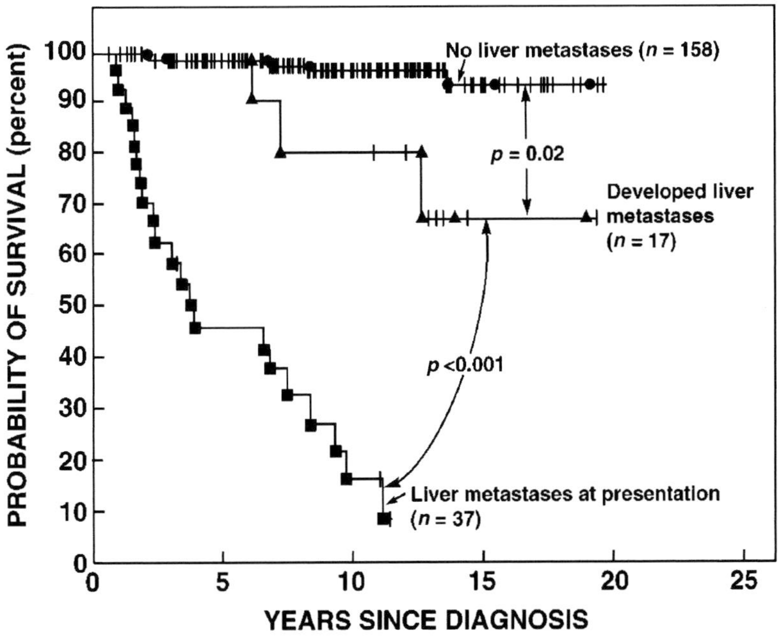

Figure 42–16. Effect of the presence of liver metastases at the initial evaluation, or the development of liver metastases on survival in patients with gastrinomas. Disease-specific survival rates are shown. Of the 158 patients with no liver metastases, 6 died during follow-up, whereas 4/17 patients who developed liver metastases died and 23/37 patients who initially had liver metastases at first evaluation, died during the follow-up period since diagnosis. (Modified from Yu F, Venzon DJ, Serrano J, et al. Prospective study of the clinical course, prognostic factors and survival in patients with longstanding Zollinger–Ellison syndrome. *J Clin Oncol* 1999;17:615–630, with permission.)

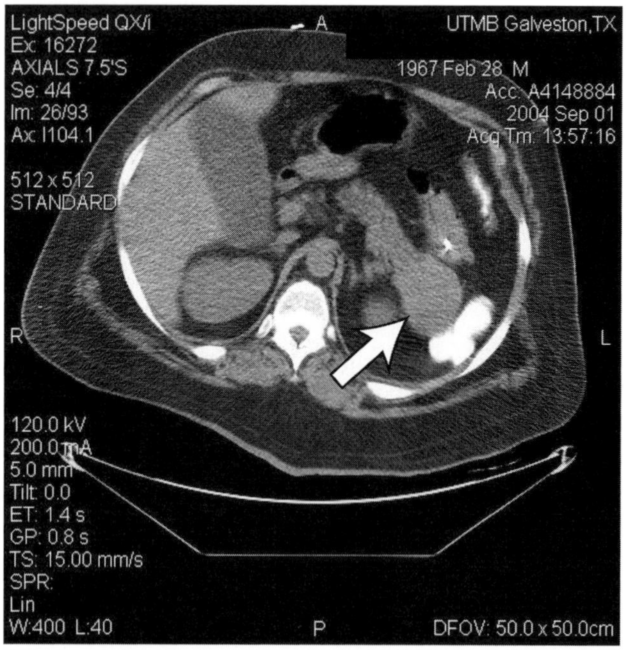

Figure 42–17. CT scan demonstrating a large VIPoma in the tail of the pancreas. (Courtesy of Aytekin Oto, M.D., The University of Texas Medical Branch.)

and metabolic acidosis (from fluid and bicarbonate loss) are common. Hypokalemia may be profound as patients can lose more than 400 mEq of potassium/day, which may lead to disturbances of cardiac rhythm, and even sudden death in extreme cases. Nearly 75% of patients have hypochlorhydria or achlorhydria and decreased levels of magnesium and phosphorus are often present. Other potential causes of diarrhea that should be considered in the differential diagnosis are ZES, laxative abuse, carcinoid syndrome, and hyperthyroidism. VIP may also vasodilate cutaneous blood vessels, causing flushing in 20% of patients.

Diagnosis of a VIPoma can be established by measuring serum levels of VIP, which are usually >150 pg/mL, in association with secretory diarrhea. Levels of VIP should be measured after an overnight fast. Localization of VIPomas is usually performed by CT scanning or SRS (Fig 42–18). When pre-operative studies are inconclusive, intra-operative ultrasound of the pancreas will localize most tumors.

Surgical treatment of VIPomas begins with aggressive pre-operative hydration and correction of electrolyte abnormalities and acid-base disturbances. Octreotide is commonly used pre-operatively to reduce diarrhea volume and facilitate fluid and electrolyte replacement. If diarrhea persists despite octreotide therapy, addition of a glucocorticoid may be helpful. Resection of the VIPoma is the treatment of choice as complete excision offers the only chance of cure. Because VIPomas tend to be invasive, simple enucleation is often inadequate and partial pancreatic resection is usually recommended. Unfortunately, complete excision is difficult, and the common presence of metastases results in only one third of patients cured after resection. Palliative resection of recurrences and metastatic foci may be helpful to control symptoms; however, improvement in overall survival is unlikely. In contrast, resection of VIP-producing ganglioneuroblastomas can yield cure rates approaching 70% in affected children. Adjuvant chemotherapy has not been shown to be beneficial.

▪ GLUCAGONOMA

Glucagonomas are exceedingly rare with an incidence of less than 1 per 1,000,000. They are 2 to 3 times more common in women than men and tend to be larger than most other pancreatic endocrine tumors, averaging 5 to 10 cm in size at the time of diagnosis. Glucagonomas are believed to arise from neoplastic alpha-cells, which normally produce glucagon to maintain glucose homeostasis. These tumors nearly always arise in the pancreas; 65–75% of these are found in the body or tail which corresponds to the normal distribution of alpha cells in the pancreas. Malignancy occurs in 50–80% of patients with a glucagonoma, as defined by metastases to regional lymph nodes or the liver. Eighty percent of patients with malignant glucagonomas have liver metastases at the time of diagnosis. Most glucagonomas are sporadic, however, 5–17% are associated with MEN-1, and these patients tend to be younger at the time of diagnosis.

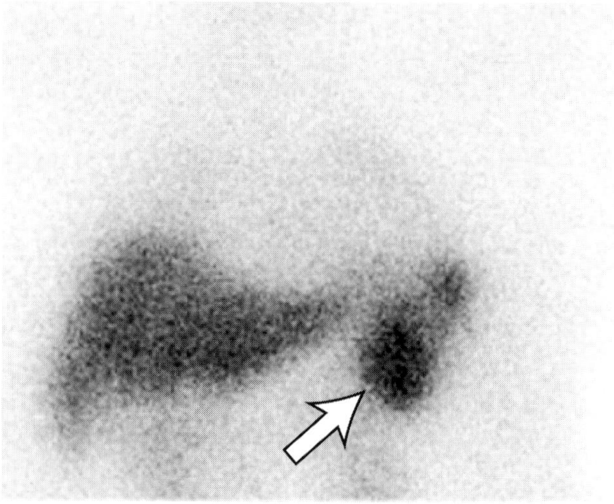

Figure 42–18. Somatostatin receptor scintigram demonstrating increased uptake in the region of the tail of the pancreas. Biochemical testing and postresection histopathology confirmed the diagnosis of VIPoma. (Courtesy of Aytekin Oto, M.D., The University of Texas Medical Branch.)

Glucagonomas release large amounts of glucagon, which induces a state of catabolism leading to clinical manifestations characteristic of the glucagonoma syndrome. The most constant finding in patients with a glucagonoma is weight loss because of metabolism of glucose, protein, and fat stores. Glucagon acts on the liver to stimulate glucose release, glycogenolysis, gluconeogenesis, and ketogenesis. Glycolysis is inhibited, which contributes to the symptoms of hyperglycemia. The circulating pool of amino acids becomes depleted as fuel for gluconeogenesis, and other protein stores from the muscle and liver are catabolized to provide more substrates for further glucose production. Lipogenesis is also inhibited and lipolysis stimulated leading to depletion of fat stores, weight loss and fat-soluble vitamin deficiency. Diabetes is present in 76–94% of patients with glucagonoma at some point during their illness and 38% of patients will demonstrate an elevated glucose level at initial presentation. Hypoaminoacidemia and normochromic normocytic anemia are also common.

The most consistent clinical finding in patients with glucagonoma is migratory necrolytic dermatitis, noted in approximately two-thirds of patients (Fig 42–19). The etiology is thought to be because of severe amino acid deficiency, although trace element deficiency and general malnutrition probably contribute. Diagnosis of a glucagonoma is often made by dermatologists, as this characteristic rash is such a constant finding in affected patients. Migratory necrolytic dermatitis begins as erythematous patches in intertriginous areas (mouth, vagina, and anus) which spread radially to form a serpiginous pattern on the trunk, extremities or face. Bullae develop, then slough, leaving crusty necrotic areas that may become superinfected with bacteria or fungi from the skin. Healing begins from the center of these lesions and takes between 2 to 3 weeks, leaving the healed skin hyperpigmented. Biopsies from the edge of these lesions will show superficial spongiosis with necrosis between the stratum corneum and the malpighian layer. Other common symptoms in patients with glucagonomas are thromboembolism, diarrhea, and vulvovaginitis.

The diagnosis of glucagonoma is established by measuring glucagon levels; a fasting glucagon level >50 pmol/L is considered diagnostic. Localization of these tumors is much easier than other pancreatic endocrine tumors, as they are typically large and can be readily seen on a CT scan. If present, metastases, especially in the liver, can be seen on CT scan. If the tumor cannot be localized by CT scan, angiography can be employed and is usually successful as glucagonomas tend to be highly vascular (Fig 42–20).

Treatment begins with medical therapy to improve the nutritional condition of these patients who have typically lost a significant amount of weight and lean body mass. Supplemental enteral nutrition in excess of basic caloric needs is often required in conjunction with high doses of octreotide (up to 1000 μg/day) to reverse the catabolic state. Prophylaxis against thromboembolism should be instituted early in the hospitalization to prevent peri-operative deep vein thrombosis and pulmonary embolism which are leading causes of death in these patients. Intravenous infusions of amino acids may be required to reverse symptoms and improve dermatitis. Once the patient's nutritional status has improved, surgical resection offers the only chance for cure. Enucleation is rarely sufficient for glucagonomas as they tend to be large and locally invasive. Distal pancreatectomy will usually suffice as most of these tumors occur in the body or tail of the pancreas. Pancreaticoduodenectomy and rarely total pancreatectomy may be required to adequately remove gross disease. Primary tumors should be resected even when metastases are present as these tumors tend to be slow growing, and tumor debulking will improve control of the catabolic state. Following resection, 5-year survival is nearly 85% if no metastases are present. Five-year survival is approximately 60% in patients with metastatic disease. Dacarbazine is uniquely effective against glucagonoma, as compared to other pancreatic endocrine tumors, and complete remission has been reported in several cases.

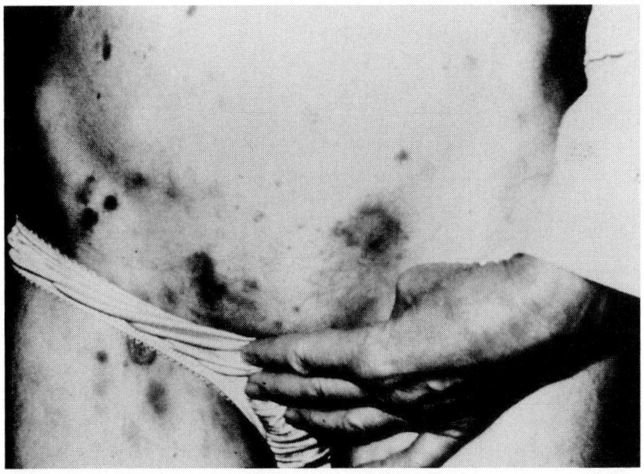

Figure 42–19. Characteristic skin rash associated with glucagonoma. This figure shows the migratory necrolytic dermatitis in a woman, 42 years of age, who has been symptomatic for 16 years. The rash had spread to involve the entire body. Note the central clearing. (Courtesy of Hugo Villar from Beauchamp RD, Thompson JC, 1997. Endocrine tumors of the pancreas. In: Zinner MJ, Schwartz SI, Ellis H (eds). *Maingot's Abdominal Operations*, 10th ed, Vol. II. Stamford, CT: Appleton & Lange, 1997:1961–1976.)

▪ SOMATOSTATINOMA

Somatostatinomas are exceedingly rare with fewer than 100 cases reported in the literature. These tumors are

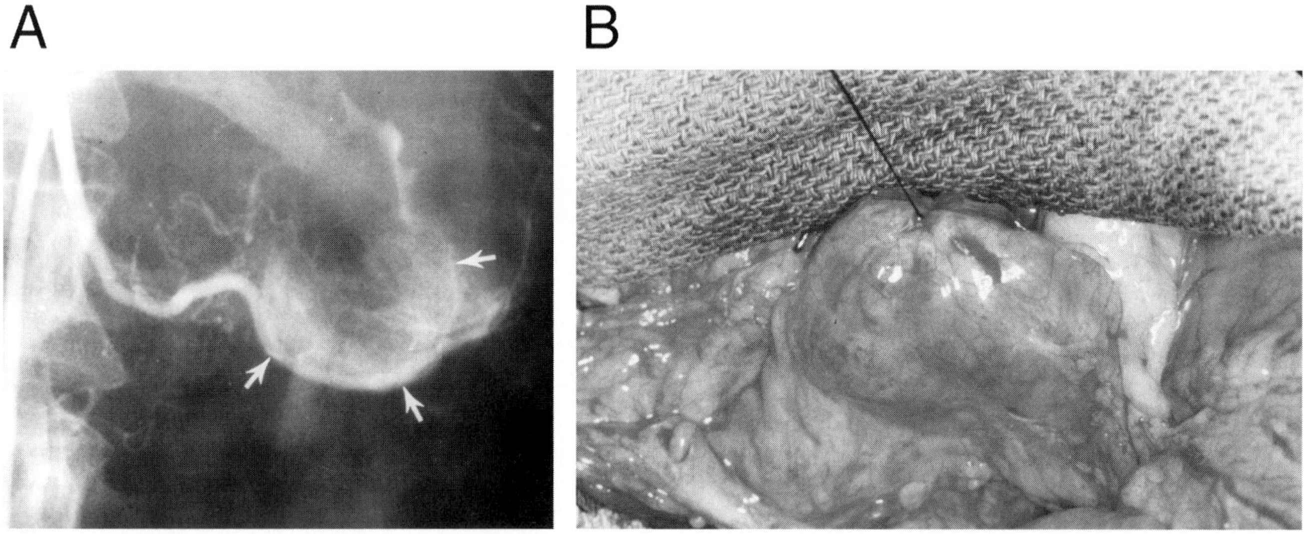

Figure 42–20. A. Angiogram showing a glucagonoma in the tail of pancreas. **B.** Appearance of the same glucagonoma in the tail of the pancreas at the time of resection. (Courtesy of Hugo Villar from Beauchamp RD, Thompson JC, 1997. Endocrine tumors of the pancreas. In: Zinner MJ, Schwartz SI, Ellis H (eds). *Maingot's Abdominal Operations,* 10th ed, Vol. II. Stamford, CT: Appleton & Lange, 1997:1961–1976.)

usually large (85% are >2 cm) and solitary. Patients are typically in their fifth or sixth decade of life at the time of diagnosis. Most somatostatinomas (68%) are found in the pancreas (usually the head) with the remainder in the duodenum or elsewhere in the small intestine. The majority are malignant with metastases to the liver or lymph nodes commonly noted at the time of diagnosis. Somatostatinomas are rarely associated with MEN-1 but may be found in conjunction with neurofibromatosis type 1 and pheochromocytomas.

Symptoms are the result of somatostatin's inhibitory effect on most GI and pancreatic functions. Somatostatin inhibits release of secretin, cholecystokinin, insulin, glucagon, gastrin, VIP, motilin, and pancreatic polypeptide. Inhibition of pancreatic enzyme secretion causes steatorrhea and gallbladder emptying is reduced, which predisposes patients to the development of cholelithiasis. Inhibition of insulin and gastrin cause diabetes and hypochlorhydria, respectively.

Diagnosis of somatostatinomas is seldom made preoperatively, but may be found during the work-up for unexplained causes of abdominal pain, jaundice, or diarrhea. The diagnosis can be confirmed by documenting an elevated fasting somatostatin level. Surgical resection of the tumor offers the only chance for cure; however, this is rarely achieved because of their large size and propensity for malignancy. If resection appears feasible, pancreaticoduodenectomy is usually required since these tumors are most commonly in the pancreatic head. If metastatic disease is present, the benefit of major pancreatic resection may be small and unlikely to improve survival.

▪ NONFUNCTIONAL TUMORS AND PPOMAS

Twenty percent of pancreatic endocrine tumors are nonfunctional. That is, hormones may be produced by these tumors but either have little biological consequence or do not produce symptoms. Nonfunctional tumors are usually diagnosed by histologic findings after a suspected pancreatic exocrine tumor has been resected, or less commonly discovered during the work-up for non-specific GI complaints. Pancreatic polypeptide (PP) secreting tumors (PPomas) are also classified as nonfunctional because even high pancreatic polypeptide levels rarely cause symptoms. On microscopic examination, nonfunctional tumors do not appear different than their functional counterparts; the endocrine origin of these tumors is usually identified by positive immunostaining for insulin. Two thirds of nonfunctional pancreatic endocrine tumors are malignant and 60–80% of malignant tumors have metastasized to distant sites at the time of diagnosis. These tumors are typically larger than their functional counterparts (4 to 5 cm vs. 1 to 2 cm, respectively) when initially discovered. Patients may present with abdominal pain and jaundice secondary to compression of adjacent structures. This is particularly common with PPomas that occur predominately within the head of the pancreas. Standard CT or MRI will usually demonstrate the location of non-functional pancreatic endocrine tumors because of their size. Surgical resection offers the only chance for cure. Unfortunately, the common presence of metastases may make complete excision impossible. The high frequency of malignancy mandates pancreaticoduodenectomy or distal pancreatectomy (not enucleation) if the intent of the pancreatic resection is curative. Even in patients with liver metastases, pancreatic resection may eliminate symptoms related to the size of the mass and improve survival. Overall, 5-year survival for nonfunctional pancreatic endocrine tumors is approximately 50%.

■ OTHER PANCREATIC ENDOCRINE TUMORS

Pancreatic endocrine tumors that produce other hormones have been described, but are extremely rare. Approximately 50 cases of pancreatic tumors that produce gastrin-releasing factor have been described, almost always in association with MEN-1. These gastrin-releasing factor-secreting tumors are usually found in the lung but the second most common location is within the pancreas. Forty percent of these patients will also have ZES and/or Cushing's syndrome. Acromegaly is often seen and the signs and symptoms of gastrin-releasing factor tumors are dependent upon whether ZES or Cushing's syndrome is also present. Adrenocorticotropic hormone (ACTH)-secreting tumors are also rare with fewer than 100 cases reported; these tumors occur in 5% of patients with ZES but 19% of patients with both ZES and MEN-1. Neurotensin-secreting tumors may produce a wide variety of symptoms (hypokalemia, weight loss, cyanosis, hypotension, flushing, and diabetes) yet it is unclear if these symptoms are a result of the effects of neurotensin itself or activation of other GI hormones. Case reports of pancreatic endocrine tumors that secrete calcitonin, enteroglucagon, CCK, gastric inhibitory peptide, luteinizing hormone, or ghrelin have also been described.

■ FUTURE DIRECTIONS

The diagnosis and treatment of pancreatic endocrine tumors remains challenging despite major advancements in the understanding of their pathophysiology and behavior. In the near future, improvements in the localization of these endocrine tumors using positron emission tomography (PET) scanning and high-resolution helical CT scanners will help to identify even small (<1 cm) tumors. Newer enzyme-linked immunoassays (ELISA) are more sensitive than older radioimmunoassays and will allow better results from serum assays and selective portal venous sampling. Early clinical trials of directed chemotherapy using radioactive drugs that bind somatostatin receptors have been shown to induce partial or minor remission in patients with somatostatin receptor positive pancreatic endocrine tumors. Laparoscopic resection of pancreatic endocrine tumors is becoming more common, especially for insulinomas where simple enucleation is adequate treatment. Distal pancreatectomy may also be performed laparoscopically allowing for adequate resection of even small malignant tumors in the pancreatic body or tail. Expanding the patient population in which laparoscopic resection is possible will depend on improvements in pre-operative localization. More extensive pancreatic resections for malignant tumors are best resected through an open approach. For patients with unresectable disease, a new somatostatin analog recently developed, lanreotide, remains biologically active for up to 2 weeks following a single injection and controls symptoms as well as octreotide which must be given three times daily.

■ SUMMARY

The management of pancreatic endocrine tumors requires a thorough understanding of the biological behavior of these tumors and the essential role of surgical intervention in providing appropriate treatment. Challenges remain in the localization of these tumors although modern imaging technology demonstrates the tumor in most cases pre-operatively. Patients with MEN-1 often have more aggressive tumors, thus surgical resection should be sufficient to account for the high likelihood of malignant and multifocal disease. Tumor resection provides an excellent chance for cure, especially for insulinomas, and debulking of even widespread disease can lead to control of debilitating symptoms, allowing for favorable long-term survival. Surgeons are uniquely qualified to care for patients with pancreatic endocrine tumors because resection of tumor burden, including recurrences, remains the most effective method to control the debilitating symptoms caused by hormone overproduction.

SUGGESTED READINGS

Altimari AF, Badrinath K, Reisel HJ, et al. DTIC therapy in patients with malignant intra-abdominal neuroendocrine tumors. *Surgery* 1987;102:1009–1017

Assalia A, Gagner M. Laparoscopic pancreatic surgery for islet cell tumors of the pancreas. *World J Surg* 2004;28:1239–1247.

Balci NC, Semelka RC. Radiologic features of cystic, endocrine and other pancreatic neoplasms. *Eur J Radiol* 2001; 38:113–119

Becker S, Kahn D, Rothman S. Cutaneous manifestations of internal malignant tumors. *Arch Dermatol Syphilis* 1942; 45:1069

Bloom SR, Polak JM, Pearse AG. Vasoactive intestinal peptide and watery-diarrhoea syndrome. *Lancet* 1973; 2:14–16

Bordi C, Azzoni C, D'Adda T, et al. Pancreatic polypeptide-related tumors. *Peptides* 2002;23:339–348.

Carty SE, Jensen RT, Norton JA. Prospective study of aggressive resection of metastatic pancreatic endocrine tumors. *Surgery* 1992; 112:1024–1031; discussion 1031–1032

De Jong M, Valkema R, Jamar F, et al. Somatostatin receptor-targeted radionuclide therapy of tumors: preclinical and clinical findings. *Semin Nucl Med* 2002; 32:133–140

Demeure MJ, Klonoff DC, Karam JH, et al. Insulinomas associated with multiple endocrine neoplasia type I: the need for a different surgical approach. *Surgery* 1991;110: 998–1004; discussion 1004–1005

Doherty GM. Multiple endocrine neoplasia type 1: duodenopancreatic tumors. *Surg Oncol* 2003; 12:135–143

Doppman JL. Pancreatic endocrine tumors—the search goes on. *N Engl J Med* 1992; 326:1770–1772

Dralle H, Krohn SL, Karges W, et al. Surgery of resectable nonfunctioning neuroendocrine pancreatic tumors. *World J Surg* 2004; 28:1248–1260

Fidler JL, Johnson CD. Imaging of neuroendocrine tumors of the pancreas. *Int J Gastrointest Cancer* 2001; 30:73–85

Frucht H, Howard JM, Slaff JI, et al. Secretin and calcium provocative tests in the Zollinger-Ellison syndrome. A prospective study. *Ann Intern Med* 1989; 111:713–722

Gibril F, Schumann M, Pace A, et al. Multiple endocrine neoplasia type 1 and Zollinger-Ellison syndrome: a prospective study of 107 cases and comparison with 1009 cases from the literature. *Medicine (Baltimore)* 2004;83:43–83

Grossman AB, Reznek RH. Commentary: imaging of islet-cell tumours. *Best Pract Res Clin Endocrinol Metab* 2005;19: 241–243

Harris GJ, Tio F, Cruz AB, Jr. Somatostatinoma: a case report and review of the literature. *J Surg Oncol* 1987;36:8–16

Hausman MS, Jr., Thompson NW, Gauger PG, et al. The surgical management of MEN-1 pancreatoduodenal neuroendocrine disease. *Surgery* 2004;136:1205–1211

Jackson JE. Angiography and arterial stimulation venous sampling in the localization of pancreatic neuroendocrine tumours. *Best Pract Res Clin Endocrinol Metab* 2005;19: 229–239

Kaczirek K, Niederle B. Nesidioblastosis: an old term and a new understanding. *World J Surg* 2004;28:1227–1230

Kahan RS, Perez-Figaredo RA, Neimanis A. Necrolytic migratory erythema. Distinctive dermatosis of the glucagonoma syndrome. *Arch Dermatol* 1977; 113:792–797

Kaltsas GA, Besser GM, Grossman AB. The diagnosis and medical management of advanced neuroendocrine tumors. *Endocr Rev* 2004;25:458–511

Krejs GJ, Orci L, Conlon JM, et al. Somatostatinoma syndrome. Biochemical, morphologic and clinical features. *N Engl J Med* 1979;301:285–292

Kurose T, Seino Y, Ishida H, et al. Successful treatment of metastatic glucagonoma with dacarbazine. *Lancet* 1984; 1:621–622

Lo CY, Chan WF, Lo CM, et al. Surgical treatment of pancreatic insulinomas in the era of laparoscopy. *Surg Endosc* 2004;18:297–302

Mansour JC, Chen H. Pancreatic endocrine tumors. *J Surg Res* 2004;120:139–161

Marynick SP, Fagadau WR, Duncan LA. Malignant glucagonoma syndrome: response to chemotherapy. *Ann Intern Med* 1980;93:453–454

McGavran MH, Unger RH, Recant L, et al. A glucagon-secreting alpha-cell carcinoma of the pancreas. *N Engl J Med* 1966;274:1408–1413

McLean AM, Fairclough PD. Endoscopic ultrasound in the localisation of pancreatic islet cell tumours. *Best Pract Res Clin Endocrinol Metab* 2005;19:177–193

Noone TC, Hosey J, Firat Z, et al. Imaging and localization of islet-cell tumours of the pancreas on CT and MRI. *Best Pract Res Clin Endocrinol Metab* 2005;19:195–211

Norton JA, Cromack DT, Shawker TH, et al. Intraoperative ultrasonographic localization of islet cell tumors. A prospective comparison to palpation. *Ann Surg* 1988;207: 160–168

Norton JA, Jensen RT. Current surgical management of Zollinger-Ellison syndrome (ZES) in patients without multiple endocrine neoplasia-type 1 (MEN1). *Surg Oncol* 2003;12:145–151

Norton JA, Jensen RT. Resolved and unresolved controversies in the surgical management of patients with Zollinger-Ellison syndrome. *Ann Surg* 2004;240:757–773

Proye CA, Lokey JS. Current concepts in functioning endocrine tumors of the pancreas. *World J Surg* 2004;28: 1231–1238

Rosch T, Lightdale CJ, Botet JF, et al. Localization of pancreatic endocrine tumors by endoscopic ultrasonography. *N Engl J Med* 1992; 326:1721–1726

Sheth S, Hruban RK, Fishman EK. Helical CT of islet cell tumors of the pancreas: typical and atypical manifestations. *AJR Am J Roentgenol* 2002;179:725–730

Sugg SL, Norton JA, Fraker DL, et al. A prospective study of intraoperative methods to diagnose and resect duodenal gastrinomas. *Ann Surg* 1993;218:138–144

Thompson JC, Hirose FM, Lemmi CA, et al. Zollinger-Ellison syndrome in a patient with multiple carcinoid-islet cell tumors of the duodenum. *Am J Surg* 1968;115:177–184

Thompson JC, Lewis BG, Wiener I, et al. The role of surgery in the Zollinger-Ellison syndrome. *Ann Surg* 1983;197: 594–607

Thompson JC, Reeder DD, Bunchman HH. Clinical role of serum gastrin measurements in the Zollinger-Ellison syndrome. *Am J Surg* 1972;124:250–261

Thompson JC, Reeder DD, Villar HV, et al. Natural history and experience with diagnosis and treatment of the Zollinger-Ellison syndrome. *Surg Gynecol Obstet* 1975;140: 721–739

Tonelli F, Fratini G, Falchetti A, et al. Surgery for gastroenteropancreatic tumours in multiple endocrine neoplasia type 1: review and personal experience. *J Intern Med* 2005;257:38–49

Udelsman R, Yeo CJ, Hruban RH, et al. Pancreaticoduodenectomy for selected pancreatic endocrine tumors. *Surg Gynecol Obstet* 1993;177:269–278

Van Hoe L, Gryspeerdt S, Marchal G, et al. Helical CT for the preoperative localization of islet cell tumors of the pancreas: value of arterial and parenchymal phase images. *AJR Am J Roentgenol* 1995;165:1437–1439

Verner JV, Morrison AB. Islet cell tumor and a syndrome of refractory watery diarrhea and hypokalemia. *Am J Med* 1958;25:374–380

Virgolini I, Traub-Weidinger T, Decristoforo C. Nuclear medicine in the detection and management of pancreatic islet-cell tumours. *Best Pract Res Clin Endocrinol Metab* 2005;19: 213–227

Whipple AO, Frantz WK. Adenoma of islet cells with hyperinsulinism: a review. *Ann Surg* 1935;101:1299

Wiesli P, Brandle M, Pfammatter T, et al. Insulin determination by specific and unspecific immunoassays in patients with insulinoma evaluated by the arterial stimulation and venous sampling test. *Eur J Endocrinol* 2004;151:123–126

Wiesli P, Brandle M, Schmid C, et al. Selective arterial calcium stimulation and hepatic venous sampling in the evaluation of hyperinsulinemic hypoglycemia: potential and limitations. *J Vasc Interv Radiol* 2004;15:1251–1256

Yalow RS, Berson SA. Some applications of isotope dilution techniques. *Am J Roentgenol Radium Ther Nucl Med* 1956; 75:1059–1067

Zhang M, Xu X, Shen Y, et al. Clinical experience in diagnosis and treatment of glucagonoma syndrome. *Hepatobiliary Pancreat Dis Int* 2004;3:473–475

Zollinger RM, Ellison EH. Primary peptic ulcerations of the jejunum associated with islet cell tumors of the pancreas. *Ann Surg* 1955;142:709–723; discussion, 724–728

X

SPLEEN

43

The Spleen

Gina Adrales ▪ Thomas R. Gadacz

▪ HISTORICAL BACKGROUND

The spleen was regarded by Galen as "an organ of mystery," by Aristotle as unnecessary, by Pliny as an organ that might hinder the speed of runners and also as an organ that produced laughter and mirth, a concept reasserted in the Babylonian Talmud. The first recorded splenectomy was performed for splenomegaly on a 24-year-old Neapolitan woman in 1549 by Adrian Zacarelli. The first successful partial splenectomy for trauma was reported by Franciscus Rosetti in 1590. Thus, partial splenectomy for trauma antedated total splenectomy for trauma, first performed by Nicolaus Matthias in 1678 in Capetown, South Africa, on a patient whose spleen protruded through a flank wound. The first splenectomy for trauma in the United States was reported by O'Brien, a Royal Navy surgeon, in 1816. In 1866, Sir Thomas Spencer Wells gave an account of the first successful splenectomy in England.

Although Bilroth reported on an 1881 autopsy that a splenic injury might have healed spontaneously, as recently as 1927 Hamilton Bailey asserted that "surgical aid is always needed." During the first two decades of the 20th century, however, proponents began to appear championing the use of judicious tamponade of the organ and suture repair was reported to be successful. Zikoff, in Russia, is credited with the first successful repair of a lacerated spleen in 1895. The first successful partial splenectomy for trauma in modern times was reported by Campos Christo in 1962.

The role of the spleen in combating infection has been considered for many years. In 1919, controlled experiments with rat plague bacillus by Morris and Bullock concluded that removal of the spleen "robs the body of its resistance." Until relatively recently, however, most physicians and surgeons felt that splenectomy did not compromise the host defense against infection. The first of the contemporary reports was that of King and Shumacker in 1952, chronicling an increased susceptibility to infection in children following splenectomy for hematologic disorders. In 1973, Singer's review of the literature emphasized the increase in postsplenectomy sepsis in infants and children.

▪ ANATOMY

The spleen arises by mesenchymal differentiation along the left side of the dorsal mesogastrium in juxtaposition to the anlage of the left gonad in the 8-mm embryo. In the healthy adult, the weight of the spleen ranges between 75 and 100 g. It resides in the posterior portion of the left upper quadrant lying deep to the ninth, tenth, and eleventh ribs, with its long axis corresponding to that of the tenth rib. Its convex, superior, and lateral surfaces are immediately adjacent to the undersurface of the left leaf of the diaphragm. The configuration of the concave, medial surface of the spleen is a consequence of impressions made by the stomach, pancreas, kidney, and splenic flexure of the colon (Fig 43–1).

The position of the spleen is, in part, maintained by several suspensory ligaments, including the gastrosplenic, splenophrenic, splenocolic, and splenorenal ligaments (Figs 43–2 and 43–3). The gastrosplenic ligament contains the short gastric vessels that course to the splenic hilum from the greater curvature while the remaining ligaments are generally avascular, except in patients with portal hypertension or myeloproliferative disorders.

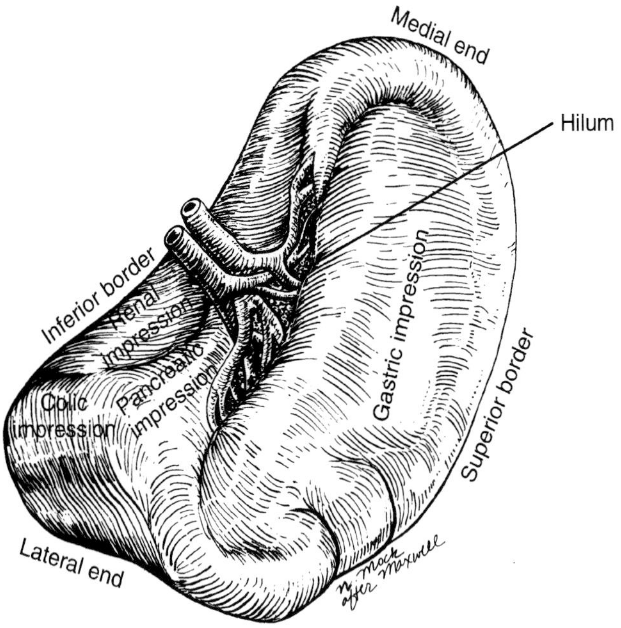

Figure 43–1. Gross anatomy of the spleen.

The splenic artery, a branch of the celiac artery, provides the spleen with arterial blood. A varying degree of branching occurs proximal to the hilus. Frequently, a branch to the inferior pole originates centrally. The major venous drainage flows through the splenic vein, which usually receives the inferior mesenteric vein centrally, and then joins the superior mesenteric vein to form the portal vein.

Accessory spleens, made of blood, sinuses, and malpighian bodies, have been classified into two types: (1) the more uncommon is a constricted part of the main organ to which it is bound by fibrous tissue, and (2) the more common is a distinct, separate mass. The latter has been reported in 14–30% of patients, with a higher incidence in patients with hematologic disorders. These accessory organs receive their blood supply from the splenic artery. They are present in decreasing order of frequency in the hilus of the spleen, the gastrosplenic ligament, splenorenal ligament, and the great omentum (Fig 43–4).

Accessory spleens may also occur in the pelvis of the female, either in the presacral region or adjacent to the left ovary, and in the scrotum in juxtaposition to the left testicle.

The spleen is made up of a capsule that is normally 1- to 2-mm thick, and trabeculae that surround and invaginate the pulp. The parenchyma (Fig 43–5) is made up of "white pulp" that functions as an immunologic organ, "red pulp" that phagocytizes particulate matter from the blood, and a marginal zone. The white pulp, which is central and surrounds a central artery, is made of lymphatic nodules with germinal centers and periarterial lymphatic sheaths that constitute a reticular network filled with lymphocytes and macrophages. Peripheral to the white pulp is the marginal zone that contains end arteries arising from the central artery and from peripheral penicilliary arteries. The marginal zone contains lymphocytes and macrophages and red blood cells (RBCs) that have exited from terminal arteries. The marginal zone also contains the marginal sinus that filters material from the centrally located white pulp. Locally produced immunoglobulins enter the marginal zone, eventually coursing to the blood stream.

Peripheral to the marginal zone is the red pulp. This pulp consists of cords and sinuses that contain cellular elements of blood in transit. Most of the blood flow passing through the spleen courses through an "open" circulation in which the blood passes from arterioles to reticular cell-lined networks of the splenic cords and to the sinuses.

▪ PHYSIOLOGY

Although the spleen is not necessary for life, it performs important functions that are generally divided into two major categories: (1) those related to cellular elements in the circulating blood and (2) those that are immunologic in nature.

The cellular functions include hematopoiesis, storage, "pitting," and "culling." Hematopoiesis, which supplies ery-

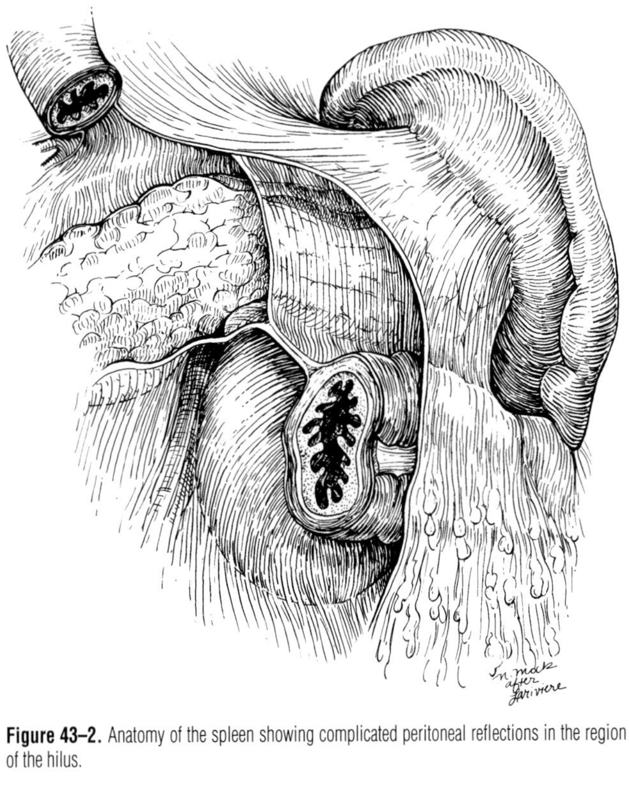

Figure 43–2. Anatomy of the spleen showing complicated peritoneal reflections in the region of the hilus.

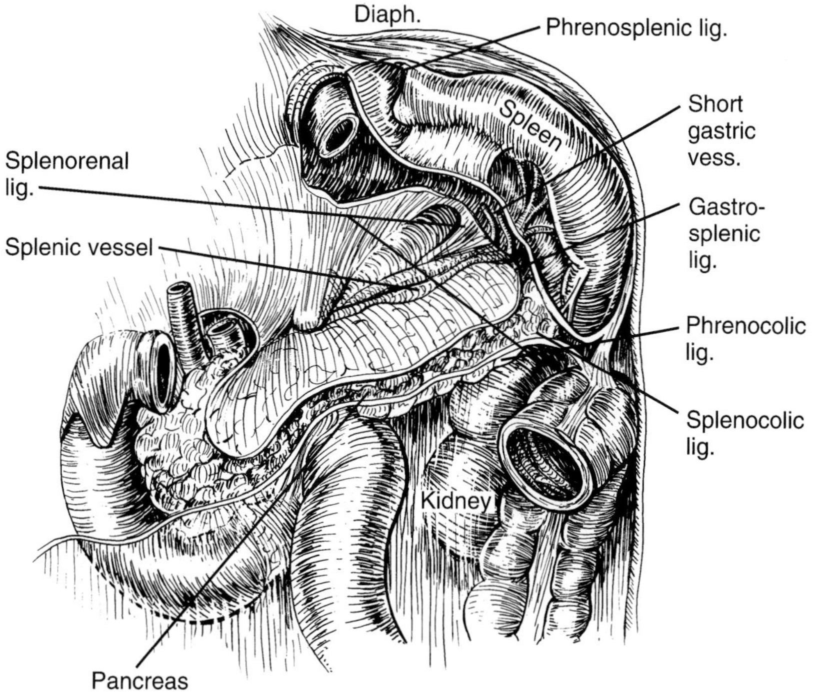

Figure 43–3. Ligaments of the spleen.

throid, myeloid, lymphoid cells, and platelets in fetal life, essentially ceases by the seventh intrauterine month. In human beings, the spleen does not serve as an important reservoir for blood cells, except platelets. At any given time, about one third of the total platelet mass is in the spleen.

Pitting refers to the removal of rigid structures such as Heinz bodies, Howell-Jolly bodies, and hemosiderin granules from red cells. The process involves the removal of nondeformable intracellular substances from deformable cells. The rigid body is phagocytized while the deformable cytoplasmic mass passes into the sinus and returns to the general circulation. The postsplenectomy blood smear is characterized by the presence of circulating erythrocytes with Howell-Jolly and Pappenheimer bodies (siderotic granules). Nucleated cells also have their nuclei removed in the same fashion.

Culling is the term applied to the spleen's ability to remove red cells that are aged or abnormal. Normally, as the red cell ages after a life span of approximately 120 days, it loses osmotic balance and membrane integrity, and therefore deformability. When these cells lose their deformability they are phagocytized by native macrophages. The spleen does not represent the only site for red cell destruction, and there is no difference in red cell survival following splenectomy. Naturally deformed cells and red cells that are affected by disease states also are removed by phagocytosis. In those circumstances in which there is a superabundance of reticulocyte formation, these cells are remodeled in the spleen and exit as mature cells. In the normal adult, the spleen is the most important site of selective erythrocyte sequestration. During its 120-day life cycle, the red cell spends an estimated minimum of 2 days within the spleen which, when normal, contains about 25 mL RBCs.

The neutrophil has a half-life of about 6 hours; hence 85% of neutrophils either emigrate at random into tissues or are destroyed within 24 hours. Although the role of the spleen in the destruction of neutrophils under normal conditions is not well quantified, the role of the spleen is amplified in some hypersplenic states, with resulting neutropenia. This augmented removal can occur because of splenic enlargement and accelerated sequestration of granulocytes or because of enhanced splenic removal of altered granulocytes, as seen in immune neotropenias.

There is significant interaction between the platelets and splenic cells. Normally, about one third of the platelet mass is pooled in the spleen, and this pool exchanges freely with the circulating platelets that have a life span of about 10 days. With splenomegaly, a large proportion of platelets is sequestered in the spleen (up to 80%) and this, coupled with accelerated platelet destruction in the spleen, accounts for thrombocytopenia. Splenic phagocytosis of platelets occurs in normal states, but in pathologic states, such as immune thrombocytopenia, it is greatly accelerated.

In addition to the phagocytosis of antibody-coated cells, the immunologic functions of the spleen include antibody synthesis (especially immunoglobulin M [IgM]), generation of lymphocytes, and production of tuftsin, opsonins, properdin, and interferon.

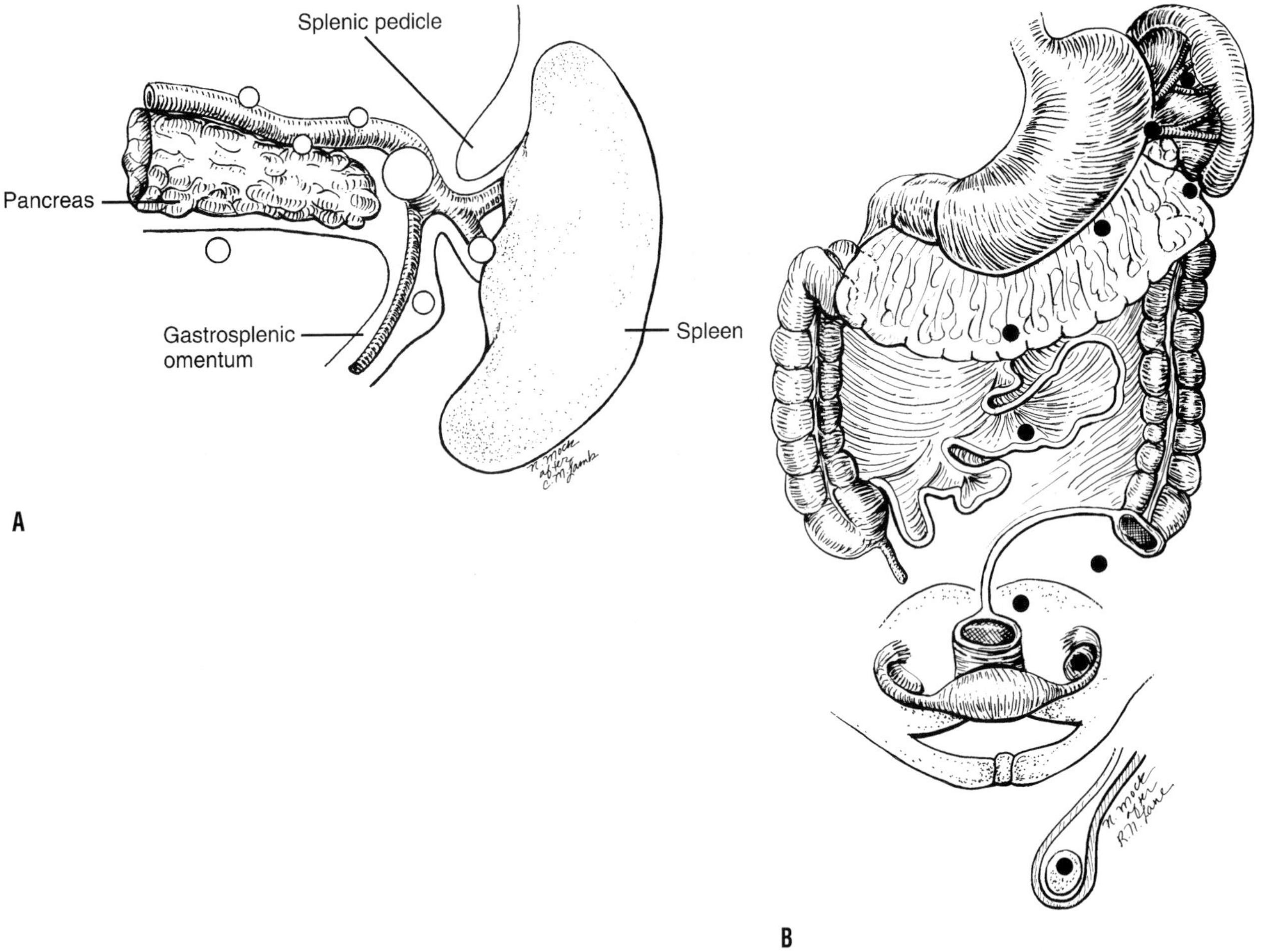

Figure 43–4. A. The more common locations of accessory spleens. Accessory spleens are also found in the left ovary, in the left testicle along the course of the left ureter, and in the lesser sac and greater omentum. **B.** Locations of accessory spleens. Note position of presacral and paraureteric splenuli.

▪ THE ASPLENIC STATE

The spleen contributes to the immune system by cell filtration, antibody and opsonin production, and phagocytic clearance of bacteria. Asplenic or hyposplenic patients are particularly susceptible to encapsulated bacteria, such as pneumococcus, and malaria. The liver may compensate for the loss of the immunologic function of the spleen but this requires an intact complement system and higher antibody production.

Overwhelming postsplenectomy sepsis (OPSS) is a rare phenomenon among adult patients after splenectomy for trauma and nonhematologic disease. A review by Cuschieri revealed that OPSS occurs in 0.9% of adults and 4.4% of children younger than 16 years of age with an attendant mortality risk of 0.8% and 2.2%, respectfully.[1] However, the mortality risk has been reported to be as high as 50–70%.[2] Reticuloendothelial dysfunction, such as that caused by hematologic disease or immunosuppression, increases the likelihood of sepsis. Young children, particularly younger than the age of 2 years, are also at increased risk because of the immaturity of the immune system.

Knowledge of the potential infection risk and patient education are fundamental to the reduction of the OPSS mortality risk. The risk persists over the patient's lifetime, with approximately 42% of cases occurring more than 5 years after splenectomy.[3] Patients should be vaccinated against encapsulated organisms with recombinant polyvalent *Streptococcus pneumonia*, *Haemophilus influenzae* type B, and *Neisseria meningitides* vaccines. These vaccines should be administered at least two weeks before planned splenectomy and as soon as possible after recovery from emergent splenectomy prior to hospital discharge. The pneumococcal vaccine should be repeated every 5 to 6 years. Pneumococcal antibody titers can be obtained to assess immunity; however, the required level of antibody protection is uncertain. Patients with immunoproliferative disorders, immunosuppressed states because of chemotherapy, and hematologic disease such as sickle cell anemia, may need

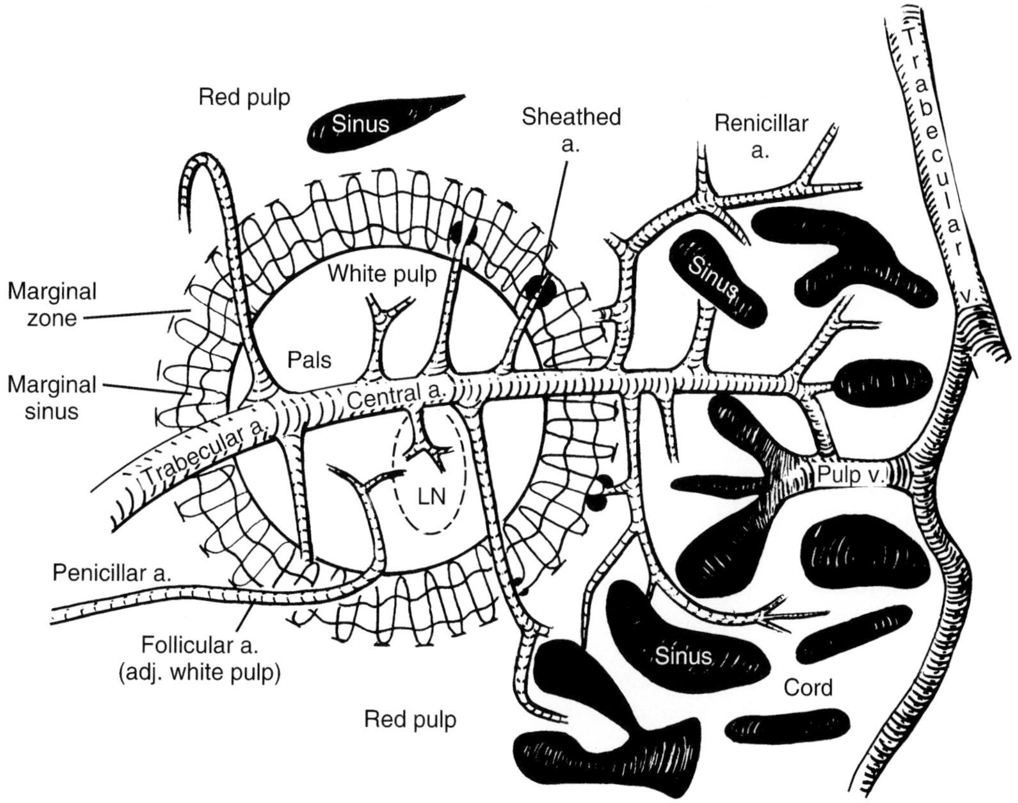

Figure 43–5. Diagram illustrating splenic compartments and potential vascular supply routes. A = artery; V = vein; LN = lymphatic nodule, which may include germinal center; PALS = periarterial lymphatic.

more frequent pneumococcal revaccination. The supporting data for meningococcal and *Haemophilus* vaccines are less defined.

Early recognition of postsplenectomy infection is key. This is particularly important as vaccination does not imply immunity and the pneumococcal vaccine is only 70% protective even in the immunocompetent host.[2] Additionally, other pneumococcal, *Haemophilus* non-type B, and meningococcus strains as well as other bacteria may cause overwhelming infection. Meningitis, particularly among children, and pneumonia are often seen. However, the initial prodrome of fever, myalgia, emesis, headache, and abdominal pain may go unrecognized without an astute awareness of the possibility of postsplenectomy sepsis. These early symptoms can quickly escalate into profound septic shock, accompanied by disseminated intravascular coagulation, and organ failure. Asplenic or hyposplenic patients should be instructed to seek immediate medical attention at the first sign of illness, with some physicians advocating a personal supply of prescribed antibiotics to have on hand. Others have advised daily penicillin prophylaxis for the first 2 years postsplenectomy, particularly for children younger than 5 years old. Lack of compliance and concern for breeding of resistant organisms have made this option less attractive.

▪ RUPTURE OF THE SPLEEN

ETIOLOGY

The causes of splenic rupture, in which the organ's parenchyma or capsule is disrupted, include penetrating trauma, nonpenetrating or blunt trauma, operative trauma, and, rarely, spontaneous rupture. Rupture of the spleen may be caused by puncture wounds because of stabbing or missiles. The trajectory of the penetrating wound may pass through the anterior abdominal wall, the posterior abdominal wall, the flank, or transthoracically, piercing the pleural space and diaphragm. Isolated splenic injury may be present, or organs in juxtaposition may be involved; this would include the stomach, left kidney, left adrenal gland, colon, pancreas, and root of the mesentery. Nonpenetrating or blunt trauma represents an increasing etiologic factor in splenic rupture.

DIAGNOSTIC STUDIES

A decrease in serial hematocrit measurements may suggest continued intraperitoneal hemorrhage. Increases in the WBC count to levels frequently greater than 15,000/

mm³ are often seen. Findings on routine abdominal films such as fractured ribs, elevated left hemidiaphragm, enlarged splenic shadow, medial gastric displacement, and widening of the space between the splenic flexure and the preperitoneal fat pad may be helpful. However, abdominal ultrasound and CT scan offer more specific information to diagnose the extent of disease or injury (Table 43–1). For instance, a contrast blush in or around the spleen on CT scan suggests active hemorrhage and may prompt angiographic embolization or splenectomy depending on the stability of the patient.

TABLE 43–1. SPLENIC ORGAN INJURY SCALE

Class I	Nonexpanding subcapsular hematoma <10% surface area.
	Nonbleeding capsular laceration with <1 cm deep parenchymal involvement.
Class II	Nonexpanding subcapsular hematoma 10–50% surface area.
	Nonexpanding intraparenchymal hematoma <2 cm in diameter.
	Bleeding capsular tear or parenchymal laceration 1–3 cm deep without trabecular vessel involvement.
Class III	Expanding subcapsular or intraparenchymal hematoma.
	Bleeding subcapsular hematoma or subcapsular hematoma >50% surface area
	Intraparenchymal hematoma >2 cm in diameter.
	Parenchymal laceration >3 cm deep or involving trabecular vessels.
Class IV	Ruptured intraparenchymal hematoma with active bleeding.
	Laceration involving segmental or hilar vessels producing major (>25% splenic volume) devascularization.
Class V	Completely shattered or avulsed spleen.
	Hilar laceration which devascularizes entire spleen.

(From Cogbill TH, Moore EE, et al. Nonoperative management of blunt splenic trauma: a multicenter experience. *J Trauma* 1989; 29:1312.)

MANAGEMENT

Penetrating injury patients and hemodynamically unstable blunt trauma patients with hemoperitoneum or peritonitis are treated with laparotomy and likely splenectomy. Splenic salvage may be attempted if hemostasis is achieved, greater than one third of the splenic mass can be preserved, and if other intraabdominal injuries, such as pancreatic trauma, do not warrant splenectomy. Splenorrhaphy and partial splenectomy were largely employed as splenic salvage techniques in the early 1990s. Nonoperative management is used increasingly in the management of splenic injury. While this practice was largely accepted in the treatment of injured pediatric patients to salvage the spleen and its immunologic function, it is only recently that nonoperative management has become established in the management of hemodynamically stable adults with blunt splenic injuries. With advances in imaging from trauma room abdominal ultrasound to spiral CT scan, more accurate and immediate grading of splenic injuries has been possible to guide therapy (Table 43–1). Grade IV and V injuries are likely to be treated with splenectomy. However, increasingly, lesser injuries are managed with close observation and serial hematocrits, and trauma centers are adopting a nonoperative approach to some grade IV injuries. Starnes and associates constructed a selection protocol based on CT grading of splenic injury.[4] Grade IV and V injuries were treated with laparotomy, while lower grade injuries were managed nonoperatively. Compared to a historical cohort of patients with blunt splenic trauma evaluated prior to implementation of the protocol, the splenic salvage rate improved from 67.9% to 72.4%. Additionally, there were no nonoperative failures after instituting the protocol.

Nonoperative failures with unpredictable and delayed splenic hemorrhage are a concern and have led to some reluctance in adopting this practice. Additionally, the concern for increased blood transfusion among patients managed nonoperatively has called this treatment strategy into question. This has not been borne out in recent literature, even in the nonoperative management of higher grade injuries.[5,6] Pachter and associates reported that 85% of 102 patients with splenic injuries managed nonoperatively did not require blood transfusion, and in fact, required less blood than the splenectomy cohort.[6]

Identification of factors that increase the risk of delayed hemorrhage after splenic trauma has been attempted in an effort to reduce nonoperative failures. Delayed hemorrhage has been linked to the presence of contrast extravasation or "blush" on CT scan.[7–10] Pseudoaneurysm and arteriovenous fistula have been reported as potential sources of delayed hemorrhage.[11,12] Admission angiography with embolization is used increasingly to manage hemodynamically stable patients with splenic trauma for splenic conservation (Fig 43–6A and 43–6B).[8,9,12–16]

Splenic salvage rates with angiographic embolization have been in the order of 87 to 95%.[9,15] Splenic embolization may be complicated by splenic abscess, infarction, and significant pain. Additionally, there are yet unanswered questions regarding the preservation of immunologic function after splenic embolization for trauma.

▪ LOCAL SPLENIC DISORDERS

ANEURYSMS OF THE SPLENIC ARTERY

Splenic artery aneurysm was first described by Baussier in 1770. St. Leger Brockman described one of the first

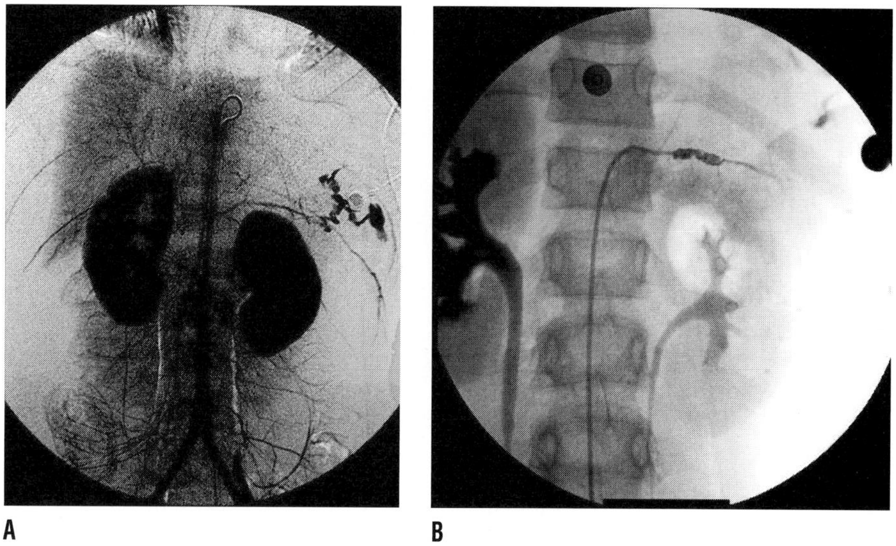

Figure 43–6. A. Contrast blush seen on angiography performed on a child who sustained blunt abdominal trauma. **B.** Splenic artery coil embolization successfully treated the splenic injury.

surgical cases in 1930. The first radiologic diagnosis was made by Lindboe in 1932.

The splenic artery is the most common visceral artery aneurysm and the second most common site of intra-abdominal aneurysms secondary to the abdominal aorta. The incidence in autopsy series ranges between 0.02% and 0.16%. Splenic artery aneurysms may occur as a complication of acute pancreatitis or pancreatic pseudocysts. An incidence as high as 10% has been reported.[17] A splenic artery aneurysm should be suspected in a patient with pancreatitis who develops gastrointestinal (GI) bleeding without an obvious source. Arteriography should be performed and is usually diagnostic as well as therapeutic. Embolization is successful in 73%.[18] In those patients with a pancreatic pseudocyst, drainage of the cysts is necessary to prevent subsequent hemorrhage.[19]

Splenic artery aneurysms may be more prevalent in women, usually as a consequence of atherosclerosis. In a series of 125 cases reported by Sherlock and Learmonth, the average diameter was 3.4 cm and the largest was 15 cm. The main splenic artery was involved in 81% of the cases, while 26% were multiple. Eighty-seven percent of splenic artery aneurysms occurred in women, and 92% of the women had been pregnant an average of 4.5 times. Rupture in the pregnant female, however, has been associated with a 70% maternal and 95% fetal mortality. Rupture during pregnancy occurs in 69% of the patients during the third trimester.

A splenic artery aneurysm usually is discovered in the sixth decade as an incidental finding. Eighty-three percent of the patients are asymptomatic at the time of diagnosis. The remainder present with epigastric, left upper quadrant, or left flank pain. The pain usually cannot be attributed conclusively to the aneurysm. The physical examination is usually normal, and a bruit is detectable in <10% of cases. A calcified lesion is noted on plain film of the abdomen in 70% of the patients (Figs 43–7A and 43–7B).

Rupture of the aneurysm is manifested by sudden abdominal pain. In 12.5% a warning hemorrhage occurs, with temporary cessation of bleeding. Rupture into the colon, stomach, and intestine may take place, but intraperitoneal rupture is by far the most common presentation. The risk of rupture in a calcified aneurysm is low, occurring in 1 of 34 patients; the patient was followed for 1 to 19 years, and that aneurysm was 7 cm in diameter. When rupture occurs in the nonpregnant female, it is usually contained in the lesser sac, resulting in a patient mortality rate of <5%.

Criteria for elective operation are not firm, but it is generally believed that removal is not required for the asymptomatic lesion that is <2 cm in diameter.[20] Symptomatic aneurysms and those greater than 2 cm should be removed if the patient is a reasonable operative risk. Lesions proximal to the hilus of the spleen can be managed by resection and primary end-to-end anastomosis or proximal and distal ligation with resection of the involved segment.[21] Proximal ligation is reasonable because the spleen will not become ischemic following central ligation of the main splenic artery. Distal lesions and multiple lesions generally require splenectomy and resection of the involved splenic artery. An aneurysm detected in a female who anticipates pregnancy should be removed and one detected during pregnancy should be removed before the third trimester.

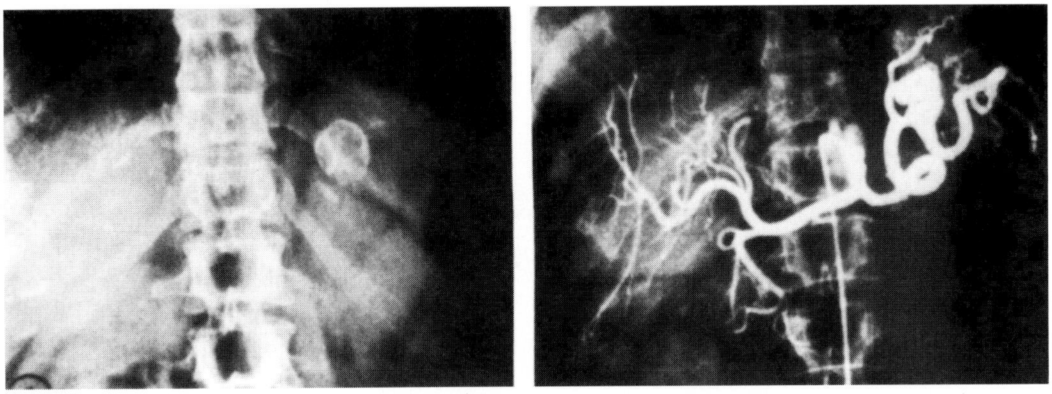

A B

Figure 43–7. A. Plain abdominal roentgenogram demonstrating "signet ring" pattern of calcification in left upper quadrant measuring 3 cm in diameter. **B.** Selective celiac arteriogram of same patient demonstrating saccular splenic artery aneurysm.

CYSTS

In 1929, Andral first described a dermoid splenic cyst at autopsy. Pean performed the first recorded splenectomy for a cyst in 1867. Cysts are generally classified as primary or secondary. Primary cysts have an epithelial lining and can be nonparasitic or parasitic (echinococcal).

Primary Cysts

Nonparasitic Cysts. This group of cysts includes simple cysts, epidermoid cysts, and dermoid cysts. Various classifications have been proposed based on whether they are lined with mesothelial, transitional, or epidermoid linings and also if they are neoplastic, traumatic or degenerative.[22]

Simple congenital cysts, lined by flattened or cuboidal cells originating from infolding of peritoneal mesothelioma during splenic development. These lesions are usually small and asymptomatic. Large simple cysts present with the same manifestations and imaging features as pseudocysts. Smaller lesions found incidentally do not require excision; larger lesions are removed by laparoscopic or open total or partial splenectomy.

About 10% of cysts are lined by squamous epithelium and are rare. These cysts are usually round and unilocular and may be very large. They are filled with yellow or brown turbid fluid. The cyst is dense and the diagnosis is established by microscopic definition of the stratified squamous lining. Examination of multiple cuts may be required to demonstrate the pathology.

Epidermoid cysts of the spleen occur in children and in young adults in 75% of the cases. About two-thirds of the patients have been female. The clinical manifestations are dependent upon the size and are similar to those of the pseudocysts, as are the imaging findings. Laparoscopic or open splenectomy or partial splenectomy is recommended for large or symptomatic cysts.

True dermoid cysts of the spleen are exceedingly rare; fewer than ten cases have met the pathological criteria of a squamous epithelium with dermal appendages such as hair follicles and sweat glands. Splenectomy is indicated.

Parasitic Cysts. Hydatid disease occurs epidemically in south-central Europe, South America, Australia, and Alaska. Two thirds or more of the splenic cysts are caused by echinococci. The parasitology of echinococcal disease is presented in the section on liver disease. Echinococcus granulosis, the most commonly implicated species, usually results in a unilocular cyst composed of an inner germinal layer (endocyst) and an outer laminated layer (ectocyst) surrounded by a fibrous capsule. Unlike the nonparasitic cysts, these are filled with fluid under positive pressure, and also contain daughter cysts and infective scolices.

Echinococcal cysts are usually asymptomatic unless they reach a size causing pressure symptoms or become secondarily infected or rupture.

As a diagnostic tool, the Casoni skin test is sensitive but not specific. The passive hemaglutination test provides the best diagnostic specificity and sensitivity and is preferable to flocculation and complement fixation tests. The abdominal films may show a partially calcified mass in the left upper quadrant. Ultrasound, CT, and MRI studies demonstrate a cystic mass that is septated and contains daughter cysts.

Careful percutaneous aspiration with irrigation with hypertonic saline to wash out the cyst and kill the protoscolices followed by irrigation with ethyl alcohol to prevent formation of cysts is one approach.[23] Splenectomy is the treatment of choice because there is no effective medical therapy. Care should be taken to avoid spilling the contents of the cyst. Intraoperatively, the lesions can be sterilized by instilling a 3% sodium chloride solution. Laparoscopic and percutaneous treatment has not been widely accepted in treating hydatid cysts because of a traditional fear of spillage and anaphylaxis.[24] If intraperitoneal spillage occurs during the dissection, anaphylactic hypotension may occur and require epinephrine to treat the shock.

Secondary Cysts

Pseudocysts do not have an epithelial lining and comprise 70–80% of splenic cysts. They are usually a result of trauma and represent resolution of a subcapsular or intraparenchymal hematoma. Malaria, infectious mononucleosis, tuberculosis, and syphilis are all predisposing factors. Pseudocysts vary in size and can be large, containing as much as 3 liters of a dark, turbid fluid. In over 80% of the cases the lesion is unilocular and the cyst wall is dense and smooth. Microscopically the wall consists of fibrous tissue without an internal epithelial lining.

Pseudocysts occur more frequently in women, children, and young adults. Many patients recall a history of trauma. One third of the patients are asymptomatic. The most frequent complaint is left upper quadrant pain radiating to the left shoulder or chest. Symptoms related to pressure on the stomach occur less frequently. Physical examination usually reveals a smooth mass in the left upper quadrant that can be seen on routine abdominal films. A focal calcification may be noted. Ultrasonography, CT, MRI, and magnetic resonance arteriography will define the cystic nature of the lesion. Laparoscopic[25] or open splenectomy is curative, and cases also have been managed by laparoscopic unroofing and draining the area, preserving the bulk of splenic parenchyma.

SPLENIC ABSCESSES

Splenic abscesses occur more frequently in the tropics, where there is a higher incidence of sickle cell anemia, with associated thrombosis of parenchymal vessels and consequent infarction.

A change in the clinical spectrum of splenic abscess was reported in 1974[26] and this has continued.[27] The major risk factors are intravenous drug use, human immunodeficiency virus disease, other hematogenous spread (endocarditis), splenic trauma, and contiguous spread. Most infections are polymicrobial and include such organisms as Staphylococcus, Salmonella, and *Escherichia coli*, *Proteus mirabilis*, Streptococcus group D, *K. pneumoniae*, Peptostreptococcus species, Bacteroides species, Fusobacterium species, Clostridium species, *Candida albicans*, and mycobacterium.

The symptoms are usually nonspecific such as malaise, weight loss, left upper quadrant pain, and fever. Most patients have a leucocytosis and an ultrasound, CT (Fig 43–8) or magnetic resonance study establishes the diagnosis of a splenic abscess. Treatment consists of

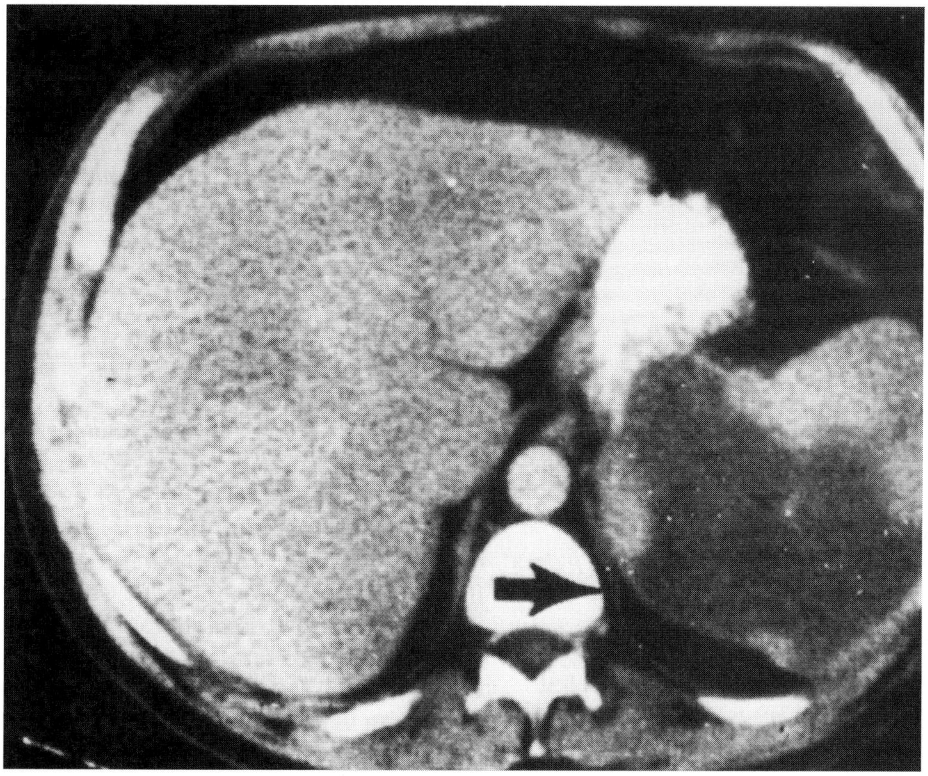

Figure 43–8. CT scan of abdomen with oral contrast demonstrating splenic abscess.

broad spectrum antibiotics and percutaneous drainage and/or laparoscopic[28] or open splenectomy. If the spleen has multiple abscesses, splenectomy is required. Many patients have multiple other abscesses and the spleen is just a part of overwhelming sepsis. Antibiotic treatment should continue until the drains or percutaneous catheters have been removed.

BENIGN NEOPLASMS

Benign splenic neoplasms are rare. These tumors generally arise from the lymphoid or vascular elements of the spleen. The most common primary neoplasm of the spleen is hemangioma. However, less than 100 cases have been described in the literature, generally in the form of individual reports and case series.[29–35] The lesion can be single or multiple. Diffuse splenic involvement is quite rare but may be complicated by splenic enlargement and severe thrombocytopenia.[36] Hemangiomas vary from well-circumscribed to irregular vascular proliferations. The majority are cavernous in nature. The potential for malignant transformation to angiosarcoma is not known but appears to be low and associated with large hemangiomas. Many splenic hemangiomas are now diagnosed incidentally during the course of imaging for other pathology. On CT scan, hemangiomas appear as homogeneous, hypodense, or multicystic lesions with variable calcification, and peripheral enhancement.[33] The hemangioma typically is seen as a round, echogenic mass on ultrasound. Angiography may also be employed to confirm the diagnosis, although this is much more invasive. On angiography, the splenic hemangioma resembles a hepatic hemangioma with the fine vascularity and "laking" effect in the capillary phase, which may be accompanied by early filling of the splenic vein.

The first successful resection of a splenic hemangioma was reported by Hodge in 1895.[37] However, the majority of splenic hemangiomas do not require surgical intervention. Splenectomy is reserved for large and symptomatic lesions. Most splenic hemangiomas are asymptomatic, with symptoms being associated with enlargement of the tumor and mass effect or rupture. In the largest series published to date, Husni reported a spontaneous rupture rate of 25%.[29] A more contemporary series from the Mayo Clinic reported no spontaneous rupture among 32 patients with splenic hemangioma; 81% were entirely asymptomatic.[35]

Littoral cell angioma has been recently described as an endothelial cell neoplasm arising from the cells lining the sinus channels of the splenic red pulp. These rare lesions express vascular and histiocyte-associated antigens.[32] While littoral cell angioma has been described as a benign neoplasm cured with splenectomy, there have been reports of associated malignant lymphomas, other visceral organ cancers, and recurrent disease identified as malignant littoral cell hemangioendothelioma.[38–40] Splenectomy and close observation is thus warranted.

Lymphangioma of the spleen is composed of a malformation of lymphatics. Microscopically, these endothelium-lined spaces are filled with lymph and blood elements. The lesion may be focal or multiple, a small or large cystic mass, or may diffusely involve the spleen. Cystic spaces of varying sizes containing clear gelatinous fluid may account for splenomegaly in the order of 2000 to 3000 g. The diagnosis is made by ultrasound or CT scan, which reveals water-density cystic lesion(s) of the spleen.[41] The lymphangioma may be isolated to the spleen or occur as a generalized lymphangiomatosis with multi-visceral involvement and a poor prognosis.[42,43] Symptoms, when present, are related to the size and mass effect of the lesion as well as bleeding, rupture, consumptive coagulopathy and hypersplenism. Splenectomy is indicated for symptomatic lesions. Partial splenectomy is reserved for small, focal symptomatic lesions.

Other benign lesions of the spleen are uncommon. Inflammatory pseudotumor of the spleen is a reactive lesion characterized by a mixture of inflammatory cells and disorganized spindle cells.[44] This tumor is typically found incidentally and is generally asymptomatic but may present with systemic symptoms such as fever, malaise, and weight loss. Inflammatory pseudotumor is infiltrative in nature and may mimic malignant lymphoproliferative disease. Splenic hamartomas are composed of irregular vascular channels lined by splenic sinus endothelium with a disorganized reticulin stroma. Splenic hamartomas are uncommon with autopsy series noting an incidence of 0.024–0.13%.[45–47] Peliosis is not a true neoplastic lesion but a blood filled cystic lesion without an endothelial lining that may be associated with focal, patchy, or diffuse involvement of the spleen. This lesion is likely reactive as it has been associated with steroids, oral contraceptives, immunosuppression medications, tuberculosis, renal disease, and malignancy. Other benign splenic tumors, such as angiomyolipoma, lipoma, hemangiopericytoma, and fibroma are rare.

PRIMARY MALIGNANT TUMORS

Primary, nonlymphoid, malignant tumors of the spleen are exceedingly rare. These include angiosarcomas, malignant fibrous histiocytomas, and plasmacytomas. Angiosarcoma is the most common nonlymphoid primary malignant neoplasm of the spleen. Histologic examination is notable for stroma with vascular channels lined by enlarged endothelial cells. There appears to be a slight male predominance but no ethnic association. Like hepatic angiosarcoma, splenic angiosarcoma is thought to be associated with exposure to a arsenic, thorium oxide (Thorotrast), and vinyl chloride although this link has not been demonstrated clearly in reported cases.[48] The clinical presentation may include abdominal pain, left upper quadrant abdominal mass, and constitutional symptoms. Metastasis is frequent and often involves the liver. Spontaneous rupture has been reported and is associated with a dismal outcome. Normocytic anemia is present in the majority of cases. Splenomegaly with hypersplenism is also seen. CT imaging often identifies a splenic lesion with central necrosis. The primary treatment is splenectomy. Cisplatin-based chemotherapy has also been used. However, even without rupture, splenic angiosarcoma holds a poor prognosis with survival measured in months.

METASTATIC TUMORS

Splenic metastasis usually represents widespread dissemination of disease. The most common primary tumors associated with splenic metastasis are lung, stomach, pancreas, breast, melanoma, and colon. Isolated splenic metastasis is unusual. This has been reported in association with colorectal, ovarian, endometrial, and renal carcinoma. Splenectomy for splenic metastasis may be justified if no other sites of disease are found on thorough evaluation; however, this is seldom the case.

LYMPHOMA

An estimated 7000 new cases of Hodgkin's lymphoma are diagnosed annually in the United States. Approximately two thirds of patients with Hodgkin's lymphoma are cured with radiation and chemotherapy.[49] Staging laparotomy was once considered the main means of determining the extent of abdominal involvement with Stage I to II supradiaphragmatic disease. Advances in imaging technology to include high-resolution spiral CT scan, technetium bone scan, and 18-fluorodeoxyglucose positron emission tomography (PET) have improved the detection of splenic and abdominal lymph node involvement. With combined modality treatment favored over extended field radiation and recent improvement in the accuracy of imaging technology, surgical staging and splenectomy for Hodgkin's lymphoma are infrequently performed. Surgical intervention may be limited to retroperitoneal lymph node sampling and splenectomy for isolated splenomegaly. The rise of minimally invasive surgery has also contributed to the evolution of the management of Hodgkin's lymphoma. The laparoscopic approach to splenectomy and staging has been shown to be feasible and associated with decreased morbidity compared to laparotomy without compromising adequate pathologic staging.[50] Laparoscopic staging for Hodgkin's lymphoma generally begins with splenectomy from the lateral approach. The patient is then moved to a supine position to complete the wedge liver biopsy, performed with ultrasonic dissection or vascular stapling devices, percutaneous core needle liver biopsies, and biopsies of portal, para-aortic, and para-iliac lymph nodes. The para-aortic sampling may also be performed from the lateral approach. Metallic clips are placed at each lymph node sampling site.

Non-Hodgkin's lymphoma is the most common malignant neoplasm of the spleen. The spleen is involved in approximately 30–40% of patients, usually as a result of spread from other sites.[50,51] Primary splenic lymphoma, that confined to the spleen, is an uncommon presentation seen in only 1% of patients with non-Hodgkin's lymphoma.[52] Some patients with isolated splenic lymphoma (Group I) will have associated splenic hilar adenopathy (Group II) or abdominal lymph node or liver involvement (Group III). Clinical presentation varies from vague constitutional symptoms to abdominal or pleuritic pain and early satiety related to splenomegaly. Thrombocytopenia, anemia, and neutropenia are associated with the disease. CT typically reveals splenomegaly with a solitary large mass but multiple masses may be seen. Splenectomy is often required to make a definitive diagnosis and resection is indicated in patients with systemic disease and splenomegaly with cytopenias.

▪ HEMATOLOGIC DISORDERS

Splenectomy addresses the role of the spleen in hematology disorders, particularly that of cellular sequestration and destruction and antibody production. In 1887, Sir Thomas Spencer Wells, the renowned gynecologist, performed a therapeutic splenectomy for what proved to be hereditary spherocytosis. The first splenectomy for autoimmune hemolytic anemia was performed in 1911 by Micheli. Six years later, Schloffer, at the suggestion of a medical student, Kaznelson, performed a splenectomy for idiopathic thrombocytopenic purpura. Today, the role of splenectomy in the management of hematologic disease has grown in parallel with the rise in laparoscopic splenectomy and its associated decreased morbidity compared to open splenectomy.

ANEMIAS

Splenectomy is indicated for specific cases of anemia. The two major categories of anemia that benefit from splenectomy are (1) intracellular defects, including membrane abnormalities, enzyme defects, and hemoglobinopathy, and (2) extracellular defects, particularly autoimmune hemolytic anemia.

HEREDITARY SPHEROCYTOSIS

This hemolytic disorder results from an inherited defect or deficiency in one of the components of the red cell cytoskeleton. It is transmitted as an autosomal dominant trait but occurs sporadically in rare instances. Hereditary spherocytosis is the most common cause of familial chronic hemolytic anemia in North America and Northern Europe, with an incidence of 1 in 5000 births or even higher if mild cases of osmotic fragility are included (1 in 2000).[53–56] Hereditary spherocytosis occurs rarely in the black population.

The defect in red cell membrane components (spectrin, ankyrin, band 3, and/or protein 4–2) weakens the structure of the red cell and changes the morphology, making it more susceptible to destruction.[53,57,58] The change results in excessive red cell trapping within the splenic pulp and hemolysis. Cells that escape the spleen on first passage are more susceptible to trapping and destruction during each successive passage. The red cells also exhibit increased osmotic fragility.

The salient clinical features include anemia, jaundice, and splenomegaly. The severity varies and may be related to the degree of red cell cytoskeleton protein deficiency, particularly spectrin shortage. Mild cases may maintain normal hemoglobin and bilirubin levels. Some may have compensated anemia with a reticulocytosis. Most have mild to moderate spleen enlargement, but splenomegaly alone is not an indication for surgery. Increases in splenic size in patients with hereditary spherocytosis may be seen in the presence of acute infection. The jaundice usually parallels the severity of anemia and generally is not intense. It is related to the increased red cell destruction resulting in abundant bile pigment that cannot be cleared by the liver. Bile pigment is not present in the urine unless there is associated biliary obstruction or hepatic damage following severe hemolytic crisis. Up to 63% of patients with hereditary spherocytosis have cholelithiasis, but this is unusual in children younger than 10 years of age.[59] The gallstones are generally pigmented. Symptomatic cholelithiasis remains a major indication for surgery in patients with hereditary spherocytosis. Periodic worsening of the associated anemia and jaundice may be seen, often following infection, emotional stress, fatigue, or prolonged exposure to cold.

Splenectomy is effective in reducing the hemolysis associated with hereditary spherocytosis. This benefit for patients with limited clinical manifestations must be balanced against the risk of postsplenectomy infectious complications. Because of the increased risk of serious postsplenectomy sepsis among young children, splenectomy is reserved preferably for patients older than the age of 6 years. Splenectomy for hereditary spherocytosis before this age should be performed only in cases of severe transfusion-dependent disease and only after the age of three.[53–60]

The severity of symptoms and associated complications of hereditary spherocytosis guide the decision for splenectomy. Children with severe hemolytic anemia and adults with moderate disease are likely to benefit from splenectomy. Additionally, those with symptomatic gallstones, including those with mild hemolysis, should be considered for splenectomy and cholecystectomy. In children without cholelithiasis, cholecystectomy is not indicated at the time of splenectomy. A limited review of patients younger than age of 18 years by Sandler and colleagues demonstrated that none developed cholelithiasis postsplenectomy over a mean follow-up of 15 years.[61]

Splenectomy is performed increasingly via laparoscopic techniques. Laparoscopic splenectomy has been established as a safe and viable option since the first reported case by Delaitre and Maignien in 1991.[62] Since that time, multiple retrospective studies have documented the benefits of shorter convalescence and hospitalization, earlier diet intake, and reduced postoperative pain over open splenectomy. Randomized controlled trials comparing the two operative techniques have not been done; this is unlikely to happen given patient preferences and referral patterns.

Hereditary Elliptocytosis

Hereditary elliptocytosis is transmitted as a simple Mendelian trait on a gene linked to the Rh blood type. It occurs in approximately 0.04% of the population. Oval erythrocytes constitute up to 25% of the total red cell population in many patients with macrocytic and hypochromic microcytic anemia. This is also true in patients with sickle cell anemia, thalassemia, and hemoglobin C disease. In patients with hereditary elliptocytosis, however, the oval- and rod-shaped forms constitute about 80–90% of the red cell population.

This disorder usually exists as a harmless trait, but in about 12% of the cases there is an active, variably compensated hemolytic anemia. The presence of hemolysis often is a familial characteristic, and it has been suggested that excessive hemolysis occurs only when the gene for elliptocytosis is present in the homozygous form, or is modified in some other way.

The majority of patients with hereditary elliptocytosis are Caucasian and the signs and symptoms are related directly to the severity of the hemolysis. Occasionally an acute hemolytic episode may be precipitated by infection. The clinical syndrome is indistinguishable from that described for hereditary spherocytosis. Gallstones are frequent, and chronic leg ulcers have been reported. The spleen is usually palpably enlarged in symptomatic cases. Diagnosis is established by the smear; Cr-51 studies in symptomatic cases demonstrate decreased red cell survival coupled with splenic sequestration. A reticulocytosis of 20% or higher occurs in patients with overt hemolysis.

Splenectomy is indicated in all symptomatic patients because removal of the organ is almost always followed by lasting effects of decreased hemolysis and corrected anemia, although the morphologic abnormality of the RBC remains unchanged. Associated cholelithiasis should be managed as in hereditary spherocytosis.

Immune Hemolytic Anemia

The first description of the disease is credited to Chauffard and Troisier who, in 1908, demonstrated autohemolysins in the serum of several patients with acute hemolytic anemia. Three years later Micheli performed the first planned, successful splenectomy, thus stimulating the application of splenectomy for hematologic disease.

Immune hemolytic anemia is a disorder in which immunoglobulin (Ig) G and/or IgM antibodies bind to erythrocyte surface antigens and stimulate erythrocyte destruction. This occurs through the complement and reticuloendothelial systems. Immune hemolytic anemia is classified as autoimmune, alloimmune, or drug-induced hemolytic anemia. Alloimmune hemolytic anemia occurs only after exposure to allogeneic erythrocytes, such as through blood transfusion, pregnancy or transplantation.[63] There is no antibody reactivity against autologous red cells. Acute hemolysis after transfusion is estimated to occur in 0.0003–0.0008%, and a delayed response is seen in 0.05–0.07%.[63–66]

Drug-induced immune hemolytic anemia occurs as drug-induced antibodies recognize intrinsic red cell antigens or erythrocyte-bound drug. Alpha-methyldopa, high-dose penicillin, second- and third-generation cephalosporins have been implicated. Drug-induced hemolytic anemia via neoantigen formation or drug adsorption is direct antiglobulin test (DAT, direct Coombs' test) positive and may be indistinguishable from warm autoimmune hemolytic anemia. Autoantibody formation may also occur. Drug-induced immune hemolytic anemia should resolve with cessation of the medication in question but may require corticosteroids and may involve a protracted recovery.

Autoimmune hemolytic anemia (AIHA) is estimated to occur in 1 to 3 per 100,000 per year.[63,67,68] IgG antibodies bind to the erythrocyte and are recognized by Fc receptors of macrophages and other phagocytic cells of the reticuloendothelial system for phagocytosis. In contrast to IgG antibodies, IgM antibodies readily activate the classical complement pathway and may lead to intravascular hemolysis. Additionally, IgM-bound erythrocytes may undergo extravascular hemolysis, particularly in the liver. Both warm and cold antibodies have been reported. Warm antibodies react best at 98.6°F (37°C) and account for the majority of cases. Secondary causes of warm AIHA have been reported, most notably, lymphoproliferative disorders such as chronic lymphocytic leukemia.[69] The presentation of warm AIHA is variable and includes vague constitutional symptoms consistent with anemia, such as weakness and dizziness. Additionally, fever, abdominal pain, cough, and bleeding may be seen. Symptoms vary with the severity of the hemolysis. Mild jaundice is often present. Splenomegaly is seen in approximately half of cases, and 25% may have associated cholelithiasis. While reticulocytopenia may occur early in the disease prior to adequate marrow response, reticulocytosis and elevated mean cell volume (MCV) is generally seen. Mild to moderate indirect hyperbilirubinemia and elevated LDH are often seen. Platelets are usually normal but occasionally AIHA and idiopathic thrombocytopenic purpura occur together (Evan's syndrome). Over 95% of warm AIHA are DAT-positive.[63] The therapy is guided by the severity of the hemolysis, with first line treatment being corticosteroids.[63,70] Prednisone therapy is maintained for one to three weeks with rapid response being the norm. After a satisfactory response, the steroid is gradually and slowly tapered to avoid relapse. Approximately 20–30% have a long-term response, with 50% requiring low-dose maintenance prednisone for months. It is estimated that 10–20% fail to respond or require toxic doses of steroids. Splenectomy should be considered for these patients, particularly if other advanced measures such as immunoglobulin therapy also fail. Splenectomy benefits approximately 60–80% of patients.

In contrast, cold agglutinin syndrome treatment is often inadequate. Primary cold agglutinin syndrome patients may only present with mild anemia and may respond favorably to cold exposure avoidance. Folic acid supplementation may be beneficial. Corticosteroids are less effective than in warm AIHA. Other immunosuppressive drugs such as chlorambucil and cyclophosphamide have demonstrated favorable results. Plasmapheresis offers a temporary response but requires concomitant immunosuppression to address cold agglutinin production. Splenectomy is ineffective in cold agglutinin syndrome.

Paroxysmal cold hemoglobinuria is an uncommon form of AIHA and is generally self-limited and treated with supportive care. Most cases occur in children, usually after a viral illness. Corticosteroids are often given to children with severe anemia but are not routinely effective.

Thalassemia

The development of intracellular hemoglobin precipitates (Heinz bodies) that damage red cells and contribute to their premature destruction can occur because of thalassemia, unstable hemoglobins, or enzyme deficiencies in the pentose phosphate pathway.

Thalassemia (Mediterranean anemia) is a congenital disorder transmitted as a dominant trait in which the anemia is primarily the result of a defect in hemoglobin synthesis. It has been referred to as Cooley's anemia, erythroblastic anemia, and target-cell anemia. As a consequence of the defect, there are intracellular precipitates that contribute to premature red cell destruction. The hemoglobin-deficient red cells are small, thin, misshapen, and have a characteristic resistance to osmotic lysis.

The disease is classified as alpha, beta, and gamma types, determined by the specific defect in the synthesis of the peptide chain. In the United States most patients suffer from beta thalassemia, and there is a quantitative reduction in the rate of beta chain synthesis, resulting in a decrease in the hemoglobin A. The characteristic feature is the persistence of Hb-F and a reduction of Hb-A. Gradations of the disease range from heterozygous thalassemia minor to severe homozygous thalassemia major. The latter is manifested by chronic anemia, jaundice, and splenomegaly.

Patients with homozygous thalassemia major usually present with clinical manifestations in the first year of life. In addition to the anemia and consequent pallor, there is usually retarded body growth and enlargement of the head. Intractable leg ulcers may be noted, and intercurrent infections are particularly common. Some patients present with repeated episodes of left upper quadrant pain related to splenic infarction. Cardiac dilatation occurs and, in advance stages, there is subcutaneous edema and effusion into serous cavities. Intercurrent infections occur frequently, often leading to death in the more severe cases. These infections may be associated with aplastic crises. Gallstones have been reported in up to 24% of cases.

Therapy is directed only at symptomatic patients, those having thalassemia major or intermedia. In these patients, transfusions are usually required at regular intervals. Because most children with thalassemia major accommodate to low hemoglobin levels, transfusions are given when the hemoglobin level is less than 10 g/dL. Although splenectomy does not influence the basic hematologic disorder, it may eliminate or reduce the hemolytic process responsible for accelerated destruction of normal donor red cells within the patient's circulation and this reduces transfusion requirements. In general the best results associated with splenectomy have been obtained in older children and in young adults with large spleens in whom excessive splenic sequestration of red cells has been demonstrated. Occasionally, splenectomy may be indicated because of mass effect symptoms associated with marked splenomegaly or repeated episodes of abdominal pain owing to splenic infarction.

Sickle Cell Disease

Sickle cell anemia is a hereditary hemolytic anemia seen predominantly in blacks, and characterized by the presence of crescent-shaped erythrocytes that, because of a lack of deformability, are trapped in the splenic cords. In this disorder, the normal hemoglobin A is replaced by hemoglobin S. Under conditions of reduced oxygen tension, hemoglobin S molecules undergo crystallization within the cell, which elongates and distorts the cell. The sickle cells increase the blood viscosity and circulatory stasis, thus establishing a vicious cycle. Sickling occurs so rapidly that blood flow through both the fast and slow compartments of the spleen is obstructed; and as a consequence, a series of microinfarcts develop. In most adult patients only a fibrous area of the spleen remains, but autosplenectomy is preceded by splenomegaly in about 75% of patients. Calcification may occur with autoinfarction (Fig 43–9).

In addition to serving as the site of destruction for damage of nondeformable erythrocytes, there are other splenic functional abnormalities in the sickle cell ane-

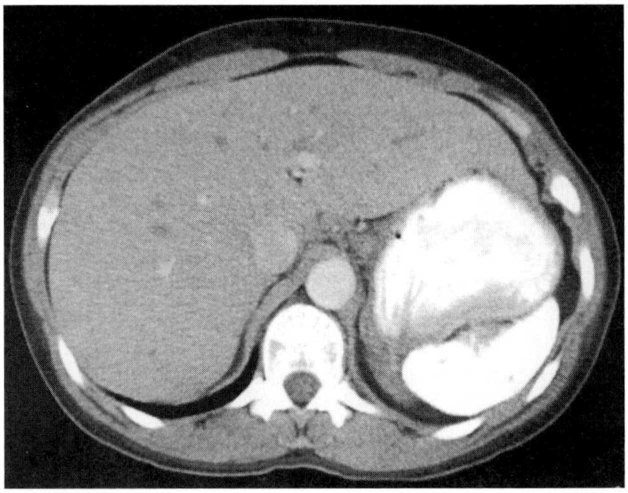

Figure 43–9. Calcified spleen in a patient with sickle cell disease causing persistent pain in left upper quadrant. Splenectomy relieved the patient's pain.

mia. These include (1) an abnormal role that the spleen plays as a red cell reservoir in these patients, (2) a reduced antibody production by the spleen, and (3) reduction in the spleen's ability to filter bacteria, especially streptococcal pneumonia.

There are two situations in sickle cell anemia where the spleen is a pathologic red cell reservoir. The first is a form of chronic hypersplenism that usually occurs in childhood or adolescence and is manifested by reduced red cell survival, leukopenia, and thrombocytopenia. In these patients, for some unknown reason, there is a failure to undergo autosplenectomy, and in this rare circumstance splenectomy will correct the leukopenia and thrombocytopenia and will also decrease the rate of red cell survival. The second abnormality has been termed acute splenic sequestration and is marked by sudden splenic enlargement associated with worsening anemia and profound hypotension. It usually occurs in the first 5 years of life in an SS child; streptococcal pneumonia infection may act as a precipitating event in these patients. The acute splenic sequestration is usually effectively treated with packed red cell transfusion. If there is a propensity for recurrence, splenectomy may be indicated.

Although the sickle cell trait occurs in approximately 9% of the black population, the majority of patients are asymptomatic. Sickle cell anemia is observed in 0.3–1.3% of blacks. Depending upon the vessels affected by vascular occlusion, the patients may have bone or joint pain, priapism, neurologic manifestations, or skin ulcers. Abdominal pain and cramps owing to visceral stasis are frequent. Rarely thrombosis of the splenic vessels may result in the complication of splenic abscess manifested by splenomegaly, splenic pain, and spiking fever.

For most patients with sickle cell anemia, only palliative therapy is available. Recent studies have shown that sodium cyanate will prevent sickling of hemoglobin S. Adequate hydration and partial exchange transfusion may help the crisis. In the circumstance of splenic abscess, incision, and drainage of the abscess cavity may be required. Splenectomy is of benefit in only a few patients in whom excessive splenic sequestration of red cells, leukocytes, or platelets can be demonstrated.

PURPURAS

Thrombotic Thrombocytopenic Purpura

First described in 1924 by Moschcowitz and later characterized as a syndrome by Singer in 1947, thrombotic thrombocytopenic purpura (TTP) is recognized as the pentad of microangiopathic hemolytic anemia, thrombocytopenia, fever, neurologic disturbance, and renal dysfunction.[71,72] Largely an idiopathic disorder, TTP also has been seen in association with bone marrow transplantation, mitomycin, cyclosporine, penicillin, and other therapeutic agents. TTP is a microvascular disorder affecting arterioles and capillaries with venule sparing. Platelet microthrombi cause partial vessel occlusion with overlying endothelial proliferation and subintimal hyalinization.[73,74] Subsequent erythrocyte damage occurs during passage through the narrowed vascular channels with abnormal forms (helmet cells, schistocytes, etc.) seen on peripheral blood smear. Marked platelet trapping occurs, namely in the spleen, with resultant thrombocytopenia ($<20 \times 10^9/L$). This may be seen as a profound decrease in platelets within hours of onset. Petechial hemorrhage and more rarely, epistaxis, retinal hemorrhage, GI and genitourinary bleeding, and hemorrhagic stroke may be seen. However, it is more usual to see no bleeding even with severe thrombocytopenia partly because of the thrombotic nature of the disease. Other clinical manifestations include, fever, general malaise and flu-like symptoms, headache, altered mental status, focal neurologic deficits, hematuria, and renal failure. The neurologic changes may be severe, such as coma, prompting emergent therapy.

Since the advent of plasmapheresis for TTP, the survival associated with the once uniformly fatal disease has improved markedly to over 90%.[73,75] Daily therapy is conducted until the hemolytic process is stabilized and the thrombocytopenic and neurologic complications subside. Plasma exchange is then tapered. Splenectomy is reserved generally for patients who are unresponsive to plasmapheresis or to reduce recurrence of disease after multiple plasma exchanges. The efficacy of splenectomy in the treatment of TTP has been controversial because of inconsistent success and the operative morbidity. More contemporary series, particularly those touting laparoscopic splenectomy, have been encouraging with decreased morbidity rates and response rates of over 50% to approximately 90%.[73,76–78]

Idiopathic Thrombocytopenic Purpura

Idiopathic thrombocytopenic purpura (ITP) is the most common hematologic indication for splenectomy. It is an acquired disorder in which platelets are destroyed by circulating IgG antiplatelet antibodies. The spleen is the source of antiplatelet antibody production as well as the major site of platelet-antiplatelet antibody complex destruction by macrophage-induced phagocytosis.

Female patients outnumber males 3:1. Most patients present with petechiae or ecchymosis. Bleeding complications such as gum bleeding, vaginal bleeding, mild GI bleeding, and hematuria may be seen. CNS bleeding occurs in 2–4% of patients and usually occurs early in the course of the disease. The spleen is typically normal size. Thrombocytopenia occurs with the platelet count generally less than 50,000/mm^3. The platelet count may approach zero and marked thrombocytopenia is associated with a prolonged bleeding time. Generally, there is no significant anemia or leukopenia unless the ITP occurs in conjunction with AIHA. ITP is often associated with other immune disorders as well, such as systemic lupus erythematosus. A bone marrow aspirate should be obtained and this will demonstrate normal to high megakaryocytes. Other causes of thrombocytopenia should be excluded.

ITP in children is typically self limited and rarely requires surgical therapy. The disease in adults is usually more persistent and requires medical and possibly surgical treatment. Corticosteroids represent the first line of therapy. Gamma globulin administration and plasmapheresis are also used. Medical therapy for adults results in a long-term response in only 15–20% compared to the sustained remission achieved in 80–90% after splenectomy. In most patients, the platelet count rises to greater than 100,000/mm^3 within 7 days. Rarely, platelet normalization is more gradual over a period of months. Splenectomy should be performed in patients who fail to respond to steroid treatment within 6 weeks, who recur after steroid taper, who respond to medical therapy but cannot tolerate the side effects, or who develop intracranial bleeding or profound GI bleeding and do not respond to intensive medical treatment. The response to splenectomy correlates with the response to IgG infusion.[79]

The laparoscopic approach to splenectomy is well-suited for ITP, because of the normal size of the spleen. Retrospective comparisons of laparoscopic and open splenectomy have demonstrated decreased blood loss, reduced postoperative pain and convalescence for the minimally invasive approach.[80–87] Hematologic outcome assessment is difficult because of the variable definitions of a complete response, limited follow-up, small sample size, and the prevalence of unmatched retrospective series. Table 43–2 compares the outcomes in five reports in which laparoscopic and open splenectomy were performed.

▪ SECONDARY HYPERSPLENISM

Splenectomy may be indicated in cases of secondary hypersplenism where mass effect symptoms or cytopenias become disabling. In addition to the effects of hypersplenism, patients may present with abdominal fullness, pain, early satiety, and constitutional symptoms. In patients with chronic lymphocytic leukemia and splenomegaly, improvement after splenectomy may be substantial even with reduced numbers of hematopoietic cells in the marrow. The hematologic response is favorable in the majority of patients with improvement in the neutropenia and thrombocytopenia. Recent studies have demonstrated that patients with chronic lymphocytic leukemia who underwent splenectomy had comparable morbidity rates and significant durable improvement in the degree of cytopenias with a possible survival advantage compared to those who received only chemotherapy.[88,89] Though the evidence is less clear, splenectomy may be performed in the treatment of chronic myelogenous leukemia for symptomatic splenomegaly, substantial transfusion requirements, and severe thrombocytopenia with limited morbidity and mortality even in the accelerated phase of the disease.[90]

Hairy cell leukemia is an indolent B cell lymphoproliferative disorder that was initially recognized by Ewald in 1923. It accounts for only 2–3% of adult leukemias.[91] The typical presentation includes cytopenia, circulating hairy cells, and splenomegaly. Treatment is considered only for symptomatic patients, including those with significant cytopenias, symptomatic splenomegaly, recurrent infection, fevers and other constitutional symptoms, painful lymphadenopathy, vasculitis, or bony involvement. Chemotherapy with purine analogs or interferon alpha is used. Splenectomy is indicated for symptomatic splenomegaly, severe thrombocytopenia, ruptured spleen, or failure to respond to chemotherapy. Approximately 40–60% of patients will have normal hematologic parameters postsplenectomy and 90% will improve in at least one parameter.[92–94]

Splenectomy may significantly improve the neutropenia in patients with Felty's syndrome characterized by splenomegaly, neutropenia, and arthralgia. Splenectomy is reserved for patients with significant neutropenia and serious or recurrent infections, increased transfusion requirements or marked thrombocytopenia. While splenectomy does not reduce the arthralgia, leg ulcers, when present, generally heal.

In patients with portal hypertension secondary to splenic vein thrombosis, splenectomy usually resolves the portal hypertension and its complications.

Splenectomy may also be indicated for symptomatic splenomegaly or severe secondary hypersplenism in patients with Gaucher's disease or sarcoidosis, although splenectomy will not alter the course of the disease.

▪ MYELOPROLIFERATIVE DISORDERS

The myeloproliferative disorders, including myeloid metaplasia and myelofibrosis, represent panproliferative

TABLE 43–2. COMPARISON OF LAPAROSCOPIC VERSUS OPEN SPLENECTOMY OUTCOMES FOR ITP

Reference	Procedure	*N*	Spleen Size	OR Time (min)	EBL (mL)	Postop Stay (days)	Morbidity	Accessory Spleen	Platelet Response
Friedman 1996	Lap	29	184 g	122	203	2.9	1	6 (21%)	27 (93%)
	Open	18	167 g	103	285	6.9	0	2 (11%)	15 (83%)
Watson 1997	Lap	13		89		2	0	2 (15%)	12 (92%)
	Open	47		84		10	9 (19%)	3 (6%)	29 (62%)
Lozano-Salazar 1998	Lap	22	10 cm			4	6	2 (9%)	87%
	Open	27	11 cm			6	10	3 (11%)	89%
Shimomatsuya 1999	Lap	14	89 g	210	560	8.9	3 (21%)	4 (29%)	13 (93%)
	Open	20	140 g	126	321	15.2	3 (15%)	4 (20%)	13 (81%)
Tanoue 1999	Lap	35	121 g	205	155	9.6	4 (11%)	4 (11%)	31(89%)
	Open	41	122 g	100	511	20.1	19 (46%)	5 (12%)	32 (78%)

processes manifested by increased connective tissue proliferation of the bone marrow, liver, spleen, and lymph nodes and a simultaneous proliferation of hematopoietic elements in the liver, spleen, and long bones. The disease is closely related to polycythemia vera, idiopathic thrombocytosis, and myelogenous leukemia. The presenting symptoms are symptomatic splenomegaly and anemia.

The laboratory hallmark is a peripheral smear that demonstrates red cell fragmentation and shows many immature forms of numerous teardrop and elongated shapes. The white blood count is in the range of 50,000/mm^3 and may reach extremely high levels. Immature myeloid cells are found in the peripheral smear. Thrombocytopenia is present in about one third of the patients and thrombocytosis, with white blood counts of >1 million, is observed in about one fourth of the patients.

Although splenectomy does not alter the course of the disease, the procedure is indicated for increasing transfusion requirements and control of anemia, leukopenia, or thrombocytopenia, or symptomatic splenomegaly. There may be massive splenic enlargement with myeloproliferative disorders. The morbidity associated with splenectomy is historically higher than that reported for other hematologic disorders with normal spleen size, although recent series are challenging that assessment. Hand-assisted laparoscopic techniques have been applied increasingly to massive splenomegaly with success.[95,96]

▪ SPLENECTOMY (ALSO SEE SECTION XI, CHAPTER 49)

PREOPERATIVE PREPARATION

In most instances, there is no specific treatment required for the preoperative management of patients undergoing splenectomy. Patients with a past history of multiple transfusions and those with auto immune hemolytic anemia may require a preoperative stay because of difficulties in blood typing and cross-matching. Platelets should not be administered preoperatively in patient with idiopathic thrombocytopenic purpura because these cells will not survive. In those patients with myeloproliferative disorders who have a tendency to develop thrombosis, it is beneficial to medicate the patient with low-dose heparin, 5000 units twice daily, and aspirin on the day before surgery and to continue this regimen for 5 days postoperatively. In elective cases, vaccines against *Streptococcus pneumonia*, *Haemophilus influenzae* type B, and *Neisseria meningitides* are administered 14 days before operation and as soon as possible for emergency cases. An orogastric tube is used during the operation to decompress the stomach and to facilitate transection of the short gastric veins.

OPERATIVE TECHNIQUE

A variety of incisions may be used, depending on the nature of the disease and the personal preference of the surgeon. A midline incision is generally applied to cases of traumatic injury because of the speed of access as well as exposure of the spleen and other possibly injured viscera. A subcostal incision also has been employed, particularly for marked splenomegaly; the thoracoabdominal approach largely has been abandoned because of its associated morbidity. Increasingly, laparoscopic techniques are applied to splenic disease, and laparoscopic splenectomy is considered to be the gold standard by current standards except perhaps for the markedly enlarged spleen.

Open splenectomy begins with mobilization of the spleen to the midline by division of the lateral and superior pole attachments. The splenocolic and splenorenal ligaments at the lower pole are also divided sharply. The short gastric vessels are divided between ligatures or clips, taking care to avoid injury to the gastric wall. Alternatively, an ultrasonic dissector may be used. The most superior short gastric vessels and gastrosplenic ligament may be quite short.

The hilar dissection should proceed carefully with isolation of the splenic vessels and gentle medial displacement of the tail of the pancreas to avoid pancreatic injury. The splenic hilum may be clamped en bloc with three clamps in the manner of Federoff (Fig 43–10) and divided and doubly ligated proximally and once distally. Some advocate individual ligation of the splenic artery and splenic vein. Alternatively, the vessels may be divided with a vascular linear stapler. Drainage is not necessary unless the pancreas has been injured.

A search for accessory spleens should be conducted during elective splenectomy. They are present in approximately 12–20% of patients and may be the source for inadequate response to splenectomy in the treatment of hematologic disease, such as ITP. The splenic hilum, gastrosplenic ligament, gastrocolic ligament, greater omentum, mesentery and presacral space are potential sites for accessory spleens, with the splenic hilum being most common.

COMPLICATIONS

Generally, the complication rate of splenectomy is fairly low for elective splenectomy, but open splenectomy for malignant disease or splenomegaly may be associated with a morbidity of 40–60%.[97–101] Early postoperative bleeding must be closely monitored, particularly in patients with thrombocytopenia or myeloproliferative disorders. In these patients it is an

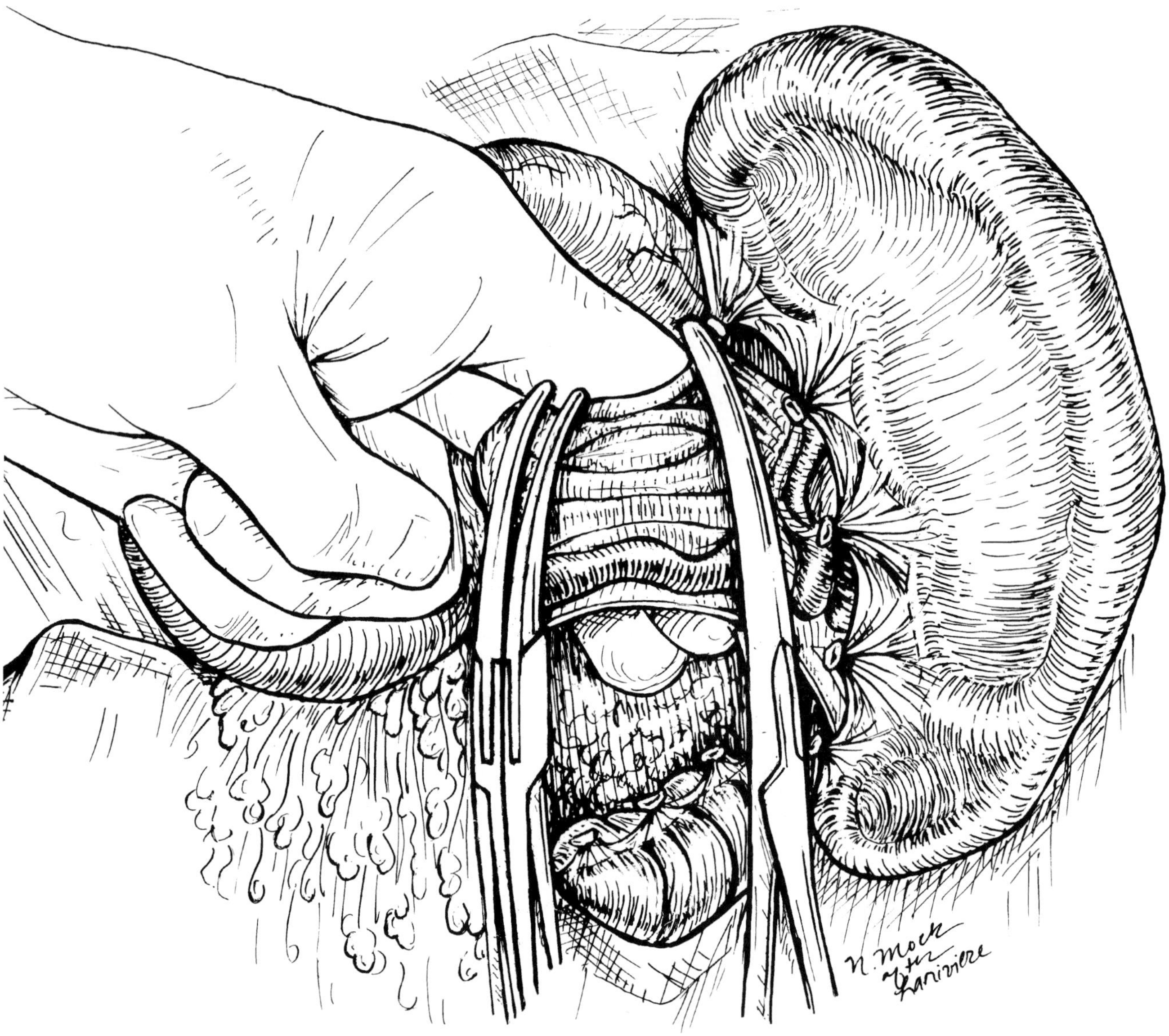

Figure 43–10. Three-clamp method of Federoff for transecting the splenic hilum. The fingers protect the tail of the pancreas while the clamps are applied.

error to indict hematologic abnormalities as the cause of bleeding, and it is generally safer to reexplore the patients early and to evacuate a hematoma to reduce the incidence of subphrenic abscess. Alternative therapy would be angiography with embolization but this may be difficult as the most common site of bleeding is a short gastric vessel. Left lower lobe atelectasis is another complication; it occurs more frequently following splenectomy, but most large series have not yet substantiated this finding. In unusual cases, the platelet count may rise to very high levels, at times greater than 2 million/mm^3, but no specific therapy other than hydration is generally indicated. If medical therapy is thought to be appropriate, a drug that inhibits platelet aggregation, such as acetylsalicylic acid can be used. Thrombosis of the splenic vein, with extension into the portal vein and superior mesenteric vein, is a rare complication, occurring mostly in patients with myeloproliferative disorders or in those with sepsis as a consequence of intra-abdominal abscess.

The increased incidence of fulminant sepsis related to Pneumococcus or to *H. influenzae* following splenectomy is an established fact but it occurs more commonly in patients who are immunosuppressed or have myeloproliferative diseases with a propensity for infection. The risk may be reduced with appropriate vaccination and early recognition as previously noted.

Injury to the tail of the pancreas is a potential risk of splenectomy, occurring in 15% or less.[102] The majority of these injuries is self-limited with hyperamylasemia and pain but may be more severe with development of a pancreatic fistula.

The complication rates for laparoscopic splenectomy have been fairly limited at less than 20%.[101,103–106] One complication that may occur during laparoscopic splenectomy that is rarely seen with open splenectomy is diaphragmatic perforation, usually related to thermal injury during mobilization of the superior pole.

■ SPLENORRHAPHY

The techniques to preserve splenic tissue and function are dictated by the extent of damage. The spleen must be mobilized carefully to allow thorough inspection of the organ. The ligamentous attachments must be divided as in splenectomy. Small lacerations can be managed by compression and the application of a hemostatic agent, such as oxidized cellulose, micronized collagen, thrombin, or fibrin glue. Significant disruptions of the splenic capsule and parenchyma can be managed generally with absorbable sutures that traverse the capsule and incorporate the parenchyma. In this circumstance, horizontal mattress sutures are advantageous because cutting through the tissue is minimized. If trauma is localized to one pole of the spleen, this area should be resected and the edges approximated with a series of mattress sutures. The omentum may be used to fill large defects or to cover the injury site to provide tamponade. A new technique has been described using radiofrequency-generated heat to perform a partial splenectomy in a patient with a tumor in the lower pole of the spleen.[107] Splenorrhaphy has largely been supplanted by the nonoperative management of relatively hemodynamically stable injured patients, with the addition of angiographic embolization when indicated.

REFERENCES

1. Holdsworth RJ, Irving AD, Cuschieri A. Postsplenectomy sepsis and its mortality rate: actual versus perceived risks. *Br J Surg* 1991;78(9):1031–1038
2. Brigden M, Pattullo A. Prevention and management of overwhelming postsplenectomy infection—an update. *Crit Care Med* 1999;27(4):836–842
3. Lynch AM, Kapila R. Overwhelming postsplenectomy infection. *Infect Dis Clin North Am* 1996:4:693–707
4. Starnes S, Klein P, Magagna L, Pomerantz R. Computed tomographic grading is useful in the selection of patients for nonoperative management of blunt injury to the spleen. *Am Surgeon* 1998;64(8):743–749
5. Goan Y, Huang M, Lin J. Nonoperative management for extensive hepatic and splenic injuries with significant hemoperitoneum in adults. *J Trauma* 1998;45(2):360–364
6. Pachter HL, Guth AA, Hofstetter SR, Spencer FC. Changing patterns in the management of splenic trauma: The impact of nonoperative management. *Ann Surg* 1998;227(5):708–719
7. Nwomeh BC, Nadler EP, Meza MP, et al. Contrast extravasation predicts the need for operative intervention in children with blunt splenic trauma. *J Trauma* 2004; 56(3):537–541
8. Davis KA, Fabian TC, Croce MA, et al. Improved success in nonoperative management of blunt splenic injuries: embolization of splenic artery pseudoaneurysms. *J Trauma* 1998;44(6):1008–1015
9. Sclafani SJ, Shaftan GW, Scalea TM, Patterson LA, Kohl L, Kantor A, Herskowitz MM, Hoffer EK, Henry S, Dresner LS, Wetzel W. Nonoperative salvage of computed tomography-diagnosed splenic injuries: utilization of angiography for triage and embolization for hemostasis. *J Trauma* 1995;39(5):818–827
10. Schurr MJ, Fabian TC, Gavant M, et al. Management of blunt splenic trauma: computed tomography contrast blush predicts failure of nonoperative management. *J Trauma* 1995;39(3):507–513

11. Cocanour CS, Moore FA, Ware DN, et al. Delayed complications of nonoperative management of blunt adult splenic trauma. *Arch Surg* 1998;133:619–625
12. Salis A, Pais SO, Vennos A, Scalea T. Superselective embolization of a traumatic intrasplenic arteriovenous fistula. *J Trauma* 1999:46:186–188
13. Haan J, Scott J, Boyd-Kranis RL, et al. Admission angiography for blunt splenic injury: advantages and pitfalls. *J Trauma* 200;51:1161–1165
14. Wahl WL, Ahrns KS, Chen S, et al. Blunt splenic injury: operation versus angiographic embolization. *Surgery* 2004;136(4):891–899
15. Dent D, Alsabrook G, Erickson BA, et al. Blunt splenic injuries: high nonoperative management rate can be achieved with selective embolization. *J Trauma* 2004; 56(5):1063–1067
16. Haan JM, Biffl W, Knudson MM, et al. Western Trauma Association Multi-Institutional Trials Committee. Splenic embolization revisited: a multicenter review. *J Trauma* 2004;56(3):542–547
17. Balsarkar DJ. Rupture of splenic artery pseudoaneurysm presenting with massive upper gastrointestinal bleed. *Am J Surg* 2002:183:197
18. Beattie GC. Evidence for a central role for selective angiography in the management of major vascular complications of pancreatitis. *Am J Surg* 2003:185:96
19. Gadacz TR, Trunkey D, Kieffer RJ, Jr. Visceral vessel erosion with pancreatitis, case reports and a review of the literature. *Arch Surg* 1978;113:1438
20. Abbas MA, Stone WM, Fowl RJ, et al. Splenic artery aneurysms: tow decades experience at Mayo clinic. *Ann Vasc Surg* 2002:16:442
21. Pulli R. Early and long-term results of surgical treatment of splenic artery aneurysms. *Am J Surg* 2001;182:520
22. Morgenstern L. Nonparasitic splenic cysts: pathogenesis, classification, and treatment. *J Am Coll Surg* 2002: 194:306
23. Gabal AM, Khawaja FI, Mohammad GA. Modified PAIR technique for percutaneous treatment of high-risk hydatid cysts. *Cardiovasc Intervent Radiol* 2005;28:200
24. Yaghan R. Is fear of anaphylactic shock discouraging surgeons from more widely adopting percutaneous and laparoscopic techniques in the treatment of liver hydatid cyst? *Am J Surg* 2004;187:533
25. Hansen MB, Moller AC. Splenic cysts. *Surg Laparosc Endosc Percutan Tech* 2004:14:316
26. Gadacz TR, Way LW, Dunphy JE. The changing clinical spectrum of splenic abscess. *Am J Surg* 1974;128:182
27. Phillips GS, Radosevich MD, Lipsett PA. Splenic abscess: another look at an old disease. *Arch Surg* 1997;132:1331
28. Carbonell AM, Kercher KW, Matthews BD, et al. Laparoscopic splenectomy for splenic abscess. *Surg Laparosc Endosc Percutan Tech* 2004;14:289
29. Husni EA. The clinical course of splenic hemangioma with emphasis of spontaneous rupture. *Arch Surg* 1961; 83:681–688
30. Goerge C, Scherk W, Goerg K. Splenic lesions: Sonographic patterns, follow-up, differential diagnosis. *Eur J Radiol* 1991;13:59–66
31. Kaplan J, Mcintosh G. Spontaneous rupture of a splenic, vascular malformation. *J R Coll Surg Edinb* 1987: 32:346–347
32. Arber DA, Strickler JG, Chen YY, Weiss LM. Splenic vascular tumors: a histologic, immunophenotypic, and virologic study. *Am J Surg Patho* 1997;21:827–835
33. Ros PR, Moser RP Jr., Cadhman AH, et al. Hemangioma of the spleen: radiologic-pathologic correlation in ten case. *Radiology* 1987;162:73–77
34. Disler DG, Chew FS. Splenic hemangioma. *AJR Am J Roentgenol* 1991;157:44
35. Willcox TM, Speer RW, Schlinkert RT, Sarr MG. Hemangioma of the spleen: Presentation , diagnosis, and management. *J Gastrointest Surg* 2000;4:611–613
36. Dufau JP, le Tourneau A, Audouin J, Delmer A, Diebold J. Isolated diffuse hemangiomatosis of the spleen with Kasabach-Merritt-like syndrome. *Histopathology* 1999; 35(4):337–344
37. Hodge GB, Jr. Angioma cavernosum of the spleen. *Med Rec* 1895;48:418
38. Dascalescu CM, Wendum D, Gorin NC. Littoral-cell angioma as a cause of splenomegaly. *N Engl J Med* 2001; 345(10):772–773
39. Ben-Izhak O, Bejar J, Ben-Eliezer S, Vlodavsky E. Splenic littoral cell haemangioendothelioma: a new low-grade variant of malignant littoral cell tumour. *Histopathology* 2001;39(5):469–475
40. Chatelain D, Bonte H, Guillevin L, Balladur P, Flejou JF. Small solitary littoral cell angioma associated with splenic marginal zone lymphoma and villous lymphocyte leukaemia in a patient with hepatitis C infection. *Histopathology* 2002;41(5):473–475
41. Komatsuda T, Ishida H, Konno K, et al. Two splenic lesions in need of clarification: hamartoma and inflammatory pseudotumor. *Semin Diagn Pathol* 2003;20(2):94–104
42. Barrier A, Lacaine F, Callard P, Huguier M. Lymphangiomatosis of the spleen and 2 accessory spleens. *Surgery* 2002;131(1):114–116
43. Dietz WH, Smart MJ. Splenic consumptive coagulopathy in a patient with disseminated lymphangiomatosis. *J Pediatr* 1977;90:421–423
44. Krishnan J, Frizzera G. Two splenic lesions in need of clarification: hamartoma and inflammatory pseudotumor. *Semin Diagn Pathol* 2003;20(2):94–104
45. Lam KY, Yip KH, Peh WCG. Splenic vascular lesions: Unusual features and a review of the literature. *ANZ J Surg* 1999;69:422–425
46. Berge TH. Splenoma. *Acta Pathol Microbiol Scand* 1965; 63:333–339
47. Silverman ML, Morton, N, MacKinney A, et al. Genetics of spherocytosis. *Am J Hum Genet* 1962;14:170–184
48. McGinley K, Googe P, Hanna W, Bell J. Primary angiosarcoma of the spleen: a case report and review of the literature. *South Med J* 1995;88(8):873–875
49. Fung HC, Nademanee AP. Approach to Hodgkin's lymphoma in the new millennium. *Hemat Oncol* 2002;20:1–15
50. Walsh RM, Heniford BT. Role of laparoscopic for Hodgkin's and non-Hodgkin's lymphoma. *Semin Surg Oncol* 1999;16:284–292

51. Lehne G, Hannisdal E, Langholm R, Nome O. A 10-year experience with splenectomy in patients with malignant non-Hodgkin's lymphoma at the Norwegian Radium Hospital. *Cancer* 1994;74:933–939
52. Brox A, Bishinsky JI, Berry G. Primary non-Hodgkin's lymphoma of the spleen. *Am J Hematol* 1991;38:95–100
53. Bolton-Maggs PH, Stevens RF, Dodd NJ, et al., General Haematology Task Force of the British Committee for Standards in Haematology. Guidelines for the diagnosis and management of hereditary spherocytosis. *Br J Haematol* 2004;126(4):455–474
54. Morton, N, MacKinney A, Kosowe N, et al. Genetics of spherocytosis. *Am J Hum Genet* 1962;14:170–184
55. Godal HC, Heisto H. high prevalence of increased osmotic fragility of red blood cells among Norwegian blood donors. *Scand J Haematol* 1981;27:30–34
56. Eber SW, Pekrun A, Neufeldt A, Schroter W. Prevalence of increased osmotic fragility of erythrocytes in German blood donors: screening using a modified glycerol lysis test. *Ann Hematol* 1992;64:88–92
57. Delaunay J, Alloisio N, Morle L, et al. Molecular genetics of hereditary elliptocytosis and hereditary spherocytosis. *Ann Genetics* 1996;39:209–221
58. Tse WT, Lux SE. Red blood cell membrane disorders. *Br J Haematol* 1999;104(1):2–13
59. Rutkow IM. Twenty years of splenectomy for hereditary spherocytosis. *Arch Surg* 1981;116:306–308
60. Gallagher P, Forget B, Lux S. Disorders of the erythrocyte membrane. In: Nathan D, Orkin S (eds). *Nathan and Oski's Hematology of Infancy and Childhood,* Volume 1. Philadelphia: Saunders; 1998:554–664
61. Sandler A, Winkel G, Kimura K, Soper R. The role of prophylactic cholecystectomy during splenectomy in children with hereditary spherocytosis. *J Ped Surg* 1999; 34:1077–1078
62. Delaitre B, Maignien B. Splenectomy by the laparoscopic approach. Report of a case. *Presse Med* 1991;20: 2263
63. Gehrs BC, Friedberg RC. Autoimmune hemolytic anemia. *Am J Hematol* 2002;69(4):258–271
64. Linden JV, Paul B, Dressler KP. A report of 104 transfusion errors in New York State. *Transfusion* 1992;32:601–606
65. Heddle NM, Soutar RL, O'Hoski PL, et al. A prospective study to determine the frequency and clinical significance of alloimmunization post-transfusion. *Br J Hematol* 1995;91:1000–1005
66. Vamvakas EC, Pineda AA, Reisner R, et al. The differentiation of delayed hemolytic and serologic transfusion reactions: incidence and predictors of hemolysis. *Transfusion* 1995:35:26–32
67. Pirofsky B. *Autoimmunization and the Autoimmune Hemolytic Anemias.* Baltimore: Williams & Wilkins; 1969
68. Bottiger LE, Westerholm B. Acquired haemolytic anaemia. *Acta Med Scand* 1973;193:223–226
69. Hill J, Walsh RM, McHam S, Brody F, Kalaycio M. Laparoscopic splenectomy for autoimmune hemolyutic anemia in patients with chronic lymphocytic leukemia: a case series and review of the literature. *Am J Hematol* 2004;75:134–138
70. Petz LD. Treatment of autoimmune hemolytic anemia. *Curr Opin Hematol* 2001;8:411–416
71. Moschcowitz E. Hyaline thrombosis of the terminal arterioles and capillaries: a hitherto undescribed disease. *Proc N Y Pathol Soc* 1924;24:21–24
72. Singer K, Bornstein F, Wiles A. Thrombotic thrombocytopenic purpura. *Blood* 1947;2:542–54
73. Nabhan C, Kwaan HC. Current concepts in the diagnosis and management of thrombotic thrombocytopenic purpura. *Hemat Oncol Clin N Am.* 2003;17(1):177–199
74. Kwaan HC. Clinicopathologic features of thrombotic thrombocytopenic purpura. *Semin Hematol* 1987;24(2): 71–81
75. Rock GA, Shumak KH, Buskard NA, et al. Comparison of plasma exchange with plasma infusion in the treatment of thrombotic thrombocytopenic purpura: Canadian Apheresis Study Group. *N Engl J Med* 1991;325:353–357
76. Schwartz J, Eldor A, Szold A. Laparoscopic splenectomy in patients with refractory or relapsing thrombotic thrombocytopenic purpura. *Arch Surg* 2001;136:1236–1238
77. Winslow GA, Nelson EW. Thrombotic thrombocytopenic purpura:indications for and results of splenectomy. *Am J Surg* 1995;170(6):558–563
78. Veltman GA, Brand A, Leeksma OC, et al. The role of splenectomy in the treatment of relapsing thrombotic thrombocytopenic purpura. *Ann Hematol* 1995;70(5):231–236
79. Chirletti P, Cardi M, Barillari P, et al. Surgical treatment of immune thrombocytopenic purpura. *World J Surg* 1992;16(5):1001–1005
80. Donini A, Baccarani, Terrosu G, et al. Laparoscopic vs open splenectomy in the management of hematologic diseases. *Surg Endosc* 1999;13:1220–1225
81. Park AE, Birgisson G, Mastrangelo MJ, et al. Laparoscopic splenectomy: outcomes and lessons learned from over 200 cases. *Surgery* 2000;128:660–667
82. Friedman RL, Hiatt JR, Korman JL, et al. Laparoscopic or open splenectomy for hematologic disease: which approach is superior? *J Am Coll Surg* 1997;185(1):49–54
83. Friedman RL, Fallas MJ, Carroll BJ, et al. Laparoscopic splenectomy for ITP. The gold standard. *Surg Endosc* 1996;10:991–995
84. Watson DI, Coventry BJ, Chin T, et al. Laparoscopic splenectomy for ITP. *Surgery* 1997;121:18–22
85. Lozano-Salazar R, Herrera MF, Vargas-Voráckovά F, et al. Laparoscopic versus open splenectomy for immune thrombocytopenic purpura. *Am J Surg* 1998;176:366–369
86. Shimomatsuya T, Horiuchi T. Laparoscopic splenectomy for treatment of patients with idiopathic thrombocytopenic purpura: comparison with open splenectomy. *Surg Endosc* 1999;13:563–566
87. Tanoue K, Hashizume M, Morita M, et al. Results of laparoscopic splenectomy for immune thrombocytopenic purpura. *Am J Surg* 1999;177:222–226
88. Cusack JC Jr, Seymour JF, Lerner S, Keating MJ, Pollock RE. Role of splenectomy in chronic lymphocytic leukemia. *J Am Coll Surg* 1997;185(3):237–243
89. Berman RS, Yahanda AM, Mansfield PF, et al. Laparoscopic splenectomy in patients with hematologic malignancies. *Am J Surg* 1999;178(6):530–536

90. Bouvet M, Babiera GV, Termuhlen PM, et al. Splenectomy in the accelerated or blastic phase of chronic myelogenous leukemia: a single-institution, 25-year experience. *Surgery* 1997;122(1):20–25
91. Goodman GR, Bethel KJ, Saven A. Hairy cell leukemia: an update. *Curr Opin Hematol* 2003;10(4):258–266
92. Van Norman AS, Nagorney DM, Martin JK, et al. Splenectomy for hairy cell leukemia. A clinical review of 63 patients. *Cancer* 1986;57(3):644–648
93. Jansen J, Hermans J. Splenectomy in hairy cell leukemia: a retrospective multicenter analysis. *Cancer* 1981; 47(8):2066–2076
94. Mintz U, Golomb HM. Splenectomy as initial therapy in twenty-six patients with leukemic reticuloendotheliosis (hairy cell leukemia). *Cancer Res* 1979;39(7 Pt 1):2366–2370
95. Kercher KW, Matthews BD, Walsh RM, et al. Laparoscopic splenectomy for massive splenomegaly. *Am J Surg* 2002;183(2):192–196
96. Borrazzo EC, Daly JM, Morrisey KP, et al. Hand-assisted laparoscopic splenectomy for giant spleens. *Surg Endosc* 2003;17(6):918–920
97. McRae HM, Yakimets WW, Reynolds T. Perioperative complications of splenectomy for hematologic disease. *Can J Surg* 1992;35:432–436
98. Aksnes J, Abdelnoor M, Mathisen O. Risk factors associated with mortality and morbidity after elective splenectomy. *Eur J Surg* 1995;161:253–258
99. Horowitz J, Smith JL, Weber TK, et al. Postoperative complications after splenectomy for hematologic malignancies. *Ann Surg* 1996;223:290–296
100. Coon W. Surgical aspects of splenic disease and lymphoma. *Curr Probl Surg* 1998.35:543–646
101. Targarona EM, Espert JJ, Bombuy E, et al. Complications of laparoscopic splenectomy. *Arch Surg* 2000;135: 1137–1140
102. Chand B, Walsh RM, Ponsky J, Brody F. Pancreatic complications following laparoscopic splenectomy. *Surg Endosc* 2001;15(11):1273–1276
103. Park AE, Birgisson G, Mastrangelo MJ, et al. Laparoscopic splenectomy: outcomes and lessons learned from over 200 cases. *Surgery* 2000;128:660–667
104. Knauer EM, Ailawadi G, Yahanda A, et al. 101 laparoscopic splenectomies for the treatment of benign and malignant hematologic disorders. *Am J Surg* 2003;186:500–504
105. Cogliandolo A, Berland-Dai B, pidoto RR, Marc OS. Results of laparoscopic and open splenectomy for nontraumatic diseases. *Surg Laparosc Endosc Percutan Tech* 2001;11(4):256–261
106. Walsh RM, Heniford BT, Brody F, Ponsky J. The ascendance of laparoscopic splenectomy. *Am Surgeon* 2001;67: 48–53
107. Habib NA, Spalding D, Navarra G, Nicholls J. How we do a bloodless partial splenectomy. *Am J Surg* 2003; 186(2):164–166

Section XI

MINIMALLY INVASIVE SURGERY

44

Fundamentals of Laparoscopic Surgery

Ashley Haralson Vernon ▪ *John G. Hunter*

Tremendous growth in the use of minimally invasive techniques has occurred over the past decade. This was made possible by developments in technology and was fueled by patient demands for less painful operations and quicker postoperative recovery.

Almost all general surgical procedures can be performed using minimally invasive techniques. The greatest benefit is achieved in operations where the trauma of access exceeds that of the procedure. Procedures in the chest, upper abdomen, and pelvis, especially those not requiring tissue removal, are ideally suited for minimally invasive techniques. Conversely, other procedures may have less obvious benefits when performed with minimally invasive techniques, especially if a large specimen is to be removed. To be a proficient *laparoscopist,* one must become familiar with a new set of techniques and instruments, as well as knowing when to apply them and when to convert to an open operation.

▪ PATIENT CONSIDERATIONS

PATIENT SELECTION

As in all surgery, choosing the right operation for the patient is the first step. Since all laparoscopic surgery of the abdomen requires the use of general anesthesia, the ability to tolerate anesthesia is an absolute requirement. Patients with impaired exercise tolerance or a history of shortness of breath will need a preoperative consultation with a cardiologist or pulmonologist. Patients with severe carbon dioxide retention can be difficult to manage intraoperatively because the use of carbon dioxide for pneumoperitoneum exacerbates the condition. By increasing the minute ventilation and decreasing the CO_2 pneumoperitoneum from 15 to 8–10 mmHg, one can control metabolic acidosis. Rarely, when these measures are ineffective at controlling hypercarbia, we have resorted to using nitrous oxide for peritoneal insufflation. While not suppressing combustion (as does carbon dioxide), nitrous oxide (N_2O) supports combustion no more than air and has been proven safe for laparoscopic use. A single blind randomized trial has demonstrated that N_2O pneumoperitoneum is associated with decreased postoperative pain compared with carbon dioxide.[1]

When deciding if a patient is a suitable candidate for a laparoscopic procedure, it is important to assess patient or procedure characteristics that will lengthen the operative time sufficiently to nullify the benefits of laparoscopy. If the laparoscopic operation takes substantially longer than the open equivalent or is more risky, then it is not prudent to proceed laparoscopically. A history of a prior open procedure or multiple open procedures can make access to the abdomen difficult and will be discussed in detail later in this chapter. Adhesions and scarring in the surgical field from prior surgery can make laparoscopic surgery very difficult and may require use of many novel dissecting and coagulating tools. Operating on patients with severe obesity is challenging specifically because torque on transabdominal ports leads to surgeon fatigue and diminishes surgical dexterity. In addition, the long distance from the insufflated abdominal wall to the abdominal organs can make laparoscopic surgery a "far reach." Special long ports and instruments are available to overcome this difficulty.

Inability to obtain an adequate working space makes laparoscopic surgery impossible. This is encountered most commonly in patients with dilation of the intestine from bowel obstruction. Often, laparoscopic lysis of adhesions for distal bowel obstruction is not technically feasible.[2] Some patients with appendicitis will have sufficient small bowel dilation that laparoscopic access to the right iliac fossa is not possible.

PATIENT POSITIONING

We rely on gravity for retraction of the abdominal contents to provide exposure. Sometimes this requires steep positional changes, and care must be taken to prevent nerve complications or neuropathies after laparoscopic surgery as in open surgery. Patients must be positioned properly at the beginning of the procedure, making certain that all pressure points are padded. Perineal nerve injury is caused by lateral pressure at the knee and may occur when the table is "airplaned" to the side with a retractor holding the patient in place. Femoral and sciatic neuropathies are similar in that they are due to compression. Padding the retractor arms and securing the patient to the table can prevent these neuropathies.

It is best if the arms can be tucked for most laparoscopic procedures so that the surgeon may move freely up and down the table in order to line up instruments and the target tissue. This is most important for procedures in the pelvis, where the surgeon will want to stand adjacent to the contralateral thorax. However, even with upper abdominal laparoscopy, tucked arms allow more optimal positioning of instrument columns and monitors. If there is a need to extend the arms on arm boards, one must be very careful to avoid a brachial plexus injury that occurs when the arm is extended greater than 90 degrees at the shoulder. Usually, at the start of a procedure the arm positioning is safe but may change as the patient slides down on the table. For this reason, when reverse Trendelenburg is expected, we place footplates at the feet. This prevents sliding on the table and does not cause any discomfort to the patient because it is much like standing. We secure the ankles as well to be sure they do not "twist" during the procedure. There are footplates available for split-leg tables that can be used when operating on the upper abdomen and steep reverse Trendelenburg is needed.

PATIENT PREPARATION

There may be an increased incidence of deep venous thrombosis after laparoscopic surgery that is due to pooling of blood in the venous system of the lower extremities. Venous return is impaired by compression of the iliac veins from the elevated intra-abdominal pressure exerted by the pneumoperitoneum. Additionally, the positional effects of placing the patient in a steep reverse Trendelenburg position lead to further distension of the venous system. All patients undergoing laparoscopic procedures in reverse Trendelenburg, even short procedures such as laparoscopic cholecystectomy, should have sequential compression devices placed before the procedure begins, although this does not improve femoral blood flow entirely.[3] Patients at high risk for developing deep venous thrombosis should be treated with subcutaneous anticoagulants as either fractionated or unfractionated heparin.[4] This includes patients undergoing lengthy procedures, obese patients, patients with a prior history of deep venous thrombosis or pulmonary embolism, and patients in whom ambulation after surgery will be delayed. Some authors recommend placement of vena caval filters in patients with a prior history of deep venous thrombosis who are undergoing lengthy laparoscopic procedures.[5]

Laparoscopic surgery is associated with a high incidence of postoperative nausea and vomiting. A recent review asserts that serotonin receptor antagonists such as ondansetron (Zofran, GlaxoSmithKline) appear to be the most effective and should be considered for routine prophylaxis.[6] Another prospective, blinded, randomized trial shows a decrease in the postoperative nausea and vomiting when low-dose steroids are given to all patients.[7] There was no increased infection rate in the group that received steroids. Other preventive measures include ensuring adequate hydration[8,9] and decompression of the stomach with an orogastric tube before the end of the procedure. Intravenous nonsteroidal anti-inflammatory drugs (NSAIDs) such as ketorolac provide superb pain relief and diminish the need for postoperative narcotics, which may help to prevent nausea and vomiting.

▪ PORT PLACEMENT

SITE SELECTION

Proper placement of ports is important to facilitate completion of the laparoscopic procedure. The location of port sites depends on the type of procedure; the primary port should be placed with this in mind. We do not always place the primary port at the umbilicus but rather judge which site is best for the camera or which is the safest site for the primary puncture in a previously operated abdomen. The first laparoscopic port can be positioned anywhere in the abdomen after pneumoperitoneum has been created. The additional or secondary ports should not be placed too close to each other. The optimal pattern of port placement should form an equilateral triangle or a diamond array around the operative field. This "diamond of success" takes into account the optimal working distance from the operative target for each instrument and the telescope (Fig 44–1). In laparoscopy, the standard instrument length is 30 cm. To produce a 1:1 translation and movement from the surgeon's hands to the operative field, the fulcrum of the instrument should be 15 cm from the target. A similar separation of the two working ports (surgeon's left and right hands) ensures that these two instruments will not be involved in "sword fighting" and that the angle between the two instruments at the target will be optimal (between 60 and 90 degrees). The secondary port site is chosen, and the abdominal wall is transilluminated to avoid large abdominal wall vessels.[10,11] The trocar is watched laparoscopically as it enters into the abdomen, and care is taken to avoid injuring the abdominal contents. During the procedure, the area beneath the primary trocar site is inspected for unexpected injuries.

PORT CHARACTERISTICS

There is a wide variety of ports, each with different characteristics, available on the market. The bladed trocars cut the abdominal wall fascia during entry. Because the nonbladed trocars do not cut the abdominal wall as much, they make smaller defects in the abdominal wall and may be less prone to hernia formation in the future. The most commonly used bladed ports have a shield that retracts as the blade is pushed through the fascia of the abdominal wall, and then it engages once inside the abdomen. When first introduced to the market, the shields were called safety shields, but they have lost that designation because the shield provides little protection. The nonbladed trocars come in many forms. One nonbladed trocar is used in the Step system (Autosuture, Norwalk, CT), a modified Veress needle that locks inside an expandable sheath. Once inside the abdomen, the Veress needle is removed, and a blunt port is passed into the sheath that guides the port by dilating radially.[12] The Ethicon nonbladed trocar has a rough edge of plastic that is twisted and pushed through the layers of the abdominal wall. None of these technologies have proven safer than the more economical reusable nonshielded bladed trocar systems made by most instrument companies (Fig 44–2).

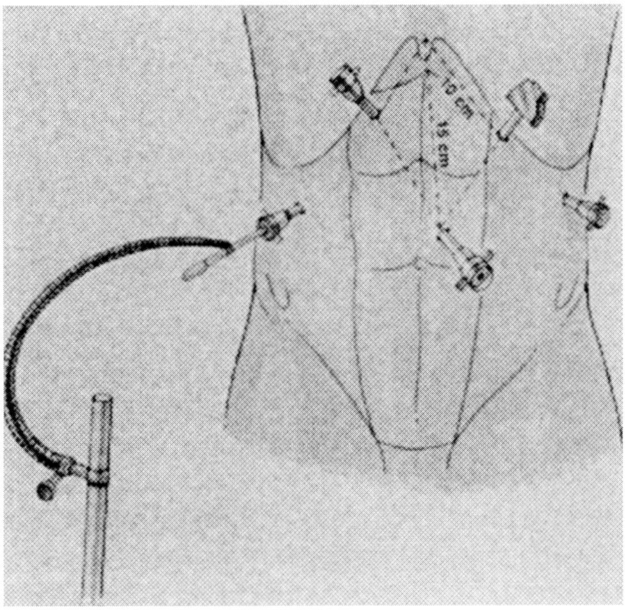

Figure 44–1. The "diamond of success" for optimal placement of laparoscopic ports. (Reprinted with permission from: Hunter JG, Trus TL, Branum GD, Waring JP. Laparoscopic Heller myotomy and fundoplication for achalasia. *Ann Surg* 1997;225:655–665.)

Important characteristics of a port need to be considered when choosing which port to use. The advantage of a port introduced with a nonbladed trocar is that the abdominal wall defect is smaller, which does not allow gas to leak from the abdomen during the procedure. Because the fascia is not cut, there is a lower risk of port-site hernia, and the fascia of most 10-mm incisions does not have to be closed. Additionally, these ports tend not to slip out of the abdominal wall during manipulation. Other considerations when choosing a port are the size of the external component, the smoothness of entry and exit of the instruments and specimens, and whether an external reducer cap is needed.

ACCESS OR PLACEMENT OF THE FIRST PORT

No single access technique has emerged as the safest and best technique.[13,14] The techniques for abdominal access include direct puncture and an open-access technique.[15] The direct-puncture technique can performed either by direct trocar insertion without pneumoperitoneum or by first obtaining pneumoperitoneum using a Veress needle and then inserting the first trocar directly. The latter technique is the performed most commonly in the United States. Each technique has a specific pattern of complications that must be considered when choosing among them.

The Veress needle access was first described in 1938.[16] This technique involves direct insertion of a needle into the peritoneum after lifting the abdominal wall with towel clips or a firm grip. The optimal site for insertion

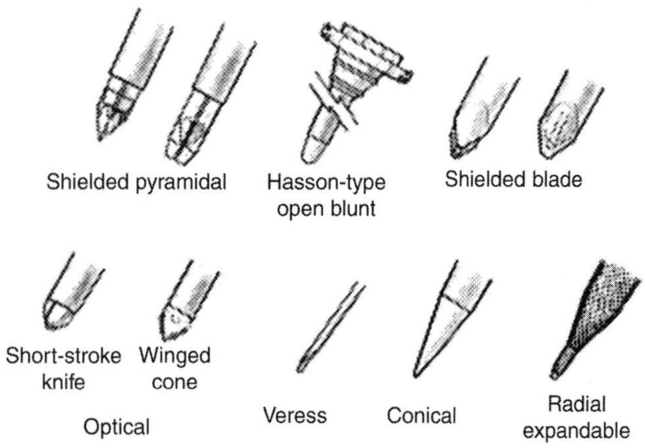

Figure 44–2. Various trocars for the introduction of laparoscopic ports through the abdominal wall. There are bladed and nonbladed types. Of the bladed trocars, there are shielded and nonshielded types. The Veress needle with a radially dilating sheath used in the Step system is an example of a nonbladed trocar. (Reprinted with permission from Chandler JG, Corson SL, Way LW. Three spectra of laparoscopic entry access injuries. *J Am Coll Surg* 2001;192:478–490; discussion 490–471.)

of the Veress needle is through the central scar at the umbilicus. One can make either a vertical skin incision through the umbilicus, hiding the incision in the base, or a curvilinear incision in an infraumbilical or supraumbilical position. Nevertheless, insertion of the Veress needle should be aimed at the central scar, where the layers of the abdominal wall are fused. This does not mean, though, that the first port inserted must be at the umbilicus. Advocates state that the benefits of this technique are the ability to place the initial port anywhere on the abdomen, that it is relatively quick, and that the skin and fascial openings are smaller, which prevents CO_2 leakage during the procedure.

For safe Veress needle insertion, one first must be certain to check the stylet and needle patency, especially when reinserting it after an unsuccessful initial pass. The Veress needle is available either as a reusable or disposable product and comes in two sizes, both long and short. The spring mechanism that pushes the stylet out, thus protecting bowel from the needle, must be tested when using the reusable Veress needle.

The safest technique requires stabilizing the abdominal wall (we prefer penetrating towel clips in nonobese patients). It is important to have control over the force and depth of insertion of the needle. This is aided by placing either your wrist against the patient's abdomen or using the nondominant hand to support the hand wielding the needle. It is sometimes necessary to raise the operating table to achieve the proper control. One must be mindful of the fact that the most common catastrophic complication from Veress needle insertion is injury to major vessels. The trajectory of the needle should not be angled toward the aorta or iliac vessels (Fig 44–3).

After placement of the Veress needle, one should perform an aspiration test by connecting a syringe filled with saline to the top of the Veress needle and aspirate. Aspiration of air, blood, or bile signifies incorrect placement and should prompt serious concern for an unexpected injury. If there is no aspirate, saline should be injected and should flow easily. The saline should flow down the Veress needle into the peritoneal cavity without pressure, a qualitative measure. Removing the plunger from the syringe and watching the saline level drop briskly may achieve a quantitative assessment of patency. If the saline flows slowly or not at all, the needle is likely in the wrong position, i.e., up against an intra-abdominal organ, or it is in the preperitoneal space. Alternatively, the tip may be occluded with fat, or the system may have an "air lock." To test this, inject a little bit of fluid again gently, and retest by removing the plunger and allowing the saline to drop into the abdomen.

The Veress needle then is connected to the insufflation tubing. The expected initial insufflation pressure, assuming proper placement, should be less than 5–6 mmHg. Abnormally high insufflation pressure is an indication that something is not right.[17] Because the insufflator is usually set to allow a maximum pressure of 15 mmHg, a value greater than this suggests that the patient is not anesthetized adequately and is contracting his or her abdominal muscles. If the insufflator records a pressure of 15 mmHg, there are a few explanations. The most ominous cause would be incorrect placement into an intra-abdominal organ. More likely, the Veress needle tip may be against omentum or is in the preperitoneal space. The insufflation line may be occluded at the stopcock, or there may be a kink in the tubing.

Direct trocar insertion without first establishing pneumoperitoneum is not used as frequently because

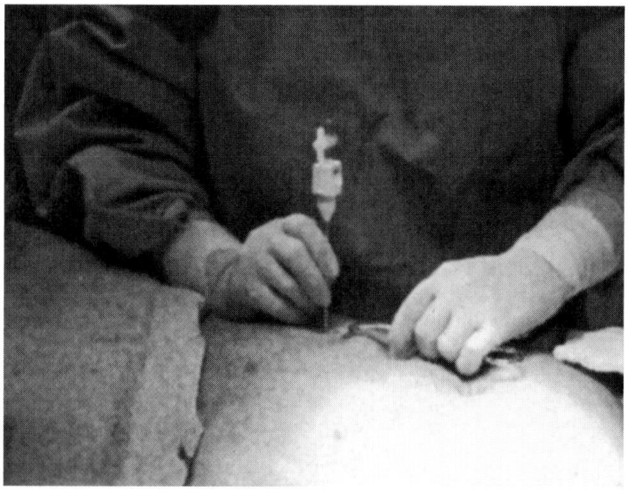

Figure 44–3. Proper Veress technique in the left upper quadrant using the dominant hand with the wrist stabilized on the patient. The nondominant hand is used to stabilize the abdominal wall.

many surgeons think that it is dangerous given that the bladed trocar must be pushed into the abdomen with significant force to penetrate the abdominal wall. Surgeons unfamiliar with the technique worry about injury to bowel and vessels when using excessive force. There are, however, many surgeons who perform this technique with no increased complication rate, confirming its safety.[18–22] Still other surgeons believe that the open-access technique that involves a "minilaparotomy" is the safest.[15,23–25]

The open, or Hasson, technique was first described in 1974.[15] A 1- to 2-cm skin incision is made at the umbilicus, and the soft tissue is divided to identify the abdominal wall. The fascia and muscles are opened with a knife, and the peritoneum is identified and grasped with Kocher or Allis clamps. A 0-0 absorbable suture is placed through the fascia, and the Hasson port is secured to the fascial sutures. Later these sutures can be used to close the abdominal wall. The insufflation tubing is attached to the sideport of the trocar, and the abdomen is inflated rapidly to 15 mmHg.

Newer trocars, called *optical trocars,* allow visualization of the tip of the trocar as it passes through the layers of the abdominal wall (Fig 44–4). A straight-viewing 0-degree scope is placed inside a clear trocar that is available with and without a bladed tip. Safe introduction of an optical trocar is a skill that requires judgment and experience and can best be learned in patients with no prior surgery after insufflation is established. Success depends on the operator's ability to see each of the layers of tissue, although visualization does not imply safety.[26] It is useful for the surgeon to have command of several access techniques because there is no single technique that is best for all circumstances.[27]

DIFFICULT ACCESS

Access can be the most challenging aspect of the procedure in some patients no matter which technique is used. This is especially true in obese patients. First, the site of the central scar often is judged inaccurately because the umbilicus is in a caudad position owing to the loose panniculus. Additionally, there is an increased distance between the skin and the abdominal wall fascia. The Veress needle may not penetrate the abdominal wall. If an open-access technique is chosen, it may be difficult to expose the abdominal wall through a small incision. Degenerated fascia in obese patients will make the abdominal wall bounce against the needle or finger, making its identification difficult. Raising the skin with penetrating towels clips does not facilitate this exposure and, in fact, distorts the anatomy, making it more difficult to identify the fascia. Sometimes a modified technique described by Vakili and Knight can be helpful.[28] This is a combination of open and Veress techniques in which a small skin incision is made in obese patients. Kochers are used to hold the abdominal wall fascia up, and a Veress needle is passed through the abdominal wall.

Access is also difficult in patients who have had prior surgery through a midline incision. In these patients, it is unsafe to perform the Hasson technique through the midline site because of the potential for adhesions of bowel to the posterior surface of the abdominal wall. Injury can occur when dividing the fascia or when sweeping adhesions away with a finger. It is difficult to perform the open technique at sites other than the umbilicus because of the multiple layers of the abdominal wall. In these patients, we prefer to place the Veress needle in the next

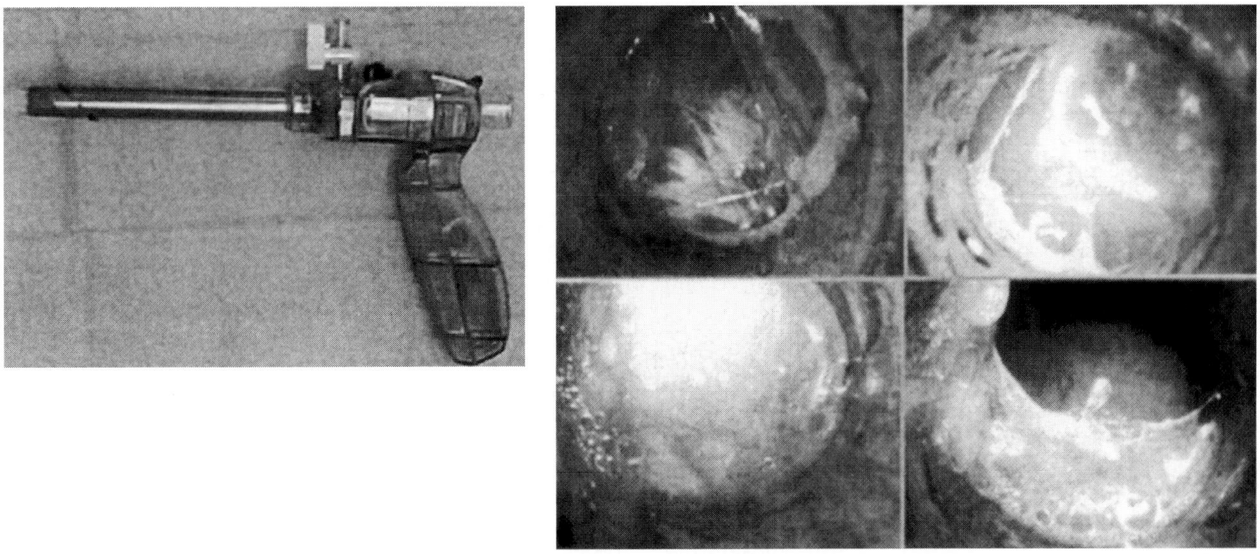

Figure 44–4. Optical trocar. (Used with pemission of Ethicon.)

safest location, which is the left upper quadrant along the costal margin. One must be certain that the table is flat because the spleen and liver are injured more easily in patients in the reverse Trendelenburg position. One must be certain that the stomach is decompressed with an orogastric tube before inserting the Veress needle in the left upper quadrant. Once insufflation is obtained, a port can be placed into the abdomen away from the previously operated field. We prefer entering with a 5-mm step port followed by a 30-degree 5-mm scope. Other surgeons recommend use of optical trocars in this situation.

FASCIAL CLOSURE

Care should be taken to prevent port-site hernias, which occur in 0.65–2.80% of laparoscopic gastrointestinal operations,[29] because they can lead to bowel obstruction, incarceration, and/or Richter's hernias. All defects created with a 10-mm or greater bladed trocar should be closed, although this is not necessary when using some of the newer nonbladed trocars that create smaller fascial defects.[30,31] Most 5-mm defects do not require fascial closure in adults, although there are reported cases of hernias at these sites.[9,32,33] Because there is always a possibility of formation of a port-site hernia, the smallest possible port always should be used. When a port is manipulated excessively or has to be replaced multiple times, there may be a larger than expected fascial defect that may require closure. Additional recommendations are to place ports lateral to the rectus muscles when possible.[34] At the conclusion of the procedure, removal of ports from the abdomen should be observed to be certain that omentum or abdominal contents are not brought up through the abdominal wall.

Fascial closure can prevent trocar-site hernia.[35] A number of port-site closure devices have been developed[36] because small laparoscopic incisions make it difficult to close the abdominal wall with round needles. The closure devices function like crochet needles, passing a suture through the abdominal wall on one side of the fascial incision. The suture end is released intra-abdominally under laparoscopic visualization, and the needle is removed. The needle is replaced (without suture) on the other side of the incision, and the free end is secured and pulled back out through the abdominal wall. A knot is then tied that closes the trocar site, as viewed laparoscopically (Fig 44–5).

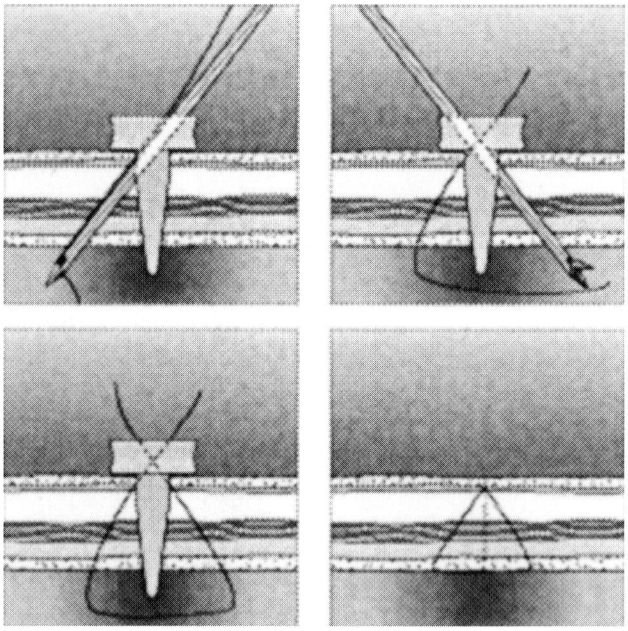

Figure 44–5. Using the Inlet device, the suture is passed through the abdominal wall on one side of the fascial incision. The suture end is released intra-abdominally under laparoscopic visualization, the suture then is pulled out on the other side of the incision using the device, and a knot is tied. (Used with permission of Inlet.)

TROCAR INJURY

The overall risk of a trocar injury to intra-abdominal structures is estimated to be between 5 in 10,000 and 3 in 1,000.[14] Almost all injuries occur during primary trocar insertion. According to Chandler and colleagues,[13] the most commonly injured organ is the small bowel (25.4%), followed by the iliac artery (18.5%), colon (12.2%), iliac vein (8.9%), mesenteric vessels (7.3%), and aorta (6.4%). All other organs were injured less than 5% of the time. The mortality from trocar injury is 13%, with 44% owing to major vessel injury, 26% to bowel injury with delayed diagnosis, and 20% to small bowel injury. Major vascular injuries are noticed immediately and require rapid conversion to laparotomy. They are managed by applying pressure when possible to allow the anesthesia team to maintain and correct volume and prepare for rapid blood loss. Then the surgeon gets control of inflow and outflow to permit repair of the injury. Unfortunately, many bowel injuries are not recognized at the time of the procedure, and nearly half are not noticed until more than 24 hours postoperatively. This obviously leads to severe sequelae and may be prevented by careful dissection and inspection at the conclusion of the procedure.

▪ EQUIPMENT

TELESCOPE

Laparoscopic and thoracoscopic telescopes come in a variety of shapes and sizes, offering several different angles of view. The standard laparoscope consists of a metal shaft 24 cm in length containing a series of quartz-rod lenses that carry the image through the length of the scope to the eyepiece. The telescope also contains parallel optical fibers that transmit light into the abdomen from the light source via a cable attached to the side of the telescope. Telescopes offer either a straight-on view with the 0 degree or can be angled at 25–30 or 45–50 degrees. The 30-degree telescope provides a total field of view of 152 degrees compared with the 0-degree telescope, which only provides a field of view of 76 degrees (Fig 44–6).

The most commonly used telescope has a diameter of 10 mm and provides the greatest light and visual acuity. The next most commonly used telescope is the 5-mm laparoscope, which can be placed through one of the working ports for an alternative view. Smaller-diameter laparoscopes, down to a 1.1-mm scope, are available and are used mostly in children. They are not used commonly in adult patients because of an inability to direct enough light into the larger abdominal cavity. The camera is attached to the eyepiece of the laparoscope for processing.

VIDEO CAMERA

A high-resolution video camera is attached to the eyepiece of the telescope and acquires the image for projection on the monitor. The video image is transmitted via a cable to a video unit, where it is processed into either an analog or a digital form. Analog is an electrical signal with a continuously varying wave or shift of intensity or frequency of voltage. Digital is a data signal with information represented by ones and zeros and is interpreted by a computer. These are the methods by which the picture is transmitted to the video monitor. The camera and cable are designed so that they can be sterilized in glutaraldehyde.

The camera iris directly controls the amount of light processed by opening the aperture of the camera. The gain controls the brightness of the image under conditions of low light by recruiting pixels to increase signal strength. Clearly, this step results in some loss of image resolution. This increases light but results in a grainy picture with poorer resolution. It also may create a loss of color accuracy owing to amplification of the noise-to-signal ratio.

LIGHT SOURCES

High-intensity light is created with bulbs of mercury, halogen vapor, or xenon. The bulbs are available in different wattages—150 and 300 W—and should be chosen based on the type of procedure being performed. Because light is absorbed by blood, any procedure in which bleeding is encountered may require more light. We use the stronger light sources for all advanced laparoscopy. Availability of light is a challenge in many bariatric procedures where the abdominal cavity is large. The light is carried to the fiberoptic bundles of the laparoscope via a fiberoptic cable. The current systems create even brightness across the field.

INSUFFLATORS

An insufflator delivers gas from a high-pressure cylinder to the patient at a high rate with low and accurately controlled pressure. Some insufflators have an internal filter that prevents contamination of the insufflator with the gas from the patient's abdomen and similarly filters any particulate matter that may be freed from the inside of an aging gas cylinder. Others require use with disposable insufflator tubing that has a filter on it. Some insufflators provide heated or humidified gas, but clinical benefit to these theoretically desirable features has not yet to be proven.

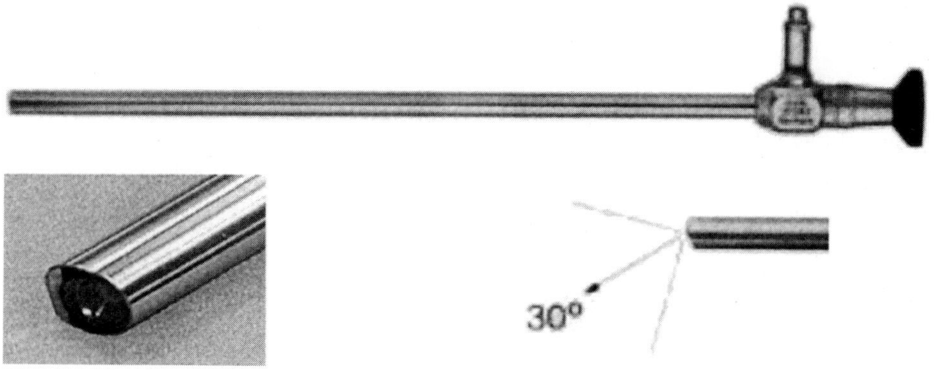

Figure 44–6. The 30-degree telescope provides a total field of view of 152 degrees compared with the 0-degree telescope, which provides a field of view of only 76 degrees. (Used with permission of Storz.)

VIDEO MONITORS

High-resolution video monitors are used to display the image. Optimal monitor size varies but ranges from 19–21 in. Smaller monitors may be used if placed close to the operative field. Larger monitors provide little advantage outside of a display setting. Cathode-ray monitors (analog) are being replaced rapidly by flat-panel (digital) displays with excellent color and spatial resolution. These monitors may be positioned optimally when hung from the ceiling on light booms.

▪ INSTRUMENTATION

The instruments used in laparoscopic surgery are similar to those of open surgery at the tips but are different in that they are attached to a long rod that can be placed through laparoscopic ports. Standard-length instruments possess a 30-cm-long shaft, but longer instruments (up to 45 cm in length) have been developed for bariatric surgery. The handles come in many varieties and must be chosen based on comfort and ergonomics, as well as the need for a locking or nonlocking mechanism. The shaft of most hand instruments is 5 mm wide; however, some specialized dissectors are available only in a 10-mm width. Pediatric laparoscopy instrumentation is generally 2–3 mm in diameter (Fig 44–7). Bowel graspers come in a wide variety with different types of teeth (Fig 44–8). The most atraumatic grasper has small, smooth teeth like a Debakey forceps. This has the advantage of not tearing the tissues and can be used on almost all organs. We use the Hunter grasper (Jarit), which, like a Debakey, can be used to grasp bowel and also can be used to grasp a needle. An additional benefit is that the tip is blunt and not prone to causing tissue trauma. Another commonly used bowel grasper is the Glassman (Storz), which is atraumatic and is slightly longer than the standard-sized Hunter grasper. It is fenestrated and cannot be used to grasp a needle. For some tissues, these instruments do not "grip" well enough, and bigger teeth or a different tip, such as those of Allis and Babcock clamps, is preferred. We reserve these larger-teethed instruments only for organs that are being removed, such as the gallbladder, or for thicker tissue, such as the stomach. The rule is to be gentle because small injuries can take a relatively long time to fix laparoscopically.

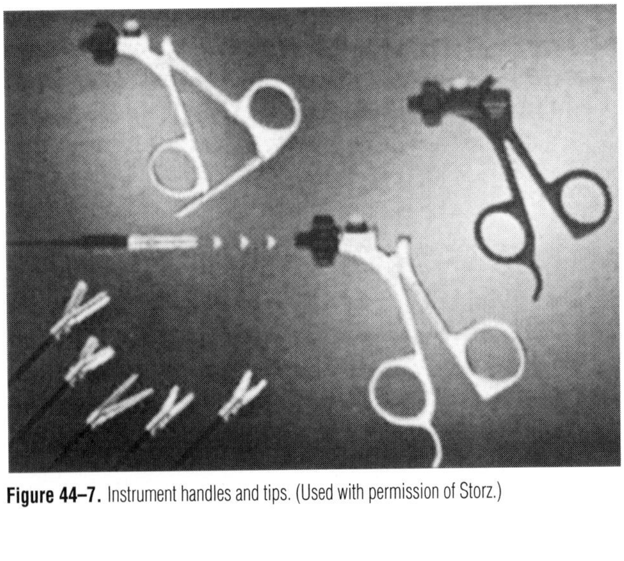

Figure 44–7. Instrument handles and tips. (Used with permission of Storz.)

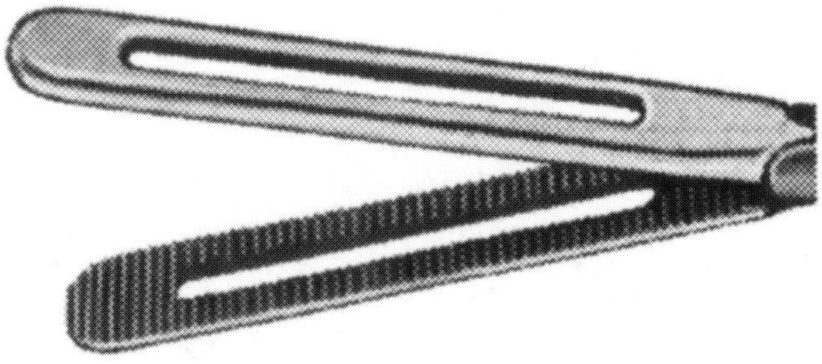

Figure 44–8. Atraumatic bowel graspers. (Used with permission of Storz.)

The most commonly used dissector is the Maryland dissector (Fig 44–9). It is useful for dissecting small ductal structures such as the cystic duct and can be used when dissecting vessels. Another use for the Maryland dissector is that it can be attached to monopolar cautery and used to grasp and cauterize a bleeding vessel (this should not be done with bowel graspers). The Maryland dissector should not be used to grasp delicate tissue because too much pressure is applied over a very small area, much like erroneously using a Kelly clamp for grasping tissue. Very delicate right-angle dissectors can be used for renal, adrenal, and splenic vessels and are less traumatic than the Maryland dissector because there are no ridges.

HEMOSTASIS

Hemostasis can be achieved using current from a monopolar electrosurgical generator applied to common instruments and controlled with a foot pedal. One of the most useful instruments for dissection is a disposable hook attached to the hand-held Bovie device for dissection (Valley Labs/Conmed and others). If a vessel has been transected and is bleeding but is too large to control with monopolar electrosurgery, a pretied lasso-like suture (Endo-loop, Ethicon Endosurgery) can be helpful. Laparoscopic clips are handy for small identifiable vessels but should not be used when a vessel is not identified. The clip is only 7 mm in length and is not useful for vessels larger than this. When the vessel is not clearly identified but the bleeding site is, ultrasonic shears and

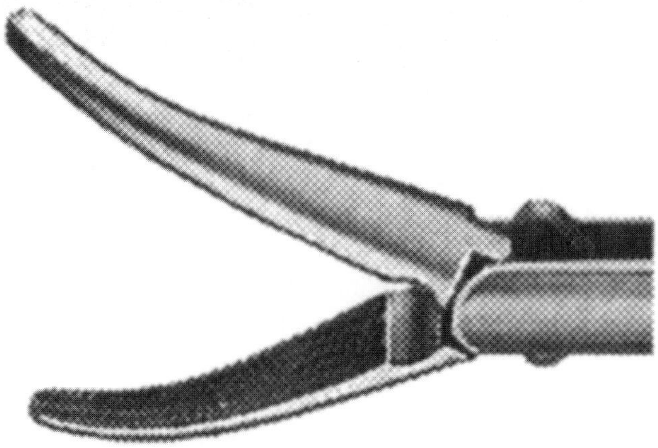

Figure 44–9. Maryland dissector. (Used with permission of Storz.)

some bipolar instruments such as the LigaSure device (ValleyLab, Boulder, CO) can be helpful. These instruments have the advantage of facilitating dissection while providing hemostasis for larger bleeding vessels.

MONOPOLAR ELECTROSURGERY

Although hemostasis is obtained using the same electrosurgical generator that is used in open surgery, there are hazards that are unique to minimally invasive surgery. The most frequently used method of delivering electrosurgery is monopolar. The desired surgical effect is hemostasis, and this is obtained by production of heat. Alternating current at 50,000 Hz (household current is 60 Hz) is generated and travels through an active electrode. The active electrode can be a Bovie tip in open surgery or, in laparoscopy, an instrument that is connected to the generator by the monopolar cord. The current passes into the target tissue at sufficiently high current density to cause a great deal of heat. Depending on tissue heating, coagulation, fulguration, or vaporization of the tissue occurs. The circuit is completed by the return of the electrons broadly spread through the tissue (insufficiently dense to cause any adverse effect) back to the generator via the return electrode (grounding pad).

In open surgery, monopolar current sometimes is passed from the active electrode (Bovie tip) to the patient via another conductive instrument, the forceps. This is called *direct coupling*. In laparoscopy, it is not prudent to touch the active electrode (an activated instrument) on or near other conductive instruments within the abdominal cavity, i.e., the laparoscope or other working instruments. Direct coupling in minimally invasive surgery always should be avoided because injury may occur out of the surgeon's field of view. It is also not prudent to activate the generator in "midair" because the current may travel out of the surgeon's field of view to a crack in the insulation of a laparoscopic instrument. This results in transfer of current to a small area that generates heat and can produce an injury. All laparoscopic instruments should be checked for cracks in the insulation before being used.

ULTRASONIC SHEARS

Before the introduction of ultrasonic shears, larger vessels had to be tied off individually. This was very tedious laparoscopically, especially with the division of short gastric vessels during fundoplication. The development of the ultrasonic shears was revolutionary, allowing surgeons to divide larger vessels quickly and dissect simultaneously. Ultrasonic energy or sound waves are used to ablate, cauterize, and cut tissues. A generator produces a 55.5-kHz (55,500 Hz) electrical signal that travels via a cable to a piezoelectric crystal stack mounted in the transducer. The crystal stack converts the electrical signal to mechanical vibration at the same frequency. The ultrasonic vibration is amplified as it traverses the length of the titanium probe that is the active blade of the scalpel. Shearing forces separate tissue and heat the surrounding tissue, thereby coagulating and sealing blood vessels without burning. Damage to adjacent tissues is low, although the active blade can become quite hot, and burn injuries can occur.

BIPOLAR ELECTROSURGERY

Bipolar electrosurgery coagulates tissue by passing a high-frequency, low-voltage electric current between two directly apposed electrodes. Laparoscopic general surgeons use it much less frequently because an additional maneuver must be made to divide the tissue. The LigaSure (ValleyLab, Boulder, CO), a newer bipolar device, coagulates larger vessels (up to 7 mm in diameter) and seals tissue and has a knife available for subsequent division of the tissue between the jaws of the forceps. The instrument makes a sound when the tissue within the jaw has been coagulated safely. The advantage is that division of larger vessels can be performed safely. Unfortunately, it is relatively slow to use as a dissecting instrument, and the tip is not very useful for dissection because it is straight and wide.[37] It does not produce a large amount of heat, and damage to surrounding tissues is low.

▪ SUTURING

Intracorporeal suturing may be out of the realm of a fundamentals of laparoscopic surgery chapter. However, obtaining this skill is critical for successful performance of many laparoscopic procedures. A fundamental skill of laparoscopic surgery is the ability to place a suture accurately and tie a knot with a needle holder and a standard surgical suture. This skill can be mastered easily with a training box. Various suture aids have been developed, such as the EndoStitch (USSC), and can be used as a substitute. However, these devices are expensive, and the range of suture and needle sizes and types is limited. Many surgeons believe that an extracorporeal knot is acceptable because it is easier to create a knot outside the patient and slide it down with a knot pusher. In most settings, this is not true because securing an extracorporeal knot creates "sawing" of the tissue as the suture is pulled through or around it. This often results in tissue tearing. For interrupted suturing, the sliding square knot is the simplest most secure knot to master (Fig 44–10).

■ THE PHYSIOLOGIC EFFECTS OF PNEUMOPERITONEUM

The pneumoperitoneum has many effects that are only partially known despite years of study in humans and in animal models. There are effects resulting from the pressure within the abdomen and effects resulting from the composition of the gas used, generally carbon dioxide.

The pressure within the abdomen from pneumoperitoneum decreases venous return by collapsing the intra-abdominal veins, especially in volume-depleted patients. This decrease in venous return may lead to decreased cardiac output. To compensate, there is an elevation in the heart rate, which increases myocardial oxygen demand. High-risk cardiopulmonary patients cannot always meet the demand and may not tolerate a laparoscopic procedure.[38] In volume-expanded healthy patients with full intra-abdominal capacitance vessels (veins), the increased intra-abdominal pressure actually may serve as a pump that increases right atrial filling pressure.[39]

Through a different mechanism associated with catecholamine release triggered by CO_2 pneumoperitoneum, heart rate rises along with systemic vascular resistance. This may lead to hypertension and impair visceral blood flow. It is not uncommon after the induction of pneumoperitoneum for the heart rate to rise along with the mean arterial pressure. This leads to a minimal effect in a young, healthy patient[40]; however, in elderly, compromised patient, the strain on the heart can lead to hypotension, end-organ hypoperfusion, and ST-segment changes.

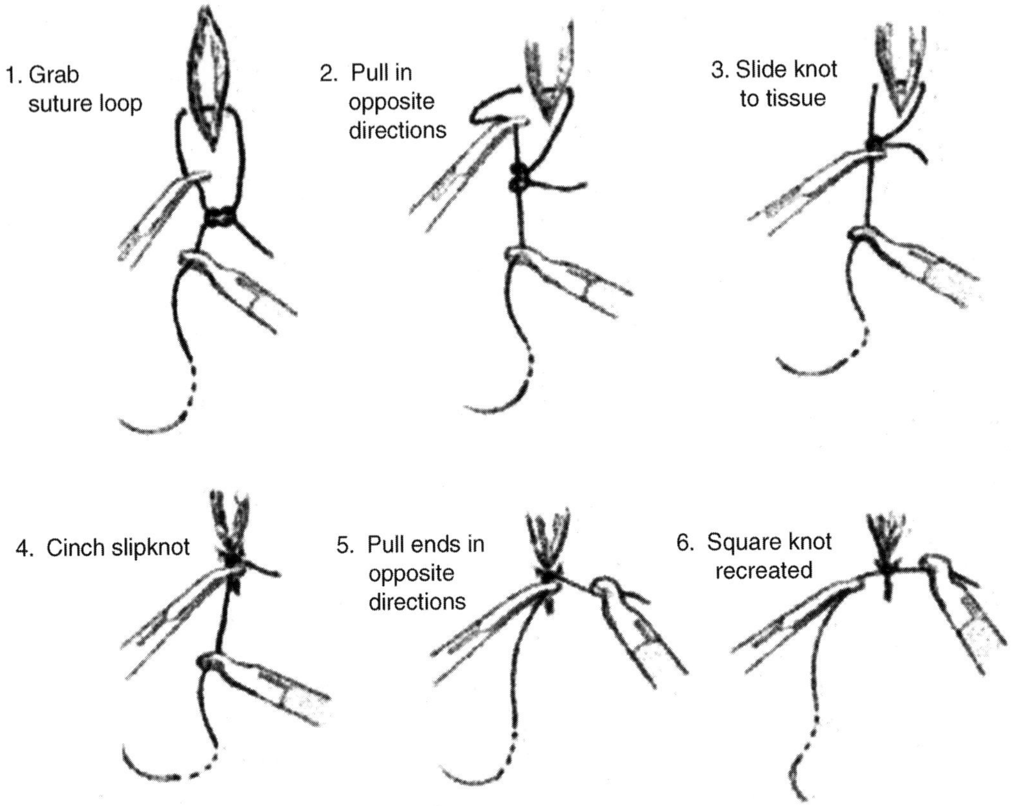
1. Grab suture loop
2. Pull in opposite directions
3. Slide knot to tissue
4. Cinch slipknot
5. Pull ends in opposite directions
6. Square knot recreated

Figure 44–10. Suturing. (Reprinted with permission from Hunter JG, Terry. Minimally invasive surgery: fundamentals. In: Cameron JL (ed). *Current Surgical Therapies.* St. Louis: Mosby.)

To minimize the cardiovascular effects of pneumoperitoneum, it is important that patients have adequate preoperative hydration. By insufflating the abdomen slowly, the vagal response to peritoneal stretching may be diminished and vagally mediated bradycardia avoided. Additionally, if cardiovascular effects are noted during insufflation or during the maintenance of pneumoperitoneum, the insufflation pressures should be lowered from the usual 15 to 12 mmHg, or pneumoperitoneum should be evacuated while the anesthesiologist sorts out the cardiovascular changes. Taking patients out of the steep reverse Trendelenburg position can help to increase venous return. Sometimes these effects can last for hours after desufflation.

The elevated intra-abdominal pressures restrict movement of the diaphragm, which reduces diaphragmatic excursion. This is represented as a decrease in functional residual capacity and pulmonary compliance and an increase in inspiratory pressure. Overall, there is no significant change in the physiologic dead space or shunt in patients without cardiovascular compromise. Bardoczky and colleagues studied seven healthy patients undergoing laparoscopy with CO_2 pneumoperitoneum.[41] After the induction of pneumoperitoneum, peak airway and plateau airway pressures increased by 50% and 81%, respectively. Bronchopulmonary compliance decreased by 47% during the period of increased intra-abdominal pressure. After desufflation, peak and plateau pressures remained elevated by 36% and 27%, respectively, for 2–6 hours. Compliance remained at 86% of the preinsufflation value.

Urine output often is diminished during laparoscopic procedures and usually is the result of diminished renal blood flow owing to the cardiovascular effects of pneumoperitoneum and direct pressure on the renal veins.[42] In addition to direct effects, elevated intra-abdominal pressure results in release of antidiuretic hormone (ADH) by the pituitary, resulting in oliguria that may last 30–60 minutes after the pneumoperitoneum is released. Aggressive fluid hydration during pneumoperitoneum increases urine output.[43] Positional changes can affect the collection of urine in the Foley catheter and must be taken into consideration if anuria is noted.

CARBON DIOXIDE–RELATED EFFECTS

Hypercapnia

Hypercapnia and acidosis are seen with pneumoperitoneum and are likely due to the absorption of carbon dioxide from the peritoneal cavity. In the ventilated patient, increasing respiratory rate or vital capacity must compensate for these changes. At extremes, increases in tidal volume may risk barotraumas, and increases in respiratory rates diminish time for gas mixing, increasing dead-space ventilation. A first steady state in $PaCO_2$ is reached around 15–30 minutes after introduction of the pneumoperitoneum. After this period, increases in $PaCO_2$ suggest that existing body buffers (>90% exist in bone) have been exhausted. Sudden increases may be related to port slippage and extraperitoneal or subcutaneous diffusion of carbon dioxide. This will resolve spontaneously once the port is repositioned.

Hypercapnia and acidosis that are difficult to control may follow, especially in elderly patients, those undergoing long operations, and patients with pulmonary insufficiency. Our response to this is to desufflate the abdomen for 10–15 minutes. If reinsufflation results in recurrent hypercapnia, then we change insufflation gases (see above) or convert to an open operation. Acidosis can persist for hours after desufflation. Other complications of pneumoperitoneum that are less frequent but may be life threatening include CO_2 embolism and capnothorax.

Carbon Dioxide Embolus

The incidence of clinically significant CO_2 embolism is very low, although recent reports using more sensitive tests suggest that tiny bubbles of gas are present commonly in the right side of the heart during laparoscopic procedures. Clinically important CO_2 embolism may be noted by unexplained hypotension and hypoxia during the operation. There is a characteristic millwheel murmur that can be detected with auscultation of the chest. This is produced by contraction of the right ventricle against the blood-gas interface. Usually the anesthesiologist notes an exponential decrease in the end-tidal CO_2, which is consistent with complete right ventricular outflow obstruction. The mainstays of treatment are immediate evacuation of the pneumoperitoneum and placement of the patient in the left lateral decubitus, head down (Durant) position. This allows the CO_2 bubble to "float" to the apex of the right ventricle, where it is less likely to cause right ventricular outflow tract obstruction. It is important to administer 100% oxygen and hyperventilate the patient during this period. Additionally, aspiration of gas through a central venous line may be performed.

Capnothorax/Pneumothorax

Capnothorax can be caused by carbon dioxide escaping into the chest through a defect in the diaphragm or tracking through fascial planes during dissection of the esophageal hiatus. It also can be due to opening of pleuroperitoneal ducts most commonly seen on the right side. Pleural tears during fundoplication can lead to pneumothorax, and additionally, the usual causes of pneumothorax, such as ruptured bullae, may be the etiology. The effects of carbon dioxide gas in the chest usually are noted as decreased O_2 saturation (a result of shunting induced by lung collapse), increased airway pressure, decreased pulmonary compliance, and increases in carbon dioxide and end-tidal CO_2. The treatment is to desufflate the abdomen and stop carbon dioxide administration, correct the hypoxemia by adjusting the ventilator, apply positive end-expiratory pressure (PEEP), if possible, and decrease the intra-abdominal pressure as much as possible. The recommendation is to avoid thoracentesis because this usually resolves with anesthetic management. We generally evacuate the capnothorax directly at the end of the procedure with a red rubber catheter placed across the diaphragm (through the pleural defect) and brought out a trocar site. The external end of the catheter is placed under water as the lung is inflated and then removed from the water when the bubbles stop. We do not obtain chest radiographs in the recovery room after these maneuvers if there is no evidence of hypoxia on 2 L/min of O_2 flow. Patients should be maintained on supplemental oxygen to help facilitate absorption of the carbon dioxide from the pleural space.

▪ CONCLUSIONS

Although minimally invasive surgery is firmly established in modern surgery, its safe performance can be ensured only with mastery of the basics. Basic skills used in laparoscopy include evaluation of a patient based on a new set of considerations, safe use of devices for abdominal access and instrumentation, and mastery of complex manual skills and intraoperative assessment of novel physiologic parameters. Laparoscopic surgery will only be employed more in the future as technical innovations allow us to care for our patients in new and better ways.

REFERENCES

1. Tsereteli Z, Terry ML, Bowers SP, et al. Prospective, randomized clinical trial comparing nitrous oxide and carbon dioxide pneumoperitoneum for laparoscopic surgery. *J Am Coll Surg* 2002;195:173–179; discussion 179–180
2. Chopra R, McVay C, Phillips E, Khalili TM. Laparoscopic lysis of adhesions. *Am Surg* 2003;69:966–968
3. Marshall NJ, Bessell JR, Maddern GJ. Study of venous blood flow changes during laparoscopic surgery using a thermodilution technique. *ANZ J Surg* 2000;70:639–643
4. Okuda Y, Kitajima T, Egawa H, et al. A combination of heparin and an intermittent pneumatic compression device may be more effective to prevent deep-vein thrombosis in the lower extremities after laparoscopic cholecystectomy. *Surg Endosc* 2002;16:781–784
5. Prystowsky JB, Morasch MD, Eskandari MK, et al. Prospective analysis of the incidence of deep venous thrombosis in bariatric surgery patients. *Surgery* 2005;138:759–763; discussion 763–755
6. Goldfaden A, Birkmeyer JD. Evidence-based practice in laparoscopic surgery: Perioperative care. *Surg Innov* 2005;12:51–61
7. Bisgaard T, Klarskov B, Kehlet H, Rosenberg J. Preoperative dexamethasone improves surgical outcome after laparoscopic cholecystectomy: A randomized, double-blind, placebo-controlled trial. *Ann Surg* 2003;238:651–660
8. Magner JJ, McCaul C, Carton E, et al. Effect of intraoperative intravenous crystalloid infusion on postoperative nausea and vomiting after gynaecological laparoscopy: Comparison of 30 and 10 mL kg^{-1}. *Br J Anaesth* 2004;93:381–385
9. Maharaj CH, Kallam SR, Malik A, et al. Preoperative intravenous fluid therapy decreases postoperative nausea and pain in high risk patients. *Anesth Analg* 2005;100:675–682
10. Epstein J, Arora A, Ellis H. Surface anatomy of the inferior epigastric artery in relation to laparoscopic injury. *Clin Anat* 2004;17:400–408
11. Hurd WW, Amesse LS, Gruber JS, et al. Visualization of the epigastric vessels and bladder before laparoscopic trocar placement. *Fertil Steril* 2003;80:209–212
12. Yim SF, Yuen PM. Randomized, double-masked comparison of radially expanding access device and conventional cutting tip trocar in laparoscopy. *Obstet Gynecol* 2001;97:435–438
13. Dabirashrafi H, Mohammad K, Tabrizi NM, et al. The use of Veress needle and 10-mm trocar (VN) versus direct trocar insertion (DTI) in the beginning of laparoscopy. *J Am Assoc Gynecol Laparosc* 1994;1:S9
14. Chandler JG, Corson SL, Way LW. Three spectra of laparoscopic entry access injuries. *J Am Coll Surg* 2001;192:478–490; discussion 490–471
15. Hasson H. Open laparoscopy: A report of 150 cases. *J Reprod Med* 1974;12:234–238
16. Veress J. Neues Instrument Zur Ausfuhrung von brustoder Bachpunktionen und Pneumonthoraybehundlung. *Deutsch Med Wochescr* 1938;64:1480–1481
17. Vilos GA, Vilos AG. Safe laparoscopic entry guided by Veress needle CO_2 insufflation pressure. *J Am Assoc Gynecol Laparosc* 2003;10:415–420
18. Dingfelder JR. Direct laparoscope trocar insertion without prior pneumoperitoneum. *J Reprod Med* 1978;21:45–47
19. Clayman RV. The safety and efficacy of direct trocar insertion with elevation of the rectus sheath instead of the skin for pneumoperitoneum. *J Urol* 2005;174:1847–1848
20. Gunenc MZ, Yesildaglar N, Bingol B, et al. The safety and efficacy of direct trocar insertion with elevation of the rectus sheath instead of the skin for pneumoperitoneum. *Surg Laparosc Endosc Percutan Tech* 2005;15:80–81
21. Agresta F, De Simone P, Ciardo LF, Bedin N. Direct trocar insertion vs Veress needle in nonobese patients undergoing laparoscopic procedures: A randomized, prospective single-center study. *Surg Endosc* 2004;18:1778–1781

22. Jacobson MT, Osias J, Bizhang R, et al. The direct trocar technique: An alternative approach to abdominal entry for laparoscopy. *JSLS* 2002;6:169–174
23. Rumstadt B, Sturm J, Jentschura D, et al. Trocar incision and closure: Daily problems in laparoscopic procedures—a new technical aspect. *Surg Laparosc Endosc* 1997;7:345–348
24. Champault G, Cazacu F, Taffinder N. Serious trocar accidents in laparoscopic surgery: A French survey of 103,852 operations. *Surg Laparosc Endosc* 1996;6:367–370
25. Saville LE, Woods MS. Laparoscopy and major retroperitoneal vascular injuries (MRVI). *Surg Endosc* 1995;9: 1096–1100
26. Sharp HT, Dodson MK, Draper ML, et al. Complications associated with optical-access laparoscopic trocars. *Obstet Gynecol* 2002;99:553–555
27. Corson SL, Chandler JG, Way LW. Survey of laparoscopic entry injuries provoking litigation. *J Am Assoc Gynecol Laparosc* 2001;8:341–347
28. Vakili C, Knight R. A technique for needle insufflation in obese patients. *Surg Laparosc Endosc* 1993;3:489–491
29. Tonouchi H, Ohmori Y, Kobayashi M, Kusunoki M. Trocar site hernia. *Arch Surg* 2004;139:1248–1256
30. Liu CD, McFadden DW. Laparoscopic port sites do not require fascial closure when nonbladed trocars are used. *Am Surg* 2000;66:853–854
31. Bhoyrul S, Payne J, Steffes B, et al. A randomized, prospective study of radially expanding trocars in laparoscopic surgery. *J Gastrointest Surg* 2000;4:392–397
32. Kwok A, Lam A, Ford R. Incisional hernia in a 5-mm laparoscopic port-site incision. *Aust NZ J Obstet Gynaecol* 2000;40:104–105
33. Reardon PR, Preciado A, Scarborough T, et al. Hernia at 5-mm laparoscopic port site presenting as early postoperative small bowel obstruction. *J Laparoendosc Adv Surg Tech A* 1999;9:523–525
34. Montz FJ, Holschneider CH, Munro M. Incisional hernia following laparoscopy: A survey of the American Association of Gynecologic Laparoscopists. *J Am Assoc Gynecol Laparosc* 1994;1:S23–24
35. Lowry PS, Moon TD, D'Alessandro A, Nakada SY. Symptomatic port-site hernia associated with a non-bladed trocar after laparoscopic live-donor nephrectomy. *J Endourol* 2003;17:493–494
36. Di Lorenzo N, Coscarella G, Lirosi F, Gaspari A. Port-site closure: a new problem, an old device. *JSLS* 2002;6: 181–183
37. Carbonell AM, Joels CS, Kercher KW, et al. A comparison of laparoscopic bipolar vessel sealing devices in the hemostasis of small-, medium-, and large-sized arteries. *J Laparoendosc Adv Surg Tech A* 2003;13:377–380
38. Gebhardt H, Bautz A, Ross M, et al. Pathophysiological and clinical aspects of the CO_2 pneumoperitoneum (CO_2-PP). *Surg Endosc* 1997;11:864–867
39. Kashtan J, Green JF, Parsons EQ, Holcroft JW. Hemodynamic effect of increased abdominal pressure. *J Surg Res* 1981;30:249–255
40. Larsen JF, Svendsen FM, Pedersen V. Randomized clinical trial of the effect of pneumoperitoneum on cardiac function and haemodynamics during laparoscopic cholecystectomy. *Br J Surg* 2004;91:848–854
41. Bardoczky GI, Engelman E, Levarlet M, Simon P. Ventilatory effects of pneumoperitoneum monitored with continuous spirometry. *Anaesthesia* 1993;48:309–311
42. Ninomiya K, Kitano S, Yoshida T, et al. Comparison of pneumoperitoneum and abdominal wall lifting as to hemodynamics and surgical stress response during laparoscopic cholecystectomy. *Surg Endosc* 998;12:124–128
43. Demyttenaere SV, Feldman LS, Bergman S, et al. Does aggressive hydration reverse the effects of pneumoperitoneum on renal perfusion? *Surg Endosc* 2006;20:274–280

45

Biliary Tract

Ketan R. Sheth ■ *Ricardo M. Bonnor* ■ *Theodore N. Pappas*

The most common biliary tract procedure currently performed is the laparoscopic cholecystectomy. This has yielded interest in management of common bile duct stones encountered during the procedure. Successful management of such stones during a laparoscopic cholecystectomy is beneficial to the patient by preventing a secondary or more invasive procedure to clear the duct. Furthermore, an all-inclusive operation may be more cost effective. Other operations on the biliary tract, including biliary resections and reconstructions can be the most technically demanding procedures a general surgeon performs. The advancement of technology and surgeon skills in the field of minimally invasive surgery has allowed for traditionally open complex biliary procedures to be attempted and successfully performed laparoscopically. This chapter focuses on minimally invasive techniques that can be commonly employed in the management of biliary tract pathology. Identification and management of common bile duct stones, choledochoscopy, and biliary bypass utilizing cholecystojejunostomy are discussed in detail. Brief mention is also made of highly advanced laparoscopic biliary tract procedures that are currently performed. While these technically advanced procedures should not be considered standard of care today, they encourage the continued advancement of minimally invasive biliary tract surgery.

■ LAPAROSCOPIC COMMON BILE DUCT EVALUATION

Common bile duct (CBD) stones are present in about 10–15% of patients with cholelithiasis. The large majority of these stones are less than 4 mm and generally pass into the duodenum without any clinical consequence.[1] Nevertheless, stones greater than 3 to 4 mm should be removed since they may cause severe complications such as pancreatitis and cholangitis. Cholangiography is the standard (along with ERCP) by which the CBD is evaluated for the presence of stones (Table 45–1). Cystic duct cholangiography can be accomplished in 90% of patients and, overall, the intraoperative cholangiogram has a sensitivity of 87% and specificity >95% for the detection of stones.[2] As it was in the era of open cholecystectomy, the use of intraoperative cholangiogram (IOC) during laparoscopic cholecystectomy remains somewhat controversial. Those that support the routine use of IOC site that this practice ensures fewer retained stones, fewer postoperative ERCPs, and a reduction of CBD injuries. Presently, the literature suggests that there is no difference in major and minor bile duct injuries whether routine or selective cholangiograms are performed.[2–5] Additionally, a large number of routine intraoperative cholangiograms have to be performed compared to a selective approach to detect missed duct injuries or extra problematic CBD stones.[5] Given this, the financial cost to diagnose a clinically significant bile duct stone that was not suspected intra-operatively has been calculated at half a million dollars.[5] Routine use of cholangiography is recommended for the relatively inexperienced surgeon or as a strategy to identify anatomy intraoperatively.

LAPAROSCOPIC CHOLANGIOGRAPHY

Once the cystic duct is identified, the proximal side is clipped as close to the gallbladder as possible, then

TABLE 45–1. INDICATIONS FOR LAPAROSCOPIC CHOLANGIOGRAM

Uncertain anatomy
Radiographic evidence of CBD stones
Abnormal liver function tests
Dilated cystic duct
Dilated CBD
Pancreatitis
Jaundice
Cholangitis
Multiple small stones in the gallbladder

using 5-mm scissors, a transverse ductotomy is made just distal to the clip. A cholangiogram catheter is then inserted via an introducer sheath or fed through a cholangiogram clamp via one of the right upper quadrant ports.[1] Once the catheter is maneuvered into the cystic duct, it is secured with a single clip or held in place with a cholangiogram clamp (Fig 45–1). Once the catheter is in place, the instruments that may interfere with a cholangiogram are removed and 50% solution of contrast material is injected under fluoroscopic guidance to obtain static and dynamic images. The management of stones found on IOC during laparoscopy is discussed later in the chapter. If still cholangiography is used, two films are required using a 5cc and 20-mL injection of diluted (50%) contrast.

LAPAROSCOPIC ULTRASOUND

Prospective trials have shown that intraoperative ultrasound (US) is comparable in terms of sensitivity and specificity to IOC in its ability to diagnose CBD stones.[6] This technique involves the use of linear-array transducer with frequency of 7.5 to 10 MHz. The image is obtained by moving the transducer first along the cystic duct and the hepatoduodenal ligament to the terminal CBD.[7,8] Potential advantages of IOUS are lower costs, lack of adverse effects, simplicity, and shorter examination times. The disadvantages are equipment availability, difficulty in visualizing the distal CBD, and operator dependency. This method of intraoperative evaluation has recently been applied and will be increasingly refined in the coming years.

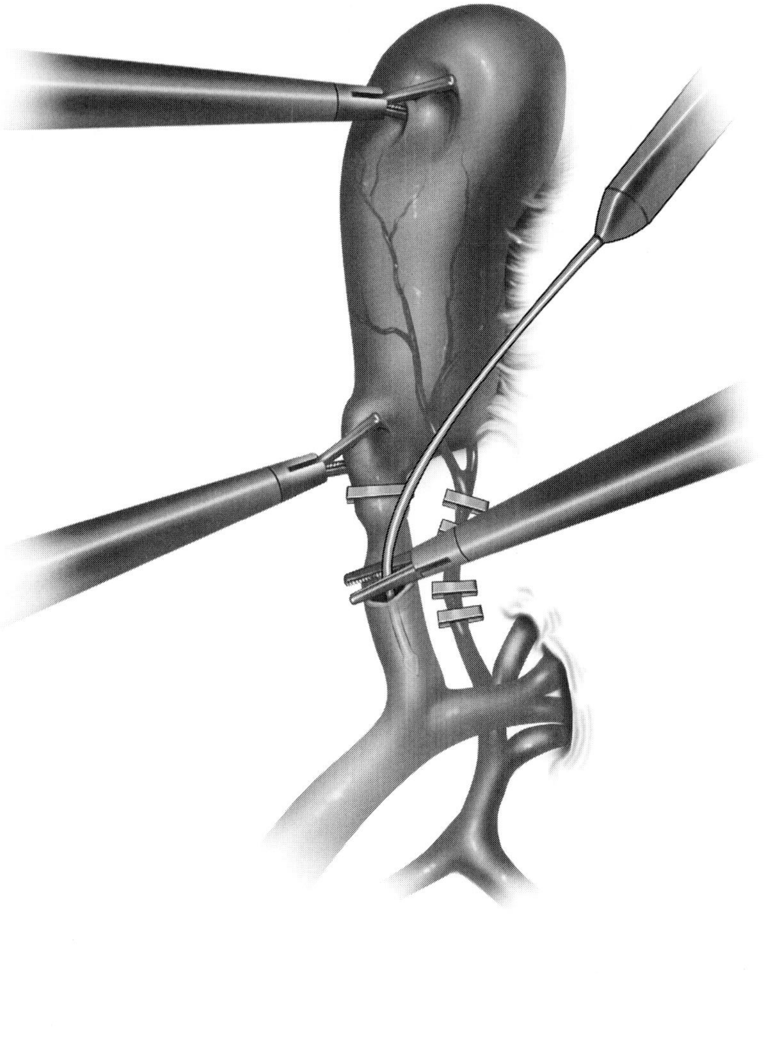

Figure 45–1. The catheter is guided into the partially transected cystic duct. When not using the cholangiogram clamp, the grasper may be used in maneuvering the catheter and secured with a single metal clip.

▪ LAPAROSCOPIC MANAGEMENT OF CHOLEDOCHOLITHIASIS

Choledocholithiasis is defined as the presence of stones in the common bile duct with the most common location of obstruction being at the narrow portion of the duct at the papilla. There are several preoperative clinical, chemical, and radiologic data that can predict the presence of common bile duct stones preoperatively (Table 45–2). Generally, there are two situations that the laparoscopic surgeon encounters when dealing with CBD stones: (1) stones documented or suspected preoperatively, (2) stones found intra-operatively. The approach of these situations is different in these two groups of patients.

For patients suspected of having CBD stones preoperatively, the clinician must decide whether to attempt common duct stone removal before operating (ERCP) or stone retrieval via laparoscopic or open methods. A number of clinical algorithms have been proposed using the objective and clinical parameters demonstrated in Table 45–2 for risk stratification inpatients with suspected CBD stones.[9] Such algorithms are not highly accurate in classifying patients who harbor CBD stones.[10]

The lack of accurate methods to predict the presence of CBD stones preoperatively is problematic because when stones are suspected on chemical and radiologic data, a normal ERCP is obtained in about 50% of the cases.[11] Since the positive predictive value of determining the presence of stones is not high, there is still controversy regarding the timing and need for ERCP.

The reported success rate of ERCP for clearing the common bile duct of stones approaches 90–95%, although this varies with the local expertise and experience of the endoscopist.[11] Similarly the laparoscopic success rate of clearing the duct is 70–90%. The choice of clearance method should be based upon several factors: the local expertise and availability of expert endoscopists with high success rate with ERCP and stone extraction, the availability of laparoscopic and choledochoscopic equipment, the surgical expertise in laparoscopic CBD surgery and the general condition of the patient. Table 45–3 suggests a strategy for selective preoperative ERCP.

When the situation arises that CBD stones are encountered intraoperatively, four options exist: (1) perform laparoscopic CBD exploration, (2) perform intraoperatively ERCP and sphincterotomy, (3) convert to open, or (4) leave the stones in place for postoperative ERCP. The third option is more costly and associated with added morbidity to the patient. The fourth option should only be used in a setting where the success of ERCP clearance of the common duct stone is very high. Although some centers have reported using intra-operative ERCP to clear the duct, this is not widely practiced since it is time consuming and cumbersome. Additionally, this may require the availability of an expert endoscopist which makes this less practical. For the patient with uncomplicated cholelithiasis, minimally invasive techniques can be applied to successfully manage the first option.

TABLE 45–2. OBJECTIVE AND INTRA-OPERATIVE CRITERIA FOR POSSIBLE PRESENCE OF CBD STONES

Clinical
Jaundice (present, recent, recurrent)
Acholic stools
Dark urine (bilirubin)
Fever
Laboratory values
Serum bilirubin >1.2 mg/dL
Serum alkaline phosphatase >250 U/L
Radiologic studies
Multiple small stones
Common bile duct diameter >6 mm
Common bile duct calculi
Intraoperative findings
Multiple small stones
Common bile duct diameter >10 mm
Cystic duct diameter 0.5 mm

TABLE 45–3. INDICATION FOR PREOPERATIVE ERCP IN PATIENTS WITH CHOLEDOCHOLITHIASIS

Clinical suspicion of CBD stones and:
Small cystic duct and/or CBD (making laparoscopic transcystic exploration difficult)
Elderly patient
High operative risk
Endoscopist with limited experience (if ERCP eventually required post-op)
Surgeon with limited experience in laparoscopic treatment of CBD stones
Strong desire of the patient to avoid open procedure

LAPAROSCOPIC TRANSCYSTIC DUCT EXPLORATION (WITHOUT CHOLEDOCHOSCOPE)

When the surgeon encounters a stone in the common bile during a positive cholangiogram, there are several treatment options available. If the duct is small and a single <3-mm stone is found, then simply instilling 1 to 2 mg of glucagon IV by the anesthetist followed by saline flushing of the duct is sometimes successful in clearing the duct (Fig 45–2).[12] Larger stones will typically not be cleared by this method.

Balloon Techniques

Low pressure balloon catheters may be introduced through a percutaneous cholangiogram sleeve into the cystic duct and then into the common bile duct. A 4F

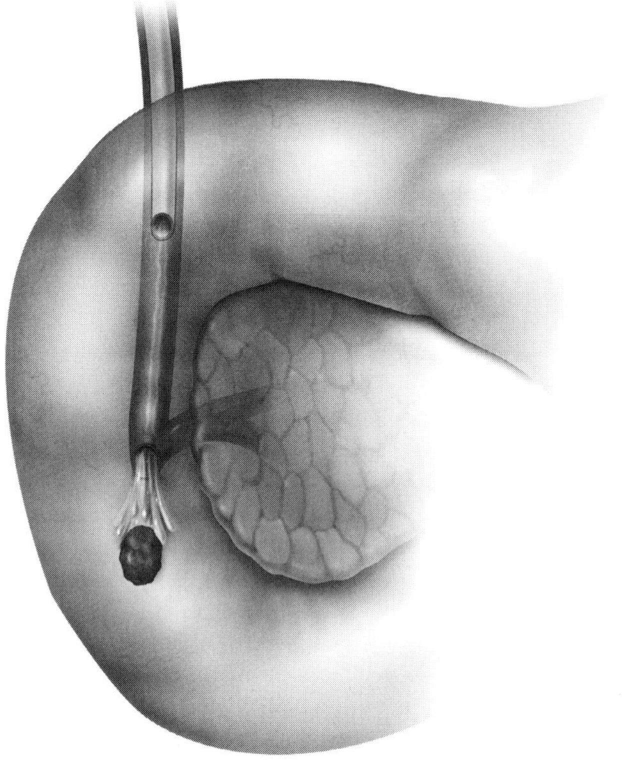

Figure 45–2. Stone forced through ampulla with saline flush. IV glucagon administration may also be used as an adjunct to flushing. Flushing may be accomplished with the cholangiocatheter or a red rubber catheter inserted via the cystic duct or common duct (if a choledochotomy has been made).

(French) Fogarty-type balloon catheter is most effective and can fit through a 12F to 14F introducer sheath placed in the abdominal wall.[13] The technique described is as follows: once the catheter tip is in the duodenum, the balloon is inflated and gently pulled back typically causing the duodenum to move with movement of the catheter; traction is stopped and the balloon deflated; then the catheter is withdrawn approximately 1 cm and the balloon is reinflated, traction is then resumed until the balloon is seen at the cystic duct cannulation site. Occasionally small stones or debris can be delivered with this method (Fig 45–3).

Another option is to use balloon dilation of the ampulla/sphincter of Oddi. Results from a few series have shown it to be a useful complementary tool for clearing common duct debris at the initial operation without embarking on the more complex bile duct exploration via a formal choledochotomy.

A 6-mm diameter balloon dilating catheter is employed over a guide wire. This is most easily accomplished using the right subcostal port site in the standard laparoscopic cholecystectomy or, alternatively, using an additional trocar in the right subcostal space. Fluoroscopy is used throughout the procedure. The wire is confirmed to be in the common bile duct and through into the duodenum. The balloon catheter is advanced over the wire and passes through the ampulla and into the duodenum. The balloon is then inflated using a dilute contrast solution. The location of the ampulla is demonstrated by the point at which the inflated balloon catheter cannot be withdrawn out of the duodenum and into the biliary system. Radiopaque markers on the balloon catheter help guide the deflated catheter so that it traverses the sphincter of Oddi. The balloon is then slowly inflated. The balloon should never be inflated larger than the diameter of the common bile duct. Dilation is held for a few minutes and then deflated. This is followed by irrigation of warm saline through the cystic duct and a completion cholangiogram. Placement of a drain is usually not necessary. Instrumentation of the ampulla may result in pancreatitis and this should be kept in mind in the postoperative period. The incidence of pancreatitis is less than 10%. Operative time is usually less than 2 hours when accompanied with a cholecystectomy with successful clearance of stones reported 85–93% of the time.[14,15]

Basket Techniques

Stone retrieval baskets may also be introduced through a 12- to 14-gauge introducer sheath. Either a helical (Dormia-type) or straight (Segura type) basket may be employed. While some authors advocate using baskets with soft filiform tips in order to avoid damage to the duct, there appears to be no difference in ductal injuries

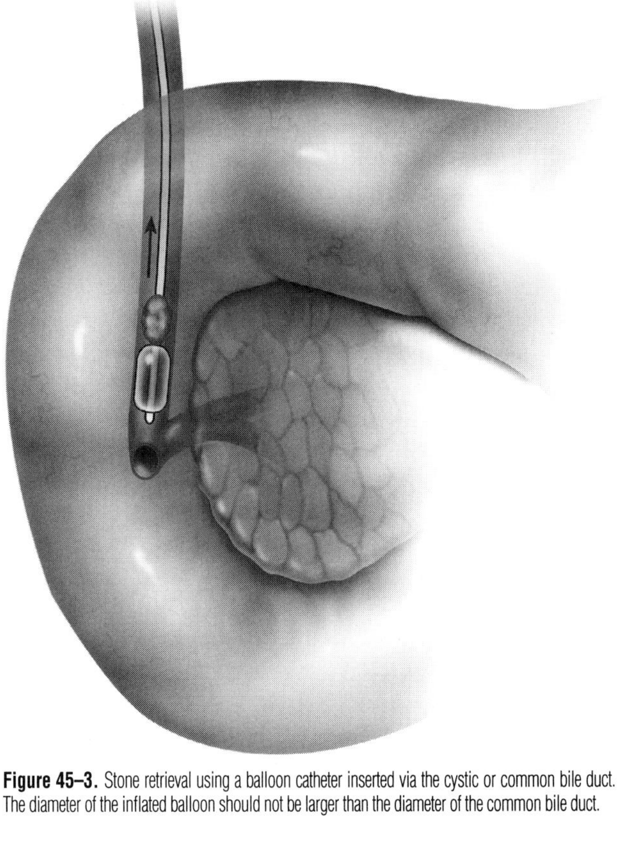

Figure 45–3. Stone retrieval using a balloon catheter inserted via the cystic or common bile duct. The diameter of the inflated balloon should not be larger than the diameter of the common bile duct.

as compared to non-filiform type baskets.[16] However, it is important to use these baskets with extreme care. There are two ways to use these baskets- with and without fluoroscopy. When using baskets with the fluoro-technique, the duct is filled with contrast material though the cholangiogram catheter that is already in place and the location of the stone is determined. The basket is then inserted through the introducer sheath into the duct and manipulated with the forceps. The position of the basket and stones is monitored with the fluoroscope (Fig 45–4). There are two disadvantages with this technique: One is the radiation exposure to the operating team and the other is the difficulty in manipulating the basket with fluoroscopic C-arm in position over the patient.

Because of these disadvantages, many have described using a nonfluoroscopic technique.[17] In order to accomplish this, several factors must be established. First, the surgeon must know the approximate length and course of the cystic duct as determined by the cholangiography. Second, the basket needs to be calibrated length-wise in order to know the location of the tip of the catheter. Lastly, the surgeon must control the handle of the basket to know when the basket is open, closed or partially closed suggesting the capture of a stone. When the basket is placed in the distal duct, the basket is gradually closed as it is withdrawn. This maneuver may have to be repeated several times. A major complication is capture of the papilla if the basket is advanced too far into the duct. This requires careful manipulation as pancreatitis or duct perforation may easily occur.

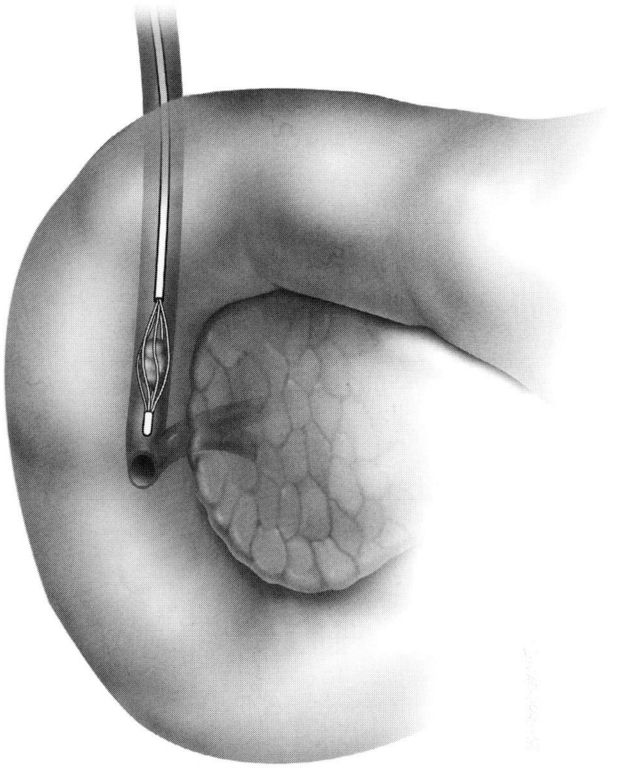

Figure 45–4. Stone retrieval using wire basket. Occasionally the basket will crush the stone. In these instances flushing and balloon sweeps may result in ductal clearance.

LAPAROSCOPIC TRANSCYSTIC EXPLORATION (WITH CHOLEDOCHOSCOPE)

Before the common bile duct is cannulated with the choledochoscope, the cystic duct must be prepared. The procedure is performed at the time of laparoscopy after cholangiography. In order to pass the scope easily and safely, the cystic duct must be large enough for this approach.[17–19] When the cystic duct is small, attempts to dilate it may be useful. Cystic duct dilation may be safely done up to 4 mm but not beyond 8 mm because of the increased risk of disruption.[17] Dilation may be performed by mechanical tapered dilators or balloon dilation. Although the most expensive way is pneumatic dilation, this is felt to be safer since radial dilatational forces exerted on the duct are safer than the shearing forced of gradual mechanical dilation. The balloon tipped catheter is passed over a 0.035-inch hydrophilic wire and dilated to approximately 6 mm (Cook, Bloomington, IN). In the situation that the cystic is very short and large enough to accept a choledochoscope, curved-tipped forceps may be inserted to expand the duct. If the cystic duct-common bile duct junction is disrupted by forceful dilation, an open repair may be required. Once the cystic duct is dilated, the scope is inserted using the hydrophilic guide wire already in place through a sheath placed as close to the cystic duct as possible. Alternatively the scope may be introduced without a guide wire as well (Fig 45–5). Careful manipulation of the scope with atraumatic forceps is extremely important as these scopes can easily be damaged. The scope can be advanced over a guide wire or freely into the cystic duct with manipulation using grasping atraumatic forceps. The most difficult part of accessing the CBD is negotiating the scope through the cystic duct. In this situation, the gallbladder should be retracted as to straighten the cystic duct as much as possible and the choledochoscope angle should be straightened as much as possible. The scope is then advanced via the cystic duct into the common bile duct under direct vision. The scope is first directed into the distal common duct and stone or stones visualized may be removed with a basket passed via the working channel of the scope. Once the stone is negotiated into the basket, both the scope and the basket are removed together through the cystic duct.

A completion cholangiogram should be performed to document clearance of both common and hepatic ducts. Because the cystic duct it dilated, it is best secured with a suture ligature rather than placing metal clips. Inspecting the proximal ductal system is rarely

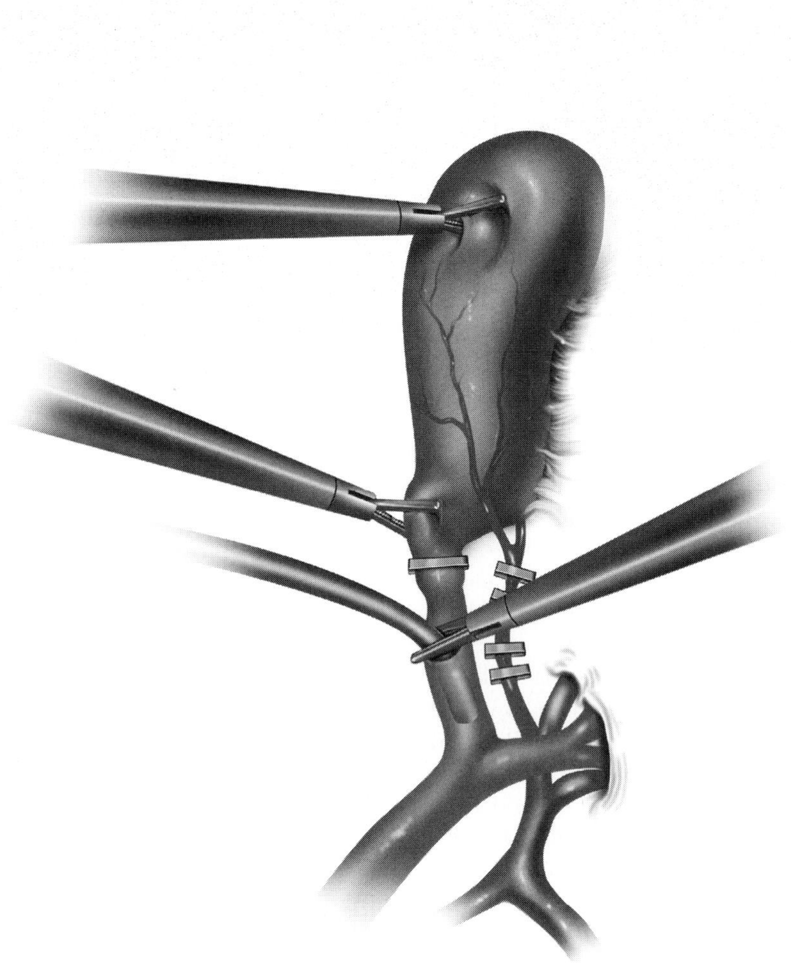

Figure 45–5. A flexible choledochoscope is passed through an introduced sheath placed in the right upper quadrant as close to the cystic duct as possible. The scope can be introduced free hand or with the use of a 0.035-inch guide wire. Care should be taken to manipulate the scope using atraumatic forceps. Using a working channel, wire baskets or balloon-tipped catheters can be passed under direct visualization for stone retrieval. To facilitate visualization, pressurized saline irrigation is used throughout the procedure to distend the common duct and clear free floating debris.

possible since it requires a short cystic duct entering at a 90-degree angle; however, proximal exploration is rarely needed. In this case the laparoscopic surgeon can attempt to clear the duct via a direct choledochotomy approach.

LAPAROSCOPIC CHOLEDOCHOTOMY

While a transcystic approach clears the duct in the majority of cases, in certain instances it will not be feasible or successful. The lumen of the duct may not dilate enough to accommodate a scope or the duct may follow a long tortuous course before joining the common bile duct. In this situation, the surgeon has the option of performing a postoperative ERCP or transductal exploration either open or laparoscopic approaches. This is a laparoscopic transductal exploration, which allows the surgeon to easily explore the proximal and distal ductal system, use a larger scope, and evacuate stones directly. A choledochotomy will require the placement of a T-tube, which has the advantage of potentially retrieving stones in the postoperative period.

The gallbladder is left in place to facilitate upward and cephalad retraction to straighten and provide tension to the common duct. Just distal to the cystic duct-common bile duct junction, a short anterior longitudinal ductotomy is created sharply. It is important to avoid vigorous dissection circumferentially around the duct and use a longitudinal incision along the axis of the duct to prevent subsequent development of ischemic strictures by inadvertent injury to the common bile duct blood supply. The choledochoscope is introduced at a right angle to the common duct and advanced under pressure saline irrigation, allowing the common duct to nicely distend and visualize any stones or strictures. The scope can also be advanced proximally to remove stones with baskets or balloon as previously described.

Upon completion of the laparoscopic common bile duct exploration via a choledochotomy, T-tube closure of the common duct is recommended. An appropriate size T tube is selected based on the size of the duct, usually a 12F or 14F T tube is sufficient. The tube is fashioned to the surgeon's preference. Filleted tubes are easier to insert. A long and short segment allow for orientation when inserted into the peritoneum and then again when inserted in the bile duct. Also, the point of entry in the abdomen to the point of entry into the duct should follow a smooth curvilinear route. The standard trocar sites do not usually allow for this and as such a separate stab incision should be used when the tube is brought out. The T tube is fully inserted into the abdomen, the horizontal limbs are compressed with a grasper and inserted into the common bile duct. The choledochotomy is then closed over the long end of the T tube, beginning at the neck and working caudally using interrupted 4-0 absorbable suture. Intracorporeal suturing is used to accomplish this (Fig 45–6). The tube is then brought out of the abdomen at a suitable location keeping to the principles highlighted above. A completion cholangiogram is recommended to ensure correct tube placement. A subhepatic closed suction drainage is then inserted and removed if there is no bile leakage around the T tube.

▪ LAPAROSCOPIC BILIARY TRACT RESECTION AND RECONSTRUCTION

Laparoscopic biliary tract resection and reconstruction is not currently widely applied because it is technically challenging even in an open setting. Nonetheless, laparoscopic cholecystojejunostomy, choledochoduodenostomy, hepaticojejunostomy, and choledochal cyst excision have been successfully performed in the hands of experienced laparoscopic surgeons.[20–25] Surgical biliary bypass to relieve malignant obstructive jaundice requires the morbidity of an operation whether it is minimally invasive or open. While minimally invasive surgery allows for less postoperative pain and more expedient recovery, the inherent risks of general anesthesia and surgical stress remain. In light of this, endoscopic stenting has gained utility especially in the palliative setting. The success of endoscopic techniques, such as stenting and sphincterotomy, in the management of malignant biliary obstruction is well documented.[26] However, recurrent jaundice and cholangitis from stent obstruction or migration necessitate changing of the stents and add to the overall morbidity and cost. Newer, self-expanding metallic wall stents have had less frequent rates of occlusion.[27] Nonetheless, patients who are younger, healthy, who might have increased survival (>6 months) or for those whom endoscopic biliary stenting is not technically possible, will be better served by a surgical biliary bypass. For benign disease, endoscopic management is not indicated as it does not achieve the long-term patency that is desirable for the treatment of benign disease. Thus, surgical biliary bypass will continue to be a valid treatment option.

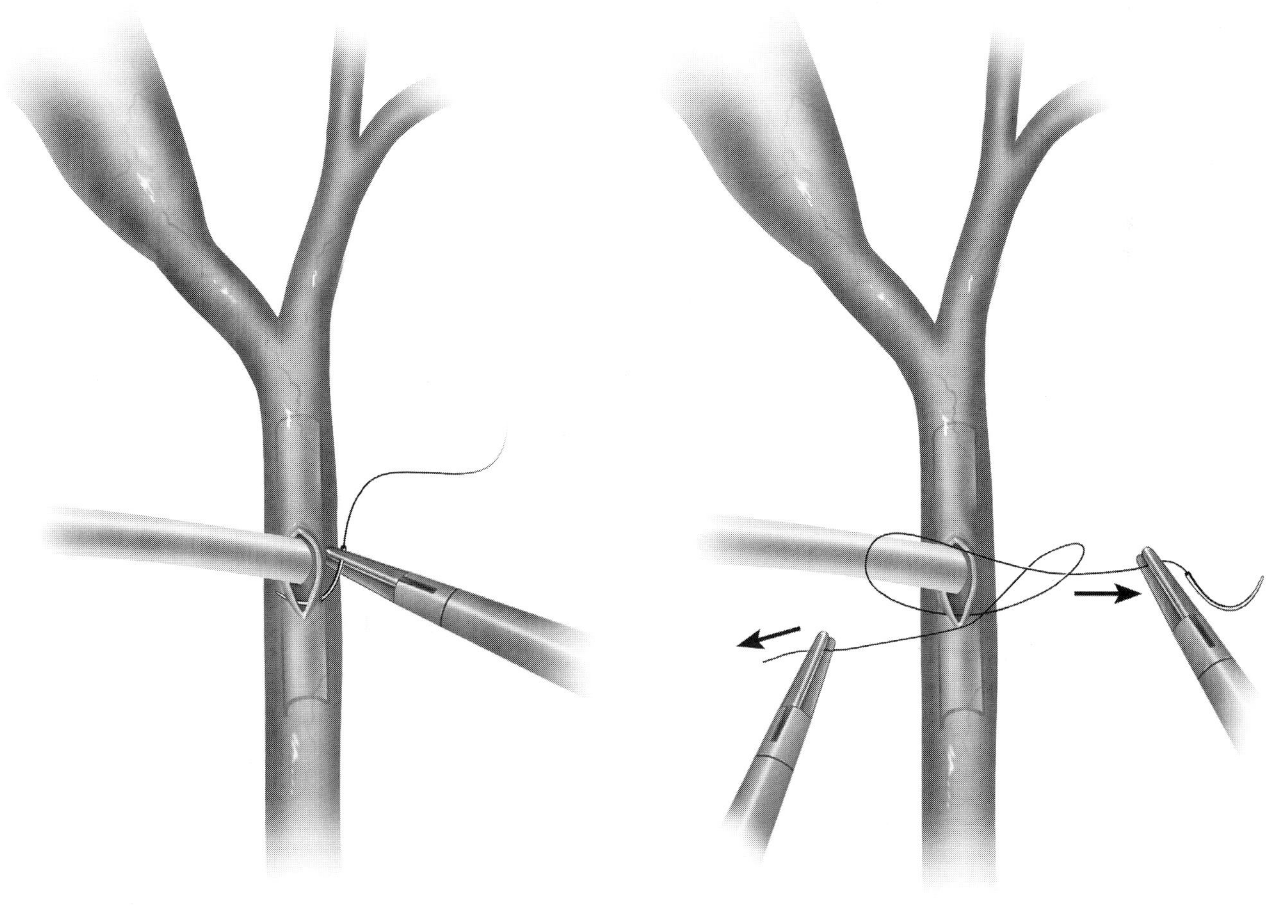

Figure 45–6. T-tube being secured in place following common bile duct exploration via a choledochotomy.

While the enthusiasm for laparoscopy has extended to complex biliary procedures, it is important to keep in mind that indications and patient selection for biliary bypass do not change with the laparoscopic modality. In fact, the technical considerations often limit rather than broaden the patient selection. Furthermore, fundamental laparoscopic principles that contraindicate its use or require discontinuation and conversion to an open procedure should always be kept in mind. It should also be emphasized that standard, accepted procedures should not have to be significantly modified to make them easier to perform in the laparoscopic setting. Conversion to an open procedure should be utilized if the goals of the operation cannot be accomplished safely through the laparoscopic technique.

TABLE 45–4. CONTRAINDICATIONS FOR LAPAROSCOPIC CHOLECYSTOJEJUNOSTOMY

Absolute
Prior cholecystectomy
Occluded cystic duct
Occluded hepatocystic junction
Hilar malignancy
Tumor encroachment within 1 cm of hepatocystic junction
Relative
Prior biliary surgery
Tumor encroachment within 2 cm of hepatocystic junction
Chronic inflammation/cholecystitis
Tumor involvement of the small bowel
Multiple small bowel adhesions

LAPAROSCOPIC CHOLECYSTOJEJUNOSTOMY

Laparoscopic cholecystojejunostomy is a safe, effective method of palliation for biliary obstruction.[28] It is relatively easy to perform when keeping with standard laparoscopic principles and can be accomplished in 45 to 60 minutes.[28,29] In patents with prior surgery and small bowel adhesions, adhesionolysis may be required to ensure that there is no tension or twisting of the bowel loop that will be utilized in the anastomosis. It should also be noted that postoperative episodes of cholangitis are more frequent with cholecystenteric bypass when compared to other bilioenteric bypasses.[30] Despite the limitations, it continues to be worthwhile in select patients.

In all instances, cholangiography, either intra-operatively or pre-operatively via ERCP, should be performed to confirm the patency of the cystic duct and hepatocystic junction. This is the Achilles heel of the operation as obstruction of either the cystic duct or hepatocystic junction will result in failure of the operation with recurrent biliary obstruction. Tumor encroachment within 1 cm of the hepatocystic junction is also a contraindication for cholecystojejunostomy. Table 45–4 lists the relative and absolute contraindications for a laparoscopic cholecystojejunostomy. A retrospective review of 218 patients from our institution revealed that only about 20% of patients that are candidates for a laparoscopic cholecystojejunostomy actually remain eligible after further testing.[22,31] Thus, this procedure is indicated for only a minority of patients. The relative ease with which it can be performed, and the palliative function that is provided without the associated morbidities of an open operation make it a valuable option in carefully selected patients.

The patient is placed supine and general endotracheal anesthesia is induced. A Hasson trocar is placed under direct visualization at the umbilicus. Pneumoperitoneum is established and a peritoneal survey is conducted to determine if the intra-abdominal anatomy will allow the safe performance of the procedure. A 12-mm port is then placed laterally on the right costal margin. This will accommodate the laparoscopic stapling device. A 5-mm port is then placed in the left upper quadrant 5 to 10 cm below the left costal margin, midclavicular line. An additional 5-mm or 10-mm port is placed just below the left costal margin to aid in retraction.

The first step is to confirm patency of the cystic duct if it has not been done by ERCP. This can be accomplished by grasping the gallbladder and needle decompressing until it is at least half-emptied. The gallbladder is then cannulated and contrast injected under fluoroscopy. The procedure should not commence if the cystic duct is occluded or if the hepatocystic duct junction is strictured from tumor involvement.

Next, a suitable loop of small bowel is grasped using an atraumatic grasping instrument and proximal and distal ends identified by tracing the loop back to the ligament of Treitz. A portion of small bowel 30 to 40 cm distal to the ligament of Treitz is selected for the anastomosis.

Sometimes the body habitus or postioning makes alignment of the bowel and gallbladder difficult. In these circumstances, the set-up for this anastomosis may be facilitated by passing a 3-0 nylon suture on a Keith needle through a separate stab incision in the right upper quadrant. The needle is expeditiously grasped once inside the peritoneal cavity to prevent inadvertent visceral injury. The needle is then passed through the gallbladder and then the antimesenteric side of the jejunum. The needle is then passed back out of the peritoneal cavity and secured extracorporeally. This suture will help manipulate the bowel and gallbladder during stapling.

An enterotomy and cholecystotomy are then made in the bowel and gallbladder, respectively, using the hook cautery device passed through the 12-mm port (Fig 45–7).

The opening should be as small as possible and a grasper can then be used to enlarge enough to permit the end of the laparoscopic stapling device to be placed through. Confirmation of intraluminal penetrance is confirmed by placing a grasper through the enterotomy and visualizing mucosa. The enterotomies are then held in apposition using the left-sided ports. Once these left-sided graspers have been placed, they should not be moved until the stapler is fired. The laparoscopic stapler (Endo GIA-30, US Surgical Corporation, Norwalk, CT) is placed through the 12-mm port. One blade of the stapler is inserted in the cholecystotomy. The enterotomy is then pulled over the second blade. The stapler is carefully closed making sure that no small bowel mesentery or adjacent structures have been caught. The stapler is fired and removed. The graspers are then used to open the anastomosis to permit

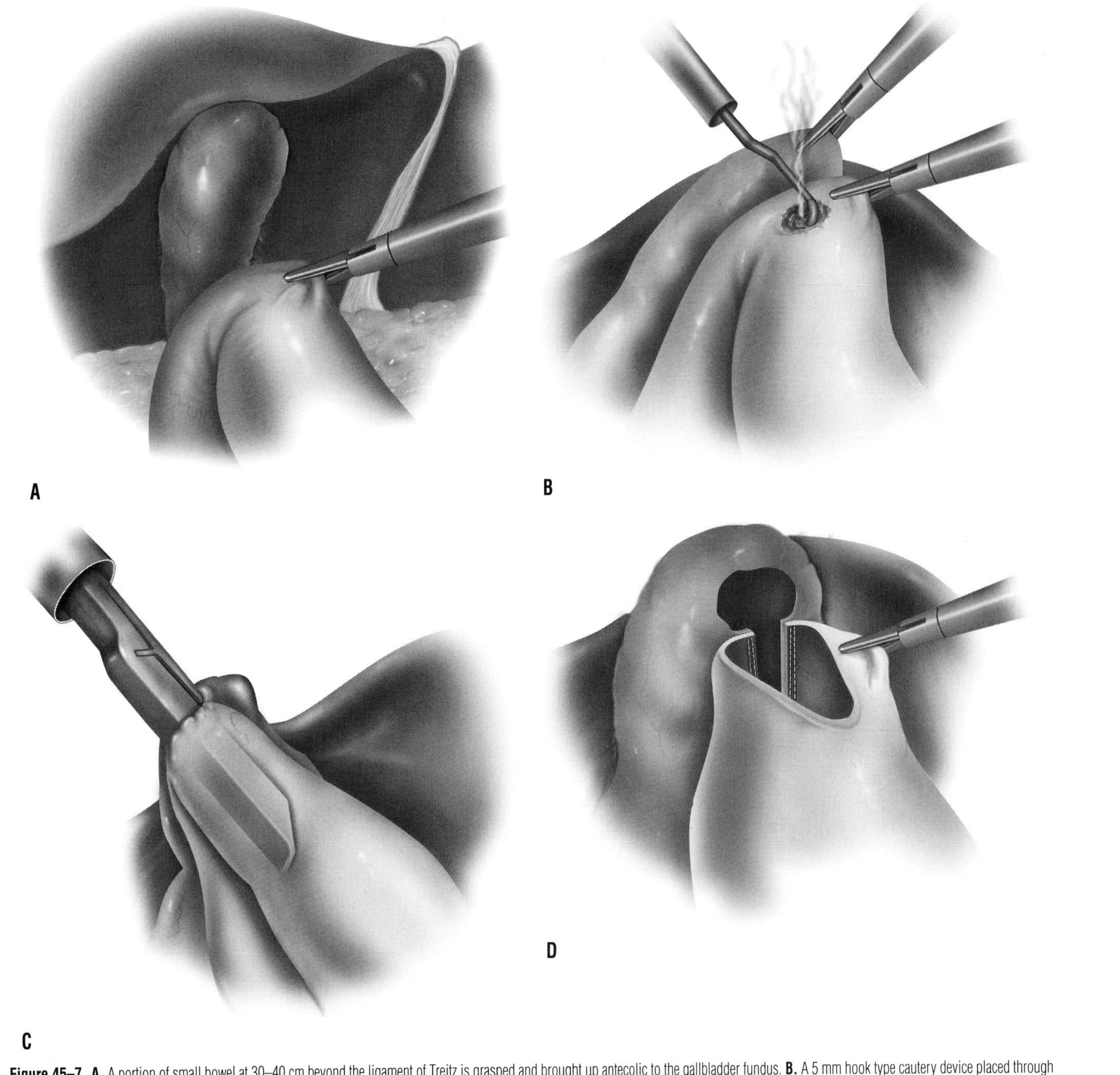

Figure 45–7. A. A portion of small bowel at 30–40 cm beyond the ligament of Treitz is grasped and brought up antecolic to the gallbladder fundus. **B.** A 5 mm hook type cautery device placed through the 12 mm right upper quadrant port is used to create a 5 mm opening in the antimesenteric portion of the small bowel. **C.** An endoscopic stapler is placed through the 12-mm right upper quadrant port. Each blade of the stapler is carefully inserted into the enterotomy and cholecystotomy, respectively. The stapler is closed and fired after proper position and freedom from surrounding structures is assured. **D.** Careful inspection of the anastomosis for integrity and hemostasis. *Continued*

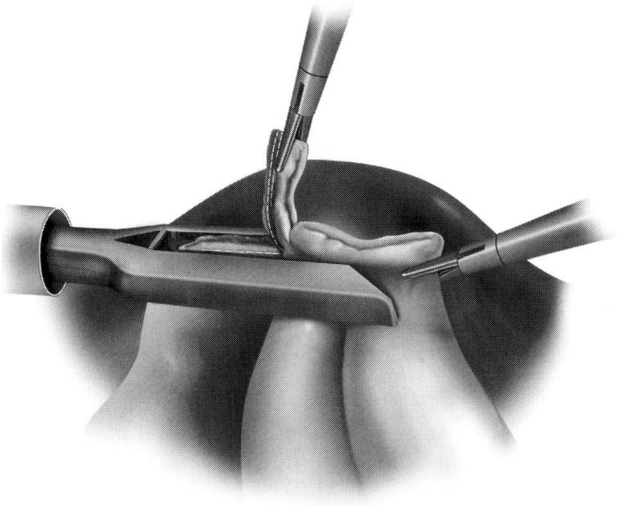

E

Figure 45–7, cont'd. E. The remaining defect is closed by transverse stapling of the anastomotic site taking care not to narrow the anastomosis.

inspection of the staple line for integrity and hemostasis. Clips may be utilized for hemostasis. The remaining defect is closed by transverse stapling of the anastomotic site taking care not to significantly narrow the newly created anastomosis. This usually requires two firings of the stapler. Finally, the stay suture is removed and the anastomosis inspected. Placement of a drain is not necessary.

A completely hand-sewn anastomosis can also be performed. The operative time for this is usually significantly greater and the patency and complication rates are not significantly different.[20,31] Hence, our bias is to perform the faster stapled anastomosis. Another variant is to staple the anastomosis between the bowel and gallbladder and then close the entero/cholecystotomies with a running intracorporal stitch using 3-0 absorbable suture. This may be useful in instances in which the stapler cannot be configured to prevent narrowing of the newly created anastomosis during closure of the defect. Another variant is to a use a Roux-en-Y reconstruction rather than a loop. In patients with benign diseases such as choledocholithiasis, inflammatory strictures, or iatrogenic bile duct injuries, the more durable choledochoduodenostomy or hepaticojejunostomy are preferred over cholecystojejunostomy.

LAPAROSCOPIC CHOLEDOCHODUODENOSTOMY AND HEPATICOJEJUNOSTOMY

The gold standard for open biliary bypass is choledochoduodenostomy or the more commonly utilized Roux-en-Y hepatico/choledochojejunostomy. Furthermore, many patients are ineligible for cholecystojejunostomy as previously mentioned. In an effort to increase the number of patients qualifying for minimally invasive biliary bypass, laparoscopic choledochoduodenostomy, choledochojejunostomy, and hepaticojejunostomy have been investigated and successfully performed. More investigations in controlled trials that examine the utility of these procedures are warranted before they are widely applied. These are considered highly advanced laparoscopic procedures and take a significant amount of time to perform. Median operative time in the hands of skilled laparoscopists is 300 minutes compared to the open median time of 180 minutes.[20,32-34] Technologic advancements have aided the surgeon in the quest for laparoscopic biliary bypass. Lapara-Tie (Ethicon) and Surgi-Wip/Endo-Stitch (U.S. Surgical) facilitate intracorporeal suturing. The temporarily endoluminally stented anastomosis (TESA) technology has been used in animal models to assist in anastomosis creation.[23,32] The basic principles remain the same, but certain variances have been adopted for successful laparoscopic performance. Commonly a transverse choledochotomy rather than the traditional longitudinal has been used for a laparoscopic choledochoduodenostomy. If a transverse choledochotomy is made, care must be taken to avoid devascularizing the bile duct as the blood supply runs parallel to the duct at the lateral and medial aspects of the duct. For a choledochoduodenostomy, the duodenum is longitudinally incised following a Kocher maneuver and a side-to-side anastomosis is created using a 4-0 polyglycolic acid suture (Fig 45–8). Laparoscopic choledochojejunostomy or Roux-en-Y hepaticojejunostomy are beginning to be performed at a few centers with a moderate amount of success being reported.[32-34] In one series of 14 patients who underwent laparoscopic hepaticojejunostomy, the

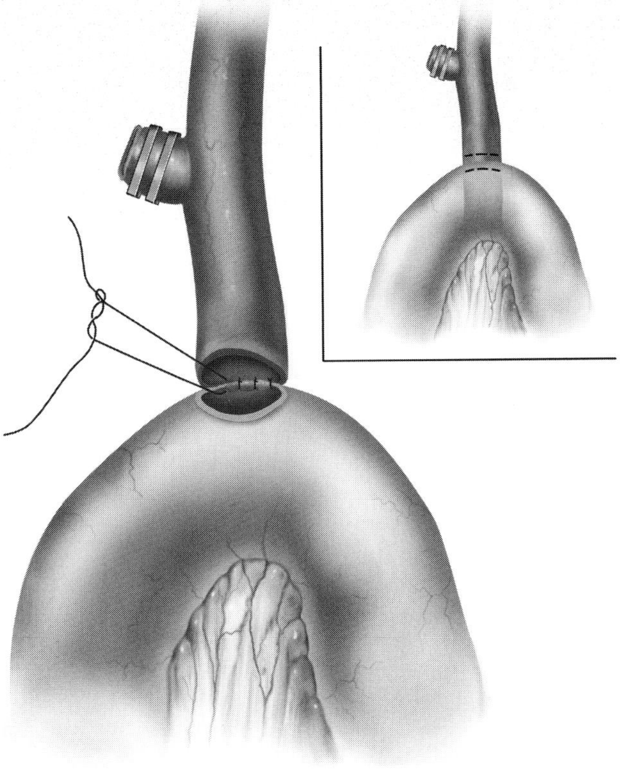

Figure 45–8. Laparoscopic choledochoduodenostomy created by placement of interrupted 4-0 absorbable sutures with intracorporeal knot tying technique.

median operative time was 129 minutes. However, the median hospital stay was 9 days.[35] Further clinical trials are needed to determine the value of these more complex biliary bypasses.

LAPAROSCOPIC CHOLEDOCHAL CYST EXCISION

Cysts of the biliary tract are rare with a majority diagnosed in childhood. They are usually treated with complete excision since they are associated with malignant degeneration. Reconstruction is performed with a Roux-en-Y hepaticojejunostomy and excellent long-term results can be achieved. Since a majority of these patients are children, a minimally invasive approach would be welcomed in hopes of limiting their absence from school and other activities important to their development. It is also cosmetically more appealing.

To date, laparoscopic excision of choledochal cysts and subsequent reconstruction have only been described in case reports.[36,37] Under laparoscopic guidance the enlarged bile duct and gallbladder (if present) are excised. A Roux-en-Y enteric anastomosis can be accomplished with a circular or linear stapler and the end-to-side bilioenteric anastomosis is created with a continuous suture. The magnified view afforded by the laparoscope and newly developed mechanical instruments for stapling and intracorporeal suturing, in addition to traditional laparoscopic advantages of less pain and faster recovery, have been cited in favor of the laparoscopic approach. The lengthy operative time and the use of costly new technical instruments to facilitate laparoscopic performance are considerable disadvantages.

■ CONCLUSION

The application of minimally invasive surgery continues to evolve and develop at a rapid pace. The success rate for removing stones among accomplished laparoscopists exceeds 90%. Unfortunately, most surgeons do not currently use a laparoscopic approach to the treatment of CBD stones. This presents significant costs (nearly double) to the patients and the health care system. In most cases, biliary tract surgeons practicing in this era should have the ability to treat benign biliary tract pathology laparoscopically in one setting.

Laparoscopic biliary reconstruction is feasible, but it demands long operative times and requires advanced laparoscopic skills as well as significant experience in hepatobiliary surgery. Nevertheless, with a careful selection of patients as well as a low threshold for conversion to an open approach, certain biliary reconstructive and resective procedures can be completed laparoscopically. The cholecystojejunostomy provides satisfactory biliary bypass in carefully selected patients and is readily accomplished through the minimally invasive technique. Further studies are necessary to accurately determine long-term patency rates and utility of more complex laparoscopic biliary-enteric anastomoses.

REFERENCES

1. Pappas TN, Chekan EG, Eubanks S. *Atlas of Laparoscopic Surgery*. Philadelphia, PA Current Medicine, Inc.; 1999: 13.6–13.12
2. Metcalfe MS, Ong T, Bruening MH, et al. Is laparoscopic cholangiogram a matter of routine? *Am J Surg* 2004;187(4):475–481
3. Dorazio RA. Selective operative cholangiography in laparoscopic cholecystectomy. *Am Surg* 1995;61:911–913
4. The Southern Surgeons Club. A prospective analysis of 1518 laparoscopic cholecystectomies. *N Engl J Med* 1991; 324:1073–1078
5. Rhodes M, Sussman L, Cohen L, et al. Randomised trial of laparoscopic exploration of common bile duct versus postoperative endoscopic retrograde cholangiography for common bile duct stones. *Lancet* 1998;351:159–161
6. Urbach DR, Khajanchee YS, Jobe BA, et al. Cost-effective management of common bile duct stones: a decision analysis of the use of endoscopic retrograde cholan-

giopancreatography (ERCP), intraoperative cholangiography, and laparoscopic bile duct exploration. *Surg Endosc* 2001;15:4–13
7. Barkun JS, Fried GM, Barkun AN, et al. Cholecystectomy without operative cholangiography: implications for common bile duct injury and retained common bile duct stones. *Ann Surg* 1993;218:371–379
8. Sugiyama M, Atomi Y. Endoscopic ultrasonography for diagnosing choledocholithiasis: a prospective comparative study with ultrasonography and computed tomography. *Gastrointest Endosc* 1997;45:143–1436
9. Kohut M, Nowakowska-Dulawa E, Marek T, et al. Accuracy of linear endoscopic ultrasonography in the evaluation of patients with suspected common bile duct stones. *Endoscopy* 2002;34:299–303
10. Deprez P. Approach of suspected common bile duct stones: endoscopic ultrasonography. *Acta Gastroenterol Belg* 2000;63:295–298
11. Jakribettuu VS, Gilliam JH, Pineau BC. Comparisons of five algorithms used to predict common bile duct stones. *Am J Gastroenterol* 2001;96:588
12. Koo KP, Traverso LW. Do preoperative indicators predict the presence of common bile duct stones during laparoscopic cholecystectomy? *Am J Surg* 1996;171:495–499
13. Phillips EH, Rosenthal RJ, Carroll BJ et al. Laparoscopic transcystic common bile duct exploration. *Surg Endosc* 1994;8(12):1389–1393
14. Appel S, Krebs H, Fern D. Techniques for laparoscopic cholangiography and removal of common duct stones. *Surg Endosc* 1992;6(3):134–137
15. Tse F, Barkum JS, Barkum AN. The elective evaluation of patients with suspected choledocholithiasis undergoing laparoscopic cholecystectomy. *Gastrointest Endo* 2004;60(3):437–448
16. Petelin J. Laparoscopic approach to common duct pathology. *Am J Surg* 1993;165:487–491
17. Fletcher DR. Common bile duct calculi at laparoscopic cholecystectomy: a technique for management. *Aust N Z J Surg* 1993;63:710–714
18. Lezoche E, Pananini AM, Carlei F, et al. Laparoscopic treatment of gallbladder and common bile duct stones: a prospective study. *World J Surg* 1996;20:535–542
19. Phillip EH, Rosenthal RJ, Carrol BJ, Falls MJ. Laparoscopic trancystic duct common bile duct exploration. *Surg Endosc* 1994;8:1389–1394
20. O'Rourke RW, Lee NN, Cheng J, et al. Laparoscopic biliary reconstruction. *Am J Surg* 2004;187:621–624
21. Fitzgibbons RJ, Gardner GC. Laparoscopic surgery and the common bile duct. *World J Surg* 2001;25:1317–1324
22. Chekan EG, Clark L, Wu J, et al. Laparoscopic biliary and enteric bypass. *Semin Surg Oncol* 1999;16:313–320
23. Schob OM, Schmid RA, Morimoto AK, et al. Laparoscopic Roux-en-Y choledochojejunostomy. *Am J Surg* 1997;173:312–319
24. Gentileschi P, Kini S, Gagner M. Palliative laparoscopic hepatico-and gastrojejunostomy for advanced pancreatic cancer. *JSLS* 2002;6(4):331–338
25. Jeyapalan M, Almeida JA, Michaelson RL, et al. Laparoscopic choledochoduodenostomy: Review of a 4-year experience with an uncommon problem. *Surg Laparosc Endosc Percutan Tech* 2002;12(3):148–153
26. Giorgio PD, Luca LD. Comparison of treatment outcomes between biliary plastic stent placement with and without endoscopic sphincterotomy for inoperable malignant common bile duct obstruction. *World J Gastroenterol* 2004;10(8):1212–1214
27. Isayama H, Komatsu Y, Tsujino T, et al. A prospective randomized study of covered versus uncovered stents for the management of distal malignant biliary obstruction. *Gut* 2004;53(5):729–734
28. Pappas TN, Chekan EG, Eubanks S. *Atlas of Laparoscopic Surgery*. Philadelphia, PA: Current Medicine, Inc., 1999
29. Raj PK, Mahoney P, Linderman C. Laparoscopic cholecystojejunostomy: a technical application in unresectable biliary obstruction. *J Laparoendosc Adv Surg Tech* 1998;7(1):47–52
30. Potts JR, Broughan TA. Palliative operations for pancreatic cancer. *Am J Surg* 1999;159(1):72–77
31. Tarnasky PR, England RE, Lail LM, et al. Cystic duct patency in malignant obstructive jaundice. *Ann Surg* 1995; 221:265–271
32. Schob O, Rothlin M, Schlumpf R. Laparoscopic biliary bypass. In Zucker KA (ed). *Surgical Laparoscopy*, 2nd ed. Philadelphia, PA: Lippincott, Williams & Wilkins; 2001: 201–210
33. Ali AS, Ammori BJ. Concomitant laparoscopic gastric and biliary bypass and bilateral thoracoscopic splanchnotomy: the full package of minimally invasive palliation for pancreatic cancer. *Surg Endosc* 2003;17(12): 2028–2031
34. Date RS, Siriwardena AK. Laparoscopic biliary bypass and current management algorithims for palliation of malignant obstructive jaundice. *Ann Surg Onc* 2004; 11(9):815–817
35. Rothlin M, Schob O, Weber M, et al. Laparoscopic gastro-and hepaticojejunostomy for palliation of pancreatic cancer. *Surg Endosc* 1999;13;1065–1069
36. Liu DC, Rodriguez JA, Meric F, et al. Laparoscopic excision of a rare type II choledochal cyst: case report and review of literature. *J Pediatr Surg* 2000;35(7):1117–1119
37. Tan HL, Shankar KR, Ford WD. Laparoscopic resection of type I choledochal cyst. *Surg Endosc* 2003;17(9):1495

46

Hernia Repair

Bardia Amirlak ■ Sumeet K. Mittal ■ Robert J. Fitzgibbons, Jr.

■ LAPAROSCOPIC ABDOMINAL WALL HERNIA REPAIR

Dr. Ralph Ger is credited with performing the first laparoscopic inguinal herniorrhaphy in the late 1970s using a prototype-stapling device to close the hernia defect from inside the abdominal cavity.[1] It was not until the advent of laparoscopic cholecystectomy, that laparoscopic inguinal herniorrhaphies began to be performed with regularity.[2,3]

Laparoscopic surgery is increasingly being used for the repair of not only inguinal but various other abdominal wall hernias. Numerous reports indicate that the laparoscopic repair of an inguinal hernia is associated with the decreased need for postoperative analgesia, shorter hospital stay, and an earlier return to normal activities.[4,5] The laparoscopic approach has not been universally accepted, however, because the operating time is longer, it costs more and there appears to be a higher risk of serious complications as a result of laparoscopic accidents compared to the open mesh repair. Many surgeons feel that laparoscopy should be reserved for recurrent, bilateral, or otherwise complicated inguinal hernias. The exact role of laparoscopy in the management of abdominal wall hernias outside of the groin is currently a subject of intense debate and further research is required to determine if benefits of minimally invasive surgery actually materialize. It may be associated with superior overall quality and strength because of the placement of the prosthesis on the abdominal side of the defect allowing intra-abdominal pressure to act as a force to keep the prosthesis in place. Conversely, in an open repair of abdominal wall hernia, intra-abdominal pressure acts as a factor predisposing to recurrence, especially when a simple onlay technique is used.

It is likely that laparoscopic surgery will take its place in the armamentarium of the abdominal wall hernia surgeon to be used on a discretionary basis. However, the purpose of this chapter is to present the current state of the art of laparoscopic surgery for abdominal wall hernias and not to compare and contrast the open counterpart.

■ ANATOMY OF THE INGUINAL REGION AND THE ANTERIOR ABDOMINAL WALL FROM A LAPAROSCOPIC PERSPECTIVE

The laparoscopic surgeon does not have the luxury of direct palpation and therefore must rely heavily on visual cues. Therefore, a detailed understanding of the anatomy of the peritoneal aspect of the anterior abdominal wall and deep inguinal region is essential for the safe and effective performance of laparoscopic hernia repairs. The anatomical descriptions that follow are presented from the abdominal perspective as would be visualized during laparoscopy. Figure 46–1 shows the laparoscopic view of the preperitoneal anatomy with the peritoneal flap elevated.

INGUINAL

The parietal peritoneum of the anterior abdominal wall forms folds on top of certain preperitoneal structures, which are referred to as ligaments. The median umbilical ligament lies in the midline, extending from the bladder fundus to the umbilicus. This struc-

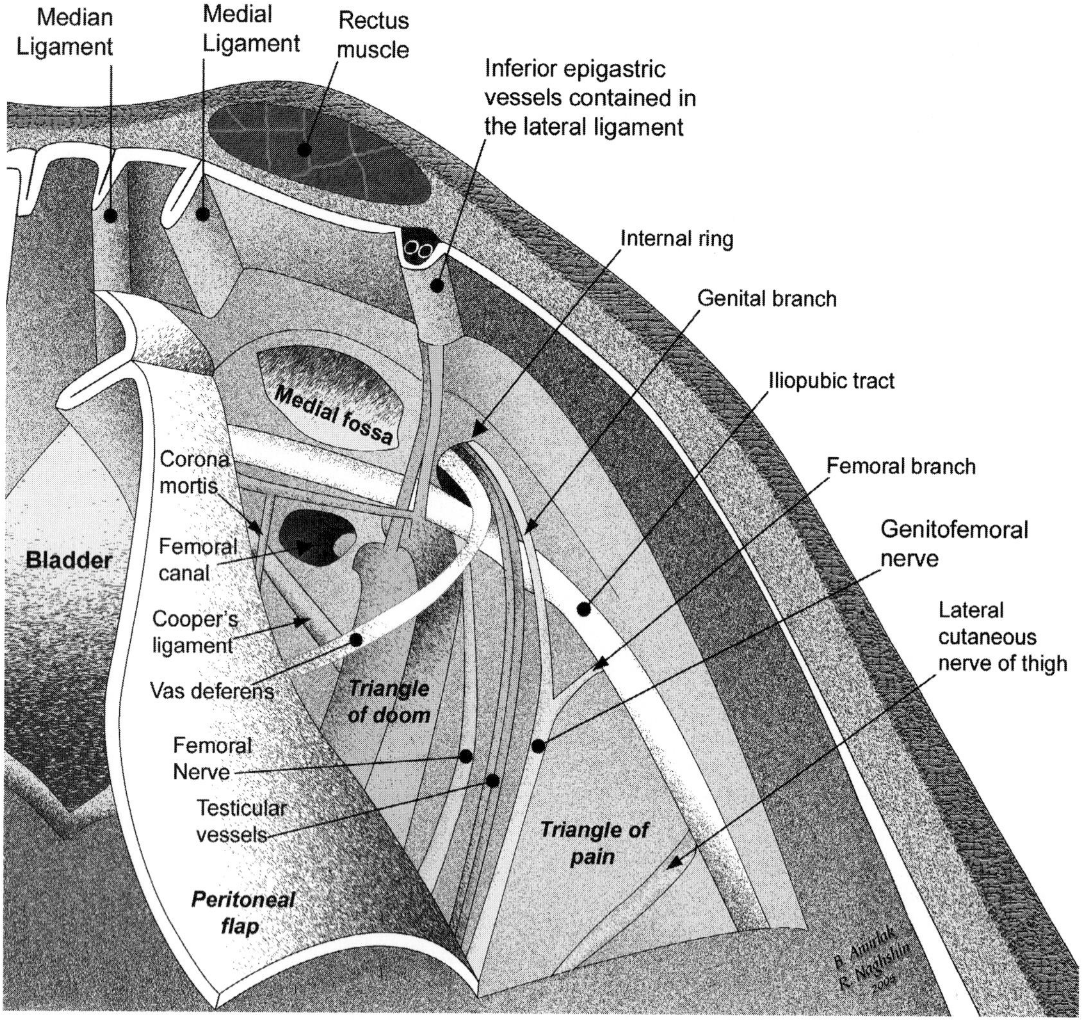

Figure 46–1. Laparoscopic view of the preperitoneal anatomy with the peritoneal flap elevated.

ture contains the urachus, which is a remnant of the fetal allantois. The obliterated fetal umbilical arteries create the paired medial umbilical ligaments on each side of the midline. Both the artery and the urachus may be patent. The lateral umbilical ligaments are formed by the underlying inferior epigastric vessels (IEV), which are enclosed by layers of transversalis fascia. Direct hernias occur in the medial fossa, which is bound by the medial and lateral umbilical ligaments. Indirect hernias occur lateral to the lateral umbilical ligament (lateral fossa) through the internal ring. Femoral hernias occur below the iliopubic tract just medial to the femoral vessels.

Deep to the peritoneum is the pre-peritoneal space. This potential space is bound by the peritoneum and the transversalis fascia and is commonly associated with two eponyms. The loose connective tissue between the pubis and the bladder/anterior abdominal wall is called the retropubic space of Retzius. Bogros' space represents the lateral extension of the space of Retzius and contains anatomical structures critical to the laparoscopic surgeon.

The transversalis fascia is next. The importance of the transversalis fascia for the laparoscopic hernia surgeon is its derivatives or analogues namely the iliopectineal arch, iliopubic tract, and crura of the deep inguinal ring. The iliopectineal arch is situated at the medial border of the iliacus muscle and is continuous with the fascia iliaca, the endoabdominal fascia covering the iliacus. The iliopectineal arch divides the vascular compartment containing the iliac vessels from the neuromuscular compartment containing the iliopsoas muscle, femoral nerve, and lateral femoral cutaneous nerve. The iliopubic tract is an aponeurotic band formed by the condensation of the anterior layer of transversalis fascia blended with the transverses abdominis aponeurosis. It attaches to the iliac crest superolaterally and inserts on the pubic tubercle medially.[6] It serves as an important landmark in a laparoscopic preperitoneal dissection. Most of the branches of the lumbar plexus nerves run inferior to this tract, and aggressive dissection or use of fastening devices such as staples, tacks, or sutures placed through or inferior to the iliopubic tract can lead to nerve or vascular injury. The superior and inferior crura of the deep inguinal ring are also derived from the transversalis fascia. Cooper's (pectineal) ligament is formed by the thickened fibrous periosteum along the pectineal line of the pubis and fibers from the iliopubic tract as they merge with the inguinal ligament.

The IEVs, which supply the anterior abdominal wall, arise from the external iliac vessels before they pass under the inguinal ligament. The IEVs enter the rectus sheath at the level of arcuate line. These vessels give rise to two major branches of concern: the external spermatic vessel and the iliopubic branch, which anastomoses via the corona mortis (found in a third of patients) (Figs 46–1 and 46–2) to the obturator artery system.[7] Damage to the corona mortis during dissection of or mesh fixation to Cooper's ligament can result in significant bleeding.

The nerve branches of the lumbar plexus that can be damaged during laparoscopic dissection vary in their course but generally lie in what is referred to as the "electrical hazard zone" (bordered medially by the spermatic cord, superiorly by the iliopubic tract, and laterally by the iliac crest). Electrocautery should not be used in this region. This area is also referred to as the "triangle of pain" by some authors, and contains (from lateral to medial) the lateral femoral cutaneous, the anterior femoral cutaneous, the femoral branch of the genitofemoral, and the femoral nerves.[8,9]

Another area in which caution should be heeded is the area referred to as the "triangle of doom" (bordered by the vas deferens medially, gonadal vessels laterally, and peritoneal edge posteriorly), containing the external iliac vessels, the deep circumflex iliac vein, the femoral nerve, and the genital branch of the genitofemoral nerve.

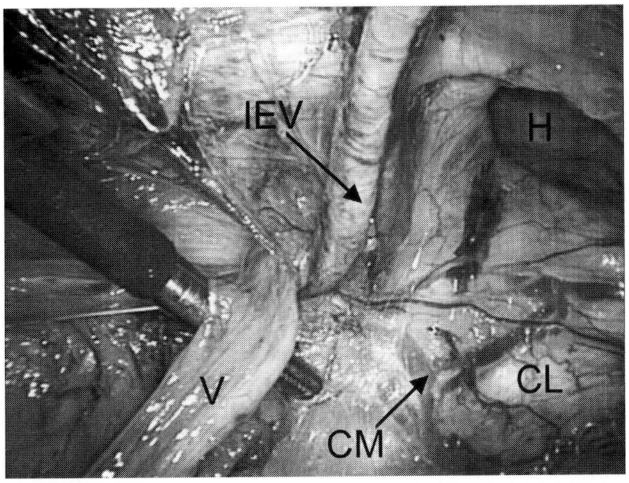

Figure 46–2. Laparoscopic view of preperitoneal space as seen during left TEP inguinal hernia repair. H, direct hernia defect; IEV, inferior epigastric vessels; CM, corona mortis; CL, Cooper's ligament; V, vas deferens.

The cord structures are formed at the internal ring when the internal spermatic vessels (pampiniform venous plexus and the testicular artery) and the genital branch of the genitofemoral nerve join the vas deferens. The identification of both the vas and the testicular vessels are important to the laparoscopic surgeon as adequate dissection of these structures is essential to assure that a large prosthesis can be placed in the preperitoneal space without the possibility of roll-up. The urinary bladder also needs to be identified where it is located medial to the medial umbilical ligament. In bilateral repairs, it is important to note that in some patients, the laparoscopic anatomy of the two sides may differ.[10,11]

ABDOMINAL WALL ANATOMY

The rectus abdominis forms the central and anchoring muscle mass of the anterior abdomen. The rectus muscle arises from the fifth to the seventh costal cartilages and inserts on the pubic symphysis and the pubic crest. The three large flat lateral muscles of the anterior abdominal wall are composed of a variable amount of muscle with a large aponeurosis. The aponeurosis is the tendon of insertion for the lateral muscles, and it also forms the sheath of the rectus abdominis. The midline decussation of the three aponeuroses forms the linea alba. The semilunar line is the slight depression in the aponeurotic fibers corresponding to the lateral edge of the rectus muscle and sheath. Fibrous tissue layers are of great importance to the hernia surgeon because of their ability to support sutures.

The external abdominal oblique muscle is the most superficial of the three lateral abdominal muscles. The external abdominal oblique arises from the posterior aspects of the lower eight ribs and interdigitates with both the serratus anterior and the latissimus dorsi at its origin. The direction of the muscle fibers varies from nearly horizontal in its upper portion to oblique in the middle and lower portions. The mostly horizontal fibers, which originate posteriorly, insert onto the anterior portion of the iliac crest. The obliquely arranged anteroinferior fibers of insertion fold upon themselves to form the inguinal ligament. The remaining portion of the aponeurosis inserts into the linea alba after contributing to the anterior portion of the rectus abdominis sheath.

The middle layer of the lateral abdominal group is the internal abdominal oblique muscle. This muscle primarily arises from the iliac fascia along the iliac crest and forms a band of iliac fascia fused with the inguinal ligament. The uppermost fibers course obliquely toward the distal ends of the lower three or four ("floating") ribs. The muscle fibers of the internal oblique fan out following the shape of the iliac crest, so that the lowermost fibers are directed inferiorly. The aponeurosis of the internal oblique muscle above the level of the umbilicus splits to envelop the rectus abdominis muscle, reforming in the midline to join and interweave with the fibers of the linea alba. Below the level of the umbilicus, the aponeurosis does not split, but rather runs anterior to the rectus muscle, continues medially as a single sheet, joins the anterior rectus sheath, and finally contributes to the linea alba. The aponeurotic portion of the internal oblique is widest at the level of the umbilicus.

The transversus abdominis muscle arises from the fascia along the iliac crest and inguinal ligament and from the lower six costal cartilages and ribs, where it interdigitates with the lateral diaphragmatic fibers. The muscle bundles of the transversus abdominis for the most part run horizontally. The lower medial fibers, however, may continue in a more inferomedial course toward the site of insertion on the crest and pecten of the pubis. The aponeurosis of the transversus abdominis joins the posterior lamina of the internal abdominal oblique, forming above the umbilicus, a portion of the posterior rectus sheath. Below the umbilicus, the transversus abdominis aponeurosis is a component of the anterior rectus sheath. The arcuate line of Douglas is formed at a variable distance caudal to the umbilicus as the result of the gradual termination of aponeurotic tissue on the posterior aspect of the rectus abdominis muscle.

The innervation of the rectus muscle comes from the seventh to the 12th intercostal nerves, which laterally pierces the aponeurotic sheath of the muscle. The lower intercostal and upper lumbar (T7 to T12, L1, L2) contribute most of the innervation to the lateral muscles as well as the overlying skin. The nerves pass anteriorly in a plane between the internal abdominal oblique and the transversus abdominis muscles. The external oblique muscle receives branches of the intercostal nerves, which penetrate the internal oblique to reach it.

The blood supply of the lateral muscles of the anterior wall is primarily from the lower three or four intercostal arteries, the deep circumflex iliac artery, and from the lumbar arteries. The rectus abdominis has a complicated blood supply derived from the superior epigastric artery (a terminal branch of the internal thoracic [internal mammary]), the inferior epigastric artery (a branch of the external iliac), and the lower intercostal arteries. The latter arteries enter the sides of the muscle after traveling between the oblique muscles. The superior and the inferior epigastric arteries enter the rectus sheath and anastomose near the umbilicus. The falciform ligament containing the obliterated umbilical vein hangs from the anterior wall from the umbilicus to the liver. If needed, the falciform ligament should be divided using harmonic shears to prevent bleeding.

▪ PROSTHESIS FOR LAPAROSCOPIC HERNIA REPAIR

The overall incidence of chronic postherniorrhaphy groin pain is lower with the use of prosthetic material in either open or laparoscopic repair, and its use has proven to be safe and effective.[12,13] The ideal prosthesis should be chemically inert, resistant to mechanical strain over the long term, and be flexible and moldable. It should not cause foreign body or allergic reactions nor be carcinogenic or prone to bacterial seeding and infection. The following is by no means intended to be a complete discussion about all the prosthetic materials available, however it should provide the reader with a concise description of various types of products so that differing properties can be highlighted.

The choice of prosthesis for laparoscopic repair varies among surgeons and institutions. They are either synthetic (preformed or composite) or non-synthetic (bioprosthesis). The most popular are polypropylene, either monofilament (Marlex, Prolene) or polyfilament (Surgipro), Dacron (Mersilene) and expanded polytetrafluoroethylene(e-PTFE) (Gore-Tex). Polypropylene and Dacron are supplied in the form of meshes, which promote fibroblast in-growth and collagen deposition, which are important in long-term fixation.[14,15] Proponents of the monofilament meshes argue that these are more resistant to infection.[16] e-PTFE is not supplied as a mesh but rather as an extruded sheet which has characteristics that are more like a membrane than a mesh. It is porous with nodes of solid PTFE (Teflon) connected by fibrils of the same material. Because e-PTFE is not a mesh, it does not promote as significant of a fibrous response as do the mesh materials and it is not so solidly incorporated into the abdominal wall. Adhesions that form to it when it is placed in contact with intra-abdominal viscera are much less tenacious than with the meshes. It is this characteristic which dictates its major indication in hernia repairs where there is any possibility of contact with intraabdominal organs. Otherwise, a mesh is preferred because of the stronger fibroblastic response.

These prosthetic materials come in many different sizes, which can then be trimmed to exact specification for a given procedure. They are also supplied in preformed shapes designed for specific operations, i.e., contoured to fit the preperitoneal space for laparoscopic herniorrhaphy.[17–19] Some are made with a memory recoil ring that allows the prosthesis to spring into place and lie flat, which makes operative manipulation easier. ePTFE, which has been modified by roughening one side or dual-sided prosthesis with polypropylene on the abdominal wall side, and ePTFE on the abdominal cavity side are available for ventral hernia surgery and may prove to be useful in laparoscopic inguinal herniorrhaphy for cases where the prosthesis cannot be completely covered by the patients own tissue or for the intraperitoneal onlay procedure. The roughened or polypropylene sides promote adhesions to the abdominal wall and the inner smooth surface decreases adhesions and may decrease fistulae to viscera. The newer biological prostheses, which remodel to human tissue made of human cadaver skin, porcine cross-linked dermal collagen or porcine small-intestinal submucosa, may also have a role in intraperitoneal placement but long-term data is lacking. Currently, they are most useful in the presence of infection where the use of any of the material prosthesis is contraindicated.[20,21]

■ FIXATION DEVICES

Some authorities feel that a complete dissection of the preperitoneal space during an inguinal herniorrhaphy, followed by insertion of a large prosthesis that results in wide overlap of the entire myopectineal orifice, makes any type of fixation unnecessary. However, most surgeons continue to practice prosthesis fixation to prevent migration or roll-up and to counteract shrinkage. The earliest fastening devices were 10-mm staplers. These devices worked well but required the surgeon to either convert one of the lateral 5-mm cannulae to a 10-mm to accommodate the stapling device, or to switch the optics back and forth between 5- and 10-mm cannulae to make it possible to always place this fastener through the umbilical site. The result was suboptimal optic angles and/or poor illumination depending upon the particular cannula switch. These inconveniences were not acceptable to most surgeons. Recent fixation devices have been designed to be used through 5-mm ports. The ends of most of these products, unlike the 10-mm staples, are not flexible. Various types of tacks can be delivered depending upon the manufacturer, including a helical coil, a key ring shape, an anchor, and so on. Counterpressure is needed during placement. These devices have also proved useful for securing the prosthesis to the abdominal wall during ventral herniorrhaphy.

The placement of full thickness sutures using a suture-passer is an excellent technique for closing small defects or attaching the prosthesis to the inner surface of the abdominal wall. Fig 46–3 illustrates the basic technique. By introducing the device through a single skin incision, but two separate musculofascial incisions, a prosthesis can be attached to the abdominal wall with a suture that incorporates the full thickness of the musculofascial elements of the abdominal wall.

■ LAPAROSCOPIC INGUINAL HERNIORRHAPHY

Groin hernias account for about three fourths of abdominal wall hernias. Indirect inguinal hernias occur twice as often as direct hernias, with femoral hernias making up a much smaller fraction. Groin hernias on the right are more frequent than those on the left.[22] The earliest laparoscopic inguinal hernia repairs (LIH) were performed by filling the hernia defect with mesh plugs.[23] Not surprisingly, the success rate was poor because Bassini's concept of complete inguinal floor reconstruction was ignored. Surgeons quickly realized that the preperitoneal space could readily be approached laparoscopically, allowing one to perform an operation quite similar to the conventional procedures popularized by Stoppa, Wantz, Nyhus, Condon, and others. The use of large, flat mesh implants in the preperitoneal space resulted in a significant drop in the recurrence rate from the early laparoscopic inguinal hernia repairs, closer to, and in some instances better than, the rate seen in open tension-free repairs.

The terminology to describe a laparoscopic inguinal hernia (LIH) can be confusing.[24] A laparoscopic preperitoneal hernia repair, in which a laparoscopy is performed and the preperitoneal space is entered with a second incision in the peritoneum, is called a transabdominal preperitoneal repair (TAPP) repair. The second general type of LIH is the totally extraperitoneal laparoscopic repair (TEP) repair. Laparoscopy, by definition, implies that the peritoneal cavity has been entered. To refer to the TEP repair as a laparoscopic technique is therefore a contradiction in terms as the peritoneal cavity is never entered intentionally. However, because a laparoscope and related instruments are used, it is fitting to discuss the extraperitoneal approach along with the other laparoscopic inguinal herniorrhaphies. An inguinal hernia repair in which prosthetic material is placed intraperitoneally over the defect under laparoscopic guidance is referred to as an intraperitoneal onlay mesh repair (IPOM repair).

Though frequently referred to as minimally invasive, laparoscopic preperitoneal inguinal hernia repairs (TAPP and TEP) require extensive dissection of and hence are better termed minimal access procedures. The intraperitoneal onlay mesh (IPOM) procedure in which the prosthesis is placed intra-abdominally avoids this radical dissection of the preperitoneal space and is therefore the only truly minimally invasive LIH.

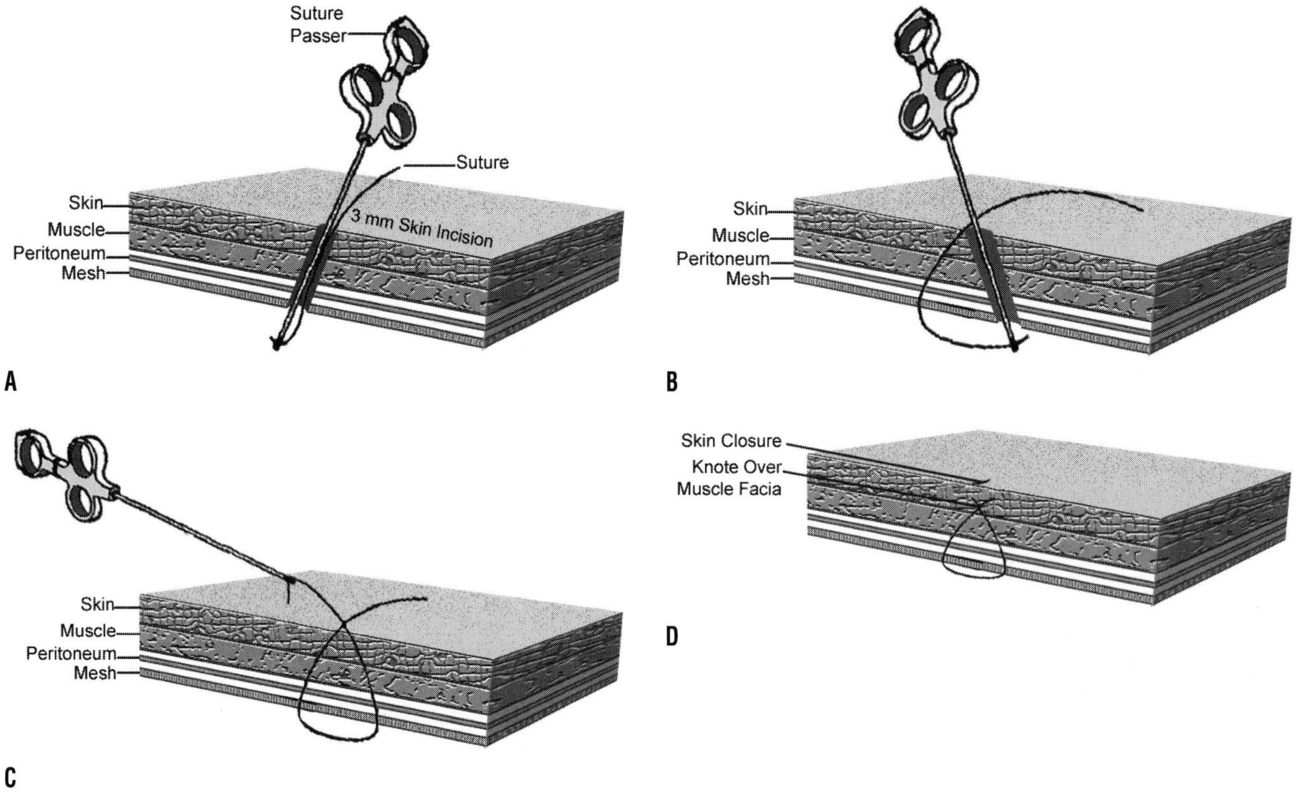

Figure 46–3. A method of placing full thickness abdominal wall sutures: (1) the sharp pointed grasper passes a suture through a 3-mm stab incision in the skin, transversing the entire abdominal wall; (2) the device is removed, leaving an end of the suture in the abdominal cavity. The suture passer is reinserted through the same skin incision but a different fascial site and the suture is grasped; (3) the suture is pulled out of the abdomen and the two ends are tied extracorporeally. (4) the suture is allowed to retract back into the subcutaneous tissue and the skin is closed over it. (For ventral hernias a slight modification is made as the two ends of the suture, which are already secured to the prosthesis, are pulled out through separate passes in the fascia but the same skin incision and tied over the fascia.)

LAPAROSCOPIC INGUINAL HERNIORRHAPHY VERSUS CONVENTIONAL

There are many different types of inguinal herniorrhaphies and significant controversy remains concerning which method is best. Review of the literature shows a clear advantage of LIH over both open tension and tension-free repairs for patient-centered outcomes such as cosmesis, postoperative discomfort, and earlier return to normal activities. Additionally, published series as well as meta-analysis of pooled patient data generally show a lower recurrence rate for LIH. However no difference between the two methods is demonstrated when the conventional prosthetic (TFR) repairs are compared separately for recurrence (Table 46–1).[12,25] The major drawbacks of LIH are the rare but nevertheless potentially devastating complications such as major vascular injury, bowel perforation, and possible adhesive complications at sites where the peritoneum is breached or prosthetic material has been placed. Supporters of the conventional (open) operation point out that the repair can be performed under local anesthesia on an outpatient basis with minimal risk of intra-abdominal injury and lower cost. The financial savings is debatable, however, if one factors in the savings associated with a shorter convalescence for LIH.

The operation remains an excellent choice for recurrent inguinal hernias if the original procedure(s) was performed in the anterior space because the preperitoneal space will not be scarred.[12,25] For bilateral hernias, the patient-centered outcomes noted above shift the risk/benefit ratio to favor laparoscopy.[26] The more contentious issue is the uncomplicated unilateral hernia. A randomized, controlled trial conducted by Fitzgibbons showed notably higher recurrence rates following laparoscopic repair than following open repair for primary inguinal hernias. Because this was a multicenter trial performed by surgeons without a subspecialty interest in inguinal herniorrhaphy, it has been felt to perhaps be more representative of the average surgeon. The results almost certainly reflect the fact that LIH is a technically difficult procedure with a lengthy learning curve. In fact, once surgeons had performed more than 250 procedures, the recurrence rate equalized. Therefore, patient selection for the procedure should depend on the surgeon's experience and skills. Surgeons with limited experience in laparoscopic

TABLE 46–1. MOST RECENT COMPARATIVE TRIALS OF LAPAROSCOPIC AND OPEN INGUINAL HERNIA REPAIR

Source	Number of Hernias LIH vs. OH	Intervention	Findings
Beets, et al. 1999[82]	37 vs. 24 (mostly recurrent)	TAPP vs. open preperitoneal	Less pain Faster recovery Higher recurrence rate Similar cost
Juul, et al. 1999[83]	138 vs. 130	TAPP vs. Shouldice	Lower analgesic requirement Earlier return to work Similar recurrences
MRC group, 1999[84]	468 vs. 460	TEP vs. mainly tension-free	Earlier return to regular activity Less long-term pain Higher recurrence rate
Picchio, et al. 1999[85]	53 vs. 52	TAPP vs. Lichtenstein	Higher pain scores Similar recovery time
Tschudi, et al. 2001[86]	51 vs. 49	TAPP vs. Shouldice	Less postop pain Earlier return to regular activity Fewer recurrences
Sarli, et al. 2001[87]	40 vs. 46	TAPP vs. Lichtenstein	Less postop pain Earlier return to work
Wright, et al. 2002[88]	145 vs. 151	TEP vs. mostly Lichtenstein	Similar recurrences Similar missed contralateral hernias
Pikoulis, et al. 2002[89]	309 vs. 234	TAPP vs. MP	Higher cost Higher recurrence rate
Mahon, et al. 2003[90]	60 vs. 60 (all bilateral or recurrent)	TAPP vs. Lichtenstein	Shorter operative time Less postop pain Earlier return to work
Andersson, et al. 2003[91]	81 vs. 87	TEP vs. Lichtenstein	Similar complication rate Earlier return to work Less postop pain Higher recurrence rate
Douek, et al. 2003[92]	122 vs. 120	TAPP vs. Lichtenstein	Less postop pain, Less frequent paresthesias Similar recurrence rate
Lal, et al. 2003[93]	25 vs. 25	TEP vs. Lichtenstein	Earlier return to work Better cosmesis Similar recurrence rate
Heikkinen, et al. 2004[94]	62 vs. 61	TAPP vs. Lichtenstein	Similar recurrence rate Less long-term groin pain
Wennstrom, et al. 2004[95]	131 vs. 130	TEP vs. Shouldice	Similar pain Similar hospital stay Similar complication rate Similar recurrence rate
Neumayer, et al. 2004[12]	862 vs. 834	TAPP/TEP vs. Lichtenstein	Less immediate postop pain Higher recurrence rate for primary hernias Similar long-term complication rate Similar recurrence rate for recurrent hernia

LIH, laparoscopic inguinal hernia repair; MP, mesh plug repair; OH, open hernia repair; Postop, postoperative; TAPP, transabdominal preperitoneal hernia repair; TEP, totally extraperitoneal repair.

hernia repair should consider open tension-free repair for primary simple unilateral inguinal hernias.

Additional indications for LIH include patients requiring laparoscopy for another reason, pain in the inguinal region not felt to be related to the hernia, as the diagnostic laparoscopy may reveal the real cause, and an acutely incarcerated groin hernia.[27] Laparoscopic inspection of intraperitoneal viscera after reduction is valuable in determining whether the incarcerated content is viable.

CONTRAINDICATIONS

Absolute contraindications of laparoscopic inguinal herniorrhaphy include intra-abdominal infection, severe illness, and irreversible coagulopathy. Previous surgery in the retropubic space, intra-abdominal adhesions, and the presence of ascites, are relative contraindications. Adhesions from previous surgeries and especially suprapubic operations make retroperitoneal dissection difficult and can result in bladder damage or peritoneal tears, leading to potential exposed mesh. A large incarcerated sliding hernia containing colon and irreducible chronic scrotal hernias are also relative contraindications due to the high risk of bowel injury during dissection.

TRANSABDOMINAL PREPERITONEAL REPAIR

This operation is performed under general anesthesia. The patient is positioned supine with arms tucked at the side to allow enough room for the surgeon to maneuver comfortably. Because a prosthesis is being used, many surgeons administer prophylactic antibiotics and/or use an iodophor-impregnated drape to reduce the risk of mesh contamination by the skin flora, though conclusive evidence of its efficacy is lacking.[28] The scrotum is not prepared into the field unless manipulation is anticipated. A urinary catheter is not necessary if the patient voids immediately before entering the operating theater. Preoperative voiding is favored since there is a higher incidence of urinary tract infection with bladder catheterization.[29]

A single video monitor is placed at the foot of the operating table, and the surgeon stands on the opposite side of the table from the hernia (Fig 46–4).

A three cannula technique is most commonly used: one 10-mm umbilical/infra-umbilical and two 5-mm placed on each side at the edge of the rectus sheath at the level of the umbilicus (Fig 46–5). A Hasson cannula is placed infraumbilically by means of the open method. The 5-mm trocar sleeves are then inserted under direct visualization. The patient is placed in the Trendelenburg position to allow the bowel to fall away from the pelvis, creating more room and providing better and safer access to the inguinal floor. An angled laparoscope greatly enhances visualization.

Once a diagnostic laparoscopy is completed, peritoneal anatomical landmarks are identified and both myopectineal orifices are inspected for additional hernias. The medial umbilical ligament can be divided if necessary but this can lead to bleeding if the umbilical vessels are patent. Fortunately, sufficient exposure can usually be obtained by dividing only the lateral side of the ligament.

The incision is continued laterally toward the anterior superior iliac spine, opening the peritoneum approximately 2 to 3 cm above the superior edge of the hernia defect. After the peritoneum has been incised, a dissection of relatively avascular preperitoneal space between the peritoneum and the transversalis fascia is commenced using posterior retraction and inferior

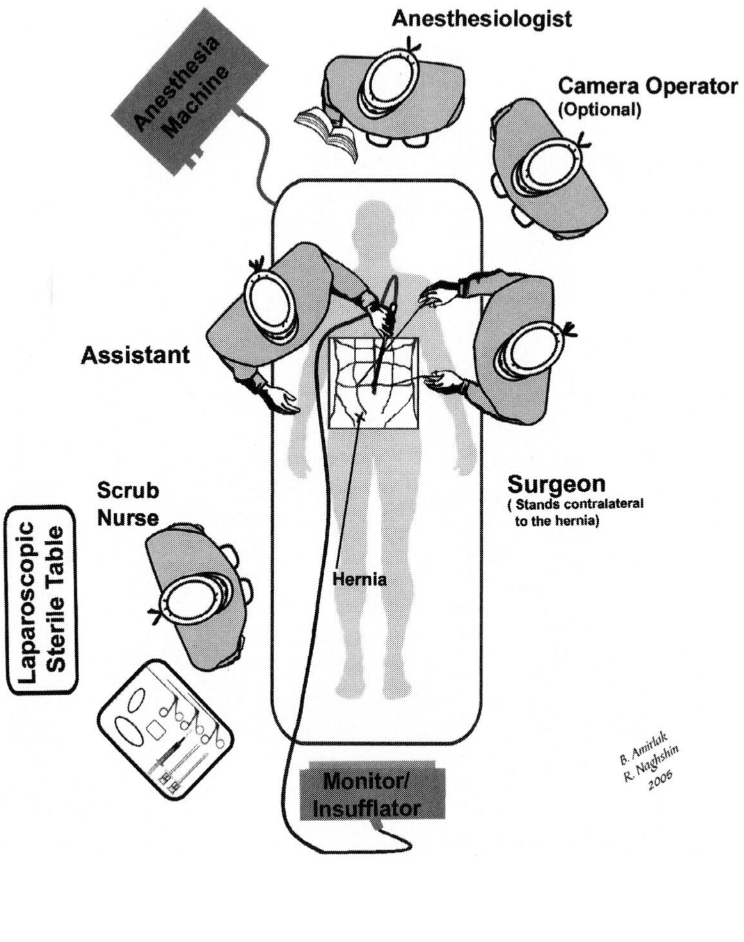

Figure 46–4. Typical operating room set up for a right sided laparoscopic inguinal hernia repair: The surgeon stands on the left side opposite the hernia. The assistant is controlling the camera.

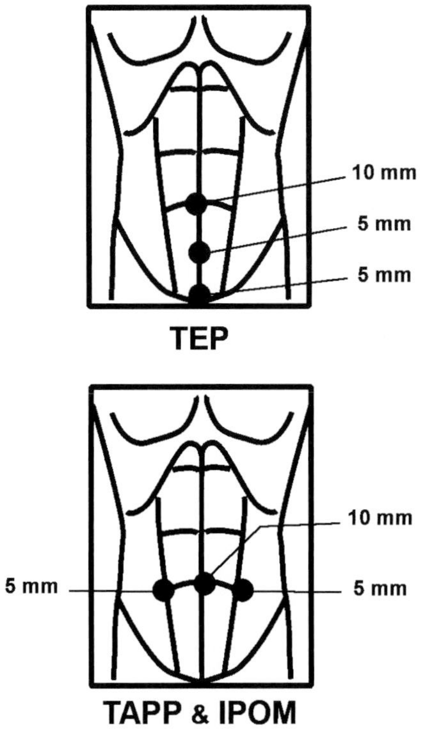

Figure 46–5. Port sites for the various laparoscopic inguinal hernia repairs.

blunt dissection. A thorough dissection with removal of preperitoneal fat allows proper identification of anatomical structures and creates space for mesh placement (Figs 46–6 and 46–7). Inadequate mobilization of the inferior peritoneal flap can result in mesh roll up when the peritoneum is closed, and has been linked to an increased chance of recurrence.[30,31] The use of an endoscopic Kittner dissector with a two-handed blunt technique works well for mobilization of the inferior peritoneal flap and lessens the likelihood of peritoneal rents produced by sharp dissection. Although extensive use of electrocautery is not needed because of the avascular nature of the proper plane, it is important to have good hemostasis since proper laparoscopic illumination is hindered by blood.

After the inferior peritoneal flap has been created, the inferior epigastric vessels, the symphysis pubis and the lower portion of the rectus abdominis muscle are identified. Medial dissection is carried out to the contralateral pubic tubercle for sufficient overlap of the myopectineal orifice. Cooper's ligament is then dissected, which serves as the inferomedial fixation point for the mesh.

When dissecting inferior to the iliopubic tract, care should be taken to prevent injury to the femoral branch of the genitofemoral nerve and the lateral femoral cutaneous nerve, which lie lateral to the spermatic vessels and usually enter the lower extremity just below the iliopubic tract. As described previously, electrocautery is not recommended in this area. Additionally, the area between the vas deferens and the spermatic vessels should be avoided since the iliac vessels and femoral nerve can be injured by staples or tacks used in this region. The dissection is completed by skeletonizing the cord structures with the least possible trauma to the vas deferens and the spermatic vessels.

For direct inguinal hernias that are located between the epigastric vessels and the pubic tubercle, the dissection is begun laterally, exposing the cord structures and the internal ring. The direct space is then dissected, reducing the sac and preperitoneal fat in the hernia orifice by gentle traction. This separates the peritoneal sac from the weakened transversalis fascia. The out-pouching of this fascia is called the pseudosac, which is allowed to retract back into the defect. It is thought that tacking or stapling a large pseudosac to Cooper's ligament may help to decrease the incidence of postoperative seroma.[32]

A small indirect sac is easily mobilized from the cord structures and reduced back into the peritoneal cavity. However, if the indirect sac is large or extends into the scrotum, it should be divided as it may be difficult to mobilize without undue trauma to the cord structures. The division should start on the opposite side of the cord structures just distal to the internal ring. The proximal sac is then dissected away from the cord structures and closed with a pretied suture. The distal sac should be opened longitudinally on the side away from the cord, as far down the cord as is convenient. Downward traction of the cord allows the surgeon to remove the excess fatty tissue attached to the cord. Fatty tissue attached to the cord or round ligament is often referred to as a lipoma.

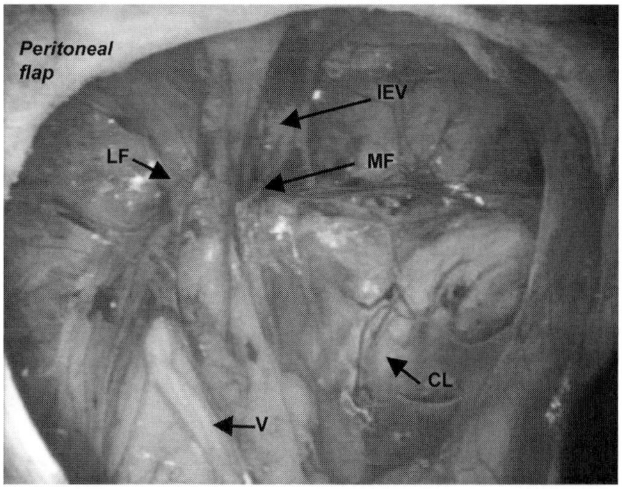

Figure 46–6. Critical anatomical landmarks are exposed during a left TAPP inguinal hernia repair. IEV, inferior epigastric vessels; MF, medial fossa containing the direct hernia; LF, lateral fossa; CL, Cooper's ligament; V, vas deferens.

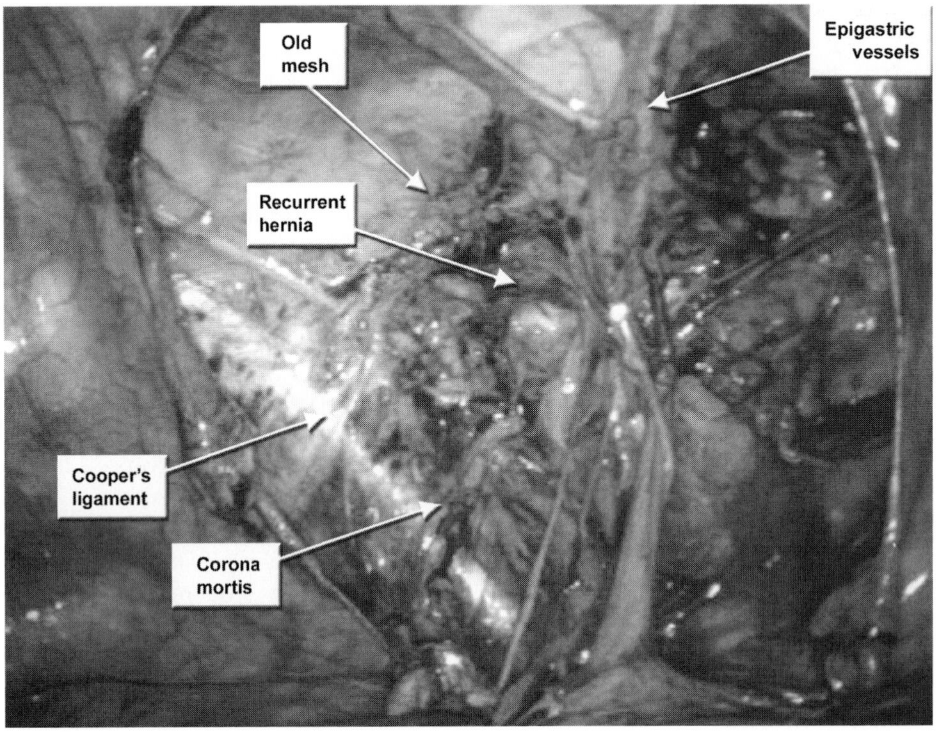

Figure 46–7. A radical dissection of the preperitoneal space for repair of recurrent right inguinal hernia with multiple previous open mesh repairs has been performed.

A missed lipoma of the cord might be mistaken as a recurrence postoperatively ("pseudorecurrence") on clinical examination. In the absence of a definite peritoneal hernia sac, cord lipomas should be treated as a hernia since they have been associated with symptoms similar to inguinal hernias.[33,34]

A large flat piece of mesh (at least 15 × 10 cm) is introduced into the abdominal cavity through the 10-mm umbilical port. Special designed preformed mesh are preferred by some (Fig 46–8). The mesh is placed over the myopectineal orifice so that it completely covers the direct, indirect, and femoral spaces with a wide overlap, spanning the space between the opposite pubic tubercle medially to anterior superior iliac spine laterally. The mesh can either be laid over the cord structures or a slit can be made to accommodate the cord. The advantage of slitting the mesh is that there is less likelihood of migration or mesh roll-up related to the anchoring effect of placing it around the cord. The disadvantage is that the size of the prosthesis is smaller and there have been reports of recurrences through such slits, presumably because the tails of the slit were not adequately approximated around the cord.[32]

The next decision deals with fixation of the prosthesis. The large prosthesis used for LIH allows the intra-abdominal pressure to act uniformly over a large area, keeping it securely in place. For this reason, some surgeons avoid using fixation all together.[19,35] This has the added advantage of preventing damage to nervous and vascular structures by staples and tacks. Most surgeons, however, have enough concern about mesh migration, roll-up, and shrinkage to use an anchoring system.[36] Disposable instruments that apply staples, helical tacks, anchors, and other mechanical fastening agents are commercially available and were discussed above. The choice is left to the surgeon. Staples along the superior border should be placed horizontally in the same direction as the ilioin-

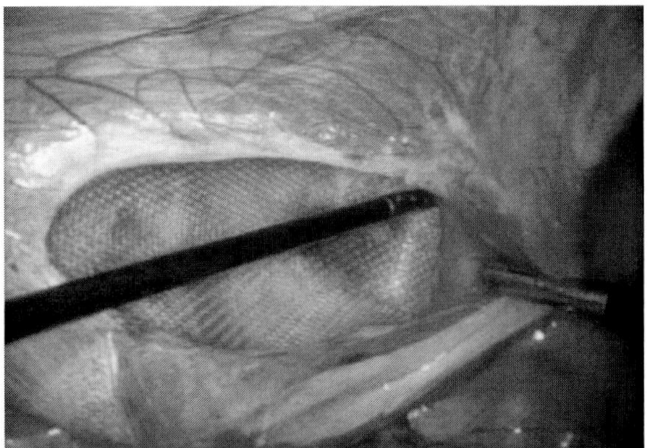

Figure 46–8. A large formed mesh is placed in the preperitoneal space during a TAPP repair of a left inguinal hernia.

guinal or iliohypogastric nerves to minimize the chance of injury to these deeper structures. Since the lateral cutaneous nerve of the thigh and the femoral branch of the genitofemoral nerve run vertically, staples on the lateral side of the prosthesis should be placed vertically. Staples along the inferolateral border of the mesh can lead to injury of these nerves and therefore should not be used here. The mesh is secured medially to the tissue adjacent to the opposite pubic tubercle, continuing fixation to the area of the ipsilateral tubercle and then Cooper's ligament. Staples and tacks should not be placed directly in the periosteum of the tubercle or Cooper's ligament as this could lead to chronic postoperative pain. Palpating the head of the anchoring device through the abdominal wall with the nondominant hand before deploying the fixator is a useful maneuver. The redundant inferior border of the mesh should be trimmed to avoid roll-up when the peritoneum is closed. Biological adhesives such as fibrin glue can also be used to fix the mesh and avoid possible damage to underlying structures. Currently, studies in humans using such adhesives are being conducted in Europe for open hernia repairs. These biodegradable adhesives have been used in laparoscopic hernia studies involving pigs with good results.[37,38]

The final step in the hernia repair is to cover the prosthesis to separate it from intra-abdominal viscera. The peritoneal flap is closed over the mesh using staples, tacks or absorbable running sutures. Decreasing the pneumoperitoneum may aid the closure. The goal should be to cover the prosthesis, isolating it from the bowel to prevent adhesions. Forceful linear re-approximation of the peritoneum should generally be avoided because undo tension can result in gaps in the peritoneal closure through which bowel can find its way causing an obstruction. Similarly, excessive tension can also result in a tenting effect leading to roll-up of the inferior edge of the prosthesis and a hernia recurrence. We do not hesitate to leave some transversalis fascia exposed as long as the mesh is covered. Another option, in cases where there is not enough peritoneal flap available, is to mobilize the omentum and secure it with staples or tacks to cover the exposed mesh. Before completing the closure, 30 mL of diluted bupivacaine anesthetic solution is placed in the preperitoneal space. It has been shown to reduce postoperative pain.[39] A technique for needle injection of local anesthetic in the preperitoneal space prior to the start of the dissection rather than at the end is felt by proponents to facilitate flap mobilization by separating the peritoneum from transversalis fascia.[40]

For bilateral hernias, the preperitoneal space over the symphysis pubis (retroperitoneal space of Retzius) is dissected so that a large common space is created between both sides. This is usually done through two separate peritoneal incisions, preserving the space between the medial umbilical ligaments. Two separate incisions as opposed to one long incision prevent inadvertent division of a patent urachus or damage to the bladder. A large prosthesis (approximately 30 × 12 cm can be secured from one anterior superior iliac spine to the other to reinforce the myopectineal orifices, in a manner not dissimilar to the Great Replacement of the Visceral Sac popularized by Stoppa in France and Wantz in the United States. Alternatively, two smaller pieces can be used which makes prosthesis manipulation simpler.[41]

Recurrent hernias are approached according to the methods of the previous repair(s). If the failed operation(s) was preperitoneal, then a conventional anterior operation is recommended. Vice versa, LIH should be chosen when the preperitoneal space has not been dissected and the earlier repair(s) was performed conventionally in the inguinal canal. The previously dissected field is thus avoided. Using the laparoscope for the repair of recurrent inguinal hernias allows complete visualization of the myopectineal orifice for the accurate identification of the nature of the recurrence, whether a result of a missed hernia (femoral or pantaloon) or inadequate mesh coverage. A large prosthesis can then be tailored to adequately cover the defect. Occasionally, the surgeon is faced with a patient who has already had both spaces dissected. If laparoscopic repair is planned, the patient should be referred to a specialized center because re-exploration of the preperitoneal space should be left to experienced surgeons. It is difficult to identify the structures in the preperitoneal space in these cases and injury to the bladder and other preperitoneal structures is common. The previously inserted mesh does not need to be removed unless it is infected. If the peritoneum covering the mesh is scarred to the point that it becomes fragmented during the dissection, a nonadherent material such as ePTFE, dual mesh, or a biological substitute should be considered for the prosthesis (Figs 46–7 and 46–9).

TOTALLY EXTRAPERITONEAL REPAIR

The rationale for the TEP procedure is to eliminate the possibility of complications such as visceral damage, adhesive intestinal obstruction, and ventral herniation by not entering the peritoneal cavity. The operating room set-up and positioning for TEP are no different than for TAPP. A similar skin incision as for the Hasson cannula (10 mm) at the umbilicus is made but this is then extended through the anterior rectus sheath on the ipsilateral side lateral to the midline. The muscle is re-

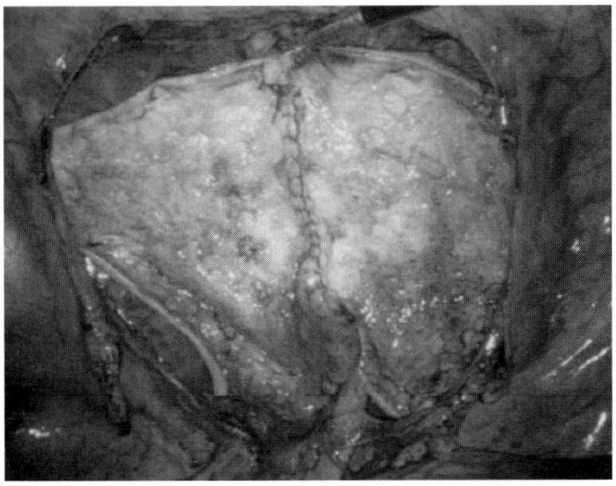

Figure 46–9. Use of AlloDerm for laparoscopic inguinal hernia repair. Two smaller pieces are sewn together using a running Prolene suture to create a larger sized biological mesh for covering the entire myopectineal orifice. Tacks are used to secure the prosthesis in place. The biological prosthesis was chosen because the peritoneum was not adequate for coverage.

tracted laterally to expose the posterior rectus sheath. Blunt dissection with a finger or a rigid laparoscope aimed toward the pubic symphysis creates a space anterior to the posterior rectus sheath. The dissection can also be accomplished under direct vision by pushing a transparent balloon-tipped cannula (Figs 46–10 and 46–11) into the space, directed toward the side of the hernia. A laparoscope is then placed in the cannula and the balloon is inflated to create extraperitoneal space for two more ports. Side-to-side movement and inflating/deflating the balloon several times facilitates the creation of this space. The pressure resulting from balloon inflation aids in hemostasis. A disadvantage of the balloon technique is a higher incidence of dissection anterior to the inferior epispastic vessels causing them to be reduced with the peritoneal flap. This can complicate exposure.

After adequate extraperitoneal room is created, a laparoscopic Hasson cannula is placed and pneumoretroperitoneum is achieved. Two additional cannulae (5 mm) are placed in the midline under direct vision: the first cannula is several centimeters above the pubic symphysis and the second is midway between the first and the umbilical cannula (Fig 46–12). An alternative is to place the cannulae on either side of the umbilicus. With either method, it is best to place them by blunt dissection with a hemostat under direct vision rather than depending exclusively on the trocar to prevent inadvertent penetration through the narrow preperitoneal space into the abdominal cavity. Once the accessory cannulae are in place, the dissection of the preperitoneal space is completed. Although the orientation is somewhat different in TEP, the remainder of the operation is carried out in a similar fashion to TAPP. Inadvertent rents in the peritoneum should be closed to facilitate maintenance of the pneumoretroperitoneum and to avoid contact of mesh with abdominal organs. Similarly, when the hernia sac is divided, the proximal portion of the sac should be closed. Carbon dioxide can escape into the peritoneal cavity during the procedure creating a competing pneumoperitoneum. If exposure is compromised, a 5-mm cannula or a Veress needle can be placed into the peritoneal cavity to reduce the pressure. We prefer the former because of our practice of routinely performing a diagnostic laparoscopy at the end to assess for unsuspected peritoneal defects. Figure 46–13 shows bowel trapped after repairing a peritoneal tear during a TEP. Without a diagnostic laparoscopy at the end of the TEP repair this would have remained unrecognized.

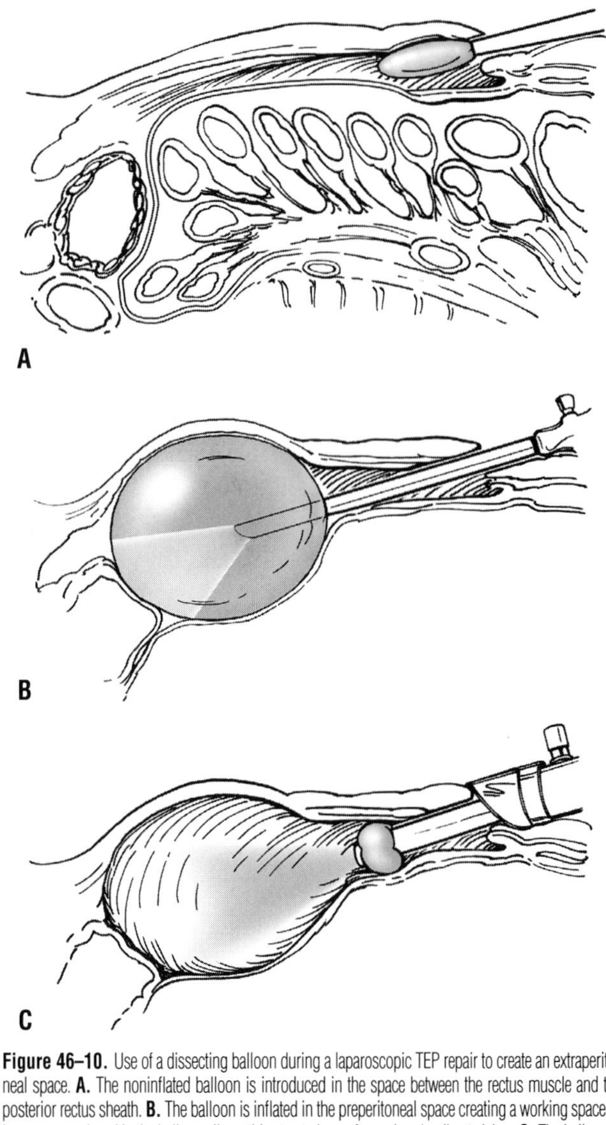

Figure 46–10. Use of a dissecting balloon during a laparoscopic TEP repair to create an extraperitoneal space. **A.** The noninflated balloon is introduced in the space between the rectus muscle and the posterior rectus sheath. **B.** The balloon is inflated in the preperitoneal space creating a working space. A laparoscope placed in the balloon allows this step to be performed under direct vision. **C.** The balloon is removed and replaced with a Hassan type cannula and CO_2 insufflation used to maintain the space.

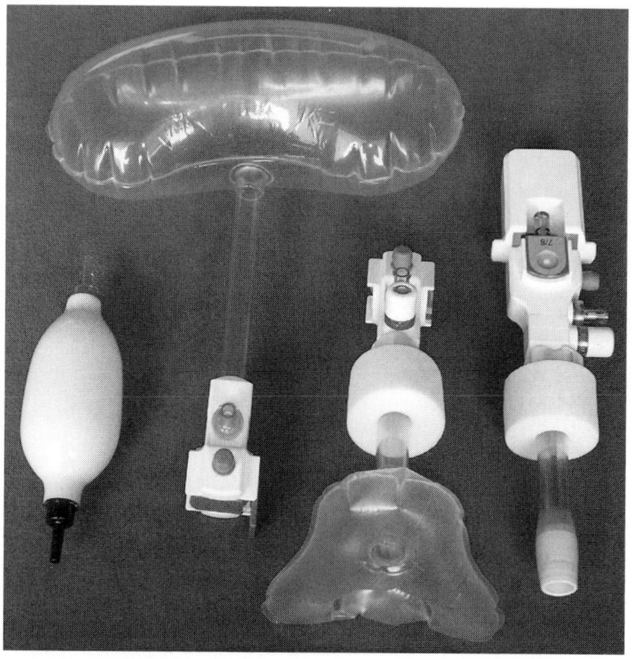

Figure 46–11. An example of a balloon dissector and specialized cannulae, which can be used for a TEP repair.

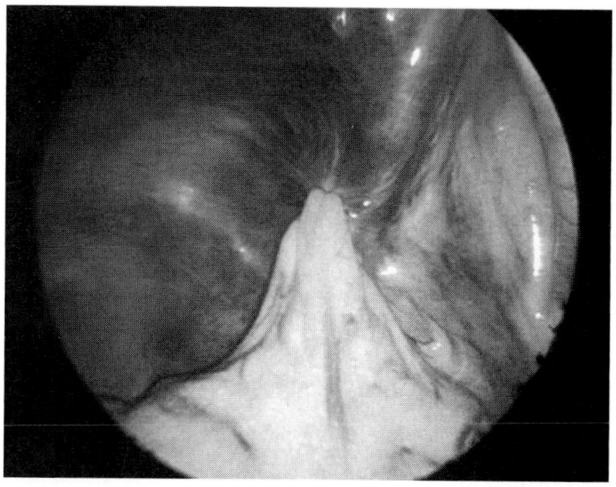

Figure 46–13. Completion Laparoscopy after TEP herniorrhaphy. During this TEP repair an inadvertent breach of the peritoneum was repaired from within the preperitoneal space with a prettied suture. A completion diagnostic laparoscopy shows bowel trapped in the repair which can only be appreciated from an abdominal perspective. The bowel was released and inspected for injury, and the peritoneal closure completed.

TAPP VERSUS TEP

There are two major criticisms of the TAPP procedure. The first is the need to enter the peritoneal cavity, resulting in the possibility of a laparoscopic accident such as injury to an intra-abdominal organ, intestinal obstruction secondary to adhesive complications, or ventral herniation. The second is the need to close the peritoneum over the prosthesis, which is time consuming and has been associated with bowel obstruction caused by herniation through gaps in the closure. The TEP operation was developed to address these concerns. The procedure is more demanding than the TAPP because of the limited working space. Most authorities believe that the laparoscopic surgeon should be comfortable with the TAPP herniorrhaphy before progressing to the TEP. Inadvertent breaches of the peritoneum are common, especially in patients with thin peritoneum or those that have scar tissue associated with previous lower abdominal surgery. The peritoneal lacerations can be difficult to recognize because they are not in the visual field of the limited working space. The consequences of these unrecognized peritoneal holes are as yet unclear. Intestinal obstruction secondary to bowel finding its way into the preperitoneal space and a death from delayed recognition of an intestinal injury have been reported.[12,42]

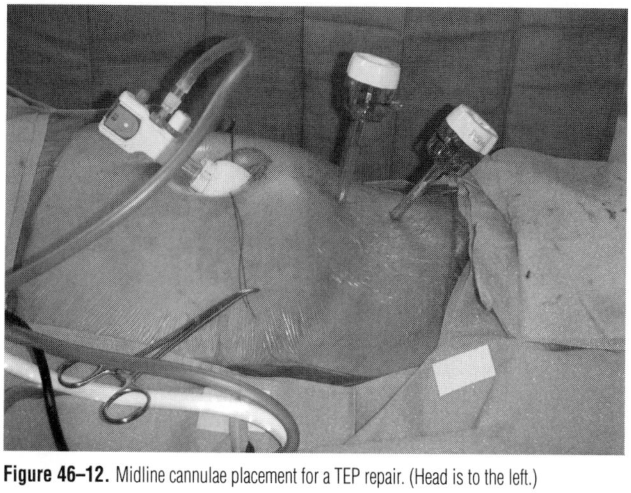

Figure 46–12. Midline cannulae placement for a TEP repair. (Head is to the left.)

INTRAPERITONEAL ONLAY MESH REPAIR

This procedure was developed to avoid the complex preperitoneal dissection used in TAPP and TEP. The theory is that the same repair should be accomplished if the prosthesis is fastened directly to the peritoneum (one thin layer beneath the preperitoneal space) using the exact same landmarks as for the preperitoneal repairs. The initial laparoscopy and port placement are the same as in the TAPP repair. A large piece of prosthetic material is introduced into the peritoneal cavity and secured using tacks, staples, or sutures. Incising the peritoneum over Cooper's ligament to aid in fixation to that structure is preferred by some surgeons. Several reports have shown reasonably good results,[24,43–46] while others have suggested a higher incidence of postoperative pain and higher recurrence rates.[47] Because of the risk of complications associated with direct contact of the mesh with intra-abdominal viscera, the

IPOM should still be considered a procedure of last resort and best reserved for patients who have contraindication to a preperitoneal dissection, e.g., previous preperitoneal repair, radiation to pelvis, and retropubic surgery.[48] The development of a mesh covered by material completely effective in eliminating the risk of intestinal adhesions or fistula formation while maintaining the properties that result in a strong synthetic mesh repair could make this operation a much more attractive option. There is minimal experience reported to date with expanded polytetrafluoroethylene (ePTFE) or the newer biological prosthesis. Further developments in synthetic nonadhesive prosthetic material or bioprosthetics may increase the applicability of this technique.

PEDIATRIC INGUINAL HERNIAS

Laparoscopic repair of inguinal hernias in pediatric patients has been reported over the past decade but is certainly not the standard of care and offers little benefit over the conventional counterpart. Although some recent series have been encouraging,[49] others have shown an increased risk of damage to the spermatic cord structures.[50–52] Perhaps the most useful role for the laparoscope is in evaluation of the opposite side during a conventional open herniorrhaphy. In children with inguinal hernias, contralateral exploration of the asymptomatic groin has been a common practice for many years. This is based on data that show a high prevalence of a patent process vaginalis on the contralateral side.[49,53] Transinguinal diagnostic laparoscopy (through the hernia sac) during open repair of inguinal hernias is a practical and safe method for evaluation of the contralateral side. A 3-mm, 70-degree-angled telescope is preferred for the examination. If an inguinal hernia or a patent processus vaginalis (Figs 46–14A and 46–14B) is identified, then a contralateral repair in the same anesthetic setting should be performed. This will spare the patient an unnecessary open groin exploration on the opposite side.

POSTOPERATIVE CARE

Postoperative follow-up and care for laparoscopic inguinal herniorrhaphy is similar to the open method. Patients are discharged to home the day of surgery if there is no urinary retention, nausea or vomiting, and pain is well controlled. They are encouraged not to lift over 15 pounds for one week as part of their pain management recommendations. After this, they are allowed to return to work and normal activity as dictated by pain tolerance. No specific restrictions are made thereafter. Patients return for follow-up at 1 week, 6 weeks, and then as needed.

▪ LAPAROSCOPIC REPAIR OF VENTRAL HERNIA

A fascial defect through the anterior abdominal wall with protrusion of an intra-abdominal organ(s) is referred to as a ventral hernia. They are most commonly secondary to fascial defects at sites of previous surgical incision (incisional hernia). Primary ventral hernias are also possible, not infrequently developing at sites of

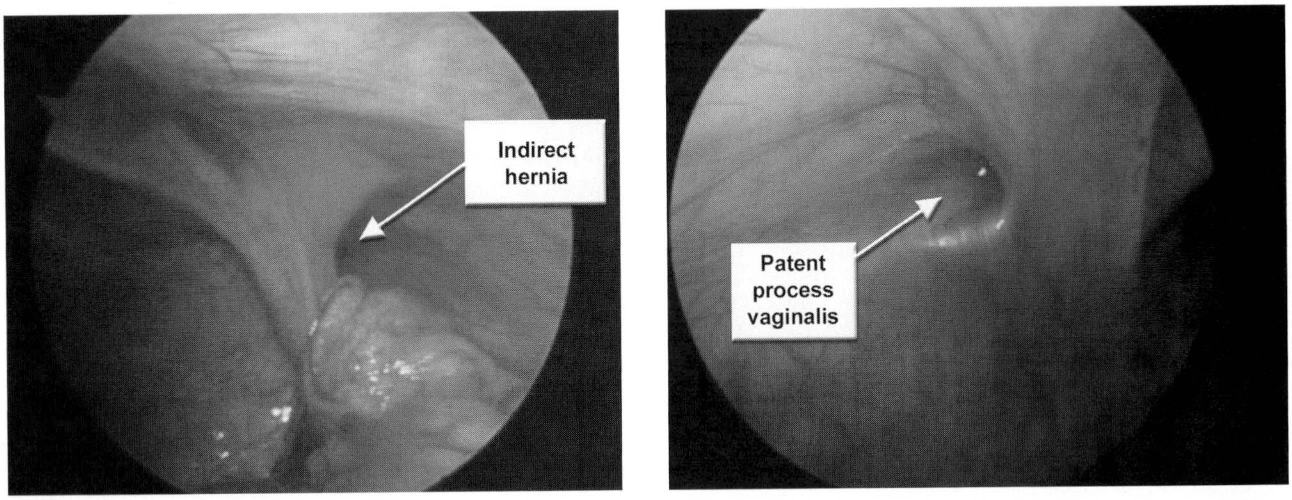

A B

Figure 46–14. A. Laparoscopic examination of the right inguinal region with the laparoscope inserted through the hernia sac during an open left herniorrhaphy in a pediatric patient. Note the indirect hernia defect with herniation of intra-abdominal content. **B.** In another patient examination of the left inguinal region during an open right inguinal hernia repair reveals a patent process vaginalis in a patient with a normal physical examination on that side.

potential weakness in the abdominal wall namely the umbilicus, epigastrium (linea alba) or linea semi-lunaris (Spigelian).

INCISIONAL HERNIA

Etiology

Between 2% and 11% of patients undergoing laparotomy develop incisional hernias with a dramatic increase if the postoperative course was complicated by wound infection. Smoking, uncontrolled diabetes, malnutrition, use of steroids, obesity, old age and antimetabolite agents among others have been implicated in an increased incidence of incisional hernias. Disease states which increase intra-abdominal pressures such as cirrhosis with ascites, obstructive uropathy, constipation, and chronic cough also predispose to incisional hernia occurrence. Additionally, incision site and the method of closure of the original wound are clearly important. Finally, basic defects in collagen metabolism are just now being defined and will probably greatly increase our knowledge of incisional hernia causation. Klinge and associates have shown that there is a decreasing collagen type I to III ratio in scar tissue with increasing number of recurrences.[54]

Clinical Presentation and Diagnosis

Ventral hernias usually present with a reducible abdominal bulge and cough impulse with or without pain. Occasionally the first presentation may be severe pain caused by incarceration. This is especially true for primary ventral hernias. The diagnosis is not always obvious, especially in obese individuals. When the diagnosis is not clear, ultrasonography, computerized axial tomography (CAT) or MRI may be helpful. The diagnostic test of choice depends upon local expertise.

Indications for Repair

There is no consensus of opinion on the role of routine ventral herniorrhaphy for the nonincarcerated, asymptomatic incisional hernia. Some surgeons feel that routine repair should be recommended for otherwise fit patients to prevent the serious complication of strangulation. Others think that the incidence is low enough that it is safe to observe a completely asymptomatic hernia. Specific risk factors that predispose to strangulation are yet to be identified.

Laparoscopic Repair

Primary surgical repair of incisional hernias have dismal outcomes as they are commonly associated with a recurrence rate of 50% or even greater.[55] Flament and Stoppa[56,57] in France, and Wantz in the Unites States described the use of a large prosthetic mesh,[58] which is placed between the rectus muscle and posterior rectus sheath. The prosthesis is secured to the full musculofascial thickness of the abdominal wall on either side of a hernia defect using a suture passer. This approach has a very low recurrence rate (3%), however, it is achieved at the expense of significantly higher morbidity because of the extensive abdominal wall dissection required to create the space for the prosthesis. The result is increased pain and significant seroma (20%) and wound infection rates. The basic principal of the repair is to use a large prosthetic mesh with 3 to 4 cm fascial overlap circumferentially.

Laparoscopic ventral hernia repair was described by Leblanc in 1993.[59] Just as the IPOM procedure was designed to avoid the extensive dissection of the preperitoneal space required for the TAPP and the TEP inguinal herniorrhaphies, the laparoscopic ventral hernia repair mimics the conventional retrorectus ventral herniorrhaphy but avoids the extensive dissection required to place the prosthesis in the abdominal wall. A large prosthesis, widely overlapping the fascial defect, is placed directly onto the peritoneum after reduction of the hernia. A suture passer is used to secure the prosthesis to the abdominal wall.

Contraindications

Laparoscopic repair can be applied to nearly all ventral hernias. However, there are a few situations where one should be cautious before proceeding with laparoscopy. These include an extensive abdominal operative history making a "frozen abdomen" possible, previous peritoneal dialysis, cirrhosis, and significant cardiopulmonary comorbidities that can lead to hemodynamic and/or respiratory compromise secondary to pneumoperitoneum. Another relative contraindication is a large ventral hernia with "loss of domain" of the abdomen, in which the viscera protrude outside the confines of the abdominal cavity to the extent that replacement followed by hernia repair might cause respiratory embarrassment and/or an abdominal compartment syndrome.

Special attention should be given to the condition of the skin, especially for large incarcerated umbilical hernias and incisional hernias in obese people. Macerated skin and even chronic ulcers are not infrequent and should be addressed prior to implanting prosthetic material for hernia repair. Caution must be used when considering the use of prosthetic material in the pediatric age group because of concerns about the relationship of the implant to surrounding tissue as the patient grows. It is considered contraindicated by many.

Preoperative Preparation

Attention is paid to mitigate the risk factors known to be associated with a ventral hernia recurrence to the greatest extent possible. Cardiopulmonary disease status should be evaluated and steps taken to assure maximum stability.

Patients are advised to take a mild laxative the day before surgery because of the possibility of enterotomy. If the colon is known to be incarcerated in the hernia, a complete mechanical and antibiotic bowel preparation is occasionally recommended. A single dose of a first generation cephalosporin is given 30 minutes prior to incision.

Surgical Technique

The patient is placed supine, preferably with both arms tucked on the side. For the initial part of the operation, the surgeon and the assistant stand on the same side of the operating table opposite to one of the monitors. The side is chosen based on the maximum distance to the hernia orifice. The further distance allows optimum angles for dissection and fastening. Only basic laparoscopic instruments including atraumatic graspers and endo-shears are required. The patient is prepped and draped and an iodophor-impregnated occlusive drape applied.

Peritoneal access should be carefully considered as, by definition, these patients have had previous abdominal surgery and therefore visceral injury is possible. An open Hasson technique at the umbilicus is useful when the hernia is located well away from the midline, but this is relatively rare. The Hassan approach is still possible away from the midline, but is more difficult especially in incisional hernia patients because they are commonly obese. Our preferred method is to use a Veress needle placed through the left 9th intercostal space to establish a preliminary pneumoperitoneum (Fig 46–15). This assumes the patient has not had previous surgery in the left upper quadrant and does not suffer from splenomegaly. The stomach is decompressed with a nasogastric tube and the left costal margin is palpated. Near the mid-clavicular line, a 2-mm incision is made just above the lower most rib (10th) and the Veress needle is inserted perpendicular to the skin. Some experience is required to recognize the characteristic "pops" as the needle penetrates first the fascia and then the peritoneum. The tenting effect as the needle penetrates the peritoneum dictates that the needle should be withdrawn 1 to 2 cm after presumed entrance into the abdominal cavity to avoid omental or mesenteric insufflation. The needle is then aspirated for blood or bile in the standard fashion but the saline drop test is not reliable in this location. Insufflation tubing is attached and gas flow started at one liter/minute. If the needle is in peritoneal space, the pressure will be low and remain low. However high initial pressure or very rapid climb indicates extraperitoneal placement and the needle should be removed and reinserted.

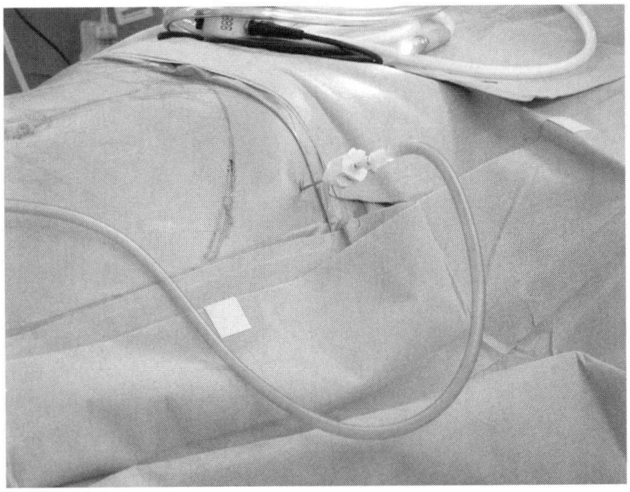

Figure 46–15. Veress needle placed through the left 9th intercostal space to establish a preliminary pneumoperitoneum.

After adequate pneumoperitoneum has been obtained, a 5-mm cannula is inserted in the left upper quadrant. Some surgeons prefer an optical trocar. A 5-mm telescope with video camera is inserted and the Veress needle insertion site and underlying viscera inspected for injury before the needle is removed. A larger 12-mm cannula, which will accommodate a larger optic and facilitate eventual prosthesis placement, is then inserted under direct vision and the original 5-mm cannula becomes an accessory port.

The decision about additional accessory cannulae are dictated by the size and location of the hernia to obtain the best ergonomic advantage. For most laparoscopic incisional hernia repairs, two or three 5-mm accessory cannulae are used but these are rotated to different locations about the periphery of the hernia during the course of the operation to maximize dissection and fastening angles. Towel clips are used to temporarily occlude unused cannula sites to prevent gas leak (Fig 46–16).

Adhesiolysis is the next step and is probably the most important in the operation as the potential for serious, even fatal complications exists if a visceral injury is not recognized. Sharp dissection is preferred. Electrocautery should be used sparingly, if at all, to avoid a transmitted burn to a hollow viscus. Abdominal distension with pneumoperitoneum suspends the viscera, stretching the adhesions. Gentle countertraction with atraumatic graspers facilitates dissection. It is important to approach the hernia from all directions. Frequently, when dissection appears difficult at one particular spot, it helps to take

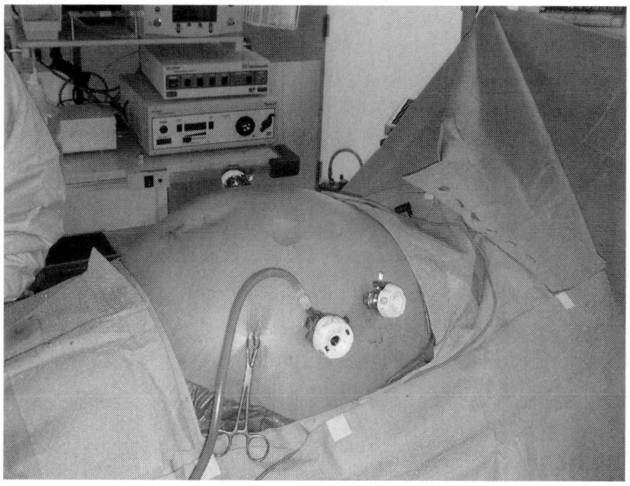

Figure 46–16. Example of cannulae placement for repair of a midline ventral hernia. Size and location of the ports may vary based upon the location and size of the hernia. The 5- and 10-mm cannulae can be rotated to different locations about the periphery of the hernia to maximize dissection and fastening angles. A towel clip is shown temporarily occluding an unused cannula site.

down other adhesions before returning. If there are truly dense adhesions, it is preferable to go outside the peritoneum. Extraperitoneal dissection should be limited to small areas as it does cause increased bleeding from the abdominal muscles. The surgeon should try to return to the intra-peritoneal plane as quickly as possible. Figure 46–17 shows the typical appearance of a large incisional hernia defect as seen from a laparoscopic perspective after the contents have been reduced. Particularly difficult is the dissection of small bowel from exposed polypropylene or Dacron mesh. Safe adhesiolysis is at times impossible as the mesh is incapsulated into the wall of the bowel. This is perhaps the most common reason for conversion to open ventral herniorrhaphy. After completing the adhesiolysis, dissected visceral organs are again inspected. The problem with unrecognized bowel injury is that it is difficult to diagnose in the postoperative period because normal pain after laparoscopic ventral herniorrhaphy is much greater than with other minimally invasive abdominal procedures. Morbidity and mortality correlates directly with the length of time such an injury is unrecognized and has considerable medicolegal consequences.

Next, an appropriate prosthesis is selected (see prosthetic materials section above). To measure the size of the defect, a marking pen is used to make a hernia "silhouette" on the skin. After the pneumoperitoneum has been evacuated, the defect is measured on the skin. The size of the prosthesis should be such that a 5-cm fascial overlap in all directions is achieved. Numbers are arbitrarily marked circumferentially on the skin adhesion barrier around the defect. The prosthesis is prepared extracorporeally by placing corresponding numbers in concert to those placed on the skin barrier, which helps with orientation later. Sutures are placed circumferentially around the periphery of the prosthesis, tied loosely and the ends left long to eventually be used as trans-fascial fixing sutures.

The prosthesis is rolled tightly (Fig 46–18) with the sutures on the inside and then introduced into the abdomen through the largest cannula site in the field (Fig 46–19A). It helps to align a 5-mm cannula opposite the insertion site. A 5-mm grasping instrument can then be placed retrograde through the larger cannula. The larger cannula is removed, leaving the tip of the grasper outside of the abdominal cavity. This allows the prosthesis to be pulled into the abdomen. The prosthesis is unrolled intra-abdominally and orientated so that the numbers on the prosthesis line up with those on the skin. Great care is taken to maintain this orientation to avoid confusion when trying to elevate the prosthesis to the anterior ab-

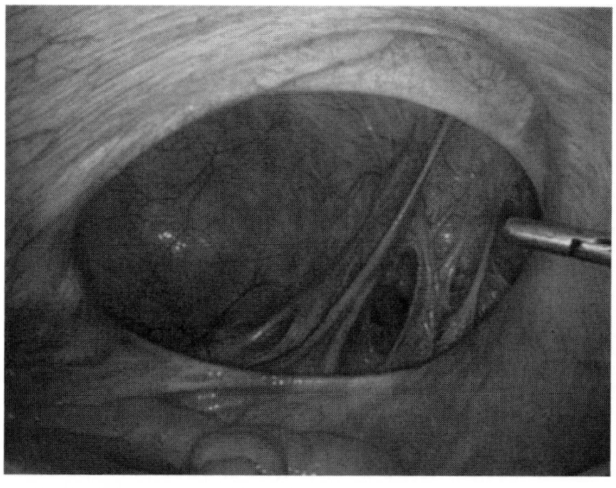

Figure 46–17. Ventral hernia defect from a laparoscopic view.

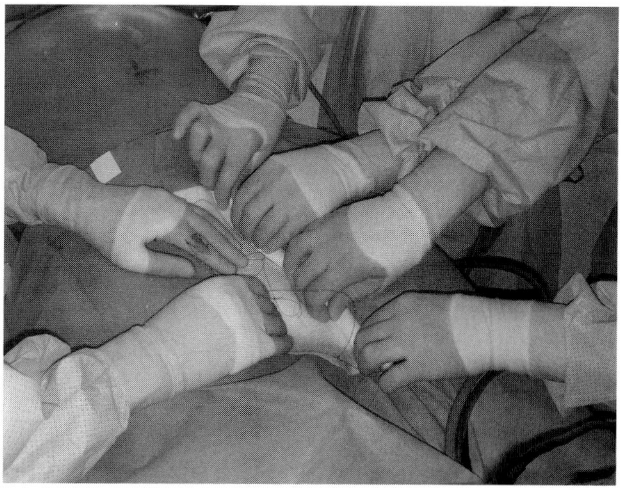

Figure 46–18. After stay sutures are placed, the prosthesis is rolled tightly prior to insertion.

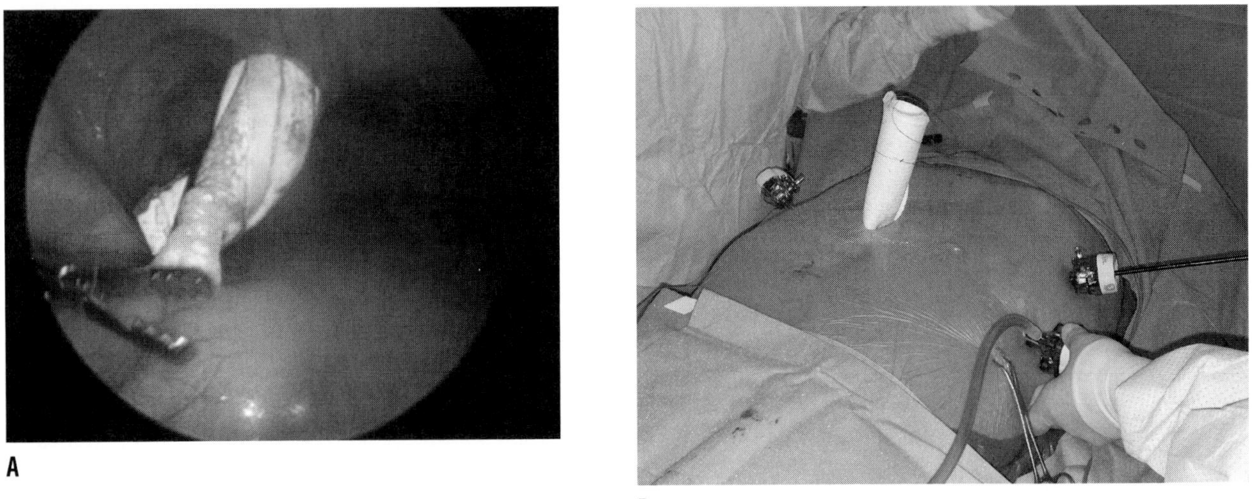

Figure 46–19. Introduction of the prosthesis into the abdomen. **A.** If the prosthesis is sufficiently small, it can be introduced through the largest cannulae site. This is facilitated by pulling with a grasper from the opposite side of the abdomen. **B.** A larger prosthesis is introduced through the center of the hernia defect by making an incision in the skin and hernia sac. The incision is then closed to prevent gas leak.

dominal wall. Using a suture passer placed through a single skin incision but separate fascial incisions, both ends of the suture are pulled outside of the abdomen. The two ends are tied with the knots residing in the subcutaneous tissue above the fascia (Fig 46–3). It is best to start tying the suture which is furthest away from the optics.

Numerous modifications on this basic theme have been described. For example, a hybrid approach in which an incision is made over the distended hernia sac after the pneumoperitoneum has been produced greatly facilitates prosthesis introduction (Fig 46–19B). Excess sac can also be removed through this incision that may help decrease seroma formation. Another example would be the use a Keith needle passed through the abdominal wall and the edge of the prosthesis instead of using a fastening device. By removing the needle and attached suture through the same skin incision but a different facial opening, the periphery of the prosthesis can be firmly sealed to the peritoneum (Fig 46–20). Frequently, a combination of these fastening methods can be used to securely attach the edges of the prosthesis to the abdominal wall, so it lies completely flat.

The repair is completed with a fastening device (see above) applied every centimeter to fix the edges to the abdominal wall, preventing roll-up (Fig 46–20). This is very important as it stops viscera from slipping between the mesh and the abdominal wall. It helps to manually deform the abdominal wall with the non-dominant hand during fixation so that the fastening device can be applied perpendicular to the abdominal wall. Figure 46–21 demonstrates a smaller prosthesis.

The procedure is completed by removing all laparoscopic cannulae and closing the fascia of any cannula site greater than 5 mm. The skin is closed with absorbable subcuticular stitches.

EPIGASTRIC HERNIAS

Epigastric hernias occur in the midline between the xiphoid process and the umbilicus. The linea alba is wider above the umbilicus, which is felt to predispose it to penetration of preperitoneal fat or a peritoneal sac with or without abdominal contents. Patients who develop epigastric hernias commonly have a single decussation of the fibers of the linea alba rather than the usual triple decussation. Epigastric hernias are considered to be acquired and are two to three times more

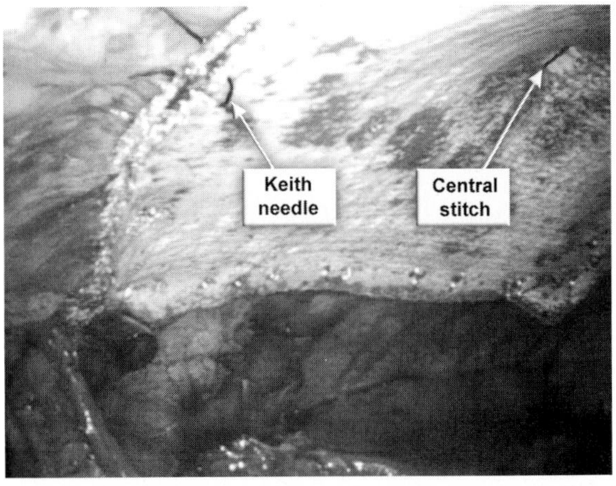

Figure 46–20. Mesh tacked to the abdominal wall, covering the ventral hernia defect. Keith needle is first used to secure the periphery of the mesh to the abdominal wall. Fastening devices are then applied every centimeter to fix the edges to the abdominal wall.

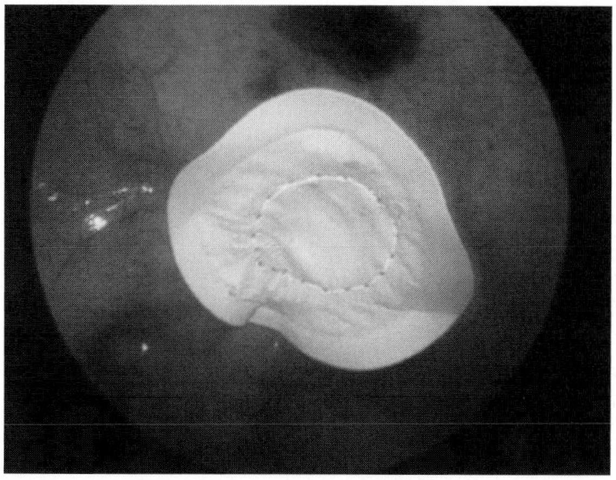

Figure 46–21. Small composite Kugel patch with memory recoil rings used for closure of small defects or laparoscopic port sites, securing with central transabdominal sutures or tacks.

common in men than in women. Twenty percent are multiple. Most are less than 1 cm and contain only incarcerated preperitoneal fat without a peritoneal sac. Patients complain of a painful nodule in the upper midline. These small hernia cannot be visualized with laparoscopy and are treated by conventional reduction of the preperitoneal fat and simple closure. However, left untreated, an epigastric hernia can become large enough for a peritoneal sac to form, into which intraabdominal contents can protrude. Laparoscopy is an excellent alternative for these larger hernias especially when the defect is close to the costal margins as the recurrence rate is quite high with primary closure.

The laparoscopic technique is similar to that described above for an incisional hernia. Frequently, the falciform ligament needs to be divided for adequate contact and overlap of the mesh with the abdominal wall. If the mesh extends beyond the costal margins, sutures should not be placed through the xiphoid or close to the ribs as these might result in prolonged postoperative pain. Fastening devices and abdominal wall sutures placed well away from bony structures is a better alternative.

UMBILICAL HERNIAS

Umbilical hernias in adults are acquired. Laparoscopic repair should be considered in patients with large defects, who are obese, or have a recurrent hernia. The laparoscopic technique is similar to that described for incisional and epigastric hernias.

POSTOPERATIVE CARE

Patients are transferred to a surgical ward and started on a clear liquid diet. Oral pain medication is usually sufficient for smaller hernias but parenteral analgesia will be required for most. Depending on extent of the adhesiolysis, a paralytic ileus might develop but it quickly resolves. Early ambulation and discharge from the hospital is the norm. No postoperative antibiotics are needed and patients are seen in follow-up in 10 to 14 days.

▪ PARASTOMAL HERNIAS

These hernias occur in more than half of patients following abdominal wall stoma formation. Para-colostomy hernias are more common than para-ileostomy hernias. Open repairs, such as primary fascial repairs, primary prosthetic repairs, and stomal relocation traditionally have been associated with a high rate of future recurrence and morbidity. Although the experience with laparoscopy in parastomal repairs is not vast, recent reports have demonstrated lower incidence of bowel injury, recurrence and infection, along with faster recovery.[60,61] Asymptomatic parastomal hernias should be managed non-operatively but bowel obstruction, strangulation, difficulty with appliance management, intractable dermatitis, pain, inability to irrigate, and cosmetic concerns frequently mandate repair.

Several laparoscopic techniques have been described. Generally, laparoscopic cannulae are placed as far as possible from the stoma site to increase the angles for instrumentation. Usually, one 10-mm and two 5-mm cannulae are used. Some authors advocate the use of a fourth port in the upper quadrant of the side with the stoma.[62] The hernia is reduced using external pressure and internal traction. Adhesions to the sac are divided to facilitate reduction. ePTFE, either as a stand alone product with the side facing the abdominal wall "roughened" to make it more adhesiogenic, or a composite of ePTFE on the visceral side and a mesh on the abdominal side are the prosthetic materials of choice. Synthetic mesh is much less expensive but visceral erosion is possible, which makes this a poor choice. Experience with the newer biological prosthesis is limited but could play a role in the future. The fascial defect is measured using transillumination of the abdominal wall from inside using the laparoscope, and a piece of suitable mesh can be sized accordingly.

There are three general methods for placement of the prosthesis although numerous modifications have been described (Fig 46–22). A slit and central circle can be cut to accommodate the bowel and the hernia defect with wide overlap. In most cases, the fascial defect around the stoma is not symmetric and therefore the prosthesis has to be prepared eccentrically. Percutaneous full thickness abdominal wall suture fixation, exclusive of skin, and circumferential metal fastenings are

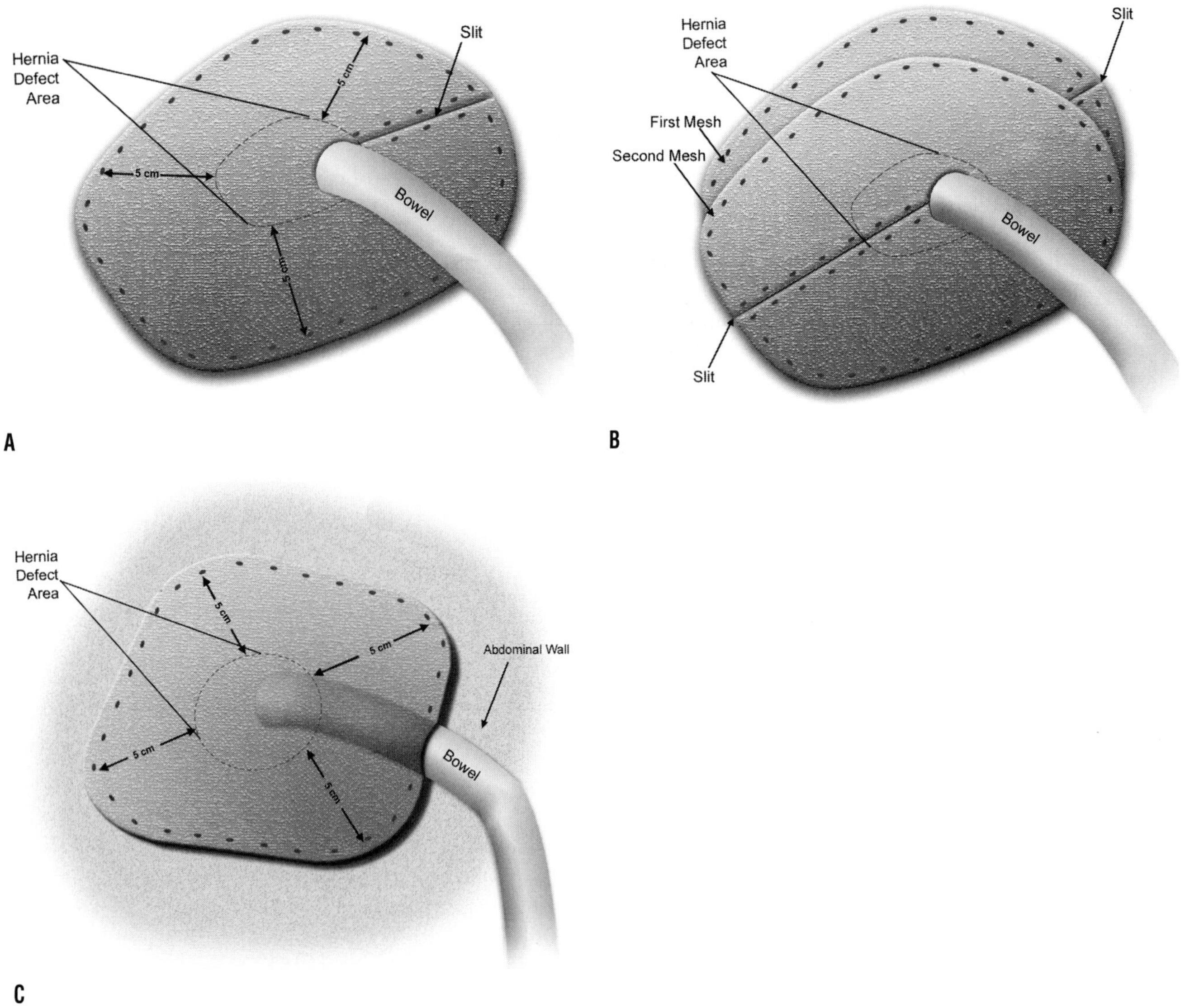

Figure 46–22. Various methods for placement of the prosthesis for para-colostomy hernia repairs. **A.** One slit and a central circle accommodates the bowel and the hernia defect. **B.** Two separate prosthesis with the slits placed 180° from each other. **C.** The prosthesis has been used to lateralize the colon and at the same time completely cover the hernia defect.

used to repair the slit around the intestine. In general, a 3- to 4-cm central circle is needed for a colostomy, and a smaller one for an ileostomy. Some authors advocate using non-absorbable sutures to secure the mesh to the seromuscular layer of intestine. Another approach is to use two separate prostheses with the slits placed 180 degrees from each other so that they are overlapping. This assures that the entire abdominal wall around the stoma will be covered with at least one layer of whole, undisturbed prosthesis, addressing the concern about recurrence through a repaired slit. A third approach is a modification of an open operation popularized by Sugarbaker.[63] The colon leading to the stoma is fixed to the lateral abdominal wall. The lateralized colon and the defect in the fascia are covered with one large sheet of ePTFE, or one of its composites, overlapping the edges of the fascial defect by at least 5 cm in all directions.

▪ LAPAROSCOPIC APPROACH TO UNUSUAL HERNIAS

Laparoscopic repair of rare abdominal wall hernias is being reported more frequently. Laparoscopy allows the surgeon to perform a tension-free herniorrhaphy on the peritoneal side of the abdominal wall resulting in a durable repair with a low rate of wound complications and short recovery time. It is not uncommon for these patients to have confusing clinical symptoms such as vague abdominal pain. Laparoscopy is particularly useful because it can be both diagnostic and therapeutic. It is also not unusual to discover these hernias during diagnostic laparoscopy for another condition. The laparoscopic method allows repair at the same setting without the need for conversion to open or return to the operating room at a later date. Figure 46–23 shows the location of a Spigelian, lumbar and obturator hernia.

A Spigelian hernia protrudes through an area of weakness in the transversus aponeurosis fascia, lateral to the rectus sheath, commonly at the arcuate line. About 20% of Spigelian hernias present with strangulation.[64] If the diagnosis is not obvious on physical examination, it should be confirmed with computed tomography or ultrasound prior to surgery.[65,66] Laparoscopy simplifies the diagnosis and pinpoints the exact location of the hernia, which can be difficult when using an open method especially when the hernia spontaneously reduces after general anesthesia is administered. Several types of repair have been described. If the hernia is small, it can be closed primarily using one of the many available trocar site fascial closing devices. Another approach is to treat it as a ventral hernia as described above and repair it with intra-abdominally placed ePTFE.[67] A totally extraperitoneal approach can also be used which has the advantage of isolating the abdominal contents from the prosthesis.[68,69] The procedure is similar to the TEP inguinal herniorrhaphy but the balloon dissector is passed more laterally to create the space needed for mesh fixation. Cannula positions include a supraumbilical port for the optics and two ports on the contralateral side of the defect. Regardless of the technique chosen, an adequate prosthetic overlap of more than 3 cm is suggested.

Lumbar hernias are rare and can be congenital or acquired. Several causes of acquired lumbar hernias

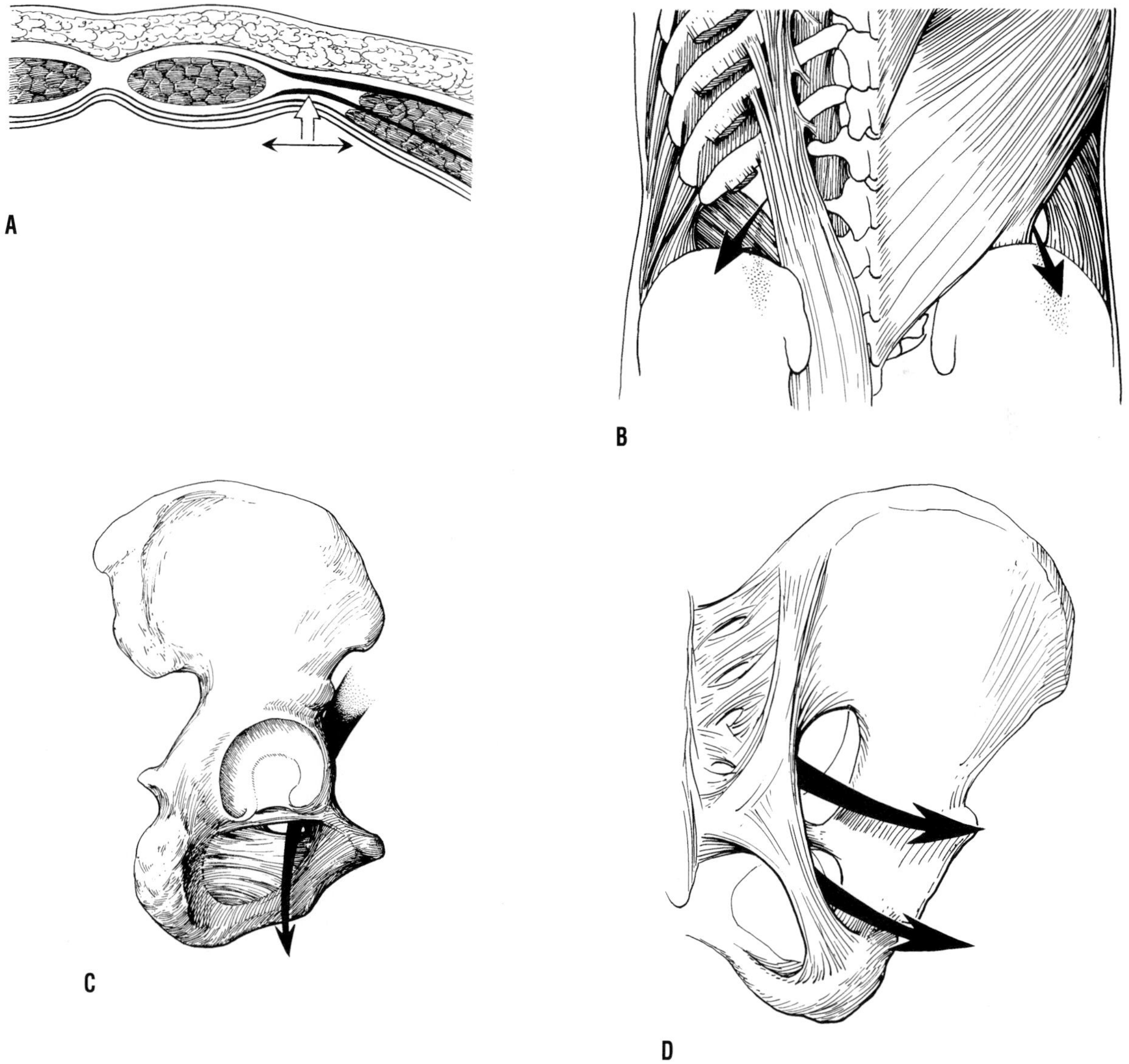

Figure 46–23. Anatomical location of several uncommon abdominal wall hernias. **A.** Spigelian Hernia, **B.** Lumbar hernia, **C.** Obturator hernia, **D.** Sciatic hernia.

include flank incisions for renal or adrenal procedures, trauma and infection. The division of lower thoracic nerves as a result of previous surgeries can cause a "pseudohernia," which has no true fascial defect but results in a bulge which is due to denervated muscle. The results of repair of these bulges is usually poor because of the lack of appreciation of the underlying pathology. The inferior lumbar triangle of Petit is bound inferiorly by the iliac crest, anteriorly by the posterior edge of the external oblique muscle, and posteriorly by the anterior border of the latissimus dorsi muscle. The superior lumbar triangle of Grynfeltt is bound in front anteriorly by the posterior border of the internal oblique muscle, superiorly by the 12th rib and serratus inferior muscle, and posteriorly by the paraspinous muscles. The floor contains the lumbodorsal fascia, which is weakened in both types of lumbar hernias. Symptoms include pain and a bulge. The diagnosis can be made by computed tomography or ultrasound. Open repairs are complicated and require large incisions and produce significant morbidity. A laparoscopic approach is particularly useful since borders of the two lumbar triangles are more easily defined from an intra-abdominal perspective, which provides an excellent field for a tension-free mesh repair with adequate overlap. In addition, there are reports that a laparoscopic approach is more cost effective than the open method.[70] The lateral decubitus position is chosen with the defect side up and ports placed anteriorly in the abdomen. Breaking the table at the junction between the iliac crest and the rib cage stretches the defect and exposes these triangles better. Adhesions should be taken down. The colon usually needs to be reflected, and with Grynfeltt's hernias the dissection is sometimes carried posterior to the kidney. A large prosthesis should be used in this case. Tacks and fascial sutures are sometimes carried all the way up to the diaphragm. Patients need to be informed that the cosmetic deformity caused by the hernia, especially the pseudohernias associated with previous flank incisions, may not be corrected by laparoscopic surgery. However, the repair does address the risk of bowel incarceration and/or strangulation.

Obturator hernias occur through the obturator canal, which is a tunnel that begins in the pelvis at a defect in the obturator membrane, passing obliquely downward to end up outside the pelvis in the obturator region of the thigh. The obturator membrane covers the obturator foramen, which is formed by the rami of the ischium and pubis. The diagnosis is occasionally made by palpation of a mass by vaginal examination or on the medial thigh. More commonly, a mass cannot be appreciated and these are found unexpectedly during laparotomy for bowel obstruction.

Femoral hernias are much less common than inguinal hernias and occur below the iliopubic tract medial to the femoral vein (Fig 46–24). Bowel obstruction is a common presentation of both types of hernia.[71] The laparoscopic approach has been used with good success in the repair of such defects.[72,73] Both TEP and TAPP have been described but the key is using a large prosthesis to cover the inguinal, femoral, and obturator orifices. The repair is the same as that for laparoscopic inguinal hernias. As with all intra-abdominal hernia repairs, if the defect cannot be covered with peritoneum, ePTFE or one of the newer biological prosthesis should be used.

Sciatic hernias are very rare and are either congenital or acquired. The defect can be through the greater sciatic foramen or the lesser sciatic foramen, above or below the piriformis muscle. Pelvic pain radiating to the buttock or posterior thigh is a common presenting symptom.[74] However, symptoms can be quite obscure depending upon the contents of the hernia. A variety of structures have been reported to be involved such as the urinary tract, small bowel, colon, omentum, fallopian tubes, ovary and even a Meckel's diverticulum.[75] The diagnosis is difficult to make by physical examination because most patients are examined in the supine position and the buttock is not normally palpated. About the only way this diagnosis can be made by physical examination is if the patient actually points it out to the physician.[76–78] Imaging studies using ultrasound or CT scan can be helpful. Laparoscopy provides a definitive way to make the diagnosis.

The laparoscopic repair is applicable to sciatic hernias as well as other rare hernias such as supravesical, perineal and perivascular hernias with the same advantages and disadvantages mentioned previously.[78–81]

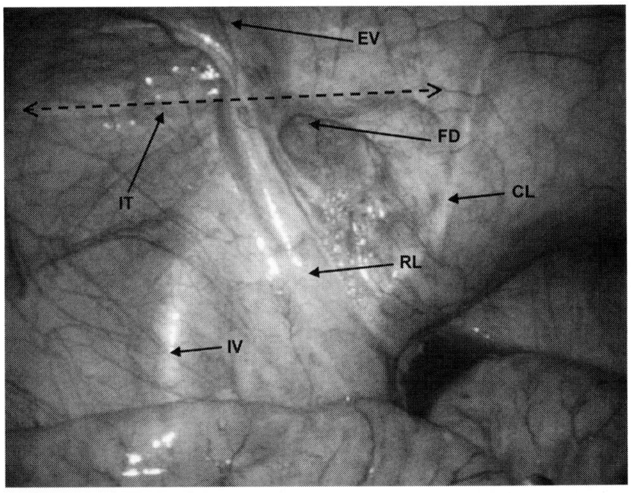

Figure 46–24. Laparoscopic view of peritoneal anatomical landmarks in a female with a femoral hernia defect. IEV, inferior epigastric vessels; IT, iliopubic tract; FD, femoral hernia defect; CL, Cooper's ligament; RL, round ligament; IV, iliac vessels.

TABLE 46–2. COMPLICATIONS OF LAPAROSCOPIC HERNIORRHAPHY

Injury	Prevention/Potential Solution
Retroperitoneal vessel injury	Leave trocars in place for tamponade and perform open laparotomy
Mesenteric and omental vessel injury	If stable, may control laparoscopically
Inferior epigastric injury	Place trocars under direct vision; suture ligation of the bleeding vessel using trocar site fascial closure devices
Gas embolism due to intravascular insufflation with Veress needle	Careful regulation of pneumoperitoneum Abort procedure with suitable resuscitation
Bowel injury with Veress needle or trocar	Leave trocars in place. If skilled laparoscopist, attempt repair without laparotomy
Bladder injury	Minor injury treated conservatively
Patent urachus disruption	Initially attempt conservative management
Hematoma	Suture ligation of the bleeding vessel with the aid of trocar site fascial closure devices
Infection	Use Ioban, prophylactic antibiotic
Trocar site hernia	Close large trocar sites using fascial closing devices or trocar site dual composite patches (Davol)
Keloid scar at trocar sites	Avoid towel clips to elevate skin in patient with history of keloid scar formation
Early vs delayed bowel obstruction	Protection of mesh with peritoneum or use of biological mesh
Respiratory embarrassment and/or abdominal compartment syndrome due to loss of domain	CT scan to determine the degree of domain loss[96] Progressive pneumoperitoneum[97,98]
Hypercapnia	Better mechanical ventilation
Phrenic nerve palsy because of the pneumoperitoneum causing stretching (Diaphragmatic dysfunction)	Transient mechanical ventilation

COMPLICATIONS

Complications unique to laparoscopic inguinal herniorrhaphy include chronic groin pain, testicular atrophy, inadvertent division of the vas deferens, disejaculation syndrome, testicular descent, bladder injury, osteitis pubis, and meshoma. Complications common to both inguinal and ventral herniorrhaphies are recurrence, wound infection, seroma, hematoma, persistent nausea and vomiting, paralytic ileus, urinary retention, aspiration pneumonia, cardiovascular complications, and perioperative respiratory insufficiency. Inordinate pain or fever should raise concern for missed visceral injury and should be appropriately investigated.

If the bowel is injured during surgery, implantation of mesh should not be considered unless the contamination was minimal. These situations may require conversion to open for visceral repair depending on the extent of injury and level of expertise. If an open repair is undertaken for ventral hernias due to this, mesh can be implanted extraperitoneally as described by Stoppa. In recent times there has been a great deal of interest in bioprosthetic materials. Although there is no evidence that they are superior to nonabsorbable material, they may have an advantage of use in a contaminated field. As with an inguinal herniorrhaphy seroma, a ventral herniorrhaphy seroma could commonly confuse the patient postoperatively, mistaking it for a recurrence.

Table 46–2 presents common complications related to the laparoscopic approach for both ventral and inguinal herniorrhaphy.

ACKNOWLEDGMENTS

Supported by a Grant from the United States Agency for Healthcare Research and Quality (5 R01 HS09860–03) and the Department of Veterans Affairs Cooperative Studies Research and Development Program (CSP # 456).

REFERENCES

1. Ger R, Mishrick A, Hurwitz J, Romero C, Oddsen R. Management of groin hernias by laparoscopy. *World J Surg* 1993;17(1):46–50
2. Schultz LS, Graber JN, Pietrafitta J, Hickok DF. Early results with laparoscopic inguinal herniorrhaphy are promising. *Clin Laser Mon* 1990;8(7):103–105
3. Schultz L, Graber J, Pietrafitta J, Hickok D. Laser laparoscopic herniorraphy: a clinical trial preliminary results. *J Laparoendosc Surg* 1990;1(1):41–45
4. Stengel D, Stengel D, Lange V. [Quality of life after inguinal hernia operation—results of a prospective study (Shouldice, Lichtenstein, TAPP)]. *Langenbecks Arch Chir Suppl Kongressbd* 1998;115:1020–1023
5. McCormack K, Scott NW, Go PM, Ross S, Grant AM. Laparoscopic techniques versus open techniques for inguinal hernia repair. *Cochrane Database Syst Rev* 2003(1): CD001785
6. Teoh LS, Hingston G, Al-Ali S, Dawson B, Windsor JA. The iliopubic tract: an important anatomical landmark in surgery. *J Anat* 1999;194 (Pt 1):137–141
7. Karakurt L, Karaca I, Yilmaz E, Burma O, Serin E. Corona mortis: incidence and location. *Arch Orthop Trauma Surg* 2002;122(3):163–164
8. Dion YM, Morin J. Laparoscopic inguinal herniorrhaphy. *Can J Surg* 1992;35(2):209–212

9. Arregui ME, Davis CJ, Yucel O, Nagan RF. Laparoscopic mesh repair of inguinal hernia using a preperitoneal approach: a preliminary report. *Surg Laparosc Endosc* 1992;2(1):53–58
10. Condon RE, Carilli S. The Biology and Anatomy of Inguinofemoral Hernia. *Semin Laparosc Surg* 1994;1(2):75–85
11. O'Malley KJ, Monkhouse WS, Qureshi MA, Bouchier-Hayes DJ. Anatomy of the peritoneal aspect of the deep inguinal ring: implications for laparoscopic inguinal herniorrhaphy. *Clin Anat* 1997;10(5):313–317
12. Neumayer L, Giobbie-Hurder A, Jonasson O, et al. Open mesh versus laparoscopic mesh repair of inguinal hernia. *N Engl J Med* 2004;350(18):1819–1827
13. Collaboration EH. Laparoscopic compared with open methods of groin hernia repair: systematic review of randomized controlled trials. *Br J Surg* 2000;87(7):860–867
14. Junge K, Klinge U, Rosch R, Klosterhalfen B, Schumpelick V. Functional and morphologic properties of a modified mesh for inguinal hernia repair. *World J Surg* 2002;26(12):1472–1480
15. Lichtenstein IL, Shulman AG, Amid PK. Use of mesh to prevent recurrence of hernias. *Postgrad Med* 1990;87(1):155–158, 160
16. Amid PK, Shulman AG, Lichtenstein IL, Hakakha M. [Biomaterials and hernia surgery. Rationale for using them]. *Rev Esp Enferm Dig* 1995;87(8):582–586
17. Bell RC, Price JG. Laparoscopic inguinal hernia repair using an anatomically contoured three-dimensional mesh. *Surg Endosc* 2003;17(11):1784–1788
18. Khajanchee YS, Urbach DR, Swanstrom LL, Hansen PD. Outcomes of laparoscopic herniorrhaphy without fixation of mesh to the abdominal wall. *Surg Endosc* 2001;15(10):1102–1107
19. Pajotin P. Laparoscopic groin hernia repair using a curved prosthesis without fixation. *Le Journal de Coelio-Chirurgie* 1998(No. 28):64–68
20. Butler CE, Prieto VG. Reduction of adhesions with composite AlloDerm/polypropylene mesh implants for abdominal wall reconstruction. *Plast Reconstr Surg* 2004;114(2):464–473
21. Edelman DS. Laparoscopic herniorrhaphy with porcine small intestinal submucosa: a preliminary study. *JSLS* 2002;6(3):203–205
22. Rutkow IM. [The socioeconomic aspects of surgical therapy. A viewpoint from the USA]. *Chirurg* 1990;61(12):874–879
23. Hawasli A. Laparoscopic inguinal herniorrhaphy: the mushroom plug repair. *Surg Laparosc Endosc* 1992;2(2):111–116
24. Fitzgibbons RJ, Jr., Camps J, Cornet DA, et al. Laparoscopic inguinal herniorrhaphy. Results of a multicenter trial. *Ann Surg* 1995;221(1):3–13
25. O'Dwyer P J. Current status of the debate on laparoscopic hernia repair. *Br Med Bull* 2004;70:105–118
26. Sarli L, Iusco DR, Sansebastiano G, Costi R. Simultaneous repair of bilateral inguinal hernias: a prospective, randomized study of open, tension-free versus laparoscopic approach. *Surg Laparosc Endosc Percutan Tech* 2001;11(4):262–267
27. Leibl BJ, Schmedt CG, Kraft K, Kraft B, Bittner R. Laparoscopic transperitoneal hernia repair of incarcerated hernias: Is it feasible? Results of a prospective study. *Surg Endosc* 2001;15(10):1179–1183
28. Fairclough JA, Johnson D, Mackie I. The prevention of wound contamination by skin organisms by the preoperative application of an iodophor impregnated plastic adhesive drape. *J Int Med Res* 1986;14(2):105–109
29. Liu SK, Rassai H, Krasner C, Braun J, Matolo NM. Urinary catheter in laparoscopic cholecystectomy: is it necessary? *Surg Laparosc Endosc Percutan Tech* 1999;9(3):184–186
30. Tetik C, Arregui ME, Dulucq JL, et al. Complications and recurrences associated with laparoscopic repair of groin hernias. A multi-institutional retrospective analysis. *Surg Endosc* 1994;8(11):1316–1322; discussion 22–23
31. Schultz LS, Cartuill J, Graber JN, Hickok DF. Transabdominal preperitoneal procedure. *Semin Laparosc Surg* 1994;1(2):98–105
32. Fitsgibbons J, Richards AT, Quinn TH. Laparoscopic inguinal herniorrhaphy. In: Cameron JL, ed. *Current Surgical Therapy*. Philadelphia, PA: Elsevier, Mosby; 2004: 1207–1214
33. Carilli S, Alper A, Emre A. Inguinal cord lipomas. *Hernia* 2004;8(3):252–254
34. Lilly MC, Arregui ME. Lipomas of the cord and round ligament. *Ann Surg* 2002;235(4):586–590
35. Beattie GC, Kumar S, Nixon SJ. Laparoscopic total extraperitoneal hernia repair: mesh fixation is unnecessary. *J Laparoendosc Adv Surg Tech A* 2000;10(2):71–73
36. Golash V. Technique of suturing the mesh in laparoscopic total extra peritoneal (TEP) repair of inguinal hernia. *Surgeon* 2004;2(5):264–272
37. Katkhouda N. A new technique for laparoscopic hernia repair using fibrin sealant. *Surg Technol Int* 2004;12:120–127
38. Katkhouda N, Mavor E, Friedlander MH, et al. Use of fibrin sealant for prosthetic mesh fixation in laparoscopic extraperitoneal inguinal hernia repair. *Ann Surg* 2001;233(1):18–25
39. Bar-Dayan A, Natour M, Bar-Zakai B, et al. Preperitoneal bupivacaine attenuates pain following laparoscopic inguinal hernia repair. *Surg Endosc* 2004;18(7):1079–1081
40. Amid PK, Shulman AG, Lichtenstein IL. Local anesthesia for inguinal hernia repair step-by-step procedure. *Ann Surg* 1994;220(6):735–737
41. Kald A, Domeij E, Landin S, Wiren M, Anderberg B. Laparoscopic hernia repair in patients with bilateral groin hernias. *Eur J Surg* 2000;166(3):210–212
42. Eugene JR, Gashti M, Curras EB, Schwartz K, Edwards J. Small bowel obstruction as a complication of laparoscopic extraperitoneal inguinal hernia repair. *J Am Osteopath Assoc* 1998;98(9):510–511
43. Franklin ME. The intraperitoneal onlay mesh procedure for groin hernias. In Fitzgibbons RJ (ed). *Nyhus and Condon's Hernia*. Philadelphia: Lippincott Williams and Wilkins; 2002

44. Layman TS, Burns RP, Chandler KE, Russell WL, Cook RG. Laparoscopic inguinal herniorrhaphy in a swine model. Third place winner of the Conrad Jobst Award in the Gold Medal paper competition. *Am Surg* 1993; 59(1):13–19
45. Toy FK, Moskowitz M, Smoot RT, Jr., et al. Results of a prospective multicenter trial evaluating the ePTFE peritoneal onlay laparoscopic inguinal hernioplasty. *J Laparoendosc Surg* 1996;6(6):375–386
46. Fitzgibbons RJ, Jr., Salerno GM, Filipi CJ, Hunter WJ, Watson P. A laparoscopic intraperitoneal onlay mesh technique for the repair of an indirect inguinal hernia. *Ann Surg* 1994;219(2):144–156
47. Kingsley D, Vogt DM, Nelson MT, Curet MJ, Pitcher DE. Laparoscopic intraperitoneal onlay inguinal herniorrhaphy. *Am J Surg* 1998;176(6):548–553
48. Schmidt J, Carbajo MA, Lampert R, Zirngibl H. Laparoscopic intraperitoneal onlay polytetrafluoroethylene mesh repair (IPOM) for inguinal hernia during spinal anesthesia in patients with severe medical conditions. *Surg Laparosc Endosc Percutan Tech* 2001;11(1):34–37
49. Chan KL, Tam PK. Technical refinements in laparoscopic repair of childhood inguinal hernias. *Surg Endosc* 2004;18(6):957–960
50. Lobe TE, Schropp KP. Inguinal hernias in pediatrics: initial experience with laparoscopic inguinal exploration of the asymptomatic contralateral side. *J Laparoendosc Surg* 1992;2(3):135–140; discussion 141
51. Gorsler CM, Schier F. Laparoscopic herniorrhaphy in children. *Surg Endosc* 2003;17(4):571–573
52. Schier F, Montupet P, Esposito C. Laparoscopic inguinal herniorrhaphy in children: a three-center experience with 933 repairs. *J Pediatr Surg* 2002;37(3):395–397
53. Yerkes EB, Brock JW, 3rd, Holcomb GW, 3rd, Morgan WM, 3rd. Laparoscopic evaluation for a contralateral patent processus vaginalis: part III. *Urology* 1998;51(3): 480–483
54. Klinge U, Zheng H, Si ZY, et al. Synthesis of type I and III collagen, expression of fibronectin and matrix metalloproteinases-1 and -13 in hernial sac of patients with inguinal hernia. *Int J Surg Investig* 1999; 1(3):219–227
55. Burger JW, Luijendijk RW, Hop WC, et al. Long-term follow-up of a randomized controlled trial of suture versus mesh repair of incisional hernia. *Ann Surg* 2004; 240(4):578–583; discussion 83–85
56. Stoppa RE. The treatment of complicated groin and incisional hernias. *World J Surg* 1989;13(5):545–554
57. Stoppa R, Henry X, Verhaeghe P. [Repair of inguinal hernias without tension and without suture using a large dacron mesh prosthesis and by pre-peritoneal approach. A method of reference for selective indication]. *Ann Chir* 1996;50(9):808–813
58. Wantz GE. Giant prosthetic reinforcement of the visceral sac. *Surg Gynecol Obstet* 1989;169(5):408–417
59. LeBlanc KA, Booth WV. Laparoscopic repair of incisional abdominal hernias using expanded polytetrafluoroethylene: preliminary findings. *Surg Laparosc Endosc* 1993;3(1):39–41
60. Kozlowski PM, Wang PC, Winfield HN. Laparoscopic repair of incisional and parastomal hernias after major genitourinary or abdominal surgery. *J Endourol* 2001; 15(2):175–179
61. Gould JC, Ellison EC. Laparoscopic parastomal hernia repair. *Surg Laparosc Endosc Percutan Tech* 2003;13(1):51–54
62. Leblanc K. Parastomal hernia repair. In: Leblanc K, ed. *Laparoscopic Hernia Surgery, an Operative Guide.* 1st ed. London: Arnold; 2003:143–149
63. Sugarbaker PH. Prosthetic mesh repair of large hernias at the site of colonic stomas. *Surg Gynecol Obstet* 1980; 150(4):576–578
64. Moreno-Egea A, Flores B, Girela E, et al. Spigelian hernia: bibliographical study and presentation of a series of 28 patients. *Hernia* 2002;6(4):167–170
65. Petronella P, Freda F, Nunziata L, Manganiello A, Antropoli M. Spigelian hernia: a rare lateral ventral hernia. *Chir Ital* 2004;56(5):727–730
66. Balthazar EJ, Subramanyam BR, Megibow A. Spigelian hernia: CT and ultrasonography diagnosis. *Gastrointest Radiol* 1984;9(1):81–84
67. Appeltans BM, Zeebregts CJ, Cate Hoedemaker HO. Laparoscopic repair of a Spigelian hernia using an expanded polytetrafluoroethylene (ePTFE) mesh. *Surg Endosc* 2000;14(12):1189
68. Moreno-Egea A, Carrasco L, Girela E, et al. Open vs laparoscopic repair of spigelian hernia: a prospective randomized trial. *Arch Surg* 2002;137(11):1266–1268
69. Tarnoff M, Rosen M, Brody F. Planned totally extraperitoneal laparoscopic Spigelian hernia repair. *Surg Endosc* 2002;16(2):359
70. Moreno-Egea A, Torralba-Martinez JA, Morales G, et al. Open vs laparoscopic repair of secondary lumbar hernias: a prospective nonrandomized study. *Surg Endosc* 2005; 19(2):184–187
71. Bergstein JM, Condon RE. Obturator hernia: current diagnosis and treatment. Surgery 1996;119(2):133–136
72. Shapiro K, Patel S, Choy C, et al. Totally extraperitoneal repair of obturator hernia. *Surg Endosc* 2004;18(6):954–956
73. Ferzli G, Shapiro K, Chaudry G, Patel S. Laparoscopic extraperitoneal approach to acutely incarcerated inguinal hernia. *Surg Endosc* 2004;18(2):228–231
74. Cali RL, Pitsch RM, Blatchford GJ, Thorson A, Christensen MA. Rare pelvic floor hernias. Report of a case and review of the literature. *Dis Colon Rectum* 1992; 35(6):604–612
75. Yu PC, Ko SF, Lee TY, et al. Small bowel obstruction due to incarcerated sciatic hernia: ultrasound diagnosis. *Br J Radiol* 2002;75(892):381–383
76. Miklos JR, O'Reilly MJ, Saye WB. Sciatic hernia as a cause of chronic pelvic pain in women. *Obstet Gynecol* 1998;91(6):998–1001
77. Kavic MS. Chronic pelvic pain in females and obscure hernias. *Hernia* 2000;4:250–254.
78. Spurbeck WW. *Prevascular and Retropsoas Hernias: Incidence of Rare Abdominal Wall Hernias.* American Hernia Society Hernia Conference; 2002 May; Tucson, AZ; 2002

79. Mehran A, Szomstein S, Soto F, Rosenthal R. Laparoscopic repair of an internal strangulated supravesical hernia. *Surg Endosc* 2004;18(3):554–556
80. Kavic MS. Chronic pelvic pain in women. In: Bendavid R, Arregui ME, ed. *Abdominal Wall Hernias Principle and Management.* New York: Springer-Verlag; 2001:636–688
81. Christine A, Arregui M. Femoral and pelvic herniorrhaphy, rare and unusual hernias. In: Leblanc K, ed. *Laparoscopic Hernia Surgery, an Operative Guide.* London: Arnold; 2003:77–81
82. Beets GL, Dirksen CD, Go PM, et al. Open or laparoscopic preperitoneal mesh repair for recurrent inguinal hernia? A randomized controlled trial. *Surg Endosc* 1999;13(4):323–327
83. Juul P, Christensen K. Randomized clinical trial of laparoscopic versus open inguinal hernia repair. *Br J Surg* 1999;86(3):316–319
84. Laparoscopic versus open repair of groin hernia: a randomised comparison. The MRC Laparoscopic Groin Hernia Trial Group. *Lancet* 1999;354(9174):185–190
85. Picchio M, Lombardi A, Zolovkins A, Mihelsons M, La Torre G. Tension-free laparoscopic and open hernia repair: randomized controlled trial of early results. *World J Surg* 1999;23(10):1004–1007; discussion 8–9
86. Tschudi JF, Wagner M, Klaiber C, et al. Randomized controlled trial of laparoscopic transabdominal preperitoneal hernioplasty vs Shouldice repair. *Surg Endosc* 2001;15(11):1263–1266
87. Sarli L, Villa F, Marchesi F. Hernioplasty and simultaneous laparoscopic cholecystectomy: a prospective randomized study of open tension-free versus laparoscopic inguinal hernia repair. *Surgery* 2001;129(5):530–536
88. Wright D, Paterson C, Scott N, Hair A, O'Dwyer PJ. Five-year follow-up of patients undergoing laparoscopic or open groin hernia repair: a randomized controlled trial. *Ann Surg* 2002;235(3):333–337
89. Pikoulis E, Tsigris C, Diamantis T, et al. Laparoscopic preperitoneal mesh repair or tension-free mesh plug technique? A prospective study of 471 patients with 543 inguinal hernias. *Eur J Surg* 2002;168(11):587–591
90. Mahon D, Decadt B, Rhodes M. Prospective randomized trial of laparoscopic (transabdominal preperitoneal) vs open (mesh) repair for bilateral and recurrent inguinal hernia. *Surg Endosc* 2003;17(9):1386–1390
91. Andersson B, Hallen M, Leveau P, Bergenfelz A, Westerdahl J. Laparoscopic extraperitoneal inguinal hernia repair versus open mesh repair: a prospective randomized controlled trial. *Surgery* 2003;133(5):464–472
92. Douek M, Smith G, Oshowo A, Stoker DL, Wellwood JM. Prospective randomised controlled trial of laparoscopic versus open inguinal hernia mesh repair: five year follow up. *BMJ* 2003;326(7397):1012–1013
93. Lal P, Kajla RK, Chander J, Saha R, Ramteke VK. Randomized controlled study of laparoscopic total extraperitoneal versus open Lichtenstein inguinal hernia repair. *Surg Endosc* 2003;17(6):850–856
94. Heikkinen T, Bringman S, Ohtonen P, et al. Five-year outcome of laparoscopic and Lichtenstein hernioplasties. *Surg Endosc* 2004;18(3):518–522
95. Wennstrom I, Berggren P, Akerud L, Jarhult J. Equal results with laparoscopic and Shouldice repairs of primary inguinal hernia in men. Report from a prospective randomised study. *Scand J Surg* 2004;93(1):34–36
96. Rubio PA, Del Castillo H, Alvarez BA. Ventral hernia in a massively obese patient: diagnosis by computerized tomography. *South Med J* 1988;81(10):1307–1308
97. Harrison D, Taneja R, Kahn D, Rush B, Jr. Repair of a massive ventral hernia in a morbidly obese patient. *N J Med* 1995;92(6):387–389
98. Raynor RW, Del Guercio LR. The place for pneumoperitoneum in the repair of massive hernia. *World J Surg* 1989;13(5):581–585

47

Small Bowel/Colon Resection

Michael M. Davies ■ Heidi Nelson

■ BACKGROUND

The use of the laparoscopic approach for colorectal surgery has developed over the last 15 years since the first laparoscopic colonic resection reported by Jacobs in 1991.[1] While laparoscopic cholecystectomy has become the standard method for resection of the gall bladder, laparoscopic small and large bowel resection have been slower to develop. This is related to the greater technical difficulties encountered because of large organ size, extensive blood supply, and wide area of dissection. These problems have gradually been overcome by modification of laparoscopic technique and development of special instruments for intracorporeal vascular ligation.

Laparoscopic small bowel and colorectal resection are now frequently used for benign disease including inflammatory bowel disease and diverticular disease.[2] In ulcerative colitis, reconstruction with ileoanal pouch formation may also be performed laparoscopically. Short term benefits of the laparoscopic approach have been demonstrated, with a faster return of gut function, leading to more rapid discharge from hospital and a faster return to normal activities. These benefits can lead to reduced costs despite the longer operating times.[3,4] Long-term benefits have also been demonstrated and these include a reduction in obstruction secondary to adhesions and reduced incidence of ventral hernia.[5]

The use of laparoscopic colorectal resection for malignant disease has developed more slowly. The results of surgery for malignancy are judged on the basis of local and distant recurrence rates in addition to surgical morbidity and mortality. Early reports suggested a significant risk of port site recurrence,[6] which discouraged the use of laparoscopic resection for malignant disease. Subsequent reports, however, have demonstrated rates, which are no different to those observed for wound recurrence in open surgery.[2] Similar short-term benefits to those demonstrated for benign disease have been achieved.[7,8] Long-term outcome data has previously been limited but we now have the results of a large, randomized trial with long-term follow-up data.[9] This has demonstrated equivalent oncological outcomes for open and laparoscopic surgery and these results are likely to promote the use of the laparoscopic colonic resection for malignant disease.

■ PRINCIPLES OF LAPAROSCOPIC SMALL BOWEL, COLON, AND RECTAL SURGERY

PATIENT SELECTION

The laparoscopic approach is applicable to the majority of patients. However, there are some contraindications to laparoscopic colorectal resection. Any condition that increases the risk of bleeding is seen as a contraindication to laparoscopic surgery because of the restricted access. Previous abdominal surgery may prevent laparoscopic surgery, but this is variable and depends on the location and extent of this previous surgery. Some abdomens are hostile to any form of surgery and laparoscopic surgery should be avoided if this is known to be the case. Otherwise laparoscopy can be attempted with the understanding that conversion may be more likely.

Morbid obesity continues to be a relative contraindication to the laparoscope-assisted approach. The increased quantity of intraabdominal fat creates difficulties with obtaining a satisfactory view and retraction of the colon, and exteriorization of the bowel. Additionally, division of a thickened mesentery is more technically difficult with increased risks of hemorrhage. A body mass index (BMI) >30 may lead to a longer operative duration, increased rate of conversion to an open procedure, and a higher morbidity rate, including increased anastomotic leakage.[10] However, as we learn from laparoscopic bariatric surgery and perform more total laparoscopic surgery, the role of laparoscopic colectomy may take on a new significance in obese patients. In addition to these general criteria, there are also some disease specific factors (discussed below), which are important in case selection.

DISEASE SPECIFIC INDICATIONS, CONTRAINDICATIONS, AND KEY POINTS

Crohn's Disease

Indications. Surgery for Crohn's disease is reserved for the management of complications of the disease and laparoscopic resection can potentially be used for any of the indications for surgery including strictures, abscesses, fistulae, and refractory disease. Procedures may include stricturoplasty, small bowel resection, segmental colonic resection, or proctocolectomy.

Contraindications. While laparoscopic resection can be used for any of the indications for surgery in Crohn's disease, there are some patients in whom an open approach may be more appropriate. Complex fistulizing disease is frequently too bulky to exteriorize through a small incision, which often obscures the local anatomy; accordingly, an open procedure is usually required. Extensive disease with multiple strictures or bulky disease due to an inflammatory mass is likely to negate the benefits of the laparoscopic approach particularly if a large wound is required to extract the resected specimen. Patients with Crohn's disease frequently require more than one procedure over time and many patients have had a number of previous laparotomies. These patients are likely to have significant adhesions that may preclude laparoscopic resection.

Key Points.

1. The extent of disease should be accurately defined preoperatively with full assessment of upper and lower gastrointestinal (GI) tracts. This ensures that the procedure can be accurately planned with assessment made for extensive, severe, or bulky disease that would prevent a successful laparoscopic procedure.
2. The extent of disease should be fully reassessed at the time of surgery. The small bowel should be completely visualized with the assistance of instruments to exclude any additional undetected disease, just like open surgery.
3. Dense adhesions or extensive disease that prevents accurate identification of vital structures and increase the risk of complications should cause the surgeon to convert early to an open procedure.

Ulcerative Colitis

Indications. Laparoscopic resection for ulcerative colitis follows the same indications as those for open surgery, which include symptomatic failure of medical therapy and dysplasia. Restorative proctocolectomy, or proctocolectomy with end ileostomy (if ileoanal pouch formation is contraindicated) can both be performed laparoscopically. In acute colitis urgent laparoscopic subtotal colectomy and end ileostomy may be performed initially as part of a two or three stage procedure. For emergency procedures including those for acute toxic megacolon, open surgery is preferred.

Contraindications. Toxic dilatation of the colon or perforation secondary to fulminant colitis are the only absolute disease specific contraindications to laparoscopic resection for ulcerative colitis.

Key Points.

1. Resection should adhere to oncological principles if the indication for surgery is dysplasia. High ligation of the vasculature, venting of the pneumoperitoneum through laparoscopic ports, wound protection, and irrigation of wounds prior to closure should be performed in case an occult malignancy is present in the resected specimen.
2. The small bowel mesentery should be fully mobilized prior to exteriorization of the colonic specimen during restorative proctocolectomy to ensure sufficient mesenteric length for ileoanal pouch formation.
3. Particular care should be taken with patients on high-dose steroids due the increased fragility of tissues. Atraumatic graspers should be used and the surgeon should avoid direct grasping of the colon.

Diverticular Disease

Indications. Laparoscopic resection can be used in the elective setting for recurrent diverticulitis. The indications for laparoscopic resection for diverticular disease are the same as those for open surgery. Current American Society of Colon and Rectal Surgeons (ASCRS) guidelines advise elective resection following two documented episodes of acute diverticulitis or after one episode if the patient is young.[11] Use of laparoscopic resection for complicated diverticulitis should be more selective.

Contraindications. Acute complications that require emergency surgery including perforation or obstruction should be managed by open surgery. Complicated diverticular disease may be associated with fistula formation that is likely to require an open procedure because of the more complex nature of the surgery required. A bulky phlegmon will require a large incision for removal of the specimen and this will negate the benefits of the laparoscopic approach.

Key Points.

1. In all cases for which a laparoscopic procedure is planned. Careful preoperative assessment with colonoscopy and CT scanning should be performed to define the nature of the disease. Evidence of complicated diverticulitis with bulky or fistulating disease should be excluded as this may preclude laparoscopic resection.
2. Placement of a ureteral stent should be considered in those cases where the left ureter may be difficult to locate as a result of inflammation of the retroperitoneum.
3. Sufficient distal mobilization of the sigmoid colon should be performed to ensure resection of the high pressure zone with anastomosis to the top of the rectum.

Colorectal Cancer

Indications. Laparoscopic resection can be performed for colon cancer with equivalent oncological outcomes to open surgery when oncological principles are practiced.[9] Results for laparoscopic rectal cancer are not yet definitive. The short-term benefits are similar to colonic resection but the results of two long-term studies[12,13] are awaited to define long term outcomes. A number of technical challenges need to be considered and mastered before laparoscopic rectal cancer resection can be recommended.

Contraindications. The only absolute contraindications to selective laparoscopic resection of cancer are T4 disease or resectable metastatic disease where surgical resection will require resection of part or all of other organs. The size of a tumor is also important and if a large incision is required to remove a bulky tumor then the benefits of the laparoscopic approach are negated and an open procedure should be performed. Urgent or emergency cases, where the bowel is perforated or obstructed should be managed with open surgery.

Key Points.

1. Full preoperative staging should be performed in a manner similar to open surgery. Colonoscopy should include tattooing of the colon if the tumor is small. This will aid localization at the time of surgery. CT scans should be reviewed to exclude locally advanced or bulky disease for which laparoscopic resection is inappropriate.
2. It is essential to perform a satisfactory oncological resection, including adequate mobilization and high vascular ligation, to ensure satisfactory lymph node harvest and resection margins. Intracorporeal ligation is usually required to achieve high vascular ligation.
3. Venting of the pneumoperitoneum via the laparoscope ports, wound protection and copious wound irrigation prior to closure should all be performed to reduce the risk of tumour implantation in wounds and port site recurrence.

CONVERSION

If difficulties are encountered during a laparoscopic procedure then conversion to an open procedure may be required. Reasons for conversion may include unexpected disease, e.g., significant adhesions or inability to identify vital structures especially ureters. A decision to convert is best made early in a procedure, if these problems are encountered, so that prolonged attempts to achieve a laparoscopic resection are not made and the increased risk of complications necessitating a later conversion are avoided. This approach will ensure that the rates of morbidity and mortality are maintained at acceptable levels.

LEARNING CURVE AND CREDENTIALING

Advanced laparoscopic skills and a solid knowledge of colorectal disease are both required to perform laparoscopic small-bowel and colon resections. There is a significant learning curve during which the length of each procedure may be longer and the rate of conversion to an open procedure may be greater, although the incidence of complications is not necessarily increased.[14] It is recommended that surgeons develop their laparoscopic skills by performing simpler procedures initially, e.g., appendicectomy, then graduating to ileocecal resections followed by sigmoid resections, prior to undertaking cancer resections. This graduated development should occur under the supervision of a more experienced laparoscopic surgeon and should be supported by attendance at training courses. The ASCRS has recommended that surgeons undertake 20 laparoscopic resections before undertaking procedures for cancer.

▪ PREOPERATIVE PREPARATION OF THE PATIENT

BOWEL PREPARATION

All patients undergoing laparoscopic bowel resection should receive a full bowel preparation. This can be given as an outpatient, the day prior to surgery and standard agents can be used, e.g., phosphosoda or GoLYTELY.

ANTIBIOTICS

Prophylactic antibiotics should be given to reduce postoperative wound infection. These may include oral antibiotics given with the bowel preparation, e.g., metronidazole and neomycin and intravenous antibiotics given at induction and postprocedure.

THROMBOEMBOLISM PROPHYLAXIS

Laparoscopic cases require routine thromboembolism prophylaxis. Surgery may be prolonged and surgeries for inflammatory bowel disease and malignancy are associated with an increased risk of thromboembolism. Use of subcutaneous heparin, thromboembolism deterrent (TED) stockings and intermittent pneumatic calf compression devices should be routine for all patients.

▪ POSTOPERATIVE CARE

The return of bowel function is more rapid following laparoscopic compared with open surgery. Therefore patients can be advanced rapidly with introduction of fluid and food as tolerated. A potential pathway would include starting liquid intake on the day following surgery and progressing onto solid diet on the second day. Opiate and oral analgesic requirements are significantly less than for open surgery.[15] Patients should be commenced on oral analgesia with the start of oral intake to reduce the need for opiate analgesia and allow early withdrawal of narcotics. Patients should be encouraged to ambulate from the first day. Urinary catheters can be removed 1 or 2 days after surgery unless a rectal resection has been performed in which case removal may be delayed. Using this "fast-track" type pathway, early discharge is frequently possible on the third postoperative day.

▪ INSTRUMENTATION (FIG 47–1)

Laparoscopic colonic resection requires use of the basic laparoscopic equipment with certain additions.

1. Video camera unit
2. Light source
3. CO_2 insufflator
4. 30-degree laparoscope (5/10 mm)
5. Suction/irrigator
6. Scissors with cautery attachment
7. Long and short Babcock graspers
8. Small graspers with cautery attachment
9. Intracorporeal vascular ligation device, e.g., LigaSure, Endoloop, or Vascular staple gun
10. Cannulas (Hassan and 10/12 or 5-mm ports)

OPTIMIZING EQUIPMENT

The list of equipment described can be used to achieve all laparoscopic colorectal procedures. Certain features can optimize the function of this equipment. Disposable scissors and suction/irrigator are preferable as these provide reliable function which is critical for laparoscopic colorectal resection, where large areas of dissection and division of multiple blood vessels are required. Cautery attachments should be on the upper side of the instruments so that this connection does not interfere with movement during dissection. A finger switch can be attached to the scissors or graspers for activation of the cautery although some operators prefer a foot pedal. The video camera unit, light source and CO_2 insufflator may be placed on a small cart so that it forms a readily mobile unit to allow optimal placement prior to and during procedures. TV monitors should also be easily mobile to allow easy position changes during the procedure and may be combined with the other equipment.

There are a wide variety of cannulas available. For all procedures (except for hand port procedures), it is recommended to use a Hassan type cannula and open insertion technique to reduce the risk of injury to intraabdominal structures. Reducing devices can then be placed if a 5mm laparoscope or instruments are used. Nonbladed cannulas can also be used at other port positions to improve safety. Short cannulas reduce the interference with view within the abdominal cavity and can be used in the majority of patients except for those with obesity. The diameter (5- or 10-mm) of cannulas

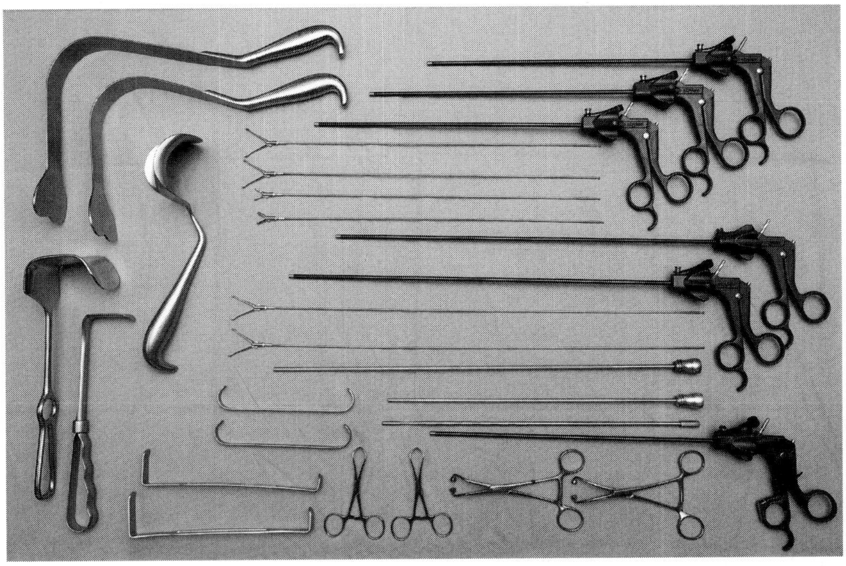

Figure 47–1. Basic equipment and instruments used for laparoscopic colon surgery.

used (other than the Hassan cannula) will depend on the procedure performed. A 5-mm or 10-mm laparoscope can also be used. The latest 5mm laparoscopes provide excellent illumination and view (although a slightly smaller field of view than the 10-mm laparoscope) and give the operator the option of moving the laparoscope to other positions without requiring larger 10-mm cannulas.

▪ PROCEDURES

LAPAROSCOPIC SMALL BOWEL RESECTION

Position

The patient is placed supine on the operating table. Both ankles are strapped to the table and a padded strap is placed across the patient's chest to prevent movement when the patient is tilted through steep angles during the procedure. A urinary catheter and a nasogastric tube are placed. The operator and assistant stand on the left side of the patient while the scrub nurse is on the patient's right. The television monitor is positioned on the side of the pathology (Fig 47–2). Maintaining an in-line alignment of the surgeons visual field, operating hands, ports and monitor ensures proper orientation of the field and elimination of reverse imaging.

Exploration

A 10- to 12-mm port is placed in the supraumbilical position using an open cutdown technique. The abdomen is then insufflated with CO_2 gas to 12 to 14 mm Hg pressure. A 30-degree laparoscope is passed through this port and the abdominal cavity assessed. Either a 5-mm or 10-mm laparoscope can be used; the size of the laparoscope will determine the size of subsequent cannulas. Placement of further ports will be determined by the site of pathology. This may already have been determined by preoperative imaging or by laparoscopic assessment. Typically a second port can be placed in the midline 2 cm above the pubic symphysis and a third port in the lower left quadrant (Fig 47–3). If the patient has had previous surgery then the operator should consider placing the first port at a distance from any previous incisions in addition to use of the open cutdown technique.

The patient should initially be positioned head down with a tilt toward the left side. An atraumatic bowel grasper should be placed through the two working ports. The ileocecal valve should be identified and then the

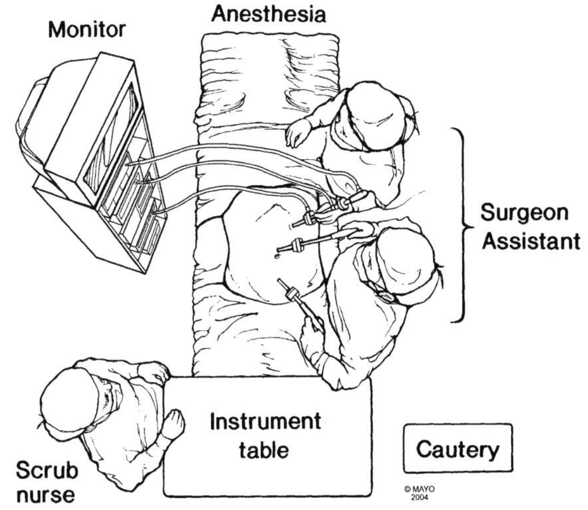

Figure 47–2. Position of equipment and the surgical team for laparoscopic small bowel resection or right hemicolectomy.

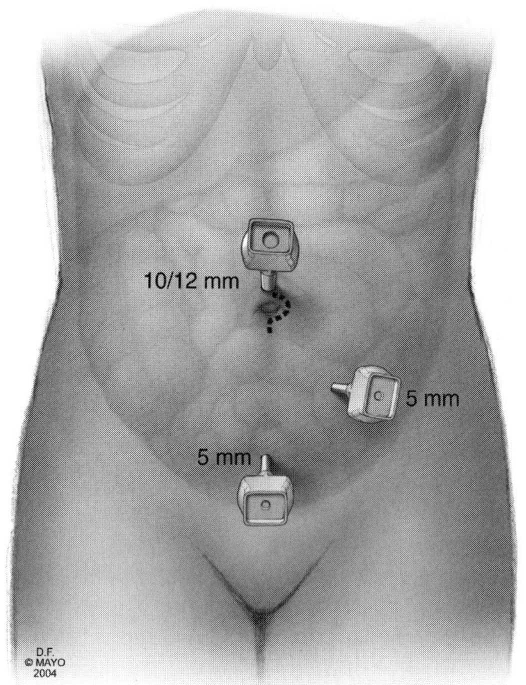

Figure 47–3. Position of laparoscope ports for small bowel resection.

small intestine can be assessed by "walking" along the bowel by passing it from grasper to grasper progressively working along the bowel to the ligament of Treitz. This can be helped by altering the position of the patient reducing the head-down tilt and then raising the head of the table as the proximal small bowel is reached.

Exteriorization, Resection, and Anastomosis

Once the area of diseased small bowel is defined, its mobility should be assessed. If the mesenteric length is sufficient then the supraumbilical port site can be extended inferiorly over a short distance, the bowel should be exteriorized and resection or strictureplasty performed using the method preferred by the operator for open procedures. In Crohn's disease the mesentery may be shortened and if resection is required then intracorporeal division of the vasculature may be required to allow exteriorization of the diseased segment of bowel. Upward tension is applied on the small bowel to display the mesenteric vessels, windows are created and the vessels are ligated with hemoclip, endoloops, or a linear vascular stapler.

The bowel is returned to the abdominal cavity following strictureplasty or resection. The fascia of the paraumbilical wound is closed. The peritoneal cavity is then re-insufflated so that it can be inspected with the laparoscope to exclude bleeding and washed with saline. The ports are then removed under vision of the laparoscope and all wounds are irrigated with sterile water. The skin is then closed.

LAPAROSCOPIC COLON AND RECTAL RESECTION

For each laparoscopic colonic procedure, a stepwise approach is followed with exploration, mobilization, vascular ligation, exteriorization, and anastomosis.

RIGHT HEMICOLECTOMY

Position

The patient is placed supine on the operating table. Both ankles are strapped to the table and a padded strap is placed across the patient's chest to prevent movement when the patient is tilted through steep angles during the procedure. A urinary catheter and a nasogastric tube are placed. The operator and assistant stand on the left side of the patient while the scrub nurse is on the patient's right. The television monitor is positioned opposite the operator on the right side of the patient (Fig 47–2).

Exploration

A 10- to 1-mm port is placed in the supraumbilical position using an open cutdown technique. The abdomen is then insufflated with CO_2 gas to 12 to 14 mm Hg pressure. A 30-degree camera is passed through this port then two 10-mm ports are then placed under direct vision, firstly in the left upper quadrant approximately one hands breadth from the umbilicus. The third port is then inserted in the midline supraumbilically (Fig 47–4).

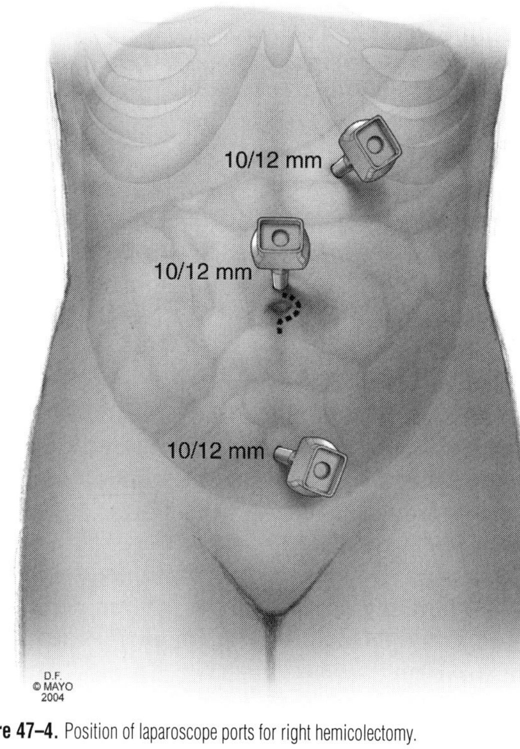

Figure 47–4. Position of laparoscope ports for right hemicolectomy.

If simple adhesions are encountered at this stage they should be divided. Then an inspection of the abdominal cavity should be performed to confirm the pathology for which surgery was indicated and to exclude other pathology. The liver is carefully inspected for metastatic disease and Babcock graspers can be used to raise each liver lobe so that all surfaces are viewed. The peritoneal surfaces should then be inspected to exclude metastases.

Mobilization of the Cecum (Fig 47–5)

Mobilization commences at the cecum. The laparoscope is moved to the left upper port. The patient is positioned in steep Trendelenburg with left side down. The pelvis is viewed to ensure that the small bowel has moved up and out of the pelvis into the abdominal cavity. If not then two graspers can be used to achieve this. If there are significant adhesions present in the pelvis, e.g., in Crohn's disease, this may not be possible and an early conversion to an open procedure is advised. If proceeding with a laparoscopic resection then it is important to identify the right ureter at the pelvic brim. The surgeon then applies traction to the tissues just lateral to the caecum. The peritoneum lateral to the colon is then incised along the white line of Toldt, with scissors attached to cautery placed through the supraumbilical port. Care should be taken to initially divide only the superficial layer of peritoneum. As the dissection proceeds toward the hepatic flexure, the pneumoperitoneum will help separate the tissue planes. The right colon is retracted toward the midline with the grasper, which is placed alongside the colon. The plane between the colon mesentery and Gerota's fascia is then developed using a combination of blunt dissection and cautery. This dissection is performed layer by layer proceeding from adjacent to the caecum toward the hepatic flexure.

To enable full mobilization of the right colon the peritoneum, which lies medial to the terminal ileum should be incised. The right ureter should be re-identified at the pelvic brim and the surgeon should be aware that it lies close behind the dissection at this point. Upward tension should be applied to the peritoneal fold medial to the terminal ileum and then careful use of cautery to incise just the superficial peritoneal layer along the pelvic brim superior and parallel to the right iliac artery. This dissection is continued up to the level of the duodenum. The lateral dissection is then advanced medially with care until the inferior vena cava caudally and the duodenum cranially are reached. These two structures indicate that the dissection has been performed as far medially as required. Once this is achieved then the area of dissection changes to mobilize the hepatic flexure.

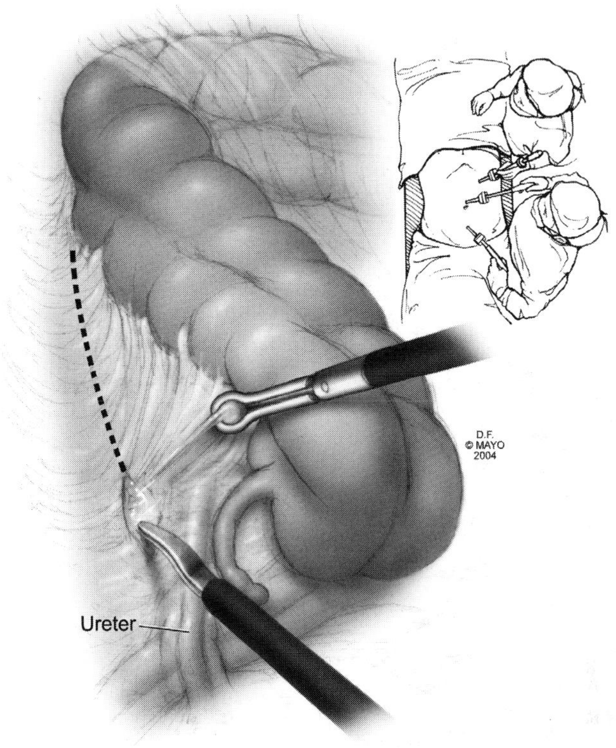

Figure 47–5. Mobilization of cecum.

Mobilization of the Hepatic Flexure (Fig 47–6)

A number of changes are required to perform this part of the procedure. The laparoscope is first moved to the lower trocar and the surgeon and assistant trade positions. The patient is now placed in reverse Trendelenburg with the left side still down. The operator changes his instrument position with a grasper through the supraumbilical port and the scissors and cautery through the left upper quadrant port. Then retraction on the colon is achieved by grasping the peritoneum just superior to the hepatic flexure inferior to the gall bladder and lifting toward the abdominal wall. A window is created by division of the superficial layer of the peritoneum at this site with the scissors. Blunt dissection is then performed to separate the underlying tissue from the peritoneum. Then the thin layer of peritoneum is lifted upward toward the abdominal wall and cauterized and divided with the scissors. Using this technique dissection then proceeds along lateral to the colon around the hepatic flexure to meet with the dissection achieved from the cecal direction. Care should be taken during this part of the dissection to not damage the duodenum. This lies superior to the initial part of the dissection and then passes medially. Careful application of the technique with gentle blunt dissection, then lifting of the peritoneum upwards to separate it from underlying tissue before cauterizing, will help ensure safety at this point.

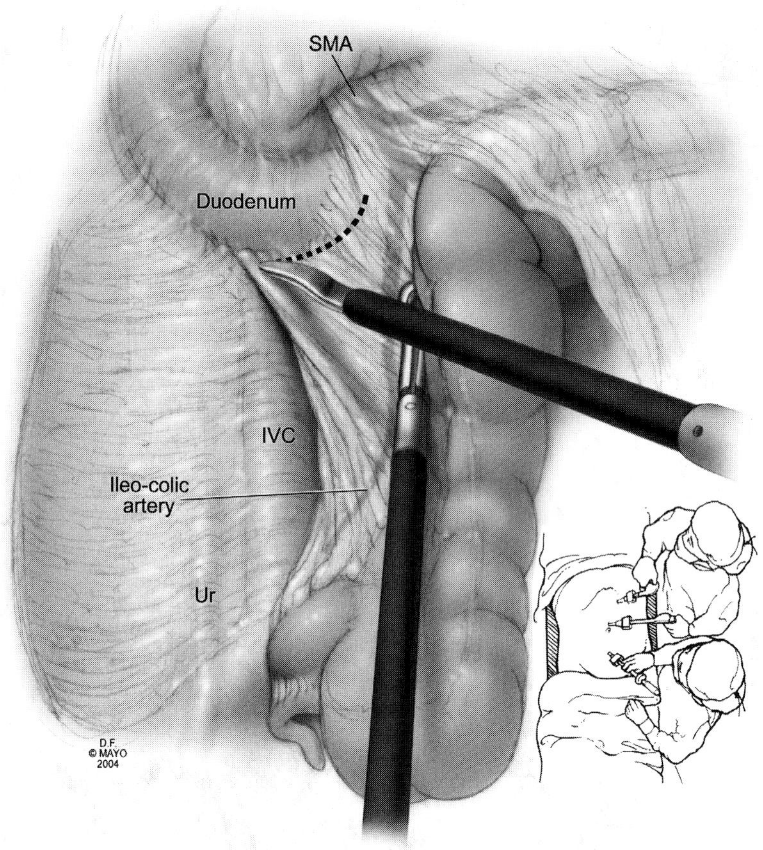

Figure 47–6. Mobilization of hepatic flexure.

Vascular Division and Exteriorization

Once sufficient mobilization is achieved, the mesenteric vessels of the section of colon to be resected should be divided. This can be performed by either intracorporeal or extracorporeal method. The intracorporeal method should be used for vascular division in malignant disease to ensure sufficiently proximal ligation of vessels. Upward tension is applied on the colon to display the ileocolic and right colic vessels. Mesenteric windows are created and the vessels are ligated with hemoclip, endoloops, or a linear vascular stapler (Fig 47–7). Once intracorporeal ligation has been completed or if extracorporeal ligation is to be performed. The patient is placed in a flat position. The camera and laparoscopic instruments are withdrawn and the gas supply turned off. The pneumoperitoneum is then released through the ports. The supraumbilical port is then removed and a 4cm vertical incision is made. The wound edges are protected with gauze or a wound guard then the bowel is exteriorized. The cecum is identified through this incision then the colon is delivered through the incision (Fig 47–8). It may be necessary to sweep the greater omentum medially and superiorly as it can fall across the distal ascending colon preventing delivery of this part of the colon. If required, extracorporeal ligation of the vasculature can then be performed in a standard manner.

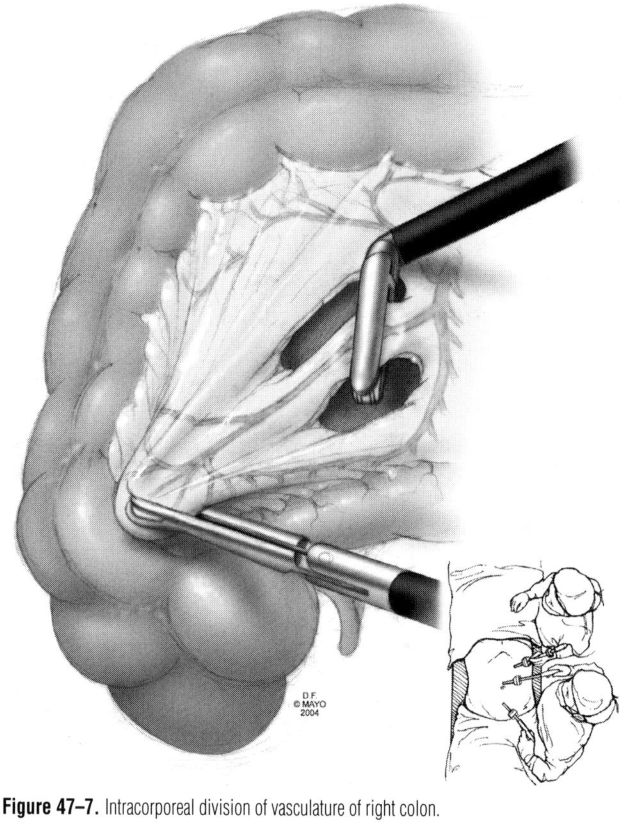

Figure 47–7. Intracorporeal division of vasculature of right colon.

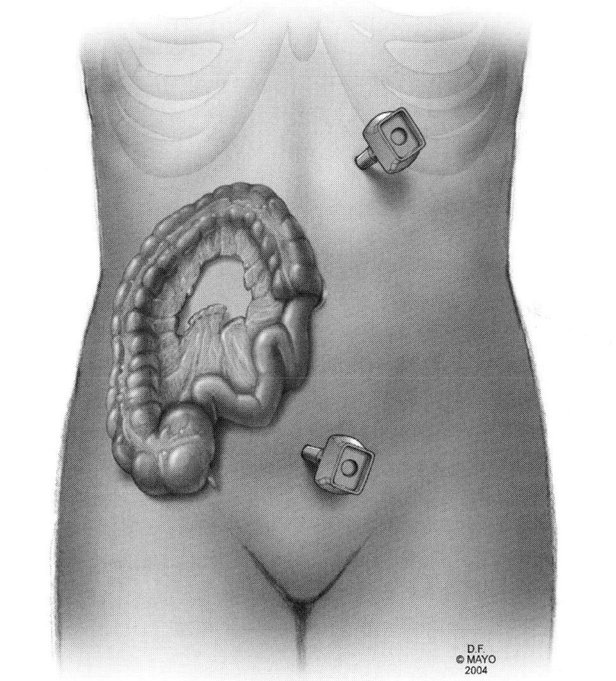

Figure 47–8. Exteriorization of right colon.

Anastomosis

Following exteriorization the bowel is resected with division of the terminal ileum and proximal transverse colon. Anastomosis is then performed with a standard stapled or hand sewn technique. The bowel is returned to the abdominal cavity. Copious irrigation of the peritoneal cavity is performed with inspection of the aspirate to ensure that this is not significantly blood stained indicating intraabdominal bleeding. The peritoneal cavity can then be inspected with the laparoscope to exclude bleeding and to wash out the peritoneal cavity. The ports are then removed under vision of the laparoscope. Copious irrigation of all wounds with sterile water is then performed. The incisions are closed in two layers, fascia and skin.

ALTERNATIVE TECHNIQUE FOR RIGHT HEMICOLECTOMY

An alternative placement of laparoscope ports can be used for right hemicolectomy. In this technique a 10-/12-mm port is initially placed in the supraumbilical position and following insufflation a 30-degree laparoscope is placed through this. Two 5-mm ports are then placed in the suprapubic and left lower quadrant positions (Fig 47–3). A grasper is placed through the left lower quadrant port and a scissors with cautery attached placed through the suprapubic port. Mobilization of the cecum and proximal ascending colon is then performed as described above. To mobilize the hepatic flexure the graspers are switched to the suprapubic port and the scissors with cautery attached are placed through the left lower quadrant port. The laparoscope remains in the supraumbilical port and is not moved unlike the previously described technique. It may be necessary to place a further 5-mm port in the right lower quadrant to allow use of a second grasper by the surgical assistant to provide countertraction during mobilization of the hepatic flexure.

This alternative technique for right hemicolectomy, avoids the need for port placement in the upper abdomen, which provides a cosmetic advantage. However there is less space for the surgeon and camera operator, particularly during mobilization of the hepatic flexure. This compromise may not suit some surgeons. The choice of technique will therefore depend on the preference of the surgeon.

LEFT HEMICOLECTOMY

Position

Resection of the left colon proceeds in a similar but mirror image to the right colon procedure. The patient is positioned in a modified lithotomy position with arms tucked to the side. The surgeon and assistant stand to the patient's right and the scrub nurse to the patient's left.

Exploration (Fig 47–9)

A four-port technique is used with ports in the supraumbilical position, midline suprapubic, right upper,

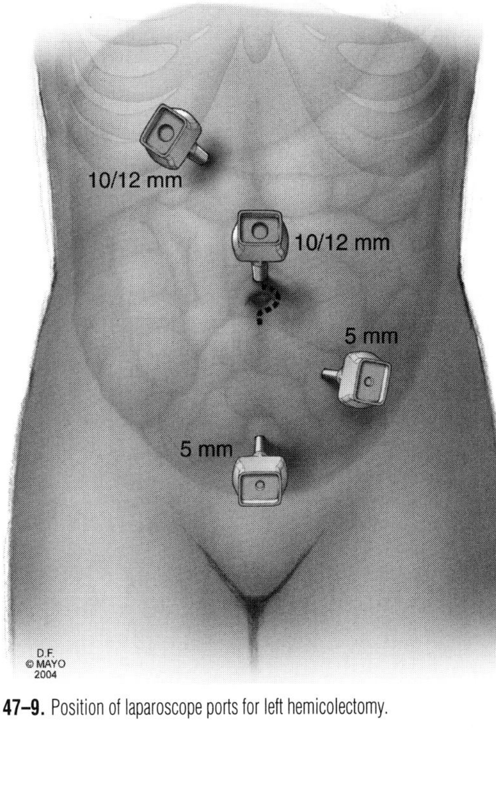

Figure 47–9. Position of laparoscope ports for left hemicolectomy.

and left lower quadrants. The laparoscope is inserted and careful assessment of the pathology and abdominal cavity is performed.

Mobilization of the Left Colon (Fig 47–10)

The patient is then placed in Trendelenburg with right side down and the small bowel is swept toward the right side of the abdominal cavity using a grasper. Dissection commences lateral to the proximal sigmoid colon. The peritoneum is grasped at this point and drawn medially with a grasper placed through the right lower quadrant port. The peritoneum is then incised to create a window using a scissors attached to cautery placed through the suprapubic port. The pneumoperitoneum will then start the dissection in this plane. The scissors can be used to extend the incision in the peritoneum in a caudal direction toward the splenic flexure along the white line of Toldt. The grasper is placed laterally along the colon with tips closed and used to retract the colon medially. The combination of this retraction and the use of scissors and cautery can be used to gradually separate the colon mesentery from Gerota's fascia. This dissection is extended towards the splenic flexure repeatedly returning to restart the dissection inferiorly so that the dissection moves further and further medially until the aorta is reached. Care should be taken with this dissection especially inferiorly to identify and protect the left ureter.

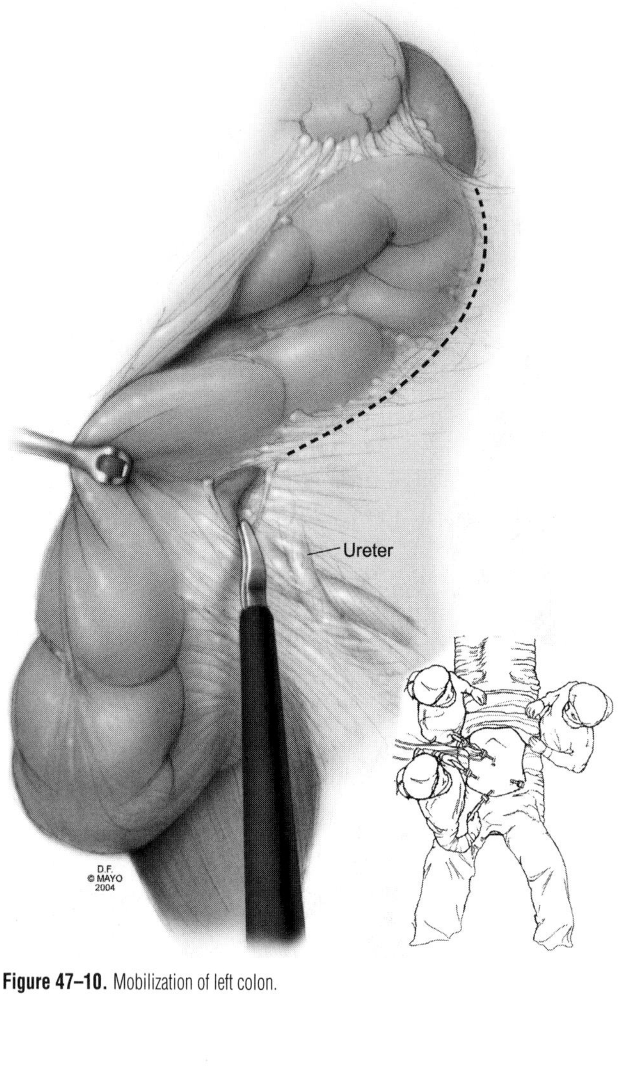

Figure 47–10. Mobilization of left colon.

Mobilization of the Splenic Flexure (Fig 47–11)

Once the lateral dissection has been performed to mobilize the left colon medially the dissection changes. The patient is placed in reverse Trendelenburg. The surgeon stands between the legs and repositions the instruments with the grasper through the suprapubic port and the scissors through the left lateral port. The assistant, standing on the patient's right, places a grasper through the right lateral port and grasps the greater omentum superior to the distal transverse colon and retracts upwards toward the abdominal wall and cranially. The surgeon applies countertraction to the assistant by grasping the peritoneum just superior to the colon and then creates a window by incising this peritoneum to enter the lesser sac. The dissection is then advanced parallel to the transverse colon to open up the lesser sac and mobilize the transverse colon. This dissection will then join up with the lateral dissection so that the splenic flexure is fully mobilized to the level of the umbilicus.

Vascular Division, Exteriorization, and Anastomosis

The vasculature of the left colon is then isolated and divided, the colon exteriorized through a midline incision and an anastomosis performed in an identical manner to that for the right colon.

SIGMOID COLECTOMY

Position

The patient is placed in a modified lithotomy position. The thighs are placed parallel to the abdomen so that they do not interfere with the movement of instruments. The surgeon and assistant stand on the right side of the patient.

Exploration (Fig 47–12)

A four-port technique is used with ports placed in the supraumbilical, suprapubic, right and left lower lateral positions. The laparoscope is placed through the supraumbilical port and inspection of the pathology and abdominal cavity performed.

Mobilization of the Proximal Sigmoid and Descending Colon

The patient is positioned in steep Trendelenburg with the right side down. The surgeon grasps the perito-

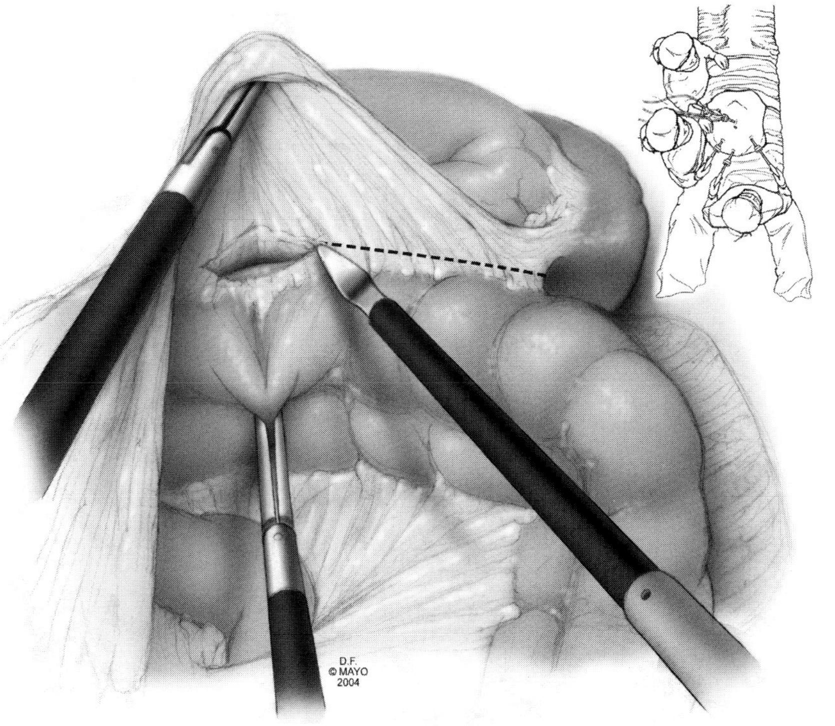

Figure 47–11. Mobilization of splenic flexure.

neum lateral to the sigmoid colon to put this on tension using a grasper passed through the right lateral port. The left ureter is identified at the pelvic brim. A scissors with cautery attached is then placed through the suprapubic port and dissection is then commenced lateral to the ureter by incising the peritoneum lateral to the sigmoid colon. The white line of Toldt is then followed up alongside the descending colon toward the splenic flexure using the same method used for a left hemicolectomy. Splenic flexure mobilization can also be performed if this is required.

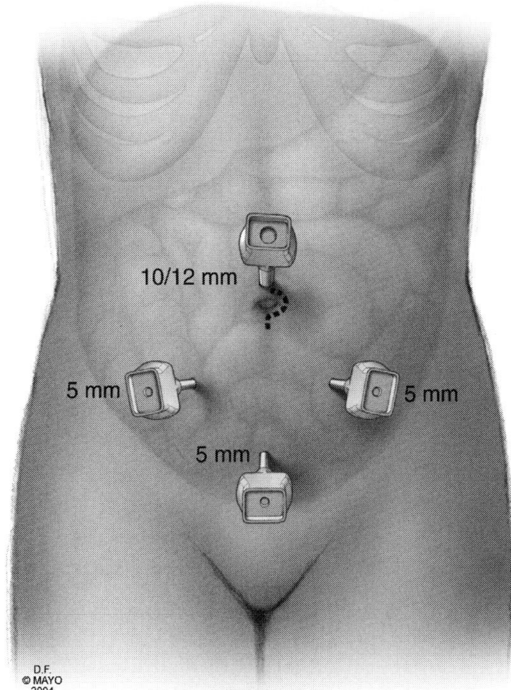

Figure 47–12. Position of laparoscope ports for sigmoid colectomy/high anterior resection.

Mobilization of the Distal Sigmoid Colon and Upper Rectum (Fig 47–13)

Mobilization is then directed caudally. The sigmoid colon is retracted cephalad and to the patient's right. The peritoneal incision is then extended distally to the midrectum entering the presacral space. Care is taken to identify and protect the left ureter and iliac vessel throughout this part of the procedure. The presacral space is developed by division of fine adhesions ensuring that the hypogastric nerves are protected and swept backwards toward the sacrum. The sigmoid colon is then retracted to the left and the right peritoneum is incised opening the presacral space from the right. This is then developed to link up with the dissection from the left side.

Vascular Ligation and Exteriorization

Ligation of the vascular pedicle is now performed. The sigmoid colon is elevated anteriorly and inferiorly to expose the mesenteric vessels, including the superior hemorrhoidal artery and the branches of the sigmoid

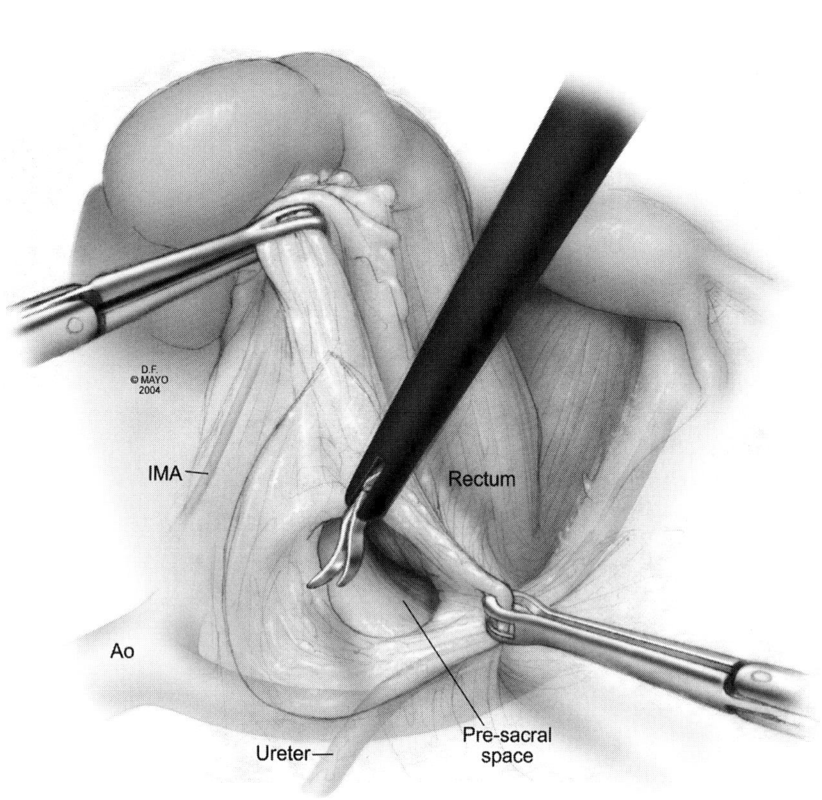

Figure 47–13. Mobilization of upper rectum.

artery. These are isolated by creating windows in the mesentery alongside the vessels. The vessels are then ligated with clips, endovascular staplers, or endoloops, and then divided.

The mobilization of the rectum is then completed by dissecting the mesentery from the upper rectum. The upper rectum is then divided using a linear cutting stapler (Fig 47–14). The mesorectum is then divided using the linear cutting stapler, harmonic scalpel, or clips. The pneumoperitoneum is then vented via the laparoscope ports. The divided proximal colon is then brought out through a low midline or Pfannenstiel incision. If the procedure is being performed for cancer, then a wound protector should be used.

Anastomosis (Fig 47–15)

The point of division of the proximal colon is defined and this is divided. A purse string is inserted and then tied around the anvil of a staple gun inserted into the lumen of the colon. This is then returned to the abdominal cavity and the fascia of the wound closed. The pneumoperitoneum is then reformed with insufflation. The shaft of the circular stapler is inserted through the anus and the spike advanced through the cross-stapled end of the proximal rectum under direct vision. The anvil is attached to the gun, which is closed and fired. The anastomotic integrity can then be assessed using a proctoscope. The pneumoperitoneum is released via the ports which are then withdrawn and the skin and fascia closed.

Rectal Resection

Resection of the rectum requires the same patient positioning and the same steps used for sigmoid colectomy, including exploration, mobilization of the proximal colon, and vascular division. The extent of proximal colonic mobilization and vascular division will depend on the indication for surgery. The following provides a description of the technique required for laparoscopic rectal resection.

Mobilization of the Rectum

Following mobilization of the distal sigmoid colon the dissection is extended into the pelvis. The patient is placed in steep Trendelenburg with a neutral left to right position. The surgeon stands on the patient's left and the assistant retracts the rectum toward the patient's right. The surgeon uses a grasper to achieve counter traction and cautery scissors are used to advance the dissection distally. The peritoneum adjacent to the rectum is incised to the peritoneal reflection. Care is taken to identify and protect the left ureter and iliac vessel throughout this part of the procedure. The presacral space is developed by division of fine adhesions to the pelvic floor, in a similar way to an open TME procedure, ensuring that the hypogastric nerves are protected and swept backwards towards the sacrum. Care should be taken to avoid penetration of the mesorectal fascia medially and damage to the pelvic nerves laterally. The peritoneum anterior to the rectum is then incised at the point

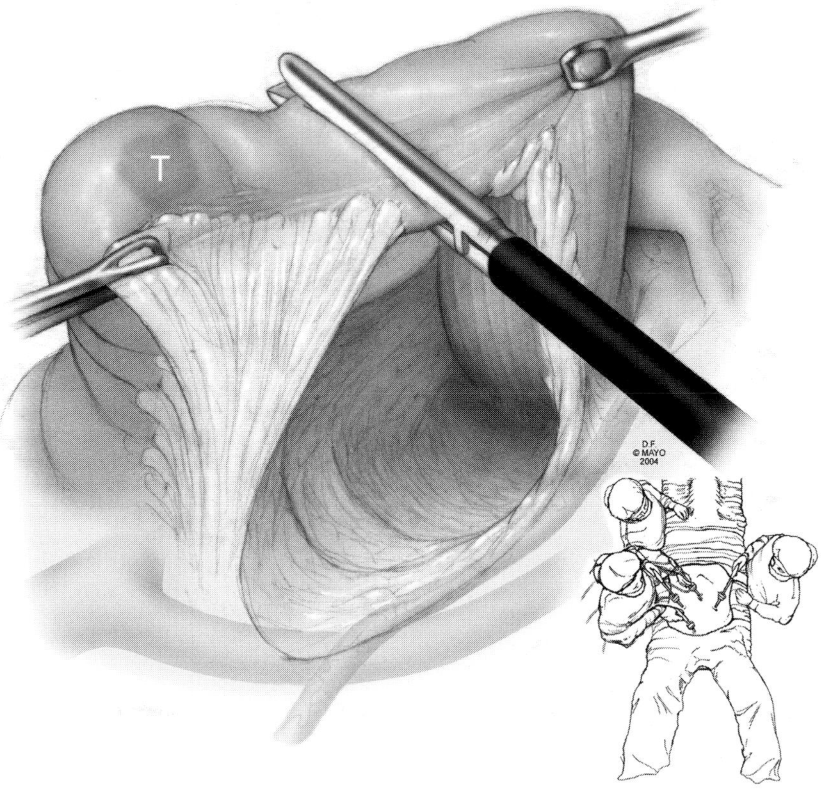

Figure 47–14. Division of upper rectum with linear stapler.

of the peritoneal reflection. The anterior rectal dissection is then performed with care not to stray out of the mesorectal plane into the seminal vesicles and prostate or vagina anteriorly. Using the combination of traction and countertraction dissection is advanced to the levators so that the rectum is fully mobilized.

Rectal Excision

Once the rectum is fully mobilized the method of exteriorization of the rectal specimen is dependent on the indication for surgery. If anastomosis is planned then the point of division of the rectum is defined and a double-stapled anastomosis is then performed (using the same method used for sigmoid colectomy) using a linear cutting staple gun to divide the rectum and then a circular stapling device to perform the anastomosis. Alternatively, if complete proctectomy is planned with excision of the anus, then once the rectum is fully mobilized to the pelvic floor the pneumoperitoneum is vented through the laparoscopic ports and the perineal dissection is performed using a standard method. Once this is complete, the rectal specimen is delivered through the perineal wound.

The wound is then closed and the abdominal cavity is insufflated. The pelvis is carefully irrigated with saline and hemostasis ensured, then a drain can is placed in the pelvis and the proximal bowel brought up to skin to form a stoma.

Laparoscopic Restorative Proctocolectomy

The patient is positioned in the synchronous position with a chest strap and a nasogastric tube and urethral catheter are placed. The rectum is then washed out with diluted povidone-iodine (Betadine). The patient is marked preoperatively for a right lower quadrant stoma.

LAPAROSCOPIC ASSISTED TECHNIQUE

Position

The surgeon and assistant stand on the patient's right side. If a defunctioning loop ileostomy is planned then the skin and subcutaneous tissue should be excised. A purse string suture is placed in the fascia and a 10-mm cannula is inserted through the stoma site using the Hassan technique. Using a reducer a 5-mm 30-degree laparoscope is placed through this port. A 5-mm port is then placed in the supraumbilical position, the laparoscope is moved to this position then two 5-mm ports are then placed in the suprapubic and left lower quadrant.

Mobilization of the Colon

The colon is mobilized sequentially starting with the left colon followed by the right colon and then the sigmoid colon as previously described.

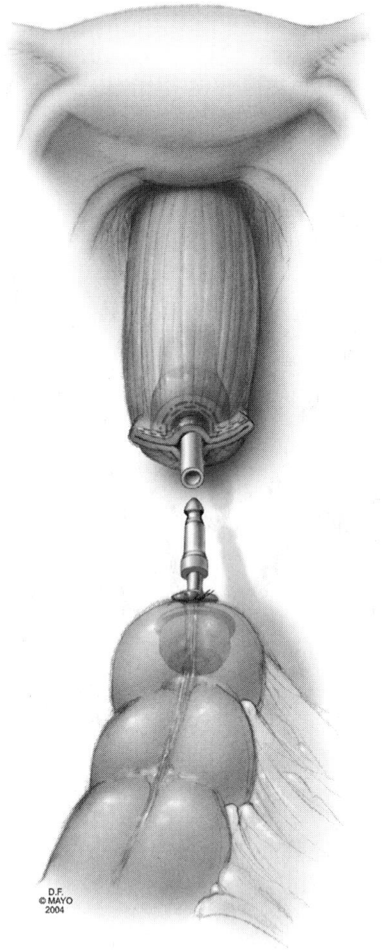

Figure 47–15. Colorectal anastomosis.

Mobilization of the Rectum and Division of the Rectum

The focus for the procedure then moves to the pelvis following full mobilization of the colon. The rectum is fully mobilized to the pelvic floor as previously described. The rectum is then divided at the pelvic floor using an endo-GIA linear cutting staple gun.

Exteriorization of the Colon and Rectum and Division of the Vasculature

The pneumoperitoneum is then vented and the supraumbilical port incision is extended for 4 to 6 cm inferiorly. The colon is delivered through this wound and the vascular pedicels ligated and divided using a standard open technique.

Formation of the Ileoanal Pouch, Anastomosis, and Formation of Loop Ileostomy

The terminal ileum is divided using a 55-mm linear cutting staple device. A J-pouch is then fashioned using a standard open technique. The pouch with the anvil of the circular staple gun in place, is put back into the abdominal cavity and the midline wound is closed. The pneumoperitoneum is then restored and the laparoscope reinserted. A circular stapling device is inserted into the anus and the pin advanced under vision (Fig 47–16). The anvil of the gun is then attached using a specially designed laparoscopic instrument ensuring that the pouch and its mesentery is lying in the correct orientation and is not twisted. The gun is then tightened and fired. Anastomotic integrity is then confirmed, and if desired, the proximal ileum can be grasped via the right lower quadrant port and brought up to skin to form a defunctioning loop ileostomy, ensuring that the orientation is clearly defined. A pelvic drain can then be placed through the suprapubic port. The pneumoperitoneum is then vented through the laparoscope port. The skin is then closed and the ileostomy matured.

ALTERNATIVE TECHNIQUES FOR RESTORATIVE PROCTOCOLECTOMY

Laparoscopic Colonic Mobilization with Open Proctectomy and Pouch Formation

Following laparoscopic colonic mobilization a small suprapubic incision (midline or Pfannenstiel) can be

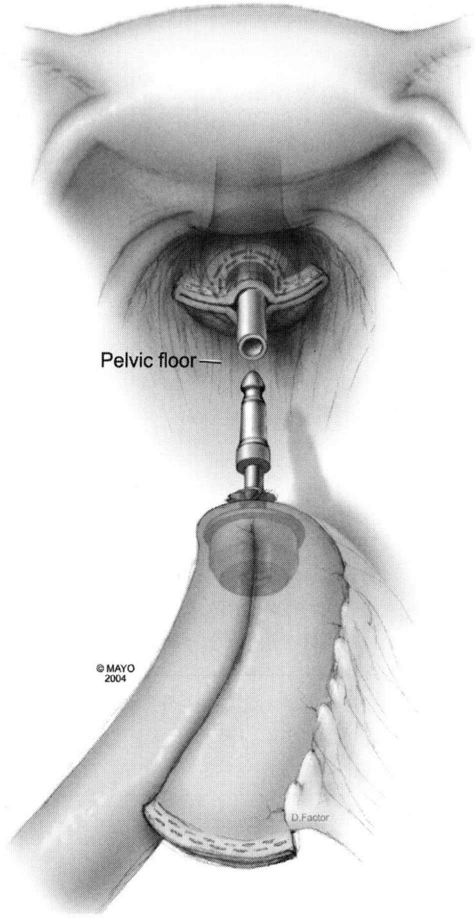

Figure 47–16. J-pouch anal anastomosis.

made to allow open rectal mobilization, proctectomy and formation of the J-pouch. It is necessary to perform intracorporeal division of the colonic vasculature using this approach. This should be performed following full colonic mobilization and can be achieved with a vascular stapling device or ligation device, e.g., LigaSure.

This approach has two main advantages. These include placement of the incision low on the abdominal wall which produces a better cosmetic result. The second advantage is that rectal mobilization and resection can be performed using an open method avoiding the requirement for laparoscopic rectal mobilization, which is technically more demanding.

Hand-Assisted Colonic Mobilization and Open Proctectomy and Pouch Formation

In this approach a hand port is placed through a low midline or Pfannenstiel incision at the start of the procedure. The colon is fully mobilized using the hand to retract the colon starting with the left, proceeding to the transverse and then the right colon and the vasculature is then divided intracorporeally. Following this the pneumoperitoneum is vented and then the rectal mobilization, excision and formation of the J-pouch are performed as open procedures through the hand port incision.

This approach is similar to the previously mentioned method but it may be quicker to mobilize the colon and divide the vasculature using hand assistance, although this will depend on operator preference and experience.

HAND-ASSISTED LAPAROSCOPIC COLORECTAL SURGERY

Hand-assisted laparoscopic surgery is a relatively new technique. It uses the advantages of laparoscopic surgery but allows use of the operator's hand to provide retraction. This technique is most useful for resection of the left and sigmoid colon. It provides the greatest advantage in subtotal colectomy where improved retraction can reduce the operating time although this is at the expense of a slightly larger incision than conventional laparoscopic-assisted colonic surgery.

HAND-ASSISTED LAPAROSCOPIC TECHNIQUE

Position and Insertion of Hand Port (Fig 47–17)

The patient is prepared as for a laparoscope-assisted procedure. For left, sigmoid and subtotal colectomy, the patient is placed in a modified lithotomy position. The thighs are placed parallel to the abdomen so that they do not interfere with the movement of instruments.

The hand port is placed in the lower abdomen either through a lower midline incision or a Pfannenstiel

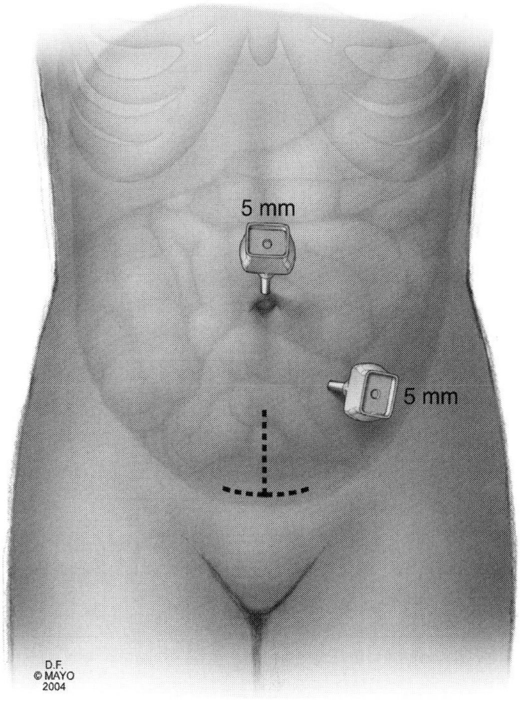

Figure 47–17. Position of incision for hand port and laparoscope ports for left colectomy or sigmoid colectomy.

incision placed 1 cm above the symphysis pubis. The incision size should be carefully measured and should be at least one half size smaller than the operator's hand. This incision is then extended through the abdominal wall and it is important to ensure that the wound length remains the same through all layers of the abdominal wall. This avoids leakage of air around the hand port. Insufflation of the abdominal cavity can then be achieved using a 5-mm canula placed under guidance from the operator's hand thorough the hand port. Once this is achieved the operator places a lubricated hand through the hand port (Fig 47–18) and uses this to guide insertion of a cannula in the supraumbilical skin. This should be 5- or 10-mm, dependent on the size of laparoscope to be used. A 30-degree laparoscope is then positioned through this cannula and a further 5-mm cannula is then placed in the left lower quadrant. A scissors with cautery attached is placed through this.

Colonic Mobilization (Fig 47–19)

The colon mobilized in the same manner as previously described except that traction is achieved by the operator's left hand. If splenic mobilization is necessary then assistance can be provided with mobilization of the splenic flexure using a grasper placed through a 5-mm cannula in the right lower quadrant, if required. If a subtotal or proctocolectomy is planned then once the splenic flexure is fully mobilized then the surgeon

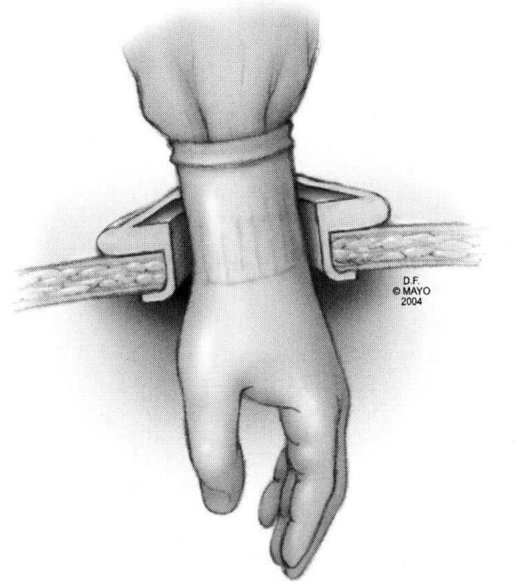

Figure 47–18. Position of hand following insertion through hand port.

progresses along the transverse colon towards the hepatic flexure, mobilizing the colon from the greater omentum. Right colon mobilization is then performed with a scissors placed through a right lower quadrant cannula (placed through the site of a defunctioning ileostomy if planned) and retraction using the operator's right hand.

Vascular Division

Once the colon is completely mobilized, the surgeon the starts division of the vasculature on the left side. Intracorporeal vascular division is performed, using a vascular stapling device or LigaSure device placed through the left lower quadrant port and used to divide the vasculature by moving progressively along the colonic mesentery to the point of colonic division. If a sigmoid resection is planned, extracorporeal division of the vasculature can be performed if the colon is sufficiently mobilized and a lower midline hand port incision is used.

Exteriorization and Anastomosis

Once the colon is fully mobilized then the colon can be exteriorized via the hand port, divided and then anastomosed using the operator's preferred technique.

Rectal Dissection and Formation of an Ileoanal Pouch

If a proctocolectomy is planned, the colon is fully mobilized and the vasculature divided and then the hand port can be removed. The rectum can then be mobilized to the pelvic floor using a standard open technique. This can then be stapled and divided. The rectum and colon is then delivered through the wound and the terminal ileum divided using a linear staple cutter. A J-pouch is then fashioned and anastomosed to the anus with circular staple gun passed through the anus. If a defunctioning loop ileostomy is planned, a loop of proximal ileum is passed through the right lower quadrant trephine, ensuring that the orientation is correct. A drain is placed into the pelvis through the left lower quadrant port.

Wound Closure

A check for hemostasis is made, then the hand port incision is closed with a sutured mass closure of deep layers and subcuticular absorbable suture to the skin and to the supraumbilical port site.

POSTPROCEDURE CARE FOLLOWING HAND-ASSISTED COLORECTAL SURGERY

Patients undergoing hand-assisted colorectal procedures have a similar post procedure recovery to those patients undergoing total laparoscopic-assisted proce-

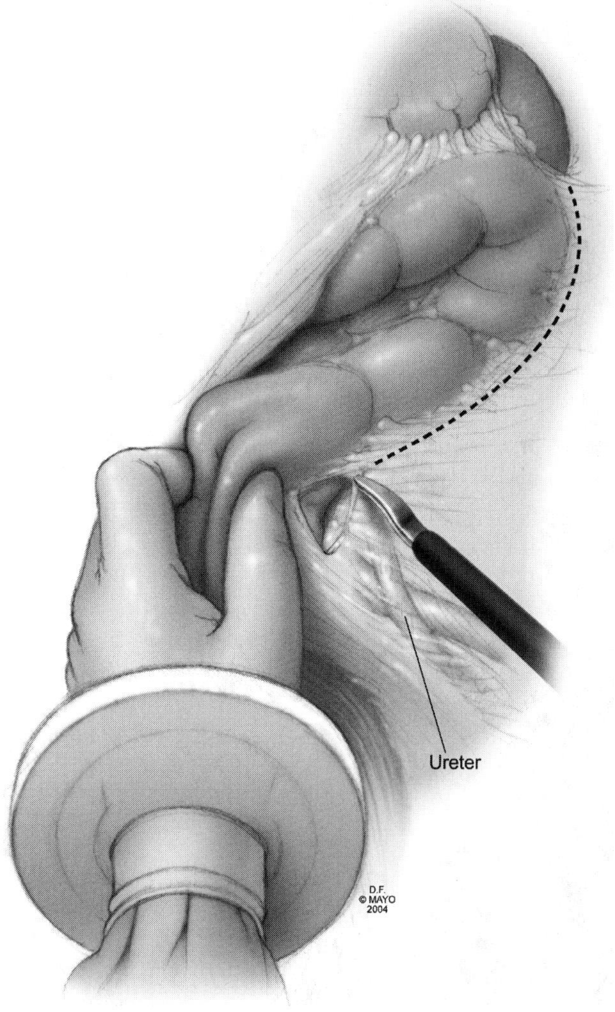

Figure 47–19. Hand-assisted mobilization of left colon.

dures. Consequently the postprocedure care should follow the same pathway as that for total laparoscopic-assisted procedures.

REFERENCES

1. Jacobs M, Verdeja JC, Goldstein HS: Minimally invasive colon resection (laparoscopic resection) *Surg Lap Endosc* 1991;1:144–150
2. Chung CC, Tsang WWC, Kwok SY, et al. Laparoscopy and its current role in the management of colorectal disease. *Colorectal Dis* 2003;5:528–543
3. Young-Fadok TM, HallLong K, McConnell EJ, et al. Advantages of laparoscopic resection for ileocolic Crohn's disease. Improved outcomes and reduced costs. *Surg Endosc* 2001;15(5):450–454
4. Delaney CP, Kiran RP, Senagore AJ, et al. Case-Matched comparison of clinical and financial outcome after laparoscopic or open colorectal surgery. *Ann Surg* 2003; 238:67–72
5. Duepree HJ, Senagore AJ, Delaney CP, et al. Does means of access affect the incidence of small bowel obstruction and ventral hernia after bowel resection? Laparoscopy versus laparotomy. *J Am Coll Surg* 2003;197(2):177–181
6. Berends FJ, Kazemier G, Bonjer HJ, et al. Subcutaneous metastases after laparoscopic colectomy (letter). *Lancet* 1994;344:58
7. Milsom JW, Bohm B, Hammerhofer KA, et al. A prospective randomised trial comparing laparoscopic versus conventional techniques in colorectal cancer surgery: a preliminary report. *J Am Coll Surg* 1998;187:46–54
8. Lacy AM, Garcia-Valdecasas JC, Delgado S, et al. Laparoscopy-assisted colectomy versus open colectomy for the treatment of non-metastatic colon cancer: a randomised trial. *Lancet* 2002;359:2224–2229
9. The Clinical Outcomes of Surgical Therapy Study Group. A comparison of laparoscopically assisted and open coleotomy for colon cancer. *N Engl J Med* 2004; 350:2050–2059
10. Senagore AJ, Delaney CP, Madboulay K, et al. Laparoscopic colectomy in obese and non obese patients. *J Gastrointest Surg* 2003;7:558–561
11. ASCRS Practice Parameters for the Treatment of Sigmoid Diverticulitis. March 2000
12. Stead ML, Brown JM, Bosanquet N, et al. Assessing the relative costs of standard open surgery and laparoscopic surgery in colorectal cancer in a randomised controlled trial in the United Kingdom. *Crit Rev Oncol Hematol* 2000;33:99–103
13. The COLOR Study Group, Hazebroek EJ. A randomised clinical trial comparing laparoscopic and open resection for colon cancer. *Surg Endosc* 2002;16:949–953
14. Schlachta CM, Mamazza J, Seshadri PA, et al. Defining a learning curve for laparoscopic colorectal resections. *Dis Colon Rectum* 2001;44:217–222
15. Milsom JW, Bohm B, Hammerhofer KA, et al. A prospective randomised trial comparing laparoscopic versus conventional techniques in colorectal cancer surgery: a preliminary report. *J Am Coll Surg* 1998;187:46–54

48

Hiatal Hernia Repair and Heller Myotomy

Ashley Haralson Vernon ■ *John G. Hunter*

■ HIATAL HERNIA

Giant hiatal hernias comprise only 5% of hernias at the diaphragmatic hiatus and are characterized by a portion of the stomach "rolling" into the chest next to the esophagus. Over the years, the descriptors that have been used for this complex anatomic problem have confused many. In 1926, Ake Akerlund named and classified hiatal hernias into three types: (1) hiatal hernia with a shortened esophagus, (2) paraesophageal hernia, and (3) hernias not included in these first two categories.[1] Later, in the 1950s, Allison classified hiatal hernias into two types: the sliding hernia and the paraesophageal or rolling hernia.[2] The configuration of the stomach within the hernia sac often has been described in terms of whether a gastric volvulus exists and whether the rotation is organoaxial or not.

More recently, hiatal hernias have been classified into four types. In type I hernias, the gastroesophageal junction "slides" into the mediastinum, pulling the stomach behind it (Fig 48–1). The majority (95%) of hiatal hernias are type I hernias. They are common and may be asymptomatic or may be associated with symptoms of gastroesophageal reflux disease (GERD). The indication for surgical repair of type I hernias depends on the severity of the symptoms and the ability to manage symptoms and/or esophageal damage with medical therapy (see Chapter 8A). In type II hernias, the gastroesophageal junction resides in the abdomen, and a portion of the gastric fundus slides into the mediastinum adjacent to the esophagus (Fig 48–2). This type of hiatal hernia is very rare, comprising fewer that 1% of all hernias. The type III hernia, the most common giant hiatal hernia, is characterized by the presence of the stomach and the gastroesophageal junction in the mediastinum (Fig 48–3). The type IV hiatal hernia is a more extensive type III hernia with other abdominal organs, such as colon, spleen, or liver, located within the chest. Another rare hiatal hernia is the parahiatal hernia, in which the stomach herniates through a small defect in the diaphragm, adjacent to the left crus of the diaphragm, anteriorly (Fig 48–4).

Hiatal hernia types II, III, and IV usually are referred to as *paraesophageal hernias.* This nomenclature may be confusing because it suggests that type II hernias come from type I hernias and lead to type III and IV hernias. This is untrue, and in fact, the natural history of hiatal hernia suggests that type III hernias evolve from type I hernias, explaining why type III hernias are much more common than type II hernias.

A simplified nomenclature suggests that we describe hiatal hernias as *giant* when they are more than 5 cm in either dimension, saving the term *paraesophageal hernia* for the rare type II hernia. Giant hernias may contain the stomach in a sliding (type I) or a rolling fashion (type III). When the majority of the stomach is in the hernia sac, this should be characterized as an intrathoracic or "upside down" stomach. The term *gastric volvulus* should be dropped because the appearance of the stomach within the sac changes with the position of the patient and because the intrathoracic stomach does not require urgent detorsion, as might be implied by the use of the term *volvulus.*

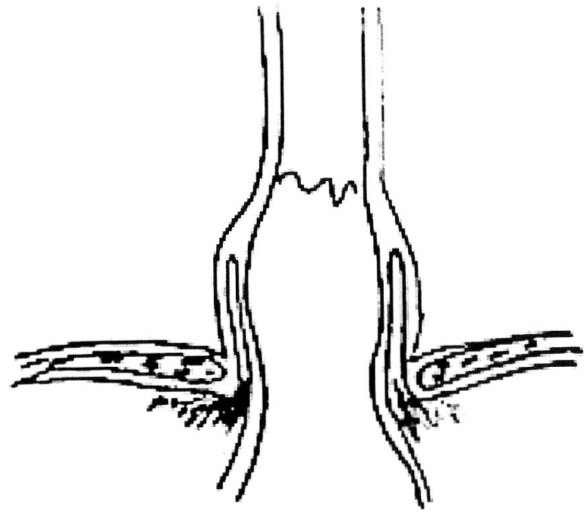

Figure 48–1. Type I "sliding" hernia. The gastroesophageal junction "slides" into the mediastinum, pulling the stomach behind it. (Reprinted with permission from Trus TL, Bax T, Richardson WS, et al. Complications of laparoscopic paraesophageal hernia repair. *J Gastrointest Surg* 1997;1:221–228.)

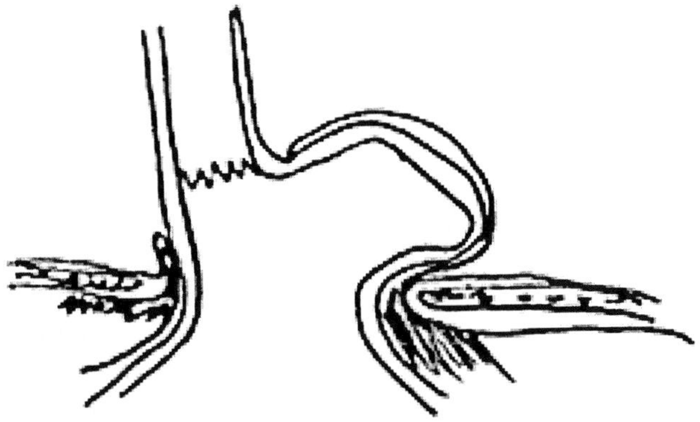

Figure 48–3. Type III "mixed paraesophageal" hernia. The stomach and the gastroesophageal junction are in the mediastinum. (Reprinted with permission from Trus TL, Bax T, Richardson WS, et al. Complications of laparoscopic paraesophageal hernia repair. *J Gastrointest Surg* 1997;1:221–228.)

NATURAL HISTORY AND PRESENTATION

As stated previously, most hiatal hernias are asymptomatic and only require surgical repair to manage symptoms of GERD. As hiatal hernias enlarge, symptoms related to the volume of stomach in the hernia sac begin to emerge. These symptoms include postprandial chest pain or pressure (often relieved by belching), dysphagia, shortness of breath resulting from gastric displacement of lung volume, and more severe GERD symptoms. If the herniated stomach rolls acutely, gastric inlet or outlet obstruction may lead to intermittent vomiting or complete foregut obstruction. Unique to the giant hernia is iron-deficiency anemia, which may be occult in nature or may be associated with gastric erosions or ulceration on the greater curvature at the point where the stomach traverses the crural opening. These ulcers, called *Cameron's ulcers,* are the result of stasis of intraluminal food, mechanical trauma, and gastric acid hypersecretion in the herniated stomach. These ulcers generally heal with proton pump inhibitors and should be treated aggressively before operative repair. The response of iron-deficiency anemia to hiatal hernia repair is dramatic, even in the absence of erosions or ulcers detected endoscopically.[3,4]

Rarely, giant hiatal hernias may result in a surgical catastrophe from incarceration or strangulation of the herniated stomach. Upper gastrointestinal bleeding and foregut obstruction are the usual associated presenting signs. Treatment of this condition requires vigorous resuscitation and urgent laparotomy.

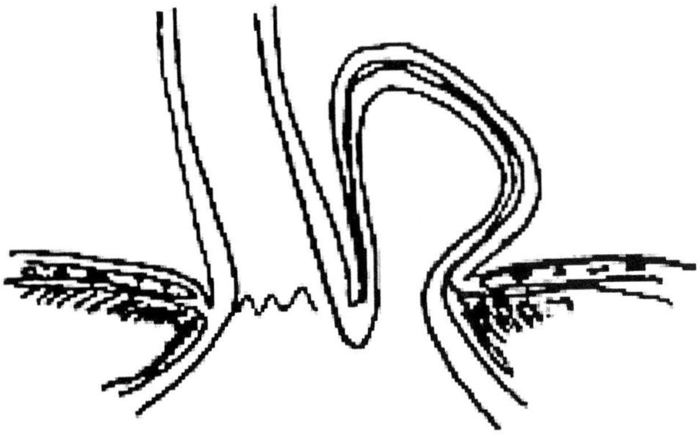

Figure 48–2. Type II "true paraesophageal" hernia. The gastroesophageal junction resides in the abdomen, and a portion of the gastric fundus slides into the mediastinum adjacent to the esophagus. (Reprinted with permission from Trus TL, Bax T, Richardson WS, et al. Complications of laparoscopic paraesophageal hernia repair. *J Gastrointest Surg* 1997;1:221–228.)

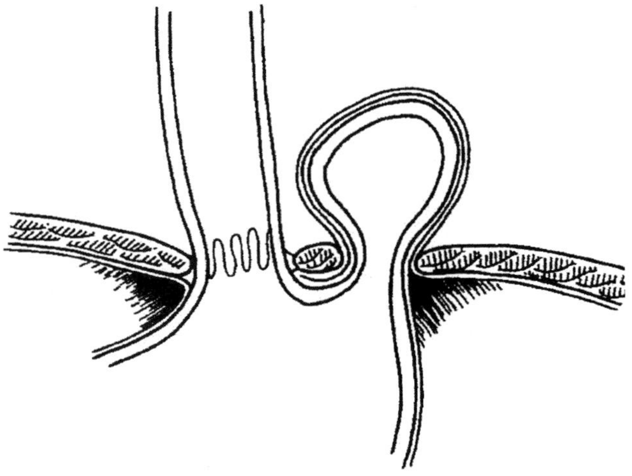

Figure 48–4. Parahiatal hernia. The stomach herniates through a small defect in the diaphragm, adjacent to the crus of the diaphragm. (Reprinted with permission from Trus TL, Bax T, Richardson WS, et al. Complications of laparoscopic paraesophageal hernia repair. *J Gastrointest Surg* 1997;1:221–228.)

Partial gastrectomy and reconstruction frequently are necessary. Mortality from this emergency presentation exceeds 20%.

INDICATIONS FOR SURGERY

Most patients with giant hiatal hernias are intermittently symptomatic, manifested by the symptoms mentioned earlier. These patients should undergo elective repair of the hiatal hernia by a laparoscopic approach if there is no contraindication. Occasionally, one encounters a patient with a giant hiatal hernia who is truly asymptomatic. While the classic teaching has been that these patients should undergo repair to avoid the risk of strangulation, the rarity of this event, combined with the known mortality of elective repair (1–2%), has led some to recommend that completely asymptomatic patients without iron-deficiency anemia be treated with watchful waiting.[5]

PATIENT PREPARATION

While patient preparation is predicated on the history and physical examination, many patients with large hiatal hernias need a broader preoperative evaluation than patients with GERD alone because of the increasing age and more frequent cardiopulmonary symptoms in the population with giant hiatal hernia. Patients with a history of shortness of breath and impaired exercise tolerance will need a preoperative consultation with a pulmonologist and pulmonary function tests. Patients with severe carbon dioxide retention can be difficult to manage intraoperatively, and one should consider using an alternative insufflating agent, such as nitrous oxide, or modifying the anesthetic technique if CO_2 is to be used.[6] When using CO_2 for creation of the pneumoperitoneum, the anesthesiologist can reduce CO_2 retention by increasing minute ventilation, and the surgeon can decrease the level of CO_2 absorption by decreasing the pneumoperitoneum pressure from 15 to10 mmHg or as necessary if carbon dioxide levels rise intraoperatively.

Mandatory preoperative evaluation includes barium swallow and endoscopy. Esophageal motility study confirms the presence of normal esophageal peristalsis. Some surgeons believe that this study may be omitted because the presence of occult motility disorders is rare in this population.[7] A 24-hour pH study is rarely necessary because the indication for repair is the presence of a symptomatic hernia and does not require proof of esophageal acid exposure.

SURGICAL MANAGEMENT

The salient features of the procedure include reduction of the hernia, excision of the hernia sac, closure of the hiatal defect, establishment of adequate intra-abdominal esophageal length, and fundoplication. We perform an antireflux procedure in most patients even if the patients do not complain of reflux symptoms preoperatively. The logic for this approach is as follows: Intraesophageal acid exposure frequently is present in type III hernias despite the absence of symptoms.[7] Over 60% of patients with type III hernias have been reported to have a hypotensive lower esophageal sphincter and abnormal 24-hour pH monitoring, and 20% of patients will have reflux symptoms postoperatively when an antireflux procedure is not performed.[8] Additionally, a fundoplication may help to maintain the gastroesophageal junction within the abdomen, especially as the hiatal repair weakens. The gastroesophageal junction can be returned to the appropriate location within the abdomen in most cases, although some will require extensive esophageal mobilization.[9] Sometimes the esophagus is shortened, and mobilization alone will not provide adequate length to return the gastroesophageal junction to the abdomen. In these cases, a surgical esophageal lengthening procedure, a Collis gastroplasty, is required.[10]

Description of Procedure

The patient is placed in the supine position on a split-leg table with the legs abducted to a 45-degree angle at the hip. Although not usually an issue with thin patients, footplates are used to secure the patient on the table and prevent sliding because most of the procedure is performed with the patient in the reverse Trendelenburg position. The arms may remain out on armboards.

A Foley catheter and orogastric tube are placed. The orogastric tube sometimes is difficult to pass. If obstruction is encountered, placement of the tube should not be forced. Instead, it is appropriate to wait until the contents of the sac have been reduced before attempting to pass it again. It usually will be necessary to decompress the stomach of air prior to taking down the short gastric vessels and creating the retrogastric window. A liver retractor is used to elevate the left lobe of the liver off the hiatus. Liver retraction can be achieved with a 5-mm "endoflex" articulated retractor attached to a flexible retractor arm ("snake") mounted to the Bookwalter post on the right side of the table. An alternative is to use the Nathanson retractor attached to the Bookwalter post on the patient's side. Advanced laparoscopic instruments are needed, including atraumatic bowel graspers such as Hunter graspers (Jarit Surgical Instruments, Hawthorne, NY), laparoscopic Metzenbaum scissors, and needle drivers.

The surgeon operates standing between the patient's legs. The abdomen is insufflated using a Veress needle at the umbilicus or in the left upper quadrant when a prior midline incision has been made. The procedure is performed through five ports—three 5-mm ports and two 10-mm ports (Fig 48–5). A 10-mm port is placed 15 cm inferior to the xiphoid process just to the left at midline. This port needs to be high on the abdomen so that visualization into the mediastinum is possible if an extended mediastinal dissection is necessary in patients with a shortened esophagus. A right lateral 5-mm port is placed, and a liver retractor is used to elevate the left lobe of the liver anteriorly to expose the hiatus. The surgeon's right-hand instruments are placed in a port that is along the left costal margin 12 cm from the xiphoid process. The surgeon's left-hand instruments are placed through a 5-mm port in the patient's right upper abdomen. An effort should be made to place this high and lateral even though a portion of the liver or the falciform ligament frequently makes this impossible. It is optimal if the camera and two operating ports form a diamond shape with the hiatus at the top corner. The assistant uses a 5-mm port in the left flank in the anterior axillary line about 4–6 cm inferior to the surgeon's right-hand port.

The operation begins by reduction of the paraesophageal hernia. The assistant gently retracts the herniated contents inferiorly so that the left crus of the diaphragm can be identified. Once the left crus of the diaphragm is clearly identified, the peritoneum overlying the left crus of the diaphragm is divided on the abdominal side of the crus. This is different from division of the gastrophrenic peritoneum separating the gastric fundus from the diaphragm done in a fundoplication. The inclination is to divide this at the mediastinal edge so that some peritoneum remains on the crus, but this will make it difficult to retrieve the edge of the sac when it retracts into the chest if released. The sac then is pulled inferiorly and medially, and the mediastinal tissues are pushed laterally. The assistant retracts either the stomach or the sac. The mediastinal pleura can be identified laterally; it is a much brighter white color than the sac. It always needs to be pushed laterally when identified, and it should be protected from being torn or entered. If it is entered, continue to proceed laparoscopically unless the patient's condition deteriorates. Do not repair it because that may create a dangerous flap that may lead to a tension pneumothorax.

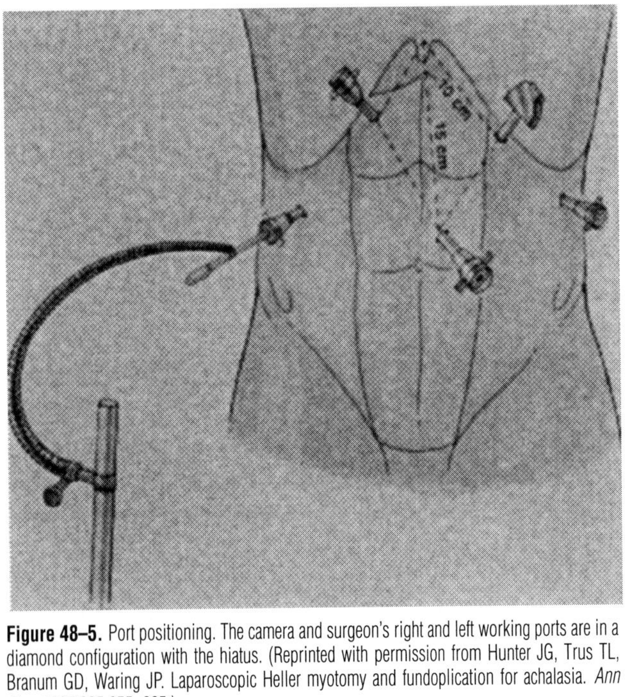

Figure 48–5. Port positioning. The camera and surgeon's right and left working ports are in a diamond configuration with the hiatus. (Reprinted with permission from Hunter JG, Trus TL, Branum GD, Waring JP. Laparoscopic Heller myotomy and fundoplication for achalasia. *Ann Surg* 1997;225:655–665.)

It is often possible to remove the entire anterior sac in one piece (Fig 48–6). It is easy to get lost in this dissection, especially on the right side of the esophagus, where the tissue planes are not as easily identified. Care should be taken to preserve the anterior vagus, which may run substantially off the esophagus to the left and may be hard to distinguish from a mediastinal band connecting the hernia sac to mediastinal tissue. Rarely is it necessary to divide the anterior vagus nerve to complete the dissection, particularly in reoperative cases. After the sac is freed from the mediastinum, the final attachments remain on the anterior surface of the gastroesophageal junction and are closely related to the anterior gastroesophageal fat pad. This is divided at a short distance away from the stomach to protect the vagus. The Harmonic scalpel (Ethicon, Cincinnati, OH) should be used to prevent bleeding.

At this point it is necessary to fully mobilize the fundus so that the posterior dissection of the gastroesophageal junction and excision of posterior sacs can be performed. The short gastric vessels are usually long in patients with giant hernias and are divided using the Harmonic scalpel. Short gastric vessel division starts approximately one-third of the way down the greater curvature. An atraumatic bowel grasper is used in the surgeon's left hand to retract the stomach near the area of initial dissection, holding it medially and anteriorly. The assistant uses an atraumatic bowel grasper and retracts the short gastric mesentery posteriorly and laterally. A hole into the lesser sac is created in an area that is avascular. Once a passage to the lesser sac is created, the surgeon's grasper is placed on the greater curve, and the assistant's grasper is placed in the opening. Again, the surgeon retracts medially and inferiorly, and the assistant retracts laterally and anteriorly, gradually mobilizing the stomach away from the spleen. This is usually not as treacherous as in the patient with a hiatal hernia because the vessels are long, and the dissection is away from the spleen.

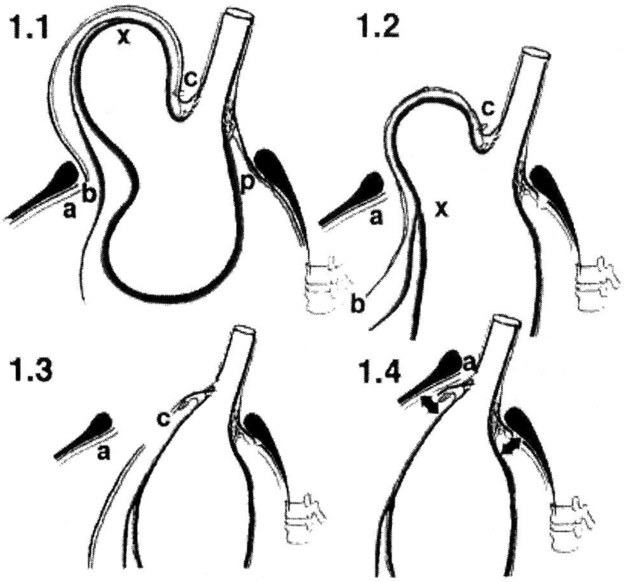

Figure 48–6. Excision of sac. Schematic view of a sagittal section through a type III paraesophageal hernia. Although superb, the depiction by illustrator Mary Brown in Allison's classic article[2] does not show the more common type III hernia with cephalad displacement of the gastroesophageal junction, nor the posterior component **p**, continuous with the lesser sac. **x** is the line of reflection of the greater omentum from the anterior wall of the stomach. Metallic clips (**c**) have been applied to the site of reflection of the peritoneal layer of the anterior (greater) sac from the prolapsed fundus. The layers of peritoneum and endoabdominal fascia are incised at the left crus, exposing crural muscle, and clamped together at **b. 1.2** The incision is carried along the edge of the hiatal defect counterclockwise toward the right crus, and the sac is teased out of the mediastinum, pulling the stomach down with it. This reduces handling of the stomach and the risk of injuring it. Liberation of both anterior and posterior elements of the sac completes circumferential mobilization of the gut tube, allowing the esophagus to lengthen and the gastroesophageal junction to lie without traction below the diaphragm. **1.3** The sac is excised by cutting external to the line of clips (**c**) to avoid the vagus and left gastric pedicle. **1.4** Crural repair creates a snug fit around the esophagus. Regardless of whether an antireflux procedure is added, the gastric fundus should be secured to the diaphragm with three to four stitches to prevent reherniation of the stomach. Arrows mark suggested sites through the stomach wall and diaphragm. (Reprinted with permission from Edye MB, Canin-Endres J, Gattorno F, Salky BA. Durability of laparoscopic repair of paraesophageal hernia. *Ann Surg* 1998;228:528–535.)

The posterior hernia sac is not as easily identified as the anterior sac. The posterior sac is reduced from the mediastinum and detached from the crura but usually not removed from the abdomen because of the intimate relation between the sac and the posterior vagus nerve. A clean posterior dissection is vital so that the crura can be closed accurately and securely, and there is no residual lead point into the chest for recurrence of the hernia.[11] At this point it is helpful to encircle the esophagus with a Penrose drain to use for retraction. An atraumatic grasper is passed behind the esophagus from the right side, and a 0.25-in Penrose drain 4 in in length is grasped and fed behind the esophagus. The limbs of the Penrose drain are secured using an Endoloop (Ethicon, Cincinnati, OH). The assistant uses the Penrose drain for traction. This allows further dissection of the retroesophageal window and later continued dissection of the mediastinum, if necessary. When the posterior vagus nerve is identified, it is left adjacent to the esophagus wrapped within the Penrose drain.

Once the short gastric vessels are divided and the retroesophageal window is established, the location of the gastroesophageal junction needs to be identified carefully. It is critical that there be at least 2 cm of intra-abdominal esophagus below the level of the crura. If the gastroesophageal junction is above this level, then an extensive mediastinal dissection needs to be carried out. If after mediastinal dissection the esophagus is short, then a Collis gastroplasty should be performed and is described below.

The large diaphragmatic defect is closed behind the esophagus with interrupted, pledgeted 0 Ethibond (Ethicon, Cincinnati, OH) or silk suture. The fundus should be free to pass behind the esophagus and remain there without traction. A 2-cm Nissen fundoplication is performed over a 56–60F dilator. The fundoplication is secured using three 2-0 nonabsorbable sutures, silk or Ethibond (Ethicon, Cincinnati, OH). Each stitch should incorporate a full thickness of stomach and partial thickness of esophagus. The sutures are tied intracorporeally. The length of the fundoplication should be 2 cm or less, and a U stitch is an acceptable alternative to simple suturing. However, failure of the U stitch will lead to failure of the fundoplication. The dilator is removed. The instruments and ports are removed from the abdomen as the CO_2 pneumoperitoneum is evacuated, and the skin is reapproximated.

Postoperative Management

The orogastric tube is removed at the end of the procedure, and many patients begin liquids on that same day. Patients with very large hernias and extensive dissections will remain NPO until a contrast material swallow study is performed on the first day after surgery. If no leak is present, the patient is advanced to a liquid diet. Most patients are discharged on the second postoperative day. The diet is advanced slowly over 3 weeks.

OUTCOMES

It has been reported that the laparoscopic repair of paraesophageal hernias is associated with higher complication and recurrence rates than the open methods of repair. We identified 136 consecutive patients who underwent laparoscopic repair of a paraesophageal hernia between 1993 and 1999. There were nine intraoperative complications, five early complications (10.2%), and three related deaths (2.2%). Three laparoscopic operations were converted to open procedures. The percentage of patients experiencing chest pain, dysphagia, heartburn, and regurgitation in the moderate to severe range preoperatively dropped from 34–47% to 5–7% ($p < 0.05$). Three patients underwent repeat laparoscopic repair for symptomatic recurrences.[12]

Using follow-up barium studies, Soper and colleagues analyzed the data for 116 patients who underwent laparoscopic paraesophageal hernia repair performed between 1992 and 2001.[13] On follow-up, 73 (76%) are asymptomatic, 11 (11%) have mild symptoms, and 12 (13%) took antacid medications. Protocol barium esophagrams were obtained in 69% of patients at 6–12 months' follow-up. Recurrence of the hiatal hernia was documented in 21 patients (22% overall and in 32% of those undergoing contrast studies). Reoperation was performed in three patients (3%). When only the patients with recurrent hiatal hernias were considered, 13 (62%) are symptomatic, but only 6 (28%) required medication for symptoms. Protocol esophagrams detect recurrences that are minimally symptomatic. The laparoscopic repair of paraesophageal hernias provides excellent long-term symptomatic relief in the majority of patients and has a low rate of symptomatic recurrence despite a relatively high incidence of recurrent hiatal abnormalities after paraesophageal hernia repair.

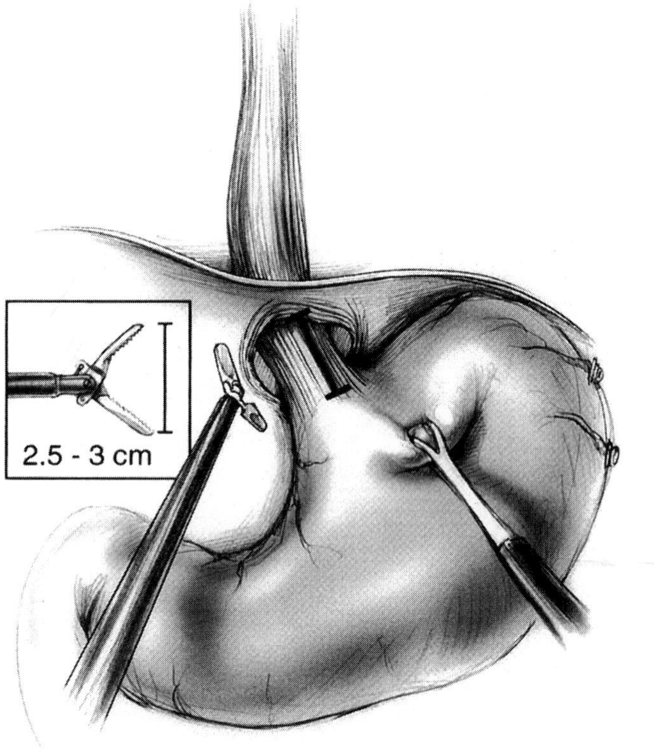

Figure 48–8. Assessment of intra-abdominal esophageal length. The laparoscopic grasper is used to assess adequate length.

MESH FIXATION

Success of the paraesophageal hernia repair depends on the integrity of the tissue and the tension needed to approximate it. It is common to repair other types of hernias using a tension-free technique with mesh, but most surgeons are reluctant to use mesh around the esophagus because of complications such as esophageal stricture, erosion, and perforation. There is currently a multicenter trial to evaluate a new type of mesh made from porcine small intestine submucosa (Surgisis, Cook Biotech, West Lafayette, IN) that serves as a temporary lattice for tissue ingrowth, leading to a strong matrix.[14] Other, newer mesh products are available, including Alloderm (LifeCell, Branchburg, NJ) and, for larger pieces of mesh, Permacol (Tissue Science Laboratories, Covington, GA). After the hiatus is closed posteriorly by approximating the right and left crus with interrupted sutures, a 7×10 cm piece of mesh is fashioned in a U-shaped configuration. The mesh will cover the crural repair completely and is secured to the diaphragm using interrupted silk sutures and/or tissue glue (Fig 48–7).

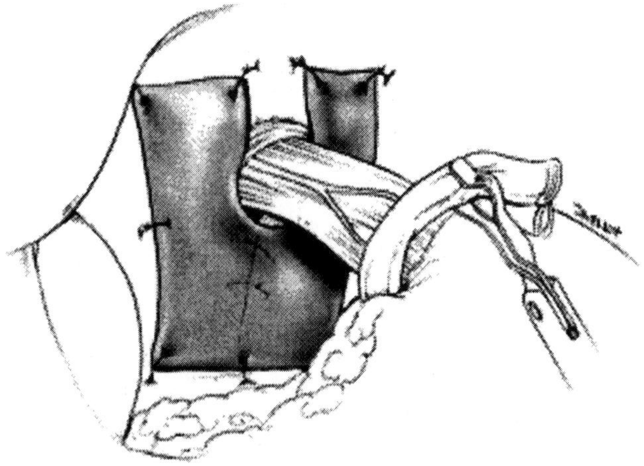

Figure 48–7. Mesh repair of the hiatus. (Reprinted with permission from Oelschlager BK, Barreca M, Chang L, Pellegrini CA. The use of small intestine submucosa in the repair of paraesophageal hernias: Initial observations of a new technique. *Am J Surg* 2003;186:4–8.)

COLLIS GASTROPLASTY

Description of Procedure

Wedge gastroplasty is performed using the same port placement as that used in the preceding description. The location of the gastroesophageal junction is identified by locating the gastroesophageal fat pad and observing the position of the cardiophrenic angle. By holding the crura together with atraumatic graspers and releasing the stomach, we assess the length of intra-abdominal esophagus (Fig 48–8). An extensive mediastinal mobilization of the esophagus (at least 4–6 cm above the gas-

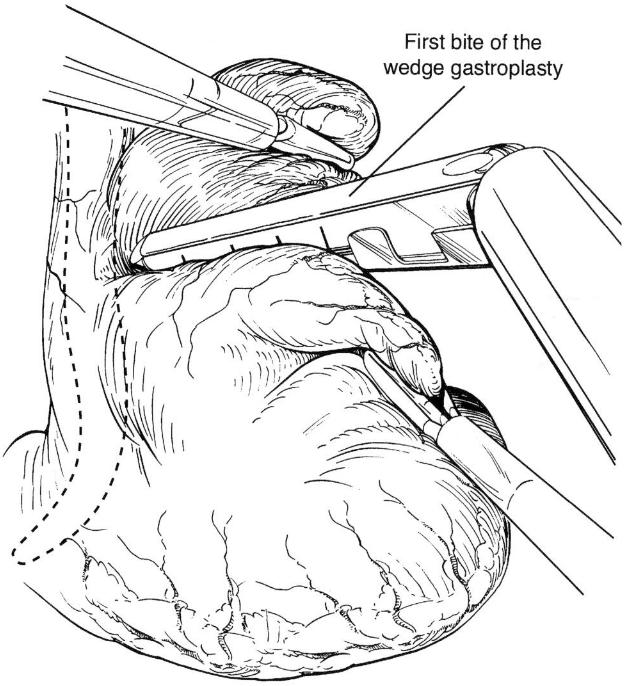
First bite of the
wedge gastroplasty

Figure 48–9. Collis gastroplasty. With the greater curvature of the stomach retracted inferiorly, the 30-mm endoscopic stapler is inserted, roticulated maximally, and fired.

troesophageal junction) is performed circumferentially in cases of shortened esophagus. If there is less than 2 cm of intra-abdominal esophageal length posteriorly, we proceed with gastroplasty. The orogastric tube is removed, and a 48F esophageal dilator is advanced under vision with the laparoscope. A point approximately 3 cm inferior to the angle of His is marked with electrocautery. The 10-mm left subcostal port is changed out for a 12-mm port, and a roticulating endoscopic 45-mm linear cutting stapler (blue load, 2.5-mm thickness) (Universal EndoGIA, USSC, Stamford, CT) is introduced into the abdomen and flexed maximally. The assistant retracts the gastric fundus inferiorly, and the surgeon maintains traction on the greater curve just below the angle of His as the stapler is advanced into position. The stapler is fired one to three times until the marked point, inferior to the angle of His, is reached (Fig 48–9). It is important that the dilator is reached with the final firing, and this is ensured when the dilator is pushed away when closing the stapler (Fig 48–10). The Penrose drain usually is removed at this point to prevent it from being entrapped in the staple line. Once the transverse staple line is complete, a vertical staple line is created. Through the same left subcostal port, the stapler is introduced and roticu-

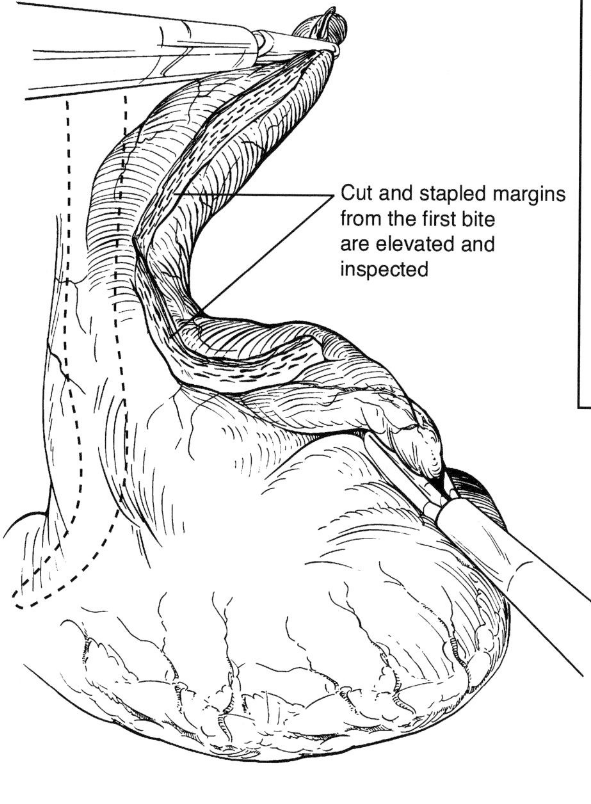
Cut and stapled margins
from the first bite
are elevated and
inspected

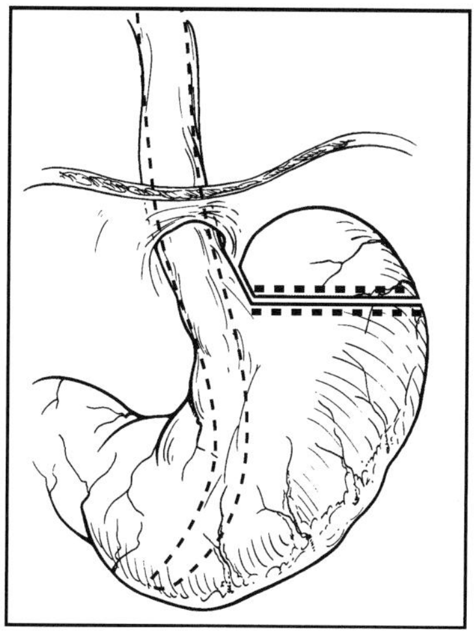

Figure 48–10. Collis gastroplasty. The endoscopic stapler is fired in series until the 48F esophageal dilator is reached.

lated (usually one or two "clicks") in the opposite direction so that it is parallel to the esophagus and abutting the dilator. It is crucial that the assistant place lateral traction on the wedge of stomach to be removed. The stapler is fired once or twice to produce a stapled wedge of stomach approximately 15 mL in volume that is removed from the abdomen (Fig 48–11). This creates a tube, or neoesophagus, that is 3–4 cm in length. The dilator is removed, and an orogastric tube is passed so that the tip is in the proximal stomach. The distal esophagus and proximal stomach are filled with 250 mL of dilute methylene blue to test the staple line and establish that there is no leak. The methylene blue is suctioned out, and we return to the usual operative conduct, including crural closure, passing the fundus behind the gastroesophageal junction, and securing the wrap for creation of a tension-free 360-degree floppy fundoplication. The staple line is oriented so that it is apposed to the stomach wall, thereby burying it. When placing the sutures of the wrap, the most cephalad suture is placed on the true esophagus just above its border with the neoesophagus (Fig 48–12) to ensure that there is no gastric mucosa above the wrap.

Outcomes

Patients treated with Collis gastroplasty and fundoplication for esophageal shortening have excellent short- and long-term outcomes with minimal morbidity.[15] In 2002, we identified 51 consecutive patients who underwent laparoscopic Collis gastroplasty with fundoplication between 1993 and 2000.[16] Two patients died of unrelated causes, and 38 of 49 (78%) of the remaining patients were able to complete a telephone query of symptoms, medical treatment, and patient satisfaction. At an average of 44 months (range 17–96 months), only 7 of 38 patients (18%) had been symptomatic, with heartburn in 4 and dysphagia in 3. All symptoms were controlled with medication. There were an additional 4 patients with no symptoms who took medication, for a total of 11 patients (29%) on therapy. Of the 18 patients who had late postoperative endoscopy, 5 had endoscopic evidence of recurrent GERD (2 with esophagitis, 2 with stricture, and 1 with both). Ninety-seven percent (37 of 38 patients) rated their outcomes as "much improved" compared with their preoperative status. While these results fall short of outcomes with laparoscopic fundoplication in patients with uncomplicated GERD, minimally invasive Collis gastroplasty provides complete symptom control in 80% of a complex set of patients at nearly 4 years of follow-up.

These patients require frequent follow-up and objective testing because the neoesophagus may contain functional gastric mucosa. In a study by Jobe and colleagues,[17] half the patients who underwent endoscopy after Collis gastroplasty had evidence of distal esophageal acid exposure. Of these patients, most had evidence by Congo red stain of acid-secreting gastric mucosa above the wrap. This resulted in esophagitis, although there was poor symptom correlation. Because of this finding, patients should undergo postoperative objective testing and use acid-suppressing medications when neoesophageal acid production is documented.

▪ ACHALASIA

From the seventeenth to the twentieth centuries, the treatment of achalasia was performed by forceful dilation, first by Thomas Willis in 1674 using a cork-tipped whalebone. In 1914, Ernest Heller described the cardiomyotomy.[18] This operation consisted of two myotomies on opposite sides of the esophagus performed via a laparotomy. A single anterior cardiomyotomy was described by Zaaiijer in 1923. Although laparotomy was the favorite approach for Heller myotomy for many years, thoracic surgeons in the United States, Canada, and Great Britain started performing this procedure through a left thoracotomy 40 years ago. The early minimally invasive procedures for achalasia duplicated this approach. It soon became clear that the laparoscopic approach was superior both for performance of an adequate myotomy onto the stomach and for performing the fundoplication. The standard of care now dictates the performance of a laparoscopic anterior Heller myotomy and partial fundoplication, either a posterior (Toupet) or anterior (Dor) fundoplication.

NATURAL HISTORY AND PRESENTATION

Achalasia is a rare disease outside of central and northern South America. In North America and Europe, idiopathic achalasia has an incidence of 0.5 per 100,000 and a prevalence of 8 per 100,000.[19] It has been described from infancy to the ninth decade; however, most patients present between the ages of 20 and 40 years, and there is no gender predilection. Most commonly, patients with achalasia present with dysphagia, regurgitation of undigested food, and weight loss. In addition, many patients complain of chest pain and/or heartburn, often a result of fermentation of food in the esophageal body. Achalasia is characterized, physiologically, by an absence of peristalsis in the esophageal body and a hypertensive nonrelaxing lower esophageal sphincter. The histologic change seen most commonly in the esophagus of achalasia patients is a decrease or loss of myenteric ganglion cells, usually associated with inflammation and fibrosis. One quarter of the patients with achalasia present with an esophageal body of normal caliber, one-half with moderate dilation of the

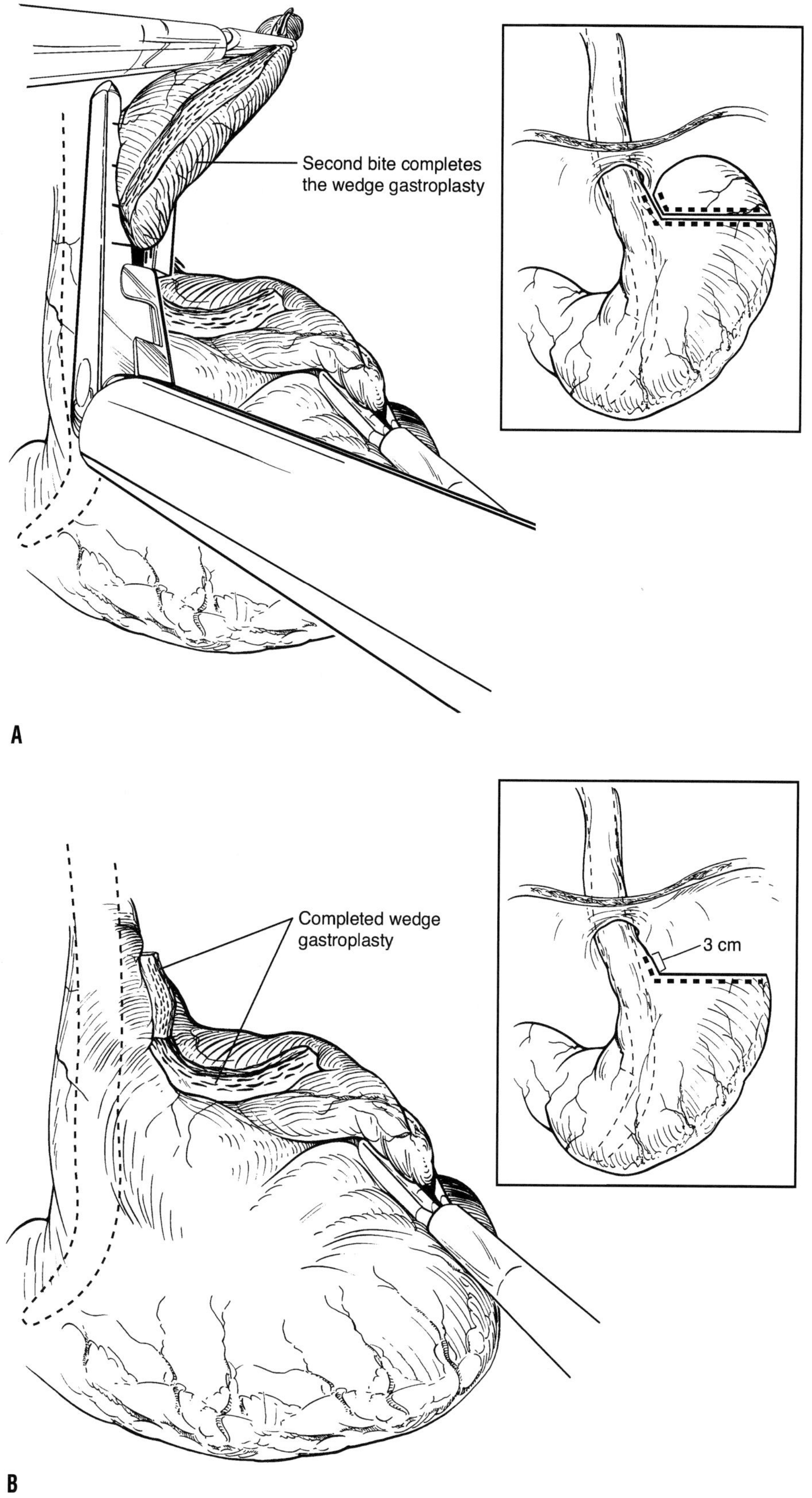

Figure 48–11. Collis gastroplasty. The endoscopic stapler is roticulated so that it can be fired adjacent and parallel to the esophageal dilator.

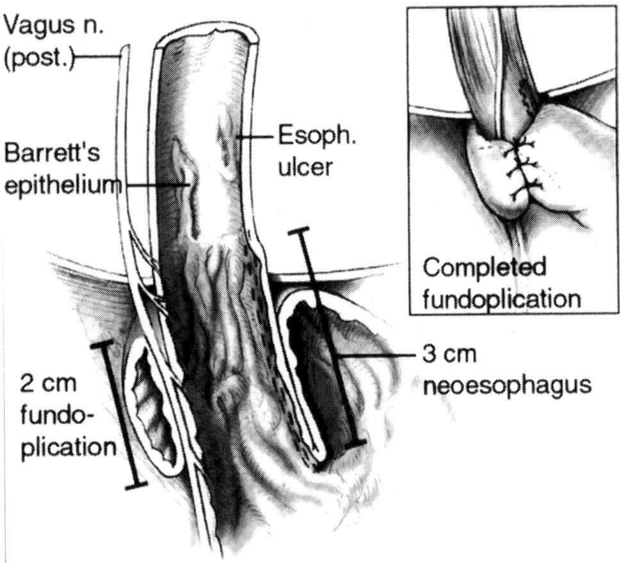

Figure 48–12. Collis gastroplasty. Creation of the 360-degree floppy fundoplication around the neoesophagus. For correct placement of the fundoplication, the superior aspect of the fundoplication should be at or above the neoesophagus. (Reprinted with permission from Jobe BA, Horvath KD, Swanstrom LL. Postoperative function following laparoscopic collis gastroplasty for shortened esophagus. *Arch Surg* 1998;133:867–874.)

esophageal body (2–5 cm), and one-quarter with a megaesophagus (esophageal body > 5 cm).

INDICATIONS FOR SURGERY

Laparoscopic Heller myotomy is indicated in any individual fit for general anesthesia who has the diagnosis of achalasia. This should be confirmed by the performance of barium swallow, esophagoscopy, and esophageal motility study. The only two groups of patients with relative contraindications to surgery are those in whom a previous Heller myotomy has been performed and the lower esophageal sphincter pressures are less than 10–15 mmHg and those patients with megaesophagus or a sigmoid esophagus. Many of these patients are subjected to esophagectomy in the Chagas' belt (South and Central America), but in North America, most first undergo myotomy to gain the benefits of the simpler procedure before proceeding to esophagectomy.

PATIENT PREPARATION

As mentioned earlier, the evaluation typically starts with a barium swallow for those who have dysphagia. The dysphagia associated with achalasia usually is insidious in onset. When it progresses to frequent regurgitation, aspiration, or weight loss, the patient usually seeks medical attention. A barium swallow demonstrates an esophageal body with diminished or absent peristalsis and a tight, "bird's beak" lower esophageal sphincter.

An esophageal motility study is critical for this diagnosis. The manometric hallmark is the absence of peristalsis in the esophageal body. Generally, the lower esophageal sphincter fails to relax with a wet swallow, and the resting pressure usually is elevated. Occasionally, one finds a high-pressure dysfunctional lower esophageal sphincter with peristalsis present; this is not achalasia. In fact, one should suspect an alternate diagnosis, such as pseudoachalasia, under these circumstances. Pseudoachalasia is an obstruction of the gastroesophageal junction by an extrinsic mass, usually a tumor, but occasionally such oddities as pancreatic pseudocysts or aortic aneurysms may cause pseudoachalasia. Rarely, pseudoachalasia is a paraneoplastic condition associated with cancer remote from the gastroesophageal junction, often in the upper airway.

Endoscopy is critical in all patients to confirm the diagnosis. Findings include food in the esophageal body or merely a very narrow, tight lower esophageal sphincter. The endoscopist typically reports that with pressure on the lower esophageal sphincter, there is a sudden yielding referred to as a "pop" that allows the scope into the stomach. This represents the relaxation of the lower esophageal sphincter under pressure. Esophageal pH studies are not useful because of presence of fermenting food in the distal esophagus.[20]

SURGICAL MANAGEMENT

Description of Procedure

As stated previously, the laparoscopic Heller myotomy and anterior or posterior fundoplication are the procedures of choice. The patient is positioned on a split-leg table with footplates, with the surgeon standing between the legs. After insufflation of the abdomen, the patient is placed in steep reverse Trendelenburg position. As described for hiatal hernia repair, five trocars are used. After elevating the left lobe of the liver, dissection commences identically to a laparoscopic Nissen fundoplication by incising the phrenoesophageal ligament. The right crus of the diaphragm is identified, and the esophagus and stomach are dissected free of the crus. This dissection is carried over the top and down the left side. Although some surgeons do not disturb the posterior esophageal attachments, it is our procedure to encircle the esophagus entirely with a Penrose drain. We retract the gastroesophageal junction inferiorly and ensure that adequate mediastinal dissection is performed. Once the esophagus is mobilized thoroughly, the epiphrenic fat pad is removed anteriorly down to the level of the muscularis propria with the Harmonic scalpel. Starting at the gastroesophageal junction, to the left of the anterior vagus, a pair of scissors is used to spread the longitudinal fibers of the esophagus. A Maryland dissector can be used as well (Fig 48–13). The scissors or an electrosurgical hook are slid beneath the circular muscle, and the plane is opened up. Once it is clear that the muscular layer of the esophagus has been separated from the mucosa, the scissors are used to divide the circular muscle. Once in the submucosal plane, it is simple to proceed superiorly, first with a blunt instrument to establish the plane and then with a pair of scissors or hook. The harmonic scalpel has been used in this region but is associated with sufficient mucosal damage that we prefer not to use it. The myotomy is carried up the esophagus approximately 4–6 cm. The myotomy then is carried down on the stomach an additional 2 cm (Fig 48–14). The collar-sling musculature is more difficult to dissect and is much thinner than the esophageal muscle layers. Great care must be used in this region not to perforate the gastric mucosa. We perform this by grasping the edges of the muscle with two atraumatic graspers and pulling them apart. On completion of the myotomy, a flexible endoscope is passed through the mouth and guided down through the myotomy to make sure that it has been carried low enough on the stomach. The upper abdomen is filled with water, and the esophagus

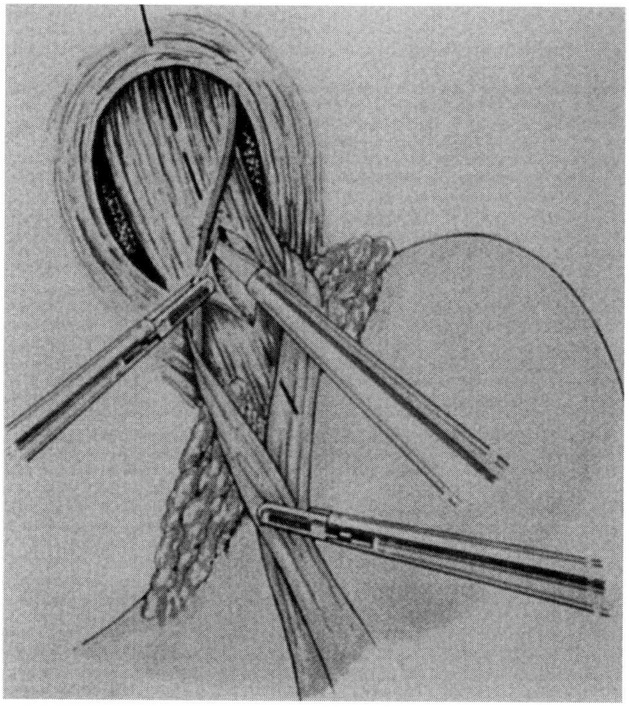

Figure 48–13. Heller myotomy is started above the gastroesophageal junction by spreading the longitudinal muscle, isolating the circular muscle, and dividing it with scissors. (Reprinted with permission from Hunter JG, Trus TL, Branum GD, Waring JP. Laparoscopic Heller myotomy and fundoplication for achalasia. *Ann Surg* 1997;225:655–665.)

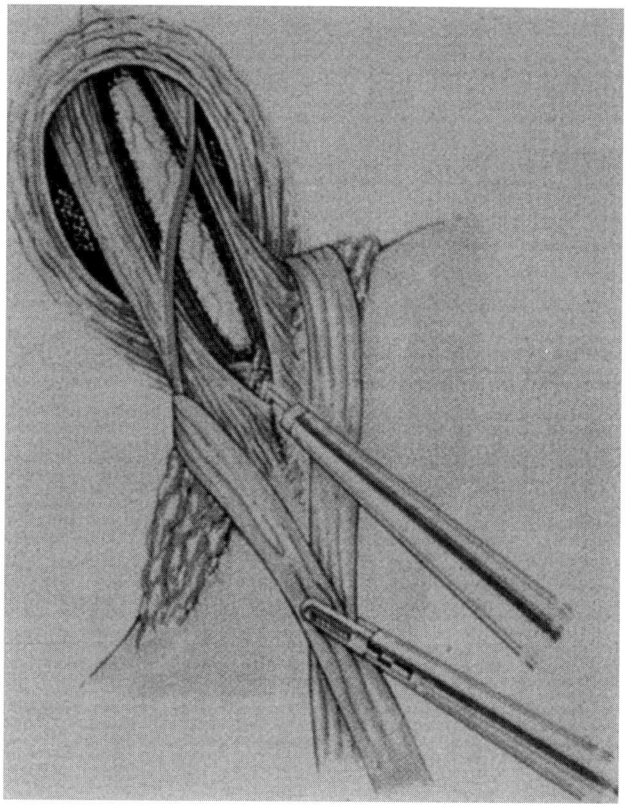

Figure 48–14. The myotomy is carried down onto the upper stomach, where the muscle layers are not as easily identified. (Reprinted with permission from Hunter JG, Trus TL, Branum GD, Waring JP. Laparoscopic Heller myotomy and fundoplication for achalasia. *Ann Surg* 1997;225:655–665.)

and stomach are filled with air to ensure that no leaks occur. The scope is then removed.

Whether we perform an anterior or posterior fundoplication, we usually mobilize the short gastric vessels. If an anterior fundoplication is to be performed, two sutures are placed to the cut edge of the muscularis on the left, three sutures are placed to the diaphragmatic arch, and two additional sutures are placed to the cut edge of the muscularis on the right. If a posterior fundoplication is to be performed (Fig 48–15), the suturing is again to the cut edges of the mucosa. Occasionally, a large diaphragmatic defect will require a crural suture be placed to avoid herniation of the fundoplication. If a small mucosal rent is made during the course of dissection, this generally can be closed with a single running suture of 4-0 Vicryl. Following closure, it is essential that the repair be tested with methylene blue or air prior to completing the operation.

Postoperative Management

It is our practice to get a barium swallow the day after surgery to ensure that no esophageal leaks have been missed. Perforations detected within the first 24 hours postoperatively can be repaired directly, but those de-

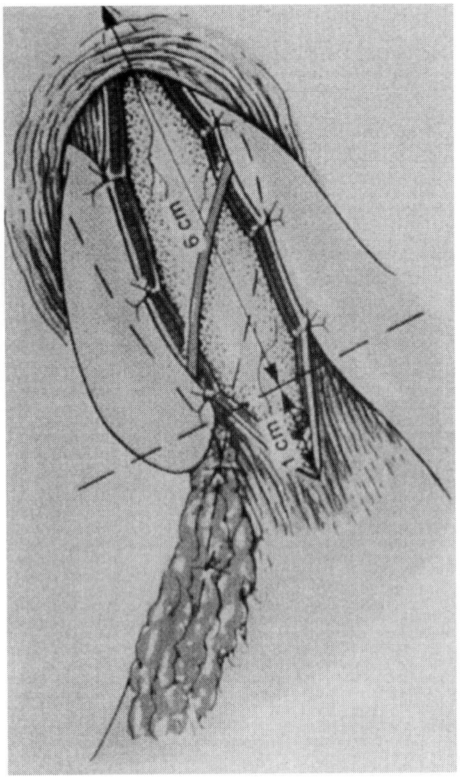

Figure 48–15. The Toupet fundoplication is sutured to the cut edge of the myotomy. (Reprinted with permission from Hunter JG, Trus TL, Branum GD, Waring JP. Laparoscopic Heller myotomy and fundoplication for achalasia. *Ann Surg* 1997;225:655–665.)

tected beyond this period will need more a more extensive procedure, from closure and patching to esophageal exclusion depending on the size of the laceration and the condition of the patient. Patients are kept on a liquid diet for 3–4 days and then advance to a soft diet while the edema resolves. They usually are discharged 1–3 days after surgery and start a regular diet 3 weeks later.

OUTCOMES

Complications of significance occur rarely for laparoscopic Heller myotomy and should be less than 5%. Death has been reported rarely and should occur in less than 1 in 500 operations. Inadvertent esophagotomy occurs infrequently (7%) during the course of the operation and cannot be predicted by preoperative therapy or duration or severity of dysphagia.[21]

A recent report by Melvin showed that robotic Heller myotomy with partial fundoplication was safe and effective in 104 patients. In this series, there were no esophageal perforations, and most patients were discharged on the first postoperative day.[22]

Laparoscopic Heller myotomy has shown to have similar intermediate- and long-term outcomes to those with open surgery.[23,24] Normal swallowing is the result in 90–95% of patients, with the remainder having to modify their diet. Khajanchee and colleagues recently published intermediate results in 121 patients undergoing laparoscopic Heller myotomy with Toupet fundoplication for achalasia.[25] After a median follow-up period of 9 months, 102 patients (84.3%) had excellent relief of dysphagia. Eight additional patients (6.6%) demonstrated a significant improvement in dysphagia scores. Only 11 patients (9.0%) had either no change or a worsening of their dysphagia. Postoperatively, all patients with manometry had a normal lower esophageal sphincter pressure and good lower esophageal sphincter relaxation. Odds of failure were greatest for patients with severe preoperative dysphagia, male patients, and patients with classic amotile achalasia. Of the 60 patients having heartburn-like symptoms preoperatively, 19 (31.7%) continued to have similar symptoms after surgery. Sixteen (33.3%) of the 48 patients having postoperative pH studies demonstrated objective reflux. Five (31.2%) of these patients had symptoms of reflux.

Dysphagia improves in most patients after laparoscopic Heller myotomy with partial fundoplication. Patients with severe preoperative dysphagia, esophageal dilation, or amotile achalasia may have greater chances of a poor outcome. These results are better than can be achieved with botulinum toxin or balloon dilation. For this reason, most gastroenterologists now prefer laparoscopic Heller myotomy to all other forms of therapy for achalasia in a patient fit for operation.

REFERENCES

1. Akerlund HO, Key E. Hernia diaphragmatica hiatus oesophagei vom anastomischen und roentgenologischen gesichtspunkt. *Acta Radiol* 1926;6:3–22
2. Allison PR. Reflux esophagitis, sliding hiatal hernia and anatomy of repair. *Surg Gynecol Obstet* 1951;92:419–431
3. Low DE, Unger T. Open repair of paraesophageal hernia: Reassessment of subjective and objective outcomes. *Ann Thorac Surg* 2005;80:287–294
4. Hayden JD, Jamieson GG. Effect on iron deficiency anemia of laparoscopic repair of large paraesophageal hernias. *Dis Esophagus* 2005;18:329–331
5. Stylopoulos N, Gazelle GS, Rattner DW. Paraesophageal hernias: Operation or observation? *Ann Surg* 2002;236:492–500; discussion 500–491
6. Tsereteli Z, Terry ML, Bowers SP, et al. Prospective, randomized clinical trial comparing nitrous oxide and carbon dioxide pneumoperitoneum for laparoscopic surgery. *J Am Coll Surg* 2002;195:173–179; discussion 179–180
7. Swanstrom LL, Jobe BA, Kinzie LR, Horvath KD. Esophageal motility and outcomes following laparoscopic paraesophageal hernia repair and fundoplication. *Am J Surg* 1999;177:359–363

8. Trus TL, Bax T, Richardson WS, et al. Complications of laparoscopic paraesophageal hernia repair. *J Gastrointest Surg* 1997;1:221–228
9. O'Rourke RW, Khajanchee YS, Urbach DR, et al. Extended transmediastinal dissection: An alternative to gastroplasty for short esophagus. *Arch Surg* 2003;138: 735–740
10. Swanstrom LL, Marcus DR, Galloway GQ. Laparoscopic Collis gastroplasty is the treatment of choice for the shortened esophagus. *Am J Surg* 1996;171:477–481
11. Edye M, Salky B, Posner A, Fierer A. Sac excision is essential to adequate laparoscopic repair of paraesophageal hernia. *Surg Endosc* 1998;12:1259–1263
12. Mattar SG, Bowers SP, Galloway KD, et al. Long-term outcome of laparoscopic repair of paraesophageal hernia. *Surg Endosc* 2002;16:745–749
13. Diaz S, Brunt LM, Klingensmith ME, et al. Laparoscopic paraesophageal hernia repair, a challenging operation: Medium-term outcome of 116 patients. *J Gastrointest Surg* 2003;7:59–66; discussion 66–57
14. Oelschlager BK, Barreca M, Chang L, Pellegrini CA. The use of small intestine submucosa in the repair of paraesophageal hernias: Initial observations of a new technique. *Am J Surg* 2003;186:4–8
15. Terry ML, Vernon A, Hunter JG. Stapled-wedge Collis gastroplasty for the shortened esophagus. *Am J Surg* 2004;188:195–199
16. Vernon AH, Jobe BA, Smith CD, Hunter JH. Long-term follow-up of laparoscopic Collis gastroplasty. Paper presented at Digestive Disease Week, San Francisco, 2002
17. Jobe BA, Horvath KD, Swanstrom LL. Postoperative function following laparoscopic collis gastroplasty for shortened esophagus. *Arch Surg* 1998;133:867–874
18. Heller E. Extramukose Karkioplastic beim chronisken Kardiospasmus mit Dilatation des Oesophagus. *Mitt Grenzgeb Med Chir* 1914;27:141–149
19. Mayberry JF Jr. Achalasia in the city of Cardiff Wales UK from 1926 to 1977. *Digestion* 1980;20:248–252
20. Smart HL, Evans DF, Slevin B, Atkinson M. Twenty-four-hour oesophageal acidity in achalasia before and after pneumatic dilatation. *Gut* 1987;28:883–887
21. Rakita S, Bloomston M, Villadolid D, et al. Esophagotomy during laparoscopic Heller myotomy cannot be predicted by preoperative therapies and does not influence long-term outcome. *J Gastrointest Surg* 2005;9:159–164
22. Melvin WS, Dundon JM, Talamini M, Horgan S. Computer-enhanced robotic telesurgery minimizes esophageal perforation during Heller myotomy. *Surgery* 2005; 138:553–558; discussion 558–559
23. Sharp KW, Khaitan L, Scholz S, et al. 100 consecutive minimally invasive Heller myotomies: Lessons learned. *Ann Surg* 2002;235:631–638; discussion 638–639
24. Patti MG, Fisichella PM, Perretta S, et al. Impact of minimally invasive surgery on the treatment of esophageal achalasia: A decade of change. *J Am Coll Surg* 2003;196: 698–703; discussion 703–695
25. Khajanchee YS, Kanneganti S, Leatherwood AE, et al. Laparoscopic Heller myotomy with Toupet fundoplication: outcomes predictors in 121 consecutive patients. *Arch Surg* 2005;140:827–833; discussion 833–824

49

Laparoscopic Splenectomy

Caprice C. Greenberg ■ Ali Tavakkolizadeh ■ David C. Brooks

Delartie and Maiguier first introduced laparoscopic splenectomy in 1991.[1] At that time, conversion rates were high, and some surgeons argued against the routine use of laparoscopic splenectomy. As experience with laparoscopic procedures has evolved in general and laparoscopic instruments and equipment have improved, laparoscopy has become the preferred technique for splenectomy. A recent article reported an increase in the number of splenectomies attempted laparoscopically from 17% in 1994 to 75% in 1998, demonstrating the prevalence of this technique today.[2] The many advantages of the laparoscopic approach can explain this increased use. These benefits include less postoperative pain, decreased length of hospital stay, faster return to full activity, a better cosmetic result, and reduced costs when compared with the open technique.[3,4]

■ PATIENT SELECTION

The indications for laparoscopic splenectomy are the same as for open splenectomy and are outlined in Table 49–1. Please refer to Chapter 43 for a full discussion of the indications for splenectomy. Most patients requiring splenectomy are candidates for a laparoscopic procedure. There are several subgroups, however, that warrant careful consideration. The absolute and relative contraindications for laparoscopic splenectomy can be divided into patient and technical factors.

PATIENT-RELATED FACTORS

There are few patients who cannot tolerate a pneumoperitoneum using today's technology. Patients with severe respiratory compromise or those who are highly dependent on their cardiac preload may not be able to tolerate the increased intra-abdominal pressure, and an open technique should be considered. Unfortunately, these patients are the most likely to benefit from the earlier mobilization and decreased postoperative pain associated with the laparoscopic approach. There have been numerous reports documenting the safety of laparoscopic splenectomy during pregnancy and childhood.

The laparoscopic approach should not be used in hemodynamically volatile patients, particularly the unstable trauma patient. The one indication for laparoscopic splenectomy in the setting of trauma is the late development of posttraumatic splenic cysts.

TECHNICAL FACTORS

The laparoscopic approach necessitates destruction of the splenic anatomy because the spleen is removed piecemeal through the small port incision. Any condition where examination of the spleen in its integrity is desired should be performed using the open or laparoscopic-assisted techniques.

A large spleen may be a relative contraindication to laparoscopy. Consensus does not currently exist regarding a prohibitive spleen size for using a laparoscopic approach. Although some surgeons consider splenic weight greater than 1000 g to be a contraindication, studies have demonstrated the feasibility of the laparoscopic approach in this subgroup of patients, recognizing limitations.[5] Two studies document the increased risks associated with laparoscopy in the setting of massive splenomegaly (>1000 g) when compared with spleens of normal size. These in-

TABLE 49–1. INDICATIONS FOR LAPAROSCOPIC SPLENECTOMY

Autoimmune disorders
Idiopathic thrombocytopenia purpura (ITP)
Thrombotic thrombocytopenic purpura (TTP)
Autoimmune hemolytic anemia
Hereditary hemolytic anemias
Spherocytosis
Elliptocytosis
Hemoglobinopathies
Hematologic malignancies
Hodgkin's disease
Non-Hodgkin's lymphoma
Leukemia (CCL, HCL)
Miscellaneous disorders
Myeloproliferative disorders
Hypersplenism
Cysts and tumors

clude longer operative time (203 versus 156 minutes and 170 versus 102 minutes), increased blood loss (600 versus 125 mL), higher conversion rates (41% versus 3% and 18% versus 5%), increased postoperative length of hospital stay (4 versus 2 days and 5 versus 3 days), and postoperative morbidity (56% versus 6%).[6,7] Neither of these studies concluded that massive splenomegaly was a contraindication for laparoscopic splenectomy but rather emphasized the need for vigilance and a low threshold for conversion to an open procedure. Besides a more challenging dissection, placement of the spleen in the removal bag following resection can be difficult. The risk of intra-abdominal rupture with subsequent splenosis also contributes to the reluctance of some surgeons to perform laparoscopic splenectomy in patients with splenomegaly. Many advocate the use of hand-assisted laparoscopic surgery in cases of splenomegaly. The technique is described later in this chapter.

▪ APPROACHES FOR LAPAROSCOPIC SPLENECTOMY

The first attempts at laparoscopic splenectomy were performed through an anterior approach. This was performed with the patient in the lithotomy position and used five laparoscopic ports. This approach was abandoned later in favor of the lateral approach (described in detail below), which is currently the preferred approach. The lateral approach was developed initially for laparoscopic adrenalectomy. The lateral position of the patient uses the weight of the spleen and gravity to gain exposure during various steps of the procedure. In addition, it facilitates dissection of the superior short gastric vessels and superior pole when compared with the traditional anterior approach.

▪ PREPARATION FOR THE PROCEDURE

Laparoscopic splenectomy, as with all advanced laparoscopic procedures, requires a number of specialized instruments and equipment to be able to perform the procedure safely and efficiently. A minimum of two monitors should be available in the room. Three or four trocars are used for the procedure: one 12-mm trocar and two or three 5-mm trocars. The use of the Veress needle or the open technique for entering the abdominal cavity is left to the individual surgeon. We prefer the Veress technique and therefore require a Veress needle and 10-mL slip-tip syringe with saline. Laparoscopic filtered insufflation tubing, a laparoscopic suction irrigator, and the monopolar cord for the cautery must be available before beginning the case. Additionally, other energy sources such as ultrasonic dissecting shears (Harmonic, Ethicon Endosurgery, Cincinnati, OH) and electrothermal bipolar vessel sealer (LigaSure, Valleylab, Boulder, CO) can be very useful. A formal open laparotomy set should be readily available in case emergent conversion to an open procedure is necessary.

Figure 49–1 illustrates the optimal room setup and patient positioning for this procedure. A monitor should be placed on each side of the patient toward the head of the operating table. The patient is supine initially for the induction of general anesthesia and placement of the Foley catheter, as well as a nasogastric tube for gastric decompression. The patient then is placed in a modified right lateral decubitus position. The optimal angle is 60 degrees between the patient's back and the operating table (see Fig 49–1). The advantage of this angle over the full lateral decubitus position relates to ease of positioning should conversion to an open procedure be necessary. Either a beanbag or roll can be used to support the patient. The patient should be taped in this position to prevent movement when the table is manipulated during the case. An axillary roll is required in the dependent axilla, and the left arm should be placed on an elevated armrest and secured in place. The legs should be padded with the left leg straight and the right leg bent to 60 degrees. The table should be broken at the level of the umbilicus to maximize the distance between the rib cage and the superior iliac spine. The sterile field should extend from the nipples to the pubic bone in the cranial-caudal position and from the right anterior axillary line to the left scapular tip. The table can be rolled to the left to flatten the abdomen for trocar placement. For the remainder of the procedure, the reverse Trendelenburg position will facilitate visualization of the spleen in the left upper quadrant.

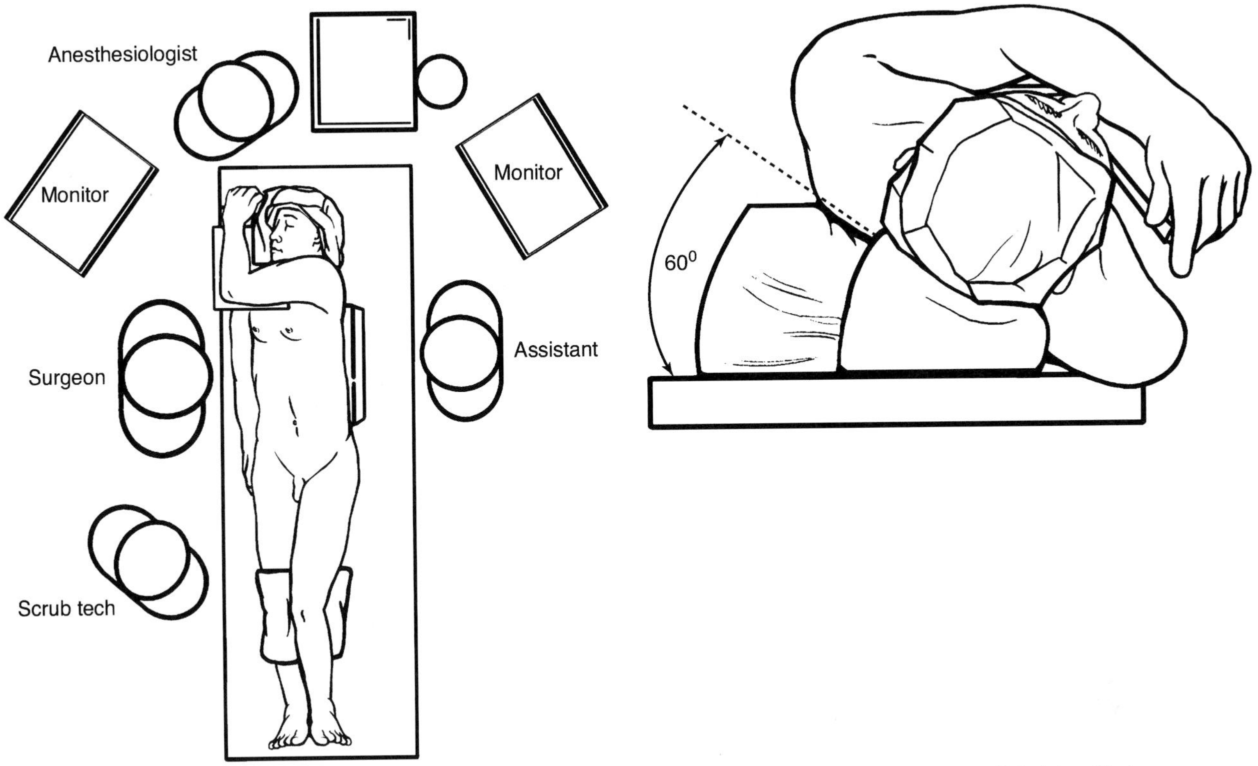

Figure 49–1. Room setup and optimal patient positioning for laparoscopic splenectomy. (Adapted from http://www.fubmc.edu/surg-sci/atlas/splenect.htm.)

■ DETAILS OF THE OPERATIVE PROCEDURE

TROCAR PLACEMENT

We have used a four-port technique traditionally; however, more recently, we have adopted a three-port technique in patients in whom adequate exposure of the splenic vessels can be obtained without an additional assistant's instrument. There are a number of possible trocar placements for laparoscopic splenectomy, and placement will need to be individualized to the patient anatomy. Figure 49–2A illustrates our usual placement for either the three- or four-port technique. The most lateral port can be omitted if the patient's anatomy permits. Figure 49–2B offers an example of an alternative approach for the three-port technique. The advantage of this second approach is that the supraumbilical midline port can be extended to permit placement of the 15-mm retrieval bag (see below). In our experience, such a midline extension is associated with less postoperative pain than the extension of the more lateral ports, which involves division of the muscle. The abdomen is entered using the Veress needle just inferior to the left costal margin in the midclavicular line. In patients in whom the spleen is large and occupies most of the left upper quadrant, there is concern for splenic injury with the Veress needle. In these patients, we revert to the open technique for placement of the camera port. Pneumoperitoneum is attained using carbon dioxide gas to a pressure of 15 mmHg. The camera port is placed to the left of the midline through the rectus muscle, taking care to avoid the epigastric vessels. A 10-mm 30-degree laparoscope is introduced into the peritoneal cavity. The remaining ports should be placed under direct visualization once the camera has been placed and the spleen has been visualized. Port placement will need to be individualized to the patient's anatomy. The camera port and two working ports should be triangulated to allow adequate manipulation. A fourth port always can be added in the lateral position near the anterior axillary line if necessary as the case progresses. We use a 12-mm camera port and two 5-mm ports initially. The 12-mm port can be used for the camera, as well as the stapling device.

DISSECTION

The procedure begins by exploring the abdomen to identify any accessory spleens. The most common sites for accessory spleens include the omentum, the splenic hilum, the tail of the pancreas, and the splenocolic and gastrosplenic ligaments. Each of these sites should be considered as the dissection continues. The dissection

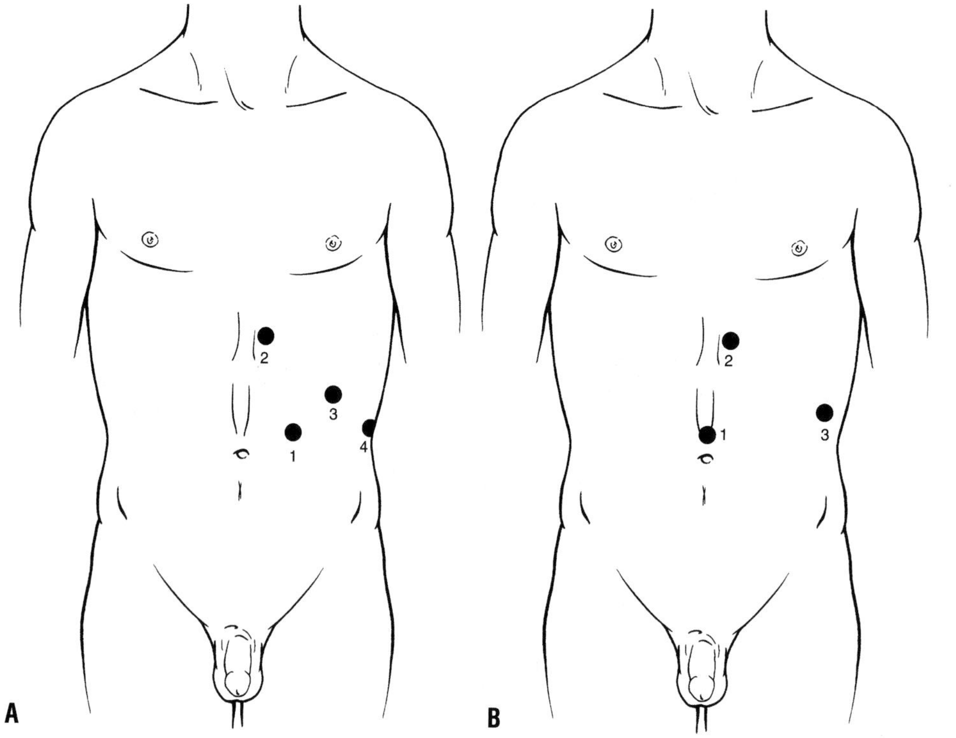

Figure 49–2. Trocar placement for laparoscopic splenectomy. **A.** Recommended trocar placement. Port 1 is 12 mm, whereas the remainder are 5-mm ports. Port 4 is omitted for the three-port technique. **B.** Alternative for trocar placement.

begins by mobilizing the splenic flexure of the colon, including the renocolic ligament, as needed to provide adequate exposure to the inferior pole of the spleen and the gastrocolic and splenocolic ligaments (Fig 49–3A). The lower pole of the spleen can be elevated with a blunt dissector. The splenocolic and phrenocolic ligaments are divided. Once the inferior pole of the spleen has been freed, attention is turned to the lower lateral splenic attachments. These are divided moving superiorly from the inferior pole using the ultrasonic shears until the dissection becomes difficult (see Fig 49–3B). Only the lower half of these attachments should be divided at this point in the operation. It is important to avoid full lateral mobilization at this point because this would result in the spleen falling medially and hindering dissection of the short gastric vessels.

Next, attention is turned to ligating the short gastric vessels (see Fig 49–3C). The first step is to enter the gastrocolic ligament through the avascular plane. Once the lesser sac has been entered, the short gastric vessels are identified and divided. Dissection should continue in a caudal to cranial direction, ligating the short gastric vessels as they are encountered. The ultrasonic dissecting shears will facilitate quicker dissection in this area, and the short gastric vessels can be coagulated with confidence using this technique. As the surgeon is mobilizing the gastrosplenic ligament, traction and countertraction should be provided by the surgeon's nondominant hand and one hand of the assistant. In the four-port technique, the assistant's other hand should be providing blunt retraction on the spleen toward the left shoulder. It is crucial that the all the short gastric vessels be divided before proceeding to avoid bleeding that can be difficult to control at a later stage. The most cranial vessels can be difficult to identify and may be immediately adjacent to the left crus of the diaphragm. Medial rotation of the stomach can help to expose these vessels and ensure complete ligation (see Fig 49–3D). Once all the short gastric vessels have been ligated, the assistant and the surgeon elevate the spleen using blunt dissectors while the surgeon divides the entire splenic hilum using an endoscopic stapling device (see Fig 49–3E). It is imperative that the stapler includes the entire hilum to avoid partial division of one of the vessels. If this is not possible, the hilum should be dissected further until the stapler fits comfortably across the hilum. We typically use a 60-mm, 2.5-mm stapler. If the hilar vessels are closely related, we prefer to use a 45-mm, 2.0-mm stapler. The smaller staples (2.0 mm) provide better hemostatic control of the vessels but are only supplied in the short length (45 mm) and thus are not suitable for all occasions. To minimize port size, we typically change to a 5-mm laparoscope at this point. The new camera then is inserted through one of the 5-mm ports, freeing the 12-mm port for introduc-

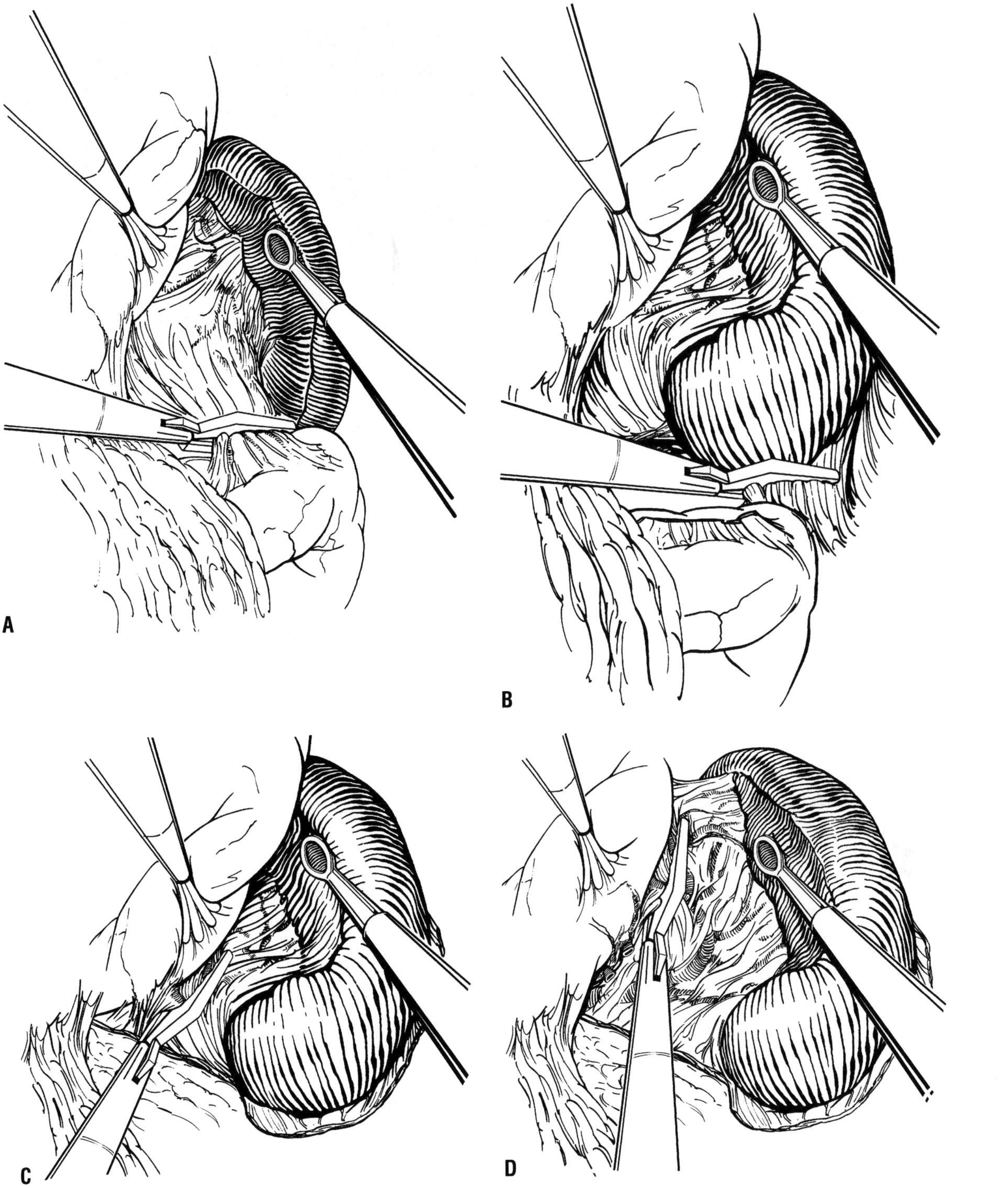

Figure 49–3. Steps in the dissection during laparoscopic splenectomy. **A.** Mobilize the splenic flexure of the colon using the ultrasonic dissecting shears (harmonic scalpel) to free the lower pole of the spleen. **B.** Free the lateral attachments of the spleen progressing superiorly from the lower pole. Leave the most superior attachments to the diaphragm intact. **C.** Ligate the short gastric vessels using the ultrasonic dissecting shears (harmonic scalpel). **D.** Medial rotation of the stomach can help to identify the most superior short gastric vessels. Special attention should be given to ensure ligation of these vessels. *Continued*

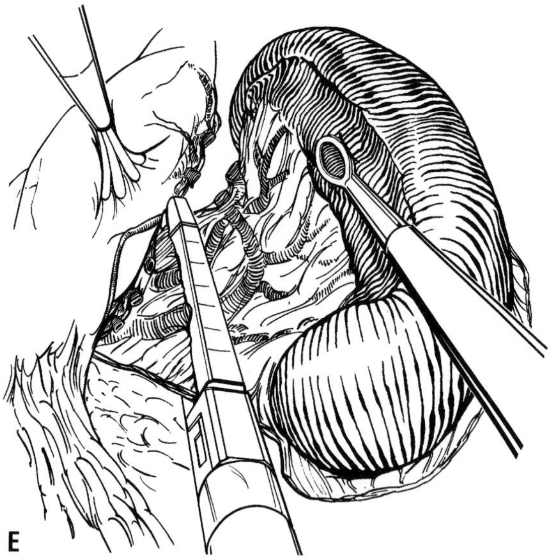

E

Figure 49–3, cont'd. E. Divide the splenic hilum. Take down the remaining superior attachments so that the entire spleen is free.

tion of the stapler. An alternative approach is to use two 12-mm ports, one for the camera and a separate one for the stapler.

REMOVAL OF THE SPECIMEN

We continue to use the 5-mm laparoscope for the remainder of the procedure. The 12-mm port should be removed, and a 15-mm endoscopic bag should be placed directly through the skin incision without a port. The spleen is placed in the endoscopic bag, and the bag is brought up through the skin. This maneuver provides a good seal at the port site and allows for reinflation of the pneumoperitoneum. The splenic bed is now inspected for hemostasis. Particular attention should be given to the splenic hilum and short gastric vessels. Iatrogenic injury to other organs, particularly the pancreatic tail, should be ruled out. The spleen then is morselized using digital disruption and removed using ring forceps until the entire bag can be removed from the abdominal cavity. Care should be taken during this part of the procedure to ensure that the ring forceps do not tear the retrieval bag and inadvertently grasp intra-abdominal contents through the bottom of the bag. This can lead to unrecognized complications, such as a small bowel enterotomy or pancreatic leak. If anatomic integrity of the spleen is required for pathologic examination, the trocar site can be extended further to allow intact removal of the organ, converting to a laparoscopic-assisted procedure.

Following removal of the specimen, the ports are reinserted, and the abdomen is examined and irrigated if necessary. If an open technique is used for the camera port, closure of this fascia may be necessary. No other port sites will require fascial closure. The skin is approximated with absorbable sutures.

VARIATIONS ON THE PROCEDURE

Hand-Assisted Laparoscopic Surgery (HALS)

Hand-assisted laparoscopic splenectomy offers an alternative to conventional laparoscopic splenectomy. The hand-assisted technique allows the surgeon to regain the sense of depth and tactile feel that is lost in the conventional laparoscopic technique. In addition, it facilitates exposure when that is limited and will allow greater manipulation of the specimen. This can be especially important in difficult cases, such as in patients with splenomegaly. Another advantage is the retrieval of the specimen in its intact state.

The hand-port incision can be placed in a variety of positions, such as the supraumbilical midline or a Pfannenstiel incision. We favor an upper midline incision. The hand port is important in maintaining the pneumoperitoneum when the operator withdraws his or her hand from the peritoneal cavity. A number of such ports have been developed and are available commercially.[8] Typically, the nondominant hand is placed in the abdominal cavity and used to assist with the surgery.

The role of HALS in splenic surgery is debated widely. Several case series suggest possible advantages for HALS in patients with splenomegaly.[9,10] This technique allows for gentler retraction of the spleen during dissection, as well as palpation and precise location of the splenic artery. No advantage is seen for hand assistance over conventional laparoscopy when the spleen is of normal size.

Individual Ligation of the Hilum

In the techniques described earlier, the hilum is divided en masse using an endoscopic vascular stapling device. Individual ligation of the artery and vein also has been described. The surgeon should be aware of this useful alternative technique. It can be particularly helpful when the hilum is bulky or the spleen is large, and safe placement of the stapler is not possible. In this technique, sharp and blunt dissection is used to dissect the peritoneal and fibrinous attachments in the hilum. A right-angle dissector is used to isolate each vessel. A silk ligature is tied using extracorporeal or intracorporeal technique on the proximal side. The specimen side can be either clipped or tied.

■ PERIOPERATIVE MANAGEMENT

VACCINATIONS

Asplenic patients are at increased risk for infection with encapsulated organisms, including *Streptococcus pneumoniae, Haemophilus influenzae* type b, and *Neisseria meningitides.* All patients undergoing laparoscopic splenectomy must receive vaccinations for these three bacteria. The ideal timing of immunization is 14 days preoperatively in elective cases and 14 days postoperatively in urgent or emergent situations. Many surgeons advocate the administration of the vaccines prior to discharge to ensure that vaccination is not neglected.

■ POSTOPERATIVE MANAGEMENT

Some surgeons advocate postoperative decompression of the stomach with a nasogastric tube to prevent hemorrhage from the short gastric vessels. We have not found this necessary and allow sips of clear liquids on the night of surgery, advancing the diet over the course of the first postoperative day. We feel that a single dose of preoperative antibiotics is sufficient and do not use postoperative antibiotics. The patient's complete blood count typically is checked on the morning after surgery. The manipulation of the stomach may lead to some early satiety in the immediate postoperative period. This will resolve in 6–8 weeks. Patients are also instructed to refrain from high-impact or jarring-type exercises for 2 weeks so that raw surfaces within the splenic fossa are allowed to heal without disturbance.

POSTOPERATIVE COMPLICATIONS

The postoperative complications following open splenectomy also occur following laparoscopic splenectomy, including bleeding, atelectasis, pneumonia, reactive pleural effusion, subphrenic fluid collections, and injury to the colon, stomach, or tail of the pancreas. In addition, portal vein thrombosis is observed more commonly following laparoscopic splenectomy.[11] The etiology is poorly understood but may relate to decreased portal blood flow during laparoscopic surgery or a hypercoagulable state following pneumoperitoneum. Patients with portal vein thrombosis will require anticoagulation.

REFERENCES

1. Delaitre B, Maignien B. Laparoscopic splenectomy: Technical aspects. *Surg Endosc* 1992;6:305–308
2. Brodsky JA, Brody FJ, Walsh RM, et al. Laparoscopic splenectomy. *Surg Endosc* 2002;16:851–854
3. Winslow ER, Brunt LM. Perioperative outcomes of laparoscopic versus open splenectomy: A meta-analysis with an emphasis on complications. *Surgery* 2003;134:647–653; discussion 54–55
4. Schlinkert RT, Mann D, Weaver A. Laparoscopic splenectomy: Reduction of hospital charges. *J Gastrointest Surg* 1998;2:278–282
5. Targarona EM, Espert JJ, Balague C, et al. Splenomegaly should not be considered a contraindication for laparoscopic splenectomy. *Ann Surg* 1998;228:35–39
6. Patel AG, Parker JE, Wallwork B, et al. Massive splenomegaly is associated with significant morbidity after laparoscopic splenectomy. *Ann Surg* 2003;238:235–240
7. Berman RS, Yahanda AM, Mansfield PF, et al. Laparoscopic splenectomy in patients with hematologic malignancies. *Am J Surg* 1999;178:530–536
8. Targarona EM, Gracia E, Rodriguez M, et al. Hand-assisted laparoscopic surgery. *Arch Surg* 2003;138:133–141; discussion 41
9. Targarona EM, Balague C, Cerdan G, et al. Hand-assisted laparoscopic splenectomy (HALS) in cases of splenomegaly: A comparison analysis with conventional laparoscopic splenectomy. *Surg Endosc* 2002;16:426–430
10. Rosen M, Brody F, Walsh RM, Ponsky J. Hand-assisted laparoscopic splenectomy vs conventional laparoscopic splenectomy in cases of splenomegaly. *Arch Surg* 2002; 137:1348–1352
11. Ikeda M, Sekimoto M, Takiguchi S, et al. High incidence of thrombosis of the portal venous system after laparoscopic splenectomy: A prospective study with contrast-enhanced CT scan. *Ann Surg* 2005;241:208–216

50

Video-Assisted Thoracic Surgery of the Esophagus

Michael S. Kent ■ *James D. Luketich*

Since the initial description of laparoscopic fundoplication in 1991,[1] many surgeons have embraced minimally invasive surgery for esophageal disease. Others, including some thoracic surgeons, were less enthusiastic about the minimally invasive approach and had concerns over compromised outcomes. In some cases, these surgeons simply lacked the technical experience required for complex laparoscopic procedures. Nonetheless, numerous reports have documented that for both gastroesophageal reflux and achalasia[2,3] the laparoscopic approach offers equal efficacy and safety as well as decreased recovery times compared with traditional open surgery. These reports and the benefits of minimally invasive surgery perceived by the general public have increased referrals to surgeons for management of these diseases, even though alternative medical therapies are available.[4,5]

Although laparoscopic approaches for many benign conditions involving the distal esophagus have now met with widespread acceptance, this is not the case for minimally invasive approaches to the thoracic esophagus or for more complex esophageal operations such as the repair of large paraesophageal hernias or esophagectomy.

However, the application of minimally invasive surgery to these complex cases may offer several potential benefits. First, open esophagectomy is associated with a significant morbidity and mortality, even in experienced centers.[6] This high complication rate along with the disappointing 25% 5-year survival rate after esophagectomy has led to an increasing debate over the role of surgery in the treatment of esophageal cancer. This has led to alternative approaches such as definitive chemoradiation alone or photodynamic therapy. Although no randomized studies of minimally invasive esophagectomy (MIE) have been performed, our experience in our first 222 patients has suggested that MIE is associated with a complication rate and mortality lower than most reports of open esophagectomy.[7] Additionally, we and others have shown that minimally invasive staging of esophageal cancer patients is superior to conventional staging by CT and endoscopic ultrasound,[8] and may allow for a better selection of patients to receive combined modality therapy. In this chapter we review our experience with minimally invasive surgery for esophageal cancer, as well as detail surgical techniques for other diseases of the thoracic esophagus, such as resection of benign esophageal tumors and thoracoscopic treatment of esophageal dysmotility. Laparoscopic approaches to other complex esophageal operations are covered elsewhere in this text.

■ ESOPHAGEAL CANCER

The optimal management of patients with potentially resectable esophageal cancer is still evolving. Although surgery remains the standard of care for early disease, several studies have suggested that definitive chemoradiation may be an acceptable alternative. This position is supported by the results of a randomized, prospective trial conducted by the Radiation Therapy Oncology Group (RTOG 8501), which compared definitive chemoradiation versus radiation therapy alone for patients with locally advanced esophageal cancer, who were not considered surgical candidates.[9] The study was closed after accrual of 121 patients, because of a clear survival benefit in the combined treatment group. The surprising finding in this study was that the 5-year survival in chemoradiation group was 27%, a rate not appreciably different from the survival following esophagectomy alone.[10] Additional support for the use of chemoradiation alone for esophageal cancer comes from the results of two, large prospective European studies. In these studies, chemoradiation followed by surgery was compared to chemoradiation alone, and both studies suggested equivalent survival between the two treatment arms.[11,12] Additionally, one of these studies reported decreased early mortality, shorter hospital stay and improved performance status in the chemoradiation only group.[13]

The impact of these reports has been to recommend nonoperative therapy for marginal surgical candidates, such as the elderly or those with multiple comorbidities. Indeed the National Comprehensive Cancer Network now considers definitive chemoradiation to be an acceptable alternative to esophagectomy in their recent guidelines.[14] It is incumbent upon esophageal surgeons, therefore, to continue to refine the technique of esophagectomy, in order to offer therapy with either lower morbidity, improved survival, or both compared to traditional esophagectomy.

STAGING FOR ESOPHAGEAL CANCER

Unlike lung cancer, in which mediastinoscopy is an accepted and proven staging technique, there is no invasive modality considered standard for staging patients with esophageal cancer. However, to date none of the noninvasive staging techniques currently available, such as CT, endoscopic ultrasound (EUS), or positron emission tomography (PET), have proven accurate enough to preclude the need for invasive staging.

The current noninvasive technology suffers from several, well-described limitations. Computed tomography, often the initial staging test performed for patients with esophageal cancer, is an appropriate tool to screen for distant disease, such as pulmonary or liver metastases. However even in this role, occult metastatic disease is missed by CT scans in 15–20% of patients.[15] Furthermore, CT is clearly unable to provide sufficient anatomic detail to accurately stage either the depth of invasion of the esophageal wall, or to determine the presence of local nodal involvement. Indeed the accuracy of CT scanning for nodal disease is only 45–60% in most series.[16,17]

PET scanning is a recently introduced technology that is based on imaging the differential uptake of radiolabeled glucose by malignant and normal cells. PET scanning has been extensively studied in the context of both lung and esophageal cancer. Indeed in some centers PET scanning has become a routine component of the pre-operative evaluation of lung cancer patients. This practice is justified by several meta-analyses that have demonstrated the superiority of PET over CT in staging nodal disease in the mediastinum.[18,19] However equal efficacy for PET scanning has not been demonstrated for esophageal cancer patients. We have found the accuracy of PET scanning to assess locoregional lymph nodes in patients with esophageal cancer to be only about 50%.[20] In our experience PET scanning has been more useful in detecting distant metastatic disease. In a series of 100 consecutive patients with potentially resectable esophageal cancer staged at our institution by PET and CT, PET identified metastatic disease in 16% of patients missed by CT.[21] The false-negative rate for PET in this series was only 10%, usually in cases of subcentimeter disease that was below the detection threshold of PET scans.

Another staging tool available in specialized centers is EUS. Although EUS is operator dependent, in experienced hands its accuracy in assessing T stage is greater than 90%, and it has an image resolution of 0.2 mm.[22] The accuracy of determining T stage increases with penetration of the esophageal wall: the accuracy for T1 tumors is 80%, T2 tumors 90%, and T3/4 tumors 95%.[23] However the accuracy of EUS to determine nodal status is far lower than its ability to determine tumor depth, and has been reported to be in the range of 65–86%.[24,25]

TECHNIQUE OF MINIMALLY INVASIVE SURGICAL STAGING

Currently, all patients at the University of Pittsburgh with a diagnosis of esophageal cancer undergo noninvasive staging with CT scans, PET scanning, and EUS. If any of these studies indicates either metastatic disease or nodal involvement (in the case of EUS), then a needle biopsy is performed. If distant metastatic disease is proven, palliative options are generally pursued. For patients without proven metastatic disease and gastroesophageal junction tumors, we then generally proceed to laparoscopic staging. Laparoscopic staging is performed with the patient in a steep reverse Trendelenburg position with the surgeon standing on the patient's right side. Usually five laparoscopic ports are used. After the first port is placed, a visual assessment is made of the peritoneal surfaces and if obvious metastatic disease is present then biopsy confirmation is obtained and the staging is complete. If no metastatic disease is seen on this initial survey, a more thorough staging is performed. The five ports generally include: a 10-mm blunt cut-down port just to the patient's right of midline midway between the xiphoid and umbilicus (for the surgeon's right hand instruments), a 5-mm port at the same level to the left of midline for the laparoscope, two additional 5-mm ports along the right costal margin (for liver retraction and dissection), and a 5-mm port on the left costal margin for countertraction by the assistant (Fig 50–1). The liver surfaces are carefully examined and any abnormalities biopsied. Ultrasound examination of the liver may then be performed, although in our experience the yield of ultrasound in patients who do not have some visual evidence of liver metastases is low.[26] Next the stomach is carefully assessed for gastric extension of the tumor to determine the suitability of the stomach for gastric pull-up. Nodal assessment is initiated by incising the gastrohepatic ligament. The lesser sac is entered and nodes along the lesser curve (level 17) and at the base of the celiac artery (level 20) are sampled (Fig 50–2). At the conclusion of the staging procedure a laparoscopic feeding tube may be placed. However, we have found that in most cases dysphagia will respond to chemotherapy, rendering a feeding tube unnecessary. If the patient has no metastatic disease and minimal or no nodal disease, we proceed to minimally invasive

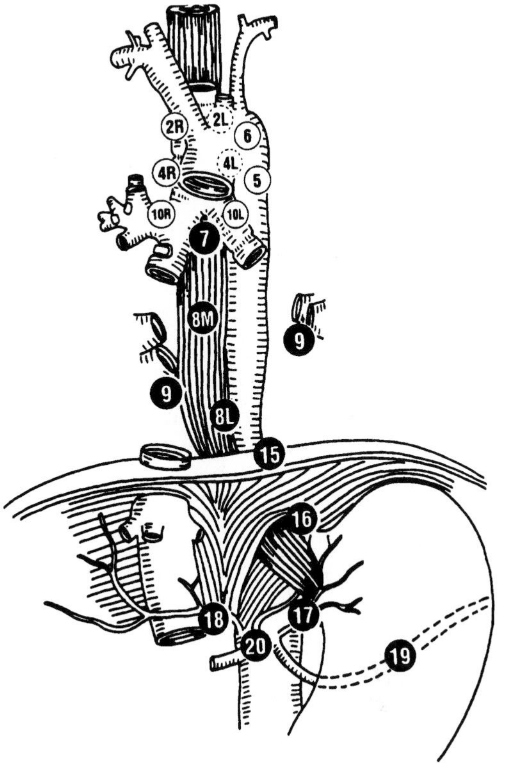

Figure 50–2. Nodes from levels 17 and 20 are harvested during laparoscopic staging. (Reprinted from: Krasna MJ, Reed CE, Nedzwiecki D, et al. CALGB 9380: a prospective trial of feasibility of thoracoscopy/laparoscopy in staging esophageal cancer. *Ann Thorac Surg* 2001; 71(4): 1073–1079, with permission from Society of Thoracic Surgeons.)

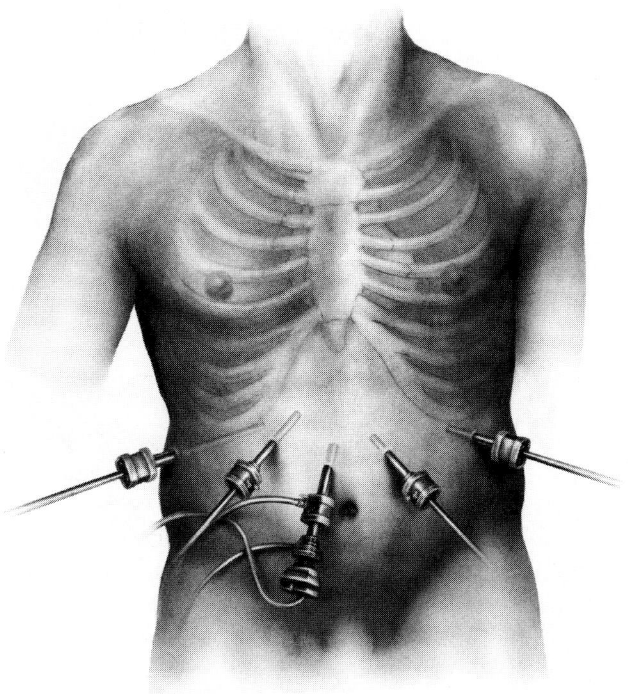

Figure 50–1. Port placement for laparoscopic staging. (Reprinted from: Alvelo-Rivera M, De Hoyos A, Luketich JD. Laparoscopic and thoracoscopic esophagectomy. Operative Techniques in Thoracic and Cardiovascular Surgery 2004; 9(2):157–176, with permission from Elsevier.)

esophagectomy. If chemotherapy is planned an infusaport is placed at the time of staging.

Thoracoscopy is used selectively for tumors of the midthoracic esophagus, once laparoscopic staging has excluded gross intra-abdominal disease. This practice is based on our prospective series of 53 patients all of whom underwent both laparoscopic and thoracoscopic staging. Of the 36 patients found to be node-positive, 31 were identified by laparoscopy.[26] Should thoracoscopy be indicated the approach is normally through the right chest, although a left-sided approach may be appropriate if suspicious pulmonary lesions are identified on that side. If thoracoscopy is indicated, four ports are used for access (Fig 50–3). The initial step is to mobilize the inferior pulmonary ligament and to sample the level 9 nodes. Next the pleura overlying the lower one third of the esophagus is opened. Once this plane is developed nodes from the peri-esophageal (level 8) and subcarinal stations (level 7) may be harvested. Lymph node dissection is continued until a positive node is found or an adequate sampling indicates benign nodes only.

Two large, prospective studies have investigated the benefits of minimally invasive staging for esophageal

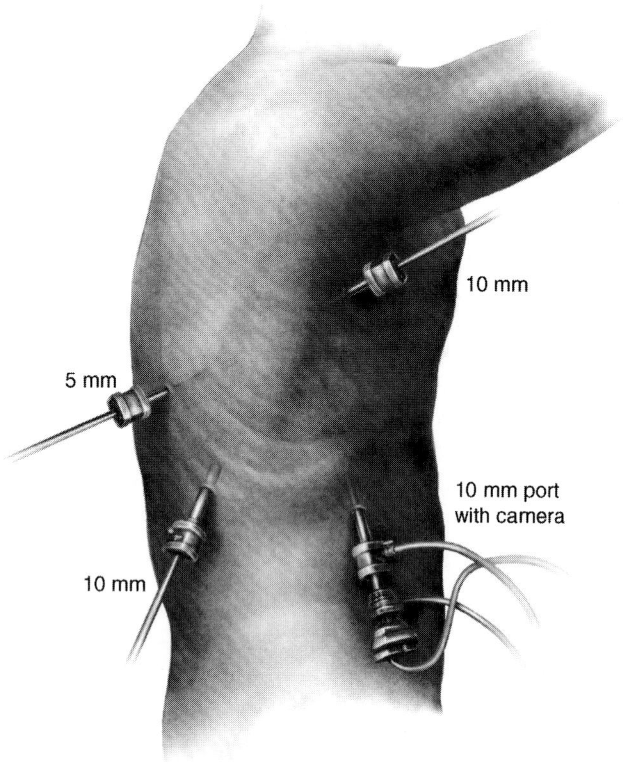

Figure 50–3. Port placement for thoracoscopic mobilization of the esophagus and thoracoscopic staging. (Reprinted from: Alvelo-Rivera M, De Hoyos A, Luketich JD. Laparoscopic and thoracoscopic esophagectomy. Operative Techniques in Thoracic and Cardiovascular Surgery 2004; 9(2):157–176, with permission from Elsevier.)

cancer. The first, from our institution, showed significant advantages for invasive staging compared with more standard modalities.[26] All 53 patients in this report underwent CT and concurrent laparoscopy and thoracoscopy. Forty-seven patients also underwent endoscopic ultrasound. The sensitivities of CT and EUS to document nodal metastases were only 33% and 63%, respectively. Even when these two modalities were combined inaccuracies in staging were seen in 32% of cases, compared with MIS. Only two complications were seen in this series: one prolonged air leak and a port site hernia that was repaired on the first postoperative day.

The second study, comprising 134 patients, was a multi-institution, NCI-sponsored study designed to determine the feasibility of MIS.[28] Successful MIS was defined as documentation of T4 or M1 disease, the procurement of at least one abdominal and three thoracic lymph nodes, or one node that documented metastatic disease. MIS was found to be successful in 73% of patients and was performed with no mortality and only minimal morbidity. Noninvasive tests, such as CT and EUS, failed to identify positive lymph nodes documented by MIS in 20% of patients. Unfortunately the true sensitivity of MIS was not determined by this study since the majority of patients underwent induction chemotherapy prior to resection.

Ultimately the role of MIS will be determined by clinical trials that demonstrate a survival advantage for patients with node-positive disease who receive induction therapy. To date, only one randomized study, with significant limitations, has demonstrated a benefit for preoperative chemoradiation.[29] However, the poor survival obtained after surgery alone assures that the neoadjuvant approach will continue to be investigated. We believe that a major flaw of the studies performed to date is that patients have not been adequately staged prior to undergoing combined modality therapy. Accurate staging may identify a subpopulation of patients who would benefit from such aggressive treatment, and studies not designed for subgroup analysis may report false-negative conclusions.

MOLECULAR STAGING OF ESOPHAGEAL CANCER

It is estimated that between 30–50% of patients who are staged as node-negative by routine histological evaluation following esophagectomy will develop a recurrence of their disease.[27] This suggests that these patients harbored micrometastatic disease that was undetected by routine histology. In an attempt to improve the staging of these patients, we have used MIS to obtain lymph nodes that are evaluated with molecular biology techniques, such as reverse transcription polymerase chain reaction (RT-PCR), to determine the presence of micrometastases.[30] In a recent report we evaluated nodes from 30 patients who were histologically staged as node-negative.[31] Among these 30 patients 11 were identified by RT-PCR as harboring micrometastatic disease. Furthermore, the quantitative expression of carcinoembryonic antigen by RT-PCR was a powerful, independent predictor of disease recurrence and death (Fig 50–4). We believe that these techniques may identify patients with early-stage disease that have a high risk of recurrence and may benefit from additional therapy.

MINIMALLY INVASIVE ESOPHAGECTOMY

The technique of MIE has evolved as our experience with other minimally invasive foregut procedures, such as laparoscopic Heller myotomy, repair of giant para-esophageal hernia, and staging for esophageal cancer has grown. To date, we have performed over 500 MIE at the University of Pittsburgh Medical Center.

Initial attempts at MIE were hybrid operations combining traditional open surgery with minimally invasive techniques. The first such report by Collard in 1993 included 12 patients who underwent thoracoscopic mobilization of the esophagus followed by lap-

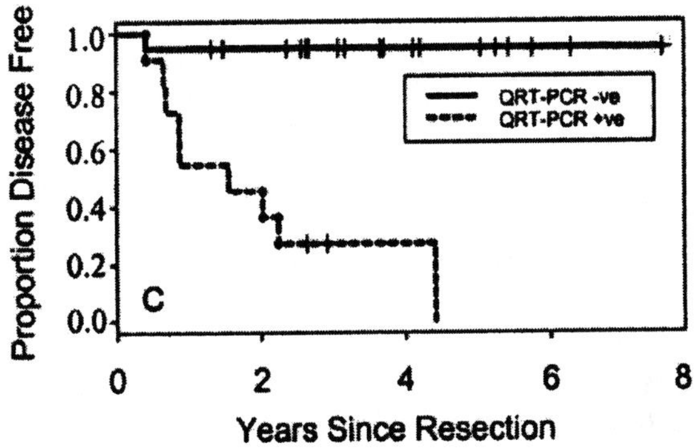

Figure 50–4. Disease-free survival of esophageal cancer patients defined as node-negative and node-positive by quantitative RT-PCR. (Reprinted from: Godfrey TE, Raja S, Finklestein SD. Prognostic value of quantitative reverse transcription-polymerase chain reaction in lymph node-negative esophageal cancer patients. *Clin Cancer Res* 2001; 7:4041–4048, with permission of the American Association for Cancer Research, Inc.)

arotomy and preparation of the gastric conduit.[32] In that series, two patients required conversion to thoracotomy for bleeding. Several subsequent reports have demonstrated the feasibility of this approach; however no definitive benefit has been shown compared to open esophagectomy.[33–35]

A completely laparoscopic transhiatal esophagectomy has also been described. The largest series, published by DePaula in 1995,[36] described 48 patients who required esophagectomy predominantly for end-stage achalasia secondary to Chagas' disease. Only two patients required conversion to laparotomy. The first experience with MIE in the United States was not reported until 1997, when Swanstrom described a carefully selected group of nine patients with small tumors, benign strictures and Barrett's disease.[37] Eight of these patients had a totally laparoscopic transhiatal esophagectomy, while one required the addition of a right VATS procedure.

Similar to these early reports, our initial efforts at minimally invasive esophagectomy were with the transhiatal approach. Advantages of a totally laparoscopic approach include single patient positioning and no need for single-lung ventilation. However, we found that the disadvantages of this approach were significant. The small working space through the hiatus allowed limited access to the middle and upper third of the esophagus, and made any thoracic lymph node dissection extremely difficult. Because of this, our current approach includes a right VATS to mobilize the thoracic esophagus followed by laparoscopy to prepare the gastric tube. Although early in our experience MIE was only offered to patients with Barrett's disease and early-stage tumors, we now offer MIE to patients with more advanced disease. Patients found to have bulky celiac nodal metastases by CT or staging laparoscopy are not felt to be candidates for MIE, and consideration is given to either an open operation, a neoadjuvant protocol, or definitive chemoradiation.

OPERATIVE TECHNIQUE

The initial step of MIE is an on-the-table esophagogastroduodenoscopy (EGD) to confirm the location of the tumor and the suitability of the stomach as a conduit for reconstruction. If clinically indicated we then perform laparoscopic staging. If the staging is negative, patients are then intubated with a double-lumen endotracheal tube and turned to a left lateral decubitus position. The surgeon stands on the right side and the assistant on the left. Four thoracoscopic ports are used, in the same positions as for thoracoscopic staging (Fig 50–3). A 10-mm camera port is placed in the 8th or 9th intercostal space, anterior to the midaxillary line. A 10-mm port is placed at the 8th or 9th intercostal space, posterior to the posterior axillary line, for the ultrasonic coagulating shears (U.S. Surgical, Norwalk, CT). A 10-mm port is placed in the anterior axillary line at the 4th intercostal space and is used to place a fan shaped retractor to retract the lung anteriorly and expose the esophagus. The last 5-mm port is placed just posterior to the tip of the scapula and is used for retraction and countertraction by the assistant. An optional initial step in exposure is to place a retracting suture (Endo-Stitch, U.S. Surgical, Norwalk, CT) through the central tendon of the diaphragm, which is brought out through the anterior chest wall near the costophrenic recess anteriorly using an Endo-close device (U.S. Surgical, Norwalk, CT). This suture retracts the diaphragm inferiorly and allows excellent visualization of the lower one third of the esophagus.

The inferior pulmonary ligament is then divided and the mediastinal pleura overlying the esophagus divided to the level of the azygos vein. The azygos vein is then ligated using an endoscopic stapler (Endo-GIA II, U.S. Surgical, Norwalk, CT). The mediastinal pleura is preserved above the azygos vein. This helps to maintain the gastric conduit in a mediastinal location and may seal the plane between the stomach and the thoracic inlet, minimizing any downward extension of a cervical anastomotic leak into the chest. The esophagus is mobilized circumferentially and all the surrounding lymph nodes and fat are resected en bloc up to 2 cm above the carina. Above this level the dissection is directly against the esophagus to avoid damage to the recurrent nerves. The thoracic duct is left intact and care is taken to clip any lymphatic attachments between the duct and the peri-esophageal tissues to minimize the risk of a chylothorax. A Penrose drain is placed around the esophagus which aids in subsequent retraction and mobilization (Fig 50–5). The entire thoracic esophagus is then mobilized from thoracic inlet to the diaphragm.

It is important not to carry the dissection too low into the peritoneal cavity, which would hinder the creation of pneumoperitoneum during laparoscopy. Also, we keep the dissection plane close to the esophagus at

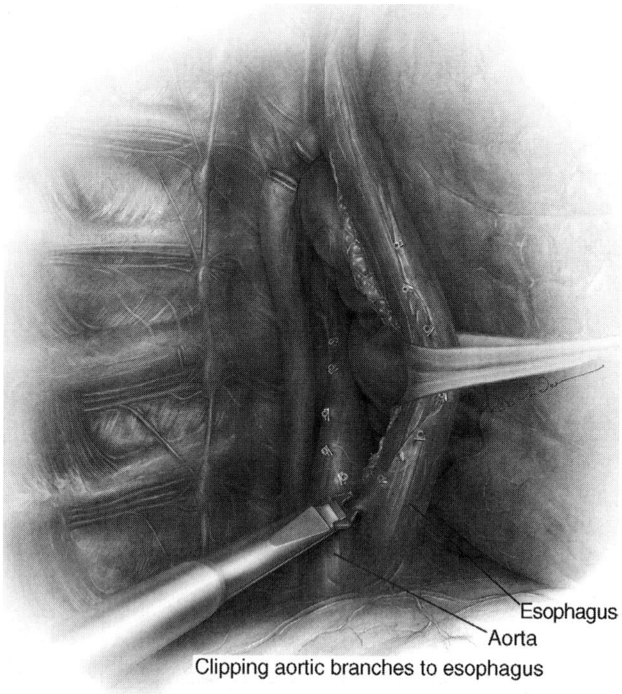

Figure 50–5. A Penrose drain is placed around the thoracic esophagus for retraction. (Reprinted from: Alvelo-Rivera M, De Hoyos A, Luketich JD. Laparoscopic and thoracoscopic esophagectomy. Operative Techniques in Thoracic and Cardiovascular Surgery 2004; 9(2):157–176, with permission from Elsevier.)

the superior extent of the dissection, to avoid injury to either the airway or the recurrent laryngeal nerves. After placement of a single 28F (French) chest tube, we inflate the lung and examine the airway and parenchymal surfaces for any air leaks. The thoracic ports are closed and the patient is turned to the supine position for laparoscopy.

The five abdominal ports used for gastric mobilization are in the same orientation as those used in laparoscopic staging (Fig 50–1). In general, the two midline ports are placed at a point approximately two thirds the distance from the xiphoid to the umbilicus. This lower position of the ports may make the hiatal dissection somewhat difficult but greatly facilitates the mobilization of the gastric tube. This emphasizes the importance of completely mobilizing the esophagus and any hiatal hernia sac circumferentially during the thoracoscopic dissection. The gastrohepatic ligament is first divided and the right and left crura are dissected. Unlike other operations of the gastroesophageal junction, we do not divide the phrenoesophageal ligament until the conclusion of laparoscopy. This allows us to maintain the pneumoperitoneum for the duration of the procedure. The stomach is then mobilized by dividing first the short gastric vessels and then the gastrocolic omentum, carefully preserving the right gastroepiploic vessels. The stomach is then retracted superiorly and the left gastric artery is divided using a vascular stapler. In our experience, performing a laparoscopic pyloromyotomy that is technically complete is difficult and thus we perform a pyloroplasty. The pyloroplasty is created by opening the pylorus with the ultrasonic shears and closing the pylorus transversely using the Endo-stitch (Fig 50–6). Once experience is gained the pyloroplasty can be performed in less than 10 minutes.

The gastric tube is then started by dividing the stomach at the lower end of the lesser curve near the incisura using a vascular load (2.5 mm) stapler, with care being taken to preserve the main right gastric vessels and one or two of the first branches entering the antral area (Fig 50–7). Next, an additional port is placed in the lower mid-right quadrant to allow the placement of an atraumatic grasper on the pyloro-antral area. One assistant places careful downward traction on the lower antral area, and a second assistant places cephalad countertraction using an atraumatic grasper placed along the greater curve near the line of the short gastrics. This countertraction is essential during each application of the staple line to avoid tethering along the lesser curve and to allow the greater curve to uncoil and lengthen as each staple application is performed. Additionally by precisely placing the cephalad grasper along the line of the short gastric vessels we avoid spiraling of the tube that would compromise the blood supply to the greater curve. Caution must be used during any application of a grasper to the gastric tube, es-

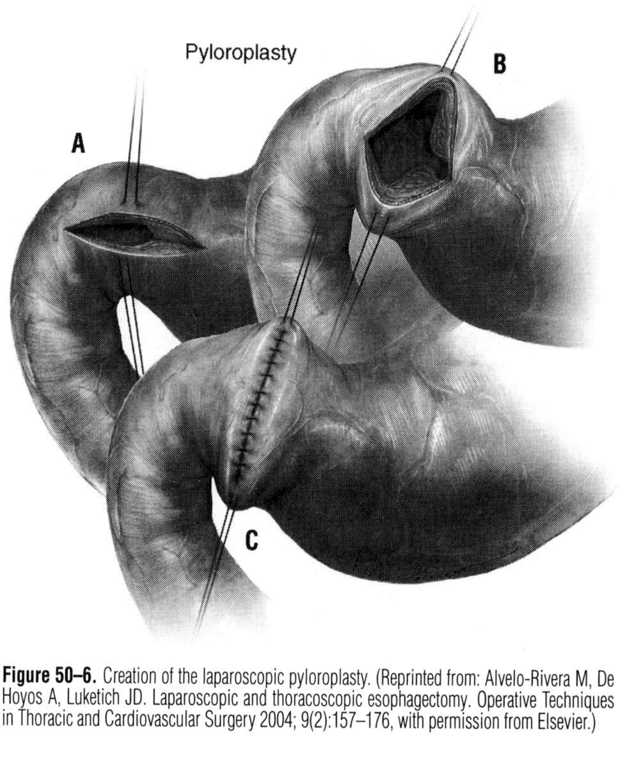

Figure 50–6. Creation of the laparoscopic pyloroplasty. (Reprinted from: Alvelo-Rivera M, De Hoyos A, Luketich JD. Laparoscopic and thoracoscopic esophagectomy. Operative Techniques in Thoracic and Cardiovascular Surgery 2004; 9(2):157–176, with permission from Elsevier.)

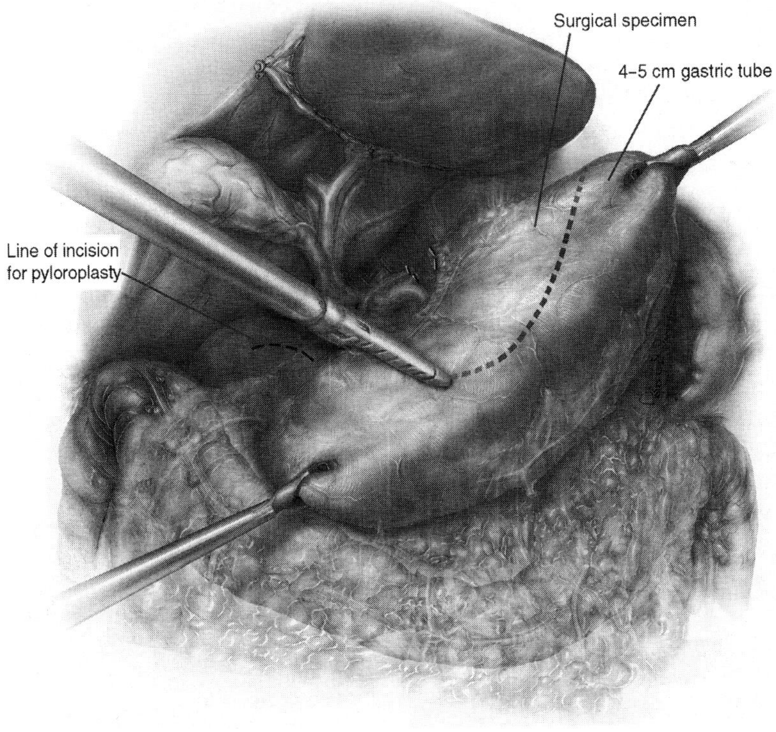

Figure 50–7. A vascular stapler is fired across the lesser curvature near the incisura to begin formation of the gastric tube. (Reprinted from: Alvelo-Rivera M, De Hoyos A, Luketich JD. Laparoscopic and thoracoscopic esophagectomy. Operative Techniques in Thoracic and Cardiovascular Surgery 2004; 9(2):157–176, with permission from Elsevier.)

pecially the mid to superior portions, and the tube must be handled gently at all times. A bruised and ecchymotic tube with multiple serosal tears will predispose to gastric tip necrosis and must be avoided. The final gastric tube is 5 to 6 cm in diameter.

Earlier in our experience we created a very narrow gastric tube of approximately 3 cm and found a significant increase in gastric tip necrosis and anastomotic leaks. Thus we modified our technique to perform a moderately narrow gastric tube of 5 to 6 cm. In over 150 consecutive operations using this 5- to 6-cm tube, we have observed a leak rate of 6% with only one gastric tip necrosis. The most superior portion of the gastric tube is then attached to the resection specimen using a single figure of eight Endo-stitch. A feeding jejunostomy is then placed using a needle catheter kit (Compact Biosystems, Minneapolis, MN). A limb of jejunum is first tacked to the anterior abdominal wall, in the left lateral mid-quadrant using an Endo-stitch. The needle and guidewire are then passed into the jejunum under laparoscopic vision. Proper positioning of the catheter is confirmed by observing distension of the jejunum as 10 mL of air is rapidly insufflated into the needle catheter. The jejunum is then circumferentially tacked to the abdominal wall covering the entrance of the needle catheter into the jejunum using several additional Endo-stitches. We then divide the phrenoesophageal membrane and partially divide the right and left crura to allow easy passage of the stomach into the mediastinum.

Next a horizontal neck incision is made to expose the cervical esophagus. We typically leave the Penrose drain around the esophagus during VATS mobilization and push this drain into the neck at the conclusion of thoracoscopy. This allows quick identification of the correct dissection plane. Next, the laparoscope is reinserted and as the esophagus is pulled out of the neck, the assistant performing the laparoscopy carefully maintains orientation of the tube to avoid twisting as it ascends through the hiatus. Additionally, care must be taken to avoid any tension on the greater curve vascular arcade during this step. In some cases, enlargement of the hiatus is necessary to allow removal of the resected specimen though the hiatus. The esophagogastric specimen is delivered into the neck and the cervical esophagus is divided 1 to 2 cm below the cricopharyngeus using the Auto-Purse String device (U.S. Surgical, Norwalk, CT), if an EEA anastomosis is to be used.

The type of anastomosis is up to the individual surgeon. In general, we prefer the EEA if the length of the gastric tube permits ample delivery into the cervical area. We then perform a side-to-end esophagogastrostomy using a 25-mm EEA stapler. The stapler is placed through a gastrotomy at the most cephalad tip of the gastric tube and the tip exits posterolaterally approximately 6 to 8 cm down from the gastrotomy site. The tip is docked to the anvil in the cervical esophagus and fired. A gloved finger is placed through the gastrotomy and a visual inspection of the staple line and EEA rings is performed. A nasogastric tube is carefully guided down to the midlevel of the gastric tube. The distal gastric tip is resected using an Endo-GIA II blue stapler.

The laparoscope is then again reinserted to ensure that there is no redundancy of the conduit above the diaphragm. This is done by placing gentle traction on the antrum until any redundancy is retrieved back into the peritoneal cavity. This step is usually completed once the gastric tube is noted to move slightly from the neck as traction is placed with the laparoscopic instruments. Finally, three tacking sutures are placed between the gastric tube and the diaphragm to prevent hiatal herniation and to maintain final orientation of the gastric tube as it enters the hiatus. Usually one suture is placed between the left crus and the stomach just anterior to the greater curve arcade, the second on the right side of the gastric tube just above the right gastric vessels and the third stitch anteriorly between the stomach and the diaphragm. Figure 50–8 illustrates the completed reconstruction.

OUTCOMES AND COMPLICATIONS FOLLOWING MIE

We have recently published our series of 222 consecutive patients who have undergone minimally invasive esophagectomy at the University of Pittsburgh.[7] Although early in the series we selectively performed MIE on patients with smaller tumors and no previous therapy, 35% of the patients in the overall series had been treated with chemotherapy and 16% with radiation. Additionally, 25% of patients had undergone prior open abdominal surgery.

MIE was completed as planned in 206 patients (93%). No emergent conversions to an open procedure were necessary for bleeding. Of the 16 cases who required nonemergent conversion, 11 required a minithoracotomy for adhesions and, in one case, oversewing of an intercostal vessel that could not be controlled by VATS.

There were three deaths in the series (mortality 1.4%). These three deaths were from post-operative pneumonia and multisystem organ failure in one patient, an MI on postoperative day five in another, and pericardial tamponade that developed 3 days after MIE. None of these deaths were in patients who developed an anastomotic leak or gastric tube necrosis. Presumably, traction injury to the pericardium during VATS was the mechanism for the development of postoperative tamponade in the third patient.[38] This very low mortality rate compares favorably with the largest series of open esophagectomy (Table 50–1). Certainly, it is not clear whether this is due to the minimally invasive approach or the fact that surgery is performed at a dedicated esophageal center with a high caseload.

The rate of anastomotic leak in this series was 11.7%. In our experience this complication was frequently related to the diameter of the gastric tube. The leak rate associated with a 3-cm diameter tube was 26% in 56 consecutive patients. In those patients who underwent creation of a larger conduit the leak rate was only 6%.

Injury to the recurrent laryngeal nerve is a complication associated with significant morbidity. Mechanisms related to this complication include excessive traction on the nerve during the neck dissection or injury during dissection of the upper one third of the esophagus. In our series vocal cord palsy occurred in 3.6% of patients. This is lower than our open experience and is in part due to enhanced visualization of the upper thoracic esophagus during VATS. Additionally, we divide the vagus nerves early in the course of the dissection to avoid traction injury on the recurrent nerve trunks. Also, we have limited our lymph node dissection above the azygos vein, to avoid injury to the nerve in this area. Other complications seen after MIE, as well as open esophagectomy, include chylothorax, delayed gastric emptying and airway injuries. All of these complications are potentially related to surgical technique. Inadequate control of small ductules that branch off of the thoracic duct or a gross tear of the main duct

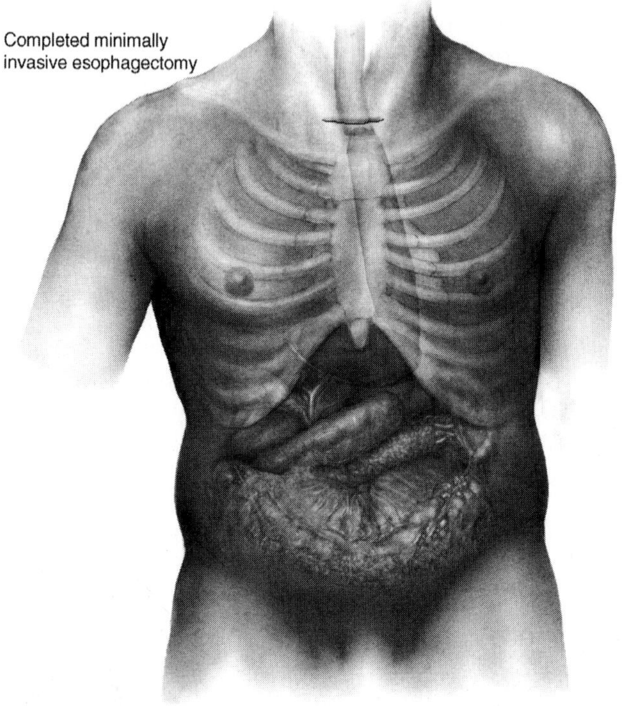

Figure 50–8. Final reconstruction following minimally invasive esophagectomy. (Reprinted from: Alvelo-Rivera M, De Hoyos A, Luketich JD. Laparoscopic and thoracoscopic esophagectomy. Operative Techniques in Thoracic and Cardiovascular Surgery 2004; 9(2):157–176, with permission from Elsevier.)

TABLE 50–1. MORTALITY AND MORBIDITY FOLLOWING MIE COMPARED TO OPEN ESOPHAGECTOMY

	Pittsburgh	Michigan	VA	Sloan-Kettering	Duke
	N = 222	*N* = 1085	*N* = 1777	*N* = 510	*N* = 379
Mortality	1.4%	4%	9.8%	4%	5.8%
Anastomotic leak	11.7%	13%	NR	21%	14%
Pneumonia	7.7%	2%	21.4%	21%	16%
Vocal cord palsy	3.6%	7%	NR	4%	NR
Gastric tube necrosis	3.2%	0.83%	NR	1%	NR
Chylothorax	3.2%	1.7%	0.02%	2.4%	NR
Myocardial infarct	1.8%	NR	1.2%	NR	NR
Delayed gastric emptying	1.8%	NR	NR	NR	NR
Tracheal tear	0.9%	0.4%	NR	NR	NR
Renal failure	0.9%	NR	2.1%	NR	NR
Splenectomy	0	3.1%	NR	NR	NR
Delayed (>30 days) diaphragmatic hernia	1.8%	NR	NR	1.2%	NR

NR = Not reported
From Schuchert MJ, Luketich JD, Fernando HC. Complications of minimally invasive esophagectomy. *Sem Thorac Cardiovasc Surg* 2004;16(2):133–141.

is typically the cause of a chylothorax. Seven patients (3%) developed this complication early in our series. Following this early experience we have liberally applied clips to even small branches emanating from the thoracic duct along the right esophageal border during VATS, and this complication has fallen to less than 1%.

Delayed gastric emptying is reported to occur in up to 10% of patients following esophagectomy. This may be because of a number of factors, including the vagotomy itself, the creation of a full-size gastric conduit that may empty poorly compared to a tubularized conduit, incomplete pyloromyotomy or pyloroplasty, spiraling of the gastric tube, excess stomach above the diaphragm leading to a sigmoid loop effect, and an inadequate crural opening. In our series, only 2% of patients developed delayed gastric emptying after MIE. The creation of a pyloroplasty rather than a pyloromyotomy, and attention to all of the details listed above has contributed to this low complication rate.

Fortunately, significant airway injuries in our experience have been exceedingly rare, occurring in only two patients. One of these injuries occurred postoperatively during reintubation for respiratory distress and one was believed to result from injury to the posterior membranous trachea from unintentional contact of the autosomic shears. In other series tracheal injury has been associated with the resection of bulky, midthoracic tumors. This is usually either due to either traction or cautery injury during esophageal mobilization. In these cases of bulky tumors we would therefore recommend a thoracotomy, particularly if the patient has received neoadjuvant radiation.

With a median follow-up of 19 months, overall survival was similar to that after open esophagectomy. Figure 50–9 illustrates survival stratified by stage. Of importance in assessing outcomes is not only overall survival, but also the quality of life following esophagectomy. We have documented this by administering a validated quality of life instrument (SF-36) and a disease-specific questionnaire (the Heartburn Related Quality of Life index, or HR-QOL) to patients before and after MIE. The HR-QOL instrument noted that dysphagia and heartburn scores following esophagectomy were excellent, and that only 4% of patients had severe, poorly controlled reflux. In addition the overall quality of life as measured by the Short-Form 36 was no different than that of age-matched controls.

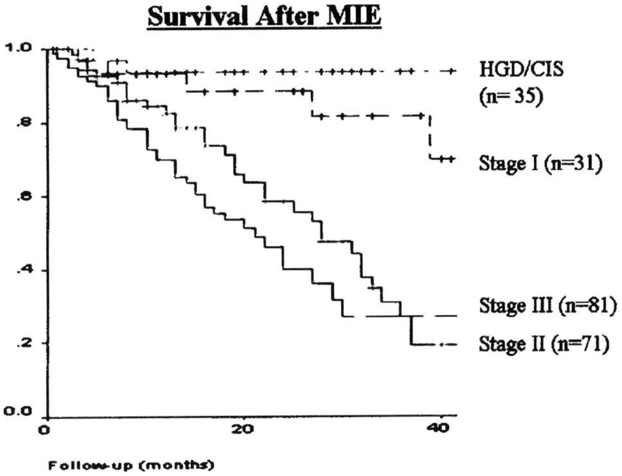

Figure 50–9. Survival following minimally invasive esophagectomy. (Reprinted from: Luketich JD, Alvelo-Rivera M, Buenaventura PO, et al. Minimally invasive esophagectomy: outcomes in 222 patients. *Ann Surg* 2003; 238(4):486–495. Copyright © 2003 Lippincott William & Wilkins.)

RESECTION OF ESOPHAGEAL LEIOMYOMA

Leiomyomas represent the most common benign tumor of the esophagus, accounting for approximately two thirds of all cases.[39] These tumors occur in the middle (33%) and lower (56%) esophagus, a distribution that parallels the degree of smooth muscle in the esophageal wall.[40] Consequently, leiomyoma are rarely found in the cervical esophagus, which is composed predominantly of skeletal muscle. The majority of these tumors arise from the muscularis propria and extend into the lumen of the esophagus. On occasion, however, they may arise from the muscularis mucosa, in which case they tend to pedunculate as a result of peristalsis.[40]

Over 85% of patients with small leiomyoma are asymptomatic. When present, symptoms are often nonspecific, such as chest pain, regurgitation, and dysphagia. On rare occasion these tumors may ulcerate and present with GI bleeding. Interestingly there does not appear to be a clear correlation between the size of the tumor and either the frequency or severity of symptoms.[41,42]

The natural history of these uncommon tumors is not well understood, and therefore the guidelines for resection of asymptomatic tumors are unclear. Certainly, resection of either symptomatic tumors or those in which a malignant histology is suspected is appropriate. In most series criteria for resection of asymptomatic lesions has been a size greater than 3 to 5 cm. However, it has been well-documented that the size of these tumors can remain stable over several years.[43] Furthermore, unlike smooth muscle tumors of the stomach, the propensity of these tumors to degenerate into leiomyosarcoma is extremely rare, and in fact only two cases have ever been documented.[44,45] What is clear is that the decision to recommend surgery will depend on the morbidity associated with the procedure.

TECHNIQUE OF RESECTION

The approach to resection depends on the location of the tumor. Leiomyoma of the midthoracic esophagus are approached at the University of Pittsburgh through a right VATS approach, and those at the GE junction with laparoscopy. Esophagoscopy is performed prior to draping to confirm location of the tumor. The scope is frequently left in place to assist the surgeon in determining where to begin the myotomy. The four thoracoscopic ports are the same used for minimally invasive esophagectomy.

Exposure of the tumor is obtained by dividing the inferior pulmonary ligament and then opening the pleura overlying the esophagus. Care must be exercised at this point to preserve the vagus trunk and its branches. The esophagus may need to be dissected circumferentially for exposure, particularly if the tumor appears to arise from the left side of the esophagus. A Penrose drain can be placed around the tumor and manipulated using an Endo-Babcock grasper (Fig 50–10). The longitudinal muscular layer is then opened sharply and the leiomyoma is exposed. Due to the firm, rubbery nature of the tumor, it is often difficult to grasp and we frequently place a stitch into the tumor for traction. The tumor is then enucleated with the ultrasonic dissector, hook electrocautery and the Endo-peanut. After the tumor is removed the esophagus is submerged under water and insufflated with air from the esophagoscope to determine mucosal integrity. The myotomy is then closed using interrupted 2-0 Surgidac stitches (Fig 50–11). Although not all surgeons feel that this step is necessary,[46] several studies have documented the occurrence of postoperative dysphagia due to the formation of a mucosal pseudodiverticulum at the myotomy site. In these cases symptoms resolved after approximation of the myotomy.[47,48]

Between 1995 and 2001 we have resected nine patients with esophageal leiomyoma, and have recently published our results.[49] In this series the tumor loca-

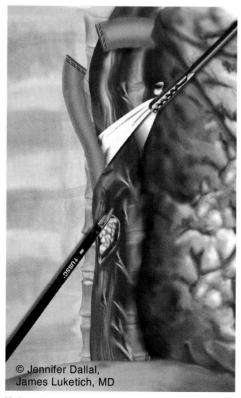

Figure 50–10. Resection of an esophageal leiomyoma is facilitated by use of a Penrose drain.

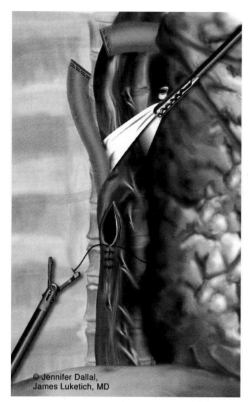

Figure 50–11. Closure of the myotomy following leiomyoma resection.

tion was evenly divided between the middle and distal third of the esophagus and the GE junction. All the patients with tumor in the thoracic esophagus were approached with a right VATS. Two patients underwent an additional Collis-Nissen procedure for significant reflux disease. There were no complications and the median hospital stay was 2.3 days. One patient was noted to have a mucosal injury at time of surgery; this was repaired using an endo-GIA stapler without complication. The mean tumor size was 2.7 cm, however we have safely resected tumors up to 8 cm in size using minimally invasive techniques.

▪ TREATMENT OF ACHALASIA

The introduction of minimally invasive techniques has revolutionized the treatment paradigm of patients with achalasia. The long-term benefits of surgery over medical management have been clearly documented for many years.[50,51] However in the past patients were often not referred for surgery due to the morbidity of the thoracotomy necessary for an esophagomyotomy. The advent of minimally invasive techniques has led to a resurgence in surgery as the primary treatment modality for this disease.[52]

Most surgeons experienced in the treatment of achalasia have adopted laparoscopy as their preferred approach (see Chapter 8). Indeed in our own series of minimally invasive esophagomyotomy 92% of patients underwent laparoscopy as opposed to thoracoscopy.[53] Similarly the initial group to describe VATS myotomy has now come to favor laparoscopy.[54] However, there are reasons to consider thoracoscopy as an acceptable alternative. During thoracoscopy the distal esophagus and GE junction are visualized without the necessity of dividing the phrenoesophageal ligament. Proponents of thoracoscopy claim, consequently, that the preservation of this ligament will prevent postoperative reflux and obviate the need for an anti-reflux procedure, which is usually added after a laparoscopic esophagomyotomy.[55]

However, there are some inherent disadvantages to thoracoscopic myotomy. First, anesthesia is complicated by the need for single-lung ventilation. In addition, thoracoscopy is more uncomfortable for the patient, particularly since a "mini-thoracotomy" access incision[56,57] and a chest tube are usually required for the procedure. More important is the concern that the myotomy may be incomplete when performed thoracoscopically. Critics of the operation cite the difficulty of working in a plane perpendicular to the esophagus and extending the myotomy adequately onto the stomach when working through the chest.[58]

Overall, thoracoscopic myotomy has been shown to provide symptomatic improvement in 76% of patients with achalasia.[58] These results do not compare favorably to laparoscopy, in which 94% of the nearly 500 patients reported in the literature have had relief of their dysphagia. In addition, a 35% rate of postoperative reflux is associated with thoracoscopy, compared with a rate of only 9% following laparoscopic myotomy and fundoplication.[59]

Most reports of thoracoscopic myotomy describe a "hybrid operation," which utilizes a mini-thoracotomy through which standard instruments are used. Additional port sites are placed to provide illumination and counter-retraction. This approach likely reflects the preferences of thoracic surgeons who may not be as familiar with techniques of laparoscopy. We favor laparoscopy, as do the vast majority of surgeons performing myotomy. In our opinion only the rare patient with a hostile abdomen from multiple prior abdominal procedures would be a potential candidate for VATS myotomy. Even in this setting, a laparoscopic approach may still be possible.

OTHER INDICATIONS

A variety of other thoracoscopic esophageal procedures have been described, though their merit is difficult to determine due to the rarity of the diseases and the small number of patients studied. For example, resection of midthoracic diverticula has been reported in series of one to three patients, in which results were described as "excellent."[60,61] However in a larger series of 11 patients from France three developed an esophageal fistula and two required reoperation.[62] The authors of that study concluded "minimally invasive surgery does not confer significant benefit compared with open surgery in the treatment of diverticula of the thoracic esophagus." We have reviewed our experience with this disease and reported a 20% leak rate after resection.[63] One patient (5%) subsequently died from complications related to a leak.

Thoracoscopic treatment of Boerhaave's syndrome[64,65] and repair of an anastomotic leak following esophagectomy[66] have also been described in case reports. A minimally invasive approach certainly merits consideration in these cases only if the surgeon feels he can make safe, and expeditious progress in these semi-urgent cases. In general, we approach the majority of these cases through an open approach.

REFERENCES

1. Dallemagne B, Weerts J, Jehaes C et al. Laparoscopic Nissen fundoplication: preliminary report. *Surg Endosc* 1991;3:138–143
2. Ackroyd R, Watson DI, Majeed AW. Randomized clinical trial of laparoscopic versus open fundoplication for gastro-oesophageal reflux disease. *Br J Surg* 2004;91: 975–982
3. Douard R, Gaudric M, Chaussade S, Couturier D. Functional results after laparoscopic Heller myotomy for achalasia: A comparative study to open surgery. *Surgery* 2004;136:16–24
4. Patti M, Fisichella P, Perretta S et al. Impact of minimally invasive surgery on the treatment of achalasia: a decade of change. *J Am Coll Surg* 2003;196:6998–6705
5. Little AG. Gastroesophageal reflux disease: a historical review of surgical therapy. *J Surg Res* 2004;117:30–33
6. Millikan K, Silverstein J, Hart V et al. A 15-year review of esophagectomy for carcinoma of the esophagus and cardia. *J Am Coll Surg* 1999;118:328–332
7. Luketich J, Alvelo-Rivera M, Buenaventura P et al. Minimally invasive esophagectomy: outcomes in 222 patients. *Ann Surg* 2003;238:486–495
8. Luketich JD, Schauer P, Landreneau R et al. Minimally invasive surgical staging is superior to endoscopic ultrasound in detecting lymph node metastases in esophageal cancer. *J Thorac Cardiovasc Surg* 1997;114:817–821
9. Al-Sarraf M, Martz K, Herskovic A, et al. Progress report of combined chemoradiotherapy versus radiotherapy alone in patients with esophageal cancer: an intergroup study. *J Clin Oncol* 1997;15:277–284
10. Hulscher JB, van Sandick JW, de Boer AG. Extended transthoracic resection compared with limited transhiatal resection for adenocarcinoma of the esophagus. *N Engl J Med* 2002;347:1662–1669
11. Bedenne L, Michel P, Bouche O, et al. Randomized phase III trial in locally advanced esophageal cancer: radiochemotherapy followed by surgery versus radiochemotherapy alone (FFCD 9102) (Abstract 519). *Proc Am Soc Clin Oncol* 2002;21:130a
12. Stahl M, Stuschke M, Lehmann N, et al. Chemoradiation with and without surgery in patients with locally advanced squamous cell carcinoma of the esophagus. *J Clin Oncol* 2005;24:2310–2317
13. Bedenne L, Michel P, Bouche O, et al. Randomized phase III trial in locally advanced esophageal cancer: radiochemotherapy followed by surgery versus radiochemotherapy alone (FFCD 9102) (Abstract 519). *Proc Am Soc Clin Oncol* 2002;21:130a
14. NCCN Guidelines. Version 1. 2003. Available at: http://www.nccn.org. Last accessed June 2005
15. Luketich J, Meehan M, Schauer P, et al. Minimally invasive staging for esophageal cancer. *Surg Endosc* 1999; 13(suppl 1):59
16. Flanagan F, Dehdashti F, Siegel B et al. Staging of esophageal cancer 18F fluorodeoxyglucose positron emission tomography. *AJR Am J Roentgenol* 1997;168:417
17. Kole A, Plukker J, Nieweg O et al. Positron emission tomography for staging of esophageal and gastroesophageal malignancy. *Br J Cancer* 1998;78:521
18. Dwamena B, Sonnad S, Angobaldo J et al. Metastases from non-small cell lung cancer: mediastinal staging in the 1990s- meta-analytic comparison of PET and CT. *Radiology* 1999;213:530–536
19. Hellwig D, Ukena D, Paulsen F et al. Meta-analysis of the efficacy of positron emission tomography with F-18 fluorodeoxyglucose in lung tumors. *Pneumologie* 2001; 55:367–377
20. Luketich J, Schauer P, Meltzer C et al. Role of positron emission tomography in staging esophageal cancer. *Ann Thorac Surg* 1997;64:765–769
21. Luketich J, Friedman D, Weigel T et al. Evaluation of distant metastases in esophageal cancer: 100 consecutive positron emission tomography scans. *Ann Thorac Surg* 1999;68:1133
22. Tytgat G, Tio T. Esophageal ultrasonography. *Gastroenterol Clin North Am* 1991;20:659
23. Saunders H, Wolfman N, Ott D: Esophageal cancer: radiologic staging. *Radiol Clin North Am* 1997;35:281
24. Luketich J, Schauer P, Landreneau R et al. Minimally invasive staging is superior to endoscopic ultrasound in detecting lymph node metastases in esophageal cancer. *J Thorac Cardiovasc Surg* 1997;114:817
25. Vickers J. Role of endoscopic ultrasound in the preoperative assessment of patients with esophageal cancer. *Ann R Coll Surg Engl* 1998;80:233
26. Luketich JD, Meehan M, Nguyen NT et al. Minimally invasive surgical staging for esophageal cancer. *Surg Endosc* 2000;14:700–702
27. Steup W, De Lyn P, Deneffe G et al. Tumors of the esophagogastric junction. Long-term survival in relation to the pattern of lymph node metastasis and a critical analysis of the accuracy or inaccuracy of pTNM classification. *J Thorac Cardiovasc Surg* 1996;111:85–94

28. Krasna MJ, Reed CE, Nedzwiecki D. CALGB 9380: a prospective trial of the feasibility of thoracoscopy/laparoscopy in staging esophageal cancer. *Ann Thorac Surg* 2001;71(4):1073–1079
29. Walsh TN, Noonan N, Hollywood D et al. A comparison of multimodal therapy and surgery for esophageal adenocarcinoma. *N Engl J Med* 1996;335:462–467
30. Kassis E, Nguyen N, Shriver S et al. Detection of occult lymph node metastases in esophageal cancer by minimally invasive staging combined with molecular diagnostic techniques. *JSLS* 1998;2:331–336
31. Godfrey T, Raja S, Finkelstein S et al. Prognostic value of quantitative reverse transcription polymerase chain reaction in lymph node-negative esophageal cancer patients. *Clin Cancer Res* 2001;7:4041–4048
32. Collard JM, Lengele B, Otte JB, et al. En bloc and standard esophagectomies by thoracoscopy. *Ann Thorac Surg* 1993;56:675–679
33. Akaishi T, Kaneda I, Higuchi N, et al. Thoracoscopic en bloc total esophagectomy with radical mediastinal lymphadenectomy. *J Thorac Cardiovasc Surg* 1996;112:1533–1540
34. Robertson GS, Lloyd DM, Wicks AC, et al. No obvious advantages for thoracoscopic two-stage oesophagectomy. *Br J Surg* 1996;83:675–678
35. Law S, Wong J. Use of minimally invasive oesophagectomy for cancer of the esophagus. *Lancet Oncol* 2002;3: 215–222
36. DePaula AL, Hashiba K, Ferreira EA, et al. Laparoscopic transhiatal esophagectomy with esophagogastroplasty. *Surg Laparosc Endosc* 1995;5:1–5
37. Swanstrom LL, Hansen P. Laparoscopic total esophagectomy. *Arch Surg* 1997;132:943–947
38. Cherian V, Divatia J, Kulkarni A et al. Cardiomediastinal tamponade and shock following three-stage transthoracic esophagectomy. *J Postgrad Med* 2001;47;185–187
39. Seremetis M, Lyons W, deGuzman V, Peabody J. Leiomyomata of the esophagus: an analysis of 838 cases. *Cancer* 1976;38:2166–2177
40. Lawrence S Lee BS, Sunil Singhal MD, Brinster C. et al. Current management of esophageal leiomyoma. *J Am Coll Surg* 2004;198:136–146
41. Hatch G, Wertheimer-Hatch L, Hatch K et al. Tumors of the esophagus. *World J Surg* 2000;24:401–441
42. Fountain S., Leiomyoma of the esophagus. *Thorac Cardiovasc Surg* 1986;3:194–195
43. Glanz I, Grunebaum M. The radiologic approach to leiomyoma of the esophagus with long term follow-up. *Clin Radiol* 1977;28:197–200
44. Biasini A. Su di un caso di fibroleiomyoma dell'esofago ipobronchiale in transformazione maligna asportazione per via transpleurodiaframmatica ed esofago-gastrostomia guarigione. *Pathologica* 1949;41:260–267
45. Calmenson M, Claggett O. Surgical removal of leiomyomas of the esophagus. *Am J Surg* 1946;72:745–747
46. Hennessy T, Cuschieri A. Tumours of the esophagus. In Hennessy T and Cuschieri A. (eds). *Surgery of the Oesophagus.* London: Butterworth-Heinemann; 1992:275–327
47. Bonavina L, Segalin A, Rosati R, et al. Surgical therapy of esophageal leiomyoma. *J Am Coll Surg* 1995;181:257–262
48. Roviaro G, M. Maciocco M, Varoli F, et al. Videothoracoscopic treatment of oesophageal leiomyoma. *Thorax* 1998; 53:190–192
49. Samphire J, Nafteux P, Luketich J. Minimally invasive techniques for resection of benign esophageal tumors. *Sem Thorac Cardiovasc Surg* 2003;15:35–43
50. Ellis F. Esophagectomy for achalasia: a 22-year experience. *Br J Surg* 1993;80:882–885
51. Ferguson M, Reeder L, Olak J. Results of myotomy and partial fundoplication after pneumatic dilation for achalasia. *Ann Thorac Surg* 1996;62:327–330
52. Patti M, Fisichella P, Perretta S, et al. Impact of minimally invasive surgery on the treatment of esophageal achalasia: a decade of change. *J Am Coll Surg* 2003;196:698–705
53. Luketich J, Fernando H, Christie N, et al. Outcomes after minimally invasive esophagomyotomy. *Ann Thorac Surg* 2001;72:1919–1913
54. Pellegrini C, Wetter L, Patti M et al. Thoracoscopic esophagomyotomy. Initial experience with a new approach for the treatment of achalasia. *Ann Surg* 1992;216:291–296
55. Codispoti M, Soon S, Pugh G, Walker W. Clincal results of thoracoscopic Heller's myotomy in the treatment of achalasia. *Eur J Cardiothorac Surg* 2003;24:620–624
56. Lee J, Wang C, Huang P, et al. Enduring effects of thoracoscopic heller myotomy for treating achalasia. *World J Surg* 2004;28:55–58
57. Kesler K, Tarvin S, Brooks J, et al. Thoracoscopy-assisted heller myotomy for the treatment of achalasia: results of a minimally invasive technique. *Ann Thorac Surg* 2004; 77:385–391
58. Abir F, Modlin I, Kidd M, Bell R. Surgical Treatment of achalasia: current status and controversies. *Dig Surg* 2004;21:165–176
59. Richards W, Torquati A, Holzman M. Heller myotomy versus Heller myotomy with Dor fundoplication for achalasia: a prospective randomized double-blind clinical trial. *Ann Surg* 2004;240:405–412
60. Dado G, Bresadola V, Terrosu G, Bresadola F. Diverticulum of the midthoracic esophagus: pathogenesis and surgical treatment. *Surg Endosc* 2002;16:871
61. Beckerhinn P, Kriwanek S, Pramhas M, et al. Video-assisted resection of pulsative midesophagus diverticula. *Surg Endosc* 2001;15:720–722
62. Levard H, Carbonnel F, Perniceni T, et al. Minimally invasive surgery for diverticula of the thoracic esophagus. Results in 11 patients. *Gastroenterol Clin Biol* 2001;25:885–890
63. Fernando H, Luketich I, Samphire I, et al. Minimally invasive operation for esophageal diverticula. *Ann Thorac Surg* 2005;80:2076–2080
64. Landen S, El Nakadi I. Minimally invasive approach to Boerhaave's syndrome: a pilot of three cases. *Surg Endosc* 2002;16:1354–1357
65. Ikeda Y, Niimi M, Sasaki Y, et al. Thoracoscopic repair of a spontaneous perforation of the esophagus with the endoscopic suturing device. *J Thorac Cardiovasc Surg* 2001;121:178–179
66. Nguyen N, Follette D, Roberts P, et al. Thoracoscopic management of postoperative esophageal leak. *J Thorac Cardiovasc Surg* 2001;121:391–392

51

Laparoscopic Adrenalectomy

Atul A. Gawande ■ Francis D. Moore, Jr.

The advent of laparoscopic adrenalectomy has brought significant benefits in reducing the morbidity of adrenalectomy. These benefits, however, should not serve as a pretext to extend the indications for adrenal resection. This technique has matured considerably since its introduction, but still incurs a substantial risk of conversion to traditional, open adrenalectomy, most often on an urgent basis for bleeding encountered during the video-guided dissection. This rate currently is approximately 1 per 20 patients undergoing the laparoscopic approach.[1–3] Thus, the candidate for laparoscopic approach must also be a candidate for a large incision.

■ ADVANTAGES TO THE LAPAROSCOPIC APPROACH

In addressing this issue, still not well quantified, one must keep the 5% conversion rate to open surgery in mind. Thus any advantage to the 19 nonconverted cases must be weighed against the possible disadvantage of urgent conversion to the 20th patient. Furthermore, there is such a breadth of patient response to equivalent injuries that this technique will present no advantage to some. Published series consistently show a subset of patients who tolerate open surgery with little morbidity and another subset of patients who do not tolerate even laparoscopic surgery without substantial morbidity and prolonged hospital stays.[4] We are presently unable to reliably predict who these patients are who will not benefit from a less-invasive technique.

Those intrinsic limitations recognized, one can assume that for most patients, the smaller incisions, lower blood loss, and lessened abdominal wall/flank trauma from divided muscles will translate to a less painful and more rapid recovery. Median hospital stay is under 3 days for laparoscopic adrenalectomy, versus 7 days or more for the open procedure.[3] In addition, one can anticipate a reduction in general morbidity, such as catheter-associated urinary tract infections, pneumonias, and deep venous thrombosis. The attraction to patients is obvious. One can counter that modern large-incision surgery has improved dramatically with the use of continuous epidural anesthesia, more rapid mobilization, and improvements in operative technique. Nonetheless, incisions for open adrenalectomy are large and morbid: subcostal incisions produce long-term limitation of rectus abdominis function; midline celiotomies result in ileus and a frequent incidence of ventral hernia; and thoracoabdominal incisions can produce pain and muscle denervation syndromes. These long-term issues are avoided almost entirely with the laparoscopic approach.

The laparoscopic approach is particularly advantageous for the patient who is disabled with Cushing's syndrome from an autonomous adrenal adenoma. Patients with this diagnosis have such reduced muscle mass and reduced defense against infection that they essentially become completely immobilized with an open adrenalectomy, with very extended recoveries and an attendant increase in general complications, including wound disruption.

Laparoscopy is also especially advantageous for the patient with Conn's syndrome and a small unilateral peripheral adrenal adenoma. These patients can undergo nodulectomy for their tumors and be back to work within days.

▪ DISADVANTAGES TO THE LAPAROSCOPIC APPROACH

The confined two-dimensional field of view and the lack of tactile feedback impose a limiting reality on this surgery: one generally must see the adrenal in order to resect it adequately. There are, however, circumstances in which the adrenal must remain unseen—in other words, it must be removed as a radical adrenalectomy with an intact capsule of surrounding perinephric and suprarenal fat. The most common circumstance is that of suspected malignancy, in which breach of the adrenal and spillage of cells can severely compromise the ultimate survival of the patient. Although laparoscopic adrenalectomy for malignancy is being performed experimentally, the technique is not established as yet.[5,6] The use of laparoscopy for potentially curable adrenal malignancy is to be condemned at this time.

The other circumstance in which a laparoscopic approach might be problematic is in patients who require bilateral adrenalectomy for ACTH-dependent Cushing's syndrome. In these patients, spillage of adrenal cortical cells in the presence of increased levels of their trophic factor, ACTH, risks reimplantation and the adrenal equivalent of splenosis. The authors are aware of such an unfortunate case. This risk is compounded by the absolute necessity to remove all adrenal tissue, a maneuver that is difficult to accomplish with certainty without laparoscopic manipulation and retraction of the adrenal itself. The adrenal gland is so friable in these cases that manipulation virtually guarantees breach of the adrenal.

Another limiting circumstance is morbid obesity. The adrenal can frequently be obscured by surrounding fat. A CT scan will provide an estimate of the amount of fat around the adrenal. Large amounts should dissuade the surgeon from choosing laparoscopy, as there already will be substantial difficulty encountered even with effective patient positioning and longer instruments. Although ultrasound can demonstrate the exact location of the adrenal in these cases, it does not readily allow the safe dissection of the adrenal vein within a field of fat that cannot be retracted.

The use of the hand-assisting ports might attenuate some of these issues, but is unproven. It could also be the case that use of an incision large enough to admit a hand or forearm could abrogate some of the advantage of laparoscopy with respect to long-term wound complications and short-term wound pain.

Bilateral adrenalectomy should likely be considered to be an open procedure due to its significant reduction in operating time compared to bilateral laparoscopic surgery.[7]

▪ COMPLICATIONS UNIQUE TO LAPAROSCOPIC ADRENALECTOMY

A 2004 meta-analysis of laparoscopic adrenalectomy series revealed a significantly lower complication rate compared to open adrenalectomy (10.9% versus 35.8%).[3] However, there are several complications specific to this procedure. These relate to the need for abdominal insufflation with carbon dioxide gas, the lack of a three-dimensional operative field, and the inability to grasp the adrenal gland atraumatically.

Pneumothorax is seen in 1–2% of patients. Both left and right adrenalectomies approach the adrenal by dissection of the diaphragm, freeing the spleen or the liver from its attachments, respectively. It appears that abdominal carbon dioxide insufflation in combination with denuding the abdominal surface of the diaphragm can allow for passage of gas into the thoracic cavity, even in the absence of a full-thickness laceration, producing ipsilateral pneumothorax. This is identified as protrusion of the diaphragm into the operative field. If there is no respiratory compromise, the surgeon generally can complete the operation as planned with the expectation that the carbon dioxide will rapidly absorb, and the pneumothorax resolve, without the need for evacuation.

Vascular injuries represent nearly half of complications,[3] and result from the limitations of visualization and the lack of tactile confirmation. On the right, the renal vein can have an oblique course and course through the inferior portion of the dissection, causing confusion with the adrenal vein. The right adrenal vein is often well visualized with laparoscopic technique, but is also of variable location in a superior-inferior plane and anterior-posterior plane. A vein with a diameter significantly smaller than the length of a standard endoscopic clip should be viewed with skepticism if thought to be the adrenal vein. A vein with a diameter significantly larger than an endoclip or that does not clearly connect to the variegated dark yellow adrenal gland is a suspect for the renal vein and should not be divided without certain identification. On the left, the tail of the pancreas is encountered and often can appear similar to the adrenal with its lobular consistency. However, the pancreas is a distinct grayish-white color in contrast to the characteristic bright coloration of the dark yellow adrenal. The granularity of the adrenal is also much finer than the lobules of the pancreas. In addition, there is often a segmental upper pole renal artery that lies just deep to the lower portion of the adrenal. The named arteries of the adrenal are all quite narrow, in the 0.5-mm range, and are often not seen during dissection. Division of an identifiable artery should therefore be very carefully considered.

There are two additional issues. First, superficial lacerations of the spleen or liver can result from either dissection or retraction. The vast majority of these are managed simply by cauterization or patience, or both. Second, there is potential of electrosurgical injury from grounding/arcing through bystander organs. The common lateral approach allows abdominal organs to drop away from contact with the instrumentation. Ultrasonic scalpels and bipolar coagulation devices are coming into more frequent use and reduce risk of this mechanism of injury.

■ INDICATIONS FOR LAPAROSCOPIC ADRENALECTOMY

It should be evident from the discussion above that the primary indications for surgery relate to small adrenal tumors that assuredly are benign (Table 51–1). The indications will be listed in order of frequency.

CONN'S SYNDROME

Primary hyperaldosteronism is characterized by suppressed plasma renin activity with a concomitant elevated or high-normal aldosterone. It usually manifests with hypertension and hypokalemia. Of the two, hypokalemia is curable, but the hypertension is often only improved, especially if long-standing. Thus patients with recent onset of hypertension and severe hypokalemia are more likely to benefit from surgery than those with long-standing hypertension that is well-controlled with spironolactone or amiloride. Cases that respond to surgery have unilateral small (<1.5 cm) lesions; there should be not even a hint of an additional nodule in either adrenal. These are essentially never malignant. In addition, the frequency of nonfunctioning adenomas is so high that the presence of a >1.5 cm adrenal nodule should raise suspicion that the large nodule is not the functional tumor in that patient. Resolution of ambiguities in the diagnosis can be based on a failure to suppress aldosterone secretion with salt loading or with selective venous sampling to establish the lateralization.[8] As aldosteronomas are solitary and benign, they can be treated with nodulectomy ("cortex-sparing") if peripheral. The exact relationship to the adrenal vein is often unclear until surgery, location in proximity to the vein being a contraindication to nodulectomy. The newer hemostatic instrumentation such as the ultrasonic scissors greatly assist nodulectomy, as it is possible to divide adrenal tissue without blood loss.

PHEOCHROMOCYTOMA

A laparoscopic approach can be considered if the patient is stable and if the lesion is benign. With respect to the former, the surgeon must envisage the scenario of uncontrolled hemorrhage in the patient and determine whether that patient could withstand an urgent conversion to open adrenalectomy in the context of uncontrolled catecholamine secretion. Part of that ini-

TABLE 51–1. INDICATIONS FOR LAPAROSCOPIC ADRENALECTOMY

Diagnosis	Indicated	Comments
Conn's syndrome (hyperaldosteronism)		
Solitary functional nodule	Yes	Nodule should be <1.5 cm on CT imaging
Hyperplasia	No	Unclear benefit to bilateral adrenalectomy
Cushing's syndrome		
Solitary functioning nodule	Yes	Only if <4 cm and no ketosteroid output
ACTH-dependent	No	Risk of implantation and recurrence
Nonfunctioning adenoma		
<5 cm	No	No indication for surgery
>5 cm	No	Possible malignancy
Pheochromocytoma		
<3 cm	Yes/No	American Society of Anesthesiologists class 1 or 2 patients, lesion lateral
>3 cm	No	Risk of malignancy; risk of local recurrence
MEN-associated	Yes/No	Only if contralateral adrenal tumor is <1 cm
Paraganglioma	No	Risk of local recurrance
Virilizing adenoma	Yes/No	Only if <2 cm
Feminizing adenoma	No	Usually malignant
Carcinoma	No	Poor ability to control margins
Cyst	Yes/No	Only if symptomatic; consider fenestration
Metastatic lesion	Unknown	Control of margins may not affect patient outcome
Myelolipoma	Yes	Often too large to remove without an incision

tial assessment should not fail to consider the possibility of susceptibility to catechol-caused tachyarrhythmias and the possibility of ventricular scarring and lack of compliance from long-standing catecholamine excess. Sufficient experience has been gained with outpatient alpha blockade and forced hydration to consider the otherwise healthy patient as able to tolerate an intraoperative emergency. It is important that an operating surgeon experienced with preoperative preparation be personally responsible for this portion of the care. The temptation of the inexperienced to add beta blockade and thus impair effective alpha blockade is profound. Beta blockade should not be used in the absence of preoperative tachyarrhythmias.

With respect to potential malignancy in the pheochromocytoma, there are several considerations. First, the lesion should be <4 cm. Second, the lesion should produce both epinephrine and norepinephrine (e.g., check urine vanillylmandelic acid and metanephrine levels). Lack of epinephrine metabolites suggests paraganglioma. Third, the lesion should clearly not be a paraganglioma on CT imaging. It should be almost perfectly round and well lateral. Oblong, medial, epinephrine-lacking lesions are a risk for paraganglioma, for which laparoscopy is contraindicated. This is because of (1) high rates of local recurrence and the need to treat with wide resection margins and (2) lack of a single draining vein and the consequent difficulty in controlling hypertension during surgery.

MEN-2 requires special consideration. The mortality of this syndrome is due now to spread of the medullary thyroid cancer, often over decades. Pheochromocytomas are benign and bilateral, but may grow at differing rates. Although bilateral adrenalectomy likely is required ultimately, many patients benefit from removal of the adrenal with the dominant lesion initially and a contralateral resection years later, when the second adrenal begins to produce biochemical abnormalities. Thus a purposeful staging of the adrenalectomies may save patients years of the inconvenience and slight mortality associated with iatrogenic addisonism.

CORTISOL-PRODUCING ADRENAL ADENOMA

The morbidity of Cushing's syndrome is so great that it is advantageous to consider these patients for surgery at the earliest possible moment. Lack of ACTH dependence must be established both by dexamethasone suppression testing and by obvious atrophy of remaining adrenal tissue by CT scan. For laparoscopy, these tumors should be small enough (<3 cm) to represent little risk of malignancy and should produce little ketosteroids. In patients who are severely afflicted, there may be so much periadrenal fat and centripetal fat redistribution that they present the same technical difficulties as the morbidly obese. Estimates of periadrenal fat extent can be made from CT scans. Commonly, young women with this condition have placed themselves on stringent diets to prevent what they perceive to be obesity. In these cases there may be little periadrenal fat despite a pronounced cushingoid body habitus.

ADRENAL CYST

These lesions are usually incidental and surgery is not indicated unless there is a solid component to the cyst wall. That is suggestive of malignancy and contraindicates a laparoscopic approach. For fear of spontaneous rupture, a few very large cysts should be excised by laparoscopic nodulectomy or subjected to fenestration of the cyst wall into the peritoneal cavity.

MYELOLIPOMA

These lesions are also generally inadvertently discovered. Their appearance can cause confusion with liposarcoma, a situation easily resolved with needle biopsy showing typical bone marrow elements. Many of these benign lesions come to laparoscopic resection based on attribution of symptoms of back/flank pain to them.

▪ TUMOR-SPECIFIC CONTRAINDICATIONS TO LAPAROSCOPIC ADRENALECTOMY

CARCINOMA

The margins of resection cannot be effectively controlled. This leads to a high local recurrence rate. These should therefore not be removed laparoscopically.

PARAGANGLIOMA

The margins of resection cannot be effectively controlled. This leads to a high local recurrence rate. These should therefore not be removed laparoscopically.

ALDOSTERONISM DUE TO HYPERPLASIA

It is unclear whether the benefit to hypertension would outweigh the harm of bilateral adrenalectomy.

INCIDENTALOMA

Small (<4 cm) nonfunctioning adrenal tumors have no known progression to malignancy, little intrinsic malignant potential, and little observed growth. Removal is not indicated. Lesions >4 cm are a risk for carcinoma, which is a contraindication to laparoscopy.

ACTH-DEPENDENT HYPERCORTISOLISM

There is a risk of adrenal breach, spillage of cells, and local implantation. Surgery for recurrence is challenging.

FEMINIZING/VIRILIZING ADENOMA

A high proportion of these are malignant and therefore generally not candidates for laparoscopy.

METASTATIC LESIONS

This is a narrowly defined situation in patients with lung cancer whose recurrence appears to be solitary and in an adrenal. A few patients will achieve long-term survival with adrenalectomy. It is not known whether local margin control is important or whether adrenalectomy would influence survival in a large trial. As this is a rare situation, we advise caution and common sense. These likely should be treated as if a primary malignancy.

■ TECHNICAL CONSIDERATIONS

There are a few general recommendations that make the laparoscopy smoother. First, any bleeding, even the most minor, substantially impairs visualization. Dissection should be gentle, patient, and every act of tissue division accompanied by a hemostatic maneuver. Second, irrigation to remove obscuring blood cannot be reliably evacuated. Irrigation generally should not be used, as it tends to accumulate over the bed of dissection and be as obscuring as the blood. Third, removal of blood by suction tends to collapse the operative field and lead to tedious adjustment of retraction. For these reasons, small neurosurgical patties are the best way to remove blood and to control minor bleeding. The use of instruments with enhanced hemostatic capability, such as ultrasonic shears or bipolar vessel sealing devices, should be considered. Fourth, manipulation of instruments through the most lateral port is impaired by patients with wide hips. It also impairing to have ports that are so close together that the instruments hit each other. Thus the details of the patient's position and the placement of the ports are not routine and should not be delegated. Finally, the adrenal itself cannot be gripped and retracted directly without rupture and bleeding. Thus retraction should be performed by leaving periadrenal fat strategically attached to the adrenal and gripping the fat or by elevation of the adrenal from beneath.

Laparoscopic evidence of potential malignancy should prompt unquestioned conversion to an open adrenalectomy. Such evidence would include findings of tumor adhesion to adjacent structures, necrosis, or significantly increased size compared with preoperative imaging. Disruption of any adrenal mass with spillage should also lead to a decision to convert.

POSITIONING

We prefer a lateral decubitus position due to the spontaneous retraction of organs away from the field of surgery by gravity (Fig 51–1). The patient should be placed with the umbilicus at the level of the break in the table, so as to be able to effectively extend the oper-

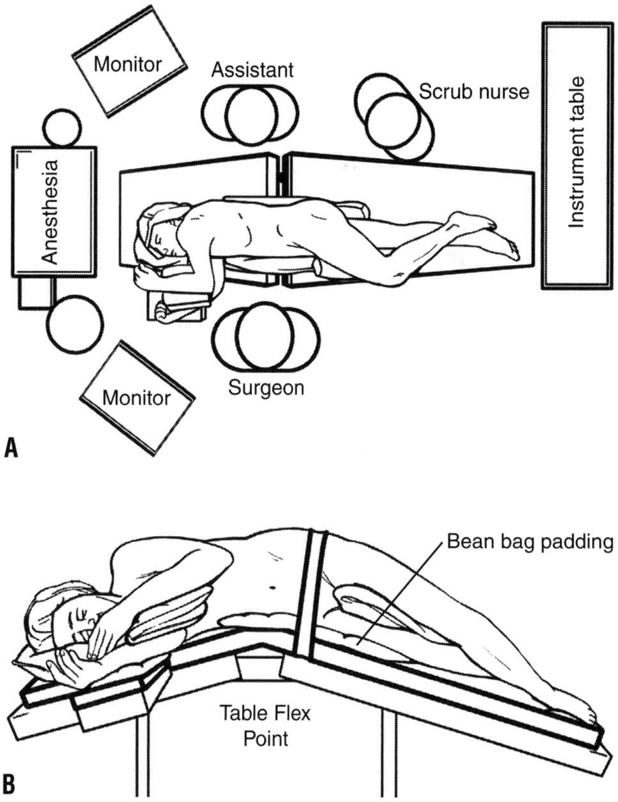

Figure 51–1. Optimal positioning of patient for a left laparoscopic adrenalectomy in the lateral decubitus position. The mid-abdomen is placed over the break in the table to optimize trunk extension and reduce interference with instrument movement by the iliac crest. The anterior abdominal wall should not be compressed.

ating table and use the kidney bar if needed. When turned into lateral position, the patient's abdomen should be at the edge of the table and unsupported. The common use of rolls or towels in front of the abdomen to perfectly stabilize the patient on the table has the effect of compressing abdominal contents up into the operative field, thus preventing the desired retraction of liver, colon, or spleen by gravity. The shoulders should be vertical, but consideration of a more oblique position of the hips should be given, for the purposes of enhancing abdominal access.

INSTRUMENTATION

We prefer 0° laparoscopes, although visualization often seems better with 30° laparoscopes. The reason for this is that the initial dissection to view the adrenal vein is not complete until it can be clearly visualized with a 0° scope. Dissection based on the view with the angled scope may lead to premature, and more hazardous, resection without adequate identification of surrounding structures. For an experienced laparoscopist, however, appreciation of this issue could make the angled scope advantageous. On the right, a liver retractor and a device to secure it to the table are needed. Flexible retractors that reshape into a triangle have less tendency to lacerate the liver than fans or wands, but also give less effective retraction. Four ports are usually required on the right and three on the left. Electrocautery scissors are useful for initial dissection of liver or spleen away from the diaphragm, as well as dissection of the splenic flexure. Ultrasonic shears or the equivalent should be used for resection of the adrenal and endoclips for securing of the adrenal vein. Grasping instrumentation used on periadrenal tissue to retract the adrenal is imperfect; the best that we have found is either the Maryland dissector, for retraction from a single point, or the Hunter grasper, for retraction across a broad base. An endoscopic clip applier should be available to control the adrenal vein.

RIGHT ADRENALECTOMY

After anesthesia and positioning, port placement is marked on the abdominal wall. Four ports arrayed from the xiphoid to the posterior axillary line along the costal margin can be designed, if entry is to be gained with a Veress needle and an angled scope is to be used. We use three ports on the costal margin with a muscle-splitting open entry through the lateral rectus for scope placement and adrenal removal (Fig 51–2). The middle port and the entry incision are placed along the line of a pos-

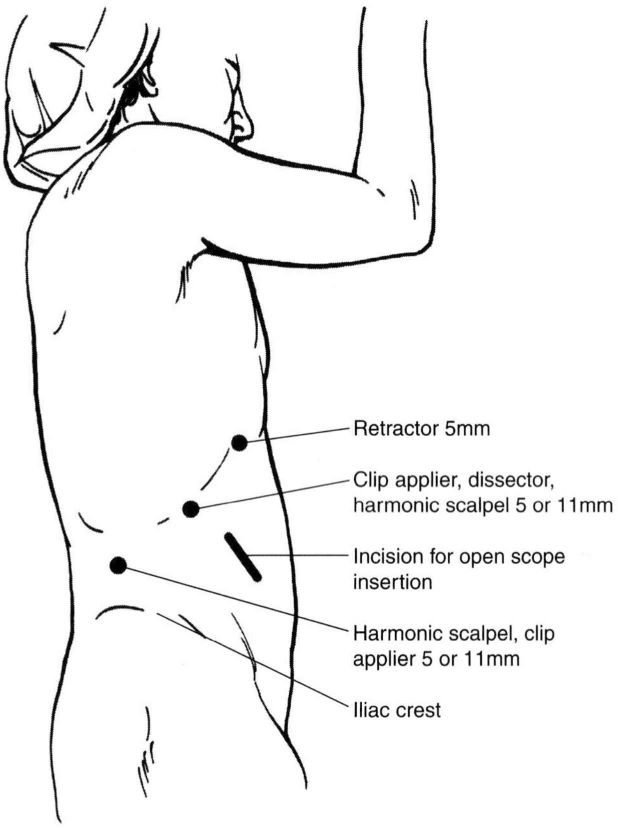

Figure 51–2. Port placement for a right laparoscopic adrenalectomy. In this example, abdominal entry is gained under direct visualization through the most medial site.

sible limited thoracoabdominal incision. In this technique, 5-mm ports are used medially and 11-mm ports at the rectus and most laterally (for the clip applier).

After safe entry is achieved, adhesions of bowel and colon in the right upper quadrant are divided for an unobstructed view (Fig 51–3). With a retractor in the middle port and electrocautery scissors in the lateral port, the diaphragmatic attachments of the right lobe of the liver are divided, until one can easily retract the right lobe superiorly and medially. This retraction should bring the top of the kidney, the lateral adrenal fat, and the subhepatic vena cava into view. Fixed liver retraction should then be set.

Dissection to expose the vena cava proceeds along the lateral sweep of the duodenum (Fig 51–4). Any obscuring hepatic flexure attachments should be divided. The peritoneum overlying the adrenal where it abuts the posterior right lobe is then divided, bringing portions of the adrenal into view (Fig 51–5). Just inferior to the liver, the adrenal is then gently swept laterally until a point of attachment to the IVC is recognized. This region is dissected especially cautiously, as it contains the adrenal vein (Fig 51–6). The vein is then freed until it has enough length to allow the placement of two or

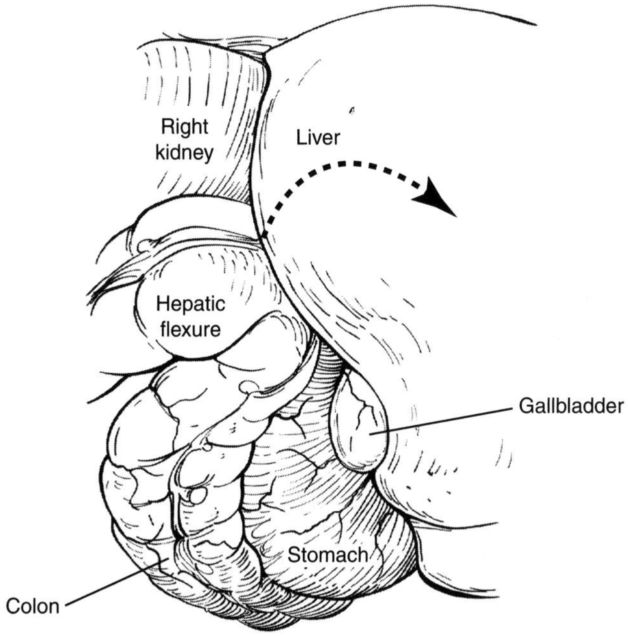

Figure 51–3. Initial view of right upper quadrant in a right laparoscopic adrenalectomy. Arrow indicates the direction of liver retraction from the epigastric port.

three clips on the caval side, definitively not on cava itself (Fig 51–7). The vein is then divided with fine scissors at the adrenal margin (Fig 51–8). A Maryland dissector is then passed though the small tissue gap left by

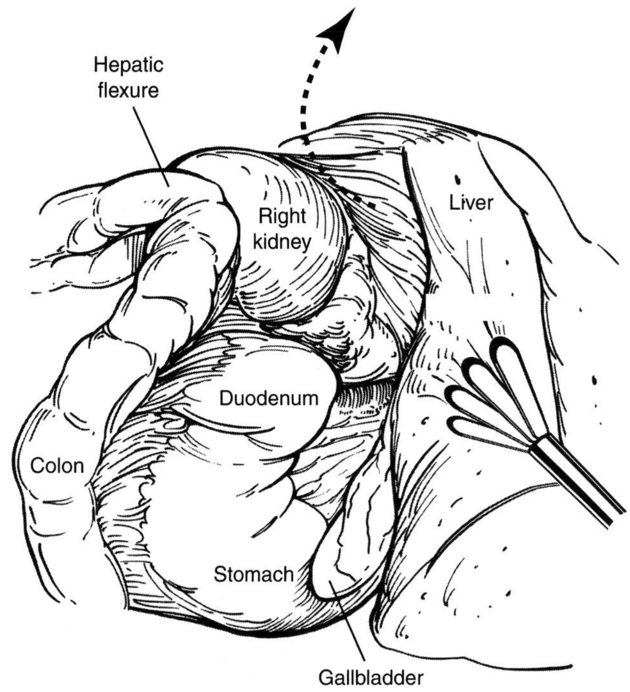

Figure 51–4. View during right laparoscopic adrenalectomy with the liver retracted from the epigastric post. Some attachments of the right lobe of the liver to the diaphragm have been divided. The *dotted line* indicates the line of further peritoneal incision to mobilize the right lobe of the liver from the diaphragm.

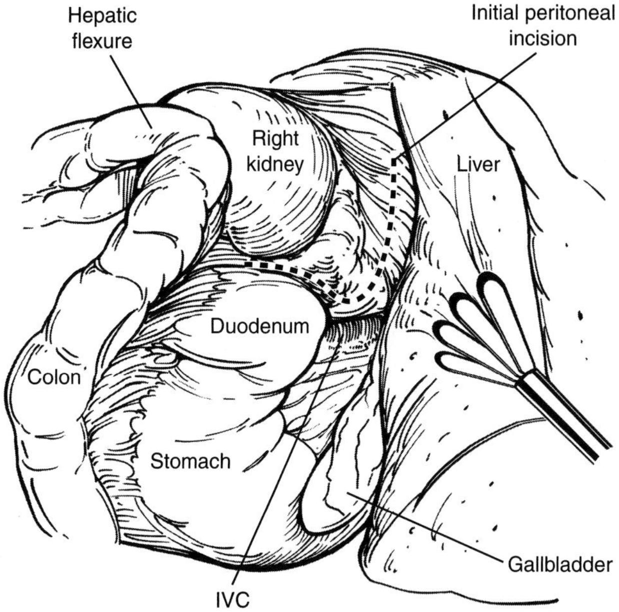

Figure 51–5. View during right laparoscopic adrenalectomy after initial dissection to mobilize the right adrenal. The *dotted line* shows the peritoneal incision under the retracted liver that exposes the adrenal.

vein division, where it will freely pass to the diaphragm. By then elevating the adrenal, circumferential resection with ultrasonic scissors is then possible with minor grasping of periadrenal fat required. The excised adrenal is then placed in a bag and removed through the rectus port. As this maneuver will usually cause all retraction to be lost, port sites and the bed of dissection should be checked for hemostasis first.

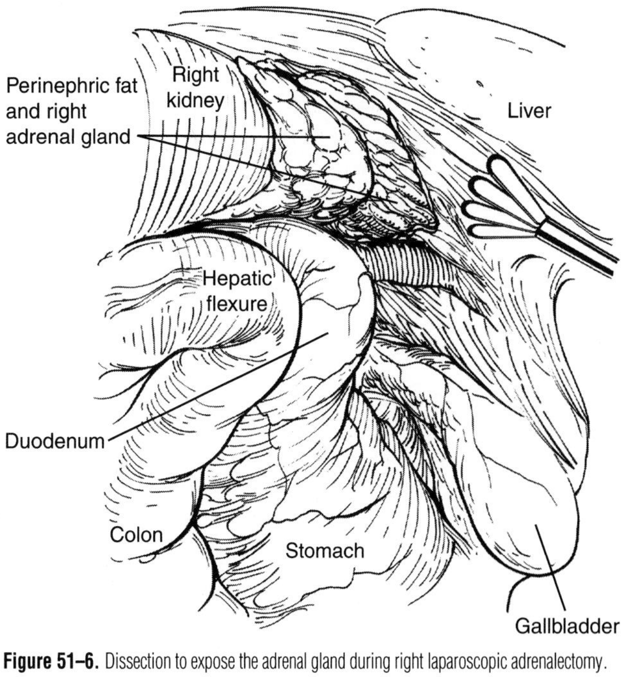

Figure 51–6. Dissection to expose the adrenal gland during right laparoscopic adrenalectomy.

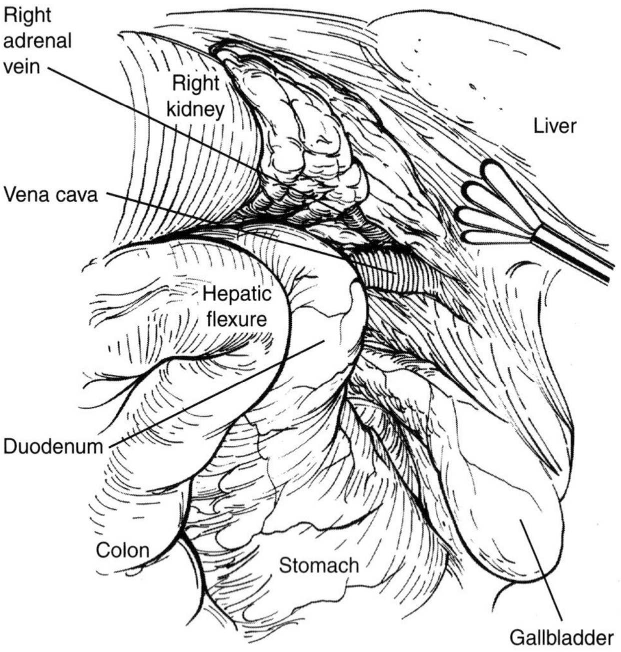

Figure 51–7. Dissection to expose the adrenal vein during right laparoscopic adrenalectomy. The length of the right adrenal vein is exaggerated in this schematic.

LEFT ADRENALECTOMY

After anesthesia and positioning, port placement is marked on the abdominal wall. Three ports are arrayed from the xiphoid to the posterior axillary line along the costal margin, if entry is to be gained with a Veress needle and an angled scope is to be used. We use two ports on the costal margin with a muscle-splitting open entry through the lateral rectus for scope placement and adrenal removal (Fig 51–9). A fourth port is not needed, as the spleen retracts with gravity. The middle port and the entry incision are placed along the line of a possible limited thoracoabdominal incision. In this technique, a 5-mm port is used medially and 11-mm ports at the rectus and most laterally (for the clip applier).

Electrocautery scissors are passed through the most medial port and used to take down the splenic flexure. This exposes the anterior lateral surface of the left kidney. Dissection is carried superiorly, using instruments in the lateral port, to separate the tail of the pancreas from the renal hilum and the spleen from the lateral abdominal wall and diaphragm (Fig 51–10). Retraction with a grasper in the xiphoid port is helpful. This dissection is carried out repetitively, dividing successive attachments to the splenic flexure of the colon and to the spleen itself, until the spleen falls from the field by gravity alone.

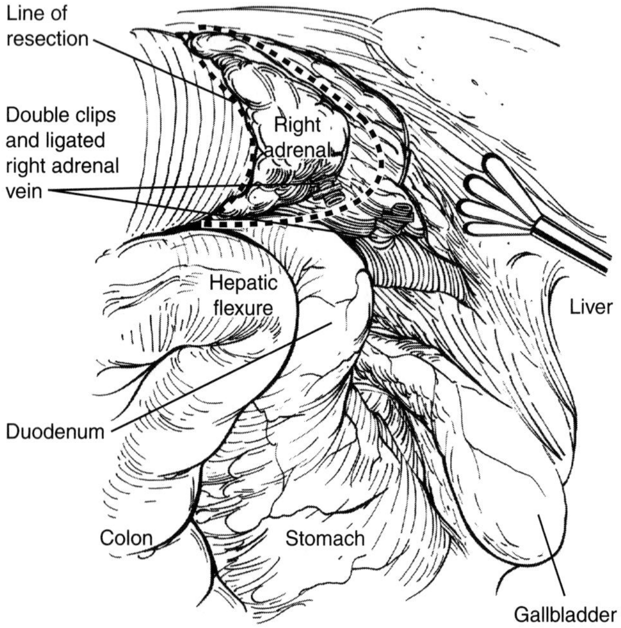

Figure 51–8. View during right laparoscopic adrenalectomy after division of the right adrenal vein with clips. The *dotted line* indicates the line of resection to complete the adrenalectomy. Retraction underneath the adrenal at the site of the severed adrenal vein is often advantageous. The length of the right adrenal vein is exaggerated in this schematic.

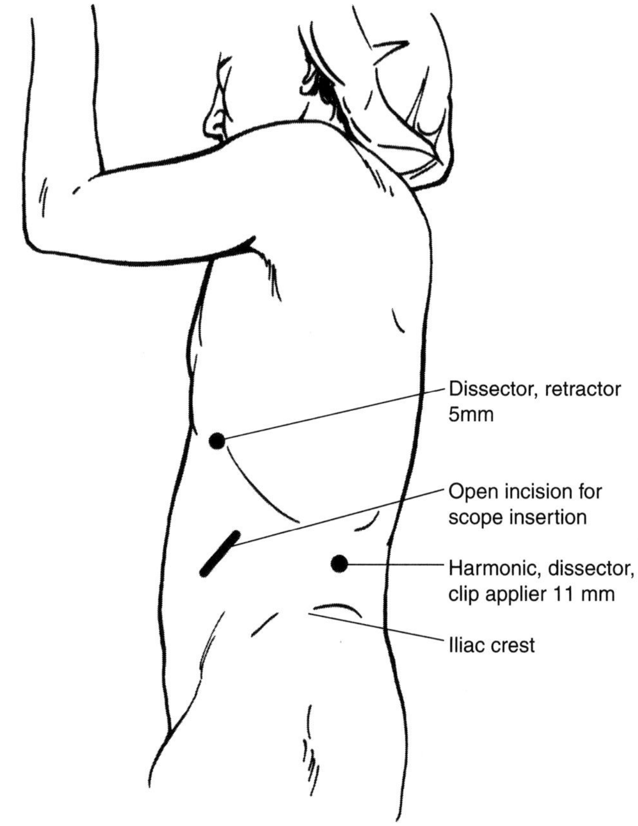

Figure 51–9. Port placement for left laparoscopic adrenalectomy in the right lateral decubitus position. In this example, initial abdominal entry is gained through a medial incision. A fourth port is often not required on the left.

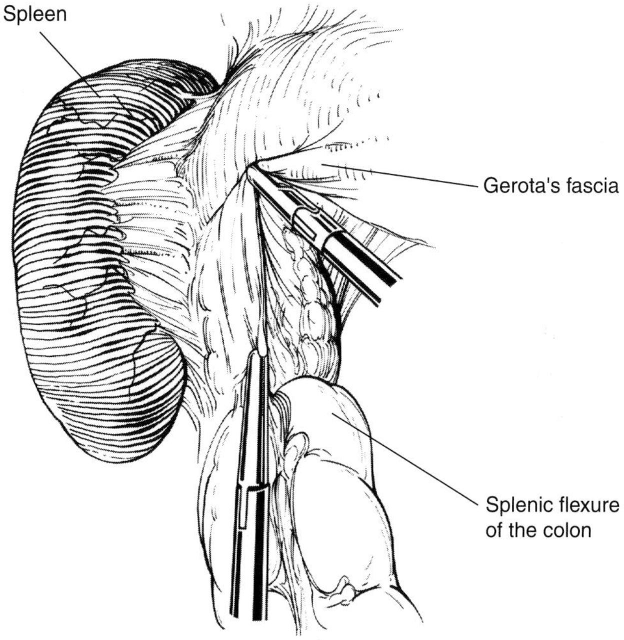

Figure 51–10. View during left laparoscopic adrenalectomy, showing division of the peritoneum over the kidney and progressive detachment of the spleen from the left diaphragm.

At this point, the adrenal should be visible as a mass that moves within its envelope of fat when gently manipulated. Laparoscopic ultrasound can be helpful when the adrenal cannot be easily localized. The inferior edge of the adrenal is then gently teased upwards and dissection carried in a medial direction until the adrenal vein is encountered (Fig 51–11). The vein is freed sufficiently to place two clips on the renal vein side and one on the adrenal side. After dividing the vein, a blunt Kittner dissector is gently passed through the space behind the vein and used to elevate the adrenal. The adrenal is then excised with an ultrasonic shear, taking care not to injure the renal vein or the adjacent segmental renal artery (Fig 51–12). Removal is accomplished as above.

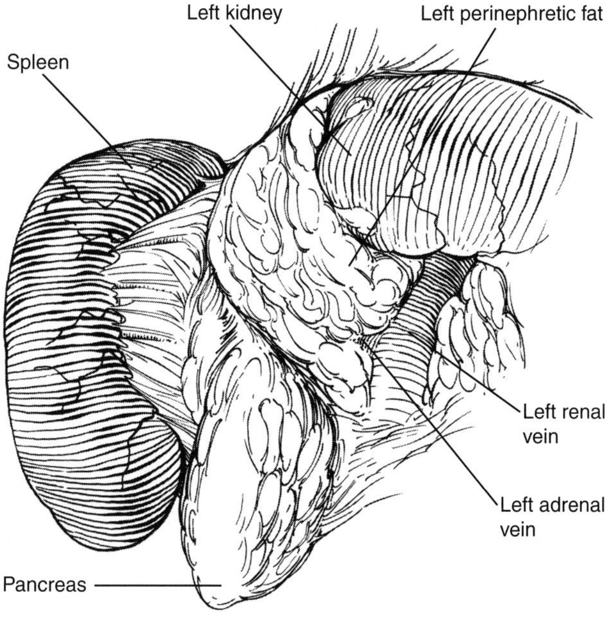

Figure 51–11. View during left laparoscopic adrenalectomy. The spleen had been partially mobilized and is retracting to the right by gravity. The separation between the posterior pancreas and the anterior surface of the left adrenal had been developed. The left renal vein is exposed, as well as the take-off of the left adrenal vein.

NOTE ON NODULECTOMY OR CORTEX-SPARING SURGERY

This excisional surgery requires that the aldosteronoma is peripheral and not lying over the adrenal vein. Equivalent exposure of the adrenal is required as for outright adrenalectomy. However, instead of identifying the adrenal vein and mobilizing from there, the lateral portion of the gland is defined and retracted forward, entering the plane along the diaphragm. When the point is reached that the nodule is visible and a probe can fit in the space between the medial edge of the nodule and the point of most medial dissection, then the adrenal can be divided with ultrasonic scissors. Final hemostasis should be accom-

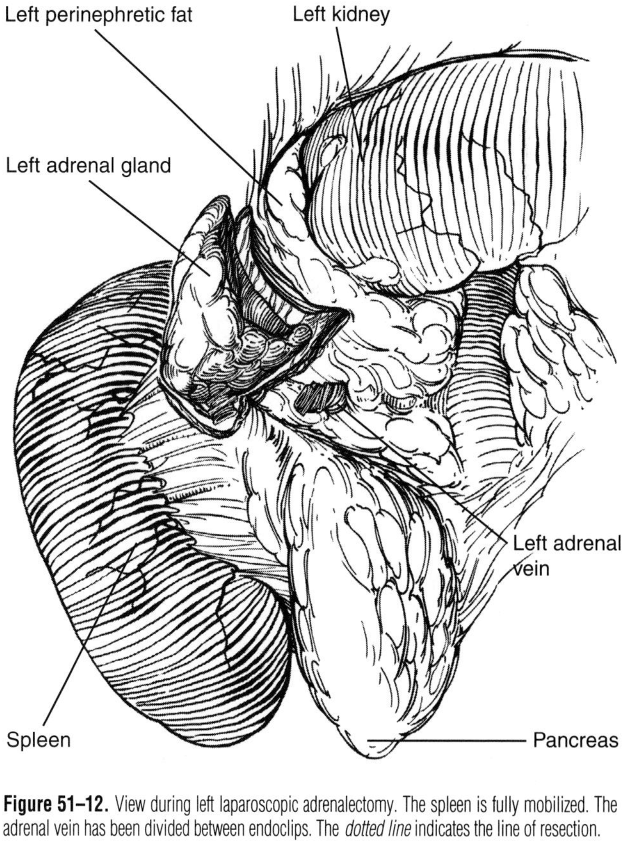

Figure 51–12. View during left laparoscopic adrenalectomy. The spleen is fully mobilized. The adrenal vein has been divided between endoclips. The *dotted line* indicates the line of resection.

plished with this exposure, prior to removal of the nodule from the abdomen.

■ CONCLUSION

At this time, laparoscopic removal of pathological adrenal glands offers significant advantages to the patient in terms of short-term recovery and incisional cosmesis. Patient selection to assure that malignant tumors are not approached without adhering to basic principles of surgical oncology and to assure that the procedure is indicated are the current imperatives. Although the latter is likely never to change, improved laparoscopic instrumentation and improved diagnosis and staging of adrenal malignancies may soon make open adrenalectomy a distinct rarity.

REFERENCES

1. Zeh HR, Udelsman R. One hundred laparoscopic adrenalectomies: a single surgeon's experience. *Ann Surg Oncol* 2003;10:1012–1017
2. Prager G, Heinz-Peer G, Passler C et al. Applicability of laparoscopic adrenalectomy in a prospective study in 150 consecutive patients. *Arch Surg* 2004;139:46–49
3. Assalia A, Gagner M. Laparoscopic adrenalectomy. *Br J Surg* 2004;91:1258–1274
4. Barreca M, Presenti L, Renzi C et al. Expectations and outcomes when moving from open to laparoscopic adrenalectomy: multivariate analysis. *World J Surg* 2003; 27:223–228
5. Porpiglia F, Fiori C, Tarabuzzi R et al. Is laparoscopic adrenalectomy feasible for adrenocortical carcinoma or metastasis? *BJU Int* 2004;94:1026
6. Henry J, Sebag F, Iacobone M et al. Results of laparoscopic adrenalectomy for large and potentially malignant tumors. *World J Surg* 2002;26:1043–1047
7. Porpiglia F, Fiori C, Bovio S et al. Bilateral adrenalectomy for Cushing's syndrome: a comparison between laparoscopy and open surgery. *J Endocrino Invest* 2004; 27:654–658
8. Young WF Jr, Stanson AW, Thompson GB et al. Role for adrenal venous sampling in primary hyperaldosteronism. *Surgery* 2004;136:1227–1235

SELECTED READINGS

Acosta E, Pantoja JP, Gamino R, Rull JA, Herrera MF. Laparoscopic versus open adrenalectomy in Cushing's syndrome and disease. *Surgery* 1999;126:1111–1116

Barnett CC, Varma DG, El-Naggar AK et al. Limitations of size as a criterion in the evaluation of adrenal tumors. *Surgery* 2000;128:973–983

Bonjer HJ, Sorm V, Berends FJ et al. Endoscopic retroperitoneal adrenalectomy: lessons learned from 111 consecutive cases. *Ann Surg* 2000;232:796–803

Brauckhoff M, Thanh PN, Gimm O et al. Functional results after endoscopic subtotal cortical-sparing adrenalectomy. *Surg Today* 2003;33:342–348

Brunaud L, Bresler L, Zarnegar R et al. Does robotic adrenalectomy improve patient quality of life when compared to laparoscopic adrenalectomy? *World J Surg* 2004;28: 1180–1185

Brunt LM, Bennett HF, Teefey SA, Moley JF, Middleton WD. Laparoscopic ultrasound imaging of adrenal tumors during laparoscopic adrenalectomy. *Am J Surg* 1999;178: 490–495

Brunt LM, Doherty GM, Norton JA et al. Laparoscopic adrenalectomy compared to open adrenalectomy for benign adrenal neoplasms. *J Am Coll Surg* 1996;183:1–10

Brunt LM, Moely JF. Adrenal incidentaloma. *World J Surg* 2001;25:905–913

Brunt LM, Moley JF, Doberty GM et al. Outcomes analysis in patients undergoing laparoscopic adrenalectomy for hormonally active adrenal tumors. *Surgery* 2001;130: 629–635

Brunt LM. The positive impact of laparoscopic adrenalectomy on complications of adrenal surgery. *Surg Endosc* 2002;16:252–257

Chavez-Rodrigues J, Pasieka JL. Adrenal lesions assessed in the era of laparoscopic adrenalectomy: a modern day series. *Am J Surg* 2005;189:581–586

Cheah WK, Clark OH, Horn JK, Siperstein AE, Duh QY. Laparoscopic adrenalectomy for pheochromocytoma. *World J Surg* 2002;26:1048–1051

Chen B, Zhou M, Cappelli MC, Wolf JS Jr. Port site, retroperitoneal and intra-abdominal recurrence after laparoscopic adrenalectomy for apparently isolated metastasis. *J Urol* 2002;168:2528–2529

Cobb WS, Kercher KW, Sing RF, Heniford BT. laparoscopic adrenalectomy for malignancy. *Am J Surg* 2005;189:405–411

Duh QY, Siperstein AE, Clark OH et al. Laparoscopic adrenalectomy: comparison of lateral and posterior approaches. *Arch Surg* 1996;131:870–876

Farres H, Felsher J, Brodsky J et al. Laparoscopic adrenalectomy: A cost analysis of three approaches. *J Laparoendosc Adv Surg Tech* 2004;14:23–26

Fernandez-Cruz L, Saenz A, Benarroch G et al. Laparoscopic unilateral or bilateral adrenalectomy for Cushing's syndrome. *Ann Surg* 1996;224:727–736

Foxius A, Ramboux A, Lefebvre Y et al. Hazards of laparoscopic adrenalectomy for Conn's adenoma: when enthusiasm turns to tragedy. *Surg Endosc* 1999;13:715–717

Gagner M, Lacroix A, Prinz RA et al. Early experience with laparoscopic approach for adrenalectomy. *Surgery* 1993; 114:1120–1125

Gagner M, Pomp A, Heniford BT, Pharand D, Lacroix A. Laparoscopic adrenalectomy: lessons learned from 100 consecutive cases. *Ann Surg* 1997;226:238–247

Guazoni G, Montorsi F, Bocciardi A et al. Transperitoneal laparoscopic versus open adrenalectomy for benign hyperfunctioning adrenal tumors: a comparative study. *J Urology* 1995;153:1597–1560

Hawn MT, Cook D, Deveney C, Sheppard BC. Quality of life after laparoscopic bilateral adrenalectomy for Cushing's disease. *Surgery* 2002;132:1064–1069

Heniford BT, Arca MJ, Walsh RM. Gill laparoscopic adrenalectomy for cancer. *Semin Surg Oncol* 1999;16:293–306

Henry JF, Defechereux T, Raffaelli M, Lubrano D, Gramatica L. Complications of laparoscopic adrenalectomy: results of 169 consecutive procedures. *World J Surg* 2000;24: 1342–1346

Hobart MG, Gill IS, Schweizer D, Sung GT, Bravo EL. Laparoscopic adrenalectomy for large-volume (> or = 5 cm) adrenal masses. *J Endourol* 2000;14:149–154

Horgan S, Sinanan M, Helton WS, Pellegrini CA. Use of laparoscopic techniques improves outcome from adrenalectomy. *Am J Surg* 1997;173:371–378

Hwang J, Shoaf G, Uchio EM et al. Laparoscopic management of extra-adrenal pheochromocytoma. *J Urol* 2004; 171:72–76

Iihara M, Suzuki R, Kawamata A et al. Adrenal-preserving laparoscopic surgery in selected patients with bilateral adrenal tumors. *Surgery* 2003;134:1066–1073

Inabet WB, Caragliano P, Pertsemlidis D. Pheochromocytoma: Inherited associations, bilaterality, and cortex preservation. *Surgery* 2000;128:1007–1012

Inabet WB, Pitre J, Bernanrd D, Chapuis Y. Comparison of hemodynamic parameters of open and laparoscopic adrenalectomy for pheochromocytoma. *World J Surg* 2000;24:574–578

Ishidoya S, Ito A, Sakai K et al. Laparoscopic partial versus total adrenalectomy for aldosterone producing adenoma. *J Urol* 2005;174:40–43

Jacobs JK, Goldstein RE, Geer RJ. Laparoscopic adrenalectomy: a new standard of care. *Ann Surg* 1997;225:495–502

Kercher KW, Novitsky YW, Park A et al. Laparoscopic curative resection of pheochromocytomas. *Ann Surg* 2005;241: 919–928

Kim JH, Ng CS, Ramani AP et al. Laparoscopic radial adrenalectomy with adrenal vein thrombectomy: technical considerations. *J Urol* 2004;171:1223–1226

Kim AW, Quiros RM, Maxhimer JB, El-Ganzouri AR, Prinz RA. Outcome of laparoscopic adrenalectomy for pheochromocytomas vs aldosteronomas. *Arch Surg* 2004;139: 526–531

Li ML, Fitzgerald PA, Price DC, Norton JA. Iatrogenic pheochromocytosis: a previously unreported result of laparoscopic adrenalectomy. *Surgery* 2001;130:10720–10727

Lucas SW, Spitz JD, Arregui ME. The use of intraoperative ultrasound in laparoscopic adrenal surgery. *Surg Endosc* 1999;13:1093–1098

MacGillivray DC, Whalen GF, Malchoff CD, Oppenheim DS, Shichman SJ. Laparoscopic resection of large adrenal tumors. *Ann Surg Oncol* 2002;9:480–485

Mobius E, Nies C, Rothmund M. Surgical treatment of pheochromocytomas: laparoscopic or conventional? *Surg Endosc* 1999;13:35–39

Mutter D, Dutson E, Marescaux J. Complications of laparoscopic adrenalectomies. *European Surgery* 2003;35:80–83

Nagesser SK, vanSeters AP, Kievit J et al. Long-term results of total adrenalectomy for Cushing's disease. *World J Surg* 2000;24:108–113

Nakada T, Kubota Y, Sasagawa I et al. Therapeutic outcome of primary hyperaldosteronism: adrenalectomy versus enucleation of aldosterone-producing adenoma. *J Urology* 1995;153:1775–1780

Nies C, Langer P. Minimally invasive adrenalectomy and malignant adrenal tumours. *European Surgery* 2003;35:76–79

Obermeyrer RJ, Knauer EM, Millie MP et al. Intravenous methylene blue as an aid to intraoperative localization and removal of the adrenal glands during laparoscopic adrenalectomy. *Am J Surg* 2003;186:531–534

Prager G, Heinz-Peer G, Passler C et al. Applicability of laparoscopic adrenalectomy in a prospective study of 150 consecutive patients. *Arch Surg* 2004;139:46–49

Prinz RA. A comparison of laparoscopic and open adrenalectomies. *Arch Surg* 1995;130:489–494

Rayan SS, Hodin RA. Short-stay laparoscopic adrenalectomy. *Surg Endosc* 2000;14:568–572

Sardi A, McKinnon WM. Laparoscopic adrenalectomy in patients with primary aldosteronism. *Surg Laparosc Endosc* 1994;4:86–91

Sarela AI, Murphy I, Coit DG, Conlon KCP. Metastasis to the adrenal gland: the emerging role of laparoscopic surgery. *Ann Surg Oncol* 2003;10:1191–1196

Schell SR, Talamini MA, Udelsman R. Laparoscopic adrenalectomy for nonmalignant disease: improved safety, morbidity, and cost-effectiveness. *Surg Endosc* 1999;13: 30–34

Shen WT, Kebebw E, Clark OH, Duh QY. Reasons for conversion from laparoscopic to open or hand-assisted adrenalectomy: review of 261 laparoscopic adrenalectomies from 1993 to 2003. *World J Surg* 2004;28:1176–1179

Shen WT, Lim RC, Siperstein AE et al. Laparoscopic vs open adrenalectomy for the treatment of primary hyperaldosteronism. *Arch Surg* 1999;134:628–632

Shen WT, Sturgeon C, Clark OH, Duh QY, Kebebew E. Should pheochromocytoma size influence surgical approach? A comparison of 90 malignant and 60 benign pheochromocytomas. *Surgery* 2005;136:1129–1137

Skaragard ED, Albanese CT. The safety and efficacy of laparoscopic adrenalectomy in children. *Arch Surg* 2005;140: 905–908

Takeda M, Go H, Imai T, Nishiyama T, Moroshita H. Laparoscopic adrenalectomy for primary hyperaldosteronism: report of initial ten cases. *Surgery* 1993;115:621–625

Tauzin-Fin P, Sesay M, Gosse P, Ballanger P. Effects of perioperative 1 block on haemodynamic control during laparoscopic surgery for phaeochromocytoma. *J Anaesth* 2004;92:512–517

Walz MK, Peitgen K, Walz M et al. Posterior retroperitoneoscopic adrenalectomy: lessons learned with five years. *World J Surg* 2001;25:728–734

Warinner SA, Zimmerman D, Thompson GB, Grant CS. Study of three patients with congenital adrenal hyperplasia treated by bilateral adrenalectomy. *World J Surg* 2000;24:1347–1352

52

Laparoscopic Surgery for Morbid Obesity

Stacy A. Brethauer ▪ Bipan Chand ▪ Philip R. Schauer

Obesity is now recognized as a major public health problem in the developed countries, affecting approximately 300 million people worldwide.[1] Obesity is defined as a Body Mass Index (BMI) >30 kg/m^2 and morbid obesity as a BMI of >35 kg/m^2 with obesity-related comorbidities or a BMI >40 kg/m^2. Table 52–1 shows classifications of obesity according to BMI and excess body weight.

This disease involves a complex interaction of metabolic, genetic, psychological, and social issues and is the second leading cause of preventable death in the United States after smoking. Obesity leads to many comorbidities that can affect every system in the body (Table 52–2). The costs of obesity include direct medical costs of treating obesity illnesses and indirect costs due to lost workdays, productivity and future income due to premature death. The total cost attributable to obesity in the United States is over $100 billion annually. Worldwide, approximately 2.5 million annual deaths occur because of obesity-related comorbidities and obesity shortens the life span of those who suffer with it. It is estimated that a man in his twenties with a BMI over 45 will have a 22% reduction (13 years) in life expectancy.[2]

The evolution of bariatric surgical procedures, particularly the more recent development of laparoscopic techniques, has led to substantial progress in the study of obesity and has attracted surgeons with interests in advanced gastrointestinal (GI) and laparoscopic surgery to the field. Between 1993 and 2003, the number of bariatric procedures performed worldwide increased from 40,000 to 146,000 and membership in the International Federation for the Surgery of Obesity increased by 121%.[3] The United States has more bariatric surgeons (850) than any other country and approximately 140,000 bariatric operations were performed in the United States in 2004. Despite the successes of bariatric surgery to date, though, only 1–2% of those eligible for bariatric surgery in the United States have undergone a weight-loss procedure.[3] Ensuring that referring physicians and patients are aware of the benefits and reasonable risk of bariatric surgery remains a challenge for bariatric surgeons.

Significant weight loss after bariatric surgery has been well established. The focus of this discipline over the last 10 years has shifted from demonstrating weight loss to evaluating the resolution of obesity-related comorbidities, the cost-effectiveness of bariatric surgery and increased life expectancy after surgery.

▪ SURGICAL TREATMENT FOR OBESITY

BARIATRIC SURGERY OUTCOMES

Weight Loss: Magnitude and Durability

Bariatric surgery is currently the most effective method to treat severe obesity. Excess weight is defined as the amount of weight above the patient's ideal body weight. The amount of excess weight loss (EWL) varies according to procedure, but there is little controversy regarding the short-term efficacy of bariatric surgery. Long-term data is now emerging that shows mainte-

TABLE 52–1. DEFINITIONS OF OBESITY ACCORDING TO BMI AND EXCESS BODY WEIGHT

Category		BMI	% Over IBW
Underweight		<18.5	
Normal		18.5–24.9	
Overweight		25.0–29.9	
Obesity	(Class 1)	30–34.9	>20%
Severe obesity	(Class 2)	35–39.9	>100%
	(Class 3)	40–49.9	
Superobesity		>50	>250%

BMI, body mass index; IBW, ideal body weight.

nance of weight loss 5 to 15 years after modern bariatric procedures. This sustained weight loss has a major impact on individual patients' health and longevity and society's costs related to obesity.

A meta-analysis by Buchwald and colleagues[4] found an average EWL of 61% among 10,172 patients who underwent bariatric surgery. Patient who underwent biliopancreatic diversion had the largest EWL (70%), followed by gastroplasty (68%), gastric bypass (62%), and gastric banding (47.5%). The follow-up periods varied among studies, but weight loss assessments at 2 years or less did not differ significantly from assessments at more than 2 years for most groups. Table 52–3 summarizes the weight loss, improvements in four major comorbidities, and mortality rates after bariatric surgery.

The Swedish Obesity Subjects (SOS) Study Scientific Group is a prospective, controlled matched pair cohort study comparing surgery to nonsurgical treatment for obesity.[5] The surgically treated patients underwent vertical banded gastroplasty, fixed or adjustable gastric banding, or gastric bypass. The nonsurgical group received interventions ranging from intense behavioral therapy to no specific treatment according to the practices of their primary care physicians. Changes in weight were analyzed at 2 and 10 years. After 2 years, analysis of 3,505 patients showed a weight increase of 0.1% in the control group and a decrease of 23.4% of initial weight in the surgical group ($p < 0.001$). Analysis at 10 years included 641 surgical and 627 nonsurgical patients. The control group had gained 1.6% of their original weight and the surgical group had a weight decrease of 16.1% overall. Among the surgical patients, those who underwent gastric bypass lost the greatest amount of weight (25% of their original weight), but only 34 gastric bypass patients have completed 10 years of the study (Fig 52–1).

In a report of long-term results after gastric bypass, White and colleagues reported good maintenance of weight loss. Average EWL at 1, 2, 5, 10, and 14 years was 88%, 87%, 70%, 75%, and 59%, respectively.[6] In this study, 76% of patients had at least 2 years of follow-up and 39% were followed for at least 5 years. Similarly, Pories and colleagues reported EWL at 2,5,10, and 14 years of 70%, 58%, 55%, and 49%, respectively with less than 3% of patients lost to follow-up.[7] These long-term studies of RYGB reveal some modest, gradual weight regain after the initial rapid weight loss in the first 18 months and the subsequent plateau period of 1 to 2 years following RYGB.

TABLE 52–2. COMORBIDITIES ASSOCIATED WITH OBESITY

Cardiovascular		
Hyperlipidemia		
Hypertension		
Coronary artery disease		
Left ventricular hypertrophy		
Heart failure		
Venous stasis ulcers/Thrombophlebitis		
Pulmonary		
Obstructive sleep apnea		
Asthma		
Obesity hypoventilation syndrome		
Endocrine		
Insulin resistance		
Type 2 diabetes		
Polycystic ovarian syndrome		
Hematopoietic		
Deep venous thrombosis		
Pulmonary embolism		
Gastrointestinal		
Gallstones		
Gastroesophageal reflux disease		
Abdominal hernia		
Genitourinary		
Stress urinary incontinence		
Urinary tract infections		
Obstetric/Gynecologic		
Infertility		
Miscarriage		
Fetal abnormalities		
Musculoskeletal		
Degenerative joint disease		
Gout		
Plantar fasciitis		
Carpal tunnel syndrome		
Neurologic/Psychiatric		
Stroke		
Pseudotumor cerebri		
Migraine headaches		
Depression		
Anxiety		
Increased Cancer Risk		
Endometrial	Prostate	Esophagus
Ovarian	Kidney	Colon
Breast	Liver	Pancreas

TABLE 52–3. WEIGHT LOSS AND REDUCTION IN COMORBIDITIES AFTER BARIATRIC SURGERY

	Gastric Banding	Gastroplasty	Gastric Bypass	BPD or DS	Total
EWL	47%	68%	62%	70%	61%
Mortality	0.1%[a]	0.1%[a]	0.5%	1.1%	NR
Resolution of DM	48%	72%	84%	99%	77%
Resolution of Hyperlipidemia	59%	74%	97%	99%	79%
Resolution of Hypertension	43%	69%	68%	83%	62%
Resolution of Sleep Apnea	95%	78%	80%	92%	86%

[a]Represents composite mortality for all restrictive procedures.
Adapted from Buchwald H, Williams SE. Bariatric surgery worldwide 2003. *Obes Surg* 2004; 14(9):1157–1164;
BPD, biliopancreatic diversion; DS, duodenal switch; EWL, excess weight loss; NR, not reported; DM, diabetes mellitus.

The Australian Safety and Efficacy Register of New Interventional Procedures-Surgical (ASERNIP-S report No. 31) analyzed the international literature on laparoscopic adjustable gastric banding (64 studies) and comparative procedures (vertical banded gastroplasty and gastric bypass, 57 studies). Three studies in this review had 4-year follow-up data for LAGB and reported EWL ranging from 44–68%.[8–10] The ranges of EWL at 4 years after RYGB and VBG were 50–67% and 40–77%, respectively. The authors concluded that RYGB results in greater weight loss than LABG up to 2 years after surgery, but current data does not indicate a significant difference in weight loss between the two procedures from 2 to 4 years and more data is necessary to determine the long-term efficacy of LAGB relative to RYGB. Several subsequent reports have shown 5- and 6-year EWL after LAGB ranging between 50–60%.[11–13]

Biliopancreatic diversion and BPD with duodenal switch (BPD/DS) provide excellent long-term weight loss. Hess and Hess have demonstrated 75% EWL in 167 patients 10 years after duodenal switch (92% follow-up).[14,15] Scopinaro reported overall EWL of 74% at 8 years and 77% at 18 years after open BPD with nearly 100% follow-up and showed no difference in long-term EWL between morbidly obese and super-obese patients.

Life Expectancy

It seems intuitive that dramatic weight reduction and resolution of major life-threatening comorbidities would prolong life, but until recently there has been little data to support this assumption. Flum and col-

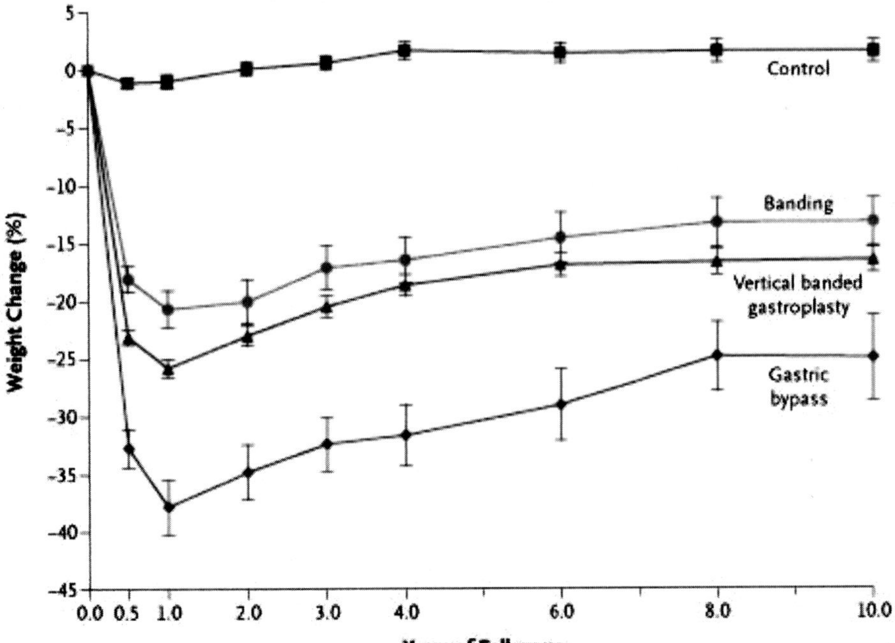

No. of Subjects									
Control	627	585	594	587	577	563	542	535	627
Banding	156	150	154	153	149	150	147	144	156
Vertical banded gastroplasty	451	438	438	438	429	417	412	401	451
Gastric bypass	34	34	34	34	33	32	32	29	34

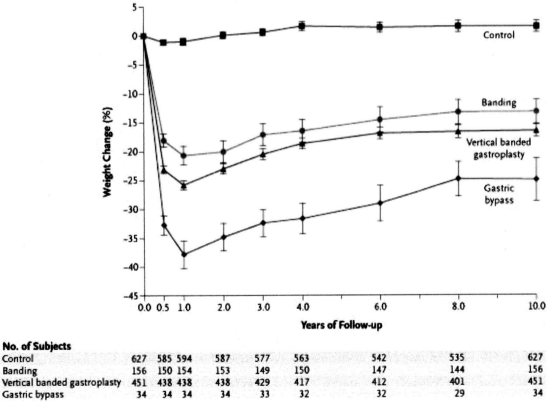

Figure 52–1. Swedish Obesity Subjects study group data of 10-year weight loss by procedure. (Sjostrom L, Lindroos AK, Peltonen M, et al. Lifestyle, diabetes, and cardiovascular risk factors 10 years after bariatric surgery. *N Engl J Med* 2004;351(26):2683–2693. Copyright 2004 Massachusetts Medical Society. All rights reserved.)

leagues evaluated survival after gastric bypass in a retrospective cohort study and found a 27% reduction in 15-year mortality in morbidly obese patients who underwent gastric bypass versus those that did not. After the surgical patients reached the first postoperative year, the long-term survival advantage increased to 33%.[16]

Christou and colleagues evaluated mortality in an observational cohort study comparing 1035 gastric bypass patients to 5746 age- and gender-matched morbidly obese controls. Five-year mortality in the surgical group was 0.68% compared to 16.2% in the medically managed patients (89% relative risk reduction) (Fig 52–2).[17] MacDonald and associates retrospectively compared obese diabetic patients who underwent gastric bypass (n = 154) to a similar group of obese diabetic patients who did not have surgery (n = 78) and found significant reductions in diabetes and mortality in the surgical group. With up to 10 years of follow-up, the mortality rate in the surgical group was 9% (including perioperative deaths) compared to 28% in the nonsurgical control group. This reduction in mortality was related to decreased cardiovascular deaths among patients who had gastric bypass.[18]

One of the major endpoints of the Swedish Obesity Subjects trial is the effects of surgical weight loss on mortality. While it is clear that the mortality rate is not increased in the surgical group (including a perioperative mortality of 0.25%) over the 10-year study period to date, data supporting a reduction in mortality in this study has not yet been released.[5]

Perioperative Mortality

Perioperative mortality rates after bariatric surgery are dependent on the procedure performed, the severity of the patient's comorbid conditions, and the surgeon's experience. Overall, pulmonary embolism is responsible for 36% of perioperative deaths, cardiac complications (myocardial infarction, heart failure) are responsible for 24%, and GI leaks account for 20% of deaths within 30 days of bariatric surgery. The remaining 20% of perioperative deaths are due to respiratory, vascular, and hemorrhagic causes.[19]

As demonstrated in Buchwald's meta-analysis, bariatric procedures that do not involve any gastrointestinal anastomoses (restrictive procedures) carry the lowest perioperative mortality rates (0.1%).[4] A systematic review of the international literature revealed a 0.05% mortality rate after laparoscopic adjustable gastric banding and this is considered the safest bariatric procedure performed today.[20] Mortality rates after gastric bypass range from 0–2% and there was no difference in mortality rates between open and laparoscopic gastric bypass in three randomized trails.[21–23] The mortality rate for gastric bypass (open and laparoscopic) in Buchwald's meta-

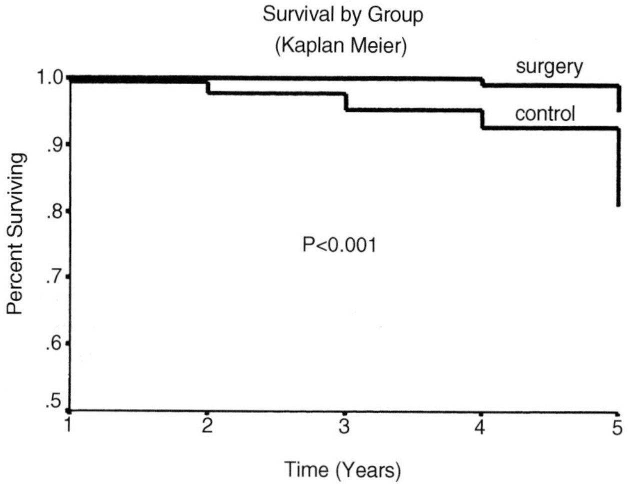

Figure 52–2. Survival by group in a matched-cohort analysis demonstrating an 89% risk reduction in mortality at five years in bariatric surgery patients versus matched controls. (From Christou NV, Sampalis JS, Liberman M, et al. Surgery decreases long-term mortality, morbidity, and health care use in morbidly obese patients. *Ann Surg* 2004;240(3):416–423; discussion 423–424 with permission.)

analysis is 0.5%.[4] Malabsorptive procedures such as biliopancreatic diversion and duodenal switch are more technically demanding and are associated with higher mortality rates than other bariatric procedures. Overall, these procedures have a 1.1% mortality rate[4] and large series of BPD and DS performed by experienced surgeons report mortality rates ranging from zero to 1.9%.[24–26] Relatively small series of laparoscopic BPD and DS report mortality rates from zero to 2.5%.[27–31] Direct comparisons of published mortality rates between procedures may be misleading, though, since mortality risk factors such as BMI, sex, age, and comorbid conditions can vary widely. For example, studies of patients undergoing BPD often have a higher BMI when compared to the LAGB series and this may, in part, account for the increased mortality rates.

In a review of Medicare patients undergoing bariatric surgery, Flum and colleagues found that patients older than 65 had a significantly higher risk of death after bariatric surgery than younger patients.[32] All-cause mortality for 16,155 Medicare patients who underwent bariatric surgery (81% RYGB) was 2% at 30 days and 2.8% at 90 days after surgery. Patients older than 65 had 4.8% 30-day and 6.9% 90-day mortality rates. The risk of early postoperative death was associated with lower surgeon volume which has also been demonstrated in other studies.[33] A larger review of 60,077 patients who underwent gastric bypass surgery in California reported mortality rates more consistent with those seen in large case series. In this review, in-hospital mortality was 0.18%, 30-day mortality was 0.33%, and 1-year mortality was 0.91%.[34]

Postoperative mortality rates after bariatric surgery compare favorably to those seen after major cardiovascular and cancer operations. A review of Medicare patients found postoperative mortality rates ranging from 2.9% to 13.8% for cancer resections, 1.8% to 5.6% for peripheral vascular procedures, and 5.3% to 14.1% for cardiac procedures.[35]

Cost-Effectiveness of Bariatric Surgery

The societal costs of obesity are high and they continue to rise as the obesity epidemic grows. Many studies have demonstrated the increased health care costs associated with obesity.[36–41] In 1995, $99.1 billion was spent on health care for obesity, $51.6 billion were direct medical costs and the remaining $47.5 billion were indirect costs relating to lost work productivity secondary to morbidity and mortality.[40] One half of the health care costs for obesity are paid by Medicaid and Medicare.[42] In 2000, the Centers for Disease Control and Prevention estimated total cost for obesity in the United States rose to $117 billion ($61 billion direct costs, $56 billion indirect costs). Most costs were related to treating chronic illnesses of obesity including diabetes, hypertension, and cardiovascular disease.

Despite the rapidly increasing costs of obesity over the last decade, there have been few reports on the cost-effectiveness of surgical weight loss until recently. Sampalis and associates[43] compared long-term direct health care costs in 1035 patients who underwent bariatric surgery to 5746 age- and gender-matched obese controls. The major operation was the open Roux-en-Y gastric bypass (79%) and the surgical group in total lost 67% of their excess body weight at 5 years follow-up. Bariatric surgery patients had higher hospitalization costs in the first year, but at 3.5 years the cost of surgery was compensated for by a reduction in total costs (Fig 52–3). At 5 years, the difference in costs between the surgical and nonsurgical cohorts was $5.7 million (Canadian) per 1000 patients, a reduction of 29% with surgery. A review of over 60,000 bariatric surgery patients in California reported an increase in hospital admissions after gastric bypass surgery compared to pre-operative admission rates. The costs related to hospital admission after bariatric surgery was higher compared to pre-operative costs and the reasons for admission were different before and after surgery. In addition to procedure-related admissions after bariatric surgery, many patients underwent elective plastic or orthopedic surgery after weight loss.[34]

The need for medication, specifically antihypertensive and diabetic medications, is reduced by as much as 77% after bariatric surgery[44] and the savings in drug costs was equal to the cost of surgery at 32 months in one study.[45] The Swedish Obese Subjects trial evaluated medication use after bariatric surgery and found that 6 years after surgery, surgical patients had a 69% and 31% reduction in cost for diabetic and cardiovascular medication, respectively compared to conventionally treated obese patients. Because of increased use of GI medications, iron, and vitamins by the surgical group, though, there was no overall difference in total medication costs.[46]

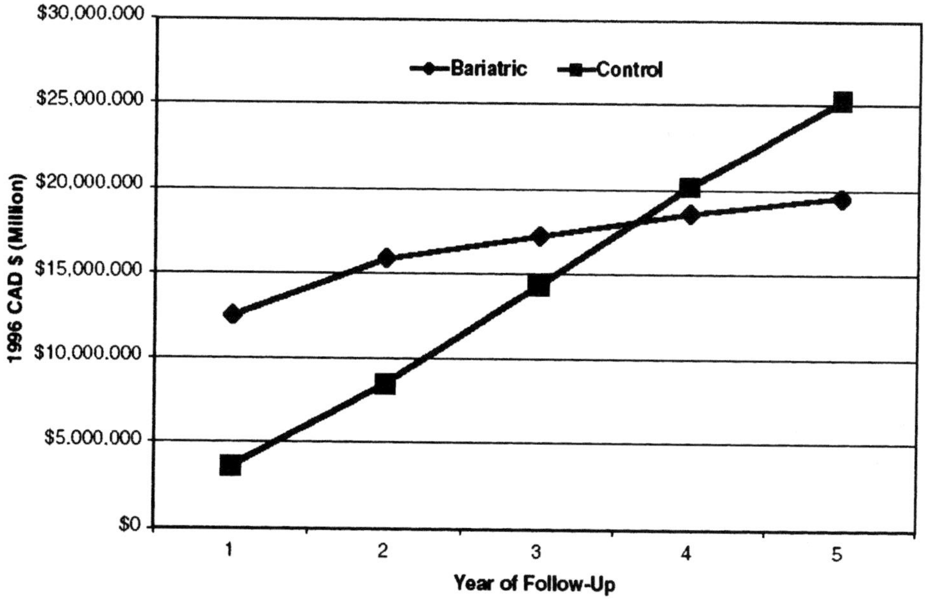

Figure 52–3. Average cumulative costs per 1,000 patients for hospitalization by group and year of follow-up. (Reproduced from Sampalis JS, Liberman M, Auger S, Christou NV. The impact of weight reduction surgery on health-care costs in morbidly obese patients. *Obes Surg* 2004;14(7):939–947 with permission from *Obesity Surgery*.)

Other cost-effectiveness analyses have demonstrated decreases in sick leave and disability claims[47] and reduction in outpatient visit costs[48] in the first year after bariatric surgery.

Assessments of quality-adjusted life-years (QALY) also favor bariatric surgery over nonsurgical treatment of obesity. Two analyses found the cost/QALY for bariatric surgery less than \$50,000 and a third study found a cost savings of \$4,000/QALY.[49] One evaluation of gastric bypass versus no treatment favored surgery in all risk subgroups (men and women aged 35 to 55 years with BMI between 40 and 50 kg/m^2) and suggested that cost-effectiveness was greatest among women and patients with higher BMIs.[50]

Despite mounting evidence that supports the cost-effectiveness of bariatric surgery, bariatric surgeons continue to encounter difficulty in receiving reimbursement for these procedures. Further comprehensive cost-effectiveness analyses will be required to convince policy makers and insurance carriers that bariatric surgery can favorably impact the costs of the obesity epidemic.[51]

RESOLUTION OF COMORBIDITIES

Metabolic Syndrome

The cluster of cardiovascular risk factors referred to as the metabolic syndrome was first described as Syndrome X by Reaven in 1988.[52] This syndrome consists of abdominal obesity, atherogenic dyslipidemia, elevated blood pressure, insulin resistance or glucose intolerance, a proinflammatory state, and a prothrombotic state. Obesity is thought to be a necessary factor for the development of the metabolic syndrome, but many obese people do not develop the metabolic syndrome. Genetic factors and age also play an important role in the patients who develop this syndrome.[53]

There are three different classification systems used to diagnose metabolic syndrome[54–56] but all are based on the same six metabolic abnormalities. Table 52–4 shows the National Cholesterol Education Program's Adult Treatment Panel III (NCEP/ATP III) criteria.[54] Using the NCEP/ATP III definition, the age-adjusted prevalence of the metabolic syndrome for U.S. adults 20 years or older is 27% and the prevalence is increased by 23.5% in adult women over the last decade. The rate of metabolic syndrome has been reported as high as 52% in patients seeking bariatric surgery.[53] The increasing prevalence of metabolic syndrome in the United States will likely lead to higher rates of diabetes and cardiovascular disease in the future.[57]

Abdominal, or central, obesity implies a higher distribution of visceral fat relative to peripheral or subcutaneous fat. Increased abdominal fat is more accurately measured by waist circumference than BMI and there is a strong correlation between abdominal fat and metabolic risk factors.[58,59]

TABLE 52–4. ATP III CRITERIA FOR METABOLIC SYNDROME[54]

Three or more of the following:	
Central obesity	
Waist circumference in men	>102 cm
Waist circumference in women	>88 cm
Hypertriglyceridemia	>150 mg/dL
Low HDL cholesterol	
Men	<40 mg/dL
Women	<50 mg/dL
High blood pressure	>130/ >85 mm Hg
Fasting blood glucose	>110 mg/dL

The exact contribution of each component of the metabolic syndrome to the overall cardiovascular risk is not known, but each provides a specific target for individual medical therapy. Bariatric surgery results in the simultaneous improvement of all the components of the metabolic syndrome. In a study by Mattar and associates, the incidence of metabolic syndrome decreased from 70% to 14% 15 months after bariatric surgery (with 60% EWL)[60] and Lee and associates demonstrated 95.6% resolution of the metabolic syndrome in 337 patients 1 year after laparoscopic VBG or laparoscopic RYGB.[53] Christou's matched-cohort study demonstrated an 82% reduction in cardiovascular risk with 67% EWL 5 years after bariatric surgery compared to medically managed obese patients.[17]

Diabetes Mellitus. Fifteen percent of morbidly obese patients have diabetes mellitus and another 15% to 25% have impaired fasting glucose.[4,61–63] Diabetes mellitus in the morbidly obese patient is a progressive disease and the duration of obesity correlates with a patient's chance of developing diabetes.[63] Bariatric surgery has a profound effect on diabetes and a meta-analysis of all procedures found resolution of this comorbidity in 77% of patients and improvement or resolution in 86% as measured by glycosylated hemoglobin, fasting glucose, and fasting insulin.[4] This effect varies according to the procedure, though. Procedures that bypass a portion of the foregut (BPD, DS, RYGB) are more effective in normalizing glucose metabolism. There are several proposed mechanisms for this rapid improvement in diabetes after certain bariatric procedures. These include limited caloric intake and the rapid development of a negative energy balance after surgery, suppression of ghrelin, a gut hormone that exerts diabetogenic effects, and increased production of incretions such as glucose-like peptide-1 (GLP-1) and glucose-dependent insulinotropic peptide (GIP) that stimulate insulin secretion in response to an enteral nutrient load.[64] The rapid delivery of nutrients to the hindgut and the exclusion of the duodenum and proximal jejunum from nutrient exposure in BPD and RYGB are possible explanations for the rapid and durable improvement in glucose metabolism seen after these operations. The precise mechanism of diabetes resolution and the interplay of gut hormones that occurs after these operations are still under investigation.

In a meta-analysis that included 3625 patients with diabetes or impaired glucose tolerance, diabetes resolved in 99% of patients after BPD, 84% after gastric bypass, 72% after gastroplasty, and 48% after gastric banding.[4] Large series of laparoscopic gastric bypass report resolution of diabetes in 83–98% of patients.[62,65,66] Laparoscopic adjustable gastric banding results in resolution of diabetes in 54–64% of patients and improved glucose control in 26–43% 5 to 6 years after surgery.[13,67] In the SOS trial, bariatric surgery patients (predominantly restrictive procedures) had significantly higher rates of diabetes resolution at 2 years than medically treated matched obese patients (72% vs. 21%) and this benefit continued at 10 years of follow-up (36% vs. 13%).[5]

Hypertension. The incidence of hypertension in the bariatric surgery population ranges from 35% to 51%.[4,63] Like many other cardiovascular risk factors, hypertension resolves or improves after surgical weight loss. Overall, 62% of patients have resolution of their hypertension after bariatric surgery and an additional 17% improve. Resolution of this comorbidity also varies with procedure. Biliopancreatic diversion had the highest rate of resolution (83%) and gastric banding had the lowest (43%) in Buchwald's meta-analysis.[4] Hypertension resolves in 52–92% of patients after laparoscopic gastric bypass.[62,65,66] Sugerman studied the relationship between diabetes, hypertension, and severe obesity and found that the longer a person remains severely obese, the higher the likelihood of developing diabetes, hypertension, or both. In his study of 1025 severely obese patients, 75% of patients with diabetes also had hypertension. Excess weight loss of 59% at 5 to 7 years resulted in resolution of hypertension in 66% of patients and diabetes in 86%.[63]

Hyperlipidemia. Dyslipidemia and hypercholesterolemia occur in 36% and 40% of the bariatric population, respectively. Bariatric surgery improves serum lipid profiles in 79% of patients and thereby decreases cardiovascular risk. The highest rates of change occur with malabsorptive (BPD) or combination (gastric bypass) procedures with improvement in hyperlipidemia in over 96% of patients. Several studies have shown similar reductions in hypertriglyceridemia with improvements in 62–100% of patients depending on the procedure.[4,5] In the SOS trial, recovery from hypertriglyceridemia and a low HDL level occurred more frequently in the surgery group than the control group over the 2- and 10-year follow-up periods, but there was no difference in hypercholesterolemia between groups at either time period.

Hypercoagulable State. Morbid obesity is associated with elevated levels of fibrinogen, factor VII, factor VIII, von Willebrand factor, plasminogen activator inhibitor and a hypercoagulable state.[68] This prothrombotic state has clinical implications in terms of cardiovascular and thromboembolic risk. Obese patients are at increased risk for cardiovascular disease[69,70] and the prothrombotic state of obesity, in combination with the other components of the metabolic syndrome, lead to progressive arterial disease in many of these patients.

The rates of DVT and PE after laparoscopic gastric bypass range from 0–1.3% and 0–1.1%, respectively.[22,65,71,72] There is a potentially higher risk of developing a DVT after open surgery (less mobility) when compared to a laparoscopic approach but no difference has been demonstrated in comparative studies. Bariatric patients are considered very high risk for a thrombotic event and receive prophylaxis with leg compression devices and low molecular weight or unfractionated heparin. The time required for the coagulation system to normalize after surgical weight loss is unknown. In our practice, patients with a BMI over 55 are discharged on extended prophylaxis. The duration of therapy is determined on an individual case basis.

Pro-Inflammatory State. Adipocytes in morbidly obese patients produce excessive amounts of pro-inflammatory cytokines and these mediators have detrimental effects on hypertension, diabetes, dyslipidemia, thromboembolic phenomena, infections, and cancer. Morbidly obese patients have elevated levels of IL-6, TNF-alpha, and C-reactive protein (CRP)[73–75] and decreased levels of IL-10 (a potent anti-inflammatory cytokine) and adiponectin (anti-inflammatory effects). A relationship has been established between the number of metabolic abnormalities in obese patients and CRP levels, and CRP levels are strongly associated with BMI.[76] Weight loss does result in a reduction of inflammatory mediators,[77] presumably by decreasing the peripheral and visceral fat stores, and resolution of this pro-inflammatory state coincides with improvement or resolution of many obesity-related comorbidities.

Pulmonary Disease

Obstructive Sleep Apnea. Obstructive sleep apnea is present in 15–60% of morbidly obese patients.[48,78] Patients presenting for bariatric surgery evaluation may already have the diagnosis of sleep apnea, however a careful evaluation is required to diagnose patients with occult sleep apnea. A missed diagnosis may put the patient at an increased perioperative pulmonary risk. Several scoring systems have been used to screen these patient pre-operatively but these do not predict the severity of the condition[48] and some authors advocate polysomnography for all bariatric patients.[78] Sleep apnea significantly improves post-operatively in most bariatric patients. In Buchwald's meta-analysis, 86% of patients had resolution of their sleep apnea after bariatric surgery.

Obesity Hypoventilation Syndrome. Obesity hypoventilation syndrome (OHS), also know as Pickwickian Syndrome, is defined as awake hypoventilation (confirmed by an elevated $PaCO_2$) and at least one feature of chronic hypoventilation such as cor pulmonale, pulmonary hypertension, or erythrocytosis. Additionally, an overnight sleep study is needed to document either an increase in PCO_2 of more than 10 mm Hg or an oxygen desaturation not explained by apnea or hypopnea. This disorder is present in approximately 8% of morbidly obese patients undergoing bariatric surgery. Sugerman and associates reported significant improvements in arterial blood gas measurements (PaO_2 from 50 to 69 mm Hg, $PaCO_2$ from 52 to 42 mm Hg) and hemodynamic measurements (pulmonary artery pressure from 36 to 23 mm Hg, pulmonary artery wedge pressure from 17 to 6 mm Hg) in 18 patients 3 to 9 months after bariatric surgery.[79] Longer follow-up (6 years) of 38 patients with OHS revealed similar improvement in blood gas measurements and complete resolution of OHS in 29 patients. Of those with OHS, 38 have been followed for 5.8 ± 2.4 y since surgery and 29 are currently asymptomatic. In this series, patients with OHS weighed more and were more often men. Operative mortality rates were higher in bariatric patients with respiratory insufficiency compared to patients without respiratory compromise (2.4% vs. 0.2%).[80]

Asthma. Asthma is a chronic inflammatory disease affecting 10–30% of the obese population. The prevalence of asthma has increased by 74% over the last two decades and the concomitant increase in obesity has led to studies in adults and children to evaluate an association between the two. Adults with asthma are more likely to be obese and seven of eight prospective studies in adults found a positive association between BMI and the development of asthma. In children, three of four prospective studies demonstrated a significant association between excess weight and the development of asthma.[81]

Bariatric surgery leads to resolution of asthma in up to 50% of patients[82] and significant improvement in symptoms and reduced medication use in 80% to 90% of patients after gastric bypass,[72] LAGB,[83] and BPD.[84]

Gastroesophageal Reflux Disease

Gastroesophageal reflux disease (GERD) is common in obese patients and occurs in 36–55% of patients.[4,85,86] Increased intra-abdominal pressure is the primary causative factor for the high incidence of GERD in this population. In addition to symptomatic reflux, there is a higher incidence of manometric abnormalities[87] and esophagitis[86] in the morbidly obese. Bariatric surgery, especially gastric bypass, is very effective in treating reflux disease. Three laparoscopic gastric bypass studies report resolution of GERD in 72–98% of patients,[65,66,72] and large series of LAGB report resolution of GERD in 76–89% of patients.[13,67] When evaluating patients for GERD, it is important to consider obesity as the underlying potential problem. Patients that suffer from reflux and are morbidly obese should be considered candidates for a weight loss operation and not a fundoplication procedure.[88]

Nonalcoholic Steatohepatitis

Nonalcoholic fatty liver disease (NAFLD) includes a spectrum of disease that begins with fatty infiltration of the liver and progresses to fibrosis and ultimately to cirrhosis in 25% of patients.[89] The prevalence of this comorbidity is increasing with the rates of obesity in western countries and is currently 2–3% overall.[90] The prevalence of NAFLD in morbidly obese patients ranges from 20–40% and surgical weight loss has a significant impact on this disease. In a study by Mattar and associates, 70 patients who underwent laparoscopic bariatric surgery had pre- and postop liver biopsies. After surgical weight loss of 59% EWL, there was marked improvement in liver steatosis (from 88% to 8%), inflammation (from 23% to 2%), and fibrosis (from 31% to 13%) with an interval of 15 ± 9 months between biopsies. Inflammation and fibrosis resolved in 37% and 20% of patients, respectively, corresponding to improvement of 82% in grade and 39% in stage of liver disease.[60] Similar improvement of fatty liver disease and metabolic syndrome have been demonstrated after biliopancreatic diversion[91] and laparoscopic adjustable gastric banding.[92]

Venous Stasis Disease

Impaired venous return from the lower extremities in morbidly obese patient is presumably secondary to increased intra-abdominal pressure and can result in lower extremity venous stasis disease and refractory ulcers. This comorbidity is associated with a higher complication rate than that seen in the general bariatric surgery population. Sugerman and colleagues reviewed 64 patients with venous stasis disease (0.3% of their patient population) and found that these patients were significantly heavier than patients without venous stasis disease and had more comorbidities. Specifically, patients with venous stasis had obesity hypoventilation syndrome, sleep apnea, hypertension, and diabetes more frequently than patients without venous stasis. The rates of pulmonary embolus (4%), anastomotic leak and peritonitis leading to death (3%), incisional hernia (38%), and overall operative mortality (8%) were significantly higher in the patients with venous stasis disease. Four years after surgery, venous stasis ulcers resolved in all but three of these patients.[93]

The indications for pre-operative vena caval filter placement in bariatric surgery are not well-defined and remain controversial. Some authors, though, recommend prophylactic preoperative placement of filters in patients with venous stasis disease, particularly in patients with a history of venous thromboembolism or in super-obese patients with venous stasis and concomitant obesity hypoventilation.[94,95]

Pseudotumor Cerebri

Idiopathic intracranial hypertension is diagnosed in the setting of pulsatile tinnitus, severe headaches, and elevated cerebrospinal fluid pressure in a patient with normal brain imaging. The most likely etiology of this phenomenon is increased intra-abdominal pressure that is transmitted to the thoracic cavity and impedes venous return from the brain. A study of 19 patients with pseudotumor cerebri who underwent bariatric surgery found resolution of headaches and pulsatile tinnitus in all but one patient within four months of surgery. Cranial nerve dysfunction and papilledema resolved in all patients with 1 year of follow-up. Interestingly, two patients with weight regain had return of their neurologic symptoms.[96]

Stress Urinary Incontinence

Morbid obesity has a negative impact on urogenital health.[97] The increased intra-abdominal pressure associated with increasing BMI correlates with stress urinary incontinence, particularly in younger, multiparous patients.[98] Bump and associates evaluated the effects of weight loss after gastric bypass on lower urinary tract function in 12 patients. Nine patients (75%) had resolution of incontinence and significant improvements in vesicle pressure and urodynamic measurements occurred after weight loss. In patients undergoing laparoscopic gastric bypass, Schauer and associates demonstrated 44% resolution and 39% improvement in stress urinary incontinence symptoms[72] and DeMaria and associates reported resolution in 29 of 33 patients (88%) 1 year postoperatively.[65]

BARIATRIC PROCEDURES

Bariatric procedures are characterized by their mechanism of weight loss: restrictive (VBG, LAGB), malabsorptive (BPD, DS), or a combination of restriction and malabsorption (RYGB). Roux-en-Y gastric bypass is the most commonly performed procedure in the United States and accounts for 80–85% of procedures performed.[99] Laparoscopic adjustable gastric banding was approved for use in the United States in 2001 and is growing in popularity. Biliopancreatic diversion and duodenal switch procedures are performed in relatively few centers in the United States, and VBG is performed by only 5% of U.S. bariatric surgeons as a result of its high re-operation rate and less than desirable weight loss.

Laparoscopic Roux-en-Y Gastric Bypass

Mechanism of Weight Loss. Roux-en-Y gastric bypass is a combination procedure that includes a restrictive component (small gastric pouch and small stoma) and a malabsorptive component with a Roux-en-Y gastrojejunostomy that bypasses the duodenum and proximal jejunum. The restrictive component restricts the amount of food intake and the intestinal bypass has physiologic effects (dumping and rapid nutrient delivery to the hindgut) that likely contribute to the long-term efficacy of the operation. Gut hormone changes after RYGB impact satiety and glucose metabolism and the precise mechanism and interplay between the specific hormones in play are actively being investigated.[64]

Technique, Linear Stapled Gastrojejunostomy. An ordered, stepwise approach to laparoscopic gastric bypass improves efficiency in the operating room and provides the assistant and technician with a predictable operative plan (Table 52–5). We place the patient in the supine position with the feet together on a footboard. Abdominal access is obtained using a 5-mm Optiview trocar (Ethicon Endosurgery, Cincinnati, OH) or a left upper quadrant Veress needle and the remaining ports are placed under direct vision after needle localization and infiltration of local anesthetic (Fig 52–4). After access is obtained, laparoscopic inspection of the peritoneal cavity is completed then the patient is placed in steep Trendelenburg position. A 5-mm liver retractor is placed and anchored to the bed.

TABLE 52–5. KEY STEPS OF LAPAROSCOPIC ROUX-EN-Y GASTRIC BYPASS

Roux Limb

1. Place transverse colon and omentum in upper abdomen with bed flat.
2. Place jejunum in "C" configuration to identify Ligament of Treitz and transect jejunum 30 to 50 cm distal to ligament.
3. Mark end of Roux limb with Penrose drain to avoid confusing it with the biliopancreatic limb.
4. Measure Roux limb using rigid measuring device and straightened bowel.
5. Create stapled enteroenterostomy and close common opening without narrowing lumen.
6. Place reinforcing sutures at both ends of jejunojejunal anastomosis to prevent twisting and obstruction.
7. Close mesenteric defect with running non-absorbable suture to prevent internal hernia.
8. Divide omentum down the middle to the level of the transverse colon to reduce tension on the Roux limb.

Gastric Pouch

1. Place patient in steep reverse Trendelenburg position when creating gastric pouch.
2. Create 15-mL vertically-oriented gastric pouch using linear stapler. Vertical staple line should end at the Angle of His.
3. Mobilize pouch off of left crus to reduce tension on the gastrojejunal anastomosis.
4. Deliver Roux limb in antecolic, antegastric position between leaves of omentum using Penrose drain for traction.
5. Bring jejunojejunal anastomosis up to transverse colon to minimize tension on the Roux limb while creating the gastrojejunal anastomosis.

Gastrojejunal Anastomosis

1. Create a 1- to 1.5-cm gastrojejunal anastomosis (GJ) using linear stapler, circular stapler, or hand-sewn technique. Use nonabsorbable sutures for inner layer.
2. Use intraoperative endoscopy to evaluate GJ anastomosis for bleeding and leaks.
3. Sew omentum over gastrojejunal anastomosis to contain potential leaks at the GJ anastomosis.
4. Place a closed-suction drain posterior to anastomosis to control potential leaks.

Final Steps

1. Sew Roux limb to gastric remnant with interrupted stitch to prevent twisting.
2. Perform core needle liver biopsy.
3. Inspect for appropriate bowel orientation, twisting, kinks, staple line bleeding or failure, and retained sponges.
4. Close ports ≥ 10 mm with fascial sutures.

The Roux limb and jejunojejunostomy are completed first (Fig 52–5). The transverse colon is passed to the upper abdomen and the ligament of Treitz is identified. The proximal jejunum is then placed in a "C" configuration to help orient the proximal and distal segments. The jejunum is then divided 30 to 50 cm distal to the ligament of Treitz using a 45-mm linear stapler (2.5 mm staples). The mesentery of the jejunum is further divided with two firings of the Echelon linear stapler (Ethicon Endosurgery, Cincinnati, OH) to provide sufficient length of mesentery for tension-free passage of the Roux limb to the gastric pouch. The Roux limb is marked by sewing a Penrose drain to the corner. The enteroenterostomy is then completed. The Roux limb is measured distally from the Penrose drain for a distance of 75 cm (150 cm for patients with BMI >50). Once the appropriate length is measured, a stay suture is placed to approximate the biliopancreatic limb and the Roux limb side by side. A side-to-side, functional end-to-end jejunojejunostomy is then created using the linear stapler and the remaining enterotomy is closed with another firing of the linear stapler, Care is taken not to narrow either lumen with this final firing of the stapler. Once this anastomosis is completed, it is inspected for kinking or obvious staple line failures and reinforcing sutures are placed. One reinforcing stitch is placed between the end of the biliopancreatic limb and the Roux limb. Another is placed proximally at the crotch between the two limbs, and a third is placed proximal to that to prevent the proximal bowel from kinking over the anastomosis. The mesenteric defect is closed with a running non-absorbable suture. To minimize tension on the Roux limb, the greater omentum is divided using ultrasound dissection and the Roux limb is passed between the leaves of the divided omentum and up to the gastric pouch in an antecolic and antegastric fashion.

Gastric dissection is started by opening a window over the caudate lobe through the pars lucida with the Harmonic Scalpel (Ethicon Endosurgery, Cincinnati, OH) and firing the 60-mm linear stapler toward the lesser curvature of the stomach (Fig 52–6). The descending branch of the left gastric artery is transected with this approach, but the main trunk of the left gastric is preserved and provides the main blood supply to the gastric pouch. Once the lesser curvature is reached, a retrogastric space is devel-

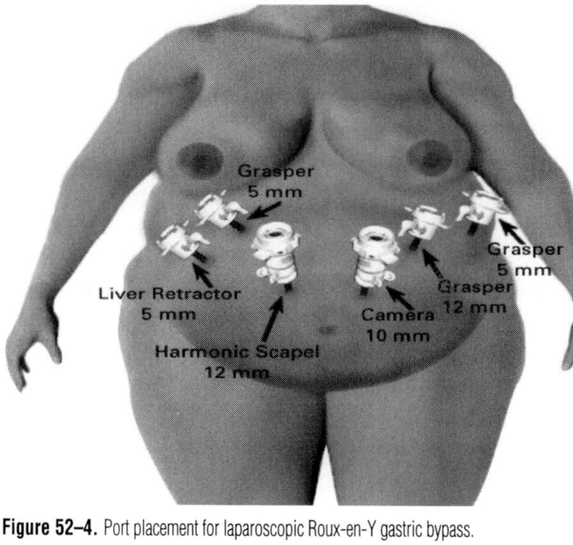

Figure 52–4. Port placement for laparoscopic Roux-en-Y gastric bypass.

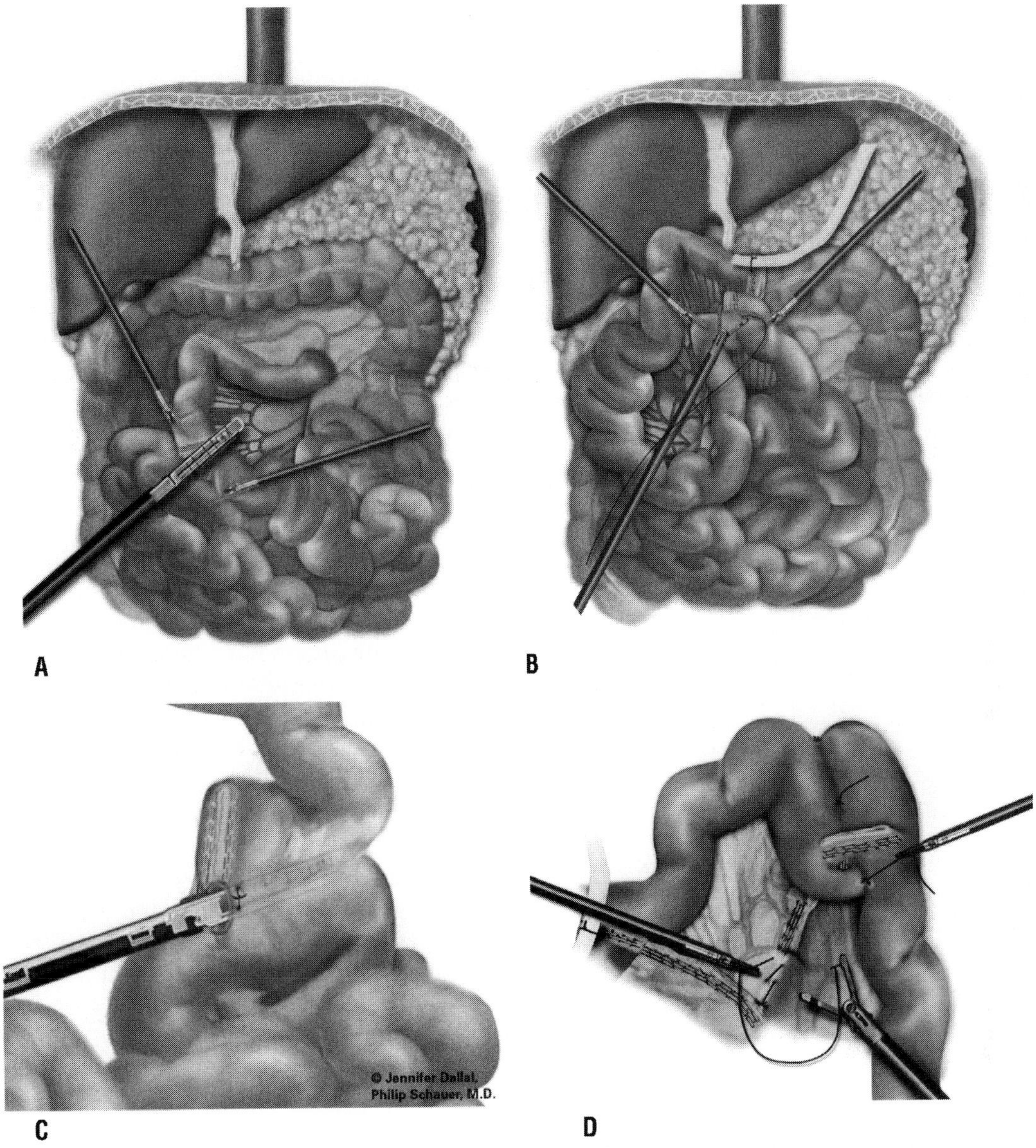

Figure 52–5. Creation of jejunojejunostomy, laparoscopic Roux-en-Y gastric bypass. **A.** The jejunum is placed in a "C" configuration and divided 30 to 50 cm distal to the ligament of Treitz. The mesentery is then divided with two firings of the linear stapler with a vascular load. **B.** The Roux limb is marked with a penrose drain and measured 75 cm (150 cm for BMI >50). **C.** The biliopancreatic and Roux limbs are approximated with a suture and the side-to-side, functional end-to-end anastomosis is created with a linear stapler. **D.** The common enterotomy is closed with a linear stapler and the mesenteric defect is closed with nonabsorbable suture.

oped to allow the passage of the linear stapler in the lesser sac. One horizontal firing of the stapler is completed 4 cm below the gastroesophageal junction and then two or three vertical firings of the 60-mm linear stapler (3.5 mm staples) are directed to the angle of His to create a 15 mL to 30 mL vertically oriented gastric pouch. The small gastric pouch and the gastric remnant are then gently dissected away from each other to minimize the chances of developing a gastro-gastric fistula. Dissection of the gastric pouch from the left crus improves mobility of the pouch and minimizes tension on the gastrojejunal anastomosis. If oozing is encountered during this dissection, we place a sponge in the abdomen and pack the area lateral to the Angle of His. This improves visualization as the pouch is mobilized.

The Roux limb is brought up to the gastric pouch in an antecolic, antegastric fashion. Prior to starting the gastrojejunal anastomosis, the entire Roux limb is delivered superiorly and the jejunojejunostomy (which can act as an anchor on the Roux limb while performing the anastomosis) is brought up to the level of the transverse colon to relieve tension. The retrocolic, antegastric or retrocolic, retrogastric placements can be used when tension on the Roux limb dictates. These techniques require more operative time and creates the need to close the mesocolic defect, a potential site for internal hernia. The Roux limb is sutured to the posterior wall of the gastric pouch using a running 2-0 absorbable suture. After a small gastrotomy and enterotomy are made adjacent to one another the linear stapler is placed 1.5 cm into each lumen, closed and fired (Fig 52–6). The remaining opening is then closed in two continuous layers of absorbable suture over an endoscope. The endoscope sizes the anastomosis to 30F (French), allows inspection for anastomotic bleeding at the time of the procedure, and provides insufflation for leak testing. A Jackson-Pratt drain is placed posterior to the anastomosis and omentum is sutured over the top of the anastomosis. The Roux limb is sutured to the gastric remnant as it passes over it to minimize the risk of twisting. We perform a core needle liver biopsy as part of every bariatric procedure. After the liver biopsy is completed, a final inspection is performed looking for bowel kinks or twists, staple line bleeding or failure, and retained sponges (if used during the gastric dissection). Port sites 10 mm or greater are then closed with absorbable suture using a suture-passer.

Circular Stapled Gastrojejunostomy, Transoral Method. The circular stapler can be used to create the gastrojejunostomy in both open and laparoscopic RYGB. In the laparoscopic bypass, the anvil for the circular stapler can be placed in the gastric pouch either transabdominally or by the transoral route (Fig 52–7). In the transoral technique popu-

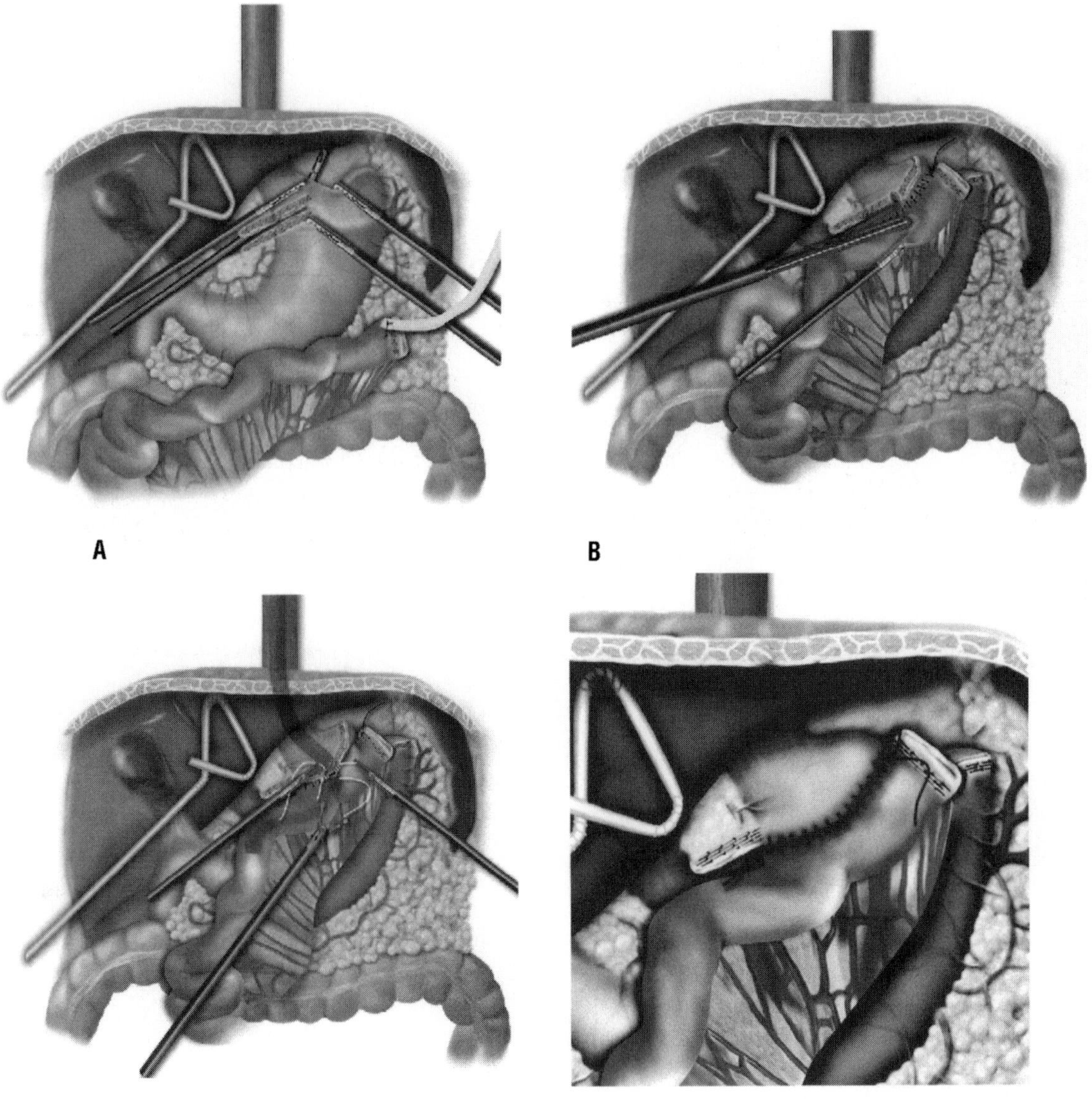

A B C D

Figure 52–6. Creation of the linear stapled gastrojejunostomy for laparoscopic Roux-en-Y gastric bypass. **A.** The 15-mL gastric pouch is created with a linear cutting stapler. The pouch and Roux limb are then approximated with a posterior suture line. **B.** A linear stapler is placed into small adjacent openings in the pouch and Roux limb and fired to create a 1.5-cm anastomosis. **C.** The common opening is closed over an endoscope using absorbable suture for the inner layer. **D.** The completed gastrojejunostomy. Omentum is used to cover the anastomosis and a closed-suction drain is placed posteriorly.

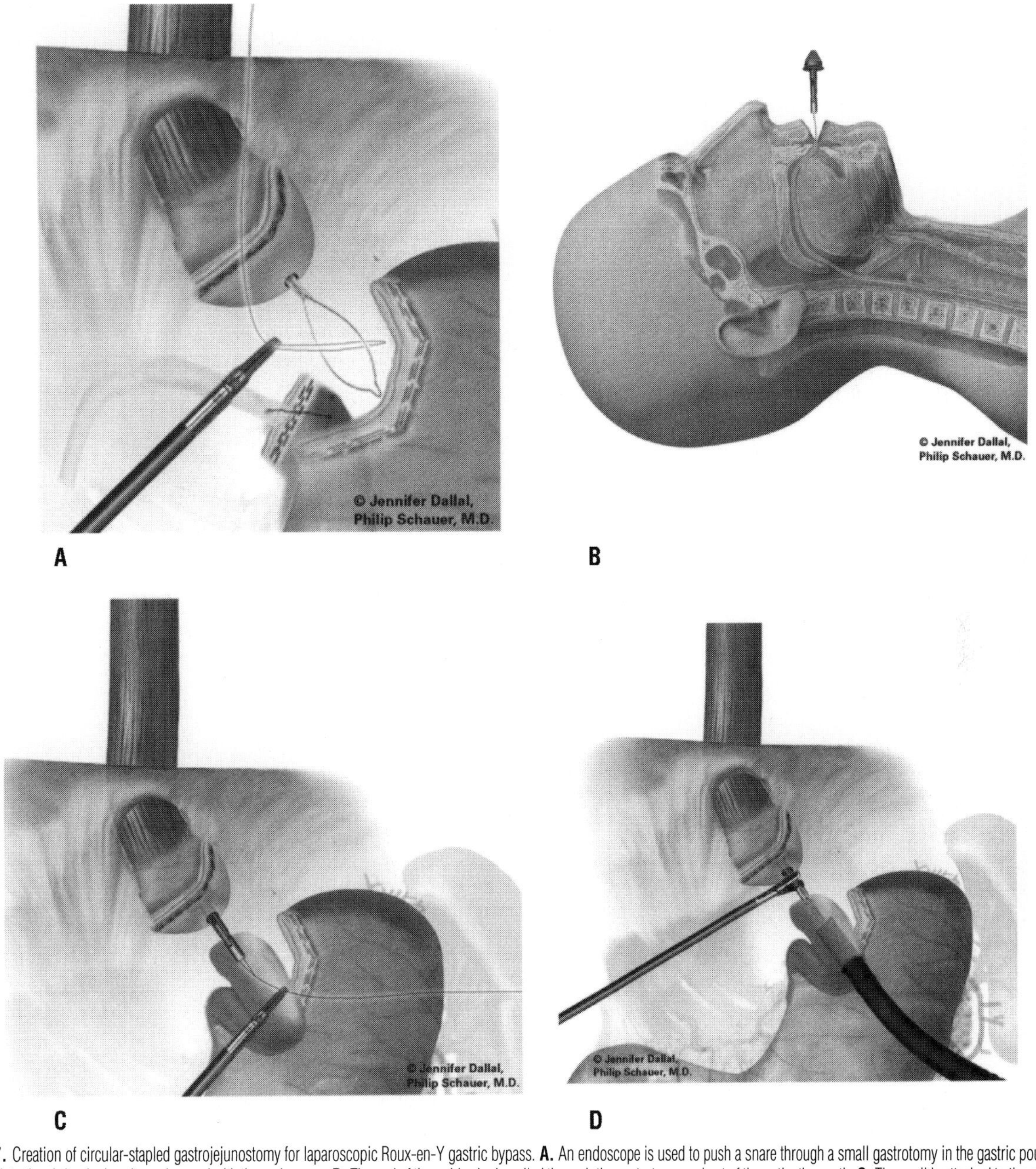

Figure 52–7. Creation of circular-stapled gastrojejunostomy for laparoscopic Roux-en-Y gastric bypass. **A.** An endoscope is used to push a snare through a small gastrotomy in the gastric pouch. A guidewire is placed into the abdominal cavity and snared with the endoscope. **B.** The end of the guidewire is pulled through the gastrotomy and out of the patient's mouth. **C.** The anvil is attached to the guidewire outside of the patient and is then pulled antegrade into the gastric pouch. **D.** The stapler is placed in the Roux limb, connected to the anvil, and fired to complete the anastomosis.

larized by Wittgrove,[66] the small gastric pouch is created using linear staplers as described above. An endoscope is placed transorally into the gastric pouch and a snare is passed through a small gastrotomy. A guidewire is placed transabdominally, snared and delivered out of the patient's mouth by withdrawing the endoscope. A 21- or 25-mm anvil is attached to the guide wire and then pulled into the gastric pouch. This can be facilitated by folding the head of the anvil parallel with the shaft and ensuring that the patient is completely paralyzed. The jaw is subluxed as the anvil is pulled into the esophagus. Once the anvil is in the pouch and the shaft is delivered through the gastrotomy, the guidewire is then cut from the anvil and removed. The Roux limb is delivered to the gastric pouch and the circular stapler is placed through a left upper quadrant port. This typically needs to be manually enlarged to allow passage of the stapling device. The end of the stapler is placed into the open end of the Roux limb or a separate enterotomy and the spike is pushed through the antimesenteric border of the Roux limb. The stapler is then attached to the anvil and is closed and fired to create the anastomosis. The open end of the Roux limb (or enterotomy) is then closed with a firing of the linear stapler. The anastomosis is tested for leaks with air or methylene blue dye. The anvil can also be tied to a nasogastric tube and passed into the gastric pouch, eliminating the need for an endoscopic guidewire.

Circular Stapled Gastrojejunostomy, Transabdominal Method. This method differs from the transoral method only in the way that the anvil is delivered into the pouch. A gastrotomy is created remote from the pouch in the body of the stomach and the anvil is placed in the lumen. The anvil is positioned in the cardia of the stomach and the shaft is delivered through a small anterior gastrotomy. The pouch can be partially completed (horizontal firing of the stapler) prior to delivering the anvil into the upper stomach. The pouch is then completed around the anvil and the circular stapled anastomosis is created as above by placing the stapler through the open end of the Roux.

Hand-Sewn Gastrojejunostomy. Completely hand-sewn anastomoses are used by many open bariatric surgeons and some laparoscopic bariatric surgeons. Higa and associates popularized the laparoscopic method of hand-sewn anastomoses.[100] This technique has the advantages of using less specialized equipment and eliminating the need to enlarge a port site for the circular stapler. This technique requires considerable skill to complete in an appropriate time. After the pouch is created, the Roux limb is delivered to the gastric pouch and a two-layer 10- to 12-mm anastomosis is created over an orogastric tube with 3-0 polyglactin sutures. Figure 52–8 shows the completed laparoscopic Roux-en-Y gastric bypass.

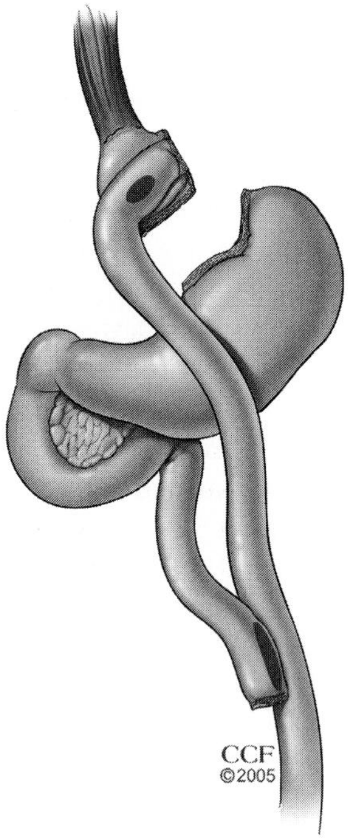

Figure 52–8. Completed Roux-en-Y gastric bypass.

Open Roux-en-Y Gastric Bypass

Technique. The abdomen is entered through an upper midline incision and a thorough exploration is completed after adequate exposure is obtained. The ligament of Treitz is identified by lifting the transverse colon and the jejunum is divided with a linear stapler 30 to 50 cm distal to the ligament. A standard length (75 cm) or long-limb length (150 cm) Roux limb is measured and a side-to-side jejunojejunostomy is created with the linear stapler. A suture is placed at the crotch of the anastomosis and another is placed more proximally between the two limbs to prevent the bowel from kinking over the anastomosis. The mesenteric defect at the jejunojejunostomy is then closed with nonabsorbable suture. The gastric pouch is created next. The anterior and lateral phrenoesophageal ligament are opened to the angle of His and the gastrohepatic ligament is opened over the caudate lobe. The mesentery between the second and third branches of the left gastric artery is divided and a retrogastric space is developed from the lesser curvature to the angle of His. A 15- to 30-mL vertically oriented pouch is formed using an articulating linear stapler. The Roux limb can be brought up to the gastric pouch retrocolic and retrogastric, retrocolic and antegastric, or antecolic and antegastric depending on the surgeon's preference and tension on the Roux limb. If the Roux limb is brought through the transverse mesocolon, the space between the jejunal and transverse colon mesenteries is closed (Peterson's space) to prevent internal herniation of small bowel. A 1- to 1.5-cm gastrojejunostomy is either hand-sewn over a 30F dilator or created with a circular or linear stapler. The anastomosis is tested with air insufflation or methylene blue through a nasogastric tube or with endoscopy.

Complications of RYGB. The overall incidence of major postoperative complications is similar between open and laparoscopic RYGB (10–15%) but the types of complications differ according to technique. Podnos and colleagues reviewed complications rates after open RYGB (n = 2771, 8 series) and Laparoscopic RYGB (n = 3464, 10 series).[71] Anastomotic leaks occur 1–5% of the time in open and laparoscopic series[22,65,67,72,100–103] and the leak rate in Podnos' review was 2.1% for laparoscopic RYGB and 1.7% for open RYGB (not significant). Leak rates, particularly with the laparoscopic technique, decrease with surgeon experience.

GI tract hemorrhage occurs 0.4–4% of the time after laparoscopic RYGB.[22,65,68,72,100–103] and the incidence is

higher in the laparoscopic group (1.9% vs. 0.6%) compared to open RYGB.[71] Postoperative GI bleeding typically occurs at the gastrojejunostomy or the gastric remnant staple line.

Marginal ulceration occurs at the gastrojejunostomy 1–16% of the time after isolated gastric bypasses[17,104] and is associated with ischemia, smoking, excessive acid exposure (gastro-gastric fistula), nonsteroidal anti-inflammatory use, and *H. pylori* infection. Marginal ulcers typically occur within 2 months after surgery.

The lower incidence of wound complications (infections and incisional hernias) is a major advantage of laparoscopic RYGB. This was demonstrated in Nguyen's randomized, controlled trial of laparoscopic versus open RYGB with a wound infection rate of 1.3% and 10.5% and incisional hernia rates of zero and 7.9%, respectively.[22] Other series of open RYGB have reported incisional hernia rates as high as 15–20%.[66,105] Wound infections occurred more frequently after open RYGB than after laparoscopic RYGB in Podnos' review as well (6.63% vs. 2.98%, $p < 0.001$).[71]

Pulmonary complications occur after open and laparoscopic RYGB, but there was no significant difference in rates of postoperative pneumonia in Podnos' review (0.33% open, 0.14% laparoscopic). Nguyen's randomized trial did show significant advantages in early postop pulmonary function and pain control with the laparoscopic approach (Figs 52–9 and 52–10).[106]

Other late complications of RYGB include bowel obstruction and anastomotic stricture. Bowel obstruction after laparoscopic RYGB most commonly results from an internal hernia and this complication occurs 1–10% of the time.[22,66,72,103,107] In a comprehensive review of the large open and laparoscopic series, the incidence of late bowel obstruction was 2.1% for open RYGB and 3.2% for laparoscopic RYGB ($p = 0.02$). Anastomotic stricture at the gastrojejunostomy occurs more frequently with laparoscopic RYGB than with open RYGB (4.7% vs. 0.7%, respectively in Podnos' review). The use of the circular stapler, particularly the 21-mm size, is associated with higher stricture rates than other techniques.[108]

Nutritional deficiencies can occur after RYGB. Deficiency of iron (6–52%), folate (22–63%) and vitamin B12 (3–37%) are common postoperatively and contribute to the development of anemia found in 54% of patients.[109,110] Routine supplementation with iron, vitamin B12, folate, and calcium following gastric bypass is recommended.

Distal gastric bypass with a 50-cm common channel results in protein-calorie malnutrition in 28.5% of patients.[111] A low serum albumin and phosphate level indicate depletion in total body protein. Excessive malabsorption in these cases may be reversed by conversion to a 150- to 200-cm common channel. It is important to provide thiamine replacement and to avoid the refeeding syndrome in these patients.[112–114]

The mortality rate for gastric bypass in Buchwald's meta-analysis was 0.5%.[4] In a review of 6235 patient who underwent gastric bypass, the mortality rate was higher in the open RYGB series (0.9%) compared to the laparoscopic group (0.2%, $p = 0.001$) but there was no difference in mortality rates between open and laparoscopic RYGB in three randomized trials.[21–23] In laparoscopic RYGB series (with >100 patients), the mortality rate ranges from zero to 0.9%.[65,66,72,103,115]

Efficacy. RYGB typically results in 65–80% EWL and maximum weight loss occurs 18 to 24 months after surgery. There is no significant difference in weight loss between the open and laparoscopic approach. In a study by Schauer and colleagues the mean excess weight loss was 83% at 1 year and 77% at 30 months.[72] Longer follow-up after RYGB reveals some weight regain with 60–70% EWL at 5 years. Fourteen-year follow-up of RYGB demonstrates EWL of 49% to 59%.[6,7] The Swedish Obese Subjects (SOS) Study demonstrated 10-year weight loss (as a percentage of initial body weight) of 25% for RYGB.[5] Weight loss in super-obese patients (BMI >50) is less with EWL of 51% to 69% at 12 to 36 months.[101,116–118]

RYGB results in significant improvement or resolution of many major obesity-related comorbidities (Table 52–6). Degenerative joint disease, hyperlipidemia, gastroesophageal reflux, hypertension, obstructive sleep apnea, depression, stress urinary incontinence, asthma, migraine headaches, venous insufficiency, congestive heart failure, and diabetes improve or resolve in the majority of patients after surgery.

Laparoscopic Adjustable Gastric Banding

Mechanism of Weight Loss. Laparoscopic adjustable gastric banding is a purely restrictive procedure. Like vertical banded gastroplasty, it creates a small proximal gastric pouch with a small outlet. This operation limits the quantity of food that can be consumed at one time, but may not have all of the same physiologic effects on gut hormones that the bypass procedures have. The advantage of LAGB over VBG is that the gastric stoma can be adjusted by filling the inner collar of the band with saline via a subcutaneous port. This allows titration of weight loss in balance with symptoms of dysphagia and satiety.

Technique. The LAGB is technically the simplest bariatric surgery to perform and requires less operating time than other bariatric procedures. As with other bariatric procedures, a stepwise approach can improve efficiency in the operating room and provide a reproducible teaching environment (Table 52–7). The patient is placed in steep reverse Trendelenburg position and six laparoscopic

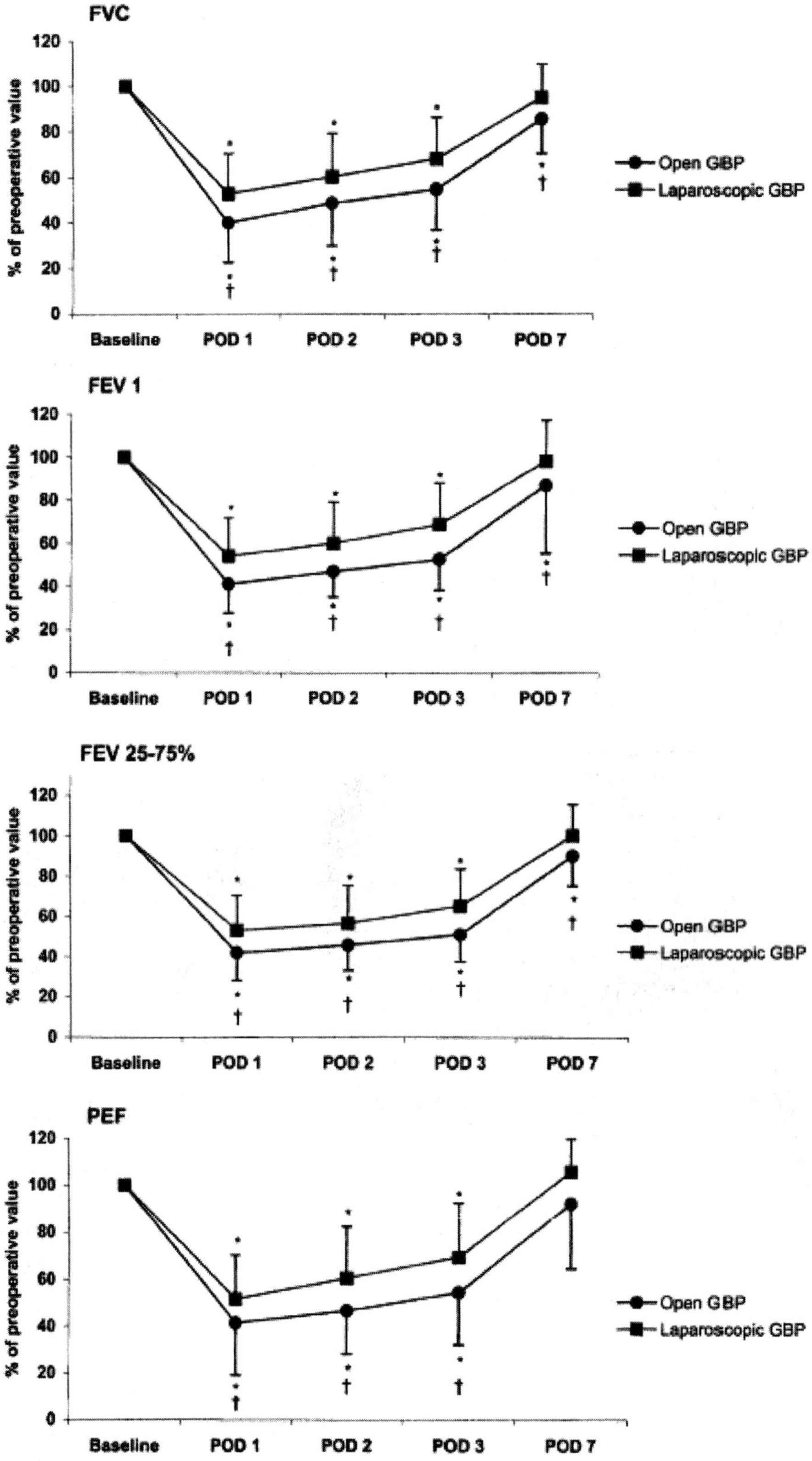

Figure 52–9. Postoperative spirometry (FVC, FEV_1, FEV 25–75%, and PEF) after laparoscopic and after open gastric bypass (GBP). *$p < 0.05$ compared with baseline value; †$p < 0.05$ compared with laparoscopic GBP. FEV_1, forced expiratory volume in 1 sec; FEV 25–75%, forced expiratory volume at mid-expiratory phase; FVC, forced vital capacity; PEF, peak expiratory flow; POD, postoperative day. (Reprinted from Nguyen NT, Lee SL, Goldman C, et al. Comparison of pulmonary function and postoperative pain after laparoscopic versus open gastric bypass: a randomized trial. *J Am Coll Surg* 2001;192(4):469–476; discussion 476–477 with permission from American College of Surgeons.)

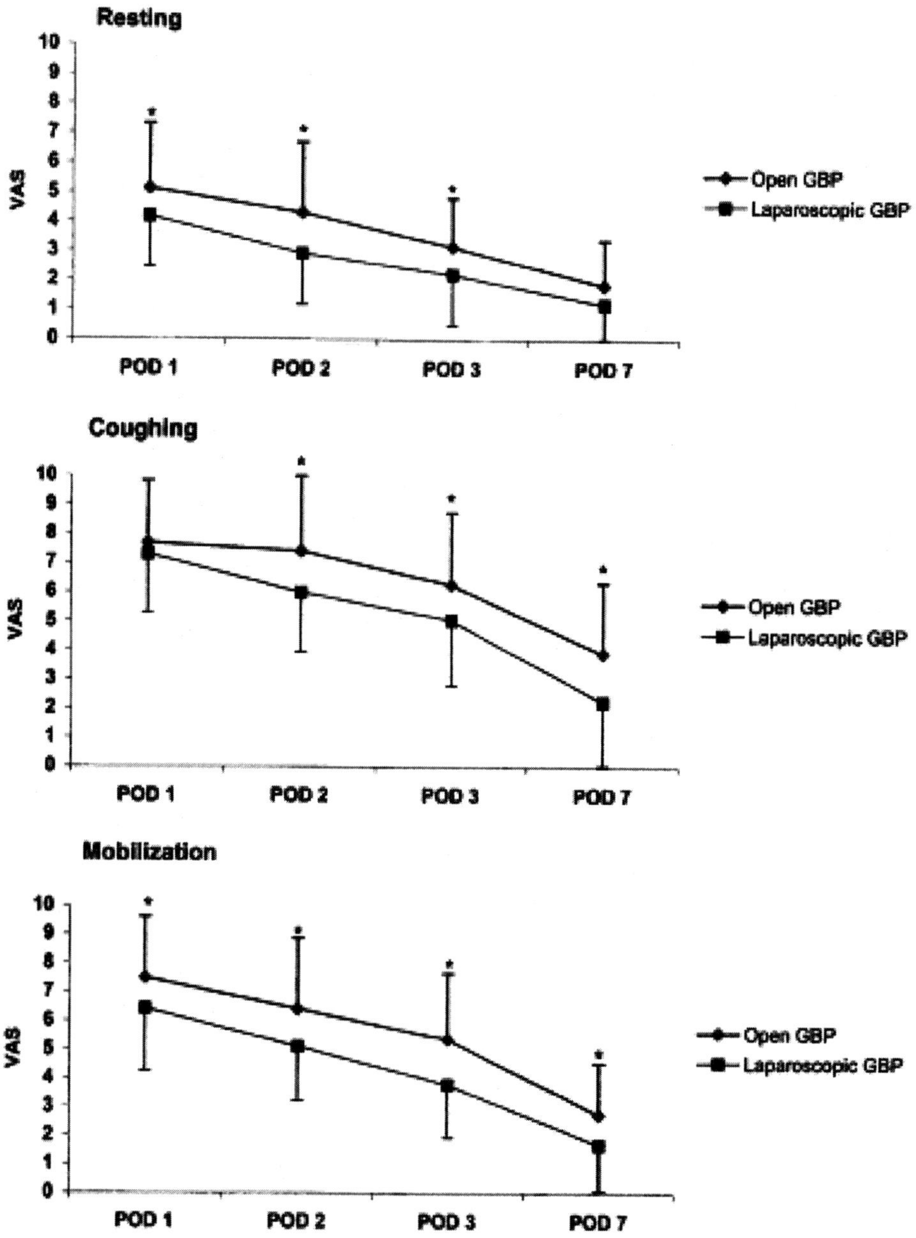

Figure 52–10. Visual analog scale (VAS) pain scores at rest, upon coughing, and during mobilization after laparoscopic and after open gastric bypass (GBP). *$p < 0.05$ compared with laparoscopic GBP. POD, postoperative day. (Reprinted from Nguyen NT, Lee SL, Goldman C, et al. Comparison of pulmonary function and postoperative pain after laparoscopic versus open gastric bypass: a randomized trial. *J Am Coll Surg* 2001;192(4):469–476; discussion 476–477 with permission from American College of Surgeons.)

ports are placed after pneumoperitoneum is established (Fig 52–11). The left lobe of the liver is retracted anteriorly to provide exposure of the gastroesophageal junction and a window is created in the clear space of the gastrohepatic ligament. The pars flaccida technique incorporates the fat along the lesser curvature in the band and has been shown to decrease the risk of prolapse. A small peritoneal opening is created at the base of the right diaphragmatic crus and at the angle of His. A blunt-tipped instrument is placed into the retrogastric space from right to left and gently directed to the angle of His. This dissection is performed blindly to avoid creating a posterior space and upward force should be avoided to prevent injury to the esophagus or stomach. Gentle pressure is applied against the anterior surface of the left crus until the instrument is visualized. The blunt instrument is pushed through the opening at the angle of His to complete the retrogastric tunnel (Fig 52–12). The band and tubing are placed in the abdominal cavity and the end of the tubing is grasped with the blunt instrument placed behind the stomach. The band is then pulled through the retrogastric tunnel. Prior to locking

TABLE 52–6. BENEFITS OF LAPAROSCOPIC BARIATRIC PROCEDURES

	Laparoscopic Gastric Bypass 6,7,21,22,65,66,72,101,103 115–117,150	Laparoscopic Adjustable Gastric Banding 13,20,67,117,118,120,151–154
Excess Weight Loss	68–80%	44–68%
EWL for BMI >50	51–66%	47–49%
Hospital Stay	2–4 days	1–2 days
Durability of Procedure	49–59% EWL at 14 years*	57% EWL at 6 years
Resolution of Comorbidities		
Diabetes	82–98%	54–64%
Hypertension	52–92%	55%
Hypercholesterolemia	63%	74%
GERD	72–98%	76–89%
Sleep Apnea	74–100%	94%
DJD	41–76%	NR
Urinary Incontinence	44–88%	NR

*Open gastric bypass.
BMI, body mass index; EWL, excess weight loss; GERD, gastroesophageal reflux disease; DJD, degenerative joint disease; NR, not reported.

the band in place, ensure that it is encircling the stomach and not the esophagus. Approximately one centimeter of stomach should be visible above the band. The tail of the band is passed through the buckle and the band is locked in place around the gastric cardia. After the band is locked, it should rotate freely back and forth. If resistance is encountered when performing this rocking motion, perigastric fat within the band should be divided until the band rotates freely. This maneuver prevents complete stomal obstruction postoperatively. Three or four interrupted sutures are placed to plicate the anterior stomach over the band to the anterior surface of the gastric pouch. This minimizes the risk of anterior prolapse. To minimize the risk of band erosion, the plication should be tension-free and not cover the buckle of the band. The tube attached to the band is brought out through a left-sided paramedian trocar site and attached to the port. The trocar incision is lengthened to provide adequate dissection down to the anterior rectus fascia. The port is then secured to the anterior rectus fascia with nonabsorbably sutures. Pneumoperitoneum is re-established and the tubing is inspected for kinks.

Patients remain in the hospital for 1 or 2 days and an upper GI study is done prior to discharge to confirm band position and patency. Anti-emetic therapy should begin in the operating room as post-operative retching can result in early prolapse of the stomach through the band. After discharge, patients are kept on a liquid diet for one month and the first band adjustment is performed 4–6 weeks postoperatively. Patients are then followed monthly for the first year to assess weight loss and symptoms and to make further adjustments if necessary. Band adjustments are usually performed in the office but can be performed using fluoroscopy. The access port is located by palpation and a noncoring needle on a 3-mL syringe is placed through the diaphragm of the port. The amount of saline added or removed depends on the patient's weight loss, satiety after meals, and symptoms associated with excessive restriction. Patients should lose 1 to 2 pounds per week after band placement and have postprandial satiety that lasts several hours.

Dysphagia can result from overeating, eating too quickly, or failing to adequately chew pieces of meat or bread. If eating habits have been addressed and dysphagia continues, a band adjustment with removal of some saline may be required. Patients should be counseled to remain on clear liquids for 24 hours after an episode of severe dysphagia as mucosal edema at the stoma may develop. A patient who presents with persistent obstruction of the band stoma after eating will complain of severe chest pain and will be unable to tolerate liquids. This will be relieved after the obstructing food is regurgitated, but if this does not occur, the band should be completely deflated to allow passage of the obstructing food. The patient should remain on a liquid diet for two or three days at which time the band can be re-adjusted.

Reflux can occur when the band is too tight but it may also be a symptom of prolapse. An esophagogram will determine the cause and guide treatment. Reflux from an over-tight band can be remedied with removal

TABLE 52–7. KEY STEPS OF LAPAROSCOPIC ADJUSTABLE GASTRIC BANDING

Dissection (pars flaccida technique)

1. Open clear space of gastrohepatic ligament, create small opening in peritoneum over base of right crus.
2. Create small opening in peritoneum over left crus at the Angle of His.
3. Pass blunt-tipped instrument blindly into retrogastric space from right to left. Pressure should be directed against anterior surface of left crus to avoid injuring the esophagus or stomach.
4. Pop through peritoneal opening at Angle of His under direct vision.

Band placement

1. Deliver band and tubing into peritoneal cavity and grasp end of tubing with blunt dissector at Angle of His.
2. Pull tube through tunnel until band is in place.
3. Prior to locking band closed, make sure band is around stomach, not esophagus. There should be approximately 1 cm of stomach visible above the band.
4. Close the band and make sure it rotates freely. If there is resistance, divide the perigastric fat inside the band until it rotates freely.
5. Starting toward the greater curvature, place three or four sutures (1 cm apart) to plicate the anterior gastric wall to the anterior wall of gastric pouch. Avoid tension or plicating over the buckle of the band.

Port and tubing

1. Deliver band tubing through left paramedian port.
2. Create adequate incision at paramedian port and dissect to anterior rectus fascia.
3. Attach tubing to port and secure port to rectus fascia with nonabsorbable sutures.
4. Replace laparoscope and check tubing for kinks.
5. Leave band deflated for 4 to 6 weeks.

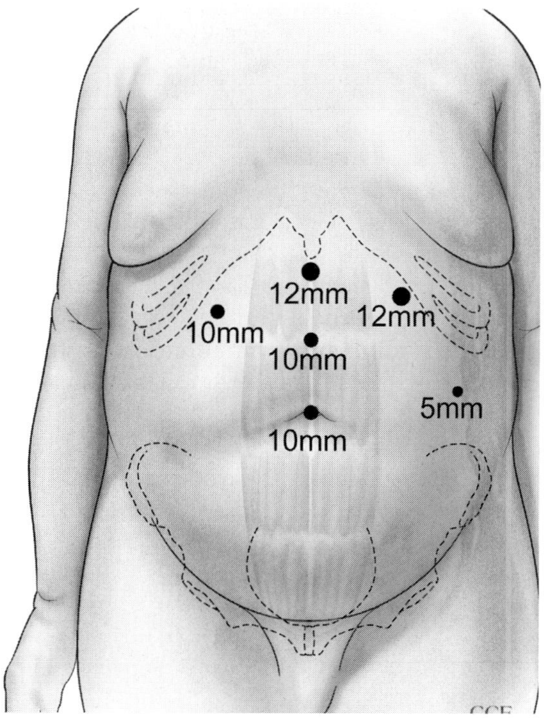

Figure 52–11. Port placement for laparoscopic adjustable gastric banding.

of some saline. Reflux secondary to gastric prolapse requires an operation to reduce the prolapse and reposition the band.

Aggressive postoperative band filling can be associated with an increase in band-associated complications. Busetto and associates[119] found that most band-related complications were controlled by simple band deflation. The average number of postoperative band adjustments after surgery was 2.3 ± 1.7 and the average maximum band filling after surgery was 2.8 ± 1.2 mL. For patients who had more than 3 mL in their band 6 months after surgery, further band inflation was associated with reduced EWL and higher band-associated complications.

Complications. Laparoscopic adjustable gastric banding has a low operative mortality (0.05%) and an 11% rate of perioperative and late complications.[20] In the Italian Collaborative Study, seven patients died (out of 1265) for a mortality rate of 0.55%.[8] Intraoperative bleeding or injury to the stomach, esophagus, or spleen occur less than 1% of the time.[20] Several studies have reported early complications including bowel perforation in 0.5% of patients, rare bleeding complications (0.1%), and thromboembolic rates (0.01% to 0.15%) lower than those seen with gastric bypass.[11,13,20] Late complications are typically band-related and include band slippage, band erosion, and tube-related problems. In a review of the international literature, tube and port malfunctions occurred in 5.4% of patients and these complications require a second operation to correct.[20] Persistent vomiting, pouch dilation, and gastroesophageal reflux can also occur as late complications.

In a study of 1250 patients, O'Brien and Dixon reported no mortalities and a 1.8% early major complication rate, most of which were access port infections. The most common late complication requiring re-operation after LAGB is gastric prolapse or slippage and this

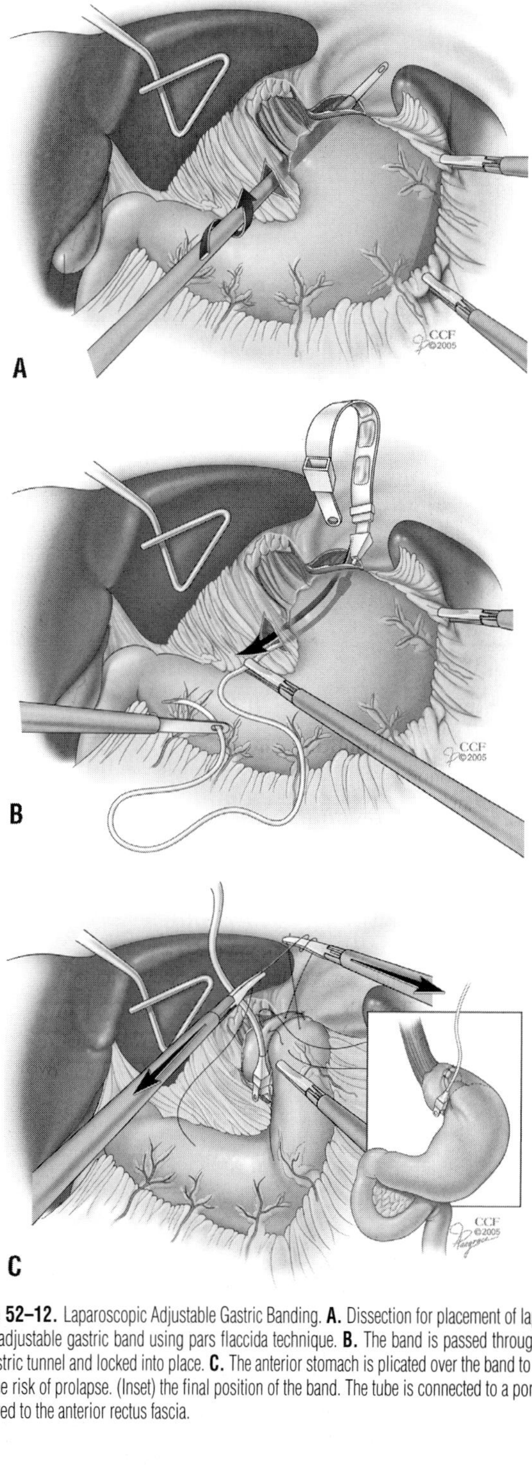

Figure 52–12. Laparoscopic Adjustable Gastric Banding. **A.** Dissection for placement of laparoscopic adjustable gastric band using pars flaccida technique. **B.** The band is passed through the retrogastric tunnel and locked into place. **C.** The anterior stomach is plicated over the band to minimize the risk of prolapse. (Inset) the final position of the band. The tube is connected to a port that is secured to the anterior rectus fascia.

complication decreased with experience (from 25% in the first 500 patients to 4.7% in the last 600 patients). Band erosion into the stomach occurred in 3% of patients early in their experience and problems with the access port occurred 5.4% of time.[67,120]

Efficacy. Excess weight loss after LAGB in the United States is typically 40–55%. Weight loss is more gradual with LAGB compared to RYGB and maximum weight loss typically occurs 2 the 3 years after the operation. Patient follow-up after LAGB plays in important role in the success of the operation. In a study by Shen and associates[118] LAGB patients who returned for more than six of their scheduled follow-up appointments in the first year after surgery (>50% compliance) had higher EWL (50%) than patients who returned for six or less appointments (42% EWL, $p = 0.005$). Compliance with follow-up appointments did not affect weight loss in gastric bypass patients followed for the same period.

O'Brien reported results on 709 patients undergoing the LAGB in Australia with a mean EWL of 57% at 72 months and major improvements in diabetes, asthma, gastroesophageal reflux, dyslipidemia, sleep apnea, depression, and quality of life.[16] Table 52–6 shows EWL and resolution rates of comorbidities for large series of LAGB. The Italian Collaborative Study Group for the Lap-Band system reviewed 1863 patients undergoing LAGB. Six-year follow-up showed a steady decrease in BMI from a preoperative average of 43 to a BMI of 32 at 72 months.[17]

Initial results with the LAGB in the United States were not as favorable as those in Europe and Australia and early series reported EWL of 35–45% and high complication and band removal rates.[10] More recent U.S. studies of LAGB have reported results that approach the success rates seen in international studies, though. Ponce et al. reported EWL of 64% at 48 months after LAGB with 75% of patients achieving >50% weight loss. This recent study also had low complications rates with seven access port problems (0.7%), 14 acute stomal obstructions (1.4%), and eight band explantations (0.8%). Changing their dissection method from the perigastric to the pars flaccida technique decreased band prolapse rates from 20.5% to 1.4%.[121] Long-term data is necessary to determine the durability of LAGB compared to RYGB and BPD, but it currently provides a safe and effective method of surgical weight loss, particularly for patients who are unwilling to accept the risks associated with other bariatric procedures.

Vertical Banded Gastroplasty

Mechanism of Weight Loss. Vertical banded gastroplasty is a purely restrictive procedure that has a small proximal gastric pouch with a fixed, banded outlet. Long-term weight loss after VBG is less than with RYGB and patients that eat sweets or consume high calorie liquids frequently fail this operation. Poor long-term weight loss and high late complication rates have caused VBG to largely fall out of favor in the United States.

Technique. The pouch is formed by completing a retrogastric dissection from the gastrohepatic ligament to the angle of His and placing the anvil of an EEA circular stapler behind the stomach. A circular stapled window is created six centimeters below the angle of his and approximately 3 cm from the lesser curvature. When performed laparoscopically, accurate placement of the anvil in the retrogastric space can be facilitated by attaching the anvil to a heavy suture on a straight needle. After the dissection is complete, the needle can be placed in the retrogastric space and passed transgastrically adjacent to a 34F Bougie. The anvil is pulled through both walls of the stomach using the suture. Once the anvil is in place, the spike is removed. A circular stapler shaft is passed through an enlarged port site, connected to the anvil and fired adjacent to the Bougie to create a circular window in the proximal stomach. Four rows of staples are then fired superiorly from the window to the angle of His to create a 50-mL pouch. A linear cutting stapler can also be used to create the vertical pouch and eliminate the risk of gastrogastric fistula through a non-divided staple line. A 1 x 6 cm strip of polypropylene mesh is then sewn to itself around the outlet channel to fix the diameter of the stoma (Fig 52–13).

Complications. Early complications after VBG are infrequent, but late complications have resulted in a 17–30% re-operation rate. The most common late complications of VBG are gastroesophageal reflux (16–38%), stomal stenosis (20%), staple line disruption (11–48%), incisional hernia (13%), band migration (1.5%) and intractable vomiting (30–50%). Because of the poor long-term weight loss and high late complication rate, VBG is rarely performed by bariatric surgeons in the United States.

Efficacy. Vertical banded gastroplasty achieves acceptable early weight loss, but has less favorable long-term weight loss than other procedures used today. Some series have reported adequate long-term success with VBG, but excess weight loss 3 to 5 years after VBG is typically 30–60%. Ten-year follow-up data shows that only 26–40% of patients maintain acceptable weight loss (>50% EWL) and one third of patients in these series returned to or exceeded their pre-operative weight.[122]

Biliopancreatic Diversion

Mechanism of Weight Loss. Biliopancreatic diversion and duodenal switch procedures are malabsorptive and

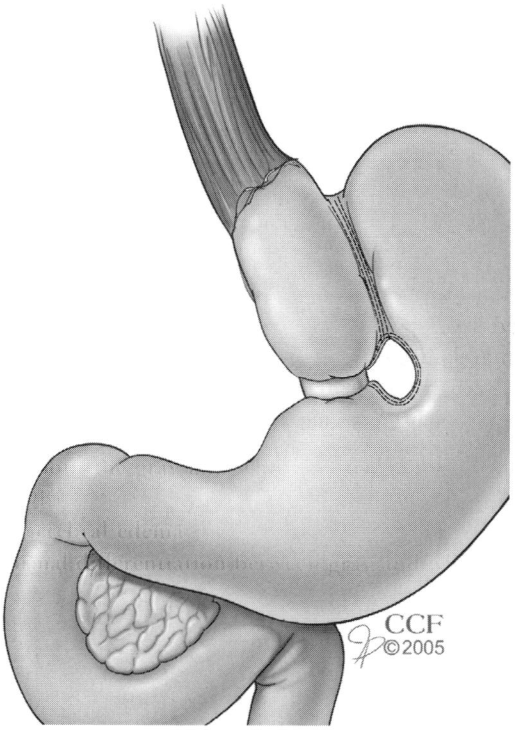

Figure 52–13. Vertical banded gastroplasty.

work by limiting intestinal energy absorption.[14,24,25] Initially, food intake is reduced because of reduction in gastric volume (partial gastrectomy or sleeve gastrectomy), but long-term, the limited absorptive area of the common channel determines weight loss. Ultimately, patients can consume excess calories (>2000 Kcal/day) without weight regain. The duodenal switch was developed to reduce the incidence of marginal ulceration, diarrhea, dumping syndrome, and protein calorie malnutrition seen with BPD. Both procedures rapidly deliver nutrients to the hindgut and alter gut hormone physiology. These changes may be partially responsible for the rapid and durable improvement in glucose metabolism and long-term weight loss after these procedures.

Technique. BPD consists of a subtotal gastrectomy leaving a proximal 200- or 400-mL pouch. The subtotal gastrectomy is intended primarily to reduce marginal ulcer rates by eliminating the gastric antrum rather than reducing gastric volume and intake. The small bowel is divided 250 cm from the ileocecal valve and a common channel is formed by completing the Roux-en-Y enteroenterostomy 50 to 100 cm from the ileocecal valve. The Roux limb is anastomosed to the gastric pouch. If present, the gall bladder is routinely removed at the time of BPD as a result of the high incidence of postoperative cholelithiasis.

The duodenal switch consists of a sleeve gastrectomy along the lesser curvature of the stomach leaving the antrum, pylorus, and the first portion of the duodenum in continuity. The remaining gastric reservoir is 150 to 200 mL. The ileum is divided 250 cm from the ileocecal valve and the proximal duodenum is then divided. A duodenoileostomy is created using a 250-cm-long alimentary limb and an enteroenterostomy is completed to form a 100-cm common channel (Fig 52–14). Both procedures have been performed laparoscopically.

Complications. In a meta-analysis that included 3030 patients who underwent BPD or DS, mortality was 1.1%. Marginal ulceration can occur up to 10% of the time, but this can be reduced to 1–3% with the duodenal switch and acid suppression therapy. Other complications include dumping syndrome, protein-calorie malnutrition and anemia in up to 12% and 40% of patients, respectively, vitamin B12 deficiency, hypocalcemia, fat-soluble vitamin deficiency, and bone demineralization (6%).[110] Problematic side effects of malabsorptive procedures include six to eight bowel movements per day and foul-smelling stools.

In Scopinaro's series of 1968 BPD patients, the overall rate of early major surgical complications (intraperitoneal bleeding, wound dehiscence, wound infection, anastomotic leak, and gastric perforation) decreased from 2.7% in his first 738 cases to 1.4% in his last 500 cases. Late complications included anemia (5%), anastomotic ulcer (3%), incisional hernia (9%), and protein calorie malnutrition in 7% of patients. Two percent of patients required reoperation to elongate the common channel. Operative mortality decreased to 0.4% in the last half of the series.[15]

The feasibility of laparoscopic BPD and DS has been demonstrated in small series by surgeons highly experienced with the procedures. Complication rates are similar to open series in this early experience with the exception of patients with a BMI >65.[30]

Efficacy. Weight loss after BPD is excellent and the results are durable. A meta-analysis demonstrated that BPD had a higher percentage of excess weight loss (70%) than other bariatric procedures.[4] Scopinaro reported overall EWL of 74% at 8 years and 77% at 18 years after BPD. In this series, there was no difference in long term EWL between morbidly obese and super-obese (>120% ideal body weight) subjects.[17] Ren and colleagues performed 40 laparoscopic BPD-DS procedures and reported EWL of 58% at 9 months.[30]

Rates of comorbidity resolution after BPD or DS equal or exceed rates for other bariatric procedures (Table 52–3) and the cardiovascular risk factors that

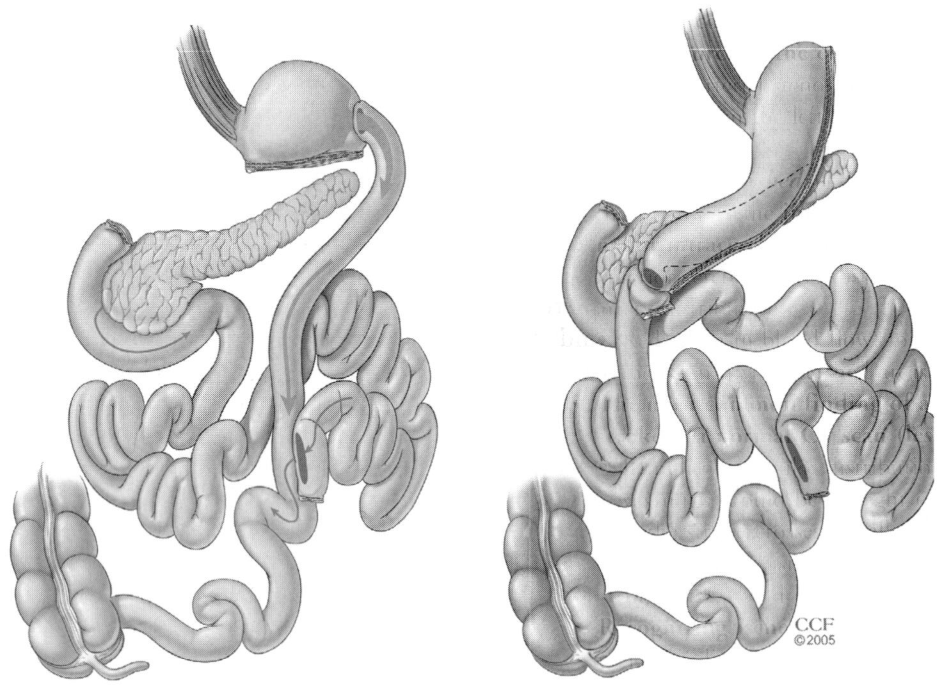

Figure 52–14. Biliopancreatic diversion (left) and biliopancreatic diversion with duodenal switch (right).

comprise the metabolic syndrome normalize in nearly all patients followed for 10 years after BPD.[123]

Other Bariatric Procedures

Implantable Gastric Stimulator. Gastric myoelectrical stimulation was developed to achieve weight loss without altering gastrointestinal anatomy and to avoid the morbidity associated with other bariatric procedures. The proposed mechanisms of action for weight loss with gastric stimulation include impaired gastric motility, gastric distension in the fasting state, and neurohumoral effects via the vagus nerve and circulating gut hormones. No clear understanding of the mechanism has been developed, however, which raises questions regarding the efficacy of this device. This investigational procedure involves implanting one or two electrodes laparoscopically along the greater curvature of the stomach 6 to 8 cm proximal to the pylorus. The electrodes are placed in a seromuscular tunnel and are then secured in place with clips or sutures. Endoscopy is performed to rule out transmural placement and the electrodes are then delivered through a trocar site and attached to a generator that is implanted in a subcutaneous pocket.

A randomized, placebo-controlled trial in the United States found a high number of lead dislodgements and no difference in weight loss between activated and nonactivated groups at six months. A subsequent open-label trial reported 23% EWL at 16 months of follow-up.[124] Overall, the implantable gastric stimulator (IGS) has resulted in 20% to 25% EWL at 15 months in initial clinical trials and this has been achieved with minimal morbidity and no long-term complications.[124–126] Greater weight loss has been achieved in carefully selected patients and these preliminary results suggest that IGS may be an appropriate weight loss option for selected patients in the future, but additional randomized controlled studies will be required for validation. This device is currently not FDA-approved for use outside of clinical trials.

Intragastric Balloon. Endoscopic placement of an intragastric balloon has resulted in modest weight loss in clinical studies. In a study by Doldi and associates, 349 intragastric balloons were placed in 303 patients. Patients in this study were also placed on a 1000 Kcal/day diet. After 4 months, patients lost an average of 14 kg (BMI reduction of nearly 5 kg/m^2) and showed improvement in diabetes and other comorbidities.[127] Balloon placement can be complicated by patient intolerance, balloon deflation, and gastric ulceration in a small number of patients. These and other authors have concluded that the optimal indication for the intragastric balloon is to achieve short-term weight loss in preparation for a more durable bariatric procedure.[128,129]

SPECIAL SITUATIONS

Pregnancy after Bariatric Surgery

Pregnancy outcomes have been evaluated after gastric bypass, gastric banding, and biliopancreatic diversion. Most patients undergoing bariatric surgery are women of childbearing age and contraception during the period of rapid weight loss should be emphasized. Pregnancies do occur during this period, though, as well as during the later weight-stable period. In fact, fertility can significantly improve after surgically induced weight loss.

Laparoscopic adjustable gastric banding has an advantage over other bariatric procedures in the pregnant patient in that it can be actively managed during the pregnancy to achieve appropriate maternal weight gain. A comparison of 79 pregnant women with a LAGB to 40 previous (pre-band) pregnancies in the same group, 79 matched obese pregnant subjects, and community outcomes demonstrated the safety of the LAGB in pregnancy. Birth weight, pregnancy-induced hypertension, and gestational diabetes rates in the LAGB group were lower than in pre-band pregnancies and the matched controls and were comparable to community norms.[130]

Weight loss after BPD improves fertility and provides benefits in terms of normalizing gestational weight changes, normalizing infant birth weight and reducing rates of fetal macrosomia. Children of mothers who conceived after BPD have normal growth patterns.[91] Delaying pregnancy until weight loss stabilizes is recommended and careful attention to nutritional parameters must occur during pregnancy in these patients.

After gastric bypass, patients becoming pregnant have fewer pregnancy-related complications than obese patients who delivered prior to gastric bypass. There was less gestational diabetes,[131] hypertension, and large for gestational-age infants in post-gastric bypass surgery pregnancies.[132] Close monitoring of nutritional status should occur with specific attention to iron, calcium, folate, and vitamin B12 supplementation.

Adolescent Bariatric Surgery

Obesity in the pediatric and adolescent population has increased significantly over the last two decades and the prevalence has nearly doubled in the last 10 years.[133] Thirty-one percent of children and adolescents age 6 to 19 are at risk for overweight or overweight (>85th percentile) and 16% are overweight (>95th percentile).[134] The 1991 NIH consensus conference did not sanction bariatric surgery in adolescents due to lack of evidence at that time. Obesity in adolescence, though, is associated with the same comorbidities seen in the adult population. The incidence of hypertension, hypercholesterolemia, type 2 diabetes, sleep apnea, pseudotumor cerebri, polycystic ovarian syndrome, nonalcoholic fatty liver disease, and musculoskeletal problems is higher in obese adolescents than normal weight adolescents. Cardiovascular risk is increased in obese children and the metabolic syndrome is present in 30% of overweight and 50% of severely obese adolescents.[135,136] Childhood and adolescent obesity is also associated with a myriad of severe psychological and social problems and significantly decreased self-esteem, lower personal expectations, and a health-related quality of life similar to children diagnosed with cancer.[137–139]

Recent small series support the safety and efficacy of RYGB[63,137,140] and LAGB[141] in carefully selected adolescents. The selection criteria for these patients are strict and the BMI criteria are generally higher than for adults (>40 with severe obesity-related comorbidity or >50 with less severe comorbidities).[57] To be considered for surgery, these patients must have achieved skeletal maturity (13 to 14 years in girls, 15 to 16 years in boys) and failed at least 6 months of a medically supervised weight loss program. Psychologic evaluations in this group of patients is important to determine emotional maturity, motivation, and family support and to identify any psychological or social contraindications to performing the surgery.[142]

Short term results with open and laparoscopic RYGB has been favorable in this group with 62% to 87% EWL and resolution of comorbidities in nearly all patients one to two years after surgery.[137,140] In a review of 33 adolescents who underwent bariatric surgery (30 were gastric bypasses), Sugerman and associates had no operative deaths and EWL of 56% at 10 years. Comorbidities resolved at 1 year except for hypertension in two patients, GERD in two patients, and joint pain in seven patients. Five patients had regained most or all of their lost weight 5 to 10 years after surgery, though, and the EWL for six patients followed to 14 years was 33%.

The laparoscopic adjustable gastric band is currently not approved for use in adolescents in the United States, but success with this procedure has been demonstrated elsewhere for this age group. Dolan and associates reported 59% EWL 24 months after surgery in 17 patients. There were only two band-related complications in this series. The LAGB is an attractive option for the adolescent population due to its reversibility, but long-term follow-up data is limited. The LAGB is purely restrictive procedure and, like the VBG, frequent intake of high-calorie liquids can defeat the operation.

Biliopancreatic diversion is the most effective bariatric procedure in terms of weight loss and durability, but the higher morbidity and mortality associated with the procedure and the high incidence of nutritional deficiencies make this operation much less attractive in the adolescent population.

Bariatric Surgery in the Elderly

As with the adolescent age group, there was insufficient evidence in 1991 for the NIH consensus conference to make recommendations about bariatric surgery for patients older than 60 years. In a cross-sectional population study, 33% of the U.S. population 60 years or older were obese and 3.9% were extremely obese (BMI >40). These patients frequently have multiple comorbidities and are generally higher risk operative candidates as a result of long-standing cardiovascular and pulmonary disease. Age older than 55 has been shown to be an independent predictor of mortality after bariatric surgery.[143] Nevertheless, carefully selected patients in this age group can benefit greatly from surgical weight loss. More important than the chronological age, the patient's physiologic age, comorbidity severity, and functional status determine how they will tolerate, and benefit from, bariatric surgery. Recent evidence supporting bariatric surgery in older patients consists of case series of open and laparoscopic RYGB,[144–146] laparoscopic gastric banding,[147,148] and biliopancreatic diversion.[149] In a series by Papasavas, 71 patients with a mean age of 59 underwent laparoscopic RYGB with 67% EWL at 24 months postoperatively with 87% resolution of diabetes, 70% resolution of hypertension, and 86% resolution of sleep apnea one year after surgery. Only three patients (4%) required rehabilitation postoperatively. Other reports have also confirmed the safety of gastric bypass in older patients but have demonstrated less weight loss and less complete resolution of comorbidities in the older patient groups.[144,146]

Gastric banding has been evaluated in patients older than 50 years of age and in a report of 68 patients, EWL was 68% at 1 year. Complications requiring reoperation occurred in 10% of patients and 97% had improvement in their obesity-related comorbidities.[148] A study comparing long-term weight loss and complication rates between older and younger patients who underwent biliopancreatic diversion demonstrated similar weight loss at 5 years, but a trend toward higher rates of protein malnutrition, anastomotic ulcer, and need for reversal in patients older than 55 years.[149]

A large retrospective cohort study evaluating the risk of early all-cause mortality among Medicare beneficiaries found advancing age to be a strong predictor of early death after bariatric surgery.[32] Highest rates of early mortality were seen in older men (19.6% 30-day mortality for men >75 years). For patients 65 years and older, the 30-day and 90-day mortality rates were 4.8% and 6.9%, respectively. These mortality rates are considerably higher than those reported in case series and further investigation will undoubtedly be conducted in this group of patients.

■ SUMMARY

The prevalence of obesity is steadily increasing in the United States and the high prevalence of childhood obesity in our society suggests an ominous future for this health crisis. Morbid obesity is a deadly disease. An adequate prevention and treatment strategy will require major changes in public policy, health care practices, and societal attitudes about this problem.

There is mounting evidence that surgical options for the treatment of morbid obesity are effective with reasonable, but not insignificant, complication and mortality rates. Despite the efficacy of surgery in reducing weight and eliminating or improving many life-threatening comorbidities, less than 2% of eligible patients in the United States are being referred for bariatric surgery. Bariatric surgery is rapidly growing as a surgical subspecialty and this increased interest will undoubtedly lead to further research focusing on the mechanisms of weight loss, surgical risk reduction, improvements in surgical techniques and durability, and new endoscopic approaches to weight loss surgery.

REFERENCES

1. *International Obesity Task Force. Call for obesity review as overweight numbers reach 1.7 billion* (press release). London, England: International Obesity Task Force, March 17, 2003. Available at: http://www.iotf.org. Accessed July 20, 2005
2. Fontaine KR, Redden DT, Wang C, et al. Years of life lost due to obesity. *JAMA* 2003;289(2):187–193
3. Buchwald H, Williams SE. Bariatric surgery worldwide 2003. *Obes Surg* 2004;14(9):1157–1164
4. Buchwald H, Avidor Y, Braunwald E, et al. Bariatric surgery: a systematic review and meta-analysis. *JAMA* 2004; 292(14):1724–1737
5. Sjostrom L, Lindroos AK, Peltonen M, et al. Lifestyle, diabetes, and cardiovascular risk factors 10 years after bariatric surgery. *N Engl J Med* 2004;351(26):2683–2693
6. White S, Brooks E, Jurikova L, Stubbs RS. Long-term outcomes after gastric bypass. *Obes Surg* 2005;15(2):155–163
7. Pories WJ, Swanson MS, MacDonald KG, et al. Who would have thought it? An operation proves to be the most effective therapy for adult-onset diabetes mellitus. *Ann Surg* 1995;222(3):339–350; discussion 350–352
8. Angrisani L, Alkilani M, Basso N, et al. Laparoscopic Italian experience with the Lap-Band. *Obes Surg* 2001; 11(3):307–310
9. O'Brien PE, Brown WA, Smith A, et al. Prospective study of a laparoscopically placed, adjustable gastric band in the treatment of morbid obesity. *Br J Surg* 1999; 86(1):113–118
10. DeMaria EJ, Sugerman HJ, Meador JG, et al. High failure rate after laparoscopic adjustable silicone gastric banding for treatment of morbid obesity. *Ann Surg* 2001;233(6):809–818

11. Belachew M, Belva PH, Desaive C. Long-term results of laparoscopic adjustable gastric banding for the treatment of morbid obesity. *Obes Surg* 2002;12(4):564–568
12. Vertruyen M. Experience with Lap-band System up to 7 years. *Obes Surg* 2002;12(4):569–572
13. O'Brien PE, Dixon JB, Brown W, et al. The laparoscopic adjustable gastric band (Lap-Band): a prospective study of medium-term effects on weight, health and quality of life. *Obes Surg* 2002;12(5):652–660
14. Hess DS, Hess DW, Oakley RS. The biliopancreatic diversion with the duodenal switch: results beyond 10 years. *Obes Surg* 2005;15(3):408–416
15. Scopinaro N, Gianetta E, Adami GF, et al. Biliopancreatic diversion for obesity at eighteen years. *Surgery* 1996; 119(3):261–268
16. Flum DR, Dellinger EP. Impact of gastric bypass operation on survival: a population-based analysis. *J Am Coll Surg* 2004;199(4):543–551
17. Christou NV, Sampalis JS, Liberman M, et al. Surgery decreases long-term mortality, morbidity, and health care use in morbidly obese patients. *Ann Surg* 2004; 240(3):416–423; discussion 423–424
18. MacDonald KG, Jr., Long SD, Swanson MS, et al. The Gastric Bypass Operation Reduces the Progression and Mortality of Non-Insulin-Dependent Diabetes Mellitus. *J Gastrointest Surg* 1997;1(3):213–220
19. Mason EE, Tang S, Renquist KE, et al. A decade of change in obesity surgery. National Bariatric Surgery Registry (NBSR) Contributors. *Obes Surg* 1997;7(3):189–197
20. Chapman AE, Kiroff G, Game P, et al. Laparoscopic adjustable gastric banding in the treatment of obesity: a systematic literature review. *Surgery* 2004;135(3):326–351
21. Lujan JA, Frutos MD, Hernandez Q, et al. Laparoscopic versus open gastric bypass in the treatment of morbid obesity: a randomized prospective study. *Ann Surg* 2004; 239(4):433–437
22. Nguyen NT, Goldman C, Rosenquist CJ, et al. Laparoscopic versus open gastric bypass: a randomized study of outcomes, quality of life, and costs. *Ann Surg* 2001; 234(3):279–289; discussion 289–291
23. Westling A, Gustavsson S. Laparoscopic vs open Roux-en-Y gastric bypass: a prospective, randomized trial. *Obes Surg* 2001;11(3):284–292
24. Scopinaro N, Adami GF, Marinari GM, et al. Biliopancreatic diversion. *World J Surg* 1998;22(9):936–946
25. Marceau P, Hould FS, Simard S, et al. Biliopancreatic diversion with duodenal switch. *World J Surg* 1998;22(9): 947–954
26. Totte E, Hendrickx L, van Hee R. Biliopancreatic diversion for treatment of morbid obesity: experience in 180 consecutive cases. *Obes Surg* 1999;9(2):161–165
27. Baltasar A, Bou R, Miro J, et al. Laparoscopic biliopancreatic diversion with duodenal switch: technique and initial experience. *Obes Surg* 2002;12(2):245–248
28. Paiva D, Bernardes L, Suretti L. Laparoscopic biliopancreatic diversion: technique and initial results. *Obes Surg* 2002;12(3):358–361
29. Rabkin RA, Rabkin JM, Metcalf B, et al. Laparoscopic technique for performing duodenal switch with gastric reduction. *Obes Surg* 2003;13(2):263–268
30. Ren CJ, Patterson E, Gagner M. Early results of laparoscopic biliopancreatic diversion with duodenal switch: a case series of 40 consecutive patients. *Obes Surg* 2000; 10(6):514–523; discussion 524
31. Scopinaro N, Marinari GM, Camerini G. Laparoscopic standard biliopancreatic diversion: technique and preliminary results. *Obes Surg* 2002;12(3):362–365
32. Flum DR, Salem L, Elrod JA, et al. Early mortality among Medicare beneficiaries undergoing bariatric surgical procedures. *JAMA* 2005;294(15):1903–1908
33. Nguyen NT, Paya M, Stevens CM, et al. The relationship between hospital volume and outcome in bariatric surgery at academic medical centers. *Ann Surg* 2004; 240(4):586–593; discussion 593–594
34. Zingmond DS, McGory ML, Ko CY. Hospitalization before and after gastric bypass surgery. *JAMA* 2005; 294(15):1918–1924
35. Goodney PP, Siewers AE, Stukel TA, et al. Is surgery getting safer? National trends in operative mortality. *J Am Coll Surg* 2002;195(2):219–227
36. Thompson D, Brown JB, Nichols GA, et al. Body mass index and future healthcare costs: a retrospective cohort study. *Obes Res* 2001;9(3):210–218
37. Thompson D, Edelsberg J, Colditz GA, et al. Lifetime health and economic consequences of obesity. *Arch Intern Med* 1999;159(18):2177–2183
38. Wolf AM. What is the economic case for treating obesity? *Obes Res* 1998;6(Suppl 1):2S–7S
39. Wolf AM. Economic outcomes of the obese patient. *Obes Res* 2002;10(Suppl 1):58S–62S
40. Wolf AM, Colditz GA. Current estimates of the economic cost of obesity in the United States. *Obes Res* 1998; 6(2):97–106
41. Finkelstein EA, Fiebelkorn IC, Wang G. National medical spending attributable to overweight and obesity: how much, and who's paying? *Health Aff (Millwood)* 2003;Suppl Web Exclusives:W3–219–26
42. Finkelstein EA, Fiebelkorn IC, Wang G. State-level estimates of annual medical expenditures attributable to obesity. *Obes Res* 2004;12(1):18–24
43. Sampalis JS, Liberman M, Auger S, Christou NV. The impact of weight reduction surgery on health-care costs in morbidly obese patients. *Obes Surg* 2004;14(7):939–947
44. Potteiger CE, Paragi PR, Inverso NA, et al. Bariatric surgery: shedding the monetary weight of prescription costs in the managed care arena. *Obes Surg* 2004;14(6):725–730
45. Snow LL, Weinstein LS, Hannon JK, et al. The effect of Roux-en-Y gastric bypass on prescription drug costs. *Obes Surg* 2004;14(8):1031–1035
46. Narbro K, Agren G, Jonsson E, et al. Pharmaceutical costs in obese individuals: comparison with a randomly selected population sample and long-term changes after conventional and surgical treatment: the SOS intervention study. *Arch Intern Med* 2002;162(18):2061–2069
47. Narbro K, Agren G, Jonsson E, et al. Sick leave and disability pension before and after treatment for obesity: a

report from the Swedish Obese Subjects (SOS) study. *Int J Obes Relat Metab Disord* 1999;23(6):619–624
48. Rasheid S, Banasiak M, Gallagher SF, et al. Gastric bypass is an effective treatment for obstructive sleep apnea in patients with clinically significant obesity. *Obes Surg* 2003;13(1):58–61
49. Salem L, Jensen CC, Flum DR. Are bariatric surgical outcomes worth their cost? A systematic review. *J Am Coll Surg* 2005;200(2):270–278
50. Craig BM, Tseng DS. Cost-effectiveness of gastric bypass for severe obesity. *Am J Med* 2002;113(6):491–498
51. Martin LF, White S, Lindstrom W, Jr. Cost-benefit analysis for the treatment of severe obesity. *World J Surg* 1998; 22(9):1008–1017
52. Reaven GM. Banting lecture 1988. Role of insulin resistance in human disease. *Diabetes* 1988;37(12):1595–1607
53. Grundy SM, Brewer HB, Jr., Cleeman JI, et al. Definition of metabolic syndrome: Report of the National Heart, Lung, and Blood Institute/American Heart Association conference on scientific issues related to definition. *Circulation* 2004;109(3):433–438
54. Third Report of the National Cholesterol Education Program (NCEP) Expert Panel on Detection, Evaluation, and Treatment of High Blood Cholesterol in Adults (Adult Treatment Panel III) final report. *Circulation* 2002;106(25):3143–3421
55. Alberti KG, Zimmet PZ. Definition, diagnosis and classification of diabetes mellitus and its complications. Part 1: diagnosis and classification of diabetes mellitus provisional report of a WHO consultation. *Diabet Med* 1998;15(7):539–553
56. Einhorn D, Reaven GM, Cobin RH, et al. American College of Endocrinology position statement on the insulin resistance syndrome. *Endocr Pract* 2003;9(3):237–252
57. Inge TH, Garcia V, Daniels S, et al. A multidisciplinary approach to the adolescent bariatric surgical patient. *J Pediatr Surg* 2004;39(3):442–447; discussion 446–447
58. Fantuzzi G. Adipose tissue, adipokines, and inflammation. *J Allergy Clin Immunol* 2005;115(5):911–919; quiz 920
59. Janssen I, Katzmarzyk PT, Ross R. Waist circumference and not body mass index explains obesity-related health risk. *Am J Clin Nutr* 2004;79(3):379–384
60. Mattar SG, Velcu LM, Rabinovitz M, et al. Surgically-induced weight loss significantly improves nonalcoholic fatty liver disease and the metabolic syndrome. *Ann Surg* 2005;242(4):610–617; discussion 618–620
61. Pories WJ, MacDonald KG, Jr., Morgan EJ, et al. Surgical treatment of obesity and its effect on diabetes: 10-y follow-up. *Am J Clin Nutr* 1992;55(2 Suppl):582S–585S
62. Schauer PR, Burguera B, Ikramuddin S, et al. Effect of laparoscopic Roux-en Y gastric bypass on type 2 diabetes mellitus. *Ann Surg* 2003;238(4):467–484; discussion 84–85
63. Sugerman HJ, Sugerman EL, DeMaria EJ, et al. Bariatric surgery for severely obese adolescents. *J Gastrointest Surg* 2003;7(1):102–107; discussion 107–108
64. Cummings DE, Overduin J, Foster-Schubert KE. Gastric bypass for obesity: mechanisms of weight loss and diabetes resolution. *J Clin Endocrinol Metab* 2004;89(6):2608–2615
65. DeMaria EJ, Sugerman HJ, Kellum JM, et al. Results of 281 consecutive total laparoscopic Roux-en-Y gastric bypasses to treat morbid obesity. *Ann Surg* 2002;235(5): 640–645; discussion 645–647
66. Wittgrove AC, Clark GW. Laparoscopic gastric bypass, Roux-en-Y-500 patients: technique and results, with 3–60 month follow-up. *Obes Surg* 2000;10(3):233–239
67. O'Brien PE, Dixon JB. Lap-band: outcomes and results. *J Laparoendosc Adv Surg Tech A* 2003;13(4):265–270
68. Mertens I, Van Gaal LF. Obesity, haemostasis and the fibrinolytic system. *Obes Rev* 2002;3(2):85–101
69. Clinical Guidelines on the Identification, Evaluation, and Treatment of Overweight and Obesity in Adults—the evidence report. National Institutes of Health. *Obes Res* 1998;6(Suppl 2):51S–209S
70. Eckel RH, Grundy SM, Zimmet PZ. The metabolic syndrome. *Lancet* 2005;365(9468):1415–1428
71. Podnos YD, Jimenez JC, Wilson SE, et al. Complications after laparoscopic gastric bypass: a review of 3464 cases. *Arch Surg* 2003;138(9):957–961
72. Schauer PR, Ikramuddin S, Gourash W, et al. Outcomes after laparoscopic Roux-en-Y gastric bypass for morbid obesity. *Ann Surg* 2000;232(4):515–529
73. Chan JC, Cheung JC, Stehouwer CD, et al. The central roles of obesity-associated dyslipidaemia, endothelial activation and cytokines in the Metabolic Syndrome—an analysis by structural equation modelling. *Int J Obes Relat Metab Disord* 2002;26(7):994–1008
74. Hotamisligil GS. The role of TNFalpha and TNF receptors in obesity and insulin resistance. *J Intern Med* 1999; 245(6):621–625
75. Visser M, Bouter LM, McQuillan GM, et al. Elevated C-reactive protein levels in overweight and obese adults. *JAMA* 1999;282(22):2131–2135
76. Ford ES. The metabolic syndrome and C-reactive protein, fibrinogen, and leukocyte count: findings from the Third National Health and Nutrition Examination Survey. *Atherosclerosis* 2003;168(2):351–358
77. Cottam DR, Mattar SG, Barinas-Mitchell E, et al. The chronic inflammatory hypothesis for the morbidity associated with morbid obesity: implications and effects of weight loss. *Obes Surg* 2004;14(5):589–600
78. O'Keeffe T, Patterson EJ. Evidence supporting routine polysomnography before bariatric surgery. *Obes Surg* 2004;14(1):23–26
79. Sugerman HJ, Baron PL, Fairman RP, et al. Hemodynamic dysfunction in obesity hypoventilation syndrome and the effects of treatment with surgically induced weight loss. *Ann Surg* 1988;207(5):604–613
80. Sugerman HJ, Fairman RP, Sood RK, et al. Long-term effects of gastric surgery for treating respiratory insufficiency of obesity. *Am J Clin Nutr* 1992; 55(2 Suppl): 597S–601S.
81. Ford ES. The epidemiology of obesity and asthma. *J Allergy Clin Immunol* 2005;115(5):897–909; quiz 910
82. Sugerman HJ, Brewer WH, Shiffman ML, et al. A multicenter, placebo-controlled, randomized, double-blind, prospective trial of prophylactic ursodiol for the prevention of gallstone formation following gastric-bypass-induced rapid weight loss. *Am J Surg* 1995;169(1):91–96; discussion 96–97

83. Dixon JB, Chapman L, O'Brien P. Marked improvement in asthma after Lap-Band surgery for morbid obesity. *Obes Surg* 1999; 9(4):385–389
84. Simard B, Turcotte H, Marceau P, et al. Asthma and sleep apnea in patients with morbid obesity: outcome after bariatric surgery. *Obes Surg* 2004;14(10):1381–1388
85. Frezza EE, Ikramuddin S, Gourash W, et al. Symptomatic improvement in gastroesophageal reflux disease (GERD) following laparoscopic Roux-en-Y gastric bypass. *Surg Endosc* 2002;16(7):1027–1031
86. Suter M, Dorta G, Giusti V, Calmes JM. Gastro-esophageal reflux and esophageal motility disorders in morbidly obese patients. *Obes Surg* 2004;14(7):959–966
87. Hong D, Khajanchee YS, Pereira N, et al. Manometric abnormalities and gastroesophageal reflux disease in the morbidly obese. *Obes Surg* 2004; 14(6):744–9
88. Schauer P, Hamad G, Ikramuddin S. Surgical management of gastroesophageal reflux disease in obese patients. *Semin Laparosc Surg* 2001;8(4):256–264
89. Youssef WI, McCullough AJ. Steatohepatitis in obese individuals. *Best Pract Res Clin Gastroenterol* 2002;16(5): 733–747
99. Neuschwander-Tetri BA, Caldwell SH. Nonalcoholic steatohepatitis: summary of an AASLD Single Topic Conference. *Hepatology* 2003;37(5):1202–1219
91. Marceau P, Kaufman D, Biron S, et al. Outcome of pregnancies after biliopancreatic diversion. *Obes Surg* 2004; 14(3):318–324
92. Dixon JB, Bhathal PS, Hughes NR, O'Brien PE. Nonalcoholic fatty liver disease: Improvement in liver histological analysis with weight loss. *Hepatology* 2004;39(6): 1647–1654
93. Sugerman HJ, Sugerman EL, Wolfe L, et al. Risks and benefits of gastric bypass in morbidly obese patients with severe venous stasis disease. *Ann Surg* 2001;234(1):41–46
94. Sapala JA, Wood MH, Schuhknecht MP, Sapala MA. Fatal pulmonary embolism after bariatric operations for morbid obesity: a 24-year retrospective analysis. *Obes Surg* 2003;13(6):819–825
95. Keeling WB, Haines K, Stone PA, et al. Current indications for preoperative inferior vena cava filter insertion in patients undergoing surgery for morbid obesity. *Obes Surg* 2005; 15(7):1009–12
96. Sugerman HJ, Felton WL, 3rd, Sismanis A, et al. Gastric surgery for pseudotumor cerebri associated with severe obesity. *Ann Surg* 1999;229(5):634–640; discussion 640–642
97. Kapoor DS, Davila GW, Rosenthal RJ, Ghoniem GM. Pelvic floor dysfunction in morbidly obese women: pilot study. *Obes Res* 2004;12(7):1104–1107
98. Bai SW, Kang JY, Rha KH, et al. Relationship of urodynamic parameters and obesity in women with stress urinary incontinence. *J Reprod Med* 2002;47(7):559–563
99. Santry HP, Gillen DL, Lauderdale DS. Trends in bariatric surgical procedures. *JAMA* 2005;294(15):1909–1917
100. Higa KD, Ho T, Boone KB. Laparoscopic Roux-en-Y gastric bypass: technique and 3-year follow-up. *J Laparoendosc Adv Surg Tech A* 2001;11(6):377–382
101. Biertho L, Steffen R, Ricklin T, et al. Laparoscopic gastric bypass versus laparoscopic adjustable gastric banding: a comparative study of 1,200 cases. *J Am Coll Surg* 2003;197(4):536–544; discussion 544–545
102. Fernandez AZ, Jr., DeMaria EJ, Tichansky DS, et al. Experience with over 3,000 open and laparoscopic bariatric procedures: multivariate analysis of factors related to leak and resultant mortality. *Surg Endosc* 2004;18(2):193–197
103. Papasavas PK, Hayetian FD, Caushaj PF, et al. Outcome analysis of laparoscopic Roux-en-Y gastric bypass for morbid obesity. The first 116 cases. *Surg Endosc* 2002; 16(12):1653–1657
104. Sapala JA, Wood MH, Sapala MA, Flake TM, Jr. Marginal ulcer after gastric bypass: a prospective 3-year study of 173 patients. *Obes Surg* 1998;8(5):505–516
105. Sugerman HJ, Kellum JM, Jr., Reines HD, et al. Greater risk of incisional hernia with morbidly obese than steroid-dependent patients and low recurrence with prefascial polypropylene mesh. *Am J Surg* 1996;171(1):80–84
106. Nguyen NT, Lee SL, Goldman C, et al. Comparison of pulmonary function and postoperative pain after laparoscopic versus open gastric bypass: a randomized trial. *J Am Coll Surg* 2001;192(4):469–476; discussion 476–477
107. Blachar A, Federle MP, Pealer KM, et al. Gastrointestinal complications of laparoscopic Roux-en-Y gastric bypass surgery: clinical and imaging findings. *Radiology* 2002;223(3):625–632
108. Nguyen NT, Stevens CM, Wolfe BM. Incidence and outcome of anastomotic stricture after laparoscopic gastric bypass. *J Gastrointest Surg* 2003;7(8):997–1003; discussion 1003
109. Brolin RE, Gorman JH, Gorman RC, et al. Are vitamin B12 and folate deficiency clinically important after roux-en-Y gastric bypass? *J Gastrointest Surg* 1998;2(5):436–442
110. Bloomberg RD, Fleishman A, Nalle JE, et al. Nutritional deficiencies following bariatric surgery: what have we learned? *Obes Surg* 2005;15(2):145–154
111. Sugerman HJ, Kellum JM, DeMaria EJ. Conversion of Proximal to Distal Gastric Bypass for Failed Gastric Bypass for Superobesity. *J Gastrointest Surg* 1997;1(6):517–525
112. DeMaria EJ, Schauer P, Patterson E, et al. The optimal surgical management of the super-obese patient: the debate. *Surg Innov* 2005;12(2):107–121
113. Mason EE. Starvation injury after gastric reduction for obesity. *World J Surg* 1998;22(9):1002–1007
114. Terlevich A, Hearing SD, Woltersdorf WW, et al. Refeeding syndrome: effective and safe treatment with Phosphates Polyfusor. *Aliment Pharmacol Ther* 2003;17(10): 1325–1329
115. Higa KD, Boone KB, Ho T. Complications of the laparoscopic Roux-en-Y gastric bypass: 1,040 patients—what have we learned? *Obes Surg* 2000;10(6):509–513
116. Farkas DT, Vemulapalli P, Haider A, et al. Laparoscopic Roux-en-Y gastric bypass is safe and effective in patients with a BMI > or = 60. *Obes Surg* 2005;15(4):486–493
117. Oliak D, Ballantyne GH, Davies RJ, et al. Short-term results of laparoscopic gastric bypass in patients with BMI > or = 60. *Obes Surg* 2002;12(5):643–647
118. Parikh MS, Shen R, Weiner M, et al. Laparoscopic bariatric surgery in super-obese patients (BMI>50) is safe and effective: a review of 332 patients. *Obes Surg* 2005; 15(6):858–863

119. Busetto L, Segato G, De Marchi F, et al. Postoperative management of laparoscopic gastric banding. *Obes Surg* 2003;13(1):121–127
120. O'Brien PE, Dixon JB. Weight loss and early and late complications—the international experience. *Am J Surg* 2002;184(6B):42S–45S
121. Ponce J, Paynter S, Fromm R. Laparoscopic adjustable gastric banding: 1,014 consecutive cases. *J Am Coll Surg* 2005;201(4):529–535
122. Ramsey-Stewart G. Vertical banded gastroplasty for morbid obesity: weight loss at short and long-term follow up. *ANZ J Surg* 1995;65(1):4–7
123. Scopinaro N, Marinari GM, Camerini GB, et al. Specific effects of biliopancreatic diversion on the major components of metabolic syndrome: a long-term follow-up study. *Diabetes Care* 2005;28(10):2406–2411
124. Shikora SA. "What are the yanks doing?" the U.S. experience with implantable gastric stimulation (IGS) for the treatment of obesity—update on the ongoing clinical trials. *Obes Surg* 2004;14(Suppl 1):S40–S48
125. Favretti F, De Luca M, Segato G, et al. Treatment of morbid obesity with the Transcend Implantable Gastric Stimulator (IGS): a prospective survey. *Obes Surg* 2004; 14(5):666–670
126. Shikora SA. Implantable Gastric Stimulation—the surgical procedure: combining safety with simplicity. *Obes Surg* 2004;14(Suppl 1):S9–S13
127. Doldi SB, Micheletto G, Perrini MN, Rapetti R. Intragastric balloon: another option for treatment of obesity and morbid obesity. *Hepatogastroenterology* 2004;51(55):294–297
128. Weiner R, Gutberlet H, Bockhorn H. Preparation of extremely obese patients for laparoscopic gastric banding by gastric-balloon therapy. *Obes Surg* 1999;9(3):261–264
129. Hodson RM, Zacharoulis D, Goutzamani E, et al. Management of obesity with the new intragastric balloon. *Obes Surg* 2001;11(3):327–329
130. Dixon JB, Dixon ME, O'Brien PE. Birth outcomes in obese women after laparoscopic adjustable gastric banding. *Obstet Gynecol* 2005;106(5):965–972
131. Wittgrove AC, Jester L, Wittgrove P, Clark GW. Pregnancy following gastric bypass for morbid obesity. *Obes Surg* 1998;8(4):461–464; discussion 465–466
132. Richards DS, Miller DK, Goodman GN. Pregnancy after gastric bypass for morbid obesity. *J Reprod Med* 1987; 32(3):172–176
133. Kimm SY, Barton BA, Obarzanek E, et al. Obesity development during adolescence in a biracial cohort: the NHLBI Growth and Health Study. *Pediatrics* 2002;110(5):e54
134. Hedley AA, Ogden CL, Johnson CL, et al. Prevalence of overweight and obesity among US children, adolescents, and adults, 1999–2002. *JAMA* 2004;291(23):2847–2850
135. Cook S, Weitzman M, Auinger P, et al. Prevalence of a metabolic syndrome phenotype in adolescents: findings from the third National Health and Nutrition Examination Survey, 1988–1994. *Arch Pediatr Adolesc Med* 2003; 157(8):821–827
136. Weiss R, Dziura J, Burgert TS, et al. Obesity and the metabolic syndrome in children and adolescents. *N Engl J Med* 2004;350(23):2362–2374
137. Strauss RS, Bradley LJ, Brolin RE. Gastric bypass surgery in adolescents with morbid obesity. *J Pediatr* 2001; 138(4):499–504
138. Falkner NH, Neumark-Sztainer D, Story M, et al. Social, educational, and psychological correlates of weight status in adolescents. *Obes Res* 2001;9(1):32–42
139. Schwimmer JB, Burwinkle TM, Varni JW. Health-related quality of life of severely obese children and adolescents. *JAMA* 2003;289(14):1813–1819
140. Stanford A, Glascock JM, Eid GM, et al. Laparoscopic Roux-en-Y gastric bypass in morbidly obese adolescents. *J Pediatr Surg* 2003;38(3):430–433
141. Dolan K, Creighton L, Hopkins G, Fielding G. Laparoscopic gastric banding in morbidly obese adolescents. *Obes Surg* 2003;13(1):101–104
142. Inge TH, Zeller M, Garcia VF, Daniels SR. Surgical approach to adolescent obesity. *Adolesc Med Clin* 2004; 15(3):429–453
143. Livingston EH, Huerta S, Arthur D, et al. Male gender is a predictor of morbidity and age a predictor of mortality for patients undergoing gastric bypass surgery. *Ann Surg* 2002;236(5):576–582
144. St Peter SD, Craft RO, Tiede JL, Swain JM. Impact of advanced age on weight loss and health benefits after laparoscopic gastric bypass. *Arch Surg* 2005;140(2):165–168
145. Papasavas PK, Gagne DJ, Kelly J, Caushaj PF. Laparoscopic Roux-En-Y gastric bypass is a safe and effective operation for the treatment of morbid obesity in patients older than 55 years. *Obes Surg* 2004;14(8):1056–1061
146. Sugerman HJ, DeMaria EJ, Kellum JM, et al. Effects of bariatric surgery in older patients. *Ann Surg* 2004; 240(2):243–247
147. Abu-Abeid S, Keidar A, Szold A. Resolution of chronic medical conditions after laparoscopic adjustable silicone gastric banding for the treatment of morbid obesity in the elderly. *Surg Endosc* 2001;15(2):132–134
148. Weiss HG, Nehoda H, Labeck B, et al. Pregnancies after adjustable gastric banding. *Obes Surg* 2001;11(3):303–306
149. Cossu ML, Fais E, Meloni GB, et al. Impact of age on long-term complications after biliopancreatic diversion. *Obes Surg* 2004;14(9):1182–1186
150. Nguyen NT, Ho HS, Palmer LS, Wolfe BM. A comparison study of laparoscopic versus open gastric bypass for morbid obesity. *J Am Coll Surg* 2000;191(2):149–155; discussion 155–157
151. Dixon JB, O'Brien PE. Selecting the optimal patient for LAP-BAND placement. *Am J Surg* 2002;184(6B):17S–20S
152. Dolan K, Hatzifotis M, Newbury L, Fielding G. A comparison of laparoscopic adjustable gastric banding and biliopancreatic diversion in superobesity. *Obes Surg* 2004;14(2):165–169
153. Kormanova K, Fried M, Hainer V, Kunesova M. Is laparoscopic adjustable gastric banding a day surgery procedure? *Obes Surg* 2004;14(9):1237–1240
154. Watkins BM, Montgomery KF, Ahroni JH. Laparoscopic adjustable gastric banding: early experience in 400 consecutive patients in the USA. *Obes Surg* 2005; 15(1):82–87

53

Laparoscopic Staging and Bypass

Kevin C. P. Conlon ■ *Angela T. Riga*

The use of minimally invasive surgical techniques for staging and palliative bypass is increasing in surgical practice for patients with intra-abdominal cancer. Experience over the last decade has suggested that not only is minimally invasive surgery (MIS) safe in the cancer patient but also that many of the advantages observed for patients with benign conditions such as gastroesophageal reflux and biliary tract disease also can be achieved for the cancer patient. As experience accumulates, an increasing number of patients are undergoing minimally invasive procedures with curative or palliative intent. This chapter will focus on the role of MIS staging and palliative surgery for patients with intra-abdominal malignancy.

■ RATIONALE FOR MIS STAGING

As the multidisciplinary management of gastrointestinal cancer has evolved over the last decade, an accurate extent of disease work-up has become essential to treatment planning. Staging procedures should accurately define the extent of disease, direct appropriate therapy, facilitate the use of adjuvant therapies, and avoid unnecessary interventions in a safe and cost-efficient fashion.

Recent advances in radiology have provided many noninvasive tools, such as multidetector computed tomographic (CT) scanning, magnetic resonance imaging (MRI), and positron-emission tomographic (PET) scanning, that have had a considerable impact on the extent of disease work-up. Unfortunately, these modalities often underestimate the extent of disease, with small-volume metastatic disease being appreciated only at open surgical exploration. For over 100 years, laparoscopy has been suggested as a means for identifying such small-volume disease. Recently, a significant amount of data has been produced to suggest that the use of laparoscopy and laparoscopic ultrasound in the staging of gastrointestinal malignancies has an impact on overall management.[1–4] The aim of laparoscopic staging is to mimic staging at open exploration while minimizing morbidity, enhancing recovery, and thus allowing for quicker administration of adjuvant therapies if indicated. Proponents believe that laparoscopic staging should be viewed as complementary and not as a replacement for other staging modalities such as CT scanning, MRI, or PET scanning. In simplistic terms, the advantages of laparoscopy are that it allows the surgeon to visualize the primary tumor, determine vascular involvement, identify regional nodal metastases, detect small-volume peritoneal/liver metastases, and obtain tissue for histologic diagnosis.

■ SURGICAL TECHNIQUE FOR LAPAROSCOPIC STAGING

The procedure usually is performed under general anesthesia with the patient positioned supine on the operating table. A warming blanket is placed underneath the patient, who is secured appropriately to the table with padding over the pressure points.

The following operative equipment is considered necessary for laparoscopic staging:

1. A 30-degree angled laparoscope either 10 or 5 mm in diameter
2. 5-mm laparoscopic instruments, including a Maryland dissector, a blunt-tip dissecting forceps, a cup/biopsy forceps, atraumatic grasping forceps, a liver retractor, and scissors
3. A 5- or 10-mm suction/irrigation device
4. A laparoscopic ultrasound probe (optional)

In general, we prefer a multiport technique for staging. Access is gained into the peritoneal cavity using a blunt port placed subumbilically by direct cutdown. By using forceps to grasp the fascial layers, retractors can be avoided and the wound size minimized. An alternative approach, particularly in patients with previous midline incisions, is to place the initial port in either the right or the left upper quadrant of the abdomen. Many surgeons prefer to use a Veress needle to achieve pneumoperitoneum prior to placing the surgical ports. In this case, care should be exercised to avoid visceral or vascular injury.

Pneumoperitoneum is achieved with CO_2 gas. Insufflation commences at a low flow rate until peritoneal entry is confirmed. An intraperitoneal pressure of 10–12 mmHg is considered optimal. However, in patients with cardiopulmonary compromise, a lower maximum pressure may be chosen. An 5- to 10-mm 30-degree angled telescope is preferred, and systematic examination of the peritoneal cavity is performed. Additional trocars then are inserted under direct vision. Placement depends on the site of the primary tumor (i.e., colonic, gastric, pancreatic, etc.) and the findings at initial inspection (i.e., whether obvious metastatic disease is present). In general, ports are placed along the planned open incision line (Fig 53–1).

Following port placement, a detailed examination of the peritoneal cavity is performed in a similar fashion to an open exploration. The primary tumor is assessed. Any extension into contiguous organs can be identified. Following an initial survey, a systematic examination of the intra-abdominal viscera is performed commencing with the liver. To facilitate hepatic examination, the patient is placed in a 20-degree reverse Trendelenberg position with 10 degrees of left lateral tilt. The anterior and posterior surfaces of the left lateral segment of the liver are examined, followed by examination of the anterior and inferior surfaces of the right lobe. Despite the absence of tactile sensation, indirect palpation of the liver surface can be achieved by using two instruments (Fig 53–2). A blunt suction device is particularly useful in compressing the liver tissue in order to detect small metastases. Improved visualization of diaphragmatic and posterior surfaces may be achieved by placing the camera in the right upper quadrant port. The

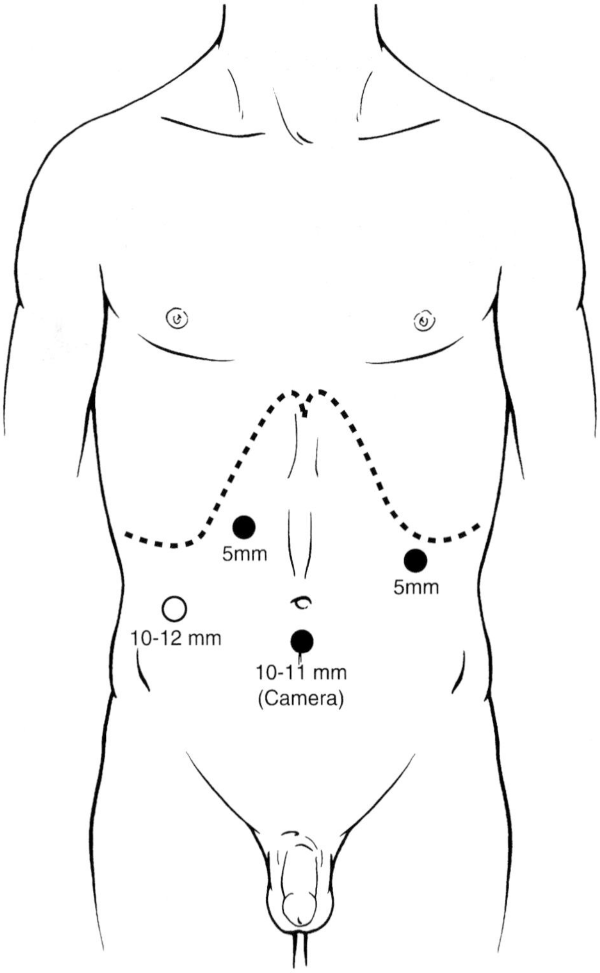

Figure 53–1. Port placement.

hilus of the liver, hepatoduodenal ligament, and foramen of Winslow then are examined. Any abnormal lymphadenopathy can be identified and biopsied using the cup forceps. In general, the duodenum is not mobilized. However, for patients with pancreatic or common bile duct tumors, close attention is paid to the presence or absence of tumor infiltration in the angle between the duodenum and the lateral aspect of the common bile duct because this may indicate significant vascular involvement.

The patient then is repositioned into a 10-degree Trendelenberg position without lateral tilt to facilitate examination of the transverse mesocolon and retroperitoneum. The omentum is retracted toward the left upper quadrant, elevating and enabling inspection of the transverse mesocolon and the ligament of Treitz. The mesocolon is inspected carefully with particular attention to the middle colic vein, which usually is visible. Any abnormal adenopathy around the middle colic vein is noted and may be biopsied. For patients with an upper gastrointestinal primary tumor, the lesser sac is

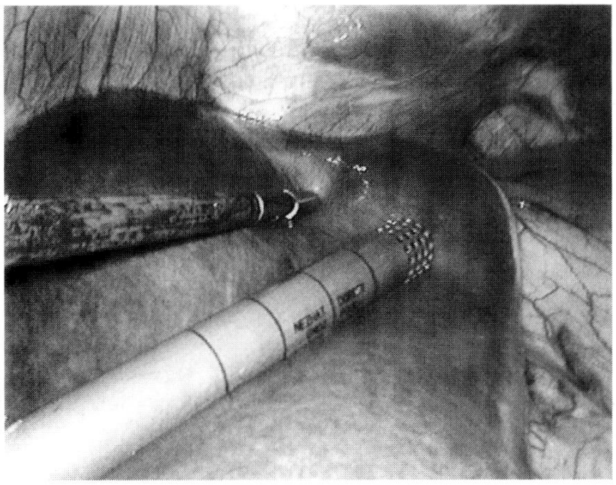

Figure 53–2. Examination of the liver.

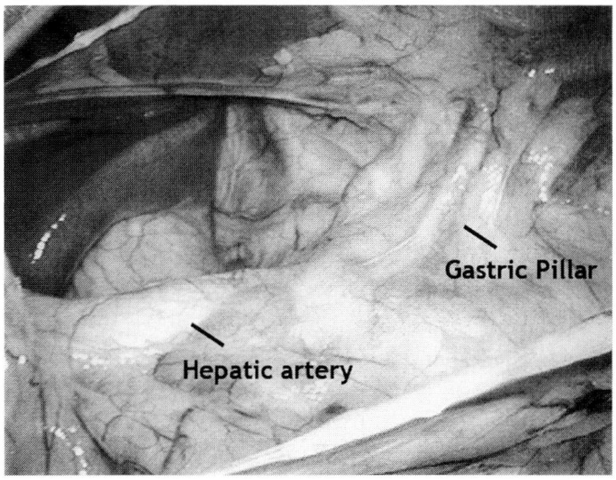

Figure 53–4. Laparoscopic exposure of the gastric pillar.

examined. To facilitate this maneuver, the patient then is returned to a supine position, the left lobe of the liver is elevated, and the gastrohepatic omentum is incised (Fig 53–3). This exposes the caudate lobe of the liver, the inferior vena cava, and the celiac axis. If present, an aberrant left hepatic artery should be identified and preserved. Often, adhesions between the stomach and the pancreas require division to allow entry into the lesser sac. By elevating the stomach, the "gastric pillar" can be clearly identified (Fig 53–4). The pillar contains the left gastric artery and vein. This structure followed down leads us to the celiac axis, and any suspicious nodal tissue can be biopsied. The hepatic artery also is identified and followed to the hepatoduodenal ligament. The anterior aspect of pancreas, hepatic artery, and left gastric artery are also seen. Any suspicious periportal, hepatic, or celiac nodes can be removed readily with the cup forceps.

For gastric and pancreatic cancers, peritoneal lavage cytology is performed. In general, the specimens are taken at the start of the laparoscopy to avoid potential contamination from tumor manipulation or dissection. Between 200 and 400 mL of normal saline is instilled into the peritoneal cavity. The abdomen is agitated gently before aspiration. In pancreatic cases, samples are taken from the right and left upper quadrants. An additional sample is taken from the pelvis in patients with gastric cancer because this has been shown to increase the diagnostic yield.

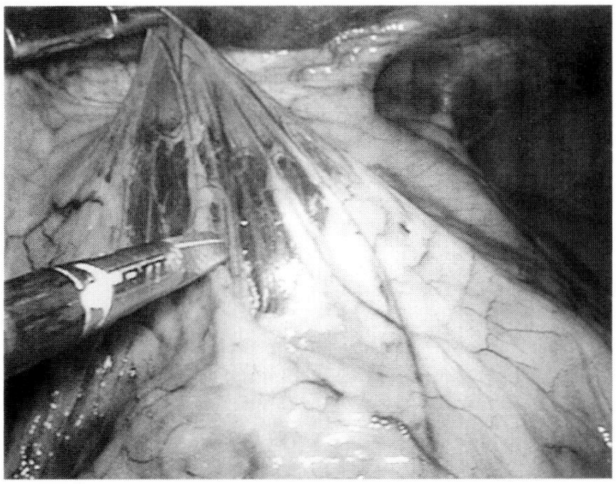

Figure 53–3. Exposure of the lesser sac.

If available, laparoscopic ultrasound (LUS) can be performed at this stage. Laparoscopy by its nature is a two-dimensional modality, with the result that appreciation of deep or subsurface lesions in solid organs is often suboptimal. LUS can partially overcome this deficiency. Transducers in clinical use employ either curved or linear-array technology and have a high-frequency performance with a range in the region of 6–10 MHz, allowing for high-resolution images to be obtained that can detect lesions from 0.2 cm in size. In addition, Doppler flow capability, if present, allows for accurate vessel identification and facilitates assessment of the tumor-vessel interface. The LUS probe is inserted via a 10- to 12-mm port, usually in the right upper quadrant.

The LUS is an invaluable tool for examination of the liver. Initially, the transducer is placed over the left lateral segment, allowing assessment of segments I, II, and III. It is important that the probe is placed in direct contact with the liver surface to maximize acoustic coupling. Examination of the right lobe commences with the probe on the dome of the liver. The vena cava is visualized at the back and as the probe is moved forward slowly to identify the hepatic and portal veins. Within the liver, these can be identified by virtue of their surrounding fibrous sheath. The remaining hepatic segments (IV, V, VI, VII, and VIII) are examined by rotating the probe over the rest of the liver. Suspicious lesions can be biopsied either by fine-needle aspiration (FNA) or by percutaneously inserted core biopsy needles under LUS guidance. With the probe over segment V, the gallbladder is assessed, and with transverse

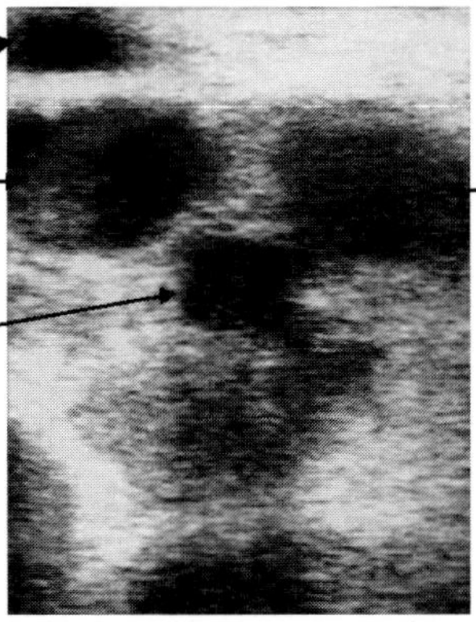

Figure 53–5. Laparoscopic ultrasound of hepatoduodenal ligament.

placement of the probe over the hepatoduodenal ligament, the common hepatic duct, common bile duct, and hepatic arteries along with the portal vein can be identified (Fig 53–5). The portal vein can be followed to its confluence with the splenic and superior mesenteric vein. The superior mesenteric artery also can be seen and its relationship to a pancreatic tumor, if present, determined. The pancreas can be examined, and any lesion can be identified.

LUS also has been used in gastric cancer staging. To facilitate examination, the stomach is distended by inserting 500 mL of warm saline via an orogastric tube. The LUS probe then is brought slowly over the serosal surface. Excellent images of the gastric wall can be obtained. However, technical constraints such as near-field loss limit the sensitivity particularly for deep T2 lesions.

▪ ESOPHAGEAL CARCINOMA

Esophageal cancer accounts for less than 5% of all gastrointestinal cancers. In 2004, approximately 14,250 patients were diagnosed with esophageal carcinoma in the United States.[5] Unfortunately, the prognosis remains poor, with an overall survival rate of approximately 5–10%. Currently in clinical practice, the histologic presentation appears to be changing. Previously, the majority of tumors were of the squamous cell type and found predominantly in the middle to upper esophagus. At present, adenocarcinoma of the gastroesophageal junction or lower esophagus is more common and appears to be increasing in incidence. Surgical resection remains the treatment of choice for all histologic subtypes, but owing to its high morbidity and mortality, resection should be reserved for patients without disseminated disease. In addition, in the last few years, there has been a significant progress in palliative nonsurgical reatment options. Therefore, accurate staging for esophageal cancer is of paramount importance.[4,6–8,10]

Common diagnostic modalities are listed in Table 53–1. These have been discussed in detail elsewhere in this book. Endoscopy remains the diagnostic gold standard. Biopsies can be obtained and an assessment of local disease extent made. In patients considered unsuitable for surgical resection, a number of palliative options such as endoscopic dilation, laser ablation, or placement of luminal stents exist.

CT scanning of the thorax and abdomen is the radiologic staging modality of choice. The primary tumor can be visualized and metastatic disease detected. However, while data suggest that current-generation high-resolution helical CT scanning is of significant value, its capacity to accurately T stage the disease and predict lymphatic and peritoneal spread remains about 60%, 60%, and 80%, respectively.[10,11] Endoscopic ultrasonography (EUS) enables detailed imaging of the esophageal wall, local lymph nodes, and contigious structures, making it the ideal tool for TNM staging.[6,7,12] The shape, pattern, and demarcated borders of nodes are examined to assess metastatic potential.[13,14] EUS appears superior to CT scanning for locoregional staging.[8,15] Harewood and Wiersema from the Mayo Clinic compared the cost of EUS FNA with CT FNA and a surgical approach in staging patients with nonmetastatic esophageal cancer. They suggested that by avoiding unnecessary surgery, primarily by detecting celiac node involvement, EUS FNA was the least costly strategy.[16] Recent work has suggested that fluorine-18-flurodeoxyglucose (FDG) PET scanning has a role for the detection of metastatic disease and for restaging after neoadjuvant therapy or evaluation of recurrence. In a prospective study by Flammen and colleagues, of 74 patients, FDG PET scanning had a significantly higher rate of detection of stage IV disease compared with the combination of CT scanning and EUS. It upstaged disease in 15% and downstaged disease in 7% of patients.[17] Other studies have reported similar results.[18–20]

Despite this increasingly sophisticated diagnostic armamentarium, up to 20% of patients will continue to have radiologically occult peritoneal, nodal, or liver

TABLE 53–1. DIAGNOSTIC MODALITIES FOR STAGING ESOPHAGEAL CARCINOMA

Clinical examination
Chest x-ray
Barium swallow
Endoscopy with biopsies
Endoscopic ultrasound (EUS)
Contrast-enhanced computed tomography (CT) of chest/abdomen/pelvis
MRI
Positron emission tomography (FDG-PET)
Laparoscopy
Laparoscopic ultrasound

metastases detected at surgical exploration. Laparoscopy has been suggested as a means to detect such disease and thus exclude this cohort of patients from potentially ineffective treatment regimens.

The yield of laparoscopic staging appears to be determined at least in part by the site of disease and histologic cell type. In an earlier review of 369 patients with carcinoma of the distal esophagus or gastric antrum, Dagnini and colleagues demonstrated occult disease in 33% at laparoscopy in patients with adenocarcinoma of either the distal esophagus or gastric cardia.[21] However, laparoscopic staging had a minimal impact for patients with squamous cell cancers in the upper third of the esophagus, changing management in only 3.5% of cases. Stein and colleagues reported similar results. At laparoscopy following radiologic staging, they found that 25% of patients with locally advanced (T3/T4) adenocarcinoma of the distal esophagus or gastric cardia had peritoneal or liver metastases.[22] Thus, for patients with squamous cell carcinoma of the esophagus, we believe that laparoscopic staging is not indicated in the absence of suspicious intra-abdominal imaging findings.

Stell and colleagues reported that laparoscopy had a superior accuracy in determining intra-abdominal disease compared with ultrasound or CT scanning (65% versus 34% or 45%, respectively).[23] Watt and colleagues compared the accuracy of laparoscopy, ultrasound, and CT scanning in detecting intra-abdominal metastases in patients with esophageal cancer and adenocarcinoma of the cardia.[24] Laparoscopy was significantly more accurate than the imaging studies, with 88% sensitivity, 100% specificity, and 96% accuracy. Ultrasound and CT scanning failed to detect peritoneal metastases, whereas laparoscopy correctly identified metastases in eight of nine patients before surgery. The added value of laparoscopic ultrasonography (LUS) to standard laparoscopy has been examined by a number of authors. Wakelin and colleagues compared the role of CT scanning, laparoscopy with laparoscopic ultrasound (LUS), and endoscopic ultrasound (EUS) in preoperative staging.[25] Locally advanced tumors (T3/T4) were identified accurately by CT scanning in 94% and by EUS in 88% of the cases. LUS was unable to identify tumors above the diaphragm, but in the locally advanced cases where the tumor could be seen, the accuracy was 83%. EUS was the best modality for assessing early tumors and locoregional nodal involvement. In addition, LUS was noted to have a greater accuracy and specificity (81% and 100%) for the detection of intra-abdominal metastases versus CT scanning (72% and 90%).[25] Whether LUS adds value to standard laparoscopic staging remains unclear. Smith and colleagues demonstrated that 18% of patients with presumed resectable disease were spared an unnecessary operation owing to laparoscopy.[26] LUS findings resulted in a further 8% avoiding open exploration. The main benefit appears to be in the assessment of nodal disease, particularly in the celiac axis, hepatoduodenal ligament, and para-aortic area. Disease in these sites accounts for more than 40% of the positive findings at laparoscopy.[27] Bonavina and colleagues also demonstrated that laparoscopy had a higher sensitivity (78%) in detecting nodal disease compared with ultrasound (11%) and CT scanning (55%).[28] Others have reported similar findings.[29–33] The yield for detecting lymphatic metastases may be increased by combining thoracoscopic and laparoscopic staging. By using such a strategy, Krasna and colleagues reported a 94% diagnostic accuracy for detecting lymph node disease.

▪ GASTRIC CANCER

Despite its apparent falling prevalence in the Western world, gastric cancer remains a significant public health problem and one of the leading causes of cancer death worldwide. The prognosis remains poor, with 50% of patients dying of the disease within 2 years of diagnosis, even in those who have undergone a potentially "curative" resection.[35,36] The poor outcome may be related in part to late presentation and inadequate staging and subsequent selection for surgery. Historically, following diagnosis and if medically fit, patients were subjected to open exploration for either resection or palliation. Pye and colleagues reviewed the operative outcome for 916 patients with carcinoma of the esophagus or stomach treated in Wales between 1995 and 1996.[37] The authors reported that 23% of the operations were exploratory alone in nature. However, with the recent development of multidisciplinary approaches to the disease, improved staging, and the establishment of less invasive palliative algorithms, the need for operative intervention has been questioned.[38]

Accurate staging is essential for patient selection. A sophisticated and complex diagnostic armamentarium exists (Table 53–2). While upper gastrointestinal endoscopy and biopsy remain the primary diagnostic tools, with multislice contrast-enhanced CT scanning, endoscopic ultrasonography (EUS), MRI, and PET scanning being used increasingly for preoperative staging, laparoscopy and laparoscopic ultrasound have an important role in the staging algorithm for gastric cancer (Fig 53–6). Proponents of laparoscopic staging suggest that laparoscopy can play a pivotal role, on the one hand, identifying patients who may benefit from surgical resection and, on the other, identifying the group of patients with disseminated or locally advanced intra-abdominal disease for whom extensive surgery would not be worthwhile.

TABLE 53–2. DIAGNOSTIC ARMAMENTARIUM FOR ASSESSING GASTRIC CANCER

Endoscopy with biopsies
Endoscopic ultrasound (EUS)
Computed tomography
Magnetic resonance imaging
Positron emission tomography
Laparoscopy
Laparoscopic ultrasound
Laparoscopic sentine node assessment

While level I evidence does not exist for the use of laparoscopic staging in gastric cancer, a number of large single-institution studies have been carried out that allow us to make a number of conclusions regarding its role in the staging algorithm. As in esophageal cancer, laparoscopy will detect radiologically occult metastatic disease in a significant number of patients. Gross and colleagues reported that laparoscopy identified metastatic disease in 57% of patients whose preoperative imaging had shown no metastases.[39] Possik reviewed 360 patients who underwent staging laparoscopy. The accuracy for detection of peritoneal and hepatic metastases was 89% and 96%, respectively.[40] Stell and colleagues carried out a prospective study comparing laparoscopy, ultrasound, and CT scanning. Laparoscopy had 99% accuracy in detecting hepatic metastases compared with 76% and 79% for CT scanning and ultrasound, respectively. The sensitivity of laparoscopy was 96% versus 37% and 53% for ultrasound and CT scanning. Laparoscopy also was superior in diagnosing peritoneal disease with an accuracy of 94% compared with 84% for ultrasound and 81% for CT scanning.[23] D'Ugo and colleagues similarly compared prospectively staging laparoscopy with CT scanning and ultrasound in a group of 100 patients with gastric cancer. Unsuspected metastatic disease was found in 21 cases. Overall TNM staging accuracy for laparoscopy was 72% compared with 38% for ultrasound and CT scanning.[41] Similar results were reported from Burke and colleagues, who demonstrated biopsy-proven metastatic disease in 37% of 110 patients considered to have localized disease by prelaparoscopic staging.[38] Lehnert and colleagues looked at 120 consecutive patients with gastric cancer.[42] In contrast with the previous studies, which suggested that laparoscopic staging should be performed in all patients with gastric cancer, these authors suggested that a more selective approach may be appropriate. Laparoscopy was preformed on only 15 patients owing to inconclusive preoperative staging. In 6 of these patients, unsuspected liver or peritoneal metastases were identified. However, at a subsequent laparotomy, 4 of the 15 were found to have small intraperitoneal deposits not identified at laparoscopy, suggesting to the authors that laparoscopy should be

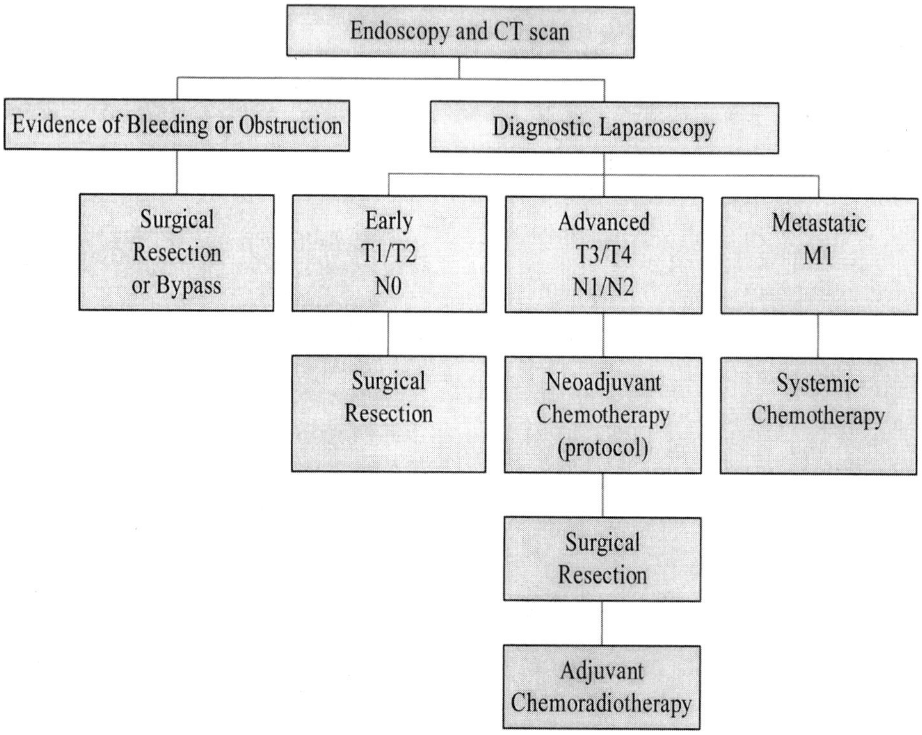

Figure 53–6. Staging algorithm for gastric cancer.

reserved for patients with an increased risk of local irresectablity or intra-abdominal metastases.

While the literature would suggest that despite currently available imaging modalities, laparoscopic staging will continue to detect small-volume metastatic disease in 20–30% of cases (Fig 53–7), the identification of occult nodal disease remains problematic. CT scanning accuracy in determining nodal disease varies in the literature from 25–70%. EUS appears somewhat better. Wakelin and colleagues have reported an overall accuracy of EUS in nodal staging for proximal or orogastric junction tumors of 72%.[25] If tumors that are nontraversable by endoscope are excluded, its accuracy increases by approximately 10%. Reported accuracy rates for laparoscopy and LUS vary from 60–90%. With LUS, direct biopsy of suspicious nodes can be obtained, which improves the utility of the modality. In distal gastric cancer, Finch and colleagues demonstrated an accuracy of 82% in T staging with the use of LUS.[43] This compares favourably with other studies looking at the use of EUS (83%) or CT scanning (66%) for T staging distal tumors.[23] In addition, the authors noted an accuracy rate of 89% for LUS in assessing lymph node status. In contrast, Wakelin noted that 38% of nodes were understaged. It would appear, therefore, that as with other ultrasound data, results are operator-dependent and reflect a willingness or not to aggressively biopsy suspicious nodes.

In this chapter we have concentrated on the role of laparoscopic staging in determining unresectability. However, the advent of minimally invasive techniques applied to early gastric cancer has raised the possibility that laparoscopic staging may have an increasing role in staging that spectrum of the disease. It has been argued that gastric cancer is one of the most suitable targets for MIS based on sentinel node status. Staging laparoscopy combined with sentinel node mapping may become a very important adjunct to laparoscopic local resection for curative treatment of sentinel-node-negative early gastric cancer.[44] More work is required before the true utility of this approach is understood.

As mentioned earlier, we routinely take peritoneal washings for cytologic examination at the time of laparoscopic staging. However, the added value of obtaining peritoneal cytology remains controversial. Recently, Sotiropoulos and colleagues reviewed the impact of laparoscopic staging following an intensive preoperative assessment that included ultrasound and helical CT scanning.[45] In 45 patients with potentially resectable disease, laparoscopy resulted in upstaging of 23 patients (51%). Laparotomy was avoided in 14 patients. Peritoneal cytology taken at the time of laparoscopy did not yield additional information. Similar results were noted by Wilkiemeyer and colleagues, who found that laparoscopic

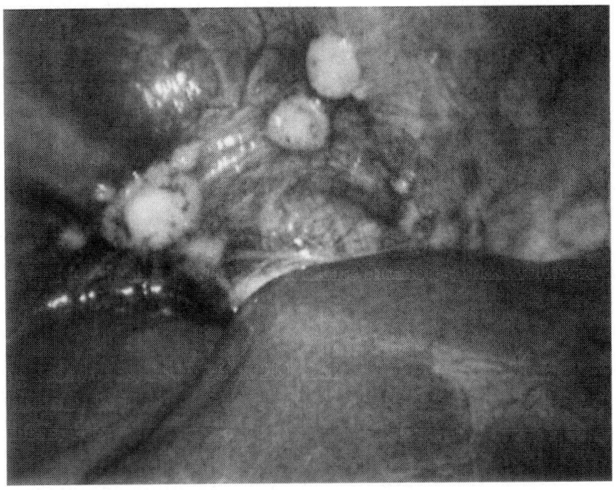

Figure 53–7. Peritoneal disease gastric cancer.

examination upstaged 53% of patients with esophagogastric cancer.[46] However, peritoneal cytology failed to identify 45% of the patients with positive laparoscopic findings and did not add any additional stage IV patients to the laparoscopy-negative group. These authors concluded that peritoneal cytology adds little to laparoscopic staging. However, while the added value of cytologic analysis may be limited in determining metastatic disease at the time of initial laparoscopy, an interesting paper from Bentrem and colleagues from Memorial Sloan-Kettering Cancer Center in New York suggests that the finding of positive peritoneal cytology at laparoscopic staging identifies a patient population at very high risk for early disease recurrence following potentially curative resection for gastric cancer.[47]

PRIMARY AND SECONDARY LIVER CANCER

At present, surgical resection is the most effective therapy for primary and metastatic disease of the liver. While there are no definitive criteria that define what constitutes resectable disease in part owing to differing therapeutic philosophies and surgical experience, most surgeons would consider extrahepatic disease, extensive bilobar disease, or the presence of extensive cirrhosis as the major factors that would preclude a potentially curative resection.

As with the other gastrointestinal malignancies, imaging modalities such as CT scanning, MRI, and PET scanning are available for preoperative staging. Despite the use of these modalities, a significant number of patients continue to have exploration without resection.[48–50] Laparoscopy therefore can serve to improve curative resection rates and decrease unnecessary laparotomy with its associated morbidity and quality-of-life issues.

Over the last decade, a number of centers have used laparoscopic staging, with reports of the detection of subradiologic disease varying from 10–60%.[51,52] The variability in part relates to the completeness and quality of preoperative imaging. Jarnagin and colleagues from Memorial Sloan-Kettering Cancer Center reviewed their experience with 186 patients who had either primary and secondary hepatic malignancies who underwent surgery at their institution.[49] Laparoscopy was attempted in 104 patients and completed successfully in 85%. Overall, 26 (25%) of these patients were noted to have unresectable disease at the time of laparoscopic staging, and although 9 patients had subsequent laparotomy for palliation, 17 patients were spared a laparotomy. More extensive hepatic disease, peritoneal disease, and extensive cirrhosis were the main laparoscopic findings that precluded resection. Difficulties were encountered determining the true extent of tumor vascular invasion or extensive biliary involvement. In addition, findings at laparoscopy had an impact on the type of resection performed in a further 10%. The authors also compared the patients undergoing laparoscopic staging with a similar nonrandomized cohort of 82 patients who did not receive laparoscopic staging but went directly to operation during the same time period. At open laparotomy, 28 (34%) of this group were noted to have unresectable disease. Although 9 patients had a palliative procedure, 19 patients had only an exploratory procedure, which the authors suggested potentially could have been avoided with laparoscopy. Comparing the two groups, laparoscopic staging was associated with increased resectability rates (83% versus 63%), shorter hospital stay (8.6 versus 11.9 days), and reduced hospital charges. A subsequent study from the same institution analyzed experience with 401 patients.[53] Prior surgery did not preclude staging because a complete laparoscopic examination was performed in 291 (73%) cases. Despite a false-negative rate of 22%, laparoscopic staging improved the overall resectability rate from 62–78%.

In an attempt to define the patients who would benefit from laparoscopic staging, the same group created a clinical risk score (CRS) based on five factors related to the primary tumor and the hepatic disease[54,55] (Table 53–3). Each criterion was assigned one point. Thus 42% of patients with a CRS score of greater than 2 had unresectable disease detected at laparoscopy versus 0% of patients with CRS scores of 0–1. Therefore, targeting laparoscopy to high-risk patients should avoid unnecessary laparoscopic staging in low-risk patients, whereas performing it in the high-risk group should prevent needless staging laparotomies and overall improve the yield from laparoscopy.

TABLE 53–3. CLINICAL RISK SCORE FOR THE DETERMINATION OF RESECTABILITY IN HEPATIC COLORECTAL DISEASE

Lymph node–positive tumor
Disease-free interval between primary colonic surgery and detection of metastatic disease less than 12 months
Number of hepatic tumors greater than one (based on preoperative imaging)
CEA greater than 200 ng/mL within 1 month of surgery
Size of the largest hepatic tumor greater than 5 cm

The history of a prior colectomy does not preclude accurate laparoscopic staging. Rahusen and colleagues performed laparoscopy in 50 patients with colorectal metastases, laparoscopy completing the examination in 94% and demonstrating unresectable disease in 38%.[56] In a more recent study reported by de Castro and colleagues,[57] staging laparoscopy was performed in 33 patients with primary tumors and 51 with colorectal liver metastases. Occult disease was noted at laparoscopy in 39% of patients in the primary group and in 12% of the patients with metastatic disease. However, the authors noted that laparoscopic staging had understaged 18% of patients in the metastatic group who were found at subsequent laparotomy to have unresectable disease. They suggested that in this group, the adhesions from the prior colon surgery may have led to a more limited staging procedure. Koea and colleagues also noted in 5 of 59 patients who had colorectal metastases to the liver that adhesions prevented laparoscopic staging.[58]

Recently, Thaler and colleagues suggested that the addition of intraoperative ultrasonography (IUS) improved the yield of laparoscopic staging. In a review of 136 patients, laparoscopic staging/IUS changed the treatment plan in 48% of patients. Surgically untreatable disease was noted in 25% owing to peritoneal metastases, nodal involvement, or diffuse hepatic disease.[59] Others have noted the added value of LUS. Foroutani and colleagues reported a greater sensitivity of LUS compared with triphasic CT scanning in detecting liver tumors.[60] LUS detected all liver tumors seen on CT scanning and in addition detected a further 10%. LUS appeared to be superior in imaging lesions less than 2 cm in diameter.[60] In a subsequent publication from the same group, the authors reported their experience with LUS and biopsy in 310 patients with 1080 primary and metastatic liver lesions.[61] Using a linear side-viewing transducer, core needle biopsies were taken using a 18-gauge spring-loaded biopsy gun. Histologic confirmation was obtained in all patients, with no bleeding complications or visceral injuries. Callery and colleagues demonstrated that the addition of LUS identified unresectable disease in 11 of 50 patients in whom standard laparoscopy was considered normal.[52] Hartley and colleagues reported that LUS was equivalent to MRI in determining resectability, particularly for primary hepatic tumors.[62] However, they and others also have noted that determining the extent of vascular and biliary involvement was problematic.[60] Rahusan and colleagues also examined the role of LUS in assessing patients with potentially resectable colorectal metastases.[56] Following standard laparoscopic assessment, 13% of patients were found to have disease that precluded resection. By adding LUS, the number increased to 25%. Overall, they found that the addition of LUS translated to an increase in resection rates from 46–71%, avoiding unnecessary laparotomy in 36%. Metcalfe and colleagues also examined a similar cohort of patients and demonstrated that laparoscopic staging in selected patients detects most unresectable disease.[63] For primary hepatocellular disease, the results appear similar.[64,65] Lo and colleagues performed staging laparoscopy with LUS in 91 patients with primary hepatocellular carcinoma (HCC), identifying unresectable disease in 16%, two-thirds of whom avoided any further surgical intervention and commenced nonoperative treatment earlier.[50]

The role of laparoscopic staging in the evaluation of noncolorectal nonneuroendocrine tumors was studied by D'Angelica and colleagues from Memorial Sloan-Kettering Cancer Center.[66] Following preoperative staging, 30 patients considered to have resectable disease underwent laparoscopy. Staging was completed in 80% and correctly identified 6 patients of the 9 finally found to have unresectable disease.

▪ PANCREATIC CANCER

Adenocarcinoma of the pancreas remains a lethal disease.[67] Despite increased awareness and improved diagnostic modalities, most patients continue to present with advanced disease at the time of diagnosis. Actual 5-year survival is between 2% and 3%, with surgical resection offering the only chance of cure. However, resection is only appropriate for a minority of patients. For the majority, the need for surgical intervention is controversial. In common with esophagogastric cancers, the notion that all patients require an operative procedure for accurate staging or palliation no longer is true. Our increased understanding of the natural history of the disease, coupled with the improvements in nonoperative palliative techniques, suggests that effective palliation does not require an open surgical procedure. Proponents of laparoscopic staging argue that the combination of dynamic contrast-enhanced CT scanning and/or MRI with laparoscopy remains the most effective means of staging, preventing needless open surgery for those who would not benefit, while not precluding resection for those who would benefit. Avoidance of unnecessary open procedures potentially will result in reduced perioperative morbidity and mortality, decreased hospital stay, shorter time to appropriate therapy, improved quality of life, and overall reduced treatment costs.

Laparoscopic staging for pancreatic cancer is not a new concept. In fact, the first published case in the United States of a minimally invasive approach to cancer staging was in a patient with pancreatic cancer. Bernheim in 1911 staged a patient of W. S. Halstead with presumed pancreatic cancer prior to laparotomy.[68] He stated that the procedure he termed *organoscopy* "may reveal general metastases or a secondary nodule in the liver, thus rendering further procedures unnecessary and saving the patient a rather prolonged convalescence." The use of laparoscopy was sporadic and not widespread until the seminal works of Alfred Cushieri from Scotland and Andrew Warshaw from the United States.[69,75–77] Both used the technique before the laparoscopic revolution and began to define the role it would have in the staging algorithm.

The yield of positive laparoscopy that avoids unnecessary laparotomy is highly dependent on the quality of the preoperative radiologic studies. The yield of laparoscopy cannot be assessed from studies that have not included state-of-the-art CT scans.[70] Currently, the standard protocol should include a contrast-enhanced thin-cut dynamic CT scan of the pancreas. Initial reports from Memorial Sloan-Kettering Cancer Center concerning laparoscopic staging of peripancreatic malignancy reported an improvement in resectability from 50% based on standard CT scanning alone to 92% when staging laparoscopy was performed.[71] Compared with previous reports, improvements in technology and better patient selection have reduced the benefit of laparoscopy. However, laparoscopy continues to consistently upstage approximately 15–20% of patients with radiologically resectable disease.[52,71–74]

Warshaw and colleagues compared the imaging modalities CT scanning, MRI, angiography and laparoscopy and found in 22 of 88 patients that CT scanning failed to demonstrate peritoneal disease revealed at laparoscopy. In this study, laparoscopy had a sensitivity of 96%.[69] The authors commented that laparoscopic staging owing to the magnification indeed may allow better assessment of the peritoneal cavity compared with palpation alone. Similar results were reported by Reddy and colleagues, who found that 29% of their patients had distant disease discovered at laparoscopy and were spared further intervention.[78] Yoshida and colleagues retrospectively analyzed 45 patients with radiologically resectable pancreatic head cancer based on preoperative helical CT scanning to clarify the role of staging laparoscopy.[79] Laparoscopy identified 4 patients (9%) with localized unresectable and 12 (27%) with metastatic disease. Fernandez-Del Castillo of Massachusetts General Hospital performed laparoscopy in 114 patients with pancreatic cancer with no evidence of metastatic disease on a preoperative CT scan.[74] Unsuspected intra-abdominal metastases were detected in 24% of the patients. None of these patients had further surgery. Staging laparoscopy missed peritoneal disease in 2 patients, resulting in a false-negative rate of 7%. The addition of cytology of peritoneal lavage upstaged a further 17% (16 of 92) of patients. At Memorial Sloan-Kettering Cancer Center over a 5-year period, 577 patients following contrast-enhanced CT scans were considered to have potentially resectable disease and underwent staging laparoscopy.[80] Unresectability was determined at laparoscopy if histologic proof was obtained of

1. Metastasis (hepatic, serosal, and/or peritoneal) (Fig 53–8)
2. Extrapancreatic extension of the tumor (i.e., mesocolic involvement)
3. Celiac or high portal node involvement
4. Invasion or encasement of the celiac or hepatic artery
5. Involvement by tumor of the superior mesenteric artery

Portal or superior mesenteric venous involvement was considered a relative contraindication to resection depending on the degree and extent of involvement.

In the MSKCC series, 366 were considered to have resectable disease after laparoscopic staging and subsequently underwent open exploration, with 92% (338 patients) being resected. The predominant sites for metastases were the liver and the peritoneal cavity. The resectability rate was compared with results from the decade before the introduction of laparoscopic staging, when 1135 patients at MSKCC were explored but only 35% were resected. In a recent prospective study reported by Doran and colleagues, 239 patients with suspected periampullary cancer underwent staging laparoscopy following dual-phase helical CT scanning.[81] CT "resectable" disease was noted in 190 patients, of whom laparoscopy correctly identified unresectable disease in 28 patients. Overall, owing to findings at laparoscopy, 15% of patients were spared a further procedure, leading the authors to conclude that when added to CT scanning, laparoscopic staging provides valuable information that improves the selection of patients for surgical or nonsurgical treatment significantly. Many other centers have reported similar results (Table 53–4).

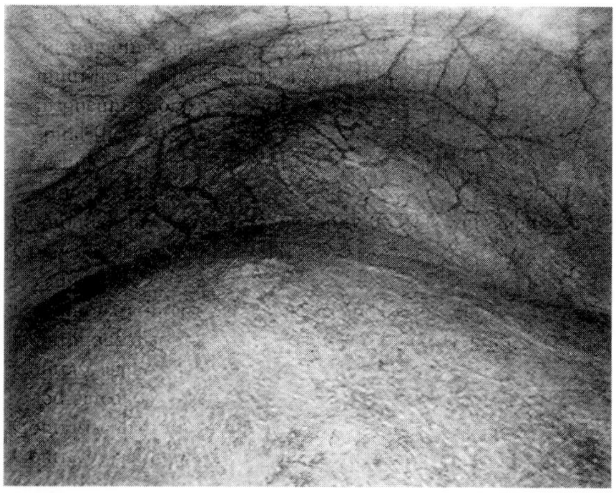

Figure 53–8. Metastic cancer.

Despite this experience, there is not uniformity around the value of laparoscopic staging. Critics argue that confining laparoscopy to the setting of determination of resectability overestimates the usefulness of laparoscopy because it fails to account for patients who require open procedures for palliation of unresectable disease.[70]

Pisters and colleagues from the MD Anderson Cancer Center reported resectabiltiy rates of 80% using high-quality CT scanning alone.[70] Based on these data, the authors proposed that the maximum positive yield of routine staging laparoscopy in patients with potentially resectable disease on high-quality CT scanning would be 20%, assuming a false-negative result of zero. This group did not perform routine staging laparoscopy but rather used selective laparoscopy at the time of planned laparotomy for tumor resection in patients with localized disease on CT scan and patients at high risk for occult M1 disease.[82,83] This is a strategy that has been advocated by others.[84] Gouma and colleagues from Amsterdam assessed the role of laparoscopic staging in patients with periampullary tumors compared with standard radiologic staging with helical CT scanning.[85] Laparoscopic staging identified biopsy-proven unresectable disease in only 13% of 297 patients, with a detection rate of 35%. Based on the findings, the authors proposed that laparoscopic staging should be performed selectively. Since their practice is to recommend a surgical bypass as palliation for patients with locally advanced unresectable disease, they believe that laparoscopic staging only adds value in the presence of metastatic disease.

It has been suggested that recent advances in CT and MRI technology may improve the diagnostic accuracy of preoperative radiologic staging. The introduction of multislice dynamic CT scanning and the ability to create high-resolution 2D and 3D imaging displays such as curved planar images, maximum and minimum image projections, and volume-rendering images have enhanced the utility of CT scanning, particularly in as-

TABLE 53–4. DETECTION OF INTRA-ABDOMINAL METASTASES AT LAPAROSCOPIC STAGING IN PATIENTS CONSIDERED TO HAVE RADIOLOGIC RESECTABLE DISEASE

Author	Year	Number of Patients	Number with Intra-Abdominal Metastases (%)
John	1995	40	14 (35%)
Fernandez-del Castello	1995	114	27 (24%)
Conlon	1996	108	28 (26%)
Holzman	1997	28	14 (50%)
Jiminez	2000	125	30 (24%)
White	2001	45	8 (18%)
Vollmer	2002	72	16 (22%)
Doran	2004	45	8 (18%)

sessing the relationship of the tumor to the peripancreatic vessels.[86,87] However, despite these advances, current studies continue to show an approximate 15–20% yield for laparoscopic staging.

LUS has been used by a number of groups in an attempt to increase the yield of laparoscopic staging.[91,92] John and colleagues showed that laparoscopy demonstrated unsuspected metastatic disease in 14 of 40 patients considered to have resectable disease.[72] However, laparoscopy had only 50% sensitivity in predicting tumor resectability. The accuracy in predicting resectability increased to 89% with the addition of LUS. Several other studies have demonstrated that the added value of LUS to standard laparoscopy is on the order of 14–25%.[52,93–95] In an early report, Murugiah and colleagues reported their experience in 12 patients with suspected resectable pancreatic head cancer.[96] Laparoscopy identified advanced disease in 4 patients. LUS detected further disease in an additional 2 patients and predicted resectable disease in 6 patients (50%). Only 1 of 6 patients submitted to laparotomy had unresectable disease owing to lymph node metastases. Further work from this group using LUS in 40 patients confirmed the reason for unresectability in 59%, provided staging information in addition to that of laparoscopy alone in 53%, and altered management in 25%. Overall, laparoscopy with LUS was more specific and accurate in predicting tumor resectability than laparoscopy alone (88% and 89% versus 50% and 65%).

Callery and colleagues analyzed the effect of routine implementation of laparoscopy with LUS, determining that the addition of LUS improved staging by identifying an additional 22% of patients with unresectable disease.[52] Minnard and colleagues reported the benefit of LUS over laparoscopy alone in evaluating the primary tumor and the presence of vascular involvement.[94] LUS findings resulted in a change in surgical treatment in 14% of patients in whom standard laparoscopic examination was equivocal (Fig 53–9). A further study by Schachter and colleagues demonstrated a change in surgical intervention in 36% of patients, with avoidance of unnecessary laparotomy in 31%.[97] Catheline and colleagues reported that LUS altered therapy in 41% of cases, avoiding open exploration in 46%.[98] This group reported a 90% sensitivity for assessing positive nodal disease and 100% for hepatic and peritoneal disease. Vollmer and colleagues similarly reported an improvement in resection rates using LUS (84% with laparoscopic staging versus 58% without).[99] Merchant and colleagues concluded that the addition of laparoscopic ultrasound during laparoscopic staging enhances the ability of laparoscopy to determine resectability and approaches the accuracy of open exploration without increasing morbidity or mortality significantly.[100]

Cytologic examination of peritoneal washing obtained at the time of laparoscopy has been suggested to enhance the sensitivity of staging laparoscopy.[101] Laparoscopy combined with peritoneal cytology is reported to upstage approximately 10% of patients.[100,102] Peritoneal recurrence is a significant site of failure following a potentially curative pancreaticoduodenectomy. Leach and colleagues studied a consecutive series of patients with suspected or biopsy-proven radiologically resectable adenocarcinoma of the pancreatic head.[103] Peritoneal washings were obtained at the time of staging laparoscopy and/or at subsequent laparotomy. Positive peritoneal cytology (PPC) was noted in 7% of patients, all of whom had overt metastatic disease at a median of 4.8 months. Merchant and colleagues examined 228 patients with radiographically resectable pancreatic adenocarcinoma who underwent laparoscopic staging.[100] Peritoneal washings were taken from both upper quadrants

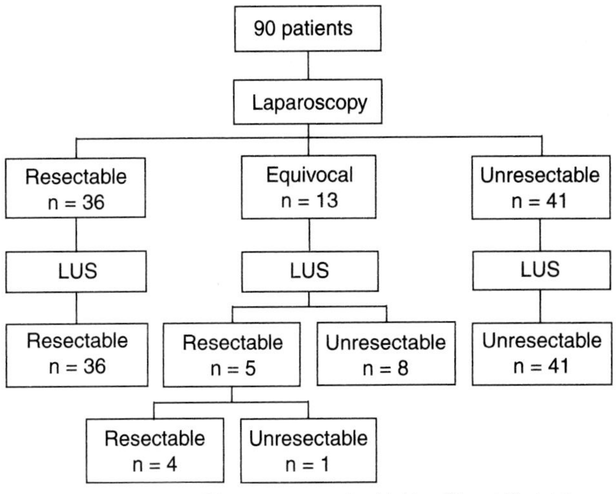

Figure 53–9. Results from LUS in pancreas cancer. Reprinted from Minnard EA, et al. Laparoscopic ultrasound enhances standard laparoscopy in the staging of pancreatic cancer. *Ann Surg* 1998;228:182–187.

at the beginning of laparoscopy. Overall survival was significantly higher in patients with negative peritoneal cytology. The authors determined that PPC had a positive predictive value of 94.1%, specificity of 98.1%, and sensitivity of 25.6% for determining unresectability.

Two recent reports have focused on the role of laparoscopic staging in patients with locally advanced unresectable disease who were considered for adjuvant chemoradiotherapy. Shoup and colleagues reviewed 100 consecutive patients with locally advanced disease who underwent laparoscopic staging.[104] Contemporary imaging studies failed to detect metastatic disease in 37% of cases. Peritoneal disease was noted in 12 cases, liver metastases in 18, and 7 patients had both (Table 53–5). Similar results were reported by Liu and Traverso, who described their experience with 74 patients, all of whom had undergone high-quality pancreas protocol CT examination prior to laparoscopic staging.[105] Occult tumor was found in 34% of patients. The authors reported that tumors situated in the body and tail of the gland were more likely than head lesions to have unsuspected metastases (53% versus 28%). Both groups suggest that in patients with locally advanced disease, laparoscopic staging be performed before combined modality therapy is initiated.

The studies cited earlier focus on invasive ductal adenocarcinoma of the pancreas. For other cell types, including neuroendocrine tumors, intraductal papillary mucinous neoplasms, and cystadenocarcinomas, the data are sparse. A review of the Memorial Sloan-Kettering experience with laparoscopy in nonfunctioning islet cell tumors by Hockwald and colleagues found a high incidence of occult metastases at laparoscopy.[106] CT scan followed by laparoscopy was significantly more sensitive than CT scan alone in predicting resectability (93% versus 50%; $p = 0.03$). This resulted from a high false-negative rate on CT scan for small-volume metastatic disease, hepatic disease being the most common site. The predictive value for tumor resectability also was much higher for CT scan followed by laparoscopy than for CT scan alone (95% versus 74%). Brooks and colleagues examined the role of laparoscopic staging in 144 patients with ampullary, duodenal, and distal bile duct tumors.[107] Patients with distal bile duct tumors also appeared to benefit from laparoscopic staging in terms of both determining resectability and avoiding unnecessary surgery. In contrast, patients with known duodenal or ampullary tumors gained little added value from laparoscopic staging.

■ OTHER INTRA-ABDOMINAL TUMORS

UROLOGIC CANCER

Over the last decade, there has been a significant expansion in urologic laparoscopic techniques. Laparoscopic nephrectomy, retroperitoneal dissection for testicular carcinoma, and laparoscopic prostectomy are performed routinely in specialized centers. However, laparoscopy for staging of disease has a limited role.

In prostate cancer, staging relies on sophisticated imaging such as ultrasound, CT scanning, and pelvic MRI in combination with histologic assessment of the tumor. Laparoscopic pelvic nodal dissection is performed selectively.[108–111] In the main, if performed, it is reserved for the poor prognostic patient who has clinically localized disease with a prostate-specific antigen (PSA) level greater than 20 ng/mL, a T3 lesion, a high-grade cancer, and a negative pelvic CT scan or MRI in whom curative local treatment is being contemplated.[112]

Laparoscopic pelvic nodal dissection also has been used in selected cases of poor prognostic invasive bladder cancer, penile cancer, and urethral cancer to confirm the presence of regional metastatic disease in patients in whom percutaneous image-guided biopsy is not possible.

Retroperitoneal lymph node dissection is still the most sensitive and specific method for the detection of lymph node metastases in stage I nonseminomatous testicular carcinoma. The laparoscopic approach, although practiced in only a few centers, has been reported to have some advantages compared with open surgery in terms of reduced blood loss, fewer intraoperative complications, and less operative time. The conversion rate is less than 10%, antegrade ejaculation can be preserved, and it provides adequate oncologic results.[113,114]

TABLE 53–5. INCIDENCE OF METASTATIC DISEASE FOUND AT LAPAROSCOPY IN PATIENTS WITH LOCAL OR ADVANCED DISEASE

	Total	No. with Liver Metastasis	No. with Peritoneal Metastasis	No. with Liver and Peritoneal Metastases	Patients with Metastatic Disease
All patients	100	18 (18%)	12 (12%)	7 (7%)	37 (37%)
Patients with pancreatic head cancers	69	15 (22%)	7 (10%)	4 (6%)	26 (38%)
Patients with pancreatic body/tail cancers	31	3 (10%)	5 (16%)	3 (10%)	11 (35%)

Reprinted from Shoup M, Winston C, Brennan MF, et al. Is there a role for staging laparoscopy in patients with locally advanced unresectable pancreatic adenocarcinoma? *J Gastrointest Surg* 2004; 8:1068–1071.

LYMPHOMA

Laparoscopy has an increasing role in staging of lymphoproliferative disease within the abdomen. Historically, staging of lymphoma involved an exploratory laparotomy, nodal sampling, liver biopsy, and splenectomy.[115,116] However, with improvements in imaging and the expansion of combination chemotherapeutic regimens, the need for surgical exploration diminished.[117] In recent years, the increasing complexity of histologic subtyping and the development of salvage therapies for recurrent disease have led to the requirement for precise diagnosis of intra-abdominal disease. Percutaneous FNA biopsy is now performed frequently. However, some difficulties arise for the pathologist in definitively distinguishing, on the one hand, low-grade lymphomas from reactive processes or, on the other, intermediate and/or high-grade lymphomas from anaplastic carcinoma. Immunohistochemistry can improve the diagnostic accuracy of FNA; however, nodal architecture is increasingly important for distinguishing indolent from aggressive lymphomas. Furthermore, cytogenic and molecular evaluation can have important prognostic significance.

Early reports have demonstrated that laparoscopy can provide adequate tissue for such analysis with lower morbidity and mortality compared with a laparotomy (Fig 53–10). Staging laparoscopy involves a thorough examination of the abdominal cavity and the retroperitoneal space, sampling of retroperitoneal lymph nodes, and liver biopsy. In female patients who are scheduled to receive radiotherapy, laparoscopic oophoropexy can be performed to reduce the risk of radiation-induced ovarian failure.[118]

Mann and colleagues reported a consecutive series of 101 laparoscopic procedures in patients with suspected lymphoma. A positive diagnosis was obtained in 62 patients, with only one false-negative result and one technical failure.[119] In another series, 118 patients had retroperitoneoscopy for retroperitoneal lymphadenopathy. An overall sensitivity of 91% was reported, but there were 9 false-negative results in the 70 cases of lymphoma. Clinical diagnosis for 34 patients was changed radically by the results of the procedure, including 30 patients suspected to have lymphoma who turned out to have a variety of benign and malignant conditions.[120] A recent prospective study examined the accuracy of laparoscopy in the diagnosis and staging of lymphoproliferative disease. Laparoscopy was completed successfully in 128 of 131 patients. Morbidity was low (2.9%), with no mortality. In all, 96.4% of the patients in whom a primary diagnosis was made and all the relapsed patients were treated on the basis of the laparoscopic findings.[121] This latter group is interesting because it is estimated that up to 40% of patients with an abdominal mass at initial diagnosis will have a residual mass following completion of therapy. An obvious concern is that there may be residual disease or that a transformation to a higher grade has occurred.[122] Percutaneous biopsy is often nondiagnostic, raising the potential that laparoscopic biopsy may have a role in assessing the true remission status. Whether functional imaging such as PET scanning will alter this need remains to be seen.

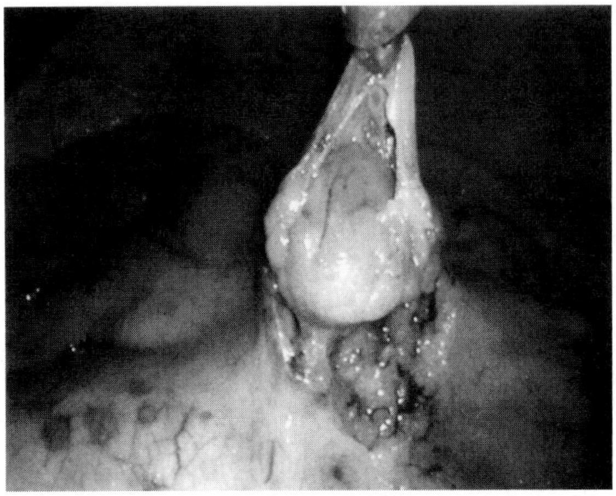

Figure 53–10. Laparoscopy in lymphoma.

▪ COMPLICATIONS OF STAGING LAPAROSCOPY

Laparoscopic staging appears safe and is associated with a low rate of major morbidity such as hemorrhage, visceral perforation, and intra-abdominal infection, which may occur in 1–2% of cases. As the use of laparoscopy increased, concern was expressed regarding the potential risk of disseminating disease at the time of pneumoperitoneum. An initial case report in 1978 by Dobronte and colleagues described a "port site" tumor implant in a patient with malignant ascites 2 weeks following laparoscopy.[123] A number of similar reports followed, again involving patients who had disseminated disease at the time of their laproscopic examination. Nieveen van Dijkum and colleagues from Amsterdam demonstrated an overall 2% port-site recurrence, with all cases having advanced peritoneal disease.[124]

Clinical experience over the last 10 years would appear to support the hypothesis that laparoscopic staging is safe from the oncologic standpoint. Pearlstone and colleagues from the MD Anderson Cancer Center described their experience with laparoscopy in 533 patients with nongynecologic intra-abdominal cancer, 339 of whom had laparoscopic procedures for upper gastrointestinal malignancies.[125] They reported port-site recurrences in 4 patients (0.88%), 3 of whom had advanced disease at the time of initial laparoscopy. Similar results were noted in a report from Memorial Sloan-Kettering Cancer Center, which reviewed a prospective database of 1650 diagnostic laparoscopic procedures performed in 1548 patients with upper gastrointestinal malignancies, in which a total of 4299 trocars were inserted.[126] The most frequent diagnosis was pancreatic cancer (51.2%). At a median follow-up of 18 months, a port-site recurrence was noted in 13 patients (0.8%). An open operation was performed in 1040 patients, of whom 9 (0.9%) developed a wound recurrence. This latter figure is similar to the 0.8% incisional recurrence rate noted by Hughes and colleagues in a review of 1600 open laparotomies for colon cancer.[127] Median time for the development of the port-site recurrence in the MSKCC study was 8.2 months. Eight occurred in patients with documented metastatic disease at the time of laparoscopy, and the remaining 5 had local or distant disease at the time of diagnosis of the port-site implant, and therefore, the recurrence did not appear to be an isolated event but rather a marker for more advanced disease. The authors concluded that laparoscopic staging appeared safe from an oncologic standpoint. This is further supported by a retrospective review of 235 patients who had laparoscopy to stage pancreatic cancer. This study demonstrated a port-site recurrence rate of 3% versus a 3.9% incisional recurrence rate in those patients who had an exploratory laparotomy alone.[128]

A number of hypotheses have been suggested to explain port-site implantation. Tumor seeding has been associated with carbon dioxide pneumoperitoneum in animal studies; however, reports that tumor growth is established more easily after open laparotomy would appear to refute this theory.[129–131] Other mechanisms, such as tissue manipulation, direct wound contamination, poor surgical technique, or immunologic effects such as changes in host immune responses, also have been suggested.[132] It appears so far, however, in most studies that port-site implantation is uncommon, differs little from open surgical incision recurrence, and is more likely to reflect the underlying biologic behavior of the disease rather than the type of surgery.

▪ LAPAROSCOPIC BILIARY AND GASTRIC BYPASS

Since the majority of patients with pancreatic cancer have unresectable disease at the time of presentation, palliation to minimize symptoms and maximize quality of life has a major role in the care of these patients. Palliation most commonly is required for one of three problems: biliary obstruction, gastric outlet obstruction, and relief of pain.

While both cholecystoenteric and choledochoenteric bypasses have been performed laparoscopically, the latter is much more difficult technically, requiring a high level of laparoscopic skills. A sufficient length of common duct needs to be exposed, and a difficult intracorporial anastomosis between the small bowel and the common duct must be performed. Cholecystojejunostomy is the more commonly performed laparoscopic procedure (Fig 53–11). Patient selection is critical. A low insertion of the cystic duct into the common bile duct or tumor impingement within 1 cm of the duct is a predictor of early technical failure. The anastomosis can be performed with either a stapled or hand-sewn technique. In patients who have experienced a prior cholecystectomy or who have a diseased gallbladder, blocked cystic duct, low insertion of the cystic duct, or tumor encroachment on the cystic duct or gallbladder, a cholecystojejunostomy is not possible; therefore, either a laparoscopic cholodochojejunostomy is performed, or the procedure is converted to open and a standard surgical bypass is performed.

Rhodes and colleagues presented in 1995 one of the first series of patients who underwent laparoscopic palliation for advanced pancreatic carcinoma. From the 16 patients, 7 underwent laparoscopic cholecystojejunostomy, 5 had laparoscopic gastroenterostomy, 3 had both procedures, and in 1 patient laparoscopic palliation failed. The median operating time was 75 minutes, the hospital stay was 4 days, the morbidity was 13%, and the median survival in 10 patients was 201 days, with the rest of the patients remaining alive at the time of the publication.[133] In 1999, Rothlin and colleagues published a case-controlled study of 28 patients with pancreatic cancer divided in two groups; in one group, laparoscopic palliation was performed, and the other group underwent conventional surgical palliation.[134] Of the 14 patients in the laparoscopic group, 7 had laparoscopic gastroenterostomy, 3

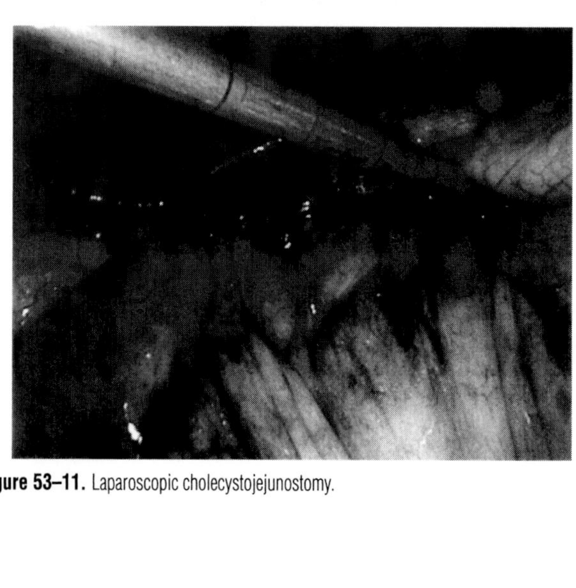

Figure 53–11. Laparoscopic cholecystojejunostomy.

had gastoenterostomy and hepaticojejunostomy, and 4 had staging laparoscopy only. Postoperative morbidity was 7% for the laparoscopic group compared with 43% for the open palliation group. There were no deaths in the laparoscopic group versus 29% mortality in the open group. Average postoperative hospital stay was 9 days for the laparoscopic group versus 21 days for the open group. Finally, the laparoscopic group required significantly less analgesia postoperatively. Recently, Choi presented a series of 78 gastrojejunostomies, 45 open and 33 laparoscopic, performed for palliation of gastric outflow obstruction caused by advanced gastric, duodenal, ampullary, and pancreatic cancers.[135] In the laparoscopic group, there was less suppression of immune function, lower morbidity, and earlier recovery of bowel function.

The true incidence of symptomatic gastric outlet obstruction (GOO) remains unclear. Historically, it was considered that more than 25% of patients would develop GOO during the course of their illness, and therefore, prophylaxic gastric bypass was recommended at the time of exploratory laparotomy. However, as the need for open exploration for staging purposes has decreased, the need for prophylaxic bypass for the majority of patients has been questioned. GOO is a late complication of advanced pancreatic cancer affecting 10–20% of patients who survive more than 15 months.[136–138] However, fewer than 3% of the patients who develop GOO require surgical bypass.[136,139,140] Most important, 60% of patients with advanced pancreatic cancer have delayed gastric emptying with no evidence of gastric or duodenal invasion. This may be explained by tumor infiltration of the celiac plexus causing gastric stasis, nausea, and vomiting.[141]

Espat and colleagues examined in a prospective but nonrandom study of 155 patients undergoing laparoscopic staging.[136] Following laparoscopy, 40 patients had locally advanced unresectable disease, and the remainder had metastatic disease. In follow-up, only 3% of patients required a subsequent open operation for biliary drainage or GOO. A subsequent update of this experience has confirmed the results, with over 90% of patients dead of disease. This low incidence of patients requiring operation for symptomatic GOO is consistent with the data seen from the nonoperative control groups in randomized trials of endoscopic biliary drainage versus surgery.

A laparoscopic gastroenterostomy is a relatively straightforward procedure. Nagy and colleagues reported a series of laparoscopic gastrojejunostomies.[142] Nine of 10 patients in this series had GOO from pancreatic malignancy. The laparoscopic method was successful in 90%. There was no postoperative morbidity or mortality associated with the surgical technique.

SURGICAL TECHNIQUE FOR BILIARY AND GASTRIC BYPASS

The patient is placed supine on the operating table in 10 degrees of reverse Tredelenberg position with 10 degrees of left lateral tilt. The placement of trocars is similar to that for the standard staging procedure. However, in order to accommodate a linear stapler, the right upper quadrant 10-mm trocar is converted into a 12- to 15-mm size. Following exploration, the ligament of Trietz is identified, and a loop of jejunum approximately 30 cm distal to the ligament of Treitz is brought in an antecolic position to the gallbladder (Fig 53–12). Using an intracorporeal suturing technique, the jejunum is approximated to the gallbladder by two 3-0 coated, braided lactomer sutures (Polysorb, U.S. Surgical, Norwalk, CT). The distended gallbladder may be decompressed using a Veress needle attached to a suction device. There is usually minimal biliary spillage owing to the raised intra-abdominal pressure consequent on the pneumoperitoneum. Small enterotomy incisions (10 mm) are made in the gallbladder and jejunum using either scissors or a device such as the ultrasonic shears (Fig 53–13). Hemostasis is achieved with electrocautery. Any spillage can be dealt with by suction device placed through the left upper quadrant port. An endoscopic 30-mm linear stapler using 3.5-mm staples is introduced through the right upper quadrant port, and the "jaws" are manipulated into the gallbladder and jejunum in a standard fashion. Often this is difficult because of the proximity of the port site to the gallbladder. A roticulating stapler facilitates this maneuver. The stapler heads are approximated, and the instrument is fired (Fig 53–14). After removing the stapler, the anastomosis is inspected, hemostasis is confirmed, and the gallbladder interior is aspirated and irrigated with saline.

The resulting enterotomy can be closed by using either a completely intracorporeal or laparoscopically assisted approach. Using an intracorporeal technique, the defect is closed with a continuous seromuscular 3-0 coated, braided lactomer suture, with knots tied using an intracorporeal technique (Fig 53–15).

An alternative method is to create a completely hand-sewn anastomosis using 3-0 coated, braided lactomer suture. If a running suture is used, the assistant should maintain tension on the suture with an atraumatic grasping forceps following placement of each stitch. Knots can be tied either using intracorporeal or extracorporeal technique.

A laparoscopically assisted method is suitable in thin patients. Two stay sutures are placed on either side of the anastomotic defect. These sutures are cut long. The 12-mm trocar is removed, and the incision is enlarged to 20 mm. Using retraction on the stay sutures, the newly created biliary-enteric anastomosis can be exteri-

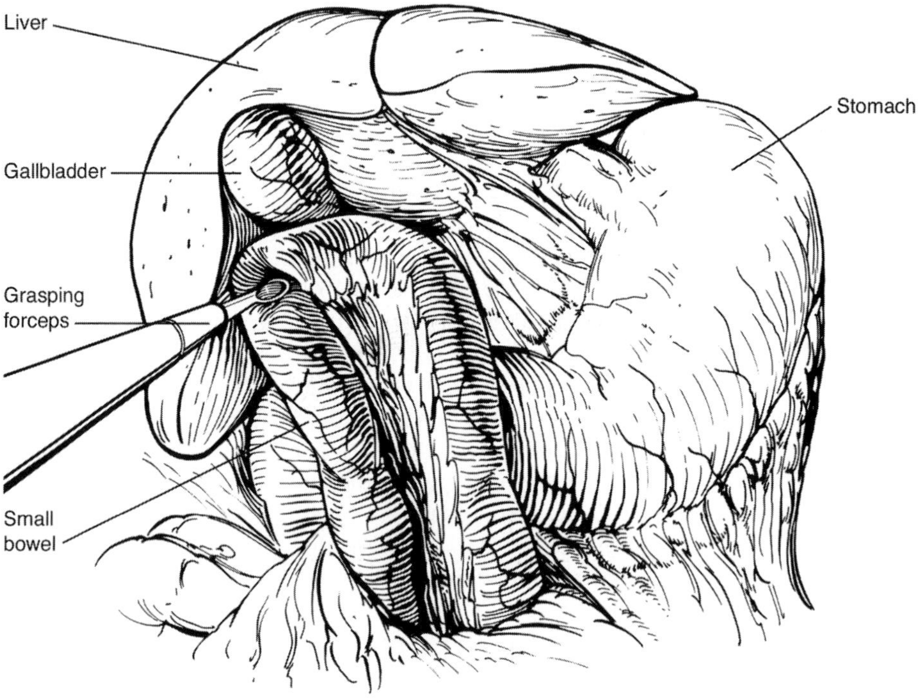

Figure 53–12. Laparoscopic cholecystojejunostomy.

orized and the enterotomy closed in a standard fashion. When this is completed, the bowel is returned to the abdominal cavity, and the wound is closed. The abdomen is reinsufflated and the anastomosis inspected. This technique allows for the construction of a 2.5-cm cholecystojejunal anastomosis without any bowel narrowing. No intra-abdominal drains are used.

The technique for fashioning a gastrojejunostomy is similar. In this case, a proximal loop of jejunum is brought in an antecolic position to the stomach. The

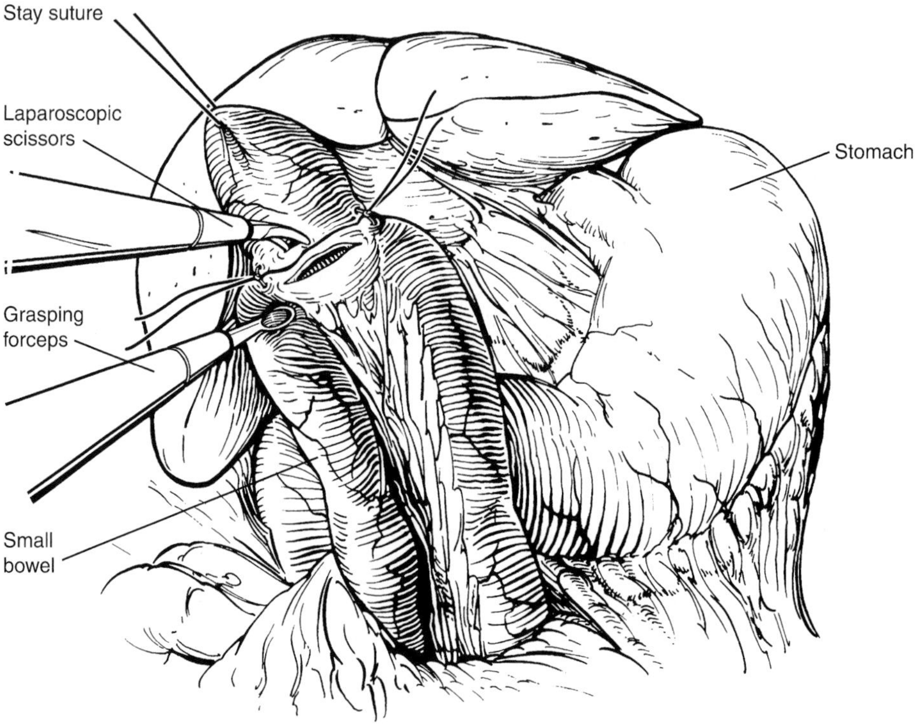

Figure 53–13. Approximation of small bowel to gallbladder, creation of enterotomy.

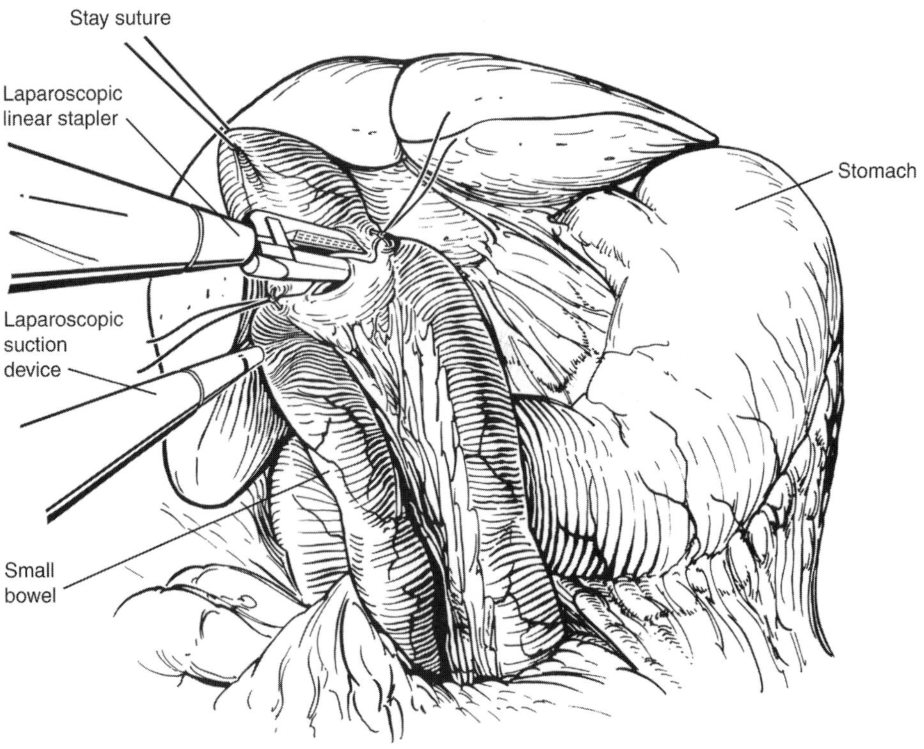

Figure 53–14. Stapled anastomosis.

left upper quadrant 5-mm laparoscopic trocar is converted to a 12-mm trocar. Two 3-0 coated, braided lactomer sutures (Polysorb, U.S. Surgical) are used to approximate the jejunum to the stomach. Enterotomies are made in both stomach and jejunum. In cases in which there has been a significant period of gastric obstruction, the gastric wall may be hypertrophied, making creation of the gastrotomy difficult.

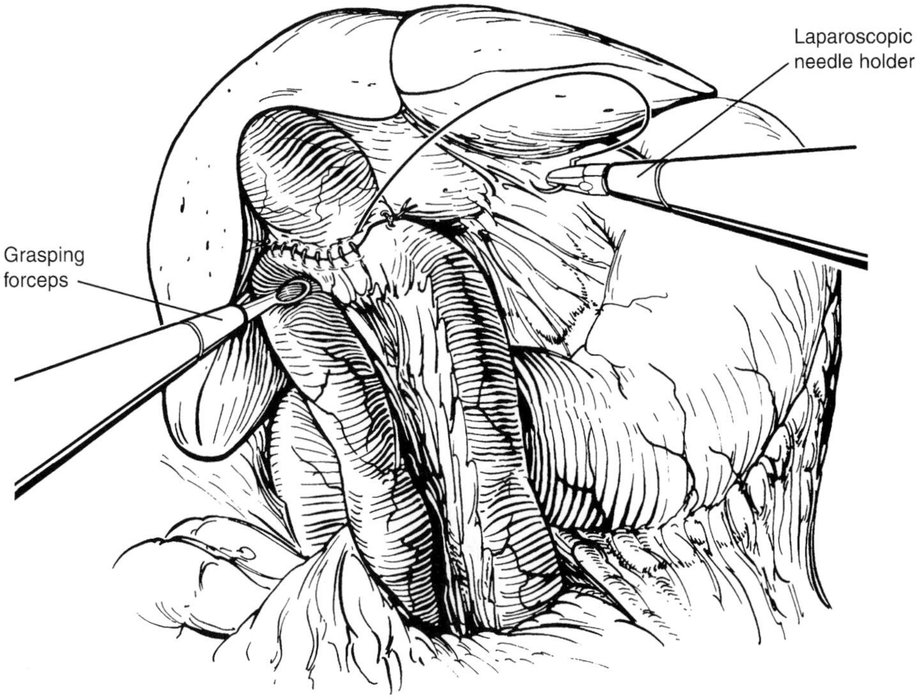

Figure 53–15. Closure of enterotomy.

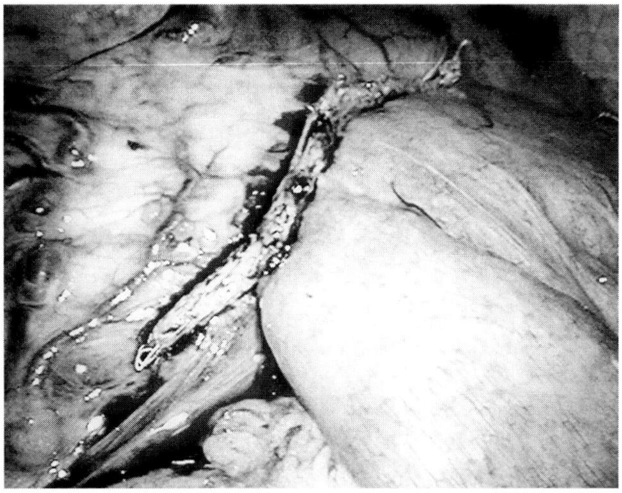

Figure 53–16. Gastrojejunostomy.

Confirmation that one is inside the stomach is required before placement of the stapler. When this is achieved, a 30-mm linear stapler is inserted through the 12-mm left upper quadrant port and manipulated into both enterotomies. The instrument is positioned and fired. The stapler is removed and reloaded, returned into the anastomosis, and refired. This creates an anastomosis approximately 5 cm in length. The anterior defect can be closed in a fashion similar to the cholecystojejunostomy (Fig 53–16). Any defects in the anastomosis can be repaired with individual 3-0 sutures.

The ideal palliative procedure for biliary or gastric obstruction should be effective in relieving jaundice or gastric outlet obstruction, have minimal morbidity, be associated with a short hospital stay, have a low symptomatic recurrence, and maintain quality of life. Laparoscopic procedures have the potential to achieve these goals, although data do not support prophylactic bypass procedures in patients who do not otherwise require surgery.

▪ SUMMARY

Laparoscopy is no longer a tool of limited use and now has widespread indications within surgical oncologic practice. It has benefit in the detection and staging of gastrointestinal malignancies, saving a small but significant number of patients with unresectable disease from unnecessary laparotomy. Its role in palliative surgery remains to be fully clarified; however, recent literature suggests that it may have a valid role and may become part of mainstream surgical practice.

REFERENCES

1. Hemming AW, Nagy AG, Scudmore CH, et al. Laparoscopic staging of intra-abdominal malignancy. *Surg Endosc* 1995;9:325–328
2. Van Delden OM, De Wit LT, Bemelman WA, et al. Laparoscopic ultrasonography for abdominal tumor staging: Technical aspects and imaging findings. *Abdom Imaging* 1997;22:125–131
3. Buyske J. Role of videoscopic-assisted techniques in staging malignant diseases. *Surg Clin North Am* 2000;80:495–503
4. Pratt Bl, Greene FL. Role of laparoscopy in the staging of malignant disease. *Surg Clin North Am* 2000;80:1111–1126
5. Romijn MG, van Overhagen H, Spillenaar Bilgen EJ, et al. Laparoscopy and laparoscopic ultrasonography in staging of oesophageal and cardial carcinoma *Br J Surg* 1998;85:1010–1012
6. Aibe T, Fuji T, Okita K, et al. A fundamental study of normal layer structure of the gastrointestinal wall visualised by endoscopic ultrasonography. *Scand J Gastroenterol* 1986;21: 6–15
7. Tio TL, Tytgat GNJ. Endoscopic ultrasonography of normal and pathologic upper gastrointestinal wall structure: Comparison of studies in vivo and in vitro with histology. *Scand J Gastroenterol* 1986;21:27–33
8. Dittler HJ, Siewert JR. Role of endoscopic ultrasonography in esophageal carcinoma. *Endoscopy* 1993;25:156–161
9. Rosch T. Endosonographic staging of esophageal cancer: a review of literature results. *Gastrointest Endosc Clin North Am* 1995;5:537–547
10. Lea JW 4th, Prager RL, Bender HW Jr. The questionable role of computed tomography in preoperative staging of esophageal cancer. *Ann Thorac Surg* 1984;38:479–481
11. Thompson WM, Halvorsen RA, Foster JR, et al. Computed tomography for staging esophageal and gastroesophageal cancer: Re-evaluation. *AJR* 1983;141:951–958
12. Kimmey MB, Martin RW, Haggit RC, et al. Histologic correlates of gastrointestinal ultrasound images. *Gastroenterology* 1989;96:433–441
13. Aibe T, Ito T, Yoshida T. Endoscopic ultrasonography of lymph nodes surrounding the upper GI tract. *Scand J Gastroenterol* 1986;21: 164–169
14. Tio TL, Cohen P, Coene PP, et al. Endosonography and computed tomography of esophageal carcinoma: Preoperative classification compared to the new TNM system. *Gastroenterology* 1989;96:1478–1486
15. Rosch T, Lorenz R, Zenker K, et al. Local staging and assessment of resectability in carcinoma of esophagus, stomach, and duodenum by endoscopic ultrasonography. *Gastrointest Endosc* 1992;38:460–467
16. Harewood GC, Wiersema MJ. A cost analysis of endoscopic ultrasound in the evaluation of esophageal cancer. *Am J Gastroenterol* 2002;97:452–458
17. Flamen P, Leurut A, Van Cutsem E, et al. Utility of positron emission tomography for the staging of patients with potentially operable esophageal carcinoma. *J Clin Oncol* 2000;18:3202–3210

18. Flanagan FL, Dehdashti F, Siegal BA, et al. Staging of esophageal cancer with ^{18}F-fluordexyglucose positron emission tomography. *AJR* 1997;168:417–424
19. Block MI, Patterson GA, Sundaresan RS, et al. Improvement in staging of esophageal cancer with addition of positron emission tomography. *Ann Thorac Surg* 1997;64: 770–776
20. Weber WA, Ott K, Becker K, et al. Prediction of response to preoperative chemotherapy in adenocarcinoma of the esophagogastric junction by metabolic imaging. *J Clin Oncol* 2001;19:3058–3065
21. Dagnini G, Caldironi MW, Marian G, et al. Laparoscopy in abdominal staging of esophageal carcinoma: Report of 369 cases. *Gastrointest Endosc* 1986;32:400–402
22. Stein HJ, Kraemer SJ, Freussner H, et al. Clinical value of diagnostic laparoscopy with laparoscopic ultrasound in patients with cancer of the esophagous or cardia. *J Gastrointest Surg* 1997;1:167–173
23. Stell DA, Carter Cr, Stewart I, Anderson JR. Prospective comparison of laparoscopy, ultrasonography and computed tomography in the staging of gastric cancer. *Br J Surg* 1996;83:1260–1262
24. Watt I, Stewart I, Anderson D, et al. Laparoscopy, ultrasound, and computed tomography in cancer of the oesophagus and gastric cardia: A prospective comparison for detecting intra-abdominal metastases. *Br J Surg* 1989; 76:1036–1042
25. Wakelin SJ, Deans C, Crofts PL, et al. A comparison of computerised tomography, laparoscopic ultrasound and endoscopic ultrasound in the preoperative staging of oesphago-gastric carcinoma. *Eur J Radiol* 2002;41:161–167
26. Smith A, Finch MD, John TG, et al. Role of laparoscopic ultrasonography in the management of patients with oesophagogastric cancer. *Br J Surg* 1999;86:1083–1087
27. Rau B, Hunerbein M, Hohenberger P, et al. Staging laparoscopy of esophageal cancer. In: Hohenberger, Conlon (eds). *Staging Laparoscopy.* Berlin: Springer; 2002:55–67
28. Bonavina L, Incarbone R, Lattuada E, et al. Preoperative laparoscopy in management of patients with carcinoma of the esophagous and of the esophagogastric junction. *J Surg Oncol* 1997;65:171–174
29. Goletti O, Buccianti P, Chiarugi M, et al. Laparoscopic sonography in screening metastases from gastrointestinal cancer: Comparative accuracy with traditional procedures. *Surg Laparosc Endosc* 1995;5:176–182
30. Grimm H, Binmoeller K, Hamper K, et al. Endosonography for preoperative locoregional staging of esophageal and gastric cancer. *Endoscopy* 1993;25:224–230
31. Kalantzis N, Kallimanis G, Laoudi F, et al. Endoscopic ultrasonography and computed tomography in preoperative (TMN) classification of esophageal carcinoma (abstract). *Endoscopy* 1992;24:653
32. Catalono MF, Sivak MV Jr, Rice T, et al. Endosonographic features predictive of lymph node metastases. *Gastrointest Endosc* 1994;409:442–446
33. Menon KV, Dehn TC. Multiport staging laparoscopy in oesophageal and cardiac carcinoma. *Dis Esophagus* 2003; 16:295–300
34. Krasna MJ, Jiao X, Mao YS, et al. Thorascopy/laparoscopy in the staging of esophageal cancer: Maryland experience. *Surg Laparosc Endosc Percutan Tech* 2002;12: 213–218
35. Karpeh MS Jr, Brennan MF. Gastric carcinoma. *Ann Surg Oncol* 1998;5:650–656
36. Brennan MF, Karpeh MS Jr. Surgery for gastric cancer: The American view. *Ann Surg Oncol* 1996;23:352–359
37. Pye JK, Crumplin MK, Charles J, et al. Hospital clinicians in Wales: One-year survey of carcinoma of the oesophagus and stomach in Wales. *Br J Surg* 2001;88: 278–285
38. Burke EC, Karpeh MS Jr, Conlon KC, et al. Laparoscopy in the management of gastric adenocarcinoma. *Ann Surg* 1997;225:262–267
39. Gross E, Bancewicz J, Ingram, G. Assessment of gastric cancer by laparoscopy. *Br Med J* 1984;288:1577
40. Possik RA, Franco EL, Pires DR, et al. Sensitivity, specificity and predictive value of laparoscopy for the staging of gastric cancer and for the detection of liver metastases. *Cancer* 1986;58:1–6.
41. D'Ugo DM, Persiani R, Caracciolo F, et al. Selection of locally advanced gastric carcinoma by preoperative staging laparoscopy. *Surg Endosc* 1997;11:1159–1162
42. Lehnert T, Rudek B, Buhl KK, et al. Impact of diagnostic laparoscopy on the management of gastric cancer: Prospective study of 120 consecutive patients with primary gastric adenocarcinoma. *Br J Surg* 2002;89:471–475
43. Finch M, John T, Garden OJ, et al. Laparoscopic ultrasonography for staging gastroesophageal cancer. *Surgery* 1997;121:10–17
44. Kitagawa Y, Fujii H, Mukai M, et al. Current status and future prospects of sentinel node navigational surgery for gastrointestinal cancers. *Ann Surg Oncol* 2004;11: 242S–244S
45. Sotiropoulos GC, Kaiser GM, Lang H, et al. Staging laparoscopy in gastric cancer. *Eur J Med Res* 2005;10: 88–91
46. Wilkiemeyer MB, Bieligk SC, Ashfaq R, et al. Laparoscopy alone is superior to peritoneal cytology in staging gastric and esophageal carcinoma. *Surg Endosc* 2004;18: 852–856
47. Bentrem D, Wilton A, Mazumdar M. The value of peritoneal cytology as a preoperative predictor in patients with gastric carcinoma undergoing a curative resection. *Ann Surg Oncol* 2005;12:339–341
48. Fortner JG, Silva JS, Cox EB, et al. Multivariate analysis of a personal series of 247 patients with liver metastases from colorectal cancer: Treatment by intrahepatic chemotherapy. *Ann Surg* 1984;199:317–324
49. Jarnagin WR, Bodniewicz J, Dougherty E, et al. A prospective analysis of staging laparoscopy in patients with primary and secondary hepatobiliary malignancies. *J Gastrointest Surg* 2000;4:24–43
50. Lo CM, Lai E, Liu CL, et al. Laparoscopy and laparoscopic ultrasonography avoid exploratory laparotomy in patients with hepatocellular carcinoma. *Ann Surg* 1998; 227:527–532

51. John TG, Greig JD, Crosbie JL, et al. Superior staging of liver tumors with laparoscopy and laparoscopic ultrasound. *Ann Surg* 1994;220:711–719
52. Callery MP, Strasberg SM, Doherty GM, et al. Staging laparoscopy with laparoscopic ultrasonography: Optimizing resectability in hepatobiliary and pancreatic malignancy. *J Am Coll Surg* 1997;185:33–39
53. D'Angelica M, Fong Y, Weber S, et al. The role of laparoscopy in hepatobiliary malignancy: Prospective analysis of 401 cases. *Ann Surg Oncol* 2003;10:183–189
54. Jarnagin WR, Conlon K, Bodniewicz J, et al. A clinical scoring system predicts the yield of diagnostic laparoscopy in patients with potentially resectable hepatic colorectal metastases. *Cancer* 2001;91:1121–1128
55. Grobmyer SR, Fong Y, DíAngelica M, et al. Diagnostic laparoscopy prior to planned hepatic resection for colorectal metastases. *Arch Surg* 2004;139:1326–1330
56. Rahusen FD, Cuesta MA, Borgstein PJ, et al. Selection of patients for resection of colorectal metastases to the liver using diagnostic laparoscopy and laparoscopic ultrasonography. *Ann Surg* 1999;230:31–37
57. de Castro SM, Tilleman EH, Busch OR, et al. Diagnostic laparoscopy for primary and secondary liver malignancies: Impact of improved imaging and changed criteria for resection. *Ann Surg Oncol* 2004;11:522–529
58. Koea J, Rodgers M, Thompson P, et al. Laparoscopy in the management of colorectal cancer metastatic to the liver. *ANZ J Surg* 2004;74:1056–1059
59. Thaler K, Kanneganti S, Khajanchee Y, et al. The evolving role of staging laparoscopy in the treatment of colorectal hepatic metastases *Arch Surg* 2005;140:727–734
60. Foroutani A, Garland AM, Berber E. Laparoscopic ultrasound versus triphasic computed tomography for detecting liver tumors. *Arch Surg* 2000;135:953–958
61. Berber E, Garland AM, Engle KL, et al. Laproscopic ultrasonography and biopsy of hepatic tumors in 310 patients. *Am J Surg* 2004;187:213–218
62. Hartley JE, Kumar H, Drew PJ, et al. Laparoscopic ultrasound for the detection of hepatic metastases during laparoscopic colorectal cancer surgery. *Dis Colon Rectum* 2000;43:320–324
63. Metcalfe MS, Close JS, Iswariah H, et al. The value of laparoscopic staging for patients with colorectal metastases. *Arch Surg* 2003;138:770–772
64. Lightdale CJ. Laparoscopy and biopsy in malignant liver disease. *Cancer* 1982;50:2672–2675
65. Jeffers L, Spieglman G, Reddy R, et al. Laparoscopically directed fine needle aspiration for the diagnosis of hepatocellular carcinoma: A safe and accurate technique. *Gastrointest Endosc* 1988;34:235–237
66. D'Angelica MD, Jarnagin WR, Dematteo RP, et al. Staging laparoscopy for potentially resectable non-colorectal nonendocrine liver metastases. *Ann Surg Oncol* 2003;9:204–209
67. Jemal A, Tiwari RC, Murray T, et al. Cancer statistics, 2004. *CA Cancer J Clin* 2004;54:8–29
68. Bernheim BM. Organoscopy. *Ann Surg* 1911;53:764–767
69. Warshaw AL, Gu ZY, Wittenberg J, et al. Preoperative staging and assessment of resectability of pancreatic cancer. *Arch Surg* 1990;125:230–233
70. Pisters PW, Lee JE, Vauthey JN, et al. Laparoscopy in the staging of pancreatic cancer. *Br J Surg* 2001;88:325–337
71. Conlon KC, Dougherty E, Klimstra DS, et al. The value of minimal access surgery in the staging of patients with potentially resectable peripancreatic malignancy. *Ann Surg* 1996;223:134–140
72. John TG, Greig JD, Carter DC, et al. Carcinoma of the pancreatic head and periampullary region: Tumor staging with laparoscopy and laparoscopic ultrasonography. *Ann Surg* 1995;221:156–164
73. Bemelman WA, et al. Diagnostic laparoscopy combined with laparoscopic ultrasonography in staging of cancer of the pancreatic head region. *Br J Surg* 1995;82:820–824
74. Fernandez-del Castillo C, Rattner DW, Warshaw AL. Further experience with laparoscopy and peritoneal cytology in the staging of pancreatic cancer. *Br J Surg* 1995;82:1127–1129
75. Warshaw AL, Tepper JE, Shipley WU. Laparoscopy in the staging and planning therapy for pancreatic cancer. *Am J Surg* 1986;151:76–80
76. Cuschieri A, Hall AW, Clark J. Value of laparoscopy in the diagnosis and management of pancreatic carcinoma. *Gut* 1978;19:672–677
77. Cuschieri A. Laparoscopy for pancreatic cancer: Does it benefit the patient? *Eur J Surg Oncol* 1988;14:41–44
78. Reddy KR, Levi J, Livingstone A, et al. Experience with staging laparoscopy in pancreatic malignancy. *Gastrointest Endosc* 1999;49:498–503
79. Yoshida T, et al. Staging with helical computed tomography and laparoscopy in pancreatic head cancer. *Hepatogastroenterology* 2002;49:1428–1431
80. Conlon KC, Brennan MF. Laparoscopy for staging abdominal malignancies. *Adv Surg* 2000;34:331–350
81. Doran HE, Bosonnet L, Connor S, et al. Laparoscopy and laparoscopic ultrasound in the evaluation of pancreatic and periampullary tumors. *Dig Surg* 2004;21:305–313
82. Abdalla EK, et al. Subaquatic laparoscopy for staging of intraabdominal malignancy. *J Am Coll Surg* 2003;196:155–158
83. Spitz FR, et al. Preoperative and postoperative chemoradiation strategies in patients treated with pancreaticoduodenectomy for adenocarcinoma of the pancreas. *J Clin Oncol* 1997;15:928–937
84. Obertop H, Gouma DJ. Essentials in biliopancreatic staging: A decision analysis. *Ann Oncol* 1999;10:150–152
85. Nieveen van Dijkum EJ, et al. Laparoscopic staging and subsequent palliation in patients with peripancreatic carcinoma. *Ann Surg* 2003;237:66–73
86. Prokesch RW, Schima W, Chow LC, et al. Multidetector CT of pancreatic adenocarcinoma: Diagnostic advances and therapeutic relevance. *Eur Radiol* 2003;13:2147–2154
87. Itoh S, et al. Assessment of the pancreatic and intrapancreatic bile ducts using 0.5-mm collimation and multiplanar reformatted images in multislice CT. *Eur Radiol* 2003;13:277–285
88. Johnson PT, Heath DG, Hofmann LV, et al. Multidetector-row computed tomography with three-dimensional volume rendering of pancreatic cancer: A complete preoperative staging tool using computed tomography angiography and

volume-rendered cholangiopancreatography. *J Comput Assist Tomogr* 2003;27:347–353
89. Merkle EM, Boll DT, Fenchel S. Helical computed tomography of the pancreas: Potential impact of higher concentrated contrast agents and multidetector technology. *J Comput Assist Tomogr* 2003;27:S17–22
90. Nino-Murcia M, Tamm EP, Charnsangavej C, et al. Multidetector-row helical CT and advanced post processing techniques for the evaluation of pancreatic neoplasms. *Abdom Imag* 2003;28:366–377
91. Cuesta MA, Meijer S, Borgstein PJ, et al. Laparoscopic ultrasonography for hepatobiliary and pancreatic malignancy. *Br J Surg* 1993;80:1571–1574
92. Ascher SM, Evans SR, Zeman RK. Laparoscopic cholecystectomy: Intraoperative ultrasound of the extrahepatic biliary tree and the natural history of postoperative transabdominal ultrasound findings. *Semin Ultrasound CT MR* 1993;14:331–337
93. John TG, et al. Laparoscopy with laparoscopic ultrasonography in the TNM staging of pancreatic carcinoma. *World J Surg* 1999;23:870–881
94. Minnard EA, et al. Laparoscopic ultrasound enhances standard laparoscopy in the staging of pancreatic cancer. *Ann Surg* 1998;228:182–187
95. Pietrabissa A, et al. Laparoscopy and laparoscopic ultrasonography for staging pancreatic cancer: critical appraisal. *World J Surg* 1999;23:998–1002
96. Murugiah M, Paterson-Brown S, Windsor JA, et al. Early experience of laparoscopic ultrasonography in the management of pancreatic carcinoma. *Surg Endosc* 1993;7:177–181
97. Schachter PP, et al. The impact of laparoscopy and laparoscopic ultrasonography on the management of pancreatic cancer. *Arch Surg* 2000;135:1303–1307
98. Catheline J, Turner R, Rizk N. The use of diagnostic laparoscopy supported by laparoscopic ultrasonongraphy in the assessment of pancreatic cancer. *Surg Endoscopy* 1999;13:239–245
99. Vollmer CM, Drebin JA, Middleton WD, et al. Utility of staging laparoscopy in subsets of peripancreatic and biliary malignancies. *Ann Surg* 2002;235:1–7
100. Merchant NB, Conlon KC, Saigo P, et al. Positive peritoneal cytology predicts unresectability of pancreatic adenocarcinoma. *J Am Coll Surg* 1999;188:421–426
101. Jimenez RE, Warshaw AL, Fernandez-del Castillo C. Laparoscopy and peritoneal cytology in the staging of pancreatic cancer. *J Hepatobil Pancreat Surg* 2000;7:15–20
102. Fernandez-del Castillo CL, Warshaw AL. Pancreatic cancer: Laparoscopic staging and peritoneal cytology. *Surg Oncol Clin North Am* 1998;7:135–142
103. Leach SD, et al. Significance of peritoneal cytology in patients with potentially resectable adenocarcinoma of the pancreatic head. *Surgery* 1995;118:472–478
104. Shoup M, Winston C, Brennan MF, et al. Is there a role for staging laparoscopy in patients with locally advanced unresectable pancreatic adenocarcinoma? *J Gastrointest Surg* 2004;8:1068–1071
105. Liu RC, Traverso W. Diagnostic laparoscopy improves staging of pancreatic cancer deemed locally unresectable by computed tomography. *Surg Endosc* 2005;19:638–642
106. Hochwald SN, Weiser MR, Colleoni R, et al. Laparoscopy predicts metastatic disease and spares laparotomy in selected patients with pancreatic non-functioning islet cell tumors. *Ann Surg Oncol* 2001;8:249–253
107. Brooks AD, Mallis MJ, Brennan MF, et al. The value of laparoscopy in the management of ampullary, duodenal, and distal bile duct tumors. *J Gastrointest Surg* 2002; 6:139–145
108. Schuessler WW, Vancaillie TG, Reich H, et al. Transperitoneal endosurgical lymphadenectomy in patients with localized prostate cancer. *J Urol* 1991;145:988
109. Griffith DP, Schuessler WW, Nickell KG, et al. Laparoscopic pelvic lymphadenectomy for prostatic adenocarcinoma. *Urol Clin North Am* 1992;19:407–415
110. Kerbl K, Clayman RV, Petros JA, et al. Staging pelvic lymphadenectomy for prostate cancer: A comparison of laparoscopic and open techniques. *J Urol* 1993;150:396–399
111. Moore RG, Partin AW, Kavoussi LR. Role of laparoscopy in the diagnosis and treatment of prostate cancer. *Semin Surg Oncol* 1996;12:139–144
112. Kava BR, Dalbagni G, Conlon KC, et al. Results of laparoscopic pelvic lymphadenectomy in patients at high risk for nodal metastases from prostate cancer. *Ann Surg Oncol* 1998;5:173–180
113. Steiner H, Peschel R, Janetschek G, et al. Long-term results of laparoscopic retroperitoneal lymph node dissection: A single-center 10-year experience. *Urology* 2004;63:550–555
114. Corvin S, Kuczyk M, Anastasiadis A, et al. Laparoscopic retroperitoneal lymph node dissection for nonseminomatous testicular carcinoma. *World J Urol* 2004;22:33–36
115. Glatstein E, Guernsey JM, Rosenberg SA, et al. The value of laparotomy and splenectomy in the staging of Hodgkin's disease. *Cancer* 1969;24:709–718
116. Veronesi U, Musumeci R, Pizzetti F, et al. The value of staging laparotomy in non-Hodgkin's lymphoma. *Cancer* 1974;33:446–459
117. Lacher MJ. Routine staging laparotomy for patients with Hodgkin's disease is no longer necessary. *Cancer Invest* 1983;1:93–99
118. Cuschieri A. Role of video-laparoscopy in the staging of intra-abdominal lymphomas and gastrointestinal cancer. *Semin Surg Oncol* 2001;20:167–172
119. Mann GB, Conlon KC, LaQuaglia M, et al. Emerging role for laparoscopy in the diagnosis of lymphoma. *J Clin Oncol* 1998;16:1909–1915
120. Porte H, Copin MC, Eraldi L, et al. Retroperitoneoscopy for the diagnosis of infiltrating retroperitoneal lymphadenopathy and masses. *Br J Surg* 1997;84: 1433–1436
121. Silecchia G, Raparelli L, Perrotta N, et al. Accuracy of laparoscopy in the diagnosis and staging of lymphoproliferative diseases. *World J Surg* 2003;27:653–658
122. Surbane A, Longo DL, DeVita VT, et al. Residual abdominal masses in aggressive non-Hodgkin's lymphoma after combination chemotherapy: Significance and management. *J Clin Oncol* 1988;6:1832–1837
123. Dobronte Z, Wittmann T, Karacsony G. Rapid development of malignant metastases in the abdominal wall after laparoscopy. *Endoscopy* 1978;10:127–130

124. Nieveen van Dijkum EJ, de Wit LT, van Delden OM, et al. Staging laparoscopy and laparoscopic ultrasonography in more than 400 patients with upper gastrointestinal carcinoma. *J Am Coll Surg* 1999;189:459–465
125. Pearlstone DB, Mansfield PF, Curley SA, et al. Laparoscopy in 533 patients with abdominal malignancy. *Surgery* 1999;125:67–72
126. Shoup M, Brennan MF, Karpeh MS, et al. Port site metastasis after diagnostic laparoscopy for upper gastrointestinal tract malignancies: an uncommon entity. *Ann Surg Oncol* 2002;9:632–636
127. Hughes ES, McDermott FT, Polglase AL, et al. Tumor recurrence in the abdominal wall scar tissue after large-bowel cancer surgery. *Dis Colon Rectum* 1983;26:571–572
128. Velanovich V. The effects of staging laparoscopy on trocar site and peritoneal recurrence of pancreatic cancer. *Surg Endosc* 2004;18:310–313
129. Bouvy ND, Marquet RL, Jeekel H, et al. Impact of gas(less) laparoscopy and laparotomy on peritoneal tumor growth and abdominal wall metastases. *Ann Surg* 1996;224:694–700; discussion 700–701
130. Jones DB, Guo LW, Reinhard MK, et al. Impact of pneumoperitoneum on trocar site implantation of colon cancer in hamster model. *Dis Colon Rectum* 1995;38:1182–1188
131. Yamaguchi K, Hirabayashi Y, Shiromizu A, et al. Enhancement of port site metastasis by hyaluronic acid under CO_2 pneumoperitoneum in a murine model. *Surg Endosc* 2001;15:504–507
132. Curet MJ. Port site metastases. *Am J Surg* 2004;187:705–712
133. Rhodes M, Nathanson L, Fielding G. Laparoscopic biliary and gastric bypass: A useful adjunct in the treatment of carcinoma of the pancreas. *Gut* 1995;36:778–780
134. Rothlin MA, Schob O, Weber M. Laparoscopic gastro- and hepaticojejunostomy for palliation of pancreatic cancer: A case-controlled study. *Surg Endosc* 1999;13: 1065–1069
135. Choi YB. Laparoscopic gastrojejunostomy for palliation of gastric outlet obstruction in unresectable gastric cancer. *Surg Endosc* 2002;16:1620–1626
136. Espat NJ, Brennan MF, Conlon KC. Patients with laparoscopically staged unresectable pancreatic adenocarcinoma do not require subsequent surgical biliary or gastric bypass. *J Am Coll Surg* 1999;188:649–657
137. Sohn TA, Lillemoe KD, Cameron JL, et al. Surgical palliation of unresectable periampullary adenocarcinoma in the 1990s. *J Am Coll Surg* 1999;188:658–669
138. Molinari M, Helton WS, Espat NJ. Palliative strategies for locally advanced unresectable and metastatic pancreatic cancer. *Surg Clin North Am* 2002;81:651–666
139. Casaccia M, Diviacco P, Molinello P, et al. Laparoscopic palliation of unresectable pancreatic cancers: Preliminary results. *Eur J Surg* 1999;165:556–559
140. Yim HB, Jacobson BC, Saltzman JR, et al. Clinical outcome of the use of enteral stents for palliation of patients with malignant upper GI obstruction. *Gastrointest Endosc* 2001;53:329–332
141. DiMango EP, Reber HA, Tempero MA. AGA technical review on the epidemiology, diagnosis, and treatment of pancreatic ductal adenocarcinoma. *Gastroenterology* 1999;117:1464–1484
142. Nagy A, Brosseuk D, Hemming A, et al. Laparoscopic gastroenterostomy for duodenal obstruction. *Am J Surg* 1995;165:539–542

INDEX

Note: Page numbers followed by *f* indicate figures; those followed by *t* indicate tables.

D

F

G

R

S

T

V